ARCHIVES OF GENERAL PSYCHIATRY

JANUARY 1997

FORTY YEARS OF LITHIUM TREATMENT

M. Schou

COMMENTARIES BY KUPFER AND FRANK, GERSHON AND SOARES, AND GITLIN AND ALTSHULER

A LINKAGE STUDY OF BIPOLAR ILLNESS
W. H. Berrettini, T. N. Ferraro, L. R. Goldin, et al

A PROSPECTIVE STUDY OF RISK FACTORS PREDICTING GRIEF INTENSITY FOLLOWING PREGNANCY LOSS
H. J. E. M. Janssen, M. C. J. Cuisinier, K. P. H. M. de Graauw, K. A. L. Hoogduin

DEPRESSION DURING MANIA: TREATMENT RESPONSE TO LITHIUM OR DIVALPROEX
A. C. Swann, C. L. Bowden, D. Morris, et al

BEHAVIOR OF BOYS IN KINDERGARTEN AND THE ONSET OF SUBSTANCE USE DURING ADOLESCENCE
L. C. Mâsse, R. E. Tremblay

NO ABNORMALITY IN THE GENE FOR THE G PROTEIN STIMULATORY α SUBUNIT IN PATIENTS WITH BIPOLAR DISORDER
A. Ram, F. Guedj, A. Cravchik, et al

PSYCHIATRIC AND SUBSTANCE USE COMORBIDITY AMONG TREATMENT-SEEKING OPIOID ABUSERS
R. K. Brooner, V. L. King, M. Kidorf, et al

CLINICAL RISK FOLLOWING ABRUPT AND GRADUAL WITHDRAWAL OF MAINTENANCE NEUROLEPTIC TREATMENT
A. C. Viguera, R. J. Baldessarini, J. D. Hegarty, et al

PSYCHIATRIC SEQUELAE OF POSTTRAUMATIC STRESS DISORDER IN WOMEN
N. Breslau, G. C. Davis, E. L. Peterson, L. Schultz

American Medical Association
Physicians dedicated to the health of America

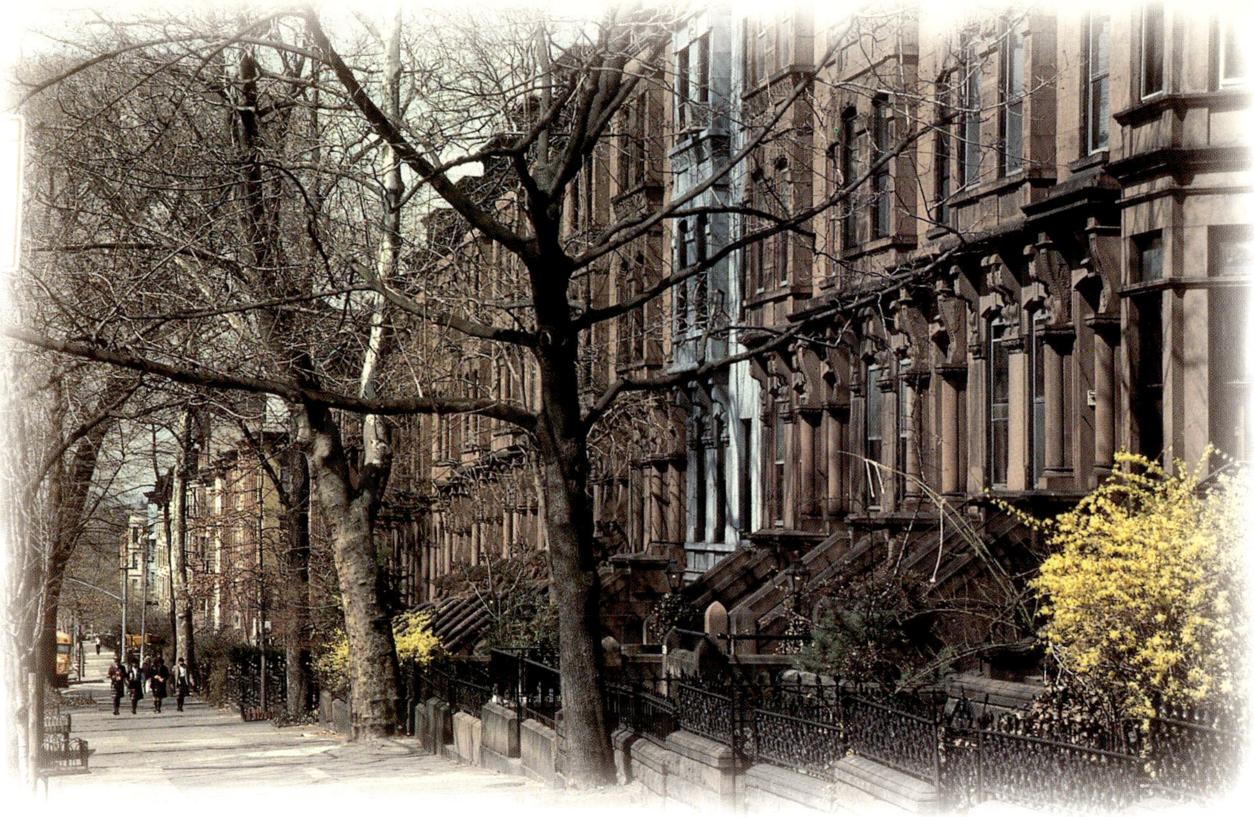

Dave has lived in this neighborhood for over 3 years.

Just this month, he joined the community.

- ☐ ***Once-a-month dosing:*** *the assurance of drug delivery for a full month*
- ☐ *Allows patients the freedom to concentrate on their lives, not their medication*
- ☐ *Total monthly haloperidol dose less than with oral HALDOL® (haloperidol)*
- ☐ *Consistent, predictable blood levels*[1]
- ☐ *Potentially fewer extrapyramidal side effects compared to the oral form*[2]

During dose adjustments or episodes of exacerbation of psychotic symptoms, therapy with HALDOL Decanoate 100 or HALDOL Decanoate 50 can be supplemented with short-acting oral forms of HALDOL. The side effects of HALDOL Decanoate 100 and HALDOL Decanoate 50 are those of oral HALDOL. The prolonged action of HALDOL Decanoate 100 and HALDOL Decanoate 50 should be considered in the management of side effects.

Please see Brief Summary of Prescribing Information on adjacent page.

A New Start

HALDOL® Decanoate 100

(HALOPERIDOL) INJECTION 100 mg/mL

ARCHIVES
OF
GENERAL PSYCHIATRY

VOL 54 NO. 1, JANUARY 7

NEWS AND VIEWS

Forty Years of Lithium Treatment 9
Mogens Schou, MD, DrMed, DrHCMult

COMMENTARIES

Forty Years of Lithium Treatment 14
David J. Kupfer, MD; Ellen Frank, PhD

Current Therapeutic Profile of Lithium 16
Samuel Gershon, MD; Jair C. Soares, MD

Unanswered Questions, Unknown Future for One of Our Oldest Medications 21
Michael J. Gitlin, MD; Lori L. Altshuler, MD

ORIGINAL ARTICLES

A Linkage Study of Bipolar Illness 27
Wade H. Berrettini, MD, PhD; Thomas N. Ferraro, PhD; Lynn R. Goldin, PhD; Sevilla D. Detera-Wadleigh, PhD; Henry Choi; David Muniec; Juliet J. Guroff, MSW; Diane M. Kazuba; John I. Nurnberger, Jr, MD, PhD; Wang-Ting Hsieh, PhD; Margret R. Hoehe, MD; Elliot S. Gershon, MD

Depression During Mania: Treatment Response to Lithium or Divalproex 37
Alan C. Swann, MD; Charles L. Bowden, MD; David Morris, PhD; Joseph R. Calabrese, MD; Frederick Petty, MD, PhD; Joyce Small, MD; Steven C. Dilsaver, MD; John M. Davis, MD

No Abnormality in the Gene for the G Protein Stimulatory α Subunit in Patients With Bipolar Disorder 44
Anca Ram, MD; Françoise Guedj, MD; Anibal Cravchik, MD, PhD; Lee Weinstein, MD; Qiuhe Cao, MD; Judith A. Badner, MD, PhD; Lynn R. Goldin, PhD; Nimrod Grisaru, MD; Husseini K. Manji, MD; Robert H. Belmaker, MD; Elliot S. Gershon, MD; Pablo V. Gejman, MD

Clinical Risk Following Abrupt and Gradual Withdrawal of Maintenance Neuroleptic Treatment 49
Adele C. Viguera, MD; Ross J. Baldessarini, MD; James D. Hegarty, MD, MPH; Daniel P. van Kammen, MD, PhD; Mauricio Tohen, MD, DrPH

American Medical Association
Physicians dedicated to the health of America

P. John Seward, MD
Executive Vice President
Kenneth E. Monroe
Deputy Executive Vice President
George D. Lundberg, MD
Editor in Chief, Scientific Information and Multimedia
James F. Rappel
Group Vice President, Business and Management Services
Robert L. Kennett
Vice President, Publishing
Michael D. Springer
Publisher, New Media
Peter L. Payerli
Associate Publisher

Mary C. Steermann
Director, Production & Distribution Division
Cheryl Iverson
Director, Editorial Processing Division
Geoffrey A. Flick
Manager, Marketing Services

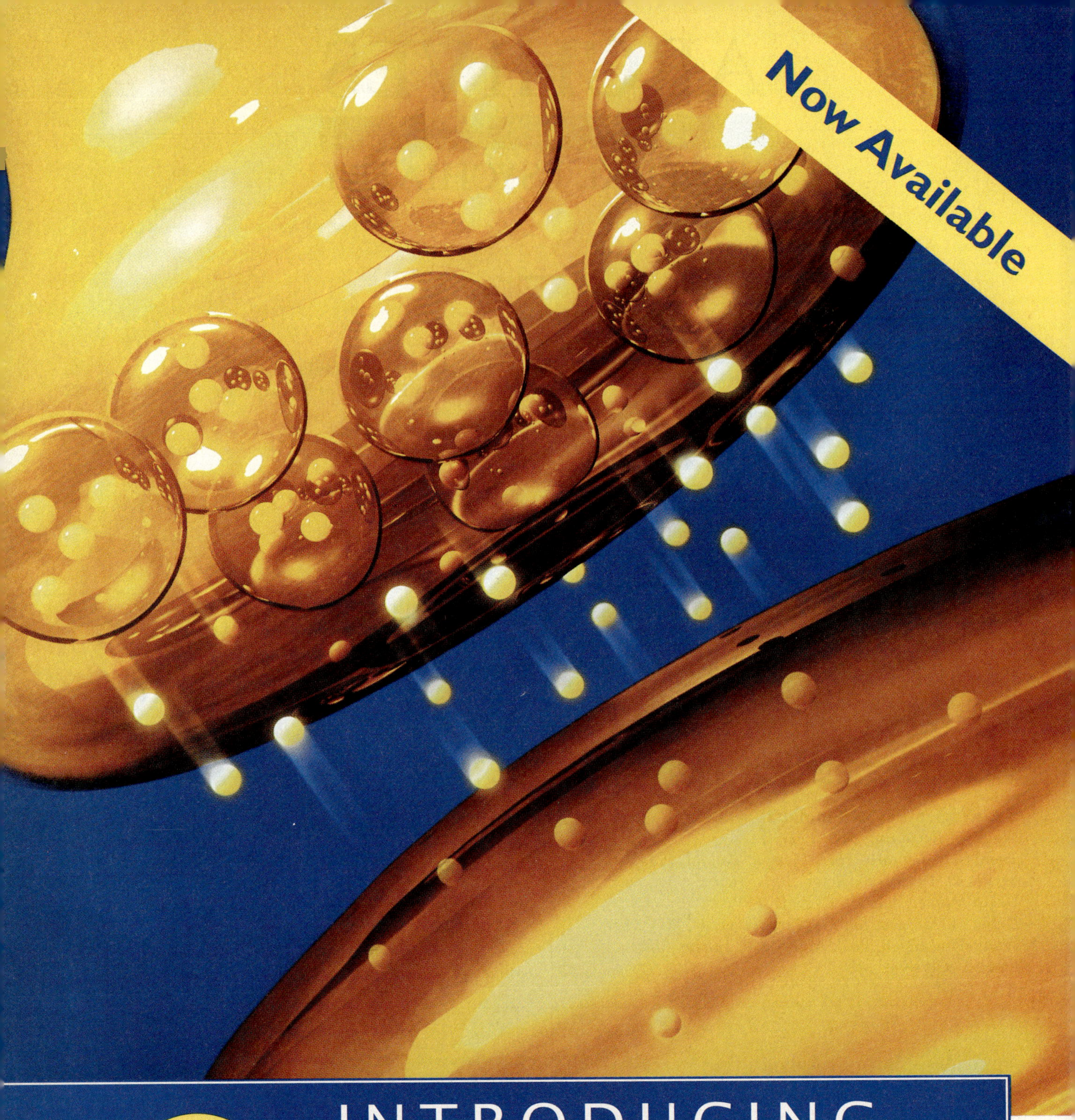
Now Available

A Prospective Study of Risk Factors Predicting Grief Intensity Following Pregnancy Loss 56
Hettie J. E. M. Janssen, PhD; Marian C. J. Cuisinier, PhD; Kees P. H. M. de Graauw, PhD; Kees A. L. Hoogduin, MD, PhD

Behavior of Boys in Kindergarten and the Onset of Substance Use During Adolescence 62
Louise C. Mâsse, PhD; Richard E. Tremblay, PhD

Psychiatric and Substance Use Comorbidity Among Treatment-Seeking Opioid Abusers 71
Robert K. Brooner, PhD; Van L. King, MD; Michael Kidorf, PhD; Chester W. Schmidt, Jr, MD; George E. Bigelow, PhD

Psychiatric Sequelae of Posttraumatic Stress Disorder in Women 81
Naomi Breslau, PhD; Glenn C. Davis, MD; Edward L. Peterson, PhD; Lonni Schultz, PhD

LETTERS TO THE EDITOR

Smoking Affects Plasma-Soluble Interleukin-2 Receptor Levels in Patients With Schizophrenia 89
Thomas Pollmächer, MD; Dunja Hinze-Selch, MD; Janet Mullington, PhD; Thomas Fenzel, MD; Florian Holsboer, PhD

In Reply 89
Rohan Ganguli, MD; Jaspreet S. Brar, MD, MPH

REGULAR DEPARTMENTS

This Month in *Archives of General Psychiatry* 8

Instructions for Authors 92

Physician Recruitment Advertising 94

ARCHIVES OF GENERAL PSYCHIATRY

THIS MONTH IN ARCHIVES OF GENERAL PSYCHIATRY

Although twin, family, and adoption studies clearly indicate heritable influences on bipolar disorder, the loci conveying risk have not been identified. In an attempt to localize bipolar susceptibility factors, **Berretini et al** (page 27) performed a genetic linkage study with 400 DNA samples from 22 pedigrees. Their results demonstrate that a bipolar susceptibility locus exists near the centromere of chromosome 18. Identification of such susceptibility loci may lead to the cloning of specific genes that convey risk for bipolar illness.

In a large placebo-controlled comparison of lithium and divalproex therapy in acute manic episodes, **Swann et al** (page 37) investigated the effect of pretreatment depressive symptoms on antimanic response. Depressive symptoms profoundly reduced antimanic response to lithium but had no effect on response to divalproex; patients without depressive symptoms responded robustly to lithium therapy. These data suggest that depression during mania is associated with poor response to lithium therapy.

The intracellular effects of many hormones, growth factors, neurotransmitters, and ions are mediated via a G protein-coupled pathway. Alterations of this pathway may represent an important mechanism underlying bipolar disorder. By mutational analysis of G_s-α exons, association, and genetic linkage **Ram et al** (page 44) tested the hypothesis that a mutation in G_s-α gene confers an increased susceptibility to bipolar illness. The present results do not support a role of the G_s-α protein gene in the genetic predisposition to bipolar illness. However, this study does not rule out the involvement of other G proteins in the pathophysiology of bipolar illness.

Abrupt discontinuation of some maintenance psychotropic medications is followed by a high risk of early relapse. **Viguera et al** (page 49) evaluated clinical data on 1200 schizophrenic patients who had been withdrawn abruptly or gradually from neuroleptic therapies. After abrupt discontinuation, relapse reached 50% within 30 weeks, and was more frequent among inpatients. Most patients who did not relapse within 6 months remained stable for up to 4 years without medication, indicating clinical heterogeneity.

In a prospective longitudinal study **Janssen et al** (page 56) investigated which risk factors could best predict women's grief intensity following pregnancy loss. A relatively long pregnancy, a more neurotic personality, more preloss psychiatric symptoms, and the absence of living children appear to be important risk factors for stronger grief responses in women following pregnancy loss.

In a longitudinal study of boys, **Mâsse and Tremblay** (page 62) assessed whether novelty seeking, harm avoidance, and reward dependence behaviors measured at age 6 years could predict the onset of cigarette smoking, alcohol abuse, and drug abuse in these boys when they were aged 10 to 15 years. Their study demonstrated that both novelty seeking and harm avoidance were useful in predicting early onset substance use.

In the largest psychiatric comorbidity study of opioid abusers to date, **Brooner et al** (page 71) found that almost half of the men and women entering drug abuse treatment had a psychiatric disorder. Antisocial personality disorder and major depression were the most common diagnoses. Psychiatric comorbidity was strongly associated with having a more long-term and severe pattern of substance use disorder.

Breslau et al (page 81) in an epidemiologic study of 801 women, found that Posttraumatic Stress Disorder (PTSD) increased the risk for first onset major depression and alcohol use disorder. In addition, preexisting major depression increased women's vulnerability to the PTSD-effects of traumatic events and women's risk of exposure to traumatic events. The causal explanation of these findings is uncertain and might involve an underlying vulnerability to major depression.

This issue also contains an article by Mogens Schou, titled "Forty Years of Lithium Treatment," with Commentaries by Kupfer and Frank; Gershon and Soares; and Gitlin and Altshuler.

New Members of the Editorial Board

The ARCHIVES is pleased to announce the addition of 3 individuals to its Editorial Board. David L. Braff, MD, professor of psychiatry at the University of California, San Diego School of Medicine, is an expert in the neurobiology of schizophrenia. Ellen Frank, PhD, professor of psychiatry and psychology at the University of Pittsburgh (Pa) School of Medicine, is an expert in the evaluation and treatment of mood disorders. Kenneth S. Kendler, MD, professor of psychiatry and human genetics at the Medical College of Virginia–Virginia Commonwealth University, Richmond, is an expert in psychiatric genetics, nosology, and epidemiology. Each has published widely and has served as an invaluable reviewer. More important, they are thoughtful, creative individuals who have tireless energy, clear minds, and senses of humor. They will add depth and breadth to our scientific mission and we welcome them.

Jack D. Barchas, MD
Editor

# ARCHIVES
OF
GENERAL PSYCHIATRY

VOL 54 NO. 2, FEBRUARY 1997

NEWS AND VIEWS

Research With Cognitively Impaired Subjects: Unfinished Business in the Regulation of Human Research 105
Richard J. Bonnie, LLB

Caring About Risks: Are Severely Depressed Patients Competent to Consent to Research? 113
Carl Elliott, MD, PhD

COMMENTARIES

Rethinking the Conduct of Psychiatric Research 117
Paul S. Appelbaum, MD

Protecting Subjects and Fostering Research: Striking the Proper Balance 121
Robert M. A. Hirschfeld, MD; William Winslade, PhD, JD; Todd L. Krause, PhD

ORIGINAL ARTICLES

Circadian Rest-Activity Disturbances in Seasonal Affective Disorder 124
Martin H. Teicher, MD, PhD; Carol A. Glod, RN, PhD; Eleanor Magnus; David Harper; Gregory Benson; Kathryn Krueger, MD; Cynthia E. McGreenery

Effects of Tryptophan Depletion on Drug-Free Patients With Seasonal Affective Disorder During a Stable Response to Bright Light Therapy 133
Alexander Neumeister, MD; Nicole Praschak-Rieder, MD; Barbara Heßelmann, MD; Marie-Luise Rao, PhD; Judith Glück, Msc; Siegfried Kasper, MD

Complex Interaction of the Sleep-Wake Cycle and Circadian Phase Modulates Mood in Healthy Subjects 145
Diane B. Boivin, MD, PhD; Charles A. Czeisler, PhD, MD; Derk-Jan Dijk, PhD; Jeanne F. Duffy, MBA; Simon Folkard, PhD, DSc; David S. Minors, PhD; Peter Totterdell, MSc; James M. Waterhouse, DPhil

Reduced Blue Cone Electroretinogram in Cocaine-Withdrawn Patients 153
Monique Roy, MD; Alec Roy, MD; John Williams, MD; Lawrence Weinberger, PhD; David Smelson, PsyD

American Medical Association
Physicians dedicated to the health of America

Auditory Working Memory and Wisconsin Card Sorting Test Performance in Schizophrenia 159
James M. Gold, PhD; Constance Carpenter, PhD; Christopher Randolph, PhD; Terry E. Goldberg, PhD; Daniel R. Weinberger, MD

Eye Tracking, Attention, and Schizotypal Symptoms in Nonpsychotic Relatives of Patients With Schizophrenia 169
Richard S. E. Keefe, PhD; Jeremy M. Silverman, PhD; Richard C. Mohs, PhD; Larry J. Siever, MD; Philip D. Harvey, PhD; Lee Friedman, PhD; Sonia E. Lees Roitman; Rachel L. DuPre; Christopher J. Smith; James Schmeidler, PhD; Kenneth L. Davis, MD

Temperance Board Registration for Alcohol Abuse in a National Sample of Swedish Male Twins, Born 1902 to 1949 178
Kenneth S. Kendler, MD; Carol A. Prescott, PhD; Michael C. Neale, PhD; Nancy L. Pedersen, PhD

LETTERS TO THE EDITOR

Phosphorus 31 Magnetic Resonance Spectroscopy in Patients With Huntington Disease 186
Peter C. Williamson, MD; Ashok Malla, MD; Len Cortese, MD; A. Jon Stoessl, MD; Dick Drost, PhD; Jeff A. Stanley, PhD;

In Reply 187
Jay W. Pettegrew, MD; Matcheri S. Keshavan, MD

Use of Methylphenidate in a Patient With Glaucoma and Attention-Deficit Hyperactivity Disorder: A Clinical Dilemma 188
Barbara Bartlik, MD; Gregory Harmon, MD; Peter Kaplan, MD

Sex Differences in Schizophrenia 189
Godfrey D. Pearlson, MD; Thomas E. Schlaepfer, MD

REGULAR DEPARTMENTS

This Month in *Archives of General Psychiatry* 104

Index to Advertisers 144

Physician Recruitment Advertising 191

**Instructions for Authors—
See January 1997 issue, page 92.**

ARCHIVES OF GENERAL PSYCHIATRY

ARCHIVES OF GENERAL PSYCHIATRY

Seasonal affective disorder (SAD) is believed to stem from a disturbance in biological rhythms that emerges in the absence of sufficient daylight. **Teicher et al** (page 124) used wrist-worn activity monitors to study the rhythms of motor activity in patients with SAD and normal adult controls in their natural environment. Patients with SAD were less active, particularly during the first 2 hours after arising. Their 24-hour circadian rhythm peaked at later times and was more variable between days. These findings confirm and extend theories about the nature of biological rhythm disturbances in depression.

There is evidence that light therapy exerts its antidepressant properties by involving serotonergic mechanisms. **Neumeister et al** (page 133) found that the beneficial effects of bright-light therapy in the treatment of patients suffering from seasonal affective disorder (SAD) are interrupted by rapid depletion of dietary tryptophan. This finding suggests that the maintenance of light therapy–induced remission from depression in patients with SAD seems to depend on the short-term availability of serotonin and that the brain serotonin system might be involved in the mechanism of action of light therapy.

Disturbances of circadian or sleep-wake–dependent parameters have been hypothesized to account for the diurnal variation of mood in humans. **Boivin et al** (page 145) demonstrated that moderate changes in the timing of the sleep-wake cycle may have profound effects on subsequent mood in healthy young adults.

Cocaine dependence may involve changes in the dopaminergic system. As the retina has a high concentration of dopamine, **Roy et al** (page 153) studied the electroretinogram (ERG) in persons with cocaine dependence. Recently withdrawn cocaine-dependent patients had significantly reduced blue cone ERG responses compared with matched normal controls. This finding suggests that dysregulation of blue cone function may be a consequence of cocaine dependence and that the ERG may be useful in future studies of cocaine-dependent patients.

Patients with schizophrenia demonstrate impairment on the Wisconsin Card Sorting Test, a complex problem-solving test. However, the specific cognitive processes that underlie the impairment have not been identified. **Gold et al** (page 159) hypothesized that working memory might be a critical determinant of test performance. They found that a novel measure of working memory was highly correlated with test performance in schizophrenia, and that patients' deficits, relative to controls, could be accounted for by working memory performance. The results suggest that failures on complex tasks may be explained by elementary cognitive processes.

Biological relatives of patients with schizophrenia demonstrate increases in schizotypal personality symptoms, eyetracking disturbances, and attentional abnormalities measured by Continuous Performance Tests (CPT), but the relationship among these potential components of a schizophrenia-related phenotype is unknown. **Keefe et al** (page 169) reported that eyetracking quality was more powerful than CPT measures in discriminating relatives of patients with schizophrenia from controls, yet only CPT errors were associated with schizotypal personality disorder symptoms. Eyetracking and CPT measures were uncorrelated in relatives. Eyetracking deficits and attentional disturbances may be separate components of a phenotype related to schizophrenia and might be considered as independent factors in genetic studies of schizophrenia.

How important are genetic vs environmental factors in the cause of alcoholism, and how stable are these factors over time? **Kendler et al** (page 178) examined temperance board registrations (TBR) from 1929 to 1974 in male-male Swedish twin pairs born from 1902 to 1949. Probandwise, concordance for TBR was 47.9% in monozygotic and 32.8% in dizygotic twins. Genetic and familial-environmental risk factors accounted for 54% and 14%, respectively, of the liability to TBR, estimates that were stable across birth cohorts. Genetic factors are of major importance in determining the cause of alcoholism in men, while familial-environmental factors appear to be less significant.

Two "News & Views" articles are also included in this issue. They are "Research on Cognitively Impaired Subjects: Unfinished Business in the Regulation of Human Research" by Richard J. Bonnie and "Caring About Risks: Are Severely Depressed Patients Competent to Consent to Research?" by Carl Elliot, along with "Commentaries" by Paul S. Appelbaum and Robert M. A. Hirschfeld et al.

ARCHIVES OF GENERAL PSYCHIATRY

VOL 54 NO. 3, MARCH 1997

PERSPECTIVES

Managed Care and the Future of Psychiatry 201
Thomas Detre, MD; Margaret C. McDonald, PhD

COMMENTARIES

Essential Roles for Psychiatry in the Era of Managed Care 206
Mark Olfson, MD, MPH; Myrna M. Weissman, PhD; John F. Gottlieb, MD

The Futures of Psychiatry 212
Steven S. Sharfstein, MD

ORIGINAL ARTICLES

Effects of Intrathecal Thyrotropin-Releasing Hormone (Protirelin) in Refractory Depressed Patients 214
Lauren B. Marangell, MD; Mark S. George, MD; Ann M. Callahan, MD; Terence A. Ketter, MD; Peggy J. Pazzaglia, MD; Todd A. L'Herrou, MA; Gabriele S. Leverich, MSW; Robert M. Post, MD

Mesolimbic Dopamine D_3 Receptors and Use of Antipsychotics in Patients With Schizophrenia: A Postmortem Study 225
Eugenia V. Gurevich, PhD; Yvette Bordelon; Raymond M. Shapiro, MD, PhD; Steven E. Arnold, MD; Raquel E. Gur, MD; Jeffrey N. Joyce, PhD

Visual Imagery and Perception in Posttraumatic Stress Disorder: A Positron Emission Tomographic Investigation 233
Lisa M. Shin, AM; Stephen M. Kosslyn, PhD; Richard J. McNally, PhD; Nathaniel M. Alpert, PhD; William L. Thompson; Scott L. Rauch, MD; Michael L. Macklin; Roger K. Pitman, MD

American Medical Association
Physicians dedicated to the health of America

Positron Emission Tomography Measurement of Cerebral Metabolic Correlates of Yohimbine Administration in Combat-Related Posttraumatic Stress Disorder 246
J. Douglas Bremner, MD; Robert B. Innis, MD, PhD; Chin K. Ng, PhD; Lawrence H. Staib, PhD; Ronald M. Salomon, MD; Richard A. Bronen, MD; James Duncan, PhD; Steven M. Southwick, MD; John H. Krystal, MD; Dayton Rich; George Zubal, PhD; Holley Dey, MD; Robert Soufer, MD; Dennis S. Charney, MD

The Course of Psychopathologic Features in Mild to Moderate Alzheimer Disease 257
D. P. Devanand, MD; Diane M. Jacobs, PhD; Ming-Xin Tang, PhD; Caridad Del Castillo-Castaneda; Mary Sano, PhD; Karen Marder, MD; Karen Bell, MD; Frederick W. Bylsma, PhD; Jason Brandt, PhD; Marilyn Albert, PhD; Yaakov Stern, PhD

The Role of Heredity in Late-Onset Alzheimer Disease and Vascular Dementia: A Twin Study 264
A. L. Mina Bergem, MD; Knut Engedal, MD, PhD; Einar Kringlen, MD, PhD

Familial Aggregation and Phenomenology of 'Early'-Onset (at or Before Age 20 Years) Panic Disorder 271
Risë B. Goldstein, PhD; Priya J. Wickramaratne, PhD; Ewald Horwath, MD; Myrna M. Weissman, PhD

Severe Stress, Depressive Symptoms, and Changes in Lymphocyte Subsets in Human Immunodeficiency Virus–Infected Men: A 2-Year Follow-up Study 279
Jane Leserman, PhD; John M. Petitto, MD; Diana O. Perkins, MD; James D. Folds, PhD; Robert N. Golden, MD; Dwight L. Evans, MD

REGULAR DEPARTMENTS

This Month in *Archives of General Psychiatry* 200

Index to Advertisers 211

Physician Recruitment Advertising 286

Instructions for Authors— See January 1997 issue, page 92.

ARCHIVES OF GENERAL PSYCHIATRY

ARCHIVES OF GENERAL PSYCHIATRY

Psychiatry's growing biological basis is making it more like other medical specialties, particularly neurology. **Detre** and **McDonald** (page 201) conclude that psychiatry and neurology should become a single discipline and that new "clinical neuroscientists" should be trained in both fields. They recommend that health care delivery system research be integrated into current academic curricula to ensure continuity of high-quality, cost-effective care for mentally ill patients. Two Commentaries about this article—by Olfson, Gotlieb, and Weissman and by Sharfstein—are also included in this issue.

To clarify the potential mood effects of thyrotropin-releasing hormone (TRH), **Marangell et al** (page 214) injected this drug directly into spinal fluid. Intrathecal TRH produced a rapid, but transient, improvement in mood and suicidality in patients with treatment-refractory depression. These findings suggest that TRH could be a positive modulator of mood and support the feasibility of direct administration of peptides into the central nervous system.

Gurevich et al (page 225) found that the density of mesolimbic D_3 dopamine receptors was increased in the brains of patients with schizophrenia who had received no antipsychotic drugs but not in those who had been treated with antipsychotic drugs. The study suggests that individuals with schizophrenia may have an increased density of D_3 receptors, and that antipsychotic drugs may work by decreasing their density.

Shin et al (page 233) used positron emission tomography to study regional cerebral blood flow in combat veterans with and without posttraumatic stress disorder (PTSD). They found increased blood flow in the anterior cingulate cortex and the right amygdala when subjects viewed or imagined combat-related scenes. These results suggest that limbic and paralimbic regions of the brain are involved in the processing of trauma-relevant stimuli in PTSD.

Bremner et al (page 246) used positron emission tomography and fludeoxyglucose F18 to measure brain metabolism with yohimbine, an agent that stimulates brain norepinephrine release, and placebo in patients with PTSD and controls. There was a notable difference in brain metabolic response to yohimbine in patients with PTSD in prefrontal, temporal, parietal, and orbitofrontal cortex compared with controls. Patients showed a tendency toward decreased brain metabolism and controls showed a tendency toward increased brain metabolism. These findings are consistent with an enhancement of norepinephrine release in the brain with yohimbine in patients with PTSD.

Patients with Alzheimer's disease (AD) often experience behavioral changes, psychosis, and depression. **Devanand et al** (page 257) followed up a large group of patients with early signs of AD for up to 5 years. Misidentification, wandering or agitation, and physical aggression increased in prevalence during follow-up. Depressed mood, accompanied by sleep and appetite disturbance, was uncommon and rarely persisted.

The role of heredity in senile dementia has been a controversial issue. In a large-scale twin study from Norway, **Bergem et al** (page 264) found that Alzheimer's disease (AD) is mainly genetically determined, whereas vascular dementia is environmentally determined. Most of the cases of AD were familial. There was an association between apolipoprotein E $\epsilon 4$ allele and AD in about 40% of the cases. Thus, there are other susceptibility genes for AD to be detected.

Early age at onset, associated with increased familial risk and a distinctive clinical presentation in many disorders, has not been well studied in panic disorder. In a direct-interview family study, **Goldstein et al** (page 271) report that onsets of panic disorder in probands at or before age 20 confer the highest risk of the disorder to relatives. Age at onset may be useful in differentiating familial subtypes of panic disorder.

In a prospective study, **Leserman et al** (page 279) found that severe stress and depressive symptoms were related to decreases of several lymphocyte subsets among men infected with human immunodeficiency virus (HIV). These findings suggest that stress and depression may negatively affect immune measures in men infected with HIV and that these psychological factors may have potential clinical implications for the course of this disease.

ARCHIVES
OF
GENERAL PSYCHIATRY

VOL 54 NO. 4, APRIL 1997

ORIGINAL ARTICLES

The Diagnostic Validity of Melancholic Major Depression in a Population-Based Sample of Female Twins 299
Kenneth S. Kendler, MD

The Cross-national Epidemiology of Panic Disorder 305
Myrna M. Weissman, PhD; Roger C. Bland, MB; Glorisa J. Canino, PhD; Carlo Faravelli, MD; Steven Greenwald, MA; Hai-Gwo Hwu, MD; Peter R. Joyce, PhD; Elie G. Karam, MD; Chung-Kyoon Lee, MD; Joseph Lellouch, PhD; Jean-Pierre Lépine, MD; Stephen C. Newman, MD; Mark A. Oakley-Browne, PhD; Maritza Rubio-Stipec, MA; J. Elisabeth Wells, PhD; Priya J. Wickramaratne, PhD; Hans-Ulrich Wittchen, PhD; Eng-Kung Yeh, MD

Lifetime Co-occurrence of *DSM-III-R* Alcohol Abuse and Dependence With Other Psychiatric Disorders in the National Comorbidity Survey 313
Ronald C. Kessler, PhD; Rosa M. Crum, MD, MHS; Lynn A. Warner, MPP; Christopher B. Nelson, PhD, MPH; John Schulenberg, PhD; James C. Anthony, PhD

Adult Major Affective Disorder After Prenatal Exposure to an Influenza Epidemic 322
Ricardo A. Machón, PhD; Sarnoff A. Mednick, PhD, DrMed; Matti O. Huttunen, MD

The Prevalence of *DSM-III-R* Diagnoses in a National Sample of Dutch Adolescents 329
Frank C. Verhulst, MD; Jan van der Ende, MS; Robert F. Ferdinand, MD; Marianne C. Kasius, MD

American Medical Association
Physicians dedicated to the health of America

NEWS AND VIEWS

Coming to Terms With the Terms of Risk 337
Helena Chmura Kraemer, PhD; Alan E. Kazdin, PhD; David R. Offord, MD; Ronald C. Kessler, PhD; Peter S. Jensen, MD; David J. Kupfer, MD

ORIGINAL ARTICLES

Detecting Personality Disorders in a Nonclinical Population: Application of a 2-Stage Procedure for Case Identification 345
Mark F. Lenzenweger, PhD; Armand W. Loranger, PhD; Lauren Korfine, AM; Cynthia Neff, PhD

Multisomatoform Disorder: An Alternative to Undifferentiated Somatoform Disorder for the Somatizing Patient in Primary Care 352
Kurt Kroenke, MD; Robert L. Spitzer, MD; Frank V. deGruy III, MD; Steven R. Hahn, MD; Mark Linzer, MD; Janet B. W. Williams, DSW; David Brody, MD; Mark Davies, MS

Positron Emission Tomography Measurement of Cerebral Metabolic Correlates of Tryptophan Depletion–Induced Depressive Relapse 364
J. Douglas Bremner, MD; Robert B. Innis, MD, PhD; Ronald M. Salomon, MD; Lawrence H. Staib, PhD; Chin K. Ng, PhD; Helen L. Miller, MD; Richard A. Bronen, MD; John H. Krystal, MD; James Duncan, PhD; Dayton Rich; Lawrence H. Price, MD Robert Malison, MD; Holley Dey, MD; Robert Soufer, MD; Dennis S. Charney, MD

Effects of Meta-chlorophenylpiperazine Infusions in Patients With Seasonal Affective Disorder and Healthy Control Subjects: Diurnal Responses and Nocturnal Regulatory Mechanisms 375
Paul J. Schwartz, MD; Dennis L. Murphy, MD; Thomas A. Wehr, MD; Diego Garcia-Borreguero, MD; Dan A. Oren, MD; Douglas E. Moul, MD, MPH; Norio Ozaki, MD; Alisa J. Snelbaker, MA; Norman E. Rosenthal, MD

BOOK REVIEWS

The Motherhood Constellation: A Unified View of Parent-Infant Psychotherapy 387
Daniel N. Stern
Reviewed by Thomas F. Anders, MD

An Unquiet Mind 388
Kay Redfield Jamison
Reviewed by James Kocsis, MD

REGULAR DEPARTMENTS

This Month in *Archives of General Psychiatry* 298

Physician Recruitment Advertising 390

Index to Advertisers 392

Instructions for Authors—
See January 1997 issue, page 92.

ARCHIVES
OF
GENERAL PSYCHIATRY

ARCHIVES OF GENERAL PSYCHIATRY

VOL 54 NO. 5, MAY 1997

NEWS AND VIEWS

The Rationale and Ethics of Medication-Free Research in Schizophrenia 401
William T. Carpenter, Jr, MD; Nina R. Schooler, PhD; John M. Kane, MD

COMMENTARIES

Medication-Free Research With Schizophrenic Patients: A European Perspective 412
Fritz A. Henn, PhD, MD; Malcolm Lader, OBE, DSc, PhD, FRCPsych; Hanfried Helmchen, MD

The Call of the Sirens: Navigating the Ethics of Medication-Free Research in Schizophrenia 415
Joseph J. Fins, MD; Franklin G. Miller, PhD

ORIGINAL ARTICLE

A Quantitative Analysis of Smooth Pursuit Eye Tracking in Monozygotic Twins Discordant for Schizophrenia 417
Robert E. Litman, MD; E. Fuller Torrey, MD; Daniel W. Hommer, MD; Allan R. Radant, MD; David Pickar, MD; Daniel R. Weinberger, MD

REPLY COMMENTARY

Smooth Pursuit Eye Tracking in Twins: A Critical Commentary 429
Philip S. Holzman, PhD; Deborah L. Levy, PhD; Steven W. Matthysse, PhD; Larry A. Abel, PhD

ORIGINAL ARTICLES

Magnetic Source Imaging Evidence of Sex Differences in Cerebral Lateralization in Schizophrenia 433
Martin Reite, MD; Jeanelle Sheeder; Peter Teale, MSEE; Matthew Adams; Douglas Richardson; Jack Simon, MD, PhD; Richard H. Jones, PhD; Donald C. Rojas, PhD

American Medical Association

Physicians dedicated to the health of America

P. John Seward, MD
Executive Vice President

Kenneth E. Monroe
Deputy Executive Vice President

George D. Lundberg, MD
Editor in Chief, Scientific Information and Multimedia

James F. Rappel
Group Vice President, Business and Management Services

Robert L. Kennett
Vice President, Publishing

Peter L. Payerli
Associate Publisher

Mary C. Steermann
Director, Production & Distribution Division

Cheryl Iverson
Director, Editorial Processing Division

Geoffrey A. Flick
Manager, Marketing Services

Psychotic Exacerbations and Enhanced Vasopressin Secretion in Schizophrenic Patients With Hyponatremia and Polydipsia 443
Morris B. Goldman, MD; Gary L. Robertson, MD; Daniel J. Luchins, MD; Donald Hedeker, PhD; Ghanshyam N. Pandey, PhD

Relapse and Rehospitalization During Maintenance Treatment of Schizophrenia: The Effects of Dose Reduction and Family Treatment 453
Nina R. Schooler, PhD; Samuel J. Keith, MD; Joanne B. Severe, MS; Susan M. Matthews; Alan S. Bellack, PhD; Ira D. Glick, MD; William A. Hargreaves, PhD; John M. Kane, MD; Philip T. Ninan, MD; Allen Frances, MD; Marc Jacobs, MD; Jeffrey A. Lieberman, MD; Rosalind Mance, MD; George M. Simpson, MD; Margaret G. Woerner, PhD

Backward Masking Performance in Unaffected Siblings of Schizophrenic Patients: Evidence for a Vulnerability Indicator 465
Michael F. Green, PhD; Keith H. Nuechterlein, PhD; Bruno Breitmeyer, PhD

Thought Disorder in Schizophrenic and Control Adoptees and Their Relatives 475
Dennis K. Kinney, PhD; Philip S. Holzman, PhD; Bjørn Jacobsen, MD; Lennart Jansson, MD; Britta Faber, MD; Wera Hildebrand, PhD; Eva Kasell; Morris E. Zimbalist

The Brain Metabolic Patterns of Clozapine- and Fluphenazine-Treated Patients With Schizophrenia During a Continuous Performance Task 481
Robert M. Cohen, PhD, MD; Thomas E. Nordahl, PhD, MD; William E. Semple, PhD; Paul Andreason, MD; Robert E. Litman, MD; David Pickar, MD

Increased Phospholipid Breakdown in Schizophrenia: Evidence for the Involvement of a Calcium-Independent Phospholipase A_2 487
Brian M. Ross, PhD; Craig Hudson, MD; Jeffrey Erlich; Jerry J. Warsh, MD, PhD; Stephen J. Kish, PhD

REGULAR DEPARTMENTS

This Month in *Archives of General Psychiatry* 399

Physician Recruitment Advertising 495

Index to Advertisers 496

**Instructions for Authors—
See January 1997 issue, page 92 or visit the Web site at http://www.ama-assn.org.**

ARCHIVES
OF
GENERAL PSYCHIATRY

ARCHIVES
OF
GENERAL PSYCHIATRY

VOL 54 NO. 6, JUNE 1997

COMMENTARY

Models to Conceptualize Risk Factors for Bulimia Nervosa 507
Katherine A. Halmi, MD

ORIGINAL ARTICLES

Risk Factors for Bulimia Nervosa: A Community-Based Case-Control Study 509
Christopher G. Fairburn, DM, MPhil, FRCPsych; Sarah L. Welch, DPhil, MRCPsych; Helen A. Doll, MSc; Beverley A. Davies; Marianne E. O'Connor

Hormonal and Subjective Responses to Intravenous *meta*-Chlorophenylpiperazine in Bulimia Nervosa 521
Robert D. Levitan, MD; Allan S. Kaplan, MD; Russell T. Joffe, MD; Anthony J. Levitt, MD; Gregory M. Brown, MD

Decreased Serotonin Function in Bulimia Nervosa 529
David C. Jimerson, MD; Barbara E. Wolfe, RN, PhD; Eran D. Metzger, MD; Dianne M. Finkelstein, PhD; Thomas B. Cooper, MA; Jeffrey M. Levine, MD

Cerebral Gray Matter Volume Deficits After Weight Recovery From Anorexia Nervosa 537
Evelyn K. Lambe, MSc; Debra K. Katzman, MD; David J. Mikulis, MD; Sidney H. Kennedy, MD; Robert B. Zipursky, MD

Psychosocial Correlates of Job Strain in a Sample of Working Women 543
Redford B. Williams, MD; John C. Barefoot, PhD; James A. Blumenthal, PhD; Michael J. Helms, MS; Linda Luecken, MA; Carl F. Pieper, DPH; Ilene C. Siegler, PhD, MPH; Edward C. Suarez, PhD

American Medical Association
Physicians dedicated to the health of America

P. John Seward, MD
Executive Vice President

Kenneth E. Monroe
Deputy Executive Vice President

George D. Lundberg, MD
Editor in Chief, Scientific Information and Multimedia

James F. Rappel
Group Vice President, Business and Management Services

Robert L. Kennett
Vice President, Publishing

Peter L. Payerli
Associate Publisher

Mary C. Steermann
Director, Production & Distribution Division

Cheryl Iverson
Director, Editorial Processing Division

Geoffrey A. Flick
Manager, Marketing Services

Quetiapine in Patients With Schizophrenia: A High- and Low-Dose Double-blind Comparison With Placebo 549
Joyce G. Small, MD; Steven R. Hirsch, MPhil, MD, FRCP, FRCPPsych; Lisa A. Arvanitis, MD; Barbara G. Miller, MS; Christopher G. G. Link, MB ChB, MPhil, MRCPsych, Dip Pharm Med, MFPM; and the Seroquel Study Group

Increased Concentrations of Presynaptic Proteins in the Cingulate Cortex of Subjects With Schizophrenia 559
Steven M. Gabriel, PhD; Vahram Haroutunian, PhD; Peter Powchik, MD; William G. Honer, MD, FRCPC; Michael Davidson, MD; Peter Davies, PhD; Kenneth L. Davis, MD

The Effects of a Selective D_4 Dopamine Receptor Antagonist (L-745,870) in Acutely Psychotic Inpatients With Schizophrenia 567
Mark S. Kramer, MD, PhD; Barbara Last; Albert Getson, PhD; Scott A. Reines, MD, PhD; and the D_4 Dopamine Antagonist Group

BOOK REVIEW

Electronic *DSM-IV* 573
Daniel Mimouni, MD; Yuval Bloch, MD

OBITUARIES

George Winokur, MD, 1925-1996 574
Samuel B. Guze, MD

Ray W. Fuller, PhD, 1936-1996 575
Marlene L. Cohen, PhD; David L. Nelson, PhD; Steven M. Paul, MD

LETTERS TO THE EDITOR

Schizophrenia After Prenatal Famine 577
Jim van Os, MSc, PhD

In Reply 578
Ezra S. Susser, MD, DrPH; Richard Neugebauer, PhD; Hans W. Hoek, MD; Alan S. Brown, MD; Shang P. Lin, PhD; Daniel Labovitz, MD; Jack M. Gorman, MD

N-Methyl-D-Aspartate Receptor Hypofunction in Schizophrenia Could Arise From Reduced Cortical Connectivity Rather Than Receptor Dysfunction 578
Ralph E. Hoffman, MD; Thomas H. McGlashan, MD

In Reply 579
John W. Olney, MD; Nuri B. Farber, MD

REGULAR DEPARTMENTS

This Month in *Archives of General Psychiatry* 506

Instructions for Authors 581

Physician Recruitment Advertising 583

Index to Advertisers 584

ARCHIVES OF GENERAL PSYCHIATRY

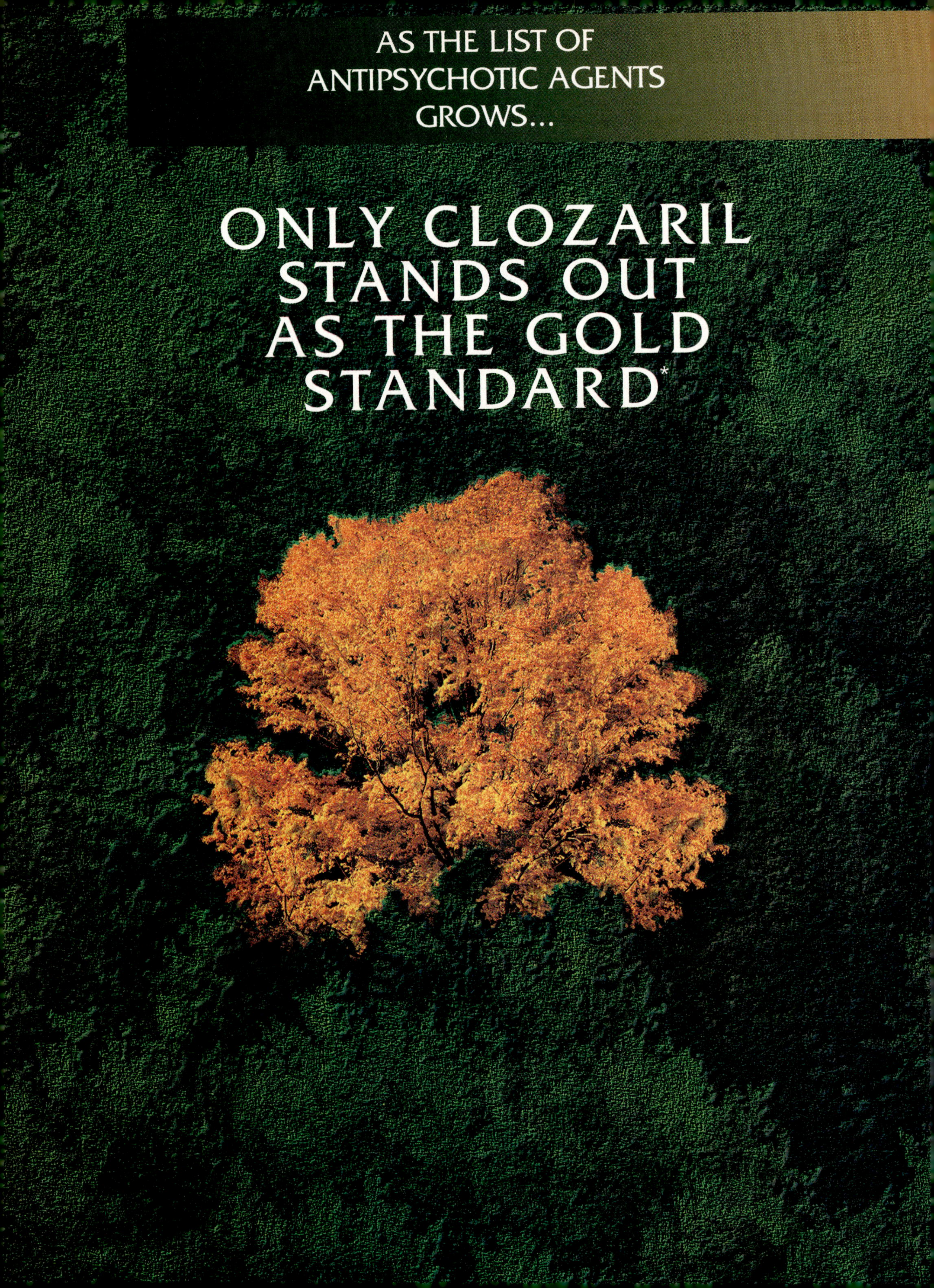

AS THE LIST OF
ANTIPSYCHOTIC AGENTS
GROWS...
ONLY CLOZARIL
STANDS OUT
AS THE GOLD
STANDARD*

ARCHIVES OF GENERAL PSYCHIATRY

VOL 54 NO. 7, JULY 1997

NEWS AND VIEWS

A Molecular and Cellular Theory of Depression 597
Ronald S. Duman, PhD; George R. Heninger, MD; Eric J. Nestler, MD, PhD

COMMENTARY

Molecular Biology of Behavior: Targets for Therapeutics 607
Robert M. Post, MD

ORIGINAL ARTICLES

A Controlled Family History Study of Childhood-Onset Depressive Disorder 613
Maria Kovacs, PhD; Bernie Devlin, PhD; Myrna Pollock, MSW; Cheryl Richards, MBA; Protap Mukerji, MS

Developmental Precursors of Affective Illness in a General Population Birth Cohort 625
Jim van Os, MSc, PhD; Peter Jones, MSc; Glyn Lewis, MSc, PhD; Michael Wadsworth, MPhil, PhD; Robin Murray, DSc

First-Episode Major Depression: Few Sex Differences in Course 633
H. Blair Simpson, MD, PhD; John C. Nee, PhD; Jean Endicott, PhD

Clinical Improvement With Fluoxetine Therapy and Noradrenergic Function in Patients With Panic Disorder 643
Jeremy D. Coplan, MD; Laszlo A. Papp, MD; Daniel Pine, MD; Jose Martinez, MA; Thomas Cooper, MA; Leonard A. Rosenblum, PhD; Donald F. Klein, MD; Jack M. Gorman, MD

American Medical Association
Physicians dedicated to the health of America

All articles published, including editorials, letters, and book reviews, represent the opinions of the authors and do not reflect the policy of the American Medical Association, the Editorial Board, or the institution with which the author is affiliated, unless this is clearly specified.

Advertising Office: J. P. Cahill & Associates, 341 S Waiola Ave, La Grange, IL 60525 (708) 352-0322. **AMA Physician Recruitment Advertising Department:** Robert Lake, Supervisor, 800-262-2260.

Disrupted Pattern of D_2 Dopamine Receptors in the Temporal Lobe in Schizophrenia: A Postmortem Study 649
Sara K. Goldsmith, PhD; Raymond M. Shapiro, MD, PhD; Jeffrey N. Joyce, PhD

Reduction of Synaptophysin Immunoreactivity in the Prefrontal Cortex of Subjects With Schizophrenia: Regional and Diagnostic Specificity 660
Leisa A. Glantz, MS; David A. Lewis, MD

Maternal Smoking During Pregnancy and the Risk of Conduct Disorder in Boys 670
Lauren S. Wakschlag, PhD; Benjamin B. Lahey, PhD; Rolf Loeber, PhD; Stephanie M. Green, MS; Rachel A. Gordon, MA; Bennett L. Leventhal, MD

LETTERS TO THE EDITOR

The Ondine Curse, False Suffocation Alarms, Trait-State Suffocation Fear, and Dyspnea-Suffocation Fear in Panic Attacks 677
Ronald Ley, PhD

In Reply 677
Steven Taylor, PhD; S. Rachman, PhD

In Reply 678
Donald F. Klein, MD

REGULAR DEPARTMENTS

This Month in *Archives of General Psychiatry* 596

Physician Recruitment Advertising 679

Index to Advertisers 680

**Instructions for Authors—
See June 1997 issue, page 581 or visit the Web site at http://www.ama-assn.org.**

ARCHIVES OF GENERAL PSYCHIATRY

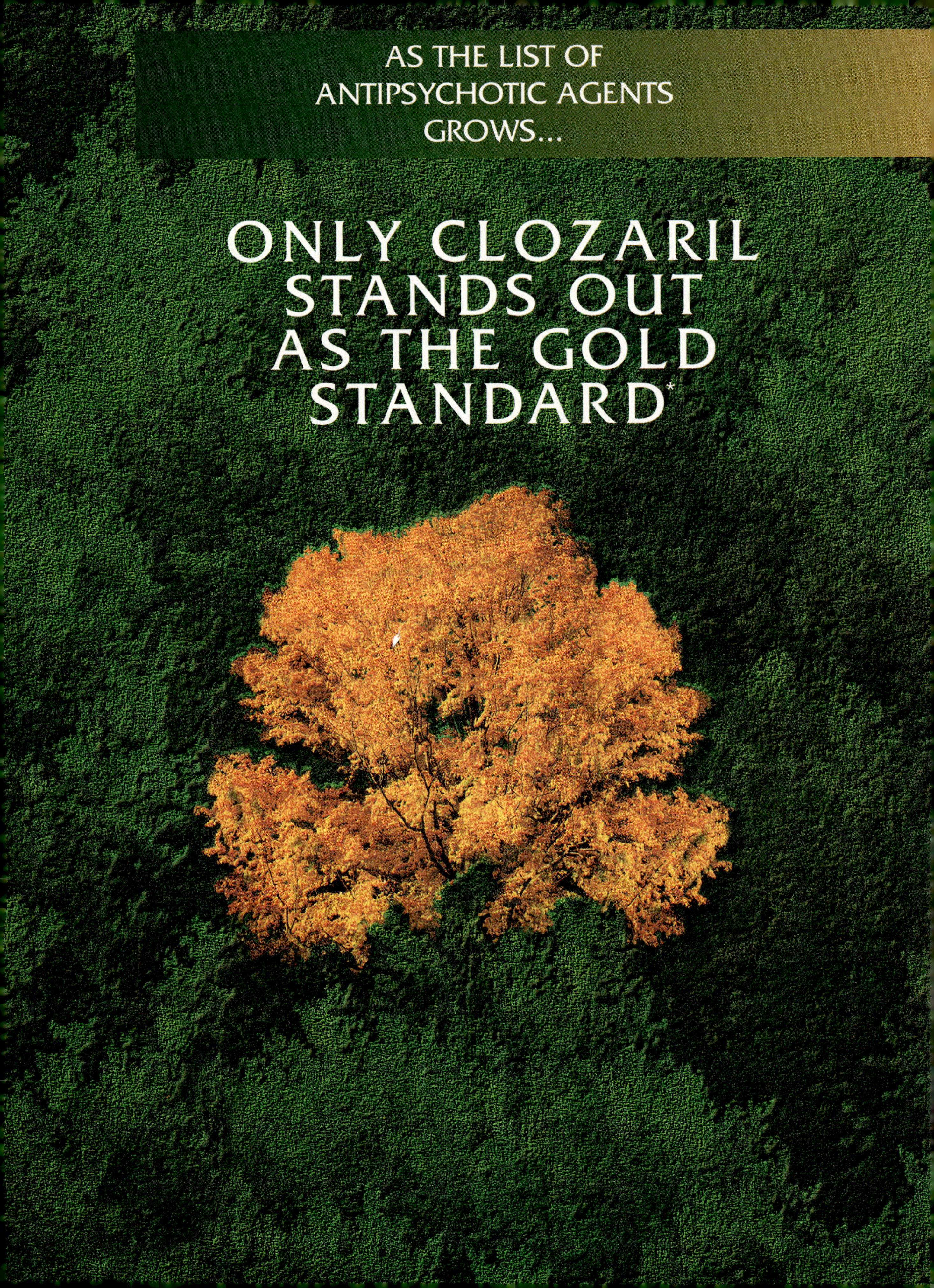
AS THE LIST OF
ANTIPSYCHOTIC AGENTS
GROWS...
ONLY CLOZARIL
STANDS OUT
AS THE GOLD
STANDARD*

ARCHIVES OF GENERAL PSYCHIATRY

VOL 54 NO. 8, AUGUST 1997

COMMENTARY

Drug Abuse and Addiction Treatment Research: The Next Generation 691
Alan I. Leshner, PhD

ORIGINAL ARTICLES

Impaired Color Vision in Cocaine-Withdrawn Patients 696
Parul Desai, MD; Monique Roy, MD; Alec Roy, MD; Stafford Brown; David Smelson, PsyD

Fluoxetine in Depressed Alcoholics: A Double-blind, Placebo-Controlled Trial 700
Jack R. Cornelius, MD, MPH; Ihsan M. Salloum, MD, MPH; Joan G. Ehler, MD; Patricia J. Jarrett, MD, PhD; Marie D. Cornelius, PhD; James M. Perel, PhD; Michael E. Thase, MD; Ann Black, MS

Prediction of Compliance With Outpatient Referral in Patients With Schizophrenia and Psychoactive Substance Use Disorders 706
Christian R. Miner, PhD; Richard N. Rosenthal, MD; David J. Hellerstein, MD; Larry R. Muenz, PhD

Buprenorphine vs Methadone Maintenance Treatment for Concurrent Opioid Dependence and Cocaine Abuse 713
Richard S. Schottenfeld, MD; Juliana R. Pakes, MEd; Alison Oliveto, PhD; Douglas Ziedonis, MD; Thomas R. Kosten, MD

SPECIAL ARTICLE

The National Institute on Drug Abuse Collaborative Cocaine Treatment Study: Rationale and Methods 721
Paul Crits-Christoph, PhD; Lynne Siqueland, PhD; Jack Blaine, MD; Arlene Frank, PhD; Lester Luborsky, PhD; Lisa Simon Onken, PhD; Larry Muenz, PhD; Michael E. Thase, MD; Roger D. Weiss, MD; David R. Gastfriend, MD; George Woody, MD; Jacques P. Barber, PhD; Stephen F. Butler, PhD; Dennis Daley, MSW; Sarah Bishop, MA; Lisa M. Najavits, PhD; Judy Lis, MSN; Delinda Mercer, MA; Margaret L. Griffin, PhD; Karla Moras, PhD; Aaron T. Beck, MD

American Medical Association
Physicians dedicated to the health of America

All articles published, including editorials, letters, and book reviews, represent the opinions of the authors and do not reflect the policy of the American Medical Association, the Editorial Board, or the institution with which the author is affiliated, unless this is clearly specified.

Information for Patients: Physicians are advised to discuss the following issues with patients for whom they prescribe CLOZARIL® (clozapine):

– Patients who are to receive CLOZARIL® (clozapine) should be warned about the significant risk of developing agranulocytosis. They should be informed that weekly blood tests are required to monitor for the occurrence of agranulocytosis, and that CLOZARIL® (clozapine) tablets will be made available only through a special program designed to ensure the required blood monitoring. Patients should be advised to report immediately the appearance of lethargy, weakness, fever, sore throat, malaise, mucous membrane ulceration or other possible signs of infection. Particular attention should be paid to any flu-like complaints or other symptoms that might suggest infection.

– Patients should be informed of the significant risk of seizure during CLOZARIL® (clozapine) treatment, and they should be advised to avoid driving and any other potentially hazardous activity while taking CLOZARIL® (clozapine).

– Patients should be advised of the risk of orthostatic hypotension, especially during the period of initial dose titration.

– Patients should be informed that if they stop taking CLOZARIL® (clozapine) for more than 2 days, they should not restart their medication at the same dosage, but should contact their physician for dosing instructions.

– Patients should notify their physician if they are taking, or plan to take, any prescription or over-the-counter drugs or alcohol.

– Patients should notify their physician if they become pregnant or intend to become pregnant during therapy.

– Patients should not breast feed an infant if they are taking CLOZARIL® (clozapine).

Drug Interactions: The risks of using CLOZARIL® (clozapine) in combination with other drugs have not been systematically evaluated.

The mechanism of CLOZARIL® (clozapine) induced agranulocytosis is unknown; nonetheless, the possibility that causative factors may interact synergistically to increase the risk and/or severity of bone marrow suppression warrants consideration. Therefore, CLOZARIL® (clozapine) should not be used with other agents having a well-known potential to suppress bone marrow function.

Given the primary CNS effects of CLOZARIL® (clozapine), caution is advised in using it concomitantly with other CNS-active drugs or alcohol.

Orthostatic hypotension in patients taking clozapine can, in rare cases (approximately 1 case per 3,000 patients), be accompanied by profound collapse and respiratory and/or cardiac arrest. Some of the cases of collapse/respiratory arrest/cardiac arrest during initial treatment occurred in patients who were being administered benzodiazepines; similar events have been reported in patients taking other psychotropic drugs or even CLOZARIL® (clozapine) by itself. Although it has not been established that there is an interaction between CLOZARIL® (clozapine) and benzodiazepines or other psychotropics, caution is advised when clozapine is initiated in patients taking a benzodiazepine or any other psychotropic drug.

Because CLOZARIL® (clozapine) is highly bound to serum protein, the administration of CLOZARIL® (clozapine) to a patient taking another drug which is highly bound to protein (e.g., warfarin, digitoxin) may cause an increase in plasma concentrations of these drugs, potentially resulting in adverse effects. Conversely, adverse effects may result from displacement of protein-bound CLOZARIL® (clozapine) by other highly bound drugs.

Cimetidine and erythromycin may both increase plasma levels of CLOZARIL® (clozapine), potentially resulting in adverse effects. Although concomitant use of CLOZARIL® (clozapine) and carbamazepine is not recommended, it should be noted that discontinuation of concomitant carbamazepine administration may result in an increase in CLOZARIL® (clozapine) plasma levels. Phenytoin may decrease CLOZARIL® (clozapine) plasma levels, resulting in a decrease in effectiveness of a previously effective CLOZARIL® (clozapine) dose.

A subset (3%-10%) of the population has reduced activity of certain drug metabolizing enzymes such as the cytochrome P450 isozyme P450 2D6. Such individuals are referred to as "poor metabolizers" of drugs such as debrisoquin, dextromethorphan, the tricyclic antidepressants, and clozapine. These individuals may develop higher than expected plasma concentrations of clozapine when given usual doses. In addition, certain drugs that are metabolized by this isozyme, including many antidepressants (clozapine, selective serotonin reuptake inhibitors, and others), may inhibit the activity of this isozyme, and thus may make normal metabolizers resemble poor metabolizers with regard to concomitant therapy with other drugs metabolized by this enzyme system, leading to drug interaction.

Concomitant use of clozapine with other drugs metabolized by cytochrome P450 2D6 may require lower doses than usually prescribed for either clozapine or the other drug. Therefore, co-administration of clozapine with other drugs that are metabolized by this isozyme, including antidepressants, phenothiazines, carbamazepine, and Type 1C antiarrhythmics (e.g., propafenone, flecainide and encainide), or that inhibit this enzyme (e.g., quinidine), should be approached with caution.

CLOZARIL® (clozapine) may also potentiate the hypotensive effects of antihypertensive drugs and the anticholinergic effects of atropine-type drugs. The administration of epinephrine should be avoided in the treatment of drug induced hypotension because of a possible reverse epinephrine effect.

Carcinogenesis, Mutagenesis, Impairment of Fertility: No carcinogenic potential was demonstrated in long-term studies in mice and rats at doses approximately 7 times the typical human dose on a mg/kg basis. Fertility in male and female rats was not adversely affected by clozapine. Clozapine did not produce genotoxic or mutagenic effects when assayed in appropriate bacterial and mammalian tests.

Pregnancy Category B: Reproduction studies have been performed in rats and rabbits at doses of approximately 2-4 times the human dose and have revealed no evidence of impaired fertility or harm to the fetus due to clozapine. There are, however, no adequate and well-controlled studies in pregnant women. Because animal reproduction studies are not always predictive of human response, and in view of the desirability of keeping the administration of all drugs to a minimum during pregnancy, this drug should be used only if clearly needed.

Nursing Mothers: Animal studies suggest that clozapine may be excreted in breast milk and have an effect on the nursing infant. Therefore, women receiving CLOZARIL® (clozapine) should not breast feed.

Pediatric Use: Safety and effectiveness in pediatric patients have not been established.

ADVERSE REACTIONS: Associated with Discontinuation of Treatment: Sixteen percent of 1080 patients who received CLOZARIL® (clozapine) in premarketing clinical trials discontinued treatment due to an adverse event, including both those that could be reasonably attributed to CLOZARIL® (clozapine) treatment and those that might more appropriately be considered intercurrent illness. The more common events considered to be causes of discontinuation included: CNS, primarily drowsiness/sedation, seizures, dizziness/syncope; cardiovascular, primarily tachycardia, hypotension and ECG changes; gastrointestinal, primarily nausea/vomiting; hematologic, primarily leukopenia/granulocytopenia/agranulocytosis; and fever. None of the events enumerated accounts for more than 1.7% of all discontinuations attributed to adverse clinical events.

Commonly Observed: Adverse events observed in association with the use of CLOZARIL® (clozapine) in clinical trials at an incidence of greater than 5% were: central nervous system complaints, including drowsiness/sedation, dizziness/vertigo, headache and tremor; autonomic nervous system complaints, including salivation, sweating, dry mouth and visual disturbances; cardiovascular findings, including tachycardia, hypotension and syncope; and gastrointestinal complaints, including constipation and nausea; and fever. Complaints of drowsiness/sedation tend to subside with continued therapy or dose reduction. Salivation may be profuse, especially during sleep, but may be diminished with dose reduction.

Incidence in Clinical Trials: The following table enumerates adverse events that occurred at a frequency of 1% or greater among CLOZARIL® (clozapine) patients who participated in clinical trials. These rates are not adjusted for duration of exposure.

Treatment-Emergent Adverse Experience Incidence Among Patients Taking CLOZARIL® (clozapine) in Clinical Trials (N = 842) (Percentage of Patients Reporting)

Body System / Adverse Event[a]	Percent
Central Nervous System	
Drowsiness/Sedation	39
Dizziness/Vertigo	19
Headache	7
Tremor	6
Syncope	6
Disturbed sleep/Nightmares	4
Restlessness	4
Hypokinesia/Akinesia	4
Agitation	4
Seizures (convulsions)	3[b]
Rigidity	3
Akathisia	3
Confusion	3
Fatigue	2
Insomnia	2
Hyperkinesia	1
Weakness	1
Lethargy	1
Ataxia	1
Slurred speech	1
Depression	1
Epileptiform movements/Myoclonic jerks	1
Anxiety	1
Cardiovascular	
Tachycardia	25[b]
Hypotension	9
Hypertension	4
Chest pain/Angina	1
ECG change/Cardiac abnormality	1

(Continued)

Treatment-Emergent Adverse Experience Incidence Among Patients Taking CLOZARIL® (clozapine) in Clinical Trials (N = 842) (Percentage of Patients Reporting)

Body System / Adverse Event[a]	Percent
Gastrointestinal	
Constipation	14
Nausea	5
Abdominal discomfort/Heartburn	4
Nausea/Vomiting	3
Vomiting	3
Diarrhea	2
Liver test abnormality	1
Anorexia	1
Urogenital	
Urinary abnormalities	2
Incontinence	1
Abnormal ejaculation	1
Urinary urgency/frequency	1
Urinary retention	1
Autonomic Nervous System	
Salivation	31
Sweating	6
Dry mouth	6
Visual disturbances	5
Integumentary (Skin)	
Rash	2
Musculoskeletal	
Muscle weakness	1
Pain (back, neck, legs)	1
Muscle spasm	1
Muscle pain, ache	1
Respiratory	
Throat discomfort	1
Dyspnea, shortness of breath	1
Nasal congestion	1
Hemic/Lymphatic	
Leukopenia/Decreased WBC/Neutropenia	3
Agranulocytosis	1[b]
Eosinophilia	1
Miscellaneous	
Fever	5
Weight gain	4
Tongue numb/sore	1

[a]Events reported by at least 1% of CLOZARIL® (clozapine) patients are included.

[b]Rate based on population of approximately 1700 exposed during premarket clinical evaluation of CLOZARIL® (clozapine).

Other Events Observed During the Premarketing Evaluation of CLOZARIL® (clozapine): This section reports additional, less frequent adverse events which occurred among the patients taking CLOZARIL® (clozapine) in clinical trials. Various adverse events were reported as part of the total experience in these clinical studies; a causal relationship to CLOZARIL® (clozapine) treatment cannot be determined in the absence of appropriate controls in some of the studies. The table above enumerates adverse events that occurred at a frequency of at least 1% of patients treated with CLOZARIL® (clozapine). The list below includes all additional adverse experiences reported as being temporally associated with the use of the drug which occurred at a frequency less than 1%, enumerated by organ system.

Central Nervous System: loss of speech, amentia, tics, poor coordination, delusions/hallucinations, involuntary movement, stuttering, dysarthria, amnesia/memory loss, histrionic movements, libido increase or decrease, paranoia, shakiness, Parkinsonism, and irritability.

Cardiovascular System: edema, palpitations, phlebitis/thrombophlebitis, cyanosis, premature ventricular contraction, bradycardia, and nose bleed.

Gastrointestinal System: abdominal distention, gastroenteritis, rectal bleeding, nervous stomach, abnormal stools, hematemesis, gastric ulcer, bitter taste, and eructation.

Urogenital System: dysmenorrhea, impotence, breast pain/discomfort, and vaginal itch/infection.

Autonomic Nervous System: numbness, polydypsia, hot flashes, dry throat, and mydriasis.

Integumentary (Skin): pruritus, pallor, eczema, erythema, bruise, dermatitis, petechiae, and urticaria.

Musculoskeletal System: twitching and joint pain.

Respiratory System: coughing, pneumonia/pneumonia-like symptoms, rhinorrhea, hyperventilation, wheezing, bronchitis, laryngitis, and sneezing.

Hemic and Lymphatic System: anemia and leukocytosis.

Miscellaneous: chills/chills with fever, malaise, appetite increase, ear disorder, hypothermia, eyelid disorder, bloodshot eyes, and nystagmus.

Postmarketing Clinical Experience: Postmarketing experience has shown an adverse experience profile similar to that presented above. Voluntary reports of adverse events temporally associated with CLOZARIL® (clozapine) not mentioned above that have been received since market introduction and that may have no causal relationship with the drug include the following:

Central Nervous System: delirium; EEG abnormal; exacerbation of psychosis; myoclonus; overdose; paresthesia; possible mild cataplexy; and status epilepticus.

Cardiovascular System: atrial or ventricular fibrillation and periorbital edema.

Gastrointestinal System: acute pancreatitis; dysphagia; fecal impaction; intestinal obstruction/paralytic ileus; and salivary gland swelling.

Hepatobiliary System: cholestasis; hepatitis; jaundice.

Hepatic System: cholestasis.

Urogenital System: acute interstitial nephritis and priapism.

Integumentary (Skin): hypersensitivity reactions: photosensitivity, vasculitis, erythema multiforme, and Stevens-Johnson Syndrome.

Musculoskeletal System: myasthenic syndrome and rhabdomyolysis.

Respiratory System: aspiration and pleural effusion.

Hemic and Lymphatic System: deep vein thrombosis; elevated hemoglobin/hematocrit; ESR increased; pulmonary embolism; sepsis; thrombocytosis; and thrombocytopenia.

Miscellaneous: CPK elevation; hyperglycemia; hyperuricemia; hyponatremia; and weight loss.

DRUG ABUSE AND DEPENDENCE: Physical and psychological dependence have not been reported or observed in patients taking CLOZARIL® (clozapine).

Store and Dispense: Storage temperature should not exceed 86°F (30°C). Drug dispensing should not ordinarily exceed a weekly supply. Dispensing should be contingent upon the results of a WBC count.

*Trademark of Medical Economics Company, Inc.

Sandoz Pharmaceuticals Corporation, East Hanover, New Jersey 07936
REV: MARCH 1997 P30118906

ORIGINAL ARTICLES

Problem-Service 'Matching' in Addiction Treatment: A Prospective Study in 4 Programs 730
A. Thomas McLellan, PhD; Grant R. Grissom, PhD; David Zanis, PhD; Mary Randall, MA; Peter Brill, MD; Charles P. O'Brien, MD, PhD

Naltrexone and Alcohol Dependence: Role of Subject Compliance 737
Joseph R. Volpicelli, MD, PhD; Karen C. Rhines; Jared S. Rhines; Laura A. Volpicelli; Arthur I. Alterman, PhD; Charles P. O'Brien, MD, PhD

Double-blindness Procedures, Rater Blindness, and Ratings of Outcome: Observations From a Controlled Trial 744
Metin Başoğlu, MD, PhD; Isaac Marks, MD, FRCPsych; Maria Livanou; Richard Swinson, MD, FRCPsych

Noradrenergic and Serotonergic Function in Posttraumatic Stress Disorder 749
Steven M. Southwick, MD; John H. Krystal, MD; J. Douglas Bremner, MD; C. A. Morgan III, MD; Andreas L. Nicolaou, PhD; Linda M. Nagy, MD; David R. Johnson, PhD; George R. Heninger, MD; Dennis S. Charney, MD

LETTERS TO THE EDITOR

Clozapine Withdrawal: Serotonergic or Dopaminergic Mechanisms? 760
Herbert Y. Meltzer, MD

In Reply 761
Ross J. Baldessarini, MD; Frank I. Tarazi, PhD; Nora S. Kula, MS; David M. Gardner, Pharm D

Philip Seeman, MD, PhD 762

Anterior Paralimbic Mediation of Procaine-Induced Emotional and Psychosensory Experiences 763
Stephen M. Saravay, MD

In Reply 764
Terence A. Ketter, MD; Paul J. Andreason, MD; Chulhee Lee, PhD; Debra S. Gill, MA; Priti I. Parekh; Mark W. Willis, MEng; Peter Herscovitch, MD; Robert M. Post, MD; Mark S. George, MD

Correction and Clarification 765
Samuel Gershon, MD; Jair C. Soares, MD

REGULAR DEPARTMENTS

This Month in *Archives of General Psychiatry* 690

Physician Recruitment Advertising 767

Index to Advertisers 768

**Instructions for Authors—
See June 1997 issue, page 581 or visit the Web site at http://www.ama-assn.org.**

ARCHIVES OF GENERAL PSYCHIATRY

Dopamine is found in high concentrations in the retina and is involved in color vision. Use of cocaine may alter dopaminergic neurotransmission. **Desai et al** (page 696) found that cocaine-dependent patients, when withdrawn from cocaine, had significantly increased error scores on color vision tests and more color vision losses than normal controls.

Cornelius et al (page 700) report the results of the first double-blind, placebo-controlled study of fluoxetine therapy in depressed alcoholics. In this study, depressive symptoms and alcohol use improved more with fluoxetine therapy than with placebo.

Many patients with schizophrenia and concurrent addictive disorders may be treated adequately as outpatients. However, some do not comply with outpatient referral. **Miner et al** (page 706) show that by considering schizophrenia syndrome typology and gender, noncompliance may be predicted before referral. Identified patients may especially benefit from assertive community outreach programs.

Problems with methadone maintenance, including high rates of cocaine abuse among patients in treatment, support the need to evaluate alternative maintenance agents, especially the mixed partial agonist/antagonist buprenorphine. **Schottenfeld et al** (page 713) found significantly less illicit opiate use at higher vs lower daily maintenance doses of buprenorphine and methadone in rates of cocaine use. The study supports the efficacy of buprenorphine as a maintenance treatment.

Developing treatments for cocaine use disorders is a high national priority. **Crits-Christoph et al** (page 721) describe the design of the National Institute on Drug Abuse Collaborative Cocaine Treatment Study—a large, multisite clinical trial for outpatients with cocaine dependence. In addition to the background for the project, this article presents the project's main aims, the rationale for the choice of treatments and patients, and a description of the research plan.

The effects of treatments may be improved if patients are "matched" to the right treatment. **McLellan et al** (page 730) tested a patient-program and a problem-service matching strategy with working, insured substance abuse patients treated within a 4-program network. It was virtually impossible to "match" patients to a particular treatment program owing to constraints imposed by geography, insurance, and patient preference. However, in all programs, patients who were randomly assigned to receive professional services prospectively matched to their admission problems had 20% to 40% better 6-month outcomes than patients treated under standard care conditions in the same programs.

Naltrexone therapy has been shown to improve the treatment of alcoholism in 2 double-blind studies. As with all medications, however, it must be taken to be effective. **Volpicelli et al** (page 737) studied a large group of alcoholics and found again that naltrexone therapy is significantly more effective than placebo in patients who comply with treatment.

A Commentary by Alan I. Leshner, PhD, titled "Drug Abuse and Addiction Treatment Research: the Next Generation," is also included in this issue.

The double-blind procedure in clinical trials aims to reduce bias in the assessment of treatment efficacy from assessors' and patients' expectations, but few researchers have reported whether blindness has actually been maintained in their study. In a double-blind, randomized controlled trial of alprazolam and exposure in panic disorder with agoraphobia, **Başoğlu et al** (page 744) found that assessor and patient blindness as to treatment condition was not maintained, but unblinding was unrelated to clinical outcome. Future reports of clinical trials need to note whether blindness has been maintained and how any unblinding affected their ratings of clinical outcome.

To test for possible neurotransmitter alterations in traumatized combat veterans with posttraumatic stress disorder (PTSD), **Southwick et al** (page 749) assessed behavioral and cardiovascular responses to intravenous yohimbine, a probe of the noradrenergic systems, and to intravenous m-chlorophenylpiperazine (m-CPP), a probe of the serotonergic systems. One group of combat veterans had a high rate of yohimbine-induced panic attacks and flashbacks while another group had a similar response to m-CPP. The data suggest 2 subgroups of patients with PTSD: one with a sensitized noradrenergic system and the other with a sensitized serotonergic system.

ARCHIVES OF GENERAL PSYCHIATRY

VOL 54 NO. 9, SEPTEMBER 1997

COMMENTARY

Child Psychiatric Disorder: Measures, Causal Mechanisms, and Interventions 785
Michael Rutter, MD, FRS

ORIGINAL ARTICLES

Adequacy of Interviews vs Checklists for Classifying Childhood Psychiatric Disorder Based on Parent Reports 793
Michael H. Boyle, PhD; David R. Offord, MD; Yvonne A. Racine, MA; Peter Szatmari, MD; Mark Sanford, MB, ChB; Jan E. Fleming, MD

The Virginia Twin Study of Adolescent Behavioral Development: Influences of Age, Sex, and Impairment on Rates of Disorder 801
Emily Simonoff, MD; Andrew Pickles, PhD; Joanne M. Meyer, PhD; Judy L. Silberg, PhD; Hermine H. Maes, PhD; Rolf Loeber, PhD; Michael Rutter, MD, FRS; John K. Hewitt, PhD; Lindon J. Eaves, Dsc

Boys' Behavioral Inhibition and the Risk of Later Delinquency 809
Margaret Kerr, PhD; Richard E. Tremblay, PhD; Linda Pagani, PhD; Frank Vitaro, PhD

A Global Scale to Measure the Quality of the Family Environment 817
Joseph M. Rey, MD, FRANZCP; Michelle Singh, MPsychol(Clin); Se-fong Hung, FHKAM(Psychiatry), MRCPsych; David R. Dossetor, MD, MRCPsych; Louise Newman, MD, FRANZCP; Jon M. Plapp, PhD; Kevin D. Bird, PhD

Frontostriatal Measurement in Treatment-Naive Children With Obsessive-Compulsive Disorder 824
David R. Rosenberg, MD; Matcheri S. Keshavan, MD; Kirsten M. O'Hearn; Elizabeth L. Dick; Werner W. Bagwell; Andrew B. Seymour; Debra M. Montrose, MSW; Joseph N. Pierri, MS, MD; Boris Birmaher, MD

Oculomotor Response Inhibition Abnormalities in Pediatric Obsessive-Compulsive Disorder 831
David R. Rosenberg, MD; David H. Averbach, MD; Kirsten M. O'Hearn; Andrew B. Seymour; Boris Birmaher, MD; John A. Sweeney, PhD

Neuroendocrine Response to Fenfluramine Challenge in Boys: Associations With Aggressive Behavior and Adverse Rearing 839
Daniel S. Pine, MD; Jeremy D. Coplan, MD; Gail A. Wasserman, PhD; Laurie S. Miller, PhD; Jane E. Fried, MD; Mark Davies, MPH; Thomas B. Cooper, MS; Laurence Greenhill, MD; David Shaffer, MD; Bruce Parsons, PhD, MD

American Medical Association
Physicians dedicated to the health of America

P. John Seward, MD
Executive Vice President

Kenneth E. Monroe
Deputy Executive Vice President

George D. Lundberg, MD
Editor in Chief, Scientific Information and Multimedia

James F. Rappel
Group Vice President, Business and Management Services

Robert L. Kennett
Vice President, Publishing

Peter L. Payerli
Associate Publisher

Vanessa Hayden
Director, Production & Distribution Division

Cheryl Iverson
Director, Editorial Processing Division

Geoffrey A. Flick
Manager, Marketing Services

Psychiatric Outcomes in Low-Birth-Weight Children at Age 6 Years: Relation to Neonatal Cranial Ultrasound Abnormalities 847
Agnes H. Whitaker, MD; Ronan Van Rossem, PhD; Judith F. Feldman, PhD; Irvin Sam Schonfeld, PhD, MPH; Jennifer A. Pinto-Martin, PhD; Carolyn Torre, RN, MA; David Shaffer, MD; Nigel Paneth, MD, MPH

Long-term Stimulant Treatment of Children With Attention-Deficit Hyperactivity Disorder Symptoms: A Randomized, Double-blind, Placebo-Controlled Trial 857
Christopher Gillberg, MD, PhD; Hans Melander, MSc; Anne-Liis von Knorring, MD, PhD; Lars-Olof Janols, MD, PhD; Gunilla Thernlund, MD; Bruno Hägglöf, MD, PhD; Lena Eidevall-Wallin, MD; Peik Gustafsson, MD; Svenny Kopp, MD

SPECIAL ARTICLE

National Institute of Mental Health Collaborative Multimodal Treatment Study of Children With ADHD (the MTA): Design Challenges and Choices 865
L. Eugene Arnold, MEd, MD; Howard B. Abikoff, PhD; Dennis P. Cantwell, MD; C. Keith Conners, PhD; Glen Elliott, MD, PhD; Laurence L. Greenhill, MD; Lily Hechtman, MD; Stephen P. Hinshaw, PhD; Betsy Hoza, PhD; Peter S. Jensen, MD; Helena C. Kraemer, PhD; John S. March, MD, MPH; Jeffrey H. Newcorn, MD; William E. Pelham, PhD; John E. Richters, PhD; Ellen Schiller, PhD; Joanne B. Severe, MS; James M. Swanson, PhD; Donald Vereen, MD; Karen C. Wells, PhD; for the MTA

NEWS AND VIEWS

Medication Development and Testing in Children and Adolescents: Current Problems, Future Directions 871
Benedetto Vitiello, MD; Peter S. Jensen, MD

ORIGINAL ARTICLE

A Clinical Psychotherapy Trial for Adolescent Depression Comparing Cognitive, Family, and Supportive Therapy 877
David A. Brent, MD; Diane Holder, MSW; David Kolko, PhD; Boris Birmaher, MD; Marianne Baugher, MA; Claudia Roth, MSW; Satish Iyengar, PhD; Barbara A. Johnson, MD

CORRECTION

Backward Masking Performance in Unaffected Siblings of Schizophrenic Patients: Evidence for a Vulnerability Indicator 846
Michael F. Green, PhD; Keith H. Nuechterlein, PhD; Bruno Breitmeyer, PhD

REGULAR DEPARTMENTS

This Month in *Archives of General Psychiatry* 783

Classified Advertising 887

Index to Advertisers 888

Instructions for Authors—
See June 1997 issue, page 581 or visit the Web site at http://www.ama-assn.org.

ARCHIVES OF GENERAL PSYCHIATRY

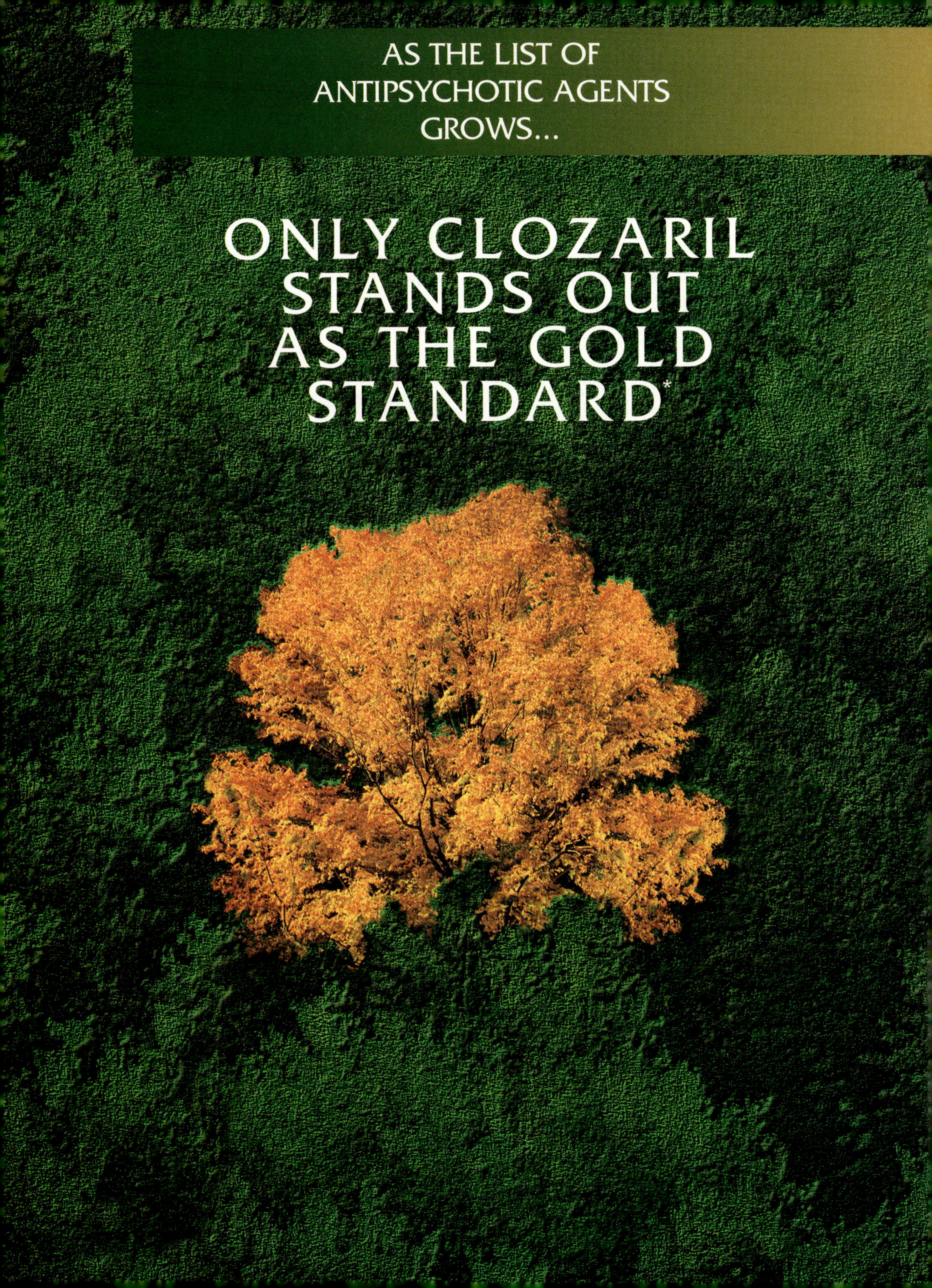
AS THE LIST OF
ANTIPSYCHOTIC AGENTS
GROWS...
ONLY CLOZARIL
STANDS OUT
AS THE GOLD
STANDARD*

ARCHIVES OF GENERAL PSYCHIATRY

VOL 54 NO. 10, OCTOBER 1997

ORIGINAL ARTICLES

Childhood-Onset Schizophrenia: Progressive Ventricular Change During Adolescence 897
Judith L. Rapoport, MD; Jay Giedd, MD; Sanjiv Kumra, MD; Leslie Jacobsen, MD; Amy Smith; Paul Lee; Jean Nelson, MHS; Susan Hamburger, MS

Autonomic Nervous System Markers of Psychopathology in Childhood-Onset Schizophrenia 904
Theodore P. Zahn, PhD; Leslie K. Jacobsen, MD; Charles T. Gordon, MD; Kathleen McKenna, MD; Jean A. Frazier, MD; Judith L. Rapoport, MD

COMMENTARY

Neurobiology and Neuroplasticity in Schizophrenia: Continuity Across the Life Cycle 913
Henry A. Nasrallah, MD; Herman A. Tolbert, MD

NEWS AND VIEWS

The 'Vascular Depression' Hypothesis 915
George S. Alexopoulos, MD; Barnett S. Meyers, MD; Robert C. Young, MD; Scott Campbell, PhD; David Silbersweig, MD; Mary Charlson, MD

Manual-Guided Psychosocial Treatment: A New Virtual Requirement for Pharmacotherapy Trials? 923
Kathleen M. Carroll, PhD

COMMENTARY

A Psychotherapeutic Context for Clinical Trials Is Promising, But Manualization Is Not 929
Donald F. Klein, MD; Lauren B. Smith

ORIGINAL ARTICLE

Offspring of Depressed Parents: 10 Years Later 932
Myrna M. Weissman, PhD; Virginia Warner, MPH; Priya Wickramaratne, PhD; Donna Moreau, MD; Mark Olfson, MD

Reduction of Synaptophysin Immunoreactivity in the Prefrontal Cortex of Subjects With Schizophrenia: Regional and Diagnostic Specificity 943
Leisa A. Glantz, MS; David A. Lewis, MD

Delayed Normalization of Central D_2 Dopamine Receptor Availability After Discontinuation of Haloperidol Decanoate: Preliminary Findings 953
Svante Nyberg, MD, PhD; Lars Farde, MD, PhD; Christer Halldin, PhD

American Medical Association
Physicians dedicated to the health of America

P. John Seward, MD
Executive Vice President

Lynn Jensen, PhD
Acting Chief Operating Officer

George D. Lundberg, MD
Editor in Chief, Scientific Information and Multimedia

Robert L. Kennett
Vice President, Publishing

Peter L. Payerli
Associate Publisher

Vanessa Hayden
Director, Production & Distribution Division

Cheryl Iverson
Director, Editorial Processing Division

Geoffrey A. Flick
Manager, Marketing Services

All articles published, including editorials, letters, and book reviews, represent the opinions of the authors and do not reflect the policy of the American Medical Association, the Editorial Board, or the institution with which the author is affiliated, unless this is clearly specified.

Measurement of Glutamate and Glutamine in the Medial Prefrontal Cortex of Never-Treated Schizophrenic Patients and Healthy Controls by Proton Magnetic Resonance Spectroscopy 959
Robert Bartha, BSc; Peter C. Williamson, MD; Dick J. Drost, PhD; Ashok Malla, MB; Tom J. Carr, MD; Len Cortese, MD; Gita Canaran, MA; R. Jane Rylett, PhD; Richard W. J. Neufeld, PhD

BOOK REVIEW

Major Theories of Personality Disorder 967
John F. Clarkin, Mark F. Lenzenweger (eds)
Reviewed by W. J. Livesley, MD, PhD

LETTERS TO THE EDITOR

Treatment of Bulimia Nervosa With Ondansetron 969
Boyd K. Hartman, MD; Patricia L. Faris, PhD; Suck Won Kim, MD; Nancy C. Raymond, MD; Robert L. Goodale, MD; William H. Meller, MD; Elke D. Eckert, MD

Patent Laws: Could Changes Enhance Drug Development? 970
Jeffrey A. Mattes, MD

The Identification and Validation of Distinct Depressive Syndromes in a Population-Based Sample of Female Twins 970
Frederic M. Quitkin, MD; Jonathan W. Stewart, MD; Patrick J. McGrath, MD; Edward V. Nunes, MD; Donald F. Klein, MD

D_2 Dopamine Receptor Occupancy: A Crossover Comparison of Risperidone With Clozapine Therapy in Schizophrenic Patients 972
Tung-Ping Su, MD; Anil K. Malhotra, MD; Kayleen Hadd, RN, MSN; Alan Breier, MD; David Pickar, MD

Sertraline and Imipramine for the Treatment of Dysthymia 973
Frans de Jonghe, MD, PhD

In Reply 973
Michael E. Thase, MD

The Idiosyncratic Definition of Nicotine Dependence 973
Naomi Breslau, PhD

In Reply 974
David M. Fergusson, PhD; Michael T. Lynskey, MSc; John L. Horwood, MSc

CORRECTIONS

Increased Concentrations of Presynaptic Proteins in the Cingulate Cortex of Subjects With Schizophrenia 912
Steven M. Gabriel, PhD; Vahram Haroutunian, PhD; Peter Powchik, MD; William G. Honer, MD, FRCPC; Michael Davidson, MD; Peter Davies, PhD; Kenneth L. Davis, MD

Reduction of Synaptophysin Immunoreactivity in the Prefrontal Cortex of Subjects With Schizophrenia: Regional and Diagnostic Specificity 950
Leisa A. Glantz, MS; David A. Lewis, MD

REGULAR DEPARTMENTS

This Month in *Archives of General Psychiatry* 896
Classified Advertising 975
Index to Advertisers 976
Instructions for Authors—See June 1997 issue, page 581 or visit the Web site at http://www.ama-assn.org.

ARCHIVES OF GENERAL PSYCHIATRY

ARCHIVES OF GENERAL PSYCHIATRY

VOL 54 NO. 11, NOVEMBER 1997

COMMENTARY

The Clinical Course of Unipolar Major Depressive Disorders 989
Lewis L. Judd, MD

ORIGINAL ARTICLES

Natural History of Diagnostic Interview Schedule/*DSM-IV* Major Depression: The Baltimore Epidemiologic Catchment Area Follow-up 993
William W. Eaton, PhD; James C. Anthony, PhD; Joseph Gallo, MD; Guojun Cai, MD; Allen Tien, MD; Alan Romanoski, MD; Constantine Lyketsos, MD; Li-Shiun Chen, MD

Recovery From Major Depression: A 10-Year Prospective Follow-up Across Multiple Episodes 1001
David A. Solomon, MD; Martin B. Keller, MD; Andrew C. Leon, PhD; Timothy I. Mueller, MD; M. Tracie Shea, PhD; Meredith Warshaw, MSS, MA; Jack D. Maser, PhD; William Coryell, MD; Jean Endicott, PhD

Treatment of Major Depression With Psychotherapy or Psychotherapy-Pharmacotherapy Combinations 1009
Michael E. Thase, MD; Joel B. Greenhouse, PhD; Ellen Frank, PhD; Charles F. Reynolds III, MD; Paul A. Pilkonis, PhD; Katharine Hurley, MS; Victoria Grochocinski, PhD; David J. Kupfer, MD

Temporal Profiles of the Course of Depression During Treatment: Predictors of Pathways Toward Recovery in the Elderly 1016
Mary Amanda Dew, PhD; Charles F. Reynolds III, MD; Patricia R. Houck, MS; Martica Hall, PhD; Daniel J. Buysse, MD; Ellen Frank, PhD; David J. Kupfer, MD

Family and Individual Therapy in Anorexia Nervosa: A 5-Year Follow-up 1025
Ivan Eisler, PhD; Christopher Dare, FRCPsych; Gerald F. M. Russell, MD; George Szmukler, MD; Daniel le Grange, PhD; Elizabeth Dodge, MSc

American Medical Association
Physicians dedicated to the health of America

A Double-blind, Randomized, Placebo-Controlled Trial of Fluoxetine in Children and Adolescents With Depression 1031
Graham J. Emslie, MD; A. John Rush, MD; Warren A. Weinberg, MD; Robert A. Kowatch, MD; Carroll W. Hughes, PhD; Tom Carmody, PhD; Jeanne Rintelmann

A Randomized Trial of Assertive Community Treatment for Homeless Persons With Severe Mental Illness 1038
Anthony F. Lehman, MD, MSPH; Lisa B. Dixon, MD; Eimer Kernan, MSW; Bruce R. DeForge, PhD; Leticia T. Postrado, PhD

Sex Differences in Posttraumatic Stress Disorder 1044
Naomi Breslau, PhD; Glenn C. Davis, MD; Patricia Andreski, MA; Edward L. Peterson, PhD; Lonni R. Schultz, PhD

PERSPECTIVES

A 'Second Life' Agenda: Psychiatric Research Issues Raised by Protease Inhibitor Treatments for People With the Human Immunodeficiency Virus or the Acquired Immunodeficiency Syndrome 1049
Judith G. Rabkin, PhD, MPH; Stephen Ferrando, MD

REGULAR DEPARTMENTS

This Month in *Archives of General Psychiatry* 986

Classified Advertising 1055

Index to Advertisers 1056

Instructions for Authors—
See June 1997 issue, page 581 or visit the Web site at www.ama-assn.org.

ARCHIVES OF GENERAL PSYCHIATRY

Forty Years of Lithium Treatment

Mogens Schou, MD, DrMed, DrHCMult

This review is based on a lecture in which I was requested to present my personal experiences and views. Since its introduction into psychiatry more than 40 years ago, lithium treatment has in most countries gained wide acceptance in the prophylaxis of unipolar and bipolar affective disorders. At one time it was feared that lithium treatment might lead to a decrease in the glomerular filtration rate, but systematically collected data indicate that even long-term treatment does not induce renal insufficiency. During treatment, regular laboratory monitoring of serum lithium and creatinine concentrations is recommended. Recent studies suggest that long-term lithium treatment does not raise the mortality of manic-depressive patients and indeed may have a mortality-lowering and antisuicidal effect. Despite the availability of alternative therapies, lithium remains the treatment of choice for the prophylaxis of recurrent manic-depressive illness.

Arch Gen Psychiatry. 1997;54:9-13

THE SITUATION IN 1950 AND TODAY

In the late 1930s, the advent of electroconvulsive treatment of manic-depressive illness was received enthusiastically; now depressions and manias could be relieved and deaths due to acute delirium prevented. Thus, the treatment of manic-depressive patients had become markedly improved, but there was still a long way to go. Of the drug treatments, only opium drops and barbiturates, both entirely unsatisfactory, were available for treating depression and mania, respectively, and electroconvulsive treatment did not, at least as then given, prevent the recurrence of manic and depressive episodes.

During the 1950s, major developments occurred. Lithium salts and neuroleptic drugs were introduced for the treatment of mania, and tricyclic antidepressants, for depression. Between 1960 and 1970 the prophylactic effect of lithium in unipolar and bipolar affective illness was observed, tested, and substantiated. Antiepileptics and antidepressants were later found to be valid prophylactic alternatives. A new era had indeed dawned for manic-depressive patients; without these developments many more would have been hospitalized or might have died.

A number of studies from recent years have shown lithium treatment carried out under "naturalistic" or "clinical practice" conditions to be markedly less effective than found in studies from research establishments. Reasons for and remedies against this phenomenon have been discussed in detail elsewhere.[1]

See also pages 14, 16 and 21

Let us now consider current problems and controversies surrounding lithium treatment.

LITHIUM PROPHYLAXIS IN UNIPOLAR AFFECTIVE ILLNESS

Today, lithium prophylaxis is universally considered the treatment of choice for recurrent bipolar illness. Trials by Baastrup et al and myself[2,3] have demonstrated that lithium is also prophylactically effective in recurrent unipolar manic-depressive ill-

From the Psychiatric Hospital, Risskov, Denmark.

ness (recurrent major affective disorder), and, in most parts of the world, lithium has been used successfully for this indication.[4] In a recent comprehensive analysis of the literature Souza and Goodwin[5] concluded: "There is no reason to doubt the efficacy of lithium in the prophylaxis of unipolar depressive illness."

However, this view does not appear to be shared by American psychiatrists. Although in the early 1970s lithium was recognized by the US Food and Drug Administration as a prophylactic agent in recurrent bipolar illness, there has not been a similar recognition in recurrent unipolar illness. Moreover, three recent reviews[6-8] by American authors dealt with long-term management of recurrent depressions, two of which described maintenance treatment with antidepressants and electroconvulsive treatment but did not mention lithium.[6,7] The third review concluded that in unipolar depressive disorder "the routine use of lithium salts instead of, or in combination with, antidepressants does not appear well-justified as a first-line maintenance treatment."[8] In the third reviewer's opinion, lithium had been shown prophylactically ineffective in two studies: British psychiatrists found no advantage of treatment with amitriptyline plus lithium over treatment with amitriptyline alone,[9] and an American study found lithium no better than placebo in patients with a severe index episode.[10]

However, the British study reveals nothing about the value of lithium alone, and it is difficult to see how a single American study (based on pooling of patients from many clinics with consequent risk for "loose" diagnoses) can outweigh the evidence of more than 15 studies carried out over the last 25 years that show the prophylactic, recurrence-preventive action of lithium to be as effective in unipolar as in bipolar affective disorder.[5,11,12]

A German randomized multicenter study of 80 patients with unipolar illness has shown prophylactic superiority of lithium over amitriptyline (W. Greil, MD, unpublished data, 1994). However, the amitriptyline doses were rather low, and there is clearly room for further trials comparing lithium and antidepressants in the treatment of unipolar illness.

In recent years American research has proved that long-term treatment with antidepressants is prophylactically effective in recurrent depressions.[13,14] Although these are fine studies, lithium prophylaxis was not mentioned. I believe that patients who suffer from recurrent depressions without obvious psychosocial precipitating factors, have symptom-free intervals, and are without deviating character features, might benefit from first-line or second-line lithium maintenance treatment. The final choice of prophylactic agent must depend on how individual patients respond to and tolerate treatment with antidepressants and with lithium.

Possible reasons why antidepressants may be preferred to lithium as prophylactic agents may be that patients treated for acute depression are likely to be prescribed the same medication for maintenance treatment and that patients usually prefer to use medication that does not require monitoring by blood tests. Moreover, the new specific serotonin reuptake inhibiting antidepressants have few side effects, and they are being marketed aggressively (even to the extent of being called "happiness pills," which they are not).

Since an extensive controlled prophylactic trial has shown lithium to be significantly more effective than carbamazepine,[15] my view is that for patients with bipolar illness, lithium should be the first-choice prophylactic agent and carbamazepine a valid alternative. For patients with unipolar illness, the new antidepressants may, for the reasons given above, be preferable as first-choice agents, but lithium should not be forgotten as an effective alternative of proven efficacy.

LITHIUM TREATMENT AND KIDNEY FUNCTION

Long-term lithium treatment was at one time feared to damage kidney function and endanger patients' lives. These fears have been allayed. Lithium treatment does affect renal concentrating ability and patients must be warned against dehydration; however, according to extensive reviews in 1988 and 1989, lithium treatment, even when administered for many years, does not lead to changes in the glomerular filtration rate or to renal failure.[16,17]

During the last 5 years there have been a few cases in which lithium-treated patients experienced renal insufficiency with no perceivable cause other than, possibly, the treatment. von Knorring and associates[18] reported that a 71-year-old woman was given hemodialysis after a gradual rise in her serum creatinine level to higher than 500 μmol/L (5.7 mg/dL) during the second decade of lithium treatment. In a study by Gitlin,[19] three of 82 patients given lithium for an average period of 4.3 years experienced renal insufficiency (defined as serum creatinine concentrations consistently higher than 176 μmol/L [2.0 mg/dL]). One of the patients, a 48-year-old man who had been taking lithium for 16 years, needed hemodialysis. I know of a further case, a 72-year-old man who showed a gradual rise of serum creatinine levels to higher than 600 μmol/L (6.8 mg/dL) after 27 years of lithium treatment and who subsequently received hemodialysis (M. Schou, MD, unpublished observations, 1994).

It is difficult to know how to interpret such rare events. They may be late and exceptional adverse effects of lithium treatment, or they may be mere coincidences. Renal insufficiency without a known cause and that requires treatment has been known to occur in the general population. The incidence of renal failure among manic-depressive patients not treated with lithium is unknown.

In terms of practical consequences I agree with Gitlin,[19] who concluded that

> these findings do not imply that lithium treatment should be withheld from appropriate patients, nor do they imply that rises in creatinine levels up to 140 mmol/L or above warrant automatic lithium discontinuation. However, regular monitoring of the creatinine levels of lithium-treated patients, eg, every 6 months to 1 year, and medical consultation if the creatinine level rises much above this threshold would seem to be warranted.

Lithium-induced polyuria and, not always fully reversible, renal concentrating deficit, are well-known side effects of lithium treatment, but investigation of patients given lithium for up to 30 years has not revealed them as harbingers of reduction of glomerular filtration rate and renal insufficiency.[20]

MONITORING OF LITHIUM TREATMENT

Clinical and laboratory monitoring of lithium treatment is important to maintain effective and safe therapy and to keep side effects to a minimum. During the past years there has been debate about the need for, and the frequency of, routine serum lithium determinations.[21-26]

My own recommendations have varied over the years. For a long time I advocated regular serum lithium determinations as a safeguard against over-dosage, under-dosage, and reduction of the renal lithium clearance. The situation changed when extensive studies indicated that lithium treatment does not lower the glomerular filtration rate or the lithium clearance. Based on these observations, I found it important to counteract exaggerated fear of lithium-induced kidney damage and suggested that serum lithium levels need not be determined routinely.[27] However, at the same time I emphasized the importance of frequent contacts between patient and physician for discussion of treatment progress and possible personal and social problems associated with the illness or the treatment. On these occasions serum lithium, serum creatinine, and thyroid-stimulating hormone values might also be determined.

In recent years I have again recommended regular determinations of serum lithium levels. The serum lithium concentration is one of the issues that patient and physician may profitably discuss; this serves a didactic purpose and improves compliance as patients are made aware of their coresponsibility for the treatment. In addition, lithium concentrations should be determined in "at-risk" situations; on suspected impending intoxication; to check for noncompliance; and at shorter intervals during initial dosage adjustment.[28] In cases of litigation, the physician's position is stronger if he or she can show that the patient has been monitored regularly.

The frequency of routine checkups is debatable. In a recent set of recommendations, Birch et al[29] suggested serum lithium and creatinine determinations every 2 to 6 months. It is natural that hospitals and clinics follow a certain routine, but the procedure should not be too rigid. I have, for example, a few patients whose serum lithium levels are determined only once or twice a year. But these patients are experienced; they know exactly which signs and symptoms to look for and under what circumstances to seek medical help.

As standard serum lithium concentrations for prophylaxis, I recommend levels of 0.5 to 0.8 mmol/L (identical in patients with bipolar and unipolar illness). This is in accordance with the study of Gelenberg et al,[30] in which serum lithium values of 0.4 to 0.6 mmol/L were found to have few side effects but also low efficacy, and values of 0.8 to 1.0 mmol/L were found to have marked efficacy but also many side effects. Concentrations lower than 0.5 mmol/L may be indicated in some elderly patients and concentrations higher than 0.8 mmol/L may be indicated in some young patients. Even within the recommended range, individual fine-tuning of dosage may be beneficial. Changes in serum lithium levels as small as 0.1 to 0.2 mmol/L, upward or downward, may substantially improve patients' quality of life during maintenance treatment.

Although I now recommend regular serum lithium and creatinine determinations (and determinations of serum thyroid-stimulating hormone once a year), I realize that certain risks are involved. Unless physicians are expressly warned when concentrations become too high or too low, or change too much (and this is not difficult with computer-controlled laboratory printouts), they may ignore routine laboratory results. Moreover, when physicians know that their patients are "under laboratory control," they may be tempted to neglect that careful observation of and attentive listening to patients is the best guarantee of safe and effective lithium treatment. Laboratory monitoring of lithium treatment is important, clinical monitoring essential.

MORTALITY OF PATIENTS GIVEN LONG-TERM LITHIUM TREATMENT

It has been demonstrated that the mortality of manic-depressive patients is markedly higher than that of the general population, and the increase is mainly, but not exclusively, caused by suicide. How does long-term lithium treatment affect this?

A number of mortality studies have been carried out on lithium-treated patients. Some are based on patients from single clinics[31-33] and others on pooled patient data from clinics in different countries, eg, those published by the International Group for the Study of Lithium-Treated Patients (IGSLI).[34-36]

With a single exception,[31] the studies have shown that the mortality of manic-depressive patients given long-term lithium treatment is markedly lower than that of patients not receiving such treatment.[32-36] In several of the studies, the mortality of the lithium-treated patients did not differ from that of the general population.

In the IGSLI studies, in which data were pooled from clinics in Risskov (Denmark), Berlin (Germany), Hamilton (Ontario), and Vienna (Austria), observations were based on a total of 5600 patient years. Standardized mortality ratios were calculated by dividing the number of observed deaths among the patients by the number of deaths expected in the general population after individual matching for sex, age, and observation period. In bipolar and unipolar manic-depressive patients, as well as in patients with schizoaffective disorder, the standardized mortality ratios did not differ from unity; in other words, the mortality ratios were not significantly higher than in the general population.

Studies of drug effects on mortality are more difficult to perform than those on morbidity. Death is such a rare event that very large numbers of patients must be treated and followed up over very long periods. Prospective mortality studies with random allocation to active drug and placebo treatment are obviously out of the question. Furthermore, while response can be studied before, during, and after treatment in the same group of patients in drug trials of morbidity, that is not possible in mortality studies, for a person can die only once. In studies without a randomized control group, subtle selection effects must be considered. For example, if patients with alcoholism or somatic illness have been excluded from prophylactic treatment, this could cause decreased mortality that need not be a result of the treatment.

The finding that the mortality of lithium-treated patients is not higher, or only moderately higher, than that of the general population does not prove, cannot prove, that lithium lowers mortality. The observation is, however, consistent with such an assumption.

Studies have also been carried out on patients who stopped taking lithium.[37-40] The mortality and suicide rates of these patients were significantly higher than those of the general population. As discontinuation of lithium treatment does not occur at random, we are again faced with the possibility that factors other than lithium treatment could have influenced mortality. I do not see how we can ever obtain conclusive evidence on this point, since seriously ill patients cannot be maintained on treatment with placebo.

However, one may compare lithium with prophylactic alternatives. In a German multicenter study, unfortunately only partly published, which lasted 2½ years, several hundred patients were randomly allocated to treatment with lithium or carbamazepine for bipolar illness and treatment with lithium or amitriptyline for unipolar illness.[41] Among the patients given the antidepressant drug, there were five suicides and no suicide attempts; among the carbamazepine-treated patients, there were four suicides and five suicide attempts; in the lithium-treated group, there were no suicides and no suicide attempts. The frequency of suicidal acts among the lithium-treated patients was significantly lower than the corresponding frequencies among those who were given antidepressants or carbamazepine (χ^2, $P<.001$ for both groups). These observations are consistent with the assumption that lithium treatment protects against suicidal behavior.

As scientists we must conclude that a mortality-lowering, antisuicidal effect of long-term lithium treatment has not been proved but remains a possibility.[42] As clinicians we must ask whether our patients and their relatives can afford that we disregard this possibility. As far as mortality is concerned, lithium seems currently the best remedy we can offer.

Let us, however, not forget what in my opinion is the most important outcome of the mortality investigations, and one on which there is agreement. All the studies have shown that long-term lithium treatment is *not* associated with *increased* mortality.

DISAPPOINTMENTS

In what ways do I feel disappointed with lithium after more than 40 years' experience?

I hoped for a long time that lithium could be rejected because something distinctly better emerged. That has not happened. I do not regard the current alternatives as generally better than lithium. They may be better for some patients and in special situations, but we are still waiting for something that is radically superior to lithium and its alternatives in terms of side effects and efficacy.

Another disappointment is that we still do not know the mechanism of action of lithium in affective illness. Many hypotheses exist, some of them ingenious and attractive, but none as yet proved correct. Moreover, in spite of what many believe, the same situation applies to antidepressants, anticonvulsants, and electroconvulsive treatment. As we do not know the pathophysiological basis of manic-depressive illness, we do not understand how treatments work; and as we do not know how treatments work, we cannot understand the pathophysiology of manic-depressive illness. The locked box with its key inside appears to present an insoluble problem. Nevertheless, in such situations a combination of perseverance and inspired guessing has before now borne fruit, and I trust that this may happen again.

PERSPECTIVES

Let us now consider various perspectives of lithium treatment. In 1969 Baastrup et al and I[3] carried out a randomized double-blind discontinuation trial to test lithium's prophylactic effect. Within 6 months, half of the patients receiving placebo relapsed, compared with none of the patients who continued taking lithium. The trial thus confirmed the prophylactic efficacy of lithium. The point I want to make, however, is that the patients all had a valid psychological explanation of why a recurrence had occurred at that particular time, eg, marital problems, transfer to a new apartment, or financial difficulties. The recurrences led to admission of the patients, and the ward staff, who apart from a single initiate did not know about the discontinuation trial, accepted unquestioningly the patients' psychological explanations.

This experience can be viewed in two ways. One can assume that recurrence in the placebo group was determined exclusively by the endogenous rhythm of the manic-depressive disease, and that lithium had corrected the anomaly. The patients' subjectively convincing psychological explanations thus represented a rationalization. On the other hand, it is conceivable that the recurrences in the placebo group were in fact provoked by environmental stress in persons with a particularly high vulnerability. In the patients given lithium, the treatment elevated the threshold for environmentally induced provocation of recurrences.

There is probably some truth in both scenarios. I find it difficult to conceive of a psychological phenomenon that is not accompanied by some biological change, neurophysiological or neurochemical. And there are presumably few biological processes that do not influence the mind, or psychological thresholds, to some extent. The day will presumably come when we succeed in finding out how our therapies work, and this may lead to new treatments with improved efficacy and even higher specificity.

What about the more distant future? If research should one day clarify the cerebral mechanisms that govern the endogenous mood level, this would raise the possibilities not only of *normalizing* mood but also of *manipulating* mood. It may, for example, become possible to adjust one's own mood, or that of others, to a particular level. This would enable people to choose spending their lives in a condition of light chronic mania, subjectively more alluring than even the most enjoyable alcohol- or crack cocaine–induced euphoria. Is this a happy vision? Or is it a frightening one? It is a possibility that forces us to ponder the central question: Should scientists under all circumstances reveal the secrets of nature, or are there doors that, because of the possible consequences, they should abstain from opening?

Another vexing question about the future is the following. If it becomes possible through gene manipulation to eradicate the disposition to manic-depressive illness, is that a desirable goal? It may be, and some Chinese legislators seem inclined to think so. Or it may not. Had eugenic measures of this kind been feasible and practiced in the past, then I myself might not have been in existence and able to express the views presented here.

Accepted for publication June 30, 1995.

This review was based on the first keynote address presented by the author at the First International Conference on Bipolar Disorder, Pittsburgh, Pa, June 23, 1994.

Reprint requests to The Psychiatric Hospital, 2 Skovagervej, DK-8240 Risskov, Denmark (Dr Schou).

REFERENCES

1. Schou M. Lithium prophylaxis: about 'naturalistic' or 'clinical practice' studies. *Lithium.* 1993;4:77-81.
2. Baastrup PC, Schou M. Lithium as a prophylactic agent: its effect against recurrent depressions and manic-depressive psychosis. *Arch Gen Psychiatry.* 1967;16:162-172.
3. Baastrup PC, Poulsen JC, Schou M, Thomsen K, Amdisen A. Prophylactic lithium: double-blind discontinuation in manic-depressive and recurrent-depressive disorders. *Lancet.* 1970;2:326-330.
4. Souza FGM, Mander AJ, Goodwin GM. The efficacy of lithium prophylaxis of unipolar depression: evidence from its discontinuation. *Br J Psychiatry.* 1990;157:718-722.
5. Souza FGM, Goodwin GM. Lithium treatment and prophylaxis in unipolar depression: a meta-analysis. *Br J Psychiatry.* 1991;158:666-675.
6. Nobler MS, Sackeim HA. Pharmacotherapy and electroconvulsive therapy for mood disorders. *Curr Opin Psychiatry.* 1993;6:10-15.
7. Kupfer DJ. Management of recurrent depression. *J Clin Psychiatry.* 1993;54(suppl 2):29-33.
8. Thase ME. Maintenance treatments of recurrent affective disorders. *Curr Opin Psychiatry.* 1993;6:16-21.
9. Johnstone EC, Owens DGC, Lambert MT, Crow TJ, Frith CD, Done DJ. Combination tricyclic antidepressant and lithium maintenance medication in unipolar and bipolar depressed patients. *J Affect Dis.* 1990;20:225-233.
10. Prien RF, Kupfer DJ, Mansky PA, Small JG, Tuason VB, Voss CB, Johnson WE. Drug therapy in the prevention of recurrences in unipolar and bipolar affective disorders. *Arch Gen Psychiatry.* 1984;41:1096-1104.
11. Goodwin FK, Jamison KR. *Manic-Depressive Illness.* Oxford, England: Oxford University Press; 1990.
12. Davis JM, Wang Z, Janicak PG. A quantitative analysis of clinical drug trials for the treatment of affective disorders. *Psychopharmacol Bull.* 1993;29:175-181.
13. Frank E, Kupfer DJ, Perel JM, Cornes C, Jarrett DB, Mallinger AG, Thase ME, McEachran AB, Grochocinski VJ. Three-year outcomes for maintenance therapies in recurrent depression. *Arch Gen Psychiatry.* 1990;47:1093-1099.
14. Kupfer DJ, Frank E, Perel JM, Cornes C, Mallinger AG, Thase ME, McEachran AB, Grochocinski VJ. Five-year outcome for maintenance therapies in recurrent depression. *Arch Gen Psychiatry.* 1992;49:769-773.
15. Greil W, Ludwig-Mayerhofer W, Steller B, Czernik A, Giedke H, Müller-Oerlinghausen B, Osterheider M, Rudolf GAE, Sauer H, Tegeler J, Wetterling T. Lithium-oder Carbamazepinprophylaxe bei affektiven Psychosen? Ergebnisse einer kontrollierten, multizentrischen Studie. In: Müller-Oerlinghausen B, Berghöfer A, eds. *Ziele und Ergebnisse der medikamentösen Prophylaxe affektiver Psychosen.* Stuttgart, Germany: Thieme; 1994:113-119.
16. Schou M. Effects of long-term lithium treatment on kidney function: an overview. *J Psychiatr Res.* 1988;22:287-296.
17. Waller DG, Edwards JG. Lithium and the kidney: an update. *Psychol Med.* 1989;19:825-831.
18. von Knorring L, Wahlin A, Nyström K, Bohman SO. Uraemia induced by long-term lithium treatment. *Lithium.* 1990;1:251-253.
19. Gitlin MJ. Lithium-induced renal insufficiency. *J Clin Psychopharmacol.* 1993;13:276-279.
20. Kallner G, Petterson U. Renal, thyroid and parathyroid function during lithium treatment: laboratory test in 207 people treated for 1-30 years. *Acta Psychiatr Scand.* 1995;91:48-51.
21. Aronson JK, Reynolds DJM. ABC of monitoring drug therapy: lithium. *BMJ.* 1992;305:1273-1276.
22. Hullin RP, Srinivasan DP, Birch NJ. Monitoring lithium treatment. *BMJ.* 1993;306:269.
23. Kehoe RF. Monitoring lithium treatment. *BMJ.* 1993;36:269-270.
24. Aronson JK, Reynolds DJM. Monitoring lithium treatment. *BMJ.* 1993;306:270.
25. Guscott R, Taylor L. Monitoring of lithium treatment. *Can J Psychiatry.* 1993;38:74.
26. Schou M. Monitoring of lithium treatment: reply to Guscott and Taylor. *Can J Psychiatry.* 1993;38:74.
27. Schou M. Relapse prevention in manic-depressive illness: important and unimportant factors. *Can J Psychiatry.* 1991;36:502-506.
28. Schou M. *Lithium Treatment of Manic-Depressive Illness: A Practical Guide.* 5th ed, revised. Basel, Switzerland: Karger; 1993.
29. Birch NJ, Grof P, Hullin RP, Kehoe RF, Schou M, Srinivasan DP. Lithium prophylaxis: proposed guidelines for good clinical practice. *Lithium.* 1993;4:225-230.
30. Gelenberg AJ, Kane JM, Keller MB, Lavori P, Rosenbaum JF, Cole K, Lavalle J. Comparison of standard and low serum levels of lithium for maintenance treatment of bipolar disorder. *N Engl J Med.* 1989;321:1489-1493.
31. Norton B, Whalley LJ. Mortality of a lithium-treated population. *Br J Psychiatry.* 1984;146:277-282.
32. Coppen A, Standish-Barry H, Bailey J, Houston G, Silcocks P, Hermon C. Long-term lithium and mortality. *Lancet.* 1990;335:1347.
33. Coppen A, Standish-Barry H, Bailey J, Houston G, Silcocks P, Hermon C. Does lithium reduce the mortality of recurrent mood disorders? *J Affect Dis.* 1991;23:1-7.
34. Müller-Oerlinghausen B, Ahrens B, Volk J, Grof P, Grof E, Schou M, Vestergaard P, Lenz G, Simhandl C, Thau K, Wolf R. Reduced mortality of manic-depressive patients in long-term lithium treatment: an international collaborative study by IGSLI. *Psychiatry Res.* 1991;36:329-331.
35. Müller-Oerlinghausen B, Ahrens B, Grof E, Grof P, Lenz G, Schou M, Simhandl C, Thau K, Volk J, Wolf R, Wolf T. The effect of long-term lithium treatment on the mortality of patients with manic-depressive or schizo-affective illness. *Acta Psychiatr Scand.* 1992;86:218-222.
36. Ahrens B, Müller-Oerlinghausen B, Schou M, Wolf T, Alda M, Grof E, Grof P, Lenz G, Simhandl C, Thau K, Vestergaard P, Wolf R, Möller H. Cardiovascular and suicide mortality of affective disorders may be reduced by lithium prophylaxis. *J Affect Dis.* 1995;33:67-75.
37. Nilsson A. Mortality in recurrent mood disorders during periods on and off lithium: a complete population study in 362 patients. *Pharmacopsychiatry.* 1995;28:8-13.
38. Müller-Oerlinghausen B, Müser-Causemann B, Volk J. Suicides and parasuicides in a high-risk patient group on and off lithium long-term medication. *J Affect Dis.* 1992;25:261-270.
39. Lenz G, Ahrens B, Denk E, Müller-Oerlinghausen B, Schratzberger-Topitz A, Simhandl C, Wancata J. Mortalität nach Ausscheiden aus der Lithiumambulanz. In: Müller-Oerlinghausen B, Berghöfer A, eds. *Ziele und Ergebnisse der medikamentösen Prophylaxe affektiver Psychosen.* Stuttgart, Germany: Thieme; 1994:49-52.
40. Felber W, Kyber A. Suizide und Parasuizide während und außerhalb einer Lithiumprophylaxe. In: Müller-Oerlinghausen B, Berghöfer A, eds. *Ziele und Ergebnisse der medikamentösen Prophylaxe affektiver Psychosen.* Stuttgart, Germany: Thieme; 1994:53-59.
41. Thies-Flechtner K, Seibert W, Walther A, Greil W, Müller-Oerlinghausen B. Suizide bei rezidivprophylaktisch behandelten Patienten mit affektiven Psychosen. In: Müller-Oerlinghausen B, Berghöfer A, eds. *Ziele und Ergebnisse der medikamentösen Prophylaxe affektiver Psychosen.* Stuttgart, Germany: Thieme; 1994:61-64.
42. Schou M. Mortality-lowering effect of prophylactic lithium treatment: a look at the evidence. *Pharmacopsychiatry.* 1995;28:1.

Conversions From Système International (SI) Units to Traditional Units (Modified From *The SI Manual in Health Care*)

System	Component	SI Reference Interval*	SI Unit	Conversion Factor (Divide by)	Traditional Reference Interval*	Traditional Unit
Serum	Lithium ion, therapeutic	0.50-1.50	mmol/L	0.001441	350-1050	μg/dL
		0.50-1.50	mmol/L	1.441	0.35-1.05	mg/dL

**These reference values are not intended to be definitive since each laboratory determines its own values. They are provided for illustration only.*

Forty Years of Lithium Treatment

THE article "Forty Years of Lithium Treatment"[1] represents a remarkable journey of 40 years by Schou, one of the pioneers in the treatment of manic-depressive illness and one of the most fervent advocates for lithium prophylaxis. Schou's article is based on a lecture given at the introductory plenary session of the First International Conference on Bipolar Disorder held in Pittsburgh, Pa, June 23-24, 1994.

The major purpose of this conference was to identify both current advances in the treatment of bipolar disorder and unresolved problems in both the short- and long-term treatment of this severe psychiatric disorder. Many of the speakers demonstrated their concern that as many as 40% of patients with bipolar disorder are not effectively treated with lithium. Since the development of alternative forms of therapy has become of increasing importance, it seems appropriate to review the current assets and liabilities of lithium treatment.

In this context, Schou's article represents a strong, articulate, and well-referenced review that is primarily focused on the positive aspects of lithium prophylaxis for bipolar and unipolar affective disorders. While he is concerned about recent studies that have suggested that there are a considerable number of people who do not respond to lithium treatment,[2,3] he is convinced that many of these studies represent naturalistic investigations, indicating lower levels of efficacy, probably as a result of compliance problems and patient selection criteria. Indeed, he is less concerned about the controversy of lithium indications in bipolar disorder than the indication for lithium in the long-term treatment of unipolar recurrent disorders. His own strong impression from the literature and his considerable clinical experience is that lithium represents a first line of treatment for unipolar prophylaxis. In contrast, some investigators have argued that lithium is not appropriate as a first-line treatment for recurrent unipolar disorders.[4] In one study, in which imipramine appeared superior to lithium in long-term prophylaxis, the initial treatment protocol necessitated successful response to the combination of imipramine and lithium and, thus, did not provide an adequate test of the question of whether patients who respond initially to lithium therapy can be maintained prophylactically on lithium regimen.[3] Perhaps, the field could use a controlled short-term and long-term trial comparing lithium vs tricyclic antidepressants vs SSRIs (selective serotonin reuptake inhibitors) in unipolar recurrent disorder. Schou does admit, however, that the ease of treatment and the increased level of compliance with routine antidepressants may lead to a greater use of alternatives to lithium in the treatment of recurrent unipolar illness.

See also pages 9, 16, and 21

Our own position is that while we would certainly agree that there are data supporting the use of lithium prophylaxis in unipolar recurrent illness, we believe that the studies on efficacy and the ease of use and adherence to either traditional tricyclic antidepressants or the newer SSRIs suggest that these agents represent a more useful alternative for the treatment of recurrent unipolar illness for both short- and long-term treatment.[5] Furthermore, in the United States, with the increasing treatment of recurrent unipolar illness by primary care practitioners, the antidepressants seem to be a more acceptable form of treatment than the use of lithium.

Turning to lithium administration, with respect to the notion of monitoring serum lithium, Schou feels that there is a need for regular determination of serum lithium only every 2 to 6 months. This recommendation represents a reduction in routine monitoring frequency compared with earlier suggestions. With respect to the appropriate dosage of lithium, Schou points to very small fine-tuning of dosage as beneficial in the long-term treatment. Therefore, the clinician has to be quite observant in examining the concentration and its effect on each patient, particularly those who are elderly.

Schou goes on to demonstrate that the use of lithium may lead to decreased mortality compared with other antidepressants. He also argues that the long-term side effects of lithium, such as kidney abnormalities, should not be of major continued concern. Schou refers to several German and Scandinavian studies[6-8] to support his argument that lithium treatment seems to be unrelated to suicide attempts and successful suicide. There are a number of areas that one would wish that Schou would have covered as important areas needing special attention in 1995. One of these areas is the treatment of bipolar depression. Clearly, neither the short- nor long-term treatment of bipolar depression is yielding the same level of efficacy as is obtained in the treatment of mania. Zornberg and Pope[9] have shown that, in contrast to the extensive data on the treatment of manic states, the paucity of data on the treatment of bipolar depression is appalling. Furthermore, the extant studies are limited or inconclusive. The major problem may be that the treatment strategies and efficacy rates do not seem to be as good as similar strategies for the treatment of unipolar depression. This has been confirmed by a number of studies by Keller and colleagues,[10] as well as in unpublished analyses of the current Pittsburgh protocol.

One key area of disappointment that we share with Schou has been that a better drug has not yet emerged. Some of this disappointment, we think, is related to the early belief that the introduction of lithium carbonate would "cure" this disorder. The reluctance of individuals to seek treatment and the stigma attached to the treatment of mood disorders have compounded the difficulty of inducing pharmaceutical companies to begin tackling the problem of finding antidepressants that would be especially useful in bipolar disorder. For that matter, even testing the antidepressants that the pharmaceutical companies are currently introducing (eg, SSRIs) to determine whether there is a specific indication for bipolar disorder has not happened. This appears to be in the face of evidence that the prevalence of bipolar depression is substantial, especially in female individuals.

Another disappointment that we share with Schou is that we still do not understand the mechanism of action of lithium in mood disorders. A very recent article on signal transduction pathways by Manji et al,[11] published in the ARCHIVES, represents an excellent review of the search for and identification of intracellular targets for lithium's action. These areas of interest, involving signal transduction pathways and, in particular, G proteins, suggest important potential breakthroughs in not only understanding the action of lithium but being in a better position to understand the action of all psychotropic agents in bipolar disorders.

The final disappointment or concern that Schou describes relates to one of ours: the future of genetics and molecular neurobiology in bipolar disorder. We believe that it is unlikely that a single gene will be found to account for all bipolar disorder, and that it is extremely likely that manic-depressive illness represents a complex polygenic genetic disorder. As such, a number of genes will ultimately be identified that contribute to the onset and development of this disorder. Both the molecular biologists and those clinicians and counselors who may eventually be involved in genetic counseling need to prepare for the period in time in which they will be put in a position of "prescribing" and counseling individuals and families with respect to bipolar illness. This represents both a set of problems and an important set of future opportunities for our field.

In closing, we believe that many of the disappointments that Schou enumerates will turn out to be the very fruits that need to be further investigated. We hope that there will be a follow-up to these very tough and important questions at the Second International Conference on Bipolar Disorder scheduled for June of 1997 in Pittsburgh.

David J. Kupfer, MD
Ellen Frank, PhD
Department of Psychiatry
University of Pittsburgh School of Medicine
Western Psychiatric Institute and Clinic
3811 O'Hara St
Pittsburgh, PA 15213

This study was supported in part by grants MH-29618 and MH-30915 from the National Institute of Mental Health and a grant from the Stanley Center for the Innovative Treatment of Bipolar Disorder.

REFERENCES

1. Schou M. Forty years of lithium treatment. *Arch Gen Psychiatry.* 1997;54:9-13.
2. Johnstone EC, Owens DGC, Lambert MT, Crow TJ, Frith CD, Done DJ. Combination tricyclic antidepressant and lithium maintenance medication in unipolar and bipolar depressed patients. *J Affect Disord.* 1990;20:225-233.
3. Prien RF, Kupfer DJ, Mansky PA, Small JG, Tuason VB, Voss CB, Johnson WE. Drug therapy in the prevention of recurrences in unipolar and bipolar affective disorders: report of the NIMH Collaborative Study Group comparing lithium carbonate, imipramine, and a lithium carbonate–imipramine combination. *Arch Gen Psychiatry.* 1984;41:1096-1104.
4. Thase ME. Maintenance treatments of recurrent affective disorders. *Curr Opin Psychiatry.* 1993; 6:16-21.
5. Frank E, Kupfer DJ, Perel JM, Cornes C, Jarrett DB, Mallinger AG, Thase ME, McEachran AB, Grochocinski VJ. Three-year outcomes for maintenance therapies in recurrent depression. *Arch Gen Psychiatry.* 1990;47:1093-1099.
6. Ahrens B, Müller-Oerlinghausen B, Schou M, Wolf T, Alda M, Grof E, Grof P, Lenz G, Simhandl C, Thau K, Vestergaard P, Wolf R, Möller H. Cardiovascular and suicide mortality of affective disorders may be reduced by lithium prophylaxis. *J Affect Disord.* 1995;33:67-75.
7. Nilsson A. Mortality in recurrent mood disorders during periods on and off lithium: a complete population study in 362 patients. *Pharmacopsychiatry.* 1995;28:8-13.
8. Schou M. Mortality-lowering effect of prophylactic lithium treatment: a look at the evidence. *Pharmacopsychiatry.* 1995;28:1.
9. Zornberg GL, Pope Jr, HG. Treatment of depression in bipolar disorder: new directions for research. *J Clin Psychopharmacol.* 1993; 13:397-408.
10. Keller MB, Lavori PW, Coryell W, Andreasen NC, Endicott J, Clayton PJ, Klerman GL, Hirschfeld RMA. Differential outcome of pure manic, mixed/cycling, and pure depressive episodes in patients with bipolar illness. *JAMA.* 1986; 255:3138-3142.
11. Manji HK, Potter WZ, Lenox RH. Signal transduction pathways: molecular targets for lithium's actions. *Arch Gen Psychiatry.* 1995;52: 531-543.

COMMENTARY

Current Therapeutic Profile of Lithium

WITH THE advent of new pharmacotherapies for bipolar disorder, it may be an opportune time to look at the course of events that initiated the possibility of specific pharmacotherapy for this disorder. It is now 48 years since Cade's original report about the effects of lithium carbonate treatment in cases of mania was published.[1] The time course of lithium therapy introduction in 1949, and its subsequent development, is concomitant with the span of the professional career of one of us (S.G.). The article by Schou[2] in this issue of the ARCHIVES raises several key points that we would like to address.

MAGNITUDE OF LITHIUM EFFECTIVENESS IN MANIA

The early studies of lithium in the treatment of acute mania reported high effectiveness. In Cade's initial open study,[1] all 10 patients with mania clearly responded to lithium administration. In subsequent, controlled studies, high (~70%-80%), effectiveness of lithium therapy was found.[3-6] Later studies suggested lower response rates in the treatment of acute mania. In some recent trials,[7-11] lithium effectiveness varying from 34% to 70% has been reported. Three recent controlled studies found lithium effectiveness varying from 59% to 91% in patients with pure mania[12-14]; in patients with mixed mania, response rates have varied from 29% to 43%.[7,12-14]

In the prophylactic treatment of bipolar disorder, the initial controlled studies accounted for effectiveness around 80% or higher during varied follow-up periods.[15-24] The reported failure rates in later studies have been substantially higher, around 50% to 60%, for comparable follow-up times.[25-30] Actually, in 1 of these studies, lithium effectiveness was as low as 33%[28] after 2 years of treatment. Recent uncontrolled naturalistic studies, in which patients were followed up for long periods, suggested that in a significant proportion of patients receiving lithium treatment their condition will not remain stable. Harrow et al[30] reported failure rates of 40% after an average of 1.7 years, not significantly different from those in patients not taking medication. O'Connell et al[31] reported that, after 1 year, only in 56% of 248 patients, bipolar disorder had not recurred. Keller et al[32] found cumulative relapse rates of 48% in 1 year and 81% in 5 years in patients with pure bipolar mania type I, with higher rates, of 57% and 91%, in patients with mixed mania and rapid cycling, respectively. Winokur et al[33] reported that, after a 10-year follow-up period, only 11% of 131 patients with bipolar disorder had not had further episodes. Peselow et al[34] reported lithium effectiveness rates of 83% in 1 year, 52% in 3 years, and 37% after 5 years. The authors suggested that these findings pose questions about the value of lithium treatment in ordinary clinical settings.

This apparent decline in lithium effectiveness in the short-term treatment and prophylaxis of bipolar disorder has caused extensive debate. The explanation is probably multifactorial. First, the profile of the samples studied may have changed. Because of more widespread lithium use, patients with more severe cases, and with more comorbid psychopathologic features, may be a significant part of those enrolling in these studies. In several of these trials, previous lithium therapy had failed in a large proportion of the patients. Additionally, increased awareness of the disorder among the public may have resulted in more patients being treated in the community, rather than in academic medical centers, where most of these trials are conducted. Thus, patients with more severe cases and with lower proportions of cases of pure bipolar disorder seem to have been included in the later lithium trials, and this is a major factor in explaining this perceived decreasing effectiveness. Second, the diagnostic category of bipolar disorder is now much broader, including some cases previously diagnosed as schizoaffective disorders or schizophrenia. A higher number of patients with atypical bipolar disorder and patients with rapid cycling who have a worse response to lithium therapy have been recruited for the more recent studies. This may be a crucial factor underlying the increase reported in failure rates. Third, the presentation and course of the disorder may have changed. Different available treatment options, which can complicate the course of the disease (eg, tricyclic antidepressant drugs), might have contributed to the decreasing effectiveness of lithium treatment.

See also pages 9, 14, and 21

The significance of medication compliance in the patients in whom prophylactic treatment failed is still an unresolved issue. Guscott and Taylor[35] suggested that poor compliance with lithium therapy may be a major factor in the discrepancy between its known prophylactic efficacy and its actual effectiveness in clinical settings. Only one third of patients in the community were estimated to remain compliant. Recent onset of noncompliance can actually be part of the early signs of manic decompensation. The magnitude of medication noncompliance among the failures to lithium prophylaxis still remains to be determined.

Thus, the perceived changes in lithium effectiveness, with decreased effectiveness rates, seem to be primarily attributed to a change in the sample population studied. What is called bipolar disorder today is a much more heterogeneous group than it was in the 1960s, without much emphasis being put on the course of the disorder to make this diagnosis nowadays. The role of more available treatment modalities in complicating the course of the disorder has to be further elucidated. In patients with the typical bipolar disorder, who have complete remission of symptoms and full recovery to preillness levels of functioning, lithium effectiveness is still high.

LITHIUM EFFECTIVENESS IN UNIPOLAR DEPRESSION

The effectiveness of lithium as a single treatment for acute and recurrent unipolar depression has been controversial for many years.[2,36-38] Most of the controlled studies showed that lithium has antidepressant actions, but not to the same extent as do the antidepressant drugs, with response rates around 30% to 40%.[39,40] Other positive studies were double blind but not placebo controlled and involved samples of patients with bipolar and unipolar depression.[41-43] Lithium therapy is more effective in bipolar than unipolar depression.[39,43] As an augmentation treatment for unipolar depression, lithium effectiveness is well recognized, and this strategy has ample acceptance in clinical practice.[44-46]

In the prophylactic treatment, 1 double-blind placebo-controlled study,[16] involving 65 patients with recurrent affective disorders who were followed up to 122 weeks, found significant benefits from lithium therapy, but no comparison with antidepressant drugs was done. One controlled prospective 2-year trial with 122 patients with unipolar and bipolar depression[17] found that both lithium and imipramine were more effective than placebo for prophylaxis in patients with unipolar depression, without significant differences between these 2 treatment modalities. A later, double-blind, placebo-controlled study involving a sample of 150 patients with unipolar depression[28] found treatment with antidepressant drugs to be more effective than with lithium for prophylaxis of unipolar depression, and it did not find additional advantages of combination lithium-antidepressant treatment over the treatment with antidepressant drugs alone. Overall, lithium therapy was found to be better than placebo in most of the studies, but not as effective as therapy with antidepressants.[39,40] Part of this evidence comes from retrospective and naturalistic studies and needs to be weighed against evidence originating from large, well-controlled, prospective trials.[28]

Despite ongoing debate about this issue, the evidence coming from well-controlled prospective studies does not support the indication of lithium as a prophylactic agent for unipolar disorder, because it is not as effective as antidepressant drugs. Combination treatment seems to offer no advantage. It has some effectiveness in the treatment of the acute episode, but is not comparable to treatment with antidepressant drugs.

MAINTENANCE REGIMEN

The best maintenance strategy in the treatment of bipolar disorder still raises some controversy. Recent trials indicate that the ideal range for the serum lithium concentration, if tolerated by patients, is 0.8 to 1.0 mmol/L. Gelenberg et al,[47] in a well-controlled study involving 94 patients, found significant benefits from higher levels over the more traditionally proposed lower ranges for the serum lithium concentrations of 0.5to 0.8 mmol/L. Keller et al[48] conducted a double-blind study of low-dose (0.4-0.6 mmol/L) vs standard-dose (0.8-1.0 mmol/L) therapy, and they found that the risk of disease recurrence was 2.6 times higher in the low-dose group. As expected, in these higher dose ranges more side effects were present. Surprisingly, few controlled studies have systematically investigated the relationship between serum lithium level and clinical response. There are suggestions that patients with more than 3 episodes of the disorder do not respond better to lithium prophylaxis at higher serum lithium levels.[49] However, until further controlled evidence challenges this assumption, the standard recommendation for patients who failed to respond to lithium prophylaxis at serum lithium levels of 0.6 to 0.8 mmol/L is to try levels higher than 0.8 mmol/L.

The measurement of in vivo brain lithium levels in patients was made with nuclear lithium-7 magnetic resonance spectroscopy, which has brought new possibilities for the investigation of the relevance of lithium levels in tissue to clinical response. Lithium levels in the brain have been determined in a few studies, and lithium levels in the brain are typically about half those in serum,[50,51] but there seems to be considerable variability in the brain lithium–serum lithium ratios in patients in whom therapeutic serum lithium levels are maintained,[52] which can underlie nonresponse to the medication. Improvement in patients with mania was better correlated with brain than with serum lithium concentrations in a small (n=14) patient sample.[53] The investigation of the lithium levels in the brain in relation to clinical response may help elucidate lithium mechanism of action, and may contribute to a better understanding of the cases of lithium treatment failure. These efforts may eventually result in newer ways to determine the most effective maintenance dose for patients with bipolar disorder.

Good compliance with lithium administration is the key for successful prophylaxis. The patient's awareness of the recurrent course of the disorder and good follow-up and monitoring of side effects are the most important factors in attempts to maximize therapeutic effects of the lithium treatment.

INFLUENCE OF LITHIUM PROPHYLAXIS ON MORBIDITY AND MORTALITY

Bipolar disorder is a recurrent condition, often accompanied by psychosocial impairment. Fewer than one fourth of the patients having disorder recurrences were found to have stable work performance.[54] The mortality rates in patients with bipolar disorder have been 2 to 3 times higher than in the general population.[55] Other authors[56] found even more dramatic, rates with a 5-fold increase. One study[57] shows higher late-life mortality associated with mania than with depression.

Suicide rates are higher in bipolar disorder, with one fourth of the patients attempting suicide during the course of their illness[58] and a high rate of suicide completion of 1 in 10 patients.[59] In another study,[60] these estimates were even higher: 48% of 67 patients with a history of suicidal attempts. It has been suggested that patients with bipolar disorder are at 7.5 times higher risk of committing suicide than are patients with unipolar disorder.[59]

Lithium prophylaxis can reduce the mortality in this patient population, by decreasing the distress and physical risks associated with disease recurrences and decreasing suicidality.[61,62] According to a recent report by the National Institute of Mental Health, Bethesda, Md,[63] lithium treatment can prolong the life expectancy of patients with bipolar disorder by an average of 7 years. Several studies[64-69] have suggested that lithium treatment decreases the rates of suicide attempts and suicide completion in patients with bipolar disorder. Retrospective studies of suicide victims with diagnosis of mood disorders have found that most of them were not receiving lithium therapy, were noncompliant, or were inappropriately treated.[70-73]

Evidence that lithium use may have significant influence on mortality from suicide in patients with bipolar disorder is, thus, extensive. Because both electroconvulsive and antidepressant therapies did not cause similar effects in mortality rates,[74] this rate decrease seems to be attributable to lithium administration. The studies on lithium prophylaxis show that it has a significant influence on patient's quality of life and prevents suicide.

LITHIUM SPECIFICITY IN BIPOLAR DISORDER

Initially, lithium was proposed to be a specific therapeutic agent for bipolar disorder. In view of accumulating studies on lithium during the past 50 years, it seems timely to reexamine this literature. Cade[1] proposed use of lithium as a specific treatment for mania, based on his observations that lithium produced significant benefits in all 10 patients with mania whom he studied. In 3 of 6 patients with dementia praecox, only a quieting effect was observed, and in 3 patients with chronic depressive psychosis, no effects were found. Gershon and Yuwiler,[75] in 1960, expanded the idea of lithium specificity, finding it to be highly effective in the treatment of patients with mania and to have minimal or no effect in several other neuropsychiatric disorders. Schou[76] also supported lithium specificity in its actions in the treatment of manic-depressive illness.

The use of lithium was investigated during the past several years in a variety of conditions other than bipolar disorder, such as schizophrenia, schizoaffective disorders, alcohol and other substance abuse and dependence, and personality disorders. It has little or no effect in these conditions,[77,78] but it is highly effective in patients with typical bipolar disorder.[8,79] In the treatment of alcoholism, after initial enthusiasm about the potential of lithium, particularly in cases associated with depressive symptoms, double-blind, controlled trials conclusively showed no effectiveness.[80] It was also found to be beneficial for paroxysmal aggression, such as impulse control disorder, and aggressiveness.[81] Controlled evidence of its effectiveness was also found in both children and adolescents with aggressive behavior in conduct disorder.[82]

The accumulated research during the last several years still strongly supports the concept of lithium as a specific treatment modality for bipolar disorder. Limited controlled evidence of its effectiveness in forms of paroxysmal aggressiveness also exists.

COMPARISON WITH NEWER THERAPEUTIC APPROACHES

Because other therapies for bipolar disorder have arisen, it is imperative to consider them in comparison with lithium therapy, which, in our view, is still the first-line therapy for bipolar disorder. The advances in clinical research in this field have begun to provide effective alternatives for the patients who either do not respond or do not tolerate lithium treatment. Two of these medications, carbamazepine and valproate, have been tested in the short-term treatment and prophylaxis of bipolar disorder, and, in some studies, they were found to have effectiveness comparable with that of lithium and overall were clearly superior to placebo.[83-87] In the prophylaxis of bipolar disorder, no adequate database exists to confirm effectiveness of carbamazepine and valproate. In some patient populations (eg, patients with dysphoric mania, mixed states, or rapid cycling) and in patients with associated neurological abnormalities, response to these 2 therapeutic agents appears to be better than to lithium,[88] favoring them as first-line treatment modalities in these cases. Another agent that has been proposed to be effective in the treatment for mania is verapamil, a calcium-channel blocker.[89,90] Larger trials should replicate these findings and examine verapamil effectiveness in prophylactic treatment. Benzodiazepines, such as lorazepam and clonazepam, have also been proposed for the short-term treatment of mania and prophylaxis of bipolar disorder,[91,92] but their action seems to be more sedating and nonspecific and not as effective as that of lithium or anticonvulsant drugs. Benzodiazepines, however, may have an important role in adjunctive treatment.

Valproate has gained more acceptance than carbamazepine because of its more benign side-effect profile, without the potential of bone marrow suppression as seen with carbamazepine. More recently, inositol has been suggested to be a potential therapeutic agent for bipolar depression (and for the side effects of lithium therapy), and beginning trials have suggested its positive effects.[93] A recently developed search for new inhibitors of the enzyme inositol monophosphatase,[94] which is thought to be a major step in the mechanism of lithium action, is a promising area of research that can potentially result in breakthroughs in this field.

Despite many years and efforts to develop treatment for bipolar disorder, lithium is still the most effective therapeutic agent, and, despite recent debate about its real effectiveness in everyday clinical settings, it has played a major role in the treatment of bipolar disorder. Recent research efforts may lead to more effective treatment alternatives for patients who fail to respond to lithium treatment.

In conclusion, we think that our commentary contributes to the thoughts presented by Schou[2] and that it underlines some of the important questions raised in his article. We also hope that the next decade will successfully address these unresolved issues.

Samuel Gershon, MD
Jair C. Soares, MD
Department of Psychiatry
Western Psychiatric Institute and Clinic
University of Pittsburgh Medical Center
3811 O'Hara St
Pittsburgh, PA, 15213

Corresponding author: Samuel Gershon, MD, Western Psychiatric Institute and Clinic, University of Pittsburgh Medical Center, 3811 O'Hara St, Pittsburgh, PA, 15213.

REFERENCES

1. Cade JFJ. Lithium salts in the treatment of psychotic excitement. *Med J Aust.* 1949;14:349-352.
2. Schou M. Forty years of lithium treatment. *Arch Gen Psychiatry.* 1997;54:9-13.
3. Spring G, Schweid D, Gray C, Steinberg J, Horwitz M. A double-blind comparison of lithium and chlorpromazine in the treatment of manic states. *Am J Psychiatry.* 1970;126:1306-1310.
4. Johnson G, Gershon S, Burdock EI, Floyd A, Hekimian L. Comparative effects of lithium and chlorpromazine in the treatment of acute manic states. *Br J Psychiatry.* 1971;119:267-276.
5. Prien RF, Caffey EM Jr, Klett CJ. Comparison of lithium carbonate and chlorpromazine in the treatment of mania: report of the Veterans Administration and National Institute of Mental Health Collaborative Study Group. *Arch Gen Psychiatry.* 1972;26:146-153.
6. Shopsin B, Gershon S, Thompson H, Collins P. Psychoactive drugs in mania: a controlled comparison of lithium carbonate, chlorpromazine, and haloperidol. *Arch Gen Psychiatry.* 1975;32:34-42.
7. Himmelhoch JM, Mulla D, Neil JF, Detre TP, Kupfer DJ. Incidence and significance of mixed affective states in a bipolar population. *Arch Gen Psychiatry.* 1976;33:1062-1066.
8. Price LH, Heninger GR. Lithium in the treatment of mood disorders. *N Engl J Med.* 1994;331:591-598.
9. Small JG, Klapper MH, Kellams JJ, Miller MJ, Milstein V, Sharpley PH, Small IF. Electroconvulsive treatment compared with lithium in the management of manic states. *Arch Gen Psychiatry.* 1988;45:727-732.
10. Small JG, Klapper MH, Milstein V, Kellams JJ, Miller MJ, Marhenke JD, Small IF. Carbamazepine compared with lithium in the treatment of mania. *Arch Gen Psychiatry.* 1991;48:915-921.
11. Bowden CL, Brugger AM, Swann AC, Calabrese JR, Janicak PG, Petty F, Dilsaver SC, Davis JM, Rush AJ, Small JG, Garza-Trevino ES, Risch SC, Goodnick PJ, Morris DD. Efficacy of divalproex vs lithium and placebo in the treatment of mania. *JAMA.* 1994;271:918-924.
12. Secunda SK, Katz MM, Koslow SH, Maas JW, Swann AC, Chang S. Sociodemographic characteristics, clinical course, and prediction of treatment response in a manic population. *J Affect Disord.* 1985;8:113.
13. Prien RF, Himmelhoch JM, Kupfer DJ. Treatment of mixed mania. *J Affect Disord.* 1988;15:9-15.
14. Dilsaver SC, Swann AC, Shoaib AM, Bowers TC, Halle MT. Depressive mania associated with nonresponse to antimanic agents. *Am J Psychiatry.* 1993;150:1548-1551.
15. Baastrup PC, Poulsen JC, Schou M, Thomsen K, Amdisen A. Prophylactic lithium: double-blind discontinuation in manic-depressive and recurrent-depressive disorders. *Lancet.* 1970;2:326-330.
16. Coppen A, Noguera R, Bailey J, Burns BH, Swani MS, Hare EH, Gardner R, Maggs R. Prophylactic lithium in affective disorders: controlled trial. *Lancet.* 1971;2:275-279.
17. Prien RF, Klett J, Caffey EM. Lithium carbonate and imipramine in prevention of affective episodes: a comparison in recurrent affective illness: report of the Veterans Administration and National Institute of Mental Health Collaborative Study Group. *Arch Gen Psychiatry.* 1973;29:420-425.
18. Prien RF, Caffey EM, Klett CJ. Prophylactic efficacy of lithium carbonate in manic-depressive illness: report of the Veterans Administration and National Institute of Mental Health Collaborative Study Group. *Arch Gen Psychiatry.* 1973;28:337-341.
19. Cundall RL, Brooks PW, Murray LG. A controlled evaluation of lithium prophylaxis in affective disorders. *Psychol Med.* 1972;2:308-311.
20. Hullin RP, McDonald R, Allsopp MNE. Prophylactic lithium in recurrent affective disorders. *Lancet.* 1972;1:1044-1046.
21. Stallone F, Shelley E, Mendlewicz J, Fieve RR. The use of lithium in affective disorders, III: a double-blind study of prophylaxis in bipolar illness. *Am J Psychiatry.* 1973;130:1006-1010.
22. Dunner DL, Fleiss JL, Fieve RR. Lithium carbonate prophylaxis failure. *Br J Psychiatry.* 1976;129:40-44.
23. Fieve RR, Kumbarachi T, Dunner DL. Lithium prophylaxis of depression in bipolar I, bipolar II, and unipolar patients. *Am J Psychiatry.* 1976;133:925-929.
24. Quitkin F, Rifkin A, Kane J, Ramos-Lorenzi JR, Klein DF. The prophylactic effect of lithium and imipramine in bipolar II and unipolar patients: a preliminary report. *Am J Psychiatry.* 1978;135:570-572.
25. Ahlfors UG, Baastrup PC, Dencker SJ, Elgen K, Lingjaerde O, Pedersen V, Schou M, Aaskoven O. Flupenthixol decanoate in recurrent manic-depressive illness. *Acta Psychiatr Scand.* 1981;64;226-237.
26. Quitkin FM, Kane JM, Rifkin A, Ramos-Lorenzi JR, Saraf K, Howard A, Klein DF. Lithium and imipramine in the prophylaxis of unipolar and bipolar II depression: a prospective, placebo-controlled comparison. *Psychopharmacol Bull.* 1981;17:142-144.
27. Kane JM, Quitkin FM, Rifkin A, Ramos-Lorenzi JR, Saraf K, Howard A, Klein DF. Prophylactic lithium with and without imipramine for bipolar I patients: a double-blind study. *Psychopharmacol Bull.* 1981;17:144-145.
28. Prien RF, Kupfer DJ, Mansky PA, Small JG, Tuason VB, Voss CB, Johnson WE. Drug therapy in the prevention of recurrences in unipolar and bipolar affective disorders: report of the NIMH Collaborative Study Group Comparing Lithium Carbonate, Imipramine, and a Lithium Carbonate-Imipramine Combination. *Arch Gen Psychiatry.* 1984;41:1096-1104.
29. Watkins SE, Callender K, Thomas DR, Tidmarsh SF, Shaw DM. The effect of carbamazepine and lithium on remission from affective illness. *Br J Psychiatry.* 1987;150:180-182.
30. Harrow M, Goldberg JF, Grossman LS, Meltzer HY. Outcome in manic disorders. *Arch Gen Psychiatry.* 1990;47:665-671.
31. O'Connell RA, Mayo JA, Flatow L, Cuthbertson B, O'Brien BE. Outcome of bipolar disorder on long-term treatment with lithium. *Br J Psychiatr.* 1991;159:123-129.
32. Keller MB, Lavori PW, Coryell W, Endicott J, Mueller TI. Bipolar I: a five-year prospective follow-up. *J Nerv Ment Dis.* 1993;181:238-245.
33. Winokur G, Coryell W, Akiskal HS, Endicott J, Keller M, Mueller T. Manic-depressive (bipolar) disorder: the course in light of a prospective ten-year follow-up of 131 patients. *Acta Psychiatr Scand.* 1994;89:102-110.
34. Peselow ED, Fieve RR, Difiglia C, Sanfilipo MP. Lithium prophylaxis of bipolar illness. *Br J Psychiatr.* 1994;164:208-214.
35. Guscott R, Taylor L. Lithium prophylaxis in recurrent affective illness: efficacy, effectiveness and efficiency. *Br J Psychiatry.* 1994;164:741-746.
36. Morris JB, Beck AT. The efficacy of antidepressant drugs: a review of research (1958-1972). *Arch Gen Psychiatry.* 1974;30:667-674.
37. Mendels J. Lithium in the treatment of depression. *Am J Psychiatry.* 1976;133:373-378.
38. Schou M. Lithium as a prophylactic agent in unipolar affective illness: comparison with cyclic antidepressants. *Arch Gen Psychiatry.* 1979;36:849-851.
39. Goodwin FK, Jamison KR. *Manic-Depressive Illness.* New York, NY: Oxford University Press; 1990.

40. Souza FGM, Goodwin GM. Lithium treatment and prophylaxis in unipolar depression: a meta-analysis. *Br J Psychiatry.* 1991;158:666-675.
41. Mendels J, Secunda SK, Dyson WL. A controlled study of the antidepressant effects of lithium carbonate. *Arch Gen Psychiatry.* 1972;26:154-157.
42. Worrall EP, Moody JP, Peet M, Dick P, Smith A, Chambers C, Adams M, Naylor GJ. Controlled studies of the acute antidepressant effects of lithium. *Br J Psychiatry.* 1979;135:255-262.
43. Baron A, Gershon ES, Rudy V, Jonas WZ, Buchsbaum M. Lithium carbonate response in depression: prediction by unipolar/bipolar illness, average-evoked response, catechol-*O*-methyl transferase, and family history. *Arch Gen Psychiatry.* 1975; 32:1107-1111.
44. de Montigny C, Grunberg F, Mayer A, Deschenes JP. Lithium induces rapid relief of depression in tricyclic antidepressant drug nonresponders. *Br J Psychiatry.* 1981;138:252-256.
45. Heninger GR, Charney DS, Sternberg DE. Lithium carbonate augmentation of antidepressant treatment: an effective prescription for treatment-refractory depression. *Arch Gen Psychiatry.* 1983; 40:1335-1342.
46. Price LH, Charney DS, Heninger GR. Variability of response to lithium augmentation in refractory depression. *Am J Psychiatry.* 1986;143: 1387-1392.
47. Gelenberg AL, Kane JM, Keller MB, Lavori P, Rosenbaum JF, Cole K, Lavelle J. Comparison of standard and low serum levels of lithium for maintenance treatment of bipolar disorder. *N Engl J Med.* 1989;321:1489-1493.
48. Keller MB, Lavori PW, Kane JM, Gelenbeg AJ, Rosenbaum JF, Walzer EA, Baker LA. Subsyndromal symptoms in bipolar disorder: a comparison of standard and low serum levels of lithium. *Arch Gen Psychiatry.* 1992;49:371-376.
49. Bowden CL. Predictors of response to divalproex and lithium. *J Clin Psychiatry.* 1995;56 (suppl 3):25-30.
50. Komoroski RA, Newton JE, Walker E, Cardwell D, Jagannathan NR, Ramaprasad S, Sprigg J. In vivo NMR spectroscopy of lithium-7 in humans. *Magnet Reson Med.* 1990;15:347-356.
51. Kato T, Takahashi S, Inubushi T. Brain lithium concentration by ^{7}Li- and ^{1}H-magnetic resonance spectroscopy in bipolar disorder. *Psychiatry Res.* 1992;45:53-63.
52. Sachs GS, Renshaw PF, Lafer B, Stoll A, Guimaraes AR, Rosenbaum JE, Gonzalez RG. Variability of brain lithium levels during maintenance treatment: a magnetic resonance spectroscopy study. *Biol Psychiatry.* 1995;38:422-428.
53. Kato T, Inubushi T, Takahashi S. Relationship of lithium concentrations in the brain measured by lithium-7 magnetic resonance spectroscopy to treatment response in mania. *J Clin Psychopharmacol.* 1994;14:330-335.
54. Goldberg JF, Harrow M, Grossman LS. Recurrent affective syndromes in bipolar and unipolar mood disorders at follow-up. *Br J Psychiatr.* 1995; 166:382-385.
55. Mueller-Oerlinghausen B, Ahrens B, Grof E, Grof P, Lenz G, Schou M, Simhandl C, Thau K, Volk J, Wolf R, Wolf T. The effect of long-term lithium treatment on the mortality of patients with manic-depressive and schizoaffective illness. *Acta Psychiatr Scand.* 1992;86:218-222.
56. Vestergaard P, Aagaard J. Five-year mortality in lithium-treated manic depressive patients. *J Affect Disord.* 1991;21:33-38.
57. Shulman KI, Tohen M, Satlin A, Mallya G, Kalunian D. Mania compared with unipolar depression in old age. *Am J Psychiatry.* 1992;149:341-345.
58. Regier DA, Boyd JH, Burke JD Jr, Rae DS, Myers JK, Kramer M, Robins LN, George LK, Karno M, Locke BZ. One-month prevalence of mental disorders in the United States: based on five Epidemiologic Catchment Area sites. *Arch Gen Psychiatry.* 1988;45:977-986.
59. Morrison JR. Suicide in a psychiatric practice population. *J Clin Psychiatry.* 1982;43:348-352.
60. Roy-Byrne PR, Post RM, Hambrick DD, Leverich GS, Rosoff AS. Suicide and course of illness in major affective disorder. *J Affect Disord.* 1988; 15:1-8.
61. Barraclough B. Suicide prevention, recurrent affective disorder and lithium. *Br J Psychiatry.* 1972; 121:391-392.
62. Coppen A, Barry-Standish H, Houston G, Silcocks P, Hermon C. Does lithium reduce the mortality of recurrent mood disorders? *J Affect Disord.* 1991;23:1-7.
63. National Institute of Mental Health. *Affective Disorders (Mood Disorders): Budget Estimate.* Bethesda, Md: National Institute of Mental Health; 1995:43-53.
64. Kay DWK, Petterson U. Mortality in manic-depressive illness: a clinical, social and genetic study. *Acta Psychiatr Scand.* 1977;56:269.
65. Glen AIM, Dodd M, Hulme EB, Kreitman N. Mortality on lithium. *Neuropsychobiology.* 1979;5: 167-173.
66. Coppen A, Standish-Barry H, Bailey J, Houston G, Silcocks P, Hermon C. Long-term lithium and mortality. *Lancet.* 1990;335:1347.
67. Muller-Oerlinghausen B, Ahrens B, Volk J, Grof P, Grof E, Schou M, Vestergaard P, Lenz G, Simhandl C, Thau K, Wolf R. Reduced mortality of manic-depressive patients in long-term lithium treatment: an international collaborative study by IGSLI. *Psychiatry Res.* 1991;36:329-331.
68. Muller-Oerlinghausen B, Muser-Causemann B, Volk J. Suicides and parasuicides in the high-risk patient group on and off lithium long-term medication. *J Affect Disord.* 1992;25:261-270.
69. Crundwell JK. Lithium and its potential benefit in reducing increased mortality rates due to suicide. *Lithium.* 1994;5:193-204.
70. Roy A. Risk factors for suicide in psychiatric patients. *Arch Gen Psychiatry.* 1982;39:1089-1095.
71. Schou M, Weeke A. Did manic-depressive patients who committed suicide receive prophylactic or continuation treatment at the time? *Br J Psychiatry.* 1988;153:324-327.
72. Isometsa E, Henriksson M, Lonnqvist J. Completed suicide and recent lithium treatment. *J Affect Disord.* 1992;26:101-104.
73. Isometsa ET, Henriksson MM, Aro HM, Lonnqvist JK. Suicide in bipolar disorder in Finland. *Am J Psychiatry.* 1994;151:1020-1024.
74. Black DW, Winokur G, Nasrallah A. Is death from natural causes still excessive in psychiatric patients? *J Nerv Mental Dis.* 1987;175:674-680.
75. Gershon S, Yuwiler A. Lithium ion: a specific psychopharmacological approach to the treatment of mania. *J Neuropsychiatry.* 1960;1:229-241.
76. Schou M. Normothymotics, 'mood-normalizers.' *Br J Psychiatry.* 1963:109:803-809.
77. Watanabe S, Ishino H, Otsuki S. Lithium ion and affective psychosis. *Folia Psychiatr Neurol Jpn.* 1974;28:267-305.
78. Schou M. Lithium in the treatment of other psychiatric and nonpsychiatric disorders. *Arch Gen Psychiatry.* 1979;36:856-859.
79. Prien RF, Potter WZ. NIMH Workshop report on treatment of bipolar disorder. *Psychopharmacol Bull.* 1990;26:409-427.
80. Lejoyeux M, Ades J. Evaluation of lithium treatment in alcoholism. *Alcohol Alcoholism.* 1993; 28:273-279.
81. Sheard MH, Marini JL, Bridges CI, Wagner E. The effect of lithium on impulsive aggressive behavior in man. *Am J Psychiatry.* 1976;133:1409-1413.
82. Campbell M, Kafantaris V, Cueva JE. An update on the use of lithium carbonate in aggressive children and adolescents with conduct disorder. *Psychopharmacol Bull.* 1995;31:93-102.
83. Coxhead N, Silverstone T, Cookson J. Carbamazepine versus lithium in the prophylaxis of bipolar affective disorder. *Acta Psychiatr Scand.* 1992;85:114-118.
84. Lusznat RM, Murphy DP, Nunn CMH. Carbamazepine vs lithium in the treatment and prophylaxis of mania. *Br J Psychiatry.* 1988;153, 198-204.
85. Freeman TW, Clothier JL, Pazzaglia P, Lesem MD, Swann AC. A double-blind comparison of valproate and lithium in the treatment of acute mania. *Am J Psychiatry.* 1992;49:108-111.
86. Pope Jr HG, McElroy SL, Keck Jr PE, Hudson JI. Valproate in the treatment of acute mania: a placebo-controlled study. *Arch Gen Psychiatry.* 1991;48:62-68.
87. Bowden CL, Brugger AM, Swann AC, Calabrese JR, Janicak PG, Petty F, Dilsaver SC, Davis JM, Rush AJ, Small JG, Garza-Trevino ES, Risch SC, Goodnick PJ, Morris DD. Efficacy of divalproex vs lithium and placebo in the treatment of mania. *JAMA.* 1994;271:918-924.
88. McElroy SL, Keck, Jr PE, Pope, Jr HG, Hudson JI. Valproate in the treatment of bipolar disorder: literature review and clinical guidelines. *J Clin Psychopharmacol.* 1992;12:42S-52S.
89. Garza-Trevino ES, Overall JE, Hollister LE. Verapamil versus lithium in acute mania. *Am J Psychiatry.* 1992;149:121-122.
90. Dubovsky SL, Franks RD, Allen S, Murphy J. Calcium antagonists in mania: a double-blind study of verapamil. *Psychiatry Res.* 1986;18:309-320.
91. Chouinard G. The use of benzodiazepines in the treatment of manic-depressive illness. *J Clin Psychiatry.* 1988;49(suppl11):15-19.
92. Sachs GS, Rosenbaum JF, Jones L. Adjunctive clonazepam for maintenance treatment of bipolar affective disorder. *J Clin Psychopharmacol.* 1990;10:42-47.
93. Benjamin J, Agam G, Levine J, Bersudsky Y, Kofman O, Belmaker RH. Inositol treatment in psychiatry. *Psychopharmacol Bull.* 1995;31:167-175.
94. Atack JR, Broughton HB, Pollack SJ. Inositol monophosphatase: a putative target for Li^{+} in the treatment of bipolar disorder. *Trends Neurosci.* 1995;18:343-349.

Unanswered Questions, Unknown Future for One of Our Oldest Medications

As ONE of the oldest pillars of modern psychopharmacology, lithium remains a treatment toward which all psychiatrists should feel a deep indebtedness. The decreased morbidity associated with its demonstrated efficacy in both the acute and maintenance phases of bipolar disorder has provided greatly needed relief and hope for patients and their families.[1] More than any other individual, Dr Mogens Schou has been responsible for demonstrating lithium's efficacy and promoting its use. Now, 40 years after lithium's introduction into psychiatry, he reviews some of the current controversies about this remarkable drug.[2]

LITHIUM AS A MAINTENANCE TREATMENT

One of Schou's concerns is the underappreciation of lithium's capacity as a maintenance treatment for bipolar disorder. He alludes to the recent naturalistic studies that suggest that lithium seems less effective in these samples than in the many controlled studies. In a previous publication,[3] he concluded that the results of these naturalistic studies

> reveal what happens to carelessly selected patients who are given long-term maintenance treatment under conditions of insufficient information, support, and supervision.

The implication of this comment, of course, is that the poorer results in the naturalistic studies should not be interpreted as evidence of lithium's failure so much as of the failure of proper delivery of the medication. Consistent with this, in the current article,[2] Schou concludes overall that, for bipolar disorder, lithium should be the "first-choice prophylactic agent."

Although the data from published studies would certainly support this conclusion, two other factors in addition to those noted by Schou would seem to explain the disparity between the controlled studies and naturalistic data: a shift in the types of bipolar disorder patients treated in clinical settings and compliance problems. Many bipolar patients evaluated in recent studies show high rates of at least one comorbid disorder such as alcohol or other drug abuse, anxiety disorders, personality disorders, and impulse control disorders.[4-11] Although more work is needed in this area, a number of studies have already demonstrated that the presence of some of these comorbid disorders, especially substance abuse, predicts a poorer response to treatment.[4,5,12] The naturalistic studies that demonstrate poorer responses to lithium may reflect the more complicated cases of bipolar disorders than are currently seen in most clinical settings. Additionally, an increasing number of patients with bipolar spectrum disorders, such as bipolar II disorder, cyclothymia, and other milder disorders, are being treated with mood stabilizers. The lack of studies on the optimal pharmacotherapy of these patients precludes any conclusion regarding the efficacy of lithium (or, in fact, any other medication) in treating them. However, these less-than-classic patients may not show the same robust response to lithium compared with the more prototypical bipolar patients treated in the original lithium studies.

See also pages 9, 14, and 16

The adverse effect profile of lithium, especially weight gain and cognitive dulling, has also diminished lithium's attractiveness to many patients and clinicians.[1,13] These adverse effects are among the most common causes of lithium noncompliance, which has been estimated as ranging between 18% and 53%, with adherence to medications especially difficult in the time-unlimited maintenance phase of the illness.[1] Compliance may be even more difficult now that alternative treatments such as divalproex sodium and carbamazepine are available. Compared with lithium, these other mood stabilizers possess different adverse effect profiles. If controlled studies with divalproex and carbamazepine demonstrate the efficacy of these drugs for maintenance treatment (as they have for the acute treatment of mania),[14-16] the treatment of choice for any individual patient may increasingly depend on adverse effect considerations.

While acknowledging that antidepressants (especially the newer agents such as the selective serotonin reuptake inhibitors) are well-documented, effective treatments for unipolar depression, Schou is also concerned that psychiatrists in the United States do not sufficiently appreciate the efficacy of lithium in the maintenance treatment of recurrent major depression. In support of his conclusion, two recent studies, including one meta-analysis, suggest the value of lithium for maintenance treatment of unipolar depression.[17,18] Schou notes that

> patients who suffer from recurrent depressions without obvious psychosocial precipitating factors, have symptom-free intervals, and are without deviating character features, might benefit from first-line or second-line lithium maintenance treatment.

Whereas a substantial number of depressed patients meet these criteria, they may represent a small percentage of the total depressed population who present for treatment and are typically considered for pharmacotherapy. Similar to the shift in the types of bipolar patients recently seen in the United States, comorbid substance abuse, dysthymia (with chronic depressive symptoms), anxiety disorders, and personality disorders are now common in depressed patients.[19-21] As a result of these more complicated depressions, classic recurrent unipolar depression seems to have become an increasingly unusual phenomenon. Therefore, even if we accept lithium's efficacy as a maintenance treatment for patients with classic unipolar depression, the clinical applicability of this finding may be relevant to a relatively small group of depressed patients seen in clinical practice.

As they do with its use in bipolar disorder, compliance problems also plague the use of lithium for patients with depressive disorders. We would guess that few among us would rather take lithium with its possibilities of weight gain, tremor, and the need for recurrent blood tests vs one of the newer antidepressants.

Lithium may be useful, however, in other clinical situations with unipolar depressive patients. One example would be its utility when switching from one antidepressant to another that requires a 2-week or longer washout between treatments (eg, a selective serotonin reuptake inhibitor to a monoamine oxidase inhibitor or a monoamine oxidase inhibitor to a variety of other antidepressants). Since lithium can be safely combined with any of these agents, therapy may be started during the tapering phase of the first antidepressant. In some cases, patients will note moderate improvement on lithium, obviating the need to begin the other antidepresssant. Even a partial response to lithium in this circumstance will ease the transition if the second antidepressant is required.

Overall, lithium's efficacy as a maintenance treatment in mood disorders is indisputable. However, its effectiveness, acceptance, and utility for patients with complicated disorders and/or those who are sensitive to adverse effects, especially when alternative medications are available, is less clear.

LONG-TERM LITHIUM TREATMENT AND RENAL FUNCTION

Schou[2] notes the observation of a few cases in which no cause other than lithium was found to explain progressive renal insufficiency due to interstitial nephritis. Without comparative data, such as what percentage of the general population and/or what percentage of bipolar patients not treated with lithium develop renal insufficiency, he wisely concludes that statements regarding lithium's etiological role remain unproved. Nonetheless, the number of reported cases of either serious renal insufficiency or simply "creeping creatinines"[22] continues to cause some concern. Other than the cases described in a previous publication,[23] we have seen three other lithium-treated patients in which serum creatinine levels gradually increased beyond 177 µmol/L (2.0 mg/dL) with no obvious cause other than the long-term ingestion of lithium. Additionally, a recent study demonstrated that 21% of patients treated with lithium for more than 15 years had reduced glomerular filtration rates.[24] Unfortunately, no predictors consistently identify a group at high risk of lithium-induced nephropathy. As noted by Schou, renal concentrating deficits do not predict decreased creatinine clearance. Until more is known about lithium's nephrotoxic capacity, we agree with Schou's conclusion that periodic checks of serum creatinine levels in lithium-treated patients (every 6 months to 1 year during maintenance therapy[25]) continue to be appropriate. However, the growing number of cases described and the lack of such cases anecdotally reported with other, more commonly prescribed psychoactive drugs (such as antidepressants) gives cause for some concern.

LIFE EVENTS AS TRIGGERS FOR BIPOLAR EPISODES

In reviewing an early study by Baastrup et al[26] of which he was a coauthor, Schou[2] alludes to the different explanations for relapses in bipolar disorder, briefly noting the controversy surrounding the role of life events as triggers for relapse. Although not central to the article, this issue and its implied clinical relevance form an increasingly important component of optimal treatment for bipolar disorder. Whatever the comparable merits of lithium, divalproex, and carbamazepine in controlled or naturalistic studies, relapses in patients who are in maintenance treatment occur far more frequently than either patients or clinicians would like. One strategy to remedy this situation would be to optimize the prescription of our current mood stabilizers and to evaluate other pharmacotherapies that might be effective. Another complementary strategy would be to develop interventions that might minimize the capacity of stressful life events to trigger episodes of mania or depression. A growing body of literature already suggests that life events are associated with relapses of bipolar disorder, even for those patients adequately treated with mood stabilizers.[27,28] Mechanisms by which these triggering events could change the course of the illness have also been proposed.[29] Given the above discussion about the large number of bipolar patients with comorbid disorders, it would seem likely that more complex psychopathological features (especially if the comorbid disorders are personality disorders) demand more complex multimodal treatments. In our efforts to define the best treatments for bipolar disorder, we must consider designing treatments for specific populations (eg, those with dual diagnoses), as well as for those with other underlying vulnerabilities (eg, those with heightened sensitivity to environmental stressors).

CONCLUSION

In what direction should we proceed toward clarifying the unresolved issues regarding lithium therapy? First, the comparative efficacies of lithium, carbamazepine, and divalproex (and the risk-benefit ratio in terms of adverse effects and compliance) in the maintenance treatment of bipolar disorder should be evaluated more systematically. Additional work on lithium's efficacy in treating acute depressive episodes for both unipolar and bipolar depressions would also be very useful. Although learning more about lithium's renal effects would help clarify some of the questions raised above and in Schou's article, this area should not be considered a top priority given our ability to monitor renal function and to switch to other agents if needed. Next, since the efficacy of pharmacotherapy alone in the maintenance treatment of bipolar disorder is less than ideal, the role of psychosocial factors in the course of bipolar disorder should be further explored. As suggested above, a corollary of these efforts would be to develop psychological and psychosocial interventions that might minimize the impact of these stresses and augment the efficacy of mood stabilizers. Finally, strategies for enhancing compliance and thereby improving outcome have not been given sufficient attention, and their study should be encouraged.[30]

With additional knowledge, we will be better able to place lithium in the appropriate context: Is it still the preeminent treatment for bipolar disorder, or, like the evolution of newer antihypertensives that have replaced reserpine, β-blockers, and other medications for most treated patients, will we ultimately view it as simply the first such effective treatment?

Michael J. Gitlin, MD
Lori L. Altshuler, MD
Department of Psychiatry
University of California
at Los Angeles
Los Angeles, CA 90024-6968

REFERENCES

1. Goodwin FK, Jamison KR. *Manic Depressive Illness.* New York, NY: Oxford University Press; 1990.
2. Schou M. Forty years of lithium treatment. *Arch Gen Psychiatry.* 1997;54:9-13.
3. Schou M. Lithium prophylaxis: about 'naturalistic' or 'clinical practice' studies. *Lithium.* 1993; 4:77-81.
4. Brady JT, Sonne SC. The relationship between substance abuse and bipolar disorder. *J Clin Psychiatry.* 1995;56:19-24.
5. Sonne SC, Brady KT, Morton WA. Substance abuse and bipolar affective disorder. *J Nerv Ment Dis.* 1994;182:349-352.
6. Winokur G, Coryell W, Akiskal HS, Maser JD, Keller MB, Endicott J, Mueller T. Alcoholism in manic-depressive (bipolar) illness: familial illness, course of illness, and the primary-secondary distinction. *Am J Psychiatry.* 1995; 152:365-372.
7. Keck PE, McElroy SL, Strakowski SM, West SA, Hawkins JM, Huber TJ, Newman RM, DePriest N. Outcome and comorbidity in first- compared with multiple-episode mania. *J Nerv Ment Dis.* 1995;183:320-324.
8. Chen Y-W, Dilsaver SC. Comorbidity of panic disorder in bipolar illness: evidence from the Epidemiologic Catchment Area survey. *Am J Psychiatry.* 1995;152:280-282.
9. Strakowski SM, Tohen M, Stoll AL, Faedda GL, Goodwin DC. Comorbidity in mania at first hospitalization. *Am J Psychiatry.* 1992;149:554-556.
10. Pica S, Edwards J, Jackson HJ, Bell RC, Bates GW, Rudd RP. Personality disorders in recent-onset bipolar disorder. *Compr Psychiatry.* 1990; 31:499-510.
11. O'Connell RW, Mayo JA, Sciutto MS. PDQ-R personality disorders in bipolar patients. *J Affect Disord.* 1991;23:217-221.
12. Tohen M, Waternaux CM, Tsuang MT. Outcome in mania: a 4-year prospective follow-up of 75 patients utilizing survival analysis. *Arch Gen Psychiatry.* 1990;47:1106-1111.
13. Gitlin M, Cochran S, Jamison K. Maintenance lithium treatment: side effects and compliance. *J Clin Psychiatry.* 1989;50:127-131.
14. Pope HG, McElroy SL, Keck PE, Hudson JI. Valproate in the treatment of acute mania: a placebo-controlled study. *Arch Gen Psychiatry.* 1991;48: 62-68.
15. Bowden CL, Brugger AM, Swann AC, Calabrese JR, Janicak PG, Petty F, Dilsaver SC, Davis JM, Rush AJ, Small JG, Garza-Trevino ES, Risch SC, Goodnick PJ, Morris DD, for the Depakote Mania Study Group. Efficacy of divalproex vs lithium and placebo in the treatment of mania. *JAMA.* 1994;271:918-924.
16. Small JG, Klapper MH, Milstein V, Kellams JJ, Miller MJ, Marhenke JD, Small IF. Carbamazepine compared with lithium in the treatment of mania. *Arch Gen Psychiatry.* 1991;48:915-921.
17. Souza FGM, Mander AJ, Goodwin GM. The efficacy of lithium in prophylaxis of unipolar depression: evidence from its discontinuation. *Br J Psychiatry.* 1990;157:718-722.
18. Souza FGM, Goodwin GM. Lithium treatment and prophylaxis in unipolar depression: a meta-analysis. *Br J Psychiatry.* 1991;158:666-675.
19. Keller MB. Diagnostic and course-of-illness variables pertinent to refractory depression. In: Tasman A, Goldfinger SM, Kaufmann CA, eds. *American Psychiatric Press Review of Psychiatry.* Washington, DC: American Psychiatric Press; 1990;9:10-32.
20. Oldham JM, Skodol AE. Personality disorders and mood disorders. In: Tasman A, Riba MB, eds. *American Psychiatric Press Review of Psychiatry.* Washington, DC: American Psychiatric Press; 1992;11:418-435.
21. Robins LN, Locke BZ, Regier DA. An overview of psychiatric disorders in America. In: Robins LN, Regier DA, eds. *Psychiatric Disorders in America.* New York, NY: The Free Press; 1991: 328-366.
22. Jefferson JW. Lithium: a therapeutic magic wand. *J Clin Psychiatry.* 1989;50:81-86.
23. Gitlin M. Lithium-induced renal insufficiency. *J Clin Psychopharmacol.* 1993;13:276-279.
24. Bendz H, Aurell M, Balldin J, Mathe AA, Sjodin I. Kidney damage in long-term lithium patients: a cross-sectional study of patients with 15 years or more on lithium. *Nephrol Dial Transplant.* 1994; 9:1250-1254.
25. American Psychiatric Association. Practice guidelines for the treatment of patients with bipolar disorder. *Am J Psychiatry.* 1994;151(suppl):1-36.
26. Baastrup PC, Poulsen JC, Schou M, Thomsen K, Amdisen A. Prophylactic lithium: double-blind discontinuation in manic-depressive and recurrent-depressive disorders. *Lancet.* 1970;2: 326-330.
27. Ellicott A, Hammen C, Gitlin M, Brown G, Jamison K. Life events and the course of bipolar disorder. *Am J Psychiatry.* 1990;147:1194-1198.
28. Hunt N, Bruce-Jones W, Silverstone T. Life events and relapse in bipolar affective disorder. *J Affect Disord.* 1992;25:13-20.
29. Post RN. Transduction of psychosocial stress into the neurobiology of recurrent affective disorder. *Am J Psychiatry.* 1992;149:999-1010.
30. Cochran S. Preventing medical noncompliance in the outpatient treatment of bipolar affective disorders. *J Consult Clin Psychol.* 1984;52:873-878.

A Linkage Study of Bipolar Illness

Wade H. Berrettini, MD, PhD; Thomas N. Ferraro, PhD; Lynn R. Goldin, PhD; Sevilla D. Detera-Wadleigh, PhD; Henry Choi; David Muniec; Juliet J. Guroff, MSW; Diane M. Kazuba; John I. Nurnberger, Jr, MD, PhD; Wang-Ting Hsieh, PhD; Margret R. Hoehe, MD; Elliot S. Gershon, MD

Background: Although genetic epidemiological studies of bipolar (BP) illness are consistent with a heritable component, inherited risk factors remain unknown. The goal of the present study is to describe the localization of BP susceptibility loci through linkage strategies, including a genome-wide search.

Methods: A linkage study of 22 BP families has been performed. These BP families include almost 400 persons, 173 of whom have been diagnosed as having BP I, schizoaffective, BP II with major depression, or recurrent unipolar illness. Using an autosomal dominant disease model with 85% or 50% age-dependent penetrance, and a recessive model with 85% penetrance, linkage analyses were performed assuming a narrow (BP and schizoaffective) or a broad (BP, schizoaffective, or unipolar) definition of the BP spectrum. Affected sibling pairs and affected pedigree member analyses were performed when positive lod scores were observed in multiple pedigrees. The present article describes linkage analysis of 310 DNA markers on chromosomes 1, 5p, 6, 8, 10q, 11q, and 12 to 18.

Results: None of the loci examined disclosed compelling evidence for linkage using lod score analyses. Model-independent analysis by multilocus affected pedigree member method in the pericentromeric chromosome 18 region disclosed statistically significant evidence ($P<.0001$) for a BP susceptibility gene in this region. Multilocus analysis by affected sibling pair method also disclosed evidence for linkage ($P<.00008$).

Conclusions: Our results imply that a BP susceptibility gene exists near the centromere of chromosome 18. Confirmation of this finding (by independent investigators studying different pedigrees) has been published, suggesting that a valid BP disease linkage may have been discovered.

Arch Gen Psychiatry. 1997;54:27-35

From the Department of Psychiatry and Human Behavior, Jefferson Medical College, Thomas Jefferson University, Philadelphia, Pa (Drs Berrettini and Ferraro and Mr Choi); the Clinical Neurogenetics Branch, National Institute of Mental Health, Bethesda, Md (Drs Goldin, Detera-Wadleigh, Hsieh, Hoehe, and Gershon, Mr Muniec, and Mss Guroff and Kazuba); and the Institute for Psychiatric Research, Department of Psychiatry, Indiana University, Indianapolis (Dr Nurnberger). Dr Hsieh is now with Abbott Research Laboratories, North Chicago, Ill, and Dr Hoehe is with the Max Delbruck Center of Molecular Medicine, Berlin, Germany.

As REVIEWED by Nurnberger et al,[1] twin, family, and adoption studies of bipolar (BP) disease are consistent with complex (nonmendelian) inheritance. Patterns of transmission of illness within families can be studied with segregation analysis to detect a particular mode of inheritance, such as a single gene with X-linked or autosomal recessive genetics. In a segregation analysis of BP families, Rice et al[2] reported that a single locus was not favored over a mixed model of transmission (including the possibility of multiple genes and an environmental effect), a result consistent with complex inheritance of BP disease.

Linkage analysis of complex (nonmendelian) diseases is difficult because of unknown mode of inheritance, genetic heterogeneity, and nongenetic factors in illness.[3-6] Nonetheless, linkage analysis has been successful in localizing disease-causing genes for subtypes of complex illnesses characterized by heterogeneous causes (osteoarthritis,[7-9] Alzheimer disease,[10-12] and breast cancer[13,14]). These successes suggest that impediments associated with complex diseases are not absolute obstacles to discovering susceptibility genes for nonmendelian illnesses.

During the past decade, linkage studies of BP disease have been conducted with molecular genetic techniques in an effort to localize vulnerability genes,[15,16] but no confirmed linkages have been established. Evidence for a BP gene on 11p15[17] has been weakened by failure to confirm the finding in numerous other pedigrees,[18-21] and by evaluation of newly ascertained persons in the

See Materials and Methods on next page

MATERIALS AND METHODS

BP PEDIGREES

Of the 22 BP pedigrees studied in this linkage investigation, diagnostic and ascertainment methods for 21 have been described previously.[32] These 21 families include about 365 informative persons (persons whose genotypes can be determined directly or indirectly). We also studied the "right extension" of Old Order Amish pedigree 110,[22] which seemed to have a unilineal pattern of illness descent similar to our pedigrees, as described elsewhere.[32] Almost all family members had a modified Schedule for Affective Disorders and Schizophrenia—Lifetime Version semistructured interview. In these 21 families, 165 members (whose genotypes can be determined) are diagnosed as having schizoaffective (SA), BP I, BP II with major depression, or recurrent unipolar (UP) illness as previously described.[32] These ill pedigree members constitute about 135 affected sibling pairs (ASPs).

Additional persons have become ill in this pedigree series since an earlier description[32] of pedigree structures. In family 1516, additional DNA samples from recently ascertained children and grandchildren of person 321 have been genotyped. These persons include 4 affected persons under affection status model II. In family 1442, person 095 has experienced recurrent UP illness. The right extension of Old Order Amish pedigree 110[22] contains 30 informative persons, 8 of whom are diagnosed as having BP spectrum illness. For the Old Order Amish pedigree segment, diagnostic research records were reviewed and diagnoses assigned consistent with our criteria.

The mean (±SD) number of pedigrees studied with each marker is 21±1. A few pedigrees were not analyzed at some loci because of technically unacceptable data. The mean (±SD) number of persons genotyped at each marker is 338±21. The mean (±SD) heterozygosity (from the literature) for the DNA markers studied is 71%±14%. There are about 135 ASPs in these 22 BP pedigrees. This pedigree series has a power greater than 90% to detect linkage under several disease models if 50% of the kindreds are linked to a single locus.[32,38]

DNA MARKERS

The loci studied include microsatellite (simple sequence repeat) polymorphisms. DNA probes identifying restriction fragment length polymorphisms and minisatellites also were studied. Most DNA probes were provided as gifts or were purchased from the American Type Culture Collection (Rockville, Md), or Collaborative Research Inc (Bedford, Mass).

DNA probes were labeled by random primer extension or nick translation with deoxycytosine triphosphate labeled with phosphorus 32 (3000 Ci/mmol) as described[32] to a specific activity of 10^9 cpm/µg. DNA samples were extracted from lymphoblastoid cell lines or from whole blood[39] and were digested with restriction endonucleases according to the manufacturer's recommendations, using 5 U/µg of DNA. Agarose gel electrophoresis (10 µg of digested DNA per lane), transfer to nylon membranes, hybridization, washing, and autoradiography were done as described.[32]

Some microsatellite primers were synthesized on a DNA synthesizer (Milligen Cyclone), cleaved with 20% ammonium hydroxide overnight at room temperature (or for 5 hours at 55°C), the supernatant was lyophilized, reconstituted in 0.5 mL of water, and used without further purification after spectroscopic quantification. Most primers were purchased from Research Genetics Inc (Huntsville, Ala). Microsatellites were studied using the polymerase chain reaction, by modifying a previously described protocol.[40] A 20-µL reaction included genomic DNA (30 ng), deoxyadenosine triphosphate, deoxyguanosine triphosphate (dGTP), deoxycytidine triphosphate, and thymine triphosphate (200 µmol/L each), tromethamine (10 mmol/L, pH 8.3), potassium chloride (50 mmol/L), primers, magnesium chloride, and 0.5 U of *Taq* polymerase. The concentrations of magnesium chloride and oligonucleotide primers were optimized empirically for each locus studied. Typically, 2.5-mmol/L magnesium chloride was used with 250-nmol/L labeled primer and 500-nmol/L unlabeled primer.

Oligonucleotide end-labeling at the 5′ position was carried out in a 125-µL reaction using a 1-nmol/L concentration of 1 primer, 250 µCi of ^{32}P-γ adenosine triphosphate (3000 Ci/mmol, 10 mCi/mL, NEG-002A, NEN Research Products, Boston, Mass), 10× forward exchange buffer (Promega, Madison, Wis), and 1 U/µL of T_4 polynucleotide kinase (Promega). This reaction produces sufficient end-labeled primer to conduct at least 100 polymerase chain reactions. The reaction was incubated at 37°C for 30 minutes and was terminated by passage of the reaction mixture through a spin column (Select-D, G-25, 5 Prime-3, Sephadex, Prime Inc, Boulder, Colo). A thermocycler (9600, Perkin-Elmer Corp, Norwalk, Conn) was programmed for a denaturation step (1 minute, 94°C) and an annealing step (30-60 seconds); there was no specific step for primer extension. The temperature of the annealing step was optimized for each locus studied, but typically was 55°C. The primary thermal program was run for 30 cycles followed by 1 cycle of a secondary thermal program with identical denaturation and annealing steps, followed by a 5-minute interval at 72°C to ensure complete synthesis.

Polymerase chain reaction products were analyzed by polyacrylamide gel electrophoresis as described.[34] Aliquots from polymerase chain reactions were added to equal volumes of 90% formamide loading buffer containing xylene cyanol (0.3%) and bromphenol blue (0.3%). This mixture was heated to 95°C for 5 minutes to fully denature DNA, and 2-µL aliquots were loaded onto 8.0% polyacrylamide

original pedigree.[22] The color vision region of Xq28 also has been linked to BP illness.[23-25] Again, however, several independent investigators have not confirmed this linkage.[26-29] Some of the original evidence for linkage to clinically assessed color blindness and G6PD deficiency in one report[25] was *not* confirmed by genotyping with relevant Xq28 DNA markers.[30] This failure of replication[30] is remarkable, because the original report[25] described a maximal lod score of 9, a profound level of statistical significance that should confer validity beyond reasonable doubt. Careful review[31] of the discrepancies between the original report[25] and the molecular failure to replicate[30] led to the conclusion that the original report[25] was flawed by questionable methods, including poor quality control of G6PD assays, failure to maintain an independence between gels (35×40 cm), cast using 64-well combs and 0.4-mm spacers. Gels were run at 75 W constant power for 3 to 4 hours. Standard-sized markers were prepared from *Hae*III- and *Msp*I-digested PBR322 fragments that were dephosphorylated using calf alkaline phosphatase (Promega) and end-labeled as described herein. After electrophoresis, gels were dried and exposed to x-ray film.

GENOTYPING

Genotypes were analyzed by persons who were unaware of all diagnoses. Genotypes were determined from autoradiograms read by 2 independent readers (familiar with the polymorphism in question) whose results were compared by computer matching to detect discrepancies. Discrepancies were resolved by reference to a third reader. Inconsistencies with pedigree structure were resolved by reinspection of the autoradiogram with reference to pedigree diagrams without diagnoses. If inconsistencies could not be resolved, the persons were considered as "genotype unknown" for that marker. Persons whose genotypes were inconsistent with the pedigree structure for more than 2 markers (from different DNA aliquots or different nylon membranes) were deleted from the study until a new source of DNA was obtained.

LINKAGE CALCULATIONS

Definition of the spectrum of BP diagnoses considered as affected is a controversial matter for linkage studies. These definitions of illness are known in genetic terminology as affection status models. Narrow definitions (eg, only BP I and SA-manic) can be useful to avoid the deleterious effects of misdiagnosis of well persons as having a mild form of the BP spectrum (eg, cyclothymia). Broader definitions (including UP diagnoses) are useful because they allow for more ill persons to be included in the linkage analysis, yielding increased power to detect linkage if the affection status model is correct. In practice, investigators often test a narrow and a broad model. Affection status models I (BP I, BP II with major depression and schizoaffective) and II (model I plus recurrent UP) were used to calculate lod scores. Persons with recurrent UP illness were considered unaffected when data were analyzed under affection status model I.

Two-point analyses (at 0%-20% recombination) were conducted with the MLINK program from the LINKAGE package (versions 5.03 and 5.10). A variable age of onset (15-50 years) was assumed with a maximal penetrance of 85% and 50% (at age 50 years) in an autosomal dominant model. A dominant model is consistent with the structures of these pedigrees, which were selected for a single source of illness transmission.[32] A disease gene frequency of 1.5% was assumed for 85% penetrance and 2.5% for 50% penetrance, because this is consistent with the prevalence of BP disease.[1] The 50% penetrance value was used to reduce the influence of genotypes from unaffected persons on the lod score.[41] At 50% penetrance, an unaffected person who has passed through the age of risk contributes only 20% of the value of an affected person. Penetrance of the normal genotype was set at 1% to allow for a small number of phenocopies.

When the true mode of transmission is unknown, as is the case for BP illness, misspecification of the analytic model as dominant (when the true mode of transmission is recessive) markedly reduces power to detect linkage.[42] Therefore, 2-point linkage analyses assuming a recessive model of transmission (85% penetrance and 15% disease gene frequency) were calculated for all regions. DNA marker allele frequencies (used to calculate lod scores) were obtained from the literature. Lod scores also were calculated using allele frequencies derived from these pedigrees, but differences were minimal (data not shown).

Two-point lod scores at each locus for individual families were examined visually to detect evidence for heterogeneity. When heterogeneity seemed possible (judging from the inspection of 2-point lod scores, some families yielded positive scores, but most were negative), the HOMOG program[43] was used to test for linkage in the presence of heterogeneity.

For chromosome 18 markers, affected pedigree member (APM) and ASP analyses were done on a chromosomal region. The APM[44] analysis requires no assumptions about a mode of transmission, penetrance, or disease allele frequencies. When pairs of ill relatives are observed to share a marker allele, the APM analysis assesses the probability that this has occurred by chance. This probability (that pairs of ill relatives share a marker allele) is a function of the population frequency of that marker allele. For the APM analyses, allele frequencies were estimated from these pedigrees using the method of Boehnke[45] or by allele counting.

The ASP statistic, another model-free method, tests whether pairs of affected siblings share a proportion of identical-by-descent (IBD) marker genes greater than the expected null hypothesis value (50%).[46] The ASP statistics were computed (using all of the available data on the sibship and their parents) with the SIBPAL program of the SAGE package.[47] These statistics are computed on all possible affected pairs. This procedure may inflate the contribution of sibships with large numbers of affecteds. To correct for this, we modified the degrees of freedom of the Student *t* test to be the number of independent affected pairs (defined per sibship as the number of affected persons −1) in the sample instead of the number of all possible pairs. The ASP analysis of chromosome 18 markers was reported elsewhere,[36] but 8 additional affected persons have been genotyped recently with chromosome 18 markers, and new analyses are reported here, including a multipoint identity-by-descent analysis of the ASPs in the sample.[48,49]

diagnosis and genotype assignment, and genotypic determinations based solely on family history. This experience leads to the conclusion that independent molecular confirmation of reported linkages must remain the standard criterion regardless of the statistical significance quoted in a single report.

We have previously described a series of 21 multiplex BP pedigrees suitable for linkage studies.[32] Using these kindreds, a systematic search for BP vulnerability genes has been conducted with linkage analysis. Previous results (using, in some cases, a smaller subset of the families) have been published on about 350 loci covering most regions of chromosome 5,[33] 1, 10q, 11q, 13, 15, and 17[34]; 57 microsatellite markers[35]; 20 markers near the centromere of chromosome 18[36]; and markers on chromosomes 2, 3, 4, 5, 7, 9, 10p, 11p, 22, and Xpter.[37]

Table 1. Heterogeneity Analyses for Genomic Screening of 22 Bipolar Pedigrees*

Chromosome No.	Unmapped Marker Loci Studied	Mapped Marker Loci Studied	Centimorgans: Examined (Mapped)	Centimorgans: Excluded	Centimorgans: Not Excluded
1	1	51	367.9	122.4	245.5
5p	0	5	46.0	2.0	44.0
6	0	28	223.0	150.1	72.9
8	0	22	224.3	110.6	113.7
10q	0	18	128.0	24.9	103.1
11q	1	22	121.9	37.0	84.9
12	0	23	188.9	97.9	91.0
13	0	23	215.0	31.2	183.8
14	0	18	160.5	97.3	63.2
15	0	22	145.0	4.0	141.0
16	0	24	162.6	68.6	94.0
17	0	25	182.0	63.6	118.4
18	6	21	174.5	84.6	89.9
Total	**8**	**302**	**2339.6**	**894.2**	**1445.4**

**Linkage analysis assuming a dominant 50% penetrance model and 50% heterogeneity is summarized for each chromosome studied, in terms of distances excluded under this model (area around each marker for which the lod score is less than −2).*

Results for chromosomes 6, 8, 12, 14, 16, and 18 are reported herein. Analyses for chromosome 18 reported herein are updated (with new diagnostic material) from those published previously,[36] by inclusion of genotypes on 14 additional persons, 8 of whom are affected. More than 75 new highly polymorphic markers have been added to the 6 chromosomes previously studied for BP linkage by Berrettini et al.[34]

RESULTS

Linkage analysis to affective illness with 310 DNA markers (covering about 50% of the genome) was performed in a series of BP pedigrees using 2-point (marker-to-illness) lod scores, under 3 inheritance models (dominant 85% and 50% penetrance and recessive 85% penetrance). This did not disclose homogeneous linkage or a subset of linked families when using HOMOG.[43] An exclusion map was prepared under a model of single locus inheritance with genetic heterogeneity and reduced penetrance, based on evidence from simulations that several models of complex and oligogenic inheritance could be detected under such an analytic model.[50] We chose a genetic model of dominant inheritance, proportion of families linked $\alpha=.5$, penetrance defined according to age-dependent liability classes with 50% penetrance at the highest age, and illness allele frequency of .025 or less. Under this model, the criterion for exclusion of linkage was a lod score, calculated using the heterogeneity parameter (α), less than −2. The results for this exclusion procedure are summarized in an unpublished exclusion map, which also shows the sum of lod scores for all pedigrees under genetic homogeneity for the dominant model described above, and for a recessive model with maximum penetrance 85% and illness allele frequency of 15% (the exclusion map will be supplied on request).

Unless a population isolate is studied, it is unreasonable to assume that BP illness is genetically homogeneous. When studying multiple outbred pedigrees, exclusion of linkage assuming genetic homogeneity is therefore a mathematical calculation of uncertain value. The exclusion procedure based on 50% heterogeneity (rather than alternative procedures[51]) was made to avoid finding exclusion for an unrealistic assumption of genetic homogeneity (or small degrees of heterogeneity). The lod score computations, including the exclusion computations, were used for heuristic purposes, because the genetic models are arbitrarily chosen. From this exclusion analysis one can choose promising chromosomal regions for further study, and one can get a sense of the amount of genetic information present from the negative value of the lod score at a given location (assuming there is no linkage). We would not, however, consider any of the locations excluded except under the genetic model used. Of 2339 cM on chromosomes 1, 5p, 6, 8, 10q, 11q, and 12 to 18 covered by these marker loci, 894 cM are excluded and 1445 cM are not excluded, under this exclusion definition of 50% heterogeneity and a 50% penetrance dominant model (**Table 1**). A considerable region of nonexclusion exists on chromosome 18. As described elsewhere,[36] of the 22 families examined for the pericentromeric chromosome 18 region, several pedigrees yielded positive lod scores (>1) in a dominant 50% penetrance analysis, and other families had similar lod scores in a recessive 85% penetrance analysis.

Using the CRI-MAP program[52] a genetic linkage map was constructed in this pedigree series (**Figure**). The map thus generated was in good agreement with a recently published map.[53] We performed the ASP analysis on all the loci on the map, and on some additional loci whose map position was equivocal in this analysis. These additional loci included markers on the q arm (D18S64 and D18S35), which is about 33 cM telomeric to D18S47.

The ASP analyses of linkage to BP illness with these chromosome 18 loci showed increased allele-sharing in the region between S62 and S56, with affection status model II most consistently positive (**Table 2**). Multilocus ASP analysis yielded $P=.0024$ for markers of 18q near the centromere (D18S40-S56; **Table 3**), and $P\leq.00008$ for markers on 18p (D18S62-S40). Multipoint APM[44] re-

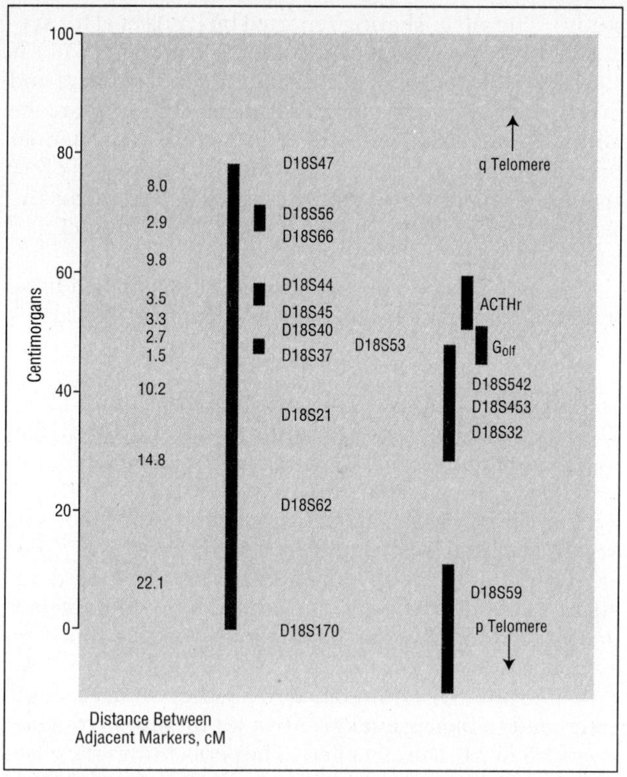

Chromosome 18 linkage map from this pedigree series. For each segment developed in a specific run, loci are added sequentially when a unique placement can be made. Other possible orders are eliminated by the criterion: log_{10} likelihood is 3 U less than the likelihood of the retained locus order. The flips option was then applied to determine whether there are adjacent loci on this map whose order can be reversed without worsening the log_{10} likelihood by 2 U. When this was the case, the ordering was considered ambiguous (indicated by a bar to the left of the loci positions). The region between S62 and S66 includes loci with affected sibling pair values of P<.01. *The 2 candidate genes (G_{olf} and ACTHr [also known as melanocortin-2]) were mapped in this pedigree series.*

sults were also consistent with linkage in this region (theoretical $P<.00001$, Table 3). Inclusion of genotypes for 8 additional affected persons increases evidence for a BP vulnerability gene, compared with previously reported results,[36] with some significance levels increasing by more than 2 orders of magnitude.

COMMENT

In a systematic search for linkage to BP disease, covering about 50% of the genome, lod score methods did not provide evidence for linkage. However, statistical evidence for a vulnerability gene near the centromere of chromosome 18 was suggested by inspection of lod scores under different modes of inheritance.[36] The APM and ASP statistics imply that inheritance of disease depends on inheritance of marker alleles. The updated ASP and APM chromosome 18 results reported here (with genotypes from 8 additional affected persons) disclose increased evidence for linkage compared with previously reported results.[36] The number of additional persons is too small to constitute a test of replication. However, the present extension of the previous article[36] (with new diagnostic and genotypic data) is important in view of reports that a few

Table 2. Affected Sibling Pair Analysis of Chromosome 18 DNA Markers*

	Affection Status Model			
	I		II	
Marker Locus	IBD Value, %	*P*	IBD Value, %	*P*
S59	54	.173	51	.369
S170	53	.28	53	.163
S62	53	.162	57	.002
S21	55	.066	57	.0013
S37	56	.029	56	.0108
S32	61	.0003	62	$<10^{-5}$
S453	53	.162	54	.063
S53	58	.0175	54	.041
S40	57	.051	58	.0046
S45	58	.0089	57	.002
S44	53	.20	55	.029
S66	58	.044	56	.028
S56	60	.0043	57	.0067
S47	53	.163	52	.159
S35	50	.99	51	.296
S64	55	.065	51	.268
S31	52	.288	50	.478
S27	51	.439	49	.99

**Affected sibling pair analysis using all information from 22 bipolar pedigrees.* P *values were adjusted for multiple sibling pairs within sibships by reducing the degrees of freedom in the* t *test to the number of independent comparisons. IBD indicates identical by descent.*

Table 3. Nonparametric Multilocus Analyses of Chromosome 18 DNA Markers*

Affected Pedigree Member Analysis				
Weighting Function	Statistic	*P*	Empirical *P*	Affected Sibling Pair Analysis, *P*
Map S62---.20---S37---.026---S53---.024---S40				
f(p)=1	1.32	.092	...	.00008
f(p)=1/√p	1.68	.046	...	
f(p)=1/p	0.87	.191	...	
Map S40---.03---S45---.035---S44---.086---S66---.033---S56				
f(p)=1	4.48	.000004	<.0001	.0024
f(p)=1/√p	3.68	.00012	.0005	
f(p)=1/p	1.38	.0832	...	

**The numbers between markers in the maps represent genetic distances in morgans. For affected sibling pair analyses, the weighting functions were used to examine the possible effect of misspecifying allele frequencies (p) on the results. The empirical* P *value is the probability of observing a simulated value as large as or larger than the actual statistic by chance, as determined by calculating 10 000 replicates of an unlinked marker on these 22 pedigrees. These results are based on 127 affected individuals (for the multipoint affected pedigree member calculations) and 72 affected sibling pairs (number being reduced by a correction for the number of independent affected pairs) for the affected sibling pair analysis.*

diagnostic changes[22] can have a marked effect on evidence for linkage.[17]

Regardless of the significance level for data suggesting a BP susceptibility gene in the pericentromeric region of chromosome 18, independent confirmation in other pedigrees is required before the evidence can be accepted as valid. Confirmation of our chromsome 18 pericentromeric BP linkage evidence has been published by

Stine et al.[54] These authors studied 28 BP kindreds collected with methods similar to those described herein. They reported data on about 100 ASPs. Their ASP results are similar to ours; at D18S37, their IBD value was 64% ($P \leq .0003$); at D18S53, IBD was 56% ($P = .02$); at D18S40, IBD was 57% ($P = .02$). Stine et al[54] reported that this increased allele-sharing was observed in pedigrees showing paternal transmission of disease alleles for these pericentromeric chromosome 18 markers. When our ASP data are analyzed by the sex of the transmitting parent, only those kindreds in which fathers transmit illness show increased allele-sharing for pericentromeric chromosome 18 markers.[55] Thus, our data confirm those of Stine et al[54] regarding paternal transmission. This observation of positive statistics in *paternal* BP kindreds for 18p markers also has been confirmed by Gilliam et al[56] in an analysis of 5 paternal BP kindreds (lod score of 2.68 at D18S53 in a recessive disease model analysis). From more than 50 BP kindreds, Gilliam et al defined 5 in which only fathers transmitted illness. These 5 BP kindreds provide confirmatory evidence of linkage to 18p markers.

Nothen et al[57] reported a maximum lod score of 2.48 for D18S453 among 61 German BP kindreds using a recessive disease model analysis. Analysis by the sex of the transmitting parent revealed that the positive statistics derived mostly from paternal kindreds, where the lod score at D18S453 was 1.91 under a recessive model. This report also provides confirmatory evidence of BP linkage to 18p markers.

THIS CONFIRMED excess paternal transmission is consistent with parental imprinting of the pericentromeric chromosome 18 BP susceptibility locus. It is strongly recommended that attempts to confirm this pericentromeric chromosome 18 linkage involve analyses of data by sex of the transmitting parent.

Wildenauer et al[58] reported a lod score of 2.56 at D18S53 in a recessive model (by ASP analysis, $P = .0023$) in 59 multiplex German and Israeli schizophrenia pedigrees, in which there were only 2 BP cases. When these data were analyzed by a multipoint IBD statistic, the maximum lod score was 3.2 at D18S53. This report did not provide an analysis of transmission by gender. The data of Wildenauer et al are consistent with the possibility that this region of 18p may contain a gene that increases the risk for psychotic disorders of varying syndromal form. Mostly negative statistics have been reported for these 18p markers among schizophrenia kindreds by DeLisi et al.[59]

Pauls et al[60] described lod score and nonparametric analyses in the Old Order Amish pedigree BP kindreds. They conclude that a major locus for BP illness does not exist among the Old Order Amish pedigree on chromosome 18. This conclusion is congruous with our observations, because a locus of minor effect is most consistent with our data and with those of Stine et al.[54] In view of our estimate that attempts at confimation be based on at least 100 ASPs, it is noteworthy that the ASP data of Pauls et al[60] are based on 12 ASPs (none of which overlap with the Old Order Amish pedigree in the current study). The allele-sharing reported by Pauls et al for several pericentromeric markers (IBD% ranges, 52-71) is similar to the degree of allele-sharing reported here and in Stine et al,[54] but the data of Pauls et al[60] do not reach nominal statistical significance in a consistent manner because the number of pairs is limited. Examples of other reports with very limited power to detect the locus described here include De bruyn et al[61] and Coon et al,[62] each with less than 50 ASPs.

When Suarez et al[63] simulated oligogenic additive inheritance (in which 6 loci independently increased risk for illness), they determined sample sizes necessary to detect linkage initially and then confirmed linkage in a second set of pedigrees. They reported that a much larger sample would be needed to confirm a specific locus than was required for the initial detection. Based on this simulation, it can be expected that some studies with adequate sample sizes will fail to confirm the chromosome 18 observations described here and in Stine et al.[54] For example, Smyth et al[64] and Kelsoe et al[65] studied adequate sample sizes from the United Kingdom, Icelandic, and North American populations, and they found no evidence of linkage.

The putative chromosome 18 susceptibility locus is estimated to increase relative risk for BP illness by a factor of 1.5 to 2.0, a minor effect. The pericentromeric chromosome 18 statistics explain a small fraction of genetic susceptibility for BP illness. Given our estimate that the chromosome 18 linkage might increase relative risk for BP illness by a factor of 1.5 to 2.0, it is essential that attempts to confirm our observations be conducted with data sets of 100 or more ASPs. Smaller data sets may not have sufficient power to detect linkage to a locus of such moderate effect.[63]

Lander and Kruglyak[66] offer criteria for significance and confirmation of linkage in complex inheritance traits. For allele-sharing methods in relative pairs, the significance threshold in a genomic scan (such as the one reported here) is $P \approx 10^{-5}$, and for confirmation at a specific locus it is $P < .01$. Our chromosome 18 results and those of Stine et al[54] seem to meet these significance criteria, with the qualification that multiple analyses have been conducted.

The addition of recurrent UP illness to the spectrum defined as affected did not decrease evidence for a susceptibility gene in the ASP analysis. If recurrent UP illness was not part of the BP spectrum in these families, one would expect that inclusion of this diagnosis in the ASP analysis would reduce evidence for a susceptibility gene, because this would have the effect of introducing phenocopies into the analysis. This locus may increase risk for recurrent UP illness when it occurs within a BP familial context.

Given the evidence for a BP vulnerability gene near these chromosome 18 markers, 2 candidate genes deserve mention. Guanosine triphosphate-binding proteins (G proteins) transduce neurotransmitter receptor activation into second messenger system changes within the cell.[67] G proteins are composed of α, β, and γ subunits. The α subunit binds GTP, possesses GTPase enzyme activity, and confers specificity for receptor and second messenger binding.[67] Lithium decreases the affinity with which the α subunit binds GTP,[68] and antidepressants modulate the expression of G-protein genes in brain.[67] A gene for an α subunit of a G protein[69] has been localized to the 18p11.2 region.[70] Immunocytochemical and northern hybridization experiments suggest that this α subunit, G_{olf}, may be expressed in nasal epithelium and in several regions of mammalian brain, including olfactory tract, bulb and tubercle, nucleus accumbens septi, striatum, and substantia nigra.[71,72] A G-protein subunit gene with expression in brain would be a plausible BP candidate gene.

Much evidence has accumulated to suggest that mood disorders are associated with various abnormalities of the hypothalamic-pituitary-adrenal axis.[73] A gene for an adrenocorticotropic hormone receptor (MC2)[74] has been localized to 18p11.2[75] and genetically mapped[76] to the region of linkage. Mutations in this gene might explain some of the hypothalamic-pituitary-adrenal axis abnormalities seen in patients with severe mood disorders.

The G_{olf} and MC2 genes deserve further study in linkage and association investigations of BP disease. In addition to the G_{olf} gene and the MC2 gene, there must be a large number of unknown genes within the linkage region. Although one of these may function as a susceptibility locus (neither necessary nor sufficient to produce disease), it may be difficult to map precisely such a gene of partial effect using a linkage paradigm in a common disease.[77] Greenberg[77] suggests that association studies may be preferable. Our results and those of Stine et al[54] suggest that BP association studies with the G_{olf} gene and the MC2 gene should be conducted, and other expressed genes in the region should be characterized.

Criteria for linkage exclusion of a nonmendelian disease remain undefined. The optimal strategy of genomic scanning for linkage, under complex inheritance, has been considered in formal analyses only recently.[78,79] In our own data, how much of the genome has been scanned in the present series of pedigrees? This would depend on the functional length of the genome (in centimorgans) and the specific model parameters. As already observed, 38% of 2333 cM scanned here are excluded under the 50% penetrance dominant model, assuming 50% heterogeneity. For a gene with small effect, little of the genome has been examined for linkage with a sufficient number of BP pedigrees and highly informative markers. This BP linkage project, which includes more than 500 loci (more than 100 000 genotypes) in a series of 22 pedigrees, has made a substantial contribution toward localization of susceptibility genes for BP illness.[33-37]

Accepted for publication April 22, 1996.

This study was supported by an Established Investigator Award (Dr Berrettini) and a Young Investigator Award (Dr Ferraro) from the National Alliance for Research on Schizophrenia and Depression, Chicago, Ill, and by grant MH 49181 from the National Institute of Mental Health, Bethesda, Md (Dr Berrettini), and a grant to the Foundation for Advanced Education in the Sciences, Bethesda, by Anita Kaskel Roe.

The laboratory of Ray White, University of Utah, Salt Lake City, provided more than 75 probes, for which we are grateful. We thank Leena Ala-Kokko, James Weber, Joan Overhauser, Conrad Gilliam, Richard Straub, Steve Gerkin, David Callen, and Jean Weissenbach for providing unpublished primer sequences for numerous microsatellites. We thank the following persons for providing probes: Ingrid Caras (DAF), Sandra Gendler (MUC1), Nicholas Dracopoli (D1S9, D1S13, D1S14, D1S15, and FGR), M. Goossens (PBGD), S. K. Karathanasis (APOA1), Clive Dickson and G. Peters (INT-2), N. K. Spurr (STMY and CDC2), E. Dietzsch (D11S29), Brian Kobilka and Robert Lefkowitz (alpha 2 C10), V. Ramesh (HOAT-1), Prof C. H. C. M. Buys (D13S11, D13S12, and D13S22), T. Dryja (RB), W. Cavenee (D13S39 and D13S41), A. E. Bale (D13S31, D13S32, and D13S35), D. Barker (D17S58, D17S40, D17S57, and D17S73), M. V. Chao (NGFR), K. K. Kidd (TK1), John Armour (D18S32, D18S31, D13S70, D8S162, D12S41, D12S42, D14S22, D14S44, D15S86, and D16S309), Gilles Vergnaud (D13S107), Jean-Louis Mandel (D18S3), Uta Francke (SSAV1), Jean-Pierre Julien (NEFL), Eliot Spindel (GRP), Stanley Prusiner (MBP), Ivan Balazs (D18S27 and D14S1), Perrin White (CYP11B1), and Carlo Croce (MYC). We thank the many investigators who made their probes available to us through the American Type Culture Collection. D12S65 was provided by the Japanese Cancer Research Resources Bank.

We gratefully acknowledge the technical assistance of Nina Harris, Chris Ballas, Amy Wagner, David Heydt, Joan Barrick, Teresa Collela, Mia Norlin, and Charles Cappellari. We thank Jessica Vaserman for her assistance in the exclusion mapping analysis, Janice Egeland, PhD, for making the Old Order Amish pedigree samples available to us through the Coriell Institute for Medical Research, where many of these cell lines are stored. The sibling pair results of this article were obtained using the program package SAGE ([1992] Statistical Analysis for Genetic Epidemiology, Release 2.1. Computer program package available from the Department of Biometry and Genetics, Louisiana State University Medical Center, New Orleans), which is supported by US Public Health Service Resource Grant 1 P41 RR03655 from the Division of Research Resources. We thank M. Elizabeth Maxwell, MSW, Anne L. Smith, MSW, Juliet J. Guroff, MSW, Diane M. Kazuba, Joel Hamovit, MSW, Susan Simmons-Alling, MSN, Carolyn York, and Marvin Brown, MD, for clinical assistance in pedigree collection. We thank the families who participated, and the National Alliance for the Mentally Ill for encouraging family participation.

Reprints: Wade H. Berrettini, MD, PhD, Thomas Jefferson University, Department of Psychiatry and Human Behavior, 1025 Walnut St, 312 College, Philadelphia, PA 19107 (e-mail: berrettiniw@jeflin.tju.edu).

REFERENCES

1. Nurnberger JI Jr, Goldin LR, Gershon ES. Genetics of psychiatric disorders. In: Winokur G, Clayton P, eds. *The Medical Basis of Psychiatry.* New York, NY: WB Saunders Co; 1986:486-521.
2. Rice JP, Reich T, Andreasen NC, Endicott J, Van Eerdewegh M, Fisherman R, Hirschfield RMA, Klerman GL. The familial transmission of bipolar illness. *Arch Gen Psychiatry.* 1987;44:441-447.

3. Lander ES, Botstein D. Strategies for studying heterogeneous genetic traits in humans by using a linkage map of restriction fragment length polymorphisms. *Proc Natl Acad Sci U S A.* 1986;83:7353-7357.
4. Risch N. Genetic linkage and complex diseases, with special reference to psychiatric disorders. *Genet Epidemiol.* 1990;7:3-16.
5. Ott J. Cutting the Gordian Knot in linkage analysis of complex human traits. *Am J Hum Genet.* 1990;46:219-221.
6. Martinez MM, Goldin LR. Power of the linkage test for a heterogeneous disorder due to two independent inherited causes. *Genet Epidemiol.* 1990;7:219-230.
7. Palotie A, Veisanen P, Ott J, Ryhanen L, Elima K, Vikkula M, Cheah K, Vuorio E, Peltonen L. Predisposition in familial osteoarthrosis linked to type II collagen gene. *Lancet.* 1989;i:924-927.
8. Knowlton RG, Katzenstein PL, Moskowitz RW, Weaver EJ, Malemud CJ, Pathria N, Jimenez SA, Prockop DJ. Genetic linkage of a polymorphism in the type II procollagen gene (COL2A1) to primary osteoarthritis associated with mild chondrodysplasia. *N Engl J Med.* 1990;322:526-530.
9. Ala-Kokko L, Baldin CT, Moskowitz RW, Prockop DJ. Single base mutation in the type II procollagen gene (COL2A1) as a cause of primary osteoarthritis associated with a mild chondrodysplasia. *Proc Natl Acad Sci U S A.* 1990;87:6565-6568.
10. St George-Hyslop P, Haines J, Rogaev E, Mortilla M, Vaula G, Pericak-Vance M, Foncin J-F, Martin JB, Gusella J. Genetic evidence for a novel familial Alzheimer's disease locus on chromosome 14. *Nat Genet.* 1992;2:330-334.
11. Van Broeckhoven C, Backhovens H, Cruts M, De Winter G, Bruyland M, Cras P, Martin JJ. Mapping of a gene predisposing to early-onset Alzheimer's disease to chromosome 14q24.3. *Nature Genet.* 1992;2:335-339.
12. Schellenberg GD, Bird TD, Wijsman EM, Orr HT, Anderson L, Nemens E, White JA, Bonnycastle L, Weber JL, Alonso ME, Potter H, Heston LL, Martin GM. Genetic evidence for a familial Alzheimer's disease locus on chromosome 14. *Science.* 1992;258:668-671.
13. Easton DF, Bishop DT, Ford D, Crockford GP, the Breast Cancer Linkage Consortium. Genetic linkage analysis in familial breast and ovarian cancer: results from 214 families. *Am J Hum Genet.* 1993;52:678-701.
14. Hall JM, Lee MK, Newman B, Morrow JE, Anderson LE, Huey B, King M-C. Linkage of early-onset familial breast cancer to chromosome 17q21. *Science.* 1990;250:1684-1690.
15. Pakstis AJ, Kidd JR, Dastiglione CM, Kidd KK. Status of the search for a major genetic locus for affective disorder in the Old Order Amish. *Hum Genet.* 1991;87:475-483.
16. Coon H, Jensen S, Hoff M, Holik J, Plaetke R, Reimberr F, Wender P, Leppert P, Byerley W. A genome-wide search for genes predisposing to manic-depression, assuming autosomal dominant inheritance. *Am J Hum Genet.* 1993;53:1234-1249.
17. Egeland JA, Gerhard DS, Pauls DL, Sussex JN, Kidd KK, Allen CR, Hostetter AM, Housman DE. Bipolar affective disorder linked to DNA markers on chromosome 11. *Nature.* 1987;325:783-787.
18. Detera-Wadleigh SD, Berrettini WH, Goldin LR, Boorman D, Anderson S, Gershon ES. Close linkage of c-Harvey-ras-1 and the insulin gene to affective disorder is ruled out in three North American pedigrees. *Nature.* 1987;325:806-808.
19. Hodgkinson S, Sherrington R, Gurling HMD, Marchbanks RM, Reeders S, Mallet J, Petursson H, Brunjolfsson J. Molecular evidence for heterogeneity in manic-depression. *Nature.* 1987;325:805-807.
20. Gill M, McKeon P, Humphries P. Linkage analysis of manic-depression in an Irish family using H-ras 1 and INS DNA markers. *J Med Genet.* 1988;25:634-637.
21. Mitchell P, Waters B, Morrison N, Shine J, Donald J, Eissman J. Close linkage of bipolar disorder to chromosome 11 markers is excluded in two large Australian pedigrees. *J Affect Disord.* 1991;20:23-32.
22. Kelsoe JR, Ginns El, Egeland JA, Gerhard DS, Goldstein AM, Bale SJ, Pauls DL, Long RT, Kidd KK, Conte G, Housman DE, Paul SM. Reevaluation of the linkage relationship between chromosome 11p loci and the gene for bipolar affective disorder in the Old Order Amish. *Nature.* 1989;342:238-243.
23. Winokur G, Clayton PJ, Reich T. *Manic-depressive Illness.* St Louis, Mo: Mosby–Year Book Inc; 1969:112-125.
24. Mendlewicz J, Fleiss JL. Linkage studies with X-chromosome markers in bipolar manic-depressive and unipolar (depressive) illness. *Biol Psychiatry.* 1974;9:261-294.
25. Baron M, Risch N, Hamburger R, Mandel B, Kushner S, Newman M, Drumer D, Belmaker RH. Genetic linkage between X-chromosome markers and bipolar affective illness. *Nature.* 1987;326:289-292.
26. Gershon ES, Targum SD, Matthysse S, Bunney WE Jr. Color blindness not closely linked to bipolar illness. *Arch Gen Psychiatry.* 1979;36:1423-1430.
27. Berrettini WH, Goldin LR, Gelernter J, Gejman PV, Gershon ES, Detera-Wadleigh S. X-chromosome markers and manic-depressive illness: rejection of linkage to Xq28 in nine bipolar pedigrees. *Arch Gen Psychiatry.* 1990;47:336-373.
28. Del Zompo M, Bocchetta A, Ruiu S, Goldin LR, Berrettini WH. Association and linkage studies of affective disorders. In: Racagni G, Brunello N, Fukuda T, eds. *Biological Psychiatry.* New York, NY: Elsevier Science Inc; 1991;2:446-448.
29. Smyth C, Kalsi G, Brynjolfsson J, Petursson H, Curtis D, Rifkin L, Murphy P, Moloney E, O'Neill J, Gurling HMD. A test of the Xq27-q28 linkage in bipolar and unipolar familes selected for absent male-to-male transmission. *Psychiatr Genet.* 1995;5(suppl):84.
30. Baron M, Freimer NF, Risch N, Lerer B, Alexander JR, Straub RE, Asokan S, Das K, Peterson A, Amos J, Endicott J, Ott J, Gilliam C. Diminished support for linkage between manic-depressive illness and X-chromosome markers in three Israeli pedigrees. *Nature Genet.* 1993;3:49-55.
31. Straub R, Gilliam C. Genetic linkage studies of bipolar affective disorder. *Genome Analysis.* 1993;6:77-99.
32. Berrettini WH, Goldin LR, Martinez MM, Maxwell T, Smith AL, Guroff JJ, Kazuba DM, Nurnberger JI Jr, Hamovit J, Simmons-Alling S, Robb AS, Gershon ES. A bipolar pedigree series for genomic mapping of disease genes: diagnostic and analytic considerations. *Psychiatr Genet.* 1991;2:125-160.
33. Detera-Wadleigh SD, Berrettini WH, Goldin LR, Martinez M, Hsieh W-T, Hoehe M, Coffman D, Rollins DY, Muniec D, Choi H, Wiesch D, Guroff J, Gershon ES. A systematic search for a bipolar predisposing locus on chromosome 5. *Neuropsychopharmacology.* 1992;6:219-229.
34. Berrettini WH, Detera-Wadleigh SD, Goldin LR, Martinez M, Hsieh W-T, Hoehe M, Choi H, Muniec D, Ferraro TN, Guroff JJ, Kazuba D, Harris N, Kron E, Nurnberger JI Jr, Alexander RC, Gershon ES. Genomic screening for genes predisposing to bipolar disease. *Psychiatr Genet.* 1991;2:191-208.
35. Gejman PV, Martinez M, Qiuhe C, Friedman E, Berrettini WH, Goldin LR, Koroulakis P, Ames C, Lerman MA, Gershon ES. Linkage analysis of 57 microsatellite loci to bipolar disorder. *Neuropsychopharmacology.* 1993;9:31-49.
36. Berrettini WH, Ferraro TN, Goldin LR, Weeks D, Detera-Wadleigh S, Nurnberger JI Jr, Gershon ES. Pericentromeric chromosome 18 DNA markers and manic-depressive illness: evidence for a susceptibility gene. *Proc Natl Acad Sci U S A.* 1994;91:5918-5921.
37. Detera-Wadleigh SD, Hsieh W-T, Berrettini WH, Goldin LR, Rollins DY, Muniec D, Grewal R, Guroff JJ, Turner G, Coffman D, Barrick J, Mills K, Murray J, Donohue SJ, Klein DC, Sanders J, Nurnberger JI Jr, Gershon ES. Genetic linkage mapping for a susceptibility locus to bipolar illness: chromosomes 2, 3, 4, 7, 9, 10p, 11p, 22, and Xpter. *Am J Med Genet.* 1994;54:206-218.
38. Boehnke M. Estimating the power of a proposed linkage study: a practical computer simulation approach. *Am J Hum Genet.* 1986;39:513-527.
39. Lahiri DK, Nurnberger JI Jr. A rapid nonenzymatic method for the preparation of HMW DNA from blood for RFLP studies. *Nucleic Acids Res.* 1991;19:5444-5449.
40. Weber JL, May PE. Abundant class of human DNA polymorphisms which can be typed using the polymerase chain reaction. *Am J Hum Genet.* 1989;44:388-396.
41. Lander ES. Mapping complex genetic traits in humans. In: Davies KE, ed. *Genome Analysis: A Practical Approach.* Washington, DC: BRL Press; 1988:171-189.
42. Clerget-Darpoux F, Bonaiti-Pellie C, Hochez J. Effects of misspecifying genetic parameters in lod score analysis. *Biometrics.* 1986;42:245-253.
43. Ott J. *Analysis of Human Genetic Linkage.* Baltimore, Md: The Johns Hopkins University Press; 1991:88-93.
44. Weeks DE, Lange K. A multilocus extension of the affected-pedigree-member method of linkage analysis. *Am J Hum Genet.* 1992;50:859-868.
45. Boehnke M. Allele frequency estimation from data on relatives. *Am J Hum Genet.* 1991;48:22-25.
46. Blackwelder WC, Elston RC. A comparison of sib-pair linkage tests for disease susceptibility loci. *Genet Epidemiol.* 1985;2:85-97.
47. Tran LD, Elston RC, Keats BJB, Wilson AF. *Sib-Pal: Sib-Pair Linkage Program: Version 2.5.* New Orleans, La: RC Elston; 1991.
48. Goldgar DE. Multipoint analysis of human quantitative variation. *Am J Hum Genet.* 1990;45:957-967.
49. Goldgar DE, Lewis CU, Gholami K. Analysis of discrete phenotypes using a multipoint identity by descent method: application to Alzheimer's disease. *Genet Epidemiol.* 1993;10:383-388.
50. Goldin LR, Weeks DE. Two-locus models of disease: comparison of likelihood and nonparametric linkage methods. *Am J Hum Genet.* 1993;53:908-915.
51. Ott J. Choice of genetic models for linkage analysis of psychiatric traits. In: Gershon ES, Cloninger CR, eds. *Genetic Approaches to Mental Disorders: Proceedings of the 82nd Annual Meeting of the American Psychopathological Association Inc.* Washington, DC: American Psychiatric Press; 1994:63-76.

52. Lander ES, Green P. Construction of multilocus genetic maps in humans. *Proc Natl Acad Sci U S A.* 1987;84:2363-2367.
53. Overhauser J, Silverman GA, Gerken S, Geurts van Kessel A. Report of the third international workshop on human chromosome 18 mapping. *Cytogenet Cell Genet.* 1995;71:105-119.
54. Stine OC, Xu J, Koskela R, McMahon FJ, Gschwend M, Friddle C, Clark CD, McInnis MG, Simpson SG, Breschel TS, Vishio E, Riskin K, Feilotter H, Chen E, Folstein S, Meyers DA, Botstein D, Marr TG, DePaulo JR. Evidence for linkage of bipolar disorder to chromosome 18 with a parent-of-origin effect. *Am J Hum Genet.* 1995;57:1384-1394.
55. Gershon ES, Badner JA, Ferraro TN, Detera-Wadleigh S, Berrettini WH. Maternal inheritance and chromosome 18 allele sharing in unilineal bipolar illness pedigrees. *Am J Med Genet.* 1996;67:202-207.
56. Gilliam TC, Knowles JA, Baron M. Genome wide search for genes predisposing to bipolar affective disorder. In: *Function and Dysfunction in the Nervous System.* Cold Spring Harbor, NY: Cold Spring Harbor Laboratory Press. In press.
57. Nothen MM, Cichon S, Craddock N, Albus M, Maier W, Lichtermann D, Weigelt B, Franzek E, Rietschel R, Korner J, Fimmers R, Propping R. Linkage studies of bipolar disorder to chromosome 18 markers. *Biol Psychiatry.* 1996;3:615.
58. Wildenauer DB, Hallmayer J, Albus M, Schwab SG, Strauss M, Hoenig S, Borrman M, Lichtermann D, Ackenheil M, Ebstein RE, Trixler M, Lerer B, Maier W. 18p—a susceptibility locus for affective and schizophrenia disorder? *Psychiatr Genet.* 1996;6:152.
59. DeLisi LE, Lofthouse R, Lehner T, Morganti C, Vita A, Shields G, Bass N, Ott J, Crow TJ. Failure to find a chromosome 18 pericentromeric linkage in families with schizophrenia. *Neuropsychiar Genet.* In press.
60. Pauls DL, Ott J, Paul SM, Allen CR, Fann CSJ, Carulli JP, Falls KM, Bouthillier CA, Gravius TC, Keith TP, Egeland JA. Ginns El. Linkage analyses of chromosome 18 markers do not identify a major susceptibility locus for bipolar affective disorder in the Old Order Amish. *Am J Hum Genet.* 1995; 57:636-643.
61. De bruyn A, Souery D, Mendelbaum K, Mendlewicz J, Van Broekhoven C. Linkage analysis of families with bipolar illness and chromosome 18 markers. *Biol Psychiatry.* 1996;39:679-688.
62. Coon H, Hoff M, Holik J, Hadley D, Fang N,Reimherr F, Wender P, Leppert M, Byerly W. Analysis of chromosome 18 DNA markers in multiplex pedigrees with manic depression. *Biol Psychiatry.* 1996;39:689-696.
63. Suarez BK, Hampe CL, VanEerdewegh PV. Problems of replicating linkage claims in psychiatry. In: Gershon ES, Cloninger CR, eds. *Genetic Approaches to Mental Disorders.* Washington, DC: American Psychiatric Press; 1994:23-46.
64. Smyth C, Kalsi G, Brynjolfsson J, Sherrington RS, O'Neill J, Curtis D, Rifkin L, Murphy P, Petursson H, Gurling HMD. Linkage analysis of manic depression (bipolar affective disorder) in Icelandic and British kindreds using markers on the short arm of chromosome 18. *Psychiatr Genet.* 1995;5(suppl):19. Abstract.
65. Kelsoe JR, Sadovick AD, Kristbjarnarson H, Bergesch P, Mroczkowski-Parker Z, Flodman P, Rapaport MH, Mirow AL, Egeland JA, Spence MA, Remick RA. Genetic linkage studies of bipolar disorder and chromosome 18 markers in North American, Icelandic, and Amish pedigrees. *Psychiatr Genet.* 1995;5: S17.
66. Lander ES, Kruglyak L. Genetic dissection of complex traits: guidelines for interpreting and reporting linkage results, *Nature Genet.* 1995;11:241-247.
67. Lesch K-P, Manji HK. Signal-transducing G proteins and antidepressant drugs: evidence for modulation of subunit gene expression in rat brain. *Biol Psychiatry.* 1992;32:549-579.
68. Avissar S, Schrieiber G. The involvement of guanine nucleotide binding proteins in the pathogenesis and treatment of affective disorders. *Biol Psychiatry.* 1992;31:435-459.
69. Jones DT, Reed RR. G_{olf}: an olfactory neuron-specific G protein involved in odorant signal transduction. *Science.* 1989;244:790-793.
70. Overhauser J, Mewar R, Rojas K, Lia K, Kline AD, Silverman GA. STS map of genes and anonymous DNA fragments on human chromosome 18 using a panel of somatic cell hybrids. *Genomics.* 1993;15:387-392.
71. Herve D, Levi-Strauss M, Marey-Semper I, Verney C, Tassin J-P, Glowinski J, Girault J-A. G_{olf} and G_s in rat basal ganglia: possible involvement of G_{olf} in the coupling of dopamine D1 receptor with adenyl cylase. *J Neurosci.* 1993;13: 2237-2244.
72. Zigman JM, Westermark GT, LaMendola J, Boel E, Steiner DF. Human G_{olf}: cDNA structure and expression in pancreatic islets and other tissues outside the olfactory neuroepithelium and central nervous system. *Endocrinology.* 1993; 133:2508-2512.
73. Stokes PE, Sikes CR. Hypothalamic-pituitary-adrenal axis in affective disorders. In: Meltzer HY, ed. *Psyhcopharmaoclogy: The Third Generation of Progress.* New York, NY: Raven Press; 1987:589-607.
74. Mountjoy KG, Robbins LS, Mortrud MT, Cone RD. The cloning of a family of genes that encode the melanocortin receptors. *Science.* 1992;257: 48-51.
75. Gantz I, Tashiro T, Barcroft C, Konda Y, Shimoto Y, Miwa H, Glover T, Munzert G, Yamada T. Localiztions of the genes encoding the melanocortin-2 (adrenocorticotropin hormone) and melanocortin-3 receptors to chromosomes 18p11.2 and 20q13.2-q13.3 by fluorescence in situ hybridization. *Genomics.* 1993;18:166-167.
76. Detera-Wadleigh S, Yoon SW, Berrettini WH, Goldin LR, Turner G, Yoshikawa T, Rollins DY, Muniec D, Nurnberger JI Jr, Gershon ES. Adrenocorticotropin receptor/melanocortin receptor 2 map within a reported susceptibility region for bipolar illness on chromosome 18. *Am J Med Genet.* 1994;55:1-8.
77. Greenberg DA. Linkage analysis of 'necessary' disease loci versus 'susceptibility' loci. *Am J Hum Genet.* 1993;32:135-143.
78. Elston RC. Hoch Award Lecture. *P* values, power, and pitfalls in the linkage analysis of psychiatric disorders. In: Gershon ES, Cloninger CR. eds. *Genetic Approaches to Mental Disorders: Proceedings of the 82nd Annual Meeting of the American Psychopathological Association Inc.* Washington, DC: American Psychiatric Press; 1994:3-22.
79. Brown DL, Gorin MB, Weeks DE. Efficient strategies for genomic searching using the affected-pedigree-member method of linkage analysis. *Am J Hum Genet.* 1993;54:544-552.

ORIGINAL ARTICLE

Depression During Mania

Treatment Response to Lithium or Divalproex

Alan C. Swann, MD; Charles L. Bowden, MD; David Morris, PhD; Joseph R. Calabrese, MD; Frederick Petty, MD, PhD; Joyce Small, MD; Steven C. Dilsaver, MD; John M. Davis, MD

Background: Little information exists from controlled studies about clinical characteristics that predict treatment response in mania. The presence of depressive symptoms during manic episodes may be associated with poor response to psychopharmacological treatments. This is an investigation of the relation between depressive symptoms and treatment response in acute manic episodes.

Methods and Design: In a parallel-group, double-blind study, 179 patients hospitalized for acute manic episodes were randomized to receive divalproex sodium, lithium carbonate, or placebo (ratio, 2:1:2). The study was carried out at 9 academic medical centers. Patients had comprehensive evaluations of behavior and symptoms before and during 3 weeks of treatment. The primary outcome measure, change in mania factor scores derived from the Schedule for Affective Disorders and Schizophrenia: Change Version, was compared in patients with and without depressive symptoms at baseline according to nurse- or physician-rated scales.

Results: Depressive symptoms were associated with poor antimanic response to lithium and with better response to divalproex. This was not due to differences in overall severity of illness, substance abuse, gender, age, or history.

Conclusions: These data suggest that even a modest level of pretreatment depression-related symptoms is a robust predictor of lithium nonresponse, and is associated with better response to divalproex. Although their overall efficacy in acute mania is similar, lithium and divalproex may be most effective in clinically and biologically distinct groups of patients.

Arch Gen Psychiatry. 1997;54:37-42

From the Department of Psychiatry, University of Texas Medical School at Houston (Drs Swann and Dilsaver); the Department of Psychiatry, University of Texas Health Science Center at San Antonio (Dr Bowden); Abbott Laboratories Inc, North Chicago, Ill (Dr Morris); the Department of Psychiatry, Case Western Reserve University, Cleveland, Ohio (Dr Calabrese); the Department of Psychiatry, University of Texas Southwestern Medical School at Dallas (Dr Petty); the Department of Psychiatry, University of Indiana School of Medicine, Indianapolis (Dr Small); and the Department of Psychiatry, University of Illinois at Chicago (Dr Davis).

THE RATIONAL treatment of manic episodes requires the identification of characteristics that influence response to specific agents. Little information directly compares predictors of the antimanic efficacy of lithium with that of other drugs. Outcome studies generally have compared only overall treatment response. A limited literature exists, however, on predictors of poor response to lithium itself. The strongest predictors of nonresponse to lithium seem to be a mixed or depressive-manic state,[1,2] rapid cycling,[3,4] mania complicated by other psychiatric or medical disorders,[5] severe or psychotic manic episodes,[2] and a sequence of depression followed by mania.[6] Of these, a mixed state, with concomitant manic and depressive syndromes, seems to be the most robust predictor of poor response to lithium.

Illness states that combine depressive and manic features are a clinical challenge. These constitute about 40% of manic episodes[7] and often are severe, associated with notable behavioral problems, and difficult to treat.[7-10] Because of the apparent poor response to lithium treatment in patients with combined mania and depression,[2] it is important to determine whether any other treatment modalities are more effective. Data from small or uncontrolled studies suggest that anticonvulsants may be useful in combined depression and mania.[11,12] The small sizes and uncontrolled nature of studies in which depression during mania was included as a variable limit the confidence with which it can be considered a general predictor of lithium nonresponse.[7] Information from controlled trials comparing treatment response with different agents in persons experiencing manic episodes with concomitant depression could prove valuable. We know of only 1 such report, in which se-

See Patients and Methods on next page

PATIENTS AND METHODS

We have described the protocol, including patients, evaluations, and treatment, in detail.[13] Herein we give the salient features.

PATIENTS

Hospitalized patients with acute manic episodes were invited to participate in the study. All participants gave informed consent before any study procedures were begun. Patients were required to meet Research Diagnostic Criteria for primary mania, based on the Schedule for Affective Disorders and Schizophrenia (SADS).[14,15] Information about previous course of illness, substance abuse, family history, and demographics was obtained using all available sources, including family members and medical records. Exclusion criteria included meeting *Diagnostic and Statistical Manual of Mental Disorders, Revised Third Edition* criteria for substance abuse within the 3 previous months, concurrent medical or psychiatric illnesses or treatments that could interfere with the efficacy with the study treatments or with the interpretation of treatment response, and previous treatment with valproate.

EVALUATIONS

Pretreatment evaluations included the SADS, demographic and treatment history, and a comprehensive medical, psychiatric, and neurologic evaluation. Patients and available relatives were interviewed and other sources of information were reviewed to obtain information about history and treatment. During and before treatment, patients periodically had evaluations, including the SADS: Change Version (SADS-C),[16] Affective Disorder Rating Scale (ADRS),[17] plasma drug levels, and evaluations of side effects. The primary efficacy measure was the SADS-C, which includes an 11-item mania factor, the Mania Rating Scale. The Mania Rating Scale comprises the 5-item Mania Syndrome Scale (affective symptoms considered specific for mania, including elevated mood and grandiosity) and a 6-item Behavior and Ideation Scale (including hostility, lack of insight, and similar items not as specific to mania but integral to manic episodes).

TREATMENT PROTOCOL

Subjects were randomized to divalproex, lithium, or placebo groups at a ratio of 2:1:2 and were treated in a double-blind manner. An unblinded investigator not involved in the patients' care or evaluation received information about drug levels and instructed treating physicians on dose changes. Treatment lasted for 3 weeks unless subjects met predetermined criteria for recovery or treatment nonresponse, or unless they or their clinicians decided on withdrawal from the study. Measures to protect patients, including rescue medication and early termination of the study, are described in detail.[13] Analyses reported herein are based on change between the baseline and final study evaluations.

STATISTICAL ANALYSIS

Statistical significance is based on 2-tailed $P<.05$. Analyses were performed using SAS (SAS Institute Inc, Cary, NC), for 3 definitions of classic and depressive mania. Pretreatment differences between patients with depressive and classic mania were analyzed using the Fisher exact test for dichotomous variables, analysis of variance (ANOVA) for age,

verity of depressed mood before treatment seemed to predict good response to valproate sodium and poor response to lithium carbonate.[12]

We have recently completed a large placebo-controlled study comparing lithium and divalproex sodium in 179 patients in acute manic episodes. Overall response to lithium and divalproex was similar.[13] The patients' pretreatment evaluations included comprehensive diagnostic and symptom scales that make it possible to assess the presence and severity of depressed mood and of syndromal depression as well as mania. We report herein the effect of depressed mood and related symptoms on response to lithium, divalproex, and placebo in acute mania.

RESULTS

Figure 1 shows the change from baseline in the mania syndrome scale of the SADS-C. The presence of depressive symptoms affected response to lithium or divalproex differently. Patients meeting the SADS-C criteria had similar response to divalproex, regardless of depressive symptoms. Response to lithium, however, was similar to placebo in patients with depressive mania but was robust in classic mania. A significant interaction was observed between effects of treatment drug and depressive presentation on response. For the narrower SADS-C/DM definition, results were similar, although response to divalproex seemed better in depressive-manic episodes.

Figure 2 shows that results were similar for the Behavior-Ideation Scale. The Behavior-Ideation Scale describes aspects of thought and behavior not specific to mania but prominent during manic episodes.

For the Mania Rating Scale, shown in **Figure 3**, the differences between lithium response in depressive and classic episodes and the interaction between treatment drug response and episode presentation were highly significant using the SADS-C criteria. With the narrower SADS-C/DM definition, a significant interaction again was observed between drug response and depressive presentation. Because the results using the ADRS plus SADS-C criteria were essentially identical to those with SADS-C criteria alone, we compared the narrowest (SADS-C including depressed mood) and broadest (SADS-C criteria without requirement for depressed mood) criteria.

A depressive presentation was associated with a poorer response to lithium, with less improvement (or even slight deterioration) in all 3 scales compared with classic mania. Depressive symptoms had no significant effect on response to divalproex, although with the more stringent criteria, a trend was observed toward more im-

and the Kruskal-Wallis test for Global Assessment Scale and symptom severity scores. Changes from baseline to final evaluation for the manic rating, manic syndrome, and behavior-ideation scores were analyzed using 2-way ANOVA. For each study drug comparison, the ANOVA included factors for the study drugs, mania subtype (classic vs depressive), and drug by subtype interaction.

DEFINITION OF MIXED OR DEPRESSIVE-MANIC STATE

Our objective was to determine the specificity of depressive symptoms as a predictor of response. Therefore, we sought criteria to determine the minimal level of depressive symptoms that would be associated with a change in treatment response. We compared 3 definitions of classic and depressive mania that varied in stringency:

1. SADS-C. Depressive mania was defined as the presence of at least 2 items of the SADS-C depression subscale (depressed mood, worry, self-reproach, negative evaluation of self, discouragement, suicidal tendencies, loss of interest, fatigue, or social withdrawal). Patients not meeting these criteria were classified as having classic mania. Each of the 9 items was scored from 0 (absent) to 5; a score of 2 or more indicates that the symptom was present.
2. SADS-C/DM. Depressive mania required a score of 1 or more on the SADS-C depressive mood item, and on at least 1 additional item from the depression subscale. These patients were the subset of those meeting the SADS-C criteria in which 1 of the positive items was depressed mood.
3. SADS-C/ADRS. Depressive mania was defined as a score of more than 2 on the ADRS (scored 0 if absent) plus a score of 2 or more on the SADS-C depression subscale.

Definitions 1 and 2 measure increasing severity of syndromal depression as rated with the SADS-C by a trained clinician. Definition 3 is a combined measurement of syndromal depression and ADRS rating of dysphoric mood. The ADRS rating is based on observation by a trained nurse of behavior during a work shift and has been shown to be a sensitive measure of depression and anxiety in patients with manic episodes.[18,19] Patients meeting definitions 2 and 3 are subsets of those meeting definition 1. Because the specific focus of this study is the role of depressive symptoms rather than of a specific but variously defined type of manic episode (such as "mixed" or "dysphoric"), we will use the term *depressive mania* for manic episodes that also had depressive symptoms.

CHARACTERISTICS OF PATIENTS IN DEPRESSIVE AND CLASSIC MANIC EPISODES

The data in **Table 1** describe patients meeting the 3 definitions for depressive-manic episodes. The SADS-C criteria, including depressed mood, were the most exclusive, with about 38% of patients classified as having depressive-manic episodes. The SADS-C criteria without requirement for depressed mood (58%), or with the additional requirement of an ADRS depression score of at least 3 (53%), were broader. Age, gender distribution, incidence of substance abuse, baseline Global Assessment Scale score, psychosis, and hallucinations did not differ between patients with depressive and classic episodes for any of the definitions. For the SADS-C and SADS-C/ADRS definitions, patients with depressive mania had significantly fewer severe delusions than did those with classic mania. The same tendency, although not reaching significance, was also present in patients with the SADS-C/DM definition.

provement in behavior-ideation and mania rating scores in depressive than in classic mania. Consistently, a significant interaction was seen between clinical presentation and treatment drug response. Subjects experiencing depressive mania had better response to divalproex than to lithium, but the reverse was true for classic mania.

Table 2 gives changes from baseline to final evaluation in patients with classic and depressive mania randomized to placebo. Change during placebo administration was similar in patients with and without depressive mania.

Table 3 gives the percentage of patients receiving each treatment who left the study before 21 days of treatment, including patients removed from the study due to lack of response.[13] The rate of dropouts due to lack of response was, as one would expect, parallel to lack of efficacy in rating scale change. Dropout rates due to intolerance were higher for lithium and were unrelated to treatment response.

That patients with classic and depressive mania were similar with respect to the demographic and illness-course characteristics given in Table 1 suggests that these characteristics did not contribute to the differential treatment response in these patients. This was confirmed by multiple regression analysis, in which treatment drug group (comparing lithium with divalproex), gender, substance abuse history, presence of psychosis, and number of previous episodes of affective illness did not contribute significantly to change in the Mania Rating Scale scores.

COMMENT

Depressive symptoms during manic episodes had contrasting effects on response to lithium and divalproex. Manic patients with depressive symptoms responded poorly to lithium; those without depressive symptoms responded well. Depressive symptoms did not significantly alter response to divalproex. Stringent criteria for mixed states were not necessary to predict poor lithium response: the presence of any 2 depressive symptoms was associated with poor response to lithium. The difference in response was not attributable to effects of substance abuse, severity of mania, or characteristics of previous episodes, because these did not differ between classic and depressive mania.

Previous studies of predictors of treatment response in manic episodes have had limitations, including small numbers of subjects, lack of control groups, and unsystematic criteria for response. Reports that lithium was ineffective in patients with mania and concomitant

Table 1. Characteristics of Patients With Depressive and Classic Mania*

Characteristic	Type of Mania	SADS-C	SADS-C/DM	SADS-C/ADRS
No. of women	Classic	75 (29)	110 (42)	83 (33)
	Depressive	103 (45)	68 (32)	95 (41)
Age, y	Classic	40.7±11.6	39.5±11.6	39.9±11.7
	Depressive	37.9±10.7	38.3±10.4	38.3±10.6
Substance abuse	Classic	19 (26)	27 (25)	21 (26)
	Depressive	30 (30)	22 (33)	28 (30)
Psychosis	Classic	9 (12)	17 (16)	12 (15)
	Depressive	21 (22)	13 (20)	18 (20)
Hallucinations	Classic	11 (15)	19 (18)	14 (17)
	Depressive	26 (27)	18 (28)	23 (26)
Delusion score	Classic	3.10±1.77	2.95±1.71	3.06±1.76
	Depressive	2.57±1.59†	2.53±1.61	2.55±1.59‡
GAS score	Classic	36.5±11.1	36.4±10.8	36.4±11.1
	Depressive	36.9±9.6	37.4±9.3	37.1±9.5

Values are given as mean (±SD) and number (percentage) of subjects. SADS-C indicates Schedule for Affective Disorders and Schizophrenia: Change Version; SADS-C/DM, patients meeting SADS-C criteria where 1 of the positive items was depressed mood; SADS-C/ADRS, a score greater than 2 on the Affective Disorder Rating Scale plus a score of 2 or greater on SADS-C; and GAS, Global Assessment Scale.

†*Kruskal-Wallis* $\chi^2=4.14$, df=1, $P<.05$.

‡*Kruskal-Wallis* $\chi^2=3.87$, df=1, $P<.05$.

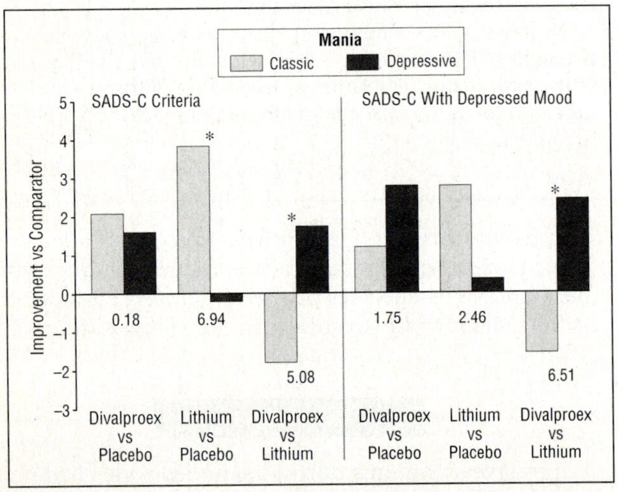

Figure 1. *Depressive symptoms and treatment response, Manic Syndrome Scale. The vertical axis shows change in rating scores; positive values indicate that the test drug was better than the comparator. Test drug is shown first and comparator second. The number near each bar is the F ratio for treatment×presentation interaction, with 1,135* df *for divalproex vs placebo, 1,103* df *for lithium vs placebo, and 1,98* df *for lithium vs divalproex. SADS-C indicates Schedule for Affective Disorders and Schizophrenia: Change Version; DVP, divalproex; PBO, placebo; and Li, lithium. Significant treatment×presentation interaction by analysis of variance; asterisk indicates* $P<.05$.

depression therefore have not been able to distinguish the role of a combined depressive and manic state from severity of mania, psychosis,[2,9] substance abuse,[20] or gender[2,21] on treatment response. Cohen et al[8] reported that poor response to lithium among patients with combined depression and mania was not attributable to severity of mania. Swann et al,[18] using multiple regression

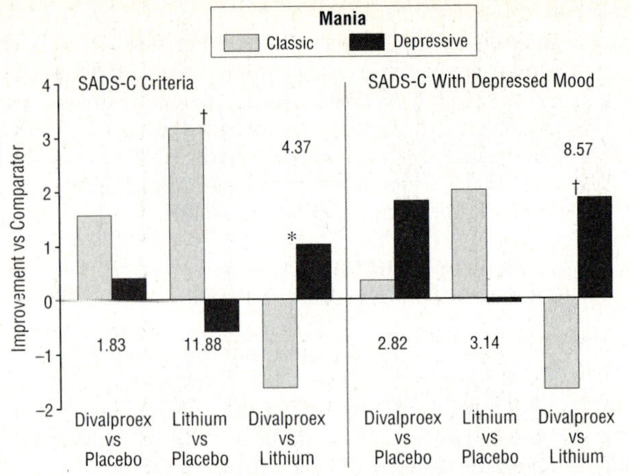

Figure 2. *Depressive symptoms and treatment response, Behavior-Ideation Scale. Explanations of data and abbreviations are given in the legend for Figure 1. Depressive and classic presentations are different by analysis of variance; asterisk indicates* $P<.005$.

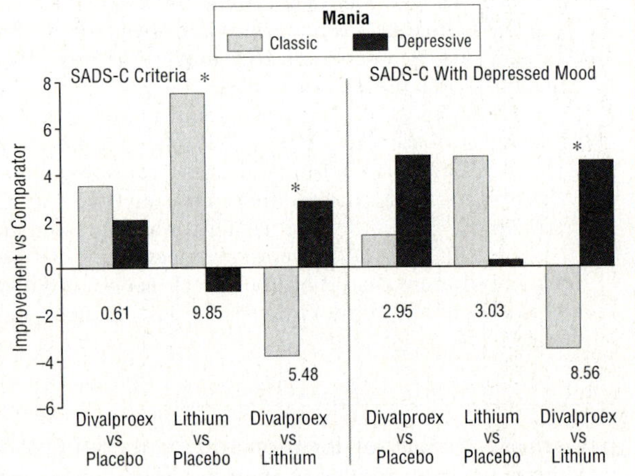

Figure 3. *Depressive symptoms and treatment response, Mania Rating Scale. Explanations of data and abbreviations are given in the legend for Figure 1. Depressive and classic presentations are different by analysis of variance; asterisk indicates* $P<.005$.

analysis, found that overall severity made a much smaller contribution to lithium nonresponse than did having combined depressive and manic syndromes.

Few controlled studies have been done of treatments other than lithium in patients with concomitant depressive and manic states. Thus it has been unclear whether the relative ineffectiveness of pharmacological agents in these patients' states was general or was specific to lithium. Post et al[10] reported that responders to carbamazepine in a crossover study of 17 patients had a trend ($P=.10$) toward higher "dysphoria" ratings than did nonresponders. Freeman et al,[12] in a double-blind comparison of lithium and valproate in 27 patients, found that patients whose mania improved during valproate treatment had higher pretreatment depression scores than did nonresponders, but the sample was too small to provide adequate power for a comparison of lithium and valproate response, and there was no placebo group. Electroconvulsive therapy may be a more effective antimanic

Table 2. Placebo Response in Classic and Depressive Mania*

Scale	Criteria: SADS-C	SADS-C/DM	SADS-C/ADRS
Mania Syndrome Scale			
Classic	1.94±6.28 (31)	3.09±7.14 (45)	2.36±6.32 (33)
Depressive	2.73±7.01 (41)	1.19±5.71 (27)	2.38±7.03 (39)
Behavior-Ideation Scale			
Classic	0.42±3.79 (31)	1.22±5.10 (45)	0.06±3.94 (33)
Depressive	2.61±5.23 (41)	1.44±4.57 (27)	2.46±5.33 (39)
Mania Rating Scale			
Classic	1.87±9.70 (31)	4.91±12.17 (45)	2.70±9.96 (33)
Depressive	5.82±12.1 (41)	2.81±9.62 (27)	5.33±12.2 (39)

**Values are given as mean±SD improvement in rating scores between baseline and the final treatment evaluation. The number of subjects is given in parentheses. Abbreviations are given in the footnote to Table 1.*

Table 3. Dropout Rates for Patients With Depressive and Classic Mania*

	Criteria			
	SADS-C		SADS-C/DM	
Treatment	Classic	Depressive	Classic	Depressive
Placebo				
Lack of effect	56	46	50	52
Intolerance	3	2	2	4
Other	6	7	7	7
Divalproex				
Lack of effect	40	26	40	15
Intolerance	0	9	2	12
Other	8	5	7	4
Lithium				
Lack of effect	24	42	29	40
Intolerance	18	11	14	13
Other	6	11	5	13
χ^2, homogeneity of odds ratio, divalproex vs lithium (*df*=1)				
Lack of effect	2.85, *P*=.09		3.84, *P*=.05	
Intolerance	2.82, *P*=.09		1.38, *P*=.24	

**Unless otherwise noted numbers are the percentage of patients who left the study before completion. Abbreviations are given in the footnote to Table 1.*

treatment than lithium when depression also is present.[22] The available data suggest that the presence of depression during mania does not predict nonresponse to carbamazepine or valproate to the degree that it does for lithium.

The effect of a depressive presentation on response to divalproex seemed to differ among criteria. Using the more inclusive SADS-C criteria, presence of a depressive-manic state had no significant effect on response to divalproex. Using the narrower criteria of SADS-C, including depressed mood, divalproex was possibly more efficacious in depressive than in classic manic episodes ($P=.08$ for behavior-ideation score and $P=.09$ for Mania Rating Scale). This is consistent with the report by Freeman et al[12] that valproate responders had higher pretreatment SADS depression factor scores than did nonresponders.

Acute mania responds similarly, overall, to lithium and to divalproex.[13] The results of our study suggest, however, that patients responding to the 2 agents have different clinical characteristics. This differential drug treatment response implies that lithium and divalproex have distinct mechanisms of action as antimanic agents, and that manic episodes are biologically heterogeneous.[23] Determination of the behavioral and biological specificities of that heterogeneity, and their relation to the mechanisms of action of pharmacological agents, could aid in the development of rational treatment strategies for acute episodes of mania.

In summary, these data suggest that (1) the presence of depressive symptoms is associated with lack of response to lithium but has little effect on response to divalproex, (2) lithium is substantially more effective in classic than in depressive mania, with even minimal depression-related symptoms associated with poor response to lithium, (3) response to divalproex does not differ between classic and depressive mania, although more pervasive depressive features may be associated with better response to divalproex, (4) minimal depressive features predict better response to divalproex than to lithium, and (5) lithium resistance in depressive mania seems to be unrelated to gender, age, substance abuse, or overall severity of illness.

Accepted for publication March 26, 1996.

This study was upported in part by Abbott Laboratories Inc, North Chicago, Ill.

Reprints: Alan C. Swann, MD, 1300 Moursund Ave, Room 270, Houston, TX 77030.

REFERENCES

1. Prien RF, Himmelhoch JM, Kupfer DJ. Treatment of mixed mania. *J Affect Disord.* 1988;15:9-15.
2. Secunda S, Katz MM, Swann AC, Koslow SH, Maas JW, Chang S, Croughan J. Mania: diagnosis, state measurement, and prediction of treatment response. *J Affect Disord.* 1985;8:113-121.
3. Kishimoto A, Ogura C, Hazama H, Inoue K. Long-term prophylactic effects of carbamazepine in affective disorder. *Br J Psychiatry.* 1983;143:327-331.
4. Kukopoulos A, Caliari B, Tondo A. Rapid cyclers, temperament, and antidepressants. *Compr Psychiatry.* 1983;24:249-258.
5. Black DW, Winokur G, Hulbert J, Nasrallah A. Predictors of immediate response in the treatment of mania: the importance of comorbidity. *Biol Psychiatry.* 1988;24:191-198.

6. Faedda GL, Baldessarini RJ, Tohen M, Strakowski SM, Waternaux C. Episode sequence in bipolar disorder and response to lithium treatment. *Am J Psychiatry.* 1991;148:1237-1239.
7. McElroy SL, Keck PE, Pope HG Jr, Hudson JI, Faedda GL, Swann AC. Clinical and research implications of the diagnosis of dysphoric or mixed mania or hypomania. *Am J Psychiatry.* 1992;149:1633-1644.
8. Cohen S, Khan A, Cox G. Demographic and clinical features predictive of recovery in acute mania. *J Nerv Ment Dis.* 1989;177:638-642.
9. Dilsaver SC, Swann AC, Shoaib AM, Bowers TC, Halle MT. Mixed mania associated with nonresponse to antimanic agents. *Am J Psychiatry.* 1993;150: 1548-1551.
10. Post RM, Uhde TW, Roy Byrne PP, Joffe RT. Correlates of antimanic response to carbamazepine. *Psychiatry Res.* 1987;21:71-83.
11. Calabrese JR, Woysheville MJ, Kasimond SE, Rapport DJ. Predictors of valproate response in bipolar rapid cycling. *J Clin Psychopharmacol.* 1993;13: 280-283.
12. Freeman TW, Clothier JL, Pazzaglia P, Lesem MD, Swann AC. A double-blind comparison of valproate and lithium in the treatment of acute mania. *Am J Psychiatry.* 1992;149:108-111.
13. Bowden CL, Brugger AM, Swann AC, Calabrese JR, Janicak PG, Petty F, Dilsaver SC, Davis JM, Rush AJ, Small JG, Garza Trevino ES, Risch SC, Goodnick PJ, Morris DD. Efficacy of divalproex vs lithium and placebo in the treatment of mania. *JAMA.* 1994;271:918-924.
14. Spitzer RL, Endicott J. *Schedule for Affective Disorders and Schizophrenia.* 3rd ed. New York, NY: New York State Psychiatric Institute Biometrics Institute; 1978.
15. Spitzer RL, Endicott J, Robins E. *Research Diagnostic Criteria for a Selected Group of Functional Disorders.* 3rd ed. New York, NY: New York State Psychiatric Institute Biometrics Institute; 1978.
16. Spitzer RL, Endicott J. *Schedule for Affective Disorders and Schizophrenia: Change Version.* 3rd ed. New York, NY: Biometrics Research, New York State Psychiatric Institute; 1978.
17. Murphy DL, Pickar D, Alterman I. Methods for the quantitative assessment of depressive and manic behavior. In: Burdoch EI, Sudilovsky A, Gershon S, eds. *Quantitative Techniques for the Evaluation of the Behavior of Psychiatric Patients.* New York, NY: Marcel Dekker Inc; 1982:355-393.
18. Swann AC, Secunda SK, Katz MM, Koslow SH, Maas JW, Chang S, Robins E. Lithium treatment of mania: clinical characteristics, specificity of symptom change, and outcome. *Psychiatry Res.* 1986;18:127-141.
19. Swann AC, Secunda SK, Katz MM, Croughan J, Bowden CL, Koslow SH, Berman N, Stokes PE. Specificity of mixed affective states: clinical comparison of mixed mania and agitated depression. *J Affect Disord.* 1993;28:81-89.
20. Himmelhoch JM, Garfinkel ME. Sources of lithium resistance in mixed mania. *Psychopharmacol Bull.* 1986;22:613-620.
21. Nunn CMH. Mixed affective states and the natural history of manic-depressive psychosis. *Br J Psychiatry.* 1979;134:153-160.
22. Small JG, Klapper MH, Kellams JJ, Miller MJ, Milstein V, Sharpley PH, Small IF. ECT compared with lithium in the management of manic states. *Arch Gen Psychiatry.* 1988;45:727-732.
23. Swann AC, Stokes PE, Casper R, Secunda SK, Bowden CL, Berman N, Katz MM, Robins E. Hypothalamic-pituitary-adrenocortical function in mixed and pure mania. *Acta Psychiatr Scand.* 1992;85:270-274.

Notice to Authors

Both our readers and reviewers prefer shorter papers. Effective immediately, the text of manuscripts submitted to the ARCHIVES, not counting the "Abstract," "Tables," and "References" must not exceed 5000 words, and ideally should be less than 4000 words. Title length must not exceed 120 characters.

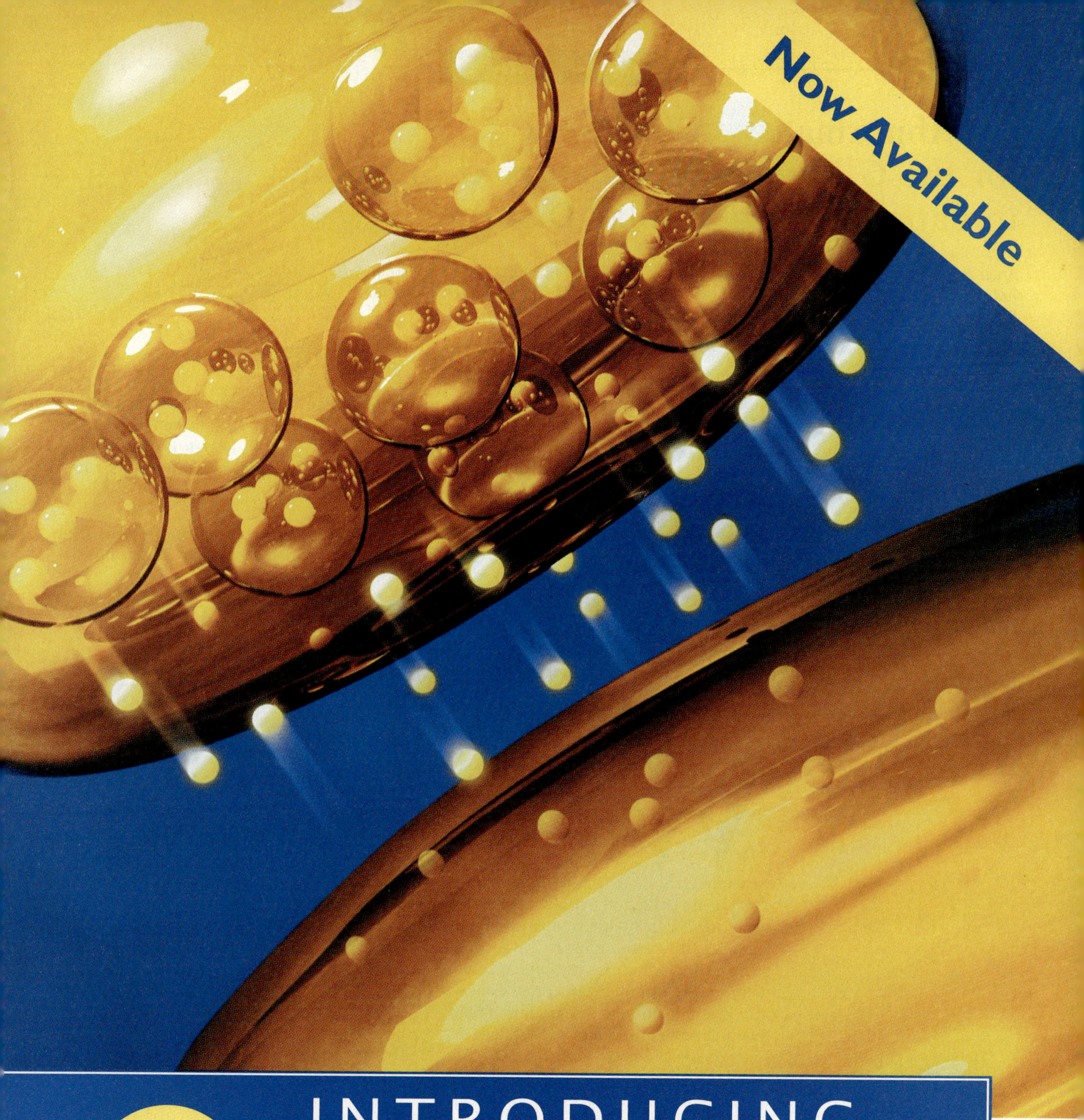

INTRODUCING

New Wellbutrin® SR

(bupropion HCl) SUSTAINED-RELEASE TABLETS 100mg/150mg

GlaxoWellcome

 Printed in USA. WEL253R0 December 1996

ORIGINAL ARTICLE

No Abnormality in the Gene for the G Protein Stimulatory α Subunit in Patients With Bipolar Disorder

Anca Ram, MD; Françoise Guedj, MD; Anibal Cravchik, MD, PhD; Lee Weinstein, MD; Qiuhe Cao, MD; Judith A. Badner, MD, PhD; Lynn R. Goldin, PhD; Nimrod Grisaru, MD; Husseini K. Manji, MD; Robert H. Belmaker, MD; Elliot S. Gershon, MD; Pablo V. Gejman, MD

Background: The available evidence for an involvement of the heterotrimeric guanine-nucleotide-binding proteins (G proteins) in bipolar disorder relies primarily on the effects of lithium salts on G protein function and on alterations in the concentration or function of G proteins (most notably G_s-α) in peripheral leukocytes and in postmortem tissues of patients with bipolar disorder.

Methods: The hypothesis that a mutation in G_s-α gene confers an increased susceptibility to bipolar disorder was tested by the following strategies: (1) mutational screening of the G_s-α subunit gene coding sequences and promoter sequences by denaturing gradient gel electrophoresis in unrelated individuals with bipolar disorder and (2) association and linkage analyses with a common silent exonic polymorphism, using genetic allelic information from American families with at least 1 affected child. For association analysis, the transmission test for linkage disequilibrium was used; for linkage analysis, nonparametric methods were used.

Results: No structural or regulatory mutations in this gene were found in bipolar disorder; the results of association and genetic linkage were negative.

Conclusion: Our results do not support the speculation that the G_s-α protein gene has a role in the genetic predisposition to bipolar disorder.

Arch Gen Psychiatry. 1997;54:44-48

WHILE THE first hypotheses suggesting an involvement of catecholamines in bipolar disorder were offered more than 30 years ago,[1] postsynaptic transduction hypotheses are relatively new. G proteins transduce signals from cell surface receptors to intracellular effectors, including enzymes and ion channels.[2] The G protein heterotrimer consists of α, β, and γ subunits. The α subunit binds guanine nucleotides and, in the inactive state, is associated with a noncovalent complex consisting of β and γ subunits. On binding ligand to its receptor, the receptor interacts with 1 or more G proteins, resulting in exchange of guanosine 5′-triphosphate (GTP) for guanosine 5′-diphosphate (GDP) on the α subunit and in dissociation from the βγ complex. The free GTP-bound α subunit may then modulate specific effectors. The α subunit has intrinsic GTPase activity, which hydrolyzes GTP to GDP, resulting in inactivation and reassociation with βγ complex. Recent evidence[3] suggests that the α, β, and γ subunits may contribute to the specificity of the interaction of G proteins with receptors and effectors. Also, agonists exhibit higher affinity for receptor–G protein complexes than for isolated receptors.[4]

It has been suggested (but not confirmed) that an interaction between lithium and G proteins exists in acute experimental paradigms.[5,6] In addition, long-term effects of lithium salts have been associated with increased adenylate cyclase activity[7-9] and a decrease in G_s, G_i-1, and G_i-2α subunit messenger RNA expression.[9-11] Schreiber et al[12] reported that coupling of muscarinic receptors and β-adrenergic receptors to G proteins was increased in patients with untreated mania, but it was normal in patients with mania treated with lithium carbonate.

Young et al[13,14] reported increased levels of G_s-α in brains of patients with bipolar disorder compared with those of unaffected controls and subjects with schizophrenia. Recently, Young et al[15]

See Subjects and Methods on next page

From the Clinical Neurogenetics Branch (Drs Ram, Guedj, Cravchik, Cao, Badner, Goldin, Gershon, and Gejman) and the Experimental Therapeutics Branch (Dr Manji), National Institute of Mental Health, and the Metabolic Diseases Branch, National Institute of Diabetes and Digestive and Kidney Diseases (Dr Weinstein), Bethesda, Md; and the Beer Sheva Mental Health Center, Ben Gurion University (Drs Grisaru and Belmaker), Beer Sheva, Israel.

SUBJECTS AND METHODS

SUBJECTS

For mutational analysis, genomic DNA samples from 26 unrelated patients with bipolar disorder were evaluated. Nine samples (from patients whose abnormalities in G protein function had been described[12]) were received from Beer Sheva Mental Health Center in Israel. Additionally, DNA from 16 unrelated individuals with familial bipolar disorder (schizoaffective disorder [n=3], bipolar type I disorder [n=8], and bipolar type II disorder with major depression [n=5]) were studied. One individual (from the Old Order Amish pedigree 110) with bipolar type I disorder was also included.[21] In addition, a DNA sample from an unaffected individual and with no known ill relatives was included in denaturing gradient gel electrophoresis (DGGE) experiments.

For association and linkage analyses, we studied 21 previously described pedigrees.[22] These families consist of 365 individuals, 159 of whom are affected. Diagnoses were based on personal semistructured interviews, medical records, and information from relatives; subjects with schizoaffective disorders and bipolar type I and type II disorders were classified as affected and included in the analysis, as supported by twin, family, and adoption studies, as discussed elsewhere.[23]

MUTATIONAL ANALYSIS

Polymerase Chain Reaction

The human G_s-α gene contains 13 exons spanning 20 kilobase pairs[24] and is located on the distal long arm of chromosome 20.[25] Exons 1 to 13, including their respective bordering intronic sequences (exons 2-13), and promoter sequences of the G_s-α gene were amplified by polymerase chain reaction (PCR) from genomic DNA, and the amplified fragments were analyzed by DGGE (see **Table 1**).

Genomic DNA (50 ng) was amplified in a 100 μL of PCR mixture containing deoxynucleotide triphosphates (200 mmol/L each), 0.01% (wt/vol) gelatin, 50-mmol/L potassium chloride, 10-mmol/L TRIS-hydrochloride (pH, 8.3), 1.5- to 2.5-mmol/L magnesium dichloride, and 2.5 U of *Taq* polymerase (Boehringer Mannheim, Indianapolis, Ind) during 37 cycles. To control for contamination, a sample with no DNA was included in PCR experiments.

The G_s-α promoter is highly rich in guanidine and cytosine (85%)[24]; therefore, it is difficult to amplify by PCR, and because of that it was not analyzed in our previous reports on Albright hereditary osteodystrophy and other potential G_s-α disorders.[26] We have succeeded in amplifying a fragment with promoter sequences from −790 to −340, including 3 guanidine-citosine boxes and 2 repeated sequences, both of them being putative transcription factors binding sites.[24]

Denaturing Gradient Gel Electrophoresis

Denaturing gradient gel electrophoresis is based on 2 principles: (1) partial denaturation of double-stranded DNA retards its mobility on gel electrophoresis and (2) thermal DNA denaturation is extremely sequence sensitive. Sequence differences are detectable as a pattern of 1 or more unique bands on the gel.

DNA Melting

Analyses of genomic fragments encompassing exons and neighboring intronic sequences, including splicing sites, were generated by a computer algorithm (Melt87)[27] that simulates the probability of melting contours of DNA as a function of temperature. Results of melting analyses are used to select the precise genomic DNA sequences to be amplified. A guanidine-cytosine clamp-attachment is used to modify the melting properties of genomic DNA during PCR; in each case, the site that predicted the most uniform low-melting domain was chosen.[28,29]

Electrophoresis

Polymerase chain reaction products were analyzed in a temperature-controlled vertical gel electrophoresis apparatus (Hoefer SE600, Hoefer Scientific Instruments, San Francisco, Calif). Gradient gels, containing 7% polyacrylamide (37.5:1 acrylamide:bisacrylamide) in 1×TAE (Tris-acetate-EDTA) buffer, were prepared from 2 stock solutions: 0%, ie, containing no denaturants, and 100%, ie, containing 7-mol/L urea and 40% (vol/vol) formamide. Gradients were prepared by a gravitational gradient former. After electrophoresis, gels were stained with silver (BioRad, Richmond, Calif).

Nucleotide Sequencing

The DNA sequencing (on solid support) was performed on samples suspected of bearing nucleotide substitutions.

ASSOCIATION ANALYSIS

Transmission Disequilibrium Test

This test considers parents who are heterozygous for an allele associated with disease and evaluates the frequency with which that allele or its alternate is transmitted to affected offspring.[30] It detects linkage between the marker locus and the disease locus only if association (attributed to linkage disequilibrium) is present (**Table 2**).

LINKAGE ANALYSIS

Affected Pedigree Method Analysis

The statistical analysis using the Affected Pedigree Method statistic tests whether affected pairs of relatives share or do not share a marker allele more often than would be expected by chance.[31]

Affected Sib-Pair Statistic

This statistic tests whether affected sib pairs have a mean proportion of marker genes identical by descent that is greater than 0.50.[32] The sib-pair statistical data were computed on all possible affected pairs (using all the available data on the sibship and their parents), using the SIBPAL program (Version 2.6, SAGE package available from the Department of Biometry and Genetics, Louisiana State University Medical Center, New Orleans).

Table 1. Polymerase Chain Reaction Primers and Conditions and Denaturing Gradient Gel Electrophoresis Gradient

Sequences	Primers	Magnesium Chloride, mmol/L	Annealing		Extension		Chemical Gradient, %
			Temp, °C*	Time, s	Temp, °C*	Time, s	
Promoter	5′CCGGGCGCGCTCCCTCCCCTTCCGCCCACCCCAG-3′ 5′CTCGGCCGGGCCCCCGCCGCCGCCCCGAGCCAAAAG-3′	2.5	66	50	75	60	30-90
Exon 1	5′ATGGGCTGCCTCGGGACAG-3′ 5′CGAGGGCCCCCGGGCCGGGGC-3′	2.5	77	50	75	50	50-100
Exon 2	5′CL+TGCCCAAAGTGTTAAAATGCCT 3′ 5′AAACTGCAGTATAAAGTCTGTTCCTCTTAC 3′	1.5	58	45	72	60	5-75
Exon 3	5′CCGAATTCTCTTGGCTGATGGTTGAGGA3′ 5′ CL+CAGTTTCCCAGTATGATCTTCA 3′	1.5	59	30	72	60	15-85
Exon 4	5 CL+CCAGTACTCCTAACTGACATGG 3′ 5 GCTACAAGACAGACAGCACAAG 3′	1.5	58	45	72	60	5-75
Exon 5	5 CL+AGCCAGTGCTGTTCCCTGACCG 3 5 CCTATATGGACACTGTGCTCAG 3	1.5	58	45	72	60	50-100
Exon 6	5′ CL+TTGCCTTTCTCTAAACTTTCTT 3′ 5′ AACTGCAGTGTCTGTTTTATGTGCTGATGG 3′	1.5	58	45	72	60	15-85
Exon 7	5 CL+GCAAATTGATGTGAGCGCTGTG 3 5 GTAGTTTGGAAAGAGGGCTCAG 3′	1.5	58	45	72	60	5-75
Exon 8	5′ TCGGTTGGCTTTGGTGAGATCCA 3′ 5′ CL+AGAAACCATGATCTCTGTTATA 3′	1.5	58	45	72	60	20-70
Exon 9	5′ AACTGCAGCCAGTCCCTCTGGAATAACCG 3′ 5′CL+AGCGACCCTGATCCCTAACAAC 3′	1.5	58	45	72	60	15-85
Exons 10 and 11	5′ AAGAATTCTTAGGGATCAGGGTCGCTGCTC 3′ 5′ CL+ATGAACAGCCAGCAAGAGTGGA 3′	1.5	58	45	72	60	15-85
Exon 12	5′ AAGAATTCGCACCCCAGCTCTGCTTGAATT 3′ 5′ CL+GAGAGGAAACTAAAGACAGGCT 3′	1.5	58	45	72	60	15-85
Exon 13	5′ CL+CGAGGGTGTCACTGACAAGTCC 3′ 5′ TATGGATCCATCATTCTTTGCTCACATTTA 3′	1.5	58	45	72	60	15-85

*Temp indicates temperature.

found a marked increase of G_s-α immunoreactivity in leukocytes of patients with bipolar disorder. In partial agreement with previous reports, Manji et al[16] noted increased G_s-α (45-kd) immunoreactivity levels in leukocytes of patients with bipolar disorder.

Two previous studies[17,18] did not reveal genetic linkage under genetic homogeneity between the *G_s-α* gene and bipolar disorder. However, the interpretation of linkage results depends on the number of families studied, the genetic model assumed, the set of parameters chosen for the analyses, its statistical power to detect linkage, and linkage and heterogeneity (which are functions of the genetic model, parameters, and sample size), and the informativeness for the used DNA marker. Association may be present when linkage is undetectable; the power to detect an association for a genetically heterogeneous disorder depends, among other factors, on the prevalence of the disease variant for which the association is important.[19] We have studied association by comparing the frequencies of alleles transmitted and not transmitted to the patients from their parents.[20] Because both the transmitted and nontransmitted alleles come from the same population, any association that is found is attributed to linkage disequilibrium. We have also tested the hypothesis that either a structural mutation in the gene (ie, a mutation in the coding region) or a regulatory mutation in the promoter (ie, a mutation changing the expression of the protein) explains the published data. Additionally, we performed nonparametric linkage in a series of families with bipolar disorder.

RESULTS

MUTATIONAL ANALYSIS

The PCR products revealed identical sizes in agarose electrophoresis for each fragment amplified and DGGE of exons 5, 7, and 13 showed patterns consistent with DNA sequence variations in several individuals with bipolar disorder (**Figure**). Direct comparison of these DGGE patterns with DGGE patterns that are specific for known nucleotide variations for exons 5, 7, and 13 revealed that they correspond to the same nucleotide substitutions. The polymorphism in exon 5 has been previously described by us, and it was used by us to map the *G_s-α* gene.[25] In exons 7 and 13, two silent sequence variations were found: ATC→ATT (Ile^{185}) and AAC→AAT (Asp^{375}), respectively. We did not detect new DNA variants in the *G_s-α* gene that predict amino acid substitutions, altered splicing sites, or changes in the amplified regulatory sequences. We also performed association and linkage analyses, using a PCR amplifiable biallelic polymorphism in exon 5, which is recognized by the restriction endonuclease Fok*I*.[25]

ASSOCIATION

We analyzed the transmission of allele 1 ($FokI^+$; frequency, 0.63) of a biallelic polymorphism located in exon 5 of *G_s-α*.[25] Seventy five patients with schizoaffective and bipolar type I and type II disorders and 68 parents of these patients were studied. An additional 11

Table 2. Transmission Disequilibrium Test for G_s-α Gene*

		Nontransmitted Alleles	
		1	2
Transmitted Alleles	1	41	36
	2	28	12

This table shows 41 parent-affected offspring combinations in which the parent is homozygous for allele 1; 64 (36+28) parent-affected offspring combinations in which the parent is heterozygous for allele 1; and 12 parent-affected offspring combinations in which the parent does not carry allele 1. Of the 64 heterozygous parent-affected transmissions, allele 1 was transmitted 36 times and not transmitted 28 times. This is not significantly different from what would be expected under no linkage or association.

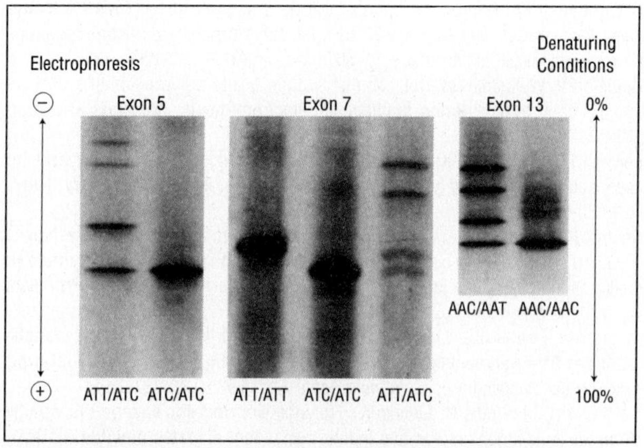

Denaturing gradient gel electrophoresis of polymerase chain reaction–amplified genomic fragments encompassing exons 5, 7, and 13. (Conditions are described in the "Polymerase Chain Reaction" and "Denaturing Gradient Gel Electrophoresis" subsections of the "Subjects and Methods" section and summarized in Table 1.) The silent DNA sequence variations are: exon 5, ATT→ATC (Ile[131]); exon 7, ATC→ATT (Ile[185]); and exon 13, AAC→AAT (Asp[371]). These polymorphisms are also found in normal populations. We did not detect new DNA variants that predict amino acid substitutions in the G_s-α gene. Gels were stained with silver.

parents had their genotypes inferred from the genotypes of several offspring for the transmission disequilibrium analysis. The observed number of transmissions of allele 1 to affected offspring is not significantly different from what would be expected under no linkage or association (χ^2=1.00, 1 *df*, *P*=.3).

LINKAGE

Nonparametric methods were applied to linkage analysis data. The affected sib-pair analysis showed that the proportion of marker alleles identical by descent was 0.53, which is not significantly different from 0.50. The Affected Pedigree Method statistic results were also not significant.

COMMENT

The evidence for an etiologic role of G protein abnormalities in bipolar disorder has been circumstantial. In our study, no mutations associated with bipolar disorder were detected in the scanning of promoter sequences, protein-coding nucleotide sequences, and splicing sites of the G_s-α gene by DGGE analysis in patients with bipolar disorder.

How can these negative data be interpreted? Did DGGE analysis fail to detect a disease-associated mutation? Denaturing gradient gel electrophoresis has been successfully applied in the detection of mutations of the G_s-α gene.[26] It is unlikely that a mutation present in 1 of the samples could have escaped detection.[26-29] Additional explanations for our negative results are as follows: (1) the existence of other, yet unrecognized, regulatory sequences in the G_s-α gene; (2) the presence of expanding trinucleotide repeats in the G_s-α locus; and (3) the presence of intronic mutations. However, results of our association and linkage analyses contradict these possibilities. Of course, our study cannot exclude a mutation in bipolar disorder in a G protein gene other than G_s-α.

The mutational analysis finding of 1 in 26 patients has a 95% confidence interval with a lower bound of 0.001 and an upper bound of 0.21,[33] ie, we can reject that more than 20% of patients with bipolar disorder have a mutation in G_s-α. However, on biological grounds, 2 facts should be noted: (1) a mutation in the G_s-α gene would have been expected to occur in our "nonrandom sample," ie, in the 9 patients with bipolar disorder from Israel who were known to have had abnormal G protein function,[12] and (2) as previous work describing alterations of G_s activity or its amount in bipolar disorder has reported, significant differences existed between affected subjects and controls, even when they have used relatively small sample sizes.[12-16] This suggests that, if the reported defect in G protein function in bipolar disorder is associated with a variation in the G_s-α gene, it has to be common. Because no mutations are noted in these patients, we conclude that the reported G protein abnormalities are not likely to be related to some underlying mutation of this gene and may, therefore, represent a state trait, as opposed to a genetic trait. Furthermore, the negative results from association and linkage studies performed on a large number of pedigrees confirm the negative results from the mutation analysis experiments. Therefore, we conclude that it is unlikely that the G_s-α gene is related to susceptibility to bipolar disorder.

Accepted for publication February 7, 1996.

We thank Carol Markey for editorial help.

Reprints: Pablo V. Gejman, MD, Unit on Molecular Clinical Investigation, Clinical Neurogenetics Branch, National Institute of Mental Health, 10 Center Dr, MSC 1274, Bethesda, MD 20892-1274 (e-mail: pgej@helix.nih.gov).

REFERENCES

1. Schildkraut JJ. The catecholamine hypothesis of affective disorders: a review of supporting evidence. *Am J Psychiatry.* 1965;122:509-522.
2. Spiegel A, Shenker A, Weinstein L. Receptor-effector coupling by G proteins: implications for normal and abnormal signal transduction. *Endocr Rev.* 1992; 13:536-565.

3. Kleuss C, Scherubl H, Hescheler J, Schultz G, Wittig B. Different β-subunits determine G-protein interaction with transmembrane receptors. *Nature.* 1992; 358:424-426.

4. Gilman A. G proteins: transducers of receptor-generated signals. *Ann Rev Biochemistry.* 1987;56:615-649.

5. Avissar S, Schreiber G, Danon A, Belmaker R. Lithium inhibits adrenergic and cholinergic increases in GTP binding in rat cortex. *Nature.* 1988;331:440-442.

6. Ellis J, Lennox R. Receptor coupling to G proteins: interactions not affected by lithium. *Lithium.* 1991;2:141-147.

7. Manji HK, Bitran JA, Masana MI, Chen GA, Hsiao JK, Risby ED, Rudorfer MV, Potter WZ. Signal transduction modulation by lithium: cell culture, cerebral microdialysis and human studies. *Psychopharmacol Bull.* 1991;27:199-208.

8. Masana MI, Bitran JA, Hsiao JK, Potter WZ. In vivo evidence that lithium inactivates G_i modulation of adenylate cyclase in brain. *J Neurochem.* 1992;59: 200-205.

9. Colin SF, Chang HC, Mollner S, Pfeuffer T, Reed RR, Duman RS, Nestler EJ. Chronic lithium regulates the expression of adenylate cyclase and G_i-protein α subunit in rat cerebral cortex. *Proc Natl Acad Sci U S A.* 1991;88:10634-10637.

10. Hsiao JK, Manji HK, Chen GA, Bitran JA, Risby ED, Potter WZ. Lithium administration modulates platelet G_i in humans. *Life Sci.* 1992;50:227-233.

11. Li PP, Tam YK, Young, LT, Warsh JJ. Lithium decreases G_s, G_i-1 and G_i-2 α subunit mRNA levels in rat cortex. *Eur J Pharmacol.* 1991;206:165-166.

12. Schreiber G, Avissar S, Danon A, Belmaker RH. Hyperfunctional G proteins in mononuclear leukocytes of patients with mania. *Biol Psychiatry.* 1991;29:273-280.

13. Young LT, Li PP, Kish SJ, Siu KP, Warsh JJ. Postmortem cerebral cortex G_s α-subunit levels are elevated in bipolar affective disorder. *Brain Res.* 1991; 553:323-326.

14. Young LT. Li PP, Kish SJ, Siu KP, Kamble A, Hornykiewicz O, Warsh JJ. Cerebral cortex G_s α protein levels and forskolin-stimulated cyclic AMP formation are increased in bipolar affective disorder. *J Neurochem.* 1993;61:890-898.

15. Young LT, Li PP, Kamble A, Siu KP, Warsh JJ. Mononuclear leukocyte levels of G proteins in depressed patients with bipolar disorder or major depressive disorder. *Am J Psychiatry.* 1994;151:594-596.

16. Manji HK, Chen G, Shimon H, Hsiao JK, Potter WZ, Belmaker RH. Guanine-nucleotide-binding proteins in bipolar affective disorder: effects of long-term lithium treatment. *Arch Gen Psychiatry.* 1995;52:135-144.

17. Gejman PV, Martinez M, Cao Q, Friedman E, Berrettini WH, Goldin LR, Koroulakis P, Ames C, Lerman MA, Gershon ES. Linkage analysis of fifty-seven microsatellite loci to bipolar disorder. *Neuropsychopharmacology.* 1993;9:31-40.

18. Le F, Mitchell P, Vivero C, Waters B, Donald J, Selbie LA, Shine J, Schofield P. Exclusion of close linkage of bipolar disorder to the G_s-α subunit gene in nine Australian pedigrees. *J Affect Disord.* 1994;32:187-195.

19. Gershon ES, Martinez M, Goldin L, Gelernter J, Silver J. Detection of marker associations with a dominant disease gene in genetically complex and heterogeneous diseases. *Am J Hum Genet.* 1989;45:578-585.

20. Falk CT, Rubinstein P. Haplotype relative risks: an easy reliable way to construct a proper control sample for risk calculations. *Ann Hum Genet.* 1987; 51:227-233.

21. Egeland JA, Gerhard DS, Pauls DL, Sussex JN, Kidd KK, Allen CR, Hostetter AM, Housman DE. Bipolar affective disorders linked to DNA markers on chromosome 11. *Nature.* 1987;325:783-787.

22. Berrettini W, Goldin L, Martinez M, Maxwell M, Smith A, Guroff J, Kazuba D, Nurnberger Jr J, Hamovit J, Simmons-Alling S, Muniec D, Choi H, York C, Robb A, Gershon E. A bipolar pedigree series for genomic mapping of disease genes: diagnostic and analytic considerations. *Psychiatr Genet.* 1991;2:125-160.

23. Gershon ES, Hamovit J, Guroff J, Dibble E, Leckman JF, Sceery W, Targum SD, Nurnberger JI Jr, Goldin LR, Bunney WE Jr. A family study of schizoaffective, bipolar I, bipolar II, unipolar, and normal control probands. *Arch Gen Psychiatry.* 1982;39:1157-1167.

24. Kozasa T, Itoh H, Tsukamoto T, Kaziro Y. Isolation and characterization of the human G_s-α gene. *Proc Natl Acad Sci U S A.* 1988;85:2081-2085.

25. Gejman PV, Weinstein LS, Martinez M, Spiegel AM, Cao Q, Hsieh WT, Hoehe MR, Gershon ES. Genetic mapping of the G_s-α subunit gene (*GNAS1*) to the distal long arm of chromosome 20 using a polymorphism detected by denaturing gradient gel electrophoresis. *Genomics.* 1991;9:782-783.

26. Gejman PV, Weinstein LS. Detection of mutations and polymorphisms of G_s α subunit gene by denaturing gradient gel electrophoresis. *Methods Enzymol.* 1994;237:308-320.

27. Lerman LS, Silverstein K. Computational simulation of DNA melting and its application to denaturing gradient gel electrophoresis. *Methods Enzymol.* 1987; 155:482-501.

28. Sheffield VC, Cox DR, Lerman LS, Myers RM. Attachment of a 40–base-pair G + C-rich sequence (GC-clamp) to genomic DNA fragments by the polymerase chain reaction results in improved detection of single-base changes. *Proc Natl Acad Sci U S A.* 1989;86:232-236.

29. Myers RM, Fischer SG, Lerman LS, Maniatis T. Nearly all single base substitutions in DNA fragments joined to a GC-clamp can be detected by denaturing gradient gel electrophoresis. *Nucleic Acids Res.* 1985;13:3131-3145.

30. Spielman R, McGinnis R, Ewens W. Transmission test for linkage disequilibrium: the insulin gene region and insulin-dependent diabetes mellitus (IDDM). *Am J Hum Genet.* 1993;52:506-515.

31. Weeks D, Lange K. The affected pedigree member method of linkage analysis. *Am J Hum Genet.* 1988;42:315-326.

32. Blackwelder WC, Elston RC. A comparison of sib-pair linkage tests for disease susceptibility loci. *Genet Epidemiol.* 1985;2:85-97.

33. Fleiss JL. *Statistical Methods for Rates and Proportions.* 2nd ed. New York, NY: John Wiley & Sons; 1981.

ORIGINAL ARTICLE

Clinical Risk Following Abrupt and Gradual Withdrawal of Maintenance Neuroleptic Treatment

Adele C. Viguera, MD; Ross J. Baldessarini, MD; James D. Hegarty, MD, MPH; Daniel P. van Kammen, MD, PhD; Mauricio Tohen, MD, DrPH

Background: Abrupt discontinuation of long-term psychotropic medication can be followed by a high risk of early relapse. This study aimed to quantify the relapse risk over time in patients with schizophrenia following discontinuation of maintenance neuroleptic treatment.

Methods: Data on the timing of relapses in patients with schizophrenia after withdrawal from neuroleptic therapy were located by a computerized literature search, combined with new data, and evaluated by survival analysis.

Results: Data were found for 1210 schizophrenic subjects: 1006 (795 inpatients and 211 outpatients) were withdrawn abruptly from oral neuroleptic therapy, and 204 discontinued treatment gradually (≥3 weeks) or stopped treatment with depot neuroleptic drugs. After abrupt discontinuation of oral medication, the risk of relapse reached 50% within 30 weeks, with remarkably little additional risk thereafter to 3.7 years; inpatients relapsed more rapidly than did outpatients (10 vs 18 weeks to a 25% relapse risk). In studies including subjects whose drug therapy was withdrawn abruptly (n=49) vs gradually (n=58), relapse was earlier after abrupt discontinuation (25% risk in 6 vs 10 weeks), with a persistent difference for at least 6 months.

Conclusions: The relapse risk was high within 6 months of discontinuing oral neuroleptic therapy, particularly in hospitalized patients. Most patients who remained stable for 6 months continued to do so for long periods without medication, indicating clinical heterogeneity. Drug-withdrawal stressors, related to long-term pharmacodynamic adaptations, are implicated. Since the risk was lower after gradually discontinuing oral neuroleptic therapy or stopping depot injections, early relapse may be spared by a slow removal of drugs.

Arch Gen Psychiatry. 1997;54:49-55

From the Consolidated Department of Psychiatry and Neuroscience Program, Harvard Medical School, Boston, Mass (Drs Viguera, Baldessarini, Hegarty, and Tohen); the General Adult Psychiatry Program and Laboratories for Psychiatric Research, Mailman Research Center, McLean Division, Massachusetts General Hospital, Belmont (Dr Baldessarini); the Department of Epidemiology, Harvard School of Public Health, Boston, Mass (Drs Viguera, Hegarty, and Tohen); and the Department of Psychiatry, University of Pittsburgh, and Highland Drive Veterans Affairs Medical Center, Pittsburgh, Pa (Dr van Kammen).

FOLLOWING THEIR introduction in the 1950s, neuroleptic drugs became the cornerstone of pharmacological treatment of psychotic disorders. The findings from many studies support their short-term efficacy and long-term benefits.[1-3] Most studies of neuroleptic maintenance have involved the interruption of treatment to compare a placebo with continued medication. Meta-analyses of such studies have found high rates of relapse in the weeks after the interruption of active treatment.[1,3] Gilbert and colleagues[3] recently concluded that the risk of psychotic relapse within 10 months was only 16% if antipsychotic medication was continued, and 53% after discontinuation.

Late adverse effects (particularly tardive dyskinesia) encourage attempts to minimize the risks without a loss of the benefits of maintenance neuroleptic therapy. Options include individual adjustment to a minimum effective dose,[4-7] as well as the use of very low or intermittent dosing,[8-10] as the search for safer and more effective antipsychotic agents continues.[11,12] Low or intermittent dosing involves the removal of neuroleptic drugs. Such procedures and, indeed, the research that supports long-term neuroleptic treatment, evidently assume that the removal of a drug does not increase the clinical risk above that associated with the natural history of untreated illness. Critical reevaluation of this assumption is encouraged by a recent

See Materials and Methods on next page

MATERIALS AND METHODS

We searched for studies that involved the abrupt or gradual discontinuation of maintenance treatment with oral antipsychotic agents or stopping injections of long-acting preparations in patients who were diagnosed as having schizophrenia. MEDLINE-computerized searching and references obtained from the resulting reports yielded 11 studies with data on the time to relapse for individuals, or survival analyses of groups, and provided 1006 subjects (795 inpatients and 211 outpatients) who were abruptly withdrawn from oral neuroleptic maintenance.[25-35] Similar new data involved 94 subjects with schizophrenia according to *DSM-III-R* criteria who were rapidly discontinued from oral haloperidol therapy at the Highland Drive Veterans Affairs Medical Center, Pittsburgh, Pa (methodological details have been reported elsewhere[36,37]) and 6 similar subjects from a study at the Massachusetts Mental Health Center, Boston, on removing an average of 85% of the initial medication (A. I. Green, MD, S. V. Faraone, PhD, W. A. Brown, MD, J. Guttierez, MD, and M. T. Tsuang, MD, DSc, PhD, oral and written communications [generously provided by Dr Green to R.J.B.], June 1995). Four studies (n=107 subjects, including 7 from Dr Green) provided additional data on gradual (>3 weeks) withdrawal of oral medication.[28,38,39] Five studies (n=83 cases, including 8 from Dr Green) involved stopping injections of a long-acting neuroleptic drug.[34,40-42] We excluded several studies that involved simultaneous or undefined mixtures of oral and depot neuroleptic medications, intermittent neuroleptic therapy, or imprecisely defined timing of drug discontinuation. Analyses are based on findings from 16 reports plus 2 unpublished data sets, yielding 1210 patients who were diagnosed as having schizophrenia and followed up after discontinuation of maintenance neuroleptic treatment.

Characteristics of the 22 cohorts that were studied[25-42] are summarized (**Table 1**); some studies failed to specify drugs and doses but did indicate when only oral or depot medication was involved. Definitions of relapse or exacerbation of illness varied but usually involved clinical assessment or the use of rating scale scores to indicate the worsening of psychotic symptoms severe enough to warrant hospitalization or reinstitution of antipsychotic treatment. Discontinuation and follow-up assessments were double-blind in 20 of the 22 cohorts (only 2 studies were open). "Abrupt" discontinuation usually involved stopping neuroleptic treatment within 1 day; "gradual" discontinuation included the tapering of oral doses over at least 3 weeks (mean±SD, 3.39±6.00 months), or no further depot neuroleptic therapy after a final injection. Treatment averaged 7.75±6.07 months and postwithdrawal follow-up after the last dose averaged 54±46 weeks (range, 10 weeks to 4 years), or 16, 20, and 17 months after discontinuing oral medication treatment abruptly or gradually, or stopping depot injections, respectively (Table 1).

The relapse risk over time after the discontinuation of neuroleptic therapy was analyzed by Kaplan-Meier and actuarial survival analysis, with variances, and compared statistically by Mantel-Cox nonparametric log rank techniques to provide a χ^2.[20,21,43,44] These values, as well as the time to a defined percent relapse±SE, were calculated with commercially available microcomputer programs (Statview/Survival Tools, Abacus Concepts, Inc, Berkeley, Calif). Unless otherwise stated, data are presented as the means±SD or rates±SE; 2-tailed statistical significance required $P<.05$ (nonsignificance, $P\geq.10$).

reconsideration of the risks involved in experimental protocols that require interruption of maintenance treatments.[13-17]

High early morbid risk follows abrupt interruption of maintenance treatments in several psychiatric disorders. In addition to early withdrawal reactions to the abrupt removal of benzodiazepines in patients with anxiety disorders,[18] and physiological symptoms associated with the removal of some antipsychotic and antidepressant agents,[19] worsening of primary disorders often follows the rapid removal of long-term psychotropic treatments. This response includes recurrence of affective episodes in a majority of patients with bipolar I or II disorders within several months of stopping successful lithium carbonate monotherapy after several years,[20-22] as well as in patients with major depression after interrupting similarly prolonged imipramine hydrochloride maintenance.[23] Moreover, after stopping lithium therapy abruptly in patients with bipolar disorders, the time to a first recurrence was much briefer than the shortest intervals between spontaneous recurrences before starting maintenance treatment.[20] The risk of recurrence of mania or depression in patients with bipolar disorders was reduced markedly by gradual discontinuation of lithium therapy, even during several weeks.[21,22] These[17,21,22] and congruent new findings[24] suggest a period of unusually high relapse risk after the removal of maintenance treatments that can be reduced, and not merely delayed, by gradual removal of medication.

Discontinuing oral neuroleptic medication, particularly abruptly, also carries a high risk of psychotic morbidity.[3,15] The hypothesis that this risk is very high within the first several months after discontinuation and less thereafter is supported by results of a preliminary analysis that indicated a 13-fold increase in relapse within 3 months of discontinuing neuroleptic treatment; this risk fell below 2-fold in the second year.[15] We predicted that slow discontinuation of orally administered neuroleptic drugs or stopping injections of long-acting agents would delay and perhaps even reduce this risk.[15] Survival analysis was used to quantify the risk over time after the interruption of neuroleptic treatment in patients with schizophrenia, based on data from previous reports as well as from studies of new subjects.

RESULTS

The survival function after abrupt discontinuation of oral neuroleptic treatment in 1006 schizophrenic patients (**Figure 1**) indicated a rapid failure of clinical stability within 3 to 6 months, reaching a relapse risk of 25% within

Table 1. Analysis of Schizophrenia Studies*

Source, y	No. of Patients	% Men†	Site‡	Diagnosis	Treated, mo§	Agents Stopped‖	Last Dose, mg/d¶	Study Design	Relapse Criteria#	Follow-up, wk**
Abruptly Discontinued From Therapy With Oral Medication (n=1006)										
Olson and Peterson,[25] 1960	117	...	I	Clinical	...	Various	...	Open	A	24
Whittaker and Hoy,[26] 1963	19	100	I	Clinical	16	Perphenazine	260	Blind, placebo	B	10
Caffey et al,[27] 1964	171	100	I	Clinical	>12	Chlorpromazine, thioridazine	375	Blind, placebo	A, B	16
Greenberg and Roth,[28] 1966	16	100	I	Clinical	>8	Chlorpromazine	500	Blind, placebo	A	24
Engelhardt et al,[29] 1967	142	...	O	Clinical	...	Various	...	Blind, placebo	C	192
Prien et al,[30] 1969	196	50	I	Clinical	>2	Chlorpromazine	1150	Blind, placebo	A	24
Leff and Wing,[31] 1971	14	(50)	O	Clinical	...	Various	200	Blind, placebo	A	46
Hogarty et al,[32] 1974	182	(50)	I	Clinical	>2	Chlorpromazine	265	Blind, placebo	C	92
Clark et al,[33] 1975	9	0	O	RDC	>3	Pimozide, thioridazine	...	Blind, placebo	A	24
Levine et al,[34] 1980	27	(50)	O	Clinical	>12	Fluphenazine	1100	Blind, placebo	A, C	15
Cheung,[35] 1981	13	(50)	O	Clinical	>3	Various	165	Blind, placebo	B, C	72
van Kammen et al,[36,37] 1994, 1997††	94	100	I	*DSM-III-R*	>6	Haloperidol	400	Blind, placebo	A	52
Green et al, 1995‡‡	6	...	O	*DSM-III*	>12	Various	...	Blind	A	24
Gradually Discontinued From Therapy With Oral Medication (n=113)										
Greenberg and Roth,[28] 1966§§	20	100	I	Clinical	≥8	Chlorpromazine	500	Blind, placebo	A	46
Branchey et al,[38] 1981‖‖	20	(50)	I	RDC	>3	Loxapine	890	Blind, placebo	A	24
Crow et al,[39] 1986¶¶	66	...	O	RDC	>1	Various	175	Blind, placebo	B, C	104
Green et al, 1995‡‡##	7	...	O	*DSM-III*	>12	Various	...	Blind	A	24
Discontinued From Therapy With Depot Medication (n=91)										
Dencker et al,[40] 1980	32	75	O	Clinical	>15	Clopenthixol decanoate, flupentixol palmitate	145, 44.4	Open	A	104
Levine et al,[34] 1980	23	(50)	O	Clinical	>1	Fluphenazine decanoate	30.9	Blind, placebo	A, C	15
Wistedt,[41] 1981	16	(50)	O	Clinical	>12	Fluphenazine decanoate, flupentixol decanoate	24.5, 20.0	Blind, placebo	A, C	24
Sampath et al,[42] 1992	12	...	O	RDC	>12	Fluphenazine decanoate	33.3	Blind, placebo	A	48
Green et al, 1995‡‡	8	...	O	*DSM-III*	>12	Fluphenazine or haloperidol decanoate	...	Blind	A	24

**These studies of cohorts for which neuroleptic maintenance treatment was discontinued involved 1210 psychotic inpatients or outpatients who were receiving long-term maintenance neuroleptic treatment in clinically stable status prior to discontinuation; diagnoses were based on unspecified clinical criteria, Research Diagnostic Criteria (RDC), or the American Psychiatric Association* DSM-III *or* DSM-III-R.

†*Gender was defined as the percentage of men; (50%) indicates approximately equal numbers of men and women subjects; approximately 69% were men.*

‡*Settings of studies were inpatient (I) units (47%) or outpatient (O) clinics (53%).*

§*Mean duration of treatment prior to discontinuation was 7.75±6.07 months or more.*

‖*Depot esters (decanoate and palmitate) were injected intramuscularly.*

¶*Doses are average chlorpromazine-equivalent milligrams per day (oral) or actual milligrams per 3 weeks (depot).*

#*Relapse criteria: A, clearly worse clinically or by ratings; B, antipsychotic re-treatment required; and C, hospitalization required.*

***Weighted (by n) mean follow-up time (months) was 15.6±16.1 (abrupt, oral), 19.5±13.9 (gradual, oral), and 17.4±11.1 (abrupt, depot).*

††*Data from van Kammen and colleagues were previously unpublished, but their methods were presented elsewhere.*[36,37]

‡‡*A. I. Green, MD, S. V. Faraone, PhD, W. A. Brown, MD, J. Guttierez, MD, and M. T. Tsuang, MD, DSc, PhD, oral and written communications from Dr Green to R. J. B., June 1995.*

§§*Gradual discontinuation time was 420 days (weighted average, 3.39±6.39 months).*

‖‖*Gradual discontinuation time was 23 days (weighted average, 3.39±6.39 months).*

¶¶*Gradual discontinuation time was 30 days (weighted average, 3.39±6.39 months).*

##*Gradual discontinuation time was 60 days (weighted average, 3.39±6.39 months).*

10.2±0.6 (±SE) weeks and 50% within 30.3±15.4 weeks. There were remarkably few additional relapses after the first 6 months without medication: the computed failure rate reached 46.0% by 6 months, and it increased only another 10.2% in the period from 6 to 24 months (**Table 2**).

Oral neuroleptic drugs were removed rapidly in 795 inpatients and 211 outpatients. Their stability after drug removal differed markedly (Mantel-Cox χ^2=28.4, P<.001 [**Figure 2**]): 25% of inpatients vs outpatients relapsed within 10.0±0.62 vs 18.0±1.65 weeks, and 50% of inpatients relapsed within 18.0±1.65 weeks, while only 40.8% of outpatients relapsed within a maximum of 3.69 years of follow-up (Figure 2). Within 6 months without medication, the relapse risk (±SE) was 49.6%±1.8% for inpatients vs 31.4%±3.2% for outpatients. Differences between hospitalized and ambulatory patients were similar when those who were undergoing gradual removal of neuroleptic drugs were included (data not shown).

The survival over time was very similar after the gradual discontinuation of oral medication over an average of 3.39±6.39 months and stopping depot injections (n=113 and n=91, respectively; χ^2=0.12; P>.10); thus, the data were pooled to provide a group of patients with gradual discontinuation of treatment. There was no significant overall difference in the resulting survival functions for those who discontinued treatment abruptly vs gradually (n=1006 and n=204, respectively; χ^2=1.70; P>.10), although the time to a 25% relapse risk tended to be shorter after abrupt discontinuation (11.0±0.3 vs 15.0±1.0

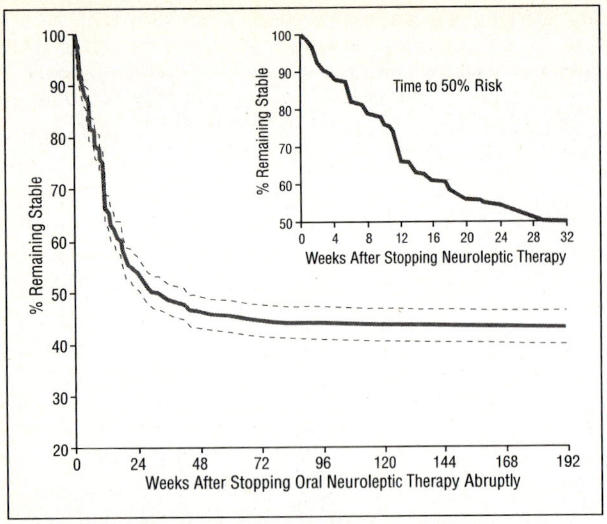

Figure 1. *Computed "survival" functions based on findings from studies that discontinued maintenance oral neuroleptic drugs in patients with schizophrenia (Table 1). Data are the percentage of patients whose conditions remained stable vs the weeks after the abrupt stoppage of treatment (n=1006). Dashed lines indicate 95% confidence intervals. Inset, The time to a 50% relapse risk (7.5 months).*

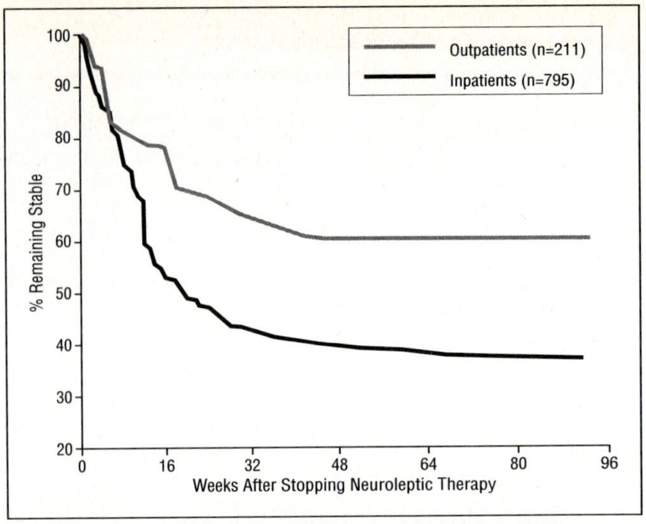

Figure 2. *Percent "survival" of schizophrenic inpatients (n=795) and outpatients (n=211) whose conditions remained stable after abrupt discontinuation of oral neuroleptic therapy. The risk was greater for inpatients (χ^2=28.4,* P*<.001), of whom 50% relapsed by 5 months; outpatients were followed up to 4 years without reaching a 50% relapse risk (data not shown).*

Table 2. Relapse Risk vs Time After Stopping Oral Neuroleptic Treatment Abruptly*

Follow-up, mo	Cumulative % Relapse (95% CI)
1	12.0 (10.0-14.1)
2	21.6 (19.1-24.2)
3	33.9 (30.9-36.8)
6	46.0 (42.9-49.1)
12	54.4 (51.2-57.5)
24	56.2 (53.1-59.3)

**CI indicates confidence interval. Based on Kaplan-Meier survival analysis, with 95% CIs, as shown in Figure 1.*

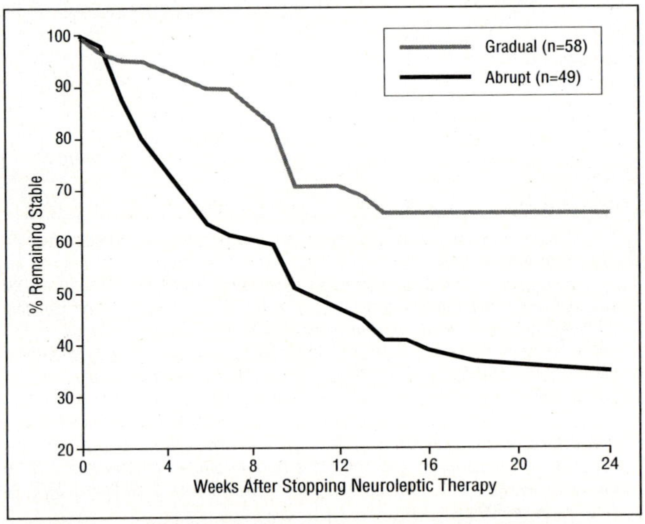

Figure 3. *Percent "survival" of schizophrenic patients whose conditions remained stable after the abrupt discontinuation of neuroleptic therapy (n=49) vs the gradual discontinuation (or stoppage of depot injections [n=58]), based on reports with data for both conditions in the same study[28,34] (A. I. Green, MD, S. V. Faraone, PhD, W. A. Brown, MD, J. Guttierez, MD, and M. T. Tsuang, MD, DSc, PhD, oral and written communications, June 1995). The risk was greater for patients who were withdrawn abruptly (χ^2=11.1,* P*<.001), of whom 50% relapsed within 2.5 months, while outpatients did not reach that level.*

weeks). Given this suggestive observation and the probable heterogeneity among studies, we further compared results from the 3 studies that were found with abrupt (n=49) and gradual (n=58) removal of neuroleptic agents within the same trial[28,34] (A.I. Green et al, oral and written communications, June 1995) (Table 1). With data pooled from these better-matched cohorts, there was a significant difference in survival functions (χ^2=11.1, *P*<.001 [**Figure 3**]). After abrupt vs gradual discontinuation, respectively, the computed time to a 25% relapse risk was 6.00±1.50 vs 10.0±1.73 weeks, and the computed probability of relapsing within 6 months was 32.5%±3.0% vs 64.9%±6.5% (a 2-fold difference).

COMMENT

The present findings from 1960 to 1995 should be interpreted cautiously owing to the variability in diagnostic criteria, lengths and methods of follow-up, and definitions of relapse, as well as the types, duration, and doses of neuroleptic drugs (Table 1). Most reports also provided little information about possibly relevant aspects of clinical history, current state, and nonpharmacological variables in aftercare. Since most data were derived from the randomized placebo cohorts of controlled trials, following substantial periods of stabilization with drug treatment, it is probable that acutely ill patients were excluded from drug withdrawal. Despite these caveats, the present analyses yield interesting information about the relapse risk over time, especially its relation to hospitalization and to the rate of drug removal.

There was a high early risk of exacerbation of psychotic symptoms soon after the abrupt interruption of ongoing oral neuroleptic maintenance. The initial relapse rate was approximately 1.7%/wk in the first 30 weeks after the abrupt discontinuation of oral neuroleptic therapy, and it was much lower at later times (Figure 1, Table 2), as noted previously.[15] Among patients whose conditions remained stable during the first several months after they stopped taking neuroleptic drugs, the later risk of relapsing was remarkably limited (Figures 1 and 2)—particularly in outpatients, only 40% of whom relapsed within 2 years (Figure 2). This finding contrasts sharply with that of similar analyses of patients with bipolar I disorder who were abruptly removed from lithium maintenance treatment, in whom the relapse risk exceeded 90% within 2 years of follow-up.[20,24]

Most of the studies concerning the abrupt removal of oral neuroleptic treatment antedate contemporary diagnoses (Table 1) and may have applied relatively broad criteria for schizophrenia.[45] Accordingly, the finding that the clinical state in 40% or more of patients remained stable without medication for several years (Figure 1) might reflect diagnostic or other clinical heterogeneity.[46,47] However, a remarkably similar mean proportion (≈40%) of persons who were diagnosed as having dementia praecox or schizophrenia during the past century have shown a favorable long-term outcome.[45] Moreover, 1 of the present studies involved the abrupt discontinuation of oral haloperidol treatment in 94 schizophrenic patients who were diagnosed by using modern *DSM-III-R* criteria (Table 1).[36] In this study, only 62% of those who were followed up for a year relapsed. These considerations suggest that the observed heterogeneity in long-term survival without medication may reflect factors other than diagnosis; however, the available data do not provide secure estimates of the proportion of schizophrenic patients who were diagnosed by using contemporary criteria and whose conditions remained stable following an initial risk period after treatment was stopped.

An essential question is whether the observed early morbidity merely reflects the natural history of untreated severe psychotic illness that reemerges without protective medication. The timing of an early relapse is generally consistent with the elimination of neuroleptic drugs from brain tissue, which may extend throughout several weeks or longer after repeated administration and accumulation in tissue.[1,2,48] However, an early relapse risk may well exceed the natural course of psychotic illness. This early risk may be related to the stress of removing treatment, which may reflect pharmacodynamic adaptations associated with prolonged drug treatment. Such changes include the induction of dopaminergic supersensitivity in the forebrain[49]; this requires 4 to 6 weeks to return to basal levels even after a single dose of a neuroleptic drug in animals,[49] or longer after repeated dosing,[50] and so may be congruent with the 4 to 24 weeks of a high relapse risk after the abrupt interruption of clinical treatment (Figure 1).[3,15] A later risk may more nearly reflect the natural history of untreated schizophrenia, albeit probably distorted by an early failure of the most vulnerable patients.

The time to a 50% relapse after the discontinuation of lithium maintenance in patients with bipolar disorders[20,24] or termination of antidepressant maintenance in patients with major depression[23] (both about 20 to 30 weeks) compares well with the 30 weeks after the abrupt withdrawal of oral neuroleptic drugs in patients with schizophrenia (Figure 1). In bipolar disorders, the early risk of recurrences following the abrupt interruption of several years of successful lithium maintenance treatment may well exceed the risk related to the natural course of untreated illness because (1) the time to a first recurrent episode was significantly earlier than predicted by spontaneous, prelithium-cycling rates[20,24] and (2) gradual discontinuation of lithium not only delayed recurrences, but *reduced* their risk during prolonged follow-up to that paralleling the untreated illness.[21,22,24]

GRADUAL REMOVAL of maintenance pharmacotherapy may also limit the relapse risk in schizophrenia (Figure 3), but since the few studies with both abrupt and gradual removal of neuroleptic drugs involved a follow-up of 6 months or less (Figure 3), it is not clear whether slow discontinuation reduced, or merely delayed, relapse. Moreover, some neuroleptic drugs have a terminal half-life of a week or more,[48] and elimination of depot neuroleptic agents requires at least 4 to 6 months[42,51] to limit further the presumably drug-free follow-up that is observed. Inderbitzen et al[6] also found that slow removal of about half of a maintenance dose of neuroleptic drugs during 5 months had little early clinical impact, although the length of follow-up was limited (<1 year), and the dose that was removed may have represented an excess. The important question of how much of a neuroleptic dose can be removed safely at what rate in psychotic patients requires further study, if clinically appropriate protocols can be defined.[13-15,17]

In addition to the rate of drug withdrawal, other factors may contribute to the risk of psychotic relapse after the discontinuation of neuroleptic therapy or abrupt reductions of dose. Early relapse may be particularly likely with certain agents (eg, after rapidly stopping treatment with clozapine or changing it to a more typical neuroleptic drug).[52] Covariance of relapse and the prior dose of a neuroleptic drug may also occur, but is probably confounded by higher clinical dosing in more severe illness.[3,15,30] Additional nonpharmacological factors associated with increased vulnerability to psychotic relapses have been suggested, including male gender, youth, early onset, a severe history, comorbid substance abuse, coarse brain disease, and metabolic or endocrinological evidence of increased arousal-distress, or psychotic activation induced by a stimulant.[3,10,36,53] Such factors could not be evaluated here but should be considered in future treatment-discontinuation studies. Discontinuation of neuroleptic therapy in hospitalized patients led to a greater risk of early relapse than in outpatients (Figure 2); however, such findings may no longer generalize if changing indications for hospitalization are blurring former symptomatic differences between hospitalized and ambulatory psychotic patients.[2,45,47]

The full implications of the present findings are limited by the typically complex and irregular course of untreated schizophrenia[46,47] to be compared with the course following discontinuation of treatment. Although clinical and possible ethical considerations now severely constrain observations of untreated psychotic patients for prolonged periods,[13,14] treatment noncompliance as well as elective clinical practice often interrupt antipsychotic treatment for varying periods. In psychotic affective disorders, intermittent-interrupted exposure to neuroleptic drugs is particularly common, and its potential contribution to clinical instability is unknown.[1,2,54,55] In addition, most experimental protocols that evaluate the long-term efficacy of neuroleptic agents and many other drugs have compared continued vs withdrawn treatment.[1-3,15-17] The results of such studies that support a therapeutic effect usually have not considered contributions of drug withdrawal to observed drug-placebo contrasts. Moreover, protocols that have been designed to study patients in a presumed drug-free state often have employed a drug "washout" that was probably too short to provide a drug-free and physiologically basal state.[1,2,48]

In conclusion, rapid discontinuation of maintenance treatment with short-acting oral neuroleptic agents in schizophrenia carried a 50% risk of relapse within 30 weeks; pharmacodynamic stress factors contributing to this risk may include supersensitivity of central dopamine receptors. Further study is required to clarify whether (1) the high morbid risk following abrupt interruption of maintenance treatment exceeds that in untreated psychotic illness and (2) gradual drug removal can reduce, and not merely postpone, relapse. In general, the present findings add to growing evidence that abrupt discontinuation of maintenance treatment with psychotropic agents is followed by a high rate of early relapses in several major psychiatric disorders. This phenomenon should be considered in the design and interpretation of research protocols as well as in clinical management, and the rates reported here should help in planning research and in counseling patients. Gradual dose reduction (with close clinical follow-up) may limit relapse risk associated with interruption of maintenance treatment, and is recommended.

Accepted for publication January 3, 1996.

This study was supported in part by grants MH-31154 and MH-47370 from the National Institute of Mental Health, Rockville, Md, and by awards from the Bruce J. Anderson Foundation and the Adam Corneel, Anonymous Donor, Vivian Temte, and Richard Whalin Psychiatric Research Funds, Boston, Mass.

Alan Green, MD, generously provided data from his studies. Mary Kelley, MS, Silvina Zarate, and Michelle Weiss, MS, assisted with data analyses.

Corresponding author: Ross J. Baldessarini, MD, Mailman Research Center 316, McLean Division, Massachusetts General Hospital, 115 Mill St, Belmont, MA 02178.

REFERENCES

1. Baldessarini RJ. *Chemotherapy in Psychiatry: Principles and Practice.* Cambridge, Mass; Harvard University Press; 1985.
2. Baldessarini RJ. Drugs and the treatment of psychiatric disorders: antipsychotic and antianxiety agents. In: Harden W, Rudin W, Molinoff PB, Rall T, eds. *Goodman and Gilman's the Pharmacologic Basis of Therapeutics.* 9th ed. New York, NY: McGraw-Hill Book Co; 1996:399-430.
3. Gilbert PL, Harris MJ, Jeste DV. Neuroleptic withdrawal in schizophrenic patients: a review of the literature. *Arch Gen Psychiatry.* 1995;52:173-188.
4. Baldessarini RJ, Cohen BM, Teicher MH. Significance of neuroleptic dose and plasma level in the pharmacological treatment of psychoses. *Arch Gen Psychiatry.* 1988;45:79-91.
5. McEvoy JP, Hogarty GE, Steingard S. Optimal dose of neuroleptic in acute schizophrenia: controlled study of the neuroleptic threshold and higher haloperidol dose. *Arch Gen Psychiatry.* 1991;48:739-745.
6. Inderbitzen LB, Lewine RRJ, Scheller-Gilkey G, Swofford CD, Egan GJ, Gloersen BA, Vidanagama BP, Waternaux C. A double-blind dosage reduction trial of fluphenazine decanoate in chronic, unstable schizophrenic patients. *Am J Psychiatry.* 1994;151:1753-1759.
7. Smith RC. Lower-dose therapy with traditional neuroleptics in chronically hospitalized schizophrenic patients. *Arch Gen Psychiatry.* 1994;51:427-429.
8. Carpenter WT, Hanlon TE, Heinrichs DW, Summerfelt AT, Kirkpatrick B, Levine J, Buchanan RW. Continuous vs targeted medication in schizophrenic outpatients: outcome results. *Am J Psychiatry.* 1990;147:1138-1148.
9. Herz MI, Glazer WM, Mostert MA, Sheard MA, Szymanski HV, Hafez H, Mirza M, Vana J. Intermittent vs maintenance medication in schizophrenia: two-year results. *Arch Gen Psychiatry.* 1991;48:333-339.
10. Jolley AG, Hirsch SR. Continuous vs intermittent neuroleptic therapy in schizophrenia. *Drug Saf.* 1993;8:331-339.
11. Baldessarini RJ, Frankenburg FR. Clozapine—a novel antipsychotic agent. *N Engl J Med.* 1991;324:746-754.
12. Meltzer HY. Atypical antipsychotic drugs. In: Bloom FE, Kupfer DJ, eds. *Psychopharmacology: the Fourth Generation of Progress.* New York, NY: Raven Press; 1995:1277-1286.
13. Rothman KJ, Michels KB. The continuing unethical use of placebo controls. *N Engl J Med.* 1994;331:294-298.
14. Taubes G. Use of placebo controls in clinical trials disputed. *Science.* 1995; 267:25-26.
15. Baldessarini RJ, Viguera AC. Neuroleptic withdrawal in schizophrenic patients. *Arch Gen Psychiatry.* 1995;52:189-192.
16. Jeste DV, Gilbert PL, McAdams LA, Harris MJ. Considering neuroleptic maintenance and taper on a continuum: need for individual rather than dogmatic approach. *Arch Gen Psychiatry.* 1995;52:209-212.
17. Baldessarini RJ, Suppes T, Tondo L. Lithium withdrawal in bipolar disorder: implications for clinical practice and experimental therapeutics research. *Am J Ther.* 1996;3:492-496.
18. Lader M. Benzodiazepines: a risk-benefit profile. *CNS Drugs.* 1994;1:377-387.
19. Dilsaver SC. Heterocyclic antidepressant, monoamine oxidase inhibitor and neuroleptic withdrawal phenomena. *Prog Neuropsychopharmacol Biol Psychiatry.* 1990;14:137-161.
20. Suppes T, Baldessarini RJ, Faedda GL, Tohen M. Risk of recurrence following discontinuation of lithium treatment in bipolar disorder. *Arch Gen Psychiatry.* 1991;48:1082-1088.
21. Faedda GL, Tondo L, Baldessarini RJ, Suppes T, Tohen M. Outcome after rapid vs gradual discontinuation of lithium in bipolar mood disorders. *Arch Gen Psychiatry.* 1993;50:448-455.
22. Suppes T, Baldessarini RJ, Faedda GL, Tondo L, Tohen M. Discontinuing maintenance treatment in bipolar manic-depression: risks and implications. *Harvard Rev Psychiatry.* 1993;1:131-144.
23. Kupfer DJ, Frank E, Perel JM, Cornes C, Mallinger AG, Thase ME, McEachran AB, Grochocinski VJ. Five-year outcome for maintenance therapies in recurrent depression. *Arch Gen Psychiatry.* 1992;49:769-773.
24. Baldessarini RJ, Tondo L, Faedda G, Floris G, Suppes T, Rudas N. Effects of the rate of discontinuing lithium maintenance treatment in bipolar disorders. *J Clin Psychiatry.* 1996;57:441-448.
25. Olson GW, Peterson DB. Sudden removal of tranquilizing drugs from chronic psychiatric patients. *J Nerv Ment Dis.* 1960;131:252-255.
26. Whittaker CB, Hoy RM. Withdrawal of perphenazine in chronic schizophrenia. *Br J Psychiatry.* 1963;109:422-427.
27. Caffey EM, Diamond LS, Frank TV, Grasberger JC, Herman L, Klett CJ, Rothstein C. Discontinuation or reduction of chemotherapy in chronic schizophrenics. *J Chronic Dis.* 1964;17:347-358.
28. Greenberg LM, Roth S. Differential effects of abrupt vs gradual withdrawal of

chlorpromazine in hospitalized schizophrenic patients. *Am J Psychiatry.* 1966; 123:221-226.
29. Engelhardt DM, Rosen B, Freedman N, Margolis R. Phenothiazines in prevention of psychiatric hospitalization: delay or prevention of hospitalization, a reevaluation. *Arch Gen Psychiatry.* 1967;16:98-101.
30. Prien RF, Cole JO, Belkin NF. Relapse in chronic schizophrenics following abrupt withdrawal of tranquilizing medication. *Br J Psychiatry.* 1969;115:679-686.
31. Leff JP, Wing JK. Trial of maintenance therapy in schizophrenia. *Br J Psychiatry.* 1971;11:599-604.
32. Hogarty GE, Goldberg SC, Schooler NR, Ulrich RF. Drug and sociotherapy in the aftercare of schizophrenic patients: two-year relapse rate. *Arch Gen Psychiatry.* 1974;31:603-608.
33. Clark ML, Huber WK, Hill D, Wood F, Costiloe JP. Pimozide in chronic schizophrenic outpatients. *Dis Nerv Syst.* 1975;36:137-141.
34. Levine J, Schooler NR, Severe J, Escobar J, Gelenberg AJ, Mandel M, Sovner R, Steinbook R. Discontinuation of oral and depot fluphenazine in schizophrenic patients after one year of continuous medication. *Adv Biochem Psychopharmacol.* 1980;24:483-495.
35. Cheung HK. Schizophrenics fully remitted on neuroleptics for 3-5 years—to stop or continue drugs? *Br J Psychiatry.* 1981;138:490-494.
36. van Kammen DP, Agren H, Yao JK, O'Connor DT, Gurklis J, Peters JL. Noradrenergic activity and prediction of psychotic relapse following haloperidol withdrawal in schizophrenia. *Am J Psychiatry.* 1994;51:379-384.
37. van Kammen DP, Kelley ME, Gurklis JA, Gilbertson MW, Yao JK, Condray R, Peters JL. Predicting duration of clinical stability following haloperidol withdrawal in schizophrenia. *Neuropsychopharmacology.* In press.
38. Branchey MH, Branchey LB, Richardson MA. Effects of neuroleptic adjustment on clinical condition in tardive dyskinesia in schizophrenic patients. *Am J Psychiatry.* 1981;138:608-612.
39. Crow TJ, MacMillan JF, Johnson AL, Johnstone EC. Randomized controlled trial of prophylactic neuroleptic treatment. *Br J Psychiatry.* 1986;148:120-127.
40. Dencker SJ, Lepp M, Malm U. Do schizophrenics well adapted in the community need neuroleptics? a depot withdrawal study. *Acta Psychiatr Scand.* 1980;61(suppl 279):64-76.
41. Wistedt B. A depot neuroleptic withdrawal study: a controlled study of the withdrawal of depot fluphenazine decanoate and depot flupenthixol decanoate in chronic schizophrenic patients. *Acta Psychiatr Scand.* 1981;64:65-84.
42. Sampath G, Shah A, Krska J, Soni SD. Discontinuation in the very stable schizophrenic patient: relapse rates and serum neuroleptic levels. *Hum Psychopharmacol.* 1992;7:255-264.
43. Cox DR. Regression models and life tables. *J R Stat Soc Ser B.* 1972;34:187-220.
44. Kahn HA, Sempos CT. *Statistical Methods in Epidemiology.* New York, NY: Oxford University Press Inc; 1989.
45. Hegarty JD, Baldessarini RJ, Tohen M, Waternaux CM, Oepen G. One hundred years of schizophrenia: a meta-analysis of the outcome literature. *Am J Psychiatry.* 1994;151:1409-1416.
46. Fenton WS, McGlashan TH. Natural history of schizophrenia subtypes. *Arch Gen Psychiatry.* 1991;48:969-977.
47. Ram R, Bromet EJ, Eaton WW, Pato C, Schwartz JE. The natural course of schizophrenia: a review of first-admission studies. *Schizophr Bull.* 1992;18: 185-207.
48. Cohen BM, Tsuneizumi T, Baldessarini RJ, Campbell A, Babb S. Differences between antipsychotic drugs in persistence of brain levels and behavioral effects. *Psychopharmacology (Berl).* 1992;108:338-344.
49. Baldessarini RJ, Tarsy D. Relationship of the actions of neuroleptic drugs to the pathophysiology of tardive dyskinesia. *Int Rev Neurobiol.* 1979;21:1-45.
50. Müller P, Seeman P. Dopaminergic supersensitivity after neuroleptics: time-course and specificity. *Psychopharmacology (Berl).* 1978;60:1-11.
51. Eklund K, Forsman A. Minimal effective dose and relapse—double-blind trial: haloperidol decanoate vs placebo. *Clin Neuropharmacol.* 1991;14(suppl 2):S7-S17.
52. Baldessarini RJ, Gardner DM, Garver DL. Conversions from clozapine to other antipsychotics. *Arch Gen Psychiatry.* 1995;52:000-000.
53. Lieberman JA, Alvir J, Geisler S, Ramos-Lorenzi J, Woerner M, Novacenko H, Cooper T, Kane JM. Methylphenidate response, psychopathology and tardive dyskinesia as predictors of relapse in schizophrenia. *Neuropsychopharmacology.* 1994;11:107-118.
54. Chou J C-Y. Recent advances in the treatment of acute mania. *J Clin Psychopharmacol.* 1991;11:3-21.
55. Sernyk MJ, Woods SW. Chronic neuroleptic use in manic depressive illness. *Psychopharmacol Bull.* 1993;29:375-381.

ORIGINAL ARTICLE

A Prospective Study of Risk Factors Predicting Grief Intensity Following Pregnancy Loss

Hettie J. E. M. Janssen, PhD; Marian C. J. Cuisinier, PhD; Kees P. H. M. de Graauw, PhD; Kees A. L. Hoogduin, MD, PhD

Background: This prospective longitudinal study investigated which selected person-oriented, social environment, demographic, and pregnancy-related risk factors could best predict women's grief intensity following pregnancy loss.

Method: In a prospective longitudinal study, 2140 pregnant women within 12 weeks' gestation answered a first questionnaire in writing. Of this sample, 227 women experienced an involuntary pregnancy loss and were followed up for a period of 18 months, during which grief was reassessed four times, using the Perinatal Grief Scale. The prospectively measured risk factors were hierarchically ordered and linked to each woman's individual grief response over time.

Results: The hypothesized risk factors, with the exception of a prior pregnancy loss, significantly related to grief intensity following the pregnancy loss and together explained 35% of the variance in grief scores among subjects. Gestational age, preloss neurotic personality, preloss psychiatric symptoms, and family composition showed the strongest relation to grief intensity following a pregnancy loss. Only psychiatric symptoms showed an interaction with time in that the women who evidenced more psychiatric symptoms before the pregnancy loss showed more intense grief shortly following the pregnancy loss. The other risk factors had a constant effect, irrespective of the time that had passed since the loss.

Conclusion: A relatively long preloss pregnancy, a more neurotic personality, more preloss psychiatric symptoms, and the absence of living children appear to be important risk factors for stronger grief responses in women following a pregnancy loss.

Arch Gen Psychiatry. 1997;54:56-61

AS A result of the supposed high risk of complicated grief reactions in the first year following pregnancy loss,[1] several studies have been performed to identify the related risk factors.[2-20] The studies retrospectively assessed different risk factors and linked them to grief intensity at the time of the study. This kind of retrospective study is flawed, however, in that a postloss assessment of the preloss situation might produce responses colored by the experience of the pregnancy loss. Toedter and colleagues[21] suggested that, ideally, a prospective study should be conducted. We decided to carry out a prospective study to test hypotheses formulated on the basis of results derived from earlier retrospective studies.

The results of previous retrospective studies of *pregnancy-related* variables showed that grief intensity was greater following loss of a pregnancy that reached a longer gestation than that following a shorter gestation.[5,11,17,18] A history of pregnancy loss was expected to increase grief following a subsequent loss,[9,14] although in several studies this relationship was not confirmed.[2,11,13,16,18,20] Studies also produce conflicting results when they examine feelings of ambivalence toward the fetus in relation to grief intensity following a pregnancy loss.[8,9,12] Although it was expected that women who had experienced difficulties in conceiving would evidence more intense grief following a pregnancy loss,[22,23] this relation was not established empirically.[6,18] With regard to *social environment* variables, researchers have noticed stronger grief reactions in women who received less support from their partners[3,6-7,9-10,12,13,18] or from their social network.[3,6,7,12,13,19] With re-

From the Department of Clinical Psychology and Personality, University of Nijmegen (Drs Janssen, Cuisinier, and Hoogduin); and Alfanumeriek, Software Development and Research, Oosterbeek (Dr Graauw), the Netherlands.

See Subjects and Methods on next page

SUBJECTS AND METHODS

STUDY DESIGN

An invitation to recently pregnant women to participate in the study was published in a popular family magazine in the Netherlands. We informed the readers that we were interested in how women coped with both normal pregnancy and delivery and with pregnancies in which complications (such as preterm birth, the loss of the baby, or maternal depression) occurred. The first 2140 women who responded by sending in their informed written consent were immediately sent a first questionnaire, followed by a second questionnaire sent in the sixth month of pregnancy and a third questionnaire at the expected time of 1 month following delivery. At each of these assessments, we asked the women to inform us if the pregnancy had ended in the loss of the baby. If this was the case, we included them in the loss sample and sent them a specific questionnaire directed at the emotional impact of the loss. In addition to the first loss questionnaire, which we sent as shortly as possible following the loss, they received a second questionnaire at 6 months, a third at 1 year, and a final questionnaire at 18 months following the loss.

SAMPLE DESCRIPTION

The women's reproductive history and sociodemographic characteristics varied considerably. Compared with the Dutch population at large, our sample contained an overrepresentation of women who already had 1 child. From the original sample, 227 women (10.6%) experienced an involuntary pregnancy loss; 6 of these women had been carrying twins, 1 of whom had died. As these women were still carrying their surviving child, they were excluded from the sample, so the loss group consisted of 221 women, most of whom (91%) had experienced an early loss, before the 20th week of gestation. For 35 women, the pregnancy loss occurred before they had been able to complete the first preloss questionnaire. Prospective data on these women were therefore missing, but because their postloss data were available, they remained in the study.

The women varied in age from 19 to 41 years (mean±SD age, 29.25±4.26). Most women (97%) were married or were in a steady cohabiting relationship; 19% of the women had achieved a basic level of education, 44% had had a secondary education, and 37% had achieved an advanced level of education. One third (32%) did not have children and 41% had experienced a previous pregnancy loss.

The first postloss questionnaire was completed at an average of 2.5 months following the loss; the second, third, and fourth postloss assessments, at an average of 6, 12, and 18 months following the loss, respectively. Of the women who had experienced a pregnancy loss, 13 dropped out, with 94% completing all 4 postloss questionnaires. No significant differences in age, marital status, education, number of living children, and history of a pregnancy loss were found between those who completed all 4 questionnaires and the women who dropped out of the study.

MEASURES

In the first preloss questionnaire, we assessed psychiatric symptoms by using the Dutch version of the Symptom Checklist–90 (SCL-90).[34,35] In the analyses, we used the total scale score minus the women's individual scores on the somatization cluster of this scale, as we expected that the pregnant women might, as a result of the pregnancy, show above-normal scores on somatization. In addition, in the preloss questionnaire, we assessed the personality characteristic neuroticism (or emotional instability), using the Dutch Personality Questionnaire (NPV),[36] which strongly corresponds to the Minnesota Multiphasic Personality Inventory factor negativism and the Norman factor emotional instability.[37] Neuroticism was measured by means of a combination of 4 subscales: low self-esteem, social inadequacy, general inadequacy, and aggrievedness, of which internal reliability coefficients

Continued on next page

gard to *person-oriented* variables, stronger grief reactions have been noticed in women who retrospectively reported more preloss psychiatric complaints[3,18] and physical symptoms.[18]

Personality characteristics have not yet been studied in relation to grief following a pregnancy loss, and they have barely been studied in relation to grief following other kinds of losses,[24,25] although they might be important predictors of grief. Those studies that have focused on personality characteristics found them to be a risk factor in bereavement outcome: "neurotic" people with low self-esteem showed a more problematic outcome.[26-28] Different *demographic* variables have been studied in relation to grief following a pregnancy loss. In general, no strong relations to grief were found. With regard to age, some researchers found lower grief intensity in relatively older women,[18] whereas others found age not to be related to grief.[2,11-13,15,19,20] As expected, some studies found that childless women experienced more grief when a pregnancy loss occurred,[8,18] whereas others did not.[7,12,13,15,19,20] Contrary to expectation, religious background and social economic status were found not to relate to grief intensity following a pregnancy loss.[6,12,13,18]

In the present study, we tested the following hypotheses. We expected more intense grief reactions in women who (1) had been pregnant for a longer time, (2) had a more neurotic personality prior to the loss, (3) evidenced more psychiatric symptoms prior to the loss, (4) had relatively more physical symptoms prior to the loss, (5) did not have living children at the time of the loss, (6) had experienced a pregnancy loss earlier in life, (7) were relatively younger, (8) had a partner relationship of relatively low quality prior to the loss, and (9) experienced relatively little support from their social network prior to the loss. All the other risk factors mentioned were investigated thoroughly.

Contrary to the suggestion that grief might remain stable over time,[29,30] recent studies have found that grief intensity decreases with the passing of time.[3,25,28,31-33] In the present study, we hypothesized that grief would decline over time and investigated whether the decrease in grief intensity was related to the aforementioned risk factors.

are sufficient to high and range from 0.60 to 0.91; test-retest reliability is good and ranges from $r=0.73$ to $r=0.82$.[36] The quality of the partner relationship was assessed by means of the Interpersonal Problem Solving Inventory (IPSI/IPOV).[38] This 17-item questionnaire is commonly used in the Netherlands and relates to Spanier's Dyadic Adjustment Scale.[38] Social support was assessed using Blake and McKay's single-item measure,[39] which is reported to be a good predictor of which women have an increased risk of illness, and which asks, "How many people do you have near whom you can readily count on for real help in times of trouble or difficulty?" Concurrent validity of this item was proven by a strong association with a general social support index.[39] With regard to physical symptoms, we asked the women to give a subjective indication of their physical health on a 5-point Likert-type scale ranging from very good health to very bad health. The women were also asked about their sociodemographic status and their pregnancy history.

All 4 postloss questionnaires contained the Perinatal Grief Scale's (PGS)[40] short 33-item form to assess grief intensity. As a total scale score, the PGS consists of 3 subscales: active grief, difficulty coping, and despair. The active grief subscale presents information on acute, common grief reactions; the latter 2 subscales are intended to measure complicated grief reactions in increasing order of intensity.[41] The PGS has a 5-point answering scale varying from strongly agree to strongly disagree. In the present study, a high score reflects intense grief reactions. The reliability of the PGS short form is excellent for both the original English version[40] and the Dutch version.[42] Internal reliability coefficients in the present study range from 0.89 to 0.96. In addition to the PGS, we included other standard measurement scales in all 4 postloss questionnaires, results from which were reported elsewhere.[43,44]

ANALYTIC STRATEGY

Repeated measures analysis was performed, with the risk factors as between-subjects factors and time since the pregnancy loss as a within-subjects factor. Each woman's exact time since the pregnancy loss was used in the analysis. We ordered the risk factors in advance, according to their expected importance for outcome. We first entered the pregnancy-related factor, followed by the person-related factors (such as preloss neuroticism). We then entered the demographic risk factors, followed by the social environment factors (**Table**). Data were analyzed using hierarchical multiple regression.[45] With regard to between sources of variance, the main effect of all risk factors taken conjointly was tested. As a specification of the total effect, each of the risk factors was also tested in order of their expected importance for outcome when controlling for the previous factor(s). In this way, we could determine whether a risk factor explained an extra part of the variance in addition to the variance already explained by the risk factors included earlier in the analysis. Within sources of variance were tested in the following order: (1) main effect of time since loss and (2) interaction between time since the loss and all risk factors taken conjointly. The interaction effects of time since the loss with each of the risk factors were tested as a specification.

A dummy variable was included in the analysis, where women for whom there were no prospective data were allocated a score of 1, and all other women were allocated a score of 0. Because women without prospective data had experienced a pregnancy loss early in the pregnancy, their lack of prospective data was not based on chance and, therefore, had to be accounted for.[45]

We performed a thorough analysis to determine whether certain other risk factors could explain an additional part of the variance in grief scores. These factors were education, (un)employment, religious background, the subjectively experienced support from the woman's religion, feelings of ambivalence at the beginning of the pregnancy, and the difficulty in conceiving.

RESULTS

On the PGS total scale, the hypothesized risk factors significantly ($P<.05$) related to grief intensity following the pregnancy loss (Table) and together explained 35% of the variance in grief scores between the subjects.

With regard to the hierarchically ordered risk factors, it was found that gestational age, preloss neurotic personality, preloss psychiatric symptoms, and family composition significantly related to grief intensity. Women with relatively longer pregnancies showed more intense grief reactions. Also, women with a more neurotic personality evidenced more intense grief, as did women who had evidenced relatively more psychiatric symptoms prior to the pregnancy loss. The women without living children subsequently showed stronger grief responses. Age also tended to be related to grief intensity, with relatively older women showing more intense grief.

Grief intensity decreased with time. When specifying the significant interaction between the combined risk factors and grief intensity, the interaction between time since the loss and psychiatric symptoms prior to the loss reached significance: those women who had more preloss psychiatric symptoms showed more intense grief reactions shortly following the loss, but over time, the difference in comparison with those in the women with fewer preloss psychiatric symptoms decreased (**Figure**).

When performing the same analysis for the PGS subscales, we found that one third of the variance (34%) in grief scores on the subscale active grief could be explained by the risk factors ($F=10.61$, $df=10,210$, $P<.001$) and one third of the variance (34%) in grief scores on the subscale difficulty coping ($F=10.63$, $df=10,210$, $P<.001$) and 29% of the variance in grief scores on the subscale despair ($F=8.56$, $df=10,210$, $P<.001$). The effect of gestational age on the PGS total score was also found for all 3 subscales: active grief ($F=55.17$, $df=1,210$, $P<.001$), difficulty coping ($F=27.03$, $df=1,210$, $P<.001$), and despair ($F=19.12$, $df=1,210$, $P<.001$). The same holds true for preloss neuroticism (active grief: $F=39.02$, $df=1,210$, $P<.001$; difficulty coping: $F=58.61$, $df=1,210$, $P<.001$; and despair: $F=49.52$, $df=1,210$, $P<.001$). The result concerning preloss psychiatric symptoms in relation to the total PGS was also found for the subscales dif-

Impact of Risk Factors and Time Since Pregnancy Loss on Grief Intensity*

Source of Variance	Proportion of Variance	*df*	F	*P*
Between Subjects				
A, all risk factors together	.3519	10	11.40	<.001
As specification of successive characteristics				
A1, length of pregnancy until loss	.1252	1	40.56	<.001
A2, no pretest†	.0002	1	0.06	.805
A3, preloss neuroticism	.1740	1	56.38	<.001
A4, preloss psychiatric symptoms	.0166	1	5.38	.02
A5, preloss physical symptoms	.0009	1	0.29	.6
A6, absence of living children	.0194	1	6.29	.01
A7, previous pregnancy loss	.0030	1	0.96	.33
A8, maternal age	.0085	1	2.76	.09
A9, preloss partner relationship	.0041	1	1.33	.25
A10, preloss social support	.0001	1	0.03	.85
Error between	.6481	210	...	...
Within Subjects				
B, time since loss (main effect)	.3069	1	278.77	<.001
B-A, interaction between time since loss and all risk factors together	.0236	10	2.14	.02
B- as specification of interaction effects				
B-A1, length of pregnancy until loss	.0014	1	1.31	.25
B-A2, no pretest†	.0008	1	.75	.39
B-A3, preloss neuroticism	.0009	1	.81	.37
B-A4, preloss psychiatric symptoms	.0140	1	12.71	.001
B-A5, preloss physical symptoms	.0010	1	.87	.32
B-A6, absence of living children	.0002	1	.17	.68
B-A7, previous pregnancy loss	.0006	1	.58	.45
B-A8, maternal age	.0015	1	1.33	.25
B-A9, preloss partner relationship	.0004	1	.35	.56
B-A10, preloss social support	.0030	1	2.64	.1
Error within	.6694	608	...	...

**Repeated measures analysis of grief intensity scored on the Perinatal Grief Scale. See the "Analytic Strategy" subsection in the "Subject and Methods" section for detailed explanation.*

†A missing data dichotomy with score 1 for the 35 women who experienced a pregnancy loss before pretest scores were assessed, and score 0 for all others (Cohen and Cohen[45 [chap 7]]).

ficulty coping (F=7.03, *df*=1,210, *P*=.008) and despair (F=5.45, *df*=1,210, *P*<.02), but not for active grief (F=0.008, *df*=1,210, *P*=.1). Childless women not only showed more intense grief on the PGS total scale but also on the subscales active grief (F=5.73, *df*=1,210, *P*<.02), difficulty coping (F=4.49, *df*=1,210, *P*=.03), and despair (F=5.93, *df*=1,210, *P*<.02). Older women, who tended to show more grief intensity on the total PGS, showed more difficulty coping with the loss (F=5.32, *df*=1,210, *P*=.02). Furthermore, it was found that women

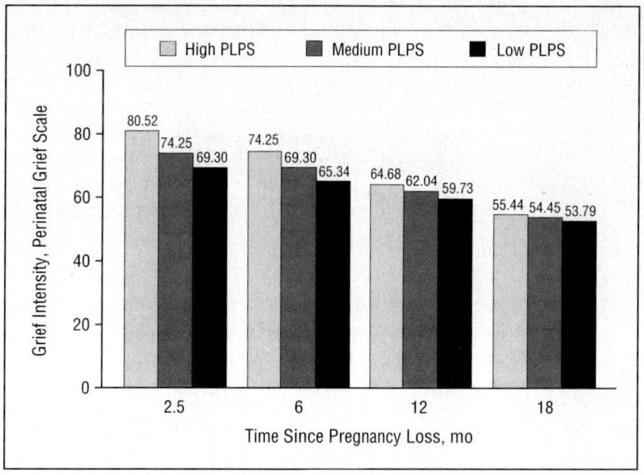

The effect of preloss psychiatric symptoms (PLPS) and time since a pregnancy loss on grief following the pregnancy loss.

with a relatively poor preloss partner relationship tended to show more despair following the loss (F=3.32, *df*=1,210, *P*=.07).

In time, active grief (F=507.07, *df*=1,608, *P*<.001), difficulty coping (F=129.82, *df*=1,608, *P*<.001), and despair (F=106.70, *df*=1,608, *P*<.001) decreased. The interaction between time since the pregnancy loss and all risk factors reached significance on 2 subscales: active grief (F=2.14, *df*=10,608, *P*=.02) and despair (F=2.52, *df*=10,608, *P*=.006). When specifying the interaction between time since the pregnancy loss and the risk factors, the effect of preloss psychiatric symptoms and time since the loss reached significance for all 3 subscales, with the women high on preloss psychiatric symptoms showing more active grief (F=14.71, *df*=1,608, *P*<.001), difficulty coping (F=8.39, *df*=1,608, *P*=.004), and despair (F=7.80, *df*=1,608, *P*=.006), particularly shortly following the pregnancy loss. The interaction between gestational age and time since the pregnancy loss only reached significance for despair (F=4.07, *df*=1,608, *P*=.04), with the women whose pregnancy had lasted longer showing relatively more despair, particularly shortly following the loss. The interaction between preloss physical symptoms and time since the loss on the despair subscale also appeared to be significant (F=5.08, *df*=1,608, *P*=.02). Women who reported having relatively more physical symptoms showed relatively more despair shortly following the pregnancy loss, but over time the difference in comparison with the other women decreased. None of the interactions with time since the pregnancy loss reached significance for any other of the risk factors.

Physical symptoms, previous pregnancy loss, preloss partner relationship, and preloss social support did not reach significance for the total PGS score in the hierarchical multiple regression analysis. However, on examination of the bivariate correlations of these risk factors to grief intensity, it appeared that only a history of a pregnancy loss did not reach the 5% significance level. All other risk factors significantly related to grief intensity as hypothesized.

When including the exploratively examined risk factors in the analysis (education, [un]employment, religious background, support from religion, ambivalence, and difficulty in conceiving), the additional variance that could be explained did not reach significance (F-change=1.32, df=16,167, P=.3).

COMMENT

In this article, we report the results of a prospective study of risk factors predicting grief intensity following a pregnancy loss. Some important risk factors, which in earlier studies were based on retrospective recall, were now prospectively assessed in pregnant women. We found that those women who had been pregnant for a relatively longer time showed more intense grief reactions following the pregnancy loss. This result supports Peppers and Knapp's[46] theory that motherly attachment to the fetus increases with length of pregnancy and, as a consequence, relates to stronger grief following a pregnancy loss. We also found that women who had relatively more preloss psychiatric symptoms, who showed a more neurotic personality, or who did not have children at the time of the loss, showed more intense grief reactions following the pregnancy loss. The result regarding neuroticism makes extra sense since, in earlier studies, because of the lack of prospective data, it was uncertain whether individuals with more neurotic personalities were predisposed to a problematic outcome.

Only in a bivariate analysis did physical symptoms, preloss partner relationship, and preloss social support prove to be significantly related to grief intensity as hypothesized. Apparently, women who have more physical symptoms and a relatively low-quality partner relationship and who receive relatively little social support are at increased risk of a problematic outcome, although other risk factors are more important. Previous pregnancy loss did not relate to grief intensity following a new loss. As was sometimes found earlier, women who have experienced a pregnancy loss earlier in life are not more prone to experience a complicated outcome following a subsequent loss. Older women experienced significantly more difficulty coping after the loss. Although one might expect this result, since older women have less time left in which to conceive and might be more fearful of increasing fertility problems, Toedter and colleagues[18] found the opposite in their study. It is unlikely that the contrasting results might be a consequence of a difference in age in both studies and, furthermore, both studies used the same grief measure. However, the contrasting results might be a product of differences in the sample selection. Toedter et al used a clinically referred loss sample, whereas pregnant women unaware of the loss to come voluntarily signed up for this study. Findings relating to age are important, however, given current trends. Older women should be informed that they can experience relatively more feelings of difficulty coping, following a pregnancy loss.

The examined risk factors together explained the 35% rate of the between-variance in grief scores. This substantial result probably means that the more important risk factors for a problematic outcome following a pregnancy loss have been highlighted. Thirty-one percent of the within-variance was explained by time since the loss and 2% by the interaction between time since the loss and the risk factors. Our study showed that grief intensity decreases with time, confirming the results of other recent studies. Only the interaction of preloss psychiatric symptoms and time since the loss appeared to be significant for both total PGS and the subscales. Any significant interaction also showed that the effect of the risk factor was the strongest shortly following the pregnancy loss and decreased with time.

Some methodological points should be considered when interpreting the results of the study. The first is that all the women signed up for the study voluntarily. One may wonder whether this type of selection could have produced biased results that might account for the differences between this study and the studies that used clinical samples.[2-8,15,18-20] It is hard to give a definitive answer to this question. Examination of the present sample suggests that the sample is a fairly good representation of the women who experience a pregnancy loss in the Netherlands. Furthermore, the dropout in this study was very low and was not selective. A potential threat to the generalizability of the results might be the seemingly high percentage of women (41%) who had experienced a previous pregnancy loss. However, since at least 1 in every 10 pregnancies fail,[47] a relatively high percentage of women in their reproductive period could be expected to have a history of a pregnancy loss. Other studies also found that large numbers of women (26%-37%) had experienced a previous pregnancy loss,[2,6,7,13,15,19-21] indicating that this is not an uncommon occurrence. Given our sample characteristics, it might well be supposed that the results are fairly generalizable to the community at large. A second point that needs further attention is that data were gathered by means of self-report. As Watson and Pennebaker[48] have shown, people with a high negative affect subjectively report more somatopsychic distress, whereas the relation to objective health status is not strong. It may be argued, therefore, that the relationship between neuroticism and intense grief found in this study might only be a result of measuring the same construct. It should be pointed out, however, that 2 completely independent scales were used to assess 2 constructs that are also theoretically thought to be different, ie, the personality trait of neuroticism and the situation-related concept of grief. What is more, using a self-report measure is a logical step because grief is a subjectively experienced reaction on which only the woman herself can report. Finally, it would have been better to have a psychiatric interview included in the study to obtain better insight into the exact occurrence of psychopathologic symptoms in women following a pregnancy loss. Because this was not done, the number of women who might actually have been diagnosed as having developed a psychiatric disorder remains unknown.

Information concerning risk factors for the more complicated grief reactions is of importance because it allows caregivers to screen, at an early stage, women at risk of developing those kinds of reaction. In cases where the pregnancy results in a premature loss, health care workers could respond in a manner geared specifically to the women's individual circumstances and could provide additional care to the women at risk to try to prevent grief disturbances in those women.

Accepted for publication March 28, 1996.

Financial support for this research was provided by the Foundation VSB (Verenigde Spaarbank) Fund, Utrecht, the Netherlands.

Reprints: Hettie J. E. M. Janssen, PhD, University of Nijmegen, Department of Clinical Psychology and Personality, Montessorilaan 3, Postbox 9104, 6500 HE Nijmegen, the Netherlands.

REFERENCES

1. Zeanah CH. Adaptation following perinatal loss: a critical review. *J Am Acad Child Adolesc Psychiatry.* 1989;28:467-480.
2. Benfield DG, Leib SA, Vollman JH. Grief response of parents to neonatal death and parent participation in deciding care. *Pediatrics.* 1978;62:171-177.
3. Cuisinier MCJ, Kuijpers JC, Hoogduin CAL, de Graauw CPHM, Janssen HJEM. Miscarriage and stillbirth: time since the loss, grief intensity and satisfaction with care. *Eur J Obstet Gynecol Reprod Biol.* 1993;52:163-168.
4. Dyregrov A, Matthiesen SB. Stillbirth, neonatal death and sudden infant death (SIDS): parental reactions. *Scand J Psychol.* 1987;28:104-114.
5. Feeley N, Gottlieb LN. Parents' coping and communication following their infant's death. *Omega.* 1988-89;19:51-67.
6. Forrest GC, Standish E, Baum JD. Support after perinatal death: a study of support and counselling after perinatal bereavement. *BMJ.* 1982;285:1475-1479.
7. Friedman T, Gath D. The psychiatric consequences of spontaneous abortion. *Br J Psychiatry.* 1989;155:810-813.
8. Graham MA, Thompson SC, Estrada M, Yonekure ML. Factors affecting psychological adjustment to a fetal death. *Am J Obstet Gynecol.* 1987;157:254-257.
9. Kennell JH, Slyter H, Klaus MH. The mourning response of parents to the death of a newborn infant. *N Engl J Med.* 1970;13:344-349.
10. LaRoche C, Lalinec-Michaud M, Engelsmann F, Fuller N, Copp M, McQuade-Soldatos L. Grief reactions to perinatal death: a follow-up study. *Can J Psychiatry.* 1984;29:14-19.
11. LaRoche C, Lalinec-Michaud M, Engelsmann F, Fuller N, Copp M, Vasilevsky K. Grief reactions to perinatal death: an exploratory study. *Psychosomatics.* 1982;23:510-518.
12. Laurell-Borulf Y. Longterm adjustment after an emotional crisis. In: *Krislosning I langtidsperspektive.* Lund, Sweden: Ed. Studenlitteratur; 1982:157-167.
13. Nicol MT, Tompkins JR, Campbell NA, Syme GJ. Maternal grieving response after perinatal death. *Med J Aust.* 1986;144:287-289.
14. Peppers LG, Knapp RJ. Maternal reactions to involuntary fetal/infant death. *Psychiatry.* 1980;43:155-159.
15. Rowe J, Clyman R, Green C, Mikkelsen C, Haight J, Ataide L. Follow-up of families who experience a perinatal death. *Pediatrics.* 1978;62:166-170.
16. Smith AC, Borgers SB. Parental grief response to perinatal death. *Omega.* 1988-89;19:203-214.
17. Theut SK, Pedersen FA, Zaslow MJ, Cain RL, Rabinovich BA, Morihisa JM. Perinatal loss and parental bereavement. *Am J Psychiatry.* 1989;146:635-639.
18. Toedter LJ, Lasker JN, Alhadeff JM. The Perinatal Grief Scale: development and initial validation. *Am J Orthopsychiatry.* 1988;58:435-449.
19. Tudehope DI, Iredell J, Rodgers D, Gunn A. Neonatal death: grieving families. *Med J Aust.* 1986;144:290-291.
20. Turner MJ, Flannelly GM, Wingfield M, Rasmussen MJ, Ryan R, Cullen S, Maguire R, Stronge JM. The miscarriage clinic: an audit of the first year. *Br J Obstet Gynaecol.* 1991;98:306-308.
21. Toedter LJ, Lasker JN, Campbell DT. The comparison group problem in bereavement studies and the retrospective pretest. *Evaluation Rev.* 1990;14:75-90.
22. Cole D. It might have been: mourning the unborn. *Psychol Today.* 1987;21:64-65.
23. Condon JT. Management of established pathological grief reaction after stillbirth. *Am J Psychiatry.* 1986;143:987-992.
24. Sanders CM. Risk factors in bereavement outcome. In: Stroebe MS, Stroebe W, Hansson RO, eds. *Handbook of Bereavement: Theory, Research, and Intervention.* New York, NY: Cambridge University Press; 1993:255-267.
25. Stroebe W, Stroebe MS. Determinants of adjustment to bereavement in younger widows and widowers. In: Stroebe MS, Stroebe W, Hansson RO, eds. *Handbook of Bereavement: Theory, Research, and Intervention.* Cambridge, Mass: University Press; 1993:208-226.
26. Meuser TM, Davies RM, Marwit SJ. Personality and conjugal bereavement in older widow(er)s. *Omega.* 1994-95;30:223-235.
27. Sanders CM. Risk factors in bereavement outcome. *J Soc Issues.* 1988;44:97-111.
28. Stroebe W, Stroebe MS, Domitter G. Individual and situational differences in recovery from bereavement: a risk group identified. *J Soc Issues.* 1988;44:143-158.
29. Shuchter SR, Zisook S. The course of normal grief. In: Stroebe MS, Stroebe W, Hansson RO, eds. *Handbook of Bereavement: Theory, Research, and Intervention.* Cambridge, Mass: University Press; 1993:23-43.
30. Wortman CB, Silver RC. The myths of coping with loss. *J Consult Clin Psychol.* 1989;57:349-357.
31. Gallagher-Thompson D, Futterman A, Farberow N, Thompson LW, Peterson J. The impact of spousal bereavement on older widows and widowers. In: Stroebe MS, Stroebe W, Hansson RO, eds. *Handbook of Bereavement: Theory, Research, and Intervention.* Cambridge, Mass: University Press; 1993:227-239.
32. Goldbach KRC, Dunn DS, Toedter LJ, Lasker JN. The effects of gestational age and gender on grief after pregnancy loss. *Am J Orthopsychiatry.* 1991;61:461-467.
33. McCrae RR, Costa PT. Psychological resilience among widowed men and women: a 10-year follow-up of a national sample. In: Stroebe MS, Stroebe W, Hansson RO, eds. *Handbook of Bereavement: Theory, Research, and Intervention.* Cambridge, Mass: University Press. 1993:196-207.
34. Arrindell WA, Ettema H. *SCL-90: Handleiding bij een Multidimensionele Psychopathologie Indicator.* Lisse, the Netherlands: Swets & Zeitlinger; 1986.
35. Derogatis LR. *SCL-90: Administration, Scoring and Procedure: Manual I for the Revised Version.* Baltimore, Md: The John Hopkins University School of Medicine; 1977.
36. Luteijn F, Starren J, van Dijk H. *Handleiding bij de Nederlandse Persoonlijkheids Vragenlijst, NPV.* Lisse, the Netherlands: Swets & Zeitlinger; 1985.
37. Evers A, van Vliet-Mulder JC, ter Laak J. *Documentatie van Tests en Testresearch in Nederland.* Assen/Maastricht, the Netherlands: Van Gorcum; 1992.
38. Lange A. *Handleiding bij de Interactionele Probleem Oplossings Vragenlijst, IPOV.* Deventer, the Netherlands: Van Loghum Slaterus; 1983.
39. Blake RL, McKay DA. A single-item measure of social support as a predictor of morbidity. *J Fam Pract.* 1986;22:82-84.
40. Potvin L, Lasker J, Toedter L. Measuring grief: a short version of the Perinatal Grief Scale. *J Psychopathol Behavior Assess.* 1989;11:24-45.
41. Lasker JN, Toedter LJ. Acute versus chronic grief: the case of pregnancy loss. *Am J Orthopsychiatry.* 1991;61:510-522.
42. Cuisinier MCJ, de Graauw CPHM, Kuijpers JC, Hoogduin CAL, van Minnen A. Meting van rouw na een zwangerschapsverlies: Eerste bevindingen met de Nederlandse versie van de Perinatal Grief Scale (PGS). *Tijdschr Psychiatrie.* 1992;34:651-656.
43. Cuisinier MC, Janssen HJ, de Graauw KP, Bakker S, Hoogduin CAL. Pregnancy following miscarriage or perinatal loss: course of grief and some determining factors. *J Psychosomat Obstet Gynecol.* In press.
44. Janssen HJEM, Cuisinier MCJ, Hoogduin CAL, de Graauw CPHM. Controlled prospective study on the mental health of women following pregnancy loss. *Am J Psychiatry.* 1996;153:226-230.
45. Cohen J, Cohen P. *Applied Multiple Regresssion: Correlation Analysis for the Behavioral Sciences.* 2nd ed. Hillsdale, NJ: Lawrence Erlbaum Assoc Publishers; 1983.
46. Peppers LG, Knapp RJ. *Motherhood and Mourning: Perinatal Death.* New York, NY: Praeger Publishers; 1980.
47. Scott JR. Spontaneous abortion. In: Scott JR, Disaia PJ, Hammond CB, Spellacy WN, eds. *Obstetrics and Gynecology.* Philadelphia, Pa: JB Lippincott; 1990; 209-220.
48. Watson D, Pennebaker JW. Health complaints, stress, and distress: exploring the central role of negative affectivity. *Psychol Rev.* 1989;96:234-254.

ORIGINAL ARTICLE

Behavior of Boys in Kindergarten and the Onset of Substance Use During Adolescence

Louise C. Mâsse, PhD; Richard E. Tremblay, PhD

Background: The purpose of this study was to assess the usefulness of personality dimensions measured at ages 6 and 10 years in predicting early onset of cigarette smoking, alcohol abuse, and other drug use in boys. In addition, the stability of the prediction between the measurements at ages 6 and 10 years was investigated.

Methods: Data from a large longitudinal study of boys were used to assess the relation between childhood personality and the onset of substance use from 10 to 15 years of age. Childhood personalities were assessed by teachers' ratings of behaviors. Self-reports of smoking cigarettes, getting drunk, and using other drugs provided the measurement of substance use. Discrete-time survival analysis was used for the statistical analyses.

Results: High novelty-seeking and low harm avoidance significantly predict early onset of substance use (eg, cigarettes, alcohol, and other drugs), but reward dependence was unrelated to any of the outcomes studied. The results also indicated that either set of predictors (ie, the personality dimensions measured at ages 6 and 10 years) could be used to predict onset of cigarette smoking, getting drunk, and other drug use, because the power of prediction was similar between the measurements at ages 6 and 10 years.

Conclusions: High novelty-seeking and low harm avoidance lead to early onset of substance use in boys. The stability of the prediction between ages 6 and 10 years suggests that the kindergarten assessments may be used for preventive efforts at school entry instead of waiting until early adolescence.

Arch Gen Psychiatry. 1997;54:62-68

From the School of Public Health, Center for Health Promotion Research and Development, University of Texas–Houston (Dr Mâsse); and the Research Unit of Children's Psycho-Social Maladjustment, University of Montréal, Montréal, Québec (Dr Tremblay).

UNDERSTANDING early onset of substance use has important implications for the development of effective prevention programs, mainly because early onset is often a marker for other persistent problems.[1-8] In recent longitudinal studies, the effects of childhood behaviors and family characteristics have been shown to predict onset of substance use among adolescents.[9-12] Although disruptive behavior and family environment have been linked to substance abuse, it has recently been suggested that basic personality dimensions are the underlying link between disruptive behavior and substance abuse.[1,13,14] In this perspective, the basic personality dimensions are hypothesized to be indirectly linked to some genetic components that may be related to the onset of substance use. Cloninger,[15] for example, suggested that alcoholism characterized by early onset of alcohol-seeking behavior (ie, type 2 alcoholism), would be predicted by a specific pattern of personality dimensions and that this pattern would differ for those who have late onset of alcohol-seeking behavior (ie, type 1 alcoholism). In Cloninger's theory, 3 personality dimensions—referred as to novelty-seeking, harm avoidance, and reward dependence—are hypothesized to be related to the behavioral activation, inhibition, and maintenance systems, respectively. More specifically, the novelty-seeking dimension refers to a heritable tendency toward exploratory activity and exhilaration that is activated by novel or appetitive stimuli. The harm avoidance dimension refers to the heritable tendency to react intensively to aversive stimuli, therefore controlling the learning mechanisms that facilitate inhibitive behaviors. Finally, the reward dependence dimension is assumed to condition the brain system responsible for onset of reward or relief of punishment. In Cloninger's

See Subjects and Methods on next page

SUBJECTS AND METHODS

SUBJECTS

The subjects (N=1034) for this study were obtained from an ongoing longitudinal study[19] that began collecting data when the boys were at the end of their kindergarten year (mean [±SD] age, 6.23±0.30 years). Subjects in this cohort were all white boys who attended 53 low socioeconomic French-speaking schools in Montréal, Québec. Subjects were retained only if both parents were born in Canada and were French-speaking. This yielded a sample that was culturally homogeneous (ie, white, French-speaking, nonimmigrant boys living in low socioeconomic areas of a large urban city). Most of the boys (67%) in this sample lived with both parents when they attended kindergarten. The mean (±SD) number of school years completed by the parents was 10.5±2.8 for the mothers and 10.7±3.2 for the fathers. At the birth of their sons, mothers were mean (±SD) 25.4±4.8 years old and fathers were 28.4±5.6 years old. Informed consent was obtained from the parents when the boys were younger than 14 years. When the boys were 14 years and older, parents and boys had to give informed consent. This study was approved by the review board for human subjects at the University of Montréal.

ATTRITION AND MISSING DATA

Subjects with incomplete data sets were eliminated from the analyses. The alcohol analyses had 784 subjects; 199 were eliminated because of missing information about alcohol abuse and 51 because of missing data on the personality variables. For the drug use analyses, 772 subjects were used, because 209 had missing information about initiation to drug use and 53 had missing information on at least 1 of the personality variables. For the cigarette analyses, the sample was reduced to 656 subjects, because 335 had missing information about cigarette use and 43 had missing information on at least 1 personality variable. The cigarette data analyses had more missing information, because questions pertaining to cigarette use started only at age 13 years.

The attritional bias was assessed by comparing the personality characteristics of the subjects included in the analyses with those who were excluded from the analyses. Because subjects had incomplete information about substance use, multiple χ^2 analyses were computed for each personality variable and substance instead of using a log-linear analysis. The results of these χ^2 analyses indicated that the subjects who were excluded from the original analyses did not differ significantly from those included in the original analyses. This finding was generalized across personality dimensions (ie, novelty-seeking, harm avoidance, and reward dependence), substances (ie, alcohol, drugs, and cigarettes), and ages (ie, personality dimensions measured at ages 6 and 10 years). These analyses indicated that the sample analyzed in this study did not differ significantly from the original sample.

INSTRUMENT

Personality Dimensions

Cloninger's personality dimensions were inferred from 2 teacher-rated questionnaires aimed at measuring childhood behavior, namely the Preschool Behavior Questionnaire[21] and the Prosocial Behaviour Questionnaire.[22] Harm avoidance, described by Cloninger as being cautious, apprehensive, and inhibited, was assessed with the following items: worries about many things, fears or is afraid of new things or new situations, and cries easily. The novelty-seeking dimension, which Cloninger defines as impulsive, excitable, and exploratory behaviors, was a composite of the following items: restless, runs about or jumps up and down and does not keep still, squirmy, and fidgety. The reward dependence dimension is defined by Cloninger as being warm, sympathetic, and sentimental, was a composite of the following 10 items: praises others, shows sympathy, helps sick child, helps hurt child, helps child in a difficult task, helps clean up mess, invites bystander, stops quarrels, helps pick up objects, and comforts upset children. Cronbach α values at age 6 years for the studied sample were as follows: .72 for harm avoidance, .89 for novelty-seeking, and .91 for reward dependence. To verify that each construct reflects these independent dimensions, the correlations among the dimensions were assessed in kindergarten. As expected, all 3 correlations (r=0.12 at age 6 years and 0.11 at age 10 years for harm avoidance and novelty-seeking, r=0.10 at age 6 years and −0.01 at age 10 years for harm avoidance and reward dependence, and r=−0.13 at age 6 years and −0.07 at age 10 years for novelty-seeking and reward dependence) were low and indicated that the dimensions were independent. To assess the stability of the personality dimensions, early childhood personality dimensions were assessed when the boys were 6 years old, and later childhood personality dimensions were measured when the boys were 10 years old.

Continued on next page

theory,[13,15,16] persons with high novelty-seeking, low harm avoidance, and low reward-dependence scores are hypothesized to predict type 2 alcoholism. This pattern was of specific interest in the present study because it is characterized by early onset of alcohol-seeking behavior.

Evidence supporting Cloninger's theory has been found in a sample of 431 Swedish males, which indicated that the 3 personality dimensions, measured at age 11 years, predicted type 2 alcoholism at age 27 years.[14] Although this study focused on alcohol intake, the theory has been used to predict other types of substances used and abused in adolescents and adults.[17,18] For example, in a cross-sectional sample of 12- to 15-year-olds, Wills et al[17] found that high novelty-seeking, low harm avoidance, and low reward dependence were significantly related to cigarette smoking and alcohol and marijuana use. In contrast, in a sample of 240 adult smokers, Pomerleau et al[18] found that persons whose scores were high on novelty-seeking and low on harm avoidance had high scores on a measure of smoking addiction. Their results, however, did not show a relation between low reward dependence and smoking addiction.

Cloninger[13] argues that the 3 personality dimensions are in part genetically determined and that these dimensions appear early in the child's development and remain stable over time. Recent studies[19,20] confirm this hypothesis: personalities at age 6 years were found useful to predict antisocial behavior[19] and personalities at

Substance Use

Information pertaining to the boys' level of substance use was assessed with a self-report questionnaire. Self-report use was obtained because it has proved to be a valid assessment of delinquent behaviors in previous studies.[23,24] This information was gathered at ages 11, 12, 13, 14, and 15 years during visits to the schools the boys attended. The questionnaire had questions pertaining to alcohol, drug, and cigarette use or abuse. To assess alcohol abuse, the boys were asked if they had been drunk in the past 12 months. The drug use questions assessed if the boys had used any drugs (ie, marijuana, crack, or other drugs) in the past 12 months. Finally, tobacco use was measured by asking the boys if they had smoked cigarettes in the past 12 months, at ages 13, 14, and 15. Because we anticipated that some boys might have experimented before we started to question them about substance use, the boys were asked each year to report when they first started to smoke cigarettes, to get drunk, or to use other drugs. This information also served to cross-validate the information provided by the boys and to identify inconsistency in the data.

STATISTICAL ANALYSIS

Discrete-time survival analyses were carried out to assess which personality variables influenced the onset of substance use. To compute the discrete-time survival analyses, the data had to be transformed. First, one variable measuring the age of the particular record (last period) had to be created as well as one that identified whether the event of interest had occurred (censored). The censored variable was a dichotomous variable that indicated whether the event occurred for the period recorded. For example, if the subject started to abuse alcohol at age 12 years, the last period would indicate the age of initiation to be 12 years for this subject and the censored variable would indicate that this subject started to abuse alcohol (ie, censored=1). For subjects unavailable for follow-up, the last period indicated the last record of this subject and the censored variable was coded as zero if the event did not occur. When these 2 variables were created, the data were converted using the Singer and Willet[25] procedure to prepare the data for computing discrete-time survival analyses with standard logistic regression software. Logistic regression analyses were computed on the transformed data, and they served to estimate the parameters of the discrete-time hazard model. These parameters were then used to recapture the fitted hazard and survival functions. The SAS[26] procedure LOGIST was used to calculate the parameters estimate. For more information on how to use this procedure see Singer and Willet.[25,27] Six discrete-time survival analyses were computed, 1 for each set of personality variables (kindergarten and later childhood personality dimensions) and each type of substance (alcohol, drugs, and cigarettes) used. The response variable for these analyses was dichotomous and measured the use or nonuse of substances and the time at which the subjects reported using or abusing the substance. The 3 personality variables (harm avoidance, novelty-seeking, and reward dependence) were evaluated as potential moderators for the risks of abusing or using substances. A hierarchical procedure was used to select the dimensions that significantly moderate the risk of substance use. The significance of the dimensions was evaluated by the Wald χ^2 statistic with the overall adequacy of the model judged by the model χ^2 statistic, and a P value less than .05 was considered significant. The accuracy of the prediction was also assessed with the Somers D_{yx} rank correlation.[28] The Somers D_{yx} rank correlation was used to determine the relation with the substance used and each of the personality dimensions. This index has a similar interpretation as the multiple correlation in linear regression, but it is a better measure of association when the dependent and independent variables are ordinal.

RELIABILITY OF RISK PREDICTION

The reliability of the kindergarten and childhood personality dimensions to predict risk of onset for use of substances was evaluated by assessing the proportion of predicted use for each substance. The number of correct, incorrect, and tied observations assessed the reliability of the tridimensional personality structure in predicting the onset of substance use and comparing the stability of the prediction. The validity of the kindergarten personality dimensions in predicting onset of substance use was assessed by comparing the contingency table from the kindergarten predictors with those of later childhood predictors. Log-linear analyses assessed whether the classification significantly differed for the 2 sets of predictors (ie, kindergarten vs later childhood personality dimensions) and verified whether the strength of the relation was the same across substances. Akaike Information Criteria,[29] in which a lower value indicates a better fit, also were used to compare overall fit between models.

age 3 years to predict adult psychiatric disorders.[20] Although the usefulness of the early personality dimensions has been shown for predicting antisocial behavior and psychiatric disorders, the stability of these predictions over time for the onset of substance use remains to be investigated.

Thus, the first aim of this study was to test, in a sample of high-risk boys, the hypothesis that high novelty-seeking, low harm avoidance, and low reward dependence measured at ages 6 and 10 years will predict early onset of cigarette use, alcohol abuse, and other drug use. The second aim of this study was to compare the effectiveness of the personality measurements at ages 6 and 10 years in predicting early onset of substance use. This latter comparison was of interest for preventive purposes, because the sooner we can identify children at risk the earlier we can implement preventive efforts.

RESULTS

AGE AT ONSET

The **Figure** shows the age at onset for getting drunk, using other drugs, and cigarette smoking. As expected, the proportion of substances used increased with age. By age 15 years, 47.5% of the boys reported being drunk in the last year, but only 30.5% said that they had used some other drugs in the last 12 months.

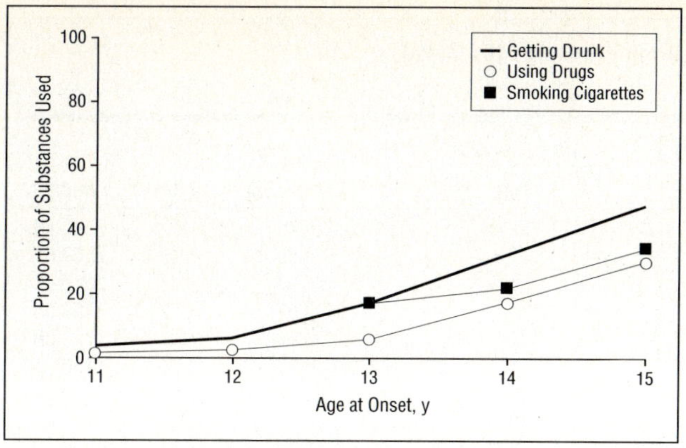

Onset of smoking cigarettes, getting drunk, and using drugs.

PERSONALITY DIMENSIONS AS PREDICTORS

The usefulness of the personality dimensions to predict substance use is shown in **Table 1**. The novelty-seeking and harm avoidance dimensions were found to predict onset of getting drunk, using drugs, and smoking cigarettes, but reward dependence was unrelated to the substances studied. The results also indicate that the predictions were the same regardless of the age at which the predictor variables were measured (ages 6 and 10 years). The parameter estimates indicate that high novelty-seeking and low harm avoidance were significantly related to the onset of use of the substances investigated. Although personality may change with experience and age, these results seem to indicate that some stability exists with these personality dimensions over time. This stability is further confirmed by the significant correlations that are found between the kindergarten and later childhood measurements (novelty-seeking, n=896, r=0.38, P<.01; harm avoidance, n=901, r=0.24, P<.01; and reward dependence, n=900, r=0.18, P<.01).

STABILITY OF PERSONALITY DIMENSIONS

The reliability of the age 6- and 10-year personality dimensions to predict onset of substance use is given in **Table 2**. These reliabilities are computed for the models, including only the significant dimensions (ie, novelty-seeking and harm avoidance). For all substances, the results indicate that the prediction of use or nonuse did not differ between the kindergarten and later childhood predictors. The percentage of correct, incorrect, and tied classifications were almost identical for the 2 sets of predictors. The Somers D_{yx} correlations also showed a similar relation between the kindergarten and age 10 years predictors. To further assess the usefulness of the personality dimensions, the reliability of the null model (ie, a model without the 3 personality dimensions but including the time indicator variables) also is given in Table 2. The results indicate that adding novelty-seeking and harm avoidance as predictors of substance use increased in all cases the accuracy of the prediction, regardless of the time at which the personality characteristics were measured. Adding these dimensions resulted in a decrease in tied predictions, which in turn resulted in a larger increase of correct predictions. Similar Akaike Information Criteria values between sets of predictors further indicate that either set of predictors may be used to predict early onset of substance use. In fact, the Akaike Information Criteria for drug use (kindergarten=1728.36 vs later childhood predictors=1730.21), cigarette smoking (kindergarten=1870.28 vs later childhood predictors=1872.82), and alcohol abuse (kindergarten=2307.61 vs later childhood predictors=2315.04) were quite similar and

Table 1. Hazard Models Predicting Onset of Alcohol Abuse, Drug Abuse, and Cigarette Smoking

Age, y	Parameter*	Parameter Estimates (SE)	Wald χ^2
	Alcohol Abuse		
6	D1	−3.36 (0.22)	240.83†
	D2	−3.06 (0.20)	230.01†
	D3	−2.31 (0.17)	180.92†
	D4	−1.36 (0.15)	79.60†
	D5	−0.90 (0.16)	33.88†
	Novelty-seeking	0.14 (0.04)	13.96†
	Harm avoidance	−0.17 (0.04)	22.02†
	Reward dependence	0.01 (0.01)	0.11
10	D1	−3.30 (0.21)	246.58†
	D2	−3.08 (0.20)	237.23†
	D3	−2.24 (0.16)	186.64†
	D4	−1.40 (0.15)	91.91†
	D5	−0.90 (0.15)	38.23†
	Novelty-seeking	0.16 (0.04)	16.83†
	Harm avoidance	−0.13 (0.04)	12.64†
	Reward dependence	−0.01 (0.01)	0.04
	Drug Abuse		
6	D1	−3.81 (0.28)	192.13†
	D2	−3.88 (0.28)	183.99†
	D3	−2.99 (0.22)	183.79†
	D4	−1.80 (0.18)	103.93†
	D5	−1.22 (0.17)	51.96†
	Novelty-seeking	0.18 (0.04)	16.75†
	Harm avoidance	−0.16 (0.04)	14.46†
	Reward dependence	0.02 (0.01)	3.01
10	D1	−3.97 (0.28)	204.83†
	D2	−4.12 (0.30)	189.38†
	D3	−3.13 (0.22)	207.87†
	D4	−1.98 (0.17)	133.75†
	D5	−1.39 (0.16)	72.68†
	Novelty-seeking	0.18 (0.04)	16.85†
	Harm avoidance	−0.13 (0.04)	10.29†
	Reward dependence	−0.01 (0.01)	0.03
	Cigarette Smoking		
6	D1	−1.89 (0.16)	136.19†
	D2	−2.31 (0.18)	169.04†
	D3	−1.69 (0.17)	105.76†
	Novelty-seeking	0.10 (0.04)	6.80†
	Harm avoidance	−0.14 (0.04)	13.45†
	Reward dependence	0.00 (0.01)	0.00
10	D1	−1.95 (0.15)	160.09†
	D2	−2.40 (0.17)	194.36†
	D3	−1.76 (0.16)	127.07†
	Novelty-seeking	0.14 (0.04)	12.28†
	Harm avoidance	−0.09 (0.04)	6.42†
	Reward dependence	−0.00 (0.01)	0.00

**D1, D2, D3, D4, and D5 are the main effects of age indicators.*
†Parameter is significant at an α of .05.

Table 2. Reliability of Prediction for the Null (N) Model, the Kindergarten Predictors (K) Model, and the Later Childhood Predictors (L) Model

Substance	Model	Classification, % Correct	Incorrect	Tied	Somers D_{xy} Correlation	AIC*
Alcohol	N	64.5	18.5	17.0	0.46	2336.43
	K	74.1	24.1	1.8	0.50	2307.61
	L	74.0	24.4	1.6	0.50	2315.04
Drugs	N	67.3	15.6	17.1	0.52	1750.05
	K	77.3	20.8	1.9	0.57	1728.36
	L	77.1	21.3	1.6	0.56	1730.21
Cigarettes	N	39.9	26.8	33.3	0.13	1884.91
	K	58.7	37.8	3.5	0.21	1870.28
	L	58.2	38.5	3.3	0.20	1872.82

*AIC indicates Akaike Information Criteria.[29]

Table 3. Survival and Hazard Functions for All Substances

Age, y	Survival* Alcohol	Drugs	Cigarettes	Hazard† Alcohol	Drugs	Cigarettes
11	.96	.98	...	.04	.02	...
12	.92	.97	...	.05	.02	...
13	.83	.93	.87	.10	.04	.14
14	.66	.81	.79	.21	.12	.09
15	.46	.65	.66	.30	.20	.16

*Probability of not using a substance.
†Probability of starting to use or abuse a substance.

did suggest that both sets of predictors were useful to predict substance use.

Table 2 also indicates that although the percentages of correct predictions were similar among the substances, the reliability of the predictions differed with the type of substance consumed. Indeed, the Somers D_{xy} correlation was smaller for cigarette use than for the other 2 substances. Further log-linear analyses, assessing differences in the number of correct, incorrect, and tied observations among the substances studied, indicated that a model including only the main effects of "substance" adequately explained the observed frequencies ($\chi^2[df=6, n=600]=.06$, $P=.99$), thus suggesting that the reliability of the prediction was the same for the 2 sets of predictors and that the prediction differed with the substance consumed. The personality dimensions were more reliable in predicting onset of getting drunk and using other drugs than they were in predicting onset of cigarette smoking.

The survival and hazard functions estimated with the 2 significant dimensions (novelty-seeking and harm avoidance) are given in **Table 3**. As expected, the probability of using any substance increased with age, and children were more likely to experiment with alcohol first. Experimenting started at age 13 years for getting drunk, but it was delayed by 1 year for other drug use. Cigarette smoking was started by age 13 years. Cigarette smoking probably started earlier, but the lack of earlier data on this variable did not allow us to confirm this hypothesis.

COMMENT

The main objective of this study was to assess the usefulness of Cloninger's personality dimensions in predicting the onset of cigarette smoking, alcohol abuse (ie, getting drunk), and other drug use. The results suggested that novelty-seeking and harm avoidance significantly predicted the onset of cigarette smoking, getting drunk, and using drugs in adolescent boys. As expected from Cloninger's theory, boys who had a high score on novelty-seeking and a low score on harm avoidance were more likely to use substances at an early age. These results only partially confirmed Cloninger's theory, because we did not find that reward dependence significantly moderated the risk of early onset of substance use. Cloninger et al,[14] however, indicated that the level of prediction for the reward dependence dimension was not as high as the other dimensions, which was also observed by Tremblay et al.[19] It is unclear why reward dependence was not found to be a predictor of substance use. It is possible that because this study focused on early onset, we could not differentiate between the experimenters and abusers. Although reward dependence was not found to be significant, it may play an important role in identifying those who will persist and maintain these behaviors. Differences also were seen in the strength of the predictions for the novelty-seeking and harm avoidance dimensions. These differences were related to the outcome predicted and the age at which the personality dimensions were measured. At age 6 years, low harm avoidance was observed to be the strongest predictor for the onset of smoking and getting drunk, but novelty-seeking was found to be a stronger predictor for the onset of other drug use. At age 10 years, novelty-seeking was found to be the strongest predictor for all outcomes studied. Because the interrelations between these 3 dimensions over time are not yet understood, future work in this area should focus on this aspect of the model.

Although novelty-seeking and harm avoidance were both found to predict the 3 outcomes studied, the prediction for cigarette use was the weakest. Our lack of data on smoking at ages 11 and 12 years might explain those differences. The most extreme cases of high novelty-seeking and low harm avoidance probably were those who started smoking before the data pertaining to smoking were first collected. It is also possible that the lower prediction may reflect that smoking is a less deviant behavior and may not be as well predicted with Cloninger's model. Further research on this issue may help clarify or interpret our findings.

This longitudinal data set also enabled us to compare the stability of the personality characteristics at ages 6 and 10 years in predicting the onset of substance use. The results indicate that early (6 years of age) and late (10 years of age) childhood personality dimensions had similar powers of prediction and that they both significantly predicted onset of substance use in adolescents. Although counterintuitive, these findings suggest that the personality traits are established as early as age 6 years. This would agree with Caspi et al,[20] who found that behavioral observations at age 3 years predict adult psychiatric disorders, and Tremblay et al,[19] who observed that personalities at age 6 years predict antisocial behaviors. From a practical point of view, these results suggest that preventive initiatives may use early childhood personality dimensions, rated by kindergarten teachers, to identify children at risk for early onset of substance use. Waiting for later or better predictions may be self-defeating, because the deviant pattern may be more crystallized and thus harder to change. Although most substance abuse prevention programs focus on early and middle adolescence,[30] there are some indications that substance abuse prevention experts are considering preschool interventions as an alternative strategy.[31] It is hoped that the findings of this study will stimulate more early interventions.

From a theoretical perspective, these results confirm that the extreme personality characteristics, which characterize most psychopathologic illnesses,[13,15] have taken form by school entry, and they seem to be stable over time.[19,32] Furthermore, the early crystallization of the personality dimensions supports the idea that they are genetically grounded.[13,15,33] Although the building blocks of the personality dimensions may be inherited, the social and mental health problems that develop from these personalities probably are influenced by the quality of the environment in the preschool years.[34] From our results, it is clear that kindergarten boys who have high novelty-seeking and harm avoidance personalities are at risk of experimenting early with cigarettes, alcohol, and other drugs; however, not all kindergarten boys with these personality characteristics will initiate these activities early, and among those who do, some will desist. There is a need to conduct studies aimed at identifying the protective factors for initiators and desistors to understand better the environmental influences interacting with the personality characteristics.

The limitations of our study should not be overlooked. Because this study operationalized Cloninger's personality dimensions from questionnaires developed to measure children's social behaviors and thus were not specifically designed to measure these dimensions, the findings deserve to be replicated. One would expect that an instrument specifically designed to measure Cloninger's personality dimensions would lead to more powerful predictions, because our instrument may be less precise than Cloninger's. However, future study comparing our personality scales with those of Cloninger may clarify this issue. In addition, this study focused on white boys from low socioeconomic areas of a specific culture, so the generalizability of our findings remains to be determined for samples that include girls and other cultures. Finally, understanding the extent to which childhood personality dimensions will predict chronic use or abuse remains to be studied with this sample. A follow-up of these subjects through adulthood will be important to answer this question.

Accepted for publication August 28, 1996.

This study was conducted at the Research Unit of Children's Psycho-Social Maladjustment, University of Montréal, and was made possible by grants from the Social Sciences and Humanities Research Council of Canada, Québec's Conseil Québéçois pour la Recherche Sociale, and Québec's Fonds pour la Formation de Chercheur et l'Aide à la Recherche funding programs.

We thank Hélène Beauchesne, MScPsEd, and Lucille David, MScPsEd, for supervising the data collection and Lyse Desmarais Gervais, MScPsEd, for managing the data bank.

Reprints: Louise C. Mâsse, Center for Health Promotion Research and Development, University of Texas–Houston, PO Box 20186, RAS E-935, Houston, TX 77225.

REFERENCES

1. Brier N. Predicting antisocial behavior in younsters displaying poor academic achievement: a review of risk factors. *J Dev Behav Pediatr.* 1995;16:271-276.
2. Brook JS, Whiteman M, Cohen P, Tanaka JS. Childhood precursors of adolescent drug use: a longitudinal analysis. *Genet Soc Gen Psychol Monogr.* 1992; 118:1995-2213.
3. Flemming JP, Kellam SG, Brown CH. Early predictors of age at first use of alcohol, marijuana, and cigarettes. *Drug Alcohol Depend.* 1982;9:285-303.
4. Friedman AS, Bransfield SA, Tomko LA, Katz S. Early childhood and maternal antecedents to drug use. *J Drug Educ.* 1991;21:313-331.
5. Gregory LW. The 'turnaround' processs: factors influencing the school success of urban youth. *J Adoles Res.* 1995;10:136-154.
6. McCord J. Relationship between alcoholism and crime over life course. In: Kaplan HB, ed. *Drugs, Crime, and Other Deviant Adaptations: Longitudinal Studies.* New York, NY: Plenum Publishing Corp; 1995:129-141. Longitudi-

nal Research in the Social and Behavioral Sciences: An Interdisciplinary Series.
7. Webb JA, Baer PE, Caid CD, McLaughlin RJ, McKelvey RS. Concurrent and longitudinal assessement of risk for alcohol use among seventh graders. *J Early Adolescence.* 1991;11:450-465.
8. White HR. Early problem behavior and later drug problems. *J Res Crime Delinquency.* 1992;29:412-429.
9. Brook JS, Cohen P. A developmental perspective on drug use and delinquency. In: McCord J, ed. *Facts, Frameworks, and Forecasts: Advances in Criminology Theory.* New Brunswick, NJ: Transaction Publishers; 1992;3: 231-251.
10. Dobkin PL, Tremblay RE, Mâsse LC, Vitaro F. Individual and peer characteristics in predicting boys' early onset of substance abuse: a 7-year longitudinal study. *Child Dev.* 1995;66:1198-1214.
11. Kellam SG, Brown CH, Rubin BR, Ensminger ME. Paths leading to teenage psychiatric symptoms and substance use: developmental epidemiological studies in Woodlawn. In: Guze SB, Earls FJ, Barrets JE, eds. *Childhood Psychopathology Development.* New York, NY: Raven Press; 1983:17-51.
12. McCord J. Alcoholism: toward understanding genetic and social factors. *Psychiatry.* 1988;51:131-141.
13. Cloninger CR. A systematic method for clinical description and classification of personality variants. *Arch Gen Psychiatry.* 1987;44:573-588.
14. Cloninger CR, Sigvardsson S, Bohman M. Childhood personality predicts alcohol abuse in young adults. *Alcohol Clin Exp Res.* 1988;12:494-505.
15. Cloninger CR. Neurogenetic adaptive mechanisms in alcoholism. *Science.* 1987; 236:410-416.
16. Cloninger CR. A unified biosocial theory for personality and its role in the development of anxiety states. *Psychiatr Dev.* 1986;3:167-224.
17. Wills TA, Vaccaro D, McNamara G. Novelty-seeking, risk taking, and related contructs as predictors of adolescent substance use: an application of Cloninger's theory. *J Subst Abuse.* 1994;6:1-20.
18. Pomerleau CS, Pomerleau OF, Flessland KA, Basson SM. Relationship of TPQ scores to smoking variables in female and male smokers. *J Subst Abuse.* 1992; 4:143-153.
19. Tremblay RE, Pihl RO, Vitaro F, Dobkin PL. Predicting early onset of male antisocial behavior from preschool behavior. *Arch Gen Psychiatry.* 1994;51:732-739.
20. Caspi A, Moffitt TE, Newman DL, Silva PA. Behavioral observations at age 3 years predict adult psychiatric disorders: longitudinal evidence from a birth cohort. *Arch Gen Psychiatry.* 1996;53:1033-1039.
21. Behar LB, Stringfield S. A behavior rating scale for the preschool child. *Dev Psychol.* 1974;10:601-610.
22. Weir K, Duveen G. Further development and validation in the Prosocial Behaviour Questionnaire for use by teachers. *J Child Psychol Psychiatry.* 1981; 22:357-374.
23. Hindelang MJ, Hirschi T, Weirs JG. *Measuring Delinquency.* Beverly Hills, Calif: Sage Publications Inc; 1981.
24. Klein MW. *Cross-national Research in Self-reported Crime and Delinquency.* Dordrecht, the Netherlands: Kluwer Academic Publishers Group; 1989.
25. Singer JD, Willet JB. It's about time: using discrete-time survival analysis to study duration and the timing of events. *J Educ Stat.* 1993;18:155-195.
26. SAS Institute Inc. *SAS/STAT User's Guide, Version 6.* 4th ed. Cary, NC: SAS Institute Inc; 1989:846.
27. Singer JD, Willet JB. Modeling the days of our lives: using survival analysis when designing and analyzing longitudinal studies of duration and the timing of events. *Psychol Bull.* 1991;110:268-290.
28. Siegel S, Castellan NJ. *Nonparametric Statistics for the Behavioral Sciences.* 2nd ed. New York, NY: McGraw-Hill Book Co; 1988.
29. Bozdogan H. Model selection and Akaike's Information Criteria (AIC). *Psychometrika.* 1987;52:345-370.
30. Botvin GJ. Substance abuse prevention: theory, practice, and effectiveness. In: Tonry M, Wilson JY, eds. *Drugs and Crime.* Chicago, Ill: University of Chicago Press; 1990:461-519.
31. Hawkins JD, Arthur MW, Catalano RF. Preventing substance abuse. In: Tonry M, Farrington D, eds. *Building a Safer Society: Strategic Approaches to Crime Prevention.* Chicago, Ill: University of Chicago Press; 1995:343-427.
32. Caspi A, Bem DJ. Personality continuity and change across the life course. In: Pervin LA, ed. *Handbook of Personality: Theory and Research.* New York, NY: Guilford Press; 1990:549-575.
33. Kagan J. Reznick JS, Snidman N. The physiology and psychology of behavioral inhibition in children. *Child Dev.* 1987;58:1459-1473.
34. Higley JD, Hasert MF, Suomi SJ, Linnoila M. Nonhuman primate model of alcohol abuse: effects of early experience, personality, and stress on alcohol consumption. *Proc Natl Acad Sci U S A.* 1991;88:7261-7265.

Psychiatric and Substance Use Comorbidity Among Treatment-Seeking Opioid Abusers

Robert K. Brooner, PhD; Van L. King, MD; Michael Kidorf, PhD; Chester W. Schmidt, Jr, MD; George E. Bigelow, PhD

Background: Major studies of psychiatric comorbidity in opioid abusers reported rates of comorbidity that far exceeded general population estimates. These studies were published more than a decade ago and reported on few women and few substance use diagnoses.

Methods: Psychiatric and substance use comorbidity was assessed in 716 opioid abusers seeking methadone maintenance. *Diagnostic and Statistical Manual of Mental Disorders, Revised Third Edition* diagnostic assessment was conducted 1 month after admission. Rates of psychiatric and substance use disorder were compared by gender, and associations were assessed between psychiatric comorbidity and dimensional indexes of substance use severity, psychosocial impairment, and personality traits.

Results: Psychiatric comorbidity was documented in 47% of the sample (47% women and 48% men). Antisocial personality disorder (25.1%) and major depression (15.8%) were the most common diagnoses. Patients had at least 2 substance use diagnoses, most often opioid and cocaine dependence. Demographics, substance use history, and personality variables discriminated between patients with vs without comorbidity. Psychiatric comorbidity also was associated with a more severe substance use disorder.

Conclusions: Psychiatric comorbidity, especially personality and mood disorder, was common in men and women. The positive associations between psychiatric comorbidity and severity of substance use and other psychosocial problems were most consistent among those with antisocial personality.

Arch Gen Psychiatry. 1997;54:71-80

Substance abusers with other psychiatric disorders pose complex diagnostic and therapeutic challenges.[1] Despite questions about the independence of many psychiatric disorders (eg, mood and personality disorders) from the substance use disorders, comorbidity often is associated with poor treatment prognosis. For example, several psychiatric diagnoses in substance abusers, especially major depression and antisocial personality, often are associated with high rates of continued substance use and greater psychosocial impairment.[2-10] The importance of these associations is most telling among intravenous opioid and cocaine abusers, in whom drug use conveys the risk of transmitting human immunodeficiency virus and other infectious diseases.[11-18]

Studies of psychiatric comorbidity in opioid abusers[3,4,19,20] have found that about 80% of patients met the criteria for at least 1 nonsubstance use psychiatric disorder, with rates of mood disorder and antisocial personality disorder far exceeding general population estimates.[21] These studies have numerous strengths (eg, operationalized diagnostic criteria) but they were published more than a decade ago.[3,4,19,20] Temporal trends in the population or in the availability of drugs and drug abuse treatment could limit their generalizability to patients entering treatment more recently.

The earlier studies have further limitations: (1) Diagnoses were made on the day of admission or at varying times before and after starting treatment. It would be preferable to make diagnostic judgments after a brief period of stabilization in treatment to reduce the influence of acute stress on psychiatric symptom reporting.[22] (2) The only substance use categories evaluated were opioid and alcohol dependence. It would be instructive to extend the evaluation to the use of cocaine and other substances commonly used by opioid abusers.[23-29] (3) Women were underrepresented.[4,19,20]

See Subjects and Methods on next page

From the Behavioral Pharmacology Research Unit, Department of Psychiatry and Behavioral Sciences, The Johns Hopkins University School of Medicine, Baltimore, Md.

SUBJECTS AND METHODS

SUBJECTS

Study participants were 716 opioid-dependent men and women consecutively admitted to our outpatient methadone maintenance clinics in Baltimore, Md, during a 5-year period (April 1, 1989, to March 31, 1994). Food and Drug Administration requirements for methadone maintenance were met along with a *Diagnostic and Statistical Manual of Mental Disorders, Revised Third Edition (DSM-III-R)* diagnosis of current opioid dependence. The 716 participants constitute 91% (716/783) of new admissions to the treatment program during the study period. Most of the 67 subjects who were excluded left treatment before completing the initial assessments (n=52) or were excluded because of incomplete diagnostic information (n=12); 3 were excluded because of severe medical problems.

Mean age was 34.8 years (SD, 6.49; range, 20-58 years); 47.2% were women; 60.2% were white, 37.7% were black, 2.1% were other races; 45.3% were never married, 37.1% were separated or divorced, 16.8% were currently married; mean years of education was 11.1 (SD, 1.99; range, 4-19 years); and 69.3% were unemployed. Women were younger than men (32.2 vs 37.2, t=10.94, df=714, P<.001), more were black (45.3% vs 34.9%, t=2.84, df=714, P=.005), and they had less education (10.9 vs 11.2, t=2.24, df=714, $P \leq .03$). The mean age at onset for any substance use (omitting nicotine) was 14.1 years (SD, 2.83 years) and the mean age at onset for opioid use was 19.8 years (SD, 4.92 years). The mean age at first substance use treatment was 26.4 years (SD, 6.52 years) and the mean age at first methadone treatment was 27.0 years (SD, 6.53).

Study enrollment required participation in a prospective evaluation of psychopathology and drug abuse treatment outcome; data given herein are from the intake assessment phase of that project. The local institutional review board approved the study. Participants provided informed consent and were compensated $40 for completing the assessments.

OVERALL DESIGN

Several procedures were used to reduce the influence of acute situational stresses and drug effects on psychiatric symptom reporting.[22] Assessment data were collected 4 to 5 weeks after admission, after stabilization on a methadone dose of 50 mg or more (range, 50-65 mg). Interviewers screened patients for evidence of drug intoxication or withdrawal (eg, slurred speech, sedation, or agitation) and cognitive impairment (ie, Mini-Mental State Examination)[30] before administering the assessments. Interviews were done only when patients scored higher than 26 on the Mini-Mental State Examination and showed no obvious signs of drug intoxication or withdrawal.

Complexities related to remaining symptom overlap were handled as follows: (1) Axis I diagnoses were rated as substance-induced if they seemed to be initiated and sustained by drug use (ie, major changes in patterns of drug use preceding syndrome onsets and offsets). For example, marked increases or decreases in amount or frequency of use several weeks before the onset and the offset of a psychiatric disorder. (2) Diagnoses were coded as independent if multiple episodes were reported and one was judged unrelated to changing patterns of substance use. (3) Diagnoses of personality disorders were made only when criteria were met early in life and remained characteristic of thought, affect, or actions, including self-reported periods of abstinence.

Reported prevalence rates include syndromes considered induced or independent. The Axis I diagnoses were current when criteria were met in the 30 days before the interview; Axis II diagnoses all were rated as current.

ASSESSMENT MEASURES

Diagnoses were made using the Structured Clinical Interview for *DSM-III-R*.[31] It provides information for making lifetime and current diagnoses for many *DSM-III-R* Axis I conditions, including those common in opioid abusers (substance use disorders and mood disorders), and the personality disorders. Studies have shown

The present study addresses these limitations. A standardized time frame after treatment entry was used for conducting diagnostic evaluation, a wider range of substance use and other psychiatric diagnoses was assessed, and a larger proportion of women was included. Results compare men and women on prevalence of substance use and other psychiatric diagnoses. Patients with and without psychiatric comorbidity are compared on demographic characteristics and dimensional indexes of substance use severity, psychosocial impairment, and personality traits.

RESULTS

RATES OF NONSUBSTANCE USE DIAGNOSES

About half (47% or 340/716) of the sample had a lifetime psychiatric diagnosis other than substance use disorder, including 48% of men and 47% of women. Among those with psychiatric comorbidity (n=340), 61.5% had 1 diagnosis (including Axis II), 21.8% had 2 diagnoses, 10.6% had 3 diagnoses, and 6.1% had 4 or more diagnoses. Prevalence rates (lifetime and current) are given in **Table 1** and **Table 2**, with ORs (95% CIs) comparing women with men. Major depression (15.8%) and antisocial personality (25.1%) were the most common lifetime diagnoses. The rate of antisocial personality equaled that of all nonsubstance use Axis I diagnoses combined (25% vs 24%, respectively). The rate of current comorbidity was 39%, with most cases involving personality disorder (34.8%); only 8% had a current Axis I diagnosis.

RATES OF SUBSTANCE USE DIAGNOSES

Table 3 gives prevalence rates (lifetime and current) for substance use disorders, with ORs comparing women with men. All patients had at least 1 substance use diagnosis beyond opioid dependence, most often good retest reliability,[32,33] including diagnoses of greatest interest in substance abusers (eg, substance dependence, major depression, and antisocial personality). Personality traits were assessed using the NEO-Personality Inventory (NEO-PI),[34,35] a self-report inventory measuring 5 personality dimensions (neuroticism, extraversion, openness to experience, agreeableness, and conscientiousness). The severity of substance abuse and psychosocial impairment was measured using the Addiction Severity Index (ASI).[36] These dimensional measures have acceptable psychometric properties.[37-40]

INTERVIEWER TRAINING

Interviewers had completed training for the master's degree in psychology. For the computer-administered measures (NEO-PI) staff were present to clarify meanings of words or read the items. Interview-based measures involved extensive didactic instruction and a 2-step corating training procedure: corating interviews done by an expert (R.K.B.) until achieving 5 consecutive cases agreeing with expert ratings (ASI, item agreement; Structured Clinical Interview, presence or absence of diagnosis), and conducting interviews until achieving 5 consecutive cases agreeing with expert coratings. To reduce "interviewer drift" on the Structured Clinical Interview, expert coratings were obtained randomly during the study period (about every 3 months). During the study period, expert coratings were obtained on 128 interviews; every diagnosis with a prevalence of 5% or greater had a κ coefficient of 0.90 or higher (median, 0.98). This procedure establishes the reliability of the ratings but not of the interview content and is limited by the absence of reinterview.

STATISTICAL ANALYSIS

Odds ratios (ORs) and confidence intervals (CIs) were calculated to compare rates of substance use and other psychiatric diagnoses in women vs men and in patients with vs without psychiatric comorbidity. Confidence intervals that do not include the value "1" are statistically significant at the $P\leq.05$ level. Demographic characteristics, ages at onset for substance use, and substance use treatment were compared using t tests (2-tailed) or χ^2 tests (Fisher exact test for small cell sizes).

Clinical and demographic characteristics of patients with vs without psychiatric comorbidity were evaluated by sorting patients into mutually exclusive groups based on psychiatric diagnostic profile: substance use disorder without other comorbidity (none), substance use disorder with antisocial personality disorder only (APD), substance use disorders with antisocial personality disorder plus other psychiatric diagnoses (mixed), and substance use disorder with other psychiatric diagnoses excluding antisocial personality (other). For descriptive purposes, means are given for each group, along with univariate analysis of variances (ANOVAs) and the Tukey post hoc tests that compare groups on demographics, substance use history, ASI scores, and NEO-PI scores.

Descriptive stepwise discriminant analyses were performed to assess multivariately the importance and independence of variables in distinguishing among the 4 groups. To maximize statistical power, the number of variables available for entry into the discriminant functions was limited to selected demographic variables (age at onset of substance use and age at onset of treatment) and NEO-PI scores that were statistically significant in the ANOVAs ($P<.001$). Minimization of the Wilks λ was used as the criterion to select variables for entry into the discriminant functions. Structure coefficients (correlation of each variable with the discriminant function) were used to assess the contributions of each variable.

Familywise error rate was controlled in t tests, ANOVAs, and χ^2 tests, using a procedure developed by Holm.[41,42] This modified Bonferroni procedure uses progressively more stringent criteria for determining statistical significance based on the relative rank of the observed P values. Reported P values are those observed before the correction procedure. Where post hoc testing was conducted, a conservative cutoff of $P\leq.01$ was used to determine statistical significance. All analyses were conducted using SPSS for the Macintosh (version 4.0.5).

cocaine dependence. The average number of lifetime diagnoses was 4.44 (3.63 dependence and 0.81 abuse diagnoses). The average number of current diagnoses was 2.11 (2.02 dependence and 0.09 abuse diagnoses).

DIAGNOSTIC PREVALENCE RATES BY GENDER

Nonsubstance Use

Axis I Diagnoses. Women were 2 to 3 times more likely than men to have a lifetime nonsubstance use Axis I diagnosis (33.4% vs 15.6%; OR, 2.14; 95% CI, 1.62-2.83), mood disorder (27.5% vs 11.4%; OR, 2.42; 95% CI, 1.74-3.37), major depression (23.7% vs 8.75%; OR, 2.71; 95% CI, 1.86-3.96), or simple phobia (5.3% vs 1.9%; OR, 2.88; 95% CI, 1.22-6.80) (Table 1). The same pattern was found for current disorders, with women 2 to 4 times as likely as men to have these diagnoses.

Axis II Diagnoses. The opposite pattern was observed for personality disorder (Table 2). Women were less likely than men to have a personality disorder (28.4% vs 40.5%; OR, 0.70; 95% CI, 0.57-0.87), although expected differences for specific diagnoses were found: women were less likely than men to have antisocial personality (15.4% vs 33.9%; OR, 0.45; 95% CI, 0.34-0.61) but 7 times more likely to have borderline personality (9.5% vs 1.3%; OR, 7.16; 95% CI, 2.82-18.16).

Substance Use Diagnoses. Gender differences in the expected direction were observed for rates of substance use diagnoses (Table 3). Compared with the men, women had fewer lifetime diagnoses (mean, 3.98 vs 4.85; t=6.40; df=714; $P<.001$). Women were less likely to have a lifetime cannabis, alcohol, or hallucinogen disorder, and less likely to have current cannabis dependence (12.1% vs 19.8%; OR, 0.61; 95% CI, 0.43-0.87) or alcohol dependence (19.5% vs 29.4%; OR, 0.67; 95% CI, 0.51-0.87).

Table 1. Axis I Nonsubstance Use Psychiatric Disorders in Male and Female Opioid Abusers

	Lifetime Rates, %				Current Rates, %			
Diagnostic Category*	Men (n=378)	Women (n=338)	Total (N=716)	Odds Ratio† (95% Confidence Interval)	Men (n=378)	Women (n=338)	Total (N=716)	Odds Ratio† (95% Confidence Interval)
Any Axis I disorder	15.6	33.4	24.0	2.14 (1.62-2.83)	5.0	11.2	8.0	2.24 (1.32-3.80)
Mood disorder	11.4	27.5	19.0	2.42 (1.74-3.37)	2.1	5.3	3.6	2.52 (1.11-5.71)
Major depression	8.7	23.7	15.8	2.71 (1.86-3.96)	1.3	5.3	3.2	4.03 (1.51-10.73)
Dysthymia	2.4	4.4	3.4	1.86 (0.83-4.20)	2.4	4.4	3.4	1.86 (0.83-4.20)
Bipolar	0.8	0.0	0.4	...	0.8	0.0	0.4	...
Anxiety disorder	6.1	10.7	8.2	1.75 (1.06-2.90)	3.4	6.8	5.0	1.98 (1.02-3.84)
Simple phobia	1.9	5.3	3.5	2.88 (1.22-6.80)	1.9	3.6	2.7	1.92 (0.76-4.81)
Social phobia	1.9	3.6	2.7	1.92 (0.76-4.81)	0.8	2.7	1.7	3.36 (0.92-12.29)
Panic	2.1	1.8	2.0	0.84 (0.29-2.39)	0.3	0.9	0.6	3.36 (0.35-32.10)
Agoraphobia	0.0	0.6	0.3	...	0.0	0.3	0.1	...
Obsessive-compulsive	0.5	0.0	0.3	...	0.5	0.0	0.3	...
General anxiety	0.3	0.0	0.1	...	0.3	0.0	0.1	...
Eating disorders	0.0	1.5	0.7	...	0.0	0.0	0.0	...
Bulimia	0.0	0.9	0.4	...	0.0	0.0	0.0	...
Anorexia	0.0	0.6	0.3	...	0.0	0.0	0.0	...
Schizophrenia	0.0	0.3	0.1	...	0.0	0.3	0.1	...

*Multiple diagnoses possible.
†Represents likelihood of disorder in women relative to men; confidence intervals that do not include the value "1" significant at $P \leq .05$.

Table 2. Personality Disorders in Male and Female Opioid Abusers

	%			
Diagnostic Category*	Men (n=378)	Women (n=338)	Total (N=716)	Odds Ratio† (95% Confidence Interval)
Any personality disorder	40.5	28.4	34.8	0.70 (0.57-0.87)
Antisocial	33.9	15.4	25.1	0.45 (0.34-0.61)
Avoidant	3.4	7.1	5.2	2.07 (1.07-3.99)
Borderline	1.3	9.5	5.2	7.16 (2.82-18.16)
Passive-aggressive	3.7	4.4	4.1	1.20 (0.59-2.45)
Paranoid	4.5	1.8	3.2	0.40 (0.16-0.99)
Dependent	0.5	3.0	1.7	5.59 (1.23-25.34)
Histrionic	0.8	2.1	1.4	2.61 (0.68-10.01)
Narcissistic	1.6	0.0	0.8	...
Obsessive-compulsive	1.1	0.3	0.7	0.28 (0.03-2.49)
Schizotypal	0.3	0.3	0.3	1.12 (0.07-17.81)
Schizoid	0.3	0.3	0.3	1.12 (0.07-17.81)

*Multiple diagnoses possible.
†Represents likelihood of disorder in women relative to men; confidence intervals that do not include the value "1" significant at $P \leq .05$.

INDEPENDENT VS SUBSTANCE-INDUCED DISORDERS

Each Axis I nonsubstance use diagnosis was rated as being independent or induced by patterns of substance use. Only 3 diagnoses had cases rated as substance-induced (major depression, dysthymic disorder, and panic disorder) .Major depression often was considered substance-induced (88 of 113 patients or 78%); lifetime prevalence of independent major depression was only 3.5% (25 of 716 patients). Dysthymic disorder was considered substance-induced 54% of the time (13 of 24 patients); lifetime prevalence of independent dysthymia was 2% (11 of 716 patients). Panic disorder was considered substance-induced 21% of the time (3 of 14 patients); lifetime prevalence of independent panic disorder was 2% (11 of 716 patients).

PATIENTS WITH VS WITHOUT PSYCHIATRIC COMORBIDITY

Associations of lifetime psychiatric comorbidity (Axis I or Axis II) to demographic and substance use variables were analyzed by comparing patients who had substance use disorder only (ie, none; n=376) with those who had substance use disorder plus any nonsubstance use diagnosis (comorbid, n=340). No significant demographic differences were seen between the comorbid and the none group on age (35.1 vs 34.6 years, t=1.09, df=714, P=.28), percent minority (38.5% vs 41.0%, χ^2=0.44, df=1, P=.51), percent men (53.5% vs 52.1%, χ^2=0.14, df=1, P=.71), percent currently married (16.2% vs 17.5%, χ^2=0.21, df=1, P=.65), or percent unemployed (72.4% vs 66.5%, χ^2=2.88, df=1, P=.09). The comorbid group had significantly less education (10.7 vs 11.4 years, t=−4.17, df=714, P<.001).

The groups differed substantially on substance use variables. The comorbid group had an earlier age at onset of any substance use than the none group (13.4 vs 14.6 years, t=5.46, df=714, P<.001), an earlier age at onset of illicit opioid use (19.2 vs 20.3 years, t=2.98, df=714, P=.003), an earlier age at onset of methadone treatment (26.3 vs 27.6 years, t=2.63, df=714, P=.009), and a greater number of lifetime substance use diagnoses (4.9 vs 4.0, t=6.55, df=714, P<.001). Odds ratios compared rates of dependence for 8 substance classes considered in the study (**Table 4**). The comorbid group was more likely than the none group to have a lifetime dependence diagnosis on these substances (6 classes) and a current dependence diagnosis (4 classes).

PSYCHIATRIC COMORBIDITY, OTHER PSYCHOPATHOLOGIC CHARACTERISTICS, AND PERSONALITY

Mutually exclusive categories of psychiatric comorbidity were created by sorting the patients with comorbidity

Table 3. Substance Use Disorders in Male and Female Opioid Abusers

Diagnostic Category*	Lifetime Rates, % Men (n=378)	Women (n=338)	Total (N=716)	Odds Ratio† (95% Confidence Interval)	Current Rates, % Men (n=378)	Women (n=338)	Total (N=716)	Odds Ratio† (95% Confidence Interval)
Opioid								
Dependence	100	100	100	. . .	100	100	100	. . .
Cocaine								
Dependence	66.1	63.0	64.7	0.95 (0.86-1.06)	39.4	41.1	40.2	1.04 (0.87-1.25)
Abuse	13.0	11.8	12.4	0.91 (0.62-1.35)	3.7	3.0	3.4	0.80 (0.36-1.77)
Cannabis								
Dependence	58.7	42.0	50.8	0.72 (0.61-0.83)	19.8	12.1	16.2	0.61 (0.43-0.87)
Abuse	17.7	11.8	14.9	0.67 (0.46-0.96)	2.6	2.1	2.4	0.78 (0.30-2.03)
Alcohol								
Dependence	56.6	43.2	50.3	0.76 (0.66-0.89)	29.4	19.5	24.7	0.67 (0.51-0.87)
Abuse	16.1	9.5	13.0	0.59 (0.39-0.88)	2.6	0.9	1.8	0.34 (0.09-1.21)
Sedative								
Dependence	47.9	40.8	44.6	0.85 (0.72-1.01)	17.2	16.6	16.9	0.96 (0.70-1.34)
Abuse	15.3	10.4	13.0	0.68 (0.46-1.00)	1.3	1.8	1.5	1.34 (0.41-4.36)
Stimulant								
Dependence	19.0	19.2	19.1	1.01 (0.75-1.37)	0.0	0.6	0.3	. . .
Abuse	15.6	7.1	11.6	0.46 (0.29-0.71)	0.0	0.0	0.0	. . .
Hallucinogen								
Dependence	21.2	14.2	17.9	0.67 (0.48-0.93)	1.1	0.3	0.7	0.28 (0.03-2.49)
Abuse	12.7	5.6	9.4	0.44 (0.27-0.74)	0.0	0.0	0.0	. . .
Other substances‡								
Dependence	15.1	12.7	14.0	0.84 (0.58-1.22)	2.6	2.7	2.6	1.01 (0.41-2.45)
Abuse	7.9	4.7	6.4	0.60 (0.33-1.08)	0.5	0.6	0.6	1.12 (0.16-7.90)

*Multiple diagnoses possible.
†Represents likelihood of disorder in women relative to men; confidence intervals that do not include the "1" significant at P≤.05.
‡Primarily inhalants, clonidine, and promethazine.

Table 4. Substance Use Disorders in Opioid Abusers With vs Without Other Comorbidity

Diagnostic Category*	Lifetime Rates, % Noncomorbid (n=376)	Comorbid (n=340)	Odds Ratio† (95% Confidence Interval)	Current Rates, % Noncomorbid (n=376)	Comorbid (n=340)	Odds Ratio† (95% Confidence Interval)
Dependence						
Opioid	100	100	. . .	100	100	. . .
Cocaine	59.0	70.9	1.41 (1.15-1.73)	32.7	48.5	1.31 (1.15-1.48)
Cannabis	47.3	54.7	1.16 (1.00-1.35)	15.7	16.8	1.01 (0.95-1.08)
Alcohol	40.7	60.9	1.52 (1.30-1.77)	18.6	31.5	1.19 (1.09-1.30)
Sedative	36.4	53.5	1.37 (1.19-1.57)	12.5	21.8	1.12 (1.05-1.20)
Stimulant	16.0	22.6	1.09 (1.01-1.17)	0.0	0.6	. . .
Hallucinogen	13.8	22.4	1.11 (1.03-1.19)	0.5	0.9	1.00 (0.99-1.02)
Other substances‡	4.8	24.1	1.25 (1.18-1.34)	0.8	4.7	1.04 (1.02-1.07)

*Multiple diagnoses possible.
†Represents likelihood of disorder in comorbid group relative to noncomorbid group; confidence intervals that do not include the value "1" significant at P≤.05.
‡Primarily inhalants, clonidine, and promethazine.

into 1 of 3 subgroups: antisocial personality only (APD, n=106), antisocial personality plus other Axis I or Axis II diagnoses (mixed, n=74), and other psychiatric diagnoses (Axis I or Axis II) excluding antisocial personality (other, n=160). **Table 5** gives demographic characteristics, rates of dependence for selected substance use classes, and scores on dimensional indexes of personality and psychopathology for each of these groups and the noncomorbid group (none). Group comparisons were made using ANOVAs, and significant main effects were evaluated with Tukey pairwise post hoc tests; all comparisons were considered significant when *P*≤.01.

Psychiatric comorbidity was associated with a greater severity of substance use and with greater psychosocial problems. Although this pattern was observed across each comorbid group compared with the none group, it was clearest in the comorbid groups with antisocial personality in which substance use and substance use problems began earlier in life. These groups differed from the none group on 13 variables; the other comorbid group differed from the none group on 9 variables.

Descriptive discriminant analyses were conducted to assess multivariately the importance of selected variables in distinguishing the 4 groups. Statistical

Table 5. Relations Between Patterns of Psychiatric Comorbidity on Demographic and Dimensional Indexes of Personality and Psychopathology*

Variable	Group Factors: None 1 (n=376)	APD 2 (n=106)	Mixed 3 (n=74)	Other 4 (n=160)	χ^2	*df*†	Overall *P*‡	Post Hoc Comparisons§
Demographic								
Age, y	34.6	36.3	34.1	34.8	2.29	(3,712)	NS	...
Education	11.4	10.8	10.2	11.0	8.75	(3,712)	<.001	1>2,3;4>3
Percent male	51.2	83.0	54.1	33.8	62.25	3	<.001	2>1,3,4
Percent unemployed	66.5	64.2	78.4	75.0	8.02	3	NS	...
Percent minority	41.0	43.4	39.2	35.0	2.33	3	NS	...
Substance use history								
Age, y								
1st substance use	14.6	13.0	12.4	14.1	17.79	(3,704)	<.001	1,4>2,3
1st treatment	27.2	25.3	24.2	26.4	5.76	(3,700)	.001	1>2,3
1st opioid use	20.3	18.5	18.3	20.1	6.62	(3,699)	<.001	1,4>2,3
1st opioid treatment	27.6	26.0	25.2	27.1	3.92	(3,702)	NS	...
No. of diagnoses‖	4.0	5.2	5.4	4.5	20.42	(3,712)	<.001	2,3>1,4
Lifetime substance dependence, %								
Cocaine	59.0	85.8	79.7	56.9	37.62	3	<.001	2,3>1,4
Alcohol	40.7	64.2	62.2	58.1	30.10	3	<.001	2,3,4>1
Cannabis	47.3	61.3	59.5	48.1	9.17	3	NS	...
Sedative	36.4	55.7	56.8	50.6	22.17	3	<.001	2,3,4>1
Addiction Severity Index composite scores								
Medical	0.13	0.15	0.22	0.18	3.20	(3,696)	NS	...
Employment	0.69	0.72	0.75	0.72	1.13	(3,696)	NS	...
Alcohol use	0.04	0.05	0.06	0.04	1.30	(3,696)	NS	...
Drug use	0.20	0.25	0.24	0.22	7.09	(3,696)	<.001	2,3>1
Legal status	0.08	0.13	0.14	0.08	4.12	(3,696)	NS	...
Family and social	0.10	0.18	0.25	0.17	15.89	(3,696)	<.001	2,3,4>1;3>4
Psychiatric	0.03	0.05	0.13	0.10	21.88	(3,696)	<.001	3,4>1,2
NEO Personality Inventory dimensions								
Neuroticism	54.9	58.7	64.3	59.5	33.06	(3,627)	<.001	2,3,4>1;3>2,4
Extraversion	50.0	50.2	47.0	47.4	6.89	(3,627)	<.001	1,2>3,4
Openness	44.1	44.4	44.4	44.8	0.35	(3,627)	NS	...
Agreeableness	39.0	34.8	31.5	35.9	10.67	(3,627)	<.001	1>2,3,4;4>3
Conscientiousness	42.6	38.7	37.0	39.2	14.83	(3,627)	<.001	1>2,3,4

None indicates substance use disorder only; APD, substance use disorder and antisocial personality; Mixed, substance use disorder, antisocial personality, and other Axis I or II disorders; Other, substance use disorder and Axis I or II disorder other than antisocial personality.

†*Sample sizes varying due to missing data (drug use history, Addiction Severity Index) or because patient refused to complete measure (NEO Personality Inventory).*

‡*Statistical significance determined using modified Bonferroni procedure to correct for multiple comparisons. Reported* P *values for significant effects are those observed before correction; NS indicates nonsignificant.*

§*Post hoc test considered significant when* $P \leq .01$.

‖*Refers to the number of lifetime abuse and dependence diagnoses.*

power was maximized by using variables significant in the ANOVAs at $P<.001$: gender and education, age at onset of any substance use, age at onset of substance use treatment, number of lifetime substance use diagnoses, and 4 NEO-PI domains (neuroticism, extraversion, agreeableness, and conscientiousness); outcome-based data (ie, ASI) were omitted from these analyses.

Comparisons were made between each of the comorbid groups and the none group, and between the 2 antisocial groups (APD vs mixed). Overall correct classification rates ranged from 65.9% (other vs none) to 79.7% (mixed vs none). **Table 6** gives correct classification rates within pairs, the canonical correlation coefficient for each analysis, and the structure matrix coefficients used to assess the contribution of each variable in discriminating groups.

In general, 8 of the 9 variables distinguished the APD group from the none group, and 6 variables distinguished the mixed and other groups from the none group. Two variables discriminated each comorbid group from the none group: education (fewer years in the comorbid groups), and gender (male gender was associated with both antisocial groups and female gender was associated with the other comorbid group). Three variables discriminated both antisocial groups from the none group: age at onset of substance use (earlier ages in antisocial groups), number of substance use diagnoses (higher number in antisocial groups), and agreeableness (lower scores in antisocial groups reflect greater antagonism and mistrust). Finally, 6 variables discriminated the 2 APD groups; the 3 strongest discriminators were gender (male gender was associated with APD), neuroticism (higher scores in mixed group), and extraversion (higher scores in APD).

Table 6. Descriptive Discriminant Function Coefficients for Selected Variables*

	Group Factors			
	APD vs None (0, 1)	Mixed vs None (0, 1)	Other vs None (0, 1)	Mixed vs APD (0, 1)
Canonical correlation coefficient	0.4375	0.5312	0.3621	0.5022
Structure matrix coefficient				
Years of education	0.2114	0.3966	0.2038	. . .
Male gender	−0.5687	−0.0656	0.4137	0.5046
Age at onset of substance use	0.4750	0.4867	. . .	0.2079
Age at onset of treatment	0.2564	. . .	. . .	. . .
Number of substance use diagnoses	−0.6013	−0.5122	−0.3703	. . .
NEO PI				
Neuroticism	. . .	−0.7191	−0.7015	−0.6525
Extraversion	−0.0279	. . .	0.4073	0.4025
Agreeableness	0.3158	0.3860	. . .	. . .
Conscientiousness	0.4533	. . .	0.5102	0.1642
Classification accuracy, %†	80/70	84/79	68/65	72/73

**APD indicates substance use disorder and antisocial personality; None, substance use disorder only; Mixed, substance use disorder, antisocial personality, and other Axis I or II disorders; Other, substance use disorder and Axis I or II disorder other than antisocial personality; NEO PI, NEO Personality Inventory. Numbers (0,1) indicate the coding assignment of each group in the discriminate analysis.*

†The percentages refer to the 2 groups being compared.

COMPARISON OF PREVALENCE RATES WITH GENERAL POPULATION RATES

Lifetime rates of nonsubstance use disorder were contrasted with rates from the Baltimore sample of the Epidemiological Catchment Area (ECA) Study.[21] Rates were compared for the any disorder category and for the 2 most common diagnoses (ie, antisocial personality and major depression). Because antisocial personality was the only Axis II diagnosis assessed in the ECA Study, comparison for the any disorder category was made after removing counts of other Axis II diagnoses from our sample.

Table 7 gives the percentages of positive cases for each diagnostic category and for each of the 3 age strata relevant to our sample. Drug abusers had a higher prevalence in each diagnostic category and each age stratum than did the ECA sample. The rate of major depression was almost 3 times greater than that of the general population, and the rate of antisocial personality was 8 times greater.

Comparing prevalence across different samples can be misleading if rates vary by age and samples differ in age distributions. Rates therefore were compared after age adjustment. The age-adjusted rates were similar to the unadjusted rates, and the population differences remained.

COMMENT

This study underscores the continued importance of psychiatric comorbidity in opioid abusers. Almost half (47%) of the sample had a lifetime nonsubstance use disorder, and 39% had a current disorder. Antisocial personality was the most common diagnosis and equaled the combined rate of all nonsubstance use Axis I diagnoses. Comorbidity rates were similar in men and women, although women had higher rates of mood disorder and borderline personality than men, and men had higher rates of antisocial personality and most substance use diagnoses. The study also confirms the expected associations between psychiatric comorbidity and substance use severity. Psychiatric comorbidity was associated with a more chronic, pervasive, and severe spectrum of substance use disorder, especially when the comorbidity included antisocial personality.

COMPARISONS WITH OTHER STUDIES OF OPIOID ABUSERS

Research in the 1970s and 1980s also documented high rates of comorbidity in opioid abusers[3,4,19,20,43] and found that most comorbidity involved mood and personality disorder. Those studies likewise reported that mood disorder was more common in women and antisocial personality was more common in men.[19,20,43] That we documented less psychiatric comorbidity than reported in previous studies deserves comment. Almost 80% of the 533 opioid abusers in the study by Rounsaville et al[19] had a comorbid diagnosis using Research Diagnostic Criteria; our rate was 47%. This difference was primarily associated with 2 diagnoses—mood disorder and personality disorder. Lifetime mood disorder in earlier studies ranged from 60%[20] to more than 70%[19]; our rate was 19%. Rates of personality disorder using *DSM-III* criteria and evaluating all possible diagnoses have ranged from 65%[20] to 68%[43]; our rate was 35%.

These differences in comorbidity rates may be associated with variations in methods and populations. For example, diagnostic evaluations in our study were made 3 to 4 weeks after admission. Other studies often assessed patients during the admission process,[2,19,20,43] a time associated with increased symptom reporting.[1,2,22,44,45] Variations in diagnostic systems may produce different rates of comorbidity, especially for mood disorders. The study by Rounsaville et al[19] used Research Diagnostic Criteria that includes diagnoses absent in the *DSM-III-R*

Table 7. Lifetime Prevalence for Nonsubstance Use Psychiatric Disorder

Diagnostic Category	Opioid Abusers		General Population ECA	
	No.	%*	No.	%†
Any nonsubstance diagnosis‡				
Overall rates§	716	42.50	2558	32.88
Age, y				
18-24	43	41.90	504	32.14
25-44	628	42.70	1212	34.65
45-64	45	40.00	842	30.76
Antisocial personality				
Overall rates§	716	25.10	2558	3.17
Age, y				
18-24	43	30.20	504	2.10
25-44	628	24.50	1212	4.50
45-64	45	28.90	842	1.90
Major depression				
Overall rates§	716	15.80	2558	5.74
Age, y				
18-24	43	11.60	504	4.10
25-44	628	16.10	1212	7.50
45-64	45	15.60	842	4.20

**Percentage satisfying* Diagnostic and Statistical Manual of Mental Disorders, Revised Third Edition *criteria.*

†*Percentage satisfying* Diagnostic and Statistical Manual of Mental Disorders, Third Edition *criteria from Baltimore, Md, sample of the Epidemiological Catchment Area Study.*[21]

‡*Personality disorders other than antisocial personality are excluded.*

§*Overall rates are based on ages 18 through 64 years only.*

(eg, minor depression and labile personality), although high rates of mood disorder also were reported in studies using the *DSM-III* system.[4,20] It is also possible that our lower rate of comorbidity is associated with greater availability of opioid substitution treatment in Baltimore (and elsewhere) during the study period. Earlier studies were conducted when this treatment was less available, potentially biasing hospital admissions toward more distressed patients with greater likelihood of having a comorbid disorder. This is consistent with the report that opioid abusers entering treatment had higher rates of mood disorder than those not seeking treatment.[46]

INDEPENDENT VS SUBSTANCE-INDUCED DISORDERS

It is well known that self-administration of many substances can produce clinical states that mimic other psychiatric syndromes.[5] Far less certain is how to distinguish these induced syndromes in substance abusers from independent forms of the disorder.[44,45] This task is especially difficult among patients with an early age of onset of unrelenting and severe substance use disorder. We addressed this problem by focusing on patterns of substance use preceding the onset and offset of comorbid syndromes rather than comparing ages at onset between the substance use disorder and other psychiatric diagnoses. Although most of the mood disorder was judged substance-induced by this approach, other psychiatric diagnoses were typically considered independent syndromes. These results are similar to other studies of substance abusers,[2,9,19,45] despite their use of the primary-secondary distinction[47] for disentangling comorbidity.

COMPARISONS WITH GENERAL POPULATION

Despite using the Baltimore sample of the ECA Study, which had a high rate of phobias (23.5%), prevalence for the any nonsubstance use disorder category was greater in our sample, although small numbers in 2 strata (18-24 and 45-64 years) raise concerns about the stability of those findings. The major difference in prevalence rates involved 2 diagnoses. We observed almost a 3-fold elevation of major depression and an 8-fold elevation of antisocial personality over the ECA sample. A similar pattern was observed in comparisons with a more recent general population survey using *DSM-III-R* criteria,[48] although their rate of lifetime major depression was similar to ours.

RELATIONS BETWEEN PSYCHIATRIC COMORBIDITY AND OTHER VARIABLES

Psychiatric comorbidity was related to severity measures of substance use and other psychosocial problems. This is consistent with previous reports of opioid abusers[2,3,6,10,49] and with many reports of alcohol abusers,[5,50] although exceptions have been reported.[51] This relation may relate to the high rates of drug use reported in treated opioid abusers with mood disorder or antisocial personality,[2-4,6] and to the greater risk of human immunodeficiency virus transmission in drug abusers with antisocial personality.[52-55] For example, one study[55] documented almost a 4-fold increase in human immunodeficiency virus infection among intravenous drug abusers with vs without antisocial personality.

The discriminant analyses disclose dimensions on which opioid abusers with comorbidity differ from those without comorbidity, and dimensions on which antisocial opioid abusers differ from those with and without other psychiatric diagnoses. Several of these dimensions were expected to differentiate groups (eg, age at onset of use), but personality trait measures were largely exploratory. It is interesting that higher neuroticism and lower agreeableness (reflecting greater antagonism) and lower conscientiousness (reflecting greater pleasure-seeking) distinguished comorbid groups from the none group. These traits may enhance vulnerability to the positive reinforcing effects of substances,[56] motivate treatment-seeking, and simultaneously confer a poor prognosis.[57]

STUDY LIMITATIONS

The study was largely retrospective and relied on self-report. Results may be influenced by recall bias, although previous work suggests that informants of drug abusers underestimate psychiatric and substance abuse problems.[58] Psychiatric comorbidity in the study may have been underestimated because of conservative requirements for symptom-coding to minimize overestimation of certain disorders. Major depression was diagnosed only when the depressed mood or loss of interest was present every day for at least 2 weeks (compared with "almost every day for 2 weeks or more"), and symptoms of personality disorder were counted only when pervasive and stable across time, including periods of abstinence. The results from our efforts to differentiate induced from independent disorders also must be viewed cautiously. This categorization is difficult even under ideal circumstances (eg, multiple informants), and especially with antisocial personality disorder.[59-62] And we did not specifically evaluate the reliability of this categorization. Generalizability of these findings to other studies probably will be influenced by methods issues (eg, nosology system used, timing of assessments relative to admission) and by population characteristics (eg, female representation).

IMPLICATIONS FOR TREATMENT

Despite subgroup differences, severe substance use disorder was evident across patients. Although methadone substitution therapy is effective in reducing illicit opioid use,[63] it has less efficacy reducing use of cocaine and other substances.[30,64-66] The problems associated with concurrent drug use in opioid abusers[30,67-69] are considerable, and several approaches have reported some success in managing them, including intensifying the counseling,[70,71] providing specialized psychotherapies,[2-4,72-76] and using behavioral incentives.[77-83] These specialized therapeutic interventions also should facilitate reduced drug use in opioid abusers with comorbid psychiatric disorder. As an example, good outcomes have been reported using specialized psychotherapies or pharmacotherapies for depressed opioid abusers,[3,73,84,85] and similar results seem possible in antisocial opioid abusers. Adding specialized psychotherapy to routine counseling significantly improved outcomes for antisocial opioid abusers with past or present mood disorder.[4] Preliminary reports from a behavioral incentive study of antisocial opioid abusers also show good results.[86]

Accepted for publication July 10, 1996.

This study was supported by US Public Health Service grants P50 DA 05273, R01 DA 05569, R18 DA 06120, and K05 DA 00050 from the National Institute on Drug Abuse, Bethesda, Md.

We gratefully acknowledge the research staff whose diligence ensured the integrity of the study, especially Kori Kindbom, MA, Jennifer Hahn, PhD, and Clay Souder, MA, who conducted most of the structured psychiatric interviews. We thank Linda Cottler, PhD, for providing additional details from the Epidemiological Catchment Area Study data and for the thoughtful review and critique. We also thank Linda Felch, MA, who provided statistical consultation and analyses.

Reprints: Robert K. Brooner, PhD, Behavioral Biology Research Center, The Johns Hopkins Bayview Medical Center, Suite 1500, 5510 Nathan Shock Dr, Baltimore, MD 21224.

REFERENCES

1. Group for the Advancement of Psychiatry. Substance abuse disorders: a psychiatric riority. *Am J Psychiatry.* 1991;148:1291-1300.
2. Rounsaville BJ, Weissman MM, Crits-Christoph K, Wilber C, Kleber H. Diagnosis and symptoms of depression in opiate addicts: course and relationship to treatment outcome. *Arch Gen Psychiatry.* 1982;39:151-156.
3. Woody GE, Luborsky L, McLellan AT, O'Brien CP, Beck AT, Blaine J, Herman I, Hole A. Psychotherapy for opiate addicts. *Arch Gen Psychiatry.* 1983;40:636-645.
4. Woody GE, McLellan AT, Luborsky L, O'Brien CP. Sociopathy and psychotherapy outcome. *Arch Gen Psychiatry.* 1985;42:1081-1086.
5. Schuckit MA. The clinical implications of primary diagnostic groups among alcoholics. *Arch Gen Psychiatry.* 1985;42:1043-1049.
6. Rounsaville BJ, Kosten TR, Weissman MM, Kleber HD. Prognostic significance of psychopathology in treated opiate addicts. *Arch Gen Psychiatry.* 1986;43:739-745.
7. Rounsaville BJ, Dolinsky ZS, Babor TF, Meyer RE. Psychopathology as a predictor of treatment outcome in alcoholics. *Arch Gen Psychiatry.* 1987;44:505-513.
8. Nace EP, Davis CW, Gaspari JP. Axis II comorbidity in substance abusers. *Am J Psychiatry.* 1991;148:118-120.
9. Rounsaville BJ, Anton SF, Carroll K, Budde D, Brigitte AP, Gawin F. Psychiatric diagnoses of treatment-seeking cocaine abusers. *Arch Gen Psychiatry.* 1991;48:43-51.
10. Rutherford MJ, Cacciola JS, Alterman AI. Relationships of personality disorders with problem severity in methadone patients. *Drug Alcohol Depend.* 1994;35:69-76.
11. Schoenbaum EE, Hartel D, Selwyn PA, Klein RS, Davenny K, Rogers M, Feiner C, Friedland G. Risk factors for human immunodeficiency virus infection in intravenous drug users. *N Engl J Med.* 1989;321:874-979.
12. Des Jarlais DC, Friedman SR, Novick DM, Sotheran JL, Thomas P, Yancovitz SR, Mildvan D, Weber J, Kreek MJ, Maslansky R, Bartime S, Spira T, Marmor M. HIV-1 infection among intravenous drug users in Manhattan, New York City, from 1977 through 1987. *JAMA.* 1989;261:1008-1012.
13. Nemoto T, Brown LS, Foster K, Chu A. Behavioral risk factors of human immunodeficiency virus infection among intravenous drug users and implications for preventive intervention. *AIDS Educ Prev.* 1990;2:116-126.
14. Haverkos HW, Lange WR. Serious infections other than human immunodeficiency virus among intravenous drug abusers. *J Infect Dis.* 1990;161:894-902.
15. Vlahov D, Anthony JC, Munoz A, Margolick J, Nelson KE, Celentano DD, Solomon L, Polk BF. The Alive Study: A longitudinal study of HIV-1 infection in intravenous drug users: description of methods. *Drug Issues.* 1991;21:759-776.
16. Metzger D, Woody GE, DePhilippis D, McLellan AT, O'Brien CP, Platt J. Risk factors for needle sharing among methadone-treated patients. *Am J Psychiatry.* 1991;148:641-643.
17. Bass JB. Tuberculosis in the 1990s. *Alcohol Clin Exp Res.* 1995;19:3-5.
18. Nelson KE, Vlahov D, Solomon L, Cohn S, Munoz A. Temporal trends of incident human immunodeficiency virus infection in a cohort of injecting drug users in Baltimore, Md. *Arch Intern Med.* 1995;155:1305-1311.
19. Rounsaville BJ, Weissman MM, Kleber, H, Wilber, C. Heterogeneity of psychiatric diagnosis in treated opiate addicts. *Arch Gen Psychiatry.* 1982;39:161-166.
20. Khantzian EJ, Treece C. *DSM-III* psychiatric diagnosis of narcotic addicts. *Arch Gen Psychiatry.* 1985;42:1067-1071.
21. Robins LN, Helzer JE, Weissman MM, Orvaschel H, Gruenbert E, Burke JD Jr, Regier DA. Lifetime prevalence of specific psychiatric disorders in three sites. *Arch Gen Psychiatry.* 1985;41:949-958.
22. Strain EC, Stitzer ML, Bigelow GE. Early treatment time course of depressive symptoms in opiate addicts. *J Nerv Ment Dis.* 1991;179:215-221.
23. Kosten TR, Gawin FH, Rounsaville BJ, Kleber HD. Cocaine abuse among opioid addicts: demographic and diagnostic factors in treatment. *Am J Drug Alcohol Abuse.* 1986;12:1-16.
24. Kolar AF, Brown BS, Weddington WW, Ball JC. A treatment crisis: cocaine use by clients in methadone maintenance programs. *J Subst Abuse Treat.* 1990;7:101-107.
25. Strain EC, Brooner RK, Bigelow GE. Clustering of multiple substance use and psychiatric diagnoses in opiate addicts. *Drug Alcohol Depend.* 1991;27:127-134.
26. Kosten TR, Morgan C, Falcione J, Schottenfeld R. Pharmacotherapy for cocaine-abusing methadone-maintained patients using amantadine or desipramine. *Arch Gen Psychiatry.* 1992;49:894-898.
27. Kidorf M, Stitzer ML. Descriptive analysis of cocaine use in methadone patients. *Drug Alcohol Depend.* 1993;32:267-275.
28. Darke S, Hall W, Ross M, Wodak A. Benzodiazepine use and HIV risk-taking behavior among injecting drug users. *Drug Alcohol Depend.* 1992;31:31-36.
29. Iguchi MY, Handelsman L, Bickel WK, Griffiths RR. Benzodiazepine and sedative use/abuse by methadone maintenance clients. *Drug Alcohol Depend.* 1993;32:257-266.
30. Folstein MF, Folstein SE, McHugh PR. Mini-Mental State: a practical method for grading the cognitive state of patients for the clinician. *J Psychiatr Res.* 1975;12:189-198.
31. Spitzer SL, Williams JBW, Gibbon M, First MB. The Structured Clinical Interview for *DSM-III-R* (SCID). *Arch Gen Psychiatry.* 1992;49:624-629.

32. Williams JBW, Gibbon M, First MB, Spitzer RL, Davies M, Borus J, Jowes MJ, Kane J, Pope HG Jr, Rounsaville BJ, Wittchen HU. The Structured Clinical Interview for *DSM-III-R* (SCID), II: multisite test-retest reliability. *Arch Gen Psychiatry.* 1992;49:630-636.
33. Perry JC. Problems and considerations in the valid assessment of personality disorders. *Am J Psychiatry.* 1992;149:1645-1653.
34. Costa PT, McCrae RR. *The NEO Personality Inventory Manual.* Odessa, Fla: Psychological Assessment Resources; 1985.
35. Costa PT, McCrae RR. *The NEO-PI/NEO-FFI Manual Supplement.* Odessa, Fla: Psychological Assessment Resources; 1989.
36. McLellan AT, Luborsky L, Woody GE, O'Brien CP. An improved diagnostic evaluation instrument for substance abuse patients: the Addiction Severity Index. *J Nerv Ment Dis.* 1980;168:26-33.
37. McCrae RR, Costa PT. Validation of the five-factor model of personality across instruments and observers. *J Pers Soc Psychol.* 1987;52:81-90.
38. Leong FTL, Dollinger SJ. NEO Personality Inventory. In: Keyser DJ, Sweetland RC, eds. *Test Critiques.* Austin, Tex: PRO-ED; 1990:527-539.
39. Kosten TR, Rounsaville BJ, Kleber HD. Concurrent validity of the Addiction Severity Index. *J Nerv Ment Dis.* 1983;171:606-610.
40. McLellan AT, Luborsky LK, Woody GE, O'Brien CP, Druley KA. Predicting response to alcohol and drug abuse treatments. *Arch Gen Psychiatry.* 1983;40:620-625.
41. Holland BS, Copenhaver MD. Improved Bonferroni-type multiple testing procedures. *Psychol Bull.* 1988;104:145-149.
42. Holm S. A simple sequentially rejective multiple test procedure. *Scand J Stat.* 1979;6:65-70.
43. Kosten TR, Rounsaville BJ, Kleber HD. *DSM-III* personality disorders in opiate addicts. *Compr Psychiatry.* 1982;23:572-581.
44. Bryant KJ, Rounsaville BJ, Spitzer RL, Williams JB. Reliability of dual diagnosis. *J Nerv Ment Dis.* 1992;180:251-257.
45. Kadden RM, Kranzler HR, Rounsaville BJ. Validity of the distinction between 'substance-induced' and 'independent' depression and anxiety disorder. *Am J Addict.* 1995;4:107-117.
46. Rounsaville BJ, Kleber HD. Untreated opiate addicts: how do they differ from those seeking treatment? *Arch Gen Psychiatry.* 1985;42:1072-1077.
47. Robins E, Guze SB. Classification of affective disorders: the primary-secondary, the endogenous-reactive, and the neurotic-psychotic concepts. In: Williams TA, Katz MM, Shields JA, eds. *Recent Advances in Psychobiology of the Depressive Illnesses: Proceedings of a Workshop Sponsored by the National Institute of Mental Health.* Washington, DC: Dept of Health, Education, and Welfare; 1972;283-293.
48. Kessler RC, McGonagle KA, Zhao S, Nelson CB, Hughes M, Eshleman S, Wittchen H-U, Kendler KS. Lifetime and 12-month prevalence of *DSM-III-R* psychiatric disorders in the United States: results from the National Comorbidity Survey. *Arch Gen Psychiatry.* 1994;51:8-19.
49. Dinwiddie SH, Reich T, Cloninger CR. Psychiatric comorbidity and suicidality among intravenous drug users. *J Clin Psychiatry.* 1992;53:364-369.
50. Hesselbrock VN, Meyer RE, Keene JJ. Psychopathology in hospitalized alcoholics. *Arch Gen Psychiatry.* 1985;42:1050-1055.
51. Longabaugh R, Rubin A, Malloy P, Beattie M, Clifford PR, Noel N. Drinking outcomes of alcohol abusers diagnosed as antisocial personality disorder. *Alcohol Clin Exp Res.* 1994;18:778-785.
52. Brooner RK, Bigelow GE, Strain E, Schmidt CW. Intravenous drug abusers with antisocial personality disorder: increased HIV risk behavior. *Drug Alcohol Depend.* 1990;26:39-44.
53. Gill K, Nolimal D, Crowley T. Antisocial personality disorder, HIV risk behavior and retention in methadone maintenance therapy. *Drug Alcohol Depend.* 1992; 30:247-252.
54. Compton WM, Cottler LB, Shillington AM, Price RK. Is antisocial personality disorder associated with increased HIV risk behaviors in cocaine users? *Drug Alcohol Depend.* 1995;37:37-44.
55. Brooner RK, Greenfield L, Schmidt CW, Bigelow GE. Antisocial personality disorder and HIV infection among intravenous drug abusers. *Am J Psychiatry.* 1993;150:53-58.
56. Khantzian EJ. The self-medication hypothesis of addictive disorders: focus on heroin and cocaine dependence. *Am J Psychiatry.* 1985;142:1259-1264.
57. Miller TR. The psychotherapeutic utility of the five-factor model of personality: a clinician's experience. *Subst Use Misuse.* 1991;57:415-433.
58. Rounsaville BJ, Wilber CH, Rosenberger D, Kleber HD. Comparison of opiate addicts' reports of psychiatric history with reports of significant other informants. *Am J Drug Alcohol Abuse.* 1981;8:51-69.
59. Alterman AI, Cacciola JS. The antisocial personality disorder diagnosis in substance abusers: problems and issues. *J Nerv Ment Dis.* 1991;179:401-409.
60. Brooner RK, Schmidt CW, Felch L, Bigelow GE. Antisocial behavior of intravenous drug abusers: implications for diagnosis of antisocial personality disorder. *Am J Psychiatry.* 1992;149:482-487.
61. Cottler LJ, Price RK, Compton WM, Mager DE. Subtypes of adult antisocial behavior among drug abusers. *J Nerv Ment Dis.* 1995;183;154-161.
62. Strain EC. Antisocial personality disorder, misbehavior, and drug abuse. *J Nerv Ment Dis.* 1995;183:162-165.
63. Institute of Medicine. In: Rettig RA, Yarmolinsky A, eds. *Federal Regulations of Methadone Treatment.* Washington, DC: National Academy Press; 1995.
64. Kosten TR, Rounsaville BJ, Kleber HD. Antecedents and consequences of cocaine abuse among opioid addicts: a 2.5-year follow-up. *J Nerv Ment Dis.* 1988; 176:176-181.
65. Arndt I, Dorozynsky L, Woody GE, McLellan AT, O'Brien C. Desipramine treatment of cocaine dependence in methadone-maintained patients. *Arch Gen Psychiatry.* 1992;49:888-893.
66. Meyer RE. New pharmacotherapies for cocaine dependence revisited. *Arch Gen Psychiatry.* 1992;49:900-904.
67. Chaisson RE, Bacchetti P, Osmond D, Brodie B, Sande MA, Moss AR. Cocaine use and HIV infection in intravenous drug users in San Francisco. *JAMA.* 1989; 261:561-565.
68. Joe GW, Simpson DD. HIV risks, gender, and cocaine use among opiate users. *Drug Alcohol Depend.* 1995;37:23-28.
69. Bux DA, Lamb RJ, Iguchi MY. Cocaine use and HIV risk behavior in methadone maintenance patients. *Drug Alcohol Depend.* 1995;37:29-35.
70. McLellan AT, Woody GE, Luborsky L, O'Brien CP, Druley KA. Increased effectiveness of substance abuse treatment: a prospective study of patient-treatment matching. *J Nerv Ment Dis.* 1983;171:597-605.
71. McLellan AT, Arndt IO, Metzger DS, Woody GE, O'Brien CP. The effects of psychosocial services in substance abuse treatment. *JAMA.* 1993;269:953-959.
72. Rounsaville BJ, Glazer W, Wilber CH, Weissman MM, Kleber HD. Short-term interpersonal psychotherapy in methadone-maintained opiate addicts. *Arch Gen Psychiatry.* 1983;40:629-636.
73. Woody GE, McLellan AT, Luborsky L, O'Brien CP, Blaine J, Fox S, Herman I, Beck AT. Severity of psychiatric symptoms as a predictor of benefits from psychotherapy: the Veterans Administration-Penn Study. *Am J Psychiatry.* 1984; 141:1172-1177.
74. Woody GE, McLellan AT, Luborsky I, O'Brien CP. Twelve-month follow-up of psychotherapy for opiate dependence. *Am J Psychiatry.* 1987;44:590-596.
75. Alterman AI, McLellan AT, Shifman RB. Do substance abuse patients with more psychopathology receive more treatment? *J Nerv Ment Dis.* 1993;181:576-582.
76. Kadden RM, Cooney NL, Getter H, Litt MD. Matching alcoholics to coping skills or interactional therapies: two-year follow-up results. *J Consult Clin Psychol.* 1991;59:598-601.
77. Stitzer ML, Iguchi MY, Felch LJ. Contingent take-home incentive: effects on drug use of methadone maintenance patients. *J Consult Clin Psychol.* 1992; 60:927-934.
78. Stitzer ML, Higgins ST. Behavioral treatment of drug and alcohol abuse. In: Bloom FE, Kupfer DJ, eds. *Psychopharmacology: The Fourth Generation of Progress.* New York, NY: Raven Press; 1994.
79. Kidorf M, Stitzer ML. Contingent access to methadone maintenance treatment: effects on cocaine use of mixed opiate-cocaine abusers. *Exp Clin Psychopharm.* 1993;1:200-206.
80. Kidorf M, Stitzer ML, Brooner RK, Goldberg J. Contingent methadone take-home doses reinforce adjunct therapy attendance of methadone maintenance patients. *Drug Alcohol Depend.* 1994;36:221-226.
81. Azrin NH, McMahon PT, Donohue B, Besalel VA, Lapinski KJ, Kogan ES, Acierno RE, Galloway E. Behavior therapy for drug abuse: a controlled treatment outcome study. *Behav Res Ther.* 1994;32:857-866.
82. Higgins ST, Budney AJ, Bickel WK, Foerg FE, Donham R, Badger GJ. Incentives improve outcome in outpatient behavioral treatment of cocaine dependence. *Arch Gen Psychiatry.* 1994;51:568-576.
83. Silverman K, Higgins ST, Brooner RK, Montoya ID, Cone EJ, Schuster CR, Preston KL. Sustained cocaine abstinence in intravenous polydrug abusers through voucher-based reinforcement therapy. *Arch Gen Psychiatry.* 1996;53:409-417.
84. Woody GE, O'Brien CP, Rickels K. Depression and anxiety in heroin addicts: a placebo-controlled study of doxepin in combination with methadone. *Am J Psychiatry.* 1975;132:447-450.
85. Titievsky J, Seco G, Barranco M, Kyle EM. Doxepin as adjunctive therapy for depressed methadone maintenance patients: a double-blind study. *J Clin Psychiatry.* 1982;43:454-456.
86. Brooner RK, Kidorf M, King VL, Bigelow GE. Preliminary results from a controlled clinical trial of behavior therapy for antisocial opioid abusers. In: Harris LS, ed. *National Institute on Drug Abuse Research Monograph: Proceedings of the 56th Annual Meeting of the College on Problems of Drug Dependence.* Washington, DC: Dept of Health and Human Services; 1995:213.

ORIGINAL ARTICLE

Psychiatric Sequelae of Posttraumatic Stress Disorder in Women

Naomi Breslau, PhD; Glenn C. Davis, MD; Edward L. Peterson, PhD; Lonni Schultz, PhD

Background: The risk for first-onset major depression, anxiety, and substance use disorders associated with prior posttraumatic stress disorder (PTSD) was estimated in a sample of women.

Methods: The National Institute of Mental Health Diagnostic Interview Schedule, revised according to *DSM-III-R*, was used to measure lifetime psychiatric disorders in a stratified random sample of 801 mothers of children, who participated in a study of cognitive and psychiatric outcomes by level of birth weight. Cox proportional hazards models with time-dependent covariates were used to calculate the hazards ratios of first onset of other disorders following PTSD.

Results: The lifetime prevalence of traumatic events was 40% and of PTSD, 13.8%. Posttraumatic stress disorder signaled increased risks for first-onset major depression (hazards ratio, 2.1) and alcohol use disorder (hazards ratio, 3.0). The risk for major depression following PTSD was of the same magnitude as the risk for major depression following other anxiety disorders. Women with preexisting anxiety and PTSD had significantly increased risk for first-onset major depression. Additional analysis showed that preexisting major depression increased women's vulnerability to the PTSD-inducing effects of traumatic events and risk for exposure to traumatic events.

Conclusions: Posttraumatic stress disorder influences the risk for first-onset major depression and alcohol use disorder. The causal explanation of these temporally secondary disorders is unclear and might involve the effect of PTSD or underlying vulnerabilities exposed by the traumatic experience.

Arch Gen Psychiatry. 1997;54:81-87

From the Departments of Psychiatry (Dr Breslau) and Biostatistics and Research Epidemiology (Drs Breslau, Peterson, and Schultz) and the Office of Academic Affairs (Dr Davis), Henry Ford Health Sciences Center, Detroit, Mich; the Department of Psychiatry, Case Western Reserve University, Cleveland, Ohio (Drs Breslau and Davis); and the Department of Psychiatry, University of Michigan, Ann Arbor (Drs Breslau and Davis).

RESEARCH ON catastrophic experiences and their signature disease, posttraumatic stress disorder (PTSD), has focused primarily on Vietnam war veterans and civilians exposed to natural disasters or other types of trauma.[1-5] Despite a growing clinical interest in PTSD as it applies to a wide range of traumatic experiences, there are limited epidemiologic data on the disorder in the general population. The available epidemiologic data indicate that PTSD is more likely to occur in women than in men, and that it is highly comorbid with other psychiatric disorders.[6-9] Little is known about the temporal order of PTSD and the psychiatric disorders with which strong lifetime associations have been noted, that is, depression, anxiety, and substance use disorders. The purpose of this investigation is to examine the psychiatric sequelae of PTSD in a large sample of women. Data were obtained from a stratified random sample of 801 mothers of children who participated in a study of cognitive and psychiatric outcomes by birth weight.

SEX DIFFERENCES IN PTSD IN THE GENERAL POPULATION

The epidemiologic findings of *DSM-III-R* PTSD in the general population were reported from 2 Epidemiologic Catchment Area study sites.[6,7] The lifetime prevalence of PTSD, measured by the National Institute of Mental Health Diagnostic Interview Schedule (NIMH-DIS), was 1% and 1.3% in the first and second sites, respectively, and was higher in women than in men, although the sex differences were not statistically significant. A survey of young adults in southeast Michigan revealed a lifetime prevalence of *DSM-III-R* PTSD, measured by the revised NIMH-DIS, of

See Subjects and Methods on next page

SUBJECTS AND METHODS

SAMPLE AND DATA

Data were obtained from a study on children's cognitive and psychiatric outcomes by birth weight, in which mothers provided information on their own psychiatric histories. A stratified random sample was drawn from the lists of newborns discharged from 2 major hospitals in southeast Michigan, one in Detroit and the other in a middle-class suburb, from January 1, 1983, to December 31, 1985. Data were gathered from January 1, 1990, to August 31, 1992, from 823 families, 75% of the target sample. Complete data for this analysis were available on 801 mothers. Detailed descriptions of the population and sample have been published elsewhere.[22,23]

Information on common psychiatric disorders in the mothers, including PTSD, was elicited by the NIMH-DIS, revised to measure *DSM-III-R* disorders, in personal interviews.[24,25] The PTSD section of the revised NIMH-DIS opens with a question in which typical PTSD events are listed and respondents are asked whether any of these events has ever happened to them. The description of traumatic events follows closely the *DSM-III-R* text, using the examples the text lists (eg, being attacked or raped, being in a fire or flood or bad traffic accident, being threatened with a weapon, or watching someone being seriously injured or killed). A respondent's report of an event that does not fit the *DSM-III-R* stressor definition (eg, severe illness, divorce, loss of job) is excluded from further inquiry, and the respondent is asked whether he or she has experienced another event of the sort described in the question. A report of a qualifying stressor is followed by questions about the occurrence of PTSD symptoms after the event. The inquiry begins with the worst event and continues up to 3 events and their PTSD sequelae. For each event, information is elicited on age at exposure and time of onset of symptoms. Because 3 events are covered, there can be up to 3 distinct PTSD episodes reported by any individual, as each qualifying event can potentially produce PTSD. Age at onset of PTSD is defined as the earliest age at which PTSD has ever occurred.

The term *secondary disorder* in this report refers to the temporal definition and does not imply causal order or clinical importance.

STATISTICAL ANALYSIS

Cox proportional hazards models for censored survival data, with age at onset of PTSD as a time-dependent covariate,[26-28] were used to calculate the hazards ratios of first onset of other disorders associated with prior PTSD (research question 1). The hazards ratio for each of the other disorders estimates the relative risk for the disorder in persons with prior PTSD compared with persons with no prior PTSD, including those who had experienced traumatic events and those who had not. Time was defined as chronological age, and all persons in whom the disorder of interest did not develop by the time of the interview were censored. Separate models were calculated for each of the following disorders: major depression, any anxiety, alcohol abuse or dependence (A/D), and illicit drug A/D. Any anxiety was defined as the occurrence of 1 or more of the anxiety disorders, excluding PTSD. Age at onset of the earliest anxiety disorder was used as the age at onset of any anxiety.

The parameter estimates (β) in the Cox proportional hazards model, as in logistic regression, are regression coefficients from which the hazards ratios can be obtained by taking the antilogarithm of the parameter estimate. The hazards ratio represents an estimate of the relative risk for an outcome in persons with the risk factor compared with persons without the risk factor. For example, the hazards ratio for major depression associated with prior PTSD compares the risk for first-onset major depression in persons

9.2%, 11.3% in women and 5.6% in men.[8] The lifetime prevalence of *DSM-III-R* PTSD in the National Comorbidity Survey (NCS) was 7.8%, 10.4% in women and 5.0% in men.[9]

The observed sex difference in the prevalence of PTSD reflects women's greater vulnerability to the PTSD-inducing effects of traumatic experiences.[8,9] Although the lifetime prevalence of traumatic events was higher in men than in women, PTSD was more likely to develop in women who were exposed to traumatic events than in men.[8,9] The sex difference in PTSD is consistent with the pattern in most anxiety disorders.[10,11]

ALTERNATIVE EXPLANATIONS FOR COMORBIDITY

All 4 general population studies reported that most persons with a history of PTSD had at least 1 other psychiatric disorder in their lifetimes. In this regard, the general population studies replicated findings from clinical samples and from the National Vietnam Veterans Readjustment Study.[12-16] It has been suggested that the high rate of comorbidity with other anxiety disorders or depression might be in part artifactual, reflecting overlapping diagnostic criteria.[13,17] A commonly held view is that psychiatric comorbidity in persons with PTSD represents a range of complications caused by distressing PTSD symptoms. Comorbid substance use disorders might be the inadvertent result of efforts at self-medication to ward off intrusive memories and other painful PTSD symptoms.[18] It has also been suggested that chronic PTSD symptoms may cause reactive depression.[14] There is little information on the chronology of multiple disorders in persons with PTSD.

Evidence that prior PTSD increases the risk for other disorders is a necessary first step in support of the notion that these other disorders might be caused by PTSD. However, such evidence might have other explanations, chief of which is the possibility of shared origins.[19-21] One potential common cause of PTSD and comorbid disorders is exposure to the traumatic events that led to PTSD.[15] To support this etiologic hypothesis, it is necessary to show that the comorbid disorders followed the exposure and were uninfluenced by PTSD. However, because the onset of PTSD, as a rule, occurs within days of the exposure, comorbid disorders that follow exposure to trauma also follow the onset of PTSD. Information on the psychiatric sequelae of traumatic events with prior PTSD with the risk in persons with no prior PTSD, at a specified time. The advantage of the Cox proportional hazards model, compared with logistic regression, is that it permits taking into account the time of the outcome variable, eg, onset of major depression, thereby taking into account differences in the period of risk across individuals. The added advantage of the proportional hazards model with time-dependent covariates is that it allows consideration of independent variables that vary over time. A time-dependent covariate is a variable whose value for any given individual may change over time. In this analysis, a person's PTSD status (as an independent variable) can change from no PTSD to PTSD at any time until the age at onset of the other (comorbid) disorder of interest or time of censoring.

Cox proportional hazards models with multiple time-dependent covariates were used to answer the other research questions in this study. To examine the role of exposure per se, apart from PTSD, in the development of other disorders (research question 2), models with 2 time-dependent covariates were used, namely, exposure to traumatic events and onset of PTSD, using those who were not exposed as reference. To compare the risk for major depression following PTSD with the risk for major depression following other anxiety disorders (research question 3), 3 time-dependent covariates were used, namely, onset of anxiety with no prior PTSD, onset of PTSD with no prior anxiety, and onset of any anxiety followed by PTSD. To estimate the risks for exposure to trauma and the risks for PTSD associated with preexisting psychiatric disorders (research question 4), 2 models with 4 time-dependent covariates were used, representing the onset of 4 specific disorders. One model predicted exposure to trauma in the total sample, and the other predicted onset of PTSD among those who were exposed to trauma. The models yielded hazards ratios for exposure and for onset of PTSD associated with each of the 4 preexisting disorders, adjusting for the others. The SAS procedure for proportional hazards regression was used.[29]

The proportional hazards model with a single time-dependent covariate used to address research question 1 is as follows:

$h_i(t)=e^{\beta Z_i(t)}h_0(t)$ where $h_i(t)$ is the hazard for individual i at time t; $h_0(t)$, the baseline hazard at time t; β, the coefficient of risk associated with PTSD; and $Z_i(t)$, 1 if the subject had PTSD prior to time t and 0 if not.

The proportional hazards model with multiple time-dependent covariates, used in the analysis for research question 3, is as follows:

$h_i(t)=e^{\beta Z_i(t)+\gamma y_i(t)+\alpha X_i(t)}h_0(t)$ where $Z_i(t)$ is 1 if the most recent event occurring before time t is PTSD with no prior anxiety and 0 if not; $y_i(t)$, 1 if the most recent event occurring before time t is anxiety with no prior PTSD and 0 if not; $X_i(t)$, 1 if the most recent event occurring before time t is PTSD with preexisting history of anxiety and 0 if not; and β, γ, and α, coefficients of risk for major depression associated with PTSD alone, anxiety alone, and PTSD following anxiety, respectively.

The proportionality assumption of the hazards ratio was tested for each of the models, using graphic techniques. We plotted log (-log [survival function]) against time. The proportional hazards model is appropriate if the curves of the strata exhibit approximately constant differences over time.[30]

In instances in which the onset of PTSD and the onset of the comorbid disorder of interest were reported to have occurred in the same year, we censored cases just prior to the year in which the 2 events occurred. The procedure avoids imposing a temporal sequence based on a priori assumptions. An assumption that PTSD or the traumatic event preceded another disorder with onset in the same year would fly in the face of evidence that preexisting psychiatric disorders predispose individuals to adversity and increase their vulnerability for PTSD.[15,19,31-33]

in exposed persons in whom PTSD did not develop might provide useful insights. If an increased risk for another disorder was found only in association with PTSD and not with exposure per se in the absence of PTSD, then the plausibility of exposure controlling the onset of comorbid disorders in persons with PTSD would be dampened.

In this report, the following questions are examined: (1) Does PTSD increase the risk for other disorders? (2) Does exposure to traumatic events increase the risk for other disorders? (3) Is the risk for depression following PTSD different from the risk for depression following other anxiety disorders? Although the focus of this report is the psychiatric sequelae of PTSD, (4) Do preexisting disorders increase the risk for PTSD?

RESULTS

DEMOGRAPHIC CHARACTERISTICS OF THE SAMPLE

The 2 strata differed markedly in racial composition, education, and marital status, with the urban stratum containing proportionately more subjects who were black, had not completed high school, and were single mothers (**Table 1**). Mean age was 33.1 years and was lower in urban than suburban women.

TRAUMATIC EVENTS AND PTSD

The lifetime prevalence of exposure to 1 or more traumatic events was 40%, 45% in urban women and 35% in suburban women. Of the 320 women who experienced traumatic events, 71.6% reported 1 event; 21.2%, 2 events; and 7.2%, 3 events. Higher proportions of urban than suburban women reported physical assault, rape, and witnessing violence toward others (**Table 2**). On other types of traumatic experiences, differences in the proportions of urban and suburban women were small. Exposure to trauma was more frequent in women who were single and had not completed high school.

The lifetime prevalence of PTSD in the total sample was 13.8%, 16.8% in urban women and 11.0% in suburban women (P=.02). Posttraumatic stress disorder was only slightly more likely to develop in urban than in suburban women following exposure (37% vs 32%, respectively); the difference in the prevalence of PTSD between the 2 subsets reflected chiefly the higher prevalence of trau-

Table 1. Demographic Characteristics of the Sample*

Characteristics	Urban Subjects (n=394)	Suburban Subjects (n=407)	Total (N=801)
Race			
Black	302 (76.6)	31 (7.6)	**333** (41.6)
White	92 (23.4)	376 (92.4)	**468** (58.4)
Education			
Some high school	99 (25.1)	29 (7.1)	**128** (16.0)
High school	104 (26.4)	124 (30.5)	**228** (28.5)
Some college	145 (36.8)	151 (37.1)	**296** (37.0)
College	46 (11.7)	103 (25.3)	**149** (18.6)
Martial status			
Married mother	165 (41.9)	332 (81.6)	**497** (62.0)
Single mother	229 (58.1)	75 (18.4)	**304** (38.0)
Mean (SD) age, y	31.7 (6.0)	34.5 (4.9)	33.1 (5.6)

**Unless otherwise indicated, data are given as number (percentage) of subjects. Percentages have been rounded and may not total 100.*

Table 2. Exposure to PTSD-Related Events*

Events	Urban Subjects (n=394)	Suburban Subjects (n=407)	Total (N=801)
Assault	66 (16.8)	33 (8.1)	**99** (12.4)
Rape	40 (10.2)	19 (4.7)	**59** (7.4)
Accident	28 (7.1)	34 (8.4)	**62** (7.7)
Disaster	24 (6.1)	24 (5.9)	**48** (6.0)
Witnessing†	49 (12.4)	30 (7.4)	**79** (9.9)
News‡	16 (4.1)	14 (3.4)	**30** (3.7)
Other§	13 (3.3)	22 (5.4)	**35** (4.4)
Any exposure∥	178 (45.2)	142 (34.9)	**320** (40.0)

**Data are given as number (percentage) of subjects. PTSD indicates posttraumatic stress disorder.*

†Includes witnessing someone being killed or seriously injured.

‡Includes news of sudden violent death or accident of a close relative or friend.

§Includes childhood neglect and/or abuse, threat, and narrow escape.

∥The proportions of persons exposed to specific events are not mutually exclusive; any exposure is the total number and percentage exposed to 1 or more events.

matic events among urban women. Events designated by respondents as the worst in their lifetime yielded 84% of the total PTSD cases, with the remaining cases detected through the extension of the inquiry into additional (ie, second and third) traumatic events. The second traumatic event increased the lifetime prevalence of PTSD in the sample from 11.6% to 13.6%, and the third, to 13.8%. Of those who met criteria for PTSD, 18% reported 2 or 3 episodes of PTSD following exposure to distinct events occurring at different times. With the exception of 1 case, PTSD symptoms began within days of exposure.

The probability of PTSD among both urban and suburban women who reported traumatic events varied by level of education and marital status, with those who had not completed high school and those who were single displaying the highest vulnerabilities.

Figure 1 displays the cumulative incidence curve of PTSD in the sample. Kaplan-Meier survival analysis,[34,35] with time defined as respondents' age, was used to estimate the cumulative incidence of PTSD from the earliest to the last case, to approximately 38 years of age. In approximately one third of the PTSD cases, onset occurred at 15 years of age or younger; in more than three quarters, onset was at 25 years of age or younger. The cumulative incidence of PTSD showed a steeper increase during the 5-year period from 18 to 22 years of age than during any earlier or later 5-year interval.

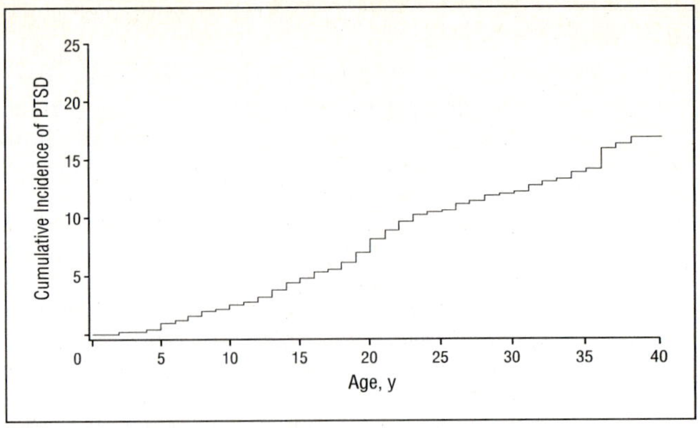

Figure 1. *Cumulative incidence of posttraumatic stress disorder (PTSD) in a sample of 801 women.*

Table 3. Lifetime Comorbidity With PTSD*

Comorbid Disorders	% of Subjects: With PTSD (n=111)	% of Subjects: Without PTSD (n=690)	OR (95% CI)
Any anxiety	55.0	26.1	3.46 (2.29-5.21)
Panic disorder	7.2	2.3	3.27 (1.37-7.84)
Agoraphobia	11.7	2.0	6.40 (2.92-14.03)
Simple phobia	36.0	16.1	2.94 (1.90-4.55)
Social phobia	26.1	13.0	2.36 (1.46-3.80)
GAD	4.5	0.7	6.46 (1.84-22.70)
Major depression	43.2	13.3	4.95 (3.21-7.65)
Alcohol A/D	21.6	8.1	3.12 (1.84-5.30)
Marijuana A/D	7.2	2.2	3.49 (1.45-8.45)
Cocaine A/D	3.6	2.0	1.80 (0.58-5.59)
Any illicit drug A/D	13.5	4.8	3.11 (1.63-5.94)
Any disorder	73.0	38.3	4.36 (2.79-6.81)

**PTSD indicates posttraumatic stress disorder; OR, odds ratio; CI, confidence interval; GAD, generalized anxiety disorder; and A/D, abuse or dependence.*

LIFETIME COMORBIDITY WITH PTSD

Table 3 provides information on lifetime comorbidity with any anxiety, specific anxiety disorders, major depression, and substance use disorders. Significant lifetime associations with PTSD were observed for all disorders except cocaine use disorder. The strongest associations were with agoraphobia, generalized anxiety disorder, and major depression. The most prevalent single comorbid disorder was major depression, with 43.2% of women with PTSD meeting criteria in their lifetimes.

PREDICTING SECONDARY DISORDERS IN PTSD

Four secondary disorders were predicted in 4 separate Cox proportional hazards models: major depression, any

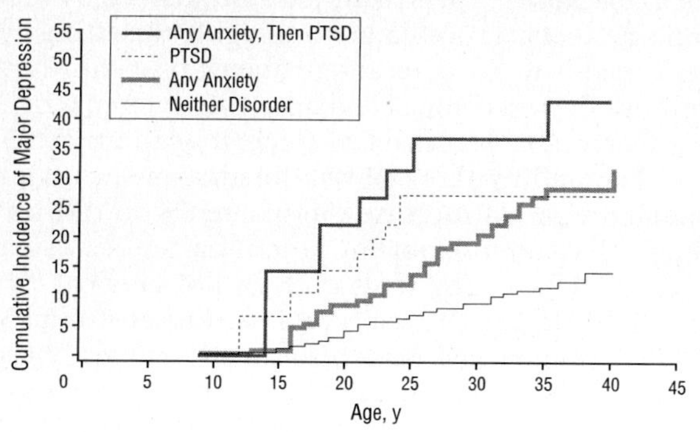

Figure 2. *Cumulative incidence of major depression by history of posttraumatic stress disorder (PTSD) and any anxiety in a sample of 801 women.*

Table 4. Hazards Ratio for Exposure and PTSD by Preexisting Disorders*

Preexisting Disorders	HR for Exposure (N=801) HR (95% CI)	P	HR for PTSD (n=320) HR (95% CI)	P
Major depression	1.9 (1.3-2.9)	.001	2.5 (1.3-4.9)	.006
Any anxiety	1.8 (1.4-2.4)	<.001	1.3 (0.8-2.1)	.27
Alcohol A/D	1.5 (0.9-2.5)	.15	1.1 (0.4-2.7)	.98
Illicit drug A/D	2.1 (1.2-3.8)	.01	0.6 (0.2-2.0)	.39

**PTSD indicates posttraumatic stress disorder; HR, hazards ratio; CI, confidence interval; and A/D, abuse or dependence. Estimates were made in 2 multiple Cox proportional hazards models with time-dependent covariates.*

anxiety disorder, alcohol A/D, and illicit drug A/D. Posttraumatic stress disorder predicted a significantly increased probability of first-onset major depression and alcohol A/D. The hazards ratio for major depression was 2.1 (95% confidence interval [CI], 1.2-3.7) and for alcohol A/D, 3.0 (95% CI, 1.7-5.6). An increased hazards ratio for illicit drug A/D of borderline statistical significance was also detected, 2.3 (95% CI, 1.0-5.4).

DOES EXPOSURE PER SE INCREASE THE RISK FOR OTHER DISORDERS?

Results of analysis with Cox proportional hazards models with 2 time-dependent covariates showed nonsignificant hazards ratios for major depression, any anxiety, or illicit drug A/D following exposure per se without PTSD. Alcohol A/D was an exception, with a significant hazards ratio of 2.1 (95% CI, 1.4-4.1).

EVALUATING THE PTSD—SECONDARY DEPRESSION ASSOCIATION

Hazards ratios for major depression were estimated for 3 mutually exclusive groups of subjects: those with PTSD and no preexisting anxiety (any anxiety), those with any anxiety and no PTSD, and those with PTSD and preexisting anxiety (any anxiety). A fourth group with neither PTSD nor any anxiety served as reference. A Cox proportional hazards model with time-dependent covariates revealed that PTSD increased the risk for secondary major depression, which was similar in size to the risk following any anxiety; hazards ratios were 2.5 (95% CI, 1.2-5.2) and 2.2 (95% CI, 1.5-3.3), respectively. When preceded by any anxiety, PTSD increased the risk for major depression, compared with any anxiety alone (hazards ratio, 1.9 [95% CI, 1.0-3.4], $P<.05$).

To illustrate these results more clearly, **Figure 2** displays the 4 cumulative incidence curves of major depression estimated in this model. These curves differ from the standard Kaplan-Meier curves in that group membership is not fixed, but instead can vary over time. Specifically, membership can change from the group with neither PTSD nor any anxiety to that with PTSD, any anxiety, or PTSD following any anxiety at any age up to the age at onset of major depression or censoring. The incidence of major depression accumulated at higher rates if PTSD occurred in the preceding years than if it did not. In addition, the incidence of major depression in women with PTSD and preexisting anxiety accumulated at higher rates than in women with only anxiety.

DO PREEXISTING PSYCHIATRIC DISORDERS INCREASE THE RISK FOR PTSD?

Preexisting disorders might increase the risk for PTSD in 2 ways: by increasing the probability of exposure to traumatic events, and by increasing the vulnerability to PTSD following exposure to trauma. In the first column of **Table 4** appear the hazards ratios for exposure associated with each of the 4 preexisting disorders, holding constant the other disorders (n=801). In the second column of Table 4 appear the corresponding hazards ratios for PTSD, calculated in the subset of exposed women (n=320). As can be seen in the first column of Table 4, preexisting major depression, any anxiety, and illicit drug A/D, each independent of the other and of prior alcohol A/D, signaled an increased risk for first exposure to traumatic events. Prior major depression, independent of its interrelationship with other disorders, also signaled an increased risk for PTSD among women exposed to traumatic events, as can be seen in the second column.

COMMENT

The key findings of this analysis are as follows: (1) The lifetime prevalence of exposure to traumatic events and PTSD in this sample of women was 40% and 13.8%, respectively. (2) Lifetime comorbidity of PTSD with any of the psychiatric disorders covered in the analysis (ie, major depression, anxiety, and substance use disorders) was 73%. (3) Posttraumatic stress disorder signaled significantly increased risks for first-onset major depression and alcohol A/D. (4) Women exposed to trauma and in whom PTSD did not develop had an increased risk for first-onset alcohol A/D but not major depression. (5) The risk for first-onset major depression in women with prior PTSD was of the same magnitude as in women with a history of 1 or more of the other anxiety disorders. Posttraumatic stress disorder in women with preexisting anxiety disorders enhanced significantly the risk for first-onset major depression. (6) Preexisting major depression increased women's vulnerability to the PTSD-inducing effects of traumatic events and risk for exposure.

The interpretation of these results should take into account several limitations. Retrospective data on lifetime history of psychiatric disorders are subject to recall errors that might bias the estimates of comorbidity. However, retrospective lifetime data are essential in research on the development of comorbidity in disorders with early age at onset, such as anxiety disorders, including PTSD.[36]

THE GENERALIZABILITY of the results is limited by the incomplete participation (75%) and by the characteristics of the sample, all of whom were mothers of children born from 1983 to 1985 in 2 major hospitals in southeast Michigan. The stratified sample represents inner-city and suburban mothers in the geographic area. The generalizability of the findings beyond this population is uncertain. Because of the young age of the women in our sample, the number of PTSD cases with age at onset later than the mid-20 years was small. As a result, the finding that PTSD increased the risk for subsequent major depression might not extend to individuals with PTSD with first onset after 25 years of age.

Although we found that the lifetime prevalence proportions of trauma and PTSD varied by marital status and level of education at the time of the interview, we did not control for either of them in the analysis. The temporal order of these factors in relation to PTSD is unclear in this study. Because single-mother status or low education might qualify as causally intervening between PTSD and major depression or another comorbid disorder, controlling for their effects can spuriously reduce any evidence of true causal associations in the data.[37,38]

The lifetime prevalence of PTSD in our sample, 13.8%, is only slightly higher than the figures previously reported for women in the study of young adults by Breslau et al[8] and in the NCS,[9] 11.3% and 10.4%, respectively. A recent national study of women by Resnick et al[39] estimated the lifetime prevalence of PTSD at 12.3%. In the study reported herein and in the study by Breslau et al, PTSD was measured by the revised NIMH-DIS, whereas in the NCS, PTSD was measured by a modified version of the revised NIMH-DIS. The principal modification in the NCS was the substitution of a list of 12 types of trauma for the single open-ended question in the NIMH-DIS, a modification designed to elicit a more complete account of traumatic events. Resnick et al also used a list of events. The lifetime prevalence of exposure in women in the NCS was 51.2% and in the study by Resnick et al, 69%. In the study reported herein and the one by Breslau et al,[8] the lifetime prevalence of exposure in women did not exceed 40%. Despite the higher lifetime prevalence of exposure in the NCS and in the study by Resnick et al,[39] the estimates of PTSD in these studies were similar to the NIMH-DIS–based estimates reported herein and by Breslau et al. The similarity across studies suggests that procedures to enhance recall might yield a higher lifetime prevalence of exposure, but that the additional events uncovered by these procedures are unlikely to have caused PTSD. Because recall is likely to be influenced by the psychologic sequelae of events, with highly upsetting events more readily recalled, recall-enhancing procedures might improve the reporting of less upsetting events, which are less memorable but also less likely to lead to PTSD.

The finding that the risk for first-onset major depression was not increased in women who did not develop PTSD after exposure to trauma replicates earlier findings of the young adult study by Breslau et al.[19] Findings of the National Vietnam Veterans Readjustment Study on lifetime comorbidity are also consistent with these observations.[16] They indicate that veterans exposed to high war-zone stress were at a markedly increased risk for PTSD and that it is only among those with PTSD (rather than those exposed to high war-zone stress) that the prevalence of co-occurring disorders reached a dramatically high level, when compared with the overall rates in all Vietnam veterans.[16]

Our results on the risk for first-onset major depression in women with PTSD but not in women without PTSD after exposure to trauma might be interpreted as evidence supporting the notion that PTSD gives rise to reactive depression, a response to the demoralization produced by PTSD symptoms. An alternative interpretation is that PTSD is not the cause of subsequent depression but instead a marker of preexisting vulnerability to major depression. The emergence of PTSD might identify a vulnerable subset among those who experienced traumatic events, and the later development of depression might result from the preexisting vulnerability, exposed and possibly exacerbated by the traumatic experience. Vulnerability to major depression might be displayed first by the development of PTSD following traumatic events, especially if exposure occurs early in life. The plausibility of this interpretation is strengthened by our finding that preexisting major depression increased the risk for development of PTSD. One might hypothesize that the increased incidence of major depression following the onset of PTSD is a manifestation of an underlying vulnerability to major depression that also increases the risk for PTSD.

Additional findings of this analysis suggest that the lifetime comorbidity between PTSD and major depression reflect 2 other processes, apart from the increased risk for secondary major depression following PTSD. Preexisting major depression predisposed subjects to traumatic events and increased the vulnerability for the PTSD-inducing effects of traumatic events. These findings are consistent with reports on the increased risk for ordinary stressful life events, as distinct from PTSD-related events, in persons with prior depression.[31,40] They also replicate results of the study by Breslau et al[19] of young adults regarding PTSD-related events. Although it is clinically accepted that preexisting psychiatric disorders influence the likelihood of PTSD following traumatic events, exposure to traumatic events is generally believed to be uninfluenced by personal attributes. Our results suggest that preexisting depression does not exert its influence merely by increasing the vulnerability to the PTSD-inducing effects of traumatic events. The way in which preexisting depression influences PTSD is in part by increasing the probability of exposure to traumatic experiences that lead to PTSD. Functional disabilities due to impairment in emotional, motivational, and cognitive capacities associated with common mental illnesses, including major depression, might increase the likelihood of exposure to stressful experiences and catastrophic events.[41-44]

Accepted for publication April 22, 1996.

Supported by grants MH-48802 and P50 MS 32399 from the National Institute of Mental Health, Bethesda, Md (Dr Breslau).

Reprints: Naomi Breslau, PhD, Department of Psychiatry, Henry Ford Health Sciences Center, 1 Ford Pl, 3A, Detroit, MI 48202-3450.

REFERENCES

1. Egendorf A, Kadushin C, Laufer RS. *Legacy of Vietnam: Comparative Adjustment of Veterans and Their Peers.* New York, NY: Center for Policy Research; 1981:5.
2. Frank E, Anderson BP. Psychiatric disorders in rape victims: past history and current symptomatology. *Compr Psychiatry.* 1987;28:77-82.
3. Kilpatrick DG, Resnick HS. Posttraumatic stress disorder associated with exposure to criminal victimization in clinical and community populations. In: Davidson JRT, Foa EB, eds. *Posttraumatic Stress Disorder: DSM-IV and Beyond.* Washington, DC: American Psychiatric Press; 1992:113-143.
4. Shore JH, Vollmer WM, Tatum EI. Community patterns of posttraumatic stress disorders. *J Nerv Ment Dis.* 1989;177:681-685.
5. Alexander DA, Wells A. Reactions of police officers to body-handling after a major disaster: a before-and-after comparison. *Br J Psychiatry.* 1991;159:547-555.
6. Helzer J, Robins L, McEvoy L. Post-traumatic stress disorder in the general population: findings of the Epidemiologic Catchment Area survey. *N Engl J Med.* 1987;317:1630-1634.
7. Davidson JRT, Hughes D, Blazer DG. Post-traumatic stress disorder in the community: an epidemiological study. *Psychol Med.* 1991;21:713-721.
8. Breslau N, Davis GC, Andreski P, Peterson EL. Traumatic events and posttraumatic stress disorder in an urban population of young adults. *Arch Gen Psychiatry.* 1991;48:216-222.
9. Kessler RC, Sonnega A, Bromet E, Nelson CB. Posttraumatic stress disorder in the National Comorbidity Survey. *Arch Gen Psychiatry.* 1995;52:1048-1060.
10. Eaton WW, Dryman A, Weissman MM. Panic and phobia. In: Robins LN, Regier DA, eds. *Psychiatric Disorders in America: The Epidemiologic Catchment Area Study.* New York, NY: Free Press; 1991:155-179.
11. Kessler RC, McGonagle KA, Zhao S, Nelson CB, Hughes M, Eshleman S, Wittchan H-U, Kendler KS. Lifetime and 12-month prevalence of *DSM-III-R* psychiatric disorders in the United States. *Arch Gen Psychiatry.* 1994;51:8-19.
12. Sierles FS, Chen JJ, McFarland RE, Taylor MA. Posttraumatic stress disorder and concurrent psychiatric illness: a preliminary report. *Am J Psychiatry.* 1983; 140:1177-1179.
13. Keane TM, Wolfe J. Comorbidity in post-traumatic stress disorder: an analysis of community and clinical studies. *J Appl Soc Psychol.* 1990;20:1776-1788.
14. Green BL, Lindy JD, Grace MC, Leonard AC. Chronic posttraumatic stress disorder and diagnostic comorbidity in a disaster sample. *J Nerv Ment Dis.* 1992; 180:760-766.
15. McFarlane AC, Papay P. Multiple diagnoses in posttraumatic stress disorder in the victims of a natural disaster. *J Nerv Ment Dis.* 1992;180:498-504.
16. Kulka R, Schlenger W, Fairbank J, Hough RL, Jordan BK, Marmar CR, Weiss DS. *Trauma and the Vietnam War Generation.* New York, NY: Brunner/Mazel; 1990:126-133.
17. Davidson JRT, Foa EB. Diagnostic issues in posttraumatic stress disorder: considerations for the *DSM-IV. J Abnor Psychol.* 1991;100:346-355.
18. Grady DA. Epilogue: 'A self-guide for Vietnam veterans'. In: Kulka R, Schlenger W, Fairbank J, Hough RL, Jordan BK, Marmar CR, Weiss DS, eds. *Trauma and the Vietnam War Generation.* New York, NY: Brunner/Mazel; 1990:276-291.
19. Breslau N, Davis GC, Andreski P, Federman B, Anthony JC. Epidemiologic findings on PTSD and comorbid disorders in the general population. In: Dohrenwend B, ed. *Adversity, Stress, and Psychopathology.* Washington, DC: American Psychiatric Press. In press.
20. Merikangas KR. Co-morbidity for anxiety and depression: review of family and genetic studies. In: Maser JD, Cloninger CR, eds. *Comorbidity of Mood and Anxiety Disorders.* Washington, DC: American Psychiatric Press; 1990:331-348.
21. Kendler KS, Neale MC, Kessler RC, Heath AC, Eaves LJ. Major depression and phobias: the genetic and environmental sources of comorbidity. *Psychol Med.* 1993;23:361-371.
22. Breslau N, DelDotto JE, Brown GG, Kumar S, Ezhuthachan S, Hufnagle KG. A gradient relationship between low birth weight and IQ at 6 years of age. *Arch Pediatr Adolesc Med.* 1994;148:377-383.
23. Breslau N, Chilcoat HG, DelDotto JE, Andreski P, Brown GG. Low birth weight and neurocognitive status at six years of age. *Biol Psychiatry.* 1996;40:389-397.
24. Robins LN, Helzer JE, Cottler L, Golding E. *NIMH Diagnostic Interview Schedule, Version III Revised.* St. Louis, Mo: Washington University; 1989.
25. American Psychiatric Association. *Diagnostic and Statistical Manual of Mental Disorders, Third Edition, Revised.* Washington, DC: American Psychiatric Press; 1987.
26. Cox DR. Regression models and life tables. *J R Stat Soc Series B.* 1974;34: 187-220.
27. Cox DR. Partial likelihood. *Biometrika.* 1975;62:269-276.
28. Breslow N. Covariance analysis of censored survival data. *Biometrics.* 1974; 30:89-99.
29. SAS Institute. *SAS Technical Report, SAS/STAT Software: The PHREG Procedure, Version 6.* Cary, NC: SAS Institute; 1991:217.
30. Kalbfleish JD, Prentice RL. *The Statistical Analysis of Failure Time Data.* New York, NY: John Wiley & Sons Inc; 1980:88.
31. Kendler KS, Kessler RC, Neale MC, Heath AC, Eaves LJ. The prediction of major depression in women: toward an integrated etiologic model. *Am J Psychiatry.* 1993;150:1139-1148.
32. Kendler KS, Neale MC, Kessler RC, Heath AC, Eaves LJ. A twin study of recent life events and difficulties. *Arch Gen Psychiatry.* 1993;50:789-796.
33. Kendler KS, Kessler RC, Walters EE, MacLean C, Neale MD, Heath AD, Eaves LJ. Stressful life events, genetic liability, and onset of an episode of major depression in women. *Am J Psychiatry.* 1995;152:833-842.
34. Kaplan EL, Meier P. Nonparametric estimation from incomplete observations. *J Am Stat Assoc.* 1958;53:457-481.
35. Kay R. Proportional hazards regression models and the analysis of censored survival data. *Appl Stat.* 1977;26:227-237.
36. Breslau N, Schultz L, Peterson EL. Sex differences in depression: a role for preexisting anxiety. *Psychiatry Res.* 1995;58:1-12.
37. Kleinbaum DG, Kupper LL, Morgenstern H. *Epidemiologic Research: Principles and Quantitative Methods.* Belmont, Calif: Lifetime Learning Publications; 1982.
38. Weinberg CR. Toward a clearer definition of confounding. *Am J Epidemiol.* 1993;137:1-8.
39. Resnick HS, Kilpatrick DG, Dansky BS, Saunders BE, Best CL. Prevalence of civilian trauma and posttraumatic stress disorder in a representative national sample of women. *J Consult Clin Psychol.* 1993;61:984-991.
40. Brown GW, Harris TO, Eales MJ. Aetiology of anxiety and depressive disorders in an inner-city population, II: comorbidity and adversity. *Psychol Med.* 1993;23:155-165.
41. Hays RD, Wells KB, Sherbourne CD, Rogers W, Spritzer K. Functioning and well-being outcomes of patients with depression compared with chronic general medical illnesses. *Arch Gen Psychiatry.* 1995;52:11-19.
42. Von Korff M, Ormel J, Katon W, Lin EHB. Disability and depression among high utilizers of health care. *Arch Gen Psychiatry.* 1992;49:91-100.
43. Broadhead WE, Blazer DG, George LK, Tse CK. Depression, disability days, and days lost from work in a prospective epidemiologic survey. *JAMA.* 1990; 264:2524-2528.
44. Ormel J, VonKorff M, Ustun B, Pini S, Korten A, Oldehinkel T. Common mental disorders and disability across cultures. *JAMA.* 1994;272:1741-1748.

Smoking Affects Plasma-Soluble Interleukin-2 Receptor Levels in Patients With Schizophrenia

Ganguli and colleagues,[1] in the August 1995 issue of the ARCHIVES, provide convincing evidence that phytohemagglutinin-induced in vitro interleukin-2 (IL-2) production is reduced in patients with schizophrenia who have never received medication compared with healthy control subjects. They note that decreased IL-2 secretion and increased systemic levels of soluble IL-2 receptors (sIL-2Rs) are robust findings that signify an alteration of immunologic functions in patients with schizophrenia. Documentation of altered IL-2 secretion in drug-naive patients is important because antipsychotic medication can influence the IL-2/IL-2 receptor system as demonstrated by clozapine-induced increases in plasma sIL-2R levels.[2]

In addition to antipsychotic medication, smoking may affect the immune system of patients with schizophrenia. In healthy smokers, phytohemagglutinin-induced lymphocyte proliferation was shown to be suppressed,[3] and systemic sIL-2R levels were reported to be increased.[4,5] The prevalence of smoking is high in patients with schizophrenia,[6] but neither the study by Ganguli et al nor the previous studies cited by these authors investigated a control group matched to the patients for smoking habits when studying IL-2 production or systemic sIL-2R levels in patients with schizophrenia.

In a sample of 39 white patients who met the diagnostic criteria for a schizophrenic or schizophreniform disorder,[7] admitted consecutively to our clinic, we measured sIL-2R plasma levels by using a commercially available enzyme-linked immunosorbent assay kit (Biermann Diagnostica, Bad Nauheim, Germany) (sensitivity, 16 U/mL; interassay and intra-assay coefficients of variation, <8%). No patient suffered from an acute infectious disease, as assessed by clinical examination, blood sedimentation rate, and white blood cell counts. No patient had received clozapine during the last 6 months; 18 patients did not receive any psychotropic medication during this period, and 21 patients received various antipsychotic agents prior to admission. Soluble IL-2 receptor levels did not differ significantly between drug-free and medicated patients (mean±SD, 325±206 vs 285±136 U/mL, $t=0.71$, $P=.48$). Eighteen patients smoked (11 men and 7 women; mean±SD age, 36.4±14.2 years), and 21 patients did not smoke (11 men and 10 women; mean±SD age, 40.7±17.2 years). The plasma sIL-2R levels were significantly higher in the patients who smoked compared with those who did not smoke (mean±SD, 365±203 vs 251±118 U/mL, $t=-2.17$, $P=.04$).

In vitro IL-2 production has not been investigated in smokers. However, decreased phytohemagglutinin-induced lymphocyte proliferation[3] and increased systemic sIL-2R levels in healthy subjects[4,5] and in patients with schizophrenia who smoke underscore that smoking may confound studies investigating the IL-2/IL-2 receptor system. Therefore, future studies investigating immune functions in patients with schizophrenia should include control groups matched for their smoking habits.

Thomas Pollmächer, MD
Dunja Hinze-Selch, MD
Janet Mullington, PhD
Thomas Fenzel, MD
Florian Holsboer, PhD
Max Planck Institute of Psychiatry
Clinical Institute
Kraepelinstrasse 10
Munich D-80804
Germany

1. Ganguli R, Brar JS, Chengappa KNR, DeLeo M, Yang ZW, Shurin G, Rabin BS. Mitogen-stimulated interleukin-2 production in never-medicated, first-episode schizophrenic patients: the influence of age at onset and negative symptoms. *Arch Gen Psychiatry*. 1995;52:668-672.
2. Pollmächer T, Hinze-Selch D, Mullington J, Holsboer F. Clozapine-induced increase in plasma levels of soluble interleukin-2 receptors. *Arch Gen Psychiatry*. 1995;52:877-878.
3. Petersen BH, Steimel LF, Callaghan JT. Suppression of mitogen-induced lymphocyte transformation in cigarette smokers. *Clin Immunol Immunopathol*. 1983;27:135-140.
4. Tollerud DJ, Weiss ST, Leung DY. Elevated soluble interleukin-2 receptors in young healthy cigarette smokers: lack of association with atopy or airways hyperresponsiveness. *Int Arch Allergy Immunol*. 1992;97:25-30.
5. Tollerud DJ, Kurman CC, Nelson DL, Brown LM, Maloney EM, Blattner WA. Racial variation in serum-soluble interleukin-2 receptor levels: a population-based study of healthy smokers and non-smokers. *Clin Immunol Immunopathol*. 1994;70:274-279.
6. de Leon J, Dadvand M, Canuso C, White AO, Stanilla JK, Simpson GM. Schizophrenia and smoking: an epidemiological survey in a state hospital. *Am J Psychiatry*. 1995;152:453-455.
7. American Psychiatric Association. *Diagnostic and Statistical Manual of Mental Disorders, Third Edition, Revised*. Washington, DC: American Psychiatric Association; 1987.

In reply

We were interested in the report by Pollmächer and colleagues indicating that sIL-2R concentrations may be influenced by smoking. The effects of smoking on sIL-2R concentrations have been previously reported in patients without schizophrenia, but Pollmächer and colleagues suggest that this effect is also found in patients with schizophrenia. Given the high prevalence of smoking among patients with schizophrenia, this is an important observation and suggests that several previous reports

Phytohemagglutinin-Stimulated Interleukin (IL)-2 Production*

	IL-2 Concentration, pg/mL	
Smoking Status	Patients (n)	Control Subjects (n)
Nonsmokers	862.8±657.0 (19)	1451.1±1255.0 (91)
Smokers	1054.1±583.0 (35)	1516.4±1212.0 (39)

*Data are given as the mean±SD.

about increased sIL-2Rs in association with schizophrenia[1-3] may need to be reanalyzed if smoking data are available for those subjects.

Decreased IL-2 production has also been consistently reported in patients with schizophrenia by several groups,[4-8] but smoking status has not been taken into account in those studies either. Pollmächer and colleagues question whether decreased IL-2 production might also be associated with smoking rather than with schizophrenia, and we would like to respond to this. We have collected smoking status data about several of the subjects who were enrolled in our earlier studies of IL-2 production, and we report those results.

Smoking data had been collected about 54 acutely ill patients with schizophrenia and 130 normal control subjects who were enrolled in an earlier study of phytohemagglutinin-stimulated IL-2 production. No difference existed in the mean age of the patients and control subjects, but a trend existed for the nonsmoking patients to be younger than the other groups. The **Table** *provides the mean IL-2 production data for each group; subjects were divided on the basis of their smoking status. No relationship existed between smoking status and IL-2 production levels, while decreased IL-2 production was associated with schizophrenia in smokers and nonsmokers. A similar analysis of patients with first-episode schizophrenia who were never medicated from a study recently reported in the* ARCHIVES[9] *also showed no effect of smoking on IL-2 production (data not shown).*

Thus, smoking status could not account for the decreased IL-2 production in our studies of this immune measure in patients with schizophrenia. Our data from control subjects also do not suggest any notable effect of smoking on IL-2 production.

Rohan Ganguli, MD
Jaspreet S. Brar, MD, MPH
Western Psychiatric Institute and Clinic
3811 O'Hara St
Pittsburgh, PA 15213-2593

1. Rapaport MH, McAllister CG, Pickar D, Nelson DL, Paul SM. Elevated levels of soluble interleukin 2 receptors in schizophrenia. *Arch Gen Psychiatry.* 1989; 46:291-292.
2. Rapaport MH, Torrey EF, McAllister CG, Nelson DL, Pickar D, Paul SM. Increased serum soluble interleukin-2 receptors in schizophrenic monozygotic twins. *Eur Arch Psychiatry Clin Neurosci.* 1993;243:7-10.
3. Rapaport MH, McAllister CG, Kim YS, Han JH, Pickar D, Nelson DL, Kirch DG, Paul SM. Increased serum soluble interleukin-2 receptors in Caucasian and Korean schizophrenic patients. *Biol Psychiatry.* 1994;35:56-60.
4. Koliaskina GI, Morozov TP, Sedirina TP, Burbayera GS. Immunological and virological studies in schizophrenia: general trends and personal data. Presented at the Second World Congress on Viruses, Immunity and Mental Health; October 6, 1988; Quebec, Canada.
5. Ganguli R, Rabin BS, Belle SH. Decreased interleukin-2 production in schizophrenic patients. *Biol Psychiatry.* 1989;26:427-430.
6. Villemain F, Chatenoud L, Galinowski A, Homo DF, Ginestet D, Loo H, Zarifian E, Bach JF. Aberrant T cell–mediated immunity in untreated schizophrenic patients: deficient interleukin-2 production. *Am J Psychiatry.* 1989;146:609-616.
7. Sirota P, Fishman P, Elizur A, Djaldetty M. Lymphokine production in schizophrenic patients. *Biol Psychiatry.* 1990;27:173A.
8. Ganguli R, Brar JS, Solomon W, Chengappa KNR, Rabin BS. Altered interleukin-2 production in schizophrenia: association between clinical state and autoantibody production. *Psychiatr Res.* 1992;44:113-123.
9. Ganguli R, Brar JS, Chengappa KNR, DeLeo M, Yang ZW, Shurin G, Rabin BS. Mitogen-stimulated interleukin-2 production in never-medicated, first-episode schizophrenic patients: the influence of age at onset and negative symptoms. *Arch Gen Psychiatry.* 1995;52:668-672.

Research With Cognitively Impaired Subjects

Unfinished Business in the Regulation of Human Research

Richard J. Bonnie, LLB

In 1978, the National Commission for the Protection of Human Subjects of Biomedical and Behavioral Research issued an important report that addressed the difficult ethical issues arising in research involving subjects with mental disabilities. However, because of irreconcilable conflicts between the scientific community and rights-oriented advocacy groups, the federal government never issued the special regulations pertaining to these issues that had been envisioned by the National Commission. Because these important ethical issues have not yet been adequately addressed by policy-making bodies, protection of cognitively impaired subjects depends too heavily on the diverse ethical sensitivities of individual investigators and on ad hoc responses of particular institutional review boards. Researchers should support a credible and authoritative process for reexamining and resolving ethical issues relating to research with cognitively impaired subjects. This can be accomplished without leading to the stalemate that doomed the National Commission's proposals. The challenge is to forge a consensus on ethical guidelines and safeguards that will most reasonably accommodate the goals of protecting the dignity and well-being of research subjects while avoiding undue impediments to valuable scientific inquiry.

Arch Gen Psychiatry. 1997;54:105-111

BACKGROUND

The ethical dangers lurking in human research have burst into public consciousness on a broad scale. Two specialty societies of German medicine recently accepted responsibility for ameliorating the consequences of the horrifying abuses perpetrated in the name of medicine and science by the Nazi doctors.[1] In so doing, they broke a disturbing, unforgotten silence by German medicine. Meanwhile, a presidential advisory committee recently issued a lengthy report on the extensive, and unethical, radiation experiments conducted in this country between 1944 and 1974, recommending that the federal government make amends by compensating the subjects of 9 experiments and apologizing to many others (*New York Times*. October 3, 1995:A19).

The juxtaposition of these 2 events vividly amplifies a point made by David Rothman, PhD, in his 1991 book, *Strangers at the Bedside*, which traces the emergence of the contemporary bioethics movement.[2] According to Rothman, the Nazi experiments documented at Nuremberg in 1945 to 1946—which led to the conviction of 16 doctors for crimes against humanity—"were not perceived by researchers or commentators to be directly relevant to the American scene. . . . " This reaction was understandable, of course—nothing in the annals of science can compare with the Nazi atrocities. Physicians forced people to drink seawater to find out how long a person might survive without fresh water. At Dachau, Russian prisoners of war were immersed in icy water to see how long a pilot might survive when shot down over the English Channel. At Auschwitz, physicians experimented with new ways to sterilize or castrate people as

See also pages 113,117, and 121

From the Institute of Law, Psychiatry, and Public Policy, University of Virginia, Charlottesville.

part of the plan to repopulate Eastern Europe with Germans. This list of infamous deeds is a long one, and one can see why American medical scientists thought that "madness, not medicine, was implicated at Nuremberg."

But German medicine *was* implicated at Nuremberg, as several recent books have amply shown,[3,4] and the German experience *was* relevant to medical research in the United States. The ultimate lesson of the Nazi experience is that protecting the autonomy and well-being of each human subject must be the preeminent ethical imperative of medical research. Yet for many years after the Nuremberg trials, it appears that many clinical researchers in the United States remained oblivious to the norms of research ethics first enunciated in the Nuremberg Code and thereafter in the World Medical Association's Helsinki Declaration in 1964. A 1961 survey of 66 medical schools revealed that only 8 had established written procedures for the conduct of human research.[5] Although the National Institutes of Health (NIH) Clinical Research Center had issued guidelines for intramural research in the 1950s, the prevailing position of NIH during this period was that extramural researchers should be guided by their own professional judgment.[6]

The modern era of research ethics began in 1966. In that year, the *New England Journal of Medicine* published an important article by Henry Beecher, MD, of Harvard Medical School that documented 22 instances of unethical research conducted by respectable investigators at responsible institutions.[7] (All of these studies had been published in major peer-reviewed scientific journals.) Also in 1966, the Food and Drug Administration adopted its first regulations on clinical drug testing, and the Surgeon General issued guidelines governing NIH-sponsored research.[6] These NIH guidelines, which established the institutional review board (IRB) system, eventually culminated in formal federal regulations issued in 1974.

It is helpful to remember that the current system of regulating human research through the IRB structure is less than 30 years old. Adoption of this innovative system had transformative historical significance—leaving behind an era of unregulated clinical discretion and ushering in the modern era of bioethics—and the IRBs have provided a workable model for "internal" review of clinical and scientific decision making by mixed bodies of laypersons and specialists. At the same time, however, we should recognize that the IRB system has remained fundamentally unchanged since it was first established, while discourse in research ethics has deepened in sophistication. It should therefore come as no surprise that the existing arrangements have recently come under critical scrutiny.

Critical attention has focused particularly on whether the current regulatory arrangements provide adequate protection for subjects with cognitive impairments. Most prominently, a study at the University of California, Los Angeles (UCLA), involving medication withdrawal from subjects with recent-onset schizophrenia was cited by the Department of Human and Health Services Office for Protection from Research Risks in 1994 for what it found to be deficiencies in the investigators' procedures for obtaining informed consent.[8] The alleged failure of the UCLA IRB to detect these deficiencies led the Office for Protection from Research Risks to require "improvement in UCLA's system for protection of human research subjects, especially potentially vulnerable research subjects, including those with severe psychiatric disorders." The remedial actions included participation of consumer representatives on the IRB and establishment of Data and Safety Monitoring Boards to oversee protocols involving overlapping responsibility for the research and the patients' ongoing clinical management.

The controversy surrounding the UCLA study called into question similar studies involving medication withdrawal from psychiatric patients.[9,10] Predictably, broad questions have been raised about the capacity of psychiatric patients and other subjects with possible cognitive impairments to provide informed consent and about the adequacy of IRB review of protocols involving these subjects.[9,10] Some critics have called for a major overhaul of the current regulatory structure. Litigation has ensued as well: in December 1996, a New York appellate court invalidated portions of the research regulations promulgated by the New York Office of Mental Health and halted a group of studies being conducted in public psychiatric hospitals in which consent had been provided by surrogates on behalf of incompetent patients; the court's concern focused particularly on studies presenting greater than minimal risk that offered little or no direct therapeutic benefit to the subjects (*T. D. v New York Office of Mental Health*, Supreme Court of New York, Appellate Division, First Department, December 5, 1996).

Many, perhaps most, ethical scientists believe that the weaknesses of the current structure have been exaggerated and are fearful that any ensuing changes will do more harm than good. And caution is most surely indicated. At the same time, however, we should not assume that the current regulatory regime is immune from legitimate criticism. To do this would be to ignore the hard lessons of experience.

Current controversies regarding research with cognitively impaired subjects should be seen, in historical context, as a reminder of unfinished business. The underlying issues include the proper balance between subject protection and methodological considerations in study design, the necessary links between administration of the research protocol and the subjects' ongoing clinical care, and means of ensuring that informed consent to research participation is provided by subjects or by their authorized surrogates. These issues have not yet been adequately addressed by policymaking bodies in a systematic and authoritative manner. As a result, protection of cognitively impaired subjects depends too heavily on the diverse ethical sensitivities of individual investigators and on ad hoc responses of particular IRBs. In my opinion, researchers would be well advised to support a credible and authoritative process for reexamining and resolving these issues. By strengthening public confidence in the ethical integrity of biomedical research, such a reexamination will be good for science and for the subjects of human research.

THE BELMONT REPORT

The underlying problem is that basic ethical issues raised by research with cognitively impaired subjects have not received systematic attention from policy-making authorities. Understanding why this is so requires a backward glance at the developmental period of regulation in research ethics. The 1966 article by Beecher[7] had put generic issues of human research on the regulatory agenda. But special attention was also directed at research involving so-called vulnerable or marginalized populations. The ethical dangers of research with vulnerable subjects were evident in the hepatitis experiment carried out at Willowbrook State Hospital in New York, in which retarded children admitted to the hospital were injected with the hepatitis virus to study the development of the disease and the effects of gamma globulin in preventing it. This investigation was exposed in 1971.[2] The next year, the public learned of a Public Health Service–sponsored investigation in Tuskeegee, Ala, in which the natural progression of syphilis was studied in a group of poor, rural, African-American subjects over a 40-year period. Many of the subjects were left untreated, even after penicillin became available. This study had been reviewed and approved by a Public Health Service review committee as late as 1969 and was discontinued only after it became exposed to the public.[2] These disclosures contributed to a growing skepticism about the ability or inclination of powerful social institutions, including science, to protect the interests of unrepresented, vulnerable, or disenfranchised social groups.

In 1974, a crescendo of public concern about the ethics of biomedical research led Congress to establish the National Commission for the Protection of Human Subjects of Biomedical and Behavioral Research (the "Commission"). The Commission was directed "to review the problems and practices associated with the protection of the rights and welfare of human subjects involved in various forms of biomedical and behavioral research." I have written in another context about the relatively modest contribution of presidential (or national) commissions to public policy on value-laden social issues.[11] However, the National Commission for the Protection of Human Subjects of Biomedical and Behavioral Research is a notable exception to a general record of underachievement. In 4 years, the Commission published 9 major reports, each of which included a detailed set of recommendations for legislative and regulatory action. As directed by Congress, the Commission gave special attention to fetal research and 3 special classes of subjects: children, prisoners, and persons "institutionalized as mentally infirm."[12]

By law, the Department of Health, Education, and Welfare (the Department of Health, Education, and Welfare and its successor, the Department of Health and Human Services, are referred to hereafter as "the Department") was required to invite public comment on the Commission's recommendations, and was directed either to implement them or to explain any decision not to do so. Eventually, in 1981, the Department issued regulations for all federally sponsored research, together with special provisions concerning fetal research and prisoner subjects. Two years later, the Department issued additional regulations on research with children. However, despite strong criticism by the President's Commission on the Study of Ethical Problems in Medicine and Biomedical and Behavioral Research, the Department declined to adopt the National Commission's recommendations—or to issue any special guidelines at all—on the particular ethical issues raised by research with persons institutionalized as mentally disabled or, more generally, persons who might have diminished capacity to provide informed consent. What accounts for this glaring deviation from the Commission's regulatory agenda? What significance does it have for the issues that we confront today? Before addressing these questions, it is necessary to review some basic ethical issues regarding research with cognitively impaired subjects, and to summarize the key features of the Commission's analysis, set forth in what has come to be known as the "Belmont Report" issued in March 1978.[12]

Permissibility of Proxy Consent

Should human research be permitted at all if the subject lacks the capacity to give informed consent? Read literally, the Nuremberg Code prohibits research without the subject's consent and does not refer to the possibility of proxy consent. However, as the Commission recognized, a categorical prohibition of proxy consent would stymie the development of knowledge regarding many severe neurological and psychiatric disorders. So it recommended that proxy consent be permitted for research with potential therapeutic benefit to the subject and for some low-risk research without therapeutic potential that would be relevant to the subject's condition.

The Ethical Significance of Institutionalization

What bearing should the fact of institutionalization have on the validity of consent? It is noteworthy, in this connection, that the Commission's charge defined the vulnerability of this subject population in terms of institutionalization rather than in terms of mental disability, per se. The reason, of course, is that institutional environments may be thought to be inherently coercive. Although this danger is readily seen for prisoner subjects, it is much more subtle for the heterogeneous populations of patients in psychiatric hospitals and in mental retardation facilities. In any case, the Commission properly concluded that the fact of institutionalization should not preclude research participation but instead should trigger careful scrutiny of the voluntariness of consent in particular cases.

The Many Shades of Autonomy

Obviously, legal and ethical requirements will differ according to whether the subject does or does not have the capacity to make an informed decision regarding research participation. However, the Commission concluded that this binary distinction between persons with and without decisional capacity was insufficient to take account of ethically relevant differences among prospective research subjects. Instead, the Commission distinguished among 4 categories of subjects: those able to give informed consent, those unable to give informed consent but nonetheless able to "assent" (ie, able to understand the procedure to be used and the right to withdraw and able to choose to participate), those unable to consent or assent but who do not object to participation, and, finally, those who object to participation.

Research Over Objection

If a competent person objects to participation in research, his or her refusal must be honored as a matter of ethical and legal principle. But what if the prospective subject's refusal is not a competent one, ie, if the subject is not capable of understanding the nature and purposes of the research or is incapable of weighing the risks and benefits in a rational manner? Should research nonetheless be prohibited on the grounds that no one, even an incompetent person, should be made an involuntary subject of a scientific experiment? The Commission concluded that research with objecting subjects should be permitted only if the research could potentially benefit the subject and is approved by a court. (In addition, if the research presents greater than minimal risk, it would be permissible only if no other beneficial treatment were available.)

Research With Nonobjecting Subjects

In an important contribution, the Commission concluded that a nonobjecting subject's inability to provide informed consent should not impede research if safeguards are adequate to protect the subject from unreasonable risk. Thus, the Commission recommended that (1) research involving less than minimal risk should be permitted as long as it is relevant to the subject's condition and (2) research presenting greater than minimal risk should be permitted with the subject's assent or, if the subject was not capable of providing assent, with the authorization of a guardian or court, if either (i) the research potentially could result in direct benefit to the subject or (ii) the research is relevant to the subject's condition, is important and presents only a minor increase over minimal risk.

Safeguards

In what turned out to be one of the most controversial features of the Commission's proposals, it recommended use of so-called consent auditors to monitor the consent process, to assess the subject's level of impairment, and to determine whether the subject was capable of providing, and had in fact provided the requisite consent or assent. Under the Commission's proposals, consent auditors would have been required for research presenting greater than minimal risk that offered no potential benefit to the subject, but otherwise would have been an optional safeguard, to be used at the discretion of the IRB.

Departmental Response

As required by law, the Department published its comments on the Belmont Report, together with proposed regulations to implement it, in November 1978.[13] In the course of its comments, the Department invited public reaction to several proposals designed to strengthen the safeguards recommended by the Commission. Most significant was its comment concerning the use of consent auditors. Whereas the Commission would have required consent auditors only for protocols presenting greater than minimal risk without potential benefit to the subject, the Department indicated that it was giving serious consideration to the possibility of requiring use of consent auditors in *all* cases involving persons institutionalized as mentally disabled, regardless of level of risk, the purpose of the research, or the use of other safeguards.[13]

In addition, the Department's comments expressed considerable uneasiness about the Commission's decision to allow research involving greater than minimal risk with (nonobjecting) subjects unable to give informed consent. Specifically, the Department indicated that it was considering proposals to require the consent of a "subject advocate" in cases of assenting subjects, and to ban research with subjects who are not capable of assenting in the absence of a potential direct benefit to the subject.

No Middle Ground

It appears that the debate about these proposed regulations within the Department divided along a classic fault line in psychiatric ethics and mental health law. On the one side, scientists were genuinely concerned that the rules and safeguards proposed by the Commission, especially the use of consent auditors and subject advocates, would seriously impede research at the very time that psychiatry stood on the threshold of major scientific advances. The ascendancy of biological psychiatry also signaled efforts to realign psychiatry with other medical specialties. In addition, the singling out of persons with mental illness perpetuates false and stigmatizing assumptions. In short, the idea of special rules for research about mental illness seemed fundamentally incompatible with the emerging self-image of modern psychiatry and with the inclusionary themes of modern mental health advocacy.

On the other side, human rights advocates were properly concerned about the special vulnerability of persons with mental disability, especially in light of the risks that can be associated with unvalidated biological treatments and subjects' diminished ability to protect themselves. The key question, from a human rights perspective, is whether clinical investigators and IRBs can be expected to give adequate attention to the desires and interests of mentally disabled subjects. The historical record of ethical insensitivity, recently punctuated by the disclosures about abuses at Tuskeegee and Willowbrook, had deepened the advocates' distrust of clinical discretion and strengthened their desire to subject clinical decision making to external controls.

The gap between these points of view was too large to be bridged in 1982. The question we now face is whether it can be bridged in 1997.

THE CONSEQUENCES OF REGULATORY SILENCE

The ethical issues surrounding the consent process did not evaporate simply because the Department regulations failed to address them. The regulations are altogether silent on impairment of decision-making capacity, the consequences of decisional impairment, the designation and duties of proxy decision makers, and the nature of safeguards that IRBs are expected to consider. The effect of regulatory silence was to leave those issues to the unguided discretion of investigators and IRBs. This is not a satisfactory solution, as the NIH recognized in 1986, when it adopted its own special guidelines for intramural research with subjects whose decision-making abilities are impaired by severe physical or mental illness.[14] In addition, the American College of Physicians published a valuable position paper in 1989 addressing ethical questions raised by research with cognitively impaired subjects.[15] In 1994, the directors of Alzheimer disease research centers published another important position paper on "Guidelines for Addressing Ethical and Legal Issues in Alzheimer Disease Research."[16] The College on Problems of Drug Dependence also published a position paper on "Human Subjects Issues in Drug Abuse Research" in 1995.[17]

I detect growing support for the idea that these issues merit reexamination in the light of experience and changed scientific and social circumstances. In October 1995, President Clinton issued an executive order establishing a National Bioethics Advisory Commission and directing the Commission to address the "protection of the rights and welfare of human research subjects" as its first priority.[18] The board of directors of the National Alliance for the Mentally Ill recently called for the development of "national standards" governing the protection of research subjects with cognitive impairments (unpublished data, National Alliance for the Mentally Ill Board of Directors, February 2, 1995). In addition, the Institute of Medicine is considering whether it might play a useful role in this unfolding process. I strongly support the concept of review by an authoritative body, not because I perceive any documented pattern of ethical misconduct, but rather because the issues have not received the systematic attention that they deserve, because the IRBs need better guidance than they have been given, and because the festering controversy surrounding these issues threatens to erode the climate of trust between researchers and consumers that sustains the social investment in scientific research.

I was amazed to discover that the existing regulations are entirely silent about impairments of decision-making capacity.[19] The only pertinent provision directs the IRB to be "particularly cognizant of the special problems of research involving vulnerable populations," including "mentally disabled persons," and to ensure that "additional safeguards" are adopted when necessary "to protect the rights and welfare of these subjects." Interestingly, however, the need for "additional safeguards" is linked exclusively to these subjects' increased susceptibility to "undue influence or coercion" rather than to concerns about impaired decisional capacity. Further, the design and implementation of these additional safeguards is left entirely to the IRB.

The regulations give no prescriptive guidance to the IRBs on the complex issues of decisional impairment and surrogate decision making addressed in the Belmont Report. The only pertinent prescriptive provision in the regulations prohibits research unless the investigator has obtained the "legally effective consent of the subject or the subject's legally authorized representative." But standing alone, this statement is both misleading and incomplete. It is misleading because it implies, erroneously, that if a prospective subject lacks the capacity to make an informed decision, consent can be provided by a duly authorized surrogate, even if the subject objects to participation. It is incomplete because the "legally authorized representative" is given no direction regarding the point of view he or she should take involving decisions about research participation—that is, whether the surrogate makes the decision that the subject would have made if competent or the decision that appears to be in the subject's best interest.

The regulations also give no guidance on the meaning of decisional capacity. The criteria of informed consent imply a demanding test of capacity because they envision a fully informed and reasoned decision by the subject. In practice, however, there is a substantial gap between the operational standard of effective consent and the idealized standard to which investigators and subjects are expected to aspire. Because many subjects do not have the *capacity* to satisfy this heroic standard, investigators are left without a realistic standard of decisional capacity that can be used in cases involving subjects with cognitive impairment. Moreover, the current regulations prescribe no safeguards to ensure that some meaningful standard is applied. As a result, IRBs are left on their own to resolve these problems, ad hoc, as they arise.

ISSUES REQUIRING ATTENTION

It is time to address the many issues that have been left unresolved by current federal regulations. I will mention a few important questions that should be explored.

Under what circumstances should IRBs consider the need for special precautions relating to subject consent? In other words, what features of a research protocol should trigger special scrutiny by the IRB?

I mentioned earlier that the Commission's proposed regulations were criticized because investigations concerning severe mental disorders were singled out for special restrictions not applicable to other biomedical research. Critics legitimately pointed out the arbitrariness of distinguishing, categorically, between subjects with mental disorders and subjects with other conditions that might also be associated with decisional impairment, and between subjects residing in institutions and subjects residing elsewhere. This point is even more pertinent today. The sites where clinical research is most naturally conducted have changed dramatically, even for cognitively impaired patients.

In the absence of coercive influences, the need for special safeguards derives primarily from a possible impairment of decisional capacity, not from the category of disorder or the site of treatment or research. This is the approach reflected in the National Institute of Mental Health intramural policy[14] and in the position statement of the American College of Physicians.[15] The federal research regulations should not include special rules for people in psychiatric hospitals, for people with mental illness, or for people with schizophrenia. Instead, the *Federal Register* should prescribe special guidelines that apply to *any* cases of decisional impairment, regardless of etiology. Institutional review boards should be directed to carefully scrutinize the consent procedures whenever the investigator proposes to include subjects known to have disorders or conditions associated with diminished cognitive functions, including dementia, Alzheimer disease, mental retardation, or schizophrenia.

What should IRBs do in such cases? What precautions should they require? First, the IRBs should require investigators to use a structured protocol for assessing decision-making capacity and for identifying subjects with a possible impairment. The scientific basis for structured competence assessment has been markedly enhanced in recent years by the work of Appelbaum and Grisso[20] and protocols for use in research settings are now available.[21] Once subjects with possible impairments have been identified, the IRB should take special precautions to ensure that valid consent (or assent) is obtained (and that it remains valid during the course of the study). The IRBs should not be required to use any single procedure. Instead, the regulations should provide a menu of safeguards, and the IRB should be directed to select the procedures that provide the best fit for the particular study, taking into account the nature and prevalence of anticipated decision-making impairments and the degree of risk presented by the study. The menu of safeguards might include specially tailored follow-up questions to assess subject understanding, videotaping or audiotaping of consent interviews, second opinions, use of consent specialists, or concurrent consent by a family member.

Should research regulations give explicit recognition to degrees of impairment of decision-making capacity? The Commission made an important contribution to the conceptual vocabulary of research ethics by drawing a distinction between "assent" and "consent" and therefore between capacity to assent and capacity to give fully informed consent. In principle, it seems sensible to adopt a variable standard of capacity according to the balance of risk and benefit in a given context. The question is whether a meaningful distinction can be drawn in practice between these levels of impairment.

I believe this approach merits careful consideration. For one thing, as I mentioned earlier, tools for structured competence assessment are now available and can easily be adapted to this task. Second, the concept of assent—and of variable standards of competence—is no longer as novel as it was in 1978 when the Commission proposed it. Indeed, something resembling the concept of assent has become the recognized standard for consent to psychiatric hospitalization.[22] Finally, the operative standard of informed consent used in everyday clinical and research practice varies according to the degree of risk. It would be sensible to bring the normative criteria into alignment with the ethical intuitions that shape everyday practice.

What are the most sensible procedures for surrogate decision making, ie, for obtaining proxy consent? As I mentioned earlier, surrogate consent (or proxy consent) is an ethically permissible procedure in the context of some—but not all—types of research involving subjects who lack the capacity to provide legally valid consent. I want to emphasize, however, that the participation of surrogate decision makers can be a useful safeguard even if the subject has the requisite capacity to provide legally valid consent. That is, surrogate decision makers can provide concurrent authorization for consenting subjects as well as proxy consent for subjects who are unable to provide consent. Use of surrogates might be especially attractive as a safeguard if research is permitted on the basis of the subject's "assent" or some other less demanding standard.

The task that lies before us is to connect the surrogate decision-making rules in research with the developing law on proxy consent for health care decision making.[23] In 1978, it was commonly believed that surrogate decision making for a person whose decisional incapacity was attributable to mental illness could be provided only by a legal guardian after an adjudication of legal incompetence. The Commission recognized that a guardianship determination was a costly and stigmatizing mechanism for responding to decisional incapacity relating to medical treatment. The Commission therefore supported the emerging concept of limited guardianship or partial incapacity—which permitted surrogate decision making for one purpose (say medical treatment) without nullifying all of the person's decision-making prerogatives, but the Commission assumed that such procedures would have to be judicial in nature.

In recent years, many states have given explicit statutory endorsement to the customary clinical practice of relying on next of kin as surrogate decision makers without any judicial appointment.[24] This can be accomplished by the patient through a durable power of attorney or other form of advance directive. Moreover, even if a person has not executed such an advance directive, the statutes of many states establish a kind of default rule—designating parents, siblings, children, or other relatives as surrogate decision makers in a specified order of priority. Most of these new surrogate decision-making statutes do not refer specifically to clinical research.[25] However, I suspect that some of them can reasonably be construed to cover research with potential therapeutic benefit that is properly linked with clinical care, and the statutes can be amended to clarify their application to research settings. Although the development of new legal tools that facilitate surrogate consent cannot solve all the problems that can arise during the consent process, such as intrafamily conflict, the many potentially useful applications of these legal innovations to clinical research should be explored.

Is it possible to use advance directives to address issues of fluctuating decisional capacity? Advance directives were virtually unknown at the time of the Belmont Report. In recent years, however, they have become part of the everyday vocabulary of medical care at the end of life, largely as a result of congressional prodding in the Patient Self-Determination Act of 1992 (Public Law No. 101-508). The use of advance directives by persons with mental disorders raises many puzzling questions, such as the validity of a so-called "Ulysses contract," in which the competent patient authorizes treatment over his or her later incompetent objections.[26,27] The applicable legal principles have not yet been fully clarified.[28] However, at least for some patients, this device could help solve some of the problems presented by medication-free investigations. For example, a presently competent subject could provide continuing consent (or empower a surrogate to authorize continued participation) in the event of later deterioration.

CONCLUSIONS

I have tried to make the case for an authoritative reexamination of the ethical issues relating to research with cognitively impaired subjects that were swept off the table a decade ago. I am confident that these issues can be addressed without leading to the stalemate that doomed the Commission's proposals. There is a large middle ground between regulatory silence and the highly intrusive regime of consent auditors, subject advocates, and judicial orders that seems to have been envisioned by some participants in the regulatory debate in 1982. Recent articles by Dresser[29] and Berg[30] have begun to explore this middle ground. The challenge ahead is to forge a consensus on the types of safeguards that will most reasonably accommodate the goals of protecting the dignity and well-being of research subjects while avoiding undue impediments to valuable scientific inquiry.

In the short run, human rights and scientific progress appear to be in tension with one another. In the long run, however, human rights and scientific progress are mutually reinforcing social aspirations. On the one hand, genuine advances in clinical understanding cannot be achieved without the cooperative participation, and trust, of research subjects and their families; moreover, the climate of trust that is necessary to sustain research depends on respect for the subjects' rights and well-being. On the other hand, the prospects for enhancing the happiness and well-being of persons with disease and disability, and of reducing disease and disability in the future, ultimately depend on a meaningful societal commitment to scientific research. It would be a sad irony indeed if shortsighted efforts to "protect" vulnerable subjects of clinical research had the effect of foreclosing opportunities for significant advances in scientific understanding and of diverting the energies of talented investigators to unimpeded fields of inquiry.

Accepted for publication November 7, 1995.

Supported by the John D. and Catherine T. MacArthur Foundation Research Network on Mental Health and the Law and by the University of Virginia Law School Foundation, Charlottesville.

Presented at the 1994 Annual Meeting of the American College of Neuropsychopharmacology, San Juan, Puerto Rico, December 13, 1994.

Reprints: Richard J. Bonnie, University of Virginia School of Law, 580 Massie Rd, Charlottesville, VA 22903-1789.

REFERENCES

1. Tufts A. Apologies for Nazi crimes. *Lancet.* 1994;344:808.
2. Rothman DJ. *Strangers at the Bedside: A History of How Law and Bioethics Transformed Medical Decision Making.* New York, NY: Basic Books Inc Publishers; 1991.
3. Annas GJ, Grodin MA. *The Nazi Doctors and the Nuremberg Code: Human Rights in Human Experimentation.* New York, NY: Oxford University Press Inc; 1992.
4. Lifton RJ. *The Nazi Doctors: Medical Killing and the Psychology of Genocide.* New York, NY: Basic Books Inc Publishers; 1986.
5. Welt LG. Reflections on the problems of human experimentation. *Conn Med.* 1961;25:75-79.
6. Benson PR, Roth LH. Trends in the social control of medical and psychiatric research. *Law Ment Health.* 1988;4:1-47.
7. Beecher HK. Ethics and clinical research. *N Engl J Med.* 1966;274:1354-1360.
8. Office for Protection from Research Risks Division of Human Subject Protections. *Evaluation of Human Subject Protections in Schizophrenia Research Conducted by the University of California Los Angeles.* Los Angeles: University of California; 1994.
9. Appelbaum PS. Drug-free research in schizophrenia: an overview of the controversy. *IRB Rev Hum Subjects Res.* 1996;18(1):1-5.
10. Katz J. Human experimentation and human rights. *St Louis Univ Law J.* 1993;38:7-54.
11. Bonnie RJ. A presidential commission on drug policy: instrument of reform or defender of the status quo? *Contemp Drug Problems.* In press.
12. Department of Health, Education, and Welfare. Research involving those institutionalized as mentally infirm: report and recommendations of the National Commission for the Protection of Human Subjects of Biomedical and Behavioral Research. *Federal Register.* March 17, 1978;43:11328-11358.
13. Department of Health, Education, and Welfare. Proposed regulations on research involving those institutionalized as mentally disabled. *Federal Register.* November 17, 1978;43:53950-53956.
14. Fletcher JC, Dommell FW Jr, Cowell DD. A trial policy for the intramural programs of the National Institute of Health: consent to research with impaired human subjects. *IRB Rev Hum Subjects Res.* 1985;7:1-6.
15. American College of Physicians. Cognitively impaired subjects. *Ann Intern Med.* 1989;111:843-848.
16. High DM, Whitehouse PJ, Post SG, Berg L. Guidelines for addressing ethical and legal issues in Alzheimer disease research: a position paper. *Alzheimer Dis Assoc Disord.* 1994;8:67-74.
17. College on Problems of Drug Dependence. Human subject issues in drug abuse research. *Drug Alcohol Depend.* 1995;37:167-175.
18. Protection of human research subjects and creation of National Bioethics Advisory Commission (executive order No. 12975). *Federal Register.* October 3, 1995;60:52063.
19. Federal policy for the protection of human subjects. *Code of Federal Regulations.* 45 §46.111 and 46.116.
20. Appelbaum PS, Grisso T. The MacArthur Treatment Competence Study, I: mental illness and competence to consent to treatment. *Law Hum Behav.* 1995;19:105-126.
21. Appelbaum PS. Patients' competence to consent to neurobiological research. *Accountability Res.* 1996;4:241-251.
22. Cournos F, Faulkner LR, Griffith EEH, Munetz MR, Winick B, Fitzgerald L. *Consent to Voluntary Hospitalization.* Washington, DC: American Psychiatric Association; 1993.
23. Buchanan AE, Brock DW. *Deciding for Others: The Ethics of Surrogate Decision Making.* New York, NY: Cambridge University Press; 1989.
24. Menikoff J, Sachs G, Siegler M. Beyond advance directives: healthcare surrogate laws. *N Engl J Med.* 1992;327:1165-1169.
25. Kapp MB. Proxy decision making in Alzheimer disease research: durable powers of attorney, guardianship, and other alternatives. *Alzheimer Dis Assoc Disord.* 1994;8:28-37.
26. Kapp MB. Implications of the Patient Self-Determination Act for psychiatric practice. *Hosp Community Psychiatry.* 1994;45:355-358.
27. Appelbaum PS. Advance directives for psychiatric treatment. *Hosp Community Psychiatry.* 1991;42:983-984.
28. Moorhouse A, Weisstub DM. Advance directives for research: ethical problems and responses. *Int J Law Psychiatry.* 1996;19:107-141.
29. Dresser R. Mentally disabled research subjects: the enduring policy issues. *JAMA.* 1996;276:67-72.
30. Berg JW. Legal and ethical complexities of consent with cognitively impaired research subjects: proposed guidelines. *J Law Med Ethics.* 1996;24:18-35.

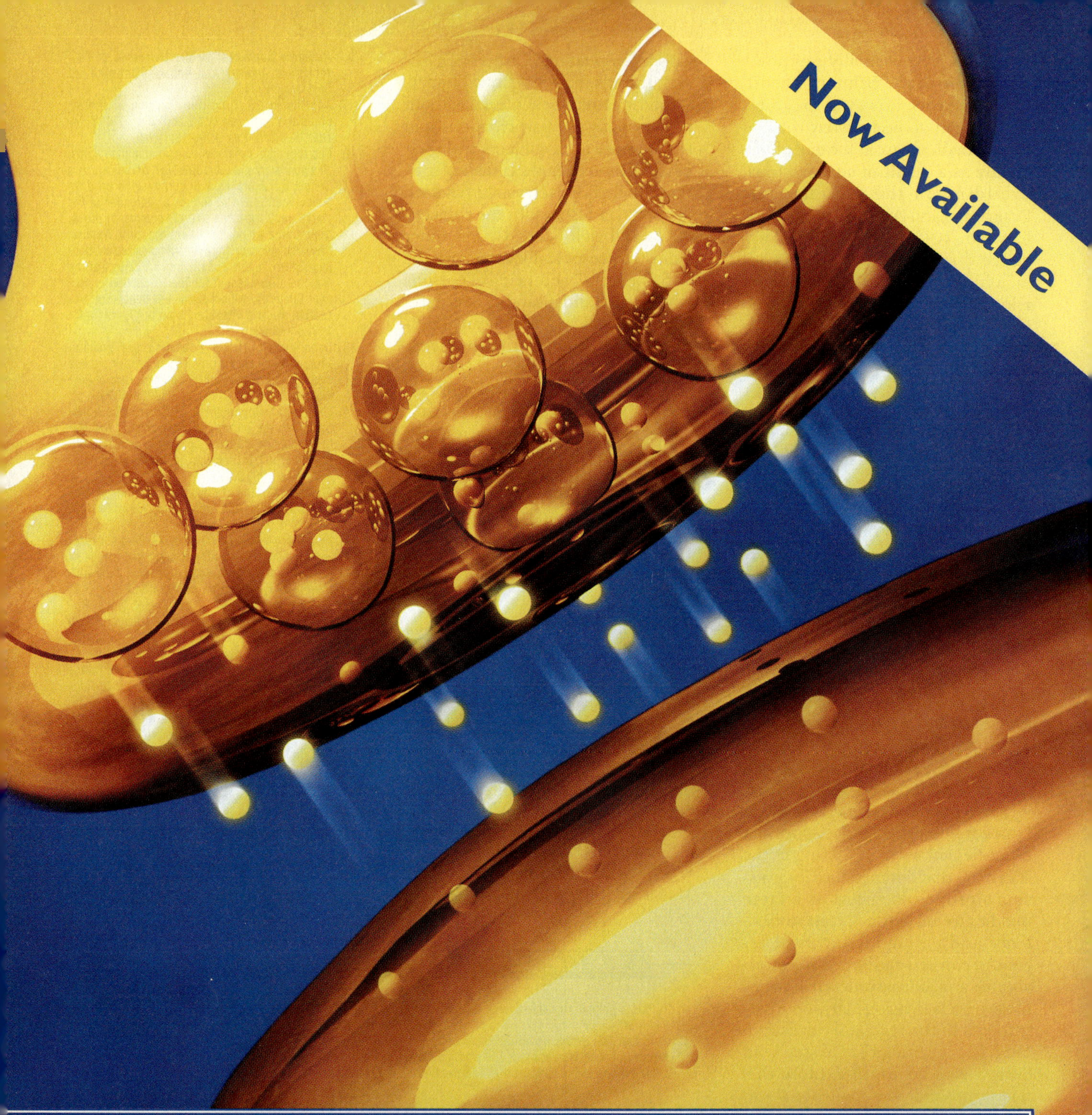
Now Available

Caring About Risks

Are Severely Depressed Patients Competent to Consent to Research?

Carl Elliott, MD, PhD

Depressed patients are often asked to take part in clinical research studies that carry risk. These patients are generally assumed to be mentally competent to consent to research, since depression often leaves a patient's cognitive abilities intact. In this article, it is argued that many severely depressed patients may not be competent to consent because they cannot be considered accountable for their decisions. The article presents 2 arguments: first, that it is unclear whether the decisions of some severely depressed patients are authentically theirs, and second, that some severely depressed patients may not have the appropriate minimal degree of concern for their own well-being. It is argued that assessments of competence must take account of emotional factors, and that, if severely depressed patients are incompetent to consent, research studies involving a poor risk-benefit ratio will be much more difficult to justify.

Arch Gen Psychiatry. 1997;54:113-116

Depressed patients are often asked to take part in clinical research, and often this research carries risks. A depressed patient might be enrolled in a protocol to evaluate a new antidepressant drug, for example, or in one that requires a washout period, in which the patient's current medication will be discontinued. Some institutional review boards continue to approve protocols that test new antidepressants against placebo controls. Any of these situations entail risks, primarily the risk that the depressed patient's condition will worsen. The potential harm can be considerable, and at the extreme end of the spectrum includes the risk for suicide.

Although the concept of competence to consent to treatment and research has been widely and thoroughly discussed,[1-5] only a few accounts give any attention to depression. Sometimes depression is not even considered a warning sign that a person's competence to consent needs to be evaluated, largely because it is not thought to be the type of disorder that would ordinarily interfere with competence. It is only the rare depressed patient who is psychotic, and while depression may often interfere with a person's memory and concentration, often this interference is not severe enough to raise any warning flags. Most accounts of competence focus on intellectual capacity and abilities to reason, and depression is primarily a disorder of mood. According to conventional thinking, depression is primarily about despair, guilt, and a loss of motivation, while competence is about the ability to reason, to deliberate, to compare, and to evaluate. Often these latter abilities are ones that depression leaves intact.

See also pages 105,117, and 121

I want to challenge this account of competence and argue that depression may well impair a patient's competence to consent to research. Most crucially, it can impair a person's ability to evaluate risks and benefits. To put the matter simply, if a person is depressed, he or she may be *aware* that a protocol carries risks, but simply not *care* about those risks. This sort of intel-

From the Biomedical Ethics Unit, McGill University, and Montreal Children's Hospital, Montreal, Quebec.

lectual impairment can be as important a part of patient competence as the more detached, intellectual understanding that most accounts of competence emphasize. If my argument is correct, then institutional review boards need to take special precautions in allowing researchers to enroll depressed patients in research protocols.

COMPETENCE AND ACCOUNTABILITY

Competence is conventionally defined as the ability to perform a task—in this case, to consent to enroll in a research protocol.[6,7] What counts as competence to consent will then depend on what one counts as the abilities relevant to the task in question. According to a widely accepted account of competence, the 1983 US President's Commission Report,[8] the relevant abilities are (1) the ability to reason and deliberate, (2) the ability to understand and communicate information, and (3) the possession of values and goals. As conceptualized within this framework, a potential research subject takes in the relevant information, weighs it according to his or her goals and values, and then reasons to an informed decision.

This account of competence, however, is incomplete. If competence to consent to research is defined simply as the ability to make a decision to enroll in a research protocol, we face the familiar problem of what *counts* as that ability—of trying to decide whether a person is incompetent by virtue of making a poor decision, or by virtue of making an irrational decision, or by virtue of coming to that decision in an unsystematic, illogical, or erratic way. Since even competent people are sometimes stubborn, obtuse, or unreasonable, we need an account of competence that explains why we sometimes believe that a person can be both competent and make bad, irrational, or even unreasonable choices.

What we really want to know when we ask if a patient is competent is whether that individual is able to make a decision *for which he or she can be considered accountable.*[9] What we want to know is whether the decisions that a person makes—whether they are good or bad, rational or irrational—are decisions for which that person can legitimately be considered responsible. This is why we define certain mental abilities as relevant: we realize that certain conditions or disorders impair a person's mental abilities such that he is not a morally responsible agent. He can make decisions, but we would not feel comfortable ascribing him with the credit or blame for that decision. If a person is making a decision that will affect his life in momentous ways, we will naturally be concerned that he makes a sound decision. But because we recognize that a person generally has the right to make even unsound decisions, a judgment about competence ensures that whatever decision a person makes, it is truly *his* decision: a decision for which he can finally be held accountable.

Once we conceptualize competence in this way, it becomes clear that it is not just intellectual ability that is relevant to competence. A person's emotional state can also affect her decisions in ways that might lead us to say that she cannot be judged fully accountable for them. The criminal law recognizes this, for example, and often grants leniency when a person acts under severe emotional distress. We often make decisions in the heat of anger or under the cold weight of despair that are uncharacteristic, that we would not have made otherwise, that we later regret, and for which we believe we should not be considered fully accountable. Likewise, we often recognize that it would be unfair to hold a person to a decision that he or she made in the face of overwhelming fear. In emotional extremes, we value, think, and behave differently—sometimes so differently that we might later believe that the decisions we have made are not decisions for which we can be held completely and unproblematically responsible.

The importance of emotion and mood for competence has not been lost on psychiatrists.[10-14] Some accounts of competence stipulate that persons must "appreciate" the consequences of their choices, rather than simply understand them factually, the term "appreciate" implying a fuller, deeper comprehension of how the decision will affect the patient's life.[15,16] A patient who can flatly recite the effects of treatment may still seem to fail to appreciate fully just how the treatment is going to affect his or her health. Nor can affect be completely divorced conceptually from cognition. Bursztajn and his colleagues[17] have pointed out how a patient's affect can influence competence by altering his or her beliefs. For example, a depressed patient, convinced that his situation will never change, may refuse treatment based on the unrealistic belief that it will not help him.

However, while some patients may have affective disorders that disrupt their cognitive, rational decision-making abilities, a slightly different sort of depressed patient presents other problems. This is the depressed patient who is capable of understanding all the facts about his illness and the research protocol in which he is enrolling, and who appreciates the risks and the broader implications of the protocol on his life, but who, as a result of his illness, is not *motivated* to take those risks into account in the same way as the rest of us. For example, these patients might realize that a protocol involves risks, but simply not *care* about the risks. Some patients, as a result of their depression, may even *want* to take risks. Roth et al[18] wonder about the competence of one such patient, a 49-year-old woman capable of fully understanding the electroconvulsive therapy for which she was being asked to consent, but who, when told that electroconvulsive therapy carried a 1 in 3000 chance of death, replied, "I hope I am the one."

Several writers have speculated about whether depression might lead patients to overestimate the side effects of interventions and underestimate the likelihood of benefit.[17,19,20] Although there are apparently no empirical studies examining the question of whether depressed patients are more likely than nondepressed patients to consent to risky or uncomfortable research, Lee and Ganzini[21,22] have studied the effects of depression and its treatment on the preferences of elderly patients for life-sustaining medical therapies. In a study of 43 depressed patients, a subgroup of 11 severely depressed patients were more likely to choose life-sustaining therapies after their depression had been treated than they were while depressed.[23] However, while this suggests that severe depression might affect the way some patients evaluate risks and benefits, it is not clear whether evaluation of life-sustaining therapy is similar enough to evaluation of research risks to bear much comparison.

Nonetheless, it seems unlikely that severely depressed patients are in the best position to make important decisions about their welfare. The Royal College of Psychiatrists in the United Kingdom is one of the few bodies to recognize this explicitly, offering the example of a patient with depressive delusions who consents to risky research because he thinks he is guilty and deserves to be punished.[24] However, given the sense of hopelessness and worthlessness that characterizes some severely depressed patients, it seems reasonable to worry about their decision making. The novelist William Styron describes his own agonizing depressive episode as

> the diabolical discomfort of being imprisoned in a fiercely overheated room. And because no breeze stirs this cauldron, because there is no escape from this smothering confinement, it is entirely natural that the victim begins to think ceaselessly of oblivion.[25]

DEPRESSION AND COMPETENCE

Although other writers have suggested that affective disorders may interfere with a patient's competence to consent to treatment, none has considered competence to consent to research, and only a few have attempted to say *why* depression impairs competence.[7] That is, while there are not many writers who would dispute that mood is a part of ordinary decision making, it is also normal for a person's mood to change from one time to another, and it is not immediately obvious why a depressed mood should invalidate a patient's competence.

There are 2 good arguments for the conclusion that some depressed patients are incompetent to consent to research, each of which is persuasive for a slightly different type of patient. The first might be called the argument from *authenticity*. When a person is caught in the grip of depression, his values, beliefs, desires, and dispositions are dramatically different from when he is healthy.[7] In some cases, they are so different that we might ask whether his decisions are truly his. A decision may not be truly his in the sense that it reflects dispositions and values that are transient and inconsistent with much more deeply ingrained traits of his character. One might say "I wasn't myself" when looking back on a time of despondency, and a caricature of the authenticity argument would hold that we should take this declaration literally: I was not myself, so that decision is not mine. Yet underneath that caricature is a grain of truth. If a person is so deeply depressed that his decisions are wildly inconsistent with his character, it seems problematic to abide by his decisions, particularly if the depression is dramatic and reversible.[26]

Here is where the notion of competence as accountability is helpful. If a person were to behave badly while mentally ill—say, in a full-blown manic episode—we would very likely think it unfair to hold him fully responsible for what he has done. His behavior was uncharacteristic; he would never have acted this way unless he was manic; his mania is temporary and reversible with lithium treatment. His actions in the manic state were not truly *his*. Similarly for the depressed patient being asked to consent to research: his mental state is such that his behavior and choices do not seem to be truly his. If something untoward were to happen to him during the research, for instance, we could not in good conscience say that he bears the full responsibility for undergoing that risk.

The authenticity argument supposes a person with a stable character and entrenched dispositions, who, while depressed, makes decisions so uncharacteristic that we feel bound to question whether those decisions were truly hers. However, sometimes this break between the depressed and predepression personality is not so dramatic. Some patients are chronically depressed, and others are depressed periodically. It would not be plausible to argue that the decisions of these depressed patients do not reflect their underlying characters—characters that are closely tied to their depression. Yet there comes a point where, if a person appears largely insensitive to her own welfare, we might believe that she is incompetent to consent to research. Why should this be so?

One answer lies in what might be called the argument from *self-interest*. Our ordinary relationships with other people are based on certain assumptions about their thoughts and behavior. One of these assumptions is that other persons have some minimal concern for their own welfare. For example, the assumption that other people ordinarily both have some minimal degree of self-interest and are best positioned to judge their own interests lies at the heart of the institution of informed consent.

However, if we have reason to believe that severely depressed patients do not have this minimal degree of concern, then a fundamental assumption underlying informed consent is undermined. We justify exposing patients to the risks of research by the assumption that the patient is evaluating that risk with some degree of concern for her welfare. A competent evaluation of risks involves taking into account one's own well-being: not necessarily taking it as an overriding or supremely important concern, but at least taking it into account. If a person is so depressed that she fails to take her interests into account in deciding whether to take a risk, then we can hardly be comfortable saying that she is accountable for taking that risk.

CONCLUSIONS

Two broad types of conclusions can be drawn from these arguments, one empirical and the other conceptual. First, more empirical research needs to be carried out to determine the ways in which severe depression might affect psychological factors relevant to competence. For example, it would be important to know the extent to which severe depression affects how much a person cares about his or her own well-being, or how it might affect a person's willingness to expose himself or herself to potential harm.

Second, these arguments suggest that we may need to alter our conventional ways of assessing competence. As I have argued, many conventional accounts of how competence should be assessed downplay the importance of emotional factors. However, if my arguments are convincing, it may not be enough for psychiatrists or researchers to evaluate competence simply by testing a person's memory and reasoning ability, such as with a Mini-Mental State Examination. Rather, it may be that evaluations should also be concerned with a person's affective and motivational state: whether a person's mood has dramatically changed recently, how concerned a patient appears to be about her own well-being, how carefully she looks at risks and benefits, and so on. Of course, sound and uniform ways of assessing these affective and motivational factors will need to be developed.

On a practical level, these arguments have potential implications for the conduct of clinical research protocols testing new treatments for major depression. For example, if it is concluded that severe depression does impair competence to consent, clinical research protocols involving subjects with depression will need to require explicitly that the competence of subjects be evaluated before entering the study. This requirement might be similar to that of psychiatric research protocols testing new antipsychotic drugs, which generally state that subjects either be competent to consent or that consent be obtained from an appropriate surrogate.

Finally, this view of competence could have practical implications for studies involving relatively poor risk-benefit ratios. Sometimes severely depressed patients are enrolled in protocols in which their depression is likely to worsen (eg, as a result of being assigned to a placebo treatment arm). Researchers argue that exposing competent adults to these sorts of risks is justified at least in part by the institution of informed consent, with the corresponding presumption that potential subjects understand the risks of the protocol, consent to them, and can be judged accountable for undertaking them.[27] But if severely depressed patients are incompetent, exposing them to the risk of having their illness worsen is much more difficult to justify.[28,29]

Accepted for publication September 29, 1995.

Acknowledgments to Fonds pour la Formation de Chercheurs et l'Aide a la Recherche (Quebec) for their financial support.

Thanks to Charles Weijer for his comments on the manuscript.

Corresponding author: Carl Elliott, MD, PhD, Biomedical Ethics Unit, McGill University, 3690 Peel St, Montreal, Quebec, Canada H3A 1W9.

REFERENCES

1. Appelbaum P, Lidz C, Meisel A. *Informed Consent: Legal Theory and Clinical Practice.* New York, NY: Oxford University Press; 1986.
2. Drane J. The many faces of competency. *Hastings Cent Rep.* 1985;15:17-21.
3. Gaylin W. The competence of children: no longer all or none. *Hastings Cent Rep.* 1982;12:33-38.
4. Lidz C, Meisel A, Zerubavel E, Carter M, Sestak R, Roth L. *Informed Consent: A Study of Decisionmaking in Psychiatry.* New York, NY: Guilford Press; 1984.
5. Jonsen A, Siegler M, Winslade W. *Clinical Ethics.* 3rd ed. New York, NY: Macmillan Publishing Co; 1992.
6. Faden R, Beauchayp T. *A History and Theory of Informed Consent.* New York, NY: Oxford University Press; 1986.
7. Buchanan AE, Brock DW. *Deciding for Others: The Ethics of Surrogate Decision Making.* Cambridge, England: Cambridge University Press; 1989.
8. US President's Commission for the Study of Ethical Problems in Medicine and Biomedical and Behavioral Research. *Making Health Care Decisions: The Ethical and Legal Implications of Informed Consent in the Patient-Practitioner Relationship.* Washington, DC: US Government Printing Office; 1983.
9. Elliott C. Competence as accountability. *J Clin Ethics.* 1991;2:167-71.
10. Culver CM, Ferrell RB, Green RM. ECT and the special problems of informed consent. *Am J Psychiatry.* 1980;137:586-591.
11. Gutheil TH, Bursztajn H. Clinician's guidelines for assessing and presenting subtle forms of patient incompetence in legal settings. *Am J Psychiatry.* 1986;143:1020-1023.
12. Fulford KWM, Howse K. Ethics of research with psychiatric patients: principles, problems and the primary responsibility of researchers. *J Med Ethics.* 1993;19:85-91.
13. Ganzini L, Lee MA, Heintz RT, Bloom JD. Is the Patient Self-Determination Act appropriate for elderly persons hospitalized for depression? *J Clin Ethics.* 1993;4:46-50.
14. Marta J. The PSDA and geriatric psychiatry: a cautionary tale. *J Clin Ethics.* 1993;4:80-81.
15. Gutheil TG, Appelbaum PS. *Clinical Handbook of Psychiatry and the Law.* New York, NY: McGraw-Hill Book Co; 1982.
16. Appelbaum P, Roth L. Competency to consent to research: a psychiatric overview. *Arch Gen Psychiatry.* 1982;39:951-958.
17. Bursztajn HJ, Harding HP, Gutheil TG, Brodsky A. Beyond cognition: the role of disordered affective states in impairing competence to consent to treatment. *Bull Am Acad Psychiatry Law.* 1991;19:383-388.
18. Roth L, Meisel A, Lidz C. Tests of competency to consent to treatment. *Am J Psychiatry.* 1977;134:279-284.
19. Ganzini L, Lee MA, Heintz RT, Bloom JD. Do-not-resuscitate orders for depressed psychiatric inpatients. *Hosp Community Psychiatry.* 1992;43:915-919.
20. Sullivan MD, Youngner SJ. Depression, competence and the right to refuse lifesaving medical treatment. *Am J Psychiatry.* 1994;151:971-978.
21. Lee MA, Ganzini L. Depression in the elderly: effect on patient attitudes toward life-sustaining therapy. *J Am Geriatr Soc.* 1992;40:983-988.
22. Lee MA, Ganzini L. The effect of recovery from depression on preferences for life-sustaining therapy in older patients. *J Gerontol.* 1994;49:15-21.
23. Ganzini L, Lee MA, Heintz RT, Bloom JD, Fenn DS. The effect of depression treatment on elderly patients' preferences for life-sustaining medical therapy. *Am J Psychiatry.* 1994;151:1631-1636.
24. Royal College of Psychiatrists. *Guidelines for Ethics of Research Committees on Psychiatric Research Involving Human Subjects.* London, England: Royal College of Psychiatrists; 1989.
25. Styron W. *Darkness Visible: A Memoir of Madness.* New York, NY: Random House; 1990.
26. Shamoo A, Irving D. The PSDA and the depressed elderly: 'intermittent competency' revisited. *J Clin Ethics.* 1993;4:74-79.
27. Roth L, Appelbaum P. Obtaining informed consent for research with psychiatric patients. *Psychiatr Clin North Am.* 1983;6:551-565.
28. Freedman B. Placebo-controlled trials and the logic of clinical purpose. *IRB Rev Hum Subjects Res.* 1990;12(6):1-6.
29. Rothman KJ, Michels KB. The continuing unethical use of placebo controls. *N Engl J Med.* 1994;331:394-398.

COMMENTARY

Rethinking the Conduct of Psychiatric Research

WHY reconsider how we conduct psychiatric research, as Bonnie[1] and Elliott[2] urge in this issue of the ARCHIVES? To be sure, several highly publicized cases have raised questions regarding the adequacy of current regulatory structures for the protection of subjects (*New York Times*. March 10, 1994:A-1 and March 4, 1995:21; *Chronicle of Higher Education*. March 31, 1995: A27). Adverse media coverage, however, even when it stimulates congressional hearings (*New York Times*. May 24, 1994:A-13), is not necessarily a sound basis on which to reopen complex issues of policy. In this case, though, there are at least 2 reasons to encourage further systematic attention to the conduct of psychiatric research.

First, doubts about whether protections are adequate to safeguard the interests of research subjects with mental illness threaten to split the alliance of family members and psychiatric researchers, a union that has become crucial for sustaining political support for research funding in psychiatry. As recent articles written by family members make clear, the perception that their relatives with mental illness are being subjected to unfair and potentially harmful research practices—whether based on reality or not—evokes a sense of anger and betrayal.[3,4] Were this perception to become widespread, one of the most potent voices for the importance of neurobiological research would be stilled, this at a time when new research techniques promise substantial insights into the pathophysiology of many forms of mental disorder.

Second, although it is impossible to gauge the nature and extent of problems in the conduct of psychiatric research from media coverage and a handful of court decisions, there are suggestions from other sources that difficulties may exist. The recently issued report of the Advisory Committee on Human Radiation Experiments (ACHRE), for example, includes results of a survey of selected human subjects research funded by the federal government.[5] Eight of the studies examined in the Committee's stratified sample of 125 projects involved cognitively impaired subjects, most with Alzheimer disease. The ACHRE found that fully half of these projects, none of which offered direct benefits to subjects, had inadequate explanations of risks and discomforts in their consent material and paid no attention to the question of how to deal with subjects who might have impaired capacities to consent to research participation. The latter finding confirms earlier indications that investigators frequently neglect issues related to subjects' competence.[6] Combined, these factors suggest that it is time to reopen formal discussion on the conduct of psychiatric research.

AREAS OF CONCERN IN PSYCHIATRIC RESEARCH

If attention is to be directed toward rethinking how we undertake psychiatric research, on what topics ought these efforts focus? Unresolved issues exist in 3 areas: methodology, informed consent, and institutional review board (IRB) oversight.

Among the most controversial issues in the methodologic area are designs that deny active medication to some or all subjects with conditions for which at least partially effective treatments exist.[7] Concerns center on both the short- and long-term consequences of relapse, especially in schizophrenia. Elliott[2] alludes to the still unresolved controversy over the use of placebos in drug treatment trials (for a balanced view see Makuch and Johnson[8]), but related questions can be raised about extended washout periods and discontinuation of medication in outpatients. Use of drugs that provoke symptoms, especially symptoms of psychosis, to tease out the mechanisms involved in psychiatric disorders is another area of contention that might benefit from careful analysis.

See also pages 105, 113, and 121

The most common rejoinder to concerns about placing research subjects at risk for harm—eg, by use of placebos—is that such practices are legitimized by the consent of subjects, who agree to accept some possibility of adverse outcomes for the sake of advancing knowledge. Because freely given informed consent is one of the ethical cornerstones of current research practices, it is troubling that some investigators' consent practices have been called into question. Projects have been criticized for failing to distinguish clearly between the benefits and risks associated with research and those that would be obtained if the potential subject sought ordinary clinical care.[9] Risks in general sometimes seem to be downplayed.[5] Both problems may be exacerbated when researchers are also in charge of subjects' clinical treatment.[10]

Practices regarding subjects with possible impairment of their decision-making capacities—an issue to which I will return shortly—have also been questioned. The lack of clarity in our current system regarding the content of consent disclosures and how to recognize and deal with patients who have impaired capacities magnifies these problems, leaving even well-meaning researchers at risk for post hoc criticism. Surrogate decision making and advance directives, widely discussed as mechanisms for addressing some of the problems related to incompetence,[11] are, as Bonnie[1] notes, infrequently used because of continuing uncertainty regarding the legitimate scope of their application. Subjects and researchers alike would benefit from clarification of these issues.

Finally, the role of IRBs in overseeing psychiatric research, and perhaps research in general, has evoked dissatisfaction from all parties involved. It is commonplace by now to bemoan IRBs' excessive and nearly exclusive focus on the content of consent forms as their primary mechanism for protecting subjects' interests. Given that existing regulations grant IRBs substantial discretion to devise other means to achieve this goal, their reluctance to do so is somewhat puzzling. Perhaps it stems from IRB members' unfamiliarity with psychiatric disorders and the particular problems they present in the research setting. Whatever the cause, discussion of ways to improve IRB performance seems amply justified.

THE PROBLEM OF COMPETENCE TO CONSENT TO RESEARCH

To encourage closer attention to problems in the conduct of psychiatric research is not to say that these issues will be easy to resolve. In addition to analytic challenges, the empirical data required to design sensible practices and regulatory approaches simply may not exist. Consideration of just one of these areas, competence to consent to research—the focus of Elliott's analysis—illustrates the complexities involved.

Dealing with subjects whose decision-making capacities may be impaired (or, in legal terms, who may be incompetent to consent to participate in research) is not an issue unique to psychiatric research. Investigators recruiting non–mentally ill geriatric, adolescent, and seriously medically ill subjects all must be concerned with whether their subjects have adequate capacities to offer valid consents. But it is difficult to avoid the conclusion that psychiatric disorders, which by definition affect mentation, raise special concerns. Indeed, a recent study of decisional capacities in the inpatient treatment context demonstrated substantial impairments in approximately 52% of schizophrenic subjects and 24% of depressed subjects, but only 12% of seriously medically ill subjects.[12] These data call into question, as Elliott's formulation suggests, the ability of these subjects to protect their own interests in making decisions about entering research projects.

Although the most significant problems seem to exist for patients with schizophrenia, I focus this discussion on patients with depression, since that is the topic of the article by Elliott.[2] It is not hard to find data suggesting that depression affects decision making. Early work suggesting that depression may help people make *better* decisions by stripping them of their optimistic illusions—the so-called depressive realism argument[13]—has since been challenged,[14] and probably was irrelevant to major depression anyway.[15] In contrast, many studies have shown cognitive impairments in depressed patients, ranging from information processing[16] to reasoning[17] to perceptions of their situation.[18]

Whether these deficits actually alter patients' decisions in clinical or research settings has not been explored extensively, although Ganzini and colleagues[19] have provided evidence that depressed patients' choices about life-sustaining treatment will be different after recovery from depression. Moreover, the consensus of clinicians seems to be that depression-related impairments can be severe enough that patients could be considered incompetent as a result.[20-22] Clinicians in 1 of the handful of studies on this point judged 21 of 96 patients referred for electroconvulsive therapy to be incompetent,[23] while, in a second study, 6 of 23 patients receiving electroconvulsive therapy were placed in that category.[24] (In neither case were standardized criteria for competence used.) The raters in the latter study also evaluated as incompetent 4 of 19 depressed research subjects.[24]

To summarize the current state of knowledge, existing evidence suggests that depression can impair cognition, sometimes so severely that a person becomes incompetent. This meager database, however, offers little guidance for those seeking to devise policies to protect research subjects. Are depressed subjects so commonly incompetent that routine mechanisms (eg, screening of all subjects before the consent process) are required for their protection? Or is this problem so infrequent that the burdens of more rigorous procedures are not warranted by the potential benefits? Is it possible to identify a subgroup of depressed subjects, perhaps those with psychotic symptoms, who are at higher risk for incompetence, so that needed protections can be focused on them alone? None of these questions can be answered at this time, yet it would be foolish to impose additional burdens on psychiatric research without knowing the answers.

Obtaining this information, however, is a complex matter in its own right. Even the question of how to determine who is competent remains open to some extent. As Bonnie[1] notes, the regulations governing federally funded research are silent on the issue of what constitutes competence. The most commonly used standards for competence embody 4 elements: the abilities to understand, appreciate, reason, and evidence a choice.[25,26] Elliott expresses the belief that this "cognitive" approach is inadequate for depressed patients, who may have deficiencies in their "affective and motivational states." He makes a persuasive case that people without the motivation to protect themselves ought to be considered incompetent to consent to research.

But beyond a few anecdotes, there are no data on the extent to which motivational impairments in depression (eg, not caring about risks) affect decisions to participate in research. Even if motivational factors turn out to be important, it may be that they act by impairing 1 or more of the traditional competence-related cognitive abilities, or that the 2 sets of impairments correlate highly. If either is the case, evaluation of competence could focus on the more easily measured cognitive factors, rather than difficult-to-assess concepts such as motivation. Agreement on issues of this sort is a prerequisite to definitive studies of competence in depression.

A second problem to be resolved before being able to ascertain the extent of incompetence in depression is the point at which a person's incapacities become sufficiently severe that he or she ought to be considered incompetent. Bonnie mentions the work that my colleague Tom Grisso and I are doing to develop practical instruments for the systematic evaluation of capacities related to competence to consent to research. These instruments are currently being field tested, and we think they hold some hope for standardizing competence assessments. The instruments themselves, however, only measure the degree of impairment in capacities; they cannot determine how much impairment we as a society are willing to tolerate before we consider someone incompetent. That task requires a normative analysis, which has yet to be undertaken.[27]

When the queries about the extent of incompetence among depressed research subjects are answered, a new set of questions will move to the fore. Given the degree of decisional problems demonstrated, what remedies are indicated? Here again, empirical data will be needed on the efficacy of the approaches suggested in identifying impaired subjects and protecting their rights. Can screening be accomplished efficiently and accurately, without unduly impeding the recruitment of subjects? Are mechanisms available to augment the decisional capacities of depressed subjects, allowing more of them to make decisions for themselves? (Some data suggest that, compared with schizophrenic subjects, patients with depression are much more likely to respond to such efforts.[28]) Can advance directives help solve some of the problem for patients with recurrent illnesses?

What should be clear from this discussion is that existing knowledge about the extent to which depression impairs competence to consent to research is so limited that no changes in policies are indicated at this point. The need for more empirical data on the scope of the problem, as well as normative analyses on the elements of competence and the point at which persons should be considered incompetent, is evident. And before new policies for dealing with incompetent subjects are implemented, it would be desirable to have experimental evidence that the policies are likely to accomplish their intended goals.

TAKING THE NEXT STEPS

How can we begin to address the issues related to methodology, informed consent, and oversight—of which competence to consent to research is just one—in a responsible manner? Finding an answer to this question is critical because of the delicate balance of interests involved. Protecting the rights and well-being of research subjects is imperative, but so too is advancing knowledge of the causes and treatments of psychiatric disorders. Even if public attention fades, the issues will remain. We ought to take advantage of the moment to develop a reasonable mechanism for tackling these dilemmas.

Bonnie argues for "a credible and authoritative process for reexamining and resolving" these issues. He notes that the new National Bioethics Advisory Commission might undertake this task. But the Commission, authorized several years ago, has been slow in getting organized, and its potential agenda of intractable ethical issues is already lengthy. Whether research issues in general, and psychiatric research in particular, would get the attention they deserve in such a process is not at all clear.

A commission focused solely on issues in the conduct of research, in itself a formidable agenda, would be better able to direct its resources to these complicated matters. Because so many of the problems identified in psychiatric research are common to medical research as a whole, the group should be charged with exploring the conundrums of research in general. Its composition should cross the usual boundaries that tend to define perspectives on ethical issues, including researchers, clinicians, ethicists, regulators, family members, and patients themselves. Federal funding for this effort might be supplemented by support from foundations that have funded medical research (sometimes neglecting the consequent ethical problems), from advocacy groups, and perhaps from the professions themselves.

Given the dearth of reliable information about many of the intricate issues involved, the success of an effort of this sort is probably linked to the group's ability to fund the collection of data essential for the formulation of reasonable policy recommendations. Both the President's Commission for the Study of Ethical Problems in Medicine and Biomedical and Behavioral Research and the more recent ACHRE demonstrated the utility of having relatively small amounts of money available to fund relevant research. For the President's Commission, this ranged from polls of public attitudes toward informed consent to reflective papers on topics relevant to the Commission's work to observational studies of consent in actual medical settings.[29] In addition to the study of a sample of recent federally funded research projects referred to above, the ACHRE conducted an informative survey of the attitudes of medical patients toward research involvement.[5] The ultimate recommendations of both groups were enhanced significantly by the availability of these data.

The temptation for those involved in psychiatric research to see questions about their practices as troublesome impediments to advancing knowledge ought to be resisted. Equally important societal interests in fairness and protection of the vulnerable are at stake here. The time is right to push for a broad consensus on these issues.

Paul S. Appelbaum, MD
Department of Psychiatry
University of Massachusetts Medical Center
55 Lake Ave N
Worcester, MA 01655

REFERENCES

1. Bonnie RJ. Research with cognitively impaired subjects: unfinished business in the regulation of human research. *Arch Gen Psychiatry.* 1997; 54:105-111.
2. Elliott C. Caring about risks: are severely depressed patients competent to consent to research? *Arch Gen Psychiatry.* 1997;54:113-116.
3. Hassner V. What is ethical? what is not? where do you draw the line? *J Calif Alliance Ment Ill.* 1994;5(1):4-5.
4. Shamoo AE, Irving DN. Accountability in research using persons with mental illness. *Accountability Res.* 1993;3:1-17.
5. Advisory Committee on Human Radiation Experiments. *Advisory Committee on Human Radiation Experiments: Final Report.* Washington, DC: US Government Printing Office; October 1995.
6. Appelbaum PS, Roth LH. The structure of informed consent in psychiatric research. *Behav Sci Law.* 1983;1:9-19.
7. Appelbaum PS. Drug-free research in schizophrenia: an overview of the controversy. *IRB Rev Hum Subjects Res.* 1996;18(1):1-5.
8. Makuch RW, Johnson MF. Dilemmas in the use of active control groups in clinical research. *IRB Rev Hum Subjects Res.* 1989;11(1):1-5.
9. Office for Protection from Research Risks. *Evaluation of Human Subject Protections in Schizophrenia Research Conducted by the University of California Los Angeles.* Washington, DC: Office for Protection from Research Risks, National Institutes of Health; May 11, 1994.
10. Katz J. Human experimentation and human rights. *St Louis Univ Law J.* 1993;38:7-54.
11. Clinical Center, National Institutes of Health. *Colloquy in Research Ethics: Issues in Biomedical Research Involving Cognitively Impaired Subjects.* Washington, DC: US Government Printing Office, National Institutes of Health; 1995.
12. Grisso T, Appelbaum PS. The MacArthur Treatment Competence Study, III: abilities of patients to consent to psychiatric and medical treatments. *Law Hum Behav.* 1995;19:149-174.
13. Alloy LB, Abramson LY. Judgment of contingency in depressed and nondepressed students: sadder but wiser? *J Exp Psychol.* 1979; 108:441-485.
14. Ackermann R, DeRubeis RJ. Is depressive realism real? *Clin Psychol Rev.* 1991;11:565-584.
15. Taylor SE. *Positive Illusions: Creative Self-Deception and the Healthy Mind.* New York, NY: Basic Books; 1989:211-226.
16. Hartlarge S, Alloy LB, Vazquez C, Dykman B. Automatic and effortful processing in depression. *Psychol Bull.* 1993;113:247-278.
17. Baker JE, Channon S. Reasoning in depression: impairment on a concept discrimination learning task. *Cognition Emotion.* 1995;9:579-597.
18. Morgado A, Smith M, Lecrubier Y, Widlocher D. Depressed subjects unwittingly overreport poor social adjustment which they reappraise when recovered. *J Nerv Ment Dis.* 1991;179:614-619.
19. Ganzini L, Lee Ma, Heintz RT, Bloom JD, Fenn DS. The effect of depression treatment on elderly patients' preferences for life-sustaining medical therapy. *Am J Psychiatry.* 1994;151:1631-1636.
20. Appelbaum PS, Grisso T. Assessing patients' capacities to consent to treatment. *N Engl J Med.* 1988;319:1635-1638.
21. Sullivan MD, Youngner SJ. Depression, competence and the right to refuse lifesaving medical treatment. *Am J Psychiatry.* 1994;151:971-978.
22. Bursztajn HJ, Harding HP, Gutheil TG, Brodsky A. Beyond cognition: the role of disordered affective states in impairing competence to consent to treatment. *Bull Am Acad Psychiatry Law.* 1991;19:383-388.
23. Bean G, Nishisato S, Rector N, Glancy G. The psychometric properties of the Competency Interview Schedule. *Can J Psychiatry.* 1994;39: 368-376.
24. Roth LH, Lidz CW, Meisel A, Soloff PH, Kaufman K, Spiker DG, Foster FG. Competency to decide about treatment or research: an overview of some empirical data. *Int J Law Psychiatry.* 1982;5:29-50.
25. Appelbaum PS, Grisso T. The MacArthur Treatment Competence Study, I: mental illness and competence to consent to treatment. *Law Hum Behav.* 1995;19:105-126.
26. Berg JW, Appelbaum PS, Grisso T. Constructing competence: formulating standards of legal competence to make medical decisions. *Rutgers Law Rev.* 1996;48:345-396.
27. Appelbaum PS. Patients' competence to consent to neurobiological research. *Accountability Res.* 1996;4:241-251.
28. Benson PR, Roth LH, Appelbaum PS, Lidz CW, Winslade WJ. Information disclosure, subject understanding and informed consent in psychiatric research. *Law Hum Behav.* 1988;12:455-475.
29. President's Commission for the Study of Ethical Problems in Medicine and Biomedical and Behavioral Research. *Making Health Care Decisions: The Ethical and Legal Implications of Informed Consent in the Patient-Practitioner Relationship.* Washington, DC: US Government Printing Office; 1982:2, 3.

COMMENTARY

Protecting Subjects and Fostering Research

Striking the Proper Balance

SHOULD institutional review boards (IRBs) provide greater oversight and guidance for researchers and research subjects with regard to informed consent for participation in research studies, especially if the subjects' cognitive or affective decision-making capacities are diminished? Bonnie[1] and Elliott[2] each raise this significant question in this issue of the ARCHIVES. Bonnie addresses cognitively impaired subjects in general. He advocates a reconsideration of the role of IRBs in assessing the decision-making capacity of all cognitively impaired research subjects. Elliott raises a more specific issue—that of the influence of mood on judgment and on informed consent. The 2 articles may be considered in terms of 4 important issues with regard to medical research: (1) the context of obtaining informed consent, (2) the question of who should make medical decisions regarding clinical care or participation in research, (3) the stigmatization of psychiatric disorders, and (4) the degree of risk to the research subject.

COMPETENCE TO CONSENT TO RESEARCH PARTICIPATION

Elliott notes that, in general, informed consent has focused on cognitive and intellectual influences on competence in terms of "ability to reason, to deliberate, to compare, and to evaluate." In this he follows the 1983 US President's Commission Report (see reference 8 in his article) for the Study of Ethical Problems in Medical and Behavioral Research. The report states that the relevant abilities for competence are "1) the ability to reason and deliberate, 2) the ability to understand and communicate information, and 3) the possession of values and goals." Elliott argues that aspects of depression, particularly severe depression, should also be considered in evaluating competence. In particular, he argues that mood, desire for punishment, guilt, and other attributes of depression may interfere substantially with competence to make a judgment.

See also pages 105, 113, and 117

Elliott argues that patients with severe depression are not competent to make their own decisions, although at times he seems to construe severe depression broadly. He also advocates the need for more empirical research about the effects of depression on competency. It is surprising that he failed to mention the comparative study of Stanley et al[3-5] regarding the consent of psychiatric patients to research. The study, which included patients with psychotic depression, found that psychiatric patients were no more likely to consent to high-risk/low-benefit experiments than were general medical patients. Further, it found that more severely affected psychiatric patients were no less able to evaluate research risk. The results of their study squarely challenge Elliott's central assumption.

In situations of extreme incapacity, the law may be invoked to appoint a guardian to assume decision-making responsibility for an incompetent person. Such a measure is taken carefully with judicial oversight. Ethical and legal traditions uphold the presumption that personal autonomy and self-determination are fundamental values. Competent individuals have the right to make their own decisions, including unwise ones. For example, competent persons may refuse beneficial medical treatment (even lifesaving care). They may also make other personal choices that are detrimental unless they have been judged to be incompetent.

We are not persuaded that we should deny a legally competent, informed person the opportunity to be voluntarily involved in research because his or her mood is disturbed. It seems to us that to respect an individual's autonomy requires us to respect the individual's choice to be involved or not in research.

MEDICAL DECISION MAKING REGARDING CLINICAL CARE AND PARTICIPATION IN RESEARCH

The concerns raised by Elliott about research could easily be extended to general clinical decision making. One could argue that treatment decisions of patients who are ill, in considerable pain, feel desperate, are in great distress, and are debilitated could be made by someone who is dispassionate, experienced, and knowledgeable, such as the clinician, or perhaps some third party who is not involved at all in the diagnosis or clinical management. It could be argued that the clinician or third party is much better able to make a reasoned, thoughtful, appropriate judgment. The third party would be uninfluenced by competing priorities, denial of illness, avoidance of unpleasant procedures, desire to avoid side effects, and so on.

Such an approach is at strong variance with prevailing opinion in the United States. For example, in a recent article, Laine and Davidoff[6] recommend strongly a "patient-centered" approach. Here, the patient and perhaps family members are actively involved in the whole process of clinical decision making, with the patient ultimately making judgments about treatment. It is the physician's responsibility to provide comprehensive and relevant information in as understandable a manner as possible to the patient and significant others.

This model can be applied to medical research, including that involving patients with psychiatric disorders. In such situations, the researcher and/or clinician must accept the responsibility for informing patients about the disorders from which they suffer, about various treatment alternatives, about the key elements of the study design, and about benefits and risks of the proposed research. Elliott's arguments serve to restrict unduly, rather than protect, the patient's right to decide for himself or herself about whether participation in a particular research study would be desirable. In a research protocol, the focus and responsibility of the researcher should be to provide comprehensive and relevant information in an understandable way about the research and the illness.

Bonnie takes a more moderate approach to informed consent. He proposes that a "menu of safeguards" be used to assess the consent of decisionally impaired research subjects. Examples of such safeguards include "follow-up questions to assess subject understanding [or] videotaping or audiotaping consent interviews." Although questions assessing subject understanding may be helpful in determining whether consent is informed, it is unclear what standard of consent Bonnie advocates. Bonnie proposes a recognition of degrees of decisional impairment. Although this proposal may have merit, it is difficult to see how degrees of impairment will be assessed and implemented.

STIGMATIZATION OF PSYCHIATRIC DISORDERS

Mental disorders have been singled out for special treatment for centuries. The overwhelming consequence of this is stigmatization and inferior treatment. Yet research in recent years has served to demonstrate that mental disorders are not different in any fundamental way from general medical illnesses. Therefore, we should strive as much as possible to treat them in the same way, and not to do things that would exacerbate stigma. Every time we make special rules for psychiatry, we increase the risk for stigmatization. Therefore, the rationale for special treatment must be compelling to outweigh the risk for stigmatization.

The arguments offered in the article by Elliott are not persuasive when viewed from this perspective, and may even be dangerous. The suggestion that a disturbed emotional state may render an individual incompetent is a serious assertion, and could lead to a return to excessive paternalism toward the mentally ill. Those of us who treat psychiatric patients, including those with depression and mania, have a difficult job. Their compliance with treatment is often problematic. Yet, we know of no one who deals with patients on an active and regular basis who would argue for taking treatment decisions out of patients' hands (with the exception of emergency situations).

DEGREE OF RISK TO THE RESEARCH SUBJECT

A key issue with regard to informed consent is the degree of risk to the subject involved in participation in a particular experiment. Concerns about competence must be heightened in experimental situations that may potentially inflict harm. In general, this is not a substantial issue in research on depression. It is rare that studies of potential new treatments for depression may result in harm to the patient. Typically, the risks are uncomfortable side effects such as sedation and gastrointestinal distress.

A more relevant issue for depression is a no-treatment comparison group, usually a placebo. The use of placebo in medical research, and in depression in particular, has recently received increased attention.[7] It is easier to demonstrate that a new medication's efficacy is not statistically different from a known standard medication than it is to demonstrate that the new medication is statistically better than nonactive treatment. To do the latter, however, involves use of a placebo, therefore withholding a known effective treatment. This is a difficult ethical issue. We believe that placebo cells should not be used with patients with depressions of moderate or worse severity.

The placebo issue is one of scientific strategy and also of ethics. The ethical question is whether the patient has been informed fully of the existence of the placebo cell and the potential consequences of participation.

SUMMARY

Bonnie reminds us of the heritage and limitations of human subjects research. He points out that over the years, the protection of human subjects in research has enjoyed progress, experienced false starts, and endured inflated expectations. Both he and Elliott call attention to the fact that IRB review rarely probes how researchers propose to deal with impairments to subjects' decision-making capacities. We agree that IRBs should be encouraged to rethink their roles. But, as Bonnie argues, this requires a systematic review of the roles and functions of IRB rather than ad hoc adjustments by individual institutional IRBs. His proposal that IRBs should be encouraged to be more vigilant and thorough in their monitoring of research is sound, especially if the subjects are vulnerable or the research is risky.

A strength of Bonnie's review is that it suggests both specific ways to test competency and a range of options for IRBs to ensure that vulnerable subjects are protected from overzealous or overreaching researchers. His historical review and normative proposals are objective, balanced, and thoughtful.

Elliott's critique seems to single out psychiatric research with depressed patients as a special problem area. Although his title emphasizes *severely* depressed patients, he sometimes appears to neglect the fact that depression ranges across a spectrum from mild to severe. Elliott's point is well taken that severely depressed patients who are clearly incompetent should not, unless proper safeguards are provided, be enrolled in research. But his analysis falters because his position does not in the end respect personal autonomy.

Robert M. A. Hirschfeld, MD
Department of Psychiatry and Behavioral Sciences
University of Texas Medical Branch at Galveston
Room 1.200, Graves Building
Galveston, TX 77555-0429
William Winslade, PhD, JD
Institute for the Medical Humanities
Department of Psychiatry and Behavioral Sciences
University of Texas Medical Branch at Galveston
Todd L. Krause, PhD
University of Houston Law Center

REFERENCES

1. Bonnie RJ. Research with cognitively impaired subjects: unfinished business in the regulation of human research. *Arch Gen Psychiatry.* 1997; 54:105-111.
2. Elliott C. Caring about risks: are severely depressed patients competent to consent to research? *Arch Gen Psychiatry.* 1997;54:113-116.
3. Stanley B, Stanley M. Psychiatric patients' comprehension of consent information. *Psychopharmacol Bull.* 1987;3:375-378.
4. Stanley B, Stanley M. Psychiatry research for psychiatric patients: protecting their autonomy. *Compr Psychiatry.* 1981;22:420-425.
5. Stanley B, Stanley M, Lautin A, Laine J, Schwartz N. Preliminary findings in psychiatric patients as research participants: a population at risk? *Am J Psychiatry.* 1981;138:669-671.
6. Laine C, Davidoff F. Patient-centered medicine: a professional evolution. *JAMA.* 1996;275:152-156.
7. Rothman KJ, Michels KB. The continuing unethical use of placebo controls. *N Engl J Med.* 1994;331:394-398.

Circadian Rest-Activity Disturbances in Seasonal Affective Disorder

Martin H. Teicher, MD, PhD; Carol A. Glod, RN, PhD; Eleanor Magnus; David Harper; Gregory Benson; Kathryn Krueger, MD; Cynthia E. McGreenery

Background: Previous studies hypothesized that seasonal affective disorder (SAD) was caused by a circadian rhythm abnormality. The purpose of this study was to ascertain whether rest-activity rhythms were phase delayed, diminished in amplitude, or more poorly entrained to the 24-hour day.

Method: Twenty healthy adult controls and 25 outpatients meeting Rosenthal–National Institute of Mental Health criteria for SAD and *DSM-III-R* criteria for major or bipolar depression with seasonal pattern had their levels of activity recorded for 72 hours (weekdays) using wrist-worn actigraphs.

Results: Subjects with SAD had activity levels that were 11% lower than controls ($P=.03$), and their levels of activity were most attenuated during the first 2 hours after arising ($P=.004$). The relative amplitude of the circadian rhythm did not differ between groups. Patients with SAD were phase delayed by 50 minutes for the entire period ($P=.02$). Analysis of each individual day indicated that patients were delayed by up to 70 minutes ($P=.007$). Interdaily stability, an index of coupling between the rhythm and its zeitgeber was reduced in SAD ($P=.01$). Compared with controls, patients with SAD had best-fit circadian periods that were 92% more deviated from 24 hours ($P=.007$) and daily acrophase (time of the peak of the fit circadian rhythm) times that were 110% more variable between days ($P<.001$).

Conclusions: Patients with SAD have circadian rest-activity rhythms that are significantly phase delayed and more poorly entrained to the 24-hour day.

Arch Gen Psychiatry. 1997;54:124-130

From the Department of Psychiatry, Harvard Medical School, Boston, Mass (Drs Teicher, Glod, and Krueger); the Developmental Biopsychiatry Research Program and Clinical Chronobiology Laboratory, McLean Hospital, Belmont, Mass (Drs Teicher, Glod, and Krueger, Mss Magnus and McGreenery, and Messrs Harper and Benson); and Northeastern University College of Nursing, Boston (Dr Glod).

SEASONAL AFFECTIVE disorder (SAD) is a recurring psychiatric disorder that affects up to 6% of the population living far from the equator.[1] Several theories have been advanced to explain the occurrence of SAD and the therapeutic response to light. From the onset, many investigators have focused on abnormalities in circadian rhythms as light is the primary zeitgeber (time giver) that entrains the circadian clock to the 24-hour day. In general, chronobiological theories of affective disorders take 2 major forms. The dominant theory has been a *phase-advance* or *phase-shift hypothesis*, most clearly articulated by Wehr et al[2] and Goodwin et al.[3] They postulate that during depression the strong circadian X oscillator (which governs core body temperature, rapid eye movement [REM] sleep propensity, and plasma cortisol secretion) is advanced in its timing relative to the weaker Y oscillator (which modulates the rest-activity cycle, propensity for slow-wave sleep, and plasma growth hormone levels). Antidepressants supposedly work by shifting and synchronizing the timing of these rhythms. Although the circadian phase-advance hypothesis is a clever and valuable heuristic, relatively few studies have been supportive.[4,5]

An alternative chronobiological theory to emerge in recent years is the *circadian dysregulation* or *attenuation* hypothesis postulated independently by Siever and Davis[6] and Schulz and Lund.[7] Briefly, they propose that circadian rhythms in depression are characterized by a loss of power or rhythmicity. This may be evidenced by a blunting of circadian amplitude, the emergence of a more noisy or chaotic presentation, or the addition of new frequency components. Antidepressants purportedly work by restoring circadian rhythmicity. There has been considerable support for this hypothesis in nonseasonal depression. Evidence for attenuated circadian amplitude has been observed in motor activity (4 of 4 studies), thyroid stimulating hormone secretion (8 of 9 studies), and melatonin secretion (9 of 12 studies).[8]

SUBJECTS AND METHODS

SUBJECTS

Locomotor activity levels and rhythms were quantified in 45 adults, including 20 healthy control subjects and 25 subjects with fall-winter SAD. All of the subjects were studied in their natural home environment, and ranged in age from 18 to 65 years. The control group consisted of 7 men and 13 women (mean±SD age, 31.9±10.8 years), and the SAD group consisted of 5 men and 20 women (mean±SD age, 38.8±12.6 years). Both control subjects and depressed patients were recruited through advertisement or self-referral. For inclusion in the study, all SAD subjects were free of psychotropic medications. For those previously treated with antidepressants, a washout period of at least 4 weeks was required (>6 weeks without fluoxetine hydrochloride). Eight patients were treated with stable doses of nonpsychotropic medications; 3 were treated with estrogen replacement, 3 received antihistamines or allergy medications (eg, terfenadine [Seldane], diphenhydramine, pseudoephedrine), 2 received treatment for hypertension with hydrochlorothiazide, and 1 patient was taking birth control pills. Control subjects were all medication free and denied any evidence of current or past psychiatric disorders.

The SAD group was studied during the fall-winter season, and the data were collected from mid-October through March, during 2 consecutive years (1989-1990, 1990-1991). The subjects were monitored during weekdays to avoid phase shifts that often occur on weekends. They resided at home, worked, or attended school, and used alarm clocks to help to maintain a normal sleep-wake schedule. Structured diagnostic interviews[23] were completed on all SAD subjects and 12 control subjects. The remaining control subjects were found to be free of *DSM-III-R* psychopathology using unstructured clinical interviews. All depressed subjects met Rosenthal–National Institute of Mental Health criteria[1] for SAD and *DSM-III-R* criteria for major depressive episode (either unipolar or bipolar) with a seasonal pattern.

After approval from the institutional review board, all of the subjects gave written informed consent. Rest and activity levels were measured using a small wrist-worn ambulatory activity monitor (MotionLogger Actigraph, Ambulatory Monitors Inc, Ardsley, NY). This device is capable of detecting accelerations greater than 0.01g (up to 10 counts per second). Activity levels were measured in 5-minute intervals over a period of 72 consecutive hours and stored in memory for later computer retrieval. The resultant data were carefully inspected to reject epochs when the monitor was not worn (eg, bathing). To be included in the study, subjects had to wear the activity monitor for at least 80% of the investigation period. Software for programming the monitor, data retrieval, and analyses was written by 1 of us (M.H.T.) for use with Macintosh computers, and is available through the distributor of the activity monitors.

DATA ANALYSIS

To answer the proposed questions, the data were analyzed in several ways. The first approach used to assess the timing and amplitude of circadian rhythm was traditional cosinor analysis,[24] in which the data were fit to a cosine function set to a frequency of 24 hours. This model yields estimates of mesor (corrected mean 24-hour activity), circadian amplitude, circadian acrophase (time of the peak of the fit circadian rhythm), and goodness of fit. In addition to circadian amplitude, the relative circadian amplitude (amplitude divided by mesor) was calculated to correct for possible differences in activity as a result of psychomotor retardation or agitation. Although traditional cosinor analysis is a time-honored procedure, there are notable inadequacies with this technique, as the duration of the daytime activity period is greater than the nighttime quiescent period. Cosinor procedures can be improved by the simultaneous fit of 2 cosine functions, 1 with a period of 24 hours and the other with a 12-hour period. This approach has been used in several contemporary studies to model circadian fluctuations in body temperature,[25,26] locomotor activity,[17,19] and hormone levels.[27] This procedure also yields estimates of the timing and amplitude of the circadian rhythm and 12-hour harmonic component.

To test for loss of circadian entrainment, 3 procedures were used. First, a more complex nonlinear dual oscillator cosinor model was used in which circadian frequency was fit as an optimized parameter.[17,28] From the fit frequency, the circadian entrainment error was calculated as the number of minutes that the best-fitting cosine function deviated from 24 hours. Second, interdaily stability was calculated as a nonparametric measure that indicates the consistency of the activity rhythm from hour to hour across days. This measure is derived from the 24-hour component of the χ^2 "periodogram." Moore-Ede et al[29] have proposed that interdaily stability reflects the amount of coupling between the circadian rhythm and the external zeitgebers (time cues) that entrain the rhythm.

Previous studies have reported weakening in interdaily stability in the locomotor activity rhythm of patients with advanced Alzheimer disease.[18,19] Finally, activity data from each successive day was fit to a fixed cosinor model to determine the daily acrophase, and to calculate the range and variability (SD) in acrophase for each subject across the 3 days of the study.

To test these hypotheses, subjects with SAD were compared with healthy control subjects using analysis of covariance procedures with age as a covariate (Systat, Evanston, Ill). There was a nearly significant difference between groups in age ($F[1,43]=3.77$; $P=.06$), and this intervening variable exerts significant effects on circadian phase and measures of entrainment. It was thus important to control for this variable to prevent spurious findings of group differences stemming from differences in age.

Calculation of mean activity, interdaily stability, and the 72-hour cosine models were performed on all of the subjects (N=45). Because of hard-drive failure, data for 2 control subjects were irretrievably lost. Calculation of daily acrophase was derived from 43 subjects, 25 with SAD and 18 controls. In this set, 1 patient with SAD and 2 control subjects had monitor removal periods of more than 6 hours on a single day, which compromised accurate assessment of daily acrophase for that day. Thus, daily acrophase measures were limited to 24 patients with SAD on day 3, and 17 control subjects on days 2 and 3. On the remaining days, data were for 25 patients with SAD and 18 control subjects.

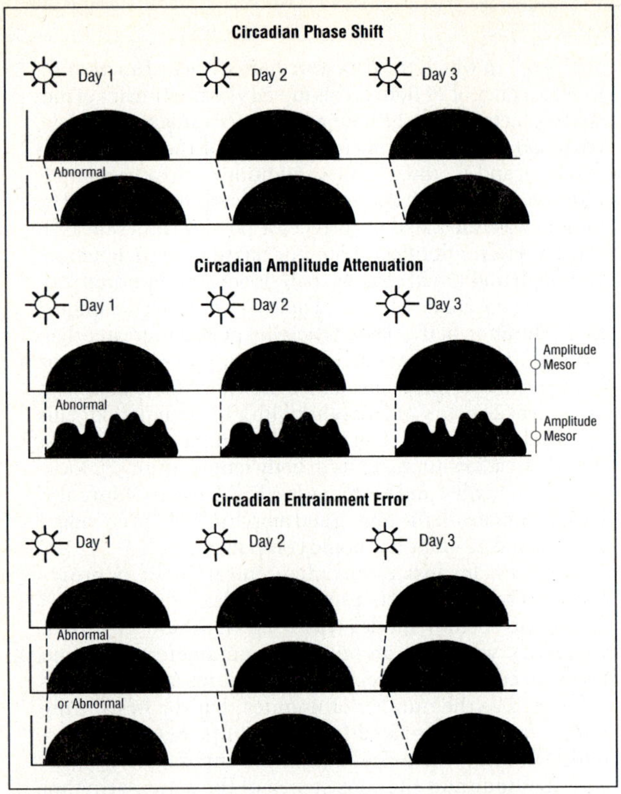

Figure 1. *Illustration of different ways in which circadian rhythms can be altered in psychiatric disorders. These include a consistent phase delay (top), weakening of circadian amplitude and rhythmicity (middle), and deviation from 24-hour entrainment (bottom).*

Lewy and Sack[9] were the first to propose a modification of the phase-shift hypothesis for SAD. Their data indicated that the timing of the circadian rhythm controlling melatonin secretion may be delayed in patients with SAD (phase-delay hypothesis), and that bright light may work by restoring the appropriate phase.[9] Similarly, Dahl et al[10] published data from a small sample that showed that the circadian rhythms of temperature and dim light melatonin onset were delayed in patients with SAD under the rigorous controlled condition of a constant routine. In contrast, Czeisler et al[11] proposed, on theoretical grounds, that the amplitude of the circadian temperature rhythm may be blunted, and hypothesized that light works by augmenting circadian amplitude. To date, we know of no published data to support the amplitude attenuation hypothesis in SAD, and preliminary studies have failed to find any evidence for blunting of either the circadian amplitude of core body temperature[12,13] or salivary melatonin secretion.[13]

Although phase shifts and amplitude attenuation have been the dominant theories in chronobiological research, there are other ways in which circadian rhythms may be abnormal. Another possibility is a lack of temporal stability of the cycle resulting from weakened entrainment to the 24-hour day. Because the primary function of the light zeitgeber is to entrain circadian rhythms to the 24-hour day, we hypothesized that the fundamental circadian disturbance to occur in SAD may be a reduction in the degree of entrainment,[14,15] and that bright artificial light may serve to re-entrain the rhythm (entrainment hypothesis).

The key differences between the phase-shift, attenuation, and entrainment hypotheses are illustrated in **Figure 1**. If a phase delay is present, then the rhythm should consistently peak at a later time in comparison with normal. Teicher et al[16] reported that the phase of the circadian rest-activity rhythm was delayed by 2 hours in geriatric patients with unipolar depression. If amplitude attenuation is present, there should be a decrease in the relative amplitude of the circadian rhythm. The strongest evidence for attenuation occurs when the amplitude of the rhythm is decreased even after correcting for differences in mean 24-hour levels. Hence, an overall reduction in activity would not necessarily blunt the amplitude of the rhythm. Teicher et al[17] reported that there was a highly significant reduction in the relative circadian activity amplitude of pediatric patients with depression. Diminished entrainment is more difficult to define. Entrainment refers to the normal tightly synchronized relationship between the timing of a rhythm and its external zeitgeber. When entrainment is diminished, the rhythm becomes less stable. Hence, the rhythm may peak at different times each day. Complete loss of entrainment would mean that the subject was "free running." These individuals could drift in and out of phase with conventional time. Persons with weakened entrainment may drift out of phase for a few days, but, when the entrainment error becomes too great, they would then correct the discrepancy. These individuals would not drift completely out of phase, and may maintain an overall 24-hour rhythm across several days, but could depart significantly from 24 hours across a few days. Witting et al[18] and Satlin et al[19] reported that patients with Alzheimer disease had evidence for weakened entrainment. Although differences between phase and period can be grasped intuitively, they are difficult to mathematically disentangle and often require complex chronobiological investigations under special conditions. The present study is a naturalistic investigation that provides preliminary insight.

The purpose of this study was to explore these chronobiological hypotheses in patients with fall-winter SAD. Locomotor activity was chosen as the dependent measure for several reasons. First, locomotor activity is a key psychobiological process that is often disturbed in patients with depression.[20] Second, activity profiles generate high-resolution time series that can be analyzed with powerful computational techniques. Third, activity monitoring provides a convenient, comfortable, and noninvasive circadian measure in the patient's natural environment. Fourth, rest-activity rhythms represent 1 of the primary physiological manifestations of the hypothesized "weak" circadian oscillators. Although activity rhythms are not a direct measure of this internal clock, and are affected by both internal and external masking factors, measures of locomotor activity provide an accepted estimate of this internal clock.[20] A constant routine paradigm was not used, as it provides data on only a single circadian cycle,[21] and weakened entrainment needs to be assessed from a number of successive cycles. Moreover, patients are deprived of sleep for 36 hours during

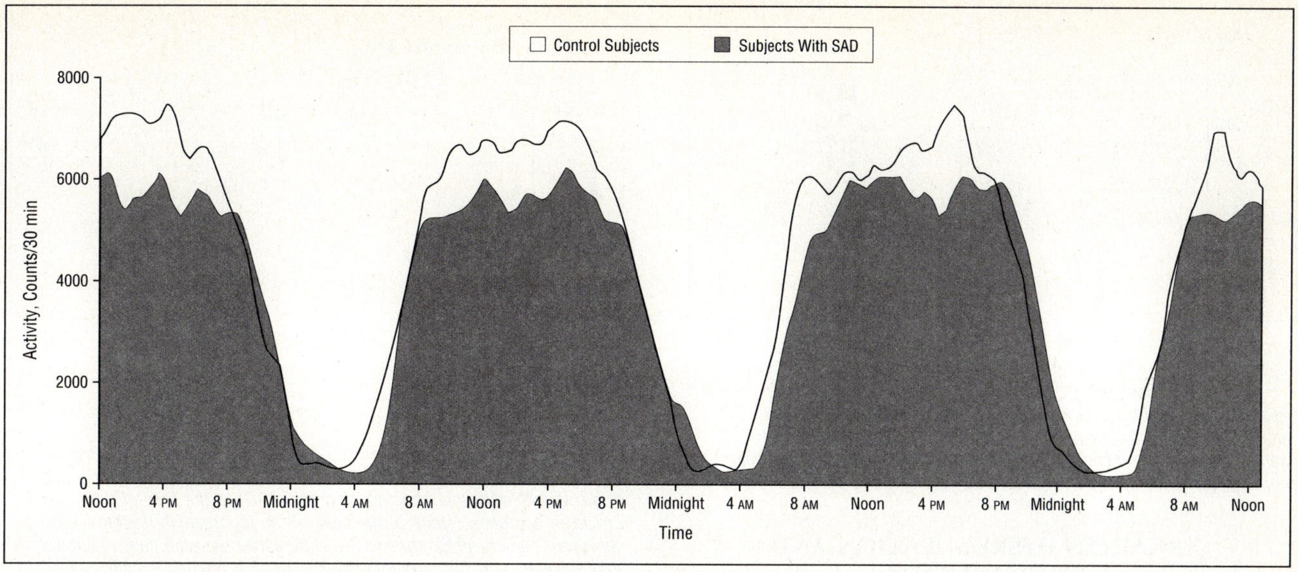

Figure 2. *Composite profiles showing 72 hours of activity (average counts per 30-minute epoch) in control subjects and subjects with seasonal affective disorder (SAD). Data were smoothed using a 3-point weighted moving average.*

the protocol, which may exert different effects on depressed patients than on control subjects[22] and thus confound interpretation of results.

RESULTS

Composite actigraph profiles are illustrated in **Figure 2**. They represent mean activity levels (actigraph counts per 30-minute epoch) over a 72-hour period. Patients with SAD had lower mean activity levels during most daytime periods. Control subjects appeared to be very consistent on a day-to-day basis in the time that their activity levels rose or fell, presumably as part of their sleep-wake cycle. As a group, the patients with SAD appeared to be slightly delayed relative to control subjects, with their activity cycles rising and falling at later clock times. However, the degree of difference varied on a daily basis. For instance, rise and fall times were only slightly delayed in patients with SAD during the second day of monitoring. There was a more pronounced delay in rise and fall times on the third day, yet there seemed to be a smaller difference in rise time during the last partial day of monitoring. In short, from the composite profiles, it appears that subjects with SAD may be less consistent in their wake and sleep times and may possibly be drifting in and out of phase relative to control subjects.

LOCOMOTOR ACTIVITY LEVELS

Quantitative analysis confirms that patients with SAD had lower overall levels of activity. Mean ($\pm$SD) 24-hour activity levels (mesor) averaged 726$\pm$78 counts per 5-minute epoch in control subjects vs 638$\pm$133 counts in patients with SAD ($F[1,42]=6.28$; $P=.02$). Differences were most consistently observed during the first few hours after arising (**Figure 3**). Control subjects averaged 1139$\pm$144 counts during the first 2 hours after awakening and leaving bed. In contrast, under the same circumstances, patients with SAD averaged only 917$\pm$259 counts ($F[1,40]=9.62$; $P=.004$).

CIRCADIAN AMPLITUDE

Using the simple cosine model, subjects with SAD had mean circadian amplitude measures that were 11% lower than those of control subjects. However, their mesor was also 11% lower. To correct for individual differences in activity, differences were assessed in relative circadian amplitude (100$\times$[amplitude/mesor]). The relative circadian amplitudes were almost identical in patients with SAD and control subjects ($F[1,42]=0.01$; $P=.92$). The same finding emerged using the dual harmonic model. Similarly, there were no differences between subjects with SAD and control subjects in amplitude after covarying for individual differences in mesor ($F[1,42]=0.31$; $P>.5$). Thus, while an overall attenuation in activity was evident in patients with SAD, there was no evidence for an attenuation in the actual amplitude of the circadian rhythm.

CIRCADIAN PHASE

On average, the rest-activity cycle of patients with SAD peaked about 50 minutes later than that of control subjects, indicating a significant phase delay ($F[1,42]=6.33$; $P=.02$). Similarly, activity acrophase was delayed by 52 minutes using the dual cosine model. Further verification of the phase delay was provided by calculating acrophase for each 24-hour period of monitoring. As shown in **Figure 4**, daily acrophase was substantially delayed in patients with SAD across the 3 days ($F[1,37]=8.07$; $P=.007$). Phase differences averaged about 50 minutes during the first and third days (day 1: $F[1,40]=5.01$; $P=.03$ and day 3: $F[1,38]=4.20$; $P=.05$), and 73 minutes on day 2 ($F[1,39]=4.76$; $P=.04$).

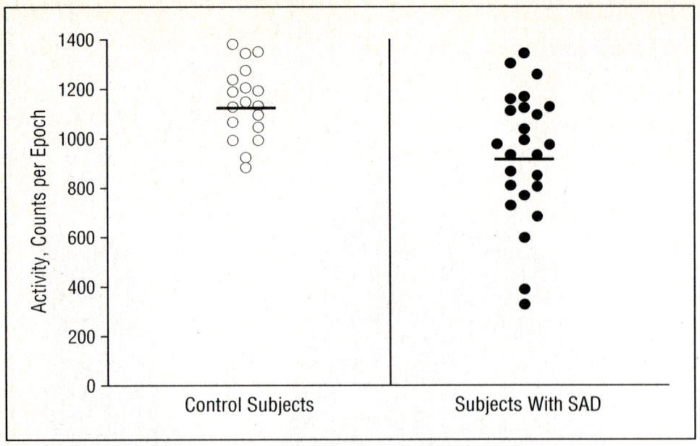

Figure 3. *Scatterplot indicating differences between control subjects and subjects with seasonal affective disorder (SAD) in mean level of activity (counts per 5-minute epoch) during the first 2 hours after arising each morning. Daily rise time was used for each subject according to sleep logs.*

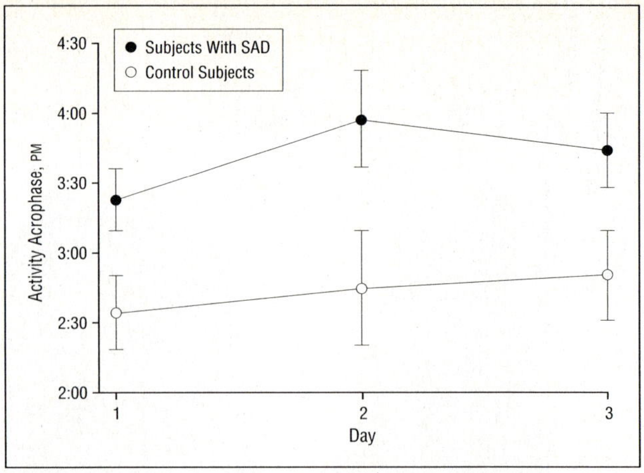

Figure 4. *Line graphs showing difference between control subjects and subjects with seasonal affective disorder (SAD) in the time of their daily circadian acrophase (time of the peak of the fit circadian rhythm). Values represent age-corrected mean±SD. Differences between control subjects and subjects with SAD were significant on each day (all* P≤*.05).*

CIRCADIAN DYSREGULATION AND ENTRAINMENT

The activity profiles of patients with SAD were more poorly fit by both the cosinor and dual harmonic models, suggesting that patients with SAD were less "circadian." Further analysis suggests that this disturbance was a result of impaired entrainment to the 24-hour day. Interdaily stability, an index of coupling between the rhythm and its 24-hour zeitgeber, was significantly reduced in patients with SAD ($F[1,41]=6.98$; $P=.01$). Similarly, fitting each subject to a more complex model in which frequency was calculated as an optimized parameter[28] revealed that the best-fit circadian period deviated from 24 hours by a 92% greater margin in patients with SAD ($F[1,42]=8.15$; $P=.007$). Finally, fitting each 24-hour period of activity to derive daily acrophase measures revealed that the timing of the daily acrophase was 110% more variable between days (SD) in patients with SAD ($F[1,40]=13.95$; $P<.001$). This was not an artifact of enhanced overall variability in patients with SAD, as they had no greater variability in their daily mesors (70.4±44.6 vs 74.5±77.8 counts, $F[1,40]=0.04$; $P=.83$).

Further analysis of the nature of the circadian rest-activity disturbance revealed that the poorer fit in SAD could be explained by weakened entrainment to the 24-hour day. Thus, patients with SAD had lower levels of interdaily stability, indicating that their hourly pattern of activity had a weaker 24-hour repeated pattern. Diminished interdaily stability implies a weakened coupling between a rhythm and its zeitgeber. It was also the case that the circadian frequency that best fit each subject's 72-hour activity time series deviated from 24 hours by a wider margin in patients with SAD. Finally, the daily acrophase of patients with SAD fluctuated more from day to day than the daily acrophase of control subjects. In short, the circadian cycle appears to be more variable across days in SAD, deviating more from 24 hours over this relatively short series, and peaking at more unstable times. This may be a consequence of less consistent resetting of the circadian clock by light. In actuality, what this basically means is that patients with SAD have more inconsistent sleep-wake times. A common pattern is to waken progressively later each day during the workweek.

COMMENT

The present study provides support for the hypothesis that patients with SAD have a disturbance in their circadian cycle. Patients with SAD were more poorly modeled by single and dual harmonic cosinor models than were control subjects, indicating that a smaller portion of their activity profile could be explained by a 24-hour rhythm. Although the degree of fit between activity profiles and cosinor model in control subjects is somewhat lower than traditionally reported for temperature[25] and cortisol rhythms,[27] it should be noted that the present results pertain to 5-minute activity epochs rather than 30- to 60-minute epochs traditionally used in studies of temperature and cortisol levels. Hourly activity measures are fit by cosine models with correlations of 0.8 to 0.95, indicating that activity is as well fit by cosine models as temperature or cortisol levels.

Weakened entrainment is a new, relatively unexplored, but intriguing hypothesis. We need to emphasize that our results also provide strong support for the more established phase-delay hypothesis. Sack et al[30] reported that dim light melatonin onset was delayed by 70 minutes at baseline in 8 subjects with SAD vs 5 control subjects. Dahl et al[10] reported that, during constant routine conditions, dim light melatonin onset was delayed by 92 minutes and rectal temperature was delayed by 146 minutes in 6 female patients with SAD vs 6 female control subjects. Wirz-Justice et al,[13] also using a constant routine, reported a nonsignificant 23-minute delay in melatonin onset, and a marginally significant 71-minute delay in the 24-hour temperature rhythm of 11 women with SAD compared with 8 female control subjects. Checkley et al,[31] however, failed to observe any significant delay in the melatonin acrophase of 20 patients with SAD and

20 control subjects when they were adapted for 4 days to an inpatient unit with scheduled sleep and wake times and low-level illumination. In the present study, the overall phase delay in SAD was from 10 patients who were more phase delayed than any control subjects. However, there were also 4 patients who were more phase advanced than control subjects, suggesting the presence of both phase-advanced and phase-delayed subtypes, as previously reported.[9,12]

Although phase delay and weakened entrainment can be thought of as 2 distinct circadian disturbances, they are interrelated. Weakened entrainment due to diminished sensitivity to the zeitgeber can produce an apparent phase delay. On the other hand, the degree of entrainment depends on the phase of the rhythm. It is interesting that serotonin has been postulated to play a pivotal role in adjusting the sensitivity of the circadian pacemaker in the suprachiasmatic nucleus to the entraining effects of light.[32] Serotonin turnover in the human hypothalamus increases as day length shortens, at least until December,[33] and serotonin levels peak in the very early morning,[33] possibly to better detect and respond to the dawn zeitgeber. Thus, seasonal fluctuations in serotonin turnover may represent a compensatory homeostatic mechanism—enhancing sensitivity in the face of an attenuated light signal. Perhaps patients with SAD have diminished retinal sensitivity[34] or inadequate serotonin compensation.[35] In any case, weakening of the entrainment relationship would cause the rhythm to become less stable, and may cause the rhythm to delay to later times when the light signal is stronger. This hypothesis could also explain discrepancies found in previous studies on the magnitude of the melatonin phase shift,[10,13,30,31] as the degree of phase delay would depend on the quality of zeitgebers provided.

Although this study provides support for both a phase shift and entrainment error, there was no evidence for an attenuation in circadian amplitude. This was not a limitation of the technique. Using the same methods, marked attenuation in relative circadian amplitude (amplitude/mesor) has been observed in pediatric patients with depression[17] and in elderly patients with Alzheimer disease.[19] The present findings are consistent with other studies that failed to observe a reduction in circadian amplitude of temperature[12,13] or melatonin[13,31] in SAD.

To our knowledge, this is the first study to directly demonstrate weakened entrainment in SAD. Goodwin and Jamison[8] raised the possibility that deficient entrainment may account for circadian phase shifts and amplitude attenuation observed in depression, but they provided no direct evidence. Similarly, Ehlers et al[36] theorized that depression may result from instability in the timing of circadian rhythms caused by weakening of social zeitgebers accompanying psychological loss. The possibility that SAD is related to weakened entrainment and circadian instability is an intuitively appealing hypothesis, as light is the primary zeitgeber that serves to entrain the rhythm.

One potential concern is that 4 patients with SAD received estrogens, which can affect circadian rhythms and melatonin secretion.[37] There were no significant differences on any circadian measure between subjects with SAD who were or were not receiving estrogen, although there was a consistent trend for patients taking estrogens to have circadian measures that were closer to normal than the other SAD subjects. Excluding these 4 patients did not alter any of the statistical effects, nor did the exclusion of all 8 subjects receiving medications.

The present study also suggests that different forms of depression, or patients in different age groups, may have different types of circadian activity disturbances. We have reported that children with depression have a markedly weakened rest-activity rhythm characterized by loss of amplitude and intrusion of higher-frequency harmonic rhythms.[17] However, they maintain normal phase and entrainment.[17] In contrast, the rest-activity pattern of geriatric patients with unipolar depression seems to be markedly phase delayed and associated with increased activity and agitation.[16] Patients with SAD have impaired circadian entrainment, a phase delay, and attenuation in overall activity levels but preserved circadian amplitude. Studies are under way to disentangle the effects of age and diagnosis.

Quantitative analysis of rest-activity lends support to the hypothesis that there is a circadian rhythm disturbance in SAD. These studies also suggest that the primary disturbance may be an abnormality in circadian phase and stability (entrainment). Further research using measures of rest-activity may aid in the differentiation of depressive subtypes and enrich our understanding of the complicated and multifaceted ways in which cyclical processes can be affected in mood disorders.

Accepted for publication June 18, 1996.

This research was supported in part by a grant from the National Institute of Mental Health (MH-48343), and from the Hall Mercer Foundation, Philadelphia, Pa, and the Snider family, Chestnut Hill, Mass.

Some data in this article were previously presented at the Society for Light Therapy and Biological Rhythms, National Institutes of Health, Bethesda, Md, April 30, 1992.

Reprints: Martin H. Teicher, MD, PhD, McLean Hospital, 115 Mill St, Belmont, MA 02178 (e-mail: teicher@warren.med.harvard.edu).

REFERENCES

1. Rosenthal NE, Sack DA, Gillin JC, Lewy AJ, Goodwin FK, Davenport Y, Mueller PS, Newsome DA, Wehr TA. Seasonal affective disorder: a description of the syndrome and preliminary findings with light therapy. *Arch Gen Psychiatry.* 1984;41:72-80.
2. Wehr TA, Muscettola G, Goodwin FK. Urinary 3-methoxy-4-hydroxphenyglycol circadian rhythm: early timing (phase advance) in manic-depressives compared with normal subjects. *Arch Gen Psychiatry.* 1980;37:257-263.
3. Goodwin FK, Wirz-Justice A, Wehr TA. Evidence that the pathophysiology of depression and the mechanism of antidepressant drugs both involve alterations in circadian rhythms. *Adv Biochem Psychopharmacol.* 1982;32:1-11.
4. Souêtre E, Salvati E, Belegou J-L, Pringuey D, Candito M, Krebs B, Ardisson J-L, Darcourt G. Circadian rhythms in depression and recovery: evidence for blunted amplitude as the main chronobiological abnormality. *Psychiatry Res.* 1989;28:263-278.

5. Wehr TA, Sack DA, Duncan WC, Mendleson WB, Rosenthal NE, Gillin JC, Goodwin FK. Sleep and circadian rhythms in affective patients isolated from external time cues. *Psychiatry Res.* 1985;15:327-339.
6. Siever LJ, Davis KL. Overview: toward a dysregulation hypothesis of depression. *Am J Psychiatry.* 1985;142:1017-1031.
7. Schulz H, Lund R. On the origin of early REM episodes in the sleep of depressed patients: a comparison of three hypotheses. *Psychiatry Res.* 1985; 16:65-77.
8. Goodwin FK, Jamison KR. *Manic Depressive Illness.* New York, NY: Oxford Press; 1990:558-560.
9. Lewy AJ, Sack RL. Light therapy and psychiatry. *Proc Soc Exp Biol Med.* 1986; 183:11-18.
10. Dahl K, Avery DH, Lewy AJ, Savage MV, Brenglemann GL, Larsen HLH, Vitiello MV, Prinz PN. Dim light melatonin onset and circadian temperature during a constant routine in hypersomnic winter depression. *Acta Psychiatr Scand.* 1993;88:60-66.
11. Czeisler CA, Kronauer RE, Mooney JJ, Anderson JL, Allen JS. Biological rhythm disorders, depression, and phototherapy: a new hypothesis. *Psychiatr Clin North Am.* 1987;10:687-709.
12. Rosenthal NE, Levendosky AA, Skwerer RG, Joseph-Vanderpool JR, Kelly KA, Hardin T, Kasper S, DellaBella P, Wehr TA. Effects of light treatment on core body temperature in seasonal affective disorder. *Biol Psychiatry.* 1990;27:39-50.
13. Wirz-Justice A, Krauchi K, Graw P, Arendt J, English J, Hetsch C, Haug H-J, Leonhardt G, Brunner DP. Circadian rhythms of core body temperature and salivary melatonin in winter SAD before and after midday light. In: Program and abstracts of the Society for Light Treatment and Biological Rhythms; June 1994; Washington, DC. Abstract 12.
14. Teicher MH, Glod CA, Harper D, Magnus E, Frank A, Benson G. Phototherapy, spectral EEG, and ambulatory activity rhythms in seasonal affective disorder. In: Program and abstracts of the Society for Light Therapy and Biological Rhythms; May 1990; New York, NY. Abstract 34.
15. Glod CA, Teicher MH, Magnus E, Harper D, Benson G, Krueger K. Circadian rest-activity disturbances in seasonal affective disorder. In: Program and abstracts of the Society of Light Therapy and Biological Rhythms; June 1992; Washington, DC. Abstract 14.
16. Teicher MH, Lawrence JM, Barber NI, Finklestein SP, Lieberman HR, Baldessarini RJ. Circadian activity rhythm disturbances in geriatric major depression. *Arch Gen Psychiatry.* 1988;45:913-917.
17. Teicher MH, Glod CA, Harper D, Magnus M, Brasher C, Wren F, Pahlavan K. Locomotor activity in depressed children and adolescents, I: circadian dysregulation. *J Am Acad Child Adolesc Psychiatry.* 1993;32:760-769.
18. Witting W, Kwa IH, Eikelenboom P, Mirmiran M, Swaab DF. Alterations in the circadian rest-activity rhythm in aging and Alzheimer's disease. *Biol Psychiatry.* 1990;27:563-572.
19. Satlin A, Teicher MH, Lieberman HR, Baldessarini RJ, Volicer L, Rheaume Y. Circadian locomotor activity rhythms in Alzheimer's disease. *Neuropsychopharmacol.* 1991;5:115-126.
20. Teicher MH. Actigraphy and motion analysis: new tools for psychiatry. *Harvard Rev Psychiatry.* 1995;3:18-35.
21. Czeisler CA, Allan JS, Strogatz SH, Ronda JM, Sanchez R, Rios CD, Freitag WO, Richardson GS, Kronhauer RE. Bright light resets the human circadian pacemaker independent of the timing of the sleep-wake cycle. *Science.* 1986; 233:667-671.
22. Wu JC, Gillin JC, Buchsbaum MS, Hershey T, Johnson JC, Bunney WE Jr, Effect of sleep deprivation on brain metabolism of depressed patients. *Am J Psychiatry.* 1992;149:538-543.
23. Spitzer RL, Williams JBW, Gibbon M, First MB. *Structured Clinical Interview for DSM-III-R—Patient Version (SCID-P, 5/1/89).* New York, NY: New York State Psychiatric Institute; 1989.
24. Nelson W, Tong IL, Lee JK, Halberg F. Methods for cosinor-rhythmometry. *Chronobiologia.* 1979;6:305-323.
25. Czeisler CA, Kronhauer RE, Allan JS, Duffy JF, Jewett ME, Brown EN, Ronda JM. Bright light induction of strong (type 0) resetting of the human circadian pacemaker. *Science.* 1989;244:1328-1333.
26. Jewett ME, Kronhauer RE, Czeisler CA. Light-induced suppression of endogenous circadian amplitude in humans. *Nature.* 1991;350:59-62.
27. Yehuda R, Teicher MH, Trestman RL, Levengood RA, Siever LJ. Cortisol regulation in post-traumatic stress disorder: a chronobiological analysis. *Biol Psychiatry.* 1996;40:79-88
28. Teicher MH, Barber NI. COSIFIT: an interactive program for simultaneous multioscillator cosinor analysis of time-series data. *Computers Biomed Res.* 1990; 23:283-295.
29. Moore-Ede MC, Sulzman FM, Fuller CA. *The Clocks That Time Us: Physiology of the Circadian Timing System.* Cambridge Mass: Harvard University Press; 1982:79-80.
30. Sack RL, Lewy AJ, White DM, Singer DM, Fireman MJ, Vandiver R. Morning vs evening light treatment for winter depression: evidence that the therapeutic effects of light are mediated by circadian phase shifts. *Arch Gen Psychiatry.* 1990;47:343-351.
31. Checkley SA, Murphy DGM, Abbas M, Marks M, Winton F, Palazidou E, Murphy DM, Franey C, Arendt J. Melatonin rhythms in seasonal affective disorder. *Br J Psychiatry.* 1993;163:332-337.
32. Morin LP, Blanchard J. Depletion of brain serotonin by 5,7-DHT modifies hamster circadian rhythm response to light. *Brain Res.* 1991;566:173-185.
33. Carlsson A, Svennerholm L, Winblad B. Seasonal and circadian monoamine variations in human brains examined post mortem. *Acta Psychiatr Scand.* 1980; 61:75-85.
34. Lam RW, Beattie CW, Buchanan A, Mador JA. Electroretinography in seasonal affective disorder. *Psychiatry Res.* 1992;43:55-63.
35. Jacobsen FM, Mueller EA, Rosenthal NE, Rogers S, Hill JL, Murphy DL. Behavioral responses to intravenous meta-chlorophenylpiperazine in patients with seasonal affective disorder and control subjects before and after phototherapy. *Psychiatry Res.* 1994;52:181-197.
36. Ehlers CL, Frank E, Kupfer DJ. Social zeitgebers and biological rhythms: a unified approach to understanding the etiology of depression. *Arch Gen Psychiatry* 1988;45:948-952.
37. Okatani Y, Sagara Y. Enhanced nocturnal melatonin secretion in women with functional secondary amenorrhea: relationship to opioid system and endogenous estrogen levels. *Horm Res.* 1995;43:194-199.

ORIGINAL ARTICLE

Effects of Tryptophan Depletion on Drug-Free Patients With Seasonal Affective Disorder During a Stable Response to Bright Light Therapy

Alexander Neumeister, MD; Nicole Praschak-Rieder, MD; Barbara Heßelmann, MD; Marie-Luise Rao, PhD; Judith Glück, Msc; Siegfried Kasper, MD

Background: A dysfunction of the serotonin system may play a major role in the pathogenesis of seasonal affective disorder. Bright light therapy has been shown to be effective in the treatment of winter depression in patients with seasonal affective disorder. Light therapy–induced remission from depression may be associated with changes in brain serotonin function.

Methods: After at least 2 weeks of clinical remission, 12 drug-free patients who had had depression with seasonal affective disorder underwent tryptophan depletion in a double-blind, placebo-controlled, balanced crossover design study.

Results: Short-term tryptophan depletion induced a significant decrease in plasma free and total tryptophan levels ($P<.001$ for both, repeated measures analysis of variance), with peak effects occurring 5 hours after ingestion of a tryptophan-free amino acid drink. It emerged that tryptophan depletion leads to a transient depressive relapse, which was most pronounced on the day after the tryptophan-depletion testing. No clinically relevant mood changes were observed in the control testing.

Conclusions: The maintenance of light therapy–induced remission from depression in patients with seasonal mood cycles seems to depend on the functional integrity of the brain serotonin system. Our results suggest that the serotonin system might be involved in the mechanism of action of light therapy.

Arch Gen Psychiatry. 1997;54:133-138

Seasonal affective disorder (SAD) is a condition characterized by annually occurring depressive episodes. Two characteristic types of seasonal mood changes have been reported: depression regularly occurring in fall and winter with full remission during the following spring and summer, which was systematically described by Rosenthal et al,[1] and the opposite pattern, recurrent depressive episodes in the summer with remission during the next fall and winter.[2,3] In the present report, we refer to SAD with fall and winter depressions.

Typical patients with SAD meet *DSM-IV*[4] criteria for major depressive disorder or bipolar disorder and fulfill for their longitudinal course the criteria of the *DSM-IV* seasonal pattern specifier. During winter depression, most of these patients complain of atypical vegetative symptoms accompanied by hypersomnia, hyperphagia, carbohydrate craving, and weight gain.[5-9] Hypotheses on the underlying mechanisms of these behavioral and neurovegetative disorders indicate that environmental variables, eg, climate, latitude, light, and changes in neurotransmitter function that naturally occur with the seasons may be important.[10-12]

The antidepressant effect of light therapy (LT) in the treatment of SAD has been widely shown.[1,13-15] Previous studies have shown that an antidepressant response in patients with SAD is contingent on the exposure of the patients' eyes to light.[16] Further important factors are the duration of daily treatment[13] and light intensity.[1,17,18] However, the role of timing of LT remains controversial.[13,19-23] The biological basis of the diverse psychological and biological changes in SAD and the underlying mechanism of action of LT are still unclear and require further study.

Numerous studies have proved that the brain serotonin (5-hydroxytryptamine [5-HT]) system might be involved in the pathogenesis of SAD and the mechanism of action of LT.[24] Human hypothalamic 5-HT shows a seasonal rhythm, with nadir values in December and January.[25] Patients with SAD often report activation after carbohydrate ingestion,[26] which may represent a behavioral-biochemical feedback loop for raising the available 5-HT content. Animal studies suggest that carbohydrate intake raises brain tryptophan (TRP) levels by

From the Department of General Psychiatry, Vienna University, Vienna, Austria (Drs Neumeister, Praschak-Rieder, Heßelmann, and Kasper and Ms Glück), and the Rheinische Friedrich-Wilhelms-University Bonn, Bonn, Germany (Dr Rao). Dr Neumeister is now affiliated with the National Institute of Mental Health, Clinical Psychobiology Branch, Bethesda, Md.

PATIENTS AND METHODS

PATIENTS

Between September 1 and December 31, 1994, 17 drug-free outpatients with depression (13 women and 4 men; mean [±SD] age, 42.0±13.5 years; range, 22-70 years) from our SAD clinic were invited to participate in a study of the behavioral effects of short-term TRP depletion after successful LT. On admission to the study, demographic and clinical information about the longitudinal course of the illness, previous treatment attempts, and other psychiatric diagnoses were obtained during a semistructured clinical interview based on *DSM-IV* criteria. The number of previous episodes and additional diagnoses were based on patient report, review of medical records, and direct contact with previous psychiatrists. All patients were diagnosed as having SAD by consensus of the authors using *DSM-IV* criteria. In addition, all patients were given a German version of the Seasonal Pattern Assessment Questionnaire.[50] Complete medical, ophthalmic, and neurologic examinations, including laboratory tests before the beginning of the trial, guaranteed that each patient was free of medical and neurologic illness. Patients with a history of substance abuse in the last 12 months before the study were ineligible for participation.

Because 5 patients (3 women and 2 men) did not complete the study protocol, their data were not analyzed. Two of them responded to dim yellow LT, 2 did not fulfill the response criteria for LT, and 1 patient refused to continue after the first part of the depletion procedure. The remaining 12 patients (**Table**) had been drug-free for at least 10 months when they entered the study.

The treatment protocol was approved by the Ethics Committee of Vienna University. Before entering the trial, all patients gave written informed consent. They were informed that a transient exacerbation of their depressive symptoms might occur during the procedure.

BEHAVIORAL RATINGS

Behavioral ratings consisted of a modified version of the 21-item Hamilton Depression Rating Scale (HDRS)[51] and 7 supplementary items (SAD Addendum [AAD]) that have been shown to have special relevance to SAD.[52] Items about sleep, weight loss, and diurnal variation of the HDRS and the AAD were omitted because these symptoms cannot be assessed during test day 2 of the TRP depletion procedure. The self-report inventory consisted of a German version of the Profile of Mood States[53] and Visual Analogue Scales (VAS) (0 mm, most ever; 100 mm, none), in which the items mood, anxiety, energy, tiredness, appetite, and general well-being were recorded. Objective ratings were obtained by the same investigator throughout the testing (N.P-R.) who was unaware of the sequence of LT and the challenge type.

LIGHT TREATMENT

All subjects received LT for the first time in their lives. The light originated from 8 neon tubes (Trulite, Durotest Corp, North Bergen, NJ) in a metal box (Theralux, type ATL-6, SML, Aachen, Germany) behind a plastic diffusing screen. The bright light condition consisted of bright, white, fluorescent light (BL), with UV screened out of the spectrum. Three thousand lux were measured at eye level, 60 cm away from the box. Dim yellow light, 100 lux at 60 cm, was used for the placebo condition. Because all patients were working, LT was administered in their homes for 2 hours between 5 and 8 PM every day.

A 1-week placebo lead-in period was administered to eliminate early placebo responders. Placebo response was defined as a 50% or greater improvement on the HDRS compared with baseline scores. While placebo responders were excluded from the study protocol, placebo nonresponders received BL therapy as described above. Treatment response was assessed weekly.

Remission was defined as proposed by Terman et al[54]: (1) pretreatment to posttreatment HDRS reduction of at least

elevating plasma TRP and lowering the plasma levels of the neutral amino acids (AAs) that compete with TRP for brain uptake.[27] Administration of the 5-HT agonist meta-chlorophenylpiperazine induces activation-euphoria in depressed patients with SAD, which was not observed after successful LT.[28] In addition, in 1 of these studies, the patients showed exaggerated prolactin and cortisol secretion after meta-chlorophenylpiperazine intake, which was normalized after LT.[29] Moreover, evidence exists that serotonergic compounds have antidepressant effects in the treatment of patients with SAD.[30-34] These studies provide evidence of a deficiency of central serotonergic transmission in SAD that may be influenced by LT.

The acute TRP depletion technique is a widely used paradigm in the investigation of the role 5-HT plays in the pathogenesis of psychiatric syndromes and their treatment. It has been reported that TRP depletion induces a rapid and substantial lowering of plasma TRP levels[35-47] and markedly reduces brain 5-HT synthesis in humans.[48] It emerged that this reduction is more pronounced in women.[48] Moreover, short-term TRP depletion causes a lowering of mood in drug-free subjects who are in remission from depression[49] and healthy subjects at genetic risk for major depressive disorder.[41] In most patients with depression who are in a selective 5-HT reuptake inhibitor–induced remission from depression, TRP depletion induces a rapid and transient depressive relapse,[36] but little change is observed in untreated patients and patients with depression.[39]

The purpose of our study was to investigate the mechanism of action of LT in patients with SAD. We hypothesized that the pathogenesis of SAD and the underlying mechanism of action of LT might depend on serotonergic mechanisms. Therefore, we studied the effect of short-term TRP depletion on drug-free patients with SAD who were in a stable, LT-induced remission from the depressive syndrome. We predicted that TRP depletion results in a transient exacerbation of depressive symptoms.

RESULTS

CHANGES IN TOTAL AND FREE PLASMA TRP LEVELS

A repeated measures ANOVA of changes in free plasma TRP levels disclosed significant effects of test dose

50% and (2) HDRS and AAD total scores of at most 12. Patients who had not met these criteria after 8 weeks of BL treatment were excluded from the study.

TRP DEPLETION PROCEDURE

Tryptophan depletion was performed after patients who were in remission had remained clinically stable for at least 14 days (mean [±SD], 25.1±7.8 days; range, 16-38 days). The effects of short-term depletion of TRP were investigated in a double-blind, placebo-controlled, balanced crossover design study. Tryptophan depletion was achieved by a 24-hour, 160-mg/d, low-TRP diet with placebo capsules taken 3 times daily (day 1), followed the next morning by ingestion of a TRP-free 15-AA drink (day 2). Control testing consisted of a 160-mg/d TRP diet supplemented with capsules containing 500 mg of L-TRP 3 times daily, followed the next morning by a 16-AA drink including 2.3 g of L-TRP. The description of the diet and the AA drinks has been documented elsewhere.[36] At day 1, patients took the diet home with them and were asked to consume it at their regular meal times. Furthermore, they were instructed to eat all of the food and to drink water or juice. Patients returned to their usual diet on day 2 at about 4 or 5 PM. No additional TRP was given to them on the evening of each test day. The TRP depletion and control tests were separated by 7 to 10 days (mean [±SD], 7.3±0.8 days; range, 7-9 days). Light therapy was continued throughout the testing, except on the evening of test day 2.

Behavioral ratings during the challenge test were performed at 8:30 AM on test day 1, 30 minutes before and 5 and 7 hours after ingestion of the AA drink (test day 2). At these time points, blood samples for free and total TRP level measurement were obtained. Ratings were obtained again between 10 and 12 AM on the day after each AA drink.

TRP MEASURES

Blood (10 mL) was sampled by means of a Venoject vacutainer tube, containing 0.1 mL edetic acid (0.38 mol/L). The blood was immediately centrifuged for 10 minutes at room temperature and 5000g. To determine total TRP, 0.5 mL of 5% sulfosalicylic acid were mixed, incubated for 10 minutes at room temperature, and centrifuged for 10 minutes at 13000g. The supernatant was frozen at −80°C until analyzed. Free TRP was determined by centrifuging 1 mL of plasma with a filter (Centrifree, Amicon, Witten, Germany) for 30 minutes at 2000g. The filtrate was frozen at −80°C until analyzed. The TRP stock solution (1 mmol/L) was prepared in water and frozen at −80°C. Total and free TRP were analyzed by high-performance liquid chromatography with electrochemical detection.

The intra-assay precision was 2.2%, the precision from day to day, 5.5%; accuracy, +1.3%; and lower limit of detection, 0.25 μmol/L.

STATISTICAL ANALYSIS

Changes in plasma free and total TRP levels and behavioral ratings were analyzed by a repeated measures analysis of variance (ANOVA) including 2 intrasubject factors: treatment (TRP depletion vs control testing) and time (free and total plasma TRP levels and behavioral ratings during the time points sampled). This allowed an investigation of the main effects of treatment and time and the interaction of treatment × time, which indicated the effect of TRP depletion in the sample as a whole. Statistically significant interactions were further examined with post hoc *t* tests to determine when the changes occurred. When statistically significant effects of ANOVAs for the total HDRS and AAD scores were obtained, ANOVAs of the individual items of the scales were used to identify which items were changing.

Depressive relapse was defined as an increase of at least 50% in HDRS score, compared with baseline, and as a score of 12 or more.

Pearson's correlations were calculated to evaluate the relation between plasma TRP levels and behavioral changes. Results were considered significant when $P<.05$. Because all tests are hypothesis-driven, we did not impose corrections on the significance level. All tests were 2-tailed. For data analysis, the SPSS/PC, V.6.01[55] was used.

(F=38.31, df=1,11; $P<.001$) and time (F=3.27, df=3,33; $P<.04$), and a significant test dose × time interaction (F=19.85, df=3,33; $P<.001$). An ANOVA of changes in total plasma TRP levels disclosed a significant main effect of test dose (F=31.13, df=1,11; $P<.001$), but not of time (F=1.79, df=3,33; $P<.17$), and a significant interaction of test dose × time (F=16.07, df=3,33; $P<.001$). As shown in **Figure 1**, peak effects occurred 5 hours after ingestion of the AA drink. Total and free plasma TRP levels decreased during TRP depletion and increased during control testing in all patients.

BEHAVIORAL EFFECTS

Mood

The most pronounced effects of TRP depletion on mood were observed on the day after ingestion of the TRP-free AA drink (**Figure 2**, top). At this time, the HDRS score was not significantly different compared with the HDRS score before the beginning of LT (t=1.1, df=11; P=.28). An ANOVA disclosed a statistically significant main effect of challenge type (F=8.54, df=1,11; $P<.02$), no significant main effect of time (F=1.98, df=3,33; $P\leq.14$), and a significant treatment × time interaction (F=5.71, df=3,33; $P<.01$). Subsequent paired t tests disclosed significantly increased HDRS scores 7 hours (t=−2.48, df=11; $P<.04$) and 24 hours (t=−2.31, df=11; $P<.05$) after ingestion of the TRP-free AA drink. No statistically significant difference was found between day 1 and day 2, 8:30 AM (t=−1.473, df=11; P=.11). Control testing produced no significant behavioral change from baseline for any subsequent time point. To identify the symptoms responsible for the change in the HDRS total score during and after TRP depletion and control testing, an ANOVA was applied on each individual item. Significant test dose × time interactions were found for "feelings of guilt" (F=2.92, df=3,33; $P<.04$), "loss of interest" (F=3.36, df=3,33; $P<.02$), "retardation of speech" (F=4.46, df=3,33; $P<.01$), "agitation" (F=3.37, df=3,33; $P<.02$), and "loss of energy" (F=2.66, df=3,33; $P<.05$). According to criteria for depressive symptom exacerbation, 6 patients experienced relapse during TRP depletion; no patient fulfilled these criteria during control testing. The behavioral effects of TRP depletion did not persist for more than 3 days after ingestion of the AA drink.

Patient Characteristics*

Patient No./ Sex/Age, y	Age at Onset, y	Diagnosis (*DSM-IV*)	*DSM-IV* Specifier	Additional Diagnosis	Score: HDRS+AAD Before Light Therapy	Score: HDRS+AAD After TRP Depletion	Score: Seasonality
1/F/49	46	MDD	Atypical	PMDD	20	16	23
2/F/35	25	BP II	Atypical	PMDD	21	18	21
3/F/49	40	MDD	Atypical	PMDD	26	26	13
4/M/38	20	MDD	Melancholic	None	27	12	12
5/F/45	30	BP II	Atypical	None	29	51	21
6/F/34	31	BP II	Atypical	None	33	30	17
7/F/41	35	MDD	Atypical	PMDD	19	4	11
8/F/43	25	BP II	Atypical	None	24	21	20
9/M/47	23	BP II	Atypical	None	26	12	18
10/F/70	37	MDD	Atypical	None	17	14	19
11/F/43	30	BP II	Atypical	None	24	13	19
12/F/27	25	MDD	Atypical	PMDD	25	25	13
Mean 43.4	30.6	...	...	...	24.3	20.2	17.3
SD 10.7	7.7	...	...	...	4.5	12.1	4.0

*DSM-IV *indicates* Diagnostic and Statistical Manual of Mental Disorders, Fourth Edition*; HDRS, modified version of the Hamilton Depression Rating Scale; AAD, seasonal affective disorder addendum for the HDRS; TRP, tryptophan; MDD, major depressive disorder; atypical, current episode meets criteria for atypical features specifier (*DSM-IV*); PMDD, premenstrual dysphoric disorder; BP II, bipolar II disorder; and melancholic, current episode meets criteria for melancholic features specifier (*DSM-IV*).*

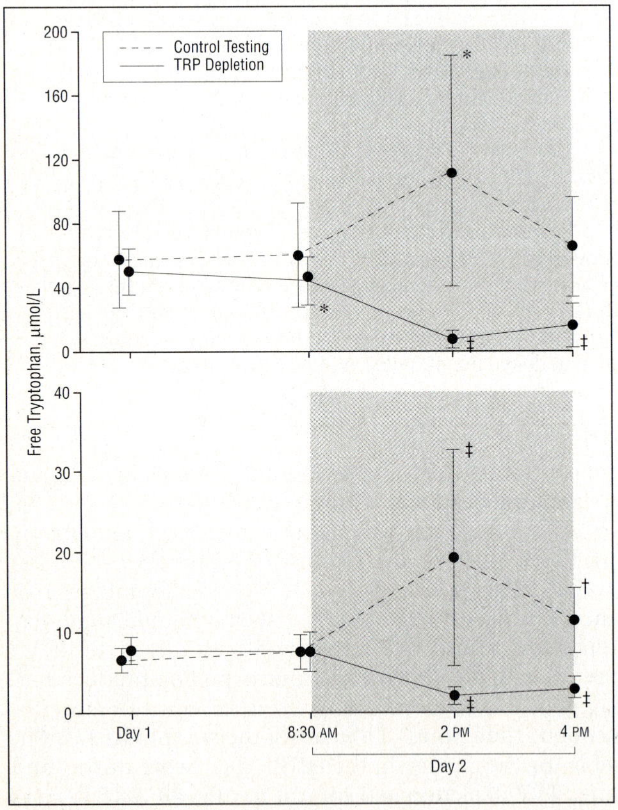

Figure 1. *Mean (±SD) total (top) and free (bottom) plasma tryptophan (TRP) levels during TRP depletion and control testing. Asterisk indicates* P<.05*; dagger,* P<.01*; and double dagger,* P<.001*; all compared with day 1, at 8:30 AM (2-tailed paired* t *test).*

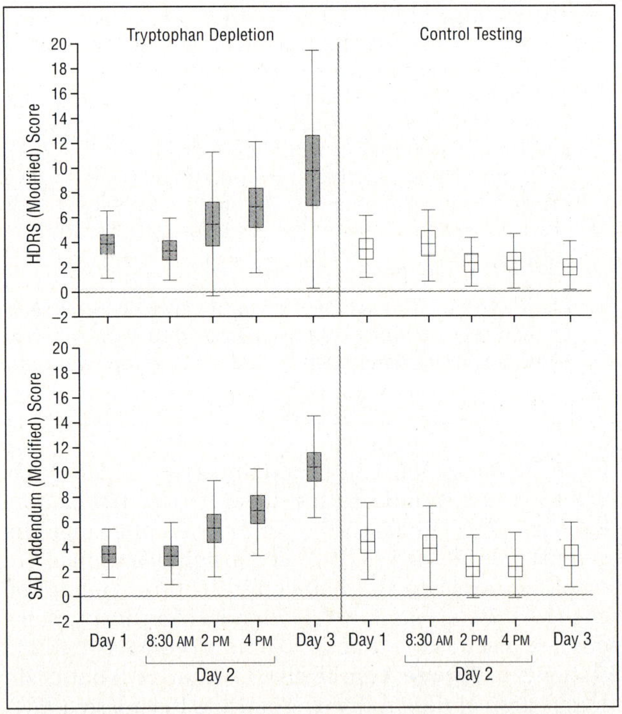

Figure 2. *Effects of tryptophan depletion and control testing in patients in remission (n=12) with seasonal affective disorder (SAD). Top, Scores on the modified version of the Hamilton Depression Rating Scale (HDRS). Bottom, Scores on the SAD Addendum (modified version). In both scales, the most pronounced effects of tryptophan depletion were observed on the day after ingestion of the tryptophan-free amino acid drink; no significant behavioral changes occurred during control testing.*

Atypical Symptoms

An ANOVA disclosed significant main effects of challenge type (F=10.04, *df*=1,11; *P*<.01), time (F=11.89, *df*=3,33; *P*<.001) and a significant interaction of challenge type × time (F=20.2, *df*=3,33; *P*<.001). The highest AAD scores were found on the day after ingestion of the TRP-free AA mixture (Figure 2, bottom). At this time point, we did not find a statistically significant difference compared with the pre-light treatment score (*t*=1.3, *df*=11; *P*=.22). Paired *t* tests identified significantly increased AAD scores 5 hours (*t*=−2.21, *df*=11; *P*<.05), 7 hours (*t*=−4.07, *df*=11; *P*<.01), and 24 hours (*t*=−5.18, *df*=11; *P*<.001) after ingestion of the TRP-deficient AA mixture in comparison with the baseline day. Statistically significant challenge type × time interactions of individual items of the AAD were noted for "fatigue" (F=4.46, *df*=3,33; $P<.005$), "social withdrawal" (F=4.12, *df*=4,44; $P<.01$), "increased appetite" (F=5.03, *df*=3,33; $P<.01$), and "carbohydrate craving" (F=3.26, *df*=3,33; $P<.02$).

Subjective Ratings

Patient self-ratings on the Profile of Mood States disclosed statistically significant challenge type × time interactions on the subscales "fatigue" (F=7.56, *df*=3,33; $P<.001$) and "mood" (F=4.3, *df*=3,33; $P<.02$). No statistically significant interactions were found for the subscales "activity" ($P=.18$) and "moroseness" ($P=.73$).

The statistically significant challenge type × time interactions on the patient-rated analogue scales of "energy" (F=3.29, *df*=3,33; $P<.04$), "general well-being" (F=3.56, *df*=3,33; $P<.03$), and "anxiety" (F=5.89, *df*=3,33; $P<.003$) indicated a marked worsening of the patients' condition after TRP depletion.

FACTORS ASSOCIATED WITH THE REOCCURRENCE OF DEPRESSION

Six of the 12 patients were randomly assigned to receive first the TRP depletion test and then the control test; the other 6 received the control test first. Ordering effects were not found. The changes in HDRS and AAD scores were unrelated to age, gender, diagnosis, day of the menstrual cycle, additional diagnosis of premenstrual dysphoric disorder, or length of remission before depletion or the seasonality score. No significant correlation was seen between the change in plasma total and free TRP levels and the change in behavioral measures on the day of or after depletion (total TRP, $r=-0.13$; free TRP, $r=-0.46$).

COMMENT

In the present study, TRP depletion, induced by a combination of a low-TRP diet and a TRP-deficient AA drink, evoked typical symptoms of depression such as impaired cognitive function, psychomotor retardation, feelings of guilt, and rumination in depressed patients in remission from SAD after LT. The effects of TRP depletion on atypical symptoms, which represent the core syndrome of SAD, were even more impressive. These symptoms returned before an increase in HDRS scores was observed. Relapse was most pronounced on the day after TRP depletion, and the extent of lowered mood was of the same magnitude as that seen in clinical depression. We did not provide our patients with a TRP replacement drink after the procedure, which probably might be helpful to observe late responses, as we did. Tryptophan depletion and control testing produced changes in plasma free and total TRP levels similar to previous studies.[35-47] Our findings pose the question whether 5-HT is a critical neurochemical transducer in LT of SAD and whether the short-term availability of 5-HT may be interpreted as a necessary condition for maintaining the antidepressant effect of LT.

Our findings somewhat differ from those of Lam et al,[56] who also investigated the effects of TRP depletion in patients with remission of SAD. Similar to our results, the beneficial effects of LT were reversed by TRP depletion, but the depressive relapse was most pronounced 5 hours after ingestion of the TRP-deficient AA mixture, and all patients recovered from the effects of TRP depletion to baseline levels by the next day. In our study, we observed a slow increase in symptoms compared with rapid changes in TRP levels. This might be due to the slow translation of lowered precursor levels into lower 5-HT in patients with SAD. An alternative explanation for the behavioral changes induced by TRP depletion might be that the reoccurrence of depression may not be caused by an abnormality of 5-HT function, but by a dysfunction of other neurotransmitter systems or brain regions modulated by 5-HT.

In the interpretation of our findings it has to be considered that the number of patients was small. We did, however, study a homogeneous group of patients by excluding placebo responders with the use of dim yellow LT at the beginning of LT. It seems unlikely that the break of LT on day 2 of the depletion procedure influenced the results. Nonspecific effects of the depletion procedure are unlikely, because patients and rater could not discriminate the TRP-free AA drink from the supplemented drink. Moreover, we do not think that the information on the possible worsening of the condition after ingestion of the AA drink had influenced the results of the investigation, because the control testing also would have induced an exacerbation of depressive symptoms in some patients, but this was not the case.

Further studies should rule out a possible influence of the brain catecholamine system on the behavioral changes we observed by comparing the effects of TRP depletion with tyrosine depletion.[57] If tyrosine depletion disclosed no effects on mood, the hypothesis that the 5-HT system plays a major role in the mechanism of action of LT would be supported.

CONCLUSION

The findings of the present study provide some evidence that serotonergic mechanisms might be involved in the effects of LT but suggest that LT does not act through primary action on 5-HT function. It would be interesting to perform this study in patients with SAD during remission in the summer. This would help to clarify whether LT corrects the underlying deficit of SAD or just compensates for it.

Accepted for publication June 18, 1996.

This study was supported in part by grant 5321 from the Jubiläumsfonds of the Austrian Federal Reserve Bank.

The analytical expertise of C. Frahnert in the field of tryptophan measurements is greatly appreciated.

Reprints: Alexander Neumeister, MD, National Institute of Mental Health, Clinical Psychobiology Branch, 9000 Rockville Pike, Building 10, Room 4S-239, Bethesda, MD 20892 (e-mail: alexn@box-a.nih.gov).

REFERENCES

1. Rosenthal NE, Sack DA, Gillin JC, Lewy AJ, Goodwin FK, Davenport Y, Mueller PS, Newsome DA, Wehr TA. Seasonal affective disorder: a description of the syndrome and preliminary findings with light therapy. *Arch Gen Psychiatry.* 1984;41:72-80.

2. Wehr TA, Sack DA, Rosenthal NE. Seasonal affective disorder with summer depression and winter hypomania. *Am J Psychiatry.* 1987;144:1602-1603.
3. Boyce P, Parker G. Seasonal affective disorder in the southern hemisphere. *Am J Psychiatry.* 1988;145:97-99.
4. American Psychiatric Association. *Diagnostic and Statistical Manual of Mental Disorders, Fourth Edition.* Washington, DC: American Psychiatric Association; 1994.
5. Rosenthal NE, Genhart M, Jacobsen FM, Skwerer RG, Wehr TA. Disturbances of appetite and weight regulation in seasonal affective disorder. *Ann N Y Acad Sci.* 1987;499:216-230.
6. Allen JM, Lam RW, Remick RA, Sadovnick AD. Depressive symptoms and family history in seasonal and nonseasonal mood disorders. *Am J Psychiatry.* 1993; 150:443-448.
7. Garvey MJ, Wesner R, Godes M. Comparison of seasonal and nonseasonal affective disorders. *Am J Psychiatry.* 1988;145:100-102.
8. Hellekson C. Phenomenology of seasonal affective disorder: an Alaskan perspective. In: Rosenthal NE, Blehar MC, eds. *Seasonal Affective Disorder & Phototherapy.* New York, NY: Guilford Press; 1989:33-45.
9. Wehr TA, Giesen HA, Schulz PM, Anderson JL, Joseph-Vanderpool JR, Kelly K, Kasper S, Rosenthal NE. Contrasts between symptoms of summer depression and winter depression. *J Affect Disord.* 1991;23:173-183.
10. Johansson G, Frakenhauser M, Lambert WW. Note on seasonal variation in catecholamine output. *Percept Mot Skills.* 1969;28:677-678.
11. Weitzman ED, de Graff AS, Sassin JF, Hansen T, Godlibsen OB, Perlow M, Hellman L. Seasonal patterns of sleep stages and secretion of cortisol and growth hormone during 24-hour periods in northern Norway. *Acta Endocrinol.* 1975;78:65-76.
12. Swade C, Coppen A. Seasonal variation in biochemical factors related to depressive illness. *J Affect Disord.* 1980;2:249-255.
13. Terman M, Terman JS, Quitkin FM, McGrath PJ, Stewart JW, Rafferty B. Light therapy for seasonal affective disorder: a review of efficacy. *Neuropsychopharmacology.* 1989;2:1-22.
14. Kasper S, Rogers SLB, Yancey A, Schulz PM, Skwerer RG, Rosenthal NE. Phototherapy in individuals with and without subsyndromal seasonal affective disorder. *Arch Gen Psychiatry.* 1989;46:837-844.
15. Society of Light Treatment and Biological Rhythms. Consensus statement on the efficacy of light treatment for SAD. *LTBR Bull.* 1990;3:5-9.
16. Wehr TA, Skwerer RG, Jacobsen FM, Sack DA, Rosenthal NE. Eye versus skin phototherapy of seasonal affective disorder. *Am J Psychiatry.* 1987;144:753-757.
17. Rosenthal NE, Sack DA, Carpenter CJ, Parry BL, Mendelson WB, Wehr TA. Antidepressant effects of light in seasonal affective disorder. *Am J Psychiatry.* 1985;142:163-170.
18. Lewy AJ, Kern HA, Rosenthal NE, Wehr TA. Bright artificial light treatment of a manic-depressant patient with a seasonal mood cycle. *Am J Psychiatry.* 1982; 139:1496-1498.
19. Wehr TA, Jacobsen FM, Sack DA, Arendt J, Tamarkin L, Rosenthal NE. Phototherapy of seasonal affective disorder: time of day and suppression of melatonin are not critical for antidepressant effects. *Arch Gen Psychiatry.* 1986;43:870-875.
20. Wirz-Justice A, Graw P, Kräuchi K, Gisin B, Jochum A, Arendt J, Fisch HU, Buddeberg C, Pöldinger W. Light therapy in seasonal affective disorder is independent of time of day or circadian phase. *Arch Gen Psychiatry.* 1993;50:929-937.
21. Meesters Y, Jansen JHC, Beersma DGM, Bouhuys AL, van den Hoofdakker RH. Light therapy for seasonal affective disorder: the effects of timing. *Br J Psychiatry.* 1995;166:607-612.
22. Lewy AJ, Sack RL, Miller S, Hoban TM. Antidepressant and circadian phase-shifting effects of light. *Science.* 1987;235:352-354.
23. Terman M, Quitkin FM, Terman JS, Stewart JW, McGrath PJ. The timing of phototherapy. *Psychopharmacol Bull.* 1987;23:354-357.
24. Kasper S, Neumeister A, Rieder N, Hesselmann B, Ruhrmann S. Serotonergic mechanisms in the pathophysiology and treatment of seasonal affective disorder. In: Holick MF, ed. *Biologic Effects of Light 1995.* Berlin, Germany: Walter de Gruyter & Co; 1996:325-331.
25. Carlsson A, Svennerholm L, Winblad B. Seasonal and circadian monoamine variations in human brains examined post-mortem. *Acta Psychiatr Scand.* 1980; 61(suppl 280):75-83.
26. Rosenthal NE, Genhart MJ, Caballero B, Jacobsen FM, Skwerer RG, Coursey RD, Rogers S, Spring BJ. Psychobiological effects of carbohydrate- and protein-rich meals in patients with seasonal affective disorder and normal controls. *Biol Psychiatry.* 1989;25:1029-1040.
27. Fernstrom JD. Carbohydrate ingestion and brain serotonin synthesis. *Appetite.* 1988;11(suppl 1):35-41.
28. Jacobsen FM, Mueller EA, Rosenthal NE, Rogers S, Hill JL, Murphy DL. Behavioral responses to intravenous meta-chlorophenylpiperazine in patients with seasonal affective disorder and control subjects before and after phototherapy. *Psychiatry Res.* 1994;52:181-197.
29. Garcia-Borreguero D, Jacobsen FM, Murphy DL, Joseph-Vanderpool JR, Chiara A, Rosenthal NE. Hormonal responses to the administration of *m*-chlorophenylpiperazine in patients with seasonal affective disorder and controls. *Biol Psychiatry.* 1995;37:740-749.
30. Ruhrmann S, Kasper S, Hawellek B, Martinez B, Höflich G, Nickelsen T, Möller HJ. Fluoxetine as a treatment alternative to light therapy in seasonal affective disorder (SAD). *Pharmacopsychiatry.* 1993;26:193.
31. Lam RW, Gorman CP, Michalon M, Steiner M, Levitt AJ, Corral MR, Watson GD, Morehouse RL, Tam W, Joffe RT. A multi-centre, placebo-controlled study of fluoxetine in seasonal affective disorder. *Am J Psychiatry.* 1995;152:1765-1770.
32. O'Rourke D, Wurtman JJ, Wurtman RJ, Chebli R, Gleason R. Treatment of seasonal affective disorder with *d*-fenfluramine. *J Clin Psychiatry.* 1989;50: 343-347.
33. Wirz-Justice A, van der Velde P, Nil R. Comparison of light treatment with citalopram in winter depression: a longitudinal single case study. *Int Clin Psychopharmacol.* 1992;7:109-116.
34. Jacobsen FM, Murphy DL, Rosenthal NE. The role of serotonin in seasonal affective disorder and the antidepressant response to phototherapy. In: Rosenthal NE, Blehar MC, eds. *Seasonal Affective Disorder & Phototherapy.* New York, NY: Guilford Press; 1989:333-341.
35. Young SN, Smith SE, Pihl RO, Ervin FR. Tryptophan depletion causes a rapid lowering of mood in normal males. *Psychopharmacology.* 1985;87:173-177.
36. Delgado PL, Charney DS, Price LH, Aghajanian GK, Landis H, Heninger GR. Serotonin function and the mechanism of antidepressant action: reversal of antidepressant-induced remission by rapid depletion of plasma tryptophan. *Arch Gen Psychiatry.* 1990;47:411-418.
37. Gessa GL, Biggio G, Fadda F, Corsini GV, Tagliamonte A. Effect of oral administration of tryptophan-free amino acid mixtures on serum tryptophan, brain tryptophan and serotonin metabolism. *J Neurochem.* 1974;22:869-870.
38. Delgado PL, Charney DS, Price LH, Landis H, Heninger GR. Neuroendocrine and behavioral effects of dietary tryptophan restriction in healthy subjects. *Life Sci.* 1989;45:2323-2332.
39. Delgado PL, Price LH, Miller HL, Salomon RM, Aghajanian GK, Heninger GR, Charney DS. Serotonin and the neurobiology of depression: effects of tryptophan depletion in drug-free depressed patients. *Arch Gen Psychiatry.* 1994; 51:865-874.
40. Barr LC, Goodman WK, McDougle J, Delgado PL, Heninger GR, Charney DS, Price LH. Tryptophan depletion in patients with obsessive-compulsive disorder who respond to serotonin reuptake inhibitors. *Arch Gen Psychiatry.* 1994; 51:309-317.
41. Benkelfat C, Ellenbogen MA, Dean P, Palmour RM, Young SN. Mood-lowering effect of tryptophan depletion: enhanced susceptibility in young men at genetic risk for major affective disorders. *Arch Gen Psychiatry.* 1994;51:687-697.
42. Salomon RM, Mazure CM, Delgado PL, Mendia P, Charney DS. Serotonin function in aggression. *Biol Psychiatry.* 1994;35:570-572.
43. Goddard AW, Sholomskas DE, Walton KE, Augeri FM, Charney DS, Heninger GR, Goodman WK, Price LH. Effects of tryptophan depletion in panic disorder. *Biol Psychiatry.* 1994;36:775-777.
44. Benkelfat C, Seletti B, Palmour RM, Hillel J, Ellenbogen M, Young SN. Tryptophan depletion in stable lithium-treated patients with bipolar disorder in remission. *Arch Gen Psychiatry.* 1995;52:154-155.
45. Weltzin TE, Fernstrom JD, McConaha C, Kaye WH. Acute tryptophan depletion in bulimia: effects on large neutral amino acids. *Biol Psychiatry.* 1994;35:388-397.
46. Weltzin TE, Fernstrom MH, Fernstrom JD, Neuberger SK, Kaye WH. Acute tryptophan depletion and increased food intake and irritability in bulimia nervosa. *Am J Psychiatry.* 1995;152:1668-1671.
47. Oldman A, Walsh A, Salkovskis P, Fairburn CG, Cowen PJ. Biochemical and behavioral effects of acute tryptophan depletion in abstinent bulimic subjects: a pilot study. *Psychol Med.* 1995;25:995-1001.
48. Benkelfat C, Nishizawa S, Young SN, Leyton M, Blier P, deMontigny C, Mzengezza S, Diksic M. Tryptophan depletion markedly reduces the rate of serotonin synthesis in healthy volunteers. Presented at the American College of Neuropsychopharmacology (ACNP) Meeting; December 11-16, 1995; San Juan, Puerto Rico.
49. Moreno F, Gelenberg AJ, Potter R, Delgado PL. Tryptophan depletion and vulnerability to depression. Presented at the American College of Neuropsychopharmacology (ACNP) Meeting 1995; December 11-16, 1995; San Juan, Puerto Rico.
50. Kasper S. Jahreszeit und Befindlichkeit in der Allgemeinbevölkerung. Eine Mehrebenenuntersuchung zur Epidemiologie, Biologie und therapeutischen Beeinflussbarkeit (Lichttherapie) saisonaler Befindlichkeitsschwankungen. In: Hippius H, Janzarik W, Müller C, eds. *Monographien aus dem Gesamtgebiete der Psychiatrie.* New York, NY: Springer-Verlag NY Inc; 1991;66:135-136.
51. Hamilton M. Development for a rating scale for primary depressive illness. *Br J Soc Psychol.* 1967;6:278-296.
52. Rosenthal NE, Genhart M, Sack DA, Skwerer RG, Wehr TA. Seasonal affective disorder. In: Hudson JI, Pope HG, eds. *Psychobiology of Bulimia.* Washington, DC: American Psychiatric Association Press; 1987:226-228.
53. McNair DM, Lorr M, Droppelmann LF. *Profile of Mood States.* San Diego, Calif: Educational and Industrial Testing Service; 1981.
54. Terman M, Terman JS, Rafferty BR. Experimental design and measures of success in the treatment of winter depression by bright light. *Psychopharmacol Bull.* 1990;4:505-510.
55. SPSS Inc. *SPSS for Windows, v.6.01.* Chicago Ill: SPSS Inc; 1994.
56. Lam RW, Zis AP, Grewal A, Delgado PL, Charney DS, Krystal JH. Effects of acute tryptophan depletion in patients with seasonal affective disorder in remission with light therapy. *Arch Gen Psychiatry.* 1996;53:41-44.
57. Miller HL, Delgado PL, Salomon RM, Berman R, Krystal JH, Heninger GR, Charney DS. Clinical and biochemical effects of catecholamine depletion on antidepressant-induced remission of depression. *Arch Gen Psychiatry.* 1996;53:117-128.

ORIGINAL ARTICLE

Complex Interaction of the Sleep-Wake Cycle and Circadian Phase Modulates Mood in Healthy Subjects

Diane B. Boivin, MD, PhD; Charles A. Czeisler, PhD, MD; Derk-Jan Dijk, PhD; Jeanne F. Duffy, MBA; Simon Folkard, PhD, DSc; David S. Minors, PhD; Peter Totterdell, MSc; James M. Waterhouse, DPhil

Background: Several studies of healthy volunteers have revealed that subjective mood may vary with the duration of prior wakefulness and with the time of day. However, in these studies, the effects of extended wakefulness and circadian phase remained confounded, and the interaction of these 2 processes could not be assessed quantitatively.

Methods: In the present study, a total of 24 healthy young subjects (16 men, 8 women) lived on a 30-hour sleep-wake schedule for 19 to 23 days or on a 28-hour sleep-wake schedule for 33 to 36 days; both schedules induced desynchrony between the subjects' sleep-wake cycle and their endogenous circadian pacemaker. Subjective mood was assessed by 2 types of visual analog scales, which were administered twice every 2 hours and every 20 minutes, respectively, during all scheduled wakefulness episodes. A circadian phase and an interval elapsed since awakening were attributed to each data point, and circadian and wake-dependent fluctuations of mood were assessed.

Results: A significant variation of mood with circadian phase was observed, but no reliable main effect of the duration of prior wakefulness was found. A statistically significant interaction of circadian and wake-dependent fluctuations was evident; when the analysis was restricted to specific circadian phases, mood improved, deteriorated, or remained stable with the duration of prior wakefulness.

Conclusions: These results indicate that, in healthy young subjects, subjective mood is influenced by a complex and nonadditive interaction of circadian phase and duration of prior wakefulness. The nature of this interaction is such that moderate changes in the timing of the sleep-wake cycle may have profound effects on subsequent mood.

Arch Gen Psychiatry. 1997;54:145-152

IT IS well established that the overt rhythms of a variety of physiological and behavioral variables, including core body temperature,[1,2] neuroendocrine secretion,[3] sleep organization and propensity,[4] subjective alertness, cognitive performance, and short-term memory,[5-9] comprise an endogenous circadian component and an evoked (eg, sleep-wake–dependent) component. Several groups have reported evidence suggesting that these processes may also modulate mood in healthy individuals. For instance, a diurnal variation in subjective measures of mood in healthy volunteers has been reported[10-14]; this variation suggests that there is an underlying circadian rhythm of mood. Moreover, a significant deterioration of mood has been noted during sleep deprivation experiments,[15-19] which suggests that time since waking is also an important component. Furthermore, there is indirect evidence to suggest the presence of a significant interaction of circadian and wake-dependent processes in the regulation of mood in healthy subjects. For instance, in the early 1970s, Taub and Berger[11,15] reported that subjective mood was influenced by altering the duration and timing of sleep episodes; they concluded that the position of sleep in the circadian cycle was important for the control of mood. Similar findings were reported by Totterdell et al,[20] who noted that the timing of sleep had a significant impact on daily mean values for mood in healthy volunteers. However, in previous studies, including constant routine protocols,[10] changes in the timing of sleep and wakefulness were confounded by simultaneous changes in the duration of wakefulness, and thus the interaction of circadian and wake-dependent fluctuations of subjective mood could not be quantified.

Given the deterioration of subjective mood rating with acute or chronic sleep deprivation in healthy subjects,[13,15-18] an experimental protocol that

From the Circadian, Neuroendocrine and Sleep Disorders Section, Division of Endocrinology, Department of Medicine, Brigham and Women's Hospital, Harvard Medical School, Boston, Mass (Drs Boivin, Czeisler, and Dijk and Ms Duffy); MRC Body Rhythms and Shiftwork Centre, University of Wales, Swansea, (Dr Folkard); School of Biological Sciences, University of Manchester, Manchester. (Drs Minors and Waterhouse); and MRC/ESRC Social and Applied Psychology Unit, University of Sheffield, Sheffield, (Mr Totterdell), England.

parcels out the relative influences of time elapsed since awakening and circadian phase must be used if this interaction is to be quantified. Previously, a nonadditive interaction of circadian and sleep-wake–dependent components in the regulation of subjective alertness, cognitive performance, and sleep propensity and organization has been demonstrated in a *forced desynchrony protocol*.[4-6,8,21] This protocol, adapted from the pioneering studies by Kleitman and Kleitman,[22] forces desynchrony between the endogenous circadian pacemaker and the sleep-wake cycle. As a result, waking episodes are initiated at virtually all phases of the endogenous circadian cycle, while variations in the duration of prior sleep episodes are minimized. This protocol allows for the analysis of endogenous circadian and wake-dependent regulation of mood and other variables, because each data point can be assigned both a circadian phase and a time since waking within the scheduled rest-activity cycle. When the forced desynchrony protocol is of sufficient duration and measurements are taken frequently, a wide range of combinations of the 2 dependent variables is realized, and an analysis of the interaction of circadian and wake-dependent regulation is possible. Using this protocol, Boivin et al[23] and Folkard[24] independently described a variation of mood with circadian phase. In the present study, the results of these 2 studies are combined and applied to an analysis of the relative contributions of circadian and wake-dependent processes to the fluctuation of subjective mood and the mutual interaction of these processes in healthy young subjects.

SUBJECTS AND METHODS

SUBJECTS AND LABORATORY PROTOCOL

Two independent sets of experiments were performed during which human subjects lived on scheduled "days" much longer than 24 hours. When the scheduled length of the day is outside the range of entrainment, these conditions induce desynchrony between the circadian timing system (which continues to oscillate according to its nearly 24-hour intrinsic period) and the imposed sleep-wake cycle. Every subject gave informed consent and none reported psychological difficulties during or after either experiment.

Throughout the experiments, core body temperature was measured by a rectal thermistor at 6-minute (experiment 1) or 1-minute (experiment 2) intervals. The phase and period of the endogenous circadian system were assessed from core body temperature series.

Experiment 1

Experiment 1 was conducted at the Temporal Isolation Unit of the School of Biological Sciences, University of Manchester, Manchester, England. The experimental protocol was approved by the local ethics committee. Fourteen healthy young volunteers (6 men and 8 women aged 18-21 years) were recruited and pronounced physically fit by a physician. All subjects had normal scores on the Eysenck Personality Inventory.[25]

Subjects lived in groups of 2 or 3 in an environment of normal indoor room light (approximately 250-300 lux) for 19 or 23 days. They controlled the lighting in the unit and had access to the time of day. On admission to the laboratory, subjects remained on a regular 24-hour schedule, with sleep episodes planned from midnight to 8 AM for 3 days (n=3) or 7 days (n=11). They were then scheduled to live on 30-hour days (20 hours of wakefulness, 10 hours of sleep/bedrest) to induce desynchrony between their endogenous circadian rhythms and their sleep-wake cycle (**Figure 1**, top).

Throughout the experiment, subjective mood was assessed twice every 2 hours, once before and once after a short (10-minute) battery of computerized psychological tests.[26] The analyses reported are based on the mean values of these 2 ratings. The results of performance tests will be reported elsewhere. A computerized unipolar visual analog scale (scale, 0-20) was used to assess the levels of subjective cheerfulness. Each rating was made in the absence of visual information on previous ratings.

Experiment 2

Experiment 2 was conducted in the Environmental Scheduling Facility of the General Clinical Research Center of Brigham and Women's Hospital, Boston, Mass. The experimental protocol was approved by the hospital's Human Research Committee. Subjective mood data from 10 healthy young men (aged 21-30 years) who participated in a forced desynchrony experiment in 1990-1991 were analyzed (see Boivin et al[27] for a description of the screening procedure). Subjects were included if their initial circadian temperature amplitude was above the fifth percentile of the population.[27]

Subjects lived individually without knowledge of the time of day for 33 to 36 days. They maintained social contacts with staff members trained to avoid communicating the time of day and the nature of the experimental conditions. On admission to the laboratory, subjects maintained their habitual 24-hour sleep-wake schedule (with 8-hour scheduled sleep episodes) for 1 day (n=1) or 3 days (n=9) under normal indoor room light (approximately 150 lux). Subjects then underwent a 40-hour constant routine followed by a 9.33-hour sleep episode. The constant routine procedure consists of a regimen of enforced semirecumbent wakefulness in constant dim light (approximately 10-15 lux) and is used to unmask the endogenous phase of the circadian pacemaker (see Czeisler et al[28] for more details). The results of the constant routine have been reported elsewhere.[5,6] After awakening from their sleep episode, the subjects were scheduled to live on a 28-hour rest-activity cycle (18.67 hours of wakefulness, 9.33 hours of sleep/bedrest). This forced desynchrony section was followed by a 50- to 65-hour constant routine. After a final recovery sleep episode, subjects were discharged from the laboratory (Figure 1, bottom).

From the start of their first constant routine to the end of the experiment, all subjects but 1 lived in an environment of dim light (approximately 10-15 lux) during periods of scheduled wakefulness; the remaining subject lived in light of approximately 40 to 60 lux. All sleep episodes took place in darkness (approximately 0.03 lux). Throughout the experiment, subjective mood was assessed every

20 minutes during periods of wakefulness using a linear, nonnumeric, 100-mm bipolar visual analog scale (sad to happy).[29] This assessment was part of a larger battery of psychological tests, the results of which have been reported elsewhere.[5,6]

STATISTICAL ANALYSIS

Experiment 1

A minimum variance procedure was used to estimate the period and phase of the endogenous circadian rhythm of core body temperature. This technique consists of 2-way analyses of variance (ANOVAs) (factors: circadian phase and duration since waking) performed over a range of successive intrinsic periods to maximize the fit to the temperature data series. The midpoint of the first 16 hours of wakefulness (ie, 8 hours after awakening) was calculated for each 30-hour day; this time was selected because subjects are usually awake for 16 hours of their 24-hour day. This midpoint was attributed a circadian phase relative to the trough of core body temperature and given a value of 0° to 360°. By definition, a complete oscillation is 360°, and phase is measured in degrees relative to the trough of the temperature cycle (0°). Results were *z*-transformed, and daily means were averaged into 4 bins (ie, 90°) according to the estimated circadian phase 8 hours after awakening. In both experiments, the bin width that provided the highest resolution while avoiding the creation of empty bins was selected for all analyses. Results were then averaged per bin across subjects and plotted (mean±SEM) as a function of circadian phase 8 hours after awakening (**Figure 2**, top). One-factor ANOVA for repeated measures was used to assess the variation of cheerfulness ratings with circadian phase.

To assess the interaction of the circadian and wake-dependent components of cheerfulness, data for the entire forced desynchrony experiment were *z*-transformed, and each individual data point was assigned values for circadian phase and time since waking. The results for each subject were averaged into 1 of 36 cells of a 2-dimensional matrix of 4 levels of circadian phase (ie, 90°) and 9 levels of time since waking (ie, each 2.22 hours of scheduled wakefulness). Two-factor ANOVA for repeated measures, with circadian phase and time since waking as the repeated factors, was used to assess the interaction of circadian phase and duration of prior wakefulness.

Experiment 2

Nonparametric spectral analysis of core body temperature data collected during the forced desynchrony section of the study was used to assess the intrinsic period of the endogenous circadian pacemaker. As for the minimum variance technique used in experiment 1, the nonparametric spectral analysis finds the best fit to the temperature data series using a range of successive intrinsic periods. The educed waveform of each subject's temperature data was then created by folding the data at this intrinsic period. For each subject, the time of the temperature minimum was determined from the midpoint between the upper and lower crossing of the mean of the educed waveform and assigned a reference value of 0°. To illustrate the endogenous circadian component of the temperature rhythm, temperature data were averaged for each subject per 15° (1 circadian hour). Next, the data were averaged over subjects and plotted as a function of circadian phase (mean±SEM) (**Figure 3**, bottom left). To illustrate the wake-dependent component of the temperature rhythm, each 28-hour day was divided into 24 bins, the first beginning at the time of waking, and for each subject the mean temperature value for each bin was found; then each bin was averaged across subjects (Figure 3, bottom right).

Average daily values for happiness were calculated as for cheerfulness in experiment 1, using the first 16 hours of every scheduled waking episode, but with 6 bins (ie, 60°) per circadian cycle (Figure 2, bottom). Smaller bin widths than in experiment 1 could be used in experiment 2 because of the shorter interval between mood assessments and the longer duration of the experiment.

To assess the circadian and wake-dependent components of mood and the interaction of these 2 processes, data for the entire forced desynchrony section were *z*-transformed, and each individual data point was assigned values for circadian phase and time since waking. The results for each subject were then averaged into 1 of 32 cells of a 2-dimensional matrix of 8 levels of circadian phase (ie, 45°) and 4 levels of time since waking (ie, each 4.7 hours of scheduled wakefulness) (Figure 3, top left and top right). Two-factor ANOVA for repeated measures, with circadian phase and time since waking as the repeated factors, was used to assess the effect of circadian phase, the effect of duration of prior wakefulness, and the interaction of these 2 components. Illustration of all levels of this interaction was possible in experiment 2 because of greater data resolution (**Figure 4**). All statistical analyses were based on the mean value per subject per bin.

RESULTS

In both experiments, the observed period of the endogenous circadian rhythm of core body temperature was slightly longer than 24 hours and much shorter than the imposed 30- or 28-hour sleep-wake cycle. As expected, this resulted in a spontaneous desynchrony between the endogenous circadian oscillations and the sleep-wake cycle (Figure 1).

Before transformation to *z* scores, absolute values for subjective cheerfulness (20-point scale) and happiness (0- to 100-mm scale) were 12.1±2.3 and 73.3±16.3 (mean±SD), respectively. The ranges of individual SDs were 1.1 to 3.8 for cheerfulness and 4.6 to 30.2 for happiness. As illustrated in Figure 2, the daily mean values for subjective cheerfulness (top panel, experiment 1) and happiness (bottom panel, experiment 2) showed rhythmic variations as a function of circadian phase 8 hours after awakening. The analysis of cheerfulness revealed a trend toward a significant fluctuation of daily mean values with circadian phase (ANOVA for repeated measures: $F_{3,39}$=2.64, P=.06), and planned comparisons showed reliable differences between 225° and 315° ($F_{1,39}$=7.48, P=.009). The fluctuation of daily mean values for subjective happiness with circadian phase was significant (ANOVA for repeated measures: $F_{5,45}$=7.78, P<.001). The pattern of this fluctuation was not exactly the same for the 2 data sets and may have been confounded by the knowledge

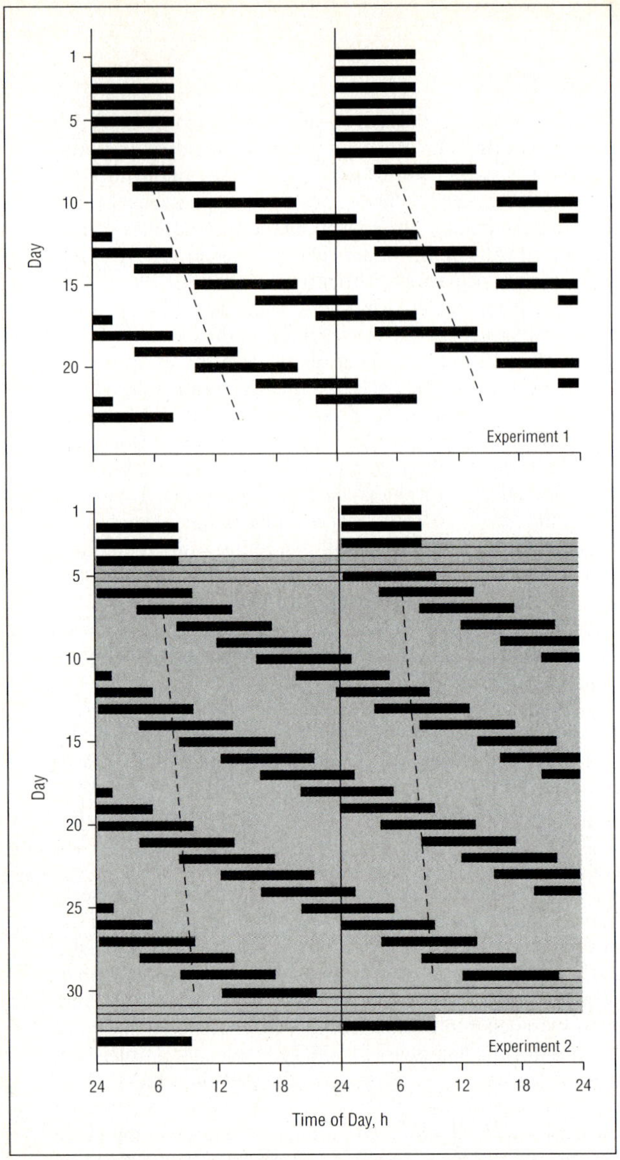

Figure 1. *Double raster plots of protocols from representative subjects from experiments 1 and 2. Black bars indicate scheduled sleep episodes; open bars, constant routines; shaded area, ambient illumination of approximately 15 lux; and dashed lines, minimum body temperature.*

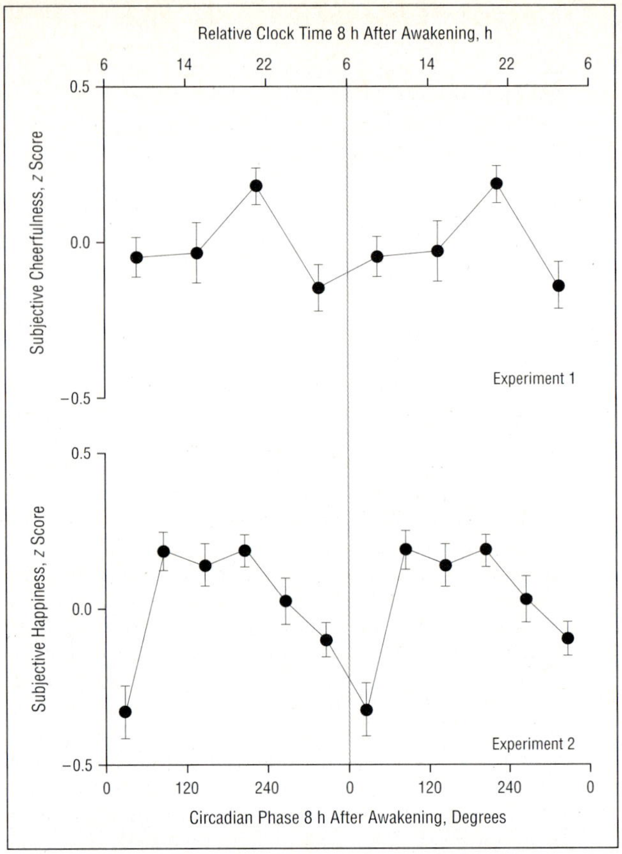

Figure 2. *Fluctuation of average daily mood against circadian phase 8 hours after awakening. Mean±SEM values were plotted at the midpoint of the bins and then double-plotted.*

of the time of day, by the shorter duration of study in experiment 1, by the difference in the mood scale used for assessment, and by the different analytic methods used to assess the intrinsic period of the temperature cycle (Figure 2). In both experiments, scores for subjective mood were lowest when the middle of the first 16 hours of wakefulness coincided with the circadian trough of the endogenous temperature rhythm (ie, 0°), which under entrained conditions corresponds to approximately 6 AM. The daily mean values for subjective measures of mood were highest when the middle of the 16-hour wakefulness episode reached a circadian phase of 120° to 240°, which under entrained conditions corresponds to approximately 2 PM to 10 PM.

The relative contributions of circadian and wake-dependent processes across the entire forced desynchrony protocol (experiment 2) are illustrated in Figure 3. The left panels show the circadian component of core body temperature and of subjective happiness averaged across all subjects. The temporal pattern of subjective happiness showed a prominent and significant circadian variation (ANOVA for repeated measures: $F_{7,63}$=8.50, $P<.001$) closely associated with another circadian rhythm, the endogenous circadian temperature cycle. Subjective mood declined with the descending limb of the circadian temperature curve and reached its lowest values at a circadian phase corresponding to the nadir of the temperature cycle. Subjective mood then improved with the ascending limb of the endogenous circadian component of the temperature cycle and reached its peak around 220° to 240°, which under entrained conditions would occur around 10 PM. As illustrated in the top right panel of Figure 3, subjective mood deteriorated with duration of prior waking, but no significant main effect was apparent on the subjective measures of mood (2-factor ANOVA for repeated measures, with circadian phase and time since waking as the factors: $F_{3,27}$=1.58, P=.22).

Figure 4 illustrates the interaction of the circadian and wake-dependent fluctuations of mood. A significant interaction of circadian phase and duration of prior wakefulness was observed in both experiments when assessed by ANOVA for repeated measures (cheerfulness: $F_{24,312}$=1.94, $P<.001$; happiness: $F_{21,189}$=2.76, $P<.001$). The fluctuation of mood associated with circadian phase was broken down into 4 durations of prior

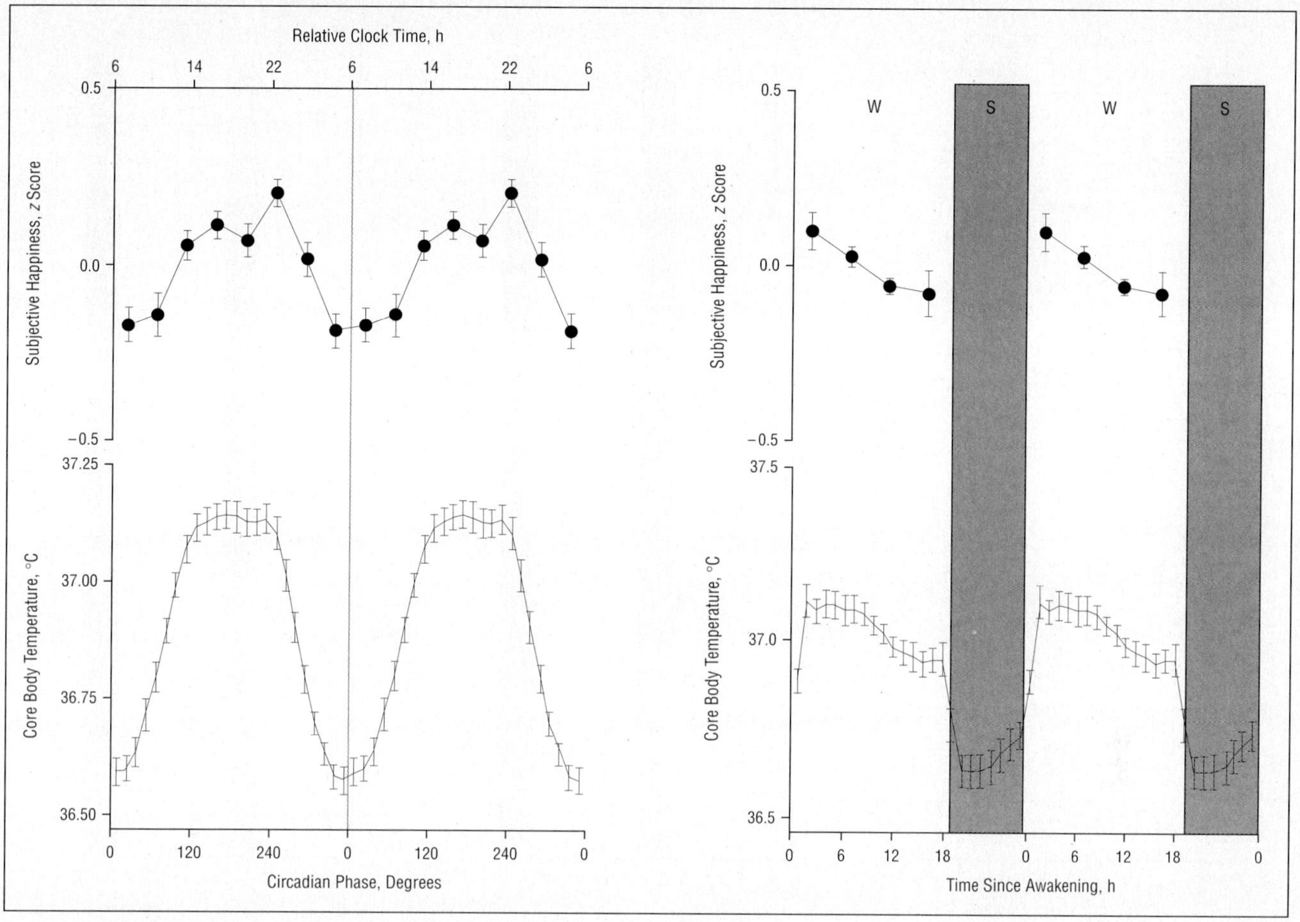

Figure 3. *Circadian and wake-dependent variations of mood and educed waveform of core body temperature (experiment 2). Mean±SEM values were plotted against circadian phase (left) or time since awakening (right). W indicates awake; S, asleep.*

wakefulness (left panels). The circadian variation of mood remained significant at each duration of prior wakefulness when evaluated by ANOVA for repeated measures, with circadian phase and prior wakefulness as the factors analyzed (0-280 minutes of prior wakefulness: $F_{7,63}$=6.20, $P<.001$; 280-560 minutes: $F_{7,63}$=4.92, $P<.001$; 560-840 minutes: $F_{7,63}$=2.67, $P=.02$; and 840-1120 minutes: $F_{7,63}$=2.93, $P=.01$). In each panel, the scores for happiness were lowest at a circadian phase corresponding to the trough of the endogenous temperature cycle, whereas the scores were highest at a circadian phase corresponding to the plateau phase of the endogenous temperature cycle. The timing of the lowest subjective happiness values moved toward later circadian phases with increasing duration of prior wakefulness (Figure 4, left). The fluctuation of mood associated with the duration of prior wakefulness was broken down into 8 circadian bins (45°). As illustrated (Figure 4, center and right), the wake-dependent fluctuation of subjective mood varied differently when analyzed at different circadian phases. Only the analyses restricted to 0° to 45, 45° to 90°, and 90° to 135° circadian revealed a significant effect of the duration of prior wakefulness on subjective mood (ANOVA for repeated measures: $F_{3,27}$=3.21, $P=.04$; $F_{3,27}$=5.49, $P=.005$; and $F_{3,27}$=10.88, $P<.001$, respectively).

COMMENT

As illustrated in Figure 1, the endogenous component of core body temperature was desynchronized from the imposed sleep-wake cycle. As demonstrated by Klerman et al,[30] the difference in period observed in these 2 individual subjects may be explained by interindividual variability in the intrinsic period, different durations of experiment, and different lighting conditions; in addition, different analytic methods were used to assess the intrinsic period of the temperature cycle. In both experiments, sleep and wakefulness were distributed over a wide range of endogenous circadian phases, a condition that allows for the quantification of endogenous circadian and wake-dependent fluctuations of subjective mood.

The present study demonstrated that endogenous circadian phase contributes to variations in subjective measures of mood, as suggested in the early 1970s by Taub and Berger.[11,15] Previous studies showed that other behavioral measures, such as subjective alertness, cognitive performance, and short-term memory, exhibit similar circadian variations.[5,6] For all these parameters, including subjective mood, the values were lowest at a circadian phase corresponding to the nadir of the endogenous circadian temperature cycle. Similarly, scores were maximal at a circadian

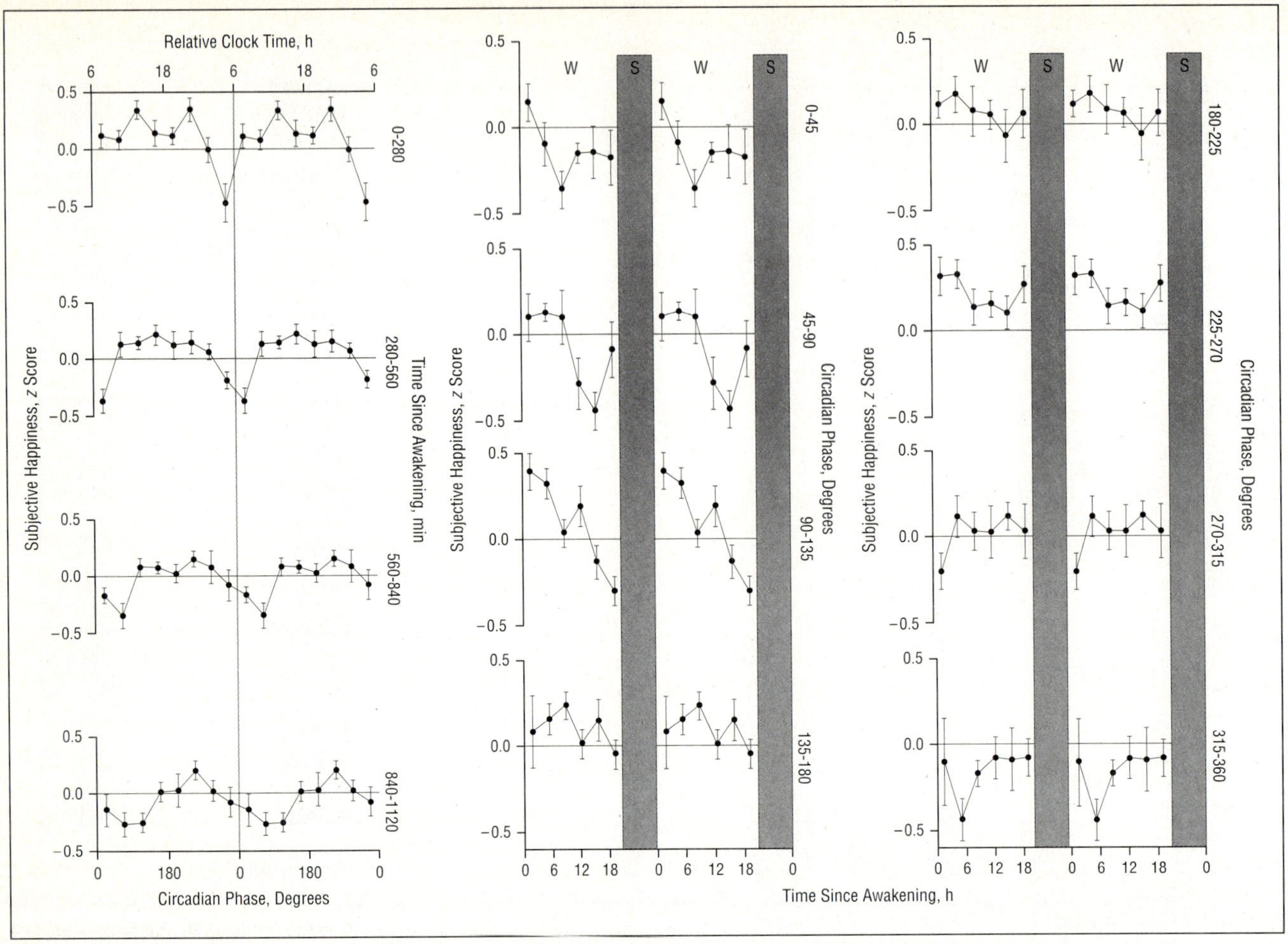

Figure 4. *Circadian variation of mood as a function of time elapsed since awakening (left) and wake-dependent variation as a function of circadian phase (right) (experiment 2). Values are mean±SEM. The analyses were restricted to specific times or phases. W indicates awake; S, asleep.*

phase coinciding with the crest of the endogenous circadian temperature cycle. These results suggest that an endogenous circadian pacemaker, presumably located in the suprachiasmatic nucleus of the hypothalamus,[31] is a determinant of observed daily variations of subjective mood, subjective alertness, cognitive performance, and short-term memory.[5,8,23] This notion is further supported by reports that, after phase shifts induced by exposure to bright or moderately bright light,[27,32] the circadian rhythms of subjective alertness and cognitive performance maintain similar temporal relationships to other reliable circadian markers. However, experimental manipulations of core body temperature similar to those used in animal research[33] are required to exclude a direct contribution of temperature to subjective mood.

Our findings are consistent with data from a number of prior experiments. Monk et al,[10] using the constant routine sleep deprivation protocol, reported that subjective measures of mood reached their lowest values close to the minimum of the core body temperature cycle. However, sleep deprivation itself has been shown to result in a deterioration of mood in healthy subjects.[12,13,15-19] Taub and Berger[11,15] and Totterdell et al[20] reported that, in sleep displacement studies, the timing of sleep had a significant impact on mean daily values for mood in healthy volunteers. However, in contrast to those studies, the design of the present experiments enabled quantification of the complex interaction of circadian and wake-dependent processes in the regulation of mood in healthy young subjects.

The present study contrasts with the previously observed significant main effect of prior wakefulness on subjective alertness and cognitive performance.[5,6] However, as suggested by the trend observed in Figure 3 (top right), our results do not allow the interpretation that prior waking has no effect on mood, since any effect may be smaller than the limits of detectability for our statistical paradigm. Indeed, when the wake-dependent component is analyzed independently of the circadian component, a significant effect of prior waking is observed (1-factor ANOVA for nonrepeated measures, with time since waking as the factor: $F_{3,7828}=13.92$, $P<.001$), even though this effect remains small.

The importance of the duration of prior wakefulness in the regulation of subjective mood became apparent in the analysis of the statistically significant interaction of prior wakefulness and circadian phase. As illustrated in Figure 4, even though the circadian variation of mood was significant at all durations of prior wakefulness, the time at which the circadian variation of mood reached its trough depended on the duration of prior wakefulness. Moreover, the analysis in which the circadian fluctuation was restricted to specific phases while prior wakefulness was varied revealed that mood improved, deteriorated, or remained stable with the duration of prior wakefulness. Systematic variation of subjective mood with the duration of prior wakefulness is therefore qualitatively different (or absent) at specific circadian phases. These results indicate that subjective mood is influenced by a complex and nonadditive interaction of circadian and wake-dependent processes and imply that the temporal alignment between the sleep-wake cycle and the endogenous circadian rhythms affects self-assessment of mood in healthy subjects. Under normally entrained conditions, subjects wake up approximately 1 to 2 hours after the endogenous minimum of the core body temperature rhythm, which occurs around 6 AM.[28] After 8 hours of wakefulness, the circadian phase is close to 120° to 130°, a situation under which, according to the present analyses, mean levels of mood during the waking day will be high. When sleep is displaced, as in shift workers,[34-36] the phase relationship between the sleep-wake cycle and the endogenous circadian pacemaker changes, and this change may alter mood during the waking episode. A high prevalence of anxiodepressive symptoms has been reported among shift workers[37-39]; our findings raise the question of whether a misalignment between the sleep-wake cycle and the endogenous circadian timing system may contribute to mood changes in that population. Figure 4, left, reveals that, with extended duration of waking, the time during which the circadian fluctuation of mood remains at its lowest values is extended. Future studies will be necessary to clarify whether chronic sleep deprivation modifies the interaction of circadian and wake-dependent processes and whether this interaction relates to anxiety and affective disorders in shift workers.

It has previously been reported that subjective alertness and cognitive performance are also determined by a nonadditive interaction of circadian phase and prior wakefulness.[6,8] These findings raise the question as to whether the changes observed in subjective mood are linked to variation in levels of alertness. However, the analysis of subjective mood differed on several points from the analysis of subjective alertness. For example, in contrast to subjective mood, subjective alertness deteriorated with an extension of prior wakefulness at all circadian phases, and the circadian variation of alertness was stronger with increasing duration of prior wakefulness. Moreover, the wake-dependent component was weaker relative to the circadian component for subjective mood than for subjective alertness.[6,8] These differences indicate that the results of the present study reflect a genuine effect of circadian phase and prior wakefulness on mood, not simply the covariation of subjective mood with subjective alertness or fatigue.

Despite the difference in affective states between healthy subjects and depressed patients, our results have implications for the analysis of the well-known phenomenon of diurnal variation of mood in endogenous depression[40-44] and the effects of sleep deprivation on affect in patients with this condition. In contrast to healthy subjects, mood often improves over the course of the waking day in depressed patients, and a further extension of wakefulness (ie, sleep deprivation) often leads to a temporary alleviation of depressive symptoms,[45-51] although both the time course of diurnal variation and the response to sleep deprivation are highly variable. These phenomena have been hypothesized to reflect a disturbance of a circadian parameter, such as a phase advance,[41,52-55] a phase delay,[56] a reduced amplitude,[57] or a disturbance of a sleep-wake dependent process (ie, the S-deficiency,[58] non–rapid eye movement sleep,[59] or rapid eye movement sleep[60,61] hypotheses), or to relate to a complex interaction of circadian and sleep-wake cycle–dependent processes[42,49,62] (for literature reviews, see Kripke,[53] van den Hoofdakker,[63] Wirz-Justice,[64] and Healy and Waterhouse[65]). Our data imply that the effects of sleep deprivation, sleep displacement, and the diurnal variation of mood can no longer be attributed to a single process but need to be interpreted as a function of the simultaneous changes in circadian phase and prior sleep-wake history and organization. Further studies will thus be necessary to clarify how circadian and wake-dependent processes specifically interact in the regulation of affective states in psychiatric disorders.

To our knowledge, this investigation is the first to quantify the complex interaction of circadian and wake-dependent fluctuation of mood in healthy young subjects. Moreover, our consistent findings (despite the differences in experimental conditions between our independent research groups) reinforce the significance of the complex interaction observed between the sleep-wake cycle and the endogenous circadian pacemaker. These results clearly demonstrate that this interaction is nonadditive, so that relatively small changes in the timing of sleep relative to the endogenous circadian pacemaker may markedly affect subjective mood during the following waking episode.

Accepted for publication April 22, 1996.

This research is supported by grants NIA-P01-AG09975 and GCRC-M01-RR02635 from the National Institutes of Health, Bethesda, Md, and by the British Medical Research Council, London, England. Dr Boivin is supported by a fellowship from the Medical Research Council of Canada, Ottawa, Ontario.

The authors are grateful to the research subjects for their participation; to the research technicians for technical assistance; to Julie Smith for data entry; and to Lisa DiFabio for editorial assistance.

Reprints: Diane B. Boivin, MD, PhD, Circadian, Neuroendocrine and Sleep Disorders Section, Division of Endocrinology, Department of Medicine, Brigham and Women's Hospital, Harvard Medical School, 221 Longwood Ave, Boston, MA 02115.

REFERENCES

1. Benedict FG. Studies in body-temperature, I: influence of the inversion of the daily routine: the temperature of night-workers. *Am J Physiol.* 1904;11:145-169.
2. Mosso U. Recherches sur l'inversion des oscillations diurnes de la température chez l'homme normal. *Arch Ital Biol.* 1887;8:177-185.
3. Weitzman ED, Czeisler CA, Moore-Ede MC. Sleep-wake, neuroendocrine and body temperature circadian rhythms under entrained and non-entrained (free-running) conditions in man. *Acta Endocrinol.* 1978;89:25.
4. Dijk D-J, Czeisler CA. Contribution of the circadian pacemaker and the sleep

homeostat to sleep propensity, sleep structure, electroencephalographic slow waves and sleep spindle activity in humans. *J Neurosci.* 1995;15:3526-3538.
5. Johnson MP, Duffy JF, Dijk D-J, Ronda JM, Dyal CM, Czeisler CA. Short-term memory, alertness and performance: a reappraisal of their relationship to body temperature. *J Sleep Res.* 1992;1:24-29.
6. Dijk D-J, Duffy JF, Czeisler CA. Circadian and sleep/wake dependent aspects of subjective alertness and cognitive performance. *J Sleep Res.* 1992;1:112-117.
7. Folkard S, Åkerstedt T. Towards the prediction of alertness on abnormal sleep/wake schedules. In: Coblentz A, ed. *Vigilance and Performance in Automated Systems.* Dordrecht, the Netherlands: Kluwer Academic Publishers; 1989:287-296.
8. Czeisler CA, Dijk D-J, Duffy JF. Entrained phase of the circadian pacemaker serves to stabilize alertness and performance throughout the habitual waking day. In: Ogilvie RD, Harsh JR, eds. *Sleep Onset: Normal and Abnormal Processes.* Washington, DC: American Psychological Association; 1994:89-110.
9. Åkerstedt T, Folkard S. Validation of the S and C components of the three-process model of alertness regulation. *Sleep.* 1995;18:1-6.
10. Monk TH, Buysse DJ, Reynolds III CF, Jarrett DB, Kupfer DJ. Rhythmic vs homeostatic influences on mood, activation, and performance in young and old men. *J Gerontol.* 1992;47:P221-P227.
11. Taub JM, Berger RJ. Effects of acute shifts in circadian rhythms of sleep and wakefulness on performance and mood. In: Scheving LE, Halberg F, Pauly JE, eds. *Chronobiology.* Tokyo, Japan: Igaku Shoin Ltd; 1974:571-575.
12. McCann UD, Penetar DM, Shaham Y, Thorne DR, Sing HC, Thomas ML, Gillin JC, Belenky G. Effects of catecholamine depletion on alertness and mood in rested and sleep deprived normal volunteers. *Neuropsychopharmacology.* 1993;8:345-356.
13. Brendel DH, Reynolds CF III, Jennings JR, Hoch CC, Monk TH, Berman SR, Hall FT, Boysse DJ, Kupfer DJ. Sleep stage physiology, mood, and vigilance responses to total sleep deprivation in healthy 80-year-olds and 20-years-olds. *Psychophysiology.* 1990;27:677-685.
14. Wood C, Magnello ME. Diurnal changes in perceptions of energy and mood. *J R Soc Med.* 1992;85:191-194.
15. Taub JM, Berger RJ. Performance and mood following variations in the length and timing of sleep. *Psychophysiology.* 1973;10:559-570.
16. Angus RG, Heslegrave RJ, Myles WS. Effects of prolonged sleep deprivation, with and without chronic physical exercise, on mood and performance. *Psychophysiology.* 1985;22:276-282.
17. Gerner RH, Post RM, Gillin JC, Bunney WE. Biological and behavioral effects of one night's sleep deprivation in depressed patients and normals. *J Psychiatr Res.* 1979;15:21-40.
18. Peeke SC, Callaway E, Jones RT, Stone GC, Doyle J. Combined effects of alcohol and sleep deprivation in normal young adults. *Psychopharmacology.* 1980;67:279-287.
19. Hendrick C, Lilly RS. The structure of mood: a comparison between sleep deprivation and normal wakefulness conditions. *J Pers.* 1970;38:453-465.
20. Totterdell P, Reynolds S, Parkinson B, Briner RB. Associations of sleep with everyday mood, minor symptoms and social interaction experience. *Sleep.* 1994;17:466-475.
21. Dijk D-J, Czeisler CA. Paradoxical timing of the circadian rhythm of sleep propensity serves to consolidate sleep and wakefulness in humans. *Neurosci Lett.* 1994;166:63-68.
22. Kleitman N, Kleitman E. Effect of non-twenty-four-hour routines of living in oral temperature and heart rate. *J Appl Physiol.* 1953;6:283-291.
23. Boivin DB, Duffy JF, Dijk D-J, Smith JA, Czeisler CA. Endogenous circadian rhythm of subjective mood in healthy young men. Presented at the Fourth Meeting of the Society for Research on Biological Rhythms; May 7, 1994; Amelia Island Plantation, Fla.
24. Folkard S. Body clock and time since sleep components of circadian rhythms in moon and performance. Presented at the Belgium Association for Sleep Studies Conference on Sleep, Alertness and Cognition; May 15, 1993; Brussels, Belgium.
25. Eysenck HJ, Eysenck SBG. *Manual of the Eysenck Personality Inventory.* London, England: University of London Press; 1964.
26. Totterdell P, Folkard S. In situ repeated measures of affect and cognitive performance facilitated by use of a hand-held computer. *Behav Res Meth Inst Comput.* 1993;24:545-553.
27. Boivin DB, Duffy JF, Kronauer RE, Czeisler CA. Sensitivity of the human circadian pacemaker to moderately bright light. *J Biol Rhythms.* 1994;9:315-331.
28. Czeisler CA, Kronauer RE, Allan JS, Duffy JF, Jewett ME, Brown EN, Ronda JM. Bright light induction of strong (type 0) resetting of the human circadian pacemaker. *Science.* 1989;244:1328-1333.
29. Aitken RCB. Measurement of feelings using visual analogue scales. *Proc R Soc Med.* 1969;62:989-993.
30. Klerman EB, Dijk D-J, Kronauer RE, Czeisler CA. Simulations of light effects on the human circadian pacemaker: implications for assessment of intrinsic period. *Am J Physiol.* 1996;270:R271-R282.
31. Klein DC, Moore RY, Reppert SM, eds. *Suprachiasmatic Nucleus: The Mind's Clock.* New York, NY: Oxford University Press; 1991.
32. Czeisler CA, Johnson MP, Duffy JF, Brown EN, Ronda JM, Kronauer RE. Exposure to bright light and darkness to treat physiologic maladaptation to night work. *N Engl J Med.* 1990;322:1253-1259.
33. Rosenthal MS, Vogel GW. The effects of a 3-day increase of ambient temperature on body temperature and REM sleep in an animal model of depression. *Sleep.* 1994;17:291-297.
34. Åkerstedt T, Gillberg M. Sleep disturbances and shift work. In: Reinberg A, Vieux N, Andlauer P, eds. *Night and Shift Work: Biological and Social Aspects.* Oxford, England: Pergamon Press Ltd; 1981:127-137.
35. Vokac Z, Lund L. Patterns and duration of sleep in permanent security night guards. *J Hum Ergol Tokyo.* 1982;11:311-316.
36. Rutenfranz J, Klimmer F, Knauth P. Desynchronization of different physiological functions during three weeks of experimental nightshift with limited and unlimited sleep. In: Colquhoun P, Folkard S, Knauth P, Rutenfranz J, eds. *Experimental Studies of Shiftwork: Proceedings of the Third International Symposium on Night- and Shiftwork Under the Auspices of the Subcommittee on Shift Work of the Permanent Commission and International Association on Occupational Health, Dortmund, October 29-31, 1974.* Opladen, Germany: Westdeutscher Verlag; 1975:74-77.
37. Gordon NP, Cleary PD, Parker CE, Czeisler CA. The prevalence and health impact of shiftwork. *Am J Public Health.* 1986;76:1225-1228.
38. Skipper JK, Jung FD, Coffey LC. Nurses and shiftwork: effects on physical health and mental depression. *J Adv Nurs.* 1990;15:835-842.
39. Healy D, Minors DS, Waterhouse JM. Shiftwork, helplessness and depression. *J Affect Disord.* 1993;29:17-25.
40. Hall P, Spear MB, Stirland D. Diurnal variaton of subjective mood in depressive state. *Psychiatr Q.* 1964;38:529-536.
41. Papousek M. Chronobiologische aspekte der zyklothymie. *Fortschr Neurol Psychiatr.* 1975;43:381-440.
42. Reinink E, Bouhuys N, Wirz-Justice A, van den Hoofdakker R. Prediction of the antidepressant response to total sleep deprivation by diurnal variation of mood. *Psychiatry Res.* 1990;32:113-124.
43. Haug HJ, Wirz-Justice A. Diurnal variation of mood in depression: important or irrelevant? *Biol Psychiatry.* 1993;34:201-203.
44. Elithorn A, Bridges PK, Lobban MC, Tredre BE. Observations on some diurnal rhythms in depressive illness. *BMJ.* 1966;2:1620-1623.
45. Pflug B, Tölle R. Disturbance of the 24-hour rhythm in endogenous depression and the treatment of endogenous depression by sleep deprivation. *Int Pharmacopsychiatry.* 1971;6:187-196.
46. Souêtre E, Salvati E, Wehr TA, Sack DA, Krebs B, Darcourt G. Twenty-four-hour profiles of body temperature and plasma TSH in bipolar patients during depression and during remission and in normal control subjects. *Am J Psychiatry.* 1988;145:1133-1137.
47. Kasper S, Kick H, Voll G, Vieira A. Therapeutic sleep deprivation and antidepressant medication in patients with major depression. *Eur Psychopharmacol.* 1991;1:107-111.
48. Wu JC, Bunney WE. The biological basis of an antidepressant response to sleep deprivation and relapse: review and hypothesis. *Am J Psychiatry.* 1990;147:14-21.
49. Bouhuys AL. Towards a model of mood responses to sleep deprivation in depressed patients. *Biol Psychiatry.* 1991;29:600-612.
50. Szuba MP, Baxter LR, Fairbanks LA, Guze BH, Schwartz JM. Effects of partial sleep deprivation on the diurnal variation of mood and motor activity in major depression. *Biol Psychiatry.* 1991;30:817-829.
51. van den Hoofdakker RH, Beersma DGM. On the contribution of sleep wake physiology to the explanation and the treatment of depression. *Acta Psychiatr Scand Suppl.* 1988;341:53-71.
52. Wehr TA, Wirz-Justice A, Goodwin FK, Duncan W, Gillin JC. Phase advance of the circadian sleep-wake cycle as an antidepressant. *Science.* 1979;206:710-713.
53. Kripke DF. Phase advance theories for affective illness. In: Wehr TA, Goodwin FK, eds. *Circadian Rhythms in Psychiatry.* Pacific Grove, Calif: Boxwood Press; 1983:41-69.
54. Souêtre E, Salvati E, Pringuey D, Plasse Y, Savelli M, Darcourt G. Antidepressant effects of the sleep/wake cycle phase advance: preliminary report. *J Affect Disord.* 1987;12:41-46.
55. Vollmann J, Berger M. Sleep deprivation with consecutive sleep-phase advance therapy in patients with major depression: a pilot study. *Biol Psychiatry.* 1993;33:54-57.
56. Lewy AJ, Sack RL, Miller LS, Hoban TM. Antidepressant and circadian phase-shifting effects of light. *Science.* 1987;235:352-354.
57. Souêtre E, Salvati E, Belugou JL, Pringuey D, Candito M, Krebs B, Ardisson JL, Darcourt G. Circadian rhythms in depression and recovery: evidence for the blunted amplitude as the main chronobiological abnormality. *Psychiatry Res.* 1989;28:263-278.
58. Borbély AA, Wirz-Justice A. Sleep, sleep deprivation and depression: a hypothesis derived from a model of sleep regulation. *Hum Neurobiol.* 1982;1:205-210.
59. Beersma DGM, van den Hoofdakker RH. Can non-REM sleep be depressogenic? *J Affect Disord.* 1992;24:101-108.
60. Vogel GW, Vogel F, McAbee RS, Thurmond AJ. Improvement of depression by REM sleep deprivation. *Arch Gen Psychiatry.* 1980;37:247-253.
61. Gillin JC. The sleep therapies of depression. *Prog Neuropsychopharmacol Biol Psychiatry.* 1983;7:351-364.
62. Wehr TA, Wirz-Justice A. Internal coincidence model for sleep deprivation and depression. In: Koella WP, ed. *Sleep 1980: Proceedings of the Fifth European Congress on Sleep Research, Amsterdam 1980.* Basel, Switzerland: S Karger AG; 1981:26-33.
63. van den Hoofdakker RH. Chronobiological theories of nonseasonal affective disorders and their implications for treatment. *J Biol Rhythms.* 1994;9:157-183.
64. Wirz-Justice A. Biological rhythms in mood disorders. In: Bloom FE, Kupfer DJ, eds. *Psychopharmacology: The Fourth Generation of Progress.* New York, NY: Raven Press; 1995:999-1017.
65. Healy D, Waterhouse JM. The circadian system and the therapeutics of the affective disorders. *Pharmacol Ther.* 1995;65:241-263.

ORIGINAL ARTICLE

Reduced Blue Cone Electroretinogram in Cocaine-Withdrawn Patients

Monique Roy, MD; Alec Roy, MD; John Williams, MD; Lawrence Weinberger, PhD; David Smelson, PsyD

Background: The main reinforcing effect of cocaine is alteration of dopaminergic neurotransmission in the brain reward systems. Since dopamine is found in high concentrations in the retina, we investigated whether cocaine dependence may be associated with abnormalities of the electroretinogram.

Methods: We compared recently withdrawn cocaine-dependent patients (n=20) with age-, sex-, and race-matched normal subjects (n=20) for responses of cone photoreceptors to light flashes on full-field electroretinograms.

Results: Cocaine-dependent patients had significantly reduced blue cone electroretinogram responses compared with matched normal subjects.

Conclusions: This result suggests that cocaine-withdrawn patients have a dysregulation of blue cone function. The electroretinogram may be useful in future studies of cocaine-dependent patients.

Arch Gen Psychiatry. 1997;54:153-156

From the Department of Ophthalmology, University of Medicine and Dentistry of New Jersey–New Jersey Medical School, Newark (Dr M. Roy), Psychiatry Service (Drs A. Roy and Williams) and Psychology Service (Drs Weinberger and Smelson), Veterans Affairs Medical Center, East Orange, NJ.

COCAINE ABUSE and dependence have become a major health problem. The main reinforcing effect of cocaine is inhibition of dopamine uptake into the presynaptic neuron, which thus increases dopaminergic neurotransmission—particularly in the nucleus accumbens and brain reward system. Self-administering studies in animals have shown that the potencies of cocainelike drugs correlate with their potencies in inhibiting tritiated mazindol binding to dopamine transporter protein.[1]

In the eye, the retina—like the brain—has a high concentration of dopamine.[2] The electroretinogram (ERG) is a neurophysiologic technique for recording electrical potentials from the retina in response to a flash of light. Depending on the state of light or dark adaptation of the retina, one can evaluate either cone or rod function.[3,4] Therefore, we decided to study the ERG in cocaine-dependent patients. We hypothesized that such patients would show ERG abnormalities when compared with matched normal subjects.

RESULTS

The 20 cocaine-dependent patients had a mean (±SD) duration of cocaine abuse of 6.7±4.2 years (range, 8 months-15 years). Their mean (±SD) age was 34.6±4.3 years, and that of the normal subjects was 34.6±6.5 years ($P<.96$). Patients were withdrawn from cocaine for a mean (±SD) of 26.1±17.4 days (range, 3-62 days).

The cocaine-withdrawn patients (n=20) showed a significantly reduced blue cone ERG response compared with normal subjects (n=20) ($P<.003$) (**Table** and **Figure**). Also, significantly more of the cocaine-withdrawn patients showed blue cone b-wave amplitudes below 0.5 μV compared with normal subjects (11 of 20 patients vs 4 of 20 normal subjects; Fisher exact test, $P<.05$), and significantly more patients had absent blue cone ERG responses (5 of 20 patients vs none of 20 normal subjects; Fisher exact test, $P<.05$). There was no significant correlation between blue cone b-wave amplitude and length of time abstinent from cocaine ($r=-0.01$, N=20).

Reproducibility of the ERG cone responses to blue and red flashes was tested in 23 normal subjects, of whom 16 were African American, 3 Hispanic, and 4 white (mean[±SD] age, 33.7±11.9 years), by repeating the ERG test twice during the same session. The ERG cone responses to blue and red flashes showed good reproducibility on test-retest ($r=0.83$, N=23, $P<.01$ and $r=0.87$, N=12, $P<.01$ for blue and red

SUBJECTS AND METHODS

A consecutive series of 20 male African-American cocaine-dependent patients admitted as inpatients to the locked Drug and Dependency Rehabilitation Unit of the East Orange (NJ) Veterans Affairs Medical Center was studied. Subjects met current *DSM-III-R*[5] criteria for cocaine dependence, reported having used at least 12 g of cocaine during the 3 months preceding their admission to the program, and had been free of medications, alcohol, and other drugs for a minimum of 3 days. Excluded were subjects who (1) were currently physically dependent on opiates, barbiturates, alcohol, or marijuana or whose principal drug dependence was not cocaine; (2) met *DSM-III-R* criteria for another current axis I disorder other than phobic or anxiety disorders, met lifetime criteria for schizophrenia or mania, or expressed marked suicidal or homicidal ideation; (3) were taking any medication; (4) had a preexisting eye condition; or (5) had clinical evidence of any cognitive impairment. Subjects were interviewed by a psychiatrist (J.W.) by means of the Structured Clinical Interview for *DSM-III-R,* Part I, to rule out major psychiatric disorder. Random weekly urinalyses were done to ensure that patients were not using illicit drugs while on the locked ward. All patients gave written informed consent.

All 20 cocaine-dependent patients were matched with normal subjects for sex, age within 5 years, and racial background. All normal subjects were medication free and gave no history of substance abuse with cocaine, other substance abuse, depression, or treatment for any psychiatric disorder. Normal subjects were recruited from among psychologists, other hospital personnel, and patients undergoing ERG because of trauma to 1 eye.

The ERG was recorded from 1 eye by means of standard methods[4] and bipolar Burian-Allen contact lens electrodes (Hansen Ophthalmic, Iowa City, Iowa). The pupil was dilated widely to at least 8 mm, and pupil diameter was measured before and after each recording session. The ERG was detected with a signal averager (model CA-1000, Nicolet Spirit, Madison, Wis) coupled to a Ganzfeld stimulator providing a relatively strong adapting field (17 000 trolands) at maximum brightness. Superimposed on this steady white-light field were flashes obtained from a strobe (model PS2; Grass Instruments, Quincy, Mass).

The flash could be modified by inserting filters into the receptacle in the strobe housing. The following filters (Kodak Wratten, Rochester, NY) were used: 98 (450 nm), 48 (471 nm), 75 (488 nm), 61 (534 nm), 21 (593 nm), and 29 (633 nm). The numbers in parentheses indicate the nominal wavelength of maximum transmission of each filter at the approximate color temperature of the strobe. The flash rate for cone ERG recording was 5.1 Hz. At least 100 responses were averaged. For the blue cone ERG, 1000 responses were averaged. With this technique, we can detect signals as low as 0.1 μV. The a- and b-wave amplitude and implicit time were measured in the standard fashion by determining the amplitude of the negative a-wave from baseline to trough and of the subsequent b-wave from the trough of the a-wave to the peak of the b-wave. The blue cone ERG appears as a separate b-wave riding on an earlier b-wave of the long and middle cone ERG. We measured the blue cone b-wave response from its initial appearance after the peak of the L and M cone b-wave to its own peak.[4] Implicit time was measured from the flash to the negative peak of the a-wave or to the positive peak of the b-wave.

In the statistical analysis, as the variances were unequal, the Wilcoxon rank sum test was used. The Fisher exact test was also used. The patients were matched in a masked fashion by one of us (A.R.) who was not involved in the ERG measurements.

flash, respectively). Four of the cocaine-withdrawn patients had the ERG repeated on a second occasion and also showed good reproducibility of blue cone b-wave amplitude (mean±SD, 0.49+0.29 μV at first test and 0.45+0.94 μV at second test; r=0.99, df=2, P<.1).

COMMENT

We found significant differences between cocaine-withdrawn patients and normal subjects for ERG responses. Cocaine-withdrawn patients had significantly reduced blue cone ERG responses. In fact, the mean amplitude of the blue cone b-wave ERG response was about half that of the normal subjects. Significantly more of the cocaine-withdrawn patients than normal subjects showed a blue cone ERG response below 0.5 μV.

The ERG responses may vary with age, sex, race, and medication status.[3] However, the results of the present study are unlikely to be explained by any of these variables, since all patients were matched for age, sex, and race with normal subjects. The cocaine-dependent patients were all drawn from a locked drug rehabilitation inpatient unit and had consistently negative random urine drug screens. None of the subjects was taking any medication. Thus, we believe that the results of the present study are best explained by the drug taken before admission of the cocaine-dependent patients. As we carefully selected only patients who were admitted for problems with cocaine, who met *DSM-III-R* criteria for cocaine dependence, who stated that cocaine was their preferred illicit drug, and who were not dependent on opiates, barbiturates, or marijuana, we believe that the findings result from the patients' recent dependence on cocaine. Although alcohol use is common among cocaine-dependent patients, the Structured Clinical Interview for *DSM-III-R,* Part I, led to the *DSM-III-R* diagnosis of alcohol abuse in only 3 of these patients, who were carefully selected to exclude those with alcohol dependence or dependence on any drug other than cocaine.

The average human retina contains 4 million to 6 million cones. Cones provide visual acuity for pattern detection as well as color vision. Color vision is mediated by 3 types of cone photoreceptors identified by their relative spectral absorption as long-, middle-, and short (blue) –wavelength–sensitive cones. Dopamine plays an essential role in primate vision.[6-9] Light—as in the ERG—stimulates retinal tyrosine hydroxylase activity, leading to the release of dopamine.[10] The primate retina contains

Electroretinogram Cone Responses in Cocaine-Dependent Patients and Normal Subjects

Electroretinogram Variable	Cocaine-Dependent Patients (n=20)	Normal Subjects (n=20)
Cone response to white flash		
a-Wave amplitude, μV	12.1±6.4	11.5±3.9
b-Wave amplitude, μV	51.1±25.7	49.0±16.9
Blue cone responses		
b-Wave amplitude, μV	0.48±0.38*	0.93±0.44
Red-green cone responses		
b-Wave amplitude, μV	3.8±3.3	3.0±1.6

**Cocaine-dependent patients had significantly smaller blue cone electroretinogram responses than normal subjects (P<.003). Data are given as mean± SD.*

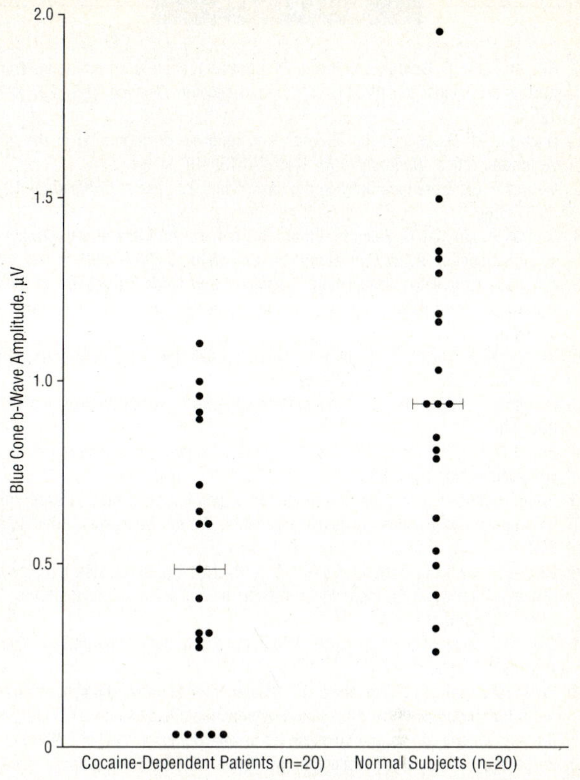

Electroretinogram blue cone b-wave amplitude in cocaine-dependent patients and matched normal subjects. Cocaine-dependent patients had significantly reduced amplitudes (Wilcoxon rank sum test, P<.003).

2 types of dopamine cells, amacrine and interplexiform cells. Dopamine amacrine cells receive presynaptic input mainly from cone bipolar cells.[8] Dopamine neurons modulate the relative weight of cone and rod inputs to common neurons[11] and directly modify the gain of photoreceptor signals.[12] D_2 and D_4 receptors have been identified on cones.[13,14] Dopamine deficiency leads to impaired retinal processing.[9]

It is noteworthy that neuroleptics[15-17] and disorders that decrease dopaminergic function decrease ERG amplitudes. For example, Takatsuna et al[18] administered 1-methyl-4-phenyl-1,2,5,6-tetrahydropyridine (MPTP), a selective neurotoxin that destroys dopamine-containing neurons, to mice and examined the ERG and retina. The ERGs were recorded before and 10, 30, and 50 days after MPTP injection. The amplitude of the ERG potentials was greatly reduced and tended to return to control levels 50 days after injection. Immunohistochemical analysis showed that 10 days after MPTP injection the number of tyrosine hydroxylase–positive dopamine-containing retinal amacrine cells was reduced by approximately 50% and that these changes lasted at least 50 days after MPTP injection. Rabbits administered MPTP also show deficiencies on the ERG.[19] Administration of MPTP induces a model of Parkinson disease in humans. Thus, patients with Parkinson disease also have a 50% decrease in retinal dopamine and show deficiencies on the ERG, particularly reduced blue cone amplitude.[20] These abnormalities normalize temporarily after treatment with levodopa. Interestingly, Kosten[21] noted minor parkinsonian symptoms in cocaine-dependent patients, which they attributed to down-regulation of striatal D_2 receptors.

That the patients in our study had been withdrawn from cocaine for a mean (±SD) of 26.1±17.4 days (range, 3-62 days) at the time of ERG testing is of note, since data increasingly suggest that cocaine has long-lasting effects on the brain. For example, Volkow et al[22-24] investigated brain glucose metabolism with positron emission tomography and fludeoxyglucose F 18 in 21 long-term cocaine abusers who were neurologically intact and 18 normal subjects. Cocaine abusers were tested 1 to 6 weeks after last use of cocaine, and 7 were retested after a 3-month drug-free period. Cocaine abusers showed significantly lower metabolic activity in 16 of 21 left frontal regions and 8 of 21 right frontal regions. These decreases persisted after 3 to 4 months of detoxification and correlated with the dose and years of cocaine used. In a second positron emission tomographic study, Volkow et al[25] used a dopamine ligand to examine D_2 receptor availability. Cocaine addicts had significant decreased dopamine D_2 receptor availability compared with normal subjects. Furthermore, these decreases persisted 3 to 4 months after detoxification and were associated with decreased metabolism in several regions of the frontal lobes.

Kosten[21] noted long-lasting decreases in cortical blood flow in cocaine-dependent patients examined with single photon emission computed tomography. They attributed this finding to the vasoconstriction effect of cocaine leading to cerebral cortical blood flow reduction. However, none of the cocaine-dependent patients in the present study had any evidence of retinal vascular lesions on detailed retinal examination, and the cone ERG response to white flash was not different between patients and normal subjects. In summary, the finding of the present study that blue cone ERG response is reduced suggests dysregulation of cone function as a consequence of cocaine dependence.

Accepted for publication January 12, 1996.

Reprints: Monique Roy, MD, University of Medicine and Dentistry of New Jersey–New Jersey Medical School, 90 Bergen St, Level 6, Room 6164, Newark, NJ 07103.

REFERENCES

1. Ritz M, Lamb R, Goldberg S, Kirhar M. Cocaine receptors on dopamine transporters are related to self-administration of cocaine. *Science.* 1987;237:1219-1223.
2. Djamgoz M, Wagner H. Localization and function of dopamine in the adult vertebrate retina. *Neurochem Int.* 1992;20:139-191.
3. Gouras P. Electroretinography: some basic principles. *Invest Ophthalmol.* 1970; 9:557-569.
4. Gouras P, MacKay C. Electroretinographic responses of the short wavelength sensitive cones. *Invest Ophthalmol Vis Sci.* 1990;30:1203-1209.
5. American Psychiatric Association. *Diagnostic and Statistical Manual of Mental Disorders, Third Edition, Revised.* Washington, DC: American Psychiatric Association; 1987.
6. Witkovsky P, Dearry A. Functional roles of dopamine in the vertebrate retina. *Prog Retina Res.* 1991;11:247-292.
7. Dowling J. Dopamine: a retinal neuromodulator? *Trends Neurosci.* 1986;9: 236-240.
8. Bodis-Wollner I, Piccolino M. *Dopaminergic Mechanisms in Vision.* New York, NY: Alan R Liss Inc; 1988.
9. Bodis-Wollner I. Visual deficits related to dopamine deficiency in experimental animals and Parkinson's disease patients. *Trends Neurosci.* 1990;13:296-302.
10. Iuvone P, Galli CL, Garrison-Gund CK, Neff NH. Light stimulates tyrosine hydroxylase activity and dopamine synthesis in retinal amacrine neurons. *Science.* 1978;202:901-902.
11. Daw NW, Jenson RJ, Brunken WJ. Rod pathways in mammalian retinae. *Trends Neurosci.* 1990;13:110-115.
12. Witkovsky P, Stone S, Tranchina D. Photoreceptor to horizontal synaptic transfer in the *Xenopus* retina: modulation by dopamine ligands and a circuit model for interactions of rod and cone inputs. *J Neurophysiol.* 1989;62:864-881.
13. Zarbin MA, Wamsley JK, Palacios JM, Kuhar MJ. Autoradiographic localization of high affinity GABA, benzodiazepine, dopaminergic, adrenergic and muscarinic cholinergic receptors in the rat, monkey and human retina. *Brain Res.* 1986;374:75-92.
14. Muresan Z, Besharse J. D_2-like dopamine receptors in amphibian retina: localization with fluorescent ligands. *J Comp Neurol.* 1993;331:149-160.
15. Muruiwa F, Kim S, Nao N, Sawada A. Effects of metoclopramide, dopamine receptor blockade, on the EOG light peak. *Nippon Ganka Gakkai Zasshi.* 1992; 96:375-380.
16. Holopigian K, Clewner L, Seiple W, Kupersmith M. The effects of dopamine blockade on the human flash electroretinogram. *Doc Ophthalmol.* 1994;86:1-10.
17. Tagliati M, Bodis-Wollner I, Kovanecz I, Stanzione P. Spatial frequency tuning of the monkey pattern ERG depends on D_2 receptor–linked action of dopamine. *Vision Res.* 1994;34:2051-2057.
18. Takatsuna Y, Adachi-Usami E, Ino H, Chiba T. Effects of MPTP on the mouse retina. *Nippon Ganka Gakkai Zasshi.* 1992;96:767-775.
19. Wong C, Ishibashi T, Tucker G, Hamasaki D. Responses of the pigmented rabbit retina to MPTP, a chemical inducer of parkinsonism. *Exp Eye Res.* 1985; 40:509-519.
20. Gottlob I, Schneider E, Heider WI, Skrandies W. Alterations of visual evoked potentials and electroretinograms in Parkinson's disease. *Electroencephalogr Clin Neurophysiol.* 1987;66:349-357.
21. Kosten T. Pharmacology of heroin and cocaine addiction. Presented at the Advances in Addiction Psychiatry Conference, Friends Hospital; fall 1994; Philadelphia, Pa.
22. Volkow ND, Fowler JS, Wolf AP, Hitzemann R, Dewey S, Bendriem B, Alpert R, Hoff A. Changes in brain glucose metabolism in cocaine dependence and withdrawal. *Am J Psychiatry.* 1991;148:621-626.
23. Volkow ND, Fowler JS, Wolf AP. Effects of chronic cocaine abuse on postsynaptic dopamine receptors. *Am J Psychiatry.* 1990;147:719-724.
24. Volkow ND, Mullani N, Gould L, Adler S, Krayewski K. Cerebral blood flow in chronic cocaine users: a study with positron emission tomography. *Br J Psychiatry.* 1988;152:641-648.
25. Volkow N, Fowler J, Wang G, Hitzemann R, Logan J, Schlyer D, Dewey S, Wolf A. Decreased dopamine D_2 receptor availability is associated with reduced frontal metabolism in cocaine abusers. *Synapse.* 1993;14:169-177.

Auditory Working Memory and Wisconsin Card Sorting Test Performance in Schizophrenia

James M. Gold, PhD; Constance Carpenter, PhD; Christopher Randolph, PhD; Terry E. Goldberg, PhD; Daniel R. Weinberger, MD

Background: Impaired Wisconsin Card Sorting Test (WCST) performance has been one critical piece of evidence suggesting frontal lobe dysfunction in schizophrenia. However, the specific cognitive processes underlying impaired performance have not been identified. Impaired WCST performance in schizophrenia might in part reflect a fundamental working memory deficit.

Method: We examined the performance of 30 normal subjects and 36 patients with schizophrenia on a neuropsychological battery including a novel measure of working memory—letter-number (LN) span.

Results: Patients with schizophrenia were impaired on LN span performance, which was also highly correlated with WCST performance ($r=0.74$). Between-group WCST differences were eliminated when we covaried LN span. Regression analyses suggested that LN span performance predicted the WCST category achieved score, whereas measures of set shifting, verbal fluency, and attention were predictive of perseveration.

Conclusion: Working memory may be a critical determinant of one aspect of WCST performance in schizophrenia.

Arch Gen Psychiatry. 1997;54:159-165

Speculation by Kraepelin[1(p219)] that in schizophrenia "the disease attacks by preference the frontal areas of the brain, the central convolutions and the temporal lobes" has been amply supported by recent neuropsychological and neuroimaging research.[2-6] Suggestive evidence of frontal lobe dysfunction in schizophrenia includes impaired Wisconsin Card Sorting Test (WCST) performance coupled with evidence of frontal lobe hypometabolism during task performance.[6,7] In this task, the subject is asked to sort a series of cards to 1 of 4 key cards that vary in shape (triangles, circles, stars, and crosses), color, and number of shapes. The subject must discover the correct matching rule using feedback (right or wrong) provided after each response. After 10 consecutive correct sorts, the experimenter shifts to reinforcing a new rule without warning. Thus, the task requires several complex cognitive operations, including concept formation, hypothesis testing, and set shifting. This cognitive complexity has taken on new importance in light of evidence of impaired WCST performance among patients with focal nonfrontal lesions or diffuse injuries.[8,9] Thus, it is likely that impairment of several different cognitive processes, perhaps mediated by different anatomic systems, can lead to performance failure on the WCST. This complicates the interpretation of WCST impairment, given evidence of widespread neuropsychological dysfunction and multiple extrafrontal anatomic abnormalities in schizophrenia.[10,11]

One approach to this interpretive complexity is to delineate the contribution of simpler, potentially more localizable, cognitive processes to WCST performance. At a minimum, successful WCST performance requires the subject to remember his or her prior response and associated feedback and to use this information to select a new response, a form of working memory. Although the ability to hold information in mind cannot guarantee a correct choice will be made, being unable to do so would preclude successful performance. Thus, we argue that working memory is a necessary but not sufficient condition for successful WCST performance.

There are multiple lines of evidence, in both humans and nonhuman primates, that the frontal cortex is a critical

From the Clinical Research Services Branch (Drs Gold and Carpenter) and the Clinical Brain Disorders Branch (Drs Goldberg and Weinberger), Intramural Research Program, National Institute of Mental Health, Washington, DC; and the Department of Psychiatry, Northwestern University Medical School, Chicago, Ill (Dr Randolph). Dr Gold is currently affiliated with the Maryland Psychiatric Research Center, Baltimore.

PATIENTS AND METHODS

PATIENTS

Thirty-six inpatient research volunteers at the National Institute of Mental Health (NIMH) Neuropsychiatric Research Hospital (Washington, DC) with a *DSM-III-R*[20] diagnosis of schizophrenia underwent testing as part of their admission clinical research evaluation. All patients underwent testing while clinically stable through use of medication, including clozapine in 4 patients and typical neuroleptics (most frequently haloperidol) in 32 patients. Adjunctive medications for the control of parkinsonian side effects were used in 24 patients, as were lithium (n=4) and benzodiazapines (n=5). Consensus research diagnosis was made by ward physicians and senior research staff following review of medical records, formal diagnostic conference, interview with the Structured Clinical Interview for *DSM-III-R* (SCID)[21] (which became standard clinical procedure during this study and was done for 14 patients), and an extended period of clinical observation. Patients received the following subtype diagnoses: undifferentiated (n=25), paranoid (n=7), and disorganized (n=4). Patients underwent medical, laboratory, neurological, and neuroimaging studies to rule out other sources of cognitive compromise and were free of a history of significant head injury, seizures, or recent substance dependence. Patients admitted to the NIMH Neuropsychiatric Research Hospital generally have a history of suboptimal response to conventional pharmacotherapy, multiple hospital admissions, and chronic functional disability. The sample had been ill, dated from first hospitalization, an average of 13.7 years (SD=7.3). Clinically, nearly every patient had evidence of both positive and negative symptoms. Fewer than 6 (17%) of 36 patients in the sample had a history of nearly continuous inpatient treatment.

NORMAL SUBJECTS

A total of 30 normal subjects were recruited from the nonprofessional staff of a local private hospital, the National Institutes of Health normal volunteer office, and a community college. All subjects denied any history of neurological or psychiatric illness on interview. Approximately one third of the sample received complete medical evaluations and formal SCID interviews. All subjects provided written, informed consent. Control subjects were paid for their participation.

PROCEDURE

All patients received a neuropsychological evaluation, including the Wechsler Adult Intelligence Scale–Revised (WAIS-R),[22] Wechsler Memory Scale–Revised (WMS-R),[23] WCST,[24] Reading subtest of the Wide Range Achievement Test–Revised (WRAT-R),[25] Verbal Concept Attainment Test (VCAT),[26] Boston Naming Test,[27] Continuous Performance Test (CPT),[28] Trail Making Test parts A and B,[29] and Controlled Oral Word Association[30] (verbal fluency). The normal subjects received an abbreviated battery, including the WRAT-R, Boston Naming Test, a short form of the WAIS-R,[31,32] and WCST, and 25 of 30 received digit span and Trail Making Test part B. All tests were administered in standard fashion except for the WCST, for which all subjects received a total of 128 cards (administered by hand).

LN SPAN TEST

Both groups received the LN span test. The task involves the auditory presentation by an examiner of a mixed series of alternating numbers and letters. The subject is asked to respond by first saying the numbers in order from the smallest to the largest, followed by saying the letters in alphabetical order. For example, a subject would hear "w7t4," and the correct answer is "47tw." Following a series of practice trials, the test involves 4 trials at each string length, beginning with 2-item strings (such as "m3") and proceeding up to 7-item strings (such as "c7g4q1s") for a total of 24 items. The total number of correct responses (of 24 possible) is presented in **Table 1** and used for the analyses. The test is terminated when a subject fails all 4 trials at any 1 string length. To assess the internal consistency of the LN span, we calculated Cronbach coefficient α and obtained a score of .85, which suggests a high degree of consistency among test items.

APPROACH TO STATISTICAL ANALYSIS

The statistical analyses addressed the following basic predictions: (1) Patients would perform poorly on the LN span. (2) The LN span and WCST would be correlated. (3) Between-group differences on the WCST would be attenuated when the impact of the LN span was statistically controlled. To assess the first prediction, the groups were first compared using the Student *t* test. We next performed Pearson correlations, separately for each group, between LN span, WCST, and other cognitive measures to assess the second prediction (correlations shown in **Table 2** and a plot of LN span and WCST category scores in the **Figure**). Given that most cognitive measures tend to be positively correlated, we next performed a series of partial correlations, examining the correlates of the LN span after the effects of full-scale IQ (FSIQ), the WMS-R Attention Index, and the WMS-R General Memory Index were removed. These variables were selected to assess if the observed LN span-WCST correlations might reflect shared variance with measures of general intellectual ability, attention, and episodic memory. To assess the third prediction, we performed a series of analyses of covariance, comparing adjusted group means on the WCST after controlling for the effect of the LN span. This analysis examines if the between-group difference on the WCST can be explained by group differences on the LN span. A parallel analysis was performed using digit span scores to examine if a measure of short-term memory would produce similar results as a proposed measure of working memory.

These prediction-driven analyses were followed by exploratory stepwise multiple regression analysis performed on LN span and WCST scores to examine the independent contribution of multiple cognitive variables, information unavailable from partial correlations.

component of the cortical networks that mediate aspects of working memory.[12-16] Cognitive models of working memory, defined as a multicomponent system that allows for the simultaneous storage and processing of information, suggest that impairments of complex problem solving may result from dysfunction in the "executive" control of working memory.[17] Kimberg and Farah[18] presented a computer simulation of the performance of patients with frontal lesions on the WCST, motor sequencing, context memory, and the Stroop Color Word Test by weakening the "association of working memory elements." Thus, it appears that elementary working memory dysfunction may lead to impairments on several complex tasks thought to be mediated by the frontal cortex.

We propose that WCST impairment in schizophrenia reflects, in part, working memory impairment. Park and Holzman[19] reported impaired visual and haptic working memory performance in schizophrenia using tasks similar to those used in the study of prefrontal cognitive function in nonhuman primates, but noted intact auditory working memory assessed by digit span. This study extends their work by relating the working memory framework to the WCST through the use of a novel auditory working memory task, letter-number (LN) span. The task was designed to fit Baddeley's[17] construct of working memory in the demand to simultaneously store and manipulate information. Standard short-term memory tests such as digit span do not require the cognitive manipulation of stored information, demanding little of the "work" implied in the concept of working memory.

We made the following predictions: (1) patients with schizophrenia will demonstrate impairment on LN span testing; (2) LN span and WCST performance will be highly correlated in patients with an attenuation of the correlation in normal subjects; and (3) between-group differences on the WCST will be attenuated when group differences on the LN span are statistically controlled. The prediction of differential correlation between LN span and the WCST in patients and normal subjects is based on the idea that working memory is a necessary but not sufficient condition for WCST success. Thus, working memory deficits in a patient group would likely enhance the relationship with the WCST.

RESULTS

As seen in Table 1, the normal subjects were significantly younger and better educated than the patient group. The groups differed significantly on all cognitive measures except the WRAT-R Reading subscale, a measure of premorbid cognitive ability ($P>.24$).

Table 1. Demographic and Cognitive Characteristics of Sample*

	Mean (SD)	
Characteristics	Controls	Patients With Schizophrenia
Education, y†	14.39 (1.9)	12.8 (1.6)
Age, y†	27.53 (7.0)	34.42 (7.8)
WRAT-R score	102.37 (14.1)	98.39 (13.3)
FSIQ†	106.13 (14.3)	86.33 (9.7)
Digit span score†	10.76 (1.9)	8.22 (2.6)
Boston Naming Test score†	54.54 (4.7)	49.89 (6.1)
Trail Making Test part B*, s†	48.44 (12.9)	140.25 (95.9)
WCST category score†	7.03 (2.4)	4.08 (3.1)
WCST % perseverative errors score†	12.08 (6.3)	24.60 (16.9)
LN span score†	15.70 (2.6)	11.25 (3.8)
WMS-R Attention Index	...	81.14 (17.0)
WMS-R General Memory Index	...	80.64 (19.0)
VCAT score	...	13.74 (4.9)
Verbal fluency score	...	35.14 (10.9)

*WRAT-R indicates Wide Range Achievement Test–Revised (Reading subtest); FSIQ, full-scale IQ; WCST, Wisconsin Card Sorting Test; LN span, letter-number span; WMS-R, Wechsler Memory Scale–Revised; and VCAT, Verbal Concept Attainment Test.
†$P<.01$, t test contrasting groups.

NEUROPSYCHOLOGICAL CORRELATES OF THE WCST AND LN SPAN

As seen in Table 2, significant correlations were observed in each group involving the LN span and WCST, and both tests correlated significantly with a wide range of tests assessing a variety of cognitive functions. The partial correlation results in the patient group suggest that the LN span-WCST categories relationship is only mildly attenuated by removing the effect of FSIQ, the WMS-R Attention Index, or the WMS-R Memory Index. Alternately, the correlation of LN span and WCST perseveration was not significant after removing the effect of FSIQ. In normal subjects, the LN span-WCST relationship was not significant after controlling for FSIQ. To summarize, these analyses demonstrate that patients with schizophrenia perform poorly on the LN span and that patient performance on the WCST, particularly the category score, covaries with patient performance on the LN span even after the effects of general intellectual competence, attention, and memory are statistically controlled.

To assess the issue of differential correlation across groups, we compared the LN span-WCST correlations using the Fisher z test. We found that the relationship with WCST category score differed between groups ($P<.05$), whereas the relationship with perseverative error did not differ ($P>.53$).

RELATIONSHIP OF LN SPAN, WCST, AND BETWEEN-GROUP DIFFERENCES

To examine the possibility that the between-group differences on the WCST are mediated by differences in working memory, we performed analyses of covariance (ANCOVA) on the WCST category and perseveration scores, covarying the LN span score. There was no interaction between group and covariate in either analysis, and the adjusted group category and perseveration mean scores did not differ significantly (adjusted category mean score in normal subjects, 6.12; in patients, 5.30 [$P>.23$]; and adjusted perseveration mean score in normal subjects, 14.35; in patients, 19.87 [$P>.14$]). Thus, there is a significant attenuation of between-group WCST differences when the contribution of the LN span is statistically controlled.

However, the obverse was not true. After covarying the WCST category score, the groups still differed significantly on LN span score (adjusted mean scores of 12.26 and 14.49 in patients and controls, respectively [$P<.01$]). We performed 2 additional ANCOVAs, covarying digit span to assess the role of more elementary short-term memory. Patients performed significantly worse than nor-

Table 2. LN Span Correlations*

	Patients With Schizophrenia						Controls			
	LN Span	WCST Category	WCST % Perseverative Errors	Part FSIQ	Part AI	Part MQ	LN Span	WCST Category	WCST % Perseverative Errors	Part FSIQ
WRAT-R	0.27	0.26	−0.28	−0.20	−0.20	0.24	0.44†	0.49‡	−0.34	0.14
FSIQ	0.58‡	0.66‡	−0.63‡	...	0.20	0.49‡	0.54‡	0.47‡	−0.52‡	...
Digit span	0.58‡	0.39†	0.16	0.37†	0.27	0.54‡	0.44†	0.34	0.03	0.32
Trail Making Test part B	−0.45‡	−0.54‡	0.73‡	−0.22	−0.30	−0.36†	−0.19	−0.02	−0.15	−0.25
Boston Naming Test	0.29	0.33†	−0.36†	−0.15	0.06	0.19	0.33	0.06	−0.33	−0.03
WCST category	0.74‡	...	−0.73‡	0.58‡	0.60‡	0.68‡	0.41†	...	−0.66‡	−0.22
WCST % perseverative errors	−0.52‡	−0.73‡	...	−0.24	−0.30	−0.40†	−0.39†	−0.66‡	...	−0.15
WMS-R AI	0.67‡	0.54‡	−0.56‡	0.45‡	...	0.61‡	...	...	...	...
WMS-R MQ	0.39†	0.50‡	−0.48‡	0.15	0.26	...	...	...	...	...
Continuous Performance Test	0.43†	0.48‡	−0.51‡	0.27	0.17	0.34†	...	...	...	...
Verbal fluency	0.42†	0.37†	−0.56‡	0.18	0.08	0.37†	...	...	...	...
VCAT	0.46‡	0.61‡	−0.54‡	0.13	0.27	0.32	...	...	...	...

**AI indicates Attention Index; MQ, General Memory Index; and Part, partial correlation with LN span and other cognitive variables, removing effects of FSIQ, AI, or MQ as specified. Other abbreviations are given in the footnote to Table 1.*
†$P<.05$.
‡$P<.01$.

mal subjects on the LN span after removing the effect of digit span (adjusted mean scores of 12.03 and 14.95 in patients and normal subjects, respectively [$P<.01$]). The groups also differed significantly on the WCST category measure after covarying digit span (adjusted mean scores of 4.59 and 6.48 in patients and controls, respectively [$P<.05$]). Thus, LN span and digit span appear to be measuring related but different dimensions of working memory.

MULTIPLE REGRESSION ANALYSES OF THE WCST AND LN SPAN

To clarify the relationship between LN span, WCST, and other neuropsychological measures, exploratory multiple regressions were performed with the patient data using WCST category, percent perseverative error, and LN span scores as dependent variables. The following additional variables were used in the regressions: FSIQ (to assess general cognitive competence); the WMS-R Attention Index and CPT (total correct detections minus total false alarms) to assess attentional functions; Trail Making Test part B, verbal fluency, and the VCAT (measures sensitive to frontal injury); and WMS-R General Memory Index (to provide a measure of episodic memory). We first performed 3 stepwise regressions, assessing the predictors of the LN span, WCST category, and WCST percent perseverative error scores. We next forced FSIQ to enter the regressions first to determine the extent to which covariance with general intellectual competence might underlie the observed relationships. This data-driven analysis was followed by a more theoretically motivated set of regressions where we examined if LN span continued to account for WCST variance after we forced the entry of the following 3 traditional measures of frontal lobe function: verbal fluency, Trail Making Test part B, and the VCAT. This last approach deals directly with the question of whether LN span incorporates a measurement dimension that is not fully explained by available "frontal" tests and that is relevant to understanding the WCST.

The stepwise regression of the WCST category score, using all the above variables with the exception of percent perseverative error score, yielded 2 significant predictors: the LN span (54% of the variance in WCST performance) and the VCAT (9% of the variance in WCST performance). No other variables were significant at $P<.05$. When FSIQ was forced to enter the regression first, it accounted for 42% of the variance in WCST performance, with LN span remaining a significant predictor contributing an additional 20% of the explained variance. No other variables were significant at $P<.05$. These results suggest that the WCST category score appears to involve 2 basic dimensions, a working memory dimension assessed by the LN span and a more conceptual-abstracting dimension assessed by the VCAT. This latter dimension appears to overlap with general cognitive ability to a great extent given the shrinkage in the contribution of VCAT when FSIQ was forced into the equation first.

The initial stepwise analysis of the WCST percent perseverative error score yielded the following 3 predictors significant at $P<.05$: Trail Making Test part B (54% of the variance), verbal fluency (an additional 11% of the variance), and the VCAT (an additional 7% of explained variance). When we forced FSIQ into the equation first, it accounted for 41% of the variance in the perseveration score, and the following 3 variables were significant at $P<.05$: Trail Making Test part B (an additional 21% of the variance), verbal fluency (6%), and the CPT (6%). Thus, the LN span does not emerge as a predictor of perseveration. Instead, a combination of ability to switch between perceptually available sets (Trail Making Test part B), to generate novel responses (verbal fluency), and to sustain selective attention (CPT) appear to be critical, as does general cognitive competence (FSIQ).

The stepwise regression for LN span yielded only 2 significant predictor variables, the WCST category score and the WMS-R Attention Index, which accounted for 54% and 11% of the variance, respectively. When FSIQ was forced into the regression first, it accounted for 34% of the variance in LN span, and both the WCST and WMS-R Attention Index remained significant individual predictors accounting for 23% and 9% of additional variance, respectively. Thus, LN span appears to involve both a passive storage, short-term memory dimension captured by the WMS-R Attention Index and a more active information manipulation dimension assessed by the WCST.

When Trail Making Test part B, verbal fluency, and the VCAT were entered as a first block, the block accounted for 51% of the variance in the WCST category score (F=10.92, $P<.001$). The LN span remained a significant predictor, entering after the first block (F=13.51, $P<.001$), accounting for an additional 15% of the variance, and bringing the combined model R^2 to 0.67 and total F value to 14.87 ($P<.001$). Thus, the LN span does appear to capture some WCST category variance beyond that accounted for by traditional frontal lobe tests. Alternately, the LN span did not account for significant variance in the WCST perseveration score after entry of the first block, which had an R^2 of 0.73.

COMMENT

Three major findings emerge from these data. First, patients with schizophrenia demonstrate deficits in auditory working memory as assessed by the LN span. Second, auditory working memory performance covaries with WCST performance in schizophrenia. Third, between-group differences in WCST category scores appear to be attributable to differences in working memory.

INTERPRETATION OF THE WCST IN SCHIZOPHRENIA

Consistent with prior studies,[33,34] these data provide further evidence that the WCST is a multidimensional task, demonstrated by significant correlations between the WCST and multiple cognitive measures. In essence, many patients with schizophrenia appear to lack the working memory capacity required by the WCST. Such a deficit likely undermines the capacity to perform more complex processes such as abstraction and hypothesis testing. Individual differences in working memory capacity above a certain threshold appear to have limited predictive value for WCST performance, as seen in the attenuated LN span-WCST correlations in the normal subjects. This may reflect the fact that the reasoning demands of the WCST are relatively modest. However, more complex reasoning tests covary with measures of working memory in normal subjects as demonstrated by Kyllonen and Christal,[35] who provocatively titled their examination

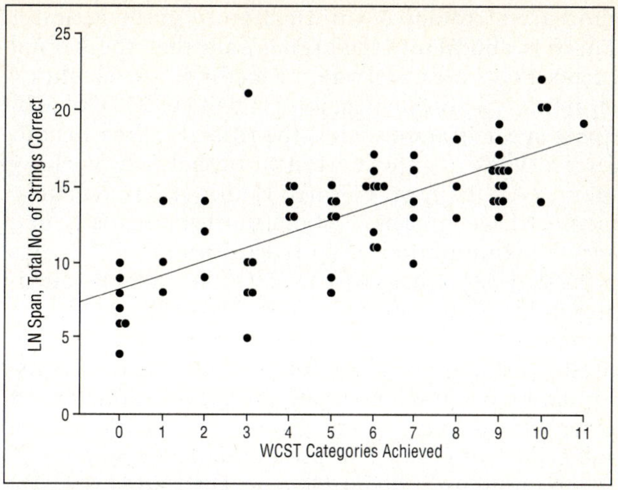

The relationship of letter-number (LN) span and Wisconsin Card Sorting Test (WCST) category scores. The line across the figure is a regression line.

of this issue "Reasoning Ability Is (Little More Than) Working Memory Capacity!"

Unexpectedly, it appears that working memory is a critical determinant of WCST success, but not of perseveration. This finding is surprising since the WCST category and perseveration scores are highly intercorrelated. Furthermore, the computer model of Kimberg and Farah[18] suggests working memory impairment has an adverse impact on both categories achieved and perseverative errors, and both scores are impaired in patients with frontal lobe lesions.[24] Thus, the present results suggesting a partial dissociation between these scores should be regarded with caution.

Clearly there are multiple ways to fail on the WCST, and being perseverative is only 1 of them. The predictors of perseveration that contributed unique variance beyond general cognitive competence include Trail Making Test part B, verbal fluency, and the CPT, measures requiring set shifting, selective attention, and response generation with little working memory demand. Possibly the severity of working memory impairment is not predictive of perseveration beyond a threshold, after which other cognitive variables become primary. Thus, the failure of the LN span to emerge as a significant independent predictor in the regressions should not be taken to mean that working memory is unrelated to perseveration. There was a significant correlation between these measures in Table 2, and the ANCOVA removing the effect of the LN span eliminated the group difference on perseveration. These preliminary data suggesting that WCST success and failure have somewhat different predictors add further evidence of the multifactorial nature of the WCST and, perhaps, of the cognitive domains that are mediated by the frontal cortex.

ASSESSMENT OF WORKING MEMORY

Despite the widespread popularity of the working memory construct, the definition of the construct varies. Research with nonhuman primates has been focused on delayed response tasks that require the short-term storage of information to guide action.[12] There is abundant converging data that the frontal cortex plays a critical role in mediating such short-term information storage, with recent evidence of anatomic specialization within the frontal cortex for different types of information to be held in working memory.[36] Human cognitive models of working memory have emphasized both short-term storage and active manipulation of stored information.[17] It has been suggested that short-term storage may be mediated by modality-specific "slave" systems, while the frontal cortex functions as an executive control system needed for more complex forms of information transformation.[17] Thus, the anatomic implications of the research on humans and nonhuman primates are somewhat different. The present data are relevant to this issue in an indirect fashion. Digit span requires passive storage, and lesion evidence suggests it is primarily mediated by posterior cortical areas.[37] Covarying digit span did not eliminate group differences in LN span or the WCST. Thus, the demand to perform multiple operations on a piece of information rather than simple storage appears to be the critical feature, the work of working memory, which is related to more complex forms of problem solving in which patients with schizophrenia demonstrate impairment.

Studies of normal subjects have documented the importance of working memory for several cognitive tasks, including reasoning and language comprehension.[17,38] Such relationships would likely be amplified in disorders that compromise working memory, and an impairment of working memory may well be responsible for some of the generalized deficit seen in schizophrenia. Indeed, the fact that an impairment of working memory should have generalized consequences is an appealing aspect of the construct for the study of schizophrenia, where a great deal of energy has been spent in attempts to demonstrate "differential deficits" and little effort has been expended on the cognitive underpinnings of generalized impairment.

The present study has a number of limitations. The NIMH Neuropsychiatric Research Hospital is a tertiary care research facility, and the present findings need to be replicated in other patient samples. Furthermore, the between-group ANCOVAs had limited power given our sample sizes. All patients underwent evaluation while receiving medication. Although there is evidence that antipsychotic medications enhance performance on measures of auditory distractibility that resemble the LN span,[39] the possibility that the observed deficits are secondary to treatment effects cannot be ruled out or tested on the basis of the present data, given nonrandom assignment of medication type and dose. We did not examine the relationship between working memory and symptomatic state, an issue that may bear on the generalizability of the current results.

The cognitive-anatomic framework we have adopted is somewhat speculative, as we do not have direct data, either from functional neuroimaging or from the study of patients with focal lesions, linking LN span performance and frontal lobe function. The fact that patients with schizophrenia perform poorly cannot be seen as direct evidence for this anatomic link, given data suggesting widespread structural and functional compromise in the illness. Furthermore, interpretation of the correlations between LN span and the WCST is complicated by the fact that the WCST is clearly not only a test of frontal lobe function. These interpretive complications can only be clarified by further normative and clinical studies. The present data suggest that the LN span and other putative tests of working memory may provide important tools for understanding the cognitive underpinnings of executive function in schizophrenia and perhaps other illness.

The poor performance of patients with schizophrenia on the categories-achieved measure of the WCST may be largely attributed to a failure in working memory as assessed by LN span. Although LN span correlated with the perseveration score, it appears that other cognitive variables are needed to account for the extent of perseveration frequently encountered in schizophrenia. An inability to simultaneously store and manipulate information likely precludes success in abstraction and hypothesis testing. Thus, an impairment of working memory may be involved in many of the cognitive deficits observed in schizophrenia that are typically attributed to frontal lobe dysfunction.

Accepted for publication February 5, 1996.

Reprints: James M. Gold, PhD, Maryland Psychiatric Research Center, PO Box 21247, Baltimore, MD 21228.

REFERENCES

1. Kraepelin E; Barclay RM, trans. *Dementia Praecox*. Edinburgh, Scotland: E & S Livingstone; 1971.
2. Kolb B, Whishaw IQ. Performance of schizophrenic patients on tests sensitive to left or right, frontal, temporal or parietal function in neurological patients. *J Nerv Ment Dis*. 1983;171:435-443.
3. Suddath RL, Christison GW, Torrey EF, Weinberger DR. Cerebral anatomical abnormalities in monozygotic twins discordant for schizophrenia. *N Engl J Med*. 1990;322:789-794.
4. Saykin AJ, Gur RC, Gur RE, Mozley D, Mozley LH, Resnick SM, Kester DB, Stafiniak P. Neuropsychological function in schizophrenia: selective impairment in memory and learning. *Arch Gen Psychiatry*. 1991;48:141-162.
5. Goldberg TE, Ragland DR, Gold J, Bigelow LB, Torrey EF, Weinberger DR. Neuropsychological assessment of monozygotic twins discordant for schizophrenia. *Arch Gen Psychiatry*. 1990;147:1066-1072.
6. Weinberger DR, Berman KF, Zec RF. Physiological dysfunction of dorsolateral prefrontal cortex in schizophrenia, I: regional cerebral blood flow (rCBF) evidence. *Arch Gen Psychiatry*. 1986;43:114-125.
7. Goldberg TE, Weinberger DR, Berman KF, Pliskin NH, Podd M. Further evidence for dementia of the prefrontal type in schizophrenia? *Arch Gen Psychiatry*. 1987;44:1008-1014.
8. Anderson SW, Damasio H, Jones RD, Tranel D. Wisconsin Card Sorting Test performance as a measure of frontal lobe damage. *J Clin Exp Neuropsychol*. 1991;13:909-922.
9. Grafman J, Jonas B, Salazar A. Wisconsin Card Sorting Test performance based on location and size of neuroanatomical lesion in Vietnam veterans with penetrating head injury. *Percept Mot Skills*. 1990;71:1120-1122.
10. Hyde TM, Casanova MF, Kleinman JE, Weinberger DR. Neuroanatomical and neurochemical pathology in schizophrenia. In: Tasman A, Goldfinger SM, eds. *Review of Psychiatry*. Washington, DC: American Psychiatric Press; 1991;10: 7-23.
11. Braff DL, Heaton R, Kuck J, Cullum M, Moranville J, Grant I, Zisook S. The generalized pattern of neuropsychological deficits in outpatients with chronic schizophrenia with heterogeneous Wisconsin Card Sorting Test results. *Arch Gen Psychiatry*. 1991;48:891-898.
12. Goldman-Rakic PS. Circuitry of primate prefrontal cortex and regulation of behavior by representational knowledge. In: Plum F, Mountcastle V, eds. *Hand-*

book of Physiology: The Nervous System. Bethesda, Md: American Physiological Society; 1987;5:373-417.
13. Funahashi S, Chafee MV, Goldman-Rakic PS. Prefrontal neuronal activity in rhesus monkeys performing a delayed anti-saccade task. *Nature.* 1993;365: 753-756.
14. Jonides J, Smith ES, Koeppe RA, Awh E, Minoshima S, Minun MA. Spatial working memory in humans as revealed by PET. *Nature.* 1993;363:623-625.
15. Gold JM, Berman KF, Randolph C, Goldberg TE, Weinberger DR. PET validation of a novel prefrontal task: delayed response alternation. *Neuropsychology.* 1996;10:3-10.
16. Petrides M, Alivisatos B, Meyer E, Evans AC. Functional activation of the human frontal cortex during the performance of verbal working memory tasks. *Proc Natl Acad Sci U S A.* 1993;90:878-882.
17. Baddeley A. *Working Memory.* New York, NY: Oxford University Press Inc; 1986.
18. Kimberg DY, Farah MJ. A unified account of cognitive impairments following frontal lobe damage: the role of working memory in complex, organized behavior. *J Exp Psychol Gen.* 1993;122:411-428.
19. Park S, Holzman PS. Schizophrenics show spatial working memory deficits. *Arch Gen Psychiatry.* 1992;49:975-982.
20. American Psychiatric Association. *Diagnostic and Statistical Manual of Mental Disorders, Third Edition, Revised.* Washington, DC: American Psychiatric Association; 1987.
21. Spitzer RL, Williams JDW. *Structured Clinical Interview for DSM-III-R.* New York, NY: New York Psychiatric Institute, Biomedical Research Division; 1985.
22. Wechsler D. *Wechsler Adult Intelligence Scale–Revised.* New York, NY: Psychological Corporation; 1981.
23. Wechsler D. *Wechsler Memory Scale–Revised.* New York, NY: Psychological Corporation; 1987.
24. Heaton RK, Chelune GJ, Talley JL, Kay GG, Curtiss G. *Wisconsin Card Sorting Test, Manual.* Odessa, Fla: Psychological Assessment Resources; 1993.
25. Jastak S, Wilkinson GS. *The Wide Range Achievement Test–Revised.* Wilmington, Delaware: Jastak Associates; 1984.
26. Bornstein RA, Leason M. Effects of localized lesions on the Verbal Concept Attainment Test. *J Clin Exp Neuropsychol.* 1985;7:421-429.
27. Kaplan EF, Goodglass H, Weintraub S. *The Boston Naming Test.* Philadelphia, Pa: Lea & Febiger; 1983.
28. Gordon Systems. *Gordon Diagnostic System.* Dewitt, NY: Gordon Systems; 1987.
29. Reitan RM, Wolfson D. *The Halstead-Reitan Neuropsychological Test Battery.* Tucson, Ariz: Neuropsychology Press; 1985.
30. Benton AL, Hamsher K deS: *Multilingual Aphasia Examination.* Iowa City, Iowa: AJA Associates, 1989.
31. Kaufman AS. *Assessing Adolescent and Adult Intelligence.* Boston, Mass: Allyn & Bacon Inc; 1990.
32. Silverstein AB. Two- and four-subtest short forms of the Wechsler Adult Intelligence Scale–Revised. *J Consult Clin Psychol.* 1982;50:415-418.
33. Sullivan EV, Mathalon DH, Zipursky RB, Kersteen-Tucker Z, Knight RT, Pfefferbaum A. Factors of the Wisconsin Card Sorting Tests as measures of frontal-lobe function in schizophrenia and chronic alcoholism. *Psychiatry Res.* 1993; 46:175-199.
34. Dehaene S, Changeux JP. The Wisconsin Card Sorting Test: theoretical analysis and modeling in a neuronal network. *Cereb Cortex.* 1991;1:62-79.
35. Kyllonen PC, Christal RE. Reasoning ability is (little more than) working memory capacity. *Intelligence.* 1990;14:389-433.
36. Wilson FAW, Scalaidhe SPO, Goldman-Rakic PS. Dissociation of object and spatial processing domains in primate prefrontal cortex. *Science.* 1993;260: 1955-1958.
37. Shallice T, Vallar G. The impairment of auditory-verbal short-term storage. In: Vallar G, Shallice T, eds. *Neuropsychological Impairments of Short-term Memory.* New York, NY: Cambridge University Press; 1990:11-53.
38. Daneman M, Carpenter PAA. Individual differences in working memory and reading. *J Verbal Learning Verbal Behav.* 1980;19:450-466.
39. Spohn HE, Strauss ME. Relation of neuroleptic and anticholinergic medication to cognitive functions in schizophrenia. *J Abnorm Psychol.* 1989;98: 367-380.

ESTABLISHED THERAPY FOR OCD

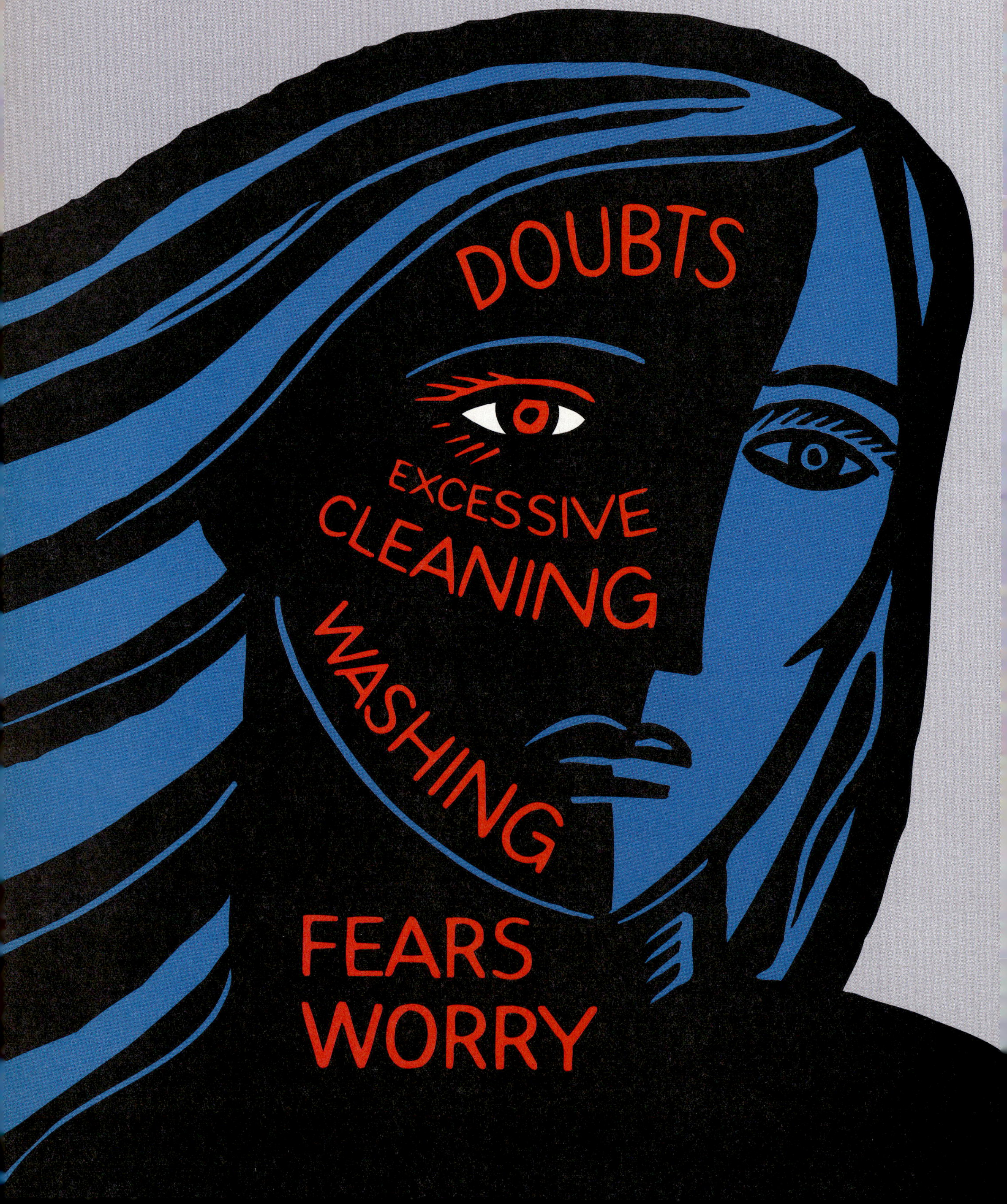

ORIGINAL ARTICLE

Eye Tracking, Attention, and Schizotypal Symptoms in Nonpsychotic Relatives of Patients With Schizophrenia

Richard S. E. Keefe, PhD; Jeremy M. Silverman, PhD; Richard C. Mohs, PhD; Larry J. Siever, MD; Philip D. Harvey, PhD; Lee Friedman, PhD; Sonia E. Lees Roitman; Rachel L. DuPre; Christopher J. Smith; James Schmeidler, PhD; Kenneth L. Davis, MD

Background: Biological relatives of patients with schizophrenia demonstrate an increased prevalence of schizotypal personality disorder symptoms, eye tracking deficits, and attentional disturbances. We investigated whether these hypothesized components of a schizophrenia-related phenotype are associated with one another or are independent in nonpsychotic relatives of patients with schizophrenia.

Methods: Eighty-three nonpsychotic first-degree relatives of 38 patients with schizophrenia and 45 control subjects without a psychiatric diagnosis underwent clinical evaluation, eye tracking evaluation, and the Continuous Performance Test (CPT) of visual attention.

Results: Eye tracking qualitative rating was more powerful than quantitative eye tracking measures or CPT measures in discriminating relatives of patients with schizophrenia from control subjects. Correlations between neurocognitive variables and *DSM-III-R* schizotypal personality disorder symptom clusters suggested that CPT errors of omission are associated with positive schizotypal symptoms. Eye tracking measures were not significantly correlated with schizotypal symptoms or CPT errors in relatives of patients with schizophrenia.

Conclusions: Eye tracking deficits in the relatives of patients with schizophrenia are unrelated to CPT deficits and schizotypal symptoms. Eye tracking deficits and disturbances in visual attention may be separate components of a schizophrenia-related phenotype and should be considered as independent factors in genetic studies of schizophrenia.

Arch Gen Psychiatry. 1997;54:169-176

FIRST-DEGREE relatives of individuals with schizophrenia have an increased risk for development of schizophrenia[1-4] or schizotypal personality disorder symptoms[1,2,5,6] and are more likely to have neurocognitive deficits such as poor eye tracking and attentional disturbances.[7-11] The familial aggregation of schizophrenia and schizotypal symptoms among relatives of patients with schizophrenia in twin and adoption studies suggests that these symptoms are partially determined by genetic factors.[1-3,5,6] Eye movement dysfunction also appears to have a substantial genetic component, as suggested by studies of twins.[12,13] If a single factor predisposes individuals to schizotypal personality disorder symptoms and to various neurocognitive deficits such as poor eye tracking and attentional disturbances, these personality and neurocognitive factors should be correlated in patients with schizophrenia and their relatives. Conversely, the independence of these factors in discriminating patients with schizophrenia and their relatives from control subjects would suggest that these factors derive from independent sources.[14]

Previous attempts to address this issue have been hampered by various methodological weaknesses, such as the assessment of schizotypal symptoms with brief clinical interviews[15,16] or questionnaires,[15] which do not measure enduring personality features and are likely to underestimate psychopathological features when compared with extensive interview procedures.[17,18] Furthermore, previous studies addressing the relationship between neurocognitive measures and schizotypal personality characteristics have not matched

From the Department of Psychiatry, Mount Sinai School of Medicine, New York, and the Bronx Veterans Affairs Medical Center, Bronx, NY (Drs Keefe, Silverman, Mohs, Siever, Harvey, Schmeidler, and Davis, Mss Lees Roitman and DuPre, and Mr Smith); and the Laboratory of Biological Psychiatry, Case Western Reserve University, Cleveland, Ohio (Dr Friedman). Dr Keefe is now affiliated with the Department of Psychiatry, Duke University Medical Center, Durham, NC.

SUBJECTS AND METHODS

SUBJECTS

All subjects were recruited, received a diagnosis, and underwent assessment at the Bronx Veterans Affairs Medical Center (Bronx, NY), Pilgrim State Psychiatric Center (West Brentwood, NY), or Mount Sinai Medical Center (New York, NY). Written informed consent was obtained from each subject before study participation. A subgroup of these subjects was included in a previous study on the performance of relatives of probands with schizophrenia on cognitive tests.[19] Fifty-four (65%) of the 83 subjects were female (χ^2=11.80).

Relatives of Patients With Schizophrenia

The family histories of all patients with schizophrenia as well as those of patients with other psychiatric disorders who are participants in our clinical research programs are routinely evaluated. Family history interviewers are unaware of proband diagnosis and have no prior knowledge of family structure. Following this initial evaluation, all available first-degree relatives from families potentially informative for genetic linkage studies of schizophrenia underwent personal evaluation. For the present study, 38 families ascertained through probands meeting *DSM-III-R*[20] criteria for chronic schizophrenia were interviewed and received a diagnosis. Twenty-four of these families were selected because family history evaluation suggested secondary cases of schizophrenia or schizotypal personality disorder. The remaining 14 families were selected randomly from all families of probands with schizophrenia evaluated at our research center who had first-degree relatives living locally. Each proband was interviewed with the Schedule for Affective Disorders and Schizophrenia–Lifetime Version[21] or the Comprehensive Assessment of Symptoms and History.[22] Patients were interviewed by 2 trained raters who observed the same interview, then made diagnoses independently. Relatives with medical illnesses with central nervous system effects were excluded from the study. Since psychosis and related factors such as long-term treatment may interfere with neurocognitive performance in a manner unrelated to familial factors,[23-26] 6 relatives with schizophrenia, 4 relatives with schizoaffective disorder, and 3 relatives with other psychotic disorders were excluded from the study. Relatives were included only if English was their first language. Eighty-three nonpsychotic first-degree relatives (29 men and 54 women) of 38 patients with schizophrenia were included in the study. The relatives consisted of 10 parents, 68 siblings, and 5 children of the probands. Nine relatives from 9 different families met criteria for schizotypal personality disorder and were included in this study.

Control Subjects

Forty-five control subjects (30 men and 15 women) were recruited from the community through newspaper advertisements. All control subjects were given medical and neurological examinations to rule out those with illnesses that might affect test performance and underwent screening for psychiatric diagnoses using the Schedule for Affective Disorders and Schizophrenia–Lifetime Version, the Personality Disorders Questionnaire,[27] and additional screening questions for assessing odd cluster and borderline personality symptoms in nonpsychiatric populations (J.M.S., Robert L. Trestman, MD, PhD, unpublished questionnaire, June 15, 1991). Subjects were included in the control group only if they had never had *DSM-III-R* Axis I or odd cluster personality disorder diagnoses. Potential control subjects were asked if any first-degree relatives had schizophrenia; only those who had no family history of schizophrenia were included in the study.

Relatives and control subjects were strictly warned not to ingest any psychoactive substances, including alcohol, for the 48 hours before testing. All subjects underwent evaluation with an interview to determine if they had used psychoactive substances, and 32 were given intoxication breath tests to evaluate blood alcohol levels. Six relatives and 1 control subject demonstrating evidence of alcohol or other substance abuse were excluded from the study. To minimize possible confounding effects of age on neurocognitive variables, subjects were included in the study only if their age ranged from 18 to 55 years.

Demographic characteristics and general intelligence factors are presented in **Table 1**. Relatives were more likely to be female and performed more poorly on the Vocabulary and Block design subtests of the Wechsler Adult Intelligence Scale–Revised.

DIAGNOSTIC METHODS AND PERSONALITY DISORDER SYMPTOM ASSESSMENT IN RELATIVES

Face-to-face interviews with all relatives were conducted using the Schedule for Affective Disorders and Schizophrenia–Lifetime Version for Research Diagnostic Criteria and *DSM-III-R* Axis I diagnosis. In addition, interviews were conducted with all nonpsychotic relatives using the Structured Interview for *DSM-III* Personality Disorders,[28] which permits the collection of detailed information regarding the relative's personality characteristics, behavior, and functioning. In studies of personality disorder using interviews conducted by the raters at our center, the instrument has shown good interrater reliability (κ=0.78) for *DSM-III-R* schizotypal personality disorder and for each of the 8 associated features (magical thinking, κ=0.86; ideas of reference, κ=0.72; social isolation, κ=0.73; recurrent illusions, κ=0.74; odd speech, κ=0.79; inadequate rapport, κ=0.67; suspiciousness or paranoia, κ=0.60; and undue social anxiety, κ=0.79). The test-retest reliability for schizotypal personality disorder is also good (κ=0.73). Informant interviews with friends or family members were used on every relative to supplement the assessment. Identical diagnostic interviews with family members of probands without schizophrenia were also conducted to maintain the raters' unawareness of proband diagnosis. At a meeting led by a diagnostic expert who was one of us (L.J.S.) and was

relatives of patients with schizophrenia and control subjects for factors such as age and general intelligence. Finally, a comparison of the relative discriminating power of qualitative ratings of eye tracking performance and quantitative measures such as smooth pursuit gain and saccadic frequency has not been made in this population.

The purposes of the present study were to deterunaware of proband diagnosis, final diagnoses and diagnostic ratings for each item associated with the Axis I and II ratings were derived in each relative.

Since schizotypal symptoms may have different heritabilities,[6,29,30] with negative schizotypal symptoms such as social isolation demonstrating a greater familial aggregation,[30] the 9 *DSM-III-R* criteria for schizotypal personality disorder were organized into the following 3 clusters of symptoms: "psychotic-like" or positive (ideas of reference, odd beliefs, unusual perceptions, and suspiciousness); "deficit-like" or negative (no close friends and constricted affect); and other (social anxiety, odd behavior, and odd speech).

NEUROCOGNITIVE TESTING PROCEDURES

The tasks described herein, administered in random order, were part of a 4-hour battery of tests that included a small battery of neuropsychological tests described in a previous report.[19] Administration of the tests described herein preceded administration of the neuropsychological tests.

Eye Tracking

An infrared light source was affixed to a set of eyeglass frames so that the source was positioned several millimeters from the surface of 1 eye just below its center. Head position was fixed with a chin and head support, and the eyeglass frames were securely attached to the subject's head to minimize head movement artifact. The eye tracking trials were run on a portable computer (software provided by Steve Flanagan, PhD, of the Beckman Research Institute, City of Hope National Medical Center, Duarte, Calif). Data were digitized at a rate of 500 Hz per channel. Stimulus presentation was on a monochrome video monitor.

Sinusoidal and constant velocity trials were presented. For the sinusoidal trials, a white X on the computer screen traversed 24° of visual angle on a horizontal line at a rate of 0.4 Hz/s (average target velocity, 19.1°/s; peak velocity, 30.1°/s). For the constant velocity trial, the same target moved at a constant velocity (19.2°/s). Four different conditions for eye tracking trials were used. The first trial was used as a practice trial to ensure that subjects understood the task and that adjustment to the task was not mistaken for legitimate eye tracking deficits. The remaining 3 trials consisted of the sinusoidal motion trial, the constant velocity trial, and a sinusoidal motion target that changed from X to O in a random, irregular sequence, during which the subject was asked to count the number of target changes.

Qualitative Rating. The degree of eye tracking impairment was assessed by 2 raters unaware of subject identification and diagnosis using global qualitative ratings from 1 (best) to 5 (worst), following exemplars produced by Shagass et al.[31] Eye blinks and periods when the subject was not tracking were not included in the assessment. Interrater reliability, determined on a subsample of eye tracking records, was high (intraclass correlation=0.85; df=1, 72; $P<.001$). Interrater reliability between our raters and Philip Holzman, PhD, was also high (intraclass correlation=0.96; df=1, 28; $P<.001$). Average performance in the 3 trials was used as a final measure of eye tracking qualitative rating. Qualitative ratings made in our laboratory have been shown to be highly correlated with ranked root mean square error (r=0.87).[32] The correlation between natural logarithm of signal-to-noise ratio and qualitative rating has also been reported to be high (0.82-0.86).[33]

Smooth Pursuit Gain. This measure was quantified in the laboratory of one of us (L.F.) who was unaware of diagnosis. Only the constant velocity trials were used. Gain was scored by methods fully described in several previous publications.[32,34-36] Briefly, gain was defined as the ratio of the eye position slope to the target position slope. Not all of the recordings were scored for gain. In 13 cases (8 relatives and 5 control subjects), artifacts such as head movement and sporadic electrophysiological noise resulted in the collection of eye tracking data that were insufficient to allow a meaningful gain calculation.

Number of Small and Large Saccades. The constant velocity trials were evaluated by 2 independent raters to determine the number of small (<5°) or large (≥5°) saccades per trial. Interrater reliability of this determination is high at our center (intraclass correlation=0.90).[35] Discrepant ratings for saccades were resolved by consensus with one of us (L.J.S.).

Continuous Performance Test

The 3-7 version of the CPT was presented on a portable computer with a monochrome video monitor.[37] A series of white digits were presented in the center of the video monitor in a quasirandom sequence. Each of 5 contiguous sets of 100 stimuli contained 10 target sequences (a 7 immediately preceded by a 3), ten 7s not preceded by a 3, and ten 3s not followed by a 7. Each digit was presented for 50 milliseconds with an interstimulus interval of 1.0 second.

To ensure that the subject fully understood the nature of the task, a brief training trial preceded the collection of test data. Data were generated concerning the number of hits, correct rejections, and errors of omission and commission.

DATA ANALYSES

To determine the appropriateness of parametric statistics for each variable, the distributions of all variables were examined within each group for significant skew, kurtosis, and heterogeneity of variance. If distributions were nonnormal or the variance was heterogeneous, standard transformations were applied. Eye tracking qualitative rating, gain, and numbers of small and large saccades required no transformation. Errors of omission and commission were transformed to $logarithm_{10}$ values; the number of schizotypal symptoms in each cluster was transformed by taking the square root of each.

mine (1) which eye tracking and Continuous Performance Test (CPT) measures best discriminate nonpsychotic relatives of patients with schizophrenia from persons without psychiatric illness who were matched for age and intelligence and (2) whether poor eye tracking, visual attentive disturbances measured by the CPT, and schizotypal symptoms measured by extensive interviews reflect independent or correlated

Table 1. Demographic Characteristics of the Sample*

	Relatives		Comparison Subjects				
	Mean (SD)	No.	Mean (SD)	No.	*t*	*df*	*P*
Age, y	35.4 (10.6)	83	35.9 (9.8)	45	0.30	126	NS
WAIS-R Vocabulary	9.9 (3.2)	78	11.5 (2.5)	37	2.66	113	<.01
WAIS-R Block design	9.8 (2.5)	38	11.3 (3.0)	36	2.31	72	<.05
Education, y	13.7 (2.5)	78	14.4 (2.3)	45	1.42	121	NS
% Female	. . .		33		. . .	1	<.001

**WAIS-R indicates Wechsler Adult Intelligence Scale–Revised; NS, not significant.*

Table 2. ET and CPT Performance in Relatives of Patients With Schizophrenia and Control Subjects*

	Relatives	Control Subjects	*t*	*df*	*P*
ET measures					
Smooth pursuit gain	0.77±0.13 (46)	0.76±0.12 (25)	0.27	69	NS
Average qualitative rating	2.64±0.46 (64)	2.28±0.64 (34)	3.20	96	.002
Small saccades	35.35±14.07 (60)	29.83±12.00 (35)	1.94	93	.06
Large saccades	7.72±6.14 (60)	8.40±7.84 (35)	0.47	93	NS
CPT measures					
$Logarithm_{10}$ errors of omission	−0.50±0.68 (74)	−0.37±0.68 (37)	−0.93	109	NS
$Logarithm_{10}$ errors of commission	−0.60±0.60 (74)	−0.80±0.43 (37)	1.76	109	.08

**Consists of unmatched samples. ET indicates eye tracking; CPT, Continuous Performance Test; and NS, not significant. Data are given as mean±SD. Numbers in parentheses indicate number of participants.*

areas of dysfunction in the nonpsychotic relatives of patients with schizophrenia.

RESULTS

ANALYSES OF THE ENTIRE SAMPLE

Analysis of Potential Confounding Variables

The proportion of subjects who smoked cigarettes on the day of testing was not significantly different in the relatives (15 [22%] of 69) and control subjects (4 [11%] of 35) (χ^2=1.65; *df*=1; NS). The proportions of subjects who habitually smoked cigarettes (18 [26%] of 69 vs 6 [17%] of 35) (χ^2=1.05; *df*=1; NS) or who drank caffeinated beverages on the day of testing were also not significantly different (36 [53%] of 68 vs 16 [46%] of 35) (χ^2=0.48; *df*=1; NS). The time of day at testing (before vs after noon) was also not significantly different between groups, as 31 (45%) of 69 relatives and 19 (54%) of 35 control subjects began testing before noon (χ^2=0.57; *df*=1; NS). Most importantly, the correlations of cigarette and caffeine use and time of day at testing with the eye tracking and CPT variables used in this study were small in the entire sample and in the separate group of relatives (range, −0.18 to 0.22), and none was statistically significant. Therefore, these potential confounding variables were not used as covariates in subsequent analyses.

Eye Tracking

Results of eye tracking were significantly worse among the relatives than the control subjects as measured by qualitative ratings, but smooth pursuit gain and number of large saccades were not significantly different between groups. There was a statistical trend for the number of small saccades to be different between groups (**Table 2**).

Continuous Performance Test

The overall error rate for relatives and control subjects was less than 1%, indicating that this was a relatively easy version of the CPT for these subjects. There was a statistical trend for relatives to make more errors of commission ($logarithm_{10}$ transformed) on the CPT than the control subjects. The number of errors of omission was not significantly different between groups.

MATCHED ANALYSES

To minimize the effect of any cluster of related individuals, 24 relatives from 24 different families of patients with

Table 3. Variance in Group Membership Accounted for by CPT and ET Variables*

Variable	R^2 Change	F Change	*df*	*P*	Total R^2	F	*df*	*P*
WAIS-R Vocabulary	0.073	3.60	1, 46	.06	0.073	3.60	1, 46	.06
ET qualitative rating	0.109	6.01	1, 45	.02	0.182	5.01	2, 45	.01
Large saccades	0.053	3.09	1, 44	.09	0.235	3.81	3, 44	.001
All other variables	0.078	1.56	3, 41	NS	0.314	3.12	6, 41	.01

**Results derived from multiple regression analysis. CPT indicates Continuous Performance Test; ET, eye tracking; WAIS-R, Wechsler Adult Intelligence Scale–Revised; and NS, not significant.*

schizophrenia were compared with 24 control subjects. These relatives and control subjects were chosen solely on the basis of a matching procedure. First, relatives and control subjects were matched by age. To covary for generalized performance deficits in the relatives, subjects were also matched on the within-group standardized score on the Wechsler Adult Intelligence Scale–Revised Vocabulary subtest.

The matched analyses produced results (expressed as mean±SD) that were very similar to those for the entire group. Again, the average qualitative rating was significantly poorer in the relatives compared with the control subjects (2.71±0.52 vs 2.28±0.60, respectively [t=2.61; df=46; P=.01). The average number of large saccades (8.75±6.97 vs 10.00±8.64, respectively [t=0.55; df=46; NS) and average smooth pursuit gain scores (0.79±0.10 vs 0.75±0.12, respectively [t=1.00; df=33; NS) did not differ significantly between groups, and there was a statistical trend for the number of small saccades to be greater in relatives than in control subjects (37.96±16.84 vs 30.79±12.23, respectively [t=1.69; df=46; P=.10). Neither logarithm_{10} CPT errors of omission nor logarithm_{10} errors of commission differentiated the groups in the matched analyses.

RELATIVE DISCRIMINATING POWER OF NEUROCOGNITIVE MEASURES

The first regression analysis was performed to determine whether significant variance in group membership was accounted for by numbers of large and small saccades and logarithm_{10} CPT errors of omission and commission beyond those accounted for by qualitative eye tracking and vocabulary scores. The order of entry into the regression equation was determined a priori; the vocabulary score was entered first, followed by the qualitative eye tracking score, followed by the other variables in hierarchical order. Since 7 of the matched subjects did not have smooth pursuit gain scores, this variable was not included in this analysis. These subjects did not differ from the rest of the sample on any of the eye tracking or CPT variables. As indicated in **Table 3**, the vocabulary score accounted for 7.3% of the between-group variance, which was at a trend level of statistical significance. Average eye tracking qualitative rating accounted for an additional 10.9% of the between-group variance. Number of large saccades accounted for an additional 5.3% of the variance in the direction of relatives having fewer large saccades than control subjects. None of the remaining variables accounted for significant additional variance. When the order of entry into the equation was reversed so that CPT variables were entered immediately after the vocabulary score, they did not account for significant variance.

Table 4. Between-Family Correlations Between *DSM-III-R* Symptoms for Schizotypal Personality Disorder and Neurocognitive Measures*

	Square Root of No. of Schizotypal Personality Disorder Symptoms		
Neurocognitive Measures	Positive	Negative	Other
Logarithm_{10} CPT errors of omission (34 families)	0.44†	0.23	0.02
Logarithm_{10} CPT errors of commission (34 families)	0.32‡	0.30‡	0.17
ET qualitative rating (33 families)	0.06	0.12	−0.07
Smooth pursuit gain (23 families)	−0.09	−0.01	0.11

**CPT indicates Continuous Performance Test; ET, eye tracking.*
†P<.01.
‡P<.10.

To determine the contribution of smooth pursuit gain to the variance in group membership, an additional regression analysis was performed excluding 7 pairs of matched subjects without gain data. In this analysis, 17 relatives and 17 matched control subjects were compared. The vocabulary score accounted for 6.2% of the between-group variance (F=2.20; df=1, 33; NS). Average eye tracking qualitative rating accounted for an additional 26.6% of the between-group variance (F=12.68; df=1, 32; P=.001), and smooth pursuit gain accounted for an additional 12.7% (F=7.20; df=1, 31; P=.01). None of the remaining variables accounted for significant additional variance. Again, when the order of entry into the equation was reversed so that CPT variables were entered immediately after the vocabulary score, they did not account for significant variance.

RELATIONSHIP OF NEUROCOGNITIVE VARIABLES TO SCHIZOTYPAL SYMPTOMS

In correlational analyses including each relative of a proband with schizophrenia, logarithm_{10} CPT errors of omission were correlated with the square root of positive schizotypal symptoms from *DSM-III-R* criteria for schizotypal personality disorder (r=0.39; df=67; P=.001). No other symptom factor was significantly correlated with logarithm_{10} CPT errors of omission or any of the other neurocognitive measures.

When the family was considered the unit of analysis, the average value of each neurocognitive measure and symptom cluster was calculated within each family, including all family members undergoing testing. The between-

Table 5. Between-Family Correlations Among Neurocognitive Measures in Relatives of Patients With Schizophrenia*

	ET Measures				CPT Measures	
Neurocognitive Measures	Qualitative Rating	Smooth Pursuit Gains	No. of Small Saccades	No. of Large Saccades	$Logarithm_{10}$ Errors of Commission	$Logarithm_{10}$ Errors of Omission
ET measures						
Qualitative rating		−0.43 (24)†	0.19 (31)	0.43 (31)†	**0.07** (30)	**−0.13** (30)
Smooth pursuit gain			−0.55 (20)†	−0.29 (20)	**−0.07** (19)	**−0.09** (19)
No. of small saccades				0.22 (31)	**−0.08** (27)	**−0.03** (27)
No. of large saccades					**0.24** (27)	**0.15** (27)
CPT measures						
$Logarithm_{10}$ errors of commission						0.53 (35)‡
$Logarithm_{10}$ errors of omission						

*ET indicates eye tracking; CPT, Continuous Performance Test. Numbers in parentheses indicate number of families in the specific analysis; between-task correlations are presented in boldface type.

†$P<.05$.

‡$P<.001$.

family correlations of schizotypal symptoms and neurocognitive measures are presented in **Table 4**. As in the between-subject analyses, $logarithm_{10}$ CPT errors of omission were significantly correlated with the square root of the number of positive symptoms. $Logarithm_{10}$ CPT errors of commission and eye tracking measures were not significantly correlated with the square root of the number of schizotypal symptoms in any of the 3 symptom factors. The square root of the total number of *DSM-III-R* schizotypal symptoms was not significantly correlated with any of the measures.

Correlational analyses were also performed based on pooled within-family data using analysis of covariance. The pooled within-family correlations support the between-family correlations. Only the pooled within-family regression coefficient between $logarithm_{10}$ CPT errors of omission and the square root of the number of positive schizotypal symptoms was statistically significant ($F=10.38$; $df=1, 33$; $P=.001$).

In sum, only the association of CPT errors of omission with the number of positive symptoms was significant by all 3 correlational techniques.

RELATIONSHIPS AMONG NEUROCOGNITIVE MEASURES IN FAMILIES AND CONTROL SUBJECTS

The between-family correlations among eye tracking and CPT measures are presented in **Table 5**. Each family's average for each measure was included in the analysis. In the families of patients with schizophrenia, none of the correlations between CPT and eye tracking measures reached statistical significance. Three correlations within tasks reached statistical significance. In contrast, in the control subjects, several of the correlations between eye tracking and CPT measures reached statistical significance (**Table 6**).

COMMENT

Qualitative ratings of eye tracking performance were the single best neurocognitive discriminator of nonpsychotic first-degree relatives of individuals with schizophrenia from control subjects without psychiatric illness matched for age and relative general intelligence. Impairments on this measure were unrelated either to schizotypal symptoms or to CPT performance. Errors of omission on the CPT, but none of the other neurocognitive measures, were positively correlated with the number of positive schizotypal symptoms in relatives. These findings are unlikely to be due to the influence of a small number of families with schizophrenia. These results suggest that abnormalities in visual attention as measured by the CPT are another manifestation of the abnormalities that are associated with schizotypal symptoms in the relatives of people with schizophrenia, yet eye tracking abnormalities are independent from schizotypal symptoms and poor visual attention in these relatives.

The superior discriminating power of poor eye tracking compared with CPT deficits in the relatives of patients with schizophrenia is consistent with the findings from studies reporting on these tasks separately. Poor eye tracking has been consistently reported in the adult relatives of patients with schizophrenia,[16,38-40] whereas CPT deficits have been reported consistently only in the children of parents with schizophrenia.[41,42] It remains to be determined whether adult relatives of patients with schizophrenia demonstrate robust attentional deficits of the type assessed by the CPT, as only 1 previous report[43] has indicated significant differences between relatives and control subjects.

Our conclusions should be tempered by a consideration of the psychometric properties of the 2 tasks. The relative discriminative power of poor eye tracking over CPT deficits in this study may be partially attributable to the fact that completing the version of the CPT that we used is easier than eye tracking, and many subjects manifest near-perfect performances. A more difficult CPT may discriminate between control subjects and relatives of probands with schizophrenia and may yield a more normal distribution of performance among relatives than that reported herein, which may allow stronger correlations with schizotypal symptoms and eye tracking variables. Data are currently being collected at our laboratory using a CPT with greater perceptual degradation and

Table 6. Correlations Among Neurocognitive Measures in Control Subjects*

Neurocognitive Measures	ET Measures				CPT Measures	
	Qualitative Rating	Smooth Pursuit Gain	No. of Small Saccades	No. of Large Saccades	$Logarithm_{10}$ Errors of Commission	$Logarithm_{10}$ Errors of Omission
ET measures						
Qualitative rating		−0.48 (24)†	0.46 (33)‡	0.34 (33)†	**0.33** (33)	**0.45** (33)‡
Smooth pursuit gain			−0.18 (25)	−0.59 (25)‡	**−0.42** (25)†	**−0.21** (25)
No. of small saccades				0.28 (35)	**0.23** (34)	**0.41** (34)†
No. of large saccades					**0.44** (34)‡	**0.11** (34)
CPT measures						
$Logarithm_{10}$ errors of commission						0.44 (37)‡
$Logarithm_{10}$ errors of omission						

**ET indicates eye tracking; CPT, Continuous Performance Test. Numbers in parentheses indicate number of subjects in the specific analysis; between-task correlations are presented in boldface type.*
†$P<.05$.
‡$P<.01$.

memory load[41] to determine how different cognitive demands affect the relations between eye tracking and CPT performance.

The qualitative rating of eye tracking performance was clearly superior to quantitative measures in discriminating relatives of patients with schizophrenia from control subjects. Quantitative measures such as smooth pursuit gain and saccadic frequency may identify specific impairments in patients with schizophrenia and their relatives.[32,39,40] However, important aspects of the eye tracking impairment found in the relatives of patients with schizophrenia may not be assessed using these measures. Qualitative and quantitative measures of eye tracking may reflect independent dimensions of disturbance.[32] Our data suggest that measures of overall eye tracking quality may be particularly sensitive to the aspects of eye tracking disturbance found in the relatives of probands with schizophrenia.

Errors of omission on the CPT were correlated with positive schizotypal symptoms in this study. The neurological relationship between attentional disturbances and schizotypal symptoms is unknown. However, CPT tasks activate regions of the frontal cortex.[44] The relatives of patients with schizophrenia, including some of our subjects,[19] perform worse than control subjects on standard neuropsychological tasks sensitive to frontal lobe dysfunction[45] and experimental tests of spatial working memory developed from models of primate prefrontal cortical function.[46] The positive symptoms of schizotypal personality disorder, such as odd beliefs and ideas of reference, may be attributable to a process whereby individuals with schizotypal symptoms and working memory deficits fill the gaps in immediately available external information with internally derived misinterpretations. Although many individuals have mild attentional deficits without the development of schizotypal symptoms, this mechanism could explain their co-occurrence in some relatives of patients with schizophrenia.

Previous studies from our center and others have reported a relationship between schizotypal personality characteristics and poor eye tracking, but these studies have focused exclusively on individuals with schizotypal symptoms ascertained from clinical populations[35,47,48] or have relied on interviews such as the Schedule for Schizotypal Personalities[49] or questionnaires such as the Chapman Scales[50,51] to assess clinical symptoms.[15,16] Our results are at apparent odds with those of previous studies, as they suggest that poor eye tracking and *DSM-III-R* schizotypal personality disorder symptom clusters may be independent factors among the relatives of patients with schizophrenia. First, it is possible that the decreased variance of schizotypal symptoms in relatives compared with clinical populations may partially account for our lower correlations. Second, our results do not rule out the possibility that schizotypal personality characteristics, when assessed as a dimension with self-report questionnaires, may be related to eye tracking deficits in the relatives of patients with schizophrenia. However, while these questionnaires produce a broad range of values, the data they produce are less directly relevant to the clinical aspects of schizotypal personality symptoms than is our comprehensive assessment of *DSM-III-R* schizotypal features throughout the entire course of adult life.

Since eye tracking deficits and schizotypal symptoms were found not to be correlated herein, they may be different schizophrenia-related phenotypes. Consequently, they could be used independently in the identification of affected patients in genetic linkage and segregation studies of schizophrenia. The Holzman-Matthysse model of an autosomal dominant gene with variable phenotypic expression as schizophrenia or eye tracking deficit has been applied to schizophrenia pedigrees.[52] The independence of eye tracking deficits and schizotypal symptoms suggests that a model of variable phenotypic expression that includes schizotypal symptoms may enhance our understanding of the mode of inheritance and expression of a schizophrenia-related gene or genes. The significant correlation between schizotypal symptoms and CPT deficits reported herein suggests that the presence of both of these characteristics in relatives of probands with schizophrenia may serve as a more narrow, and possibly more refined, phenotypic expression that is unrelated to eye tracking disturbance.[9]

Accepted for publication March 26, 1996.

Supported by young investigator awards from the National Alliance for Research on Schizophrenia and Depression, (Dr Keefe); merit review awards from the

Department of Veterans Affairs, Washington, DC (Drs Mohs and Siever); Family Study Core program project grant 45212 from the National Institute of Mental Health, Rockville, Md (Dr Silverman); a schizophrenia research grant from the Benevolent Council Foundation (Scottish Rite), Lexington, Mass (Dr Silverman [principal investigator]); grant 42827-03 from the National Institutes of Health, Bethesda, Md (Dr Siever); and a schizophrenia biological research center grant from the General Medical Research Service of Veterans Affairs, Washington (Bronx Veterans Affairs Medical Center and Dr Davis [principal investigator]).

Reprints: Richard S. E. Keefe, PhD, Department of Psychiatry, Duke University Medical Center, Box 3270, Durham, NC 27710 (email: rsekeefe@acpub.duke.edu).

REFERENCES

1. Kety SS, Rosenthal D, Wender PH. Mental illness in the biological and adoptive families of adopted individuals who have become schizophrenic: a preliminary report based on psychiatric interviews. In: Fieve R, Rosenthal D, Brill H, eds. *Genetic Research in Psychiatry.* Baltimore, Md: The Johns Hopkins University Press; 1975:47-165.
2. Rosenthal D, Wender PH, Kety SS, Welner J, Schulsinger F. The adopted-away offspring of schizophrenics. *Am J Psychiatry.* 1971;128:307-311.
3. Gottesman II, Shields J. Contributions of twin studies to perspectives on schizophrenia. In: Maher BA, ed. *Contributions to the Psychopathology of Schizophrenia.* Orlando, Fla: Academic Press Inc; 1977:169-266.
4. Kety SS, Wender PH, Jacobsen B, Ingraham LJ, Jansson L, Faber B, Kinney DK. Mental illness in the biological and adoptive relatives of schizophrenia adoptees. *Arch Gen Psychiatry.* 1991;51:442-455.
5. Kendler KS, Gruenberg AM, Strauss JS. An independent analysis of the Copenhagen sample of the Danish adoption study of schizophrenia, II: the relationship between schizotypal personality disorder and schizophrenia. *Arch Gen Psychiatry.* 1981;38:982-984.
6. Kendler KS, Ochs AL, Gorman AM, Hewitt JK, Ross DE, Mirsky A. The structure of schizotypy: a multitrait twin study. *Psychiatry Res.* 1991;36:19-36.
7. Holzman PS. Recent studies of psychophysiology in schizophrenia. *Schizophr Bull.* 1987;13:49-75.
8. Nuechterlein KH, Dawson ME. Information processing and attentional functioning in the developmental course of schizophrenic disorders. *Schizophr Bull.* 1984;10:160-203.
9. Keefe RSE, Silverman JM, Siever LJ, Cornblatt BA. Refining phenotype characterization in genetic linkage studies of schizophrenia. *Soc Biol.* 1991;38:197-218.
10. Cornblatt BA, Keilp JG. Impaired attention, genetics, and the pathophysiology of schizophrenia. *Schizophr Bull.* 1994;20:31-46.
11. Levy DL, Holzman PS, Matthysse S, Mendell NR. Eye tracking and schizophrenia: a selective review. *Schizophr Bull.* 1994;20:47-62.
12. Holzman PS, Kringlen E, Levy DL, Haverman S. Deviant eye tracking in twins discordant for psychosis: a replication. *Arch Gen Psychiatry.* 1980;37:627-631.
13. Iacono WG, Lykken DT. Electro-oculographic recording and scoring of smooth-pursuit and saccadic eye tracking: a parametric study using monozygotic twins. *Psychophysiology.* 1979;16:94-107.
14. Meehl PE. Schizotaxia revisited. *Arch Gen Psychiatry.* 1989;46:935-944.
15. Grove WM, Lebow BS, Clementz BA, Cerri A, Medus C, Iacono WG. Familial prevalence and coaggregation of schizotypy indicators: a multitrait family study. *J Abnorm Psychol.* 1991;100:115-121.
16. Clementz BA, Grove WM, Iacono WG, Sweeney JA. Smooth-pursuit eye movement dysfunction and liability for schizophrenia: implications for genetic modeling. *J Abnorm Psychol.* 1992;101:117-129.
17. Andreasen NC, Endicott J, Spitzer RL, Winokur G. The family history method using diagnostic criteria: reliability and validity. *Arch Gen Psychiatry.* 1977; 34:1229-1235.
18. Bernstein DP, Kasapis C, Bergman A, Weld E, Mitropoulou V, Horvath T, Klar HM, Silverman JM, Siever LJ. Assessing Axis II disorders by informant interview. *J Personality Disord.* In press.
19. Keefe RSE, Silverman JM, Roitman SEL, Harvey PD, Duncan MA, Alroy D, Siever LJ, Davis KL, Mohs RC. Performance of nonpsychotic relatives of schizophrenic patients on cognitive tests. *Psychiatry Res.* 1994;53:1-12.
20. American Psychiatric Association. *Diagnostic and Statistical Manual of Mental Disorders, Revised Third Edition.* Washington, DC: American Psychiatric Press; 1987.
21. Endicott J, Spitzer RL. A diagnostic review: the Schedule for Affective Disorders and Schizophrenia. *Arch Gen Psychiatry.* 1978;35:837-844.
22. Andreasen NC, Flaum MA, Arndt S. The Comprehensive Assessment of Symptoms and History (CASH): an instrument for assessing psychopathology and diagnosis. *Arch Gen Psychiatry.* 1992;49:615-623.
23. Keefe RSE. *The Relations Among Backward Masking, Continuous Performance Test, and Eye Tracking Deficits in Schizophrenia.* New York, NY: New York University; 1990. Dissertation.
24. Blackwood DHR, St Clair DM, Juir WJ, Duffy JC. Auditory P300 and eye tracking dysfunction in schizophrenia pedigrees. *Arch Gen Psychiatry.* 1991;48: 899-909.
25. Katsanis J, Iacono WG. Clinical, neuropsychological, and brain structural correlates of smooth-pursuit eye tracking performance in chronic schizophrenia. *J Abnorm Psychol.* 1991;100:526-534.
26. Neale JM, Oltmanns TF, Harvey PD. The need to relate cognitive deficits to specific behavioral referents of schizophrenia. *Schizophr Bull.* 1985;11:286-291.
27. Hyler S, Rieder R, Spitzer R, Williams J. *The Personality Disorders Questionnaire (PDQ).* New York: New York State Psychiatric Institute; 1992.
28. Stangl D, Pfohl B, Zimmerman M, Bower W, Corenthal C. A Structured Interview for the *DSM-III* Personality Disorders. *Arch Gen Psychiatry.* 1985;42: 591-596.
29. Dworkin RH, Lenzenweger MF. Symptoms and the genetics of schizophrenia: implications for diagnosis. *Am J Psychiatry.* 1984;14:1541-1546.
30. Maier W, Lichtermann D, Minges J, Heun R. Personality disorders among the relatives of schizophrenia patients. *Schizophr Bull.* 1994;20:481-493.
31. Shagass C, Amadeo M, Overton DA. Eye tracking performance in psychiatric patients. *Biol Psychiatry.* 1974;4:245-260.
32. Friedman L, Jesberger JA, Siever LJ, Thompson P, Mohs R, Meltzer HY. Smooth pursuit performance in patients with affective disorders or schizophrenia and normal controls: analysis with specific oculomotor measures, RMS error and qualitative ratings. *Psychol Med.* 1995;25:387-403.
33. Lindsey DT, Holzman PS, Haberman S, Yasillo NJ. Smooth-pursuit eye movements: a comparison of two measurement techniques for studying schizophrenia. *J Abnorm Psychol.* 1978;5:491-496.
34. Friedman L, Jesberger JA, Meltzer HY. A model of smooth pursuit performance illustrates the relationship between gain, catch-up saccade rate and catch-up saccade amplitude in normal controls and patients with schizophrenia. *Biol Psychiatry.* 1991;30:537-556.
35. Siever LJ, Friedman L, Moskowitz J, Mitropoulou V, Keefe RSE, Roitman SL, Merhige D, Trestman R, Silverman J, Mohs RC. Eye movement impairment and schizotypal psychopathology. *Am J Psychiatry.* 1994;151:1209-1215.
36. Friedman L, Abel LA, Jesberger J, Malki A, Brar R, Meltzer HY. A methodology for the assessment of smooth pursuit dysfunction. *Int J Meth Psychiatr Res.* 1992;2:209-216.
37. Harvey PD, Keefe RSE, Moskowitz J, Mohs RC, Putnam KM, Davis KL. Attentional markers of vulnerability to schizophrenia: performance of medicated and unmedicated patients and normals. *Psychiatry Res.* 1990;33:179-188.
38. Holzman PS, Proctor LR, Levy DL, Yasillo NJ, Meltzer HY, Hurt SW. Eye tracking dysfunctions in schizophrenia patients and their relatives. *Arch Gen Psychiatry.* 1974;31:143-151.
39. Grove WM, Clementz BA, Iacono WG, Katsanis J. Smooth pursuit ocular motor dysfunction in schizophrenia: evidence for a major gene. *Am J Psychiatry.* 1992;149:1362-1368.
40. Iacono WG, Moreau M, Beiser M, Fleming JAE, Lin T. Smooth-pursuit eye tracking in first-episode psychotic patients and their relatives. *J Abnorm Psychol.* 1992;101:104-116.
41. Cornblatt BA, Erlenmeyer-Kimling L. Global attentional deviance as a marker of risk for schizophrenia: specificity and predictive validity. *J Abnorm Psychol.* 1985;94:470-486.
42. Nuechterlein KH. Signal detection in vigilance tasks and behavioral attributes among offspring of schizophrenic mothers and among hyperactive children. *J Abnorm Psychol.* 1983;92:4-28.
43. Steinhauer SR, Zubin J, Condray R, Shaw DB, Peters JL, van Kammen DP. Electrophysiological and behavioral signs of attentional disturbance in schizophrenics and their siblings. In: Tamminga CA, Schulz SC, eds. *Schizophrenia Research: Advances in Neuropsychiatry and Psychopharmacology.* New York, NY: Raven Press; 1991;1:169-278.
44. Buchsbaum MS, Nuechterlein KH, Haier RJ, Wu J, Sicotte N, Hazlett E, Asarnow R, Potkin S, Guich S. Glucose metabolic rate in normals and schizophrenics during Continuous Performance Test assessed by positron emission tomography. *Br J Psychiatry.* 1990;156:216-227.
45. Kremen WS, Seidman LJ, Pepple JR, Lyons MJ, Tsuang MT, Faraone SV. Neuropsychological risk indicators for schizophrenia: a review of family studies. *Schizophr Bull.* 1994;20:103-119.
46. Park S, Holzman PS, Goldman-Rakic PS. Spatial working memory deficits in the relatives of schizophrenia patients. *Arch Gen Psychiatry.* 1995;52:821-828.
47. Keefe RSE, Siever LJ, Mohs RC, Peterson AE, Mahon TR, Bergman RL, Davis KL. Eye tracking, schizophrenic symptoms, and schizotypal personality disorder. *Eur Arch Psychiatry Clin Neurosci.* 1989;239:39-42.
48. Siever LJ, Keefe RSE, Bernstein DP, Coccaro EF, Klar HM, Zemishlany Z, Peterson AE, Davidson M, Mahon T, Horvath TB, Mohs RC. Eye tracking impairment in clinically identified patients with schizotypal personality disorder. *Am J Psychiatry.* 1990;147:740-745.
49. Baron M, Asnis L, Gruen R. The Schedule for Schizotypal Personalities (SSP): a diagnostic interview for schizotypal features. *Psychiatry Res.* 1981;4:213-228.
50. Chapman LJ, Chapman JP, Raulin ML. Scales for physical and social anhedonia. *J Abnorm Psychol.* 1976;85:374-382.
51. Chapman LJ, Chapman JP, Raulin ML. Body-image aberration in schizophrenia. *J Abnorm Psychol.* 1978;87:399-407.
52. Holzman PS, Kringlen E, Matthysse S, Flanagan S, Lipton RB, Cramer G, Levin S, Lange K, Levy DL. A single dominant gene can account for eye tracking dysfunctions and schizophrenia in offspring of discordant twins. *Arch Gen Psychiatry.* 1988;45:641-647.

Temperance Board Registration for Alcohol Abuse in a National Sample of Swedish Male Twins, Born 1902 to 1949

Kenneth S. Kendler, MD; Carol A. Prescott, PhD; Michael C. Neale, PhD; Nancy L. Pedersen, PhD

Background: Temperance boards were established in Sweden to register and follow up individuals who were seen in legal or medical settings with problems of alcohol abuse. These records, available in a large epidemiologic twin population, have provided an objective and validated measure of alcohol abuse.

Methods: We examined Swedish temperance board registrations from 1929 to 1974 (n=2516 individual twins) in all male-male Swedish twin pairs of known zygosity from the population-based Swedish Twin Registry; these twin pairs were born from 1902 to 1949 (n=8935 pairs).

Results: The lifetime prevalence and probandwise concordance rates for temperance board registrations were 13.2% and 47.9%, respectively, in monozygotic twins and 14.6% and 32.8%, respectively, in dizygotic twins. Model fitting suggested that genetic and familial-environmental risk factors accounted for 54% (95% confidence interval [CI], 47%-61%) and 14% (95% CI, 8%-19%) of the liability to temperance board registration, respectively; these estimates were stable across birth cohorts. High genetic liability was reflected by large numbers of temperance board registrations and registrations for criminal alcohol use. Elevated familial-environmental liability was indicated by an early age at first registration.

Conclusions: Genetic factors are of major etiologic importance for alcohol abuse in men, while familial-environmental factors play a significant but less important role. The etiologic importance of these factors has remained constant in Sweden for men who were born in the first half of the 20th century.

Arch Gen Psychiatry. 1997;54:178-184

IN THE FIRST systematic twin study of alcoholism, Kaij[1] ascertained 310 male twins in southwestern Sweden through temperance boards (TBs), which were established to register and follow up individuals who were seen in legal or medical settings with problems that were related to alcohol abuse.[2-4] Subsequent twin studies of alcoholism have used other information sources, including personal interviews, questionnaires, and medical or disability records.[5-9]

While having advantages, questionnaire or interview assessments of alcohol-related problems—used particularly in recent twin studies[7-9]—also have limitations. Individuals with alcoholism are difficult to contact and refuse to participate at increased rates.[10,11] The assessment of alcoholism in community samples by personal interview is only moderately reliable.[12-14]

In this report, we return to the method of examining temperance board registration (TBR), pioneered by Kaij,[1] in a much expanded sample. Assuming that alcohol abuse in Swedish men can be functionally defined by TBR, we address the following questions: (1) What is the relative importance of genetic and environmental factors in the etiology of alcohol abuse? (2) Has the etiologic role of genetic and environmental factors changed in successive birth cohorts in Sweden during the first half of the 20th century? (3) What characteristics of TBR reflect the familial risk to alcohol abuse, and do these characteristics specifically index genetic vs familial-environmental risk factors?

From the Departments of Psychiatry (Drs Kendler, Prescott, and Neale) and Human Genetics (Dr Kendler), Medical College of Virginia/Virginia Commonwealth University, Richmond, and the Institute of Environmental Medicine, Karolinska Institute, Stockholm, Sweden (Dr Pedersen).

RESULTS

TEMPERANCE BOARD REGISTRATION

Of the 17 870 twins from the 8935 pairs who were born from 1902 to 1949, 2516 or 14.1% were registered with the TB. Rates of TBR were slightly higher in DZ twins (1676/11 500=14.6%) than in MZ twins (840/6370=13.2%). Of those registered, less than half were registered once while one fifth were registered 5 or more times (**Table 1**). Drunkenness was the most common reason for registration, followed by "driving under the influence of alcohol" and "committing a crime in connection with alcohol."

MATERIALS AND METHODS

TEMPERANCE BOARD REGISTRATION

Temperance boards were officially established in Sweden in 1916,[2] but TBRs were not reliably recorded until 1929.[3] National records after 1974 are unavailable. While any individual could report someone to the TB, most registrations occurred through physicians, police, and public prosecutors.[4] All cases of "disorderliness and other offenses under the influence of alcohol" and driving "under the influence of alcohol" had to be reported to the TB.[4] Except under special circumstances, physicians were obliged to report cases of known alcoholism to the TB. The TB had to investigate each case, and an individual's record would follow him throughout life. The TBs did not have authority in cases of "occasional use of alcohol without obvious injury to himself or others."[4] The probability of TBR was related to ". . . the degree of severity of the alcohol abuse and the social injury caused."[3] The TB records were available to us only for males and included the age at first registration, the number of total registrations, and the following reason(s) for registration: (1) drunkenness, (2) illegal manufacture or sale of alcohol, (3) driving under the influence of alcohol, or (4) committing a crime "in connection with alcohol." Twins who were registered solely for illegal manufacture or sale (n=98) were excluded from analyses.

SAMPLE

The old Swedish Twin Registry[15] consisted of more than 95% of same-sex twin pairs who were born from 1886 to 1925 where both members were alive in 1959 and responded to a questionnaire in 1960. The new registry[16] consisted of more than 99% of all twins who were born from 1926 to 1958 where both members were alive in 1971. As TBR was available only for 1929 to 1974, we examined lifetime prevalence of TBR by 4-year birth cohorts from 1886 to 1958. Rates of TBR were low in those persons who were born before 1902, as individuals whose problems with alcohol occurred before 1929 were undetected (**Figure**). Rates of TBR were relatively stable for birth years 1902 to 1949, but fell sharply for birth years 1950 to 1958, as individuals whose alcohol abuse began after 1975 were not registered. We restricted our analyses to twins who were born from 1902 to 1949, where ascertainment of TBR was likely to be more complete. All major analyses were repeated on the entire cohort. Similar results were obtained.

Zygosity was determined by responses to self-report questionnaires that were shown to be 94% accurate.[17] After excluding 16 pairs with different birth dates, this sample consisted of twin pairs where zygosity information was available from both twins (n=7790) and 1 twin (n=1145). For cohort analyses, we divided the birth years from 1902 to 1949 into 4 groups that contained similar numbers of monozygotic (MZ) twins: 1902 to 1917, 1918 to 1930, 1931 to 1942, and 1943 to 1949.

A hospital diagnosis of alcoholism was obtained from the Swedish Psychiatric Twin Registry,[18] which provides complete coverage of all psychiatric contacts in mental hospitals and in-patient psychiatric departments of general hospitals[19] for the years 1968 to 1983. According to the *International Classification of Diseases, Eighth Revision*,[20] we defined alcoholism by a hospital diagnosis of alcoholism (*ICD* 303) or alcoholic psychosis (*ICD* 291).[20]

Self-report questionnaires completed in the old and new registries contained information on levels of alcohol consumption. These were converted to the average current monthly consumption of alcohol.

PRESENTATION OF RESULTS FROM TWIN STUDIES

We present results by using probandwise concordance (the proportion of co-twins of proband twins who are themselves affected), tetrachoric correlation (or "correlation of liability"), and risk ratio (RR). Probandwise concordance

Continued on next page

CONCORDANCE AND COX HAZARD MODELS

Probandwise concordance (±SE) for TBR in MZ and DZ twins was 402/840=47.9%±1.7% and 550/1676=32.8%±1.1%, respectively. By using a Cox model, the RR (defined as the increase in the hazard rate for registration in the co-twin associated with a history of TBR in the twin) equaled 7.88 in MZ twins (χ^2=559.0, *df*=1, *P*<.001) and 3.30 in DZ twins (χ^2=367.2, *df*=1, *P*<.001). The RR in MZ twins was significantly greater than the RR in DZ twins (χ^2=66.96, *df*=1, *P*<.001).

As seen in **Table 2**, concordance rates in both MZ and DZ twins were relatively stable in the 4 birth cohorts from 1902 to 1949, ranging from 43.8% to 50% in MZ twins and 29.3% to 35.5% in DZ twins. No linear trends in concordance rates over time were evident in either zygosity group.

TETRACHORIC CORRELATIONS AND MODEL FITTING

The tetrachoric correlation for TBR in the entire sample was estimated at +0.67 for MZ and +0.41 for DZ twins. The ACE model fit well (**Table 3**) (χ^2=5.05, *df*=3, *P*=.17, AIC=−0.95). A model that postulated that all twin resemblance for TBR was due to familial-environmental effects (the CE model), fit much worse, and could be strongly rejected compared with the ACE model (χ^2=50.09, *df*=1, *P*<.001). A model that postulated that all twin resemblance was due to genetic effects (the AE model) also fit relatively poorly and could be rejected against the ACE model (χ^2=5.84, *df*=1, *P*=.02). Therefore, the best-fitting model for TBR in the entire sample was the ACE model, which yielded parameter estimates (and 95% confidence intervals [CIs]) of a^2=0.54 (CI, 0.47-0.61), c^2=0.14 (CI, 0.08-0.19), and e^2=0.33 (CI, 0.30-0.35).

When the sample was divided into 4 birth cohorts, the tetrachoric correlations for TBR were relatively stable across cohorts, ranging from +0.60 to +0.70 in MZ and from +0.29 to +0.36 in DZ twins (Table 2). We first fit models, separately to each of the 4 cohorts, which permitted parameter estimates to *differ* across cohorts (Table 3, second row). Next, we fit models in which the parameter estimates were constrained to be *equal* in all 4 cohorts (Table 3, third is inefficient in an epidemiologic sample as it ignores twin pairs where neither is affected. The tetrachoric correlation assumes that underlying the observed dichotomous distribution of TBR, there exists a continuous, latent liability. The tetrachoric correlation represents the correlation between the underlying liability distributions.[21,22]

Both probandwise concordances and tetrachoric correlations examine only the presence or absence of a lifetime history of TBR, ignoring information about age at first TBR and age at censoring (due to death or termination of TBR data). To include these, we applied the Cox proportional hazard models (PHREG procedure in SAS[23]) that, controlling for year of birth, predict the hazard rate for TBR in the co-twin from the presence of TBR in the twin.

STATISTICAL ANALYSIS

We used Mx[24] to calculate tetrachoric correlations and fit models to contingency tables by using the method of maximum likelihood.[25] As outlined elsewhere,[25,26] resemblance in twins is assumed to result from 2 sets of latent factors: additive genes (A) and family or "common" environment (C)—factors such as a rural vs an urban upbringing or parental attitudes, which make members of a twin pair *similar* for their liability to alcoholism. In addition, the model contains individual specific environment (E), which reflects, along with measurement error, environmental experiences that make members of a twin pair *different* for liability to alcoholism.

We fit ACE, AE, and CE models. The AE model assumes that all familial aggregation results from additive genetic effects. The CE model assumes that all observed familial aggregation is the result of shared environmental influences.

The goal in model fitting is to explain the observed data well and parsimoniously. We operationalize this goal by using the information criterion of Akaike (AIC),[27] defined as χ^2 minus twice the *df*. By seeking the model with the minimum AIC, we hope to select the model that best reflects the balance of goodness of fit and simplicity.[28] In addition, it is possible to compare directly the CE or AE model with the ACE model by a χ^2 difference test with 1 *df*.

The final step of twin analysis is to estimate, based on the best-fitting model, the proportion of variance in liability due to individual specific environment (e^2), additive genetic factors (a^2), and common environment (c^2). The proportion of variance in liability due to additive genetic effects is often termed *heritability*.

These data also afford us an opportunity to examine the relative importance of genetic and environmental risk factors for alcohol abuse throughout historical time. We first fit standard twin models jointly to 8 groups: MZ and dizygotic (DZ) twin pairs from each of the 4 birth cohorts. Then, we fit models to the same 8 groups, by constraining the parameter estimates to be equal across birth cohorts. If the etiologic importance of genetic or environmental factors differs significantly across cohorts, the constrained models should fit poorly relative to the initial models. If genetic and environmental factors are relatively stable across cohorts, the constrained models should fit relatively well. All models assumed the same threshold of illness in both members of the twin pair, in MZ and DZ twins, and in different birth cohorts.

Finally, we examined 3 features of TBRs as "indexes" of the genetic or familial-environmental liability to illness: number of TBRs, presence of a criminal registration, and age at first registration. We examined the hazard rate for TBRs separately in MZ and DZ co-twins of registered twins,[23] looking for 3 possible patterns—that the variable (1) does not reflect liability to TBR (so does not predict TBR in MZ or DZ co-twins), (2) reflects the familial-environmental risk to TBR (so equally predicts TBR in MZ and DZ twins), and (3) reflects the genetic risk to TBR (so predicts TBR more strongly in MZ than in DZ co-twins). Statistical results and *P* values are reported, where appropriate, based on SEs corrected both for the nonindependence of observations in members of twin pairs and for "double counting" of concordant pairs.[29]

row). The ACE model fit best in both analyses. However, as indicated by the AIC score, the simpler models that assumed constant genetic and environmental effects across cohorts provided consistently better explanations of the data. The overall best-fitting "cohort model," namely, the ACE model with values of A, C, and E set equal across cohorts, produced parameter estimates that were identical to those obtained with the entire sample.

PREDICTION OF RISK OF REGISTRATION IN THE CO-TWIN

We used a Cox proportional hazard model to examine characteristics of TBR in 1 twin that predicted the risk of registration in his co-twin (**Table 4**). The age at first registration was significantly and inversely related to the hazard rate of registration in co-twins; the strength of this relationship was identical in MZ and DZ twins (RR, 0.97/year of birth in both zygosity groups). The number of registrations also significantly predicted the hazard rate of registration in the co-twin, but the predictive power was substantially greater in MZ (RR=1.33) than in DZ (RR=1.20) twins. A similar pattern was seen with criminal registration (RR=1.97 in MZ and RR=1.41 in DZ twins). A formal test for the difference in these RRs in MZ vs DZ twins revealed them to be significantly different for the number of registrations and criminal registration, but not for the age at first registration.

COMMENT

HERITABILITY OF ALCOHOLISM

Our first goal was to examine the etiologic role of genetic and environmental factors in alcohol abuse as assessed by TBR in this large epidemiologic sample of Swedish male twins. By using concordances or RRs in Cox regression models, the similarity in twins for TBR registration was significantly greater in MZ than in DZ twins. These results suggest a substantial role for genetic factors in the etiology of alcohol abuse.

This was confirmed by twin model fitting, where the best model indicated that twin resemblance

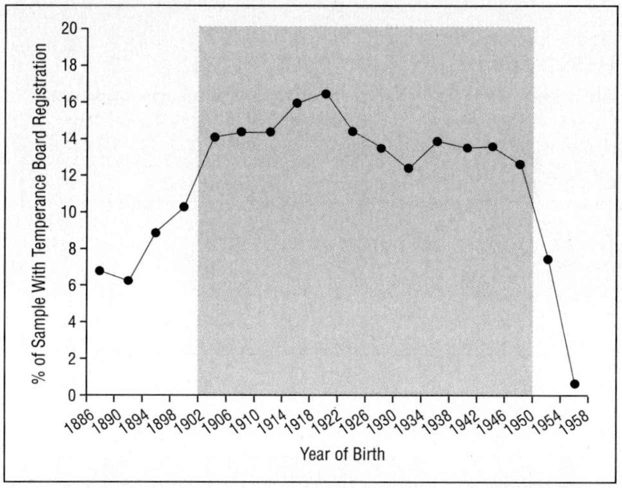

The percentage of male twins in Sweden, born from 1886 to 1958, who were registered with temperance board authorities from 1929 to 1974. The data are presented in 4-year cohorts, so that all twins who were born from 1886 to 1889 are represented by the point midway between 1886 and 1890. The shaded area indicates the period of relatively stable registration rates, representing the birth years 1902 to 1949.

Table 1. Number and Reasons for Temperance Board Registration (TBR) in Swedish Male Twins, Born 1902 to 1949*

Variable	No. (%)
No. of TBR*	
1	1139 (45.5)
2	480 (19.2)
3	246 (9.8)
4	126 (5.0)
≥5	514 (20.5)
Reasons for registration†	
Drunkenness	2171 (86.7)
Driving	912 (36.4)
Criminal	888 (35.4)

**Numbers sum to 2505, as data are missing on 11 twins.*
†Numbers sum to greater than 2505 because some twins were registered for multiple reasons.

resulted from both genetic and familial-environmental factors, with the former accounting for nearly 4 times as much variance in liability (54%) as the latter (14%). The remaining variance in liability was due to environmental factors that were not shared by members of a twin pair.

How do these results compare with findings from previous twin studies of alcoholism? The observed concordance rates (48% in MZ and 33% in DZ twins) were higher than those observed in veteran males from the National Academy of Sciences–National Research Council epidemiologic twin registry[6] and in the hospitalized sample of Gurling et al,[5] but lower than those found in the other clinical samples.[7-9] Our heritability estimate (54%) is well within the range of those reported in other modern twin studies of males: (1) Hrubec and Omenn,[6] 57%; (2) Pickens et al,[7] *DSM-III* alcohol abuse, only 38%, and alcohol abuse or dependence, 36%; (3) Caldwell and Gottesman,[9] *DSM-III* alcohol abuse or dependence, 70%; and (4) McGue et al,[8] *DSM-III* alcohol abuse or dependence, 54%. In agreement with our findings, all 3 prior twin studies that used model-fitting methods also found that familial-environmental factors contributed to twin resemblance for liability to alcoholism in men.[7-9] The number of pairs with affected twins in this study (n=2040) is nearly 3 times that of the next largest twin study of alcoholism in men (n=715[6]) and 10 to 50 times larger than those of other prior samples: (n=205[1]), (n=35[5]), (n=114[7]), (n=181[8]), and (n=54[9]).

STABILITY OF HERITABILITY OF ALCOHOL ABUSE OVER TIME

Rarely are data available to examine the etiologic role of genetic and environmental factors in a complex human trait like alcohol abuse through historical time. The period that was covered in Sweden (birth years 1902-1949) is a particularly interesting one as the general economic level of the country improved dramatically with a 6-fold increase in per capita income.[30] Large changes in per capita alcohol intake also occurred.[31]

Most interestingly, this period also saw major changes in governmental control of access to alcohol.[32] In 1917, Sweden adopted a nationwide alcohol rationing system that strictly limited the amount of alcohol that an individual was permitted to purchase. An individual's official limit varied according to sex, age, and financial situations, and was, for men older than 25 years, usually between 1 and 3 L of hard liquor per month.[33] This rationing system was abolished in 1955.

Despite our large sample size, we were unable to detect evidence that the importance of genetic and environmental factors in the etiology of alcohol abuse changed in males who were born in Sweden from 1902 to 1949. We know of no comparable study that has examined alcoholism through historical time in a genetically informative sample. Large changes in socioeconomic status and significant alterations in laws that govern access to alcohol can apparently occur without having any substantial impact on the overall importance of genetic and environmental factors in the etiology of alcohol abuse. While extrapolation from a single study is problematic, these results suggest that the heritability of alcohol abuse may be a relatively stable population characteristic that is not easily altered by social change. Our results provide no information about whether more drastic social experiments (eg, the US adoption of nationwide prohibition) might have more profound effects.

INDEXES OF GENETIC OR ENVIRONMENTAL RISK FOR ALCOHOL ABUSE

Alcoholism is a clinically heterogeneous syndrome, and many subtyping typologies have been proposed.[34,35] Recent interest has focused on attempts to define a highly heritable or "familial" form of alcoholism.[8,35-37] Cloninger et al,[37] working from TBR and other official records in a Swedish adoption sample, proposed a highly heritable "male-limited" form of alcoholism characterized by an early age at onset, recurrent illness, and criminality in biologic fathers. A history of antisocial personality or

Table 2. Sample Size, Prevalence, Probandwise Concordance, and Tetrachoric Correlation for TBR in Swedish Monozygotic and Dizygotic Male-Male Twin Pairs by Birth Cohort*

	Monozygotic Twins				Dizygotic Twins			
Birth Years†	No. of Pairs	Prevalence	Probandwise Concordance	*r*	No. of Pairs	Prevalence	Probandwise Concordance	*r*
1902-1949	**3185**	0.132	0.479	+0.669	**5750**	0.146	0.328	+0.409
1902-1917	799	0.128	0.500	+0.701	1500	0.159	0.347	+0.418
1918-1930	791	0.141	0.502	+0.688	1534	0.147	0.293	+0.340
1931-1942	842	0.138	0.438	+0.603	1507	0.136	0.323	+0.421
1943-1949	753	0.120	0.478	+0.688	1209	0.140	0.355	+0.470

**TBR indicates temperance board registration;* r, *tetrachoric correlation.*
†Line 1 represents the entire birth cohort, and lines 2-5, individual birth cohorts.

Table 3. Model Fitting for Entire Sample and for 4 Birth Cohorts With Parameters Allowed to Differ and Constrained to Be Equal Across Cohorts*

	ACE				CE				AE				Parameters of Best-Fitting Model		
Sample	χ^2	*df*	*P*	AIC	χ^2	*df*	*P*	AIC	χ^2	*df*	*P*	AIC	a^2	c^2	e^2
Entire sample	5.05	3	.17	−0.95†	55.14	4	.00	+47.14	10.89	4	.03	+2.89	0.536	0.139	0.325
Differing parameters across 4 cohorts‡	20.39	15	.16	−9.62	73.63	19	.00	+35.63	29.55	19	.06	−8.45	...	...	...
Equal parameters across 4 cohorts§	26.47	21	.19	−15.53†	76.55	22	.00	+32.55	32.31	22	.07	−11.70	0.536	0.139	0.325

**A indicates additive genetic effects; C, common or familial environment; E, unique or individual specific environment; AIC, information criterion of Akaike[27]; a^2, additive genetic effects; c^2, common environment; and e^2, individual specific environment.*
†Best-fitting model.
‡Parameters permitted to differ across 4 birth cohorts (1902-1917, 1918-1930, 1931-1942, 1943-1949).
§Parameters constrained to be equal across all 4 birth cohorts.

criminality[35] or an early age at onset[8] may also define genetically meaningful subtypes of alcoholism.[35]

We found that age at onset, the number of registrations, and criminal registration in a registered twin all significantly predicted the risk of TBR in the co-twin. These 3 predictors, however, behaved quite differently in MZ vs DZ twin pairs. Both the number of registrations and criminal registration were significantly stronger predictors of risk of TBR in MZ than in DZ co-twins, as expected if they reflected the genetic liability to alcohol abuse. By contrast, age at first registration was equally strong at predicting TBR in the co-twin in DZ as in MZ twins; this is the expected pattern if age at onset was an index of the familial-environmental liability to alcohol abuse. These results, consistent with some, but not all previous findings,[8,35,37] indicate the power of the twin design in clarifying differences in measures of "familial" alcoholism.

EQUAL ENVIRONMENT ASSUMPTION

Twin studies assume that MZ and DZ twin pairs are equally correlated for exposure to disease-predisposing environments. If MZ twins are more highly correlated than DZ twins for exposure to environmental risk factors for alcohol abuse, then our estimates of the heritability of alcohol abuse will be biased upward. Information to test this hypothesis—although limited to the frequency of contact in twin pairs in adulthood—was available from self-report questionnaires that were obtained from the new Swedish Twin Registry. As seen in other samples,[38,39] MZ twins were in significantly closer contact with one another than DZ twins (t=15.1; df=7356; P<.001). Furthermore, twins in more frequent contact with one another were more similar in their probability of TBR. However, this relationship was a weak one. Tetrachoric correlations for TBR in MZ and DZ twins, respectively, as a function of their level of contact were as follows: low contact, +0.61 and +0.39; intermediate contact, +0.67 and +0.49; and high contact, +0.66 and +0.46.

To examine what impact this violation of the equal environment assumption could have on our heritability estimates, we applied a structural equation model that included the standard parameters plus the frequency of contact as an additional source of twin resemblance.[40] The fit of the model, as assessed by AIC, was not improved by adding the "frequency of contact" parameter. If this parameter were included, it accounted for 8% of the variance in liability to TBR; estimates of a^2 and c^2 declined only very slightly. The increased frequency of contact in adulthood in MZ vs DZ twins was not likely to represent a significant violation of the equal environment assumption for TBR.

POTENTIAL LIMITATIONS

This report should be interpreted in the context of 5 methodologic limitations. First, how valid is TBR registration as a measure of alcohol abuse? Dahlberg[41] reviewed 1162 men who were registered with the TB in Malmö, Sweden, between 1929 and 1938. In only 78 (6.7%) of them was

Table 4. Prediction of Hazard Rate in Co-twin for First TBR in MZ and DZ Twins for Age at First Registration, Criminal Registration, and Number of Registrations*

	MZ Twins				DZ Twins				Interaction With Zygosity	
Predictor Variable	**RR**	**95% CI of RR**	**χ^2**	***P***	**RR**	**95% CI of RR**	**χ^2**	***P***	**χ^2**	***P***
Age at first registration	0.97	0.96-0.99	9.8	.001	0.97	0.96-0.98	16.9	<.001	0.4	.53
No. of registrations	1.33	1.25-1.41	67.2	<.001	1.20	1.14-1.26	41.3	<.001	3.8	.05
Criminal registration	1.97	1.59-2.37	33.5	<.001	1.41	1.18-1.67	12.5	.004	4.0	.05

**TBR indicates temperance board registration; MZ, monozygotic; DZ, dizygotic; RR, relative risk; and CI, confidence interval. By Cox proportional hazard model for birth years 1902 to 1949, controlling for year of birth. Of note, while the Cox models in MZ and DZ twins test whether the observed association is owing to chance, the test for interaction examines whether the predictive power of the Cox model differs significantly in MZ vs DZ twins. The RR for age at first registration is per year, for number of registrations per category (1, 2, 3, 4, and ≥5), and for criminal registration simply the presence or absence of a registration for committing a crime in connection with alcohol. Statistical results are corrected for the "double counting" of registered twins in pairs concordant for TBR.*

there doubt whether they were "addicted to abuse of alcohol," which Dahlberg defined as " . . . intoxicated almost daily, involving also incapability on his part to execute his social duties." Åmark[3] examined 407 men who were registered with the TB in Stockholm in 1945 and 1946 and concluded that 87.7% had either chronic alcoholism or alcohol addiction. In a population study, Kaij[42] compared men with alcoholism who had vs had not been registered and noted few differences between them.

We validated TBR against hospital diagnoses of alcoholism and self-report alcohol consumption. Compared with unregistered individuals, a twin with a TBR had a significant, 9.4-fold increased risk of admission to a psychiatric facility with a diagnosis of alcoholism (χ^2=429.3, *df*=1, *P*<.001). Individuals with a history of TBR reported current consumption of alcohol 2 to 3 times greater than those without such a history (*t*=20.77; *df*=11 638; *P*<.001). In the new registry, information was also available on maximum prior alcohol consumption. This was more than twice as great in those with vs without a history of TBR (*t*=18.86; *df*=6210; *P*<.001).

A second potential methodologic limitation is that, while substantial data support the validity of TBR as a measure of alcohol abuse, we know less about its sensitivity. In the Stockholm adoption sample, Cloninger et al[43] found that 58% of men with a psychiatric diagnosis of alcoholism had 1 or more TBRs. Of the 440 twins who were psychiatrically hospitalized with a diagnosis of alcoholism in our national data, 257 (58.4%) had 1 or more TBRs; this is a lower bound estimate, as the period of ascertainment for psychiatric hospitalization and TBR only partially overlapped. Given the validity of TBR as a measure of alcohol abuse, its substantial prevalence in this sample (14.1%) provides indirect evidence of its sensitivity.

How might our results be biased if a significant proportion of individuals affected with alcohol abuse go undetected by TBRs? Neither the concordance-based nor the model-based analyses of twin data assume that all cases of illness are ascertained. However, these methods do assume that the probability of ascertainment is independent in twin pairs. If ascertainment is correlated in twin pairs (eg, TBR in 1 twin increases the probability of TBR in the co-twin), and if the degree of correlation is similar in MZ and DZ twins, the correlations must be relatively extreme to bias parameter estimates substantially.[44]

More problematic is the possibility that ascertainment is correlated, and the degree of correlation is greater in MZ than in DZ twins. In his initial study of TBR, Kaij[1] investigated this possibility and concluded that correlated ascertainment was not a source of significant bias. If registration in one twin increased the probability of registration in the co-twin, and this effect was stronger in MZ than in DZ twins, then age at first TBR should be much more highly correlated in MZ than in DZ twins. However, this was not the case—correlation in age at first TBR was very similar in MZ (+0.60) and DZ (+0.57) twins (difference test: *z*=0.49, *P*=.62).

To examine this further, we simulated 2 models of correlated ascertainment for TBR,[44] assuming the probability of registration for a twin with alcohol abuse was 40% if his co-twin was unregistered. In model 1 (correlated ascertainment, equal in MZ and DZ twins), this increased to 80% if the co-twin was registered in both twin types. In model 2 (correlated ascertainment, greater in MZ than in DZ twins), having the co-twin registered increased the probability of registration to 60% in DZ and 80% in MZ twins. Estimates of the heritability of liability to TBR were unchanged in the first model and reduced moderately (54%-44%) in the second. Correlated ascertainment is unlikely to be a major source of bias in our twin study of TBR.

Third, to be included in the old and new registries, both twins had to be alive in 1959 and 1971, respectively. A bias might exist in the registries against twins with alcoholism sufficiently severe to increase substantially the risk for premature death. Such a bias would more likely deflate than inflate estimates of heritability.

Fourth, variation likely existed in both time and space in the application of the guidelines for TBR. We cannot rule out the possibility that such variation significantly influenced the results that were obtained although such an effect would tend to bias estimates upwardly for familial environment and not genetic factors.[25]

Fifth, zygosity information, obtained by mailed questionnaire, was necessary for inclusion in this sample. Prior studies suggest that individuals with alcohol problems cooperate with such surveys at reduced rates.[10,11] By using a co-twin control design, we could estimate that the probability of selection into our sample was 37% lower in individuals with vs without a history of TBR. Applying to these data a model that corrects for such sampling bias[45] resulted in a slight increase in the heritability of TBR and no change in the role of common environment. A bias associated with cooperation might also predict differences in TBR concordances in twins where both vs only 1 member returned questionnaires. This, however, was seen neither in MZ (46.6% vs 53.6%, respectively; χ^2=2.46, *df*=1, *P*=.12) nor in DZ twins (32.4% vs 34.6%, respectively; χ^2=0.64, *df*=1, *P*=.42).

By presenting results that were first based solely on TBR data and then on diagnoses that were based on registration records, personal interviews, and information from relatives, Kaij[1] provided us with a global test for most biases in Swedish registration data. The fitting of twin models to these 2 sets of results produced nearly identical estimates of the importance of genetic and environmental risk factors in the etiology of alcohol abuse in Swedish male twins.

Accepted for publication March 26, 1996.

This study was supported in part by a Research Scientist Award (grant MH01277) from the National Institutes of Health (Dr Kendler), and by grant AA09095 from the National Institute on Alcohol Abuse and Alcoholism, Bethesda, Md. The Swedish Twin Registry is administrated through the Institute of Environmental Medicine of the Karolinska Institute, Stockholm, and is supported by grants from the John D. and Catherine T. MacArthur Foundation, Chicago, Ill, and the Swedish Council for Planning and Coordination of Research, Stockholm.

Stephen Easter, MS, assisted in the statistical analysis. This study is dedicated to the memory of Lennart Kaij, MD.

Reprints: Kenneth S. Kendler, MD, Department of Psychiatry, PO Box 980710, Richmond, VA 23298-0710.

REFERENCES

1. Kaij L. *Alcoholism in Twins.* Stockholm, Sweden: Almqvist & Wiksell International; 1960.
2. Tienari P. Psychiatric illnesses in identical twins. *Acta Psychiatr Scand.* 1963; 39(suppl 171):1-195.
3. Åmark C. A study in alcoholism: clinical, social-psychiatric and genetic investigations. *Acta Psychiatr Neurol Scand.* 1951;(suppl 70):1-283.
4. Hjortzberg-Nordlund H. Abuse of alcohol in middle-aged men in Göteborg: a social psychiatric investigation. *Acta Psychiatr Scand.* 1968;44(suppl 199):1-127.
5. Gurling HMD, Oppenheim BE, Murray RM. Depression, criminality and psychopathology associated with alcoholism: evidence from a twin study. *Acta Genet Med Gemellol (Roma).* 1984;33:333-339.
6. Hrubec Z, Omenn GS. Evidence of genetic predisposition to alcoholic cirrhosis and psychosis: twin concordances for alcoholism and its biological end points by zygosity among male veterans. *Alcohol Clin Exp Res.* 1981;5:207-215.
7. Pickens RW, Svikis DS, McGue M, Lykken DT, Heston LL, Clayton PJ. Heterogeneity in the inheritance of alcoholism. *Arch Gen Psychiatry.* 1991;48:19-28.
8. McGue M, Pickens RW, Svikis DS. Sex and age effects on the inheritance of alcohol problems: a twin study. *J Abnorm Psychol.* 1992;101:3-17.
9. Caldwell CB, Gottesman II. Sex differences in the risk for alcoholism: a twin study. Presented at the 21st Annual Meeting of the Behavior Genetics Association; June 7, 1991; St Louis, Mo.
10. Allgulander C. Psychoactive drug use in a general population sample, Sweden: correlates with perceived health, psychiatric diagnoses, and mortality in an automated record-linkage study. *Am J Public Health.* 1989;79:1006-1010.
11. Cottler LB, Zipp JF, Robins LN, Spitznagel EL. Difficult-to-recruit respondents and their effect on prevalence estimates in an epidemiologic survey. *Am J Epidemiol.* 1987;125:329-339.
12. Prusoff BA, Merikangas KR, Weissman MM. Lifetime prevalence and age of onset of psychiatric disorders: recall 4 years later. *J Psychiatr Res.* 1988;22:107-117.
13. Rice JP, Rochberg M, Endicott J, Lavori PW, Miller C. Stability of psychiatric diagnoses: an application to the affective disorders. *Arch Gen Psychiatry.* 1992; 49:824-830.
14. Rubio-Stipec M, Freeman DH Jr, Robins LN, Shrout P, Canino G, Bravo M. Response error and the estimation of lifetime prevalence and incidence of alcoholism: experience in a community survey. *Int J Meth Psychiatr Res.* 1992;2:217-224.
15. Cederlof R. *The Twin Method in Epidemiological Studies on Chronic Disease.* Stockholm, Sweden: University of Stockholm; 1966. Thesis.
16. Medlund P, Cederlof R, Floderus-Myrhed B, Friberg L, Sorensen S. A Swedish twin registry. *Acta Med Scand.* 1977;(suppl 600).
17. Cederlof R, Friberg L, Jonsson E, Kaij L. Studies on similarity diagnosis in twins with the aid of mailed questionnaires. *Acta Genet Stat Med.* 1961;11:338-362.
18. Kendler KS, Pedersen NL, Johnson L, Neale MC, Mathe AA. A pilot Swedish twin study of affective illness, including hospital- and population-ascertained subsamples. *Arch Gen Psychiatry.* 1993;50:699-706.
19. National Central Bureau of Statistics. *Psychiatric In-patient Care 1977.* Stockholm, Sweden: Statistiska Centralbyran; 1981.
20. World Health Organization. *International Classification of Diseases, Eighth Revision.* Geneva, Switzerland: World Health Organization; 1968.
21. Pearson K. Mathematical contributions to the theory of evolution, VIII: on the correlation of characters not quantitatively measurable. *Proc R Soc Lond.* 1901; 66:241-244.
22. Falconer DS. The inheritance of liability to certain diseases, estimated from the incidence among relatives. *Ann Hum Genet.* 1965;29:51-76.
23. SAS Institute. *SAS/STAT User's Guide, Version 6.* 4th ed. Cary, NC: SAS Institute Inc; 1990;1 and 2.
24. Neale MC. *Mx: Statistical Modeling.* 2nd ed. Richmond, Va: Department of Psychiatry; 1994.
25. Neale MC, Cardon LR. *Methodology for Genetic Studies of Twins and Families.* Norwell, Mass: Kluwer Academic Publishers; 1992.
26. Kendler KS. Twin studies of psychiatric illness: current status and future directions. *Arch Gen Psychiatry.* 1993;50:905-915.
27. Akaike H. Factor analysis and AIC. *Psychometrika.* 1987;52:317-332.
28. Williams LJ, Holahan PJ. Parsimony-based fit indices for multiple-indicator models: do they work? *Struct Equat Model.* 1994;1:161-189.
29. Kish L, Frankel MR. Inferences from complex samples. *J R Stat Soc Ser B.* 1974;36:1-37.
30. National Central Bureau of Statistics Sweden. *Living Conditions, Report No. 6: Development and Present Situation According to Statistics Available 1976.* Stockholm, Sweden: LiberForlag; 1977.
31. Swedish Council for Information on Alcohol and Other Drugs. *Trends in Alcohol and Drug Use in Sweden, Report 93.* Stockholm, Sweden: National Institute of Public Health; 1993.
32. Grant M. *Alcohol Policies: (WHO Regional Publications, European Series, No. 18).* Copenhagen, Denmark: World Health Organization; 1985.
33. Hibell B. *Alcohol Policy in Sweden: a Short Review.* Stockholm, Sweden: Swedish Council for Information on Alcohol and Other Drugs; 1986.
34. Sher KJ. *Children of Alcoholics: a Critical Appraisal of Theory and Research.* Chicago, Ill: University of Chicago Press; 1991.
35. Hesselbrock MN. Genetic determinants of alcoholic subtypes. In: Begleiter H, Kissin B, eds. *The Genetics of Alcoholism.* New York, NY: Oxford University Press Inc; 1995:40-69.
36. Goodwin DW. Studies of familial alcoholism: a review. *J Clin Psychiatry.* 1984; 45:14-17.
37. Cloninger CR, Bohman M, Sigvardsson S. Inheritance of alcohol abuse: cross-fostering analysis of adopted men. *Arch Gen Psychiatry.* 1981;38:861-868.
38. Kendler KS, Heath AC, Martin NG, Eaves LJ. Symptoms of anxiety and depression in a volunteer twin population: the etiologic role of genetic and environmental factors. *Arch Gen Psychiatry.* 1986;43:213-221.
39. Kendler KS, Heath AC, Neale MC, Kessler RC, Eaves LJ. A population-based twin study of alcoholism in women. *JAMA.* 1992;268:1877-1882.
40. Kendler KS, Neale MC, Kessler RC, Heath AC, Eaves LJ. A test of the equal environment assumption in twin studies of psychiatric illness. *Behav Genet.* 1993;23:21-27.
41. Dahlberg G. The occurrence of alcoholics and their treatment: a social-statistical analysis for the town of Malmö 1929-1938. *Acta Med Scand.* 1942;111:325-358.
42. Kaij L. Biases in a Swedish social register of alcoholics. *Soc Psychiatry Psychiatr Epidemiol.* 1970;5:216-218.
43. Cloninger CR, Bohman M, Sigvardsson S, von Knorring AL. Psychopathology in adopted-out children of alcoholics: the Stockholm Adoption Study. In: Galanter M, ed. *Recent Developments in Alcoholism.* New York, NY: Plenum Publishing Corp; 1985;3:37-51.
44. Kendler KS, Eaves LJ. The estimation of probandwise concordance in twins: the effect of unequal ascertainment. *Acta Genet Med Gemellol (Roma).* 1989;38: 253-270.
45. Kendler KS, Holm NV. Differential enrollment in twin registries: its effect on prevalence and concordance rates and estimates of genetic parameters. *Acta Genet Med Gemellol (Roma).* 1985;34:125-140.

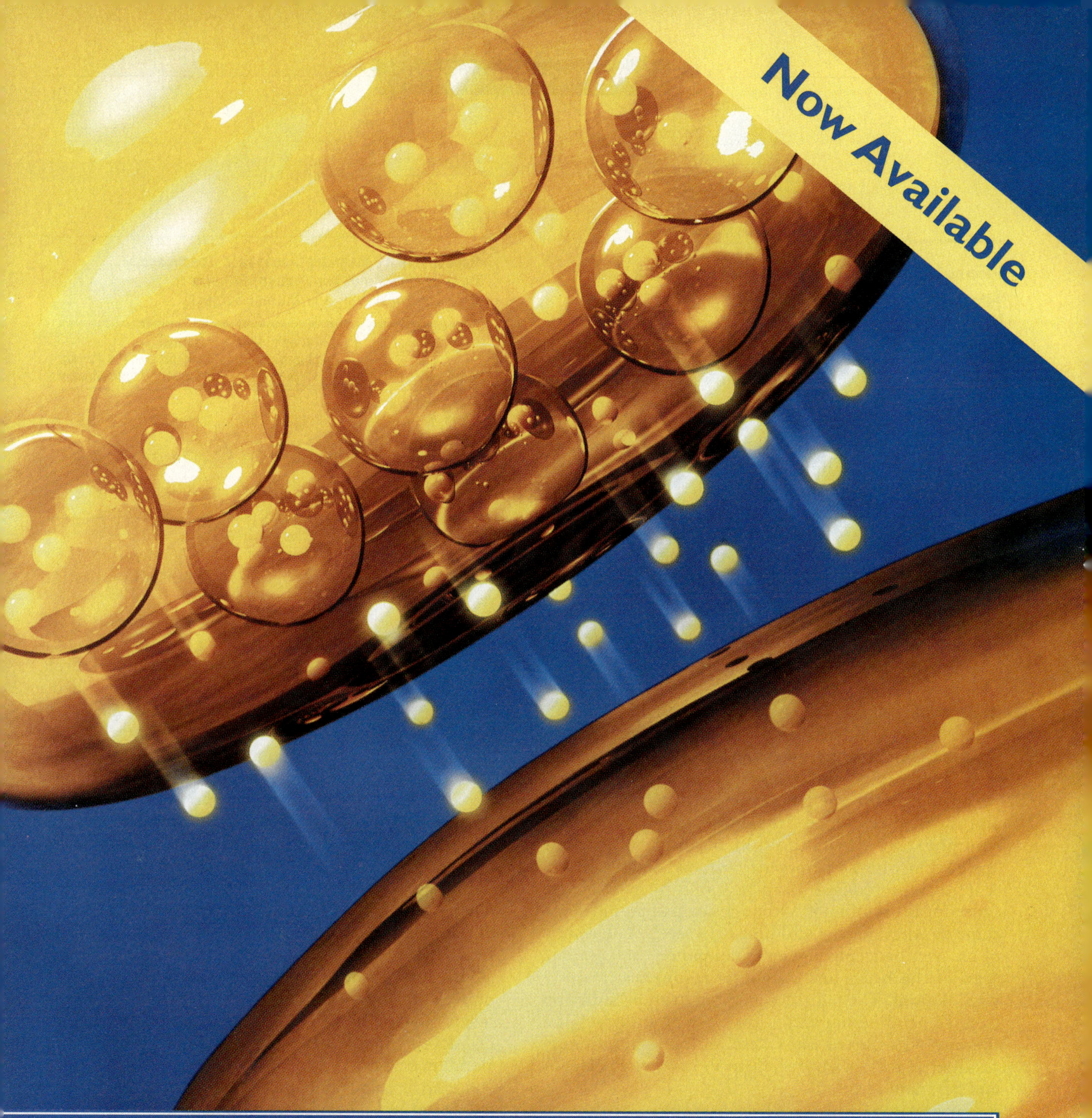
Now Available

Phosphorus 31 Magnetic Resonance Spectroscopy in Patients With Huntington Disease

Phosphorus 31 magnetic resonance spectroscopy (MRS) provides in vivo information about membrane phospholipid and high-energy phosphate metabolism in the brain.[1] We recently described ^{31}P MRS findings in never-treated patients with schizophrenia compared with matched control subjects.[2] These patients were found to have lower concentrations of phosphomonoesters and increased concentrations of phosphodiesters and calculated intracellular magnesium in the prefrontal region compared with matched control subjects. We report a case of Huntington disease (HD) that was inadvertently included in our ^{31}P MRS study in the never-treated group with schizophrenia.[2]

Report of a Case. A 19-year-old man had a 3- to 4-year history of deterioration in general functioning, increased social withdrawal, positive symptoms, and a recent history of bizarre purposeless behavior and poor judgement. The patient reported alien thoughts and ideas of reference. He demonstrated poverty of thought, flat affect, thought blocking, and poor abstraction with no perceptual or mood abnormalities. A neurologic consultation revealed no neurologic cause for his symptoms, although the patient did show some facial grimacing and unusual speech. The results of an electroencephalogram, a computed tomographic scan of the head, and magnetic resonance imaging were normal. The patient was thought to be suffering from schizophrenia, and a low dose of antipsychotic therapy was started after observation. This therapy resulted in a slight improvement in his social behavior and paranoid ideation.

Neuropsychological assessment conducted approximately 5 months after he was first seen revealed a low average verbal intelligence quotient and borderline performance on the intelligence quotient test. The neuropsychological test results suggested bilateral, frontal, and temporal lobe impairment, possibly worse in the right hemisphere, and bilateral parietal lobe impairment. The pattern of results on neurologic examination suggested a subcortical degenerative process. The antipsychotic medication was discontinued because of a problem with coordination and limited improvement of the initial symptoms. Magnetic resonance imaging 1 year after he was initially seen revealed a slight prominence of the frontal horns of both lateral ventricles but no caudate atrophy. The results of an electromyogram and nerve conduction studies were normal.

Phosphorus 31 Magnetic Resonance Spectroscopy Data in the Patient We Studied, Patients With Schizophrenia, and Normal Subjects

Metabolite	Patients With Schizophrenia* (n=10)	Normal Subjects* (n=11)	The Patient We Studied
Phosphomonoesters, mol %	12.0±0.9	14.9±1.0	9.8
Phosphodiesters, mol %	40.5±1.9	38.3±1.9	37.8
Calculated intracellular magnesium, μmol/L	420.0±94.0	318.0±31.0	393.0

Values are given plus or minus the SD.

The patient had been adopted by his parents at the age of 7 years. Only limited information about his biological parents became available, despite a careful search. The patient's biological mother was found to have had a history of recurrent seizures, severe mood disorder, withdrawal, and an inability to cope independently. The patient's biological maternal grandfather also had a history of seizures, while the biological maternal grandmother was reported to have suffered from dementia while still in her early 50s. The patient's maternal aunt had suffered from a longstanding undefined psychiatric illness. A sister from the same biological mother showed minor neurologic abnormalities during her early childhood, along with some speech difficulties. The birth and early development of the patient were unremarkable for the first 3 years. Moderately severe neurotic behavior, such as nail biting, social anxiety, and interpersonal withdrawal, became apparent during latency years after many foster home placements. After a period of adequate social development during his early teens, a notable deterioration began at the age of 16 years, in addition to longstanding learning problems.

A second neurologic opinion was obtained 1 year after the initial consultation. Diagnostic possibilities of a storage disorder, a mitochondrial disorder, or juvenile HD were considered. The storage disorder and the mitochondrial disorder were excluded after biochemical tests and biopsies of the muscle and skin were performed. Investigations for juvenile HD were pursued, and eventually HD was confirmed by genetic testing.

The **Table** provides the metabolic data of the patient when he was first seen. This patient is within the never-treated group with schizophrenia range on concentrations of phosphomonoesters but within the normal range on concentrations of phosphodiesters. His concentrations of calculated intracellular magnesium are also in the range reported for the group with schizophrenia.

Comment. Phosphomonoesters are precursors of cell membranes.[3] Our finding of decreased phosphomonoesters in patients with schizophrenia and this patient with HD may reflect a loss of dendritic proliferation in the prefrontal cortex. This could be related to increased prefrontal neuronal density, as reported by Selemon et al[4] in patients with schizophrenia, a schizoaffective disorder, and HD on postmortem examination. Because HD is associated with psychotic symptoms,[5] it is possible that both disease processes affect the same final common pathway. Tissue loss in the basal ganglia in HD[6] could lead to metabolic or histological abnormalities or both in the prefrontal cortex because of the connections between these 2 parts of the brain.[7] It is possible that similar abnormalities in patients with schizophrenia might be related to subcortical lesions at an earlier neurodevelopmental stage.

Peter C. Williamson, MD
Department of Psychiatry
University Hospital
339 Windermere Rd, Box 5339
London, Ontario
Canada N6A 5A5
Ashok Malla, MD
Len Cortese, MD
A. Jon Stoessl, MD
Dick Drost, PhD
London, Ontario
Jeff A. Stanley, PhD
Pittsburgh, Pa

This study was supported by grant MT12078 from the Medical Research Council of Canada, Ottawa, Ontario; and grant R01 MH50768 from the National Institute of Mental Health, Rockville, Md.

1. Cady EB. *Clinical Magnetic Resonance Spectroscopy*. New York, NY: Plenum Publishing Corp; 1990.
2. Stanley JA, Williamson PC, Drost DJ, Carr T, Rylett J, Malla A, Thompson RT. In vivo prefrontal ^{31}P magnetic resonance spectroscopy in schizophrenic patients. *Arch Gen Psychiatry*. 1995;52:399-406.
3. Pettegrew JW, Kopp SJ, Padok J, Minshew NJ, Feliksik JM, Glonek T, Cohen MM. Chemical characterization of a prominent phosphomonoester resonance from mammalian brain: ^{31}P and ^{1}H NMR analysis at 4.7 and 14.1 tesla. *J Magn Reson*. 1986;67:443-450.
4. Selemon LD, Rajkowska G, Goldman-Rakic PS. Abnormally high neuronal density in the schizophrenic cortex. *Arch Gen Psychiatry*. 1995;52:805-818.
5. McHugh PR, Folstein MF. Psychiatric symptoms of Huntington's chorea: a clinical and phenomenological study. In: DF Benson, D Blumer, eds. *Psychiatric Aspects of Neurologic Disease*. New York, NY: Grune & Stratton Inc; 1975.
6. Purdon SE, Mohr E, Ilivitsky V, Jones BDW. Huntington's disease: pathogenesis, diagnosis and treatment. *J Psychiatry Neurosci*. 1994;19:359-367.
7. Alexander GE, De Long MR, Strick PL. Parallel organization of functionally segregated circuits linking basal ganglia and cortex. *Ann Rev Neurosci*. 1986;9:357-381.

In reply

This is an interesting and informative case report that demonstrates changes in brain membrane phospholipid metabolism in a young subject with HD. The changes observed in the subject with HD are similar to the changes previously reported in subjects with schizophrenia.[1-3] The in vivo ^{31}P MRS findings in the subject with HD are consistent with earlier in vitro ^{31}P MRS findings on autopsy brain samples of subjects with HD that revealed changes in membrane phospholipid metabolism.[4] The young subject with HD had clinical and molecular features that were similar to young subjects with schizophrenia.

The findings of decreased phosphomonoester concentrations in this subject with HD and the previously reported subjects with schizophrenia probably reflect changes in the neuropil. These changes could be due to the following: (1) reduced neuropil development (ie, an early neurodevelopmental insult), (2) exaggerated synaptic pruning of a normal neuropil (ie, a late neurodevelopmental insult occurring during late childhood or adolescence), (3) a combination of reduced neuropil development and exaggerated pruning (ie, early plus late insults), and (4) early neurodegeneration of the neuropil.

The previous in vivo ^{31}P MRS studies and the recent histological findings of Selemon et al[5] of reduced neuropil and increased neuronal packing density in schizophrenia and HD would be compatible with any of these 4 possibilities.

In this subject with HD and in subjects with first-episode, never-medicated schizophrenia, there are MRS-detectable metabolic and molecular abnormalities in the frontal cortex without discernible magnetic resonance imaging abnormalities in either the cortex or subcortical regions. This suggests that molecular changes occurring in the frontal cortex precede discernible anatomical changes that have been demonstrated to occur in either cortical or subcortical structures in subjects with HD and schizophrenia. Carefully designed longitudinal studies assessing clinical, MRS, and magnetic resonance imaging measures will be needed to further address these findings.

In addition, the HD case illustrates the importance of data from cases excluded from schizophrenia cohorts in research studies, as these patients may represent phenocopies of disorders that mimic schizophrenia and potentially illuminate the pathophysiological features of this heterogeneous syndrome. Similarly, cases excluded from normal control cohorts can be equally revealing, such as a subject who was studied by ^{31}P MRS in the preclinical state in whom schizophrenia then eventually developed, giving the opportunity to examine MRS data before the onset of this illness.[6]

In summary, this HD case report provides insights about HD and schizophrenia at the molecular and metabolic levels. It is anticipated that MRS studies will continue to provide molecular insights about these and other psychiatric disorders.

Jay W. Pettegrew, MD
Matcheri S. Keshavan, MD
Department of Psychiatry
Western Psychiatric Institute and Clinic
3811 O'Hara St
Pittsburgh, PA 15213

1. Pettegrew JW, Keshavan MS, Panchalingam K, Strychor S, Kaplan DB, Tretta MG, Allen M. Alterations in brain high-energy phosphate and phospholipid metabolism in first-episode, drug-naive schizophrenia: a pilot study of the dorsal prefrontal cortex by in vivo ^{31}P NMR spectroscopy. *Arch Gen Psychiatry*. 1991;48:563-568.
2. Kato T, Shiori T, Murashita J, Hamakawa H, Inubushi T, Takahashi S. Lateralized abnormality of high-energy phosphate and bilateral reduction of phos-

phomonoester measured by phosphorus-31 magnetic resonance spectroscopy of the frontal lobes in schizophrenia. *Psychiatry Res.* 1995;61:151-160.
3. Stanley JA, Williamson PC, Drost DJ, Carr TJ, Rylett J, Malla A, Thompson RT. An in vivo study of the prefrontal cortex of schizophrenic patients at different stages of illness via phosphorus magnetic resonance spectroscopy. *Arch Gen Psychiatry.* 1995;52:399-406.
4. Pettegrew JW, Minshew NJ, Cohen MM, Kopp SJ, Glonek T. P-31 NMR changes in Alzheimer's and Huntington's disease brain. *Neurology.* 1984;34(suppl 1): 281. Abstract.
5. Selemon LD, Rajkowska G, Goldman-Rakic PS. Abnormally high neuronal density in the schizophrenic cortex. *Arch Gen Psychiatry.* 1995;52:805-818.
6. Keshavan MS, Pettegrew JW, Panchalingam K, Kaplan D, Bozik E. Phosphorus 31 magnetic resonance spectroscopy detects altered brain metabolism before onset of schizophrenia. *Arch Gen Psychiatry.* 1991;48:1112-1113.

Use of Methylphenidate in a Patient With Glaucoma and Attention-Deficit Hyperactivity Disorder: A Clinical Dilemma

Methylphenidate hydrochloride (Ritalin), the drug of choice for attention-deficit hyperactivity disorder (ADHD), is contraindicated in patients with glaucoma on a theoretical, class-labeling basis. As methylphenidate had been, until recently, primarily prescribed to children, the consideration of prescribing it to patients with glaucoma rarely has arisen. However, as ADHD is being diagnosed and treated in more adults, this is becoming a treatment issue.

Moreover, stimulants are being used for the treatment of drug-induced and other sexual dysfunctions on an as-needed basis.[1-3] When used cautiously in conjunction with glaucoma medications and regular ophthalmologic monitoring, methylphenidate and other psychostimulants may be safe in patients with well-controlled, open-angle glaucoma. The following is an example, as well as a practical solution, to this problem.

Report of a Case. A 55-year-old male writer with primary open-angle glaucoma was receiving methylphenidate hydrochloride, 25 mg per day, for ADHD. Although his IQ placed him in the gifted range, he had experienced repeated academic and career failure throughout his life. Over the years, he had taken numerous tricyclic selective serotonin reuptake inhibitor and antidepressant medications with questionable results. A new psychiatrist, an expert in ADHD, diagnosed the condition and prescribed methylphenidate, unaware of the patient's history of glaucoma.

Ophthalmologically, the patient displayed intact visual fields and no evidence of damage to the optic nerve. The intraocular pressure in the left eye had always been within normal limits, but before glaucoma medication, the intraocular pressure in the right eye was slightly elevated to 28 mm Hg. After the initiation of 0.5% pilocarpine hydrochloride, 4 times per day, and 0.5% betaxolol hydrochloride (Betoptic), 4 times per day, the intraocular pressure in both eyes was found to be within normal limits at 17 mm Hg. The patient was scrupulous about taking his glaucoma medications as prescribed. A subsequent examination while he was receiving methylphenidate revealed no increase in intraocular pressure.

After 1 year of methylphenidate therapy, the patient's symptoms of distractibility and impatience improved significantly with impressive gains in both his personal and professional life. Another psychiatrist whom the patient consulted about sexual symptoms associated with ADHD questioned the safety of methylphenidate in a patient with glaucoma because of the contraindication listed in the *Physician's Desk Reference*. When the patient's ophthalmologist learned of the methylphenidate therapy, he felt compelled to recommend discontinuation of the drug based on the contraindication, although there was no elevation in intraocular pressure. The psychiatrist who prescribed the methylphenidate recommended that the patient return to a prescription of an antidepressant medication. The patient, having experienced none of these improvements while receiving antidepressants, was naturally distressed.

Comment. In the aforementioned case, the patient's glaucoma was well controlled and showed no exacerbation with the addition of methylphenidate therapy. Despite clear improvement in the patient's symptoms of ADHD, both the psychiatrist and the ophthalmologist were uncomfortable with its continuation. The contraindication appears to be a theoretical one, as there are no reports in the scientific literature of actual cases involving the use of methylphenidate in patients with glaucoma. Stimulants can cause a transient elevation of intraocular pressure in patients with glaucoma.[4] Because of their weak anticholinergic effect, these stimulants potentially can cause closure of the angle and precipitate an acute glaucomatous attack in patients with narrow-angle glaucoma. However, with frequent monitoring of intraocular pressure and gonioscopic examinations, the attacks may be avoided.

Rather than deny stimulants altogether to patients with well-controlled glaucoma, particularly those with uncomplicated open-angle glaucoma, it is advisable and safe to administer them, when indicated, in a carefully monitored manner. Intraocular pressures should be measured at frequent intervals, before and after the initiation of stimulants. If intraocular pressures remain within normal limits, it should be safe to continue stimulants in patients who require them for control of symptoms. This is particularly true when stimulants are used in low dosages (< 15 mg), on an occasional, as-needed basis, as has been reported for the treatment of antidepressant-induced sexual dysfunction.

As with many medications known to elevate marginally intraocular pressure, the contraindication listed in the *Physician's Desk Reference* does not necessarily mean that it is unsafe in every circumstance to administer the medication to patients with a particular condition. In ophthalmologic practice, it is common for patients with glaucoma who require systemic medications such as steroids and atropinelike drugs to take them as long as the glaucoma is well monitored and under good control. Because most forms of glaucoma are usually responsive to treatment, it is only necessary to discontinue a clinically indicated medication in the unlikely case of poor intraocular pressure control.

Barbara Bartlik, MD
Department of Psychiatry
Human Sexuality Program
New York Hospital-Cornell Medical Center
525 E 68 St, Box 147
New York, NY 10021
Gregory Harmon, MD
Peter Kaplan, MD
New York

1. Bartlik B, Kaplan P, Kaplan HS. Psychostimulants apparently reverse sexual dysfunction secondary to selective serotonin reuptake inhibitors. *J Sex Marital Ther*. 1995;21:264-271.
2. Bartlik B, Kaplan P, Kocsis J. Effects of antidepressants on sexuality. *Prim Psychiatry*. 1995;2:13.
3. Roeloffs C, Bartlik B, Kaplan P, Kocsis J. Methylphenidate and SSRI-induced sexual dysfunction. *J Clin Psychiatry*. 1996;57:11.
4. Oshika T. Ocular adverse effects of neuropsychiatric agents. *Drug Safety*. 1995; 12:256-263.

Sex Differences in Schizophrenia

Sex differences in schizophrenia, including variation in clinical symptoms, onset age, risk factors, response to treatment, and putative biological risk markers, are widely recognized to exist, yet are hard to explain by any pathogenetic mechanism.[1,2] In his discussion of Olney and Farber's *N*-methyl-D-aspartate receptor hypothesis, Crow[3] compares various (eg, neurohumoral, anatomical, physiological) theories of the pathogenesis of schizophrenia. He further examines these theories for their ability to explain various known features of the disorder, eg, clinical symptoms, brain changes, and epidemiological characteristics. Among these epidemiological features, he includes the sex differences discussed earlier. He recognizes only 2 hypotheses, the corpus callosum change model and the abnormal language lateralization model, as being able to account successfully for sex differences in schizophrenia.

Of the theories he compares, Crow expresses the opinion that the heteromodal association cortex model only "doubtfully explains" such sex differences. We believe that in fact this model's explanatory value is high. We have presented evidence elsewhere[4,5] that heteromodal association cortex is disproportionately involved in the pathophysiology of schizophrenia regarding specific local gray matter reductions. In addition, in the normal human brain, heteromodal neocortex is strikingly sexually dimorphic,[6] in that females have proportionately more gray matter (23%) in the frontal lobe and 13% more gray matter in the superior temporal gyrus, which is consistent with sexual dimorphism previously observed for regional blood flow.[7] We have speculated elsewhere[8] that this normal female gray matter advantage may act as a protective "buffer" in schizophrenia.

Thus, we conclude that the observation that schizophrenia expresses itself differently in men and women may be due to an interaction of pathology with innate cortical differences between male and female brains.

Godfrey D. Pearlson, MD
Thomas E. Schlaepfer, MD
The Johns Hopkins Medical Institutions
Division of Psychiatric Neuroimaging
Department of Psychiatry and Behavioral Sciences
600 N Wolfe St
Meyer 3-166
Baltimore, MD 21287-7362

1. Loranger AW. Sex difference in age at onset of schizophrenia. *Arch Gen Psychiatry*. 1984;41:157-161.
2. DeLisi LE, Dauphinais ID, Hauser P. Gender differences in the brain: are they relevant to the pathogenesis of schizophrenia? *Compr Psychiatry*. 1989;30: 197-208.
3. Olney JW, Farber NB. Cited by: Crow TJ. Constraints on concepts of pathogenesis: language and the speciation process as the key to the etiology of schizophrenia. *Arch Gen Psychiatry*. 1995;52:1011-1014.
4. Schlaepfer TE, Harris GJ, Tien AY, Federman EB, Peng LW, Lee S, Pearlson GD. Pattern of decreased regional cortical gray matter volume using magnetic resonance imaging in schizophrenia. *Am J Psychiatry*. 1994;151:842-848.
5. Pearlson GD, Petty RG, Ross CA, Tien AY. Schizophrenia: a disease of heteromodal association cortex? *Neuropsychopharmacology*. 1996;14:1-17.
6. Schlaepfer TE, Harris GJ, Aylward EH, McArthur JC, Peng LW, Lee S, Pearlson GD. Structure differences in the cerebral cortex of normal male and female subjects. *Psychiatry Res*. 1995;61:129-135.
7. Gur RC, Gur RE, Obrist WD, Hungerbuhler JP, Younkin D, Rosen AD, Skolnick BE, Reivich M. Sex and handedness differences in cerebral blood flow during rest and cognitive activity. *Science*. 1982;217;659-661.
8. Pearlson GD, Pulver AE. Sex, schizophrenia and the cerebral cortex. In: Ancill RJ, Holliday S, Higenbottam J., eds. *Schizophrenia: Exploring the Spectrum of Psychosis*. New York, NY: Wiley Publishing Co; 1994; 344-362.

Managed Care and the Future of Psychiatry

Thomas Detre, MD, Margaret C. McDonald, PhD

IN 1987,[1] one of us (T.D.) issued 3 predictions about the future of psychiatry, all of which have come true: (1) The promiscuous use of psychiatry to address a world of problems that are not biomedical and are unrelated to individual patients or their families has diluted the specialty's focus and made it what it should not be—a proposed solution to social ills. (2) The routinization of complex clinical tasks has inevitably resulted in downward decentralization, enabling lower-level professionals to take over responsibilities that were once the purview of physicians. (3) New knowledge about the brain and the mind have made it mandatory for psychiatry and neurology to mate for life to assure the future of both.

These comments may have been considered gratuitous baiting of colleagues until managed care entered our lives, accelerating a process that would have occurred anyway but at a slower pace. In a way, psychiatry has been under managed care for the past 25 years, as it has routinely operated under different reimbursement criteria than those for other medical illnesses.[2] However, under the old managed care, everyone on the "multidisciplinary treatment team" got paid. Today, the psychiatrist, being the most expensive team member, is precisely the one insurers would prefer not to pay.[3]

None of these changes are unexpected. Industries, the federal government, and a growing number of states have long been experimenting with some form of managed care. The federal government was not ready to take more serious action, however, until we reached the point at which nearly 14% of the gross domestic product went to health care but still left more than 35 million persons uninsured or underinsured.[4]

With the defeat of President Clinton's proposed Health Security Act, the doors were suddenly wide open to market forces. Although that legislation addressed fundamental health care inequities, the measure failed because both the public and Congress believed it was too ambitious, too costly, and too bureaucratic. Instead of getting managed care, we got unmanaged competition from the for-profit sector of the health insurance world, which cuts costs by using primary care physicians and nurse practitioners to control access to specialists but reinvests none of its profits in education or research.

See also pages 206 and 212

The current consensus is that eventually 50% of all physicians will or should be in primary care.[5] However, it is likely that the exponential growth of new knowledge will mandate greater rather than lesser use of at least some specialists and a redefinition of primary care. The crucial task of coordinating the care of patients with complex problems that require input from several specialists will pass into the hands of well-trained and computer-literate general internists, pediatricians, and family physicians. Nurse practitioners and physician assistants will work side-by-side with physicians in caring for patients with chronic illnesses—much the same way they are already doing with patients who have cancer. (Psychiatry, by the way, was one of the earliest specialties to use a multidisciplinary team to care for chronically ill patients.) These midlevel practitioners will also take over the management of common con-

From the Health Sciences, University of Pittsburgh, Pittsburgh, Pa.

ditions and much preventive care. The number of tertiary care centers will diminish sharply as the health care provision system becomes both vertically integrated and decentralized, leaving only the most complex care in academic medical centers or, in their absence, regional centers of excellence.

DIMINISHING RETURNS

The role of psychiatrists will also change. Contrary to what academic psychiatry's political pundits would have us believe, psychiatry is not, has never been, and never will be a primary care specialty. What psychiatry is and will continue to be is a consulting specialty. Psychiatrists will assist those who provide primary care, treating directly only patients whose illnesses are refractory to traditional therapies or otherwise difficult to manage. Instead of operating in a single setting, consultant psychiatrists will "circuit-ride" among the various components of an integrated system, which will include outpatient clinics, satellites, affiliated hospitals, and home care facilities.[6] This consulting role need not be considered a consolation prize; recent studies have shown that treatment outcomes are improved when mental health care is supervised by psychiatrists and administered according to databased protocols.[7]

Current estimates, however, indicate that if 100% of the population were in managed care, as many as half of the nation's 36 000 psychiatrists would no longer be needed (*American Medical News.* March 6, 1995:1, 27, 28). The trend in managed care is to employ 1 psychiatrist for every 25 000 enrolled lives, as these firms, including those that contract exclusively for psychiatric services, employ a large number of psychologists, social workers, and other nonmedical health professionals to offer their subscribers "mental health care." In fact, the managed care companies that have been formed around mental health "carve outs" are particularly regressive because they separate psychiatric disorders from other medical disorders just when the country is moving toward having 1 primary care provider manage all of a patient's problems and just when the evidence of the biological basis of most major psychiatric illnesses has reached the point of indisputableness.

DESPECIALIZATION

Psychiatry's turf is under siege from 2 emerging fronts.[8] First, the specialty's growing biological basis makes it more like the rest of medicine, and particularly more like neurology.[9] New pharmacologic therapies are something that generalist physicians can relate to and, therefore, feel competent to provide. Second, as other providers have earned the right to practice psychotherapy without supervision from a psychiatrist,[10] a medical education is no longer mandatory for students who are interested in human behavior.

If we were to examine dispassionately what most psychiatrists are trained to do and what others do equally well, we would conclude that there is a wide range of problems—from autism to dementiform disorders—for which neurologists who have been trained in the assessment of the central nervous system using increasingly accurate electrodiagnostic and imaging methods have a clear advantage over psychiatrists. Psychiatrists still have full responsibility for so-called functional psychoses, but this exclusivity is primarily attributable to neurologists' lack of interest in managing such difficult, time-consuming problems. In response to increasing financial pressures, some neurologists (at least a convenience sample of our colleagues) have already begun to treat middle-aged and elderly patients with depression, feeling that affective changes often occur concomitantly with or secondary to other neurologic disorders and, thus, are an inherent treatment consideration.

Much of what traditionally constituted psychiatric outpatient care, including the treatment of anxiety disorders and the detoxification and psychosocial rehabilitation of patients with substance abuse, is now in the hands of nonphysicians, though psychiatrists provide consultation for pharmacological management (*The Wall Street Journal.* December 21, 1995:1, 4).[3] However, even this distinction is threatened as psychologists and nurse practitioners push state legislatures for prescription and hospital admission privileges.[10]

Psychiatrists also have to recognize that what they call the art of psychopharmacology and defend as their exclusive domain is no great intellectual challenge. Witness the No. 2 status of fluoxetine hydrochloride (Prozac; Dista Products Corp, Indianapolis, Ind) on the nation's top 10 prescription drug list—a level of use that certainly is not attributable to prescriptions from psychiatrists alone (*Clinical Psychiatry News.* August 1995:1).[11] While the prowess of primary care physicians in prescribing psychopharmacological medications can—and has—been debated, the higher tolerance ranges of the drugs in use today, combined with well-documented treatment guidelines, make the prescription of these drugs by nonpsychiatrists a more reasonable proposition. Moreover, with the exception of clozapine, current psychotropic drugs are neither more specific nor more effective than the early phenothiazines and tricyclic antidepressants; thus, all physicians, whether they are psychiatrists or primary care physicians, still have an arsenal of rifle-shot rather than well-targeted magic bullets. Under these circumstances, any knowledgeable clinician can follow protocols based on data from controlled clinical trials to use these relatively nonspecific agents. The trick for the nonpsychiatrist, if there is one, is to administer these agents in sufficient doses to determine their efficacy and to avoid the temptation of polypharmacy. If the patient does not respond within a finite period, then a drug from the next group is tried, by which time there is also a good chance for a spontaneous remission. Since psychiatric nosology offers few well-defined course markers to signal a patient's stage of illness, maintenance treatment is routinely prescribed for patients who relapse frequently or whose symptoms are sufficiently disruptive to place them or society at risk. The only other requirement for competent pharmacological management is access to an up-to-date drug information system that would enable the clinician to check drug-drug and drug-disease interactions.

Since psychosurgery has limited indications and, in any case, was always the domain of neurosurgeons, electroconvulsive therapy is the only remaining biological treatment that is still administered by psychiatrists. But again, the placement of the electrodes and the pushing of the button on automated equipment to deliver a predetermined amount of electricity are far less hazardous than defibrillating patients—a task that emergency medical technicians do routinely. The only true medical task is that of the anesthesiologist, but even that could be done by a nurse anesthetist.

What we are left with is psychotherapy. In a 1994 editorial,[12] psychotherapy was reported to account for "only" 8% of the total annual expenditure for ambulatory medical care; thus, to quote the editorial: "The probability is not so enormous that it will overwhelm reasonable efforts to provide and manage it." To be sure, a growing number of well-controlled studies have demonstrated that certain forms of psychotherapy are effective in a variety of conditions, either alone or in combination with pharmacotherapy. However, the most thoroughly tested of these (ie, cognitive-behavioral therapy and interpersonal psychotherapy) have been standardized and manualized, enabling any reasonably intelligent, well-motivated "generic therapist" to administer them; although long-term, so-called intensive therapy has been dying for decades, some of our profession's leaders cling fiercely to the illusion that it works and that only psychiatrists can do it. However, since we have proof only of its high cost and not of its effectiveness, psychiatry's reluctance to admit that the emperor is indeed naked only increases public skepticism.

Even in those instances in which psychotherapy shows some incremental benefits, given the costs, the following question is increasingly asked: "Does the difference really make a difference?" Our society long ago accepted the position of insurance companies that plastic surgery for a disfiguring lesion is reimbursable while getting a better-looking nose is not; we should now get used to the idea that the only way to receive treatments that make us feel just a little bit better is to pay for them out of our own pocket, if we can afford it. Although the term "medical necessity" implies scientific definability, the definitions are shaped considerably by prejudice and politics. In psychiatry, clear lines are being drawn between seriously and chronically mentally ill patients and the "worried well." Care for the latter is clearly not a medical necessity, and even the former must sometimes fight to prove that they are in need of sustained treatment.

REINVENTING PSYCHIATRY

As an academic specialty and as a component of the academic health center in its managed care variation, psychiatry will have increasing difficulty being an independent specialty unless it assumes a role akin to that of physiatry, which concerns itself with the rehabilitation and maintenance of patients' functional status and evaluation of treatment outcome. Academic psychiatry could, likewise, relegate itself to a clinical and clinical research role. However, traditionally, the best of our profession have devoted their careers to understanding the etiology and pathogenesis of major psychiatric illnesses, not just to treating them. Because of recent remarkable advances in basic neuroscience, continued pursuit of this quest leads psychiatrists and neurologists onto a converging path. Given that the locus of this research role remains the academic health center, the choice of university-based psychiatrists is both forced and obvious.

We believe more strongly than ever that the time has come for psychiatry and neurology to become a single discipline. As was pointed out in 1987, the current definition of psychiatric disorders is arbitrary, based largely on the presence of psychological and behavioral changes and the absence of neurologic, neuroradiological, or laboratory findings or other external validators. Unless the changes in psychological functioning and behavior that are considered pathological are, in reality, expressions of altered brain functioning, however, psychiatry can no longer be considered a *medical* specialty—and, if it is not, then what is it? This conceptualization does not deny the importance of adverse psychological and psychosocial events in the pathogenesis of disorders, nor does it minimize their role in the "pathoplasticity" of symptoms, meaning the manner in which the presentation of symptoms is molded by culture and personal experiences. It does assert that exogenous factors must produce changes in the central nervous system, expressed partially as the alterations in behavior, mood, and cognition on which psychiatric diagnoses rest and partially as other biological changes, which cannot yet be measured.

Medicine should again consider breeding a new type of physician who, for lack of a better term, may be called a "clinical neuroscientist." Such individuals should be trained to make optimal use of recent advances in neurosciences, neuropharmacology, and metabolic and functional imaging in their diagnosis and management of patients. Once they have received their basic training in both neurology and psychiatry and learned what every clinician needs to know about genetics and epidemiology and what neuropsychology can contribute to the assessment of brain functioning, these physicians could then subspecialize in one of many areas, whether it be demyelinating diseases, neuromuscular disorders, or psychoses. We would not need too many of such specialists, most of whom would practice in tertiary care centers. However, every patient in a managed care plan should have access to the expert diagnostic skills and treatment recommendation abilities of a clinical neuroscientist, should they be needed.

The established leaders of academic psychiatry, even if they agreed with this proposal, would still object on the grounds that the training of such physicians would be too lengthy and too expensive. That may be so. However, given what will be a substantial reduction in the educational component of Medicare and the steadily expanding use of nonpsychiatric professionals, it is academic medicine's moral responsibility to think through carefully who will be trained, how many of them, and how to educate them in a manner that will fill a need in our health care system. As recently touted through cover articles in several weekly news magazines, the 1990s have accurately been labeled the "decade of the brain." Medical science has finally developed the tools to get to the bottom of some of the most challenging and refractory disorders—to identify their causes and to develop effective treatments. In the long term, this new knowledge will save both lives and money. However, we must have people with the training to do the work, and we must find the "venture capital" to invest in the research and development that will eventually lead to the payoff. Responsibility for this investment must be spread among all health care providers who stand to benefit, not just among the academic medical centers at which research is carried out, and clinical neuroscientists must lead the charge.

At the same time, there is an urgent need to integrate the study of the health care provision system into our academic curriculum. Psychiatry pioneered team-based care that included nurses, social workers, and, in mental health centers, community workers some 35 years before it became fashionable. Rather than being defensive, it should now conduct outcome studies to determine what tasks psychiatrists (or clinical neuroscientists) must personally perform and what tasks can be assigned to others to ensure the continuity of high-quality, cost-effective care for mentally ill patients—most of whom suffer from chronic disorders. Since the emerging vertically integrated health care provision system will have several components without being concentrated in a single geographic location, a well-organized and user-friendly information system will be essential. This development, as well as the increased use of electronic medical records, will mandate computer literacy for all participating physicians. Remarkably, however, while the residency review committee for psychiatric training tends to criticize or outright disapprove of programs that do not dedicate sufficient time to long-term psychodynamically oriented psychotherapy, to our knowledge, it has never censured any department for not teaching the skills that all clinicians will require to function effectively not just in an integrated health care system but one that relies almost exclusively on an integrated information system.

We also need to consider collaborative ventures that would enhance opportunities for clinical research. Already in many academic medical centers, neurologists, neurosurgeons, and psychiatrists attend jointly to brain-injured patients, whether they are victims of trauma, stroke, or tumor surgery. It would be logical for psychiatrists to assume patient care responsibilities jointly in other areas as well—particularly in the care of those disorders that lie at the 2 ends of the age spectrum: the very young and the very old. And if psychiatrists and neurologists go so far as to learn one another's languages, they might find that they are actually able to do a better job caring for particular patients than they could "flying solo" and that their disciplines have far more in common than their self-imposed isolation had previously allowed them to acknowledge.[13] Finally, if psychiatrists are brave enough to recognize that there is nothing neurologic or psychiatric about neuroscience and neuropharmacology, the profession may even conclude that in this difficult fiscal climate where only 10% to 15% of research proposals are funded by the National Institutes of Health, Bethesda, Md, psychiatry should find alliances not just with departments of neurology but also with those of neurobiology, molecular genetics, and pharmacology instead of desperately trying to become its own university.

There is no question that psychiatry is undergoing its own version of apoptosis. If there is any doubt, recent "match day" figures have provided an appropriate reality check about the popularity of the specialty, with psychiatry garnering the lowest proportion (3%) of graduating medical students since 1929.[8] Ironically, this dimunition of interest comes at a time when new, noninvasive exploratory techniques have exposed the brain-mind continuum to clear view, if not immediate understanding.

The profession of psychiatry is like the 1 remaining daughter in a long family line who clings fiercely to her maiden name as the last family member to bear it. If psychiatry cohabits with—or even chooses to marry—neurology, only the name reverts. Psychiatry's intellectual heritage remains intact and combines in new ways to assure the long-term survival of its essential core.

Accepted for publication July 11, 1996.

Reprints: Thomas Detre, MD, Health Sciences, University of Pittsburgh, 3811 O'Hara St, Pittsburgh, PA 15213.

REFERENCES

1. Detre T. The future of psychiatry. *Am J Psychiatry.* 1987;144:621-625.
2. Dorwart RA. Managed mental health care: myths and realities in the 1990s. *Hosp Community Psychiatry.* 1990;41:1087-1091.
3. Lazarus A. A proposal for psychiatric collaboration in managed care. *Am J Psychother.* 1994:48:600-609.
4. Burner ST, Waldo DR. National health expenditure projections. *Health Care Financ Rev.* 1995;16:221-242.
5. Health Security Act (draft), 103rd Cong, 1st Sess (1993).
6. Olfson M, Pincus AH, Dial TH. Professional practice patterns of US psychiatrists. *Am J Psychiatry.* 1994;151:89-95.
7. Sturm R, Wells KB. How can care for depression become more cost-effective? *JAMA.* 1995;273:51-58.
8. Sierles FS, Taylor MA. Decline of U.S. medical student career choice of psychiatry and what to do about it. *Am J Psychiatry.* 1995;152:1416-1426.
9. Kay J. The influence of the curriculum in psychiatry residency education. *Psychiatr Q.* 1991;62:95-104.
10. Cummings NA. The credentialing of professional psychologists and its implication for the other mental health disciplines. *J Counsel Dev.* 1990;68:485-490.
11. Beardsly RS, Gardocki GJ, Larson DB, Hidalso J. Prescribing of psychotropic medications by primary care physicians and psychiatrists. *Arch Gen Psychiatry.* 1988;45:1117-1119.
12. Sledge WH. Psychotherapy in the United States: challenges and opportunities. *Am J Psychiatry.* 1994;151:1267-1270.
13. Starr A, Sporty LD. Similar disorders viewed with different perspectives, a challenge for neurology and psychiatry. *Arch Neurol.* 1994;51:977-980.

Essential Roles for Psychiatry in the Era of Managed Care

DURING THE past few years, managed care has moved aggressively from inpatient to outpatient psychiatric care and from the private to public sector.[1] One consequence of these developments is that psychiatrists are now at risk of losing several of their traditional clinical roles to less highly paid nonmedical mental health professionals. Some psychiatrists have responded by emphasizing their professional roots within medicine and their intellectual roots within biology and the neurosciences. In this issue of the ARCHIVES, the prescription urged by Detre and McDonald[2] that psychiatry should join neurology as a single discipline carries this response to its logical extreme.

See also pages 201 and 212

We question the wisdom and necessity of such a union. We believe that the future of psychiatry will be best served not by merging with neurology but by concentrating on the assessment and treatment of patients with major psychiatric disorders who present with diagnostic difficulties or who have not responded to simple pharmacological or psychological interventions. These patients receive care in a variety of treatment settings where they challenge and often frustrate their primary clinicians.

The economics of managed care has refined and distilled the essential clinical roles of psychiatry. Detre and McDonald[2] are right in their assertion that managed care is making psychiatry into a consulting specialty. However, this does not lead us to conclude that psychiatry should exclusively focus on the neurodiagnostic assessment of brain disorders. Psychiatry has a broader role to play in managing the large number of patients who have complicated or comorbid psychiatric disorders.[3] Psychiatrists are the only health professionals with the knowledge and ability to integrate and apply the full range of biopsychosocial interventions to manage such difficult cases.

MANAGEMENT OF COMPLEX CASES

Rational treatment and rehabilitation planning depends on an accurate diagnosis. Psychiatrists, by virtue of their medical training and interviewing skills, are uniquely prepared to perform this clinical task. Paranoid psychosis, for example, is associated with several street drugs and prescribed medications, focal central nervous system diseases, neurodegenerative diseases, and infectious diseases, as well as with a number of psychiatric disorders. Nonmedical mental health professionals do not have the training to evaluate such medical illnesses and select, order, and interpret the appropriate laboratory and radiological tests. By contrast, neurologists and other nonpsychiatrist physicians are not trained to elicit the clinical information that is needed to distinguish psychiatric disorders that commonly involve paranoid ideation (eg, borderline personality disorder, schizoaffective disorder, or schizophrenia) or to treat these disorders. An accurate psychiatric diagnosis of a personality disorder as opposed to that of a psychotic disorder may influence the extent to which psychological as opposed to pharmacological interventions are considered for the treatment of acute paranoia.

Managed care organizations value the efficient treatment of unstable psychiatric patients who are at risk of extensive service utilization.[4] These patients typically present with comorbid psychiatric disorders and often run a volatile clinical course. At different times, they may require emergency hospitalization, urgent pharmacological interventions, management of suicidal, assaultive, or impulsive behaviors, detoxification, or psychosocial interventions to prevent the loss of social supports, housing, or occupational opportunities. Psychiatrists are especially well equipped to assess these patients and select and integrate the appropriate range of services. A promising treatment model involves psychiatrist-led multidisciplinary community-based treatment teams.[5] Psychiatrists who are trained to lead such treatment teams will be highly valued by managed care plans.

There is now general agreement that managed care has been effective in reducing or at least slowing the growth of mental health costs.[6,7] This has been achieved largely through reducing the use of expensive hospital care. The treatment of relatively unstable patients in less restrictive settings places greater emphasis on symptom control and coordination of necessary mental health and social services. Psychiatrists have an essential role to play in each of these areas.

Under capitated managed care plans, there are strong financial pressures to shift the costs of treating illness-related social and occupational problems outside of the medical care financing system. While psychiatrists may not be extensively involved in the direct provision of social and occupational rehabilitative services, psychiatrists should resist efforts to narrow the mission and responsibility of the mental health services system.

An important distinguishing characteristic of psychiatry is its interest and concern with how patients function in all aspects of life. The high indirect or societal costs associated with mental and addictive disorders, including the impact on the family and children, underscore the wide-ranging effects of mental illness on social function.[8] A commitment to long-term social and occupational rehabilitative goals must not be lost in the market-driven rush to reduce mental health expenditures.

The promise of reducing inefficient practice patterns has fueled a recent surge of interest in practice guidelines. Detre and McDonald[2] suggest that simple treatment protocols will soon reduce the need for highly trained clinical judgment and thereby decrease the need for psychiatrists. However, the appropriate implementation of psychiatric treatment guidelines requires considerable clinical skill. Prevailing circumstances may require that clinicians adapt, modify, and sometimes even contradict guideline-based practice. While treatment guidelines help inform clinical decision making, they seldom substitute for mature clinical judgment. This may be particularly true in the management of patients with complex or comorbid disorders. For example, the co-occurrence of personality disorders with Axis I disorders may complicate the physician-patient alliance and thereby limit the application of treatment guidelines. Attempts to short-circuit a case-by-case approach to patient care may carry a very high price.

Evidence from research on a variety of medical procedures indicates that treatments that incorporate individual clinical judgment often outperform standardized care.[9-12] An illustration of this principle was recently provided by Saitz et al[13] who found that individualized treatment of alcohol withdrawal was far more efficient than a commonly used standardized approach to the administration of benzodiazepine. The individualized symptom-triggered therapy reduced the mean duration of treatment from 68 to 9 hours and cut in quarter the amount of chlordiazepoxide hydrochloride that was prescribed.

Several patient characteristics, including age, health status, ethnicity, and personal habits, can alter the absorption, distribution, and metabolism of psychotropic medications.[14,15] Such interindividual variation complicates simple algorithmic approaches to clinical psychopharmacology. Management of medication compliance adds further complexity as it involves intricate issues of illness denial, dysphoric drug reactions, stigma, family pressures, and negative aspects of the therapeutic alliance.[16,17] Medication management, particularly because of the connection between noncompliance and rehospitalization,[18-20] will remain a cornerstone of psychiatric practice for the foreseeable future.

CONSULTATION WITH OTHER HEALTH CARE PROFESSIONALS

The proliferation of managed care provides psychiatrists with opportunities to forge new collaborations with primary care physicians. In managed care arrangements, primary care physicians often serve as gatekeepers to specialized mental health services.[21] To prosper in such practice environments, psychiatrists will need to make themselves readily accessible to primary care physicians and their patients. Psychiatrists will be most valued if they are willing to travel to primary care clinics, focus on the patient's chief complaint, arrive at an accurate diagnosis, respond to emergency situations, offer rapid feedback to the referring physician, and provide concrete treatment suggestions.

Psychiatry has an important role to play in the care of primary care patients who have failed to respond to simple psychotropic or counseling interventions. In the case of depression that persists following antidepressant prescription, for example, a psychiatric consultation may uncover medication noncompliance, inadequate antidepressant dosing, occult substance abuse, long-term marital conflict, complicated bereavement, steroid use, or any of a variety of other conditions that may account for the poor treatment responses, and it may point to new management strategies. The benefits of primary care physician–psychiatrist collaborative management have been recently demonstrated in a randomized controlled clinical trial.[22]

Psychiatrists also have an important role to play in consulting with nonmedical mental health professionals. When a patient who is under the care of a nonmedical mental health professional reaches an impasse, a psychiatrist can assess the adequacy of the psychological treatment and the need for a psychopharmacological intervention. Such consultation may improve the efficiency of mental health care provision.

OVERVIEW

The suggestion that psychiatry should move closer to or join with neurology as a means of survival in the era of managed care overlooks fundamental differences in the training, skills, and strengths of the 2 specialties. Psychiatrists are concerned with the management of illnesses that, for the most part, become apparent only through direct interactions with the patient or through listening to others describe the patient's feelings, thoughts, and actions.[23] As such, psychiatrists have become highly proficient in clinical interviewing. Neurologists and the other medical specialists have much less expertise, skill, and interest in this mode of clinical observation.

The considerable uncertainty that surrounds the basic etiology of the major mental disorders does not diminish the value of clinical psychiatry. Moreover, progress in the fundamental biology of major depression, schizophrenia, panic disorder, and other psychiatric disorders will not secure our future. To thrive in the era of managed care, psychiatrists will need to concentrate their efforts on patients with complicated and difficult to treat disorders. These patients may have the most to benefit from the unique combination of medical training, interviewing skills, and knowledge of differential therapeutics that distinguish psychiatrists from their medical and mental health colleagues.

Mark Olfson, MD, MPH
Myrna M. Weissman, PhD
Department of Psychiatry
College of Physicians and Surgeons
Columbia University and New York State Psychiatric Institute
722 W 168th St
New York, NY 10032
John F. Gottlieb, MD
Northwestern University Medical School
Chicago, Ill

REFERENCES

1. Iglehart JK. Managed care and mental health. *N Engl J Med.* 1996:334:131-135.
2. Detre T, McDonald MC. Managed care and the future of psychiatry. *Arch Gen Psychiatry.* 1997; 54:201-204.
3. Kessler RC, McGonagle KA, Zhao S, Nelson CB, Hughes M, Eshleman S, Wittchen H-U, Kendler KS. Lifetime and 12-month prevalence of *DSM-III-R* psychiatric disorders in the United States: results from the National Comorbidity Survey. *Arch Gen Psychiatry.* 1994;51:8-19.
4. Meyer RE, Sotsky SM. Managed care and the role and training of psychiatrists. *Health Aff (Millwood).* 1995;14:65-77.
5. Burns BJ, Santos AB. Assertive community treatment: an update of randomized trials. *Psychiatr Serv.* 1995;46:669-675.
6. Callahan J, Shepard D, Beinecke RH, Larson MJ, Cavanaugh MD. Mental health/substance abuse treatment in managed care: the Massachusetts Medicaid experience. *Health Aff (Millwood).* 1995; 14:173-184.
7. Mechanic D, Schlesinger M, McAlpine DD. Management of mental health and substance abuse services: state of the art and early results. *Milbank Q.* 1995;73:19-55.
8. Rice DP, Kelman S, Miller LS. The economic burden of mental illness. *Hosp Community Psychiatry.* 1992;43:1227-1232.
9. Lerman C, Lustbader E, Rimer B, Daly M, Miller S, Sands C, Balshem A. Effects of individualized breast cancer risk counseling: a randomized trial. *J Natl Cancer Inst.* 1995;87:286-292.
10. Prochaska JO, DiClemente CC, Velicer WF, Rossi JS. Standardized, individualized, interactive and personalized self-help programs for smoking cessation. *Health Psychol.* 1993;12: 399-405.
11. Käser O, Castaño y Almendral A. Cancer of the endometrium stage I—standardized or individualized treatment. *Eur J Obstet Gynecol Reprod Biol.* 1984;18:329-334.
12. Dice JE, Burckart GJ, Woo JT, Helms RA. Standardized versus pharmacist-monitored individualized parenteral nutrition in low-birth-weight infants. *Am J Hosp Pharm.* 1981;38: 1487-1489.
13. Saitz R, Mayo-Smith MF, Roberts MS, Redmond HA, Bernard DR, Calkins DR. Individualized treatment of alcohol withdrawal: a randomized double-blind controlled trial. *JAMA.* 1994; 272:519-523.
14. Rudorfer MV. Pharmacokinetics of psychotropic drugs in special populations. *J Clin Psychiatry.* 1993;54(suppl):50-54.
15. Bond WS. Ethnicity and psychotropic drugs. *Clin Pharmacol Ther.* 1991;10:467-470.
16. Weiden P, Rapkin B, Mott T, et al. Rating of Medication Influences (ROMI) scale in schizophrenia. *Schizophr Bull.* 1994;20:297-310.
17. Frank AF, Gunderson JG. The role of therapeutic alliance in the treatment of schizophrenia. *Arch Gen Psychiatry.* 1990;47:287-235.
18. Kent S, Yellowlees P. Psychiatric and social reasons for frequent rehospitalization. *Hosp Community Psychiatry.* 1994;45:347-350.
19. Sullivan G, Wells KB, Morgenstern H, Leake B. Identifying modifiable risk factors for rehospitalization: a case-control study of seriously mentally ill persons in Mississippi. *Am J Psychiatry.* 1995;152:1749-1756.
20. Merken PA, Stanislav SW, Lacombe S, Pierce C, Hornstra R, Sommi RW. Profile of a sample of subjects admitted to an acute care psychiatric facility with manic symptoms. *Psychopharmacol Bull.* 1992;28:201-205.
21. Hurley RE, Freund DA, Gage BJ. Gatekeeper effects on patterns of physician use. *J Fam Pract.* 1991;32:167-174.
22. Katon W, Von Korff M, Lin E, Walker E, Simon GE, Bush T, Robinson P, Russo J. Collaborative management to achieve treatment guidelines: impact on depression in primary care. *JAMA.* 1995: 273:1026-1031.
23. Klerman GL. Resolved: the psychiatrist of the future will have to be a neurologist: the negative view? Presented at the 138th annual meeting of the American Psychiatric Association; May 20, 1985; Dallas, Tex.

Abnormal thyroid function tests (see **PRECAUTIONS**).

Pancreatic: Acute pancreatitis including fatalities.

Metabolic: Hyperammonemia (see **PRECAUTIONS**), hyponatremia, and inappropriate ADH secretion.

There have been rare reports of Fanconi's syndrome occurring chiefly in children.

Decreased carnitine concentrations have been reported although the clinical relevance is undetermined.

Hyperglycinemia has occurred and was associated with a fatal outcome in a patient with preexistent nonketotic hyperglycinemia.

Genitourinary: Enuresis and urinary tract infection.

Special Senses: Hearing loss, either reversible or irreversible, has been reported; however, a cause and effect relationship has not been established. Ear pain has also been reported.

Other: Edema of the extremities, lupus erythematosus, bone pain, cough increased, pneumonia, otitis media, bradycardia, cutaneous vasculitis, and fever.

OVERDOSAGE

Overdosage with valproate may result in somnolence, heart block, and deep coma. Fatalities have been reported; however patients have recovered from valproate levels as high as 2120 μg/mL.

In overdose situations, the fraction of drug not bound to protein is high and hemodialysis or tandem hemodialysis plus hemoperfusion may result in significant removal of drug. The benefit of gastric lavage or emesis will vary with the time since ingestion. General supportive measures should be applied with particular attention to the maintenance of adequate urinary output.

Naloxone has been reported to reverse the CNS depressant effects of valproate overdosage. Because naloxone could theoretically also reverse the antiepileptic effects of valproate, it should be used with caution in patients with epilepsy.

Ref. 03-4668-R3-June, 1996 (Bipolar)

ABBOTT LABORATORIES
NORTH CHICAGO, IL 60064, U.S.A.

701-731-8121A **MASTER**

PRINTED IN U.S.A.

INDEX TO ADVERTISERS

Abbott Laboratories
Depakote-Bipolar 1997 . . . . 208A-B, 209-211

Glaxo Wellcome, Inc.
Wellbutrin SR 223, 245

Hoffmann-Laroche, Inc.
Klonopin 255-256

McNeil Pharmaceuticals
Haldol Decanoate . . . . Cover 2-193

Lilly
Prozac 256A-B

Searle
Ambien 224A-B

SmithKline Beecham
Paxil 195-196

Solvay Pharmaceuticals
Luvox 242-244

U.S. Pharmaceuticals, Pfizer Inc.
Aricept 200A-H
Zoloft . . . . 232A-B, Cover 3-Cover 4

While every precaution is taken to ensure accuracy, we cannot guarantee against the possibility of an occasional change or omission in the preparation of this index.

COMMENTARY

The Futures of Psychiatry

DETRE AND McDonald[1] provide a clear and incisive explanation for the current effect of managed care on psychiatry. We are under siege. Either by design or default, market forces are being used to ration medical care and reduce costs in the United States. Market forces, embodied by for-profit managed care imperatives, give primary care clinicians a competitive edge over higher-cost specialists. Nonmedical mental health professionals compete aggressively for patients in an unbridled marketplace. In the absence of good outcome or cost-effectiveness data, those clinicians or systems that can promise good enough care at the lowest cost thrive—highly specialized systems or practitioners who focus exclusively on quality suffer. This is different in various parts of the country, with the marketplace being most ferocious in California, Minnesota, Massachusetts, Maryland, and more recently in New York.

See also pages 201 and 206

Detre and McDonald propose a solution to this crisis that would redefine psychiatry, limiting its focus to the neurosciences. The new psychiatrist would be an expert clinical neuroscientist. There would be fewer psychiatrists, better trained in a more circumscribed field. This, I believe, is an excessively limited scenario for our medical specialty. Over the centuries, medicine has been the craft or art of taking care of suffering individuals (ie, patients). Medical care has been increasingly based on scientific and public health principles that include data and theories alike. Individuals do not pursue medicine to become scientists; they want to care for the diseased and disabled. This is the fundamental business of medicine, and increasingly we have turned to demand and supply forces through managed care to determine how this business should work to balance access, quality, and cost. This new medical marketplace is a reality that must be understood if psychiatrists will adapt and survive in the next millenium.

Although psychiatrists are challenged to cope and adapt to today's managed care era, they seem to be meeting the challenge well. In the *American Medical News* last spring, psychiatry was characterized as a "good times specialty"[2] with few psychiatrists unable to find full-time work. Psychiatry ranked close to family practice, obstetrics and gynecology, and emergency medicine. This was in contrast with other medical specialties, such as pathology and reconstructive surgery, in which 10% of the specialists were without full-time jobs in their specialties.[2]

Psychiatry is still in demand, and various opportunities are available nationwide. Many geographic areas desperately need general psychiatrists. In addition, subspecialization within the field provides various roles in which the demand for this expertise is high. These include subspecializations in the addictions, severe personality disorders, child and adolescent psychiatry, geropsychiatry, and forensics. An important niche that remains underfilled is psychiatric leadership in the care and treatment of the severely and persistently mentally ill. The medical, social, and economic problems of this patient population require strong leadership, and the psychiatrist who can be the principle physician for these patients is in demand. Although psychiatry cannot consider itself a primary care specialty, the medical background of psychiatrists allows them to provide basic primary care medicine to patients with chronic mental illness. As managed care expands into the public sector, a need for such psychiatric leadership in health maintenance organizations and community mental health centers is compelling. In short, psychiatrists compete well in today's marketplace. They are flexible, adaptable, and an excellent "value," to use business language. Many niches exist for psychiatrists in medical and nonmedical marketplaces across our economy.

The decline of American medical students choosing psychiatry as a specialty will likely reverse itself, provided we do not overly restrict the definition of a psychiatrist. The recent decline is a direct result of the shift to primary care. As jobs become scarce in primary care, which is already beginning in aggressive managed care markets, many clinicians will retrain in psychiatry. Supply and demand will rule, and psychiatry will attract more medical students and general physicians within the next decade.

As long as we do not forget the value of psychiatrists, the marketplace is our friend, not our enemy. The demand for psychiatrists will shift in proportion to the demand for humane and expert diagnosis and treatment for patients with mental illness and crippling emotional distress. In addition to the mainstream of third-party financing with the growth of managed care, there is the substantial market of out-of-pocket payments for psychiatric specialty consultations and ongoing treatment. Psychiatrists compete for these fee-paying patients on the basis of value: the best quality for a reasonable price. Psychotherapy will continue to be provided by psychiatrists, with many patients paying for most of this treatment themselves. In these situations in which the patient is the paying customer, the psychiatrist will be chosen on the basis of his or her ability to move between the biomedical and psychotherapeutic frameworks with expertise, flexibility, and assurance.

The role of clinical neuroscientist will be one new opportunity for some psychiatric specialists, but it is not the exclusive future for the field. Academic psychiatry should prepare physician professionals for various futures with a focus on the ever-evolving new medical marketplace.

Steven S. Sharfstein, MD
Sheppard Pratt Health System
6501 N Charles St
Baltimore, MD 21285-6815

REFERENCES

1. Detre T, McDonald MC. Managed care and the future of psychiatry. *Arch Gen Psychiatry.* 1997;54:201-204.
2. Mitka M. Some new doctors can't find jobs. *American Medical News.* 1996;39:1.

ORIGINAL ARTICLE

Effects of Intrathecal Thyrotropin-Releasing Hormone (Protirelin) in Refractory Depressed Patients

Lauren B. Marangell, MD; Mark S. George, MD; Ann M. Callahan, MD; Terence A. Ketter, MD; Peggy J. Pazzaglia, MD; Todd A. L'Herrou, MA; Gabriele S. Leverich, MSW; Robert M. Post, MD

Background: Therapeutic effects of the tripeptide protirelin (thyrotropin-releasing hormone) have been postulated in the affective disorders, but direct assessment in humans has been hindered by poor blood-brain barrier permeability.

Methods: Eight medication-free inpatients with refractory depression received 500 μg of protirelin via a lumbar intrathecal injection and an identical sham lumbar puncture procedure, separated by 1 week, in a double-blind crossover design.

Results: Five of eight patients responded to intrathecal protirelin, defined as a 50% or greater reduction in an abbreviated Hamilton Rating Scale for Depression score. Suicidality also was reduced significantly ($P<.05$). Responses were rapid and clinically robust, but short-lived.

Conclusion: Administration of protirelin by an intrathecal route induced a rapid improvement in mood and suicidality in these refractory depressed patients, supporting the hypothesis that thyrotropin-releasing hormone could be a positive modulator of mood.

Arch Gen Psychiatry. 1997;54:214-222

THYROTROPIN-releasing hormone (TRH; protirelin) is a hypothalamic tripeptide-releasing hormone that stimulates the pituitary to secrete thyrotropin (TSH) and thereby regulates the production of thyroid hormones. In addition, TRH has direct effects on the central nervous system (CNS) that are independent of pituitary or thyroid stimulation.[1-3] High-affinity TRH receptors are found throughout the brain in humans, with the highest density in the amygdala and hippocampus.[4] The behavioral effects of TRH are state-dependent; TRH has been demonstrated to modulate both hyperactive and hypoactive states as assessed by cerebral glucose metabolism and motor activity.[5,6] Arousal from hibernation is selectively produced by protirelin administration to the hippocampus but not the hypothalamus. Thyrotropin-releasing hormone modulates the effects of serotonin and dopamine[7,8]; in addition, both TRH and its analogues are effective in many animal models of depression.[3,9] Moreover, some treatments for mood disorders increase endogenous TRH levels.[10-14] These observations, among others, suggest that TRH may be relevant to understanding the pathophysiology and treatment of mood disorders.

Although some early studies supported the antidepressant efficacy of intravenously administered protirelin, most subsequent controlled studies did not confirm these findings.[15,16] Protirelin is rapidly degraded in the periphery with a mean (±SEM) serum half-life of 5.3±0.5 minutes.[17] Estimates of the amount of protirelin that crosses the blood-brain barrier after intravenous administration range from 0.2% to 2.75%.[18] Given these data, it is possible that in prior studies of affective disorders, parental administration produced inadequate CNS TRH availability. In contrast, the half-life of protirelin in cerebrospinal fluid (CSF) is 54±5.4 minutes.[19] Circulation to rostral portions of the CNS is likely to occur, because it has been demonstrated that lipid-insoluble substances injected into the lumbar spinal fluid reach the base of the brain in approximately 60 minutes and then circulate cortically.[20] Investigators of amyotrophic lateral sclerosis demonstrated the safety and feasibility of intrathecal (IT) administration of protirelin,[19,21-24] although these studies did not address putative mood effects. The IT route of administration has produced therapeutic gains in

From the Biological Psychiatry Branch, National Institutes of Mental Health, Bethesda, Md (Drs Marangell, George, Callahan, Ketter, Pazzaglia, and Post and Messrs L'Herrou and Leverich); the Department of Psychiatry, Baylor College of Medicine, Houston, Tex (Dr Marangell); the Department of Psychiatry, Medical University of South Carolina, Charleston (Dr George); the Department of Psychiatry, Mount Sinai Medical Center, New York, NY (Dr Callahan); the Electronic Village Systems, Centreville, Va (Mr L'Herrou); the Department of Psychiatry, Stanford School of Medicine, Stanford, Calif (Dr Ketter); and the Department of Psychiatry, University of Mississippi Medical School, Jackson (Dr Pazzaglia).

PATIENTS AND METHODS

Although 9 patients received IT protirelin, the first patient was omitted because the study design was modified. Data are therefore presented from the subsequent 8 subjects, 5 women and 3 men (mean age, 45.6 years), who were inpatients at the National Institutes of Health Clinical Center, Bethesda, Md, between 1992 and 1994. All of the patients met *DSM-III-R*[28] criteria for a mood disorder without psychotic features (4 unipolar and 4 bipolar II, depressed), confirmed by a research psychiatrist using the life-charting method.[29] All of the patients were free of comorbid medical, endocrine, or neurologic disorders, which was confirmed by history, physical examination, laboratory testing, and brain imaging studies at the time of study. All of the patients had negative antithyroid antibody screens, normal serum cortisol levels, and normal cortisol suppression after taking 1 mg of dexamethasone.

Patient characteristics and prior antidepressant treatments are shown in **Table 1**. All of the patients had received at least 5 unsuccessful antidepressant trials, considered to be of adequate dose and duration, including at least 3 distinct classes of antidepressant medications and at least 1 attempt at augmentation. All but 1 patient received electroconvulsive therapy. Partial responses to some agents are noted, but all trials were eventually considered to be inadequate. All of the patients also received at least 1 unsuccessful trial of anticonvulsants as part of our other research protocols.

Patients gave oral and written informed consent and the study was approved by the Human Subjects Review Board of the National Institutes of Health Clinical Center. Patients were carefully monitored on the inpatient unit and, although many of the subjects had significant suicidal ideation, none was considered to be at acute risk for suicidal behavior at the time of the study.

Patients were medication-free for at least 2 weeks before the procedures. The double-blind crossover design consisted of a protirelin condition and a sham-control condition, separated by 1 week. Each condition consisted of a baseline day, a procedure day, and a follow-up day. Procedures were performed between 8 AM and 9 AM. The treatment order was determined in a semirandomized, balanced design. Protirelin was administered via a standard lumbar puncture, performed in the lateral decubitus position following overnight bed rest and fasting. After the usual CSF sample was drawn, a bolus injection of 500 μg of preservative-free protirelin (Relefact-TRH, Hoechst-Roussel Pharmaceuticals, Somerville, NJ), specific gravity of 0.998%±1.2%, was administered via the lumbar puncture needle. This dose was based on an estimation of maximum CNS effects and tolerability, as per previous IT studies in patients with amyotrophic lateral sclerosis.[19,21-24]

The sham condition was identical except that after the initial skin preparation and local anesthetic administration, the needle was inserted into the subcutaneous tissue but did not penetrate the dural sac and protirelin was not given. The "blind" was maintained by simulated spinal fluid collection and infusion procedures. To further control for variability, the same physician performed all of the procedures. We chose to perform the sham procedure to control for a patient undergoing a potentially anxiety-provoking procedure without imposing an additional lumbar puncture. The physicians directly involved with the procedures were the only participants aware of the patients' procedure status.

A physician-rated (blinded research psychiatrist) abbreviated Hamilton Rating Scale for Depression[30] (ModHam) and patient-rated Beck Depression Inventory (BDI)[31] were performed at 8 AM, noon, and 4 PM on the procedure days, and at 8 AM and 4 PM on the baseline and follow-up days. The ModHam rating was the primary outcome measure. The research psychiatrist who performed the blind ratings did not see the patient until several hours after the procedures, to further minimize the likelihood that he or she would be aware of side effects and therefore compromise

Continued on next page

other nonpsychiatric CNS disorders.[25-27] Thus, based on its demonstrated safety, better CNS access, and longer half-life of action, we thought that assessment of the potential effects on mood of IT administration of protirelin would be of theoretical and clinical import.

We present the results of a double-blind crossover pilot study in which 8 patients with refractory depressive illness received protirelin (500 μg) IT via a standard lumbar puncture, separated by 1 week from a sham-control procedure. The goal of this study was to clarify the potential mood effects of an acute infusion of protirelin in patients with refractory mood disorders using the IT route to help ensure delivery of the peptide to the CNS.

RESULTS

MOOD IMPROVEMENT

Five of 8 patients responded to IT protirelin, as defined by a 50% or greater decrease in ModHam ratings following IT protirelin. Four patients responded on the procedure day and 1 patient responded on the day after the protirelin procedure. After the termination of this acute protocol, the patient who showed a second-day response continued to exhibit this pattern of delayed improvement on each of several subsequent administrations of protirelin (A.M.C., Mark A. Frye, MD, L.B.M., et al, unpublished observations, September 1994). Improvement in depression appeared to be associated with protirelin treatment since 3 patients did not achieve the criterion response after receiving the sham procedure and the other 2 had more prolonged responses to protirelin.

Figure 1 and **Figure 2** depict each subject's mood response to IT protirelin and the sham procedure using the AUC analyses (see "Patients and Methods" section) as measured by ModHam and BDI scales. The AUC analysis also shows a pattern of greater improvement with protirelin than with the sham procedure on all other rating measures (**Table 2**). The difference between the 2 conditions reached statistical significance on both self- and physician ratings (BDI $t=2.68$, $P<.05$; ModHam $t=2.58$, $P<.05$). The SDs in the AUC analysis were noted to be high, the variability in part due to worsening of sympthe blind. The ModHam consisted of items 1 through 3, 8 through 10, 15, 17, 19 through 21, and 23 from the Hamilton Rating Scale for Depression. Items that were not assessable because of protocol conditions were excluded. Although this particular subset of the Hamilton Rating Scale items has not been independently validated, there is precedent in the literature for excluding items that are not assessable because of study parameters.[32,33]

Secondary outcome measures, in addition to the BDI, included a patient-rated mood analog scale, side-effect self-ratings , and Bunney-Hamburg nurse ratings[34] for depression (the Bunney-Hamburg ratings were performed every 2 hours until 11 PM). These ratings were performed hourly for the first 8 hours after the procedures. The side-effect self-rating consisted of 31 items scored on a 4-point scale (available on request).

In addition, a semistructured quantitative suicide assessment[35] was performed on the baseline day and again after the procedure (on either the procedure day or the follow-up day) by a clinical social worker (G.S.L.) who was unaware of the procedures. This interview and rating scale was added after clinical observation of a remarkable decrease in suicidal thoughts following one of the procedures that was not adequately reflected in our other rating instruments; therefore, results on this rating are available only in 7 of 8 patients.

Blood samples for measurement of TSH and prolactin (PRL) were collected every 15 minutes for the first hour after each procedure and then every hour for 8 hours and twice daily on the baseline and follow-up days. Blood samples for triiodothyronine (T_3), thyroxine (T_4), and free T_4 were collected at 8 AM, noon, and 4 PM on the procedure days and twice daily on the preprocedure and postprocedure days. The TSH level was measured with an immunoradiometric assay (Serano Diagnostics, Rome, Italy), which incorporates 2 high-affinity monoclonal antibodies. This TSH assay has a detection limit of 0.02 mU/L, an interassay coefficient of variation (CV) of 4% to 5%, and an intra-assay CV of 1.6% to 3.1%. The PRL level was measured with a microparticle enzyme immunoassay (Abbott Laboratories, North Chicago, Ill). The PRL assay has a detection limit of 0.6 μg/L, an interassay CV of 4.2%, and an intra-assay CV of 2.7%.

Serum T_3 and T_4 levels were measured by radioimmunoassay (Quanticoat, Kallestad Diagnostics, Chaska, Minn), with detection limits of 0.2 nmol/L and 13 nmol/L, respectively. The T_3 assay has an interassay CV of 5% to 7% and an intra-assay CV of 2.6%. The T_4 assay has an interassay CV of 4.6% and an intra-assay CV of 2.6%. Free T_4 was measured by radioimmunoassay (GammaCoat, Incstar Corporation, Stillwater, Minn), and has a lower detection limit of 1 pmol/L, an interassay CV of 3.8%, and an intra-assay CV of 4.23%. The CVs for T_3, T_4, and free T_4 are from our clinical laboratory and represent data from midrange samples that are applicable to the patient group used in this study.

Treatment response was defined as a 50% decrease in the ModHam score within 32 hours after the procedures. Maximal change (Δ_{max}) was defined as the difference between baseline ratings (the morning of the procedure) and postprocedure ratings (including both the procedure day and the follow-up day) for each instrument. Paired *t* tests (2-tailed, α=.05) were used to compare Δ_{max} values between each condition (protirelin vs sham). An area-under-the-curve analysis (AUC) was performed to quantify the amplitude and the duration of improvement. The boundaries for the AUC analysis for each condition were defined as the first mood change from baseline (8 AM on the procedure day) until mood ratings returned to baseline, or truncated at the end of study. Since the suicide assessment consisted of only single preprocedure and postprocedure measures, paired *t* tests were used to compare improvement between the protirelin and sham conditions. Additionally, peak level (Δ_{max}), time to Δ_{max}, and duration of increase above baseline for TSH and PRL were assessed. Spearman correlations were used to explore relationships between response, side effects, and endocrine variables.

Table 1. Patient Characteristics*

Patient No./ Sex/Age, y	Diagnosis	Length of Illness, y	No. of Prior Hospitalizations	Antidepressant Response History†	Serum Cortisol Level, nmol/L‡
1/F/50	BP2	8	7	TCA, SSRI,§ MAOI,§ Atyp,§ Aug (3), ECT§	552
2/M/50	UP	10	1	TCA (5), SSRI (3), MAOI (2), Atyp (2), Aug (4), ECT§	392
3/F/46	UP	5	4	TCA,§ SSRI (2),§ MAOI, Atyp, Aug (3), ECT§	419
4/M/24	BP2	9	4	TCA (2),§ SSRI,§ Atyp, Aug (2), ECT, Aug (2)	350
5/M/53	BP2	25	4	TCA (2),§ SSRI (2),§ Atyp,§ Aug (2), ECT	635
6/F/43	UP	2	2	TCA, SSRI, Atyp (2), Aug, ECT	549
7/F/50	BP2	5	1	TCA, SSRI (3), MAOI (2), Atyp, Aug	519
8/F/49	UP	25	0	TCA (5), SSRI (2),§ MAOI,§ Atyp (2), Aug (4), ECT	273

**BP2 indicates type II bipolar disorder; UP, unipolar disorder; TCA, tricylic antidepressants; SSRI, selective serotonin reuptake inhibitors; Atyp, atypical antidepressants (bupropion hydrochloride, venlafaxine hydrochloride); MAOI, monoamine oxidase inhibitors; Aug, augumentation with lithium carbonate, thyroid, or stimulants; and ECT, electroconvulsive therapy.*

†Antidepressant response history expressed as medication class (number of trials).

‡Serum cortisol level (reference range, 193-690 nmol/L) in the week before the study.

§Response or partial response to at least 1 agent in the class with the development of tolerance, hypomania, rapid cycling, or other complications (see text for discussion).

toms in the sham condition; however, the variance of the IT protirelin and sham conditions were not significantly different (Hartley $F_{max[2,7]}$=3.358).

Table 3 compares the 8 AM preprocedure ratings with the postprocedure rating, showing the maximum degree of symptom improvement after protirelin and sham

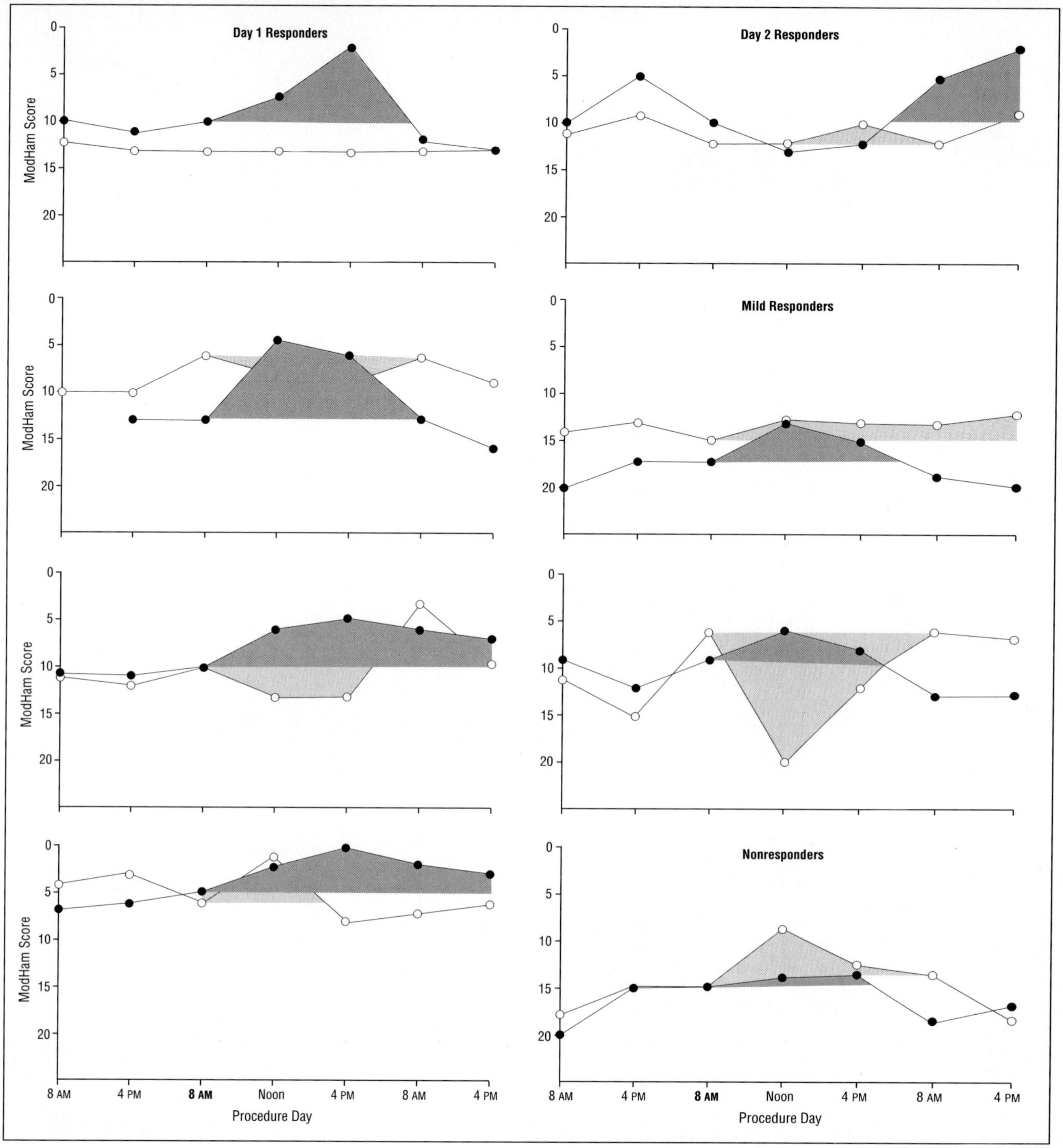

Figure 1. *Individual mood response to intrathecal protirelin (thyrotropin-releasing hormone) (closed circles) and sham (open circles) procedures, as assessed by the physician-rated abbreviated Hamilton Rating Scale for Depression (ModHam). Lower ModHam scores reflect an improvement in mood. Boldfaced time represents the time the procedure was performed. Shading represents area under the curve (see text).*

procedures. These measures reflect improvement on either the procedure day or the follow-up day. Although all depression rating scales reflected a greater improvement in the protirelin condition than in the sham condition, the differences reached statistical significance only with the BDI (t=2.46, P<.05).

Suicidal ideation was reduced significantly (P<.05) and, in some cases, dramatically following the protirelin procedure but not the sham procedure. Comparison of the change in suicidal ideation ratings between the 2 conditions showed a trend toward greater improvement after the protirelin procedure (**Figure 3**; t=2.04, P<.09).

Clinically robust antidepressant effects were reported by several patients to a degree that may not be adequately reflected in the mean ratings. One patient, who had a history of severe refractory depression and prior rapid medication-induced mood switches to mania, reported feeling "normal" for the first time in 2 years. He had a return of affective range, clarity of thought, sense of humor, and libido as well as complete resolution of

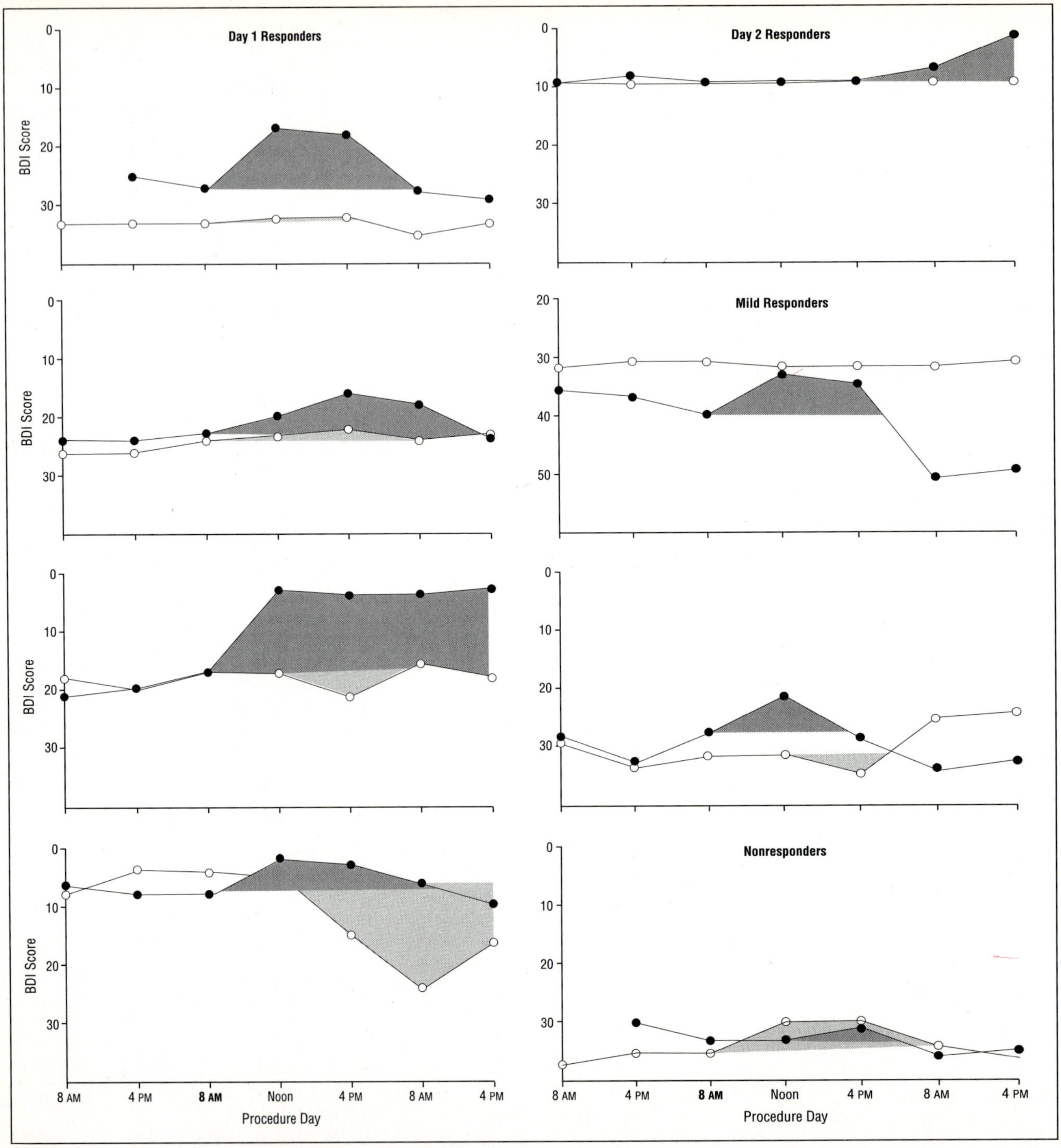

Figure 2. *Individual mood response to intrathecal protirelin (thyrotropin-releasing hormone) (closed circles) and sham (open circles) procedures, as assessed by the patient-rated Beck Depression Inventory (BDI). Lower BDI scores reflect an improvement in mood. Shading represents area under the curve (see text). Boldfaced time represents the time the procedure was performed.*

psychomotor retardation. This response was corroborated by his family members. Two other patients reported a marked improvement in mood after receiving protirelin to a degree that they had not experienced in 5 and 8 years, respectively. One of these patients experienced a remission of depressive symptoms, including long-standing carbohydrate craving, for 5 days (which was beyond the rating period of this protocol). A fourth subject reported that his long-standing anxiety was completely eliminated following the protirelin infusion. This response lasted 5 days with a gradual return toward baseline; no such change in anxiety was reported with the sham procedure.

Baseline depression severity tended to correlate positively with the degree of mood improvement following IT protirelin (Δ_{max}: mood analog scale r=0.97, P<.001; ModHam r=0.60, P=.12; Bunney-Hamburg depression rating r=0.63, P<.09). These relationships were not significant with the sham condition (r=0.42, r=0.31, and r=0.44, respectively).

There was no evidence of order or gender effects on measures of mood improvement. No patient exhibited mania or hypomania following IT protirelin.

ENDOCRINE RESPONSES

The mean serum TSH and PRL measures are shown in **Figure 4**, and individual endocrine responses to IT protirelin are shown in **Table 4**. The mean serum TSH level following IT protirelin infusion increased from a baseline level of 3.0 to 22.9 mU/L (Δ_{max} TSH=19.9 mU/L at 3 hours). One hour later, the mean serum TSH level remained elevated because of a longer duration of TSH response than is seen following intravenous protirelin and a large late TSH peak in 2 patients. The mean serum PRL level increased from a baseline value of 11.9 to 25.2 μg/L (Δ_{max} PRL=14.1 μg/L at 30 minutes). The mean TSH and PRL curves (Figure 4) include patients with both early and late peaks. There was no correlation between the degree of clinical response and serum TSH, T_3, or T_4 levels either at baseline or in response to IT protirelin.

SIDE EFFECTS

The side effects whose mean peak values on the protirelin procedure day exceeded mean peak values on the sham procedure day included shaking ($t[7]=2.52$, $P<.05$), sweating ($t[7]=2.52$, $P<.05$), restlessness ($t[7]=2.83$, $P<.05$), and shivering ($t[7]=2.76$, $P<.05$). Peak shaking and shivering both occurred 1 hour after protirelin infusion, whereas peak sweating and restlessness occurred after 2 hours. The mean duration of shaking was 4.1 hours (range, 2-16 hours); of shivering, 4.8 hours (range, 2-11 hours); of sweating, 2.1 hours (range, 0-6 hours); and of restlessness, 5.4 hours (range, 1-11 hours). There were no consistent correlations between side effects and measures of clinical improvement. The most robust correlations were negative, ie, increased duration of shaking was associated with less improvement on the self-rated mood analog scale AUC ($r=0.69$, $P<.06$) or Bunney-Hamburg nurse ratings ($r=-0.77$, $P<.05$). Systolic and diastolic blood pressure were maximally increased 15 minutes following IT protirelin from a baseline mean of 120/68 mm Hg (SD, 14.16/11.51 mm Hg) to 146/82 mm Hg (SD, 19.62/14.22 mm Hg) (systolic $t=2.457$, $P<.05$; diastolic $t=2.117$, $P=.07$) and gradually returned to baseline within 1 hour after infusion. These differences were significantly greater than those after the sham condition. There was no significant change in heart rate after either the protirelin or the sham procedure. There was no correlation between changes in systolic or diastolic blood pressure and clinical response to IT protirelin.

Table 2. Effects of Protirelin on Mood: Area-Under-the-Curve Analysis*

Rater	Instrument	Mean (SD) Protirelin Condition	Mean (SD) Sham Condition	Mean (SD) Difference	*t*
Physician	ModHam	26.5 (16.4)	−4.7 (30.1)	31.2 (34.2)	2.58†
Self	BDI	14.5 (13.8)	−2.2 (12.3)	16.7 (17.6)	2.68†
	MAS	24.5 (28.9)	9.6 (30.1)	14.9 (46.9)	0.90
Nurse	BHD	20.4 (16.0)	7.9 (43.4)	12.6 (51.1)	0.69

*Methods for calculation are described in the text. Higher area-under-the-curve values reflect greater improvement on all assessment measures. ModHam indicates abbreviated Hamilton Rating Scale for Depression; BDI, Beck Depression Inventory; BHD, Bunney-Hamburg depression rating; and MAS, mood analog scale.

†$P<.05$ from paired 2-tailed *t* test (df=7).

COMMENT

Protirelin administered into the lumbar CSF produced clinically robust, but short-lived, improvement in mood in these 8 patients with refractory unipolar and bipolar depression. Significant, and at times dramatic, decreases in suicidal ideation also were observed. In all mood ratings, improvement was greater following protirelin infusion than after the sham procedures; this difference was statistically significant for both the blind physician-rated ModHam and the self-rated BDI, as assessed by AUC analysis. The fact that several measures reached statistical significance is remarkable given the low statistical power because of the small number of patients studied.

The consistent pattern of improvement in mood following protirelin administration supports the hypothesis that the putative increases in TRH (as reported in the CSF of a subset of depressed patients[36-38]) could represent an endogenous compensatory mechanism rather than a primary pathophysiological process.[39] The fact that no pa-

Table 3. Effects of Protirelin on Mood: Maximal Change From Baseline (Δ_{max})*

Rater	Instrument	Protirelin Pre	Protirelin Post	Protirelin *t*	Sham Pre	Sham Post	Sham *t*	Δ_{max} Protirelin	Δ_{max} Sham	Δ_{max} *t*
Physician	ModHam	11.1 (3.8)	5.8 (5.1)	5.48†	10.4 (4.0)	7.4 (4.2)	3.00§	−5.3 (2.8)	−3.0 (2.8)	1.39
Self	BDI	23.1 (11.3)	15.6 (12.8)	6.12†	23.6 (11.0)	19.8 (11.9)	2.73§	−7.5 (3.5)	−3.8 (4.0)	2.46§
	MAS	6.5 (2.7)	9.3 (3.5)	4.66‡	6.1 (2.4)	8.3 (3.2)	2.69§	2.8 (1.7)	2.2 (2.2)	1.67
Nurse	BHD	6.9 (2.0)	4.0 (2.6)	4.71‡	6.4 (1.4)	4.5 (1.9)	3.91‡	−2.9 (1.7)	−1.9 (1.4)	1.47

*Pre (rating procedure morning) and post (rating most reflective of improvement following protirelin or sham procedures) ratings are given as mean (SD). ModHam indicates abbreviated Hamilton Rating Scale for Depression; BDI, Beck Depression Inventory; BHD, Bunney-Hamburg depression rating; and MAS, mood analog scale (higher numbers are associated with improved mood).

†$P<.001$ from paired *t* tests (df=7).

‡$P<.01$ from paired *t* tests (df=7).

§$P<.05$ from paired *t* tests (df=7).

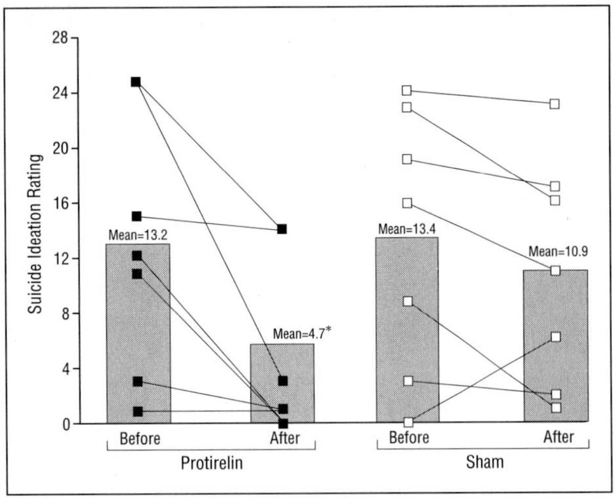

Figure 3. *Suicidal ideation before and after intrathecal protirelin (thyrotropin-releasing hormone) and sham procedures, with ratings ranging from 0 (no ideation) to 38 (severe ideation).*

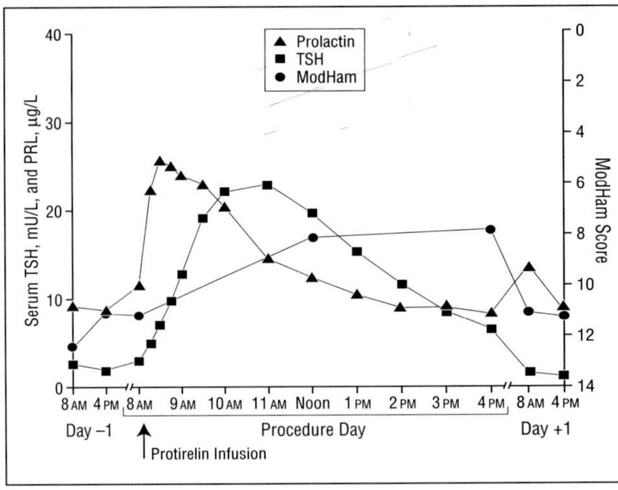

Figure 4. *Time course of mean serum thyrotropin (TSH) levels, prolactin (PRL) levels, and abbreviated Hamilton Rating Scale for Depression (ModHam) scores following intrathecal protirelin (thyrotropin-releasing hormone) procedure (N=8). Lower ModHam scores reflect improved mood (0=euthymia, 14=more depressed).*

Table 4. Summary of Individual Responses to Intrathecal Protirelin*

Patient No.	Protirelin Response‡	Response to IV Procaine Hydrochloride	TSH,§ mU/L	Hours to Δ_{max} TSH	PRLI,§ μg/L	Hours to Δ_{max} PRL	Δ_{max} Systolic BP, mm Hg	T_3,§ nmol/L	T_4,§ nmol/L	Shaking, Max/Dur‖	Shivering, Max/Dur‖
1	+	Anxiety, VH	59.8/6.4	3	32.5/9.4	2	−6	4.6/3.0	175/138	3/3	2/3
2	+	Minimal	50.3/4.4	3	16.3/4.4	3	13	2.8/1.8	98/78	4/16	4/11
3	+	Mild euphoria, VH	15.9/1.3	1.5	79.9/16.1	.5	27	4.3/2.3	145/98	2/2	3/4
4	+	Anxiety	2.4/0.2	2	25.4/11.1	.5	24	2.6/1.7	121/112	3/3	3/2
5†	+	Minimal	14.9/4.2	1.5	6.9/4.6	1	29	2.7/1.9	107/90	4/2	4/7
6	−	Anxiety, VH	14.6/2.4	1.5	55.4/21.2	.75	21	2.2/1.2	130/98	3/3	3/4
7	−	Mild anxiety, VH	7.3/0.9	3	20.0/10.0	1	42	2.9/1.4	126/98	4/2	2/2
8	−	Anxiety, euphoria, VH	31.8/4	2	26.2/10.1	1.5	24	3.4/2.0	107/85	2/2	3/5

IV indicates intravenous; TSH, thyrotropin; Δ_{max}, maximal change from baseline; PRL, prolactin; BP, blood pressure; T_3, triiodothyronine; T_4, thyroxine; and VH, visual hallucination.

†*Patient 5 was day 2 responder.*

‡*Defined as a 50% reduction in the abbreviated Hamilton Rating Scale for Depression score (see text for discussion).*

§*Δ_{max}/baseline value.*

‖*Maximum symptom severity (1-4 scale)/duration in hours.*

tient showed such an exacerbation of depression, which would have been predicted if increased TRH was part of the pathophysiology of depression, is compelling. Moreover, the consistent lack of negative affective responses may partially offset questions regarding the validity of these results because of the small sample size. It should be noted, however, that although these preliminary results are provocative, they may not be generalizable to all depressed populations. The patients in this study were a refractory subgroup who were relatively late in their course of illness (see Table 1), and as such, their neurobiology and pharmacological responses may be different from those with a less severe or shorter course of illness.

Several additional factors need to be considered in interpreting these data. Although most aspects of the protirelin condition were duplicated in the sham condition, actual penetration of the dura and collection of CSF did not occur. However, lumbar punctures are routinely performed on our unit and we have not noted any effect on mood following these procedures, nor are we aware of any reports of improved mood following a lumbar puncture procedure and the withdrawal of CSF. In general, patients were unable to distinguish whether they had received a real or sham lumbar puncture. Of greater concern is potential compromise of the blind by the distinct side effects associated with protirelin, such as shaking and shivering. However, several factors argue against a side effect–mediated placebo response to the protirelin procedure in this data set. Correlations between side effects and mood response tended to be negative; patients rated their mood as less improved the more they experienced shaking. This inverse relationship between side effects and clinical response is the opposite of what would be predicted if a positive mood response were a placebo response occurring as a result of experiencing a unique pattern of side effects. Moreover, these patients were accustomed to participating in a variety of procedures, such as positron-emission tomography with arterial line placement and pharmacologic challenges, as part of other protocols conducted by our group. For instance, all of the subjects in this study received intravenous procaine hydrochloride,[40,41] and the most common responses were anxiety and visual hallucinations (Table 4). Two of the patients in our study experienced euphoria in response to procaine; 1 was a responder and the other a nonresponder to IT protirelin, further indicating that the occurrence of prominent and novel side effects in this population is not necessarily associated with a positive placebo response.

The kinetics of TRH suggest that lumbar-IT protirelin reaches the brain. The delayed peak in serum TSH following IT protirelin administration is distinctly different from the TSH response typically seen following intravenous administration. Similar delayed endocrine responses to lumbar-IT protirelin have been previously reported.[24]

State-dependent effects of TRH were demonstrated by Stanton et al,[5] who found that centrally administered protirelin increased activity in sleeping ground squirrels but when administered to active ground squirrels, caused decreased activity. Huey et al[42] reported a positive response to intravenous protirelin in 4 manic men. It appears that in animals (and perhaps in humans), TRH may be capable of modulating deviations in activity level in either direction. Although definitive conclusions cannot be drawn from the current single-dose study, it is noteworthy that none of our patients exhibited symptoms of mania in response to protirelin, despite the fact that 5 of 8 had a history of antidepressant-induced hypomania or mania (Table 1). Also consistent with state-dependent properties, TRH effects on mood in this study were greatest in those with the most severe depression at baseline. While it could be argued that this is an artifact of regression to the mean, the phenomenon was less pronounced during the sham procedure. State-related modulatory effects may be particularly relevant to the bimodal changes in psychomotor activity and mood seen in bipolar disorder.

Although further studies are needed to definitively rule out possible side effect–mediated placebo effects, these preliminary results support the antidepressant efficacy of administering IT protirelin to refractory depressed patients and support the potential feasibility of direct administration of hydrophilic peptides into the CNS to assess their effects in serious psychiatric disorders. If replicated, these data suggest that further studies to investigate methods for extending the effects of TRH and also other strategies targeting CNS TRH systems may be warranted. Long-term IT administration of a variety of agents has been successfully employed in other nonpsychiatric CNS disorders.[25,43,44] One such strategy utilizes surgically implanted pumps that deliver agents from an externally accessible reservoir to the lumbar CSF at a programmable and adjustable rate. Direct comparison with parenteral administration is also warranted and has been preliminarily explored.[45] Other strategies targeting CNS TRH systems include the use of long-acting TRH analogues, development of nonpeptide agents that cross the blood-brain barrier and are active at TRH receptors, novel carrier or delivery systems to subvert the blood-brain barrier, or inhibitors of TRH degradation enzymes.

The rapid onset of large but short-lived antidepressant effects with associated improvement in suicidal ideation, without the induction of mania, in this small group of patients with extremely refractory unipolar and bipolar illness represents a novel but preliminary finding. Further study to assess the reliability of these findings and to discern whether these acute effects could ultimately be sustained for therapeutic purposes appears warranted.

Accepted for publication March 26, 1996.

Presented in part at the 19th Collegium Internationale Neuro-psychopharmacologicum Congress, Washington, DC, June 30, 1994.

Reprints: Robert M. Post, MD, National Institutes of Health, Bldg 10, Room 3N212, 9000 Rockville Pike, Bethesda, MD 20892.

REFERENCES

1. Breese GR, Mueller RA, Mallman RB, Frye GD. Effects of TRH on central nervous system functions. In: Liss AR, ed. *The Role of Peptides and Amino Acids as Neurotransmitters.* New York, NY: Alan R Liss Inc; 1981:99-116.
2. Loosen PT. TRH: behavioral and endocrine effects in man. *Prog Neuropsychopharmacol Biol Psychiatry.* 1988;12(suppl):S87-S117.
3. Plotnikoff NP, Prange AJ, Breese GR, Anderson MS. Enhancement of DOPA activity by a hypothalamic hormone, thyrotropin releasing hormone, TRH. *Science.* 1972;178:417-418.
4. Manaker S, Eichen A, Winokur A, Rhodes CH, Rainbow TC. Autoradiographic localization of thyrotropin releasing hormone receptors in human brain. *Neurology.* 1986;36:641-646.
5. Stanton TL, Beckman AL, Winokur A. Thyrotropin-releasing hormone effects in the central nervous system: dependence on arousal state. *Science.* 1981;214:678-681.
6. Maurelli M, Tartara A, Marchioni E, Savoldi F. The spectrum of actions of thyrotropin-releasing hormone on the CNS: a polygraphic study on rabbits. *Neurosci Lett.* 1984;46:85-90.
7. Rips R, Boschi G. Interactions between TRH and catecholamines serotonin, acetylcholine and other neuromodulators. *Prog Neuroendocrinol.* 1985;1:261-271.
8. Crespi F, Keane PE, Morre M. In vivo evaluation by differential pulse voltammetry of the effect of thyrotropin-releasing hormone (TRH) on dopaminergic and serotoninergic synaptic activity in the striatum and nucleus accumbens of the rat. *Exp Brain Res.* 1986;62:329-334.
9. Metcalf G. Regulatory peptides as a source of new drugs: the clinical prospects for analogues of TRH which are resistant to metabolic degradation. *Brain Res Rev.* 1982;4:389-408.
10. Meyerhoff JL, Bates VE, Kubek MJ. Elevated TRH levels in pyriform cortex after partial and fully generalized kindled seizures. *Brain Res.* 1990;525:144-148.
11. Kubek MJ, Meyerhoff JL, Hill TG, Norton JA, Sattin A. Effects of subconvulsive and repeated electroconvulsive shock on thyrotropin-releasing hormone in rat brain. *Life Sci.* 1985;36:315-320.
12. Kubek MJ, Sattin A. Effect of electroconvulsive shock on the content of thyrotropin-releasing hormone in rat brain. *Life Sci.* 1984;34:1149-1152.
13. Sattin A, Hill TG, Meyerhoff JL, Norton JA, Kubek MJ. The prolonged increase in thyrotropin-releasing hormone in rat limbic forebrain regions following electroconvulsive shock. *Regul Pept.* 1987;19:13-22.
14. Marangell LB, George MS, Bissette G, Pazzaglia P, Huggins T, Post RM. Carbamazepine increases CSF thyrotropin-releasing hormone in affectively ill patients. *Arch Gen Psychiatry.* 1994;51:625-628.
15. Itil TM, Patterson CD, Polvan N, Bigelow A, Bergey B. Clinical and CNS effects of oral and IV thyrotropin-releasing hormone in depressed patients. *Dis Nerv Sys.* 1975;2:529-536.
16. Prange AJ Jr, Lara PP, Wilson IC, Alltop LB, Breese GR. Effects of thyrotropin-releasing hormone in depression. *Lancet.* 1972;2:999-1002.
17. Bassiri RM, Utiger RD. Metabolism and excretion of exogenous thyrotropin-releasing hormone in humans. *J Clin Invest.* 1973;52:1616-1619.
18. Brooks BR, Kalin N, Beaulieu DA, Barksdale C, Sufit RL, Dills DG. Thyrotropin releasing hormone uptake into serum and cerebrospinal fluid following intravenous or subcutaneous administration. *Neurol Res.* 1988;10:236-238.
19. Munsat TL, Taft J, Jackson IMD. Pharmacokinetics of intrathecal thyrotropin-releasing hormone. *Neurology.* 1987;37:597-601.

20. Di Chiro G. Movement of the cerebrospinal fluid in human beings. *Nature.* 1964; 204:290-291.
21. Stober T, Schimrigk K, Dietzsch S, Thielen T. Intrathecal thyrotropin-releasing hormone therapy of amyotrophic lateral sclerosis. *J Neurol.* 1985;232:13-14.
22. Munsat TL, Taft J, Kasdon D. Intrathecal thyrotropin-releasing hormone in amyotrophic lateral sclerosis. *Neurol Clin.* 1987;5:159-170.
23. Munsat TL, Taft J, Jackson IM, Andres PL, Hollander D, Skerry L, Ordman M, Kasdon D, Finison L. Intrathecal thyrotropin-releasing hormone does not alter the progressive course of ALS: experience with an intrathecal drug delivery system. *Neurology.* 1992;42:1049-1053.
24. Vigneri R, Pezzino V, Filetti S, Squatrito S, Corso A, Maricchiolo M, Polosa P, Scapagnini U. Thyrotropin and prolactin response to intraspinal TRH administration in man. *Neuroendocrinology.* 1977;23:171-180.
25. Coffey YJ, Cahill D, Steers W, Parks TS, Ordla J, Meythaler J, Herman R, Shetter AG, Levy R, Gill B. Intrathecal baclofen for intractable spasticity of spinal origin: results of a long-term multicenter study. *J Neurosurg.* 1993;78:226-232.
26. Loubser PG, Narayan RK, Sandin KJ, Donovan WH, Russell KD. Continuous infusion of intrathecal baclofen: long-term effects on spasticity in spinal cord injury. *Paraplegia.* 1991;29:48-64.
27. Hasle H, Helgestad J, Christensen JK, Jacobsen BB, Kamper J. Prolonged intrathecal chemotherapy replacing cranial irradiation in high-risk acute lymphatic leukaemia: long-term follow up with cerebral computed tomography scans and endocrinological studies. *Eur J Pediatr.* 1995;154:24-29.
28. American Psychiatric Association. *Diagnostic and Statistical Manual of Mental Disorders, Third Edition, Revised.* Washington, DC: American Psychiatric Association; 1987.
29. Post RM, Roy-Byrne PP, Uhde TW. Graphic representation of the life course of illness in patients with affective disorder. *Am J Psychiatry.* 1988;145:844-848.
30. Hamilton M. A rating scale for depression. *J Neurol Neurosurg Psychiatry.* 1960;12:56-62.
31. Beck AT, Ward C, Mendelson M, Mock J, Erbough J. An inventory for measuring depression. *Arch Gen Psychiatry.* 1961;4:561-571.
32. Abrams R, Taylor MA, Faber R, Ts'o TO, Williams RA, Almy G. Bilateral versus unilateral electroconvulsive therapy: efficacy in melancholia. *Am J Psychiatry.* 1983;140:463-465.
33. Strouse TB, Szuba MP, Baxter Jr LR. Response to sleep deprivation in three women with postpartum psychosis. *Am J Clin Psychiatry.* 1992;53:204-206.
34. Bunney WEJ, Hamburg DA. Methods for reliable longitudinal observation of behavior. *Arch Gen Psychiatry.* 1963;9:280-294.
35. Beck AT, Kovacs M, Weissman A. Assessment of suicidal intention: the scale for suicide ideation. *J Consult Clin Psychol.* 1979;47:343-352.
36. Banki CM, Bissette G, Arato M, Nemeroff CB. Elevation of immunoreactive CSF TRH in depressed patients. *Am J Psychiatry.* 1988;145:1526-1531.
37. Kirkegaard C, Faber J, Hummer L, Rogowski P. Increased levels of TRH in cerebrospinal fluid from patients with endogenous depression. *Psychoneuroendocrinology.* 1979;4:227-235.
38. Roy A, Wolkowitz OM, Bissette G, Nemeroff CB. Differences in CSF concentrations of thyrotropin-releasing hormone in depressed patients and normal subjects: negative findings. *Am J Psychiatry.* 1994;151:600-602.
39. Post RM. Transduction of psychosocial stress into the neurobiology of recurrent affective disorders. *Am J Psychiatry.* 1992;149:999-1010.
40. Kellner CH, Post RM, Putnam F, Cowdry R, Gardner D, Kling MA, Minichiello MD, Trettau JR, Coppola R. Intravenous procaine as a probe of limbic system activity in psychiatric patients and normal controls. *Biol Psychiatry.* 1987;22: 1107-1126.
41. Ketter TA, Andreason PJ, George MS, Lee C, Gill DS, Parekh PI, Willis MW, Herscovitch P, Post RM. Anterior paralimbic mediation of procaine-induced emotional and psychosensory experiences. *Arch Gen Psychiatry.* 1996;53:59-69.
42. Huey LY, Janowsky DS, Mandell AJ, Judd LL, Pendery M. Preliminary studies on the use of TRH in manic states, depression, and the dysphoria of alcohol withdrawal. *Psychopharmacol Bull.* 1975;11:24-27.
43. Lazorthes Y, Sallerin-Caute B, Verdie JC, Bastide R. Advances in drug delivery systems and applications in neurosurgery. *Adv Tech Stand Neurosurg.* 1991; 18:143-192.
44. Chambers FA, MacSullivan R. Intrathecal morphine in the treatment of chronic intractable pain. *Ir J Med Sci.* 1994;163:318-321.
45. Callahan AM, Frye MA, Marangell LB, George MS, Ketter TA, Kimbrell TA, L'Herrou T, Pazzaglia PJ, Post RM. Differential mood and endocrine effects of intravenous vs intrathecal TRH. *Biol Psychiatry.* 1995;37:609. Abstract.

Mesolimbic Dopamine D_3 Receptors and Use of Antipsychotics in Patients With Schizophrenia

A Postmortem Study

Eugenia V. Gurevich, PhD; Yvette Bordelon; Raymond M. Shapiro, MD, PhD; Steven E. Arnold, MD; Raquel E. Gur, MD; Jeffrey N. Joyce, PhD

Background: The pharmacological properties and distribution of a recently cloned member of the dopamine D_2 receptor subfamily, the D_3 receptor, has led directly to the hypothesis that it may be the target of antipsychotic action.

Methods: To quantify D_3 receptors, we characterized the conditions for selective binding of the radioligand iodine 125-labeled (R)-*trans*-7-hydroxy-2-[*N*-propyl-*N*-(3′-iodo-2′-propenyl)-amino]tetralin ([^{125}I]*trans*-7-OH-PIPAT) to the human D_3 receptor. We then measured by quantitative autoradiography in postmortem tissue the concentration of D_3 receptors in the caudal and rostral basal ganglia regions in patients with schizophrenia and control subjects.

Results: We found about 2-fold elevations in the number of D_3 receptors in the basal ganglia and ventral forebrain of long-term hospitalized patients with schizophrenia who received no antipsychotic drugs for at least a month before death (n=7) compared with matched control subjects (n=15). Patients with schizophrenia receiving antipsychotic drugs less than 72 hours before death (n=8) had levels similar to those of control subjects. There were no differences in the binding characteristics or affinity of [^{125}I]*trans*-7-OH-PIPAT binding to D_3 receptors between control subjects and patients with schizophrenia.

Conclusion: In contrast to the previously detected elevation of D_2 and D_4 receptor levels in schizophrenia, elevation of D_3 receptor levels in limbic striatum and its efferents observed in patients with schizophrenia may be reduced by antipsychotic drugs.

Arch Gen Psychiatry. 1997;54:225-232

From the Departments of Psychiatry (Drs Gurevich, Shapiro, Arnold, Gur, and Joyce) and Pharmacology (Ms Bordelon and Dr Joyce), University of Pennsylvania School of Medicine, Philadelphia. Drs Gurevich and Joyce are now at the William T. Christopher Center for Parkinson's Disease Research, Sun Health Research Institute, Sun City, Ariz.

THE DOPAMINE (DA) hypothesis of schizophrenia has been based largely on evidence that pharmacological manipulations of DA systems either augment or alleviate the symptoms of schizophrenia.[1,2] Postmortem studies of the brains of patients with schizophrenia have found that levels of D_2-like receptors are elevated in the striatum compared with levels in age-matched control subjects.[3-5] In spite of these data, there is limited evidence in support of the hypothesis that the actions of antipsychotic drugs at D_2 receptors in the striatum modulate symptoms of schizophrenia. Typical antipsychotic drugs can induce behavioral and neurochemical changes in the striatum through actions at D_2 receptors, but the atypical antipsychotic drugs, which possess a lower likelihood of inducing extrapyramidal side effects, appear to be much less efficacious at striatal D_2 receptors.[6-8] Blockade of D_2 receptors within the striatal targets of the nigrostriatal system is likely responsible for their extrapyramidal side effects, while the actions mediated through the mesolimbic DA system appear to be implicated in the antipsychotic characteristics of DA antagonists.[6-10] The cloning of the D_3 receptor has provided a site within the mesolimbic DA system that may be directly involved in the pharmacological actions of antipsychotic drugs.[11,12] It is possible that elevated levels of D_2-like receptors observed in the limbic striatum in schizophrenia reflect modifications in the D_3 receptor thought to be the primary target of the mesolimbic DA system.[11,13,14]

Direct studies of the concentration and distribution of the D_3 receptor in the brains of patients with schizophrenia would examine the hypothesis that the D_3 receptor is involved in schizophrenia and the pharmacological actions of antipsychotic drugs. Characterization of D_3 receptors has been hampered by the absence of selective ligands, for commonly used radioligands label both D_2 and D_3 receptors. The radioligand iodine 125–labeled (R)-*trans*-7-hydroxy-2-[*N*-propyl-*N*-(3′-iodo-2′-propenyl)amino]tetralin ([^{125}I]*trans*-7-OH-PIPAT) has been developed recently,[15] and conditions for selective labeling of D_3 re-

SUBJECTS AND METHODS

CASE MATERIAL

Brain tissue was obtained at autopsy from the Hospital of the University of Pennsylvania, Philadelphia (John Trojanowski, MD, PhD, director of Medical Pathology, Department of Pathology and Laboratory Medicine). Tissue from 10 control subjects was obtained under the auspices of the University of Pennsylvania's Alzheimer Disease Center Core. Tissue from other control subjects was obtained as described in the **Table**. Review of all available medical records indicated no history of neurological or psychiatric disease and no exposure to antipsychotic drugs. Tests for the presence of alcohol and other psychoactive substances in plasma samples were routinely performed for all control subjects.

Tissue from patients with schizophrenia was derived from long-term institutionalized patients. These individuals met *DSM-III-R* criteria[18] for a primary diagnosis of schizophrenia for all of their adult lives, established by standardized chart review and caretaker interviews.[19] Gross and microscopic neuropathologic examination in brain tissue of control subjects and patients with schizophrenia confirmed the absence of neurological abnormalities in the control tissue. Assorted abnormalities were noted in 5 of the 15 patients with schizophrenia (Table). Antipsychotic drug treatment is presented in chlorpromazine equivalents (milligrams)[20] for comparison purposes. Drug treatment history was determined by standardized chart review as well as physician notes and daily nursing notes for the 30-day period immediately before death and every month for 1 year before death. Although all patients with schizophrenia had been treated with antipsychotic drugs at some point during their illness, we divided these subjects into the antipsychotic drug–free group (n=7; received no antipsychotic medication for at least 1 month before death) and the antipsychotic drug–treated group (n=8; had received antipsychotics within 72 hours of death). Chart review of a subset of the patients with extensive chart histories for the 5 years preceding death established that monthly reviews for 1 year accurately reflected the 5-year history of exposure to antipsychotic drugs. No patient had received depot neuroleptic drugs. No tardive dyskinesia was observed in these patients during the year before death or noted in the medical charts. There were no statistically significant differences in age between control subjects and patients with schizophrenia, between antipsychotic drug–free and drug–treated groups, or between either group with schizophrenia and control subjects ($F[2,27]=1.69$; $P=.2$). Neither group with schizophrenia differed significantly from control subjects or from each other in postmortem interval (PMI) ($F[2,27]=2.2$; $P=.1$). There was a significant difference between the antipsychotic drug–treated and drug–free groups in age at onset of schizophrenia ($F[1,13]=5.0$; $P=.04$), with the antipsychotic drug–free group displaying slightly earlier onset of illness.

MEMBRANE-BINDING STUDIES

Striatal tissue from frozen blocks was homogenized in 10 vol (wt/vol) of buffer containing 50-mmol/L Tris[hydroxymethyl]aminomethane hydrochloride (Tris HCl) (pH, 7) and 2-mmol/L ethylenediaminetetraacetic acid (EDTA), centrifuged at 30 000g for 20 minutes, resuspended in the same buffer, and centrifuged at the same speed. The pellet was resuspended in 0.5-mol/L sucrose buffered by 50-mmol/L Tris HCl and centrifuged at 40 000g for 1 hour. The supernatant containing myelin was discarded, and the pellet was resuspended in the Tris HCl/EDTA buffer, incubated at 37°C for 20 minutes, and centrifuged at 30 000g for 20 minutes. The resulting pellet was resuspended in the buffer to achieve the concentration of 10 mg of wet weight per milliliter (at the concentration of 10 mg/mL) in the incubation buffer that contained 50-mmol/L Tris HCl (pH, 7.4), 40-mmol/L sodium chloride, 2-mmol/L magnesium

ceptors in rat brain have been determined.[16,17] Our postmortem study reports the characterization of the binding of [^{125}I]trans-7-OH-PIPAT to the D_3 receptor in the brains of control subjects and patients with schizophrenia. We also studied D_3 receptors in the limbic striatum of patients with schizophrenia who had received antipsychotic drugs (antipsychotic drug–treated group) within 72 hours of death compared with those withdrawn from antipsychotic therapy for at least 1 month (in most patients, for >6 months) at time of death (antipsychotic drug–free group) and age-matched control subjects.

RESULTS

CHARACTERIZATION OF BINDING TO D_3 RECEPTORS

Saturation experiments with [^{125}I]*trans*-7-OH-PIPAT binding to membranes isolated from mouse fibroblasts expressing human D_3 receptors showed that the binding to the D_3 receptor is minimally affected by GTP (**Figure 1**, top). Saturation experiments in the absence and presence of GTP with membrane from 2 control subjects revealed that in the absence of GTP, [^{125}I]*trans*-7-OH-PIPAT binding is best described by a single-site model, with dissociation constants (K_d) of 7.9 and 7.5 nmol/L, respectively. In the presence of GTP, there was an increase in affinity (K_ds of 4.8 and 3.2 nmol/L) and 44% and 42.8% reductions in the maximum number of binding sites (B_{max}) for [^{125}I]*trans*-7-OH-PIPAT binding (Figure 1, center). Competition experiments showed that compounds with differing selectivity for D_2, D_3, and D_4 receptors displaced [^{125}I]*trans*-7-OH-PIPAT in the presence of GTP from a single site, with inhibition constants (K_i) expected for the D_3 receptor (**Figure 2**, top).

Saturation isotherms performed on tissue sections from 3 control subjects demonstrated that the ligand labeled a homogeneous population of binding sites with similar affinity in 4 brain regions examined. Competition experiments for [^{125}I]*trans*-7-OH-PIPAT binding in the presence of GTP with tissue sections showed that the displacement was from a single site with an order of potency consistent with that for the D_3 receptor (Figure 2, bottom). The [^{125}I]*trans*-7-OH-PIPAT binding followed a distinct pattern in the rostral basal ganglia (**Figure 3**, **Figure 4**, and **Figure 5**, top and center). There was relatively low binding in the dorsal caudate and putamen and chloride$_2$, and 5-μmol/L 1,3-di(2-tolyl)guanidine (to block ς-receptors). Membranes prepared from mouse fibroblasts transfected with the human D_3 receptor were purchased from Research Biochemicals International (Natick, Mass).

For [^{125}I]*trans*-7-OH-PIPAT binding, 60 μL of membrane suspension or 1 μL of membranes containing human recombinant D_3 receptor was added to assay tubes containing the radioligand in appropriate concentrations with or without 300-μmol/L guanosine triphosphate in a final volume of 100 μL. Nonspecific binding was determined with 10-mmol/L 7-hydroxy-dipropylaminotetraline (7-OH-DPAT). The tubes were incubated at room temperature for 90 minutes. The reaction was terminated by filtration through glass microfiber filters (Whatman International Ltd, Maidstone, England) presoaked in 0.3% polyethylenimide. Filters were then washed with 20 mL of ice-cold 50-mmol/L Tris HCl (pH, 7.5), placed into tubes, and counted in an LKB gamma counter (Wallac, Turku, Finland). For competition studies, an 0.8- to 0.9-nmol/L [^{125}I]*trans*-7-OH-PIPAT concentration was used.

AUTORADIOGRAPHIC EXPERIMENTS

For all autoradiographic experiments, 20-μm-thick sections containing either rostral basal ganglia (caudate, putamen, and nucleus accumbens) or caudal basal ganglia (tail of caudate, putamen, and external and internal segments of the globus pallidus) were used. The coronal levels were matched for their rostral-caudal position in all control subjects and patients with schizophrenia. Preliminary experiments determined optimal conditions for [^{125}I]*trans*-7-OH-PIPAT binding to the striatal sections. Equilibrium was reached by 80 minutes, and remained stable for 120 minutes. The sections were preincubated at 30°C for 30 minutes in buffer containing 50-mmol/L Tris HCl (pH, 7.4), 100-mmol/L sodium chloride, and 300-μmol/L guanosine triphosphate (GTP). One milliliter of the buffer containing 50-mmol/L Tris HCl (pH, 7.4), 0.3-nmol/L [^{125}I] *trans*-7-OH-PIPAT, 40-mmol/L sodium chloride, 5-μmol/L 1,3-di(2-tolyl)guanidine, and 300-μmol/L GTP was layered on each section for 90 minutes. Nonspecific binding was defined as that in the presence of 10-μmol/L 7-OH-DPAT. The sections were then washed in the same buffer without GTP 3 times at 4°C for 1 hour, dipped into ice-cold deionized water, and dried. The sections were laid against 3H-Hyperfilm (Amersham, Arlington Heights, Ill) along with ^{3}H-labeled standards (American Radiolabeled Chemicals, St Louis, Mo) for 24 hours. For the saturation studies, the caudal striatal sections from 3 control subjects and 3 patients with schizophrenia and 0.03- to 2-nmol/L [^{125}I]*trans*-7-OH-PIPAT were used. Competition experiments were performed on caudal striatal sections from 3 control subjects. Four sections for total binding and 2 sections for nonspecific binding were processed in all studies.

STATISTICAL ANALYSIS

Competition and saturation curves were analyzed using nonlinear curve-fitting software (FITCOMP program of Prophet, BBN Systems and Technologies, Cambridge, Mass).[21] The autoradiographic data were analyzed separately for the rostral and caudal basal ganglia by repeated measures analysis of variance (SuperANOVA, Abacus Concepts, Inc, Berkeley, Calif) with group (control antipsychotic drug–free and drug-treated groups of patients with schizophrenia) as the main effect, and brain region as a within-group factor. Sex, age, and PMI were treated as covariates. To compare binding in the individual brain areas, 1-way ANOVA with group as a main factor was used for each area. Post hoc comparisons were made using Duncans new multiple range test at the 95% confidence level. Multiple linear regression analysis using multivariate analysis of variance (MANOVA) was performed to evaluate possible correlation of the binding values in different brain areas with the doses of antipsychotic drugs received by patients at 3 times and with the age at onset of disease (Table).

more than a 2-fold enrichment in the ventral putamen and nucleus accumbens (ventral striatum). There was significantly less [^{125}I]*trans*-7-OH-PIPAT binding in the caudal part of the basal ganglia. At this level, binding was higher in the dorsal and ventral putamen than in the caudate nucleus and the globus pallidus. The ventral pallidum and the nucleus basalis of Meynert showed significantly lower binding, approximately 30% of that of the putamen.

STUDIES WITH TISSUE FROM PATIENTS WITH SCHIZOPHRENIA

We analyzed D_3 receptors labeled with [^{125}I]*trans*-7-OH-PIPAT using autoradiography in the basal ganglia of 15 patients with schizophrenia and 15 age- and PMI-matched control subjects. We found no significant correlation between the dose of antipsychotic drugs received (Table) at 3 times before death and concentration of D_3 receptors (P=.01). However, when the concentration of D_3 receptors was compared among the groups of control subjects, antipsychotic drug–treated (n=8) and drug–free (n=7) patients with schizophrenia, the drug–free group had 55% to 110% higher levels of D_3 receptors in rostral and caudal basal ganglia than control and antipsychotic drug–treated groups. There was a significant interaction between group and brain region for the rostral striatum ($F[2,10]=3.292$; $P<.001$). In the caudal striatum, the interaction effect of group by region was not significant ($F[2,10]=0.816$; $P=.61$), and the increase in concentration of D_3 receptors was more uniform among regions (Figure 5, center).

The effects of age, PMI, and sex were not significant in caudal or rostral basal ganglia, and no significant interactions of these variables with the group factor were found. Neurological abnormalities found in 5 patients with schizophrenia had no significant effect on concentrations of D_3 receptors. Early onset of schizophrenic symptoms was associated with higher concentrations of D_3 receptors in the caudal basal ganglia ($F[6,9]=3.95$; $P=.03$ with Wilks Λ test) in both antipsychotic drug–treated and drug–free groups. Among individual brain areas, the negative correlation of age at onset of symptoms with the concentration of D_3 receptors was significant in the dorsal putamen ($F[1,14]=7.4$; $r=0.602$; $P=.02$) and caudate nucleus ($F[1,14]=4.8$; $r=0.507$; $P=.05$).

Since it has been reported that patients with schizophrenia exhibit a deficit in the GTP regulation of D_2-like

Record of Patient Characteristics, Cause of Death, and Drug Treatment*

Subject	Sex	Age, y	PMI, h	Hemisphere	Age at Onset of Disease, y	Cause of Death	Antipsychotic Treatment at Intervals Before Death† At Death	1 mo	1 y	Drug Status
						Control Subjects‡				
GRC 071	F	83	22.0	L	...	Sepsis, cancer	...	...	...	
SHC 071	M	76	2.0	R	...	Congestive heart failure	...	...	...	
UCI 061	M	89	9.0	L	...	Cardiac arrest	...	...	...	
UCI 072	F	64	8.0	R	...	Myocardial infarction	...	...	...	
UCI 073	F	76	4.5	R	...	Myocardial infarctions	...	...	...	
HPC 051	F	51	4.5	R	...	Respiratory failure	...	...	...	
HPC 062	M	54	2.0	R	...	Pneumonia, sepsis	...	...	...	
HPC 063	M	57	8.0	L	...	Peritonitis, pneumonia	...	...	...	
HPC 064	M	67	8.0	L	...	Cardiopulmonary arrest	...	...	...	
HPC 075	M	79	3.0	L	...	Aspiration pneumonia	...	...	...	
HPC 076	F	65	11.0	R	...	Respiratory failure	...	...	...	
HPC 077	M	61	15.0	R	...	Sepsis	...	...	...	
HPC 078	F	98	15.0	L	...	Septic shock, leukemia	...	...	...	
HPC 080	F	89	7.0	L	...	Coronary arrest	...	...	...	
HPC 089	F	46	16.5	R	...	Coronary artery disease	...	...	...	
						Patients With Schizophrenia§				
UPS 005	M	78	19.0	L	21	Aspiration pneumonia	0	0	0	Drug-free
UPS 009	M	84	7.0	R	32	Aspiration pneumonia	0	0	150	Drug-free
UPS 011	F	74	15.0	R	18	Cardiac arrest	0	600	600	Drug-free
UPS 013	M	79	7.0	R	22	Pneumonia	0	0	250	Drug-free
UPS 014	F	82	7.0	L	20	Cardiac arrest	0	25	0	Drug-free
UPS 019	M	99	10.5	L	23	Congestive heart failure	0	0	0	Drug-free
UPS 023	F	67	8.5	R	16	Acute renal failure	0	700	900	Drug-free
UPS 004	F	75	11.0	L	33	Congestive heart failure	300	300	250	Drug-treated
UPS 006	F	76	18.0	L	34	Sepsis	300	300	200	Drug-treated
UPS 007	F	79	8.0	R	24	Cardiac arrest	200	200	200	Drug-treated
UPS 010	F	72	11.5	L	27	Perforated bowel	250	300	0	Drug-treated
UPS 012	M	71	12.0	L	21	Septic shock	300	1350	1000	Drug-treated
UPS 015	M	74	14.0	R	23	Pneumonia	100	100	100	Drug-treated
UPS 016	F	75	15.5	R	27	Pneumonia	250	250	100	Drug-treated
UPS 024	F	78	20.0	L	30	Bilateral pulmonary thrombosis	150	150	150	Drug-treated

**PMI indicates postmortem interval; GRC, control subject from Graduate Hospital, Philadelphia, Pa; SHC, control subject from Sun Health Research Institute, Sun City, Ariz; UCI, control subject from Brain Tissue Repository, University of California, Irvine; HPC, control subject from Hospital of the University of Pennsylvania, Philadelphia; UPS, patient with schizophrenia from University of Pennsylvania Registry; drug-free, had not received antipsychotic drugs for more than 1 month before death; and drug-treated, had received antipsychotic drugs in the last 72 hours before death.*

†Antipsychotic drugs were given in daily chlorpromazine equivalents in milligrams.[38]

‡Mean±SD age was 70.3±15.4 years; mean±SD PMI, 9.0±1.5 hours.

§Mean±SD age was 77.5±4.8 years; mean±SD PMI, 12.3±1.2 hours; and mean±SD age at onset of disease, 24.7±1.4 years. For drug-free patients, mean±SD age was 80.4±3.7 years; mean±PMI, 10.6±1.8 hours; and mean±SD age at onset of disease, 21.7±1.9 years. For drug-treated subjects, mean±SD age was 75.0±1.0; mean±SD PMI, 13.8±1.4 hours; and mean±SD age at onset of disease, 27.4±1.7 years (significantly different from drug-free patients, 1-way analysis of variance; $F[1,13]=5.0$; $P=.04$). Assorted abnormalities were noted on gross and microscopic neuropathologic examinations in 5 of the 15 patients with schizophrenia. UPS 004 had a resolving left occipital infarct and pigmented neuron loss in medial substantia nigra; UPS 005, status post right frontal lobe shunt and diffuse Lewy body disease; UPS 014, right cerebellar infarct, small bilateral posterior fossa meningioma, and left cerebellopontine angle schwannoma; UPS 015, right caudate lacunar infarct; and UPS 016, status post bifrontal leukotomies. No incidence of tardive dyskinesia was observed in the patients with schizophrenia.

receptors,[9] we performed saturation experiments with $[^{125}I]$*trans*-7-OH-PIPAT in the presence and absence of GTP in membranes isolated from 2 antipsychotic drug–free patients with schizophrenia to determine if the binding was GTP sensitive. In the absence of GTP, the saturation curves were best fit assuming a single-site model, with K_ds of 26.7 and 11 nmol/L. Inclusion of GTP reduced the K_ds to 6.7 and 5.9 nmol/L, respectively, and decreased the B_{max} by 49.6% and 27% (Figure 1, bottom). These data show that in antipsychotic drug–free patients with schizophrenia, the binding of $[^{125}I]$*trans*-7-OH-PIPAT was regulated by GTP in the same manner as in control subjects. Saturation isotherms (Figure 5, bottom) performed on tissue sections from 3 patients with schizophrenia demonstrated that the ligand labeled a homogeneous population of sites with a similar affinity in 4 brain regions examined. The K_ds were not different from those in control subjects.

COMMENT

Our results show that levels of D_3 receptors are elevated in the rostral and caudal basal ganglia structures of antipsychotic drug–free patients with schizophrenia compared with matched control subjects and antipsychotic drug–treated patients with schizophrenia.

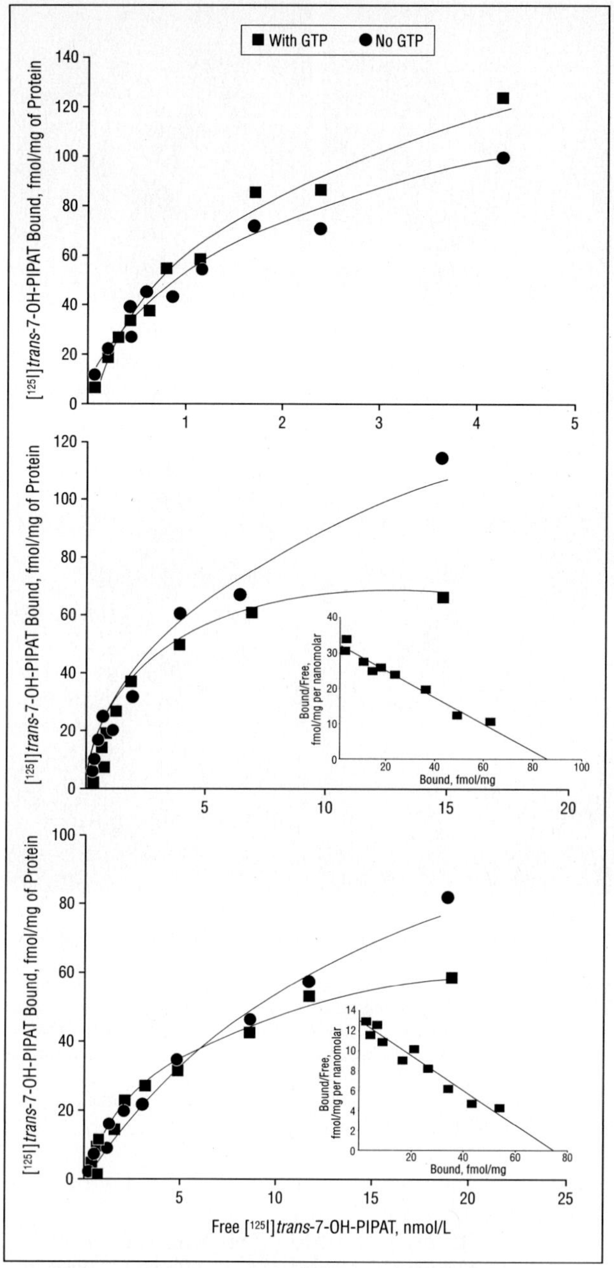

Figure 1. *The saturation isotherms of the iodine 125–labeled (R)-*trans*-7-hydroxy-2-[*N*-propyl-*N*-(3′ iodo-2′-propenyl)-amino]tetralin ([^{125}I]*trans*-7-OH-PIPAT) binding with human D_3 receptor. Top, [^{125}I]*trans*-7-OH-PIPAT binding to membranes isolated from mice fibroblasts expressing human D_3 receptor. In the absence of guanosine triphospate (GTP), the saturation data were best fit by a single-site model, with a dissociation constant (K_d) of 1.25 nmol/L and a maximum number of binding sites (B_{max}) of 120.9 fmol/mg. In the presence of GTP, the saturation data were best fit by a single-site model, with a K_d of 2.1 nmol/L and a B_{max} of 178.6 fmol/mg. Center, [^{125}I]*trans*-7-OH-PIPAT binding to membranes isolated from brain tissue of control subjects. Bottom, [125I]*trans*-7-OH-PIPAT in membranes isolated from brain tissue of patients with schizophrenia in the presence and absence of GTP. The binding experiments were performed as described in the "Subjects and Methods" section of the text. The inserts in the top and center parts show Scatchard plots for binding in the presence of GTP.*

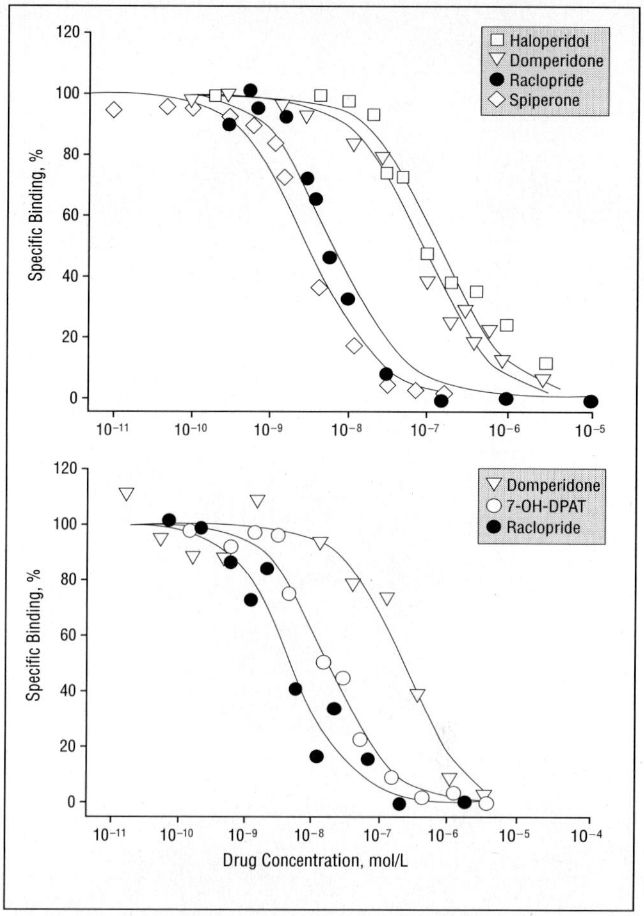

Figure 2. *The competition curves for iodine 125–labeled (R)-*trans*-7-hydroxy-2-[*N*-propyl-*N*-(3′ iodo-2′-propenyl)-amino]tetralin ([^{125}I]*trans*-7-OH-PIPAT) binding with putamen membranes (top) or sections of the caudal basal ganglia (bottom) in control subjects. Competition experiments were analyzed by nonlinear-curve-fitting software. Top, Domperidone displaced [^{125}I]*trans*-7-OH-PIPAT from membranes with IC_{50} (concentration of a drug that inhibits a function by half) of 84 nmol/L, 6.7-nmol/L raclopride, 7.8-nmol/L spiroperidol, and 138-nmol/L haloperidol. Bottom, Competition analysis for [^{125}I]*trans*-7-OH-PIPAT binding in the putamen showed that it is displaced with high affinity by raclopride (IC_{50}, 4.7 nmol/L) and 7-hydroxy-dipropylaminotetraline (IC_{50}, 17 nmol/L), and with lower affinity by domperidone (IC_{50}, 220 nmol/L).*

CHARACTERIZATION OF BINDING

Previous studies in cell lines and in membrane preparations from rat brain outlined conditions for specific labeling of D_3 receptors with [^{125}I]*trans*-7-OH-PIPAT.[15-17] The method is based on the low sensitivity of D_3 receptors and the high sensitivity of D_2 receptors to GTP.[11,16,22] In the presence of GTP, the affinity of [^{125}I]*trans*-7-OH-PIPAT to D_2 receptors (as well as to D_4 receptors and serotonin [5-HT_{1A}]) is 1000-fold lower than its affinity to D_3 receptors, and labeling becomes selective for the D_3 receptor. We showed that [^{125}I]*trans*-7-OH-PIPAT labeled 1 site on the membranes of human putamen in the absence of GTP and exhibited a reduction in the B_{max} and a decreased K_d in the presence of GTP. The most likely interpretation of these data is that in the absence of GTP, [^{125}I]*trans*-7-OH-PIPAT labels the D_3 receptor and the high affinity state of the D_2 receptor, with perhaps slightly lower affinity to the latter than to the former. In the presence of GTP, D_2 receptors were no longer labeled, resulting in an apparent decrease in B_{max} and an increase in affinity. The binding of [^{125}I]*trans*-7-OH-PIPAT to the D_3 receptor–expressing mouse fibroblast cell line was, as expected, minimally GTP sensitive, and the K_d for [^{125}I]*trans*-7-OH-PIPAT in the presence of GTP was close to that determined with mem-

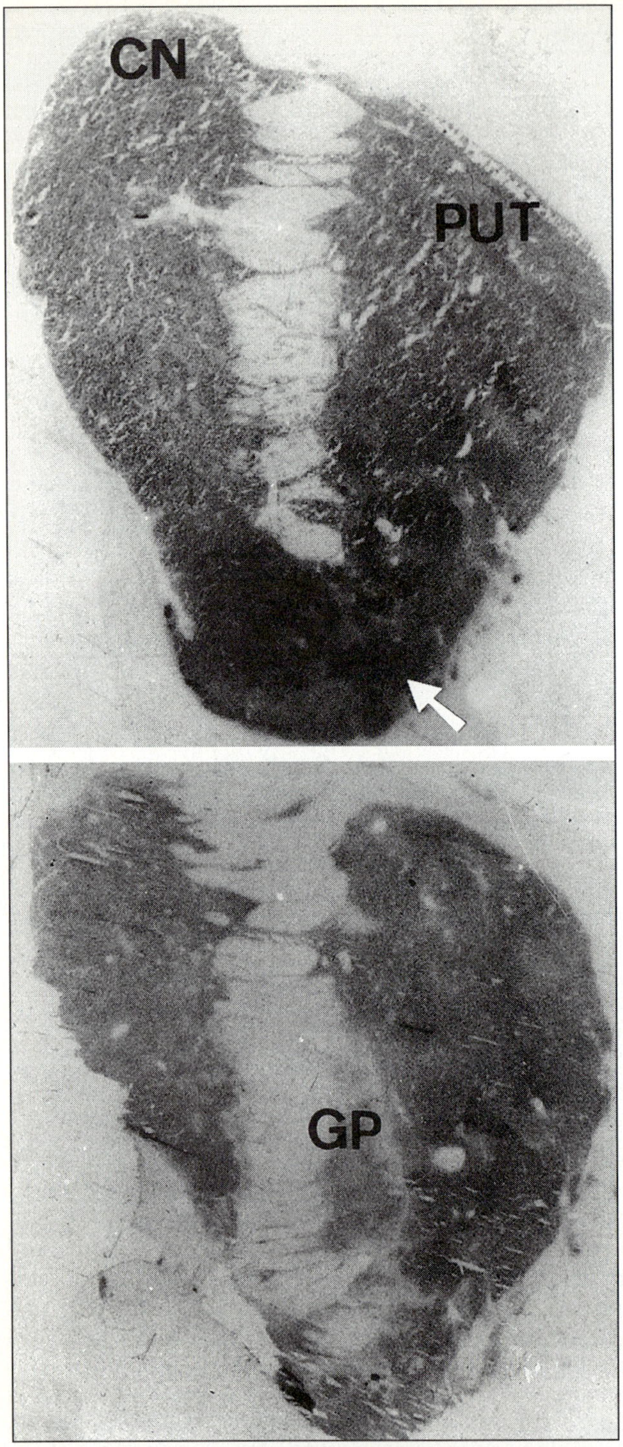

Figure 3. *Photomicrograph of iodine 125–labeled (R)-*trans*-7-hydroxy-2-[*N*-propyl-*N*-(3′ iodo-2′-propenyl)-amino]tetralinth ([^{125}I]*trans*-7-OH-PIPAT) binding to D_3 receptors at 2 different levels of the rostral striatum. Top, There was higher concentration in the ventral striatum, including the nucleus accumbens and ventral putamen (arrow), than in the caudate nucleus (CN) and dorsal putamen (PUT). Bottom, There was significantly less [^{125}I]*trans*-7-OH-PIPAT binding in the caudal part of the basal ganglia. At this level, the binding was higher in the dorsal and ventral putamen than in the caudate nucleus and the globus pallidus (GP).*

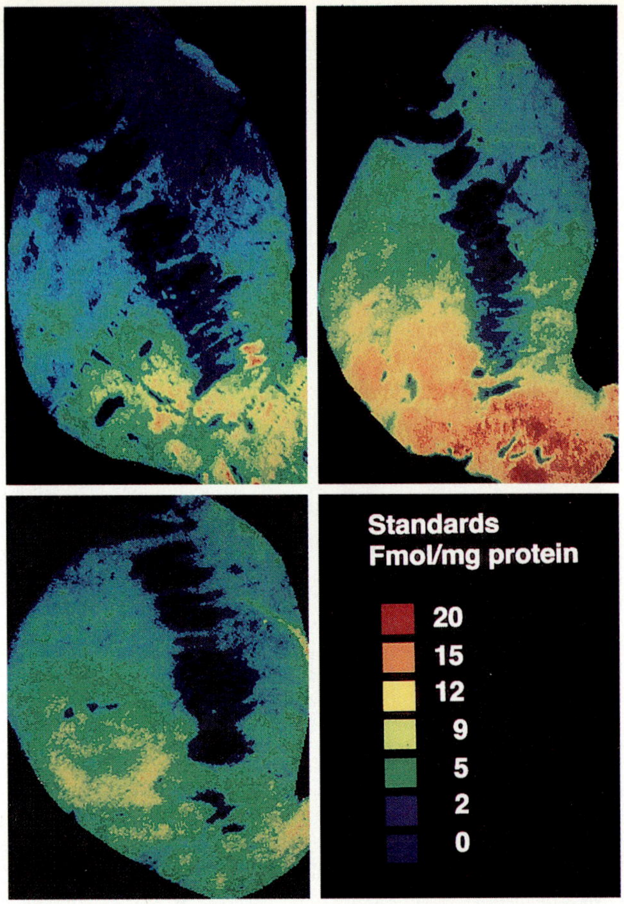

Figure 4. *Pseudocolor images of levels of iodine 125–labeled (R)-*trans*-7-hydroxy-2-[*N*-propyl-*N*-(3′ iodo-2′-propenyl)-amino]tetralin ([^{125}I]*trans*-7-OH-PIPAT) binding in the rostral striatum of a control subject (top left) and patients with schizophrenia not receiving antipsychotic drugs at time of death (top right) and those receiving antipsychotic drugs at time of death (bottom left) (scale is shown in the bottom right corner). Levels of binding were higher in the caudate nucleus, dorsal putamen, and ventral striatum (nucleus accumbens and ventral putamen) of the antipsychotic drug–free patient with schizophrenia and lower in the antipsychotic drug–treated patient.*

branes derived from human putamen. Moreover, competition experiments with D_2/D_3 antagonists for [^{125}I]*trans*-7-OH-PIPAT binding in the presence of GTP in membrane preparations and tissue sections showed displacement from a single site, resulting in K_is that are consistent with those of the D_3 receptor.

The [^{125}I]*trans*-7-OH-PIPAT binding sites were enriched in the limbic striatum and its efferents. This included the ventral striatum, with the patches particularly enriched, the ventral putamen, and GPi. The distribution was quite different from that of D_2 receptors[23] but compared well with the distribution of the binding of the D_2/D_3 antagonist ^{125}I-epidepride to D_3 receptors[11] and with [^{3}H]7-OH-DPAT.[13] The distribution of [^{125}I]*trans*-7-OH-PIPAT binding is also consistent with the distribution of D_3 messenger RNA (mRNA) and differs from that of D_2 mRNA.[14] This supports our conclusion that D_2 and D_3 receptors are segregated to different striatal-pallidal-thalamic circuits, with the D_2 receptor associated with the "motor" loop and the D_3 receptor with the "limbic" loop.[11]

MODIFICATIONS IN SCHIZOPHRENIA

An almost 2-fold increase was identified in the antipsychotic drug–free group, but not in the antipsychotic drug–treated group. The differences between the patients with

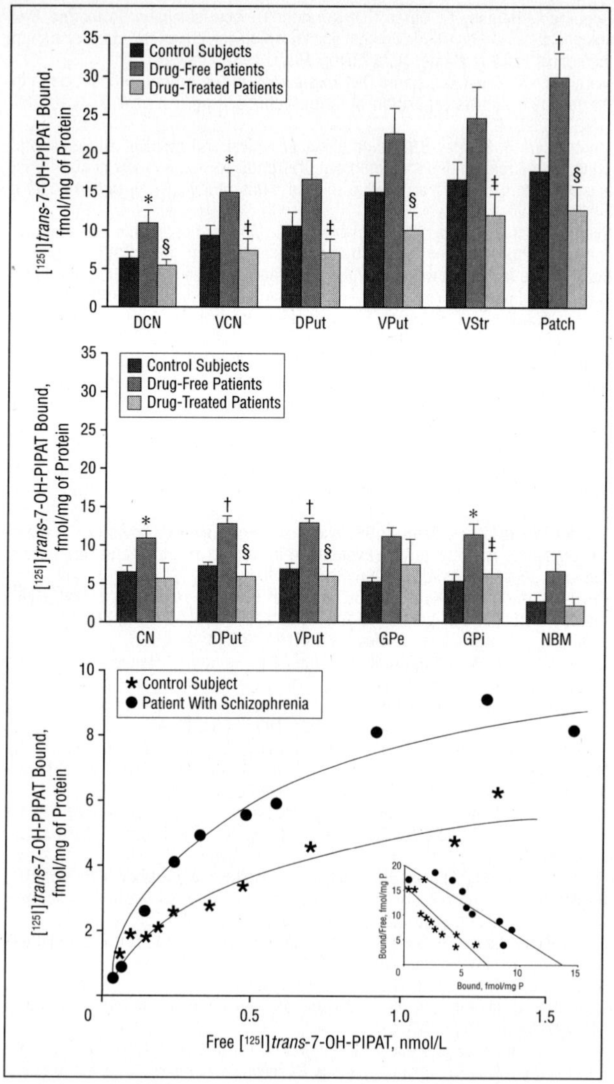

Figure 5. *Bar graphs depicting mean±SEM levels of iodine 125–labeled (R)-*trans*-7-hydroxy-2-[*N*-propyl-*N*-(3′iodo-2′-propenyl)-amino]tetralin ([^{125}I]*trans*-7-OH-PIPAT) binding in regions of the rostral striatum (top) and caudal striatum and ventral forebrain (center) from the control group, patients with schizophrenia who were not receiving antipsychotic drugs at time of death (drug-free patients), and those who were receiving antipsychotic drugs at time of death (drug-treated patients). Top, In the rostral striatum, D_3 receptors were elevated in the dorsal caudate nucleus (DCN), ventral striatum (nucleus accumbens and most ventral part of the putamen) (VStr), and patches in antipsychotic drug–free patients with schizophrenia compared with the control subjects (as shown by 1-way analysis of variance and post hoc Duncan test). In all other regions, the antipsychotic drug–treated group was different from the antipsychotic drug–free group (post hoc Duncan test). Center, For the caudal striatum, the binding values in the antipsychotic drug–free group of patients with schizophrenia were significantly higher in the CN, dorsal putamen (DPut), ventral putamen (VPut), and internal segment of the globus pallidus (GPi), compared with control subjects and the antipsychotic drug–treated group. Bottom, Representative saturation isotherms for the putamen obtained with the caudal sections of basal ganglia from control subjects and patients with schizophrenia. Insert shows Scatchard transformation of the binding data. The obtained dissociation constants (K_ds) were not different between control subjects and patients with schizophrenia. In control subjects, the mean±SD K_d for the CN was 0.87±0.36 nmol/L; for the putamen, 0.54±13 nmol/L; for the external segment of the globus pallidus (GPe), 0.99±0.37 nmol/L; and for the GPi, 0.65±0.22 nmol/L. In patients with schizophrenia, the mean±SD K_d for the CN was 0.78±0.52 nmol/L; for the putamen, 0.7±0.35 nmol/L; for the GPe, 0.71±0.2 nmol/L; and for the GPi, 0.58±0.18 nmol/L. VCN indicates ventral caudate nucleus; NBM, nucleus basalis of Meynert; asterisk, P<.05 compared with control subjects; dagger, P<.01 compared with control subjects; double dagger, P<.05 compared with the other group of patients with schizophrenia; and section mark, P<.01 compared with the other group of patients with schizophrenia.*

schizophrenia and the control subjects were not due to different properties of D_3 receptors in schizophrenic tissue. The binding of [^{125}I]*trans*-7-OH-PIPAT in membranes of control and schizophrenic putamen was best fit to 1 site in the presence or absence of GTP, with a 2-fold reduction in the apparent K_d and a significant reduction of the B_{max} in the presence of GTP. In antipsychotic drug–free group, the binding of [^{125}I]*trans*-7-OH-PIPAT was regulated by GTP in the same manner as in control subjects. Saturation isotherms demonstrated that the ligand labeled a homogeneous population of binding sites with similar affinity in the 4 brain regions examined in all groups. Furthermore, the binding of [^{125}I]*trans*-7-OH-PIPAT did not correlate with the dose of antipsychotic drug at any time, and the elevation of the binding in the antipsychotic drug–free group was strictly region specific.

Thus, it seems unlikely that the lower binding in the antipsychotic drug–treated group than in the antipsychotic drug–free group was due to the presence of residual drugs in the tissue. This is supported additionally by the fact that the binding of [^{125}I]*trans*-7-OH-PIPAT observed in 2 subjects, UPS 011 and UPS 024, who had not received antipsychotic drugs for the shortest period before death were in the range of the other patients identified as antipsychotic drug–free.

The most attractive interpretation of these data, although not necessarily the only one, is that antipsychotic drugs down-regulate D_3 receptors in patients with schizophrenia who otherwise have a higher density of these receptors in specific mesolimbic structures. This interpretation is supported, in part, by the observations that long-term antipsychotic drug treatment in rats does not lead to an elevation in D_3 receptor mRNA levels or receptor numbers as it does for D_2 and D_4 receptor mRNA.[24-29] Alternatively, these differences between antipsychotic drug–treated and drug–free patients with schizophrenia may be due to a selection factor that led to continuation of treatment in 1 group and withdrawal of treatment in the other, and this treatment decision perhaps reflects intrinsic differences in neurochemical systems in the patients. We could not identify any selection factor (eg, tardive dyskinesia), but our results need to be evaluated in an independent sample of patients.

The evidence for an altered organization of D_2-like, β-adrenergic, and 5-HT_2 receptors and serotonin transporter sites within the ventral striatum of patients with schizophrenia has been discussed previously.[30] The normally well-defined compartmental organization of all these systems is disturbed in schizophrenia. Our current data add to that conceptualization. The elevated levels of D_3 receptors observed in the antipsychotic drug–free group is restricted to several specific areas. The only structures in the rostral striatum where D_3 receptor density is increased are in the ventral striatum. Moreover, D_3 receptor density tends to be elevated most in patches of dense binding found in the ventral striatum, likely associated with the striosomal compartment.[11] These regional effects are regulated by antipsychotic medication. The interpretation that the D_3 receptor levels are normally elevated in patients with schizophrenia and that the D_3 receptor is a target of antipsychotic drugs that down-regulate it depends on an understanding of the circuitry of the basal ganglia. Two distinct DA systems are believed to exist within the basal ganglia, the nigrostriatal and mesolimbic, each linked to segregated cortico-striato-pallidal-thalamo-cortical circuits.[31] The mesolimbic DA system projects to the ventral striatum and has as its primary target the D_3 receptor. The efferents of the ventral striatum remain segregated from the nigrostriatal DA system, which acts through the D_2 receptor. The ventral striatum receives limbic cortical input and projects to the ventral pallidum (and GPi), which, in its turn projects to the mediodorsal and anteroventral thalamic nuclei and, ultimately, the anterior prefrontal cortex.[9,29] The mesolimbic system is thought to act as a gate that is under the control of DA for modulating efferents from a number of other regions in the brain that are disturbed in schizophrenia.[9,32,33]

Oversimplified as this scheme may be, it is very useful in evaluating the data available on the chemical neuroanatomy of the basal ganglia in schizophrenia. The increased number of D_3 receptors in the ventral striatum and efferents observed in our studies may lead to altered neural processing in their output through the striato-pallidal-thalamo-cortical limbic loop.[5,29] Down-regulation of the D_3 receptor–mediated limbic loop by antipsychotic drugs may provide a means of resolving the imbalance in this loop. The elevation of D_2-like receptors within the motor subdivision of the striatum and its efferents that other laboratories have observed is likely the result of long-term antipsychotic drug treatment and related to the extrapyramidal effects of these drugs.[3,4,34] The mechanisms responsible for antipsychotic regulation of the systems through different DA receptors need to be further evaluated.

Accepted for publication May 15, 1996.

Supported by an award from Scottish Rite Benevolent Foundation's Schizophrenia Research Program, Northern Masonic Jurisdiction, Lexington, Mass; grants MH55144, MH43852, MH43880, AG09215, and AG10124 from the Public Health Service, Washington, DC; and an award from the American Federation for Aging Research, New York, NY (Ms Bordelon).

The [^{125}I]trans-7-OH-PIPAT was a generous gift from Hank F. Kung, PhD, and Mei-Ping Kung, PhD, Department of Radiology, University of Pennsylvania School of Medicine, Philadelphia.

Reprints: Jeffrey N. Joyce, PhD, Willliam T. Christopher Center for Parkinson's Disease Research, Sun Health Research Institute, PO Box 1278, Sun City, AZ 85372.

REFERENCES

1. Lieberman JA, Kinon BJ, Loebel AD. Dopaminergic mechanisms in idiopathic and drug-induced psychoses. *Schizophr Bull.* 1990;16:97-110.
2. Seeman P, Chau-Wong M, Tedesco J, Wong K. Brain receptors for antipsychotic drugs and dopamine: direct binding assays. *Proc Natl Acad Sci U S A.* 1975;72:4376-4380.
3. Seeman P, Bzowej NH, Guan HC, Bergeron C, Reynolds GP, Bird ED, Riederer P, Jellinger K, Tourtellote WW. Human brain D_1 and D_2 dopamine receptors in schizophrenia, Alzheimer's, Parkinson's and Huntington's disease. *Neuropsychopharmacology.* 1987;1:5-15.
4. Seeman P, Guan H-C, Van Tol HHM. Dopamine D_4 receptors elevated in schizophrenia. *Nature.* 1993;365:441-445.
5. Joyce JN, Lexow N, Bird E, Winokur A. Organization of dopamine D_1 and D_2 receptors in human striatum: receptor autoradiographic studies in Huntington's disease and schizophrenia. *Synapse.* 1988;2:546-557.
6. Hogberg T, Ramsby S, Ogren SO, Norinder U. New selective dopamine D-2 antagonists as antipsychotic agents: pharmacological, chemical, structural, and theoretical considerations. *Acta Pharm Suec.* 1987;24:289-328.
7. Merchant KM, Dobie DJ, Dorsa DM. Expression of the proneurotensin gene in the rat brain and its regulation by antipsychotic drugs. *Ann N Y Acad Sci.* 1992;668:54-69.
8. Moghaddam B, Bunney BS. Acute effect of typical and atypical antipsychotic drugs on the release of dopamine from prefrontal cortex, nucleus accumbens, and striatum of the rat: an in vivo microdialysis study. *J Neurochem.* 1990; 54:1755-1760.
9. Csernansky JG, Murphy GM, Faustman WO. Limbic/mesolimbic connections and the pathogenesis of schizophrenia. *Biol Psychiatry.* 1991;30:383-400.
10. Louilot A, Le Moal M. Lateralized interdependence between limbicotemporal and ventrostriatal dopaminergic transmission. *Neuroscience.* 1994;59:495-500.
11. Murray AM, Ryoo H, Gurevich E, Joyce JN. Localization of dopamine D_3 receptors to mesolimbic and D_2 receptors to mesostriatal regions of human forebrain. *Proc Natl Acad Sci U S A.* 1994;91:11,271-11,275.
12. Sokoloff P, Giros B, Martres M-P, Bouthenet M-L, Schwartz J-C. Molecular cloning and characterization of a novel dopamine receptor (D_3) as a target for neuroleptics. *Nature.* 1990;347:146-151.
13. Herroelen L, De Backer J-PD, Wilczak N, Flamez A, Vauquelin G, De Keyser J. Autoradiographic distribution of D_3-type dopamine receptors in human brain using [^{3}H]7-hydroxy-*N,N*-di-n-propyl-2-aminotetralin. *Brain Res.* 1994;648: 222-228.
14. Meador-Woodruff JH, Damask SP, Wang J, Haroutunian V, Davis KL, Watson SJ. Dopamine receptor mRNA expression in human striatum and neocortex. *Neuropsychopharmacology.* 1996;15:17-29.
15. Foulon C, Kung M-P, Kung HF. Synthesis of (R,S)-2′-*trans*-7-hydroxyl-2-[*N*-n-propyl-*N*-(3′-iodo-2′-propenyl0-amino]tetralin (*trans*-7-OH-PIPAT): a new D_3 dopamine receptor ligand. *J Med Chem.* 1993;36:1490-1500.
16. Burris KD, Filtz TM, Chumpradit S, Kung M-P, Foulon C, Henseler JG, Kung HF, Molinoff PB. Characterization of [^{125}I](R)-*trans*-7-hydroxy-2-[*N*-propyl-*N*-(3′-iodo-2′-propenyl)amino]tetralin binding to dopamine D_3 receptors in rat olfactory tubercle. *J Pharmacol Exp Ther.* 1994;268:939-942.
17. Kung M-P, Chumpradit S, Frederick D, Garner S, Burris K, Molinoff PB, Kung HF. Characterization of binding sites for [^{125}I]R(+)*trans*-7-OH-PIPAT in rat brain. *Naunyn Schmiedebergs Arch Pharmacol.* 1994;350:611-617.
18. American Psychiatric Association. *Diagnostic and Statistical Manual of Mental Disorders, Third Edition, Revised.* Washington, DC: American Psychiatric Association; 1987.
19. Arnold SE, Gur RE, Shapiro RM, Fisher KR, Moberg PJ, Gibney MR, Gur RC, Blackwell P, Trojanowski JQ. Prospective clinicopathological studies of schizophrenia: accrual and assessment. *Am J Psychiatry.* 1995;152:731-737.
20. Kane JM. In: Kaplan HI, Sadock BJ, eds. *Comprehensive Textbook of Psychiatry.* 5th ed. Baltimore, Md: Williams & Wilkins; 1989:777-792.
21. McGonigle P, Neve KA, Molinoff PB. A quantitative method of analyzing the interaction of slightly selective radioligands with multiple receptor subtypes. *Mol Pharmacol.* 1986;30:329-337.
22. Sokoloff P, Andrieux M, Besançon R, Pilon C, Martres M-P, Giros B, Schwartz J-C. Pharmacology of human dopamine D_3 receptor expressed in a mammalian cell line: comparison with D_2 receptor. *Eur J Pharmacol.* 1992;225:331-337.
23. Joyce JN, Sapp DW, Marshall JF. Human striatal dopamine receptors are organized in patches. *Proc Natl Acad Sci U S A.* 1986;83:8002-8006.
24. Egan MF, Hurd Y, Hyde TM, Weinberger DR, Wyatt RJ, Kleinman JE. Alterations in mRNA levels of D_2 receptors and neuropeptides in striatonigal neurons of rats with neuroleptic induces dyskinesias. *Synapse.* 1994;18:178-189.
25. Fishburn CS, David C, Carmon S, Fuchs S. The effect of haloperidol on D_2 dopamine receptor subtype mRNA levels in the brain. *FEBS Lett.* 1994;339:63-66.
26. Laruelle M, Jaskiw GE, Kipska BK, Kolachana B, Casanova MF, Kleinman JE, Weinberger DR. D_1 and D_2 receptor modulation in rat striatum and nucleus accumbens after chronic haloperidol treatment. *Brain Res.* 1992;575:47-56.
27. Lévesque D, Martres M-P, Diaz J, Griffon N, Lammers CH, Sokoloff P, Schwartz J-C. A paradoxical regulation of the dopamine D_3 receptor expression suggests the involvement of an anterograde factor from dopamine neurons. *Proc Natl Acad Sci U S A.* 1995;92:1719-1723.
28. Schoots O, Seeman P, Guan H-C, Paterson AD, Van Tol HHM. Long-term haloperidol elevates dopamine D_4 receptors by 2-fold in rats. *Eur J Pharmacol.* 1995; 289:67-72.
29. Damask SP, Bovenkerk KA, de la Pena G, Hoversten KM, Peters DB, Valentine AM, Meador-Woodruff JH. Differential effects of clozapine and haloperidol on dopamine receptor mRNA expression in rat striatum and cortex. *Mol Brain Res.* 1996;41:241-249.
30. Joyce JN. The dopamine hypothesis of schizophrenia: limbic interactions with serotonin and norepinephrine. *Psychopharmacology.* 1993;112(suppl):S16-S34.
31. Alexander GE, Crutcher MD. Functional architecture of basal ganglia circuits: neural substrates of parallel processing. *Trends Neurosci.* 1990;13:266-271.
32. Amalric M, Koob GF. Functionally selective neurochemical afferents and efferents of the mesocorticolimbic and nigrostriatal dopamine system. *Prog Brain Res.* 1993;99:209-226.
33. Mogenson GJ, Yang CR, Yim CY. Influence of dopamine on limbic inputs to the nucleus accumbens. *Ann N Y Acad Sci.* 1988;537:86-100.
34. Mackay AVP, Iversen L, Rossor M, Spokes E, Bird E, Arregui A, Creese I, Snyder SH. Increased brain dopamine and dopamine receptors in schizophrenia. *Arch Gen Psychiatry.* 1982;39:991-997.

ORIGINAL ARTICLE

Visual Imagery and Perception in Posttraumatic Stress Disorder

A Positron Emission Tomographic Investigation

Lisa M. Shin, AM; Stephen M. Kosslyn, PhD; Richard J. McNally, PhD; Nathaniel M. Alpert, PhD; William L. Thompson; Scott L. Rauch, MD; Michael L. Macklin; Roger K. Pitman, MD

Background: Relative regional cerebral blood flow (rCBF) changes were measured in Vietnam combat veterans with and without posttraumatic stress disorder (PTSD) during exposure to combat-related stimuli.

Methods: Positron emission tomography was used to measure rCBF in 7 combat veterans with PTSD (PTSD group) and 7 healthy combat veterans (control group) who viewed and generated visual mental images of neutral, negative, and combat-related pictures.

Results: Unlike control subjects, subjects with PTSD had increased rCBF in ventral anterior cingulate gyrus and right amygdala when generating mental images of combat-related pictures; when viewing combat pictures, subjects with PTSD showed decreased rCBF in Broca's area.

Conclusions: Results suggest that ventral anterior cingulate gyrus and right amygdala play a role in the response of combat veterans with PTSD to mental images of combat-related scenes. Reexperiencing phenomena of PTSD, which often involve emotional visual mental imagery, may be likewise associated with increased rCBF in these regions.

Arch Gen Psychiatry. 1997;54:233-241

From the Department of Psychology, Harvard University, Cambridge, Mass (Drs Shin, Kosslyn, and McNally and Mr Thompson); Departments of Neurology (Dr Kosslyn), Radiology (Drs Alpert and Rauch), and Psychiatry (Dr Rauch) Massachusetts General Hospital, and Department of Psychiatry (Drs Rauch and Pitman), Harvard Medical School, Boston, Mass; and the Veterans Affairs Research Service, Manchester, NH (Mr Macklin and Dr Pitman).

COMBAT VETERANS with posttraumatic stress disorder (PTSD) are physiologically more reactive to combat-related stimuli than are combat veterans without PTSD.[1-4] Pitman and colleagues[3] found that combat veterans with PTSD had greater skin conductance and lateral frontalis electromyographic responses during imagery of combat-related traumatic events than did combat veterans without PTSD. Many studies have replicated the finding of increased physiologic reactivity in combat veterans with PTSD; in contrast, we know little about brain activity in these individuals during exposure to combat-related stimuli.

Rauch and colleagues[5] recently reported the results of a positron emission tomographic (PET) study of symptom provocation in 8 individuals with PTSD. In separate scans, subjects imagined their own traumatic and neutral events. Increased blood flow was found in limbic and paralimbic regions (including amygdala, anterior cingulate gyrus, orbitofrontal cortex, and insular cortex) during the traumatic condition, relative to the neutral condition.

We describe a PET study of relative regional cerebral blood flow (rCBF) in Vietnam combat veterans with PTSD (PTSD group) and without PTSD (control group). In separate conditions, subjects viewed and generated visual mental images of neutral, negative, and combat-related pictures while they inhaled oxygen 15–labeled carbon dioxide ($^{15}O-CO_2$). We were particularly interested in examining rCBF changes in the limbic system because some of these structures appear to be involved in emotion and in the processing of stimuli with affective significance.[6-8] Furthermore, recent PET studies of other anxiety disorders have shown increased rCBF in limbic and paralimbic regions during symptom provocation.[9,10] In our study, limbic and paralimbic regions of interest (ROIs) included the amygdala, anterior cingulate gyrus, hippocampus, insular cortex, orbitofrontal cortex, and parahippocampal gyrus. Although the hippocampus and parahippocampal gyrus are more involved in memory than emotion per se, given that PTSD involves memories for traumatic events, these regions were of interest.

We expected combat-related pictures, both seen and visualized, to carry more affective significance for combat veterans with PTSD than for those without PTSD. Accordingly, we expected to find

SUBJECTS, MATERIALS, AND METHODS

SUBJECTS

Fourteen white male Vietnam combat veterans, who provided written informed consent and received payment for their participation, were recruited from a group of volunteers who had participated in previous studies at the Veterans Affairs Research Service in Manchester, NH. A doctoral-level clinician used the Clinician-Administered Posttraumatic Stress Disorder Scale (CAPS)[12] and the Structured Clinical Interview for *DSM-III-R*[13] to establish diagnoses. The PTSD group consisted of 7 combat veterans with current chronic PTSD; 2 had current major depression, 2 had past panic disorder, 3 had past alcohol dependence, and 4 had past major depression. Six of the subjects with PTSD had been taking psychoactive medication and underwent a supervised drug washout for at least 2 weeks before scanning. The control group consisted of 7 psychiatrically healthy combat veterans who had never had PTSD. One control subject had past major depressive disorder and past alcohol dependence. The other 6 control subjects had no history of psychiatric disorders. None of the subjects had a major nonpsychiatric medical illness or head injury with prolonged loss of consciousness. All subjects were right-handed, as determined by the Edinburgh Inventory.[14] This study was approved by the Subcommittee on Human Studies at the Massachusetts General Hospital, Boston, the Committee on the Use of Human Subjects in Research at Harvard University, Cambridge, Mass, and the Manchester VA Medical Center.

The extent of combat exposure was assessed with the Combat Exposure Scale.[15] Symptoms of PTSD were assessed with the Mississippi Scale for Combat-Related PTSD.[16] Immediately before scanning, each subject completed the Beck Depression Inventory,[17] the State-Trait Anxiety Inventory (STAI),[18] and a general medical history questionnaire. Subjects also completed the Vividness of Visual Imagery Questionnaire,[19,20] an instrument that assesses imagery for ordinary scenes (eg, faces or sunsets), unrelated to combat. Scores range from 16 to 80, with lower scores indicating more vivid imagery.

The subjects with PTSD were younger than control subjects (mean±SD age, 45.4±2.0 years vs 50.0±2.6 years; $t[12]=3.66$, $P=.003$), consistent with epidemiological data.[21] Mean±(SD) Combat Exposure Scale scores did not differ between subjects with PTSD and control subjects (28.1±4.4 vs 24.7±9.3; $t[12]= 0.88$, $P=.40$). Mean(±SD) scores on the Vividness of Visual Imagery Questionnaire did not differ between subjects with PTSD and control subjects (28.2±9.8 vs 26.0±7.2; $t[11]=0.46$, $P=.66$). (A Vividness of Visual Imagery Questionnaire score was missing for 1 subject with PTSD.) Not surprisingly, the subjects with PTSD scored significantly higher than control subjects on the following scales: Mississippi Scale for Combat-Related PTSD (129.1±18.7 vs 56.3±9.9; $t[12]=8.54$, $P<.001$), the Clinician-Administered Posttraumatic Stress Disorder Scale (72.7±15.6 vs 3.3±5.2; $t[12]=11.17$, $P<.001$), STAI-State (59.9±10.2 vs 26.9±4.5; $t[12]=7.83$, $P<.001$), STAI-Trait (61.1±7.4 vs 28.0±8.8; $t[12]=7.64$, $P<.001$), and Beck Depression Inventory (27.3±5.3 vs 2.1±2.2; $t[12]=11.63$, $P<.001$).

MATERIALS

Subjects viewed 3 types of color pictures: neutral (neutral in valence and unrelated to combat in Vietnam), negative (negative in valence and unrelated to combat in Vietnam), and combat (negative in valence and related to combat in Vietnam). The set of neutral pictures consisted of 30 affectively innocuous scenes (eg, a truck, buildings). The set of negative pictures consisted of 30 disturbing scenes (eg, a baby with a facial tumor, a funeral). Some of the negative and neutral pictures were from the set[22] validated for affective content by Lang and Greenwald.[23] Finally, the combat pictures consisted of 30 color photographs taken during the Vietnam war (eg, a sniper, a bodybag). Many of these pictures were used in a previous study[24] and were found to increase self-reported anxiety, anger, and sadness in combat veterans.

All pictures were scanned into a personal computer (Macintosh, Apple Corp, Cupertino, Calif) using a color scanner (Scanmaker 600ZS, Microtek, Redondo Beach, Calif) and were converted into color PICT (picture) files (300 dots per inch, 16 bits per pixel). Each picture was scaled to measure 10 × 10 cm and was displayed in the center of a blank (white) screen on a 14-in color monitor. The monitor was located on a metal gantry, approximately 50 cm from each subject's head. Pictures were presented sequentially, using the MacLab program[25] on a Macintosh computer (LC II).

Prior to the study, all pictures were rated by 15 nonveterans on 7-point scales of valence (negative to positive) and arousal (low to high). These ratings were used to ensure that stimuli assigned to different conditions were equated on these measures. The Spearman-Brown aggregate reliability of the 15 judges' ratings was 0.95 for valence and 0.91 for arousal. The estimated reliability of the average individual judge (mean Pearson r) was 0.58 for valence ratings and 0.39 for arousal ratings.

Each picture was presented with a recorded, spoken single word; eg, a picture of a wounded American soldier was accompanied by the spoken word, "wounded." The spoken words served as "tags" to help subjects distinguish between the pictures. For each picture, we also recorded a statement that referred to its content; eg, the statement corresponding to the wounded soldier picture was "The soldier has a bandage below his knee." Half of the statements correctly described their corresponding pictures, and half did not; later, subjects had to determine which of these statements were true and which were false (see the "Task Procedure" subsection within this section for details). This statement evaluation task was implemented to ensure that the subjects actually attended to the pictures. The statements contained an average of 6.4 words (range, 5-10 words). All auditory stimuli were recorded in the same male voice, using the SoundEdit (Macromedia, San Francisco, Calif) program and a standard plug-in microphone (Macintosh, Apple Corp).

TASK PROCEDURE

Each subject participated in 7 conditions. In a baseline condition, subjects were instructed to keep their eyes closed, relax, and think of nothing in particular In 3 of the remaining 6 conditions, the subjects viewed and evaluated stimuli (perception conditions), and in the other 3 conditions, they visualized and evaluated stimuli (imagery conditions); separate blocks of neutral, negative, and combat stimuli were presented in the perception and imagery conditions. The stimuli assigned to the perception and imagery conditions were rated as being roughly equal in valence and arousal; eg, the stimuli in the combat perception condition were as negative in valence and as arousing as the stimuli in the combat imagery condition.

Order of condition was counterbalanced across subjects. Four subjects per group received the "neutral-negative-combat" order, and the remaining 3 subjects per group received the reverse order. In addition, 4 subjects per group participated in the perception conditions before the imagery conditions, and the remaining 3 subjects per group received the reverse order.

Within each condition, subjects participated in a study session, followed by practice trials, and then experimental trials. Positron emission tomographic scanning occurred only during the experimental trials. In the study session, the subjects received 15 sequentially presented picture-word pairs (eg, subjects saw a picture of soldiers carrying a bodybag and simultaneously heard the word "bodybag"). Subjects were instructed to remember each picture in as much detail as possible, and they were told that they would be tested on their recall of the pictures. After subjects studied all 15 pictures twice, they were given 3 practice trials, followed by 12 experimental trials.

In the perception condition, subjects saw a previously studied picture and heard its corresponding word (eg, "bodybag"). Two seconds later, subjects heard a statement about the picture (eg, "The bodybag lies on the pavement"). While viewing the picture, the subjects determined whether the statement was true or false and then pressed 1 of 2 foot pedals (the left pedal for true, and the right pedal for false). The next trial began 500 milliseconds after a response.

The imagery task closely paralleled the perception task, except that no picture was presented and subjects' eyes were closed. In the imagery condition, subjects heard a previously studied word and generated a visual mental image of the corresponding picture. Two seconds after hearing the word, subjects heard a statement regarding their visual mental image. They inspected their mental image, determined whether the statement was true or false, and then pressed 1 of 2 foot pedals (the left pedal for true, and the right pedal for false). The next trial began 500 milliseconds after a response.

Error rates and response times were recorded by the computer. The statement evaluation task was implemented to ensure that subjects were indeed viewing or visualizing each picture. Error rates were checked to confirm that each subject was performing the task correctly.

PET PROCEDURES

The PET data were gathered by a 15-slice, whole-body tomograph (Scanditronix PC 4096, General Electric, Milwaukee, Wis) (in stationary mode) located at the Massachusetts General Hospital. The camera produced contiguous slices with a center-to-center distance of 6.5 mm (axial field, 97.5 mm). Axial resolution was 6.0 mm (full-width half maximum). The images were reconstructed using a measured attenuation correction and a Hanning-weighted reconstruction filter set to allow for 8.0-mm in-plane spatial resolution (full-width half maximum). During reconstruction, corrections were made for scattered radiation, random coincidences, and counting losses resulting from dead time in the camera electronics.

Each subject was fitted with a thermoplastic custom-molded face mask to prevent excessive head movement, and the subject's head was aligned relative to the canthomeatal line. The subject was fitted with nasal cannulae, which delivered the $^{15}O\text{-}CO_2$, and an overlying face mask attached to a vacuum. The concentration of the $^{15}O\text{-}CO_2$ was 2960 MBq/L; the flow rate was 2 L/min.

Image Acquisition and Transformation

Before scanning, several transmission measurements were made using an orbiting pin source. Within each data acquisition run, 15 measurements were made: the first 3 lasted 10 seconds each, and the remaining 12 lasted 5 seconds each. After reconstruction, measurements 4 through 15 were summed to form images of relative blood flow.

Fifteen seconds after the data acquisition started, subjects began the behavioral task. Fifteen seconds later, $^{15}O\text{-}CO_2$ administration began. Sixty seconds later, scanning and gas administration ceased. Scans were separated by approximately 10 minutes to allow for radiation decay.

Terminal count rates were between 100 000 and 200 000 events per second. No arterial lines were necessary because previous work with arterial cannulation in our laboratory has demonstrated that integrated counts over periods of up to 90 seconds are a linear function over the flow range of 1 to 130 mL/min per 100 g (N.M.A., unpublished data, 1991).

The PET data were transformed to the coordinate system of Talairach and Tournoux,[26] using procedures that have been described previously.[9,27]

PET Analyses

For each run, the mean concentration was the area-weighted sum of the concentration in each slice, adjusted to a nominal value of 50 mL/min per 100 g. The images were smoothed and scaled using a 2-dimensional gaussian filter, which was approximately 20 mm wide (full-width half maximum). For each subject within each group, the images of 1 condition were subtracted from the images of another condition (as in a paired t test) and these difference scores were averaged across subjects within each group. This process yielded images of mean differences, SDs, number of subjects, and t statistics for each subtraction. The t statistic images were converted (by integral transformation) into z-score images, called statistical parametric maps.[28]

The z-score images were inspected for foci of activation. Foci with z scores of 3.0 or higher are reported. A z score of 3.0 corresponds to $P<.001$ uncorrected for multiple comparisons (ie, multiple pixels in a given ROI). A z score of 3.75 corresponds to $P<.0001$ uncorrected for multiple comparisons and, conservatively, $P<.05$ corrected for multiple comparisons (ie, corrected for approximately 3000 comparisons, which is the number of pixels in the largest brain slice).

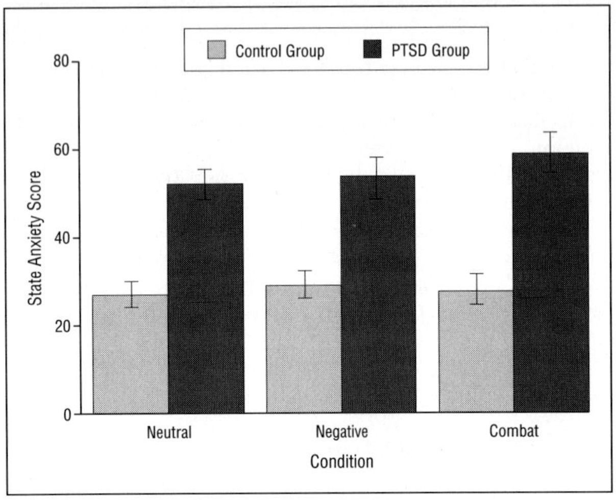

Figure 1. *Change in state anxiety, as measured by the Spielberger State-Trait Anxiety Inventory–State Form, across neutral, negative, and combat conditions in combat veterans with posttraumatic stress disorder (PTSD group) and combat veteran controls (control group). Error bars indicate SEM. The linear increase in state anxiety across conditions was significant only in the PTSD group (*P*=.02).*

rCBF increases in limbic and paralimbic ROIs during exposure to combat-related stimuli in combat veterans with PTSD, but not in healthy combat veterans. We included imagery conditions in this study because of the important role of imagery in the reexperiencing symptoms of PTSD.[11] However, we were uncertain whether the number of rCBF increases in limbic and paralimbic ROIs would differ between subtractions involving combat imagery and those involving combat perception in the PTSD group.

RESULTS

ANXIETY CHANGE

The STAI-State Form (STAI-S) was administered after the neutral, negative, and combat conditions. (Two subjects with PTSD were not given the STAI-S, 1 control subject was missing a STAI-S score for the neutral condition, and another control subject was missing a STAI-S score for the negative condition.) A 2 (group: PTSD, control) × 3 (stimulus valence: neutral, negative, combat) repeated measures analysis of variance (ANOVA) revealed that the PTSD group had higher STAI-S scores than the control group across all valence conditions ($F[1,10]=26.02$; $P=.001$) (**Figure 1**). In addition, STAI-S scores increased across the neutral, negative, and combat conditions ($F[2,18]=4.40$; $P=.03$). An interaction between group and stimulus valence indicated that the PTSD group had greater increases across valence conditions than did the control group ($F[2,18]=4.07$; $P=.03$). Linear contrasts revealed a significant linear increase in STAI-S scores across the neutral, negative, and combat conditions in the PTSD group ($F[1,8]=7.84$; $P=.02$), but not in the control group ($F<1$).

We also examined the significant group × stimulus valence interaction by computing paired *t* tests between valence conditions within each group. Because of the missing data noted above, data from only 5 subjects with PTSD and 5 control subjects could be included in these analyses. In the PTSD group, self-reported anxiety tended to increase from the negative to combat conditions ($t[4]=2.54$; $P=.06$) and from the neutral to the combat conditions ($t[4]=2.17$; $P=.10$); there was no significant increase from the neutral to the negative condition ($t[4]<1$). In the control group, there were no significant changes in anxiety for any of the comparisons ($t<1$).

STIMULUS RATINGS

After the scanning session, subjects rated all stimuli on 3 different dimensions: valence (−3 to +3), arousal (1 to 7), and personal relevance (1 to 7). (Ratings were not obtained from 1 subject with PTSD and 1 control subject.)

Ratings of valence, arousal, and personal relevance were analyzed using 3 separate 2 (group: PTSD, control) × 3 (stimulus valence: neutral, negative, combat) repeated measures ANOVAs. The analysis of valence ratings revealed only that both groups gave increasingly negative scores to the neutral, negative, and combat stimuli ($F[2,20]=18.30$; $P<.001$).

The PTSD group gave higher arousal ratings to all types of stimuli than did the control group ($F[1,10]=6.64$; $P=.03$). In addition, both groups gave increasingly higher arousal ratings to the neutral, negative, and combat stimuli ($F[2,20]=78.87$; $P<.001$). Finally, the 2 groups differed in their arousal ratings of the different types of stimuli ($F[2,20]=16.06$; $P<.001$). Follow-up *t* tests revealed that subjects with PTSD considered the combat pictures to be more arousing than did control subjects ($t[10]=3.99$; $P=.003$).

The analysis of personal relevance ratings revealed only that both groups gave increasingly higher scores to the neutral, negative, and combat stimuli ($F[2,20]=26.34$; $P<.001$).

According to the ratings of all subjects, stimuli used in the perception and imagery conditions (within each valence condition) did not differ significantly on measures of valence, arousal, or personal significance ($P>.1$). When the ratings were examined within each group, stimuli in the combat perception and combat imagery conditions did not differ on measures of valence, arousal, or personal relevance ($P>.1$).

BEHAVIORAL RESULTS

Response times were analyzed with a 2 (group: PTSD, control) × 3 (stimulus valence: neutral, negative, combat) × 2 (stimulus type: perception, imagery) repeated measures ANOVA. The subjects required different amounts of time in different valence conditions ($F[2, 24]=5.32$; $P=.01$). Post hoc paired comparisons indicated that all subjects responded more quickly in the neutral condition than in the negative ($t[13]=2.78$; $P=.02$) and combat ($t[13]=2.67$; $P=.02$) conditions; in contrast, subjects required comparable amounts of time in the negative and combat conditions ($t<1$). In addition, subjects generally responded more quickly in the perception condition than in the imagery condition ($F[1,12]=4.73$; $P=.05$). No other effects or interactions approached significance.

Table 1. Coordinates and *z* Scores of Structures With rCBF Changes: Combat Perception Minus Neutral Perception*

Area	Coordinates, mm† x	y	z	*z* Score
PTSD Group				
Increases, none				
Decreases				
Middle frontal gyrus	−24	+47	+12	3.04
Anterior cingulate gyrus	−13	+43	+4	3.64
Control Group				
Increases				
Midcingulate gyrus	+10	−30	+40	3.46
Posterior cingulate gyrus	+3	−54	+16	3.77
Area 19	+40	−79	+24	3.64
Middle frontal gyrus	−33	+39	+8	4.68
Broca's area	−35	+31	+4	3.47
Postcentral gyrus	−47	−21	+20	3.76
Superior temporal gyrus	−54	−41	+8	3.51
Supramarginal gyrus	−45	−46	+24	3.10
Decreases, none				

*rCBF indicates regional cerebral blood flow; PTSD, posttraumatic stress disorder.

†Coordinates are expressed in millimeters. On the x-axis, positive values indicate locations in the right hemisphere and negative values indicate locations in the left hemisphere. On the y-axis, positive values indicate locations anterior to the anterior commissure and negative values indicate locations posterior to the anterior commissure. On the z-axis, positive values indicate locations superior to the anterior commissure-posterior commissure (AC-PC) plane and negative values indicate locations inferior to the AC-PC plane.

Table 2. Coordinates and *z* Scores of Structures With rCBF Changes: Combat Imagery Minus Neutral Imagery*

Area	Coordinates, mm† x	y	z	*z* Score
PTSD Group				
Increases				
Anterior cingulate gyrus	+1	+23	−8	3.40
Decreases				
Inferior parietal cortex	+55	−45	+40	3.14
Superior temporal gyrus	−55	−21	+4	3.03
Control Group				
Increases				
Posterior cingulate gyrus	+6	−49	+24	4.28
Area 18	+3	−77	−4	3.11
Precuneus	−16	−62	+36	3.18
Area 19	−21	−69	+32	3.27
Decreases, none				

*rCBF indicates regional cerebral blood flow; PTSD, posttraumatic stress disorder.

†Coordinates are expressed in millimeters. On the x-axis, positive values indicate locations in the right hemisphere and negative values indicate locations in the left hemisphere. On the y-axis, positive values indicate locations anterior to the anterior commissure and negative values indicate locations posterior to the anterior commissure. On the z-axis, positive values indicate locations superior to the anterior commissure-posterior commissure (AC-PC) plane and negative values indicate locations inferior to the AC-PC plane.

Error rates were analyzed with a 2 (group: PTSD, control) × 3 (stimulus valence: neutral, negative, combat) × 2 (stimulus type: perception, imagery) repeated measures ANOVA. Subjects generally made fewer errors in the perception condition than in the imagery condition ($F[1,12]=20.08$; $P=.001$). No other effects or interactions approached significance.

PET RESULTS

We compared pairs of PET images by subtracting one from another. Only foci of activation with *z* scores above 3.0 are reported. We expected to find increased rCBF in limbic and paralimbic ROIs in the combat conditions, relative to the neutral and negative conditions. Furthermore, we expected to see these rCBF increases in the PTSD group, but not in the control group. A comparison of the negative and neutral conditions in control subjects is reported elsewhere.[29]

Combat Perception Minus Neutral Perception

As shown in **Table 1**, there were no rCBF increases in the PTSD group; however, rCBF decreases occurred in left middle frontal gyrus and left anterior cingulate gyrus.

In the control group, increased rCBF occurred in several areas: right midcingulate gyrus, right posterior cingulate gyrus, right area 19, left middle frontal gyrus, Broca's area (Brodmann area 45), left postcentral gyrus, left superior temporal gyrus, and left supramarginal gyrus. There were no rCBF decreases in the control group.

Combat Imagery Minus Neutral Imagery

Anterior cingulate gyrus was the only area of increased rCBF in the PTSD group (**Table 2** and **Figure 2**, top). This focus of activation was located in the ventral portion of anterior cingulate gyrus (approximately Brodmann areas 24 and 32). Although the area associated with the greatest *z* score (3.40) was located in right anterior cingulate (1 mm to the right of the anterior commissure–posterior commissure line), portions of left anterior cingulate also had *z* scores above 3.0. In the PTSD group, rCBF decreases occurred in right inferior parietal cortex and left superior temporal gyrus.

In the control group, increased rCBF occurred in right posterior cingulate gyrus, right area 18, left precuneus, and left area 19. There were no areas of decreased rCBF in the control group.

Combat Perception Minus Negative Perception

In the PTSD group, increased rCBF was found in right posterior cingulate gyrus and right precuneus; decreased rCBF occurred in right middle temporal gyrus, Broca's area (Brodmann area 44), and left supramarginal gyrus (**Table 3** and Figure 2, center).

In the control group, areas of increased rCBF included right posterior cingulate gyrus, right area 19, left middle frontal gyrus, left precentral gyrus, left parahippocampal gyrus, and left area 17. Also in the control group, decreased rCBF occurred in left medial frontal gyrus and left amygdala.

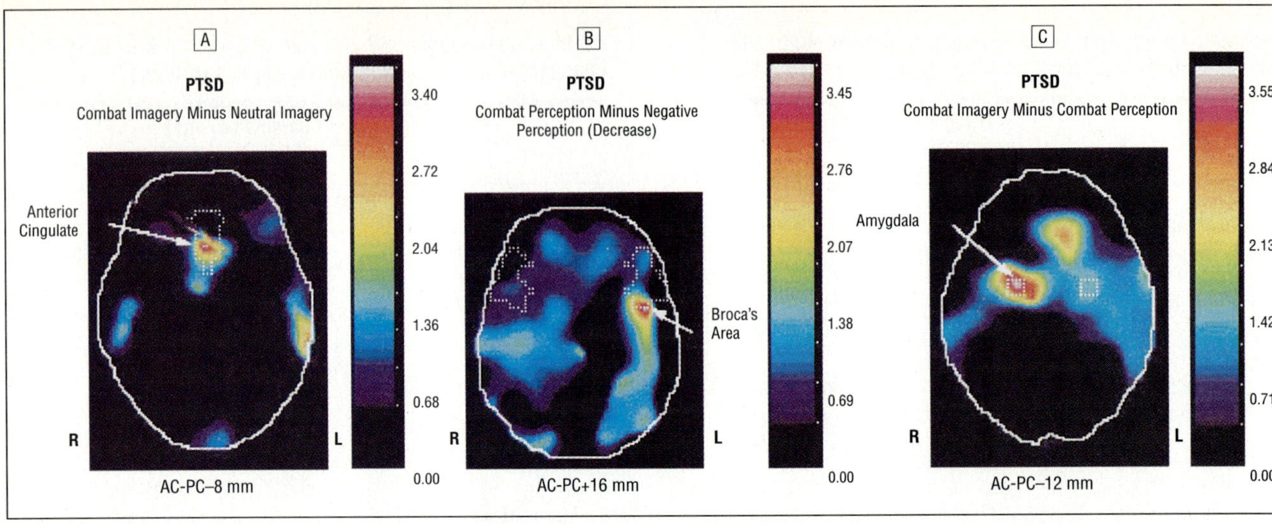

Figure 2. *Statistical parametric maps of 3 different subtractions in the posttraumatic stress disorder (PTSDI) group (n=7 in A and B; n=6 in C). The displayed images are transverse slices parallel to the anterior commissure–posterior commissure plane; the distance from the AC-PC plane is displayed (in millimeters) below each slice. The top and bottom of each slice corresponds to anterior and posterior brain regions, respectively. Left and right are reversed, as displayed. The z score associated with the focus of activation in each subtraction is displayed at the top of each Sokoloff color scale. The images show foci of activation with z scores above 3.0 in anterior cingulate gyrus (A), Broca's area (B) (decreased rCBF), and amygdala (C) in the PTSD group. In the control group, corresponding subtractions revealed no foci of activation with z scores above 3.0 in these regions.*

Table 3. Coordinates and *z* Scores of Structures With rCBF Changes: Combat Perception Minus Negative Perception*

Area	Coordinates, mm†			*z* Score
	x	y	z	
PTSD Group				
Increases				
Posterior cingulate gyrus	+3	−48	+24	3.15
Precuneus	+3	−60	+16	3.47
Decreases				
Middle temporal gyrus	+58	−41	−4	3.40
Broca's area	−47	+5	+16	3.45
Supramarginal gyrus	−49	−32	+24	3.17
Control Group				
Increases				
Posterior cingulate gyrus	+8	−34	+40	3.97
Area 19	+29	−78	+20	3.59
Middle frontal gyrus	−34	+37	+8	3.16
Precentral gyrus	−55	−2	+44	3.67
Parahippocampal gyrus	−21	−41	0	3.52
Area 17	−16	−90	0	3.11
Decreases				
Medial frontal gyrus	−8	+54	−8	3.04
Amygdala	−22	−7	−8	3.16

**rCBF indicates regional cerebral blood flow; PTSD, posttraumatic stress disorder.*

†Coordinates are expressed in millimeters. On the x-axis, positive values indicate locations in the right hemisphere and negative values indicate locations in the left hemisphere. On the y-axis, positive values indicate locations anterior to the anterior commissure and negative values indicate locations posterior to the anterior commissure. On the z-axis, positive values indicate locations superior to the anterior commissure-posterior commissure (AC-PC) plane and negative values indicate locations inferior to the AC-PC plane.

Table 4. Coordinates and *z* Scores of Structures With rCBF Changes: Combat Imagery Minus Negative Imagery*

Area	Coordinates, mm†			*z* Score
	x	y	z	
PTSD Group				
Increases				
Middle temporal gyrus	−54	−40	−4	3.31
Inferior temporal gyrus	−49	−41	−8	3.76
Decreases				
Medial frontal gyrus	+2	+43	+24	3.22
Precuneus	−21	−56	+36	3.77
Area 18	−18	−83	+12	3.13
Area 17	−13	−88	+8	3.24
Control Group				
Increases				
Area 17	−21	−93	−4	5.04
Decreases				
Inferior frontal gyrus	+43	+34	+4	3.48
Precuneus	+11	−55	+32	3.09
Area 17	+2	−69	+12	3.86
Anterior cingulate gyrus	−3	+39	+8	4.99
Middle frontal gyrus	−40	+3	+32	3.17

**rCBF indicates regional cerebral blood flow; PTSD, posttraumatic stress disorder.*

†Coordinates are expressed in millimeters. On the x-axis, positive values indicate locations in the right hemisphere and negative values indicate locations in the left hemisphere. On the y-axis, positive values indicate locations anterior to the anterior commissure and negative values indicate locations posterior to the anterior commissure. On the z-axis, positive values indicate locations superior to the anterior commissure-posterior commissure (AC-PC) plane and negative values indicate locations inferior to the AC-PC plane.

Combat Imagery Minus Negative Imagery

In the PTSD group, rCBF increases were found in left middle temporal and left inferior temporal gyri; rCBF decreases were found in right medial frontal gyrus, left precuneus, left area 18, and left area 17 (**Table 4**).

In the control group, rCBF increases occurred in left area 17 only, whereas rCBF decreases occurred in right

Table 5. Coordinates and z Scores of Structures With rCBF Changes: Combat Imagery Minus Combat Perception*

Area	Coordinates, mm† x	y	z	z Score
PTSD Group				
Increases				
Amygdala‡	+22	−4	−12	3.55
Lenticulate	+20	−7	−4	3.85
Middle frontal gyrus	−34	+48	+20	3.75
Anterior cingulate gyrus	−6	+30	−8	3.00
Supramarginal gyrus	−49	−36	+24	3.68
Decreases				
Area 18	+13	−78	0	4.51
Area 17	−2	−87	+8	4.00
Control Group				
Increases				
Middle frontal gyrus	+27	+57	+4	3.61
Superior frontal gyrus	+10	+51	+16	3.34
Inferior frontal gyrus	+50	+11	+24	3.09
Medial frontal gyrus	−1	+49	−4	3.21
Orbitofrontal cortex‡	−16	+30	−16	3.55
Anterior cingulate gyrus	−6	+25	+32	4.28
Thalamus	−11	−7	+4	3.14
Precentral gyrus	−44	−8	+8	3.11
Precuneus	−16	−49	+40	3.10
Decreases				
Anterior cingulate gyrus	+3	+40	+8	3.53
Area 18	+25	−82	+8	5.30
Area 17	+15	−85	0	5.30
Area 18	−7	−87	+16	5.17

*rCBF indicates regional cerebral blood flow; PTSD, posttraumatic stress disorder.

†Coordinates are expressed in millimeters. On the x-axis, positive values indicate locations in the right hemisphere and negative values indicate locations in the left hemisphere. On the y-axis, positive values indicate locations anterior to the anterior commissure and negative values indicate locations posterior to the anterior commissure. On the z-axis, positive values indicate locations superior to the anterior commissure-posterior commissure (AC-PC) plane and negative values indicate locations inferior to the AC-PC plane.

‡Data from 1 subject were missing from this region on this slice.

inferior frontal gyrus, right precuneus, right area 17, left anterior cingulate gyrus, and left middle frontal gyrus.

Combat Imagery Minus Combat Perception

In the PTSD group, increased rCBF occurred in right amygdala, right lenticulate, left middle frontal gyrus, left ventral anterior cingulate gyrus, and left supramarginal gyrus (**Table 5**, Figure 2, bottom). However, data from 1 subject with PTSD were missing from the amygdala; hence, the *z* score of 3.55 (for right amygdala) is based on data from 6 subjects with PTSD. Decreased rCBF occurred in right area 18 and left area 17 in the PTSD group.

In the control group, areas of increased rCBF included right middle frontal gyrus, right superior frontal gyrus, right inferior frontal gyrus, medial frontal gyrus, left orbitofrontal cortex, left dorsal anterior cingulate gyrus, left thalamus, left precentral gyrus, and left precuneus. However, blood flow data from 1 control subject were missing from the orbitofrontal cortex; thus, the *z* score of 3.55 (for orbitofrontal cortex) is based on data from 6 control subjects. In the control group, rCBF decreases were found in right anterior cingulate gyrus, right area 18, right area 17, and left area 18.

Across all subtractions, statistically significant foci of activation reflected rCBF changes ranging from 1.29% to 23.78%; however, most of rCBF changes were between 2% and 7%. The SEs associated with significant foci of activation ranged from 0.10 to 1.46 normalized blood flow units, although most SEs were between 0.1 and 0.6 normalized blood flow units.

Although this study was not designed for a direct between-groups analysis, we conducted three 2 (group)×2 (condition) repeated measures ANOVAs on normalized blood flow values in each of the following regions: anterior cingulate (combat imagery minus neutral imagery), amygdala (combat imagery minus combat perception), and Broca's area (combat perception minus negative perception). None of these ANOVAs revealed significant effects; however, the effect sizes[30] for the group×condition interactions were relatively large (r=0.40 [anterior cingulate], r=0.39 [amygdala], and r=0.43 [Broca's area]), suggesting that the interactions failed to reach conventional significance levels because of the small number of subjects studied.

COMMENT

In summary, we found greater rCBF in ventral portions of anterior cingulate gyrus in the combat imagery condition than in the neutral imagery condition, but only in combat veterans with PTSD. In the PTSD group, rCBF in right amygdala was greater in the combat imagery condition than in the combat perception condition. Furthermore, in the PTSD group, we found decreased rCBF in Broca's area in the combat perception condition, relative to the negative perception condition. Our predictions were only partially supported by the results, ie, subjects with PTSD did have rCBF increases in limbic and paralimbic ROIs during combat conditions, but this occurred in only 2 of 6 ROIs. Each of the major findings in this study is discussed below.

ANTERIOR CINGULATE

In the PTSD group, we found both increased rCBF in anterior cingulate gyrus during the combat imagery condition relative to the neutral imagery condition and decreased rCBF in anterior cingulate gyrus during the combat perception condition relative to the neutral perception condition. These 2 results suggest that increased blood flow in anterior cingulate is associated with *mental imagery* of combat-related pictures, but not with perception of those pictures.

In our PTSD group, foci of activation were located in ventral anterior cingulate gyrus, an area that may play a role in emotion and autonomic responding.[31,32] Increased rCBF in anterior cingulate gyrus also has been found in subjects with phobia during exposure to their feared objects[10] and in individuals with PTSD during visualization of their traumatic events.[5]

Alternatively, increased rCBF in anterior cingulate gyrus in our PTSD group could be attributed to increased attention or response selection[33] in the combat imagery condition, relative to the neutral imagery condition. However, if this were the case, one might expect to find foci of activation in more dorsal[33,34] regions of anterior cingulate gyrus in the PTSD group.

AMYGDALA

In the PTSD group, we found rCBF increases in right amygdala in the combat imagery condition relative to the combat perception condition. The control group had rCBF *decreases* in left amygdala in the combat perception condition, relative to the negative perception condition.

The amygdala is a subcortical temporal lobe structure implicated in fear conditioning and the processing of emotionally significant stimuli.[6,35] Cellular recording studies of monkeys and cats have shown that some neurons in the amygdala respond to aversive stimuli.[36,37] In humans undergoing surgery for intractable epilepsy, stimulation of temporal lobe limbic areas has produced reports of fear and memory recall.[38] Increased rCBF in the right amygdala has been reported in individuals with PTSD during trauma-related imagery.[5]

In PTSD subjects, the reason for increased rCBF in the amygdala during the combat imagery condition, relative to the combat perception condition, is unclear. Given that the stimuli in the combat imagery and combat perception conditions were rated by the PTSD subjects as having similar valence, arousal, and personal significance, any blood flow difference between the conditions is unlikely to have resulted from stimulus differences on these 3 dimensions.

OTHER PARALIMBIC AREAS

In the control group, we found increased rCBF in left parahippocampal gyrus in the combat perception condition, relative to the negative perception condition. In 6 of the control subjects, we found increased rCBF in orbitofrontal cortex in the combat imagery condition, relative to the combat perception condition. Increased rCBF in orbitofrontal cortex has been reported during mild dysphoria[39] and during symptom provocation in PTSD and other anxiety disorders[5,9,10]; however, the reason for such an increase in our control group is unclear. Combat exposure alone may account for orbitofrontal activation in response to imagery of combat stimuli. If this were true, then increased orbitofrontal rCBF should be seen in the PTSD group as well. Although there was such an increase in the PTSD group in this subtraction, the z score associated with it (2.71) failed to exceed our threshold.

BROCA'S AREA

In the control group, we found rCBF increases in Broca's area (Brodmann area 45) during the combat perception condition, relative to the neutral perception condition. In the PTSD group, we found rCBF decreases in Broca's area (Brodmann area 44) during the combat perception condition, relative to the negative perception condition. In a separate study, decreased rCBF in Broca's area was found in subjects with PTSD during trauma-related imagery.[5]

Given the role of Broca's area in language function,[40-42] decreased rCBF in this region may be consistent with diminished linguistic processing while subjects with PTSD viewed and evaluated combat pictures. However, we have no direct evidence to support or refute this possibility.

LIMITATIONS

Limitations of this study include the small number of subjects in each group and the absence of concurrent peripheral psychophysiologic assessment. Future studies should measure psychophysiologic responses and determine whether they correlate with rCBF changes in limbic regions. In addition, although we did assess state anxiety after each condition, we did not measure other aspects of PTSD-related emotions, such as anger and sadness. Furthermore, most of the PTSD subjects had taken psychoactive medication in the past, 3 PTSD subjects and 1 control subject had past alcohol dependence, and 2 PTSD subjects had comorbid depression at the time of testing; it is unclear what effects, if any, these variables may have had on the PET results. Missing data points (from the STAIS-S and stimulus ratings analyses) were also problematic. Finally, limitations of the PET procedures themselves should be mentioned. Error in precise localization can result from unavoidable head movement, error in movement-correction procedures, or stereotaxic transformation. In addition, although the practice of normalizing whole-brain blood flow renders a P_{CO_2} correction unnecessary, it also prevents us from detecting any whole brain blood flow changes between conditions.

Both our study and that of Rauch et al[5] found increased rCBF in anterior cingulate gyrus and right amygdala and decreased rCBF in Broca's area in subjects with PTSD. However, Rauch et al[5] also found increased rCBF in other limbic and paralimbic areas. The fact that more limbic and paralimbic structures were activated in the latter study probably reflects greater emotional responsiveness of patients with PTSD to personalized narratives of actual traumatic events than to generalized trauma-related pictures and images.

In summary, we found rCBF increases in ventral anterior cingulate gyrus and right amygdala in combat veterans with PTSD, specifically during mental imagery of combat-related stimuli. The results of this study are consistent with the notion that visual imagery of traumatic material may be mediated in part by the anterior cingulate and amygdala. However, our results are in need of replication and should be interpreted cautiously at this time. If the results are replicated, future studies should help determine more specifically the roles that these structures might play in the maintenance of PTSD.

Accepted for publication June 21, 1996.

This study was supported in part by grants N00014-93-1-0720 from the Office of Naval Research, Arlington, Va (Dr Kosslyn), and 91010703 from the John D. and Catherine T. MacArthur Foundation, Chicago, Ill (Dr Kosslyn). Dr Rauch was supported by a Young Investigator Award from The National Alliance for Research on Schizophrenia and Depression, Chicago; grant K20

MH01215 from the National Institute of Mental Health, Rockville, Md; and the Pfizer-sponsored Harvard–Massachusetts Institute of Technology Clinician Investigator Training Program, Cambridge.

Presented, in part, at the 10th Annual Meeting of the International Society for Traumatic Stress Studies, Chicago, Ill, November 8, 1994.

We thank Natasha Lasko, Avis Loring, and Steve Weise for their technical assistance. In addition, we thank all the veterans who participated in this study.

Reprints: Lisa M. Shin, AM, Department of Psychology, Harvard University, 33 Kirkland St, Cambridge, MA 02138.

REFERENCES

1. Blanchard EB, Kolb LC, Gerardi RJ, Ryan P, Pallmeyer TP. Cardiac response to relevant stimuli as an adjunctive tool for diagnosing post-traumatic stress disorder in Vietnam veterans. *Behav Ther.* 1986;17:592-606.
2. Orr SP, Pitman RK, Lasko NB, Herz LR. Psychophysiological assessment of posttraumatic stress disorder imagery in World War II and Korean combat veterans. *J Abnorm Psychol.* 1993;102:152-159.
3. Pitman RK, Orr SP, Forgue DF, de Jong JB, Claiborn JM. Psychophysiologic assessment of posttraumatic stress disorder imagery in Vietnam combat veterans. *Arch Gen Psychiatry.* 1987;44:970-975.
4. Orr SP. An overview of psychophysiological studies of PTSD. *PTSD Q.* 1994; 5:1-7.
5. Rauch SL, van der Kolk BA, Fisler RE, Alpert NM, Orr SP, Savage CR, Fischman AJ, Jenike MA, Pitman RK. A symptom provocation study of posttraumatic stress disorder using positron emission tomography and script-driven imagery. *Arch Gen Psychiatry.* 1996;53:380-387.
6. LeDoux JE. Emotion and the amygdala. In: Aggleton JP, ed. *The Amygdala: Neurobiological Aspects of Emotion, Memory, and Mental Dysfunction.* New York, NY: Wiley-Liss Inc; 1992:339-351.
7. MacLean PD. *The Triune Brain in Evolution: Role in Paleocerebral Functions.* New York, NY: Plenum Press; 1990.
8. Papez JW. A proposed mechanism of emotion. *Arch Neurol Psychiatry.* 1937; 38:725-733.
9. Rauch SL, Jenike MA, Alpert NM, Baer L, Breiter HCR, Savage CR, Fischman AJ. Regional cerebral blood flow measured during symptom provocation in obsessive-compulsive disorder using oxygen 15–labeled carbon dioxide and positron emission tomography. *Arch Gen Psychiatry.* 1994;51:62-70.
10. Rauch SL, Savage CR, Alpert NM, Miguel EC, Baer L, Breiter HC, Fischman AJ, Manzo PA, Moretti C, Jenike MA. A positron emission tomographic study of simple phobic symptom provocation. *Arch Gen Psychiatry.* 1995;52:20-28.
11. Brett EA, Ostroff R. Imagery and posttraumatic stress disorder: an overview. *Am J Psychiatry.* 1985;142:417-424.
12. Blake DD, Weathers FW, Nagy LM, Kaloupek DG, Klauminzev G, Keane TM. Rating scale for assessing current and lifetime PTSD: the CAPS-I. *Behav Therapist.* 1990;13:187-188.
13. Spitzer RL, Williams JBW, Gibbon M, First M. *Structured Clinical Interview for DSM-III-R (SCID).* Washington, DC: American Psychiatric Press; 1990.
14. Oldfield RC. The assessment and analysis of handedness: The Edinburgh Inventory. *Neuropsychologia.* 1971;9:97-113.
15. Keane TM, Fairbank JA, Caddell JM, Zimering RT, Taylor KL, Mora CA. Clinical evaluation of a measure to assess combat exposure. *Psychol Assess J Consult Clin Psychol.* 1989;1:53-55.
16. Keane TM, Caddell JM, Taylor K. Mississippi Scale for Combat-Related Posttraumatic Stress Disorder: three studies in reliability and validity. *J Consult Clin Psychol.* 1988;56:85-90.
17. Beck AT, Steer RA. *Beck Depression Inventory Manual.* San Antonio, Tex: The Psychological Corp; 1987.
18. Spielberger CD, Gorsuch RL, Lushene R, Vagg PR, Jacobs GA. *Manual for the State-Trait Anxiety Inventory.* Palo Alto, Calif: Consulting Psychologists Press; 1983.
19. Marks DF. Individual differences in the vividness of visual imagery and their effect on function. In: Sheehan WP, ed. *The Function and Nature of Imagery.* New York: Academic Press; 1972:83-108.
20. Marks DF. Visual imagery differences in the recall of pictures. *Br J Psychol.* 1973;64:17-24.
21. Kulka RA, Schlenger WE, Fairbank JA, Hough RL, Jordan BK, Marmar CR, Weiss DS. *Trauma and the Vietnam Generation: Report of Findings From the National Vietnam Veterans Readjustment Study.* New York, NY: Brunner/Mazel; 1990.
22. Lang PJ, Öhman A, Vaitl D. *The International Affective Picture System (Photographic Slides).* Gainesville, Fla: The Center for Research in Psychophysiology, University of Florida; 1988.
23. Lang PJ, Greenwald MK. *The International Affective Picture System Standardization Procedure and Initial Group Results for Affective Judgments: Technical Report 1A.* Gainesville, Fla: The Center for Research in Psychophysiology, University of Florida; 1988.
24. McNally RJ, Litz BT, Prassas A, Shin LM, Weathers FW. Emotional priming of autobiographical memory in post-traumatic stress disorder. *Cogn Emotion.* 1994; 8:351-367.
25. Costin D. MacLab: A Macintosh system for psychology labs. *Behav Res Instrum Comput.* 1988;20:197-200.
26. Talairach J, Tournoux P. *Co-Planar Stereotaxic Atlas of the Human Brain.* Stuttgart, Germany: Georg Thieme Verlag; 1988.
27. Alpert NM, Berdichevsky D, Weise S, Tang J, Rauch SL. Stereotactic transformation of PET scans by nonlinear least squares. In: Uemura K, Lassen NA, Jones T, Kanno I. *Quantification of Brain Function: Tracer Kinetics and Image Analysis in Brain PET.* Amsterdam, the Netherlands: Elsevier Science Publishers; 1993:459-463.
28. Friston KJ, Frith CD, Liddle PF, Frakowiak RSJ. Comparing functional (PET) images: the assessment of significant change. *J Cereb Blood Flow Metab.* 1991; 11:690-699.
29. Kosslyn SM, Shin LM, Thompson WL, McNally RJ, Rauch SL, Pitman RK, Alpert NM. Neural effects of visualizing and perceiving aversive stimuli: a PET investigation. *Neuro Report.* 1996;7:1569-1576.
30. Rosenthal R, Rosnow RL. *Essentials of Behavioral Research: Methods and Data Analysis.* New York, NY: McGraw Hill International Book Co; 1991.
31. Laitinen LV. Emotional responses to subcortical electrical stimulation in psychiatric patients. *Clin Neurol Neurosurg.* 1979;81:148-157.
32. Pool JL, Ransohoff J. Autonomic effects on stimulating rostral portion of cingulate gyri in man. *J Neurophysiol.* 1949;12:385-392.
33. Petersen SE, Fox PT, Posner MI, Mintun M, Raichle ME. Positron emission tomographic studies of the processing of single words. *J Cogn Neurosci.* 1989; 1:153-170.
34. Vogt BA, Finch DM, Olson CR. Functional heterogeneity in cingulate cortex: the anterior executive and posterior evaluative regions. *Cereb Cortex.* 1992;2: 435-443.
35. LeDoux JE. Cognitive-emotional interactions in the brain. *Cogn Emotion.* 1989; 3:267-289.
36. Nishijo H, Ono T, Nishino H. Topographic distribution of modality-specific amygdalar neurons in the alert monkey. *J Neurosci.* 1988;8:3556-3569.
37. Ono T, Fukuda M, Nishino H, Sasaki K, Muramoto K-I. Amygdaloid neuronal responses to complex visual stimuli in an operant feeding situation in the monkey. *Brain Res Bull.* 1983;11:515-518.
38. Gloor P, Olivier A, Quesney LF, Andermann F, Horowitz S. Limbic system in experiential phenomena of temporal lobe epilepsy. *Ann Neurol.* 1982;12:129-144.
39. Pardo JV, Pardo PJ, Raichle ME. Neural correlates of self-induced dysphoria. *Am J Psychiatry.* 1993;150:713-719.
40. Kertesz A, Harlock W, Coates R. Computer tomographic localization, lesion size, and prognosis in aphasia and nonverbal impairment. *Brain Lang.* 1979;8:34-50.
41. Ojemann GA. Brain organization for language from the perspective of electrical stimulation mapping. *Behav Brain Sci.* 1983;2:189-230.
42. McCarthy G, Blamire AM, Rothman DL, Gruetter R, Shulman RG. Echo-planar magnetic resonance imaging studies of frontal cortex activation during word generation in humans. *Proc Natl Acad Sci U S A.* 1993;90:4952-4956.

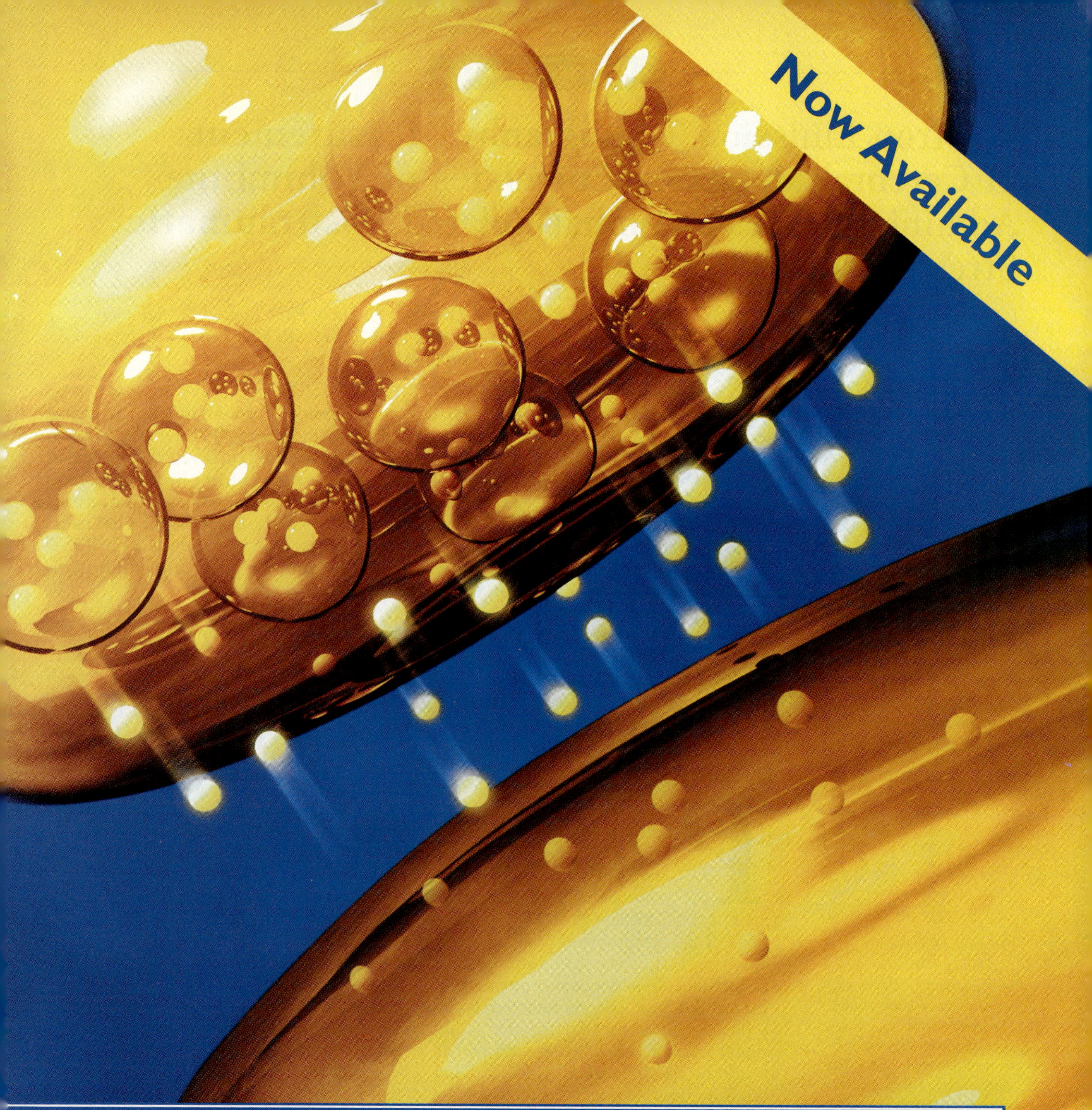
Now Available

Positron Emission Tomography Measurement of Cerebral Metabolic Correlates of Yohimbine Administration in Combat-Related Posttraumatic Stress Disorder

J. Douglas Bremner, MD; Robert B. Innis, MD, PhD; Chin K. Ng, PhD; Lawrence H. Staib, PhD; Ronald M. Salomon, MD; Richard A. Bronen, MD; James Duncan, PhD; Steven M. Southwick, MD; John H. Krystal, MD; Dayton Rich; George Zubal, PhD; Holley Dey, MD; Robert Soufer, MD; Dennis S. Charney, MD

Background: We have previously reported an increase in symptoms of anxiety in patients with posttraumatic stress disorder (PTSD) following administration of the β_2-antagonist yohimbine, which stimulates brain norepinephrine release. Preclinical studies show decreased metabolism in the neocortex and the caudate nucleus with high-dose yohimbine-induced norepinephrine release, but low levels of norepinephrine release result in an increase in metabolism in these areas.

Methods: We used positron emission tomography and fludeoxyglucose F 18 to measure brain metabolism in Vietnam combat veterans with PTSD (n=10) and healthy age-matched control subjects (n=10), following administration of yohimbine (0.4 mg/kg) or placebo in a randomized, double-blind fashion.

Results: Yohimbine resulted in a significant increase in anxiety in the patients with PTSD, but not in healthy subjects. There was a significant difference in brain metabolic response to yohimbine in patients with PTSD compared with healthy subjects in prefrontal, temporal, parietal, and orbitofrontal cortexes. Metabolism tended to decrease in patients with PTSD and increase in healthy subjects following administration of yohimbine.

Conclusion: These findings are consistent with our previous hypothesis of enhanced norepinephrine release in the brain with yohimbine in patients with PTSD.

Arch Gen Psychiatry. 1997;54:246-254

From the Departments of Psychiatry (Drs Bremner, Innis, Salomon, Southwick, Krystal, and Charney) and Diagnostic Radiology (Drs Bremner, Ng, Staib, Bronen, Duncan, Zubal, Dey, and Soufer), Yale University School of Medicine, New Haven, Conn; and the National Center for Posttraumatic Stress Disorder (Drs Bremner, Innis, Southwick, Krystal, and Charney), West Haven Veterans Affairs Medical Center (Drs Bremner, Innis, Ng, Salomon, Southwick, Krystal, Dey, Soufer, and Charney and Mr Rich), and the Yale/Veterans Affairs Positron Emission Tomography Center (Drs Ng, Dey, and Soufer and Mr Rich), West Haven, Conn.

PSYCHIATRISTS HAVE long hypothesized that alterations in noradrenergic function may underlie the symptoms of combat-related posttraumatic stress disorder (PTSD).[1-3] Observations of the symptoms of combat veterans from earlier wars, including sleep disturbance, hypervigilance, physiological arousal, and exaggerated startle response, led to the use of terms such as "irritable soldier's heart" to describe what would be classified today as PTSD. This syndrome was believed to be related to alterations in catecholamine levels. Several recent investigations have provided evidence for the idea that alterations in catecholamine levels, including norepinephrine levels, may underlie symptoms of PTSD.

Preclinical studies also support a role for norepinephrine in stress.[4-6] Norepinephrine cell bodies, primarily located in the locus caeruleus, release neurotransmitter centrally in cortical and subcortical structures.[7-12] Animal models of stress showed increased firing of the locus caeruleus and increased turnover and release of norepinephrine in these regions,[11,13-28] but increased release of norepinephrine was shown in chronically stressed animals following administration of the α_2-antagonist idazoxan, which stimulates brain norepinephrine release through blockade of the presynaptic α_2-receptor. At the level of the postsynaptic receptor, norepinephrine has a stimulatory effect with binding to α_1-receptors, an inhibitory effect with postsynaptic α_2-receptors, and excitatory and inhibitory effects with binding to postsynaptic β-receptors.[29-32] Pharmacological studies in nonhuman primates using agents that stimulate brain norepinephrine release, including the α-adrenergic blocker phentolamine, and phenylethylamine, showed a dose-dependent effect. These agents increased cerebral blood flow at lower doses, and decreased cerebral blood flow at higher doses.[33,34] Administration to animals of high doses of the α_2-antagonist yohimbine resulted in a decrease in brain metabolism in the frontal, parietal, temporal, postcentral (sensory), and occipital cortex, the caudate nucleus,[35,36] the olfactory cortex, and the sulcal cortex.[35] Electrical stimulation of the

SUBJECTS AND METHODS

SUBJECT SELECTION

The patient group was comprised of 10 Vietnam veterans with a history of combat-related PTSD who were admitted to an inpatient unit for PTSD during a 2-year period who gave informed consent for participation, met the criteria for PTSD based on the Structured Clinical Interview *DSM-III-R* (SCID)[65] (available in 9 of 10 patients), and had a score of more than 107 (consistent with the diagnosis of PTSD) on the Mississippi Scale for Combat-Related PTSD, an instrument for the measurement of PTSD symptoms.[66] Combat exposure was documented using the Combat Exposure Scale, a self-report instrument for the quantitation of level of combat exposure that has documented reliability and validity. Although the Combat Exposure Scale relies on self-report, studies showing a correlation between the score on the Combat Exposure Scale and the level of PTSD symptoms support the validity of this instrument as a measure of combat exposure.[67] That patients had been exposed to combat in Vietnam also was confirmed by the official military record of service in the Vietnam theater when these were available. In the few cases in which they were unavailable, an attempt to verify combat status was made by corroborating history obtained from family members, interviews with experienced psychiatrist clinicians, and a review of the patient's medical records. Patients were excluded if they had a history of meningitis, traumatic brain injury, neurologic disorder, current alcohol abuse, schizophrenia based on *DSM-III-R* criteria, shrapnel or other foreign bodies, human immunodeficiency virus infection, or loss of consciousness for more than 10 minutes. None of the patients had a history of loss of consciousness within the last year. Patients were observed for a 2-month period with frequent toxicology screens for validation of substance- and alcohol-free status. Patients had been medication-free for 4 weeks or more at the time of the study.

Healthy subjects (n=10) were recruited through newspaper advertisements to match the patients for age and sex. Healthy subjects included men between the ages of 18 and 65 years who were physically healthy and without psychiatric disorder as assessed with the SCID for nonpatients or psychiatric interview using SCID-based criteria. Subjects were excluded if they had a history of psychiatric disorder, exposure to extreme psychological stressor based on psychiatric interview, or the exclusion criteria described for the patients. An extreme psychological stressor was defined in accordance with the *DSM-III-R* criteria as an event beyond the range of normal human experience that would be distressing to almost anyone.

There were no differences in demographic variables between the patients and the controls. Mean (±SEM) age of the patients with PTSD was 46.7±0.54 years; in the controls, it was 44.1±2.5 years. All of the patients with PTSD were white; 7 of 10 controls were white and 3 of 10 were black (this difference was not statistically significant). All patients and controls were male and right-handed.

Patients were evaluated with the SCID for comorbid psychiatric diagnoses. The SCID data were available for 9 of 10 patients. In the patients for whom SCID data were available, 1 patient met criteria for a lifetime history of major depression and 3 for a current history of major depression. One patient met criteria for a lifetime history of dysthymia and 1 for a current history of dysthymia. None of the patients met criteria for a lifetime or current history of bipolar disorder. One patient met criteria for a lifetime history of hypomania, and none for a current history of hypomania. Three patients met criteria for a lifetime and current history of panic disorder with agoraphobia; 1 for a lifetime and current history of panic disorder without agoraphobia. One patient met criteria for a lifetime and current history of agoraphobia without panic disorder, 2 for a lifetime and current history of social phobia, 2 for a lifetime and current history of OCD, 1 for a lifetime and current history of simple phobia, and none for a lifetime or current history of GAD. No patients met criteria for a lifetime or current history of schizophrenia; 2 patients met criteria for a lifetime history and 1 for a current history of psychotic disorder not otherwise specified. Seven patients met criteria for a lifetime history of alcohol dependence and 1 for alcohol abuse; 1 for sedative, hypnotic, or anxiolytic dependence and none for abuse; 5 for cannabis dependence and none for cannabis abuse; 1 for stimulant dependence and 1 for stimulant abuse; none for opiate dependence or abuse, 1 for cocaine dependence and 2 for cocaine abuse; 2 for hallucinogen or phencyclidine hydrochloride dependence and 1 for abuse; and 1 for polydrug dependence and none for abuse.

BEHAVIORAL ASSESSMENTS

Mean (±SEM) score on the Mississippi Scale for Combat-Related PTSD in the patients with PTSD was 140.4±15.1, which indicates high levels of PTSD symptoms. Mean (±SEM) score on the Combat Exposure Scale in the patient group was 32.4±7.8 (a high level of combat exposure).

Patients also were evaluated at baseline and 20 minutes after yohimbine administration or placebo injection for anxiety symptoms with the Hamilton Anxiety Scale; panic attack symptoms with the Panic Attack Symptom Scale (PASS), clinician and patient versions; and PTSD symptoms with the PTSD Symptom Scale, clinician and patient versions. Panic attacks and flashbacks were defined using previously described criteria.[56] In 2 situations, subjects did not meet criteria for panic attacks using the full criteria but were judged clinically by 2 investigators (S.M.S. and D.S.C.) blinded to study conditions as having experienced a panic attack.

POSITRON EMISSION TOMOGRAPHY (PET) SCANNING METHODS

All subjects underwent 2 days of testing in a randomized, double-blind design with administration of yohimbine or placebo. Subjects were scanned at the Yale/Veterans Affairs Positron Emission Tomography Center, West Haven, Conn, with a 21-slice camera (Posicam 6.5, Positron Corp, Houston, Tex), with 5.125-mm interslice distance. The resolution of the camera in-plane is 5.8 mm and 11.9 mm in the z-axis.[68] The sensitivity of the camera measured in a 20-cm-diameter cylinder phantom can be expressed as the system sensitivity (165 000 kcounts/s per

Continued on next page

microcurie per cubic centimeter); slice sensitivity (9.5 kcounts/s per microcurie per cubic centimeter); or the sensitivity/axial cm (8.0 kcounts/μCi per cubic centimeter per axial centimeter). An intravenous line was inserted in the hand and warmed with heating pads for measurement of arterialized venous blood samples. Subjects received yohimbine (0.4 mg/kg) or placebo intravenously for 10 minutes immediately followed by injection of 5 mCi of FDG in a single intravenous bolus and scanning with eyes open in a dimly lit room. A PET image was reconstructed 30 to 50 minutes after injection to determine brain tissue activity. Brain and tissue time-activity curves were then combined for measurement of cerebral glucose metabolic rate in milligrams per minute per 100 mL using the fixed rate constant approach of Sokoloff et al.[69] Separate kinetic rate constants were used for gray and white matter.[70] Images were attenuation-corrected based on a transmission scan performed with a ^{67}Ga/^{68}Ge rotating rod source and reconstructed using a spatially varying convolution scatter subtraction technique and a Butterworth filter. A 20-cm cylindrical fluid-filled phantom was scanned on the same day as each study to obtain a calibration factor for each of the 21 slices.

PET-MRI COREGISTRATION

Magnetic resonance imaging scans were obtained in all subjects for coregistration with PET (**Figure 1**). Magnetic resonance imaging scans of 3-mm contiguous slices were obtained with a 1.5-T scanner (Signa, General Electric, Milwaukee, Wis). Axial images were acquired with a spoiled gradient recall acquisition in the steady state sequence with repetition time=25 ms, echo time=5 ms, number of excitations=2, flip angle=30°, matrix=256×256, field of view=24 cm. The PET and MRI scans were transferred using a computer network to a SUN Sparc10 Workstation (SUN Microsystems, Mountain View, Calif). Analyze[71] was used for coregistration of PET and MRI scans using a surface-matching algorithm.[72] The MRI was then resliced to obtain 21 MRI slices, each of which corresponded to 1 of the 21 PET slices.

MEASUREMENT OF REGIONS OF INTEREST

Regions of interest measurements on resliced MRI were performed by a blinded investigator using specific criteria developed in conjunction with a neuroradiologist (R.A.B.). These criteria were developed for reproducibility of measurements between observers and to have criteria based on an anatomical atlas that allows for the use of a common terminology and that is available to general access.[73] We have shown high levels of agreement between 2 raters using these criteria (J.D.B., Gabriel De Erasquin, MD, Eric Vermetten, MD, et al, unpublished data, March 15, 1996) (available on request). Templates for regions of interest drawn on the MRI were transferred to the PET by the Analyze computer program. These included the neocortical regions and the caudate nucleus (**Table 1**), which were hypothesized to change based on the aforementioned preclinical studies. Pons, midbrain, and white matter were not anticipated to change with yohimbine administration and were selected as comparison regions to assess the specificity of the effect of yohimbine. The other regions were examined on an exploratory basis because they have noradrenergic innervation (Table 1). Global brain metabolism was calculated by obtaining the mean of bilateral posterior white matter measurements and the mean of all gray matter measurements, with a 50% weighting to gray matter and a 50% weighting to white matter.

DATA ANALYSIS

Three-way repeated measures analysis of variance (ANOVA) with drug (yohimbine vs placebo) as the repeated measure and diagnosis and laterality (left vs right) as factors was used to examine the effects of yohimbine on metabolism in patients vs controls for specific regions of interest. Hypothesized regions of interest (Table 1), based on animal studies of areas that have been shown to decrease in metabolism with yohimbine administration, were initially combined in a single model and compared with all nonhypothesized regions for the effects of yohimbine on metabolism in patients and controls. We also compared metabolic response to yohimbine in patients vs controls in individual brain regions, including hypothesized and nonhypothesized regions. Possible asymmetries were assessed by including left and right sides for each region and conducting a 3-way ANOVA for each of the regions given in Table 1 with hemisphere (left vs right) as a factor in the ANOVA.

Exploratory analyses included univariate analyses to compare patients who had PTSD with controls at baseline (placebo day), and to compare placebo and yohimbine days within the control subjects. The Bonferroni correction (dividing the α value of .05 by the number of comparisons [18], or $P=.05/18=.003$) was used to adjust the level of significance for the potential confounder of multiple comparisons for all exploratory analyses.

Behavioral data (Hamilton Anxiety Scale and PASS clinician scores) were analyzed using nonpaired 2-tailed t tests to compare scores at baseline with scores 20 minutes after infusion of yohimbine or placebo (**Table 2**). The relation between behavioral data (the difference between baseline-subtracted anxiety scores (measured with the PASS clinician, PASS patient, and Hamilton Anxiety Scale) with yohimbine and baseline-subtracted anxiety scores with placebo and placebo-subtracted metabolism with yohimbine (a subtraction of brain metabolism on the placebo day from brain metabolism on the yohimbine day) was analyzed using Pearson product correlations. Results are reported as mean (±SEM).

locus caeruleus resulted in a decrease in brain metabolism[37] and blood flow[38-40] in several cortical and subcortical regions, but lesions of the locus caeruleus had the opposite effect.[41-43] In summary, high levels of norepinephrine release cause a decrease in blood flow and metabolism in brain areas that receive noradrenergic innervation, but low levels of norepinephrine release increase blood flow and metabolism.

Evidence for alterations in noradrenergic brain system function in patients with PTSD[44] includes (1) increased resting heart rate and blood pressure,[3,45] and increases in heart rate and systolic blood pressure with reminders of combat trauma,[46-49] (2) increased urinary norepinephrine and epinephrine in some studies[50,51] but not others,[52] (3) increased plasma epinephrine[48] and norepinephrine[53] following exposure to traumatic remind-

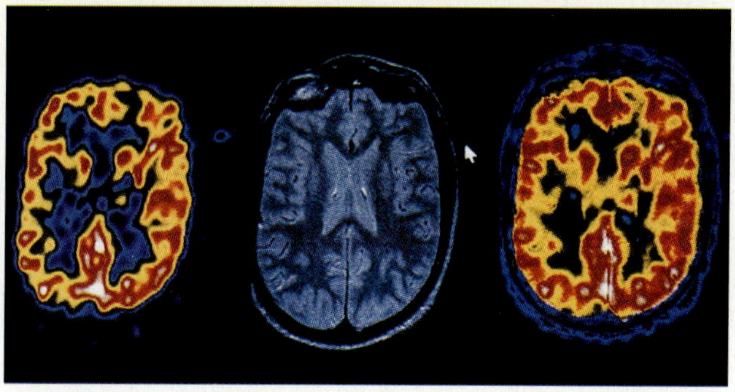

Figure 1. *Positron emission tomography (PET) and magnetic resonance imaging (MRI) coregistration using the Chamfer surface-matching technique. The images represented include a PET fludeoxyglucose F18 scan of a patient with PTSD at baseline (left), an MRI resliced to correspond to the PET (center), and a fused PET and MRI image (right). A fiducial marker, filled with fludeoxyglucose F 18, is also visualized (arrow), which was used to check for head movement during the scan.*

ers but not baseline plasma norepinephrine,[53,54] (4) decreased adrenergic receptors on platelets,[55] and (5) increased methoxyhexene phenylglycol after yohimbine administration and flashbacks in 40% and panic attacks in 70% of patients.[56] Yohimbine administration also resulted in an increase in panic attacks and plasma methoxyhexene phenylglycol in patients with another anxiety disorder, panic disorder,[57,58] but not in patients with generalized anxiety disorder (GAD),[59] depression,[60] obsessive-compulsive disorder (OCD),[61] or schizophrenia.[62] We hypothesized[5,6,56] that PTSD is associated with an increase in responsiveness to the noradrenergic agent yohimbine, which results in patients with PTSD "seeing" higher levels of yohimbine than the controls. One would predict that yohimbine causes high levels of norepinephrine release in the brain of subjects with PTSD, which results in decreased metabolism, and lower levels of norepinephrine release in controls, with increased metabolism.

Little is known about central brain function in patients with PTSD. We previously reported a decrease in right hippocampal volume as measured with magnetic resonance imaging (MRI) with associated deficits in short-term verbal memory[63,64] in Vietnam combat veterans with PTSD compared with controls. The purpose of this study was to use PET fludeoxyglucose F 18 (FDG) in the measurement of cerebral metabolism following administration of yohimbine and placebo in Vietnam combat veterans with PTSD and in healthy subjects. We hypothesized that yohimbine administration in patients with PTSD would be associated with a decrease in brain metabolism compared with controls in brain regions that have been shown to decrease in metabolism with yohimbine in preclinical studies, namely neocortical areas and the caudate nucleus.

RESULTS

BEHAVIORAL EFFECTS OF YOHIMBINE

Six of 10 patients with PTSD had a panic attack with yohimbine administration, compared with none of the controls, and 3 of 10 patients with PTSD had a flashback with yohimbine administration compared with none of the controls. Patients with PTSD had a significant increase from baseline to 20 minutes after yohimbine administration in anxiety as measured by the Ham-D (9.3±1.9 vs 20.3±2.4) (t=3.6, df=18; P<.01) and panic attack symptoms as measured by the PASS-clinician (30.7±1.4 vs 39.5±1.9) (t=3.7, df=18; P<.01) and PASS patient (31.9±1.8 vs 41.2±2.4) (t=3.1, df=18; P<.01). Controls did not have an increase in anxiety or panic symptoms with yohimbine. Neither patients nor controls had an increase in anxiety or panic symptoms on the placebo day (Table 2). These findings are similar to our previous reports.[56]

EFFECTS OF YOHIMBINE ON REGIONAL CEREBRAL METABOLISM

Two-way analysis of variance (ANOVA) with repeated measures for drug administration (placebo vs yohimbine) showed a significant difference in yohimbine response between the patients with PTSD and the controls when all regions that were hypothesized to change based on preclinical studies (neocortical regions and the caudate nucleus) were combined in a single model (main effect for drug, F[1,438]=90.65, P<.001; drug by diagnosis interaction, F[1,438]=29.05, P<.001). As predicted, patients with PTSD had a decrease in metabolism with yohimbine administration compared with placebo (t=2.09, df=238; P=.02), while controls had an increase in metabolism with yohimbine administration compared with placebo (t=5.27, df=238; P<.001). When hypothesized regions were examined individually, significant differences between patients and controls were observed for orbitofrontal cortex (main effect for drug, F[1,78]=5.18, P<.05; main effect for diagnosis, F[1,78]=13.10, P<.001; drug by diagnosis interaction, F[1,78]=12.71, P≤.006) (**Figure 2**), temporal cortex (main effect for diagnosis, F[1,78]=37.94, P<.001; drug by diagnosis interaction, F[1,78]=5.30, P<.05), prefrontal cortex (main effect for drug, F[1,78]=5.98, P<.05; main effect for diagnosis, F[1,78]=25.1, P<.001; drug by diagnosis interaction, F=5.69, P<.05), and parietal cortex (main effect for diagnosis, F[1,78]=16.07, P<.001; drug by diagnosis interaction, F[1,78]=4.29, P<.05), but not occipital cortex or postcentral gyrus (sensory cortex) (Table 1). Healthy subjects had an increase in metabolism with yohimbine administration compared with placebo in orbitofrontal cortex (t=3.79, df=39; P≤.005) and prefrontal cortex (t=3.18, df=39; P≤.003).

Repeated measures ANOVA showed a significant difference between patients and controls when all nonhypothesized regions (Table 1) were combined in a single model (main effect for diagnosis, F[1,438]=34.5, P<.001; drug by diagnosis interaction, F[1,438]=25.32, P<.001). In the patients with PTSD, metabolism decreased with yohimbine administration compared with placebo (t=3.91, df=238; P<.001), but in the controls, metabolism increased with yohimbine administration compared with placebo (t=3.29, df=238; P=.001). When these regions were examined individually, however, a difference in yohimbine response between patients and controls was observed in only 1 region, globus pallidus (main effect for diagnosis, F[1,38]=7.96, P<.01; drug by diagnosis interaction, F[1,38]=7.36, P<.05), which was not significant after correction for multiple comparisons. When patients

Table 1. Metabolic Rates With Yohimbine Administration in Patients With Posttraumatic Stress Disorder and Controls*

Brain Region	Controls (n=10) Placebo	Controls (n=10) Yohimbine	Patients With PTSD (n=10) Placebo	Patients With PTSD (n=10) Yohimbine	3-Way Analysis of Variance Drug by Diagnosis Interaction F	*P*
Hypothesized Region†						
Orbitofrontal cortex	7.60 (0.25)	10.20 (0.46)	7.40 (0.21)	6.80 (0.31)	12.71	<.001§
Parietal cortex	10.00 (0.34)	11.20 (0.41)	9.00 (0.23)	8.40 (0.21)	4.29	.04
Prefrontal cortex	11.30 (0.43)	11.90 (0.44)	9.50 (0.26)	8.60 (0.30)	5.69	.02‖¶
Temporal cortex	10.80 (0.31)	11.90 (0.32)	9.20 (0.20)	8.60 (0.24)	5.30	.02#
Postcentral gyrus	9.70 (0.37)	10.60 (0.35)	8.20 (0.22)	7.60 (0.22)	1.29	.26
Occipital cortex	9.70 (0.31)	9.80 (0.29)	8.60 (0.23)	8.20 (0.25)	0.26	.61
Caudate nucleus	11.10 (0.41)	11.50 (0.41)	9.70 (0.26)	8.60 (0.31)	2.28	.14
Nonhypothesized Region‡						
Putamen	11.50 (0.45)	12.90 (0.38)	10.20 (0.31)	9.40 (0.34)	2.59	.12
Globus pallidus	6.70 (0.27)	8.30 (0.38)	6.20 (0.27)	5.20 (0.18)	7.36	.01
Thalamus	8.00 (0.27)	9.10 (0.35)	7.20 (0.30)	6.50 (0.30)	2.09	.15
Cingulate	10.90 (0.33)	11.90 (0.41)	9.10 (0.33)	8.80 (0.25)	1.10	.30
Parahippocampal	7.60 (0.32)	8.40 (0.41)	6.20 (0.26)	5.40 (0.24)	3.53	<.07
Hippocampus	7.00 (0.27)	6.90 (0.39)	6.60 (0.18)	5.00 (0.24)	2.15	.15**
Amygdala	6.30 (0.23)	6.40 (0.33)	5.60 (0.17)	5.00 (0.23)	0.54	.47
Cerebellum	8.80 (0.31)	10.90 (0.33)	8.10 (0.26)	8.10 (0.27)	2.71	.10††
Midbrain	5.40 (0.29)	5.90 (0.27)	4.80 (0.22)	4.30 (0.21)	1.28	.26
Pons	5.80 (0.24)	5.20 (0.29)	4.90 (0.23)	3.80 (0.23)	0.46	.50
Global metabolism	7.00 (0.31)	8.20 (0.33)	7.00 (0.22)	6.10 (0.18)	2.60	.12

*Regional metabolic rates are given as mean (SEM) milligrams per minute per 100 mL of glucose. PTSD indicates post-traumatic stress disorder.

†Hypothesized regions include those found to change with yohimbine administration in unconflicted animal studies; significant main effects for diagnosis were found in all hypothesized regions.

‡Nonhypothesized regions include those not found to change with yohimbine in animal studies; significant main effects for diagnosis (P<.05) were found in all nonhypothesized regions except hippocampus and global metabolism.

§Increase in metabolism within the control group with yohimbine vs placebo administration (P<.001).

‖Decrease in metabolism for PTSD group vs control group on placebo day (P=.02).

¶Increase in metabolism within the control group with yohimbine vs placebo administration (P<.003).

#Decrease in metabolism in PTSD group vs control group on placebo day (P<.003).

**Decrease in metabolism within PTSD group with yohimbine vs placebo administration (P=.006).

††Increase in metabolism within control group with yohimbine vs placebo administration (adjusted P=.003).

with PTSD were considered alone, there was a significant decrease on the yohimbine administration day compared with the placebo day in the hippocampus (t=3.08, df=19; P=.006) (Table 1). Global metabolism with yohimbine administration did not differ between patients and controls. When an additional analysis was performed for each region (Table 1) using 3-way repeated measures ANOVA with hemisphere (right vs left) entered as a factor (in addition to drug [yohimbine vs placebo] and diagnosis [PTSD vs controls]), there was no significant main effect for hemisphere for any of the individual regions.

Exploratory univariate analyses also were performed to examine differences in metabolism at baseline between patients and controls. Patients with PTSD had a significant decrease in metabolism at baseline (placebo day) compared with controls, which was significant after correction for multiple comparison (18) (ie, P=.05/18=.0029) for temporal cortex (F[1,78]=9.63; P≤.003), but not prefrontal cortex (F[1,78]=6.05; P≤.02).

RELATION BETWEEN BEHAVIORAL MEASURES OF ANXIETY AND REGIONAL CEREBRAL METABOLISM

A relation did not exist between the difference between baseline-subtracted anxiety scores on the yohimbine and placebo days and placebo-subtracted metabolism with the yohimbine day in patients or controls for any brain region in this study. Of the patients who met criteria for panic disorder without agoraphobia, 2 of 3 had a panic attack with yohimbine administration, but the patient who met criteria for panic disorder with agoraphobia did not have a panic attack with yohimbine administration, and 3 of 5 patients without panic disorder had a panic attack with yohimbine administration. The single patient for whom the SCID was unavailable had a panic attack with yohimbine administration. No statistically significant differences were observed in placebo-subtracted metabolism with yohimbine administration in patients with PTSD who had a panic attack with yohimbine administration (n=6) compared with patients with PTSD who did not have a panic attack with yohimbine (n=4). A pattern of a decrease in placebo-subtracted metabolism with yohimbine administration was observed in the patients who had a panic attack compared with those who did not have a panic attack, with the magnitude of the difference being greatest for orbitofrontal cortex (−1,73±0.89 vs 0.03±0.94) and hippocampus (−2.14±1.02 vs −0.74±0.47). The lack of a statistically significant difference may be due to the small number of subjects in each subgroup.

Table 2. Scores on Behavioral Ratings Following Administration of Yohimbine and Placebo*

Behavioral Rating	Patients With PTSD (n=10) Baseline	Patients With PTSD (n=10) +20 Minutes	Controls (n=10) Baseline	Controls (n=10) +20 Minutes
Placebo				
Hamilton Anxiety Scale	11.3 (1.4)	12.4 (2.2)	1.3 (0.4)	0.8 (0.5)
Panic Attack Symptom Scale				
Clinician	32.9 (1.0)	32.8 (1.9)	27.5 (0.2)	27.8 (0.4)
Patient	33.9 (2.2)	34.9 (3.0)	27.5 (0.3)	28.0 (0.4)
PTSD Symptom Scale				
Clinician	22.1 (1.5)	19.1 (1.6)	...	...
Patient	22.1 (2.0)	20.6 (1.8)	...	...
Yohimbine				
Hamilton Anxiety Scale	9.3 (1.9)	20.3 (2.4)†	2.0 (0.7)	5.0 (1.6)
Panic Attack Symptom Scale				
Clinician	30.7 (1.4)	39.5 (1.9)†	27.3 (0.2)	28.8 (0.8)
Patient	31.9 (1.8)	41.2 (2.4)†	27.3 (0.2)	30.3 (1.5)
PTSD Symptom Scale				
Clinician	20.6 (2.2)	19.7 (0.9)	...	...
Patient	21.3 (1.9)	22.0 (1.8)	...	...

*Values are given as mean (SEM). PTSD indicates posttraumatic stress disorder.
†P<.01.

COMMENT

Administration of the α_2-antagonist yohimbine, which results in an increase in anxiety in patients with PTSD but not in healthy subjects, was associated with a significantly different metabolic response pattern in patients with PTSD compared with healthy subjects in neocortical brain regions that were hypothesized to change based on preclinical studies, including temporal, prefrontal, parietal, and orbitofrontal cortex. There was a tendency for yohimbine to be associated with a decrease in metabolism in the patients with PTSD and an increase in metabolism in the healthy subjects, with significant decreases in the hippocampus in patients with PTSD and significant increases in prefrontal and orbitofrontal cortex in the controls. These findings may be explained by a dose-dependent effect of norepinephrine on brain metabolism. Pharmacological studies[33,34] showed that high levels of norepinephrine release in the brain are associated with a decrease in brain metabolism, and lower levels result in an increase in brain metabolism. Yohimbine administration in normal controls may be associated with lower levels of norepinephrine release in central brain regions than in patients with PTSD, which results in increased metabolism. Consistent with this, a study with another α_2-antagonist, idazoxan, has shown an increase in prefrontal and occipital metabolism measured with PET FDG in healthy human subjects.[74] A large increase in norepinephrine in patients with PTSD, on the other hand, may lead to decreased metabolism. We are positing that patients with PTSD are in effect "seeing" higher doses of yohimbine than the controls, due to an increased sensitivity to yohimbine in PTSD.

Alterations in specific noradrenergic receptors (α_1, α_2, and β) in the brain[55,75,76] in patients with PTSD compared with controls also may account for our findings. One might speculate that in patients with PTSD, the primary effect of yohimbine on α_2-receptors is presynaptically at the level of the locus caeruleus, with a greater release of norepinephrine centrally in the brain compared with controls, which is associated with decreased neuronal function (and therefore metabolism). Conversely, in healthy subjects, the effects might be primarily on postsynaptic α_2-receptors, with blockade resulting in a release of postsynaptic α_2-receptor–mediated inhibition of cortical neuronal function. Consistent with the idea of a dose-dependent effect of norepinephrine on metabolism, PET studies in healthy subjects showed that mild degrees of stress increased cerebral blood flow, but severe stress decreased blood flow,[77] with an inverse correlation between metabolism in frontal and temporal cortex shown.[78,79]

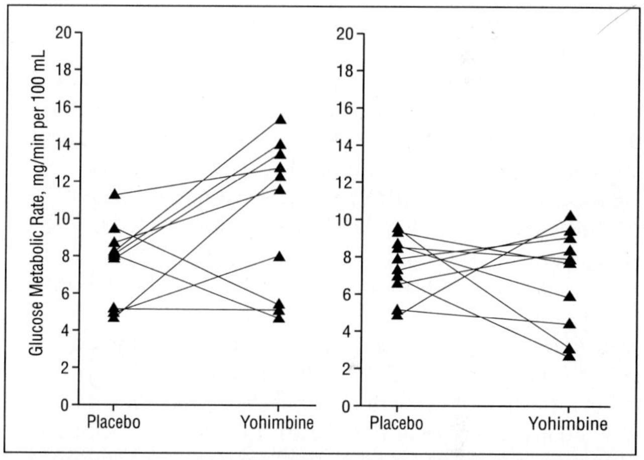

Figure 2. *Regional glucose metabolism in orbitofrontal cortex with placebo and yohimbine administration in controls (left) and patients with posttraumatic stress disorder (right). Symbols represent metabolism in individual subjects on the days of placebo and yohimbine administration. Analysis of variance with repeated measures for drug showed a significant interaction between drug and diagnosis in orbitofrontal cortex.*

We considered the possibility that yohimbine affects brain metabolism through effects on the cerebral vasculature.[80] Studies of intracarotid injection of norepinephrine in dogs[81] and humans[82] have not shown an effect of norepinephrine on brain blood flow. We have conducted preliminary studies using the Patlak Plot method,[83] in which the rate constant parameter K_1, which reflects FDG uptake from the blood into the brain and is hence influenced by blood flow, is not fixed as it is in the Sokoloff method. Preliminary results from these analyses suggest that similar results are obtained from the Patlak Plot and Sokoloff methods.

One might question whether our results are secondary to comorbid disorders in the Vietnam veterans with PTSD. Vietnam combat veterans with PTSD have high rates of comorbidity with other psychiatric disorders, ranging from 62% to 88%, most commonly depression, anxiety disorders, and alcohol and substance abuse and dependence.[84] Exclusion of patients with PTSD with comorbidity, however, would represent a highly atypical and potentially biased sample. The question of comorbidity with OCD, GAD, panic disorder, depression, and other disorders has been carefully assessed in the biological studies that have been performed in patients with PTSD.[85] These studies, using psychophysiological responsivity,[86] startle response,[49] dexamethasone suppression test,[87] and hippocampal volume,[64] did not show a difference between patients with PTSD with and without comorbid disorders that included OCD, GAD, panic disorder, depression, and alcohol and substance abuse disorders. Our previous studies have shown an exaggerated behavioral and biochemical responsiveness to yohimbine in patients with PTSD[56] and panic disorder,[57,58] but not patients with GAD,[59] depression,[60] OCD,[61] or schizophrenia.[62]

These studies did not resolve, however, whether our findings might be due to the presence of comorbid panic disorder. Previous PET and single photon emission computed tomography studies in patients with anxiety disorders, including panic disorder,[88-98] showed alterations in similar brain regions to the current study, including a blunting of cortical blood flow to lactate[92] and yohimbine[93] in panic disorder. Patients with PTSD, with and without comorbid diagnoses of panic disorder, often experience panic anxiety, often in the context of flashbacks,[99] and symptoms of panic disorder and PTSD have been linked temporally with exposure to the trauma of war in Vietnam combat veterans.[100] In our experience, patients with primary diagnoses of combat-related PTSD and comorbid panic disorder are not clinically equivalent to our patients with primary panic disorder. Findings suggest, however, that PTSD and panic disorder share alterations in noradrenergic system function. Our previous studies showed high rates of yohimbine-induced panic attacks in PTSD, and an increase in plasma levels of the metabolite of norepinephrine, methoxyhexene phenylglycol, following administration of yohimbine, in patients with PTSD with a yohimbine-induced panic attack compared with patients with PTSD without a yohimbine-induced panic attack.[56] We attempted to examine the relation between panic anxiety and brain metabolic response to yohimbine in the current study by comparing patients with PTSD with and without a yohimbine-induced panic attack. Patients with a yohimbine-induced panic attack (which occurred in 60% of patients) had a pattern of a greater reduction in metabolism with yohimbine administration than did patients without a yohimbine-induced panic attack, a difference that did not reach statistical significance, possibly due to the small sample size. In summary, questions remain about the relation between the neurobiological characteristics of PTSD and panic disorder that are not answered by our findings. Future studies are required to investigate the relation between the neurobiological characteristics of PTSD and the neurobiological characteristics of panic disorder.

Accepted for publication April 22, 1996.

This work was supported by a grant from the National Center for Posttraumatic Stress Disorder and a Veterans Affairs Research Career Development Award (Dr Bremner).

We thank Sandi Capelli, RN, Angie Genovese, RN, and Pat Barry, RN, for crucial assistance in conducting the study. We also thank Lannie Wong for expert technical advice; Hedy Sarofin for assistance in MRI scanning; George Aghajanian, MD, and Gary Aston-Jones, PhD, for useful discussions; Samuel M. Mazza, PhD, for synthesis of radioligand; Dick Hitchins, PhD, of Positron Corp, John Markey, PhD, of Yale University, Richard Carson, PhD, and Steven Bacharach, PhD, of the National Institutes of Health, Bethesda, Md, for assistance in positron emission tomography physics and quantification of signal.

Reprints: J. Douglas Bremner, MD, West Haven Veteran Affairs Medical Center (116a), 950 Campbell Ave, West Haven, CT 06516.

REFERENCES

1. Kardiner A. *The Traumatic Neuroses of War. Psychosomatic Monograph II-III.* Washington, DC: National Research Council; 1941.
2. Grinker RR, Spiegel JP. *Men Under Stress.* Philadelphia, Pa: Blakiston; 1945.
3. Kolb LC. The post-traumatic stress disorder of combat: a subgroup with a conditioned emotional response. *Mil Med.* 1984;149:237-243.
4. Chrousos GP, Gold PW. The concepts of stress and stress system disorders. *JAMA.* 1992;267:1244-1252.
5. Charney DS, Deutch AY, Krystal JH, Southwick SM, Davis M. Psychobiologic mechanisms of posttraumatic stress disorder. *Arch Gen Psychiatry.* 1993; 50:294-299.
6. Bremner JD, Davis M, Southwick SM, Krystal JH, Charney DS. The neurobiology of posttraumatic stress disorder. In: Oldham JM, Riba MG, Tasman A, eds. *Reviews of Psychiatry.* Washington, DC: American Psychiatric Press; 1993; 12:182-204.
7. Aghajanian G, Cedarbaum J, Wang R. Evidence for norepinephrine-mediated collateral inhibition of locus coeruleus neurons. *Brain Res.* 1977;136:570-577.
8. Aghajanian G. Tolerance of locus coeruleus neurons to morphine and suppression of withdrawal response by clonidine. *Nature.* 1978;276:186-188.
9. Cederbaum JM, Aghajanian GK. Activation of locus coeruleus neurons by peripheral stimuli: modulation by a collateral inhibitory mechanism. *Life Sci.* 1978;23:1383-1392.
10. Aston-Jones G, Bloom FE. Norepinephrine-containing locus coeruleus neurons in behaving rats exhibit pronounced responses to non-noxious environmental stimuli. *J Neurosci.* 1981;1:887-900.
11. Aston-Jones G, Chiang C, Alexinsky T. Discharge of noradrenergic locus coeruleus neurons in behaving rats and monkeys suggests a role in vigilance. In: Barnes CD, Pompeiano O, eds. *Progress in Brain Research.* Amsterdam, the Netherlands: Elsevier Science Publishers; 1991:501-519.
12. Heal DJ, Marsden CA. *The Pharmacology of Noradrenaline in the Central Nervous System.* New York, NY: Oxford University Press Inc; 1990.
13. Korf J, Aghajanian GK, Roth RH. Increased turnover of norepinephrine in the

rat cerebral cortex during stress: role of the locus coeruleus. *Neuropharmacology.* 1973;12:933-938.
14. Tanaka M, Kohno Y, Nakagawa R, Ida Y, Takeda S, Nagasaki N. Time-related differences in noradrenaline turnover in rat brain regions by stress. *Pharmacol Biochem Behav.* 1982;16:315-319.
15. Anisman H, Zacharko RM. Behavioral and neurochemical consequences associated with stressors. *Ann N Y Acad Sci.* 1986;467:205-225.
16. Irwin J, Ahluwalia P, Anisman H. Sensitization of norepinephrine activity following acute and chronic footshock. *Brain Res.* 1986;379:98-103.
17. Tanaka M, Kohno Y, Tsuda A, Nakagawa R, Ida Y, Iimori K, Hoaki Y, Nagasaki N. Differential effects of morphine on noradrenaline release in brain regions of stressed and non-stressed rats. *Brain Res.* 1983;275:105-115.
18. Abercrombie ED, Keller RW Jr, Zigmond MJ. Characterization of hippocampal norepinephrine release as measured by microdialysis perfusion: pharmacological and behavioral studies. *Neuroscience.* 1988;27:897-904.
19. Nissenbaum LK, Zigmond MJ, Sved AF, Abercrombie E. Prior exposure to chronic stress results in enhanced synthesis and release of hippocampal norepinephrine in response to a novel stressor. *J Neurosci.* 1991;11:1478-1484.
20. Cassens G, Roffman M, Kuruc A, Schildkraut JJ. Alterations in brain norepinephrine metabolism induced by environmental stimuli previously paired with inescapable shock. *Science.* 1980;209:1138-1140.
21. Glavin G, Tanaka M, Tsuda A, Kohno Y, Hoaki Y, Nagasaki N. Regional rat brain noradrenaline turnover in response to restraint stress. *Pharmacol Biochem Behav.* 1983;19:287-290.
22. Nissenbaum LK, Abercrombie ED. Presynaptic alterations with enhancement of evoked release and synthesis of norepinephrine in the hippocampus of chronically cold stressed rats. *Brain Res.* 1993;608:280-287.
23. Rasmussen K, Morilak DA, Jacobs BL. Single-unit activity of locus coeruleus in the freely moving cat, II: during naturalistic behaviors and in response to simple and complex stimuli. *Brain Res.* 1986;371:324-334.
24. Levine ES, Litto WJ, Jacobs BL. Activity of cat locus coeruleus noradrenergic neurons during the defense reaction. *Brain Res.* 1990;531:189-195.
25. Abercrombie ED, Jacobs BL. Single-unit response of noradrenergic neurons in the locus coeruleus of freely moving cats, II: acutely presented stressful and nonstressful stimuli. *J Neurosci.* 1987;7:2837-2843.
26. Redmond DE. New and old evidence for the involvement of a brain norepinephrine system in anxiety. In: Fann WE, ed. *Phenomenology and Treatment of Anxiety.* Jamaica, NY: Spectrum Publications Inc; 1979.
27. Grant SJ, Redmond DE. Neuronal activity of the locus coeruleus in awake *Macaca arctoides. Exp Neurol.* 1984;84:701-708.
28. Aston-Jones G. The locus coeruleus: behavioral function of locus coeruleus derived from cellular attributes. *Physiol Psychol.* 1985;13:118-126.
29. Lomasney JW, Cotecchia S, Lefkowitz RJ, Caron MG. Molecular biology of α-adrenergic receptors: implications for receptor classification and for structure-function relationships. *Biochim Biophys Acta.* 1991;1095:127-139.
30. Segal M. The action of norepinephrine in the rat hippocampus: intracellular studies in the slice preparation. *Brain Res.* 1981;206:107-128.
31. Hoffer BJ, Siggins GR, Oliver AP, Bloom FE. Activation of the pathway from locus coeruleus to rat cerebellar Purkinje neurons: pharmacological evidence of noradrenergic central inhibition. *J Pharmacol Exp Ther.* 1973;184:553-569.
32. Foote SL, Freedman R, Oliver AP. Effects of putative neurotransmitters on neuronal activity in monkey auditory cortex. *Brain Res.* 1975;86:229-242.
33. Raichle ME, Hartman BK, Eichling JO, Sharpe LG. Central noradrenergic regulation of cerebral blood flow and vascular permeability. *Proc Natl Acad Sci U S A.* 1975;72:3726-3730.
34. McCulloch J, Harper AM. Factors influencing the response of the cerebral circulation to phenylethylamine. *Neurology.* 1979;29:201-207.
35. Savaki HE, Kadekaro M, McCulloch J, Sokoloff L. The central noradrenergic system in the rat: metabolic mapping with α-adrenergic blocking agents. *Brain Res.* 1982;234:65-79.
36. Inoue M, McHugh M, Pappius HM. The effect of α-adrenergic receptor blockers prazosin and yohimbine on cerebral metabolism and biogenic amine content of traumatized brain. *J Cereb Blood Flow Metab.* 1991;11:242-252.
37. Abraham WC, Delanoy RL, Dunn AJ, Zornetzer SF. Locus coeruleus stimulation decreases deoxyglucose uptake in ipsilateral mouse cerebral cortex. *Brain Res.* 1979;172:387-392.
38. De la Torre JC, Surgeon JW, Walker RH. Effects of locus coeruleus stimulation on cerebral blood flow in selected brain regions. *Acta Neurol Scand Suppl.* 1977;64:104-105.
39. Katayama Y, Ueno Y, Tsukiyama T, Tsubokawa T. Long lasting suppression of firing of cortical neurons and decrease in cortical blood flow following train pulse stimulation of the locus coeruleus in the cat. *Brain Res.* 1981; 216:173-179.
40. Goadsby PJ, Duckworth JW. Low frequency stimulation of the locus coeruleus reduces regional blood flow in the spinalized cat. *Brain Res.* 1989; 476:71-77.
41. Bates D, Weinshilboum RM, Campbell RJ, Sundt TM. The effect of lesions in the locus coeruleus on the physiological responses of the cerebral blood vessels in cats. *Brain Res.* 1977;136:431-443.
42. Schwartz WJ. 6-Hydroxydopamine lesions of rat locus coeruleus alter brain glucose consumption, as measured by the 2-deoxy-D-[^{14}C]glucose technique. *Neurosci Lett.* 1978;7:141-150.
43. Savaki HE, Graham DI, Grome JJ, McCulloch J. Functional consequences of unilateral lesion of the locus coeruleus: a quantitative [^{14}C]2-deoxyglucose investigation. *Brain Res.* 1984;292:239-249.
44. Murburg MM, ed. *Catecholamine Function in Posttraumatic Stress Disorder: Emerging Concepts.* Washington, DC: American Psychiatric Press; 1994.
45. Blanchard EB, Kolb LC, Pallmeyer TP, Gerardi RJ. A psychophysiological study of post-traumatic stress disorder in Vietnam veterans. *Psychiatr Q.* 1982;54:220-229.
46. Blanchard EB, Kolb LC, Gerardi RJ, Ryan P, Pallmeyer TP. Cardiac response to relevant stimuli as an adjunctive tool for diagnosing post-traumatic stress disorder in Vietnam veterans. *Behav Ther.* 1986;17:592-606.
47. Pitman RK, Orr SP, Forgue DF, de Jong JB, Claiborn JM. Psychophysiologic assessment of posttraumatic stress disorder imagery in Vietnam combat veterans. *Arch Gen Psychiatry.* 1987;44:970-975.
48. McFall ME, Murburg MM, Ko GN, Veith RC. Autonomic responses to stress in Vietnam combat veterans with posttraumatic stress disorder. *Biol Psychiatry.* 1990;27:1165-1175.
49. Shalev AY, Orr SP, Peri T, Schreiber S, Pitman RK. Physiologic responses to loud tones in Israeli patients with posttraumatic stress disorder. *Arch Gen Psychiatry.* 1992;49:870-874.
50. Kosten TR, Mason JW, Ostroff RB, Harkness L. Sustained urinary norepinephrine and epinephrine elevation in posttraumatic stress disorder. *Psychoneuroendocrinology.* 1987;12:13-20.
51. Mason JW, Giller EL, Kosten TR, Harkness L. Elevation of urinary norepinephrine/cortisol ratio in posttraumatic stress disorder. *J Nerv Ment Dis.* 1988;176: 498-502.
52. Pitman R, Orr S. Twenty-four hour urinary cortisol and catecholamine excretion in combat-related posttraumatic stress disorder. *Biol Psychiatry.* 1990; 27:245-247.
53. Blanchard EB, Kolb LC, Prins A, Gates S, McCoy GC. Changes in plasma norepinephrine to combat-related stimuli among Vietnam veterans with posttraumatic stress disorder. *J Nerv Ment Dis.* 1991;179:371-373.
54. McFall ME, Veith RC, Murburg MM. Basal sympathoadrenal function in posttraumatic stress disorder. *Biol Psychiatry.* 1992;31:1050-1056.
55. Perry BD, Giller EJ, Southwick SM. Altered platelet α_2-adrenergic binding sites in posttraumatic stress disorder. *Am J Psychiatry.* 1987;144:1324-1327.
56. Southwick SM, Krystal JH, Morgan CA, Johnson D, Nagy LM, Nicolaou A, Heninger GR, Charney DS. Abnormal noradrenergic function in posttraumatic stress disorder. *Arch Gen Psychiatry.* 1993;50:266-274.
57. Charney DS, Heninger GR, Breier A. Noradrenergic function in panic anxiety: effects of yohimbine in healthy subjects and patients with agoraphobia and panic disorder. *Arch Gen Psychiatry.* 1984;41:751-763.
58. Charney DS, Woods SW, Goodman WK, Heninger GR. Neurobiological mechanisms of panic anxiety: biochemical and behavioral correlates of yohimbine-induced panic attacks. *Am J Psychiatry.* 1987;144:1030-1036.
59. Charney DS, Woods SW, Heninger GR. Noradrenergic function in generalized anxiety disorder: effects of yohimbine in healthy subjects and patients with generalized anxiety disorder. *Psychiatry Res.* 1987;27:173-182.
60. Heninger GR, Charney DS, Price LH. α_2-adrenergic receptor sensitivity in depression: the plasma MHPG, behavioral, and cardiovascular responses to yohimbine. *Arch Gen Psychiatry.* 1988;45:718-726.
61. Rasmussen SA, Goodman WK, Woods SW, Heninger GR, Charney DS. Effects of yohimbine in obsessive-compulsive disorder. *Psychopharmacology.* 1987;93:308-313.
62. Glazer WM, Charney DS, Heninger GR. Noradrenergic function in schizophrenia. *Arch Gen Psychiatry.* 1987;44:898-904.
63. Bremner JD, Scott TM, Delaney RC, Southwick SM, Mason JW, Johnson DR, Innis RB, McCarthy G, Charney DS. Deficits in short-term memory in posttraumatic stress disorder. *Am J Psychiatry.* 1993;150:1015-1019.
64. Bremner JD, Randall PR, Scott TM, Bronen RA, Delaney RC, Seibyl JP, Southwick SM, McCarthy G, Charney DS, Innis RB. MRI-based measurement of hippocampal volume in posttraumatic stress disorder. *Am J Psychiatry.* 1995; 152:973-981.
65. Spitzer RL, Williams JBW, Gibbon M. Structured Clinical Interview for *DSM-III-R.* New York, NY: New York State Psychiatric Institute, Biometrics Research Department; 1987.
66. Keane TM, Caddell JM, Taylor KL. Mississippi Scale for Combat-Related Post-

Traumatic Stress Disorder: three studies in reliability and validity. *J Consult Clin Psychol.* 1989;56:85-90.
67. Keane TM, Fairbank JA, Caddell JM. Clinical evaluation of a scale to measure combat exposure. *Psychol Assess.* 1989;1:53-55.
68. Mulaney NA, Gould LK, Hartz RK, Hitchens RE, Wong WH, Bristow D, Adler S, Philippe EA, Bendrien B, Sanders M, Gibbs B. Design and performance of Posicam 6.5 BGO Positron camera. *J Nucl Med.* 1990;31:610-616.
69. Sokoloff L, Reivich M, Kennedy C, Des Rosiers MH, Patlak CS, Pettigrew KD, Sakurada O, Shinohara M. The [^{14}]deoxyglucose method for the measurement of local cerebral glucose utilization: theory, procedure, and normal values in the conscious and anesthetized albino rat. *J Neurochem.* 1977;28: 897-916.
70. Huang S, Phelps ME, Hoffman EF, Kuhl DE. Error sensitivity of fluorodeoxyglucose method for measurement of cerebral rate of glucose. *J Cereb Blood Flow Metab.* 1981;1:391-401.
71. Robb RA, Hanson DP, Karwoski RA, Larson AG, Workman EL, Stacy MC. Analyze: a comprehensive, operator-interactive software package for multidimensional medical image display and analysis. *Comput Med Imaging Graph.* 1989;13:433-454.
72. Jiang H, Robb RA, Holton KS. A new approach to 3-D registration of multimodality medical images by surface matching. In: *Proceedings of the 2nd Conference on Visual Biomedical Computing.* 1992;1808:196-213.
73. Duvernoy H. *The Human Brain: Surface Three-Dimensional Anatomy and MRI.* New York, NY: Springer Publishing Co Inc; 1991.
74. Schmidt ME, Matochik J, Zametkin A, Risinger R, Hsiao J, Cohen R, Potter WZ. Acute effects of IV idazoxan on regional cerebral metabolism. *Am Coll Neuropharmacol Abstracts.* 1992:20.
75. McCormick DA. Cellular mechanisms underlying cholinergic and noradrenergic modulation of neuronal firing in the cat and guinea pig dorsal lateral geniculate nucleus. *J Neurosci.* 1992;12:278-289.
76. Hirsch JC, Fourment A, Marc ME. Sleep-related variations of membrane potential in the lateral geniculate body relay neurons of the cat. *Brain Res.* 1983; 259:308-312.
77. Gur RC, Gur RE, Resnick SM, Skolnick BE, Alavi A, Reivich M. The effect of anxiety on cortical cerebral blood flow and metabolism. *J Cereb Blood Flow Metab.* 1987;7:173-177.
78. Reivich M, Gur R, Alavi A. Positron emission tomographic studies of sensory stimuli, cognitive processes and anxiety. *Hum Neurobiology.* 1983;2:25-33.
79. Rodriguez G, Cogorno P, Gris Am Marenco S, Mesiti C, Nobili F, Rosadini G. Regional cerebral blood flow and anxiety: a correlation study in neurologically normal patients. *J Cereb Blood Flow Metab.* 1989;9:410-415.
80. Edvinsson L, Lindvall M, Nielsen KC, Owman CH. Are brain vessels innervated by central (nonsympathetic) adrenergic neurons? *Brain Res.* 1973;63: 496-499.
81. MacKenzie ET, McCulloch J, Harper AM. Influence of endogenous norepinephrine on cerebral blood flow and metabolism. *Am J Physiol.* 1976;231: 489-493.
82. Olesen J. The effect of intracarotid epinephrine, norepinephrine, and angiotensin on the regulation of cerebral blood flow in man. *Neurology.* 1972;22: 978-981.
83. Patlak CS, Blasberg RG. Graphical evaluation of blood to brain transfer constants from multiple time uptake data: generalizations. *J Cereb Blood Flow Metab.* 1985;5:584-590.
84. Fairbank JA, Schlenger WE, Saigh PA, Davidson JRT. An epidemiologic profile of post-traumatic stress disorder: prevalence, comorbidity, and risk factors. In: Friedman MJ, Charney DS, Deutch AY, eds. *Neurobiological and Clinical Consequences of Stress: From Normal Adaptation to PTSD.* Philadelphia, Pa: JB Lippincott; 1995:415-427.
85. Friedman MJ, Yehuda R. Posttraumatic stress disorder and comorbidity: psychobiological approaches to differential diagnosis. In: Friedman MJ, Charney DS, Deutch AY, eds. *Neurobiological and Clinical Consequences of Stress: From Normal Adaptation to PTSD.* Philadelphia, Pa: JB Lippincott; 1995:429-445.
86. Pitman RK, Orr SP, Forgue DF, Alfman B, de Jong JB, Herz LR. Psychophysiologic responses to combat imagery of Vietnam veterans with posttraumatic stress disorder versus other anxiety disorders. *J Abnorm Psychol.* 1990; 99:49-54.
87. Yehuda R, Southwick SM, Krystal JH, Bremner JD, Charney DS, Mason J. Enhanced suppression of cortisol with low dose dexamethasone in posttraumatic stress disorder. *Am J Psychiatry.* 1993;150:83-86.
88. Nordahl TE, Semple WE, Gross M, Mellman TA, Stein MB, Goyer P, King AC, Uhde TW, Cohen RM. Cerebral glucose metabolic differences in patients with panic disorder. *Neuropsychopharmacology.* 1990;3:261-271.
89. Reiman EM, Raichle ME, Butler FK, Herscovitch P, Robins E. A focal brain abnormality in panic disorder: a severe form of anxiety. *Nature.* 1984;310: 683-685.
90. Reiman EM, Raichle ME, Robins E, Mintun MA, Fusselman MJ, Fox PT, Price JL, Hackman KA. Neuroanatomical correlates of a lactate-induced anxiety attack. *Arch Gen Psychiatry.* 1989;46:493-500.
91. Drevets WC, Videen TO, MacLeod AK, Haller JW, Raichle ME. PET images of blood flow changes during anxiety: correction. *Science.* 1992;256:1696.
92. Stewart RS, Devous MD, Rush AJ, Lane L, Bonte FJ. Cerebral blood flow changes during sodium-lactate–induced panic attacks. *Am J Psychiatry.* 1988; 145:442-449.
93. Woods SW, Koster K, Krystal JH, Smith EO, Zubal IG, Hoffer PB, Charney DS. Yohimbine alters regional cerebral blood flow in panic disorder. *Lancet.* 1988; 2:678.
94. Mountz JM, Modell FG, Wilson MW, Curtis GC, Lee MA, Schmaltz S, Kuhl DE. Positron emission tomographic evaluation of cerebral blood flow during state anxiety in simple phobia. *Arch Gen Psychiatry.* 1989;46:501-504.
95. Wik G, Fredrikson M, Ericson K, Eriksson L, Stone-Elander S, Greitz T. A functional cerebral response to frightening visual stimulation. *Psychol Res.* 1992;50:15-24.
96. Frederikson M, Wik G, Greitz T, Eriksson L, Stone-Elander S, Ericson K, Sedvall G. Regional cerebral blood flow during experimental phobic fear. *Psychophysiology.* 1993;30:126-130.
97. Wu JC, Buchsbaum MS, Hershey TG, Hazlett E, Sicotte N, Johnson JC. PET in generalized anxiety disorder. *Biol Psychiatry.* 1991;29:1181-1199.
98. Buchsbaum MS, Wu J, Haier R, Hazlet E, Ball R, Katz M, Sokoloski K, Lagunas-Solar M, Langer D. Positron emission tomography assessment of the effect of benzodiazepines on regional glucose metabolic rate in patients with anxiety disorder. *Life Sci.* 1987;40:2392-2400.
99. Mellman TA, Davis GC. Combat-related flashbacks in posttraumatic stress disorder: phenomenology and similarity to panic attacks. *J Clin Psychiatry.* 1985;46:379-382.
100. Mellman TA, Randolph CA, Brawman-Mintzer O, Flores LP, Milanes FJ. Phenomenology and course of psychiatric disorders associated with combat-related posttraumatic stress disorder. *Am J Psychiatry.* 1992;149:1568-1574.

ORIGINAL ARTICLE

The Course of Psychopathologic Features in Mild to Moderate Alzheimer Disease

D. P. Devanand, MD; Diane M. Jacobs, PhD; Ming-Xin Tang, PhD; Caridad Del Castillo-Castaneda; Mary Sano, PhD; Karen Marder, MD; Karen Bell, MD; Frederick W. Bylsma, PhD; Jason Brandt, PhD; Marilyn Albert, PhD; Yaakov Stern, PhD

Background: The onset and course of the psychopathologic features of Alzheimer disease have not been established in prospective, longitudinal studies.

Methods: Two hundred thirty-five patients with early, probable Alzheimer disease were recruited at 3 sites and observed naturalistically for up to 5 years. At 6-month intervals, the Columbia University Scale for Psychopathology in Alzheimer's Disease was administered. Markov analyses were used to predict the probability of a specific symptom developing or being maintained at the next visit. For each symptom category, the maximum frequency of occurrence at 4 consecutive points (duration, 2 years) was calculated.

Results: Misidentification, wandering or agitation, and physical aggression increased during follow-up. At any visit, the likelihood of a new symptom developing was greatest for behavioral disturbance, intermediate for paranoid delusions and hallucinations, and least for depressed mood with vegetative features. Wandering or agitation occurred at 3 or more of 4 consecutive visits (duration, 2 years) in the majority of patients, paranoid delusions and hallucinations were intermediate in their degree of persistence, and depressed mood with vegetative signs rarely persisted.

Conclusions: Behavioral disturbance, particularly agitation, is common and persistent in patients with Alzheimer disease. Psychotic symptoms are less common and show moderate persistence over time. Depressed mood with vegetative signs is uncommon and rarely persists. These findings suggest leads about the optimal treatment duration for specific subtypes of psychopathologic features.

Arch Gen Psychiatry. 1997;54:257-263

From the Memory Disorders Clinic in the New York State Psychiatric Institute, the Center for Alzheimer's Disease Research in New York City, and the Departments of Psychiatry (Drs Devanand and Stern) and Neurology (Drs Jacobs, Tang, Sano, Marder, Bell, and Stern and Ms Del Castillo-Castaneda) and the Gertrude H. Sergievsky Center (Drs Jacobs, Tang, Sano, Marder, Bell, Stern, and Ms Del Castillo-Castaneda), College of Physicians and Surgeons of Columbia University, New York, NY; the Department of Psychiatry and Behavioral Sciences, The Johns Hopkins University, Baltimore, Md (Drs Bylsma and Brandt); and the Departments of Psychiatry and Neurology, Massachusetts General Hospital, Harvard Medical School, Boston (Dr Albert).

BEHAVIORAL complications that are distressing to patients and caregivers, that are often treated with psychotropic medications, and that may increase the risk of institutionalization commonly develop in patients with Alzheimer disease (AD).[1-4] Agitation may occur in up to half of the patients with AD in outpatient clinics[5,6] and nursing homes[7,8]; physical aggression is less common.[6,9,10] Common delusions in patients with AD include the belief that people are stealing their possessions and misidentification (eg, one's living place is not one's home).[1] The prevalence of delusions, which are more often isolated symptoms than diagnosable psychotic disorders, ranges from 0% to 50% in different samples.[11-16] The prevalence of psychosis and behavioral disturbance increases with disease progression and may herald a poor prognosis.[2,14,17-19] Hallucinations, more often visual than auditory, rarely manifest early in the illness but may be more common in severe dementia.[14,16,20,21] Approximately 10% to 30% of the patients with AD meet the diagnostic criteria for major depression, but it remains unclear if depression is characteristic of any stage of the illness.[22-26]

The symptoms of AD are known to fluctuate over time.[2,5,13,14] However, the onset and course of these symptoms have not been established in prospective, longitudinal studies.[27,28] This lack of knowledge about the likely "episode duration" of specific symptoms has led to uncertainties about the prediction of the clinical course and the optimal duration of treatment. The latter is important because psychotropic medication use is associated with increased side effects in the elderly (eg, neuroleptic-induced extrapyramidal signs and tardive dyskinesia).[29,30]

We reported single-site, cross-sectional data on the development and use of the Columbia University Scale for Psychopathology in Alzheimer's Disease (CUSPAD), a short semistructured instrument that can be administered by clinicians or trained research technicians.[16] As

SUBJECTS AND METHODS

SUBJECTS

A cohort of patients with early, probable AD was recruited at 3 sites: Columbia University (CU), New York, NY; The Johns Hopkins University School of Medicine (JHU), Baltimore, Md; and Massachusetts General Hospital (MGH), Boston. Informed consent was obtained from the patient and an informant (ie, a family member, close friend, or health aide) who also served as a patient advocate. No intersite differences were noted for most demographic and clinical features, including sex, ethnicity, educational level, and severity of dementia.[31] Patients at MGH were older (age, 77.5±9.5 years) compared with those at CU (age, 71.0±8.0 years) and JHU (age, 72.3±7.8 years); ages are given as the mean±SD.

Detailed neurologic, psychiatric, and neuropsychological examinations were conducted initially and at 6-month intervals. Baseline laboratory tests included relevant blood studies, a computed tomographic or magnetic resonance imaging scan of the brain, and electroencephalogram and cerebrospinal fluid studies, if indicated. Patients met *DSM-III-R* criteria for primary degenerative dementia of the Alzheimer type[32] and National Institute of Neurological Disorders and Stroke–Alzheimer's Disease and Related Disorders Association criteria for probable AD.[33] Entry criteria required an expanded modified Mini-Mental State Examination (mMMSE) score of 30 or more of 57 (approximately equivalent to ≥16 on the original Mini-Mental State Examination).[34,35]

Exclusion criteria were a history of schizophrenia or schizoaffective disorder, electroconvulsive therapy within the preceding 2 years or a history of 10 or more electroconvulsive therapy treatments in any one course, alcohol or drug dependence during the preceding 5 years, primary affective disorder within 1 year before the onset of dementia, and evidence of other causes of dementia. Patients with a history or clinical signs of stroke, radiological evidence of cortical lesions or focal cortical atrophy secondary to an infarct, or other vascular lesions 2 cm or more in diameter in any 1 computed tomographic or magnetic resonance imaging slice were excluded.[31]

Patients receiving thyroid replacement therapy (ie, 3.4%) were euthyroid. At the initial examination, 9% of the patients were participating in placebo-controlled research drug trials, including trials for oral physostigmine, piracetam, acetyl-L-carnitine, selegiline hydrochloride, and tetrahydroaminoacridine. A similar proportion of patients participated in these trials during follow-up.

COLUMBIA UNIVERSITY SCALE FOR PSYCHOPATHOLOGY IN ALZHEIMER'S DISEASE

A trained research technician administered the CUSPAD to the informant at the initial examination and at 6-month intervals. The frame of inquiry was the month before examination. Most CUSPAD items are scored dichotomously (ie, present or absent).

The 5 items for behavioral disturbance were wandering, agitation (ie, restlessness or increased motor activity), verbal outbursts, physical aggression (including threatening behavior), and sundowning (ie, increased agitation in the evening compared with the daytime). The items for depression were depressed mood, difficulty sleeping (ie, insomnia or hypersomnia), and change in appetite (ie, decreased or increased).

For delusions, the categories were any type (overall category), paranoid (including the belief that people were stealing things), misidentification (including the belief that the patient's house was not his or her home), somatic, and abandonment. For each delusion, the broad definition was met when the patient did not accept the caregiver's correction of the false belief, while a narrow definition was met when the patient did not accept the caregiver's correction of the false belief and the symptom occurred more than 3 times per week. Hallucinations were rated as vague or clear in each of 4 sensory modalities (ie, auditory, visual, tactile, and olfactory).

The analyses used the broad definition of a delusion and the presence of either a vague or clear hallucination (any sensory modality) for the following reasons. First, many clinicians can identify whether a broadly defined delusion or hallucination is present. Second, if a patient switches from meeting narrow to broad criteria for a delusion, use of the narrow definition results in the patient being misclassified as switching from delusional to nondelusional (ie, a type II error). Similarly, a restriction to only clear hallucinations is problematic if patients switch from clear to vague (or vice versa) during follow-up.

ANALYSIS PLAN

The presence of any 1 symptom within a category led to a positive score for that category. The following symptom categories were evaluated as dichotomous variables (ie, present or absent): delusions (any type), paranoid, misidentification, somatic, and abandonment delusions, hallucinations (any type), behavioral disturbance, insomnia, and depressed mood. Analyses were also conducted for specific symptoms of a priori interest, ie, wandering or agitation (a positive score for either item), physical aggression, and depressed mood with vegetative signs (ie, sleep and appetite disturbance).

Markov analyses were conducted to evaluate the course of the psychopathologic features. In this model, the current symptom status and relevant risk factors were used to predict the probability of transition to specified outcomes (ie, developing or maintaining the symptom) at the next visit (after the 6-month interval). Separately, to assess the persistence of symptoms during follow-up, the maximum frequency of occurrence of each symptom category at any 4 consecutive points (duration, 2 years), regardless of when it was first manifested, was calculated.

The main descriptive and related analyses were restricted to the first 3 years of follow-up because the number of subjects decreased further with longer follow-up. For the Markov analyses and evaluation of the persistence of symptoms, all available points (maximum, 5 years of follow-up) were used. Given the large sample size, a conservative $P<.01$ was used as the threshold criterion for significance in all analyses. All data are given as the mean±SD.

Table 1. Prevalence (Percentage) of Psychopathologic Features at 6-Month Intervals During 3 Years of Follow-up

Psychopathologic Feature	Time, y: Intake (n=235)	0.5 (n=198)	1.0 (n=188)	1.5 (n=177)	2.0 (n=157)	2.5 (n=156)	3.0 (n=137)	Test of Linearity, *P*
Any type of delusion	23.9	27.8	31.9	32.8	33.1	35.3	31.4	<.05
Paranoid	14.5	21.7	19.1	18.6	14.6	17.9	18.2	.94
Misidentification	10.2	11.1	13.3	18.6	21.7	22.4	18.3	<.005
Somatic	1.3	0.5	2.7	2.8	2.5	4.5	2.2	.06
Abandonment	1.3	1.5	4.3	4.0	0.6	1.9	2.9	.66
Hallucinations	8.1	8.1	11.6	17.0	11.3	19.8	12.2	.31
Behavior disturbance	51.9	51.5	62.2	61.0	66.9	71.2	65.7	<.001
Wandering or agitation	38.7	39.9	47.3	50.9	52.2	62.2	56.9	<.001
Physical aggression	6.4	8.6	9.6	11.3	19.8	20.5	19.0	<.001
Depressed mood	25.1	20.2	26.6	23.3	21.7	19.9	22.6	.65
Insomnia	13.6	9.7	8.9	14.6	9.3	13.3	11.3	.73
Depressed mood with vegetative signs	6.8	7.1	6.4	6.8	8.3	7.7	4.4	.89

part of a prospective, longitudinal, multicenter study, the CUSPAD was used to evaluate the course of the psychopathologic features in patients recruited at the stage of early, probable AD.[31]

RESULTS

DEMOGRAPHIC AND CLINICAL FEATURES

Of the 235 patients, 94 were from CU, 80 were from JHU, and 61 were from MGH. The number of patients decreased during the study period (**Table 1**). During the first 3 years, reasons for unavailability for follow-up included death (n=53), severe medical illness (n=9), change of residence (n=13), and other causes, including refusal (n=23).

At the initial examination, the age of the patients was 73.1±8.9 years; 82.1% were aged 65 years or older. The duration of the illness was 4.0±2.6 years, and the educational attainment of the patients was 13.1±3.7 years. Most patients were women (ie, 59.1%); the ethnic breakdown of the patients was 89.8% non-Latino white, 3.4% Latino, 6.4% African American, and 0.4% other (ie, 1 patient of African American, Irish, and Native American origin). At the initial examination, 91.1% lived at home, 6.8% lived in a nursing home, 1.3% lived in a retirement home, and 0.9% had other living situations. At the 3-year follow-up, 26.8% resided in a nursing home.

The duration of follow-up was 3.0±2.5 years. The mMMSE score (maximum score, 57) decreased from 37.9±5.6 at the initial examination to 32.2±9.8 at 1 year, 27.2±12.7 at 2 years, and 20.6±15.0 at 3 years (test of linearity: F=429.8, $P<.001$). The Blessed Functional Activity Scale (BFAS) score (from 0=no impairment to 17=severe impairment)[36,37] increased from 3.5±1.9 at the initial examination to 5.0±2.6 at 1 year, 6.6±3.6 at 2 years, and 8.2±4.3 at 3 years (test of linearity: F=476.6, $P<.001$). These changes are consistent with prior reports[17,36] about the rate of cognitive and functional decline in mild to moderate AD.

At the initial examination, most informants reported frequent contact with the patient (contact during the previous year, 287.7±124.8 days), and 63.6% of them lived with the patient. The bulk of informants comprised spouses (ie, 56.9%) and adult children (ie, 31.9%). The informant rarely changed during follow-up: spouses, 57.4% at 1 year, 60.0% at 2 years, and 61.0% at 3 years; adult children, 31.7% at 1 year, 31.5% at 2 years, and 31.5% at 3 years.

A history of a psychiatric disorder (any type) before the onset of AD was reported in 19.9% of the patients, among whom 70% had a history of depression (subtype unspecified). Antidepressant use did not change notably during follow-up: 9.4% at the initial examination, 12.6% at 1 year, 9.6% at 2 years, and 14.3% at 3 years. Neuroleptic use increased during follow-up: 0.4% at the initial examination, 6.3% at 1 year, 16.6% at 2 years, and 18.5% at 3 years. Sedative or hypnotic use also increased during follow-up: 5.5% at the initial examination, 5.2% at 1 year, 7.6% at 2 years, and 16.0% at 3 years. Overall, the proportion of patients receiving psychotropic medications (any type) increased during follow-up: 14.0% at the initial examination, 20.9% at 1 year, 27.4% at 2 years, and 38.7% at 3 years.

RELIABILITY, DIVERGENT VALIDITY, AND INTERSITE COMPARISONS

We have reported interrater reliability for the major symptom categories between the principal scale developer (D.P.D.) and a research technician (trained by D.P.D.), whether concurrently rating a single interview (κ=0.74-1.00) or conducting separate interviews (κ=0.53-0.73).[16] These 2 raters trained the research technicians at the other sites and provided ongoing consultation when patients were difficult to rate.

At the initial examination, moderate associations were noted among paranoid delusions, misidentification delusions, and behavioral disturbance (χ^2, 10.6-12.0; $df=1$; $P<.01$). These 3 symptom categories showed no notable associations with either hallucinations or depressed mood, extending the strong divergent validity previously reported from the CU site alone.[16]

At the initial examination, no intersite differences

Table 2. Baseline Relations Between Symptom Categories and Cognitive and Functional Deficits*

Symptom	Prevalence	mMMSE Mean	mMMSE SD	t	P<	BFAS Mean	BFAS SD	t	P<
Any type of delusion	Present	36.4	4.5	2.3	.02	4.1	1.7	2.6	.01
	Absent	38.4	5.8			3.4	1.9		
Paranoid	Present	38.1	5.7	1.4	.20	3.9	1.7	1.1	.30
	Absent	36.6	4.7			3.5	1.9		
Misidentification	Present	35.4	3.8	3.2	.01	4.6	1.8	2.6	.01
	Absent	38.2	5.7			3.4	1.9		
Hallucinations	Present	35.9	5.1	1.6	.20	3.7	1.5	0.4	.70
	Absent	38.0	5.6			3.5	1.9		
Behavior disturbance	Present	37.0	4.7	2.6	.01	3.8	1.9	2.0	.05
	Absent	38.8	6.3			3.3	1.8		
Wandering or agitation	Present	36.9	4.9	2.2	.05	3.9	2.1	2.4	.02
	Absent	38.5	5.9			3.3	1.7		
Physical aggression	Present	36.8	4.4	0.8	.40	4.5	1.9	2.0	.05
	Absent	37.9	5.6			3.5	1.9		
Depressed mood	Present	36.0	4.8	3.0	.01	3.9	1.8	1.6	.20
	Absent	38.5	5.7			3.4	1.9		
Insomnia	Present	36.7	5.7	1.0	.30	4.5	2.1	3.0	.01
	Absent	37.9	5.6			3.4	1.8		
Depressed mood with vegetative signs	Present	35.1	5.1	2.1	.05	4.6	2.6	2.4	.02
	Absent	38.1	5.6			3.5	1.8		

*mMMSE indicates modified Mini-Mental State Examination; BFAS, Blessed Functional Activity Scale, part 1; and *t*, 2-tailed Student *t* test.

for the prevalence of psychotic and depressive features were noted. Behavioral disturbance differed in prevalence at the 3 sites (CU, 62.8%; JHU, 52.5%; and MGH, 34.4%) (χ^2=11.9, $P<.005$), primarily because of differences in the prevalence of agitation or wandering (CU, 51.1%; JHU, 36.3%; and MGH, 23%) (χ^2=12.6, $P<.005$).

PREVALENCE OF SYMPTOMS

At the initial examination, 64.3% of the patients had 1 or more psychopathologic symptom. During the first 3 years of follow-up, only 8.5% of the patients remained free of all symptoms of psychosis, behavioral disturbance, and depression. Misidentification delusions and behavioral disturbance were the only symptom categories that significantly increased during follow-up. Wandering or agitation and physical aggression contributed to the increase in behavioral disturbance (Table 1). Similar results were obtained when the sample was restricted to the 156 patients who completed 3 years of follow-up. Somatic and abandonment delusions were rare at all points and were not analyzed further.

RELATION OF SYMPTOM CATEGORIES TO CLINICAL VARIABLES AT THE INITIAL EXAMINATION

At the initial examination, sex, ethnicity, age, duration of illness, years of education, and history of psychiatric disorder were not associated with the presence of any symptom category. Greater cognitive impairment (ie, low mMMSE score) occurred in patients with misidentification delusions, behavioral disturbance, and depressed mood. Increased functional impairment (ie, a high BFAS score) occurred in patients with delusions (any type), misidentification delusions, and insomnia. Associations between the other symptom categories, mMMSE scores, and BFAS scores were either at the trend level or not significant (**Table 2**).

MARKOV ANALYSES

Markov analyses were conducted to evaluate the transition probabilities for the onset (ie, absent at 1 point but present at the next point) and persistence (ie, present at 1 point and at the next) of specific symptoms (**Table 3**). For the onset of new symptoms, the transition probability was greatest for behavioral disturbance (ie, .36, which means that 36% of the patients without a behavioral disturbance at 1 visit manifested a behavioral disturbance at the next visit) and its subcategory of wandering or agitation and lowest for depressed mood with vegetative signs and insomnia. Hallucinations and paranoid and misidentification delusions showed intermediate transition probabilities. For persistence of symptoms, behavioral disturbance had the highest and depressed mood with vegetative signs had the lowest transition probability. The results of the Markov analyses were similar at each of the 3 sites.

Psychiatric history (covariate, present or absent) did not significantly alter the transition probabilities for any symptom category. A history of depression showed trend-level associations for current depressed mood (Wald test, $P<.05$). Neuroleptic use did not significantly decrease the transition probability for persistence of psychotic or behavioral symptoms, antidepressant use did not decrease the transition probability for persistence of depressed mood, and benzodiazepine use did not decrease the transition probability for persistence of behavioral disturbance or insomnia. The main Markov analyses were performed again after restricting the sample to patients who did not receive psychotropic medications at any time

Table 3. Markov Analyses: Transition Probabilities for Onset and Persistence of Symptoms (at the Next 6-Month Interval) During Follow-up (Up to 5 Years)

Psychopathologic Feature	Transition Probabilities* (n=1181)†	
	Onset of New Symptom	Persistence of Symptom
Any type of delusion‡	.17	.59
Paranoid	.11	.45
Misidentification	.10	.56
Hallucinations	.09	.52
Behavior disturbance	.36	.80
Wandering or agitation	.31	.74
Physical aggression	.10	.53
Depressed mood	.14	.47
Insomnia	.06	.41
Depressed mood with vegetative signs	.05	.28

*Transition probabilities range from 0 to 1. A transition probability of .11 for the onset of paranoid delusions indicates that 11% of the patients without a paranoid delusion manifested a paranoid delusion at the next visit (after the 6-month interval). A transition probability of .45 for the persistence of paranoid delusions indicates that 45% of the patients with a paranoid delusion again manifested a paranoid delusion at the next visit (after the 6-month interval).

†*n* indicates the number of subjects times the number of points at which the symptom was assessed.

‡*n*=1180.

Table 4. Persistence of Symptoms in Patients With Alzheimer Disease at 6-Month Intervals (5-Year Follow-up)

Psychopathologic Feature	Maximum Frequency*				
	Absent	1 of 4	2 of 4	3 of 4	4 of 4
Any delusion	30.6	20.0	17.8	18.9	12.8
Paranoid	46.1	23.9	13.9	12.2	3.9
Misidentification	54.4	17.2	14.4	8.3	5.6
Hallucinations	60.0	18.9	11.1	4.4	5.6
Behavior disturbance	8.3	9.4	14.4	21.7	46.1
Wandering or agitation	14.4	14.4	16.7	21.7	32.8
Physical aggression	61.1	14.4	12.8	8.9	2.8
Depressed mood	41.1	23.9	17.2	9.4	8.3
Insomnia	64.4	17.2	10.6	5.6	1.7
Depressed mood with vegetative signs	71.7	19.4	7.8	0.0	1.1

*Maximum frequency for the presence of each symptom category at any 4 consecutive points, regardless of when the symptom was first manifested. All values are percentages.

point, and similar results were obtained. The use of experimental drugs to enhance cognition in AD (covariate, present or absent) did not significantly alter the transition probability for any symptom category.

The presence of delusions, hallucinations, behavioral disturbance, or depressed mood at the initial examination was unassociated with an increased risk of dropout 6 months later. Similarly, the presence of these symptom categories at 12 months did not affect dropout at 18 months.

Additional Markov analyses for the onset of new symptoms were conducted with mMMSE (dichotomized around the mean of 38, mild impairment) and BFAS (dichotomized around the median of 5) scores included as covariates. Patients with low mMMSE scores had a higher transition probability (ie, .20 or 20%) for the development of delusions (any type) at the next visit than patients with high mMMSE scores (transition probability, .12 or 12%; Wald test, $P<.01$). Patients with low mMMSE scores had a higher transition probability for the development of misidentification delusions (low vs high mMMSE score, .10 vs .04; Wald test, $P<.01$) and hallucinations (low vs high mMMSE score, .23 vs .03; $P<.005$) but not paranoid delusions (low vs high mMMSE score, .13 vs .10). Blessed Functional Activity Scale scores did not affect the transition probability for the development of any psychotic symptom. Patients with low mMMSE scores had a higher transition probability of behavioral disturbance developing (low vs high mMMSE score, .69 vs .27; $P<.001$), including the subcategories of wandering or agitation (low vs high mMMSE score, .57 vs .20; $P<.005$) and physical aggression (low vs high mMMSE score, .19 vs .03; $P<.001$). High BFAS scores increased the transition probability of physical aggression only developing (high vs low BFAS score, .07 vs .03; $P<.01$). Neither mMMSE nor BFAS scores affected the likelihood of developing depressed mood or depressed mood with vegetative features.

PERSISTENCE OF SYMPTOMS AT 6-MONTH INTERVALS DURING FOLLOW-UP

The persistence of specific symptoms was evaluated by using all available follow-up points (up to 5 years). The maximum frequency of symptoms at any 4 consecutive visits, regardless of when the symptom was first manifested, was calculated. A total of 180 patients completed a minimum of 4 consecutive visits (duration, 2 years).

Paranoid delusions, hallucinations, and misidentification delusions usually did not persist for 4 consecutive visits (**Table 4**). However, misidentification delusions doubled in frequency during the first 3 years of follow-up (Table 2), and even longer follow-up may have revealed greater persistence of this symptom. Behavioral disturbance was the most persistent symptom category, with wandering or agitation largely accounting for this effect. Wandering or agitation was present at 3 or more of 4 consecutive visits in the majority (ie, 54.5%) of the sample, but physical aggression rarely persisted (ie, 2.8% at 4 consecutive visits). Depressed mood was present at 4 consecutive visits in 8.3% of the sample, and depressed mood with vegetative signs was the least persistent (1.1% at ≥3 of 4 visits) of all the symptoms examined (Table 4).

During these 4 consecutive visits with maximum symptom frequency, neuroleptic use was associated with paranoid delusions (χ^2=17.5, *df*=4, $P<.002$), misidentification delusions (χ^2=21.0, *df*=4, $P<.001$), hallucinations (χ^2=20.5, *df*=4, $P<.001$), and behavioral disturbance (χ^2=26.7, *df*=4, $P<.001$). Antidepressant use tended to be associated with depressed mood (χ^2=11.1, *df*=4, $P<.05$). Benzodiazepine use tended to be associated with the presence of behavioral disturbance (χ^2=12.2, *df*=4,

$P<.02$) but not with insomnia (a low-frequency symptom), depressed mood, or any psychotic feature.

COMMENT

In this multicenter, prospective study, the prevalence of specific types of psychopathologic features was consistent with findings from other studies of outpatients with AD.[5,13,15,21,38-41] Behavioral disturbance, particularly wandering or agitation, occurred in half the sample. Paranoid and misidentification delusions and hallucinations were less common. Somatic and abandonment delusions were rare.[14] Depressed mood occurred in one quarter of the sample, but depressed mood with vegetative signs was rare.

The prospective, longitudinal data are novel and have implications for clinicians and caregivers. Behavioral disturbance was common and often persistent, primarily because of the symptom of agitation.[42] Physical aggression was infrequent and persisted for 2 years or more in only 2.8% of the sample. However, Markov analyses indicated a 53% probability for physical aggression to persist from one visit to the next, and this symptom tripled in frequency from the initial examination to the 3-year follow-up examination. Therefore, physical aggression may show greater persistence in more advanced stages than those evaluated in this study.[2,9] Misidentification delusions doubled in frequency during follow-up, suggesting that this symptom may become more persistent in advanced stages. Paranoid delusions and hallucinations did not increase notably during the study period. These symptoms showed moderate persistence from one visit to the next and rarely persisted for 4 consecutive visits.[15,21]

The prevalence of depressed mood did not change during the study. Depressed mood with vegetative signs was uncommon at all points and rarely persisted. However, prior studies indicate that 10% to 30% of patients with AD meet the diagnostic criteria for major depression.[14,22] Nonspecific symptoms in patients with AD (eg, psychomotor change, apathy or lack of interest, sleep difficulties, and poor concentration) may artificially raise prevalence rates for major depression.[26,43,44] Three methodological caveats should be noted: patients with early AD who often manifest depression may have been missed because of the entry criteria,[45] antidepressant treatment may have altered symptom presentation in this naturalistic study, and the informant's mood state is known to influence reporting of depression in the patient with AD.[46]

During follow-up, strong associations existed between specific subtypes of target psychopathologic feature and the use of psychotropic medications. However, Markov analyses also indicated that these medications did not notably decrease the likelihood of symptom persistence. These data about psychotropic medications have limitations. Treatment was based on the physician's choice, and optimal dosing and patient compliance were not ensured. The CUSPAD was developed primarily to study phenomenological featues and not to assess change in treatment trials, and most items lack quantitative ratings of severity. Therefore, medication-induced reductions in symptom severity, without symptom remission, would have been missed with this instrument.[16]

Nevertheless, the persistent nature of agitation indirectly suggests that treatment of this target behavior may need to be prolonged. Paranoid delusions and hallucinations were somewhat less persistent, indicating that not all patients need long-term neuroleptic treatment for these symptoms. The evanescent nature of depressed mood with vegetative features suggests that short-term treatment strategies may be appropriate.[47] These speculations need to be tested by empirical research.

The baseline data and the longitudinal analyses indicated that most psychotic features and behavioral disturbances were associated with greater cognitive impairment, except for paranoid delusions.[48,49] Functional impairment did not show notable associations with measures of psychosis in the longitudinal data set, but high BFAS scores did increase the likelihood of the onset of physical aggression. The lack of association between depressive symptoms and either cognitive or functional impairment suggests that depression may not be characteristic of any specific stage in patients with mild to moderate AD.[14]

In summary, this prospective, longitudinal study of a multicenter cohort of outpatients with AD provided new information about the likely duration and persistence of psychopathologic symptoms. Behavioral disturbance, particularly agitation, is common and persistent in patients with AD. Psychotic symptoms are less common and show moderate persistence over time. Depressed mood with vegetative signs is uncommon and rarely persists. These naturalistic data suggest leads about the optimal treatment duration for specific subtypes of psychopathologic features, an issue that needs to be tested by empirical research.

Accepted for publication April 22, 1996.

This work was supported in part by federal grants AG07370, AG08702, and RR00645 from the National Institute on Aging and MH44176 and MH50038 from the National Institute of Mental Health, Bethesda, Md; and the Charles S. Robertson Memorial Gift for Alzheimer Disease Research.

Reprints: Yaakov Stern, PhD, Sergievsky Center, 19th Floor, 630 W 168th St, New York, NY 10032.

REFERENCES

1. Reisberg B, Borenstein J, Salob SP, Ferris SH, Franssen E, Georgotas A. Behavioral symptoms in Alzheimer's disease: phenomenology and treatment. *J Clin Psychiatry.* 1987;48:9-15.
2. Rubin E, Drevets W, Burke WJ. The nature of psychotic symptoms in senile dementia of the Alzheimer type. *J Geriatr Psychiatry Neurol.* 1988;1:16-20.
3. Devanand D, Sackeim H, Brown R, Mayeux R. A pilot study of haloperidol treatment of psychosis and behavioral disturbance in Alzheimer's disease. *Arch Neurol.* 1989;46:854-857.
4. Schneider LS, Pollock VE, Lyness SA. A meta-analysis of controlled trials of neuroleptic treatment in dementia. *J Am Geriatr Soc.* 1990;38:553-563.
5. Teri L, Larson EB, Reifler BV. Behavioral disturbance in dementia of the Alzheimer's type. *J Am Geriatr Soc.* 1988;36:1-6.
6. Devanand DP, Brockington CD, Moody BJ, Brown RP, Mayeux R, Endicott J, Sackeim HA. Behavioral syndromes in Alzheimer's disease. *Int Psychogeriatr.* 1992;4:161-184.
7. Chandler JD, Chandler JE. The prevalence of neuropsychiatric disorders in a

nursing home population. *J Geriatr Psychiatry Neurol.* 1988;1:71-76.
8. Cohen-Mansfield J, Marx MS, Rosenthal AS. A description of agitation in a nursing home. *Gerontology.* 1989;3:M77-M84.
9. Swearer JM, Drachman DA, O'Donnell BF, Mitchell AL. Troublesome and disruptive behaviors in dementia. *J Am Geriatr Soc.* 1988;36:784-790.
10. Haller E, Binder RL, McNeil DE. Violence in geriatric patients with dementia. *Bull Am Acad Psychiatry Law.* 1989;17:183-188.
11. Bucht G, Adolfsson R. The comprehensive psychopathological rating scale in patients with dementia of Alzheimer type and multi-infarct dementia. *Acta Psychiatr Scand.* 1983;68:263-270.
12. Mayeux R, Stern Y, Sano M. Psychosis in patients with dementia of the Alzheimer type. *Ann Neurol.* 1985;18:184-187.
13. Reisberg B, Franssen E, Sclan SG, Kluger A, Ferris SH. Stage-specific incidence of potentially remediable behavioral symptoms in aging and Alzheimer's disease: a study of 120 patients using the BEHAVE-AD. *Bull Clin Neurosci.* 1989;54:95-112.
14. Wragg RE, Jeste DV. Overview of depression and psychosis in Alzheimer's disease. *Am J Psychiatry.* 1989;146:577-587.
15. Burns A, Jacoby R, Levy R. Psychiatric phenomena in Alzheimer's disease, I: disorders of thought content. *Br J Psychiatry.* 1990;157:72-76.
16. Devanand DP, Miller L, Richards M, Marder K, Bell K, Mayeux R, Stern Y. The Columbia University Scale for Psychopathology in Alzheimer's Disease. *Arch Neurol.* 1992;49:371-376.
17. Stern Y, Mayeux R, Sano M, Hauser WA, Bush T. Predictors of disease course in patients with probable Alzheimer's disease. *Neurology.* 1987;37:1649-1653.
18. Drevets WC, Rubin EH. Psychotic symptoms and the longitudinal course of dementia of the Alzheimer type. *Biol Psychiatry.* 1989;25:39-48.
19. Rosen J, Zubenko GS. Emergence of psychosis and depression in the longitudinal evaluation of Alzheimer's disease. *Biol Psychiatry.* 1991;29:224-232.
20. Haddad PM, Benbow SM. Visual hallucinations as the presenting symptom of senile dementia. *Br J Psychiatry.* 1992;161:263-265.
21. Burns A, Jacoby R, Levy R. Psychiatric phenomena in Alzheimer's disease, II: disorders of perception. *Br J Psychiatry.* 1990;157:76-81.
22. Greenwald BS, Kramer-Ginsberg E, Marin DB, Laitman LB, Hermann CK, Mohs RC, Davis KL. Dementia with coexistent major depression. *Am J Psychiatry.* 1989;146:1472-1478.
23. Rovner BW, Broadhead J, Spencer M, Carson K, Folstein MF. Depression and Alzheimer's disease. *Am J Psychiatry.* 1989;146:350-353.
24. Reifler BV, Larson E, Hanley R. Coexistence of cognitive impairment and depression in geriatric outpatients. *Am J Psychiatry.* 1982;139:623-626.
25. Ballard CG, Cassidy G, Bannister C, Mohan RNC. Prevalence, symptom profile, and aetiology of depression in dementia sufferers. *J Affect Disord.* 1993;29:1-6.
26. Forsell Y, Jorm AF, Fratiglioni L, Grut M, Winblad B. Application of *DSM-III-R* criteria for major depressive episode to elderly subjects with and without dementia. *Am J Psychiatry.* 1993;150:1199-1202.
27. Raskind M, Risse S, Lampe T. Dementia and antipsychotic drugs. *J Clin Psychiatry.* 1987;48:16-18.
28. Devanand DP. Role of neuroleptics in treatment of behavioral complications. In: Lawlor BA, ed. *Behavioral Complications in Alzheimer's Disease.* Washington, DC: American Psychiatric Press; 1995:131-151.
29. Casey DE. Neuroleptic drug-induced extrapyramidal syndromes and tardive dyskinesia. *Schizophr Res.* 1991;4:109-120.
30. Jeste DV, Lacro JP, Gilbert PL, Kline J, Kline N. Treatment of late-life schizophrenia with neuroleptics. *Schizophr Bull.* 1993;19:817-830.
31. Stern Y, Folstein M, Albert M, Richards M, Miller L, Bylsma F, Lafleche G, Marder K, Bell K, Sano M, Devanand DP, Loreck D, Wootten J, Bello J. Multicenter study of predictors of disease course in Alzheimer disease (the 'predictors study'), I: study design, cohort description, and intersite comparisons. *Alzheimer Dis Assoc Disord.* 1993;7:3-21.
32. American Psychiatric Association. *Diagnostic and Statistical Manual of Mental Disorders, Third Edition, Revised.* Washington, DC: American Psychiatric Association; 1987.
33. McKhann G, Drachman D, Folstein M. Clinical diagnosis of Alzheimer's disease: report of the NINCDS-ADRDA Work Group under the auspices of Department of Health and Human Services Task Force on Alzheimer's Disease. *Neurology.* 1984;34:939-944.
34. Mayeux R, Stern Y, Rosen J, Leventhal J. Depression, intellectual impairment and Parkinson's disease. *Neurology.* 1981;31:645-650.
35. Folstein M, Folstein S, McHugh P. 'Mini-Mental State': a practical method of grading the cognitive state of patients for clinicians. *J Psychiatr Res.* 1975;12:189-198.
36. Blessed G, Tomlinson BE, Roth M. The association between quantitative measures of dementia and of senile change in the cerebral grey matter of elderly subjects. *Br J Psychiatry.* 1968;114:797-811.
37. Stern Y, Andrews H, Pittman J, Sano M, Tatemichi T, Lantigua R, Mayeux R. Diagnosis of dementia in a heterogeneous population: development of a neuropsychological paradigm-based diagnosis of dementia and quantified correction for the effects of education. *Arch Neurol.* 1992;49:453-460.
38. Rubin EH, Kinscherf DA, Morris JC. Psychopathology in younger versus older persons with very mild and mild dementia of the Alzheimer type. *Am J Psychiatry.* 1993;150:639-642.
39. Cohen D, Eisdorfer CG, Paveza G, Luchins DJ, Freels S, Ashford JW, Semal T, Levy P, Hirschman R. Psychopathology associated with Alzheimer's disease and related disorders. *J Gerontol.* 1993;48:M255-M260.
40. Tariot PN, Mack JL, Patterson MB, Edland SD, Weiner MF, Fillenbaum G, Blazina L, Teri L, Rubin E, Mortimer JA, Stern Y. The Behavior Rating Scale for Dementia of the Consortium to Establish a Registry for Alzheimer's Disease. *Am J Psychiatry.* 1995;152:1349-1357.
41. Teri L, Truax P, Logsdon R, Uomoto J, Zarit S, Vitaliano P. Assessment of behavioral problems in dementia: the Revised Memory and Behavior Problems Checklist. *Psychol Aging.* 1992;7:622-631.
42. Wagner AW, Teri L, Orr-Rainey N. Behavior problems among dementia residents in special care units: changes over time. *J Am Geriatr Soc.* 1995;43:784-787.
43. Burke WJ, Rubin EH, Morris JC, Berg L. Symptoms of 'depression' in dementia of the Alzheimer type. *Alzheimer Dis Assoc Disord.* 1988;2:356-362.
44. Cummings JL. Dementia and depression: an evolving enigma. *J Neuropsychiatry Clin Neurosci.* 1989;1:236-242.
45. Devanand DP, Sano M, Tang M-X, Taylor S, Gurland BJ, Wilder D, Stern Y, Mayeux R. Depressed mood and the incidence of Alzheimer's disease in the elderly living in the community. *Arch Gen Psychiatry.* 1996;53:175-182.
46. Mackenzie TB, Robiner WN, Knopman DS. Differences between patient and family assessments of depression in Alzheimer's disease. *Am J Psychiatry.* 1989;146:1174-1178.
47. Reifler BV, Teri L, Raskind M, Veith R, Barnes R, White E, McLean P. Double-blind trial of imipramine in Alzheimer's disease patients with and without depression. *Am J Psychiatry.* 1989;146:45-49.
48. Bylsma FW, Folstein MF, Devanand DP, Richards M, Bello J, Albert M, Stern Y. Delusions and patterns of cognitive impairment in Alzheimer's disease. *Neuropsychiatr Neuropsychol Behav Neurol.* 1994;7:98-103.
49. Jeste DV, Wragg RE, Salmon DP, Harris MJ, Thal LJ. Cognitive deficits of patients with Alzheimer's disease with and without delusions. *Am J Psychiatry.* 1992;149:184-189.

The Role of Heredity in Late-Onset Alzheimer Disease and Vascular Dementia

A Twin Study

A. L. Mina Bergem, MD; Knut Engedal, MD, PhD; Einar Kringlen, MD, PhD

Background: This study compares the relative importance of heredity and environment in the development of Alzheimer disease and vascular dementia. The relationship between apolipoprotein E and dementia is also tested.

Methods: A total of 23 000 cognitively impaired subjects from Norwegian institutions for the elderly were identified, and their files were checked against the records of 26 000 twin pairs from the Norwegian Twin Register. A sample of 72 twin pairs was selected and thoroughly investigated clinically. The mean age of the sample was 80 years.

Results: The pairwise concordance rate for Alzheimer disease was 78% (7/9) among monozygotic and 39% (9/23) among dizygotic twin pairs. The probandwise concordance rate was 83% (10/12) among monozygotic and 46% (12/26) among dizygotic twin pairs. There was no significant difference in the rate of apolipoprotein E $\epsilon 4$ allele between twin pairs concordant and discordant for Alzheimer disease. By using tetrachoric correlations, the estimated heritability was approximately 0.6. Environmental factors shared by cotwins seemed to explain most of the remaining variance. In vascular dementia, there was no significant difference in pairwise concordance rates among monozygotic (1/6 [17%]) and dizygotic (4/16 [25%]) twin pairs or in probandwise concordance rates among monozygotic (2/7 [29%]) and dizygotic (5/17 [29%]) twin pairs.

Conclusion: Heredity is the major causal factor in late-onset Alzheimer disease, whereas environmental factors dominate in vascular dementia.

Arch Gen Psychiatry. 1997;54:264-270

DEMENTIA IS common in the elderly. Its prevalence increases with age, from approximately 1.5% at 65 to 69 years of age, to 13% at 80 to 84 years, to 30% at 90 years and older.[1] Alzheimer disease (AD) and vascular dementia (VaD) are the most frequent subtypes of dementia.

In general, there is a great variability in age at onset among persons with AD. Approximately 10% of all cases have an early onset, ie, younger than 65 years. In these cases, familial factors are generally noted. Current literature indicates that both familial and sporadic manifestations occur in late-onset AD.[2-4] There is general agreement that apolipoprotein E (APOE) $\epsilon 4$ allele plays a significant role in the association with AD, since approximately 50% of the total AD cases express this allele.[5-10] However, there are reasons to believe that this is not the only causal factor in the entire spectrum of late-onset AD.

The present study investigates the relative importance of heredity and environment in the development of AD and VaD, using the twin concordance method and tetrachoric correlations. If genetic factors play a causal role in the development of either disease, the concordance rate should be significantly higher in monozygotic (MZ) than in dizygotic (DZ) twin pairs.

The few available twin studies of dementia are inconclusive, primarily because of small and selected samples.[11-17] In the study of Kallmann from 1956,[11] both zygosity and clinical diagnostic criteria are uncertain. The follow-up study by Jarvik et al[12] in 1980 suffers from small numbers. The low number of DZ twins is a problem in the study of Nee et al[13] from 1987. This subject has previously been discussed thoroughly by Breitner et al[18] and Bergem.[4]

We know of 2 other twin studies of dementia that are in progress, in which the twins have been ascertained from twin registers. Preliminary findings from the study by Pedersen et al[19] show a concordance rate of 57% in 7 MZ and 27% in 15 DZ twin

From the Department of Psychiatry, Vinderen, University of Oslo (Drs Bergem and Kringlen), and the Department of Geriatric Medicine, Ullevål Hospital (Dr Engedal), Oslo, Norway.

SUBJECTS AND METHODS

SUBJECTS

From more than 23 000 cognitively impaired subjects residing in long-term institutions for the elderly throughout Norway, we selected a twin sample, born between 1895 and 1925, by cross-checking the names with the Norwegian Twin Register,[21] which lists over 26 000 twin pairs in this age group. One hundred fifty-one index cases were thus identified. Seventy-two index cases (probands) and their cotwins remained after exclusion of 79 index cases. Reasons for exclusion were death of one or both of the twins (n=43), refusals (n=30), and erroneous diagnosis (n=6).

The 72 remaining twin probands and their cotwins were classified into groups based on type of dementia, described later in the "Diagnostic Classification" section. Using this classification, there were 38 AD, 24 VaD, 5 mixed, and 5 miscellaneous (eg, Parkinson dementia, Huntington disease dementia, Creutzfeldt-Jakob disease, alcoholic dementia) probands. Among the 72 twin pairs, there were 101 cases of dementia of all types. Ninety percent of the AD sample were 75 years or older. There were no significant differences between the groups in mean age.

The zygosities of the same-sex twins were determined by DNA fingerprinting[22] after DNA was prepared from peripheral blood samples by standard procedures. This method, superior to questionnaires, especially in the elderly, yielded 51 DZ pairs that consisted of 34 (67%) same-sex pairs. The proportion of MZ to DZ twins in this sample, 29% MZ (21/72), corresponds to figures from the general population.[23,24] Exclusion because of death of cotwins did not alter the MZ/DZ rate.

From the DNA fingerprinting, the APOE isoforms were also obtained, partly as a zygosity control and partly to compare APOE isoforms in concordant and discordant twin pairs.

The total twin sample consisted of 105 (72.9%) women and 39 (27.1%) men, which is the expected sex distribution for this age group, since men have a shorter average life expectancy than women (Norwegian figures, 72 years vs 79 years). Among the 51 DZ twin pairs, there were 34 (67%) same-sex pairs and 17 (33%) opposite-sex pairs. There was a smaller proportion of opposite-sex pairs vs same-sex pairs, probably because of fewer surviving men. **Table 1** presents the age distribution of the sample with regard to concordance, zygosity, and gender for AD and VaD twin probands. There was no significant age difference among MZ and DZ AD probands. The men were slightly younger than the women. Similarly, there was no significant difference in age between MZ and DZ VaD probands, but the concordant pairs were slightly older than the discordant group. The SDs of the age distributions were about the same in the AD and the VaD groups, 6.6 and 5.8, respectively.

DIAGNOSTIC CLASSIFICATION

Each twin was investigated clinically and classified according to *DSM-III-R*[25] and the National Institute of Neurological and Communicative Disorders and Stroke (NINCDS) and the Alzheimer's Disease and Related Disorders Association (ADRDA)[26] criteria by 2 well-trained psychiatrists (A.L.M.B. and K.E.). A standardized test battery was used to provide information for the diagnosis of each twin's condition. These instruments included The Mini-Mental State Examination[27] and the modified Geriatric Mental Status Examination–Community Survey version,[28,29] the Hamilton Rating Scale for Depression,[30] and the Dementia Mood Assessment Scale.[31] The Norwegian version of the Eysenck Personality Questionnaire[32] was administered to nondemented cotwins and siblings. The Eysenck Personality Questionnaire results will be published later. Assessment of activities of daily living using the Katz index,[33] clinical examination, medical history, and Hachinski Ischemia Scale[34] were performed. Cerebral computed tomography was also performed to support the subgroup classification of dementia. The clinical examination included physical and neurological examination and appropriate laboratory tests. A complete life and family history of the individual twin was also obtained from nondemented family members.

Conventionally, AD has been grouped into familial and sporadic cases. However, the classification of sporadic cases might be attributed to lack of information or early death of relatives.[4] If 2 or more first-degree relatives of the AD twin pair in our sample had possible or probable AD, the disease was classified as definite familial AD. If only 1 first-degree AD relative had been identified, the cases were classified as probable familial cases. If both the parents and all the siblings had been registered as being nondemented 5 or more years after the mean age of onset, the AD cases were registered as sporadic.

The stage of AD was determined according to the Brief Cognitive Rating Scale,[35] the Global Deterioration Scale,[36] and the Functional Assessment Stage.[37] The diagnoses have been confirmed by cerebral postmortem autopsy in 16 cases so far. Results of 13 of the 16 autopsies conformed fully to the clinical diagnoses, 2 conformed partly, and 1 did not conform.

Continued on next page

pairs. Breitner et al,[18,20] who studied 14 MZ and 16 DZ twin pairs with AD, found concordance rates of 35% and 0%, respectively.

RESULTS

CONCORDANCE RATES AND FAMILY HISTORY

In the total sample of 72 twin pairs, without regard to type of dementia, the probandwise concordance was 57% (12/21) among MZ twins and 33% (17/51) among DZ twins. The relative risk between MZ and DZ was 1.71, with a 95% confidence interval of 1.00 to 2.93 (P=.05).

Table 2 presents the concordance rates for the sample of AD and VaD twin pairs. Thirty-eight twin probands with AD were identified. The probandwise concordance rate was 83% among MZ and 46% among DZ twin pairs. As can be observed, both the pairwise and the probandwise methods lead to almost identical figures. The AD concordance rates are substantially higher than the population prevalence for AD of about 10% for this age group. Among the 16 twin pairs discordant for AD, 5 (31%) cotwins had VaD. There were no age and sex dif-

To obtain reasonable reliability in clinical diagnoses, 2 clinicians (A.L.M.B. and K.E.) assessed all twins, using the information in the above-listed scales. To minimize bias in the estimation of concordance rates, the second clinician was kept unaware with regard to the zygosity status of the twin pairs and with regard to the clinical ratings by the first clinician. The interrater reliability between the first and second clinicians with respect to diagnoses was 0.93, using the κ statistic.[38] Most AD cases were late-stage cases, and thus relatively easy to classify.

From the total of 60 twins with AD, there were 47 cases of probable AD and 13 cases of definite autopsy-confirmed AD, according to the NINCDS-ADRDA criteria.

CONCORDANCE FIGURES

We counted a twin pair as completely concordant if both twins had the same subtype of dementia. The classic twin method of relative risk in concordance rates (both twins affected) among MZ and DZ twins was applied to estimate the heritability of dementia.

Concordance figures may be expressed in several ways. Most common are the pairwise and the probandwise methods.[39,40] The pairwise method is simple: the calculation of the percentage of concordant pairs in the sample. In the probandwise method, a pair of twins concordant for disease is counted twice if each of them is ascertained independently. Probandwise concordance expresses concordance in terms of the risk for the cotwin of an affected twin to develop the disease. In this study, both pairwise and probandwise concordance rates are presented.

TETRACHORIC CORRELATIONS

Any significant difference between concordance rates in MZ and DZ twin pairs can be ascribed to genetic factors. However, this difference alone does not provide sufficient information for a precise estimation of the proportion of the variation that is attributable to genetic differences in the total population. The estimation of heritability, defined as the fraction of genetic variance to the total variance, requires dimensional rather than dichotomous data from MZ and DZ pairs. Such data can be obtained from tetachoric correlations, which are based on a bivariate distribution of the dichotomous variables, assuming an underlying bivariate normal distribution (liability of developing the disease). The expected values of such tetrachoric correlations are identical with the expectation of the Pearson correlations between the corresponding hypothetical underlying variables (liability). Tetrachoric correlations were computed by the PRELIS computer program,[41] which also estimates asymptotic SEs. To estimate correlations, it was necessary to construct a 2×2 table for MZ and for DZ twin pairs, where the number of concordant nondemented twins was based on the estimated prevalence of the population, corrected for the age and sex in the twin sample. Drawing from the general twin population, one would have expected to find (100−X) percent of persons with no dementia, when X is equal to the prevalence. The assumed prevalence is based on a Norwegian prevalence study by Engedal and Haugen[42] and the European Community Concerted Action Epidemiology and Prevention of Dementia (EURODEM) prevalence study[43]; these studies report a population prevalence of 10% for AD in a population with the same age distribution as the actual twin sample. This prevalence is applied as the basis for the tetrachoric correlation estimates.

Besides estimating the proportion of nondemented pairs, it was necessary to adjust the proportion of discordant pairs. The reason for this is that concordant pairs are more likely to be selected than discordant pairs, because both twins are eligible as probands. The probands were mainly selected from nursing homes. About 50% of twins with dementia reside in nursing homes. The other 50%, who are less demented, still live at home. Approximately 80% of the demented nursing home residents were identified. The twin sample thus represents approximately 40% of the total population of demented twins in Norway. If the probability for a case to be included is .4, the probability for a discordant pair to be included is also .4, whereas the probability for a positive concordant pair to be included is .64 (ie, [.4+.4]−[.4×.4]).[44] To adjust for differential probability of inclusion, the total concordant-discordant proportion was changed by the ratio .64:.4, keeping the total number of pairs unchanged. The tetrachoric correlations were estimated from the 2×2 tables, where discordant pairs were equally distributed in the 2 diagonal cells.

The estimated MZ correlation is the sum of heritability and shared environment ($r_{MZ}=h^2+c^2$), and the DZ correlation is half the heritability with the shared environment added ($r_{DZ}=\frac{1}{2}h^2+c^2$). Thus, the formula for estimating the heritability is to double the difference between correlations for MZ and DZ ($h^2=2[r_{MZ}-r_{DZ}]$).[45] The remaining population variation is equal to environmental factors, which comprise shared environment (c^2) and nonshared environment (e^2). Shared environment includes both common effects of rearing and correlated environments, and might be computed as the difference between the MZ correlation and heritability. The parameter for nonshared environment, e^2, is the remaining proportion of the variation.

ferences between the concordant and discordant pairs (Table 1).

In 68% (26/38) of all AD pairs there was a known positive family history of AD. There was no significant difference between concordant and discordant DZ twin pairs with regard to the number of familial AD cases. Further, there was no difference among MZ and DZ concordant twins. However, the numbers are small.

There was information available on the parents of 22 of these 26 familial pairs. Among the remaining 12 pairs (32%) with no known positive family history of AD, there was lack of parental information in 3 cases. Further, the siblings had died of "competing" diseases before the possible age at onset of AD, or the relatives provided insufficient information on the siblings. Thus, 11 of these pairs could not be classified as sporadic cases (no family history of AD). Only 1 discordant AD case in a DZ pair was identified as sporadic, although the father died at the age of 74 years without dementia.

With respect to the 24 VaD twin pairs, the probandwise concordance rates were identical for MZ and DZ sets (Table 2). Both concordance rates were slightly lower than the comorbidity rate between AD and VaD twins, but still higher than the expected prevalence in the general population. There were no sex differences between the concordant and discordant VaD twins, but the discordant twins were slightly, but not significantly, younger (Table 1).

APOE GENOTYPES

The APOE genotypes were analyzed in 17 AD twin pairs. The $\epsilon 4$ allele frequency was 33% (8/24) in concordant DZ pairs and 31% (5/16) in discordant DZ pairs. In the discordant DZ pairs, the $\epsilon 4$ allele frequency was 38% (3/8) in affected twins and 25% (2/8) in nonaffected cotwins. None of these differences were statistically significant. Among the 18 familial AD cases analyzed for APOE, there were 8 twins (44%) without the $\epsilon 4$ allele. The $\epsilon 4$ allele frequency was 42% (15/36) among the familial cases.

Table 1. Age Distribution With Regard to Concordance, Zygosity, and Gender in Alzheimer Disease and Vascular Demented Probands

Categories of Twins	Alzheimer Disease: No. of Probands	Alzheimer Disease: Mean (Range) Age, y	Vascular Dementia: No. of Probands	Vascular Dementia: Mean (Range) Age, y
Concordant	22	80 (66-91)	7	85 (80-92)
Discordant	16	77 (66-89)	17	79 (69-88)
Monozygotic	12	77 (66-87)	7	80 (74-88)
Dizygotic	26	79 (66-91)	17	81 (69-92)
Same-sex females	25	78 (66-89)	12	81 (75-92)
Same-sex males	4	75 (66-84)	6	79 (74-85)
Opposite sex	9	80 (69-91)	6	79 (69-88)
Total	**38**	79 (66-91)	**24**	81 (69-92)

AGE AT ONSET

There was no significant difference in age at onset between MZ and DZ concordant or discordant AD twin pairs (**Table 3**). Of the 60 cases, the age range at onset was 54 to 86 years, with a mean of 72.7 years. As expected, only 5 twins in 4 pairs (8%) were younger than 65 years at onset. By excluding early-onset cases, there was practically no change in the estimates of relative risk for AD (Table 2).

The mean level of AD was 5.3 according to the Brief Cognitive Rating Scale and 5.6 according to the Global Deterioration Scale, where 1 indicates no dementia and 7, complete dementia. The mean intrapair difference in age at onset was 3.1 years (range, 0-7 years) within concordant MZ pairs and 4.4 years (range, 0-10 years) within concordant DZ pairs.

In the 16 discordant pairs, the average duration of AD in the index twin was 3.0 years (range, 2-4 years) among the 2 MZ pairs and 7.0 years (range, 0-15 years) among the 14 DZ pairs.

CORRELATIONS

Correlations were estimated only in the AD group, where there was a significant difference between relative risks for MZ and DZ twins. **Table 4** shows the correlations based on population prevalences of 10%. The intrapair correlation for MZ is very high (0.96-0.97). Most of the variance is caused by genetic factors and shared environment, leaving only 2% to 4% to the nonshared environment. Since the DZ correlation is also rather high (0.65-0.69), shared environment is considerable (0.35-0.42). Still, heritability is the major factor, as the model

Table 2. Concordance Rates of Alzheimer Disease and Vascular Dementia in Twin Pairs*

Type of Concordance Estimate	No. of Twin Pairs: Concordant	No. of Twin Pairs: Discordant	Concordance Rate, %	RR (95% CI)	*P*
		Alzheimer Disease			
Pairwise					
MZ	7	2	78	1.99 (1.07-3.69)	.03
DZ	9	14	39		
Late-onset pairwise					
MZ	6	1	86	2.00 (1.12-3.57)	.02
DZ	9	12	43		
Probandwise					
MZ	10	2	83	1.81 (1.11-2.4)	.02†
DZ	12	14	46		
Late-onset probandwise					
MZ	9	1	90	1.80 (1.15-2.82)	.01
DZ	12	12	50		
		Vascular Dementia			
Pairwise					
MZ	1	5	17	0.67 (0.09-4.83)	.69
DZ	4	12	25		
Probandwise					
MZ	2	5	29	0.97 (0.24-3.88)	.98†
DZ	5	12	29		

**RR indicates relative risk (concordance rate$_{MZ}$/concordance rate$_{DZ}$); CI, confidence interval; MZ, monozygotic; and DZ, dizygotic. All* P *values are 2-tailed.*
†In the estimation of these P *values, some individuals are counted twice because of the probandwise method.*

Table 3. Age at Onset of Alzheimer Disease Cases

Categories of Twins	No. of Cases	Age, y		
		Mean	Range	SD
Concordant				
MZ proband	10	72.3	55-81	7.9
MZ cotwin*	10	71.8	55-82	11.7
DZ proband	12	73.7	65-86	6.4
DZ cotwin*	12	75.7	65-80	4.0
Discordant				
MZ proband	2	69.5	62-77	10.6
DZ proband	14	71.3	54-83	8.4
Total	**60**	72.7	54-86	7.5

Because the cotwins in 3 monozygotic (MZ) and 3 dizygotic (DZ) concordant pairs also were index cases, they are listed among the probands and among the cotwins. This is adjusted for in the calculation of mean age at onset. Among the discordant pairs all cases are probands, as the cotwins are not demented.

Table 4. Alzheimer Disease Twin Correlations, Heritability, and Environmental Effects for Different Probability Percentages of Positive Cases Included in the Sample When the Prevalence Is 10%*

Inclusion of Positive Cases	r_{MZ}	r_{DZ}	h^2	c^2	e^2
50%	0.97	0.69	0.55	0.42	0.02
40%	0.97	0.68	0.58	0.39	0.03
30%	0.96	0.65	0.61	0.35	0.04

Tetrachoric correlation between monozygotic (MZ): $r_{MZ}=h^2+c^2$; tetrachoric correlation between dizygotic (DZ): $r_{DZ}=\frac{1}{2}h^2+c^2$; heritability: $h^2=2(r_{MZ}-r_{DZ})$; common environment: $c^2=r_{MZ}-h^2$; and nonshared environment: $e^2=1.0-r_{MZ}$.

estimates the range of genetic factors to be 0.55 to 0.61 of the total variance. None of the parameters varied substantially with different probability percentages (30%, 40%, and 50%) for positive cases included in the sample.

The SEs are not listed in the table. Since there are some assumptions made to simulate general population data, the SE cannot be estimated precisely. A crude estimate of the SE of the heritability, based on the estimated SE of the tetrachoric correlations by the PRELIS program (approximately 0.05 for MZ correlations and 0.1 for DZ correlations), is 0.2 to 0.3. We cannot determine the precision of the estimates of the environmental factors.

COMMENT

The data indicate that genetic factors contribute strongly to the development of AD, whereas such factors are absent in VaD. Genes are obviously important in both early- and late-onset AD, regardless of APOE isoforms. We think that the data are robust, since we have been able to avoid some of the common methodological weaknesses related to sampling, zygosity, clinical diagnoses, and age correction.

SAMPLING AND ZYGOSITY

Sampling errors have been common in previous twin studies. The Nordic countries are at an advantage here, since national twin registers are available. The sampling in our study is based on cross-checking cognitively impaired cases with the Norwegian Twin Register established by Kringlen in 1962.[21] This register covers the total Norwegian population, and should be complete for all those born after 1905. By relying on twin cases reported from institutions, without a systematic check of the twin register, there is a risk of ascertaining relatively more concordant than discordant pairs. In the United States, advertising for volunteers has been the method used in several studies.[11-13] In several such samples, approximately two thirds of the twins are usually MZ, whereas in the general population only one third of twins are MZ.[23,24] Volunteers also more frequently tend to be women. In our study, both the MZ/DZ ratio and the sex ratio correspond to the ratios in the general population. Because the concordant cases have a higher chance of being included in the sample,[44] the pairwise concordance rates in both zygosity groups are likely to be considered as maximum figures. This is adjusted for in the estimation of tetrachoric correlations, as described earlier. If this also is adjusted for in the estimation of concordance rates, the rates should be 77% in MZ and 36% in DZ pairs,[44] which does not alter the conclusions of the findings.

Further, Table 4 demonstrates that there is practically no difference in estimated heritability, regardless of this twin sample representing 30%, 40%, or 50% of the total number of demented twin pairs in the population.

Since DZ pairs on the average share half their genes, it is necessary to sample a sufficient number of twins to obtain a "true" estimate of the genes involved. In several previous samples of demented twins, the number of DZ pairs is extremely low. In the study by Nee et al,[13] there was a slight difference in MZ and DZ concordance, but the number of DZ twins was too small to draw any conclusions. In our twin sample, one third of the twins are MZ and two thirds are DZ, which corresponds to the distribution in the general population. To our knowledge, ours is the only study in which opposite-sex DZ twin pairs have also been included.

CLINICAL DIAGNOSES

When both twins have definite dementia, the concordance is complete. When one twin has a clear-cut diagnosis of AD and the cotwin is somewhat cognitively impaired, the concordance is incomplete. In such cases, it is likely that the cotwin will manifest dementia later on. In our study, a twin pair is counted as concordant only if both twins have displayed the same subtype of dementia. We were very strict about the AD criteria. If there was any doubt about the cause of dementia in addition to AD, the case was assigned to the mixed dementia group. Thus, the AD group is "pure."

As the majority of cases were nursing home patients, most of the cases had moderate or severe dementia, which might be an advantage with regard to the estimation of concordance rates. According to Heston et al,[3] 10% to 20% of clinically diagnosed cases of AD are false positive. The proportion of false negatives is not known. A definite diagnosis of AD has to be based on a neuropathological diagnosis according to NINCDS-ADRDA criteria.[26] With refinements of the clinical diagnostics, the correlation between clinical diagnoses and autopsy results currently ranges from 70% to 100%.[46] So far, 15 of the diagnosed cases in this study have been confirmed by autopsy, and the agreement with clinical diagnoses is 94% (15/16).

AGE OF SAMPLE AND AGE AT ONSET

Since AD is an age-dependent disease,[47,48] persons with late onset with pathologic genes are likely to die of competing causes before AD is expressed. Thus, many of these individuals might falsely be considered to be sporadic cases, even if the relatives possess the pathologic genes. The fact that family members die of other diseases before they develop AD lowers risk estimates. On the other hand, relatives of index cases might become affected because of the high population risk in the older age groups, without sharing the gene with the proband. To estimate concordance rates in late-onset cases, all twins in the sample should have exceeded the mean age at onset by several years. The mean age of the sample is considerably higher in our study than in previous studies. Younger age of subjects and small sample sizes might explain why previous twin studies have observed considerably lower MZ and DZ concordance rates.

Even if AD were completely determined by genes and the diagnostic accuracy was 100%, MZ concordance rates would still be below 100%, because in some cases AD most likely would express itself in extreme old age.[48] There are examples of onset variations of more than 10 years within individual families,[49] and even within MZ pairs the age at onset may vary by several years.[13] If the mean sample age is lower than the expected mean age at onset, concordance rates are expected to be considerably lower, which might be the case in other studies. The age of the sample in any twin study of AD should be higher than the average age at onset, otherwise the sample is not representative. In the twin studies by Breitner et al[20] and Nee et al,[13] mean age is quite young with regard to late-onset cases, compared with the samples by Pedersen et al[19] and the present study.

HERITABILITY IN AD

The concordance rates and the relative risks are almost independent of pairwise or probandwise ascertainment in this sample. We have previously argued that our findings are relatively robust for several reasons. The correlation data support the interpretation of the concordance rates. The heritability based on the correlations is rather high, but may reflect random fluctuation as well as biases due to violation of some assumptions. We do not know the exact proportion of the demented twins included in the sample vs the total population of demented twins, but 40% is the most likely proportion. Estimates based on 30%, 40%, and 50% do not vary much (Table 4). As the sample size is small, the estimates of genetic and environmental effects based on tetrachoric correlations have large SEs.

It is interesting to note that the family history of AD was not stronger among concordant compared with discordant DZ twins. Seventy-five percent (9/12) of the concordant and 71% (10/14) of the discordant AD DZ probands displayed a family history of AD. If AD was divided into familial and sporadic cases, one would expect higher concordance among familial cases. This is not confirmed by our data. Only 1 case was classified as sporadic. In about 29% of the cases, there was not sufficient information about the families to classify them as familial or sporadic. Since AD is an age-dependent disease,[47,48] it is probable that some of these relatives might have carried the gene (or genes) for late-onset AD and died of competing causes before AD was expressed.

The 14 nondemented unaffected DZ cotwins showed no evidence of AD, probably because most of them do not share the genes of the index twin, although the genes are in the family. With older age, it is likely that a few discordant pairs in our sample may eventually become concordant, if they share the same genes. The 2 discordant MZ pairs have been discordant for just a few years, and the cotwins are still at high risk of developing the disease.

Just as for family history, there was no difference in APOE $\epsilon4$ frequency among concordant and discordant twins. About 70% of all twin pairs have a positive family history of dementia, but, nevertheless, 44% of the familial cases have no APOE $\epsilon4$. The difference between concordant and discordant pairs is not explained by family history or by APOE, which indicates that the classification of AD in familial and sporadic cases might be artificial and that there are other unknown genetic risk factors for AD than APOE $\epsilon4$.

SHARED AND NONSHARED ENVIRONMENT

In the AD group, the value of the shared environment (c^2) appears to be around 0.4. This is high considering that these twin pairs have lived most of their lives apart. None of the MZ or DZ twin pairs have lived together in adult life. Since the sample size is small, the true value might vary between 0 and 0.5. According to our results, nonshared environment explains only a negligible part of the environmental variance.

The concordance rates in VaD are similar in MZ and DZ twin pairs, which suggests that heredity might be excluded as a causal factor. Because of the relatively small number of pairs, the SEs and the 95% confidence intervals of the concordance rates are large. From these data, shared environment cannot be identified as a statistical risk factor at the .05 level, but as they stand, the data suggest that both shared and nonshared environment are probable risk factors in the development of VaD.

CONCLUSION

In this twin study, there was a significant difference in concordance between MZ and DZ twin pairs with regard to AD. Heritability of liability of developing AD, based on the most plausible assumption for prevalence, was estimated to be 0.6. These observations indicate that heredity plays a major role in the cause of AD.

No difference in MZ and DZ concordance was observed for VaD, a finding that supports an environmentally determined causation.

Accepted for publication July 10, 1996.

This study was supported by grants from the Norwegian Research Council for Science and the Humanities and the Norwegian Council for Mental Health. Grants were also received from the legacies of Anders Jahre, Solveig and Johan P. Sommer, Hans Evensen, Mr and Mrs Johan Petter Ebbel, Thordis and Johannes Gahr, Morten Dedekam Harboe, and Wilhelm Wilhelmsen.

We acknowledge Kristian Tambs, PhD, for statistical assistance and Philip S. Holzman, PhD, and Barry Reisberg, MD, for useful comments and criticism.

Reprints: A. L. Mina Bergem, MD, Department of Psychiatry, Vinderen, University of Oslo, PO Box 85 Vinderen, 0319 Oslo, Norway.

REFERENCES

1. Hofman A, Rocca WA, Brayne C, Breteler MB, Clarke M, Cooper B, Copeland JR, Dartigues JF, da Silva Droux A, Hagnell O, Heeren TJ, Engedal K, Jonker C, Lindesay J, Lobo A, Mann AH, Mølså PK, Morgan K, O'Connor DW, Sulkava R, Kay DWK, Amaducci F, for the EURODEM Prevalence Research Group. The prevalence of dementia in Europe: a collaborative study of 1980-1990 findings. *Int J Epidemiol.* 1991;20:736-748.
2. Heyman A, Wilkinson WE, Hurwitch BJ, Schmechel DE, Sigmon AH, Weinberg T, Helms MJ, Swift M. Alzheimer's disease: genetic aspects and associated clinical disorders. *Ann Neurol.* 1983;14:507-515.
3. Heston LL, Mastri AR, Anderson VE, White J. Dementia of the Alzheimer type: clinical genetics, natural history and associated conditions. *Arch Gen Psychiatry.* 1981;38:1085-1090.
4. Bergem ALM. Heredity in dementia of the Alzheimer type. *Clin Genet.* 1994; 46:144-149.
5. Saunders AM, Schmader K, Breitner JCS, Benson D, Brown WT, Goldfarb L, Goldgaber D, Manwaring MG, Szymanski MH, McCown N, Dole KC, Schmechel DE, Strittmatter WJ, Pericak-Vance MA, Roses A. Apolipoprotein E ε4 allele distributions in late-onset Alzheimer's disease and in other amyloid-forming diseases. *Lancet.* 1993;342:710-711.
6. Corder EH, Saunders AM, Strittmatter WJ, Schmechel DE, Gashell PC, Small GW, Roses AD, Haines JL, Pericak-Vance MA. Gene dose of apolipoprotein E type 4 allele and the risk of Alzheimer's disease in late onset families. *Science.* 1993;261:921-923.
7. Poirier J, Davignon J, Bouthillier D, Kogan S, Bertrand P, Gauthier S. Apolipoprotein E polymorphism and Alzheimer's disease. *Lancet.* 1993;342:697-699.
8. Brousseau T, Legrain S, Berr C, Gourlet V, Vidal O, Amouyel P. Confirmation of the ε4 allele of the apolipoprotein E gene as a risk factor for late-onset Alzheimer's disease. *Neurology.* 1994;44:342-344.
9. Lannfeldt L, Lilius L, Nastase M, Viitanen M, Fratiglioni L, Eggertsen S, Berglund L, Angelin B, Linder J, Winblad B, Basun H. Lack of association between apolipoprotein E allele ε4 and sporadic Alzheimer's disease. *Neurosci Lett.* 1994; 169:175-178.
10. van Duijn CM, de Knijff P, Crutz M, Whenert A, Havekes LM, Hofman A, van Broeckhoven C. Apolipoprotein E ε4 allele in a population-based study of early-onset Alzheimer's disease. *Nature Genet.* 1994;7:74-78.
11. Kallmann FJ. Genetic aspects of mental disorder in later life. In: Kaplan OJ, ed. *Mental Disorders in Later Life.* 2nd ed. Stanford, Calif: Stanford University Press; 1956:chap 3.
12. Jarvik LF, Ruth V, Matsuyama SS. Organic brain syndrome and ageing: a six-year follow-up of surviving twins. *Arch Gen Psychiatry.* 1980;37:280-286.
13. Nee LE, Eldridge R, Sunderland T, Thomas CB, Katz D, Thompson KE, Weingartner H, Weiss H, Julian C, Cohen R. Dementia of the Alzheimer type: clinical and family studies of 22 twin pairs. *Neurology.* 1987;37:359-363.
14. Kumar A, Schapiro MB, Grady CL, Matocha MF, Haxby JV, Moore AM, Luxenberg JS, St George-Hyslop PH, Robinette CD, Ball MJ. Anatomic, metabolic, neuropsychological and molecular genetic studies of three pairs of identical twins discordant for dementia of the Alzheimer's type. *Arch Neurol.* 1991;48:160-168.
15. Creasey H, Jorm A, Longley W, Broe GA, Henderson AS. Monozygotic twins discordant for Alzheimer's disease. *Neurology.* 1989;39:1474-1476.
16. Hunter R, Dayan AD, Wilson J. Alzheimer's disease in one monozygotic twin. *J Neurol Neurosurg Psychiatry.* 1972;35:707-710.
17. Renvoize EB, Mindham RHS, Stewart M, McDonald R, Wallace RD. Identical twins discordant for presenile dementia of the Alzheimer type. *Br J Psychiatry.* 1986;149:509-512.
18. Breitner JCS, Gatz M, Bergem ALM, Christian JC, Mortimer JA, McClearn GE, Heston LL, Welsh KA, Anthony JC, Folstein MF, Radebaugh TS. Use of twin cohorts for research in Alzheimer's disease. *Neurology.* 1993;43:261-267.
19. Pedersen NL, Gatz M, Winblad B, Pearson CG, Berg S. Dementias in Swedish twins. *Prog Clin Biol Res.* 1989;317:217-222.
20. Breitner JCS, Welsh KA, Magruder-Habib KM, Churchill CM, Robinette CD, Folstein MF, Murphy EA, Priolo CC, Brandt J. Alzheimer's disease in the National Academy of Sciences Registry of ageing twin veterans, I: pilot investigations. *Dementia.* 1990;1:297-303.
21. Kringlen E. Norwegian Twin Registers. *Prog Clin Biol Res.* 1978;24,PtB:185-187.
22. Jeffreys AJ, Wilson V, Thein SL. Individual-specific 'fingerprints' of human DNA. *Nature.* 1985;316:76-79.
23. Lykken DT, McGue M, Tellegen A. Recruitment bias in twin research: the rule of two-thirds reconsidered. *Behav Genet.* 1987;17:343-362.
24. Emery AEH. *Methodology in Medical Genetics: An Introduction to Statistical Methods.* Edinburgh, Scotland: Churchill Livingstone; 1976.
25. American Psychiatric Association. *Diagnostic and Statistical Manual of Mental Disorders, Third Edition, Revised.* Washington, DC: American Psychiatric Association; 1987.
26. McKhann G, Drachman D, Folstein M, Katzman R, Price D, Stadlan EM. Clinical diagnosis of Alzheimer's disease: report of the NINCDS-ADRDA Work Group under the auspices of Department of Health and Human Services Task Force on Alzheimer's Disease. *Neurology.* 1984;34:939-944.
27. Folstein MF, Folstein SE, McHugh PR. 'Mini Mental State': a practical method for grading the cognitive state of patients for the clinician. *J Psychiatr Res.* 1975;12:189-198.
28. Henderson AS, Duncan-Jones P, Finlay-Jones RA. The reliability of the Geriatric Mental State Examination: Community Survey version. *Acta Psychiatr Scand.* 1983;67:281-289.
29. Engedal K, Haugen PK, Gilje K, Laake P. Efficacy of short mental tests in the detection of mental impairment in old age. *Compr Gerontol A.* 1988;2:87-93.
30. Hamilton M. A rating scale for depression. *J Neurol Neurosurg Psychiatry.* 1960;23:56-62.
31. Sunderland T, Alterman IS, Yount D, Hill JL, Tairot PN, Newhouse PA, Mueller EA, Mellow AM, Cohen RM. A new scale for the assessment of depressed mood in demented patients. *Am J Psychiatry.* 1988;145:955-959.
32. Eysenck SBG, Tambs K. Cross-cultural comparison of personality: Norway and England. *Scand J Psychol.* 1990;31:191-197.
33. Katz S, Ford AB, Moskowitz RW, Jackson BA, Jaffe M. Studies of illness in the aged: the index of ADL: a standardized measure of biological and psychosocial function. *JAMA.* 1963;185:914-919.
34. Hachinski VC, Iliff LD, Zilhka E, Du Boulay GH, McAllister VL, Marshall J, Russel RW, Symon L. Cerebral blood flow in dementia. *Arch Neurol.* 1975;32: 632-637.
35. Reisberg B, Ferris SH. Brief Cognitive Rating Scale (BCRS). *Psychopharmacol Bull.* 1988;24:629-636.
36. Reisberg B, Ferris SH, de Leon MJ, Crook T. Global Deterioration Scale (GDS). *Psychopharmacol Bull.* 1988;24:661-663.
37. Reisberg B. Dementia: a systematic approach to identifying reversible causes. *Geriatrics.* 1986;41:30-46.
38. Bartko J, Carpenter WT. On the methods and theory of reliability. *J Nerv Ment Dis.* 1976;163:307-317.
39. Kringlen E. *Heredity and Environment in the Functional Psychoses: An Epidemiological-Clinical Twin Study.* Oslo, Norway: Universitetsforlaget; 1967.
40. Allen G, Harvald B, Shields J. Measures of twin concordance. *Acta Genet Stat Med.* 1967;17:475-481.
41. Jöreskog KG, Sörbom D. *PRELIS: A Preprocessor for LISREL.* Mooresville, Ind: Scientific Software; 1988.
42. Engedal K, Haugen PK. The prevalence of dementia in a sample of elderly Norwegians. *Int J Geriatr Psychiatry.* 1993;8:565-569.
43. Rocca WA, Hofman A, Brayne C, Breteler MMB, Clarke M, Copeland JR, Dartigues JF, Engedal K, Hagnell O, Heeren TJ, Jonker C, Lindesay J, Lobo A, Mann AH, Mølså PK, Morgan K, O'Connor DW, da Silva Droux A, Sulkava R, Kay DWK, Amaducci L, for the EURODEM Prevalence Research Group. Frequency and distribution of Alzheimer's disease in Europe: a collaborative study of 1980-1990 prevalence findings. *Ann Neurol.* 1991;30:381-390.
44. Kringlen E. Twins: still our best method. *Schizophr Bull.* 1976;2:429-433.
45. Falconer DS. *Introduction to Quantitative Genetics.* 2nd ed. London, England: Longman Scientific & Technical; 1981.
46. Jellinger K. Morphology of Alzheimer's disease and related disorders. In: Maurer K, Beckmann H, Riederer P, eds. *Alzheimer's Disease: Epidemiology, Neuropathology, Neurochemistry and Clinics.* Vienna, Austria: Springer; 1990:61-77.
47. Breitner JCS, Murphy EA, Folstein MF. Familial aggregation in Alzheimer dementia, II: clinical genetic implications of age-dependent onset. *J Psychiatr Res.* 1986;20:45-55.
48. Breitner JCS, Folstein MF, Murphy EA. Familial aggregation in Alzheimer dementia, I: a model for the age-dependent expression of an autosomal dominant gene. *J Psychiatr Res.* 1986;20:31-43.
49. Bird TD, Sumi SM, Nemens EL, Nochlin D, Schellenberg G, Lampe TH, Sadovnick A, Chui H, Miner GW, Thinklenberg J. Phenotypic heterogeneity in familial Alzheimer's disease: a study of 24 kindreds. *Ann Neurol.* 1989;25:12-25.

Familial Aggregation and Phenomenology of 'Early'-Onset (at or Before Age 20 Years) Panic Disorder

Risë B. Goldstein, PhD; Priya J. Wickramaratne, PhD; Ewald Horwath, MD; Myrna M. Weissman, PhD

Background: While early age at onset has been associated with increased familial risk, increased clinical severity, and distinctive patterns of comorbidity in a range of psychiatric disorders, it has received limited attention in panic disorder, both in family studies and with respect to clinical presentation.

Methods: A family study of 838 adult first-degree relatives of 152 probands in 3 diagnostic groups (panic disorder with or without major depression, subdivided by age at onset at or before 20 and after 20 years, and screened normal controls) was used to examine familial aggregation of panic disorder by proband age at panic disorder onset. Phenomenology of panic disorder in ill probands and their affected adult first-degree relatives was investigated as a function of proband panic disorder onset at or before 20 vs after 20 years of age.

Results: Compared with adult first-degree relatives of normal controls, the risks of panic disorder in adult first-degree relatives of probands with panic disorder onset at or before 20 and after 20 years of age were increased 17-fold and 6-fold, respectively. These findings were not explained by the numerous potential confounding factors that we tested. Age at panic disorder onset did not appear to be specifically transmitted within families. The clinical presentation of panic disorder differed little in either probands or affected relatives by proband age at onset.

Conclusion: The strikingly elevated risk of panic disorder in relatives of probands with panic disorder onset at or before 20 years of age suggests that age at onset may be useful in differentiating familial subtypes of panic disorder and that genetic studies of panic disorder should consider age at onset.

Arch Gen Psychiatry. 1997;54:271-278

From the Department of Psychiatry, College of Physicians and Surgeons of Columbia University, and Division of Clinical-Genetic Epidemiology, New York State Psychiatric Institute, New York. Dr Goldstein is an Aaron Diamond Foundation Postdoctoral Research Fellow at Columbia University.

EARLY AGE at onset in a range of psychiatric disorders is associated with increased familial risk, including major depression (MDD),[1-7] bipolar disorder,[8-12] schizophrenia,[13] and obsessive-compulsive disorder (OCD).[14] Early onset also tends to be associated with increased clinical severity and distinctive patterns of comorbidity in MDD,[15] bipolar disorder,[10-12] and OCD.[16] However, age at onset of panic disorder (PD) has received limited attention as a subtype in family studies, in part because the epidemiology of PD, including the occurrence of onsets in childhood and adolescence, has only recently been characterized.[17-19]

Battaglia et al[20] recently reported an association in a family history study between increased familial risk of PD with agoraphobia and early age at onset of PD in probands ascertained from an anxiety clinic. In addition, some evidence exists that early-onset PD may represent a specific subtype with respect to clinical presentation, including distinctive patterns of comorbidity and panic symptoms. Wittchen and Perkonigg,[21] in an epidemiologic sample, found "early" onset (age ≤25 years) of panic to be associated with increased risks of agoraphobia, social phobia, and depression. By contrast, "late" onset (age >25 years) carried increased risks of substance abuse and the occurrence of multiple comorbid disorders. Age at onset also was associated with differences in panic symptom patterns: individuals with early onset less often experienced dyspnea, smothering sensations, and fear of dying.

The characterization of differences in familial aggregation by age at onset could further the understanding of patterns of familial transmission of PD. In addition, clear differences in the phenomenology of PD by age at onset could have implications for the treatment of this disorder. Herein, we used family study data to ex-

METHODS

PROBAND SELECTION

The overall purpose of the study was to obtain comprehensive data by direct interview and family history on the FDRs of probands with early-onset (at ≤30 years of age) MDD, PD with and without MDD, and of normal controls with no history of mental illness. The study methodology has been described in detail elsewhere.[22] Potential probands were ascertained from treatment clinics for anxiety disorders and depression at Yale University and from the New Haven site of the Epidemiologic Catchment Area (ECA) study. By design, about two thirds of the ill probands were selected from the clinics and one third from the ECA; all normal controls were ascertained from the ECA. This sampling strategy was deliberate to determine whether clinically ascertained probands had an overrepresentation of ill relatives. Probands were white and 18 to 70 years of age; they initially met diagnostic criteria for 1 of 4 study cells: PD without MDD, PD with MDD, early-onset MDD without PD, and no mental illness. After giving informed consent, potential probands were blindly reinterviewed by a member of the research team using the Schedule for Affective Disorders and Schizophrenia–Lifetime Version for Anxiety Disorders (SADS-LA).[23] The SADS-LA generated Research Diagnostic Criteria (RDC) and was modified to incorporate *DSM-III*[24] and *DSM-III-R*[25] criteria as well.

DIAGNOSTIC CRITERIA FOR PROBANDS

Potential probands were excluded from all groups if they met criteria for schizophrenia, mania, Briquet syndrome, antisocial personality disorder, or anorexia nervosa. Substance abuse was not exclusionary if it was chronologically secondary to the inclusion diagnosis, primary but mild, or followed by a substantial interval of recovery prior to the onset of the inclusion diagnosis. In this study, we focus on probands with PD with or without comorbid MDD and their FDRs, and compare them with probands with no mental illness and their FDRs. Probands with early-onset MDD and no PD were excluded from these analyses. The diagnostic criteria for probands with PD and probands who had no mental illness were as outlined below.

PD With or Without MDD

Probands were required to meet *DSM-III* criteria for PD. Those in the comorbid group were additionally required to meet the RDC, modified to require an illness of at least 4 weeks and impairment of functioning in the major social role, for MDD. Potential probands were excluded from the PD without MDD group if they reported any evidence of MDD during their lifetimes by any diagnostic criteria at any level of certainty.

Controls With No Mental Illness

Probands were included if they had received no lifetime psychiatric diagnoses during any of the 3 waves of ECA interviews based on the Diagnostic Interview Schedule (DIS)[26] nor on reinterview for this study with the SADS-LA.

ASSESSMENT OF FDRs

After the proband was accepted into the study, all FDRs, living or dead, who were 6 years of age or older were enumerated systematically from the proband using the Pedigree Collection Form,[27] and permission to contact FDRs was obtained from each proband. All consenting adult (defined by study protocol as ≥17.5 years old) FDRs were interviewed directly with the SADS-LA by clinically trained interviewers blind to proband diagnoses. Family history data were then obtained from all interviewed subjects on all FDRs, including the proband, using a modified version of the Family History Method for Research Diagnostic Criteria (FH-RDC).[28] Details of interviewer training and interrater reliability are given elsewhere.[22]

amine age at onset in probands as a predictor of rates of PD in relatives. A secondary aim was to examine the association between age at PD onset in probands and the clinical presentation of the disorder in probands and their affected first-degree relatives (FDRs).

RESULTS

This report focuses on 152 probands (107 with PD with or without comorbid MDD, and 45 who had no mental illness) and their 838 FDRs aged 17.5 years and older. The proportions of probands in the 2 ill groups with comorbid MDD were identical at 72%. Of the 672 adult FDRs in the 3 proband groups who were alive at the time data were collected, we directly interviewed a total of 347 (52%): 62 (55.4%) of 112 in the early-onset, 191 (51.9%) of 368 in the later-onset, and 94 (49.0%) of 192 in the no mental illness group; percentages of directly interviewed FDRs did not differ significantly by proband group (P=.55).

DEMOGRAPHIC CHARACTERISTICS OF PROBANDS

The demographic characteristics of the sample as a whole have been described in detail elsewhere.[22] They are summarized in **Table 1** for probands stratified on age at onset of PD and for normal controls. Ill probands with PD onset at or before 20 years of age were significantly younger than the probands with no mental illness. Both early- and late-onset ill probands were significantly more likely to be female than were normal controls. However, the groups did not differ in socioeconomic status defined by the Hollingshead index, marital status, highest level of education completed, or current religious affiliation. There were no

BEST-ESTIMATE DIAGNOSES

Best-estimate diagnoses were made by a psychiatrist or PhD clinical psychologist on each proband and FDR based on all available information from direct interviews, family history, and medical records.[29] Diagnosticians were blind to proband diagnostic group and to the status as probands or relatives of individuals being diagnosed. Diagnoses were made according to RDC, *DSM-III*, and *DSM-III-R* criteria and assigned 1 of 3 levels of certainty: possible, probable, or definite. Age at onset and severity of impairment due to each disorder were also estimated. Diagnostic hierarchies were not applied. Reliability of best-estimate diagnoses in this sample has been reported by Weissman et al.[22]

STATISTICAL ANALYSIS

Crude lifetime rates of PD in FDRs were compared by proband age at onset using χ^2 tests. Methods of survival time analysis were used to determine familial aggregation and to identify peak age of incidence of PD among FDRs while accounting for the fact that not all FDRs have passed through the full period of risk for PD. The cumulative survival function was used to determine familial aggregation.[5] The null hypothesis of homogeneity in the cumulative survival curves was tested using the log-rank test.[30] The hazard function, which can be interpreted as the age-specific incidence rate, was used to identify the peak age of incidence among FDRs in each subset of the analysis sample formed by stratifying on age at onset in probands.[31]

In family studies, higher rates of most disorders have been found among interviewed than not interviewed relatives[32]; in epidemiologic studies, the risk of PD has been shown to be higher in females than males and among younger than older individuals.[17] Therefore, these variables were included in a proportional hazard (PH) model[33] to control simultaneously for the potentially confounding effects of sex, interview status, and age of FDRs. In addition, while we have previously shown that proband ascertainment source is not associated with familial risk for PD in general,[34] we had not previously had occasion to examine the effect of this factor on the association between proband age at PD onset and rates in relatives. We, therefore, controlled for proband source in the PH model as well. The PH model is a quasi-parametric multivariable model that applies the multiple regression method to a survival distribution or other onetime event, such as the onset of a disorder. The PH procedure yields a ratio of the hazards, or age-specific incidences, of the outcome variable, such as onset of PD in FDRs, adjusted for the effects of the control variables.

In the examination of phenomenology of PD, crude lifetime rates of comorbid disorders and proportions of probands and FDRs with specific panic symptoms were compared by proband age at onset using χ^2 or, where 25% or more of expected cell counts were less than 5, two-tailed Fisher exact tests. Continuous variables such as number of symptoms experienced during panic attacks were compared using *t* tests.

In this article, we describe familial aggregation and phenomenology of probable and definite onsets of *DSM-III-R* PD in adult FDRs of probands with PD onsets at or before 20 and after 20 years of age. We had originally intended to examine familial aggregation of PD in adult relatives by decade of age at proband onset, but we had too few probands with onsets before their middle teens or after 40 years of age, as well as too few affected FDRs, to do this. We, therefore, began the data analysis using 3 proband age-at-onset groups (≤20, 21-30, and >30 years, respectively) and found no differences either in familial aggregation or in phenomenology between the two later-onset groups. Because of the lack of differences in our outcome variables and the relatively small number of affected FDRs, we then combined these 2 groups. Initial analyses stratified on proband diagnostic group (PD with vs without MDD) revealed very similar patterns of results across the 2 diagnostic groups. Therefore, we combined these 2 groups to increase sample size and statistical power.

differences between the 2 ill groups in proportions ascertained from any of the 3 recruitment sources (depression clinic, anxiety clinic, and ECA [P=.84]).

PHENOMENOLOGY OF PD IN PROBANDS BY AGE AT ONSET

Early-onset probands were significantly more likely than later-onset probands to manifest agoraphobia (96.0% vs 76.8%, P=.04) and OCD (16.0% vs 1.2%, P=.01). However, the number of probands with these comorbid conditions was small. The 2 groups did not differ in prevalence of other lifetime comorbid disorders. As shown in **Table 2**, early-onset probands were significantly more likely to have sought professional help specifically for PD. However, the 2 groups did not differ in symptom patterns or other clinical characteristics.

AGGREGATION OF PD IN ADULT FDRs BY PROBAND AGE AT ONSET

Unadjusted and Cumulative Age-Corrected Rates

Unadjusted and cumulative age-corrected lifetime rates per 100 of PD in FDRs by proband age at onset are given in **Table 3**. First-degree relatives of probands with onset at or before 20 years of age showed strikingly higher rates of PD compared with FDRs of later-onset ill probands and FDRs of normal controls. Rates of PD among FDRs of ill probands with PD onset after 20 years of age were also highly significantly increased compared with FDRs of normal controls. The pattern of results in the age-corrected rates was similar to that in the unadjusted rates. When we restricted the sample to interviewed FDRs, the same patterns of results were observed, although the actual rates of PD were higher.

Table 1. Demographic Characteristics of Probands by Group*

Characteristic	PD Onset ≤20 y (n=25)	PD Onset >20 y (n=82)	Never Mentally Ill (n=45)	*P*
	Proband Group			
Age, y, mean±SD†	40.4±10.4	43.6±9.8	48.0±10.5	<.001
Female,‡ %	72.0	80.5	44.4	
Social class,§ %				
I and II, highest	32.0	29.3	51.1	.08
III	28.0	41.5	22.2	
IV and V, lowest	40.0	29.3	26.7	
Marital status, %				
Married/cohabiting	68.0	74.4	75.6	.37
Separated/divorced	12.0	13.4	4.4	
Widowed	0.0	3.7	6.7	
Never married	20.0	8.5	13.3	
Highest level of education, %				
Graduate/professional	16.0	9.8	22.2	.20
College graduate	16.0	22.0	22.2	
High school graduate	48.0	59.8	51.1	
<High school	20.0	8.5	4.4	
Current religious affiliation, %				
Catholic	64.0	54.9	68.9	.14
Protestant	16.0	23.2	15.6	
Jewish	4.0	6.1	13.3	
Other/none	16.0	15.9	2.2	
Ascertainment source, %				
Depression clinic	8.0	12.2	0.0	
Anxiety clinic	72.0	69.5	0.0	
Community, ECA	20.0	18.3	100.0	

**PD indicates panic disorder; ECA, Epidemiologic Catchment Area.*
†$F(2, 149)=5.17$, P<.001; never mentally ill vs PD onset at ≤20 y (P<.05) by Scheffé test.
‡$\chi^2=17.65$, df=2, P<.001; PD onset at ≤20 y vs never mentally ill, P<.05; PD onset at >20 y vs never mentally ill, P<.001.
§Defined by the Hollingshead index.

Age-Specific Rates of PD in FDRs Stratified on Age at Onset in Probands

Examination of the hazard functions for PD by proband age-at-onset group (not shown here) revealed that, while age at onset in probands is strongly inversely related to risk of PD in FDRs, age at onset of PD does not appear to be specifically transmitted within families. In particular, the peak incidence of PD was observed between the ages of 31 and 40 years among FDRs of probands with PD onset at or before 20 years of age; among FDRs of probands with later PD onset, the peak incidence was observed between 21 and 30 years of age. However, since the numbers of affected FDRs were small in these categories of proband age at onset, these results should be interpreted with caution.

Risks of PD in FDRs by Age at Onset in Probands, Controlling for Current Age, Sex, and Interview Status of FDRs, and Ascertainment Source of Probands

After these potential confounders were controlled for, FDRs of probands with onset of PD at or before 20 years of age were at a 16.9-fold (95% confidence interval, 4.4-64.3, *P*<.001) and FDRs of probands with onset after 20 years of age were at a 5.6-fold (95% confidence interval 1.5-20.8, *P*=.01) increased risk of developing PD compared with FDRs of normal controls. Increasing age was independently protective, while sex and proband source were not independently associated with risk. However, removing proband source from the PH model resulted in a decrease in the hazard ratio from 16.9 to 14.5 for

Table 2. Clinical Characteristics of Panic Disorder (PD) in Ill Probands by Age at PD Onset

Characteristic	PD Onset at ≤20 y (n=25)	PD Onset at >20 y (n=82)	*P*
	Proband Group		
Buildup of panic attacks usually within 10 min, %	92.0	92.5	1.00
Frequency of panic attacks during worst episode, %			
< Weekly	12.0	24.4	.23
> Weekly, < daily	44.0	28.1	
At least daily	44.0	47.6	
Maximum No. of anxiety symptoms, mean±SD	9.9±3.4	10.0±3.0	.90
Moderate or severe impairment due to panic disorder, %	68.0	56.1	.29
Individual panic symptoms, %			
Shortness of breath	84.0	85.0	.90
Palpitations	92.0	97.5	.21
Chest pain/discomfort	64.0	51.3	.26
Choking feelings	48.0	52.5	.69
Smothering feelings	64.0	62.5	.89
Dizziness/lightheadedness/unsteadiness	92.0	86.3	.45
Derealization	48.0	43.8	.71
Paresthesias	52.0	57.5	.63
Hot or cold flashes	64.0	75.0	.28
Sweating	76.0	77.5	.88
Faintness/fear of passing out	68.0	78.8	.27
Abdominal cramps/nausea/diarrhea	60.0	46.3	.23
Trembling/shaking	80.0	76.3	.70
Fear of dying	56.0	53.8	.84
Fear of going crazy or losing control	76.0	64.6	.29
Professional help sought for panic, %	80.0	95.0	.02
Took medication for panic, %	88.0	82.5	.52
Hospitalized for panic, %	12.0	8.8	.63
Missed work due to panic, %	56.0	44.0	.30
Problems with friends due to panic, %	56.0	52.5	.76
Problems with family due to panic, %	32.0	46.3	.21
Help-seeking behavior during attacks, %			
None (bears it alone)	40.0	45.0	.82
Asks friends or family	36.0	36.3	
Asks strangers	4.0	2.5	
Demands help	4.0	7.5	
Makes unreasonable demands	16.0	8.8	
Emergency behavior during attacks, %			
Never	56.0	51.3	.45
At least once	16.0	27.5	
More than once but not usual	20.0	18.8	
Usual	8.0	2.5	
Interruption of function during attacks, %			
None	12.0	10.0	.59
Brief interruption	16.0	26.3	
Withdrawal from activity	20.0	25.0	
Flight	52.0	38.8	
No. of lifetime episodes of PD, mean±SD	3.1±6.4	6.7±21.0	.18

FDRs of early-onset probands, while leaving the hazard ratio for relatives of later-onset probands essentially unchanged. The results were similar when the analysis sample was restricted to interviewed FDRs.

CONSIDERATION OF POSSIBLE CONFOUNDING FACTORS

Given the large number of factors that may confound the results of family studies,[5,35,36] we undertook additional analyses to search for possible confounders that might explain our results.

Sociodemographic and Clinical Characteristics

As given in Table 1, probands differed by group in current age, and ill probands were significantly more likely to be female than were normal controls. However, age at onset distributions for PD did not differ by gender, and, within proband group, rates of PD did not differ by any of these demographic characteristics. Ill probands did not differ by age at onset in number of episodes of PD, nor in rates of most comorbid diagnoses. The effects of agoraphobia as a possible familial risk factor were examined separately and were shown not to explain the increased rates of PD among relatives of early-onset probands. Comorbid OCD in probands also did not explain the increased risk to relatives of early-onset probands; however, there were only 4 early-onset probands and 1 later-onset proband with comorbid OCD.

Generation and Birth Cohort

An unequal distribution by generation (parents, siblings, and offspring) or birth cohorts of FDRs by age at onset in probands could also have confounded our findings if the FDRs of early-onset probands tended to be younger than FDRs of later-onset probands and if earlier onset of PD occurred in FDRs of early-onset probands, ie, if there were specificity of transmission of age at onset. However, we observed no evidence of specificity of transmission of age at PD onset, so it does not appear that birth cohort or generation effects could confound these results.

Family Size

To determine if a few large families accounted for the results, we examined the proportion of probands with at least 1 affected FDR by proband age at onset. As such, each family with at least 1 FDR affected was counted only once. Fifty-six percent of early-onset, 23.2% of later-onset, and 3.6% of normal probands had at least 1 FDR affected with PD (overall $\chi^2 = 28.07$, $df=2$, $P<.001$). Our results, therefore, could not be explained by a few large families.

Nonrandom Mating

To determine whether nonrandom mating confounded our findings, we excluded the offspring of probands and repeated the previously described analyses for parents and siblings of probands only. The results (not shown here) were essentially the same as those for the sample as a whole. Nonrandom mating did not bias the overall results of the survival analyses.

Table 3. Unadjusted and Cumulative Age-Corrected Lifetime Rates/100 of PD in Adult First-Degree Relatives by Proband Group

	Proband Group*		
Variable	PD Onset at ≤20 y (n_p=25, n_r=134)	PD Onset at >20 y (n_p=82, n_r=449)	Never Mentally Ill (n_p=42, n_r=155)
Rates of PD			
Unadjusted†	17.2	6.7	1.2
Age-corrected‡	21.7	8.2	1.9

*PD indicates panic disorder; n_p, No. of probands; and n_r, No. of relatives.

†Overall χ^2=36.01, df=2, $P<.001$; proband PD onset at ≤20 y vs >20 y and at ≤20 y vs never mentally ill, $P<.001$; proband PD onset at >20 y vs never mentally ill, $P=.001$.

‡Overall log-rank log-rank χ^2=40.78, df=2, $P<.001$; proband PD onset at ≤20 y vs >20 y and at ≤20 y vs never mentally ill, $P=.001$; proband PD onset at >20 y vs never mentally ill, $P<.001$.

Length of Coresidence of FDRs With Probands

To determine whether longer coresidence with symptomatic probands by FDRs in the early-onset group could account for our findings (eg, by a behavioral modeling effect), we computed the length of coresidence of each interviewed FDR with his or her proband, following the proband's PD onset. Because this information is derived from the SADS-LA interview, it by definition could not be determined for uninterviewed FDRs. We then refit the multivariable models, restricting the analysis sample to directly interviewed FDRs. First-degree relatives of early-onset probands reported longer coresidence following probands' onset of PD. However, control for this variable did not alter the patterns of our results and only slightly altered the actual hazard ratios for PD among interviewed FDRs in each proband age-at-onset group compared with FDRs of normal controls. Thus, length of exposure to symptomatic probands did not account for our findings of dramatically increased risks in FDRs of probands with the earliest onsets.

PHENOMENOLOGY OF PD IN AFFECTED FDRs OF EARLY- AND LATE-ONSET PROBANDS

Compared with affected FDRs of probands with onset of PD after 20 years of age, affected FDRs of probands with earlier onset did not differ in lifetime prevalence of any comorbid disorders, total number of comorbid lifetime diagnoses, or proportions with multiple comorbid diagnoses (data available on request). However, as shown in **Table 4**, affected FDRs of early-onset probands more often reported choking feelings, derealization, and faintness or fear of passing out than did affected FDRs of later-onset probands. Affected FDRs of early-onset probands also reported significantly more severe interruption of

Table 4. Clinical Characteristics of PD in Affected Adult First-Degree Relatives of III Probands by Proband Age at PD Onset

Characteristic	Proband Group*: PD Onset at ≤20 y (n_p=25, n_{ar}=23)	PD Onset at >20 y (n_p=82, n_{ar}=30)	*P*
Buildup of panic attacks usually within 10 min, %	81.3	88.9	.66
Frequency of panic attacks during worst episode, %			
< Weekly	56.5	30.0	.15
> Weekly, < daily	26.1	43.3	
At least daily	17.4	26.7	
Maximum No. of anxiety symptoms, mean±SD	9.3±3.0	7.6±3.3	.11
Moderate or severe impairment due to PD, %	34.8	33.3	.91
Individual panic symptoms, %			
Shortness of breath	87.5	63.0	.16
Palpitations	75.0	88.9	.39
Chest pain/discomfort	43.8	44.4	.97
Choking feelings	56.3	25.9	.05
Smothering feelings	62.5	40.7	.17
Dizziness/lightheadedness/unsteadiness	81.3	77.8	1.00
Derealization	56.3	25.9	.05
Paresthesias	43.8	37.0	.66
Hot or cold flashes	56.3	63.0	.66
Sweating	81.3	59.3	.14
Faintness/fear of passing out	81.3	33.3	.002
Abdominal cramps/nausea/diarrhea	50.0	40.7	.56
Trembling/shaking	68.8	51.9	.28
Fear of dying	43.8	55.6	.45
Fear of going crazy or losing control	66.7	53.9	.42
Professional help sought for panic, %	93.8	70.4	.12
Took medication for panic, %	66.7	48.2	.25
Hospitalized for panic, %	6.3	3.7	1.00
Missed work due to panic, %	37.5	25.9	.50
Problems with friends due to panic, %	37.5	25.9	.50
Problems with family due to panic, %	31.3	18.5	.46
Help-seeking behavior during attacks, %			
None (bears it alone)	62.5	59.3	.50
Asks friends or family	31.3	37.0	
Asks strangers	0.0	3.7	
Demands help	6.3	0.0	
Makes unreasonable demands	0.0	0.0	
Emergency behavior during attacks, %			
Never	68.8	59.3	.57
At least once	12.5	29.3	
More than once but not usual	18.8	11.1	
Usual	0.0	3.7	
Interruption of function during attacks, %			
None	12.5	44.4	.05
Brief interruption	31.2	37.0	
Withdrawal from activity	37.5	14.8	
Flight	18.8	3.7	
No. of lifetime episodes of PD, mean±SD	2.5±3.0	1.1±0.7	.09

PD indicates panic disorder; n_p, No. of probands; and n_{ar}, No. of affected relatives.

function during panic attacks than did those of later-onset probands, but other clinical characteristics of PD in affected FDRs did not differ by proband age at PD onset. Affected FDRs of early-onset probands reported an average of 1.7 more symptoms per attack than affected FDRs of later-onset probands, but this difference did not reach statistical significance due to small sample size and limited power.

Because of our finding of significantly higher rates of agoraphobia in early-onset probands, we assessed the specificity of transmission of agoraphobia within the groups of early- and late-onset probands. In the early-onset group, 50.0% of the affected FDRs of nonagoraphobic and 61.9% of the affected FDRs of agoraphobic probands met criteria for agoraphobia (P=1.00). In the later-onset group, 22.2% of the affected FDRs of nonagoraphobic and 42.9% of the affected FDRs of agoraphobic probands carried diagnoses of agoraphobia (P=.42). In neither group were these differences statistically significant; thus, we observed no evidence for specificity of transmission of agoraphobia. However, the numbers of nonagoraphobic probands, particularly in the early-onset group, were small, and our power to detect specificity of transmission was consequently limited.

COMMENT

FAMILIAL AGGREGATION OF PD

To our knowledge, ours is the first study that used direct interviews with probands and FDRs to report an association between age at onset of PD in probands and risk to relatives. While we observed PD to be familial irrespective of age at onset in probands, our results indicate that the earliest onsets, ie, those before age 20 years, confer particularly high risks to relatives. These findings were not explained by current age of probands or relatives, phenomenology of PD or comorbid MDD in probands, nonrandom mating, or length of coresidence of relatives with symptomatic probands. As has been suggested in relation to mood disorders,[2,3,6,10,12,37,38] OCD,[14] and, most recently, in a family history study of PD,[20] the earliest onsets of PD in probands may represent cases with the highest genetic loading. Alternatively, early-onset cases may occur in families with more shared environmental risk factors. If the earliest onsets of PD in probands reflect the highest genetic loading, it might also be expected that age at onset would be specifically transmitted within families, which it was not in our sample. Perhaps the propensity to manifest PD over a lifetime is determined by one set of factors, while other factors influence age at onset. The family study design we used could not differentiate the relative importance of genetic vs nongenetic factors in the familiality of PD.

PHENOMENOLOGY OF PD IN PROBANDS

Our finding of increased prevalence of agoraphobia in early-onset probands is consistent with results reported by Wittchen and Perkonigg.[21] Noyes et al[39] have suggested that panic with agoraphobia represents a more severe variant of the disorder. As such, early onset may be a marker for increased clinical severity of PD, as it is for a range of other disorders.[10-12,16] This argument is strengthened by our finding that early-onset probands had more often sought professional help for PD than later-onset probands, but it is weakened by the lack of differences by age at onset in symptom patterns, best-estimate ratings of impairment, and most forms of comorbidity. Further, the increased propensity of early-onset probands to seek professional help for PD may reflect their longer duration, rather than increased severity, of illness.

Our measures of clinical severity consisted of symptom counts, subjects' self-reported level of interruption of function during and emergency and help-seeking behavior in response to attacks, and global ratings of impairment due to PD. Because we did not collect multidimensional assessments of the clinical severity of PD, such as the State-Trait Anxiety Inventory,[40] the Beck Anxiety Inventory,[41] or the Sheehan panic and disability scales,[42] we are unable to examine this issue in further detail. However, our largely negative findings pertaining to phenomenology, which contrast with those reported by Wittchen and Perkonigg[21] from a community sample, may also reflect the uniformly high levels of clinical severity that would be expected from a sample in which more than 80% of the probands with PD were recruited from tertiary-care treatment clinics. When the probands with PD were subdivided on age at onset, there were too few in each group to test this explanation definitively.

PHENOMENOLOGY OF PD IN AFFECTED FDRs

While modest in magnitude, our findings of more total symptoms per attack, greater frequencies of several specific symptoms, and more severe self-reported interruption of function during panic attacks among affected FDRs of early-onset probands suggest that the earliest onsets of PD in probands may be associated with increased clinical severity in affected FDRs as well as with increased familial risk for the disorder. If this is true, the lack of more striking phenomenologic differences in affected FDRs by proband age at onset may result in part from the comparatively small numbers of affected relatives and limited statistical power. However, this interpretation is weakened by the fact that affected FDRs of early-onset probands were not rated by best-estimate diagnosticians as more impaired due to PD than affected FDRs of later-onset probands. Because we did not collect multidimensional assessments of the clinical severity of PD, we are unable to examine this issue in further detail.

Alternatively, our results may reflect greater awareness of PD among affected relatives of early-onset probands. As noted previously, longer exposure of FDRs to symptomatic probands did not explain the elevated risk of developing PD in the early-onset group. However, it might have affected relatives' awareness of the disorder and of the availability of treatment. Consequently, affected FDRs of early-onset probands may have been more willing to report symptoms than those of later-onset probands.

LIMITATIONS OF THE STUDY

The 107 ill and 45 normal probands and their 838 adult FDRs (583 of ill and 255 of normal probands) constitute a comparatively large sample; however, only 53 FDRs of probands with PD were affected with PD themselves. The small number of affected FDRs constrains the precision of the rates and hazard ratios for PD within proband age-at-onset groups. Therefore, our findings of no specificity of transmission of age at PD onset in particular should be considered tentative. As noted earlier, the small number of affected FDRs may also limit the ability to detect phenomenologic differences as a function of proband age at onset. In addition, the small number of ill probands within each age-at-onset subgroup who were ascertained from the community prevented us from testing whether patterns of phenomenologic differences by proband age at onset were similar or different between clinic and community probands. Variations in patterns of phenomenology by proband ascertainment source might account for the divergence of our results from those reported by Wittchen and Perkonigg[21] exclusively from a community sample. Attempts at replication of our results in larger samples of families which afford greater power are essential.

Another limitation arises from our assessment of clinical severity of PD. The use of more specifically targeted multidimensional assessments could have revealed more marked differences in clinical severity both in probands and in affected FDRs. If early-onset probands were more severely ill than later-onset probands, this difference could have accounted for some of the increased risk of PD in their FDRs.

In addition, the study relied of necessity on retrospective recall of lifetime events, some of which may have occurred many years previously. Recall biases might be of particular concern with respect to phenomenology both in probands and in their affected FDRs. Because of their greater duration of illness, early-onset probands might have been more likely to forget symptoms than later-onset probands. If this were the case, however, the results of our analyses would be biased in the direction of reducing the observed differences between proband age-at-onset groups.

In summary, the highly significant increase in risk of PD among relatives of probands with PD onset at or before age 20 years suggests that proband age at onset is a potentially useful factor in differentiating subtypes of PD and that genetic studies of PD should consider age at onset. However, our results concerning the association between proband age at onset and clinical presentation, especially in affected FDRs, are more equivocal. The ability to demonstrate an association between proband age at onset and prospectively assessed course of illness, either in probands or in their affected FDRs, would be of value in clarifying the association between age at onset and clinical characteristics of PD.

Accepted for publication May 15, 1996.

An earlier version of this article was presented as a poster at the 19th Congress of the Collegium Internationale Neuropsychopharmacologicum, June 27 through July 1, 1994, Washington, DC.

This study was supported by grants MH-28274 and MH-30906 from the National Institute of Mental Health, Rockville, Md.

We thank Susan E. Hodge, DSc, Jeremy Coplan, MD, and Steven Greenwald, MA, for their invaluable comments on drafts of this article.

Reprints: Risë B. Goldstein, PhD, Department of Psychiatry, College of Physicians and Surgeons of Columbia University, and New York State Psychiatric Institute, Division of Clinical-Genetic Epidemiology, 722 W 168th St, Unit 14, New York, NY 10032.

REFERENCES

1. Bland RC, Newman SC, Orn H. Recurrent and nonrecurrent depression: a family study. *Arch Gen Psychiatry.* 1986;43:1085-1089.
2. Gershon ES, Bunney WE, Leckman JF, Van Eerdewegh M, DeBauche BA. The inheritance of affective disorders: a review of data and of hypotheses. *Behav Genet.* 1976;6:227-261.
3. Mendlewicz J. The age factor in depressive illness: some genetic considerations. *J Gerontol.* 1976;31:300-303.
4. Moldin SO, Reich T, Rice JP. Current perspectives on the genetics of unipolar depression. *Behav Genet.* 1991;21:211-242.
5. Weissman MM, Wickramaratne P, Merikangas KR, Leckman JF, Prusoff BA, Caruso CA, Kidd KK, Gammon GD. Onset of major depression in early adulthood: increased familial loading and specificity. *Arch Gen Psychiatry.* 1984; 41:1136-1143.
6. Weissman MM, Warner V, Wickramaratne P, Prusoff BA. Early-onset major depression in parents and their children. *J Affect Disord.* 1988;15:269-277.
7. Winokur G, Cadoret R, Baker M, Dorzab J. Depression spectrum disease versus pure depressive disease: some further data. *Br J Psychiatry.* 1975;127: 75-77.
8. Pauls DL, Morton LA, Egeland JA. Risks of affective illness among first-degree relatives of bipolar I Old-Order Amish probands. *Arch Gen Psychiatry.* 1992; 49:703-708.
9. Rice JP, Reich T, Andreasen NC, Endicott J, Van Eerdewegh M, Fishman R, Hirschfeld RMA, Klerman GL. The familial transmission of bipolar illness. *Arch Gen Psychiatry.* 1987;44:441-447.
10. Strober M, Morrell W, Burroughs J, Lampert C, Danforth H, Freeman R. A family study of bipolar I disorder in adolescence. *J Affect Disord.* 1988;15: 255-268.
11. Taylor M, Abrams R. Manic states: a genetic study of early and late onset affective disorders. *Arch Gen Psychiatry.* 1973;28:656-658.
12. Taylor MA, Abrams R. Early- and late-onset bipolar illness. *Arch Gen Psychiatry.* 1981;38:58-61.
13. Pulver AE, Brown CH, Wolyniec P, McGrath J, Tam D, Adler L, Carpenter T, Childs B. Schizophrenia: age at onset, gender, and familial risk. *Acta Psychiatr Scand.* 1990;82:344-351.
14. Bellodi L, Sciuto G, Diaferia G, Ronchi P, Smeraldi E. Psychiatric disorders in the families of patients with obsessive-compulsive disorder. *Psychiatry Res.* 1992;42:111-120.
15. Kovacs M, Paulauskas S, Gatsonis C, Richards C. Depressive disorders in childhood, III: a longitudinal study of comorbidity with and risk for conduct disorders. *J Affect Disord.* 1988;15:205-217.
16. Minichiello WE, Baer L, Jenike MA, Holland A. Age of onset of major subtypes of obsessive-compulsive disorder. *J Anxiety Disord.* 1990;4:147-150.
17. Eaton WW, Dryman A, Weissman MM. Panic and phobia. In: Robins LN, Regier DA, eds. *Psychiatric Disorders in America: The Epidemiologic Catchment Area Study.* New York, NY: The Free Press; 1991:155-179.
18. Moreau D, Weissman MM. Panic disorder in children and adolescents: a review. *Am J Psychiatry.* 1992;149:1306-1314.
19. VonKorff MR, Eaton WW, Keyl PM. The epidemiology of panic attacks and panic disorder: results of three community surveys. *Am J Epidemiol.* 1985; 122:970-981.
20. Battaglia M, Bertella S, Politi E, Bernardeschi L, Perna G, Gabriele A, Bellodi L. Age at onset of panic disorder: influence of familial liability to the disease and of childhood separation anxiety disorder. *Am J Psychiatry.* 1995;152:1362-1364.
21. Wittchen H-U, Perkonigg A. Panikattacken mit frühen und spätem Beginn: Unterschiedliche pathogenetische Mechanismen? *Verhaltenstherapie.* 1993;3:296-303.
22. Weissman MM, Wickramaratne P, Adams PB, Lish JD, Horwath E, Charney D, Woods SW, Leeman E, Frosch E. The relationship between panic disorder and major depression: a new family study. *Arch Gen Psychiatry.* 1993;50:767-780.
23. Mannuzza S, Fyer AJ, Klein DF, Endicott J. Schedule for Affective Disorders and Schizophrenia–Lifetime Version (modified for the study of anxiety disorders): rationale and conceptual development. *J Psychiatr Res.* 1986;20:317-325.
24. American Psychiatric Association. *Diagnostic and Statistical Manual of Mental Disorders, Third Edition.* Washington, DC: American Psychiatric Association; 1980.
25. American Psychiatric Association. *Diagnostic and Statistical Manual of Mental Disorders, Third Edition, Revised.* Washington, DC: American Psychiatric Association; 1987.
26. Robins LN, Helzer JE, Croughan J, Ratcliff K. The NIMH Diagnostic Interview Schedule: its history, characteristics, and validity. *Arch Gen Psychiatry.* 1981; 38:381-389.
27. Thompson WD, Kidd JR, Weissman MM. A procedure for the efficient collection and processing of pedigree data suitable for genetic analysis. *J Psychiatr Res.* 1979;15:291-303.
28. Andreasen NC, Endicott J, Spitzer RL, Winokur G. The family history method using diagnostic criteria: reliability and validity. *Arch Gen Psychiatry.* 1977; 34:1229-1235.
29. Leckman JF, Sholomskas D, Thompson WD, Belanger A, Weissman MM. Best estimate of lifetime psychiatric diagnosis: a methodologic study. *Arch Gen Psychiatry.* 1982;39:879-883.
30. Mantel N. Evaluation of survival data and two new rank order statistics arising in its consideration. *Cancer Chemother Rep.* 1966;50:163-170.
31. Wickramaratne PJ, Prusoff BA, Merikangas KR, Weissman MM. The use of survival time models with nonproportional hazard functions to investigate age of onset in family studies. *J Chron Dis.* 1986;39:389-397.
32. Andreasen NC, Rice J, Endicott J, Reich T, Coryell W. The family history approach to diagnosis: how useful is it? *Arch Gen Psychiatry.* 1986;43:421-429.
33. Cox DR. Regression models and life tables. *J R Stat Soc.* 1972;34:187-220.
34. Wickramaratne PJ, Weissman MM, Horwath E, Adams PB. The familial aggregation of panic disorder by source of proband ascertainment. *Psychiatr Genet.* 1994;4:125-133.
35. Weissman MM, Gershon ES, Kidd KK, Prusoff BA, Leckman JF, Dibble E, Hamovit J, Thompson WD, Pauls DL, Guroff JJ. Psychiatric disorders in the relatives of probands with affective disorders. *Arch Gen Psychiatry.* 1984;41:13-21.
36. Weissman MM, Kidd KK, Prusoff BA. Variability in rates of affective disorders in relatives of depressed and normal probands. *Arch Gen Psychiatry.* 1982; 39:1397-1403.
37. Baron M, Mendlewicz J, Klotz J. Age-of-onset and genetic transmission in affective disorders. *Acta Psychiatr Scand* 1981;64:373-380.
38. Gershon ES, Mark A, Cohen N, Belizon N, Baron M, Knobe KE. Transmitted factors in the morbid risk of affective disorders: a controlled study. *J Psychiatr Res.* 1975;12:283-299.
39. Noyes R, Crowe RR, Harris EL, Hamra BJ, McChesney CM, Chaudhry DR. Relationship between panic disorder and agoraphobia: a family study. *Arch Gen Psychiatry.* 1986;43:227-232.
40. Spielberger C, Gorsuch A, Lushene R. *The State-Trait Anxiety Inventory.* Palo Alto, Calif: Consulting Psychologist Press; 1970.
41. Beck AT, Steer RA. Relationship between the Beck Anxiety Inventory and the Hamilton Anxiety Rating Scale with anxious outpatients. *J Anxiety Disord.* 1991; 5:213-223.
42. Leon AC, Shear MK, Portera L, Klerman GL. Assessing impairment in patients with panic disorder: The Sheehan Disability Scale. *Soc Psychiatry Psychiatr Epidemiol.* 1992;27:78-82.

ORIGINAL ARTICLE

Severe Stress, Depressive Symptoms, and Changes in Lymphocyte Subsets in Human Immunodeficiency Virus–Infected Men

A 2-Year Follow-up Study

Jane Leserman, PhD; John M. Petitto, MD; Diana O. Perkins, MD; James D. Folds, PhD; Robert N. Golden, MD; Dwight L. Evans, MD

Background: This study examined how severe stress and depressive symptoms were related to changes in immune measures during a 2-year period in a sample of gay men with human immunodeficiency virus (HIV) infection. These analyses follow up our initial cross-sectional observations that severe stress was correlated with lower levels of natural killer (NK) cells and $CD8^+$ T lymphocytes in these men.

Methods: Data were collected in North Carolina as part of an ongoing, longitudinal study, the Coping in Health and Illness Project. Sixty-six HIV-infected gay men, who were asymptomatic at baseline, were assessed systematically at 6-month intervals.

Results: Severe stress and depressive symptoms were independently related to decreases on immune measures from entry to 2-year follow-up, that is, declines in $CD8^+$ T cells and $CD56^+$ and $CD16^+$ NK cell subsets. Subjects most likely to have decreases on these immune measures were those who scored above the median on both stress and depressive symptoms.

Conclusions: Our findings are among the first prospective data showing that stress and depressive symptoms, especially when they occur jointly, are associated with decreased number of NK and $CD8^+$ T lymphocytes in HIV-infected men. Since these immune cells may play a protective role in the progression of HIV infection, our data suggest that stress and depressive symptoms may have clinical implications for the course of this disease.

Arch Gen Psychiatry. 1997;54:279-285

RELATIONSHIPS OF stress and depression with cell-mediated immune measures have been shown in several populations.[1-3] Our previous findings among asymptomatic human immunodeficiency virus (HIV)–infected gay men have shown that those with severe stress had lower cellular immune counts on several lymphocyte subsets at study entry.[4] Because these data are cross-sectional, further insight could be provided by examining these relations over time. Thus, in the same subjects, the present study focuses on how stress and depressive symptoms may be related to change in lymphocyte subsets during a 2-year period.

Although findings of the psychoneuroimmune literature in healthy subjects have been somewhat mixed, meta-analyses have shown that stress and depression are associated with moderate decreases in immune variables, including natural killer (NK) cell function, $CD8^+$ T cells, and to a lesser degree, $CD4^+$ T-helper cells.[2,3] The more limited number of psychoneuroimmune studies among HIV-infected subjects have focused on $CD4^+$ and $CD8^+$ T cells.

In a large study, HIV-infected gay men who reported depressive symptoms at study entry had greater declines in $CD4^+$ cell counts during a 5-year period.[5] A similar study of HIV-infected gay men did not find that baseline depressive symptoms correlated with declines in $CD4^+$ cell counts after 8 years.[6] Studies for shorter periods (≤1 year), and cross-sectional studies in HIV-infected samples, have not shown a relation of depression or depressed mood with changes in $CD4^+$ or $CD8^+$ lymphocyte counts.[7-10] Depression may have a less measurable effect on $CD4^+$ cell counts compared with other immune markers in HIV-infected samples because this cell population is affected early and profoundly in the course of HIV infection.[11]

Our cross-sectional findings among asymptomatic HIV-infected gay men showed that severe stress during the previous 6 months was robustly related to lower NK cell counts and lower $CD8^+$ T

From the Departments of Psychiatry (Drs Leserman, Perkins, and Golden), Medicine (Dr Leserman), and Microbiology (Dr Folds), University of North Carolina School of Medicine, Chapel Hill; and the Departments of Psychiatry (Drs Petitto and Evans), Neuroscience (Drs Petitto and Evans), Pharmacology (Dr Petitto), and Medicine (Dr Evans), University of Florida College of Medicine, Gainesville.

SUBJECTS AND METHODS

STUDY GROUP

Data were collected in North Carolina as part of an ongoing, longitudinal study, the Coping in Health and Illness Project. The study was approved by the University of North Carolina (Chapel Hill) School of Medicine Committee for the Protection of the Rights of Human Subjects, and all subjects provided written informed consent. The study group included 66 HIV-infected gay men who were asymptomatic at study entry and were assessed at 6-month intervals for a 2-year period. We recruited volunteers from rural and urban areas of the state from February 20, 1990, to July 22, 1992.

We excluded volunteers with less than 10 years of education, ages younger than 18 years and older than 50 years, previous injecting drug use as a risk factor for HIV, notable medical or neurological illness (eg, heart, lung, kidney, liver, thyroid, and gastrointestinal disease; diabetes, arthritis, cancer, head injury, stroke, seizures, attention-deficit hyperactivity disorder; loss of consciousness; surgery in last 6 months; deafness; and blindness), past treatment of alcoholism or current heavy alcohol consumption (>60 drinks per month), present or past heavy recreational drug use (eg, marijuana, phencyclidine hydrochloride, cocaine, or lysergic acid diethylamide), use of zidovudine or other antiretroviral medications, and those meeting the 1987 Centers for Disease Control (CDC) criteria for acquired immunodeficiency syndrome (AIDS) or AIDS-related complex (eg, night sweats, herpes zoster, oral candidiasis, hairy leukoplakia, shingles, unexplained fever or diarrhea, or unexplained weight loss or fatigue in the presence of other symptoms).[25] Thus, initially all men were asymptomatic, meeting the 1987 CDC definition[25] and the 1993 CDC criteria for clinical stage A (asymptomatic).[26] At 2 years, only 14 subjects (21%) had HIV symptoms consistent with the 1993 definition of clinically symptomatic (11 had stage B and 3 had stage C).

PROCEDURE

Subjects were evaluated every 6 months for 2 years, undergoing systematic medical, neurological, neuropsychological, and psychiatric assessments performed by specialists in these areas. All subjects were asked to be free of medications known to affect immune response, recreational drugs, and any alcohol consumption for at least 2 weeks before each study visit.

At each visit, subjects took nothing by mouth starting at midnight before blood drawing the following morning. Subjects were recumbent and an intravenous line was started at 8 AM in an antecubital vein, which was maintained patent with a slow, normal saline drip. To control for circadian effects and possible acute stress reaction (eg, from insertion of an intravenous line), blood was drawn after 70 minutes of rest following intravenous line placement.[27]

MEASUREMENT

Stressful Life Events

To obtain information about stressful life events and difficulties, we used a semistructured interview, the Psychiatric Epidemiology Research Interview,[28] modified to include stresses relevant to our population. The subjects indicated which of the 111 stresses listed on the interview they had experienced during the preceding 6 months. Using trained interviewers, we questioned subjects in detail about the events and difficulties experienced, and later rated these stresses using a method similar to that developed by Brown and Harris[29] and modified by Patterson et al[15] and Grant et al.[30] Two raters were trained in the rating method by the HIV Neurobehavioral Research Center in San Diego.[15] Based on this training, we developed a manual containing a detailed set of norms and vignettes for rating each of the 111 stresses. The stress ratings were designed to measure objectively stressful life events and difficulties by accounting for the contextual aspects of each stress. Thus, norms for each stress were based on the degree of threat that most people would experience given the particular circumstances (eg, financial impact, degree of control, life threat, and personal involvement). The contextual threat rating was made independently of the subject's rating and his way of coping with the stress.

One of 2 trained raters (previously shown to have high interrater reliability)[4] used the manual to rate the long-term effect of each stressful event and difficulty from 0 (no threat) to 4 (severe threat). Subjects were then given a stress score based on the total sum of severe stress ratings (those rated 3 or 4). The following are examples of severe stresses: breaking up with a long-term committed partner, and death of a close confidant or parent. Counting only severe stresses was consistent with our previous findings[4] and those of others.[15,30,31]

We removed from the stress scores the stresses that we knew were likely to be caused by disease progression (eg, onset of AIDS, drop in $CD4^+$ count, and retirement due to HIV worsening). Furthermore, the contextual threat rating, independent of the subject's rating, helps reduce the possibility that worsening disease may lead to poorer coping and higher stress scores.

Because stresses were rated at each visit for the previous 6 months, "preceding 1-year stress" covered the year before the 2-year immune assessment, ie, the sum of stresses rated during the 18-month and 2-year visits. Likewise, "preceding 2-year stress" was the sum of stresses rated during the 6-month, 1-year, 18-month, and 2-year visits.

Depression and Depressive Symptoms

To determine major depression for the past 6 months at each visit, all subjects underwent a structured psychiatric interview (a modified Structured Clinical Interview for *DSM-III-R*)[32] administered by a trained clinician. All psychiatric diagnoses were assigned at consensus diagnostic conferences as described previously.[33]

Severity of depressive symptoms was measured with the interviewer-based 17-item Hamilton Depression Rating Scale (HDRS-17).[34] Higher scores indicated more symptoms. At each visit, trained psychiatric clinicians administered the interview to assess symptoms for the past week. Interrater reliability was excellent, with an intraclass correlation coefficient of 0.99. An 11-item HDRS (HDRS-11) also was computed by eliminating the medical symptoms that overlapped with symptoms of HIV disease. This was done to help avoid confounding the depressive-symptoms measure with HIV disease progression. The following medical symptoms were excluded from the HDRS-11: gastrointestinal symptoms, weight loss, general somatic symptoms, somatic anxiety symptoms, hypochondriasis, and retardation. Items included in the HDRS-11 were depressed mood; anhedonia; loss of libido (not performance); early, middle, and late insomnia; guilt; suicide; psychic anxiety; insight; and agitation. Preliminary analysis showed that the Spearman rank correlations between the HDRS-17 and HDRS-11 ranged from 0.87 to 0.94 at each of the visits. Therefore, only findings of the HDRS-11 scores with immune data have been reported herein.

Because at each visit depressive symptoms have been rated for the past week, "preceding 1-year depressive symptoms" refers to the sum of the previous week's symptoms for the 18-month and 2-year visits. Likewise, "preceding 2-year depressive symptoms" is the sum of the previous week's symptoms for the 6-month, 1-year, 18-month, and 2-year visits.

Health-Related Variables

Enzyme-linked immunosorbent assay screening with Western blot confirmation was performed during the first visit. We assessed whether subjects received any antiviral medications at any of their visits during the 2-year period (1=yes and 0=no). We also determined the presence or absence of the following potential immune confounders: (1) long-term use of antibiotics and/or antifungals, (2) other possible immune-altering medications during the 2 weeks before the 2-year study visit (eg, use of psychotropics, antihistamines, nonsteroidal anti-inflammatory drugs, short-term antibiotics, or substance abuse), and (3) infection with a "common cold"/influenza virus during the 2 weeks before the study visit. Cigarette smoking at the 2-year visit was measured in half-pack increments from "do not smoke" (score =0) to "3 or more packs a day" (score =6).

Monoclonal Antibody and Flow Cytometry Techniques

The flow cytometric assays were performed in the Psychoneuroimmunology Laboratory of our Mental Health Clinical Research Center. To reduce assay variance, fresh internal control samples were obtained from normal healthy controls and assayed for the monoclonal antibody determinations. Peripheral blood samples were collected into heparinized specimen (Vacutainer) tubes. The Leu series of monoclonal antibodies (Becton Dickinson, Mountain View, Calif) was used to measure the predominant reactivity to the lymphocyte subsets. All studies were performed by a dual-labeling (double staining) technique, using the combination of fluorescein isothiocyanate and phycoerythrin-conjugated antibodies. These included enumeration of the following lymphocyte subsets: $CD57^+/CD8^{+/-}$, $CD16^+/CD3^-$, $CD56^+/CD3^{+/-}$, $CD4^+/CD3^+$, and $CD8^+/CD3^+$. Whole blood was incubated with premixed fluorochrome-conjugated monoclonal antibodies for 15 minutes at room temperature in the dark. Erythrocytes were lysed with a lysing reagent (FACS Lysing Solution, Becton-Dickinson Immunocytometry Systems). The resulting fluorochrome-labeled leukocytes were then washed with Dulbecco phosphate-buffered saline and sodium azide and fixed by the addition of 1% paraformaldehyde. Stained cell preparations were stored in the dark at 4°C until examination by flow cytometry using a FACScan (Becton-Dickinson) flow cytometer. Background controls for nonspecific staining consisted of anti-IgG1 fluorescein isothiocyanate and anti-IgG2 phycoerythrin, and the combination of anti–CD45-positive (pan-leukocyte) and anti-CD14 (monocytes) was used to ensure proper gating of the cell populations. Reference ranges were determined by evaluation of normal peripheral blood controls for the lymphocyte subsets examined. (Absolute lymphocyte subset counts were derived from lymphocyte subset percentages × total lymphocyte counts ×100.)

STATISTICAL METHODS

Because data on depressive symptoms, stress, and immune variables were highly skewed and contained outliers, nonparametric statistics were used for all analyses. We have reported descriptive statistics for the distribution of scores in the 25% (lowest), median, and 75% (highest) quartiles. All statistical analyses have used 2-tailed tests with level of significance at $\alpha=.05$.

To examine change on immune variables, we performed Spearman rank correlations between measures over time (indicating the amount of individual fluctuation), and the Wilcoxon signed-rank test of the median difference between 2-year minus baseline immune values (indicating change in the group as a whole).

To test our main hypotheses, we computed partial Spearman rank correlations of severe stress and depressive symptoms measures with immune counts at 2 years, adjusted for immune counts at entry and controlling for the following 6 variables: age, education, race, helper count at entry (a rough approximation of disease stage), tobacco use, and use of any antiviral medications during the 2 years. Although the latter 6 control variables did not alter most of the reported relations, they were retained in equations because 2 correlations were moderately affected by their inclusion. We attempted to control for long-term antibiotic use (5 subjects), colds (2 subjects), alcohol use (≥1 drink per day, 2 subjects), and other possible immune confounding medications (7 subjects) at the 2-year visit; these did not seem to affect our analyses, but the lack of variance made it difficult to evaluate their potential influence.

We further explored the aforementioned change model using multiple regression with ranked variables to test for interactions between stress and depressive symptoms and to examine stress and depressive symptoms during the preceding and first study year. An analysis of covariance with the same change model using ranked immune variables was performed to test differences between 3 stress-depressive symptoms groups (below median on both, above median on 1, above median on both). We also performed the Wilcoxon signed-rank test of the median differences between 2-year and baseline immune values for each of the 3 stress-depressive symptoms groups.

Table 1. Sample Characteristics*

Characteristic	Value
Race, %	
White	71
Black	29
Asymptomatic, %†	
Entry	100
2 y	79
Mean (±SD) age at entry, y	30.2 (5.8)
Mean (±SD) education at entry, y	14.4 (2.4)
Scores, 25th/median/75th quartiles‡	
Severe stress	
Preceding year	0/0/3
Preceding 2 y	0/3/6
Depressive symptoms	
HDRS-17	
Preceding year	1/4/11
Preceding 2 y	4/10/18
HDRS-11	
Preceding year	0/3/6
Preceding 2 y	2/6/11

**N=66 for all variables except n=63 for the preceding 2-year stress and depressive symptoms measures due to missing data. HDRS indicates Hamilton Depression Rating Scale.*

†Asymptomatic based on Centers for Disease Control clinical stage A.

‡Preceding 1 year is the sum of the 18-month and 2-year visits. The preceding 2 years is the sum of the 6-month, 1-year, 18-month, and 2-year visits. Numbers indicate the scores at each quartile in the distribution, with 25% indicating the lowest quartile (eg, least stressed).

lymphocytes but uncorrelated with CD4$^+$ T cells.[4] Antoni et al[12] found that a cognitive behavioral stress management intervention was associated with less distress and an increase in NK cell counts (CD56$^+$) among seropositive gay men exposed to the stress of HIV status notification. Other studies of stress and immune status have not examined NK cell markers, although Sahs et al[13] found no cross-sectional relation between depression or depressive symptoms and CD56$^+$ NK cell counts among 27 asymptomatic and 46 symptomatic HIV-seropositive men. Furthermore, other studies have not shown an association of stress with change in CD4$^+$ and CD8$^+$ cell counts over time.[7,8,14] In addition to not testing NK cell subsets, these studies tended to be limited due to the use of short follow-up periods (6 months to 1 year) during which time little change might be expected, use of unreliable methods to assess number of life stresses, and not controlling for variables known to affect immune measures (eg, medication and smoking).

Using a similar interview-based stress rating to that used in the present study, the HIV Neurobehavioral Research Center in San Diego, Calif, found that those who reported no severe life stress and few depressive symptoms had less decline in percentage of CD4$^+$ lymphocytes after 6 months compared with those who had higher scores on these psychological risk factors.[15] This study has raised the possibility that stress and depression combined may be an important predictor of immune change.

The present study examines the relation of stress and depressive symptoms with change in lymphocyte subsets from study entry to 2-year follow-up among HIV-infected gay men. We hypothesize that subjects scoring higher on stress and depressive symptoms during the preceding year and preceding 2 years will have greater decreases in NK cell subsets and CD8$^+$ T cells. We have chosen these specific immune markers because our group and others have shown reduced NK cell and CD8$^+$ T lymphocytes in stress and depression,[2-4,16,17] because NK cells have the capacity to lyse HIV-1 infected lymphocytes and may be important in the control of HIV-1 infection,[18] and because subsets of CD8$^+$ T cells may play an important role in the host defense against HIV-1, including the control of viral replication.[19-24] Like previous research, the present study examines the relation of stress and depressive symptoms with CD4$^+$ T cells.

RESULTS

Table 1 gives descriptive information about the study group. Most subjects were rated low on depressive symptoms (HDRS-17) at each visit, with only 3 (5%) to 7 (11%) scoring 10 and above at any 1 visit. Eight subjects (12%) met criteria for a major depressive episode during the preceding year, with 14 subjects (21%) meeting these criteria during the preceding 2 years. Severe life stress (≥1 incidents) was experienced by 28 subjects (42%) in the previous year and 40 subjects (63%) in the preceding 2 years. The most common stresses included deaths of family members or close friends, life-threatening or deteriorating health of close family members or friends (caretaking usually involved), and breaking up of love relationships.

Table 2 gives the distributions of the immune variables at entry and at 2-year follow-up, with the median differences between scores (signed rank test) and Spearman rank correlations (r_s). As a group, subjects tended not to change on CD4$^+$, CD8$^+$, and CD57$^+$ lymphocyte counts over time, although there was some individual fluctuation on these measures. Furthermore, subjects tended to decrease on CD16$^+$ and CD56$^+$ NK cell counts from entry to follow-up, with some individual fluctuation.

We next examined whether higher levels of severe stress and depressive symptoms were related to reductions in lymphocyte subsets (**Table 3**). Severe stress was significantly associated with moderate reductions on 2 immune variables, CD16$^+$ NK cells and CD8$^+$ T cells. These relations held for both time intervals (preceding year and preceding 2 years), with the exception that there was only a trend with CD8$^+$ T cells during the preceding 2-year interval.

Depressive symptoms were related to moderate reductions in CD16$^+$ NK cells, CD56$^+$ NK cells, and CD8$^+$ T cells using the previous-year and 2-year visits. Although not shown, the HDRS-17 (original scale with possible confounding medical symptoms) performed essentially the same as the HDRS-11. Stress and depressive symptoms were not significantly associated with CD57$^+$ lymphocytes or CD4$^+$ cells.

We further examined the contributions to our model of stress and depressive symptoms measured during the previous year (18-month and 2-year visits) compared with these variables assessed during the first study year (6-month and 1-year visits). Scores on stress and depressive symptoms for the first study year did not significantly predict immune change over and above these

Table 2. Quartiles, Signed Rank Test, and Spearman Rank Correlations of Immune Variables*

	Baseline			2 y			Signed-Rank Test		
Cell	25%	Median	75%	25%	Median	75%	Value	P	r_s
CD8+ T	0.53	0.71	0.87	0.53	0.67	0.96	16	.92	0.74
CD4+ T-helper	0.26	0.36	0.44	0.24	0.33	0.46	−144	.33	0.77
CD16+ NK	0.96	0.13	0.17	0.66	0.10	0.14	−580	<.001	0.71
CD56+ NK	0.13	0.17	0.26	0.11	0.14	0.22	−536	<.001	0.63
CD57+	0.23	0.32	0.44	0.23	0.32	0.48	220	.16	0.69

**N*=66 for all variables. Immune variables are given as lymphocyte counts, 10^9/L. NK indicates natural killer cells.*

Table 3. Spearman Rank Partial Correlations of Stress and Depressive Symptoms With 2-Year Immune Counts, Controlling for Immune Counts at Entry*

	CD8+ T		CD4+ T-Helper		CD16+ NK		CD56+ NK		CD57+	
Variable	r_s	P	r_s	P	r_s	P	r_s	P	r_s	P
Severe stress										
Preceding 1 y	−0.27	.04	−0.15	.27	−0.30	.02	−0.20	.14	−0.13	.34
Preceding 2 y	−0.24	.08	−0.17	.20	−0.28	.04	−0.14	.31	−0.08	.54
Depressive symptoms (HDRS-11)										
Preceding 1 y	−0.26	.04	−0.09	.47	−0.29	.02	−0.34	.009	−0.12	.35
Preceding 2 y	−0.29	.03	−0.16	.24	−0.30	.02	−0.34	.01	−0.24	.07
Stress/depressive symptoms scale†										
Preceding 1 y	−0.35	.007	−0.12	.38	−0.44	<.001	−0.37	.004	−0.20	.13
Preceding 2 y	−0.29	.03	−0.10	.45	−0.32	.02	−0.28	.03	−0.17	.20

**N*=66 for all variables except n=63 for the preceding 2-year stress and depressive symptoms measures due to missing data. All partial correlations control for immune count at entry, age, education, race, helper count at entry, tobacco use, and antiviral medication. NK indicates natural killer cells; HDRS, Hamilton Depression Rating Scale.*

†Scale created by dividing subjects at the median on the HDRS-11 and the median on severe stress using the preceding year (sum of 18-month and 2-year visits) and preceding 2 years (sum of 6-month, 1-year, 18-month, and 2-year visits) to create the following scale: (1) below the median on both stress and depressive symptoms, (2) above the median on either stress or depressive symptoms, and (3) above the median on both stress and depressive symptoms.

variables measured during the year before the 2-year visit. The significant immune effects of stress and depressive symptoms during the preceding 2 years seem to be due to the more proximal effects of these variables.

We found no significant interactions between stress and depressive symptoms on immune variables in our change model. Significant relations emerged, however, when we tested a combined model, looking at the effect on immune variables of a 3-category stress-depressive symptoms measure (below median on both stress and depressive symptoms [n=22], above the median on stress or depressive symptoms [n=25], and above the median on both stress and depressive symptoms [n=19]). The group scoring above the median on both stress and depressive symptoms during the preceding year had the following characteristics: 19 (100%) had at least 1 severe stress, 9 (47%) had more than 1 severe stress, 7 (37%) had at least 1 HDRS-17 score above 10, and 9 (47%) had at least 1 HDRS-11 score of 6 or higher. Table 3 gives fairly large correlations of the combined stress-depressive symptoms measure with reduced $CD16^+$ NK cells, $CD56^+$ NK cells, and $CD8^+$ T cells.

Analysis of covariance also showed that the 3 stress-depressive symptoms groups significantly differed on the immune change model. The group above the median on both stress and depressive symptoms had become significantly lower (1) on $CD16^+$ NK cells (t=2.8; P=.006), $CD56^+$ NK cells (t=2.5; P=.01), and $CD8^+$ T cells (t=2.3; P=.03) compared with the middle stress-depressive symptoms group; and (2) on $CD16^+$ NK cells (t=3.7; P<.001), $CD56^+$ NK cells (t=3.0; P=.004), and $CD8^+$ T cells (t=2.8; P=.007) compared with the low stress-depressive symptoms group. The middle stress-depressive symptoms category was not significantly different from the lowest group on this immune change model ($CD16^+$ NK cells [t=1.13; P=.26]; $CD56^+$ NK cells [t=.68; P=.50]; and $CD8^+$ T cells [t=.71; P=.48]).

To examine the absolute decline in immune variables, we also computed the Wilcoxon signed rank test on the median difference between raw immune measures at 2-year follow-up and baseline for each stress-depressive symptoms group. The group above the median on both stress and depressive symptoms showed large significant reductions on $CD16^+$ NK cells (median=−53; P<.001), $CD56^+$ NK cells (median=−48; P<.001), and $CD8^+$ T cells (median=−164; P=.004). The middle (−8, −29, and +54) and low (−5, −16, and +54) stress-depressive symptoms groups did not significantly decrease on these same immune variables, respectively. To put these decreases in perspective, the group above the median on both stress and depressive symptoms showed a drop from one half to two thirds of an SD on immune measures from baseline. The 3 stress-depressive symptoms groups did not significantly differ on median immune values at study entry.

COMMENT

To our knowledge, this study is among the first longitudinal reports to show that stress and depressive symptoms are related to alterations in lymphocyte subsets in persons infected with HIV. We have shown that stress and depressive symptoms, independently and in combination, are related to decrements in immune status during a 2-year assessment period. Especially important in explaining immune change are stresses and depressive symptoms that have occurred in close proximity to the 2-year study visit. Those above the median on both stress and depressive symptoms during the preceding year are more likely to have their immune counts decrease on 2 NK cell subsets and on $CD8^+$ T cells. This is consistent with the findings from a study using a similar interview-based assessment of stress that has shown that HIV-infected subjects scoring low on both stress and depressive symptoms have the least immunological decline during a 6-month period.[15]

Our findings extend our initial baseline observations that stress was related to decrements in NK cells and $CD8^+$ T lymphocytes.[4] In the present longitudinal analysis, we did not find that $CD57^+$ lymphocytes (a population comprising a subset of NK and T cells) were related to stress or depressive symptoms. Although there was a trend for $CD57^+$ lymphocytes to be negatively related to the stress-depressive symptoms scale, it is unclear why this cell population was not consistently affected. In the present study, we further found no relation of stress and depressive symptoms with $CD4^+$ T-helper cells, which is consistent with the findings in our previous study[4] and other studies.[7-10,14] Psychosocial factors may have less measurable effect on the number of $CD4^+$ T cells compared with NK markers in HIV-infected subjects, because this cell population is affected early and profoundly in the course of HIV infection.[11]

Our HIV-infected subjects showed a moderate (15%-20%) decline in $CD16^+$ and $CD56^+$ lymphocytes during a 2-year period. Although these subsets have been shown to be lower in those infected with HIV,[13,20,35-38] and men with AIDS have considerably lower $CD16^+$ NK cells than those with asymptomatic infection,[36,38] we know of no longitudinal studies that have examined how these measures change over time.

Although we have made an attempt to examine stress and depressive symptoms preceding immunological change, we cannot determine exactly when the immune changes occurred relative to the depressive symptoms and the stressful events. Because we made an attempt to exclude stresses caused by HIV disease progression, and ratings were made independent of subject's coping, we tried to reduce the chance that disease progression (hence immune change) might have resulted in more stresses. We cannot rule out the possibility that certain stresses, such as death of mate, might indicate that the subject has been infected with a more virulent strain of HIV. Furthermore, although we excluded depressive symptoms associated with HIV disease, we cannot determine the direction of the relation between immune change and depressive symptoms. Psychoneuroimmune studies in HIV have been further hindered by not knowing the date of seroconversion.

What is the clinical relevance of the immune changes? In the current study, change in $CD8^+$ T cells was highly correlated with change in $CD4^+$ T cells (r_s=0.43, P<.001, df=65), and the 14 subjects who became clinically symptomatic had lower 2-year $CD8^+$ T cells (t=1.96, P=.05, df=13,51), $CD16^+$ NK cells (t=2.07, P=.04, df=13,51), and CD56 NK cells (t=2.96, P=.004, df=13,51) than the 52 who remained asymptomatic. $CD8^+$ cytotoxic T lymphocytes, specific for HIV-1, have been suggested to be involved in inhibiting HIV-1 replication.[19,21,22,39] Although $CD8^+$ T cells are composed predominately of cytotoxic T lymphocytes, only a small fraction of cytotoxic T cells show HIV specific cytotoxicity when tested in vitro.[40] In addition to the nonselective cytotoxic activity of NK cells, there is evidence that HIV-1 infected $CD4^+$ T-cell lines are susceptible to NK cell–mediated cytotoxicity.[41,42] Although alterations of these cells due to stress or depressive symptoms may have clinical relevance, no published data indicate that clinical outcome will be modified by the magnitude of the stress and depressive symptoms effects shown in this study.

In conclusion, our findings are among the first longitudinal evidence that stress and depressive symptoms may decrease the number of NK cells and T-cytotoxic lymphocytes in HIV-positive men. If NK and $CD8^+$ T lymphocytes help to protect patients with HIV infection, the lowering of these cell populations due to stress and depressive symptoms may have clinical implications for the course of HIV infection.

Accepted for publication September 5, 1996.

Supported in part by grants MH-44618 and MH-33127 from the National Institute of Mental Health and by grant RR-00046 from the National Institutes of Health, Bethesda, Md.

We thank Jeffery Longmate, PhD, and Keith E. Muller, PhD, for discussions of statistical issues.

Reprints: Jane Leserman, PhD, Research Associate Professor, Department of Psychiatry, CB #7160, University of North Carolina School of Medicine, Chapel Hill, NC 27599-7160.

REFERENCES

1. Evans DL, Leserman J, Golden RN, Lewis MH, Folds JA, Ozer H. Immune correlates of stress and depression. *Psychopharmacol Bull.* 1989;25:319-324.
2. Herbert TB, Cohen S. Stress and immunity in humans: a meta-analytic review. *Psychosom Med.* 1993;55:364-379.
3. Herbert TB, Cohen S. Depression and immunity: a meta-analytic review. *Psychol Bull.* 1993;113:472-486.
4. Evans DL, Leserman J, Perkins DO, Stern RA, Murphy C, Tamul K, Liao D, van der Horst CM, Hall CD, Folds JD, Golden RN, Petitto JM. Stress-associated reductions of cytotoxic T lymphocytes and natural killer cells in asymptomatic HIV infection. *Am J Psychiatry.* 1995;152:543-550.
5. Burack JH, Barrett DC, Stall RD, Chesney MA, Ekstrand ML, Coates TJ. Depressive symptoms and CD4 lymphocyte decline among HIV-infected men. *JAMA.* 1993;270:2568-2573.
6. Lyketsos CG, Hoover DR, Guccione M, Senterfitt W, Dew MA, Wesch J, Van-

Raden MJ, Treisman GJ, Morgenstern H. Depressive symptoms as predictors of medical outcomes in HIV infection. *JAMA.* 1993;270:2563-2567.
7. Perry S, Fishman B, Jacobsberg L, Frances A. Relationships over 1 year between lymphocyte subsets and psychosocial variables among adults with infection by human immunodeficiency virus. *Arch Gen Psychiatry.* 1992;49:396-401.
8. Rabkin JG, Williams JBW, Remien RH, Goetz RR, Dertzner R, Gorman JM. Depression, distress, lymphocyte subsets, and human immunodeficiency virus symptoms on 2 occasions in HIV-positive homosexual men. *Arch Gen Psychiatry.* 1991;48:111-119.
9. Lipsitz JD, Williams JBW, Rabkin JG, Remien RH, Bradbury M, el Sadr W, Goetz R, Sorrell S, Gorman JM. Psychopathology in male and female intravenous drug users with and without HIV infection. *Am J Psychiatry.* 1994;151:1662-1668.
10. Williams JBW, Rabkin JG, Remien R, H., Gorman JM, Ehrhardt AA. Multidisciplinary baseline assessment of homosexual men with and without human immunodeficiency virus infection. *Arch Gen Psychiatry.* 1991;48:124-130.
11. Stein M, Miller AH, Trestman RL. Depression, the immune system and health and illness. *Arch Gen Psychiatry.* 1991;48:171-177.
12. Antoni MH, Baggett L, Ironson G, LaPerriere A, August S, Klimas N, Schneiderman N, Fletcher MA. Cognitive-behavioral stress management intervention buffers distress responses and immunologic changes following notification of HIV-1 seropositivity. *J Consult Clin Psychol.* 1991;59:906-915.
13. Sahs JA, Goetz R, Reddy M, Rabkin JG, Williams JBW, Kertzner R, Gorman JM. Psychological distress and natural killer cells in gay men with and without HIV infection. *Am J Psychiatry.* 1994;151:1479-1484.
14. Kessler RC, Foster C, Joseph J, Ostrow D, Wortman C, Phair J, Chmiel J. Stressful life events and symptom onset in HIV infection. *Am J Psychiatry.* 1991;148:733-738.
15. Patterson TL, Semple SJ, Temoshok LR, Atkinson JH, McCutchan JA, Straits-Troster K, Chandler JL, Grant I. Stress and depressive symptoms prospectively predict immune change among HIV-seropositive men. *Psychiatry.* 1995;58:299-312.
16. Evans DL, Pedersen CA, Folds JD. Major depression and immunity: preliminary evidence of decreased natural killer cell populations. *Prog Neuropsychopharmacol Biol Psychiatry.* 1988;12:739-748.
17. Evans DL, Folds JD, Petitto J, Golden RN, Pedersen CA, Corrigan M, Gilmore JH, Silva SG, Quade D, Ozer H. Circulating natural killer cell phenotypes in males and females with major depression: relation to cytotoxic activity and severity of depression. *Arch Gen Psychiatry.* 1992;49:388-395.
18. Tyler DS, Stanley SD, Nastala CA, Austin AA, Bartlett JA, Stine KC, Lyerly HK, Bolognesi DP, Weinold KJ. Alterations in antibody-dependent cellular cytoxicity during the course of HIV-1 infection: humoral and cell defects. *J Immunol.* 1990;144:3375-3384.
19. Pantaleo G, DeMaria A, Koenig S, Butini L, Moss B, Baseler M, Lane HC, Fauci AS. $CD8^+$ T lymphocytes of patients with AIDS maintain normal broad cytolytic function despite the loss of human immunodeficiency virus-specific cytotoxicity. *Proc Natl Acad Sci U S A.* 1990;87:4819-4822.
20. Vanham G, Kestens L, Gigase P, Colebunders M, Vandenbruaene M, Brijs L, Ceuppens JL. Evidence for circulating activated cytotoxic T cells in HIV-infected subjects before the onset of opportunistic infections. *Clin Exp Immunol.* 1990;82:3-9.
21. Walker BD, Plata F. Cytotoxic T lymphocytes against HIV. *AIDS.* 1990;4:177-184.
22. Jassoy C, Harrer T, Rosenthal T, Bradford AN, Worth J, Johnson RP, Walker BD. Human immunodeficiency virus type 1-specific cytotoxic T lymphocytes release gamma interferon, tumor necrosis factor alpha (TNF-alpha), and TNF-beta when they encounter their target antigens. *J Virol.* 1993;67:2844-2852.
23. Ho HN, Hultin LE, Mitsuyasu RT, Matud JL, Hausner MA, Bockstoce D, Chou CC, O'Rourke S, Taylor JM, Giorgi JV. Circulating HIV-specific $CD8^+$ cytotoxic T cells express CD38 and HLA-DR antigens. *J Immunol.* 1993;150:3070-3079.
24. Fauci AS. Mulfifactorial nature of human immunodeficiency virus disease: implications for therapy. *Science.* 1993;262:1011-1018.
25. Centers for Disease Control. Revision of the CDC surveillance case definition for acquired immunodeficiency syndrome. *MMWR Morb Mortal Wkly Rep.* 1987;36(suppl 1):1-5.
26. Centers for Disease Control. 1993 Revised classification system for HIV infection and expanded surveillance case definition for AIDS among adolescents and adults. *MMWR Morb Mortal Wkly Rep.* 1992;41:1-15.
27. Petitto JM, Folds JD, Ozer H, Quade D, Evans DL. Altered diurnal variation in natural killer cell phenotypes and cytotoxic activity in major depression. *Am J Psychiatry.* 1992;149:694-696.
28. Dohrenwend BS, Krasnoff L, Askenasy AR, Dohrenwend BP. Exemplification of a method for scaling life events: the PERI Life Events Scale. *J Health Soc Behav.* 1978;19:205-229.
29. Brown GW, Harris T. *Social Origins of Depression: A Study of Psychiatric Disorder in Women.* New York, NY: Free Press; 1978.
30. Grant I, Brown GW, Harris T, McDonald WI, Patterson TL. Severely threatening events and marked life difficulties preceding onset or exacerbation of multiple sclerosis. *J Neurol Neurosurg Psychiatry.* 1989;52:8-13.
31. Ramirez AJ, Craig TJK, Watson JP, Fentiman IS, North WRS, Rubens RD. Stress and relapse of breast cancer. *BMJ.* 1989;298:291-293.
32. Perkins DO, Dickison JA, Evans DL. SCID-RDC: *DSM-III-R* and RDC Integrated Interview. In: *Proceedings of the American Psychiatric Association.* New York, NY: American Psychiatric Association; 1990:75. Abstract.
33. Perkins DO, Stern RA, Golden RN, Murphy C, Naftolowitz D, Evans DL. Mood disorders in HIV infection: prevalance and risk factors in a non-epicenter of the AIDS epidemic. *Am J Psychiatry.* 1994;151:233-236.
34. Hamilton M. A rating scale for depression. *J Neurol Neurosurg Psychiatry.* 1960;23:56-62.
35. Vuillier F, Bianco NE, Montagnier L, Dighiero G. Selective depletion of low-density $CD8^+$, $CD16^+$ lymphocytes during HIV infection. *AIDS Res Hum Retroviruses.* 1988;4:121-129.
36. Mansour I, Doinel C, Rouger P. $CD16^+$ NK cells decrease in all stages of HIV infection through a selective depletion of the $CD16^+$ $CD8^+$ $CD3^-$ subset. *AIDS Res Hum Retroviruses.* 1990;6:1451-1457.
37. Margolick JB, Scott ER, Odaka N, Saah AJ. Flow cytometric analysis of T cells and natural killer cells in HIV-1 infection. *Clin Immunol Immunopathol.* 1991;58:126-138.
38. Cai Q, Huang XL, Rappocciolo G, Rinaldo CR Jr. Natural killer cell responses in homosexual men with early HIV infection. *J Acquir Immune Defic Syndr Hum Retrovirol.* 1990;3:669-676.
39. Walker BD, Flexner C, Paradis TJ, Fuller TC, Hirsch MS, Schooley RT, Moss B. HIV-1 reverse transcriptase is a target for cytotoxic T lymphocytes in infected individuals. *Science.* 1988;240:64-66.
40. Pantaleo G, De Maria A, Koenig S, Butini L, Moss B, Baseler M, Lane HC, Fauci AS. $CD8^+$ T lymphocytes of patients with AIDS maintain normal broad cytolytic function despite the loss of human immunodeficiency virus-specific cytotoxicity. *Proc Natl Acad Sci U S A.* 1990;87:4818-4822.
41. Bandyopadhyay S, Ziegner U, Campbell DE, Miller DS, Hoxie JA, Starr SE. Natural killer cell-mediated lysis of T cell lines chronically infected with HIV-1. *Clin Exp Immunol.* 1990;79:430-435.
42. Tanneau F, McChesney M, Lopez O, Sansonetti P, Montagnier L, Riviere Y. Primary cytotoxicity against the envelope glycoprotein of human immunodeficiency virus-1: evidence for antibody-dependent cellular cytotoxicity in vivo. *J Infect Dis.* 1990;162:837-843.

Physician Recruitment

Psychiatry
Multiple Specialties/Group Practice
Locum Tenens Wanted
Graduate Training/Residencies/Fellowships
Chiefs/Department Heads/Directors
Academic/Faculty
CME Corner
Courses/Symposia/Seminars
Practices For Sale
Notices

Psychiatry

WEST HAVEN: VA Connecticut Healthcare System is actively recruiting for Psychiatrist to serve as an Attending in the Primary Care Psychiatric Firm. The position involves providing primary medical care and psychiatric care in the Primary Care Psychiatric Clinic and in the Psychiatric Emergency Room. This position also involves teaching Yale Psychiatric residents and medical students. The position requires 25 hours per week including weekends and applicants should be board-eligible in Psychiatry, board eligible in Primary Care Medicine and trained in emergency psychiatry. West Haven VA is affiliated with Yale University School of Medicine, and the position requires an appointment to Yale University at the rank of instructor. Position is available in July 1997. Please send CV and letters of reference to Mark Bain, Human Resources, VA Connecticut Healthcare System, 950 Campbell Ave, West Haven, CT 06516.

GERIATRIC PSYCHIATRIST: with ABPN qualifications is sought by The University of Chicago for a full-time position with clinical and teaching responsibilities. A demonstrated record of scholarly productivity is required. Academic appointment and salary commensurate with experience. Reply to Neil H. Pliskin, PhD, Department of Psychiatry, The University of Chicago, 5841 South Maryland Ave, MC3077, Chicago, IL 60637. EOE.

PSYCHIATRIST, IOWA: Unique opportunity for a BC/BE general psychiatrist to join a busy in/out-patient, biologically-based practice within a 69-physician, multispecialty clinic. Mason City Clinic serves a 14-county area with a 250,000 population base. Full range of medical specialties and support services. Mason City offers small-town, Midwestern living, abundant outdoor recreational and cultural amenities, and convenient access to metropolitan areas. Our school systems are ranked on top both at state and national levels. Generous compensation program. Submit CV to: Ralph A. Wolf, Sr VP/Chief Administrative Officer, Mason City Clinic, PC, 250 S Crescent Dr, Mason City, IA 50401. 515-421-6574 or (toll free) 800-622-1411. Fax: 515-421-6593. You may e-mail your response to JJacksonMD@aol.com

TEXAS, the SOUTHEAST, and the SUNBELT STATES. There are Excellent Private Practice Opportunities Available in Psychiatry. Major Cities and Rural Communities Are Available.

Call 1-800-284-4560/Houston 281-493-2797

Or send CV to:
P.O. Box 42314
Houston, TX 77242-2314

FAX 281-493-2234
Reuben Bronstein
& Associates

When responding to a **Reply Box**, please send your response to *Archives of General Psychiatry*, Box___, c/o *PSY*, 515 N State St, Chicago, IL 60610.

Graduate Training/Residencies/Fellowships

POSTDOCTORAL FELLOWSHIP IN PET/SPECT/MRI IMAGING: Unique opportunity for postdoctoral training in functional brain imaging research. Emphasis on psychopharmacology and neuropsychiatric imaging. Special training in quantification techniques, research methods, and clinical applications. Didactic lectures, variety of projects, excellent mix of clinical and basic research. MD or MD/PhD and clinical credentials required. Position to start as early as MAY/JUNE 1997. Send applications to Dean F. Wong, MD, PhD, Johns Hopkins Medical Institutions, Radiology-JOHC Bldg, Room 3245, 601 N Caroline St, Baltimore, MD 21287-0807. E-mail: dfwong@rad.jhu.edu

Courses/Symposia/Seminars

LOS ANGELES, NIMH-FUNDED FACULTY SCHOLARS PROGRAM IN MENTAL HEALTH SERVICES RESEARCH (KENNETH WELLS, MD, DIRECTOR): This program develops careers in mental health services research for 6 junior to mid-career academic psychiatrists from institutions lacking a strong research base. The program offers two years of intensive research training at UCLA, followed by 2-3 years of support upon return to the home institution. Training emphasizes research on outcomes and quality of care under managed care and services for vulnerable populations (children, severely mentally ill, HIV). Applicants must be board certified and have a full-time academic appointment in psychiatry at the applicant's institution. The program covers 3/4 and the home institution 1/4 of the salary and benefits. Applications available now for start dates of July 1, 1997 or July 1, 1998 (for 3 positions). Ethnic minorities are encouraged to apply. For information, contact Jean Geisburg, (Administrator) at UCLA/NPI, 760 Westwood Blvd, Los Angeles, CA 90024, or call 310-825-4893, FAX 310-825-4560. E-mail: geisberg@ucla.edu.

Chiefs/Department Heads/Directors

CHIEF OF STAFF: The Department of Veterans Affairs Medical Center in Battle Creek, Michigan has an immediate opening for a physician with experience in the administration of managed care and demonstrated leadership skills to guide the clinical services. S/he must be eligible for appointment to an affiliated university. We currently operate 439 neuropsychiatric beds, 191 nursing home care unit beds and an outpatient clinic. The total annual outpatient visits for the Medical Center and Clinic exceeds 144,000. Benefits package includes Health Insurance, Life Insurance, Leave and Retirement Plan. Applicants may be subject to drug screening test. Interested candidates should forward CV to Dr Walter Grabowski, Chairperson, Chief of Staff Search Committee (11), VA Medical Center, 5500 Armstrong Road, Battle Creek, MI 49016 or call 616-966-5600, extension 6117. Equal Opportunity Employer.

Reply Box Service is available for an additional $20 per insertion.

THIS MONTH IN

ARCHIVES OF GENERAL PSYCHIATRY

Is melancholic depression *quantitatively* more severe than or *qualitatively* distinct from the nonmelancholic type? **Kendler** (page 299) found that in epidemiologically sampled female twins, melancholia predicted increased comorbidity with anxiety disorders, more episodes, more impairment, lower levels of neuroticism, and an increased risk of major depression (MD) in co-twins. However, within twin pairs concordant for MD, no resemblance was found for melancholia. While *DSM-IV* melancholia is a valid subtype of MD that identifies a subset of affected individuals with distinct clinical features and a high familial liability, differences between melancholic and nonmelancholic MD seem more quantitative than qualitative.

The universality of panic disorder has been challenged. **Weissman et al** (page 305) report data from epidemiologic studies conducted independently in 10 countries (the United States, Canada, Puerto Rico, France, Germany, Italy, Lebanon, Taiwan, Korea, and New Zealand). They conclude that panic disorder is relatively consistent in rates and patterns across the diverse countries studied.

Kessler et al (page 313), using retrospective age of onset data from a large national population survey, found that when a lifetime *DSM-III-R* alcohol disorder occurred with another *DSM-III-R* disorder, the alcohol disorder began at an older age. These results cannot be considered definitive because of the retrospective design of the study, but they raise the possibility that primary mental disorders are important risk factors for alcoholism.

Is schizophrenia the only psychiatric disorder that may have a neurodevelopmental origin? **Machón et al** (page 322) investigated this question in the context of the 1957 influenza epidemic in Helsinki, Finland. They report an increase in major affective disorder (particularly unipolar depression) among those who, as fetuses, were exposed to the influenza epidemic in their second trimester.

Verhulst et al (page 329) found that among 13- to 18-year-olds from the Dutch general population, the most common disorders diagnosed were anxiety and conduct disorders. Many of those who received a psychiatric (*DSM-III-R*) diagnosis functioned quite well, however, a small percentage also had overall poor functioning.

Terms such as *risk, risk factor,* and especially *cause* are often inconsistently and imprecisely used, which fosters scientific miscommunication. **Kraemer et al** (page 337) propose a paradigm to label risk factors in ways that suggest the roles they play in the etiology of a disorder and that are suggestive of what research strategies are necessary to document those roles.

Lenzenweger et al (page 345) explored the feasibility of using a PD screen and a 2-stage method in which only individuals that were screened positive for personality disorder would be interviewed by clinicians. In a nonclinical population, the screen detected all individuals who subsequently received a definite diagnosis on interview. This 2-stage method might substantially reduce the number of people requiring interview in a major epidemiologic study of PDs and could probably decrease the cost of such a study.

Using data from the Primary Care Evaluation of Mental Disorders 1000 study, **Kroenke et al** (page 352) examined the validity of multisomatoform disorder, a new diagnosis defined as 3 or more medically unexplained, currently bothersome physical symptoms, and a chronic history (≥2 years) of somatization. Disability, health care use, and patient difficulty equaled or exceeded that found with mood and anxiety disorders. Establishment of the criteria for multisomatoform disorder may be an improved means of identifying clinically significant somatization in primary care.

Bremner et al (page 364) used depressed patients as their own controls, examining brain metabolism with positron emission tomography. Patients with tryptophan depletion–induced depressive relapse (but not the nonrelapsing patients) had a decrease in brain metabolism in the prefrontal cortex, orbitofrontal cortex, and thalamus during tryptophan depletion in comparison with placebo, which was correlated with increased depression.

Schwartz et al (page 375) administered the serotonergic agent meta-chlorophenylpiperazine (m-CPP) to patients with seasonal affective disorder (SAD) and healthy controls before and after 2 weeks of light treatment and found that patients with SAD showed abnormal behavioral and neuroendocrine responses. Recovery from depression correlated with the reduction in nocturnal core temperatures following light treatment. The abnormal behavioral responses to m-CPP constitute a replicated state-marker of SAD; the reduction in nocturnal core temperatures reflects a property of light treatment that is common in other effective antidepressant treatments.

ORIGINAL ARTICLE

The Diagnostic Validity of Melancholic Major Depression in a Population-Based Sample of Female Twins

Kenneth S. Kendler, MD

Background: Although the diagnosis of melancholia is among the oldest in psychiatry, the validity of the melancholic subtype of major depression (MD) is still debated. If melancholia is a valid subtype of depression, is it *quantitatively* more severe than or *qualitatively* distinct from nonmelancholic depression?

Methods: The lifetime history of MD and melancholia, defined by *DSM-IV* criteria, was assessed at interview in 1902 female twins selected from a population-based register. Patterns of comorbidity and the relationship between melancholia and risk for MD in the co-twin were assessed by logistic regression and Cox proportional hazards models, respectively.

Results: In those with a lifetime history of MD, melancholia was associated with the following: (1) increased comorbidity with anxiety disorders and nicotine dependence but not alcohol dependence or bulimia; (2) greater number of episodes, more impairment, and help seeking; (3) lower levels of neuroticism; and (4) an increased risk of MD in co-twins—greater in monozygotic than in dizygotic pairs. Within twin pairs concordant for MD, no resemblance was found for melancholia. A multiple threshold model in which melancholic MD represented a quantitatively more severe form of depressive illness fitted the data well.

Conclusions: Melancholia, defined by *DSM-IV* criteria, is a valid subtype of MD and identifies a subset of affected individuals with distinct clinical features and a particularly high familial liability to depressive illness. However, from a familial perspective, the differences between melancholic and nonmelancholic MD are quantitative, not qualitative. ie, melancholic MD is more severe than, but is *not* etiologically distinct from, nonmelancholic MD.

Arch Gen Psychiatry. 1997;54:299-304

Although the concept of melancholia—a biologically based, severe depressive syndrome, can be traced back to antiquity,[1] the diagnostic validity of this construct remains uncertain. In particular, it has been long debated whether melancholic and nonmelancholic depression represent 2 etiologically distinct syndromes or 1 syndrome, differing only in severity.[2-5]

Given the importance of familial factors in the etiology of depression,[6] a psychiatric genetic perspective on this issue might be illuminating. In this article, we examine melancholic MD, defined by *DSM-IV* criteria,[7] as assessed in a population-based sample of female twins. From an epidemiologic perspective, we address 2 questions: (1) In those with lifetime MD, does personality type or clinical or historical features of the illness distinguish those with and without the melancholic subtype? (2) Are patterns of comorbidity different in those with melancholic vs nonmelancholic MD?

From a genetic-epidemiologic perspective, we evaluate 2 etiologic models for melancholic and nonmelancholic MD: (1) Do the 2 disorders differ *quantitatively*, ie, is melancholic MD a more severe subtype of the same disorder that, in milder form, gives rise to nonmelancholic MD? (In this context, severity is defined from a familial perspective and means "associated with an increased risk of illness in relatives.") (2) Alternatively, are melancholic and nonmelancholic MD *qualitatively* different disorders with distinct etiologies? From a familial perspective, this would predict—in pairs of relatives both affected with MD—a high degree of concordance for the melancholic vs nonmelancholic subtypes of illness.

From the Departments of Psychiatry and Human Genetics, Medical College of Virginia, Virginia Commonwealth University, Richmond.

SUBJECTS AND METHODS

POPULATION-BASED SAMPLE OF FEMALE TWINS

The white same-sex (female) twins selected for this study are part of a population used in a longitudinal study of genetic and environmental risk factors for common psychiatric disorders.[8] The twins, ascertained from the population-based Virginia Twin Registry, were eligible to participate in this study if both members of the pair had previously responded to a mailed questionnaire, to which the individual response rate was 64%. In our first personal interview, we succeeded in interviewing 92% of the eligible individuals (n=2163). Of these interviews, 90% were completed face to face, and 10% by telephone. Neither mode of interview nor the cooperation status of the co-twin was related to the risk for MD.[8] Zygosity was determined blindly by standard questions[9]; photographs; and, when necessary, by DNA.[10]

Since this original interview, we have completed 2 additional waves of interviews, both by telephone, that succeeded in interviewing 2001 (92.5%) and 1902 (87.9%) of the original sample, respectively. The mean (±SD) number of months between the first and third interviews was 61.3±5.1. In the third interview, we assessed both members of 849 pairs, 496 of whom were monozygotic (MZ) and 353 of whom were dizygotic (DZ). The mean (±SD) age of the twins who participated in the third wave of interviews was 34.6±7.5 years (range, 22-59 years). All interviews were conducted blind to information about the co-twin.

METHODS

Measures

Using adaptations of the *Structured Clinical Interview for DSM-III-R*,[11] our first personal interview assessed lifetime diagnoses of MD, generalized anxiety disorder (GAD), panic disorder, bulimia, phobias, and alcohol dependence. In addition, past-year MD and GAD were assessed during the second and third waves of telephone interviews. During the third interview, we again assessed a lifetime history of MD; this time with the addition of questions reflecting all the criteria for melancholic subtype by *DSM-IV*.[7] Criterion B5 (significant weight loss) was defined as episode-related loss of 4.5 kg or more.

Diagnoses of MD and alcohol dependence were assigned, by computer algorithm, using *DSM-III-R* criteria.[12] For GAD, we used the symptomatic criteria from *DSM-III-R*, but followed *DSM-III*[13] requiring 1-month minimum duration. *Phobia* was defined as the presence of 1 of 17 specific fears that the respondent considered to be irrational and that produced objective behavioral interference with the respondent's life.[14] To maximize the statistical power of our study, we used broader definitions of bulimia and panic disorder, for which previous analyses have shown that the additional "possible" cases of illness were on the same continuum of liability as those diagnosed with greater certainty.[15,16] Individuals who reported being, at some point in their life, regular smokers, were asked to retrospectively rate the Fagerstrom Tolerance Questionnaire[17] for their time of heaviest cigarette consumption. We defined as "nicotine dependent" any individual with a history of regular smoking and a Fagerstrom Tolerance Questionnaire score of 7 or greater. Melancholia was diagnosed by computer algorithm using *DSM-IV* criteria.[7]

At their first interview, twins were given a self-report questionnaire containing 12 and 8 items from the neuroticism and extraversion scales, respectively, derived from the Eysenck Personality Questionnaire.[18,19] As assessed by these items, the test-retest reliabilities (assessed by product-moment correlation) in this sample

RESULTS

CLINICAL AND HISTORICAL PREDICTORS, COMORBIDITY, AND PERSONALITY

Among the 568 individual twins who reported a lifetime history of MD, 285 (50.2%) met *DSM-IV* criteria for melancholia during their worst lifetime episode. Neither year of birth (χ^2=3.07, P=.08 [not significant]) nor zygosity (χ^2=0.00, P=.99[not significant]) distinguished melancholic from nonmelancholic MD. Compared with individuals with nonmelancholic MD (**Table 1**), those with melancholic MD had a similar age at onset and duration of longest episode but had significantly more episodes, met more *DSM-IV* "A" criteria for MD for their worst episode, were more likely to be incapacitated from their depression, and sought professional help more frequently.

Table 2 depicts comorbidity between nonmelancholic and melancholic MD and 6 other psychiatric or substance-use disorders. Two of the disorders, alcohol dependence and bulimia, had nonsignificantly higher odds ratios with nonmelancholic than with melancholic MD. The remaining 4 disorders: nicotine dependence, generalized anxiety disorder, panic disorder, and phobia, all had significantly greater levels of comorbidity with melancholic than with nonmelancholic MD.

Five years prior to the interview at which we assessed melancholia, the twins who at that time were not actively or recently depressed were assessed for neuroticism and extraversion. By logistic regression, neuroticism predicted those subjects with lifetime MD (n=502) who would *not* qualify for melancholia in the most recent interview (χ^2=8.73, df=1, P=.003). A *decrease* of 1 SD in neuroticism was associated with an *increase* in risk for melancholia of 1.31. No significant relationship was found between extraversion and melancholia in subjects with MD (χ^2=0.92, df=1, P=.34).

PREDICTION OF RISK OF MD IN CO-TWIN

To assess whether melancholia indexed familial severity of depressive illness, we examined whether the presence of melancholia in twins with a history of MD increased the hazard rate for MD in the co-twin. It did with an RR of 1.52 (χ^2=6.93, P=.008). Was this because melancholia specifically reflected familial severity of illness or because melancholia was only a nonspecific index of clinical severity that, in turn, reflected familial severity of MD? We addressed this question by repeating this analysis adding 4 potential meaover 17 months were +0.69 and +0.78 for neuroticism and extraversion, respectively.[20]

Statistical Analysis

Differences in clinical or historical characteristics of individuals with melancholic vs nonmelancholic MD were assessed by *t test* or χ^2 analysis. Differences in the patterns of comorbidity in the 2 depressive subtypes were examined by logistic regression in all twins with MD, testing whether a dummy independent variable, ie, melancholic vs nonmelancholic depression, predicted risk for the comorbid disorder. These analyses controlled for zygosity and year of birth.

The relationship between melancholia in 1 twin and the risk for MD in the co-twin was assessed using the Cox proportional hazards model, as operationalized in the PHREG (proportional hazards regression) procedure in *SAS/STAT User's Guide, Version 6*.[21] These analyses examine co-twins of twins with a lifetime history of MD. A predictor variable reflecting additive genetic effects should, in Cox regression, produce a regression coefficient that is approximately twice as great in MZ as in DZ twins. Because the relative risk (RR) is an exponentialized form of the regression coefficient, if melancholia reflected the *genetic* risk to MD, the RR in MZ twins should be approximately the square of the RR in DZ twins.

Correction is required in the regression analyses for assuming independence of the observations from the doubly counted twin pairs. If *T* was the total number of observations, *N* the number of doubly counted twin pairs, and *P* the number of parameters in our model, we multiplied the SEs obtained by $[(T\text{-}P)/(T\text{-}N\text{-}P)]^{1/2}$. This approximate correction is conservative as it assumes that twins are perfectly correlated for the relevant variables.[22] All significances reported are based on our corrected SEs.

Twin model fitting was performed using the computer program Mx.[23] (More details of twin model fitting can be found elsewhere.[24,25]) Our major goal here was to test "the multiple threshold model."[26] This model tests whether, from a familial perspective, 2 or more syndromes reflect different levels of severity on a single dimension of liability or syndromes with independent etiologies. In this case, we fit a multiple threshold liability model to two 3×3 tables, one each in MZ and DZ twins, cross-classifying each member of the twin pair into unaffected, nonmelancholic MD, and melancholic MD. A χ^2 goodness of fit test is available for testing this model.

We also attempted to partition the variance in the liability to MD into that due to the following parameters: genetic effects (a^2), familial-environmental effects (c^2), and environmental experiences unique to the individual (plus measurement error) (e^2). We began by fitting, to the two 3×3 contingency tables, a full or *ACE* model that contains all 3 parameters, and then fitted 2 simpler models: the *CE* model (which postulates that familial resemblance for depression is attributable solely to familial-environmental effects) and the *AE* model (which postulates that familial resemblance for depression is attributable solely to additive genetic effects). We then reported parameter estimates from the best fitting model, which was chosen using the Aikake information criterion (AIC).[27,28] The relative fit of nested models was compared by using the χ^2 difference test.

We found a small number of extreme values for the number of depressive episodes and the duration of the longest episode. To reduce the influence of these outliers, we truncated the number of episodes at 100; the duration of longest episode was truncated at 5 years. All reported *P* values are 2-tailed. All results of χ^2 from logistic and Cox regression analyses have 1 *df*.

sures of clinical severity as control variables: age at onset, number of episodes, duration of longest episode, and degree of impairment. The association between melancholia and risk for MD in the co-twin was unchanged (RR=1.55, χ^2=6.66, *P*=.009). To test this hypothesis more stringently, we added the number of criterion A symptoms endorsed as a further control. This resulted in an *increase* in the ability of melancholia in 1 twin to predict the risk of MD in the co-twin (RR=1.75, χ^2=7.81, *P*=.005).

We then examined the ability of individual *DSM-IV* criteria for melancholia to predict the risk of MD in the co-twin. Of the 8 criteria, 6 predicted an increased risk of MD in co-twin (all but A3 [early morning awakening] and A5 [significant anorexia or weight loss]). However, this relationship reached statistical significance for only 2 criteria: A2 (lack of reactivity) (RR=1.41, χ^2=4.64, *P*=.03) and B1 (distinct quality of depressed mood) (RR=1.66, χ^2=5.05, *P*=.02). While the presence of criterion B2 (depression regularly worse in the morning) did not significantly predict an increased risk of MD in the co-twin (RR=1.18, χ^2=0.37, *P*=.54), the twin's endorsement of a reverse circadian mood pattern (depression worse in the evening) strongly and significantly predicted a decreased risk of MD in the co-twin (RR=0.58, χ^2=7.84, *P*=.005).

When year of birth was controlled, melancholia in 1 twin was predictive of the risk for total MD (melancholic plus nonmelancholic subtypes) in the co-twin considerably more strongly in MZ pairs (RR=1.69, χ^2=6.30, *P*=.01) than in DZ pairs (RR=1.30, χ^2=1.15, *P*=.29). While this difference was not statistically significant (χ^2=0.91, *df*=1, 1-tailed *P*=.18), it is exactly the ratio predicted under the model of additive genetic effects (eg, $RR_{MZ}=[RR_{DZ}]^2$, see earlier). The same pattern was seen when these analyses were repeated controlling for the clinical severity of MD (ie, for MZ pairs, RR=1.72, χ^2=5.96, *P*=.01; for DZ pairs, RR=1.32, χ^2=1.10, *P*=.30).

MODEL FITTING

The multiple threshold model assumes a single continuum of liability to MD, in which, from a familial perspective, melancholic MD is the "severe" and nonmelancholic MD is the "mild" subtype. This model fitted our results well in both MZ (χ^2=0.73, *df*=3, *P*=.87) and DZ twins (χ^2=2.70, *df*=3, *P*=.44) and estimated the polychoric correlations (±SE) to be +0.44±0.06 and +0.18±0.08, respectively. The *ACE* model fitted the data very well (χ^2=5.10, *df*=10, *P*=.88, AIC=−15.49). The *AE* model, which assumes that all familial resemblance for the liability to MD is genetic

Table 1. Clinical Characteristics of Female Twins With Nonmelancholic vs Melancholic Major Depression (MD)

	MD Subtype					
	Nonmelancholic*		Melancholic†			
Characteristics	Mean	SD	Mean	SD	*t* or χ^2 (*df*)	*P*
Age at onset, y	23.4	7.8	24.0	9.0	0.95‖ (566)	.34
No. of episodes‡	5.4	10.1	8.7	16.7	2.80‖ (459.6)#	.005
Duration of longest episode,§ d	172.9	308.4	212.3	343.8	1.44‖ (566)	.15
No. of A criterion symptoms	5.9	0.8	7.3	1.2	16.47‖ (514.8)#	<.001
Incapacitated, %	20.8		46.1		40.65¶ (1)	<.001
Help seeking, %	38.3		55.1		16.05¶ (1)	<.001

*n=281-283.
†n=281-285.
‡Number of episodes truncated at 100.
§Longest episode truncated at 1825 days (5 years).
‖*t* Test.
¶χ^2 Test.
#Degrees of freedom for *t* test corrected for unequal variances.

in origin, fitted just as well, but had a better AIC because of greater parsimony (χ^2=5.10, *df*=11, AIC = -16.90). By contrast, the *CE* model, which hypothesizes that familial transmission of the liability to MD is entirely environmental, fitted the data considerably less well (χ^2=11.43, *df*=11, AIC=−10.57) (χ^2 difference test vs the *ACE* model, χ^2=6.33, *df*=1, *P*=.01). Heritability of liability to MD (a^2) was estimated from the best fitting *AE* model at +0.43.

Our sample contained a total of 107 twin pairs concordant for lifetime MD (MZ, 65; DZ, 42). Among these pairs, no significant association was seen for melancholic vs nonmelancholic subtypes) (χ^2=2.01, *df*=1 [not significant]). A similar pattern was seen when the MZ pairs (χ^2=0.12, *df*=1, *P*=.16, *P*=.73 [not significant]) and DZ pairs were analyzed separately (χ^2=3.20, *df*=1, *P*=.07 [not significant]). To explore this further, we examined correlations for the total of endorsed melancholic criteria in pairs concordant for MD. This was not significant in all twins (*r*=+0.08, *P*=.44), MZ twins (*r*=+0.03, *P*=.80), or DZ twins (*r*=+0.15, *P*=.33).

COMMENT

EPIDEMIOLOGIC APPROACHES

A recent review, focusing on treated samples, concluded that melancholia had "some clinical utility and some validity" and should be retained as a subtype of MD in *DSM-IV*.[5,7] Our results, from an epidemiologic sample, support and complement this conclusion.

Consistent with prior evidence, women from a birth certificate–based twin registry with a lifetime history of MD who reported having had melancholia also described having had more depressive episodes, a greater number of symptoms, more impairment, and more frequent help seeking. However, neither age at onset nor duration of episodes differed in individuals with melancholic and nonmelancholic MD.

While patterns of comorbidity can be informative in the evaluation of subtyping schemas, their interpretation in clinical samples can be problematic.[29] Examining an epidemiologic sample circumvents these difficulties. Nicotine dependence, GAD, panic disorder, and phobias all co-occurred significantly more frequently with melancholic than with nonmelancholic MD. By contrast, alcohol dependence and bulimia co-occurred more frequently, albeit nonsignificantly, with nonmelancholic MD.

Consistent with several diagnostic systems for melancholic or endogenous MD,[5] and with prior studies in clinical samples,[30-34] we found significantly lower levels of neuroticism, assessed outside of depressive episodes, in individuals with melancholic than in those with nonmelancholic MD. Consistent with some,[33] but not other clinical studies,[30,34] we found similar levels of extraversion in the 2 depressive subtypes.

In this twin sample, a substantial correlation is found in the genetic risk factors for MD and neuroticism.[20] Neuroticism may be a better index of the genetic risk for nonmelancholic than for melancholic MD.

GENETIC APPROACHES

We applied genetic strategies to address the underlying etiologic relationship between melancholic and nonmelancholic depression. In particular, we wanted to determine whether these 2 syndromes differed *quantitatively* or *qualitatively*. Consistent with most,[5,35-40] but not all,[41,42] reports, we found that, in twins with MD, the presence of a melancholic subtype in 1 twin substantially increased the risk for MD in her co-twin.

This finding led to 3 further questions.

First, given that patients with melancholic MD are clinically more severely ill than those with nonmelancholic MD, are we seeing a *general* effect that clinical severity correlates with familial severity[43] or is there a *specific* effect of melancholic features? The answer clearly is the latter. Controlling for a range of indexes of clinical severity only *strengthened* the association between melancholia in 1 twin and increased risk for MD in her co-twin.

Second, which individual criterion for melancholia identified twins with a high familial liability to MD? Two criteria stood out: "lack of reactivity" and "distinct quality of depressed mood." In prior studies examining individual criteria for melancholic MD,[4,5,44,45] these have usually been among the best discriminators. In a large-scale clinical study of MD,[45] "lack of reactivity" was the strongest predictor of the autonomous subtype. The predictive power of these symptoms was remarkable, as they are recalled retrospectively from episodes often years prior to interview. By contrast, psychomotor changes and guilt, often noted as strong predictors of melancholia,[5,44] were nonsignificant predictors of risk of illness in co-twins (RRs of 1.11 and 1.07, respectively). Circadian changes in mood significantly predicted illness in the co-twin, but only when operationalized as "mood worse in evening" (predicting a *reduced* risk in co-twin), rather than the traditional "mood worse in morning."

Third, given that melancholia reflected the familial vulnerability to depressive illness, did it index familial-environmental or genetic risk? If melancholia reflected familial-environmental risk factors, it should predict risk of MD in co-twin equally strongly in MZ and DZ pairs; if it reflected genetic factors, it should predict risk of MD more strongly in MZ than in DZ twins. Although the patterns of results were those predicted by the genetic model, the RR in MZ and DZ twins did not differ significantly. Despite the large twin sample, we had insufficient power to detect such differences.[46] Melancholia is an index of the familial liability to MD. Consistent with a recent clinical twin sample,[40] our results suggest, but do not prove, that melancholia specifically reflects the underlying genetic liability to affective illness.

TESTING ETIOLOGIC MODELS

While the above results are consistent with the concept that, from a familial-genetic perspective, melancholic and nonmelancholic MD differ *quantitatively*, this hypothesis can be explicitly tested by a multiple threshold model. Separately, in both MZ and DZ twins, this model fit our data very well.

We also could evaluate, using a genetic strategy, the hypothesis that melancholic and nonmelancholic MD represented *qualitatively* distinct disorders. This theory would predict, within twin pairs concordant for MD, substantial concordance for the melancholic and nonmelancholic subtypes. However, in all twin pairs and in MZ or DZ twins examined separately, the degree of concordance did not approach statistical significance.

Within the statistical power available, the pattern of findings in this twin sample suggests that melancholic and nonmelancholic MD differ quantitatively but not qualitatively. The 2 disorders are reflections of the same underlying liability to illness and not the result of 2 distinct etiologic processes.

COMPARISON WITH PREVIOUS LATENT CLASS ANALYSIS

A latent class analysis of symptoms of depression reported in the last year in this sample produced 3 subtypes of clinical depression: mild typical, atypical, and severe typical.[47] Unlike the current findings, substantial subtype resemblance was seen for these syndromes in twin pairs concordant for MD. However, subtype assignment in 1 twin did *not* significantly predict risk of MD in the co-twin.

The 1-year prevalence section of our interview does not contain melancholic symptoms; so, we cannot rigorously compare these 2 typologies for MD. Overall, these 2 analyses suggest that melancholic and atypical vegetative features may provide complementary for MD. Melancholia indexes the genetic liability to MD, while atypical vegetative features do not. However, typical-atypical vegetative features strongly "run" in concordant twin pairs, suggesting qualitatively different etiologic processes, while melancholia does not.

Table 2. Pattern of Comorbidity in Melancholic and Nonmelancholic Major Depression (MD)

Disorder	Odds Ratios With: Nonmelancholic MD	Odds Ratios With: Melancholic MD	Difference,§ *P*
Alcohol dependence	2.13*	1.81*	.56
Bulimia	2.08*	1.87‡	.70
Nicotine dependence	1.82*	3.10†	.03
Generalized anxiety disorder	3.22†	5.42†	.004
Panic disorder	2.17*	4.03†	.02
Phobia	1.10†	2.62†	.001

P<.01.*
†P<*.001.*
‡P<*.05.*
§*Difference assessed in a logistic regression in twins with major depression whether the presence of melancholia predicted risk for the comorbid disorder.*

HERITABILITY OF LIABILITY TO MD

Although not the focus on this study, we calculated the heritability of the liability to MD indexed by 3 classes of increasing liability: unaffected, nonmelancholic MD, and melancholic MD. This estimate, ie, 43%, is remarkably similar to the 42% derived from a lifetime history of total MD assessed at personal interview in this sample 5 years earlier.[8] At neither assessment did twin modeling reveal any evidence for a significant impact of the familial environment on risk of MD. These heritability estimates, however, confound true individual specific environment and measurement error. Correcting for errors of measurement may result in a substantial increase in the heritability of MD.[48]

LIMITATIONS

The results presented herein should be interpreted in the context of 3 potential limitations. First, the sample is restricted to women, mostly in early and middle adult life. While most studies of clinical subjects find no differences in rates of melancholic MD in men and women,[39,45] the large gender differences in overall population rates for MD[49,50] suggest caution in extrapolating results for affective illness from women to men.

Second, in this study, melancholic symptoms were assessed retrospectively by self-report during telephone interviews. Most clinical studies have evaluated current symptoms, using both self-report and clinician observation. Our assessment of symptoms like psychomotor retardation might differ from those used in clinical studies, where ratings were based largely on clinical assessment. Prior studies of self-report symptoms of MD suggest substantial unreliability.[51] While such measurement error is more likely to attenuate than exaggerate true relationships, the possibility that biased recall produced artifactual findings cannot be excluded. While both we[8] and other researchers[52] have found little difference in rates of MD by mode of interview, it remains possible that different results would have been obtained using face-to-face, rather than telephone, interviews.

Third, our multiple threshold model analyses and our estimations of heritability are based on the assumptions of the liability-threshold model. As previously outlined in this journal,[25] these assumptions, although unlikely to be precisely correct, remain plausible for complex human traits such as MD.

Accepted for publication August 28, 1996.

This work was supported by grant MH-40828 from the National Institutes of Health, Bethesda, Md, and the Rachel Brown Banks Endowment Fund, Richmond, Va. Dr Kendler is supported by the Research Scientist Award MH-01277 from the National Institute of Mental Health, Bethesda. The Virginia Twin Registry, established and maintained by W. Nance, MD, PhD, and L. Corey, PhD, is supported by grants HD-26746 and NS-31564 from the National Institutes of Health

I gratefully acknowledge Charles Gardner, PhD, for his assistance in the data analysis and my colleagues Lindon Eaves, PhD, Carol Prescott, PhD, Michael Neale, PhD, Andrew Heath, PhD, and Ronald Kessler, PhD, for their contribution to this study.

Reprints: Kenneth S. Kendler, MD, Psychiatric Genetics Research Program, Department of Psychiatry, PO Box 980126, Richmond, VA 23298-0126 (e-mail: kendler@gems.vcu.edu).

REFERENCES

1. Jackson SW. *Melancholia and Depression: From Hippocratic Times to Modern Times.* New Haven, Conn: Yale University Press; 1986.
2. Kendell RE. The classification of depressions: a review of contemporary confusion. *Br J Psychiatry.* 1976;129:15-28.
3. Farmer A, McGuffin P. The classification of the depressions: contemporary confusion revisited. *Br J Psychiatry.* 1989;155:437-443.
4. Zimmerman M, Spitzer RL. Melancholia: from *DSM-III* to *DSM-III-R. Am J Psychiatry.* 1989;146:20-28.
5. Rush AJ, Weissenburger JE. Melancholic symptom features and *DSM-IV. Am J Psychiatry.* 1994;151:489-498.
6. Tsuang MT, Faraone SV. *The Genetics of Mood Disorders.* Baltimore, Md: Johns Hopkins University Press; 1990.
7. American Psychiatric Association. *Diagnostic and Statistical Manual of Mental Disorders, Fourth Edition.* Washington, DC: American Psychiatric Association; 1994.
8. Kendler KS, Neale MC, Kessler RC, Heath AC, Eaves LJ. A population-based twin study of major depression in women: the impact of varying definitions of illness. *Arch Gen Psychiatry.* 1992;49:257-266.
9. Eaves LJ, Eysenck HJ, Martin NG, Jardine R, Heath AC, Feingold L, Young PA, Kendler KS. *Genes, Culture and Personality: An Empirical Approach.* London, England: Oxford University Press; 1989.
10. Spence JE, Corey LA, Nance WE, Marazita ML, Kendler KS, Schieken RM. Molecular analysis of twin zygosity using VNTR DNA probes. *Am J Hum Genet.* 1988;43:A159.
11. Spitzer RL, Williams JB, Gibbon M. *Structured Clinical Interview for DSM-III-R.* New York, NY: Biometrics Research Department, New York State Psychiatric Institute; 1987.
12. American Psychiatric Association. *Diagnostic and Statistical Manual of Mental Disorders, Revised Third Edition.* Washington, DC: American Psychiatric Association; 1987.
13. Kendler KS, Neale MC, Kessler RC, Heath AC, Eaves LJ. Generalized anxiety disorder in women: a population-based twin study. *Arch Gen Psychiatry.* 1992; 49:267-272.
14. Kendler KS, Neale MC, Kessler RC, Heath AC, Eaves LJ. The genetic epidemiology of phobias in women: the inter-relationship of agoraphobia, social phobia, situational phobia and simple phobia. *Arch Gen Psychiatry.* 1992;49:273-281.
15. Kendler KS, MacLean CJ, Neale MC, Kessler RC, Heath AC, Eaves LJ. The genetic epidemiology of bulimia nervosa. *Am J Psychiatry.* 1991;148:1627-1637.
16. Kendler KS, Neale MC, Kessler RC, Heath AC, Eaves LJ. Panic disorder in women: a population-based twin study. *Psychol Med.* 1993;23:397-406.
17. Fagerstrom K-O, Schneider NG. Measuring nicotine dependence: a review of the Fagerstrom Tolerance Questionnaire. *J Behav Med.* 1989;12:159-182.
18. Eysenck HJ, Eysenck SBG. *Manual of the Eysenck Personality Questionnaire.* London, England: Hodder and Stoughton; 1975.
19. Heath AC, Neale MC, Kessler RC, Eaves LJ, Kendler KS. Evidence for genetic influences on personality from self-reports and from informant ratings. *J Pers Soc Psychol.* 1992;63:85-96.
20. Kendler KS, Neale MC, Kessler RC, Heath AC, Eaves LJ. A longitudinal twin study of personality and major depression in women. *Arch Gen Psychiatry.* 1993;50:853-862.
21. SAS Institute. *SAS/STAT User's Guide, Version 6.* 4th ed. Cary, NC: SAS Institute Inc; 1990:1, 2.
22. Kish L, Frankel MR. Inferences from complex samples. *J R Stat Soc [B].* 1974; 36:1-37.
23. Neale MC. *Statistical Modelling With Mx.* Virginia Commonwealth University, Department of Psychiatry, Richmond, Va: 126-0126.
24. Neale MC, Cardon LR. *Methodology for Genetic Studies of Twins and Families.* Dordrecht, the Netherlands: Kluwer Academic Publishers BV; 1992.
25. Kendler KS. Twin studies of psychiatric illness: current status and future directions. *Arch Gen Psychiatry.* 1993;50:905-915.
26. Reich T, James JW, Morris CA. The use of multiple thresholds in determining the mode of transmission of semi-continuous traits. *Ann Hum Genet.* 1972; 36:163-184.
27. Akaike H. Factor analysis and AIC. *Psychometrika.* 1987;52:317-332.
28. Williams LJ, Holahan PJ. Parsimony-based fit indices for multiple-indicator models: do they work? *Struct Equation Model.* 1994;1:161-189.
29. Berkson J. Limitations of the application of fourfold table analysis to hospital data. *Biometr Bull.* 1946;2:47-53.
30. Kendell RE, DiScipio WJ. Eysenck Personality Inventory scores of patients with depressive illnesses. *Br J Psychiatry.* 1968;114:767-770.
31. Matussek P, Feil WB. Personality attributes of depressive patients. *Arch Gen Psychiatry.* 1983;40:783-790.
32. Davidson J, Miller R, Strickland R. Neuroticism and personality disorder in depression. *J Affect Disord.* 1985;8:177-182.
33. Abou-Saleh MT, Coppen A. Classification of depressive illnesses: clinico-psychological correlates. *J Affect Disord.* 1984;6:53-66.
34. Benjaminsen S. Primary non-endogenous depression and features attributed to reactive depression. *J Affect Disord.* 1981;3:245-259.
35. Gillespie RD. The clinical differentiation of types of depression. *Guy's Hosp Rep.* 1929;9:306-344.
36. Slater E, Shields J. Genetical aspects of anxiety. *Br J Psychiatry, Special Publication.* 1969;3:62-71.
37. Leckman JF, Weissman MM, Prusoff BA, Caruso KA, Merikangas KR, Pauls DL, Kidd KK. Subtypes of depression: family study perspective. *Arch Gen Psychiatry.* 1984;41:833-838.
38. Torgersen S. Genetic factors in moderately severe and mild affective disorders. *Arch Gen Psychiatry.* 1986;43:222-226.
39. Grove WM, Andreasen NC, Young M, Endicott J, Keller MB, Hirschfeld RMA, Reich T. Isolation and characterization of a nuclear depressive syndrome. *Psychol Med.* 1987;17:471-484.
40. McGuffin P, Katz R, Watkins S, Rutherford J. A hospital-based twin register of the heritability of *DSM-IV* unipolar depression. *Arch Gen Psychiatry.* 1996;53: 129-136.
41. Shapiro RW. A twin study of non-endogenous depression. *Acta Jutland.* 1970; XLII:2.
42. von Knorring L. Morbidity risk for psychiatric disorders in relatives of patients with neurotic-reactive depression. In: Racagni G, Smeraldi E, eds. *Anxious Depression: Assessment and Treatment.* New York, NY: Raven Press; 1987.
43. Kendler KS, Neale MC, Kessler RC, Heath AC, Eaves LJ. The clinical characteristics of major depression as indices of the familial risk to illness. *Br J Psychiatry.* 1994;165:66-72.
44. Nelson JC, Charney DS. The symptoms of major depressive illness. *Am J Psychiatry.* 1981;138:1-13.
45. Nelson JC, Charney DS, Quinlan DM. Characteristics of autonomous depression. *J Nerv Ment Dis.* 1980;168:637-643.
46. Wahlsten D Insensitivity of the analysis of variance to heredity-environment interaction. *Behav Brain Sci.* 1990;13:109-161.
47. Kendler KS, Eaves LJ, Walters EE, Neale MC, Heath AC, Kessler RC. The identification and validation of distinct depressive syndromes in a population-based sample of female twins. *Arch Gen Psychiatry.* 1996;53:391-399.
48. Kendler KS, Neale MC, Kessler RC, Heath AC, Eaves LJ. The lifetime history of major depression in women: reliability of diagnosis and heritability. *Arch Gen Psychiatry.* 1993;50:863-870.
49. Weissman MM, Bruce ML, Leaf PJ, Florio LP, Holzer C. Affective disorders. In: Robins LN, Regier DA, eds. *Psychiatric Disorders in America: The Epidemiologic Catchment Area Study.* New York, NY: The Free Press; 1991:53-80.
50. Kessler RC, McGonagle KA, Zhao S, Nelson CB, Hughes M, Eshleman S, Wittchen H-U, Kendler KS. Lifetime and 12-month prevalence of *DSM-III-R* psychiatric disorders in the United States: results from the National Comorbidity Survey. *Arch Gen Psychiatry.* 1994;51:8-10.
51. Bromet EJ, Dunn LO, Connell MM, Dew MA, Schulberg HC. Long-term reliability of diagnosing lifetime major depression in a community sample. *Arch Gen Psychiatry.* 1986;43:435-440.
52. Sobin C, Weissman MM, Goldstein RB, Adams P, Wickramaratne P, Warner V, Lish J. Diagnostic interviewing for family studies: comparing telephone and face-to-face interview methods for the diagnosis of lifetime psychiatric disorders in a family study. *Psychiatr Genet.* 1993;3:227-233.

ORIGINAL ARTICLE

The Cross-national Epidemiology of Panic Disorder

Myrna M. Weissman, PhD; Roger C. Bland, MB; Glorisa J. Canino, PhD; Carlo Faravelli, MD; Steven Greenwald, MA; Hai-Gwo Hwu, MD; Peter R. Joyce, PhD; Elie G. Karam, MD; Chung-Kyoon Lee, MD; Joseph Lellouch, PhD; Jean-Pierre Lépine, MD; Stephen C. Newman, MD; Mark A. Oakley-Browne, PhD; Maritza Rubio-Stipec, MA; J. Elisabeth Wells, PhD; Priya J. Wickramaratne, PhD; Hans-Ulrich Wittchen, PhD; Eng-Kung Yeh, MD

Background: Epidemiological data on panic disorder from community studies from 10 countries around the world are presented to determine the consistency of findings across diverse cultures.

Method: Data from independently conducted community surveys from 10 countries (the United States, Canada, Puerto Rico, France, West Germany, Italy, Lebanon, Taiwan, Korea, and New Zealand), using the Diagnostic Interview Schedule and *DSM-III* criteria and including over 40 000 subjects, were analyzed with appropriate standardization for age and sex differences among subjects from different countries.

Results: The lifetime prevalence rates for panic disorder ranged from 1.4 per 100 in Edmonton, Alberta, to 2.9 per 100 in Florence, Italy, with the exception of that in Taiwan, 0.4 per 100, where rates for most psychiatric disorders are low. Mean age at first onset was usually in early to middle adulthood. The rates were higher in female than male subjects in all countries. Panic disorder was associated with an increased risk of agoraphobia and major depression in all countries.

Conclusions: Panic disorder is relatively consistent, with a few exceptions, in rates and patterns across different countries. It is unclear why the rates of panic and other psychiatric disorders are lower in Taiwan.

Arch Gen Psychiatry. 1997;54:305-309

WHILE THE symptoms of panic disorder have been well described for centuries, diagnostic criteria for panic disorder as a separate entity, distinct from other anxiety disorders, first appeared in the official American Psychiatric Association's *Diagnostic and Statistical Manual of Mental Disorders, Third Edition* in 1980.[1] Since then, a considerable amount of information has appeared on familial risk, pathogenesis, morbidity, and treatment of panic disorder.[2-5]

The epidemiology of panic disorder, its prevalence, demographic variations, and comorbidity with other psychiatric disorders have been well described in the United States based on a community survey of 18 571 adults living in 5 US communities in the 1980s and a more recent US national survey of 8098 adults.[6-9]

In this article, we present epidemiological data on panic disorder from community surveys conducted in 10 countries around the world using similar diagnostic methods to determine the consistency of findings across diverse cultures.

The affiliations of the authors appear in the "Acknowledgment" section at the end of the article.

RESULTS

PREVALENCE, AGE AT ONSET, AND SEX DIFFERENCES

The annual rate of panic disorder ranged from 1.7 per 100 in West Germany to 0.2 per 100 in Taiwan (**Table 2**), a country that has low rates of all psychiatric disorders.[21] The lifetime rate ranged from 2.9 per 100 in Florence to 0.4 per 100 in Taiwan. The rates are consistently higher in female compared with male individuals in every country. The age at onset of panic disorder is usually the early to middle 20s, with later onset in West Germany (age at onset, 35.5 years) and Korea (age at onset, 32.1 years). In the Beirut study, there were 5 persons with panic disorder, all within the past 6

METHODS

DESCRIPTION OF CROSS-NATIONAL SITES

A detailed description of the cross-national sites has been previously published.[10] This cross-national collaboration included investigators from 10 countries who had conducted epidemiological community surveys based on the Diagnostic Interview Schedule, Version III,[11,12] and the *DSM-III* criteria.[1] The sites span diverse geographical, political, and cultural areas in North America, the Caribbean, Europe, the Middle East, the Orient, and the Pacific Rim. The translation, modification, and piloting of the Diagnostic Interview Schedule were made by the investigators in each country as appropriate, and details on the translations plus the methods used are included in the references.

The data from the National Institute of Mental Health Epidemiological Catchment Area Study (ECA)[13] were derived from 5 US communities (New Haven, Conn; Baltimore, Md; St Louis, Mo; the Piedmont County region of North Carolina; and Los Angeles, Calif). The Edmonton Survey of Psychiatric Disorders[14,15] was conducted in the city of Edmonton, Alberta. The Puerto Rico Study of Psychiatric Disorders[16] included persons living in a household throughout Puerto Rico, in addition to those household members temporarily away and those in institutions. The French Study of Psychiatric Disorders[17] was conducted in Savigny, a newly built city located near Paris. The Munich Follow-up Study from West Germany[18] was a 7-year follow-up investigation of a stratified random general population sample drawn from the adult population of the former Federal Republic of Germany (West Germany) in 1974. The Florence Community Survey of Anxiety Disorders from Italy[19] included 1100 persons who were randomly selected from the lists of persons registered with 6 general medical practitioners living in 3 districts of Florence. The Beirut War Events and Depression Study[20] was conducted in Lebanon and included the assessment of panic disorder in the second wave of interviews. Four communities with differential exposure to acts of war were studied: 2 communities within the city of Beirut (Ashrafieh and Ain Remmaneh), and 2 communities outside Beirut proper (Kornet Shehwan and Bejjeh). The Taiwan psychiatric epidemiology project[21] sampled 3 population areas representing metropolitan Taipei and township and rural areas throughout Taiwan. The Korean Epidemiologic Study of Mental Disorders[22,23] sampled persons in urban Seoul and scattered rural regions across the Republic of Korea. The Christchurch Psychiatric Epidemiology Study[24,25] included adults living in Christchurch in the South Island of New Zealand, oversampling young female individuals.

For comparison purposes, data from the National Comorbidity Survey (NCS),[8] a representative sample of 8098 persons aged 15 to 54 years living in the 48 coterminous US states and conducted during 1990-1992, were included. These data are considered separately because different diagnostic assessment was done using the Composite International Diagnostic Interview,[26] on whose basis *DSM-III-R* criteria–based diagnoses were made.[27]

Table 1 gives sample size, response rate, age, and sex distribution of each study.

SAMPLING DESIGN

The ECA, Edmonton, Puerto Rico, and Christchurch sites were household probability samples; the remaining sites, except for West Germany, were drawn as simple random samples constructed so that each household member had the same probability of selection. Because of unequal selection probability of a respondent in the United States, Edmonton, Puerto Rico, and Christchurch, a design weight was computed. For those sites drawn as random samples, the design weight was set at 1.0 for each respondent.

The stratification method used for the phase II 1981 follow-up in West Germany included all subjects who had high scores on the clinical self-rating scales at the phase I investigation in 1974, plus 40% of the sample who were randomly drawn from among the subjects successfully interviewed in phase I. The design weight for West Germany was computed by weighting back to the original 1974 sample by correcting for the proportion of high and low scorers in that sample.[18]

STATISTICAL ANALYSIS

To make valid comparisons of rates across sites, the rates of panic disorder at each site were standardized to the age and sex distribution of the 1980 US census. Analyses are reported only for the 18- to 64-year-old group, with values for West Germany based on ages 26 to 64 years. Data in the NCS included ages 18 to 54 years as no one older than 54 years was sampled.

The design-weighted rates for the ECA, Edmonton, Puerto Rico, West Germany, and Christchurch, and the raw rates for the other sites have been standardized to the 1980 US census. The standardization was done according to methods described by Breslow and Day.[28(pp52-57)] Prevalence rates weighted in this manner give estimates as if each site has the same age and sex distribution of the 1980 US census. Comparisons of the age at onset across sites were standardized in a similar manner. Because the focus of the comorbidity analysis was the association of panic disorder with agoraphobia and major depression within each site (rather than between sites), the proportions computed for comorbidity were weighted to the design characteristics of each sample.

The data for the NCS were weighted to the national population characteristics defined by the 1989 US National Health Interview Survey[29] and not standardized to the ECA.

All analyses were done with Statistical Analysis System software.[30] The FREQ procedure[30] was used when determining rates and proportions. The UNIVARIATE procedure[30] was used to determine the age at onset. To determine statistical association between panic disorder and another psychiatric disorder, logistic regression was used (PROC LOGIST),[30] weighted to the design characteristics of each sample and adjusted by age and sex, and an odds ratio with its 95% confidence interval was derived from logit procedures.[31]

months, which explains why the annual and lifetime rates are the same. The prevalence rates of panic disorder are higher in the NCS than in the other countries or the ECA; however, the sex ratio and age at onset are comparable to those in the other sites.

COMORBIDITY

As reported in numerous clinical studies,[2] panic disorder is significantly associated with increased risk of both major depression and agoraphobia at every cross-

Table 1. Demographic Characteristics Across Sites

Characteristics	ECA*	Edmonton, Alberta	Puerto Rico	Savigny,† France	West Germany	Florence, Italy	Beirut, Lebanon	Taiwan	Korea	Christchurch, New Zealand	NCS‡
	Site										
No. of study participants	18 571	3258	1513	1746	481§	1100	234	11 004	5100	1498	8098
Study period	1980-1984	1983-1986	1984	1987-1988	1981	1984	1987-1989	1982-1985	1984	1986	1990-1992
Response rate, %	76	72	91	63	76	100	77	90	83	70	84
Female, %	59	59	57	62	52	54	58	48	52	66	52
Age, y, at interview, %‖											
18-25	14	22	22	13	. . .¶	9	17	25	20	20	19
26-45	33	46	50	71	55	36	47	43	49	55	59
46-64	21	21	28	14	45	35	31	24	30	24	16

*Five US sites (New Haven, Conn; Baltimore Md; St Louis, Mo; Piedmont County, North Carolina; Los Angeles, Calif) from the Epidemiologic Catchment Area (ECA) study.
†Suburb of Paris.
‡Forty-eight coterminous US states; participants' ages, 18-54 years, from the National Comorbidity Survey (NCS).
§Drawn, in 1981, from 1366 subjects in 1974.
‖In raw percent, percents may not add to 100 for age because of missing values.
¶No subjects in this category.

Table 2. Prevalence Rates and Age at Onset for Panic Disorder Across Sites: Age 18-64 Years*

Site	Rate per 100 (SE)						Mean Age at Onset, y (SD)
		Lifetime					
			Sex				
	Annual	Total	F	M	F/M Ratio		
ECA†	1.0 (0.11)	1.7 (0.14)	2.3 (0.22)	1.0 (0.15)	2.3 (0.18)		24.8 (9.1)
Edmonton, Alberta	0.9 (0.19)	1.4 (0.24)	1.9 (0.38)	0.9 (0.28)	2.1 (0.37)		23.7 (10.4)
Puerto Rico	1.1 (0.30)	1.7 (0.37)	1.8 (0.54)	1.4 (0.50)	1.3 (0.45)		27.3 (9.6)
Savigny,‡ France	0.9 (0.30)	2.2 (0.46)	3.0 (0.74)	1.3 (0.50)	2.3 (0.47)		25.4 (8.6)
West Germany	1.7 (0.67)	2.6 (0.84)	3.8 (1.38)	1.4 (0.88)	2.7 (0.73)		35.5 (12.5)
Florence, Italy	1.3 (0.45)	2.9 (0.83)	3.9 (0.96)	1.2 (0.70)	3.2 (0.62)		26.1 (9.6)
Beirut, Lebanon	2.1 (0.99)	2.1 (0.99)	3.1 (1.65)	1.1 (1.02)	2.8 (1.09)		27.8 (3.6)
Taiwan	0.2 (0.04)	0.4 (0.06)	0.6 (0.10)	0.2 (0.07)	3.0 (0.37)		24.2 (8.9)
Korea	1.5 (0.17)	1.7 (0.19)	2.9 (0.34)	0.5 (0.15)	5.8 (0.32)		32.1 (10.3)
Christchurch, New Zealand	1.3 (0.34)	2.1 (0.43)	3.3 (0.74)	0.7 (0.37)	4.7 (0.55)		23.2 (7.8)
NCS§	2.2 (0.24)	3.5 (0.30)	5.1 (0.50)	1.9 (0.32)	2.7 (0.19)		25.5 (6.9)

*All values, except for the National Comorbidity Survey (NCS), standardized to the age and sex distribution of the 1980 US census.
†Five US sites (New Haven, Conn; Baltimore, Md; St Louis, Mo; Piedmont County, North Carolina; Los Angeles, Calif) from the Epidemiologic Catchment Area (ECA) study.
‡A suburb of Paris.
§Forty-eight coterminous US states; ages 18-54 from the NCS. Data weighted according to national population characteristics defined by the 1989 US National Health Interview Survey.[29]

national site and in the NCS (**Table 3**). Based on lifetime rates, the odds ratios for comorbidity of panic disorder with agoraphobia range from 7.5 in the ECA to 21.4 in Puerto Rico, and those of panic disorder with major depression range from 3.8 in Savigny to 20.1 in Edmonton. In the NCS, the odds ratio is 10.6 for agoraphobia and 5.7 for major depression.

COMMENT

The major findings from these epidemiological studies are, with a few exceptions, the consistency of rates and patterns (sex ratios, age at onset, and comorbidity) of panic disorder across diverse countries and the consistency with the clinical description of panic disorder.[2]

The limitation of the cross-national data must be acknowledged. While more than 40 000 subjects are included from 11 studies, the samples are very small for some sites (West Germany, Beirut). Moreover, the West German study is a follow-up and has an older sample, so the age at onset should be interpreted with caution in relation to the other sites. Data on comorbidity were not available in Florence. The NCS did not include anyone older than 54 years. Possible medical causes of panic disorder that may vary across sites were not ruled out. The biases introduced by use of a highly structured interview are unknown. Finally, no data are presented or are available using comparable design and diagnostic methods from most other parts of the world.

Table 3. Comorbidity of Panic Disorder With Lifetime Agoraphobia and Major Depression Across Sites: Age 18-64 Years*

	Comorbidity With					
	Agoraphobia			Major Depression		
Site	In Persons With Panic, %	In Persons Without Panic, %	OR (95% CI)	In Persons With Panic, %	In Persons Without Panic, %	ORs (95% CI)
ECA†	33.3	5.5	7.5 (5.6-10.1)	32.8	4.7	8.7 (6.4-11.7)
Edmonton, Alberta	31.8	2.7	15.1 (7.6-29.9)	68.2	9.2	20.1 (10.4-38.8)
Puerto Rico	58.2	6.0	21.4 (9.2-50.2)	38.2	3.7	15.3 (6.4-36.6)
Savigny,‡ France	48.9	6.5	12.7 (6.8-24.0)	48.9	17.3	3.8 (2.1-7.1)
Taiwan	22.5	1.4	17.2 (8.0-37.2)	22.5	1.3	19.6 (9.1-42.1)
Korea	34.7	2.1	17.2 (10.6-27.8)	28.4	2.5	13.2 (8.0-21.6)
Christchurch, New Zealand	29.5	3.4	9.4 (4.2-21.2)	40.8	11.2	4.6 (2.2-9.4)
NCS§	38.8	5.1	10.6 (7.3-15.5)	54.5	16.0	5.7 (4.0-8.1)

**Proportions are weighted to the design characteristics of each site, except for the National Comorbidity Survey (NCS). Odds ratios (ORs) with 95% confidence intervals (CIs) are weighted to the design characteristics of the sample and adjusted by age and sex within each site. Data were not available from Florence, Italy. West Germany and Beirut, Lebanon, were excluded because of small sample size.*

†Five US sites (New Haven, Conn; Baltimore, Md; St Louis, Mo; Piedmont County, NC; Los Angeles, Calif) from the Epidemiologic Catchment Area (ECA) study.

‡A suburb of Paris.

§Forty-eight coterminous US states; ages 18-54 from the NCS. Data weighted according to national population characteristics defined by the 1989 US National Health Interview Survey.[29]

While the patterns are similar to those in other countries, the rates of panic disorder (as well as most other disorders studied) were lower in Taiwan than in the other countries. The reasons for these differences are unclear and have been examined independently by others.[32] The Taiwanese investigators[32] noted that the *DSM-III* is widely used in Taiwan, so these were not new criteria. The Taiwan study[32] had a higher proportion of rural settings than the other ECA sites; however, rural-urban comparisons of rates between the ECA and Taiwan still resulted in lower rates in Taiwan. Another analysis[33] showed that the rates of cognitive impairment and generalized anxiety disorders (both of which emphasize somatic symptoms and are less stigmatized disorders in Taiwan) were more comparable to the rates of these disorders in some of the ECA sites. This comparability suggests that social stigma and cultural reluctance to endorse mental symptoms may account for some, but not all, of the differences.[33] This factor is unlikely to explain the lower rates of panic disorder that manifest mainly in somatic symptoms. A study of the rates of psychiatric disorders in Chinese living in the United States and in the Peoples' Republic of China would be useful in determining whether the lower rate of panic and other disorders is uniquely Chinese on a cultural or genetic basis. The older age at onset in West Germany could result from the older age of the sample and possibly less accurate dating of the age at onset, a birth cohort effect, or variability attributable to small sample size. The reason for the close female-male ratio in Puerto Rico is unclear.[16]

The NCS has the highest lifetime rates of panic disorder, which is twice as high as the rate in the ECA (3.5 per 100 and 1.7 per 100, respectively). These differences may be caused by a period effect with increasing rates between the ECA conducted in the early 1980s and the NCS conducted in the early 1990s. It could also be caused by differences in the *DSM-III* and *DSM-III-R* criteria for panic disorder; *DSM-III* requires 3 panic attacks in a 3-week period, while the *DSM-III-R* criteria used in the NCS are broader than the *DSM-III* criteria because they include persistent worry about having another attack rather than having 4 in 4 weeks. This means that some people make criteria for panic disorder in the NCS even if they only had 1 attack in their life as long as they worried about having another one for a month after the attack. The *DSM-III-R* also includes an additional symptom (nausea or abdominal distress) as one of the criteria. Finally, the difference in rates between the ECA and NCS could be a result of the difference in the diagnostic assessment. The diagnostic interview used in the NCS, the Composite International Diagnostic Interview,[26] included memory probes that could have increased recollection and led to higher rates. The reasons for the higher rates for most disorders in the NCS compared with those in the ECA have been under study by the National Institute of Mental Health in collaboration with Ronald Kessler, PhD. Interestingly, while we also find higher rates of panic disorder in the NCS, there was similarity in age at onset, sex ratios, and comorbidity compared with the other cross-national sites.

Accepted for publication September 16, 1996.

From the Department of Psychiatry, College of Physicians and Surgeons of Columbia University, and Division of Clinical and Genetic Epidemiology, New York State Psychiatric Institute (Drs Weissman and Wickramaratne and Mr Greenwald), New York, NY; the Department of Psychiatry, University of Alberta, Edmonton (Drs Bland and Newman); Behavioral Sciences Research Institute, University of Puerto Rico, San Juan (Dr Canino and Ms Rubio-Stipec); Department of Neurology and Psychiatry, Florence University Medical School, Florence, Italy (Dr Faravelli); Departments of Psychiatry, National Taiwan University Hospital (Drs Hwu and Yeh) and Taipei Medical College (Dr Yeh), Taipei, Taiwan; Departments of Psychological Medicine (Drs Joyce and Oakley-Browne) and Public Health and General Practice (Dr Wells),

Christchurch School of Medicine, Christchurch, New Zealand; Department of Psychiatry and Psychology, St George Hospital and American University of Beirut, and St Joseph University, Beirut, Lebanon (Dr Karam); Keyo Psychiatric Institute, Kyongii-Do, Korea (Dr Lee); Institut National de la Santé et de la Recherche Médicale, Unité 169, Villejuif (Dr Lellouch), and Hôpital Fernand Widal, Paris (Dr Lépine), France; and Max Planck Institute for Psychiatry, Clinical Institute, Munich, Germany (Dr Wittchen).

These analyses were supported by grants MH37592 and MH30906 from the National Institute of Mental Health, Rockville, Md.

Reprints: Myrna M. Weissman, PhD, College of Physicians and Surgeons of Columbia University, Division of Clinical and Genetic Epidemiology, New York State Psychiatric Institute, 722 W 168th St, Unit 14, New York, NY 10032 (E-mail: weissman@child.cpmc.columbia.edu).

REFERENCES

1. American Psychiatric Association, Committee on Nomenclature and Statistics. *Diagnostic and Statistical Manual of Mental Disorders, Third Edition.* Washington, DC: American Psychiatric Association; 1980.
2. Klerman GL, Hirschfeld RMA, Weissman MM, Pellicier Y, Ballenger JC, Costa e Silva JA, Judd LL,Keller, MB. *Panic Anxiety and Its Treatments.* Washington, DC: American Psychiatric Press; 1993.
3. Markowitz JS, Weissman MM, Ouellette R, Lish JD, Klerman GL. Quality of life in panic disorder. *Arch Gen Psychiatry.* 1989;46:984-992.
4. Klerman GL, Weissman MM, Ouellette R, Johnson J, Greenwald S. Panic attacks in the community: social morbidity and health care utilization. *JAMA.* 1991;265:742-746.
5. Weissman MM, Klerman GL, Markowitz JS, Ouellette R. Suicidal ideation and suicide attempts in panic disorder and attacks. *N Engl J Med.* 1989;321:1209-1214.
6. Eaton WW, Dryman A, Weissman MM. Panic and phobias. In: Robins LN, Regier DA, eds. *Psychiatric Disorders in America: The Epidemiologic Catchment Area Study.* New York, NY: The Free Press; 1991:155-179.
7. Horwath E, Johnson J, Hornig CD. Epidemiology of panic disorder in African-Americans. *Am J Psychiatry.* 1993;150:465-469.
8. Kessler RC, McGonable KA, Zhao S, Nelson CB, Hughes M, Eshleman S, Wittchen HU, Kendler KS. Lifetime and 12-month prevalence of *DSM-III-R* psychiatric disorders in the United States: results from the National Comorbidity Survey. *Arch Gen Psychiatry.* 1994;51:8-19.
9. Eaton WW, Kessler RC, Wittchen HU, Magee WJ. Panic and panic disorder in the United States. *Am J Psychiatry.* 1994;151:413-420.
10. Weissman MM, Bland R, Canino G, Faravelli C, Greenwald S, Hwu HG, Joyce PR, Karam EG, Lee CK, Lellouch J, Lépine JP, Newman S, Rubio-Stipec M, Wells JE, Wickramaratne P, Wittchen HU, Yeh EK. Cross-national epidemiology of major depression and bipolar disorder. *JAMA.* 1996;276:293-299.
11. Robins LN, Helzer JE, Croughan JL. The NIMH diagnostic interview schedule: its history, characteristics, and validity. *Arch Gen Psychiatry.* 1981;38:381-389.
12. Robins LN, Orvaschel H, Anthony J, Blazer D, Burnam A, Burke J. The Diagnostic Interview Schedule. In: Eaton WW, Kessler LG, eds. *Epidemiologic Field Methods in Psychiatry: The NIMH Epidemiologic Catchment Area Program.* Orlando, Fla: Academic Press; 1985.
13. Robins LN, Regier DA, eds. *Psychiatric Disorders in America: The Epidemiologic Catchment Area Study.* New York, NY: The Free Press; 1991.
14. Orn H, Newman SC, Bland RC. Design and field methods of the Edmonton survey of psychiatric disorders. *Acta Psychiatr Scand Suppl.* 1988;77:17-23.
15. Bland RC, Orn H, Newman SC. Lifetime prevalence of psychiatric disorders in Edmonton. *Acta Psychiatr Scand.* 1988;77(suppl 338):24-32.
16. Canino GJ, Bird HR, Shrout PE, Rubio-Stipec M, Bravo M, Martinez R, Sesman M, Guevara,LM. The prevalence of specific psychiatric disorders in Puerto Rico. *Arch Gen Psychiatry.* 1987;44:727-735.
17. Lépine JP, Lellouch J, Lovell A, Teherani M, Ha C, Verdier-Taillefer MH, Rambourg N, Lemperiere T. Anxiety and depressive disorders in a French population: methodology and preliminary results. *Psychiatr Psychobiol.* 1989;4: 267-274.
18. Wittchen HU, Essau CA, von Zerssen D, Krieg JC, Zaudig M. Lifetime and six-month prevalence of mental disorders in the Munich follow-up study. *Eur Arch Psychiatry Clin Neurosci.* 1992;241:247-258.
19. Faravelli C, Degl'Innocenti BG, Aiazzi L, Incerpi G, Pallanti S. Epidemiology of anxiety disorder in Florence. *J Affect Disord.* 1989;19:1-5.
20. Karam E. Dépression et guerres du Liban: méthodologie d'une recherche. *Ann Psychol SciEduc, Univ St Joseph (Beyrouth).* 1992:99-106.
21. Hwu HG, Yeh EK, Chang LY. Prevalence of psychiatric disorders in Taiwan defined by the Chinese diagnostic interview schedule. *Acta Psychiatr Scand.* 1989;79:136-147.
22. Lee CK, Kwak YS, Yamamoto J, Rhee H, Kim YS, Han JH, Choi J, Lee YH. Psychiatric epidemiology in Korea, I: gender and age differences in Seoul. *J Nerv Ment Dis.* 1990;178:242-246.
23. Lee CK, Kwak YS, Yamamoto J, Rhee H, Kim YS, Han JH, Choi J, Lee YH. Psychiatric epidemiology in Korea, II: urban and rural differences in Seoul. *J Nerv Ment Dis.* 1990;178:247-252.
24. Wells JE, Bushnell JA, Hornblow AR, Joyce PR, Oakley-Browne MA. Christchurch psychiatric epidemiology study, I: methodology and lifetime prevalence for specific psychiatric disorders. *Aust N Z J Psychiatry.* 1989;23:315-326.
25. Oakley-Browne MA, Joyce PR, Wells JE, Bushnell JA, Hornblow AR. Christchurch psychiatric epidemiology study, II: six month and other period prevalences for specific psychiatric disorders. *Aust N Z J Psychiatry.* 1989;23:327-340.
26. World Health Organization. *Composite International Diagnostic Interview (CIDI), Version 1.0.* Geneva, Switzerland: World Health Organization; 1990.
27. American Psychiatric Association, Committee on Nomenclature and Statistics. *Diagnostic and Statistical Manual of Mental Disorders, Third Edition,Revised.* Washington, DC: American Psychiatric Association; 1987.
28. Breslow NE, Day NE. *Statistical Methods in Cancer Research.* Lyon, France: International Agency for Research on Cancer; 1987;2.
29. US Department of Health and Human Services. *National Health Interview Survey: 1989.* Hyattsville, Md: National Center for Health Statistics; 1992.
30. SAS Institute Inc. *SAS Procedures Guide, Version 6.* 3rd ed. Cary, NC: SAS Institute Inc; 1990.
31. Kleinbaum DG, Kupper LL, Morgenstern H. *Epidemiologic Research: Principles and Quantitative Methods.* Belmont, Calif: Wadsworth Inc; 1982.
32. Compton WM, Helzer JE, Hwu, HG, Yeh EK, McEvoy L, Tipp JE, Spitznagel EL. New methods in cross-cultural psychiatry: psychiatric illness in Taiwan and the United States. *Am J Psychiatry.* 1991;148:1697-1704.
33. Yeh EK, Hwu HG, Yeh YL, Chang LY, Yamamoto J, Golding JM. *Life Change Events, Social Support and Mental Disorders: Taiwan-US Cross-cultural Study.* Taipei, Taiwan: Chiang Ching Kuo Foundation for International Scholarly Exchange; June 1994. Research Report Monograph (RG 010-9).

ESTABLISHED THERAPY FOR OCD

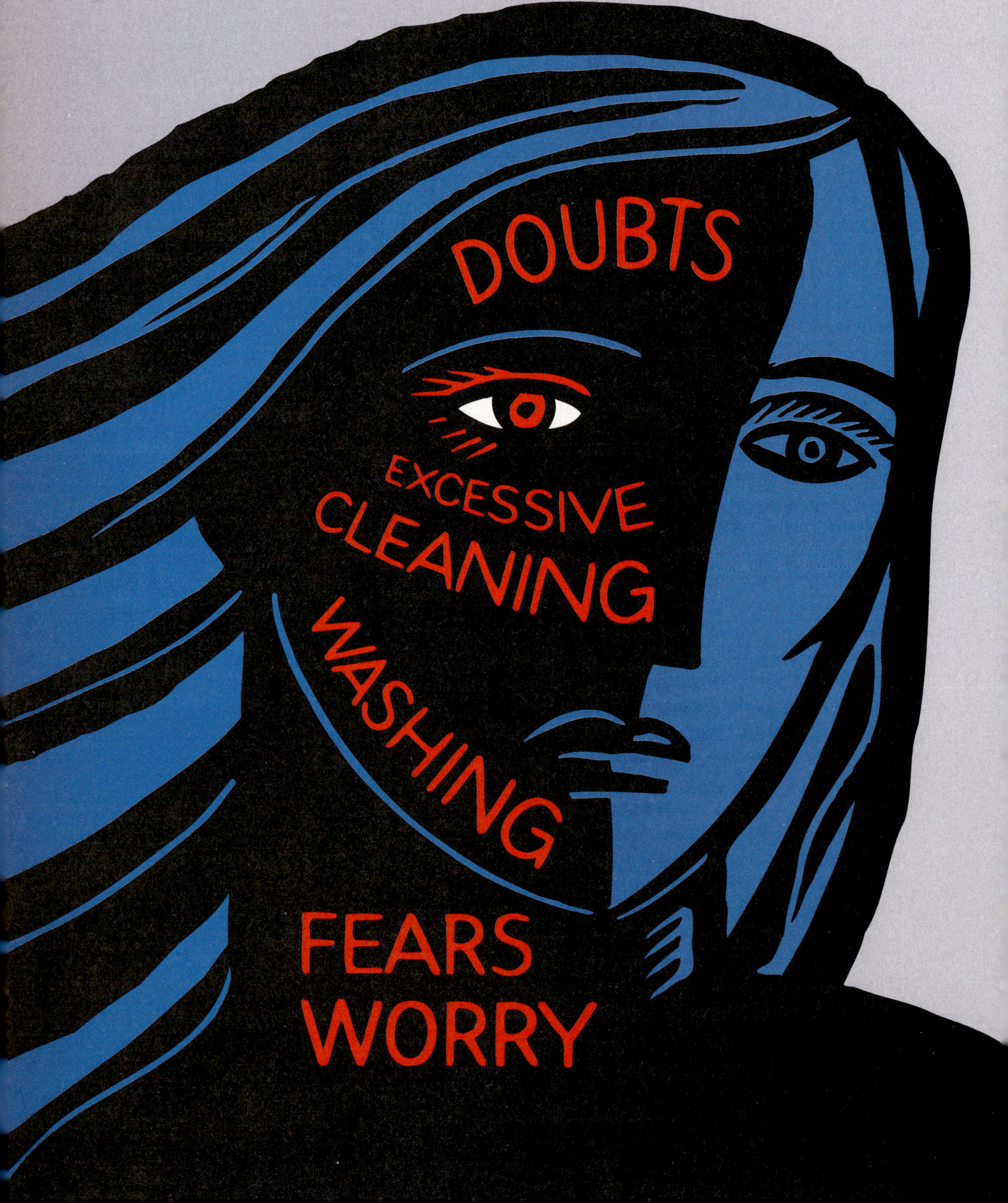

ORIGINAL ARTICLE

Lifetime Co-occurrence of *DSM-III-R* Alcohol Abuse and Dependence With Other Psychiatric Disorders in the National Comorbidity Survey

Ronald C. Kessler, PhD; Rosa M. Crum, MD, MHS; Lynn A. Warner, MPP; Christopher B. Nelson, PhD, MPH; John Schulenberg, PhD; James C. Anthony, PhD

Objective: To study patterns of co-occurrence of lifetime *DSM-III-R* alcohol disorders in a household sample.

Methods: Data came from the National Comorbidity Survey (NCS), a nationally representative household survey. Diagnoses were based on a modified version of the Composite International Diagnostic Interview.

Results: Respondents with lifetime NCS/*DSM-III-R* alcohol abuse or dependence had a high probability of carrying at least 1 other lifetimeNCS/*DSM-III-R* diagnosis. Retrospective reports have suggested that most lifetime co-occurring alcohol disorders begin at a later age than at least 1 other NCS/*DSM-III-R* disorder. Earlier disorders are generally stronger predictors of alcohol dependence than alcohol abuse and stronger among women than men. Lifetime co-occurrence is positively, but weakly, associated with the persistence of alcohol abuse among men and of alcohol dependence among both men and women.

Conclusions: Caution is needed in interpreting the results due to the fact that diagnoses were made by nonclinicians and results are based on retrospective reports of the age at onset. Within the context of these limitations, though, these results show that alcohol abuse and dependence are often associated with other lifetime *DSM-III-R* disorders and suggest that, at least in recent cohorts, the alcohol use disorders are usually temporally secondary. Prospective data and data based on clinically confirmed diagnoses are needed to verify these findings.

Arch Gen Psychiatry. 1997;54:313-321

THE CO-OCCURRENCE of alcoholism with other psychiatric disorders has been widely recognized,[1,2] with the most consistently documented co-occurring disorders being other substance use,[3] mood,[4] anxiety,[5] and schizophrenic[6] disorders. In treatment settings, these patients with "dual diagnoses" can be challenges to the clinician, as they may not respond as well to treatment as other patients, may have greater relapse, attrition, and readmission rates, and may manifest symptoms that are more severe, chronic, and refractory in nature.[2]

There are several possible explanations for these co-occurrences. They may be due to a common causal pathway (eg, a genetic predisposition).[7] One disorder may be causally secondary to the other, as when individuals self-medicate with alcohol to mask or reduce psychiatric symptoms,[8] or there may be methodological determinants (eg, unmeasured common causes or selection biases in some clinical studies).[9]

The goals of this report are 4-fold: (1) to examine the lifetime patterns of the co-occurrence of *DSM-III-R* alcohol abuse (AA) and alcohol dependence (AD) with other psychiatric disorders in a large household sample, (2) to study the reported temporal ordering between first onset of alcohol disorders and other psychiatric disorders in these data, (3) to investigate with retrospective reports of age at onset whether earlier disorders predict the subsequent first onset of AA and AD, and (4) to evaluate the role of lifetime co-occurrence in predicting the persistence of AA and AD.

RESULTS

ESTIMATED PREVALENCES OF ALCOHOL DISORDERS

Table 1 reproduces the NCS prevalence estimates for lifetime AA and AD that have been reported previously in the ARCHIVES.[10] The 12-month prevalence estimates differ from those reported previously because we used a less conservative

From the Department of Health Care Policy, Harvard Medical School, Boston, Mass (Dr Kessler); the Departments of Epidemiology (Dr Crum), Psychiatry (Dr Crum), and Mental Hygiene (Drs Crum and Anthony), School of Hygiene and Public Health, and the Department of Psychiatry and Behavioral Sciences, School of Medicine (Drs Crum and Anthony), The Johns Hopkins University, Baltimore, Md; Department of Sociology (Ms Warner), and Institute for Social Research (Dr Schulenberg), School of Social Work, University of Michigan, Ann Arbor; and the Max Planck Institute of Psychiatry–Clinical Institute, Munich, Germany (Dr Nelson).

METHODS

STUDY POPULATION

The study is based on data from the National Comorbidity Survey (NCS), a nationally representative household survey designed to study patterns and correlates of psychiatric morbidity and comorbidity. The NCS interviewed 8098 respondents between the ages of 15 and 54 years. The response rate was 82.4%. Interviews were carried out face-to-face in the homes of the respondents. A more detailed description of NCS field procedures has been presented previously in the ARCHIVES.[10]

DIAGNOSES

The diagnostic portion of the NCS was based on a modified version of the Composite International Diagnostic Interview (CIDI),[11] a fully structured diagnostic interview designed for use by lay interviewers that was developed by the World Health Organization, Geneva, Switzerland, and the US Alcohol, Drug Abuse, and Mental Health Administration, Rockville, Md.[12] Diagnoses that were made by use of *DSM-III-R*[13] were generated with the use of the CIDI diagnostic program.[14] The CIDI organic exclusion rules were used, but diagnostic hierarchy rules were not used, in defining cases.

Prior studies have found acceptable reliability and validity for all the CIDI diagnoses that are considered here.[15] Furthermore, disorder-specific validity studies in the NCS of respondents who were either diagnosed as having that lifetime disorder by the modified CIDI or who endorsed the diagnostic stem question but were not classified as a case found that the majority of CIDI cases were confirmed by a blind Structured Clinical Interview for *DSM-III-R*[16] reinterview[17-20] and that the diagnostic thresholds used in the NCS were not lower than those used in the Structured Clinical Interview for *DSM-III-R*. In the case of alcohol use disorders, 92% of the CIDI respondents classified as either abusers or dependent on alcohol were confirmed by the Structured Clinical Interview for *DSM-III-R*.

The age at onset plays an important part in the current report. This was assessed for anxiety and affective disorders by asking respondents if they could remember their exact age at the first time that they had an episode. Respondents who could not remember their exact age were asked about the earliest age that they could clearly remember a specific occasion of having the syndrome. The response to this question was used as a conservative upper-bound estimate of the age at onset of the disorder. Based on this approach, the median ages at onset for mental disorders are estimated to range between 11 (simple phobia) and 25 (generalized anxiety disorder) years. It is conceivable that these reports systematically underestimated the ages at onset if respondents focused on the first age of having a memorable period of sadness or a memorable fear even if this was prior to their age of meeting full diagnostic criteria. However, a comparison of retrospective reports among NCS respondents older than 19 years regarding the prevalence of primary anxiety disorders and mood disorders in the age range of 15 to 19 years with current reports of NCS respondents in the age range of 15 to 19 years found no evidence of retrospective overestimation.

A different approach to dating the age at onset was used for substance use disorders. Respondents were asked separately to date the age at onset of each of the 9 criterion A symptoms of dependence for each of the 9 classes of substances (ie, alcohol, 4 types of prescription medications, and 4 types of illicit drugs). The age at onset was defined as the age when the respondent first reported the persistence of the disturbance for at least 1 month or repeatedly

definition of 12-month disorder previously: patients with lifetime cases who reported at least 1 symptom in the past year. The lifetime and 12-month prevalences of AA are estimated to be 9.4% and 2.5%, respectively, while the lifetime and 12-month prevalences of AD are estimated to be 14.1% and 4.4%, respectively. Men are significantly more likely than women to be classified as having both lifetime disorders (for AA: $z=6.1$; $P<.001$; for AD: $z=9.7$; $P<.001$) and 12-month disorders (for AA: $z=4.0$; $P<.001$; for AD: $z=5.8$; $P<.001$).

CO-OCCURRENCE OF LIFETIME ALCOHOL DISORDERS WITH OTHER *DSM-III-R* DISORDERS

As presented in **Table 2**, the majority of respondents with a diagnosis of either lifetime AA or AD have a history of at least 1 other disorder. Alcohol dependence generally has a stronger pattern of positive associations than AA with other disorders, with the single exception being the larger odds ratio (OR) of AA than AD with drug abuse. The largest ORs of alcohol disorders are with drug disorders among both men and women, followed by conduct disorder and antisocial personality disorder, and anxiety disorders and affective disorders. While many of the ORs that involve AA are significantly larger for women than men, the sex differences that involve AD are generally not significant.

TEMPORAL PRIORITIES BETWEEN LIFETIME ALCOHOL DISORDERS AND OTHER PSYCHIATRIC DISORDERS

Table 3 shows that co-occurring alcohol disorders were usually reported as having a later age at onset than at least 1 other NCS/*DSM-III-R* disorder. Significant sex differences appear in the retrospective temporal ordering of AA and other disorders, with men more likely to report their AA as either pure ($z=3.6$; $P<.001$) or temporally primary ($z=2.2$; $P=.03$) and women more likely to report it as either same-year ($z=1.1$; $P=.27$) or temporally secondary ($z=4.1$; $P<.001$). A larger proportion of men than women with lifetime AA reported prior conduct disorder or adult antisocial behavior ($z=1.9$; $P=.06$), while larger proportions of women than men with AA reported prior anxiety disorders ($z=5.2$; $P<.001$), affective disorders ($z=5.4$; $P<.001$), and drug use disorders ($z=2.0$; $P=.05$).

Parallel results are reported in **Table 4** for AD. As initial symptoms of AD often occur a number of years during a longer period. The age at onset of dependence was defined as the age at which the third qualifying symptom occurred. When defined in this way, the median ages at onset are 19 years for AA without dependence, 18 years for AD, 18 years for illicit drug abuse, and 19 years for drug dependence. The use of a classification scheme that does not require the clustering of symptoms in a single year for a diagnosis of dependence introduces an overestimation of lifetime prevalence and an underestimation of the age at onset if, as in *DSM-IV*,[21] true cases are conceptualized as those in which the symptoms have to cluster in time. However, the CIDI did not assess the clustering of symptoms for alcohol or drug disorders. We did require a clustering of 3 or more criterion A symptoms in the 12 months before the interview for a diagnosis of 12-month dependence, though, so this problem is avoided in the analysis of recent disorders.

WEIGHTING PROCEDURES

The data were weighted to adjust for undersampling of new construction households and for only 1 respondent who was being interviewed in each household regardless of the household size. A random subsample of initial NCS nonrespondents were recontacted and administered a brief screening interview to assess lifetime and recent CIDI disorders. Consistent with findings from previous studies,[22,23] higher estimated prevalences of several CIDI disorders were found among initial NCS nonrespondents than respondents. The main study data were weighted to compensate for this bias. Finally, a weight was used to adjust for differences between the distributions in the sample and in the total US population on the cross-classification of a number of sociodemographic variables. These weighting procedures improve the validity of population projections, although a parallel analysis of results with and without weights shows that most results do not change substantially. A more detailed description[24] and an analysis of the consequences of the NCS weighting procedure[10] are presented elsewhere.

DATA ANALYSIS

The SEs of proportions were estimated using the Taylor series linearization method[25] with the PSRATIO program in OSIRIS.[26] The SEs of logistic regression coefficients were estimated using the method of balanced repeated replication[27] with a commercially available software package (SAS macro, SAS Institute Inc, Cary, NC).[28] Bivariate survival models were used to analyze comorbid conditions as predictors of alcohol disorder onset. This was done by converting the person-level data file into a separate person-year file for each outcome disorder in which separate observational records were created for each year of each person's life up to and including the year of first onset of the outcome disorder. A dichotomous outcome variable was created to discriminate the year of first onset of the outcome disorder (coded 1) from years prior to the onset of the outcome disorder (coded 0). These data files were analyzed using logistic regression models that included controls for person-year and cohort. Time-varying predictors were included for prior onset of other disorders. The logits can be interpreted as discrete-time survival coefficients for the associations of earlier disorders with subsequent onset of AA and AD.[29] Person-level data were used in logistic models to evaluate the bivariate lifetime comorbidities of AA and AD with each of the other NCS/*DSM-III-R* disorders, as well as to examine the effects of the prior onset of other psychiatric disorders on the persistence of AA and AD. All models were estimated separately for men and women, and the significance of sex differences was evaluated in pooled models.

prior to the onset of the full syndrome, the age at onset of AD was defined here as the age at onset of the first symptom of either abuse or dependence among respondents who subsequently met criteria for NCS/*DSM-III-R* AD. Even with this adjustment, though, the majority of NCS respondents with both AD and some other disorder reported that their AD was temporally secondary. Higher proportions of men than women reported that their AD was pure (z=2.6; P=.007) or temporally primary (z=3.3; P<.001), whereas higher proportions of women than men reported that their AD was same-year (z=0.3; P=.84) or temporally secondary (z=5.5; P<.001). A larger proportion of men than women with AD reported prior conduct disorder or adult antisocial behavior (z=3.7; P<.001), while larger proportions of women than men with AD reported prior anxiety disorders (z=7.4; P<.001), affective disorders (z=5.2; P<.001), and drug use disorders (z=1.4; P=.13).

Table 1. Lifetime and 12-Month Prevalences of NCS/ *DSM-III-R* Alcohol Abuse and Dependence, by Sex*

	Lifetime Prevalence				12-Month Prevalence			
Disorder	**%**	**SE**	**No.**	**No.$_w$**	**%**	**SE**	**No.**	**No.$_w$**
Alcohol abuse								
Men	12.5	0.8	482	503	3.4	0.4	141	138
Women	6.4	0.6	299	261	1.6	0.2	67	65
Total	9.4	0.5	**781**	**764**	2.5	0.2	**208**	**204**
Alcohol dependence								
Men	20.1	1.0	838	806	6.6	0.7	272	265
Women	8.2	0.7	374	336	2.2	0.3	91	91
Total	14.1	0.7	**1212**	**1142**	4.4	0.4	**363**	**356**

**NCS indicates National Comorbidity Survey; No., the unweighted number of respondents in the numerators of the prevalence estimates (the prevalence estimates, in comparison, are based on weighted data); and No.$_w$, the weighted number of respondents in the numerators of the prevalence estimates.*

PREDICTION OF FIRST ONSET OF ALCOHOL DISORDERS

The results in **Table 5** are based on a separate bivariate survival model for the prediction of either AA or AD from each prior disorder. Prior disorders are more powerful predictors of subsequent AD than AA. The majority of the prior disorders are stronger predictors among women than men. While the cross-sectional ORs in Table 2 are

Table 2. Lifetime Co-occurrence of Alcohol Abuse and Alcohol Dependence With Other Lifetime NCS/*DSM-III-R* Disorders, by Sex*

	Alcohol Abuse						Alcohol Dependence					
	Men			Women			Men			Women		
Lifetime Disorders	%†	OR	95% CI	%†	OR	95% CI	%†	OR	95% CI	%†	OR	95% CI
Anxiety												
GAD	2.6	0.67	0.32-1.38	8.4	1.31	0.62-2.77	8.6	3.86‡	2.27-6.58	15.7	3.01‡	1.70-5.32
Panic	1.6	0.79	0.31-2.01	7.3	1.55	0.73-3.28	3.6	2.27‡	1.11-4.64	12.0	2.98‡	1.74-5.09
Agoraphobia	5.1	1.27	0.60-2.66	9.3	1.03	0.55-1.94	6.5	1.82‡	1.04-3.20	18.5	2.53‡	1.69-3.80
Social phobia	10.8	0.97	0.66-1.41§	24.1	1.81‡	1.26-2.58	19.3	2.41‡	1.76-3.31	30.3	2.62‡	2.00-3.43
Simple phobia	5.9	0.85	0.54-1.31§	28.2	2.24‡	1.56-3.21	13.9	3.11‡	2.29-4.22	30.7	2.63‡	1.84-3.77
PTSD	2.5	0.45‡	0.23-0.88§	10.5	1.01	0.64-1.60	10.3	3.20‡	1.86-5.48	26.2	3.60‡	2.56-5.05
Any	22.7	0.95	0.69-1.31§	48.8	1.78‡	1.31-2.41	35.8	2.22‡	1.67-2.95	60.7	3.08‡	2.20-4.30
Affective												
Depression	9.0	0.65‡	0.45-0.94§	30.1	1.65‡	1.15-2.37	24.3	2.95‡	2.21-3.93	48.5	4.05‡	2.99-5.48
Dysthymia	3.6	0.71	0.37-1.36	10.1	1.33	0.68-2.59	11.2	3.81‡	2.37-6.10	20.9	3.63‡	2.55-5.18
Mania	0.3	0.15	0.06-0.36§	3.8	2.32	0.47-11.54	6.2	12.03‡	4.79-30.22	6.8	5.30‡	2.63-10.69
Any	10.2	0.64‡	0.45-0.90§	34.5	1.78‡	1.25-2.55	28.1	3.16‡	2.40-4.16	53.5	4.36‡	3.30-5.76
Drug												
Drug abuse	16.6	5.00‡	3.47-7.22	15.5	6.72‡	4.03-11.21	11.1	2.97‡	1.98-4.44	12.4	5.16‡	3.36-7.92
Drug dependence	13.1	1.59	1.00-2.51§	17.8	4.09‡	2.55-6.57	29.5	9.81‡	7.21-13.34	34.7	15.75‡	9.59-25.86
Any	29.7	2.96‡	2.08-4.20§	33.3	6.00‡	4.16-8.66	40.6	7.73‡	5.99-9.98§	47.1	14.12‡	9.33-21.36
Other												
Conduct disorder	25.3	1.45‡	1.10-1.90	13.5	2.53‡	1.31-4.88	41.6	4.29‡	3.56-5.17	22.8	5.83‡	3.62-9.38
AAB	8.8	1.01	0.59-1.72§	8.0	4.20‡	1.87-9.43	24.5	7.16‡	4.93-10.40	13.9	11.98‡	6.78-21.24
ASPD	6.1	1.20	0.62-2.34	2.1	2.09	. . .‖	16.9	8.34‡	5.40-12.87	7.8	17.01‡	6.41-45.12
Any	27.1	1.24	0.98-1.56§	19.6	3.05‡	1.76-5.27	49.7	5.01‡	4.11-6.13	28.9	6.10‡	3.88-9.58
Aggregate												
Any	56.8	1.59‡	1.20-2.10§	72.4	2.92‡	2.03-4.20	78.3	5.85‡	4.57-7.48	86.0	7.38‡	4.82-11.28
1	26.1	1.58‡	1.12-2.23	21.0	1.98‡	1.30-3.02	25.4	3.53‡	2.59-4.80	18.9	3.61‡	2.13-6.12
2	16.8	2.07‡	1.35-3.18	19.0	3.06‡	1.87-5.01	18.7	5.87‡	4.17-8.25	20.3	6.81‡	4.32-10.73
3	13.9	1.24	0.89-1.72§	32.3	4.07‡	2.63-6.30	34.2	11.43‡	8.09-16.15	46.8	13.60‡	8.51-21.72

**NCS indicates National Comorbidity Survey; OR, odds ratio; CI, confidence interval; GAD, generalized anxiety disorder; PTSD, posttraumatic stress disorder; AAB, adult antisocial behavior; and ASPD, antisocial personality disorder.*

†The entries in the "%" columns are the prevalences of the disorders represented in the rows among respondents with a lifetime diagnosis of the alcohol disorder. For example, the 2.6% in the upper left cell of the table represents lifetime prevalence of GAD in the subsample of men who have a lifetime history of alcohol abuse. On a weighted base of 503 men in this subsample (from Table 1), 2.6% is equivalent to 13 men with lifetime co-occurrence of alcohol abuse and GAD.

‡The OR is significant at the .05 level, 2-tailed test.

§The sex difference in the OR is significant at the .05 level, 2-tailed test.

‖The simulation of the SE did not converge.

much larger for drug use disorders, conduct disorder, and adult antisocial behavior than for anxiety disorders or mood disorders, this is not true in Table 5.

The NCS/*DSM-III-R* disorders that are significant predictors of subsequent AA among men all have ORs less than 1.0, indicating that these disorders are associated with a decreased risk of subsequent onset of AA. All 3 remained significant in a subsequently estimated additive multivariate model that included all significant bivariate predictors. Among women, 13 of the 22 coefficients are significant and all are positive predictors of AA. Four of these disorders—social phobia, simple phobia, depression, and drug dependence—remained significant among women in a subsequently estimated multivariate model. All the earlier disorders are positive and, for the most part, significantly associated with AD among both men and women, although many of these coefficients are significantly larger among women than men. Five of these coefficients remained significant among men (social phobia, simple phobia, mania, conduct disorder, and adult antisocial behavior), and 6 of these coefficients remained significant among women (social phobia, simple phobia, depression, drug abuse, drug dependence, and conduct disorder) in subsequently estimated multivariate models.

These results are all based on additive models. Given the strong relationships that have been documented in treatment samples between conduct disorder and antisocial personality disorder on the one hand and alcohol problems on the other, a question could be raised whether the significant predictors of AA and AD reported here only have effects in the context of co-occurring conduct disorder or antisocial personality disorder. To evaluate this issue, we estimated an interactive model in which separate predictors of subsequent AD were included for profiles of prior classes of NCS/*DSM-III-R* disorders. We also explored the possibility of estimating a model with profiles of individual disorders, but the precision of estimates was too low for this to be done. As given in **Table 6**, there is consistent evidence for significantly increased odds of AD associated with pure disorders—defined as having 1 or more of the NCS/*DSM-III-R* disorders in 1 and

Table 3. Retrospectively Reported Temporal Ordering of Ages at Onset of Alcohol Abuse and Other NCS/*DSM-III-R* Disorders, by Sex*

	Men								Women							
	Pure		Primary		Same-Year		Secondary		Pure		Primary		Same-Year		Secondary	
Lifetime Disorder	%	SE	%	SE	%	SE	%	SE	%	SE	%	SE	%	SE	%	SE
Anxiety																
GAD	97.4	0.9	1.5	0.6	0.1	0.1	1.0	0.7	91.4	2.7	4.4	1.5	0.1	0.1	4.1	2.3
Panic	98.3	0.7	1.0	0.4	0.0	. . .	0.7	0.5	92.6	2.4	6.0	2.5	0.3	0.3	1.0	0.4
Agoraphobia	94.8	1.7	1.2	0.9	0.5	0.4	3.5	1.4	90.5	2.1	4.2	1.7	0.4	0.4	4.9	1.7
Social phobia	89.1	1.8	1.8	0.8	0.7	0.4	8.4	1.6	75.9	3.2	1.2	0.6	0.5	0.5	22.4	3.1
Simple phobia	94.0	1.2	1.1	0.5	0.2	0.1	4.7	1.1	71.4	3.6	4.2	1.5	0.5	0.4	23.9	3.8
PTSD	97.5	0.7	0.9	0.3	0.2	0.1	1.5	0.6	89.5	1.8	3.1	1.2	0.1	0.1	7.3	2.0
Any	77.3	2.7	4.9	1.4	1.2	0.5	16.6	2.5	51.2	3.5	8.1	2.2	1.0	0.6	39.7	3.7
Affective																
Depression	90.7	1.6	6.8	1.3	0.6	0.3	1.9	0.5	69.4	3.6	10.5	2.2	1.9	0.7	18.2	2.9
Dysthymia	96.4	1.0	2.2	0.8	0.3	0.2	1.2	0.5	89.6	2.9	5.7	2.6	0.7	0.4	3.9	1.6
Mania	99.7	0.2	0.1	0.1	0.1	0.1	0.1	0.1	96.2	2.2	2.5	2.1	1.3	0.7	0	. . .
Any	89.3	1.7	7.1	1.3	0.7	0.4	2.8	0.8	62.5	4.0	15.0	3.5	2.3	0.7	20.2	3.1
Drug																
Drug abuse	83.2	2.4	7.7	2.0	6.1	1.4	3.0	1.2	85.0	2.9	1.5	0.7	7.8	2.6	5.7	1.2
Drug dependence	86.5	2.5	9.4	2.1	2.4	0.8	1.7	0.7	81.8	3.1	8.4	1.7	5.0	2.2	4.9	2.2
Any	69.7	3.2	17.1	2.3	8.5	1.5	4.7	1.4	66.8	4.0	9.9	2.0	12.8	3.3	10.5	2.6
Other																
Conduct disorder	75.4	2.1	1.4	1.1	0.8	0.5	22.4	2.3	86.2	3.4	0.7	0.3	1.4	1.4	11.7	2.9
AAB	91.2	1.7	4.4	1.1	1.8	0.8	2.6	1.0	92.0	2.6	2.0	0.9	1.7	0.9	4.3	2.5
ASPD	93.7	1.4	3.0	0.9	1.4	0.8	2.0	0.9	97.9	1.0	0	. . .	1.3	0.8	0.9	0.4
Any	72.9	2.1	2.8	1.3	1.2	0.5	23.1	2.3	80.4	3.7	2.7	0.9	1.7	1.4	15.1	3.5
Aggregate																
Any (≥1)	43.3	3.4	14.2	2.4	5.7	1.3	36.8	3.0	27.6	2.8	8.0	1.5	9.3	3.1	55.0	3.3
≥2	69.4	2.4	4.6	1.5	2.6	0.8	23.5	2.3	48.6	3.4	2.4	0.8	4.3	2.6	44.6	3.6
≥3	85.4	1.9	1.7	1.0	1.3	0.6	11.6	1.8	67.7	3.7	0.7	0.5	1.9	1.3	29.7	3.7

**NCS indicates National Cormorbidity Survey; Pure, the proportion of persons with lifetime alcohol abuse who have never had the disorder represented by the row; Primary, the proportion of persons with lifetime alcohol abuse who had a first onset of the disorder represented by the row after the onset of alcohol abuse; Same-Year, the proportion of persons with lifetime alcohol abuse who had a first onset of the disorder represented by the row in the same year as the onset of alcohol abuse; Secondary, the proportion of persons with lifetime alcohol abuse who had a first onset of the disorder represented by the row prior to the onset of alcohol abuse; GAD, generalized anxiety disorder; PTSD, posttraumatic stress disorder; AAB, adult antisocial behavior; and ASPD, antisocial personality disorder. The weighted numbers of respondents in each cell of the table can be computed by multiplying the base of 503 men and 261 women with lifetime alcohol abuse (from Table 1) by the proportions. For example, the 97.4% of men whose alcohol abuse is pure with respect to GAD is equivalent to 490 weighted cases.*

only 1 of the 4 broad classes considered here (ie, anxiety disorders, affective disorders, drug use disorders, and conduct disorder or adult antisocal behavior). The ORs are considerably larger for pure drug use disorders and pure conduct disorder or adult antisocial behavior than for pure anxiety or pure affective disorders and even larger for profiles defined by the co-occurrence of multiple classes of disorders.

PREDICTION OF THE PERSISTENCE OF ALCOHOL DISORDERS

We also explored the possibility that lifetime co-occurrence is associated with the persistence (12-month prevalence) of alcohol disorders. **Table 7** contains the results of bivariate logistic regression analyses. The predictors are dichotomous measures of whether the respondent had each of the other NCS/*DSM-III-R* disorders prior to the age at onset of the alcohol disorder, while the outcomes are measures of 12-month prevalence of AA and AD. The fact that the analyses are carried out in the subsamples of respondents with lifetime AA and AD rather than the total sample leads to low statistical power, as indicated in the observation that several large ORs in Table 7 are not significant. As a result, we focus on the sign patterns as well as significance in interpreting results. No sign pattern exists among men in predicting the persistence of AA. There is a consistent positive sign pattern, in comparison, among women in predicting AA. A stronger pattern is seen among men and women in predicting the persistence of AD. Results were similar when we examined multivariate rather than bivariate associations.

COMMENT

LIMITATIONS

The results have to be interpreted in the context of 3 limitations. First, we relied on lay interviewers and fully structured diagnostic interviews. Although yielding acceptable reliability and validity,[15] it is unrealistic to expect that they will match the accuracy of diagnostic classifications of trained clinicians who interview patients repeatedly, interview family, and use clinical data in reaching diagnostic decisions. In addition, some participants

Table 4. Retrospectively Reported Temporal Ordering of Ages at Onset of Alcohol Dependence (Timed According to First Symptom Onset) and Other NCS/*DSM-III-R* Disorders, by Sex*

	Men								Women							
	Pure		Primary		Same-Year		Secondary		Pure		Primary		Same-Year		Secondary	
Lifetime Disorder	%	SE	%	SE	%	SE	%	SE	%	SE	%	SE	%	SE	%	SE
Anxiety																
GAD	91.1	1.8	6.8	1.7	0.2	0.1	1.9	0.5	84.2	3.0	9.0	2.3	1.8	1.7	5.1	1.9
Panic	96.3	8.5	2.8	0.8	0.3	0.2	0.6	0.2	87.9	2.3	5.4	1.2	0.5	0.3	6.2	2.1
Agoraphobia	93.3	1.4	2.8	0.9	0.8	0.5	3.0	1.1	81.3	2.8	6.1	1.6	0.9	0.6	11.7	2.7
Social phobia	80.6	2.2	5.6	1.6	1.2	0.4	12.6	1.7	69.6	3.0	6.0	1.5	0.2	0.1	24.2	3.1
Simple phobia	85.9	1.7	4.8	1.1	0.9	0.6	8.4	1.3	69.1	3.3	3.1	1.7	0.3	0.3	27.5	2.6
PTSD	89.7	1.6	5.5	1.1	0.5	0.3	4.3	1.3	73.8	2.6	9.2	1.5	4.3	1.8	12.7	2.4
Any	64.2	2.5	11.6	2.1	2.4	0.7	21.8	2.3	39.3	3.4	8.8	1.4	2.2	0.9	49.7	3.0
Affective																
Depression	75.2	2.5	15.3	2.0	3.3	1.0	6.2	1.4	51.3	3.6	22.6	3.3	4.7	1.1	21.3	3.6
Dysthymia	88.6	1.6	7.8	1.3	1.5	0.5	2.2	0.9	79.1	2.9	12.9	2.9	1.3	0.6	6.7	1.4
Mania	93.8	1.3	4.2	1.1	0.2	0.1	1.8	0.8	93.3	1.6	3.4	1.2	1.2	0.6	2.2	1.7
Any	70.2	2.5	18.5	2.1	4.3	1.1	7.1	1.5	45.8	3.1	22.6	2.9	5.0	0.9	26.6	3.4
Drug																
Drug abuse	89.1	1.4	7.3	1.2	2.5	0.5	1.2	0.3	87.6	2.0	6.7	1.7	4.0	1.2	1.7	0.7
Drug dependence	69.8	2.2	25.6	2.2	3.7	0.7	0.9	0.3	65.3	3.5	20.0	2.6	11.2	2.7	3.5	1.9
Any	58.9	2.4	32.8	2.3	6.2	0.9	2.0	0.4	52.9	3.6	26.8	2.8	15.1	2.8	5.2	2.1
Other																
Conduct disorder	58.1	2.3	6.4	1.3	5.1	1.2	30.5	2.4	77.2	3.6	5.3	2.0	2.3	0.8	15.2	2.6
AAB	75.5	1.9	18.3	1.9	2.6	0.6	3.5	0.8	86.1	2.6	8.7	1.8	0.6	0.3	4.6	1.5
ASPD	83.2	1.7	12.5	1.6	2.2	0.6	2.1	0.7	92.2	2.5	5.8	1.7	0.1	0.1	1.9	1.1
Any	50.3	2.1	12.2	1.6	5.5	1.0	32.0	2.4	71.1	3.6	8.2	2.2	2.8	0.8	17.9	2.9
Aggregate																
Any (≥1)	21.7	1.8	24.3	2.1	7.9	1.2	46.0	2.2	14.0	2.3	14.4	2.2	8.5	1.7	63.1	2.2
≥2	47.1	3.0	10.3	1.3	5.0	1.0	37.6	2.6	32.9	3.2	5.6	1.6	5.4	1.3	56.1	2.9
≥3	63.4	2.7	5.5	1.0	2.1	0.6	28.9	2.4	53.2	3.0	2.2	0.8	3.5	1.1	41.2	2.7

**NCS indicates National Comorbidity Survey; Pure, the proportion of persons with lifetime alcohol dependence who have never had the disorder represented by the row; Primary, the proportion of persons with lifetime alcohol dependence who had a first onset of the disorder represented by the row after the onset of AD; Same-Year, the proportion of persons with lifetime alcohol dependence who had a first onset of the disorder represented by the row in the same year as the onset of alcohol dependence; Secondary, the proportion of persons with lifetime alcohol dependence who had a first onset of the disorder represented by the row prior to the onset of alcohol dependence; GAD, generalized anxiety disorder; PTSD, posttraumatic stress disorder; AAB, adult antisocial behavior; and ASPD, antisocial personality disorder. The weighted numbers of respondents in each cell of the table can be computed by multiplying the base of 838 men and 374 women with lifetime alcohol dependence (from Table 1) by the proportions. For example, the 91.1% of men whose alcohol dependence is pure with respect to GAD is equivalent to 763 weighted cases.*

might conceal disorders from lay interviewers, and this factor would lead to the underestimation of prevalences and biased estimation of ORs.[30]

A second limitation is that the survival model used here implicitly assumed that the effects of earlier disorders are constant throughout the life course of the respondent no matter what the age at onset of the earlier disorders, the age at onset of the subsequent alcohol use disorder, or the difference in these ages, and that there are no cohort differences in these effects. More complex modeling is currently under way. Although the results will not change the conclusion that the average overall associations of prior disorders with subsequent AA and AD are positive and statistically significant, it is likely that they will show that the average effects reported here do not hold in all parts of the age range and in all cohorts.

A third limitation is that the investigation of temporal priorities relied on retrospective reports of the age at onset. Prospective studies have shown that respondents' rates of forgetting their previous disorders is problematic in population surveys.[31] As a result, caution must be exercised in interpreting results based on lifetime reports. A related problem is that there might be systematic errors in retrospective recall of ages at onset[32]; this could create a false impression of temporal priority of mental disorders over alcohol use disorders. Two points related to this limitation are worth making. First, the finding that the median age at onset of AD is lower than that of AA is implausible at the individual level. However, the median age at onset of AA is based on respondents who never went on to dependence, who have comparatively late onsets of abuse compared with people who go on to dependence. Second, the median ages at onset are low compared with those found in samples with unrestricted age ranges due to the fact that the NCS is based on a young sample.

LIFETIME CO-OCCURRENCE

Within the context of these limitations, the results are consistent with those of prior studies in finding that the majority of people with an alcohol disorder have at least 1 of the other psychiatric disorders evaluated in the NCS.[1] There is much stronger evidence for lifetime co-occurrence with AD than AA. Our finding that co-occurrence is stronger among women than men is con-

Table 5. Prior Lifetime Disorders as Bivariate Predictors of the Onset of *DSM-III-R* Alcohol Abuse and Alcohol Dependence, by Sex*

Prior Lifetime Disorders	Alcohol Abuse				Alcohol Dependence			
	Men		Women		Men		Women	
	OR	95% CI	OR	95% CI	OR	95% CI	OR	95% CI
Anxiety								
GAD	0.80	0.10-6.37	1.54	0.30-7.91	3.70†	2.54-5.39	2.83†	2.11-3.79
Panic	1.04	0.05-22.05	0.51	0.19-1.40	2.63†	1.43-4.84	4.16†	1.89-9.16
Agoraphobia	1.30	0.53-3.17	0.93	0.50-1.72	1.54†	1.09-2.19‡	2.73†	1.79-4.17
Social phobia	0.97	0.62-1.51‡	2.16†	1.55-3.01	2.04†	1.78-2.35	2.57†	2.06-3.21
Simple phobia	0.89	0.58-1.35‡	2.44†	1.66-3.58	2.54†	2.01-3.22	2.81†	2.31-3.43
PTSD	0.50	0.24-1.05	1.00	0.58-1.74	2.67†	2.10-3.40	3.37†	2.45-4.63
Any	1.07	0.74-1.54‡	1.83†	1.38-2.44	2.20†	1.87-2.60‡	3.09†	2.73-3.50
Affective								
Depression	0.32†	0.17-0.59‡	2.26†	1.48-3.45	2.67†	2.07-3.46‡	4.10†	3.22-5.22
Dysthymia	0.56	0.26-1.22	1.18	0.58-2.39	3.17†	2.18-4.63	3.53†	2.68-4.66
Mania	0.11†	0.03-0.49‡	1.83	0.71-4.73	8.05†	4.48-14.48	4.73	0.79-28.16
Any	0.41†	0.25-0.68‡	2.20†	1.47-3.30	3.12†	2.51-3.87‡	4.79†	3.71-6.19
Drug								
Drug abuse	1.36	0.64-2.89‡	3.22†	2.20-4.71	2.20†	1.73-2.80‡	3.06†	2.60-3.60
Drug dependence	0.31†	0.13-0.77‡	1.88	0.51-6.94	2.96†	2.66-3.30‡	6.52†	5.44-7.80
Any	0.61	0.32-1.14‡	2.55†	1.32-4.90	2.74†	2.39-3.13‡	4.88†	4.19-5.70
Other								
Conduct disorder	1.26	0.95-1.66	1.80†	1.06-3.06	3.37†	2.94-3.87	3.63†	2.99-4.42
AAB	0.50	0.22-1.14‡	3.23	0.56-18.80	3.66†	2.98-4.51‡	5.90†	4.83-7.21
ASPD	0.57	0.22-1.51	1.14	0.48-2.67	3.92†	2.98-5.16‡	5.42†	3.72-7.88
Any	1.18	0.89-1.55‡	2.21†	1.27-3.83	3.51†	3.07-4.01	4.15†	3.53-4.87
Aggregate								
Any (≥1)	1.13	0.88-1.47‡	2.37†	1.79-3.12	3.55†	3.17-3.98‡	4.26†	3.80-4.79
≥2	1.37	0.93-2.04	2.32†	1.59-3.38	4.52†	3.76-5.43	4.67†	4.34-5.01
≥3	0.39†	0.19-0.81‡	3.19†	1.93-5.26	6.33†	5.08-7.89‡	9.65†	7.56-12.31

**OR indicates odds ratio; CI, confidence interval; GAD, generalized anxiety disorder; PTSD, posttraumatic stress disorder; AAB, adult antisocial behavior; and ASPD, antisocial personality disorder. Prior lifetime disorders are those with restrospectively reported ages at onset earlier than the onset of the alcohol disorder. Each OR was estimated in a separate discrete-time survival model in which prior onset of 1 disorder was the only substantive predictor. Controls were also included for person-year and age at interview (cohort). The weighted numbers of respondents with each of the prior disorders and subsequent alcohol disorders can be computed from the proportions in Tables 3 and 4, along with the bases in Table 1.*

†The OR is significant at the .05 level, 2-tailed test.

‡Significant sex difference in the OR at the .05 level, 2-tailed test.

Table 6. Prior Lifetime Disorder Profiles as Multivariate Predictors of the Onset of *DSM-III-R* Alcohol Dependence, by Sex*

Prior Lifetime Disorder Profiles†	Men			Women		
	OR	95% CI	$No._w$	OR	95% CI	$No._w$
None	1.00	. . .	216	1.00	. . .	69
Anxiety only	1.85‡	1.28-2.66	44	2.23‡	1.48-3.37	9
Affective only	1.83	0.92-3.61	8	2.72‡	1.41-5.27	39
Drug only	6.42‡	3.87-10.65	32	3.44‡	1.52-7.76	4
Other only	4.07‡	3.24-5.12	130	5.47‡	3.13-9.58	18
Anxiety-affective	4.02‡	1.65-9.80	16	9.11‡	5.76-14.41	41
Anxiety-drug	5.81‡	2.41-14.01	5	10.04‡	4.70-21.43	10
Anxiety-other	5.76‡	4.21-7.90	53	4.77‡	2.78-8.21	10
Affective-drug	3.97	0.97-16.29	2	6.98	0.20-238.60	3
Affective-other	11.99‡	6.31-22.79	14	14.29‡	5.69-35.84	4
Drug-other	3.85‡	1.81-8.19	17	22.37‡	10.82-46.24	5
Anxiety-affective-drug	2.52	0.87-7.30	1	12.57‡	5.19-30.44	6
Anxiety-affective-other	13.70‡	8.41-22.32	30	21.57‡	8.87-52.47	15
Anxiety-drug-other	4.44‡	2.07-9.54	8	17.86‡	5.08-62.75	6
Affective-drug-other	10.77‡	4.39-26.40	3	79.38‡	34.83-180.87	4
Anxiety-affective-drug-other	4.62‡	1.45-14.68	3	26.50‡	8.50-82.59	5

**OR indicates odds ratio; CI, confidence interval.*

†Prior disorder profiles are defined as the multivariate combination of disorders with retrospectively reported ages at onset before the onset of alcohol dependence. The ORs are based on a single discrete-time survival model for each sex-specific subsample in which dummy variables for each profile were included as predictors of first onset of alcohol dependence. Controls were also included for person-year and age at interview (cohort). The weighted numbers of respondents with each prior lifetime disorder profile and subsequent alcohol dependence ($No._w$) are also reported due to the fact that these numbers cannot be derived from any of the results in earlier tables.

‡Significant at the .05 level, 2-tailed test.

Table 7. Prior Lifetime Co-occurring Disorders as Bivariate Predictors of the Persistence (12-Month Prevalence) of NCS/*DSM-III-R* Alcohol Abuse and Alcohol Dependence, by Sex*

	Alcohol Abuse				Alcohol Dependence			
	Men		Women		Men		Women	
Prior Lifetime Disorders	OR	95% CI	OR	95% CI	OR	95% CI	OR	95% CI
Anxiety								
GAD	0.11	0.01-1.42	0.59	0.08-4.57	1.33	0.27-6.52	1.87	0.24-14.47
Panic	. . .	. . .	0.45	0.06-3.36	7.17†	1.62-31.80‡	0.55	0.11-2.78
Agoraphobia	0.34	0.05-2.09	4.91	0.56-43.15	2.74	0.94-7.97	1.01	0.37-2.73
Social phobia	0.57	0.23-1.42	2.53	0.63-10.16	1.18	0.75-1.86	1.24	0.63-2.43
Simple phobia	0.42	0.15-1.17	1.06	0.35-3.19	2.44†	1.43-4.18‡	0.93	0.41-2.07
PTSD	5.75	0.97-33.98	2.89	0.59-14.12	1.14	0.49-2.67	1.46	0.64-3.35
Any	0.54	0.25-1.15	1.65	0.44-6.11	1.79†	1.02-3.14	1.03	0.59-1.82
Affective								
Depression	0.71	0.18-2.87	1.30	0.41-4.07	1.81	0.74-4.46	0.88	0.41-1.91
Dysthymia	0.38	0.07-2.19	6.03	0.84-43.46	1.11†	0.29-4.33	1.27	0.25-6.31
Mania	. . .	. . .	1.41	0.10-18.99	4.99	1.31-19.04	1.69	0.41-6.93
Any	0.57	0.16-2.02	1.78	0.66-4.82	1.73	0.83-3.61	0.76	0.35-1.69
Drug								
Drug abuse	2.07	0.51-8.34	0.89	0.37-2.14	1.24	0.87-1.77	1.31	0.65-2.62
Drug dependence	1.90	0.14-25.99	1.05	0.13-8.24	0.96	0.40-2.31	0.97	0.27-3.42
Any	2.31	0.34-15.61	0.83	0.28-2.44	0.96	0.58-1.59	1.30	0.50-3.37
Other								
Conduct disorder	1.02	0.51-2.04	1.99	0.36-11.01	1.75†	1.19-2.56	1.96	0.95-4.03
AAB	3.81	0.62-23.46	1.29	0.10-17.58	0.92	0.51-1.63	1.09	0.27-4.41
ASPD	2.23	0.21-23.37	2.54†	1.12-5.76	0.89	0.45-1.78	0.85	0.10-6.94
Any	1.15	0.57-2.33	1.79	0.43-7.48	1.73†	1.18-2.53	1.90	0.95-3.79
Aggregate								
Any (≥1)	0.74	0.41-1.34	1.91	0.61-15.96	1.94†	1.17-3.22	1.53	0.79-2.96
≥2	1.14	0.50-2.59	1.27	0.35-4.63	2.05†	1.00-4.18	1.63	0.64-4.17
≥3	1.50	0.21-10.56	3.95	0.64-24.26	2.17†	1.04-4.52	1.45	0.68-3.06

**OR indicates odds ratio; CI, confidence interval; Prior Lifetime Disorders, those with retrospectively reported ages at onset earlier than the onset of the alcohol use disorder (each OR was estimated in a separate logistic regression model in which prior onset of one lifetime disorder was the only substantive predictor of 12-month alcohol use disorder in the subsample of respondents with the lifetime alcohol use disorder); GAD, generalized anxiety disorder; PTSD, posttraumatic stress disorder; AAB, adult antisocial behavior; and ASPD, antisocial personality disorder. The data used in the analyses are the subsamples of respondents with each of the lifetime alcohol use disorders, as given in Table 1. The proportions with each of the prior lifetime disorders can be obtained from Table 5 by using the procedures described in the footnote to that table.*

†The OR is significant at the .05 level, 2-tailed test.

‡Significant sex difference in the OR at the .05 level, 2-tailed test.

sistent with other recent research, as is the finding that the anxiety and affective disorders constitute the largest proportion of lifetime co-occurring cases among women, while the substance disorders, conduct disorder, and antisocial personality disorder account for the majority of co-occurrence among men.[33,34]

PREDICTION OF FIRST ONSET OF ALCOHOL DISORDERS

Although the finding that the majority of people with lifetime co-occurrence reported that at least 1 other disorder occurred at an earlier age than their alcohol use disorder is consistent with previous retrospective studies,[35,36] as well as with previous prospective studies of conduct disorder,[37] it is inconsistent with previous prospective studies of anxiety disorders and affective disorders.[38] As most of the latter studies were carried out some time ago, it might be that the NCS finding is due to a new risk of substance use disorders from prior anxiety and depression in recent cohorts. This possibility is consistent with a finding in the Epidemiologic Catchment Area Study of an increasing risk of substance use disorders among respondents in the age range of 18 to 30 years who reported the prior existence of an anxiety disorder.[39]

PREDICTION OF THE PERSISTENCE OF ALCOHOL DISORDERS

Although a generally positive pattern of associations was found between lifetime co-occurrence and persistence of AA among men and between both AA and AD among women, these results were weak. This weakness is superficially inconsistent with the strong association between episode comorbidity and the persistence of alcohol-related problems typically found in clinical studies.[40] However, the latter evaluate current comorbidity; this means that while concurrent comorbidity can be indicative of a more severe illness, alcohol disorders that have onsets after some other psychiatric disorder do not differ markedly in persistence from pure or primary disorders.

Accepted for publication October 10, 1996.

The NCS is a collaborative epidemiologic investigation of the prevalence, causes, and consequences of psychiatric morbidity and comorbidity in the United States

Survey Group

The National Comorbidity Survey Group, Collaborating National Comorbidity Survey Sites and Investigators: The Addiction Research Foundation, Toronto, Ontario: Robin Room, PhD. Duke University Medical Center, Durham, NC: Dan Blazer, MD, PhD; Marvin Swartz, MD. The Johns Hopkins University, Baltimore, Md: James C. Anthony, PhD; William Eaton, PhD; Philip Leaf, PhD. Max Planck Institute of Psychiatry, Munich, Germany: Hans-Ulrich Wittchen, PhD. Medical College of Virginia, Virginia Commonwealth University, Richmond: Kenneth Kendler, MD. University of Michigan, Ann Arbor: Lloyd Johnston, PhD; Harvard Medical School, Boston, Mass: Ronald C. Kessler, PhD. New York University, New York, NY: Patrick Shrout, PhD. State University of New York–Stony Brook: Evelyn Bromet, PhD. University of Miami, Coral Gables, Fla: R. Jay Turner. Washington University School of Medicine, St Louis, Mo: Linda Cottler, PhD.

supported by grant R01 MH46376 from the US Alcohol, Drug Abuse, and Mental Health Administration, with supplemental grant 90135190 from the W. T. Grant Foundation, New York, NY (Dr Kessler, principal investigator). Preparation for the report was also supported by Research Scientist Development Award K01 MH00507, National Institute of Mental Health (Dr Kessler) and Scientist Development Award for Clinicians K20 AA00168, National Institute for Alcohol and Alcohol Abuse (Dr Crum), Rockville, Md.

Corresponding author: Ronald C. Kessler, PhD, Department of Health Care Policy, Harvard Medical School, 25 Shattuck St, Boston, MA 02115.

REFERENCES

1. Regier DA, Farmer ME, Rae DS, Locke BZ, Keith SJ, Judd LL, Goodwin FK. Comorbidity of mental disorders with alcohol and other drug abuse: results from the Epidemiologic Catchment Area (ECA) Study. *JAMA.* 1990;264;2511-2518.
2. Sheehan MF. Dual diagnosis. *Psychiatr Q.* 1193;64:107-134.
3. Carroll KM, Rounsaville BJ, Bryant KJ. Alcoholism in treatment-seeking cocaine abusers: clinical and prognostic significance. *J Stud Alcohol.* 1993;54:199-208.
4. Bromet EF, Parkinson DK, Curtis EC, Schulberg HC, Blane H, Dunn LO, Phelan J, Dew MA, Schwartz JE. Epidemiology of depression and alcohol abuse/dependence in a managerial and professional work force. *J Occup Environ Med.* 1990;32:989-995.
5. McCusker CG, Brown K. The cue-responsivity phenomenon in dependent drinkers: 'personality' vulnerability and anxiety as intervening variables. *Br J Addict.* 1991;86:905-912.
6. Soyka M, Albus M, Kathmann N, Finelli A, Hofstetter S, Holzbach R, Immler B, Sand P. Prevalence of alcohol and drug abuse in schizophrenic inpatients. *Eur Arch Psychiatry Clin Neurosci.* 1993;242:362-372.
7. Luthar SS, Merikangas KR, Rounsaville BJ. Parental psychopathology and disorders in offspring: a study of relatives of drug abusers. *J Nerv Ment Dis.* 1993;181:351-357.
8. Kalodner CR, Delucia JL, Ursprung AW. An examination of the tension reduction hypothesis: the relationship between anxiety and alcohol in college students. *Addict Behav.* 1989;14:649-654.
9. Searles JS, Alterman AI. Differential attrition rates alcohol abusing and nonabusing schizophrenic inpatients: a methodological note. *Alcohol Clin Exp Res.* 1992;16:705-707.
10. Kessler RC, McGonagle KA, Zhao S, Nelson CB, Hughes M, Eshleman S, Wittchen HU, Kendler KS. Lifetime and 12-month prevalence of *DSM-III-R* psychiatric disorders in the United States: results from the National Comorbidity Survey. *Arch Gen Psychiatry.* 1994;51:8-19.
11. World Health Organization. *Composite International Diagnostic Interview (CIDI, Version 1.0).* Geneva, Switzerland: World Health Organization; 1990.
12. Robins LN, Wing J, Wittchen HU, Helzer JE. The Composite International Diagnostic Interview: an epidemiologic instrument suitable for use in conjunction with different diagnostic systems and in different cultures. *Arch Gen Psychiatry.* 1988;45:1069-1077.
13. American Psychiatric Association. *Diagnostic and Statistical Manual of Mental Disorders, Third Edition, Revised.* Washington, DC: American Psychiatric Association; 1987.
14. World Health Organization. *Composite International Diagnostic Interview Computer Programs (Version 1.1).* Geneva, Switzerland: World Health Organization; 1990.
15. Wittchen HU. Reliability and validity studies of the WHO-Composite International Diagnostic Interview (CIDI): a critical review. *J Psychiatr Res.* 1994;28:57-84.
16. Spitzer RL, Williams JBW, Gibbon M, First MB. *Structured Clinial Interview for* DSM-III-R: *Patient Edition (SCID-P, Version 1.0).* Washington, DC: American Psychiatric Press; 1990.
17. Blazer DG, Kessler RC, McGonagle KA, Swartz MS. The prevalence and distribution of major depression in a national community sample: the National Comorbidity Survey. *Am J Psychol.* 1994;151:979-986.
18. Kessler RC, Rubinow DR, Holmes C, Abelson JM, Zhao S. The epidemiology of *DSM-III-R* bipolar I disorder in a general population survey. *Psychol Med.* In press.
19. Wittchen HU, Kessler RC, Zhao S, Abelson J. Reliability and clinical validity of UM-CIDI *DSM-III-R* generalized anxiety disorder. *J Psychiatr Res.* 1995;29: 95-110.
20. Wittchen HU, Zhao S, Abelson JM, Abelson JL, Kessler RC. Reliability and procedural validity of UM-CIDI *DSM-III-R* phobic disorders. *Psychol Med.* In press.
21. American Psychiatric Association. *Diagnostic and Statistical Manual of Mental Disorders, Fourth Edition.* Washington, DC: American Psychiatric Association; 1994.
22. Allgulander C. Psychoactive drug use in a general population sample, Sweden: correlates with perceived health psychiatric diagnoses, and mortality in an automated record-linkage study. *Am J Public Health.* 1989;79:1006-1010.
23. Eaton WW, Anthony JC, Tepper S, Dryman A. Psychopathology and attrition in the Epidemiologic Catchment Area Study. *Am J Epidemiol.* 1992;135:1051-1059.
24. Kessler RC, Little RJA, Groves RM. Advances in strategies for minimizing and adjusting for survey nonresponse. *Epidemiol Rev.* 1995;17:192-204.
25. Woodruff RS, Causey BD. Computerized method for approximating the variance of a complicated estimate. *J Am Stat Assoc.* 1976;71:315-321.
26. University of Michigan. *OSIRIS VII.* Ann Arbor: Institute for Social Research, University of Michigan; 1981.
27. Kish L. Frankel MR. Balanced repeated replications for standard errors. *J Am Stat Assoc.* 1970;65:1071-1094.
28. SAS Institute. *SAS Language Guide (Release 6.03 Edition).* Cary, NC: SAS Institute Inc; 1988.
29. Allison PD. *Event History Analysis.* Beverly Hills, Calif: Sage Publications; 1984.
30. Mertens TE. Estimating the effects of misclassification. *Lancet.* 1993;342:418-421.
31. Wilhelm K, Parker G. Sex differences in lifetime depression rates: fact or artifact? *Psychol Med.* 1994;24:97-111.
32. Kessler RC, Mroczek DK, Belli RF. Retrospective adult assessment of childhood psychopathology. In: Shaffer D, Richters J, eds. *Assessment in Child Psychopathology.* New York, NY: Guilford Press. In press.
33. Nestadt G, Romanoski AJ, Samuels JF, Folstein MF, McHugh PR. The relationship between personality and *DSM-III* Axis I disorders in the population: results from the epidemiological survey. *Am J Psychiatry.* 1992;149:1228-1233.
34. Rounsaville BJ, Anton SF, Carroll K, Budde D, Prusoff BA, Gawin F. Psychiatric diagnoses of treatment-seeking cocaine abusers. *Arch Gen Psychiatry.* 1991;48:43-51.
35. Lewis CE, Helzer J, Cloninger CR, Croughan J, Whitman BY. Psychiatric diagnostic predispositions to alcoholism. *Compr Psychiatry.* 1982;23:451-461.
36. Weiss KJ, Rosenberg DJ. Prevalence of anxiety disorder among alcoholics. *J Clin Psychiatry.* 1985;46:3-5.
37. Dembo R, Allen N, Farrow D, Schmeidler J, Burgos W. A causal analysis of early drug involvement in three inner-city neighborhod settings. *Int J Addict.* 1985;20:1213-1237.
38. Schuckit MA, Hesselbrock V. Alcohol dependence and anxiety disorders: what is the relationship? *Am J Psychiatry.* 1994;151:1723-1734.
39. Bukstein OG, Brent DA, Kaminer Y. Comorbidity of substance abuse and other psychiatric disorders in adolescents. *Am J Psychiatry.* 1989;146:1131-1141.
40. Ellis D, McClure J. In-patient treatment of alcohol problems: predicting and preventing disease. *Alcohol Alcohol.* 1992;27:449-456.

ORIGINAL ARTICLE

Adult Major Affective Disorder After Prenatal Exposure to an Influenza Epidemic

Ricardo A. Machón, PhD; Sarnoff A. Mednick, PhD, DrMed; Matti O. Huttunen, MD

Background: We have previously reported an increase in schizophrenia diagnoses in a population exposed during the second trimester to the 1957 influenza epidemic. These basic findings together with a fair number of replications have been interpreted as supporting a neurodevelopmental contribution to the origins of schizophrenia. Recent neuroimaging findings suggest that affective illness may also have a neurodevelopmental origin. We examined the hypothesis that exposure to an influenza epidemic during the second trimester would increase the risk for adult major affective disorder.

Methods: The subjects had been exposed as fetuses to the type A_2/Singapore influenza epidemic in greater Helsinki, Finland. Control subjects were born in the 6 years before the epidemic.

Results: We found a significant ($P<.001$) increase in the proportion of hospital diagnoses for major affective disorder for individuals exposed to the influenza epidemic during their second trimester of fetal development compared with control subjects (13% vs 2%). This second-trimester effect seems somewhat stronger in men (16% vs 2%) ($P<.001$), although the rates of major affective disorder in women (8% vs 3%) ($P>.05$) were similar. The second-trimester effect remained when we estimated population-based rates (2.1 vs 0.6 per 1000) ($P<.05$) of major affective disorder. Additional analyses revealed that the increase of major affective disorder among subjects in the index group who were exposed during the second trimester was due to a significant ($P<.002$) elevation of unipolar forms, although a similar though not significant ($P>.05$) elevation was observed for the bipolar forms of major affective disorder.

Conclusions: These data are consistent with the hypothesis concerning the possible neurodevelopmental contribution to the origins of some forms of major affective disorder, especially unipolar depressive disorder. These encouraging findings, if replicated, may suggest that some mental disorders may stem, in part, from a disturbance in the development of the fetal brain during the second trimester.

Arch Gen Psychiatry. 1997;54:322-328

WE HAVE previously reported an increase in schizophrenia diagnoses in a Finnish population exposed during their second trimester of gestation to the 1957 influenza epidemic.[1] These basic findings have been replicated in several studies.[2-10] In addition, investigators[7,11-13] have also reported a second-trimester effect for influenza epidemics other than the one in 1957. Morris et al[14] have reported a third-trimester effect in Ireland for a period of 50 years. Fewer studies[15-19] have failed to replicate these findings. This literature[20,21] has sparked much discussion and debate (S.A.M., P. Voldsgaard, MD, B. Rodgers, PhD, H. Christensen, MD, S. Bredkjaer, MD, and F. Schulsinger, MD, Dr Med, unpublished data, 1996).

The findings described, as a whole, have been interpreted as supporting a neurodevelopmental origin of schizophrenia.[8,22] This hypothesis posits that at least 1 form of schizophrenia results from a disruption of normal brain development during a critical risk period in the second trimester. By the fifth month of gestation, almost all of the neurons slated to compose the human neocortex have been generated, but many have not yet migrated to their target structures and become positioned and synaptically connected. Early in the second trimester, the mesolimbic system, the thalamus, and the entorhinal region are experiencing rapid growth. Disturbances occurring during active development of these brain areas may produce incomplete or inappropriate migration, incorrect positioning, failures of connection, misconnections, or all of the

From the Department of Psychology, Loyola Marymount University (Dr Machón), and the Social Science Research Institute, University of Southern California (Dr Mednick), Los Angeles, Calif; and Departments of Psychiatry, University of Helsinki, and Mental Health, National Health Institute of Finland (Dr Huttunen).

METHODS

THE 1957 INFLUENZA EPIDEMIC

The 1957 "Asian" influenza epidemic is thought to have originated in northern China at the beginning of the year; it was established in Singapore in the early spring months and spread to Europe later in the summer months. The disease was found to be caused by the A_2/Singapore virus, and the first antibody rise against its antigen was observed in a complement fixation test at the end of August 1957. The first virus isolation succeeded in Helsinki on September 26, 1957, from throat washings. Finnish health officials estimated the peak of the epidemic, based on the rate of sickness absenteeism in personnel under observation in the city of Helsinki, as lasting from the second week of October and continuing for 5 weeks.[38,39]

DEFINITION OF INDEX AND CONTROL GROUPS

Thus, for this study, we defined the period of the epidemic as lasting from October 8, 1957, to November 14, 1957, in greater Helsinki, Finland. The index year cohort consisted of all children (1) born in the county of Uusimaa, Finland, (2) from November 15, 1957, to August 14, 1958, (3) who were admitted before the age of 29 years 10 months as inpatients to 1 or more of the 8 psychiatric hospitals (ie, Hesperia, Lapinlahti, Tammiharju, Kellokoski, Nikkilä, Paloniemi, Kevätkumpu, and Veikkola) serving the county of Uusimaa. The control subjects for the study comprised all children (1) born in the county of Uusimaa, (2) from November 15, 1951, to August 14, 1957, (3) who were admitted before the age of 29 years 10 months as inpatients to these same psychiatric hospitals.

The index year cohort and control subjects were paired by month of birth. Index year subjects born from November 15, 1957, to December 14, 1957, were in their ninth month of fetal life when exposed to the epidemic; the corresponding control subjects were born from November 15 to December 14 in the years 1951 through 1956. Those born from November 15, 1957, to February 14, 1958, were defined as having been exposed to the epidemic during their third trimester of fetal development. Those born from February 15, 1958, to May 14, 1958, were defined as having been exposed to the epidemic during their second trimester of fetal development. Those born from May 15, 1958, to August 14, 1958, were defined as having been exposed to the epidemic during their first trimester of fetal development. The trimesters for the control subjects were formed using similar dates as for the index group but for the years from 1951 to 1957.

Because the type A_2/Singapore influenza virus appeared for the first time in Europe in the fall of 1957, it is impossible for the control subjects to have suffered a type A_2/Singapore influenza infection during their fetal development.

PSYCHIATRIC DIAGNOSES

For the period during which the index and control groups were at risk for a psychiatric disorder (ie, up to 1988), the psychiatric hospital diagnoses in Finland were based on an adaptation of the World Health Organization classification system, *ICD-8*.[40] In *ICD-8*, the code (ie, 296.x) corresponding to the *DSM-IV*[41] "Mood Disorders" (ie, 296.x) was called "Psychoses mano-depressiva." This main code of manic depressive psychosis was divided into 5 subtypes:

Continued on next page

above.[22] Disruptions in these neural processes, in turn, increase the probability of adult schizophrenia.

Convergent evidence for this neurodevelopmental interpretation of the origins of schizophrenia has been provided by other lines of investigation, including neuropathologic studies[23-28] and hand ectoderm (ie, fingerprint ridge) studies.[29-31] More convincing evidence for the influenza-schizophrenia relationship has been recently provided by our analyses of reports from 1957 to 1958; these reports of obstetrical nurses in antenatal clinics indicate that those subjects with schizophrenia who had been exposed to influenza during the second trimester had, indeed, incurred greater rates of documented influenza infection (eg, reported symptoms of high temperatures, cough, or runny nose during pregnancy, at a time close to the actual infection) compared with those exposed during the first or third trimester.[32]

Is schizophrenia the only psychiatric disorder that may have a neurodevelopmental origin? Recent magnetic resonance imaging findings, particularly the presence of medial temporal lobe (ie, hippocampus or amygdala complex) hypoplasia and reduction of total cerebral volume, have been interpreted as providing support for a neurodevelopmental etiology for bipolar affective disorder.[33-35] These neurostructural findings parallel those for schizophrenia.

Two previous studies have examined the possible relationship between the 1957 influenza type A_2/Singapore epidemic and affective illness. Crow and Done[15] studied the admissions to psychiatric hospitals of patients of a cohort drawn from the British Perinatal Mortality Survey and National Child Development Study, all of whom were born in England, Scotland, and Wales during the week of March 3 to 9, 1958. They found a slight but not significant ($P=.11$) increase in patients with affective illness for whom maternal infection during the second trimester (5 observed, 1.9 expected) compared with the first (1 observed, 0.5 expected) or third (1 observed, 1.3 expected) trimester was reported at the time of delivery. Brown et al,[36] in a cohort drawn from the Dutch psychiatric registry, recently reported a significant ($P<.01$) decrease in the risk for affective psychosis in female but not male patients who were in gestational months 2 to 3 and 7 to 8 at the time of the 1957 influenza epidemic, compared with control subjects born in similar months but in the 2 previous and 2 following years. The authors interpreted their findings as suggesting a possible protective effect of prenatal influenza on the risk of developing affective psychosis.

One other study, by Takei et al,[13] examined the relationship between exposure to influenza epidemics between the years 1938 and 1965 in England and Wales and the development of later affective psychosis (and

296.1 (manic-depressive psychosis [MDP], manic type), 296.2 (MDP, depressed type), 296.3 (MDP, circular type), 296.8 (MDP, other type), and 296.9 (MDP, unspecified). It is, thus, important to note that the *ICD-8* code of 296.x consisted of unipolar and bipolar major affective disorders.[37] Likewise, the concept of psychosis in the *ICD-8* affective disorder sense is unspecific and does not have the more exact *DSM-IV* definition of severe major depression with psychotic features (code 296.x4).

In our analyses, the subjects in whom *ICD-8* codes 296.2, 296.8, and 296.9 were diagnosed were classified as having unipolar major affective disorder (severe major depressive disorder, *DSM-IV*: codes 296.23, 296.24, 296.33, and 296.34), and the subjects with at least 1 admission in whom *ICD-8* codes 296.1 or 296.3 were diagnosed were classified as suffering from bipolar major affective disorder (*DSM-IV* bipolar I disorders: codes 296.03, 296.04, 296.40, 296.43, 296.44, 296.63, 296.64, 296.53, 296.54, 296.73, and 296.74). The classification of the depressive episodes as severe is based on the fact that the subjects actually incurred a psychiatric hospitalization. The subtyping of the episodes of unipolar major depressions into types without or with psychotic features in *DSM-IV* terms is not possible on the basis of the available psychiatric hospital diagnosis.

We included in this study only admissions to 8 greater Helsinki psychiatric hospitals by Helsinki residents. It is possible that some unknown proportion of subjects may have been admitted to hospitals in counties outside of Uusimaa. One would expect that the possible selection effects of this emigration would be equally distributed among those born in the 3 trimester periods across the 7 years studied.

For each admission of a member of the index or control group to any of the 8 psychiatric hospitals, we recorded all primary and up to 3 additional diagnoses, dates of admission and discharge, postal code for place of birth, and sex. The data were recorded by clerical and administrative personnel of the 8 hospitals who were not aware of the hypotheses of the study.

The youngest subjects in the study were born on August 14, 1958. At the time of the last check of the medical records (ie, June 1988), individuals born on that day were 29 years 10 months of age. To equate the entire study population for period of risk for psychiatric admission, admissions beginning after a subject reached the age of 29 years 10 months were not considered in the analyses.

Individuals with at least 1 lifetime hospital diagnosis of affective psychosis (*ICD-8* code 296.x) were considered to have a major affective disorder for the purposes of this study. Subjects with a history of any lifetime diagnosis of schizophrenia were excluded from these analyses.

STATISTICAL ANALYSES

All statistical analyses, including the Fisher exact test and a χ^2 test, were performed using the Statistical Analysis System (SAS Version 6, SAS Inc, Cary, NC) for the Unix operating system.[42] Separate χ^2 or Fisher exact tests (depending on the expected cell-size calculations) were performed for each of the 3 trimesters, testing the dependence of group status (ie, index and control) on psychiatric outcome (ie, major affective disorder and not major affective disorder).

schizophrenia). They found increased population death rates from influenza being followed 5 months later by a significant ($P<.01$) increase in births of patients with schizophrenia and a concurrent decrease in births of patients with affective psychosis. This overall pattern was evident only among the female and not the male patients.

Our original article[1] about subjects in Helsinki was based on a survey of psychiatric hospital admissions through 1984 at a time when the youngest subjects were 26.2 years of age. We noted that the second-trimester effect was specific to schizophrenia. No such increase was observed for other psychiatric diagnoses; in part, this may have been due to the relatively few subjects being accorded other psychiatric diagnoses. For example, there were a total of 5 subjects with major affective disorder (2 who had been exposed to influenza during trimester 1; 3, trimester 2; and 0, trimester 3) among the index group available for analysis at that time. By age 26, only less than half of lifetime diagnoses of major affective disorder would be evident.[37] We have collected psychiatric admission data for an additional 4 years through 1988, when the youngest subjects were almost 30 years old. At this age, a greater proportion of lifetime diagnoses for major affective disorder would be evident.

In this article, we examine the hypothesis that exposure to the 1957 influenza epidemic during the second trimester of gestation would increase the risk for adult major affective disorders compared with control subjects born in the same months of the year but in the preceding 6 years before the 1957 epidemic.

RESULTS

TOTAL GROUP ANALYSES

We examined the distribution of major affective disorders, comparing index and control groups separately by the 3 trimesters. These results are given in **Table 1**. For those exposed during trimesters 1 or 3, major affective disorder was diagnosed in a similar proportion of subjects in the index and control groups. Among those exposed during their second trimester of fetal life, subjects in the index group had a significantly elevated proportion of major affective disorders (13%) relative to total psychiatric admissions compared with control subjects (2%) (2-tailed Fisher exact test, $P<.001$).

ANALYSES BY SEX

We then examined these data separately for men and women, and the results are given in Table 1. No significant ($P>.05$) differences were observed for men or women in the index and control groups who were

Table 1. Percentage of Psychiatric Admissions With Major Affective Disorders Distributed by Index and Control Groups and Trimester Grouping

Group Status*	Trimester Grouping† 1	2	3
Total sample			
Index	2 (1/51)	13 (7/56)‡	4 (2/56)
Control	3 (13/383)	2 (9/442)	4 (14/390)
Males			
Index	0 (0/30)	16 (5/32)‡	3 (1/30)
Control	3 (7/228)	2 (4/247)	3 (7/233)
Females			
Index	5 (1/21)	8 (2/24)	4 (1/26)
Control	4 (6/155)	3 (5/195)	4 (7/157)

*Index subjects were born between 1957 and 1958; control subjects were born in the preceding 6 years of the October to November 1957 epidemic, from 1951 and 1952 through 1956 and 1957.

†Trimester grouping 1 indicates subjects born between May 15 and August 14, 1958; 2, those born between February 15 and May 14, 1958; and 3, those born between November 15 and February 14, 1958. All data are given as the percentage of subjects (number of subjects/total number in that category).

‡$P<.001$, 2-tailed Fisher exact test. All other comparisons were nonsignificant.

Table 2. Population-Based Rates of Major Affective Disorder (MAD) for City of Helsinki, Finland, Born Index and Control Subjects by Trimester Grouping

Group Status	Trimester Grouping* 2	1+3
Index		
No. affected by MAD	4	3
No. of births	1902	3494
MAD rate	2.1 per 1000	0.86 per 1000
Controls†		
No. affected by MAD	7	18
No. of births	11 206	20 899
MAD rate	0.62 per 1000	0.86 per 1000

*Trimester grouping 2 indicates subjects born between February 15 and May 14, 1958; 1+3, those born between May 15 and August 14, 1958, plus those born between November 15 and February 14, 1958.

†Control subjects were born in the same months as index subjects but in the preceding 6 years, from 1951 and 1952 through 1956 and 1957.

exposed during either the first or third trimesters. Among those exposed during their second trimester of fetal life, men in the index group had a significantly elevated proportion of major affective disorders compared with men in the control group (16% vs 2%; 2-tailed Fisher exact text, $P<.001$). Second trimester–exposed women in the index group did not significantly differ from women in the control group (8% vs 3%; 2-tailed Fisher exact test, $P>.05$), although their proportion of major affective disorders showed the same trend.

POPULATION-BASED RATES OF MAJOR AFFECTIVE DISORDERS

We were able to identify a subsample of subjects with major affective disorder who were born in Helsinki by postal code of birth to estimate population-based rates of major affective disorder. We also obtained the number of live births in Helsinki by month for the years from 1951 to 1958. Population-based major affective disorder rates were obtained by dividing the number of subjects with major affective disorder who were born in Helsinki by the total number of people born in their respective period. **Table 2** provides these results. We combined trimesters 1 and 3 because they had not differed in the analyses previously described and because of the relatively few subjects with major affective disorder in these cells (1 in trimester 1 and 2 in trimester 3 for the subjects in the index group). The rate of major affective disorder for those exposed in their second trimester of fetal development was 2.1 per 1000; in comparison, the rate of major affective disorder for second-trimester control subjects was 0.62 per 1000. These differences were statistically significant ($\chi^2=4.24$, $df=1$, $P<.05$). The rate of major affective disorder for those exposed in the combined first and third trimesters (0.86 per 1000) did not differ from that of the respective control subjects (0.86 per 1000) ($\chi^2<1.0$, $df=1$, $P>.05$). For subjects in the index group, the rate of major affective disorder for those exposed during their second trimester (2.1 per 1000) did not differ from the rate for those exposed during the combined first and third trimesters (0.86 per 1000) ($\chi^2=1.5$, $df=1$, $P>.05$), although the expected trend was noted.

GENERAL PSYCHOSES ANALYSES

The results previously described show a second-trimester effect for major affective disorders, thus extending the basic findings of our original article,[1] which showed a similar effect for schizophrenia. We then posed the question of whether the second-trimester effect would likewise be observed among the general psychoses. We were able to identify and classify in the cohort the presence of any *ICD-8* lifetime diagnoses of codes 290 to 299. We then tested whether the second-trimester effect would also be found among those in whom a general psychosis had been diagnosed. These results are given in **Table 3**. Subjects in the index group who were exposed to influenza during the second trimester show a significant elevation of general psychoses compared with control subjects (58% vs 45%; $\chi^2=5.4$, $df=1$, $P<.02$). Subjects in the index group who were exposed during either the first or third trimester did not significantly differ from control subjects ($\chi^2<1.0$, $df=1$, $P>.05$).

It was possible that this statistically significant increase in general psychoses in those exposed during the second trimester was due to the previously cited increase in schizophrenia and major affective disorder diagnoses. We removed the subjects with the *ICD-8* diagnoses of codes 295 and 296 from these analyses. These results are given in Table 3. The previously observed second-trimester effect disappeared, suggesting that the observed increase in general psychosis among those exposed during the second trimester was due specifically to the increase in schizophrenia and major affective disorder diagnoses only.

Table 3. Percentage of Psychiatric Admissions With General Psychoses Distributed by Index and Control Groups and Trimester Grouping*

Group Status†	Trimester Grouping‡ 1	2	3
All psychoses			
Index	52 (37/71)	58 (52/89)§	43 (32/74)
Control	46 (230/505)	45 (268/592)	48 (259/540)
All psychoses excluding schizophrenia (code 295) and major affective disorder (code 296)			
Index	25 (15/59)	24 (12/49)	22 (12/54)
Control	26 (95/370)	25 (109/433)	25 (95/376)

*Psychoses indicates ICD-8 codes 290 to 299.
†Index subjects were born between 1957 and 1958; control subjects were born in the preceding 6 years of the October to November 1957 epidemic, from 1951 and 1952 through 1956 and 1957.
‡Trimester grouping 1 indicates subjects born between May 15 and August 14, 1958; 2, those born between February 15 and May 14, 1958; and 3, those born between November 15 and February 14, 1958. All data are given as the percentage of subjects (number of subjects/total number in that category).
§$P<.02$, $\chi^2=5.4$, df=1. All other comparisons were nonsignificant.

Table 4. Frequency of Major Affective Disorder Diagnoses by Group Status and Trimester Grouping

Group Status*	Trimester Grouping† 1	2	3
Index			
296.1 Manic depression, manic	0	2	2
296.2 Manic depression, depressed	1	1	0
296.3 Manic depression, circular	0	1	0
296.8 Manic depression, other	0	1	0
296.9 Manic depression, unspecified	0	2	0
Controls			
296.1 Manic depression, manic	9	5	5
296.2 Manic depression, depressed	1	0	2
296.3 Manic depression, circular	2	2	3
296.8 Manic depression, other	0	0	1
296.9 Manic depression, unspecified	1	2	3

*Index subjects were born between 1957 and 1958; control subjects were born in the preceding 6 years of the October to November 1957 epidemic, from 1951 and 1952 through 1956 and 1957. The ICD-8 codes are given, as are the diagnoses.
†Trimester grouping 1 indicates subjects born between May 15 and August 14, 1958; 2, those born between February 15 and May 14, 1958; and 3, those born between November 15 and February 14, 1958. All data are given as the number of subjects affected in each grouping.

UNIPOLAR VS BIPOLAR FORMS OF MAJOR AFFECTIVE DISORDER

As previously noted, the *ICD-8* diagnosis of code 296 includes unipolar and bipolar forms of affective disorder. **Table 4** provides a distribution of individual subdiagnoses of major affective disorder by group status and trimester grouping. Thus, we also conducted a series of analyses in which we examined whether the observed increase in major affective disorders among the second-trimester group would be equally observed among the bipolar (manic and circular, *ICD-8* codes 296.1 or 296.3) and unipolar (depressed, other, and unspecified, *ICD-8* codes 296.2, 296.8, or 296.9) forms of affective illness. Subjects in the index group who were exposed during the second trimester had a significantly higher proportion of unipolar forms of major affective disorder (4 [7.1%] of 56) compared with control subjects (2 [0.5%] of 442) (Fisher exact test, $P<.002$). Subjects in the index group who were exposed during the second trimester did not have a significantly different proportion of bipolar forms of major affective disorder (3 [5.4%] of 56) compared with control subjects (7 [1.6%] of 442) (Fisher exact test, $P>.05$), although the same trend as noted for the unipolar form was seen.

COMMENT

We have found an increase in the rate of hospital diagnoses for major affective disorder for individuals exposed to a large influenza epidemic during their second trimester of fetal development. This second-trimester effect seems somewhat stronger in men, although the rates of mood disorders in women were similar. The second-trimester effect remained when we examined population-based rates of major affective disorders. Additional analyses revealed that the increase of major affective disorder among those in the index group who were exposed during the second trimester was due to a statistically significant elevation of unipolar forms, although a similar though not statistically significant elevation was observed for bipolar major affective disorder as well. Our previous work has provided support for a neurodevelopmental origin of schizophrenia at a critical period during the second trimester of fetal life. The findings from this study also provide suggestive evidence for a neurodevelopmental genesis for a subgroup of major affective disorders in the second trimester as well.

Several limitations of this study are noted. The size of the sample is regrettably modest and, thus, these results should be interpreted with caution. One additional limitation is the fact that the outcome measure (ie, the psychiatric diagnosis) is based on clinical hospital diagnoses, not created for research purposes. This might potentially lower the reliability and, ultimately, the validity of the major affective disorder diagnoses. However, the fact that we excluded from the analyses all cases with a lifetime diagnosis of schizophrenia would tend to increase the validity of our major affective disorder diagnoses. Finally, the classification of subjects in the index group by trimester, based on the overlap of their birthdates with the epidemic, was the criterion for determining exposure to the influenza epidemic. We do not know which of these subjects were in fact infected, making a statement about causality tentative.

Our results differ from those of Crow and Done[15] and Brown et al.[36] The validity of the findings by Crow and Done is difficult to assess in light of the serious unreliability of maternal recall at the time of delivery (S.A.M., P. Voldsgaard, MD, B. Rodgers, PhD, H. Christensen, MD, S. Bredkjaer, MD, and F. Schulsinger, MD, Dr Med, unpublished data, 1996), the exceptionally low number of psychotic cases identified, and the underdetection of influenza infection in the cohort.[21] The findings by Brown et al[36] showed a decrease in the risk for affective psychosis in female but not male patients who were in gestational months 2 to 3 and 7 to 8 at the time of the 1957 influenza epidemic. The study by Brown et al[36] and 2 of the negative studies of schizophrenia and influenza are from the Netherlands,[17,18] all 3 of which employed the Dutch Psychiatric Registry. As Selten and Slaets[17] note, the Dutch registers only include more severe, perhaps negative symptom forms of psychotic disorders, including schizophrenia. Our own data, however, show that the subtypes of schizophrenia largely associated with influenza-related second-trimester exposure tend to be more delusional and paranoid (R.A.M., S.A.M., and M.O.H., unpublished data, 1996). Thus, the subtype of psychotic disorders associated with second-trimester influenza may be less likely ascertained in these 3 Dutch Registry studies.

Murray et al[43] and Takei et al[13] have noted a sex difference for the second-trimester effect for schizophrenia. They report that a second-trimester influenza effect is associated with a statistically significant greater increase in women with schizophrenia. Murray et al suggest that the increase in women with schizophrenia may be a consequence of women who would have been diagnosed with major affective disorder being diverted into schizophrenia by the second-trimester influenza. Our own data suggest that in this Finnish population the second-trimester influenza increases the risk of major affective disorder and schizophrenia in men and women. It is true, however, that the increase for men is greater than the increase for women and that the effect seems stronger for unipolar forms than bipolar forms of major affective disorder. Regrettably, the number of cases in this study does not permit a valid test of the hypothesis of Murray et al.

If we had analyzed all psychiatric illnesses reported as of 1988 in Helsinki and only found a statistically significant effect for major affective disorders, this finding might be attributed to chance. The analysis was motivated, however, by the article published by Nasrallah[33]; at this time, no other specific diagnoses beside schizophrenia and major affective disorders have been examined for the 1988 data set.

In a study based on ratings of psychiatric hospital medical records, we have reported that a distinguishing clinical feature of schizophrenia associated with second-trimester influenza is delusional symptomatology and absence of formal thought disorder (R.A.M., S.A.M., and M.O.H., unpublished data, 1996). In a comprehensive review of 26 studies based on more than 3800 subjects, Goodwin and Jamison[37] have noted that among subjects with affective psychosis (ie, those with manic depression) the presence or history of delusions was more than 3 times as likely as the history or presence of hallucinations. Moreover, only 1 in 5 subjects with manic depression is reported to have a history of formal thought disorder. At this time, we do not have clinical data on the presence of delusional symptoms among the subjects we studied with major affective disorder who were exposed to influenza during the second trimester of gestation. It is conceivable that second-trimester neural developmental disturbance is associated with an increased likelihood of delusional symptomatology and absence of formal thought disorder and that the decompensation may take the form of schizophrenia or major affective disorder. Perhaps genetic, precise timing of the teratogen or postnatal factors may determine which form of mental disorder (eg, schizophrenia, unipolar forms of major affective disorders, and perhaps others) is ultimately manifested.

Accepted for publication August 28, 1996.

This study was supported by a research grant from Loyola Marymount University, Los Angeles, Calif (Dr Machón); and Research Scientist Award MH00619 and grant MH37692 from the National Institute of Mental Health, Bethesda, Md (Dr Mednick).

We thank the anonymous reviewers whose valuable comments and recommendations served to strengthen this article.

Reprints: Ricardo A. Machón, PhD, Department of Psychology, Loyola Marymount University, 7900 Loyola Blvd, Los Angeles, CA 90045-8405.

REFERENCES

1. Mednick SA, Machón RA, Huttunen MO, Bonett D. Adult schizophrenia following prenatal exposure to an influenza epidemic. *Arch Gen Psychiatry.* 1988; 45:189-192.
2. O'Callaghan E, Sham P, Takei N, Glover G, Murray RM. Schizophrenia after prenatal exposure to 1957 A_2 influenza epidemic. *Lancet.* 1991;337:1248-1250.
3. Kendell RE, Kemp IW. Maternal influenza in the etiology of schizophrenia. *Arch Gen Psychiatry.* 1989;46:878-882.
4. Mednick SA, Machón RA, Huttunen MO, Barr CE. Influenza and schizophrenia: Helsinki vs Edinburgh. *Arch Gen Psychiatry.* 1990;47:875-876.
5. Kunugi H, Nankos S, Takei N. Influenza and schizophrenia in Japan. *Br J Psychiatry.* 1992;160:274-275.
6. Waddington JL. The declining incidence of schizophrenia controversy: a new approach in a rural Irish population. Presented at the annual meeting of the Royal College of Psychiatrists; July 24, 1992; Dublin, Ireland.
7. Welham JL, McGrath JJ, Pemberton MR. Schizophrenia: birthrates and three Australian epidemics. *Schizophr Res.* 1993;9:142.
8. Machón RA, Mednick SA. Adult schizophrenia and early neurodevelopmental disturbances. In: *Confrontations Psychiatriques: Épidémiologie et Psychiatrie.* Paris, France: Specia Rhône-Poulenc Rorer; 1994;35:189-215.
9. Fahy TA, Jones PB, Sham PC, Takei N, Murray RM. Schizophrenia in Afro-Caribbeans in the UK following prenatal exposure to the 1957 A2 influenza pandemic. *Schizophr Res.* 1993;9:132.
10. Beckmann J. Neuropathology findings in schizophrenics. Presented at NATO's Advanced Science Institute, Neural Development in Schizophrenia: Theory and Research; September 24, 1993; Tuscany, Italy.
11. Barr CE, Mednick SA, Munk-Jorgenson P. Exposure to influenza epidemics during gestation and adult schizophrenia: a 40-year study. *Arch Gen Psychiatry.* 1990;47:869-874.
12. Sham PC, O'Callaghan E, Takei N, Murray GK, Hare H, Murray RM. Schizophrenia following prenatal exposure to influenza epidemics between 1939 and 1960. *Br J Psychiatry.* 1992;160:461-466.
13. Takei N, O'Callaghan E, Sham P, Glover G, Murray RM. Does prenatal influenza divert susceptible females from later depressive psychosis to schizophrenia? *Schizophr Res.* 1993;9:141.
14. Morris M, Cotter D, Takei N, Walsh D, Larkin C, Waddington JL, O'Callaghan E. An association between schizophrenic births and influenza deaths in Ireland in the years 1921-1971. *Schizophr Res.* 1993;9:137.
15. Crow TJ, Done DJ. Prenatal exposure to influenza does not cause schizophrenia. *Br J Psychiatry.* 1992;161:390-393.
16. Bowler AE, Torrey EF. Influenza and schizophrenia: Helsinki vs Edinburgh. *Arch Gen Psychiatry.* 1990;47:876-877.
17. Selten J-P, Slaets JPJ. Evidence against maternal influenza as a risk factor for schizophrenia. *Br J Psychiatry.* 1994;164:674-676.

18. Susser E, Lin SP, Brown AS, Lumey LH, Erlenmeyer-Kimling L. No relation between risk of schizophrenia and prenatal exposure to influenza in Holland. *Am J Psychiatry.* 1994;151:922-924.
19. Cannon M, Cotter D, Sham PC, Larkin C, Murray RM, Coffey VP, O'Callaghan E. Schizophrenia in a Irish sample following prenatal exposure to the 1957 influenza epidemic: a case-controlled, prospective follow-up study. *Schizophr Res.* 1994;11:95.
20. Crow TJ. Prenatal exposure to influenza as a cause of schizophrenia: there are inconsistencies and contradictions in the evidence. *Br J Psychiatry.* 1994;164: 588-592.
21. O'Callaghan E, Sham P, Takei N, Glover G, Murray RM. Schizophrenia and influenza. *Lancet.* 1991;337:118-119.
22. Mednick SA, Cannon TD, Barr CE, Lyon M. *Fetal Neural Development and Adult Schizophrenia.* New York, NY: Cambridge University Press; 1991.
23. Akbarian S, Bunney Jr WE, Potkin SG, Wigal SB, Hagman JO, Sandman CA, Jones EG. Altered distribution of nicotinamide-adenine dinucleotide phosphate-diaphorase cells in frontal lobe of schizophrenic implies disturbances of cortical development. *Arch Gen Psychiatry.* 1993;50:169-177.
24. Akbarian S, Vinuela A, Kim JJ, Potkin SG, Bunney Jr WE, Jones EG. Distorted distribution of nicotinamide-adenine dinucleotide phosphate-diaphorase neurons in temporal lobe of schizophrenics implies anomalous cortical development. *Arch Gen Psychiatry.* 1993;50:178-187.
25. Bogerts B. The neuropathology of schizophrenia: pathophysiological and neurodevelopmental implications. In: Mednick SA, Cannon TD, Barr CE, Lyon M, eds. *Fetal Neural Development and Adult Schizophrenia.* New York, NY: Cambridge University Press; 1991:153-173.
26. Kovelman JA, Scheibel AB. A neurohistological correlate of schizophrenia. *Biol Psychiatry.* 1984;19:1601-1621.
27. Conrad AJ, Abebe T, Austin R, Forsythe S, Scheibel A. Hippocampal pyramidal cell disarray in schizophrenia as a bilateral phenomenon. *Arch Gen Psychiatry.* 1991;48:413-417.
28. Jakob J, Beckmann H. Prenatal developmental disturbances in the limbic allocortex in schizophrenics. *J Neural Transm.* 1986;65:303-326.
29. Bracha HS, Torrey EF, Bigelow LB, Lohr JB, Linington BB. Subtle signs of prenatal maldevelopment of the hand ectoderm in schizophrenia. *Biol Psychiatry.* 1991;30:719-725.
30. Mellor CS. Dermatoglyphic evidence of fluctuating asymmetry in schizophrenia. *Br J Psychiatry.* 1992;160:467-472.
31. Trent M, Kruger S, Perkins DO, Galernter J. Dermatological asymmetry in schizophrenia. *Schizophr Res.* 1993;9:141.
32. Mednick SA, Huttunen MO, Machón RA. Prenatal influenza infections and adult schizophrenia. *Schizophr Bull.* 1994;20:263-267.
33. Nasrallah HA. Neurodevelopmental aspects of bipolar affective disorder. *Biol Psychiatry.* 1991;29:1-2.
34. Olsen SC, Bogerts B, Coffman JA, Schwarzkopf SB, Nasrallah HA. Medial-temporal and ventricular abnormalities by MRI: comparing major psychoses. *Biol Psychiatry.* 1990;27:59A-60A.
35. Nasrallah HA. Brain structure and functions in schizophrenia: evidence for fetal neurodevelopmental impairment. *Curr Opin Psychiatry.* 1990;3:75-78.
36. Brown AS, Susser ES, Lin SP, Gorman JM. Affective disorders in Holland after prenatal exposure to the 1957 A_2 influenza epidemic. *Biol Psychiatry.* 1995; 38:270-273.
37. Goodwin FK, Jamison KR. *Manic-Depressive Illness.* New York, NY: University Press; 1990.
38. Saxé L, Hjelt L, Sjöstedt JE, Hakosalo J, Hakosalo, H. Asian influenza during pregnancy and congenital malformations. *Acta Pathol Microbiol Scand.* 1960; 49:114-126.
39. Hirvensalo M, Kinnunen O. Effect of Asian influenza on fetal development. *Ann Paediatr Fenn.* 1962;8:256-268.
40. Medicinalstyrelsen. *Classificatio Morborum et Causarum Mortis.* Helsinki, Finland: Medicinalstyrelsen; 1969.
41. American Psychiatric Association. *Diagnostic and Statistical Manual of Mental Disorders, Fourth Edition.* Washington, DC: American Psychiatric Association; 1994.
42. SAS Inc. *Statistical Analysis System: SAS/STAT User's Guide, Version 6, Fourth Edition.* Cary, NC: SAS Inc; 1990.
43. Murray RM, Takei N, Sham P, O'Callaghan E, Wright P. Prenatal influenza, genetic susceptibility and schizophrenia. *Schizophr Res.* 1993;9:137-138.

ORIGINAL ARTICLE

The Prevalence of *DSM-III-R* Diagnoses in a National Sample of Dutch Adolescents

Frank C. Verhulst, MD; Jan van der Ende, MS; Robert F. Ferdinand, MD; Marianne C. Kasius, MD

Background: We estimated the 6-month prevalence of psychiatric disorders among Dutch adolescents, using standardized, internationally available, and replicable assessment procedures, and assessed sex differences and comorbidity of diagnoses.

Methods: In phase 1, the parent, self-report, and teacher versions of the Child Behavior Checklist screened a sample representative of 13- to 18-year-olds from the Dutch general population. In phase 2, the parent (P) and child (C) versions of the Diagnostic Interview Schedule for Children (DISC) provided *DSM-III-R* diagnoses for a selected subsample of 780 subjects.

Results: The prevalence of any disorder was 21.5% for the DISC-C and 21.8% for the DISC-P. There was little overlap between subjects identified as having a disorder by the DISC-P and the DISC-C; only 4% met the criteria for any disorder on both. The most common disorders were simple phobia, social phobia, and conduct disorder. The most frequent comorbid diagnoses were anxiety and mood disorders.

Conclusions: Although prevalences of more than 21% for DISC-C– and DISC-P–derived diagnoses seem high, many adolescents with *DSM-III-R* diagnoses functioned quite well. The prevalence of any *DSM-III-R* diagnosis based on the DISC-C or DISC-P, in combination with the criterion for a definite case, was 7.9%.

Arch Gen Psychiatry. 1997;54:329-336

PREVALENCE STUDIES of psychiatric disorder in children and adolescents should ideally provide information on the number of children and adolescents in the general population at a given time who need some kind of intervention. This kind of information may aid in the planning of mental health facilities and setting of public health priorities.

Five previously published community surveys used standardized assessment procedures and refined probability sampling techniques to determine the prevalence of *DSM-III*[1] diagnoses[2-5] or diagnoses that resembled those of *DSM-III*.[6] These studies, published between 1985 and 1990, were the most recently available community surveys that provided *DSM-III* diagnoses for children and adolescents. The ages covered by these studies ranged from 4 to 16 years. The prevalences of psychiatric disorders defined in a more or less comparable way across the 5 studies were 17.6%, 17.9%, 18.1%, 22%, and 26%.

Although roughly similar, the 5 studies differed considerably in methods, including assessment procedures and the ways they coped with discrepant information from multiple informants such as parents, teachers, and adolescents (self-reports). The 5 prevalence studies also differed considerably in their choice and operationalization of morbidity criteria, hampering replicability and comparability across studies.

The primary objective of our study was to estimate the prevalence of psychiatric disorder among Dutch adolescents aged 13 to 18 years, using the most recent versions of standardized, internationally available assessment procedures. Instead of making forced choices with respect to the source of information or the morbidity criterion, we determined prevalence estimates based on different assessment approaches and different morbidity criteria. Thus, we allowed for empirical testing of different morbidity criteria. In this way, we used diagnostic methods that can be replicated by other researchers.

From the Department of Child and Adolescent Psychiatry, Sophia Children's Hospital/Erasmus University Rotterdam, Rotterdam, the Netherlands.

RESULTS

SENSITIVITY AND SPECIFICITY OF THE SCREENING PROCEDURE

Parent, teacher, and self-reports on adolescents' problem behaviors often show

SUBJECTS AND METHODS

SAMPLE AND PROCEDURE

Our study involves a 2-phase procedure, with the parent, self-report, and teacher versions of the Child Behavior Checklist (CBCL)[7] to screen a sample representative of 13- to 18-year-old adolescents from the Dutch general population in the first phase (screening phase), and the parent (P) and child (C) versions of the Diagnostic Interview Schedule for Children (DISC), version 2.3,[8] to obtain *DSM-III-R*[9] diagnoses for a selected subsample in the second phase (clinical interview phase).

This study was an extension of a study aimed at determining the frequencies of questionnaire-based parent-, teacher-, and (from 11 years of age onward) self-reported problems. Because the initial sampling procedure involved subjects aged 4 to 18 years, we will describe the selection of subjects for our study by first describing the selection of the original sample.

Screening Phase

The target population consisted of all 4- to 18-year-old children and adolescents of Dutch nationality, living in the Netherlands, a country comprising more than 15 million people. A stratified multistage cluster and random sampling design was used. The population was stratified according to 4 country regions and 4 degrees of urbanization. The sampling fraction was 1 of 5929 (2550 of 15 118 571).

A 2-stage sampling procedure was followed, with a selection of clusters in the first stage, followed by a selection of individuals in the second stage. The lower limit of a cluster was 25 subjects (1% of the desired sample size). For each stratum, the number of clusters to be selected was determined. Based on the cluster size and the sampling fraction, 8 cities with more than 148 225 (25×5929) inhabitants were selected. Other municipalities were randomly selected within each of the 16 strata with a probability of selection that was proportional to size. In this way, 81 municipalities, in addition to the 8 largest cities, were selected. Municipalities were requested to send names and addresses of a specified number of randomly selected subjects aged 4 to 18 years on January 1, 1993, equally divided across both sexes.

Of the 89 selected municipalities, 72 participated. Of the 17 municipalities who refused to cooperate, 6 could be replaced by selecting a municipality of similar degree of urbanization. Already selected municipalities of similar degrees of urbanization replaced the 11 remaining municipalities.

From April through June 1993, 82 trained lay interviewers with previous survey experience contacted the parents of selected children by mailing a letter describing the interview. The interviewer visited or telephoned the parent (preferably the mother) to make an appointment. If parents were not initially reached, interviewers called back at least 5 times on different days and at different times of the day.

A sample of 2916 subjects aged 4 to 18 years was selected; 57 of these were excluded because they were mentally retarded or had a serious physical illness or handicap or if no Dutch-speaking parent or parent surrogate was available for the interview. Of the total sample, 62 subjects were untraceable. No informant could be reached after 5 attempts for 88 subjects. Of the 2709 subjects for whom informants were reached, parent interviews were completed for 2227 (82.2%). Comparison between responders vs nonresponders revealed that the proportion of boys vs girls did not differ significantly (χ^2=1.09; *df*=1; *P*=.30). However, there were significantly more responders in the 4- to 10-year-old group (response rate, 86.1%) vs the 11- to 18-year-old group (response rate, 78.2%) (χ^2=28.26; *df*=1; *P*<.001).

After a short introduction, the youths were instructed to complete the Youth Self-Report (YSR)[10] in a room separate from where the parent was interviewed.

The parent was given a copy of the CBCL.[7] The interviewer read aloud each CBCL question and wrote down the parent's answer.

At the end of the interview, the interviewer checked the YSR and answered questions the youth had. Next, the interviewer asked the parent and youth for permission to send the Teacher's Report Form (TRF)[11] to the teacher who was the most familiar with the youth's functioning. Reminders were sent to nonresponders. Teachers who did not respond the second time were telephoned.

Clinical Interview Phase

In this phase, we focused on subjects aged 13 to 18 years. We obtained 853 CBCLs and 848 YSRs for 13- to 18-year-olds. Because not all subjects attended school, not all parents and youths gave permission to approach the teacher, and not all teachers cooperated, we obtained 568 TRFs.

Because we wanted to maximize the combined information contained by the CBCL, YSR, and TRF, we converted the total problem scores for each instrument to separate *z* scores. Next, we computed each subject's multisource score by averaging the *z* scores. All 3 sources of information were available for 566 subjects. For the 282 subjects for whom there was 1 source missing, we used the scores of the CBCL and YSR to compute the average. For 3 subjects, there was only a CBCL score available.

Of the 853 subjects with CBCLs, 780 (91.4%) consented to be reapproached. The clinical interview stage analysis consisted of separating the 200 subjects whose mean *z* scores on the CBCL, YSR, and TRF were above the 75th percentile of the cumulative frequency distribution for all

discrepancies in classifying subjects as disordered vs normal. Because no informant is intrinsically superior to another in identifying disordered subjects under all circumstances,[26-28] we combined the parent, self-report, and teacher scores in the screening phase. We took the 75th percentile of the cumulative frequency distribution of the mean *z* scores computed from the total problem scores across the CBCL, YSR, and TRF as the cutoff score to identify the deviant subjects. Sensitivity and specificity reflected the ability of the screening procedure to correctly identify disordered and normal subjects in the interviewed sample, which consisted of subjects with *z* scores greater than the 75th percentile and a random selection of subjects with scores less than the 75th percentile. Because there are no unequivocal criteria to define psychiatric disorder, **Table 1** shows the sensitivity and specificity computed

13- to 18-year-old participants (screen-positive subjects) and separating the 112 subjects randomly selected from the screening phase sample of 13- to 18-year-olds whose mean z scores on the CBCL, YSR, and TRF were below the 75th percentile for all 13- to 18-year-old participants (screen-negative subjects).

Twenty-six interviewers were trained to administer the DISC-P and DISC-C.[8] The DISC training was given in the standard 3-day training conference[12] by 3 of us (J.vdE., R.F.F., and M.C.K.) who were trained at the Columbia University (New York, NY) DISC Training Center. A total of 546 interviews were administered. For 274 (87.8%) of the 312 eligible subjects, we obtained a DISC-P, and for 272 (87.2%) of 312 subjects, we obtained a DISC-C. For the DISC-P, the compliance rate for the screen-negative subjects (87.5%) did not differ significantly from that for the screen-positive subjects (88.0%) (χ^2=0.02; df=1; P=.89). Similarly, for the DISC-C, the compliance rate for the screen-negative subjects (85.7%) did not differ significantly from that for the screen-positive subjects (88.0%) (χ^2=0.34; df=1; P=.56).

After completion of the DISC, the interviewer scored the nonclinician version[13] of the Children's Global Assessment Scale (CGAS).[14] We obtained separate CGAS scores after completion of the DISC-C and the DISC-P.

The mean interval between completion of the CBCL and administration of the DISC interviews was 118 days (SD, 29 days).

SCREENING INSTRUMENTS

The CBCL,[8] TRF,[11] and YSR[10] were used to obtain standardized parent, teacher, and self-reports of children's problem behaviors. The good reliability and validity established by Achenbach[7,10,11] were confirmed for the Dutch translations.[15-18]

PSYCHIATRIC INTERVIEWS

Diagnostic Interview Schedule for Children, Version 2.3

The National Institute of Mental Health DISC, version 2.3, is a highly structured diagnostic interview designed to be administered by well-trained interviewers who need not have formal clinical training. The DISC was especially designed to be used in epidemiological studies and contains questions that address diagnostic criteria for 40 *DSM-III-R* diagnoses and a psychosis screen. The DISC has 2 parallel forms, the DISC-C administered directly to the child or adolescent and the DISC-P administered to the parent or caregiver. Unless otherwise specified, the time frame of the DISC is the past 6 months. Earlier versions of the DISC, from which version 2.3 was derived, showed adequate test-retest reliability for subjects aged 11 to 17 years,[19] acceptable interrater reliability, and acceptable validity.[20-22]

The *DSM-III-R* diagnoses were derived from DISC scores by applying the algorithms provided by the authors of the DISC,version 2.3. Version 2.3 was translated into Dutch with the help of a linguist. We did not assess the reliability or validity of the Dutch translation. However, because we followed the original text as closely as possible, and because we instructed the interviewers according to the standard procedure, we relied on the psychometric properties as reported in the literature.

Children's Global Assessment Scale

The DISC includes questions on overall impairment for most diagnostic categories. These impairment scores are not incorporated in the diagnostic criteria. Because these impairment measures are of unknown validity, we preferred an overall impairment measure with satisfactory psychometric properties, the CGAS.[14] At the end of the interview, the interviewer scored the nonclinician version of the CGAS, an adaptation of the CGAS to be scored by lay interviewers.[13] The CGAS was designed to reflect the lowest level of functioning for a child or adolescent during a specified period. The original CGAS descriptors were simplified to provide an instrument that could be scored by a nonclinician with some knowledge of child and adolescent psychiatric disorders. The interrater, test-retest reliability, and validity measures for the original CGAS were satisfactory[14,23,24] and were replicated for the nonclinician version.[13] The nonclinician CGAS scores based on the parent and the child interview were significantly correlated with the mean CGAS scores of 2 clinical interviewers who independently interviewed the parent and the child.[13]

Shaffer et al[14] recommended the use of a cutoff score of 71 for the original CGAS to discriminate between normality and abnormality on conceptual grounds. Bird et al[24] investigated the discriminative power of the CGAS and concluded that a cutoff score of 61 can be used to identify subjects with "definite" disorders, and a cutoff score of 71 can be used to identify subjects with "probable" disorders.

Cutoff scores for the CGAS should not be regarded as definitive measures of impairment but as conventions based on criteria such as use of mental health services, need for services, and school performance, which are highly variable. Therefore, we will present findings for both CGAS cutoff scores (61 and 71) in this study, instead of selecting 1 cutoff score as the sole criterion.

STATISTICAL ANALYSIS

Prevalences, their SEs, and sex differences in prevalence were computed with commercially available software (SUDAAN).[25] In this way, we took account of the complex survey design and weighted for unequal sampling probabilities of the screen-positive and screen-negative subjects.

against different criteria for a case. Subjects were considered to have a disorder if they met *DSM-III-R* criteria for any diagnosis based on the DISC-P or the DISC-C. In addition, the diagnostic criteria were combined with 2 alternative criteria for global impairment, ie, a CGAS score of less than 61 or less than 71. Table 1 also gives the sensitivity and specificity computed against criteria based on the CGAS without DISC diagnosis.

The screening procedure yielded high sensitivity when subjects were classified as having a disorder if they met criteria for *DSM-III-R* diagnoses in combination with the CGAS criteria for impairment. The screening procedure was highly sensitive in identifying subjects with definite disorders (subjects with CGAS scores less than 61 and *DSM-III-R* diagnoses). For example, if a case was defined as the presence of 1 or more *DSM-III-R* diagnoses

Table 1. Sensitivity and Specificity for the 75th Percentile of the Mean *z* Scores of Total Problem Scores of the CBCL, YSR, and TRF by Different Diagnostic Criteria*

Diagnostic Test	Sensitivity	Specificity
DISC-P	0.51	0.82
CGAS-P <71	0.75	0.83
CGAS-P <61	0.90	0.79
DISC-P with CGAS <71	0.77	0.80
DISC-P with CGAS <61	0.87	0.78
DISC-C	0.50	0.81
CGAS-C <71	0.74	0.83
CGAS-C <61	0.89	0.79
DISC-C with CGAS <71	0.91	0.80
DISC-C with CGAS <61	1.00	0.78
DISC-P or DISC-C	0.44	0.85
CGAS-P or CGAS-C <71	0.68	0.86
CGAS-P or CGAS-C <61	0.92	0.81
DISC-P or DISC-C with CGAS <71	0.78	0.83
DISC-P or DISC-C with CGAS <61	0.90	0.80
DISC-P and DISC-C	0.81	0.77
CGAS-P and CGAS-C <71	0.91	0.81
CGAS-P and CGAS-C <61	0.83	0.77
DISC-P and DISC-C with CGAS <71	1.00	0.76
DISC-P and DISC-C with CGAS <61	1.00	0.76

**CBCL indicates Child Behavior Checklist; YSR, Youth Self-Report; TRF, Teacher's Report Form; DISC-P, Diagnostic Interview Schedule for Children, parent version; CGAS-P, Children's Global Assessment Scale, scored by lay interviewer on the basis of parent information; DISC-C, Diagnostic Interview Schedule for Children, child version; and CGAS-C, Children's Global Assessment Scale, scored by lay interviewer on the basis of child information.*

based on the DISC-P *or* DISC-C, combined with a CGAS score of less than 61, the sensitivity was 0.90, whereas the accompanying specificity of 0.80 was still reasonable. The CGAS score on its own yielded higher sensitivity than DISC diagnoses on their own. In terms of the sensitivity of the screening procedure to identify subjects with a disorder, the DISC diagnosis as morbidity criterion added little to the use of CGAS criteria. However, this does not imply that DISC information is not important, since we need information on the type of disorder in addition to information on the level of impairment.

6-MONTH PREVALENCE OF *DSM-III-R* DISORDERS

Table 2 shows the 6-month prevalences and SEs for the majority of DISC-derived specific diagnoses, the most prevalent diagnoses collapsed into major diagnostic groupings, and any disorder. Prevalences for *DSM-III-R* diagnoses are based on the DISC-P and DISC-C separately and in combination.

The prevalence of any disorder based on the DISC-P (21.8%) was quite similar to that based on the DISC-C (21.5%). We also combined DISC information on the diagnostic level. From the much lower prevalence of any disorder generated by the DISC-C and the DISC-P (4.0%) and the much higher prevalence of any disorder generated by the DISC-C or the DISC-P (35.5%), it can be concluded that there was minimal overlap between subjects who fulfilled criteria for *DSM-III-R* diagnoses based on the DISC-P vs the DISC-C.

We also determined the prevalence of *DSM-III-R* disorders in subjects who were functionally impaired according to a CGAS score of less than 71 (possible disorder) or less than 61 (definite disorder).

Table 3 shows the prevalences for 2 CGAS scores applied to subjects meeting criteria for different combinations of DISC-derived *DSM-III-R* diagnoses. We only report prevalences for 5 relatively prevalent diagnoses, 3 major diagnostic groupings, and any disorder. Table 3 also shows the prevalences for subjects with scores of less than 61 or less than 71 on the CGAS, irrespective of whether criteria for *DSM-III-R* diagnoses were met. As can be seen, a large proportion of subjects whose CGAS scores indicated impairment did not meet the criteria for a *DSM-III-R* disorder.

SEX DIFFERENCES

Tables 2 and 3 also indicate the significant ($P<.05$) differences in prevalences for boys and girls. Girls received more diagnoses of simple phobia (according to the DISC-P and the DISC-C) and social phobia (according to the DISC-C) than boys. Boys received more DISC-C diagnoses of mania, conduct disorder, any disruptive disorder, and substance use disorder than girls. According to the DISC-P, boys received more diagnoses of any tic disorder, conduct disorder, and any disruptive disorder. According to the DISC-P or DISC-C, boys received more diagnoses of conduct disorder, any disruptive disorder, and any substance use disorder than girls. For the combination of the DISC-P and DISC-C, no significant sex differences in prevalence were found.

For the testing of sex differences, we took account of the complex sampling design and unequal sampling probabilities of the screen-positive and screen-negative subjects. It is possible that differences in age distribution for boys vs girls may have affected sex differences in prevalence rates. However, the proportion of subjects in the 2 groups aged 13 to 15 years and 16 to 18 years did not differ across both sexes, both for the screen-positive (χ^2=0.0074; df=1; P=.93) and for the screen-negative subjects (χ^2=0.2609; df=1; P=.61).

COMORBIDITY

To determine the co-occurrence, or comorbidity, of diagnoses, we collapsed diagnostic categories into the following 6 groupings: anxiety disorders, tic disorders, mood disorders, attention-deficit hyperactivity disorder (ADHD), conduct-oppositional defiant disorder, and substance use disorders. **Table 4** shows the prevalences for multiple diagnoses based on these diagnostic groupings. Many subjects had only 1 diagnosis. Table 4 also lists the prevalences for multiple diagnoses for subjects who, in addition, obtained a CGAS score of less than 71 or 61. As can be seen, the effect of CGAS scores on the prevalences decreased as the number of diagnoses increased, indicating that comorbidity was associated with greater impairment.

We also inspected the numbers of subjects in the interviewed sample with different combinations of DISC-P and DISC-C disorders. The most frequent combination of disorders was anxiety disorder and mood disorder, both

Table 2. Six-Month Weighted Prevalence of *DSM-III-R* Diagnoses by Source of Information*

Diagnosis	Prevalence, % (SE)			
	DISC-P	DISC-C	DISC-P or DISC-C	DISC-P and DISC-C
Simple phobia	9.2† (2.5)	4.5 (1.5)	12.7† (2.9)	0.9 (0.4)
Social phobia	6.3 (1.6)	3.7† (1.1)	9.2 (2.0)	0.7 (0.4)
Agoraphobia	1.9 (0.8)	0.7 (0.4)	2.6 (0.9)	...
Panic disorder	0.3 (0.2)	0.2 (0.2)	0.4 (0.3)	...
Separation anxiety disorder	0.6 (0.3)	1.4 (0.8)	1.8 (0.9)	0.2 (0.2)
Avoidant disorder	3.0 (1.1)	1.4 (0.8)	4.0 (1.3)	0.3 (0.2)
Overanxious disorder	1.5 (0.5)	1.8 (0.9)	3.1 (1.0)	0.2 (0.2)
Generalized anxiety disorder	0.7 (0.3)	0.6 (0.3)	1.3 (0.5)	...
Obsessive-compulsive disorder	0.2 (0.2)	0.9 (0.4)	1.0 (0.4)	...
Any anxiety disorder	16.5 (3.0)	10.5 (2.1)	23.5 (3.6)	1.9 (0.7)
Bulimia nervosa	...	0.3 (0.2)	0.3 (0.2)	...
Anorexia nervosa	0.3 (0.2)	0.2 (0.2)	0.3 (0.2)	0.2 (0.2)
Enuresis	1.1 (0.8)	0.8 (0.8)	1.1 (0.8)	0.8 (0.8)
Encopresis	0.2 (0.2)	...	0.1 (0.1)	...
Chronic motor tic disorder	0.9 (0.8)	0.6 (0.3)	1.5 (0.8)	...
Chronic vocal tic disorder	0.3 (0.2)	...	0.3 (0.2)	...
Tourette disorder	0.2 (0.2)	...	0.1 (0.1)	...
Transient tic disorder	1.2 (0.8)	1.1 (0.8)	2.2 (1.1)	...
Any tic disorder	2.5‡ (1.1)	1.7 (0.9)	4.0 (1.4)	...
Major depression	1.3 (0.6)	2.8 (1.1)	3.6 (1.2)	0.4 (0.3)
Dysthymia	1.2 (0.5)	1.5 (0.6)	2.3 (0.8)	0.3 (0.2)
Mania	1.1 (0.8)	0.9‡ (0.4)	1.9 (0.9)	...
Hypomania	...	0.9 (0.8)	0.9 (0.8)	...
Any mood disorder	3.1 (1.1)	4.6 (1.4)	7.2 (1.7)	0.4 (0.3)
Attention-deficit hyperactivity disorder	1.8 (0.6)	1.3 (0.5)	2.6 (0.8)	0.4 (0.3)
Oppositional-defiant disorder	0.6 (0.3)	0.7 (0.4)	1.3 (0.5)	...
Conduct disorder	1.2‡ (0.4)	5.6‡ (1.6)	6.0‡ (1.6)	0.6 (0.3)
Any disruptive disorder	2.5‡ (0.7)	6.7‡ (1.8)	7.9‡ (1.8)	0.9 (0.4)
Any substance use disorder	0.4 (0.3)	3.3‡ (1.1)	3.5‡ (1.1)	0.2 (0.2)
Any disorder	21.8 (3.5)	21.5 (3.4)	35.5 (4.1)	4.0 (1.2)

**Diagnostic test abbreviations are described in the footnote to Table 1.*
†Girls show higher prevalence than boys (P<.05).
‡Boys show higher prevalence than girls (P<.05).

for the DISC-P and DISC-C. For the 6 major diagnostic categories derived from the DISC-P, the number of subjects with a particular diagnosis that occurred in combination with 1 or more other diagnoses vs the total number of subjects with that particular diagnosis were 15 vs 67 for anxiety disorders, 13 vs 17 for mood disorders, 4 vs 9 for tic disorders, 8 vs 10 for conduct-oppositional defiant disorder, 8 vs 12 for ADHD, and 3 vs 3 for substance use disorder. For the DISC-C, these numbers were 20 vs 46 for anxiety disorders, 11 vs 23 for mood disorders, 12 vs 24 for conduct-oppositional defiant disorder, 4 vs 7 for tic disorders, 8 vs 9 for ADHD, and 10 vs 14 for substance use disorder.

COMMENT

In determining the prevalence of psychiatric disorders, the key question is how we define such disorders. If we count each subject who met the criteria for 1 or more *DSM-III-R* diagnoses as having a disorder, our findings yield a 35.5% prevalence for Dutch 13- to 18-year-olds. This prevalence rate is lower than the 49.5% of 4- to 16-year-old children from Puerto Rico who met criteria for *DSM-III* diagnoses on the basis of DISC-C or DISC-P answers.[3] The higher prevalence rate obtained in the Puerto Rico study may be ascribed to the fact that DISC-C and DISC-P information was combined by the clinician on a symptom level, whereas in our study information from the 2 sources was combined on the diagnostic level. If the parent's and the child's responses in the Puerto Rico study conflicted, a psychiatrist made a clinical decision as to whose information carried the greater weight. Because there is no validated procedure on how to handle information from different sources, we chose not to combine the information on a symptom level.

If we consider the information from 1 source only, the prevalence of any disorder in the present study was 21.5% for the DISC-C and 21.8% for the DISC-P. These prevalences are similar to the 22% found for *DSM-III* diagnoses based on an adaptation of the DISC-C in New Zealand 15-year-old adolescents.[4]

Although the response rate in our study was reasonable, we do not know what the effect of nonparticipation is on the prevalence rates that we found.

INCLUSION OF IMPAIRMENT RATING

The prevalences discussed so far pertain to subjects who met criteria for a *DSM-III-R* diagnosis. It is not self-evident that *DSM-III-R* criteria can be used to identify functional impairment. Given the high prevalences based on DISC-derived *DSM-III-R* criteria, it

Table 3. Six-Month Weighted Prevalence of *DSM-III-R* Diagnoses by Different Diagnostic Criteria*

	Prevalence, % (SE)							
	DISC-P		DISC-C		DISC-P or DISC-C		DISC-P and DISC-C	
	CGAS <61	CGAS <71	CGAS <61	CGAS <71	CGAS <61	CGAS <71	CGAS <61	CGAS <71
Any anxiety disorder	4.1 (1.1)	7.5 (1.7)	2.2 (0.7)	3.8 (1.0)	5.3 (1.4)	9.7 (2.1)	0.6 (0.4)	1.0 (0.5)
Any tic disorder	0.4 (0.3)	0.7 (0.3)	0.4 (0.3)	1.4 (0.8)	0.9 (0.4)	1.9 (0.9)	...	...
Major depression	1.2 (0.5)	1.3 (0.6)	1.5 (0.6)	1.9 (0.7)	2.2 (0.8)	2.7 (0.9)	0.4 (0.3)	0.4 (0.3)
Dysthymia	1.0 (0.4)	1.0 (0.4)	1.2 (0.5)	1.5 (0.6)	1.9 (0.7)	2.2 (0.7)	0.3 (0.2)	0.3 (0.2)
Attention-deficit hyperactivity disorder	1.2 (0.5)	1.5 (0.6)	0.7 (0.3)	1.3 (0.5)	1.6 (0.5)	2.3 (0.7)	0.3 (0.2)	0.4 (0.3)
Oppositional-defiant disorder	0.6 (0.3)	0.6 (0.3)	0.6 (0.3)	0.7 (0.4)	1.2 (0.4)	1.3 (0.5)	...	...
Conduct disorder	1.2† (0.4)	1.2† (0.4)	1.5† (0.5)	2.0† (0.7)	2.0† (0.6)	2.6† (0.7)	0.6 (0.3)	0.6 (0.3)
Any substance use disorder	0.4 (0.3)	0.4 (0.3)	1.2 (0.4)	1.5 (0.5)	2.9 (0.8)	1.7† (0.6)	0.2 (0.2)	0.2 (0.2)
Any disorder	5.9 (1.5)	9.7 (2.1)	4.8 (1.3)	8.4 (2.1)	7.9 (1.9)	14.1 (2.8)	1.8 (0.7)	2.4 (0.8)
CGAS‡	7.3 (1.2)	15.3 (2.9)	7.0 (1.9)	15.4 (3.2)	9.6 (2.3)	21.4 (3.7)	4.6 (1.4)	9.1 (2.2)

**Diagnostic test abbreviations are described in the footnote to Table 1.*
†Boys show higher prevalence than girls (P<.05).
‡Numbers in this row indicate the prevalence of subjects with a CGAS score below the respective cutoff score on the basis of the parent or child interview and for the combination of the 2 interviews.

Table 4. Six-Month Prevalence Rates of Multiple Diagnoses for 6 Major Diagnostic Groupings by Different Diagnostic Criteria*

	Prevalence, % (SE)					
	DISC-P			DISC-C		
No. of Diagnoses	All CGAS	CGAS <61	CGAS <71	All CGAS	CGAS <61	CGAS <71
≥1	20.8 (3.4)	5.9 (1.5)	9.6 (2.1)	20.6 (3.3)	4.7 (1.3)	8.2 (2.0)
≥2	3.7 (1.0)	2.5 (0.7)	3.7 (1.0)	5.2 (1.5)	2.0 (0.6)	3.1 (0.9)
≥3	0.9 (0.4)	0.9 (0.4)	0.9 (0.4)	1.2 (0.4)	1.0 (0.4)	1.2 (0.4)
≥4	0.3 (0.2)	0.3 (0.2)	0.3 (0.2)	0.3 (0.2)	0.3 (0.2)	0.3 (0.2)
≥5	0.2 (0.2)	0.2 (0.2)	0.2 (0.2)	0.2 (0.2)	0.2 (0.2)	0.2 (0.2)

**Diagnostic groupings are described in the "Comorbidity" subsection of the "Results" section of the text. Diagnostic test abbreviations are described in the footnote to Table 1.*

was anticipated that not all subjects who received *DSM-III-R* diagnoses would be impaired with respect to their everyday functioning. Conversely, not all subjects who were impaired were expected to receive a *DSM-III-R* diagnosis. Because we were interested in the prevalence not only of *DSM-III-R* disorders but also of impairment, we combined CGAS ratings with DISC diagnoses. We thus obtained prevalences that reflect both the *DSM-III-R* criteria and impairment. The prevalences obtained when the CGAS score was less than 61 or 71, in addition to a *DSM-III-R* diagnosis, were much lower than those based on the presence of a *DSM-III-R* diagnosis alone.

Bird et al[3] reported a drop in prevalences of *DSM-III* disorders in 4- to 16-year-old children and adolescents from Puerto Rico from 49.5% to 33.9% when combined with a CGAS score of less than 71, and to 17.9% when combined with a CGAS score of less than 61. These prevalences were still much higher than those for corresponding CGAS scores in combination with either DISC-P or DISC-C diagnoses found in our study. However, in the study by Bird et al,[3] *DSM-III* diagnoses were based on the clinician's judgment of information elicited by both the DISC-C and the DISC-P. It may seem advantageous to incorporate clinical judgment to handle information derived from structured interviews, especially when information from different sources seems conflicting. However, unless scoring rules and decisions are made explicit and replicable, the results of such a procedure may be hard to replicate by others.

Prevalences based on CGAS scores, irrespective of whether a subject met the criteria for a *DSM-III-R* diagnosis, were somewhat higher than prevalences based on the combination of the CGAS and DISC.

We did not obtain reliability or validity measures of the nonclinical version of CGAS scores in this study. Although the nonclinical version yielded scores comparable to those of the clinical version and were correlated with other measures of impairment,[13] this does not automatically mean that the cutoff scores for the clinical version have the same meaning as the cutoff scores for the nonclinical version. However, cutoff scores should not be regarded as fixed criteria but as conventions that aid communication and comparability among researchers and clinicians.

COMBINING PARENT REPORTS AND ADOLESCENT SELF-REPORTS

Compared with single-source prevalences, the prevalence of any disorder decreased considerably if we consider as disordered those subjects who met *DSM-III-R* criteria on the DISC-P and DISC-C (3.3% with any disorder). We must therefore conclude that there is very little overlap between subjects with a *DSM-III-R* diagnosis identified by parent report and adolescent self-report. Evidently, although the prevalences based on the DISC-P and DISC-C separately were nearly identical (21.8% and 21.5%), each instrument identified different subjects in most cases. Different instruments and tapping information from different informants led to vastly different results. Discrepancies between prevalences based on information from parent vs youth were greatest for conduct disorder and any substance use disorder, with significantly higher prevalences for diagnoses based on the DISC-C vs the DISC-P. Parents of youths aged 13 to 18 years probably are largely unaware of the youth's antisocial activities and substance use, whereas, apparently, many youths were willing to report these activities to an interviewer. There was a tendency for parents to report more anxiety disorders, compared with self-reports among youths, and youths showed a tendency to report more depression and dysthymia, compared with their parents. However, these differences were not significant.

As expected, those subjects who met criteria for a DISC-P and a DISC-C diagnosis showed the most impairment. This can be concluded from the fact that the CGAS cutoff scores had little effect on the prevalences of DISC-P and DISC-C diagnoses.

Most prevalence studies have combined information from different sources in different ways. The idiosyncratic rules for handling conflicting information from different sources make it especially hard to compare the results of previous studies. We therefore combined parent and youth information in ways that are easily replicable by other investigators.

SEX DIFFERENCES

Sex differences in prevalence were for conduct disorder and any disruptive and substance use disorder, with boys having a higher prevalence than girls. Boys also obtained a higher prevalence of any tic disorder (DISC-P) and mania (DISC-C). Girls had a higher prevalence of simple phobia (DISC-P) and social phobia (DISC-C) than boys. These sex differences are consistent with those reported in other community studies.[29]

COMORBIDITY

In many subjects, criteria for only 1 diagnosis were met. For the DISC-P, in 21 (31%) of the 67 subjects with at least 1 diagnosis, the criteria for more than 1 diagnosis were met. For the DISC-C, this was the case for 27 (47%) of the 57 subjects. The prevalence of 2 or more DISC-P diagnoses was 3.7% and of 2 or more DISC-C diagnoses was 5.2%. Subjects with multiple diagnoses were regarded as more disturbed by the interviewers, because combining diagnostic criteria with CGAS cutoff scores reduced the prevalences for multiple diagnoses only slightly.

The most frequent comorbid diagnoses were anxiety and mood disorders. Thirteen of the 17 subjects who met criteria for a DISC-P mood disorder met criteria for other diagnoses as well. In 9 subjects, mood disorders were comorbid with anxiety disorders. Of the 23 subjects who met criteria for DISC-C mood disorders, 11 met criteria for other diagnoses. In 10 of these 11 subjects, the comorbid disorders included anxiety disorder. These results underscore the frequency with which the same youths meet criteria for both mood and anxiety disorders and raise the question of whether the *DSM-III-R* criteria really discriminate between separate mood and anxiety disorders.

Substance use disorder and ADHD were seldom diagnosed in subjects who did not meet the criteria for other diagnoses. In most subjects, ADHD was comorbid with conduct-oppositional defiant disorder, often in combination with a third, and, in a few subjects, a fourth or fifth diagnosis. Conduct-oppositional defiant disorder frequently occurred in combination with 2 or more other diagnoses; diagnoses in 5 of the 10 subjects with this disorder were derived from the DISC-P, and 8 of the 24 subjects with a DISC-C diagnosis of conduct-oppositional defiant disorder met criteria for 2 or more other diagnoses.

Our study provides prevalences of *DSM-III-R* disorders in adolescents aged 13 to 18 years from the general population. There was very little overlap between subjects who met criteria for *DSM-III-R* diagnoses based on the DISC-P vs the DISC-C. The vast majority of subjects who were identified by 1 informant were not identified by another. In interpreting findings from single-source studies, it should thus be realized that, despite the fact that prevalences based on parent information are similar to those based on self-reported information, both sources of information identify different subjects as disturbed.

There was a considerable reduction in prevalences when, in addition to meeting *DSM-III-R* criteria, subjects also had to meet CGAS impairment criteria, which implies that many adolescents in the community with *DSM-III-R* diagnoses functioned quite well in everyday life. Subjects who met criteria for more than 1 diagnosis and subjects who met criteria for a diagnosis on the DISC-P and the DISC-C were the most disturbed.

Accepted for publication July 10, 1996.

Supported by the Dutch Ministry of Welfare and Health, Rijswÿk, the Netherlands, and the Sophia Foundation of Medical Research, Rotterdam, the Netherlands.

Presented in part at the 13th International Congress of the International Association for Child and Adolescent Psychiatry and Allied Professions, San Francisco, Calif, July 24, 1994.

We thank Tom Achenbach, PhD, Hans Koot, PhD, and Kaija Puura, MD, for their helpful comments.

Corresponding author: Frank C. Verhulst, MD, Department of Child and Adolescent Psychiatry, Erasmus University/Sophia Children's Hospital Rotterdam, Dr Molewaterplein 60, 3015 GJ Rotterdam, the Netherlands.

REFERENCES

1. American Psychiatric Association. *Diagnostic and Statistical Manual of Mental Disorders, Third Edition.* Washington, DC: American Psychiatric Association; 1981.
2. Anderson JC, Williams S, McGee R, Silva PA. *DSM-III* disorders in preadolescent children. *Arch Gen Psychiatry.* 1987;44:69-76.
3. Bird HR, Canino G, Rubio-Stipec M, Gould MS, Ribera J, Sesman M, Woodbury M, Huertas-Goldman S, Pagan A, Sanchez-Lacay A, Moscoso M. Estimates of the prevalence of childhood maladjustment in a community survey in Puerto Rico: the use of combined measures. *Arch Gen Psychiatry.* 1988; 45:1120-1126.
4. McGee R, Feehan M, Williams S, Partridge F, Silva PA, Kelly J. *DSM-III* disorders in a large sample of adolescents. *J Am Acad Child Adolesc Psychiatry.* 1990;29:611-619.
5. Verhulst FC, Berden GFMG, Sanders-Woudstra JAR. Mental health in Dutch children, II: the prevalence of psychiatric disorder and relationship between measures. *Acta Psychiatr Scand.* 1985;72(suppl):342.
6. Offord DR, Boyle MH, Szatmani P, Rae-Grant NI, Links PS, Cadman DT, Byles JA, Crawford JW, Munroe Blum H, Byrne C, Thomas H, Woodward CA. Ontario Child Health Study, II: six-month prevalence of disorders and rates of service utilization. *Arch Gen Psychiatry.* 1987;44:832-836.
7. Achenbach TM. *Manual for the Child Behavior Checklist/4-18 and 1991 Profiles.* Burlington: University of Vermont, Dept of Psychiatry; 1991.
8. National Institute of Mental Health. *Diagnostic Interview Schedule for Children (DISC), Version 2.3.* New York: New York State Psychiatric Institute, Division of Child and Adolescent Psychiatry; 1992.
9. American Psychiatric Association. *Diagnostic and Statistical Manual of Mental Disorders, Third Edition, Revised.* Washington, DC: American Psychiatric Association; 1987.
10. Achenbach TM. *Manual for the Youth Self-Report and 1991 Profiles.* Burlington: University of Vermont, Dept of Psychiatry; 1991.
11. Achenbach TM. *Manual for the Teacher's Report Form and 1991 Profiles.* Burlington: University of Vermont, Dept of Psychiatry; 1991.
12. Fisher P, Parra MT, Wicks J, Reyland S, Shaffer D. *Diagnostic Interview Schedule for Children (NIMH DISC, Version 2.3).* New York: New York State Psychiatric Institute, Division of Child and Adolescent Psychiatry; 1992.
13. Bird HR, Gould MS. The use of diagnostic instruments and global measures of functioning in child psychiatry epidemiologic studies. In: Verhulst FC, Koot JM, eds. *The Epidemiology of Child and Adolescent Psychopathology.* Cambridge, Mass: Oxford University Press; 1995:86-103.
14. Shaffer D, Gould MS, Brasic J, Ambrosini P, Fisher P, Bird H, Aluwahlia S. A Children's Global Assessment Scale. *Arch Gen Psychiatry.* 1983;40:1228-1231.
15. Verhulst FC, Akkerhuis GW, Althaus M. Mental health in Dutch children, I: a cross-cultural comparison. *Acta Psychiatr Scand.* 1985;72(suppl):323.
16. Verhulst FC, Van der Ende J. Assessment of child psychopathology: relationships between different methods, different informants and clinical judgment of severity. *Acta Psychiatr Scand.* 1991;84:155-159.
17. Verhulst FC, Prince J, Vervuurt-Poot C, De Jong J. Mental health in Dutch adolescents: self-reported problems for ages 11-18. *Acta Psychiatr Scand.* 1989; 80(suppl):356.
18. Verhulst FC, Akkerhuis GW. Mental health in Dutch children, III: behavioral-emotional problems reported by teachers of children aged 4-12. *Acta Psychiatr Scand.* 1986;74(suppl):330.
19. Schwab-Stone M, Fisher P, Piacentini J, Shaffer D, Davies M, Briggs M. The Diagnostic Interview Schedule for Children–Revised Version (DISC-R), II: test-retest reliability. *J Am Acad Child Adolesc Psychiatry.* 1993;32:651-657.
20. Shaffer D, Schwab-Stone M, Fisher P, Cohen P, Piacentini J, Davies M, Conners K, Regier D. The Diagnostic Interview Schedule for Children–Revised Version (DISC-R), I: preparation, field testing, interrater reliability, and acceptability. *J Am Acad Child Adolesc Psychiatry.* 1993;32:643-650.
21. Piacentini J, Shaffer D, Fisher P, Schwab-Stone M, Davies M, Gioia P. The Diagnostic Interview Schedule for Children–Revised Version (DISC-R), III: concurrent criterion validity. *J Am Acad Child Adolesc Psychiatry.* 1993;32:658-665.
22. Fisher P, Shaffer D, Piacentini JC, Lapkin J, Kafantaris V, Leonard H, Herzog DB. Sensitivity of the Diagnostic Interview Schedule for Children, 2nd edition (DISC-2.1) for specific diagnoses of children and adolescents. *J Am Acad Child Adolesc Psychiatry.* 1993;32:666-673.
23. Bird HR, Canino G, Rubio-Stipec M, Ribera J. Further measures of the psychometric properties of the Children's Global Assessment Scale. *Arch Gen Psychiatry.* 1987;44:821-824.
24. Bird H, Yager TJ, Staghezza B, Gould MS, Canino G, Rubio-Stipec M. Impairment in the epidemiological measurement of childhood psychopathology in the community. *J Am Acad Child Adolesc Psychiatry.* 1990;29:796-803.
25. Babubhai SH, Barnwell BG, Bieler GS. *SUDAAN User's Manual: Software for Analysis of Correlated Data, Release 6.40.* Research Triangle Park, NC: Research Triangle Institute; 1995.
26. Achenbach TM, McConaughy SH, Howell CT. Child/adolescent behavioral and emotional problems: implications of cross-informant correlations for situational specificity. *Psychol Bull.* 1987;101:213-232.
27. Loeber R, Green SM, Lahey BB. Mental health professionals' perception of the utility of children, mothers and teachers as informants on childhood psychopathology. *J Clin Child Psychology.* 1990;19:136-143.
28. Rutter M, Tizard J, Whitmore K. *Education, Health and Behaviour.* White Plains, NY: Longman Publishing; 1970:174-177.
29. Verhulst FC. A review of community studies. In: Verhulst FC, Koot JM, eds. *The Epidemiology of Child and Adolescent Psychopathology.* Cambridge, Mass: Oxford University Press; 1995:146-177.

Coming to Terms With the Terms of Risk

Helena Chmura Kraemer, PhD; Alan E. Kazdin, PhD; David R. Offord, MD; Ronald C. Kessler, PhD; Peter S. Jensen, MD; David J. Kupfer, MD

Terms such as *risk*, *risk factors*, and especially the term *cause* are inconsistently and imprecisely used, fostering scientific miscommunication and misleading research and policy. Clarifying such terms is the essential first step. We define risk and a risk factor (protective factor) and their potency, set out the conceptual basis of the methods by which risk factors are identified and potency demonstrated, and propose criteria for establishing the status of a risk factor as a fixed or variable marker or a *causal* risk factor. All definitions are based on the state of scientific knowledge (empirical documentation), rather than on hypotheses, speculations, or beliefs. We discuss common approaches and pitfalls and give a psychiatric research example. Imprecise reports can impede the search for understanding the cause and course of any disease and also may be a basis of inadequate clinical or policy decision-making. The issues in risk research are much too important to tolerate less than precise terminology or the less than rigorous research reporting that results from imprecise and inconsistent terminology. *Arch Gen Psychiatry. 1997;54:337-343*

During the past 15 years, the field of risk-factor research has grown rapidly. Findings from this burgeoning literature are used to guide clinical and policy decision-making concerning management of risk. We focus in this report on critical scientific methods and appropriate terminologies that need to be considered to ensure that scientists communicate more accurately and consistently among themselves, with clinicians and policymakers, and to the broader public so that their research data are not misunderstood or misapplied. The methods underlying such communications are standard in epidemiology and biostatistics. The language used (risk or hazard) connotes an unwelcome outcome (disease onset, relapse, death, or disability), but the methods apply to welcome outcomes as well (prevention, remission, or recovery), that is, to protective factors as well as risk factors. For convenience in discussion of risk estimation, we will refer to all of these terms generically as *risk factors*. Herein, the term *risk* will always mean a probability of an outcome within a population of subjects (as in "the risk of lung cancer among smokers"). The term *risk factor* will be used to indicate an agent or exposure (as in "cigarette smoking is a risk factor for lung cancer").

The emphasis is on empirical evidence, not on theory, although theory guides and informs every step of the process. Moreover, potential clinical and policy implications play a major role in what is proposed, so that, while we encourage measurement of risk factors at any level and dimensionality, we have restricted the outcome to be binary, because the most crucial medical decisions tend to be binary in nature. The physician decides whether the patient is at high risk of a disorder or actually has a disorder, thus requiring medical intervention, or not. Policymakers decide to provide a particular intervention in a par-

From the Department of Psychiatry and Behavioral Sciences, Stanford University, Stanford, Calif (Dr Kraemer); the Department of Psychology, Yale University, New Haven, Conn (Dr Kazdin); Chedoke-McMaster Hospitals and Faculty of Health Sciences, McMaster University, Hamilton, Ontario (Dr Offord); the Department of Health Care Policy, Harvard Medical School, Boston, Mass (Dr Kessler); the Child and Adolescent Disorders Research Branch, National Institute of Mental Health, Rockville, Md (Dr Jensen); and the Department of Psychiatry, University of Pittsburgh School of Medicine and the Western Psychiatric Institute and Clinic, Pittsburgh, Pa (Dr Kupfer).

ticular community, or to certain people in a certain community, or not. The task of predicting dimensional outcomes is an important research goal but is distinct, we believe, from the specific task of risk estimation.

BASIC CONCEPTS OF RISK

A risk factor is a measurable *characterization* of each *subject* in a specified *population* that precedes the *outcome* of interest and which can be used to divide the population into 2 groups (the high-risk and the low-risk groups that comprise the total population).[1] The subject may be an individual person, but it might also be a family, a class, a school, or a community. The characterization may be of the individual subject (the age of a person or the size of a city) or of the context of the subject (the number of siblings in the person's family or the annual budget of the state in which the city is located). The probability of the outcome in the high-risk group of subjects must be shown to be greater than the probability of the outcome in the low-risk group. Typically, there are many ways a risk factor can be used to define high- and low-risk groups. All that is required by the definition is that at least one be explicitly demonstrated.

To demonstrate that a characterization is a risk factor requires obtaining its measure on the subjects in a sample free of the outcome of interest, then distinguishing those who do from those who do not subsequently have the outcome of interest. Minimally, the null hypothesis that the characteristic and the outcome are independent of each other must be rejected, ie, a statistically significant association between factor and outcome must be established. Requiring statistical significance is fundamentally asking that the sample size be sufficiently large and the research design and measurement adequate to document nonrandom association between the characteristic and the outcome.[2] Merely demonstrating statistical significance, however, is not enough. Claiming that some characterization is a risk factor is incomplete without specification of at least 1 definition of high and low risk based on that characterization and an indication of its potency based on that definition.

We define the term *potency* of a risk factor as the maximal discrepancy achievable using that risk factor to dichotomize the population into high- and low-risk groups. Many statistical summary measures of potency are available and commonly used (eg, odds ratio, risk ratio, relative risk, attributable risk, κ, ϕ, and γ), as well as methods for their point and confidence interval estimation.[3]

It is difficult to find 2 variables that are absolutely independent of each other. Without considering some notion of potency in the assessment, given a large enough sample size, virtually every factor could be demonstrated to be a risk factor for every outcome that follows it. That would trivialize the concept of a risk factor. The requirement in risk estimation that potency be demonstrated essentially is a requirement that every statistically significant result be supported by empirical evidence that could be evaluated for clinical or policy significance.

The following are several requirements for evaluating risk:

1. Define the outcome clearly and completely and measure it validly and reliably.
2. Define the population and sample it properly.
3. Define the risk factor, establish that it defines a characteristic that occurs before the outcome, and measure it validly and reliably.
4. Use analytic procedures that lead to definitions of high- and low-risk groups and establish that a statistically significant difference exists in the risks of these 2 groups.
5. Use analytic procedures that lead to meaningful demonstrations of potency to establish that a clinically significant or policy-significant difference exists in the risks of high- and low-risk groups.

As an example, consider the hypothesis that early sexual maturation among high school girls is a risk factor for having a panic attack. This is complex, first, because having a panic attack is episodic. A subject may have 1 panic attack in her lifetime or have attacks frequently and severely enough to have panic disorder. Whether each subject had a panic attack in the last 3 months is a different outcome from whether each subject ever had a panic attack, had a panic attack before age 15 years, or has frequent panic attacks.

The risk factor here, too, is complex. Early sexual maturation might be determined using the age of menarche. However, it might not be menarche but the physical manifestation of sexual maturation, more adequately tapped by Tanner staging,[4] that is the potent risk factor. In either case, to determine the timing of sexual maturation would require observing each girl over time, beginning long before menarche, hence not a cross-sectional study. The risk factor that would result would not be binary but ordinal: the age of menarche or the age when some physical milepost is reached. To show statistical significance, one would test the null hypothesis that the age of menarche and onset of panic attacks are independent. Once statistical significance is demonstrated, to demonstrate potency, 1 or more cut points would have to be proposed and the probability of panic as the outcome would be compared between the 2 groups.

Figure 1 shows what might result in a population of adolescent girls who at the time of entry to the study had never had a panic attack, who were then followed up for up to 5 years prospectively to observe the outcome of having 1 or more panic attacks. The age at which each girl first reached Tanner stage 3 was estimated from longitudinal data. Earlier-than-average maturers, defined as those who reached Tanner stage 3 earlier that 12.5 years,[5] is one definition of a high-risk group by which to demonstrate potency. In Figure 1, a series of outcomes is considered, defined as having a panic attack before age 12, 13, 14, and 15 years. The potency at the various ages after entry is indicated by the separation between the 2 curves.

THE IMPORTANCE OF TIME IN DEFINING OUTCOME

Crucial to the definition of the risk factor is the requirement that it precede the outcome of interest.[1] In practice, the safest course would be the measurement of the risk factor in subjects without the outcome, who are then followed up to the outcome (prospective longitudinal studies). In risk-factor assessment studies, time can be measured in various ways, the most obvious of which are calendar time, chronological age (time since birth), or time since onset of some disorder (in which the outcome is remission or recovery) or some other event (eg, time of menarche, entry to school, or entry to study). In risk-factor assessments, it is important to be precise about how time is measured, especially about what is time zero, and the units in which time is measured (the scale), for different choices produce different results.

In an incidence study at time T (eg, birth to T is age 15 years), subjects free of the outcome at time 0 are studied. The incidence at T is the probability that a subject in the population has the outcome of interest before time T. The probability that a subject does not have the outcome before time T is called the *survival probability* at time T. The graph of these probabilities as a function of T is called a *survival curve*.[6] All survival curves begin at 1 and are nonincreasing functions of T. Figure 1 shows 2 such survival curves.

In contrast, a prevalence study at time T is a study in which subjects are assessed to determine whether they are experiencing the outcome at that time. In this type of study, the prevalence of the outcome at T (eg, at age 15 years) is the probability that subjects in the population have the outcome at time T. A graph of these probabilities for varying values of T is called a *prevalence curve*.

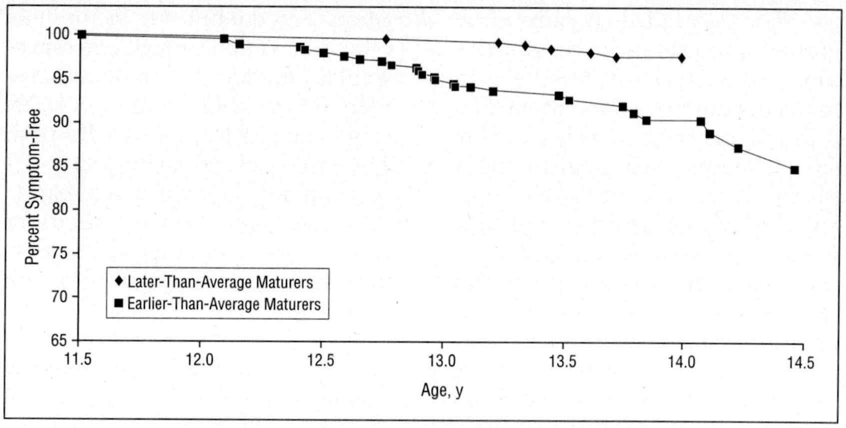

Figure 1. *Timing of maturation as a risk factor for first panic attack in a population who at entry to the study at age 12 years had never had a panic attack (Stanford Center for Research in Disease Prevention data, Stanford, Calif).*

With a birth-onset, nonepisodic, reliably measured disorder (eg, color-blindness, Down syndrome, or hemophilia), a prevalence curve will be flat as a function of age, and survival curves are uninformative, because all who will ever have the disorder have it at birth. Among psychiatric disorders, autism might fit this category.

With a later-onset but chronic and unremitting disorder, consistently and reliably diagnosed (eg, Huntington disease), the prevalence curve will increase as a function of time and will equal the complement of the survival curve for onset. The steepness of the curve depends on the heterogeneity of onset times in the population. The longer the time span over which onsets occur, the more gradual the change in the prevalence and survival curves. With such a disorder, it makes no difference whether prevalence or incidence is studied. Among psychiatric disorders, Alzheimer disease fits this category.

With an episodic disorder (eg, hypertension or arrhythmia), the prevalence curve can take on any shape. In such a situation, what one learns from a prevalence study may be inconsistent with what one learns from an incidence study, or even from other prevalence studies done at different time points. Many of the psychiatric disorders of greatest interest are those such as depression, schizophrenia, alcoholism, and panic disorder, later and variable in onset and episodic in nature.[7] When prevalence is assessed for such a disorder, the time the question is asked changes the answer. The answer depends on that subject's time of onset relative to the time at which the question is asked, whether there is or is not remission after onset, the number and duration of bouts and remissions, and other features of the course of the disorder after onset. What predicts the time of onset, what predicts time to remission, recovery, or other features of time course all may be different sets of risk factors.

In designing psychiatric risk research studies, it would be preferable to separate different such outcomes, seeking (1) the risk factors for onset in the general population, (2) the risk factors for remission or recovery in the postonset subpopulation, and (3) the risk factors for relapse among the subpopulation of those who experience remission. The answers in such a staged strategy would then relate more clearly to informing (1) strategies for prevention, (2) strategies for treatment, and (3) strategies for maintenance.

Much more problematic than prevalence studies are studies in which time is ignored or dealt with poorly. A commonly used outcome is that obtained by the answer to the question "Does the subject have the disorder?" (prevalence), but with different times (eg, ages) mixed together. What results is a mixture of prevalences. Equally problematic is the outcome determined by the answer to the question "Has the subject ever had the disorder?" (lifetime prevalence) when time is ignored. The subject is supposed to answer yes if onset has occurred before the time at which the question is asked. If all the respondents are at the same point in time when the question is asked, what results is the incidence (not prevalence). If respondents are not at the same time, what results is an uninterpretable mixture of incidences.

In both of the aforementioned cases, the nature of the mixture of prevalences or incidences is determined by the age distribution of the subjects sampled, which would foster inconsistencies of results across various studies with different age distribution of subjects.

The issue of time gains even greater importance in view of the time specificity of some risk factors for an outcome in a population. For example, marriage is a risk factor for suicide among teenage girls, and a protective factor among adult women.[8-11] Survival curves for high- and low-risk groups may cross, and, at the time of that crossing point, the definitions of high- and low-risk groups reverse. Even when they do not cross, different survival curves (as in Figure 1) are always more disparate at some times than at others. Thus, the potency of any risk factor, however measured, is likely to be quite different for one value of time than for another.

For all these reasons, in a risk-assessment study, time needs to be well defined and measured as part of the definition of the outcome. If the subjects are assessed at varying times, analyses and conclusions cannot be mixed together but should be assessed separately for different values of time (as in the prevalence or survival curves).

POPULATION SPECIFICITY OF RISK FACTORS

If a population is homogeneous in the outcome (everyone in the population has the outcome or everyone does not) or if the population is homogeneous in a factor, then that factor cannot be demonstrated to be a risk factor for that outcome in that population, because one cannot then define a high- and low-risk group with different probabilities of the outcome (as per the basic definition). A certain degree of heterogeneity of both the factor and the outcome is necessary to demonstrate that the factor is a risk factor. The more homogeneous the population for either the factor or the outcome, the more difficult it is to document that the factor is a potent risk factor. At the very least, large sample sizes will be needed to have the statistical power to detect differences.

Moreover, populations may be defined in different ways: the general population, the population of California, or white females. Just as a factor need not be an equally potent risk factor for all possible choices of time, a factor that is a potent risk factor for an outcome in one population need not be a risk factor in all other populations, much less one of similar potency. For these reasons, there is a need for caution in referring to the risk factors for a disorder. The profile of risk factors may depend on population characteristics.

The population specificity of risk factors is an especially important issue in multisite studies. Site may be itself a risk or protective factor for certain outcomes. Site differences arise from differences in the sociodemographic characteristics of the subjects at each site and from the differences in environment or in social or medical practices at each site. This is yet another explanation of disparities of results among risk research studies.

RISK FACTORS: A TYPOLOGY

The aforementioned considerations begin the process of defining a vitally important typology of risk factors. To begin, the outcome and the population need to be well and consistently defined. Then, by definition, a factor can be any characterization of a subject. No limitations are placed on the level of measurement of a factor (binary [eg, sex], categorical [eg, race], ordinal [eg, level of education]), on the distribution of factor measures, or on the number of items used to define the factor (ie, univariate vs multivariate).

Any characterization measured concomitantly with or after the outcome may potentially be a result or consequence of the outcome (a symptom or a scar). A characterization that satisfies all other requirements for a risk factor but precedence might be called a *correlate* of the outcome. Thus, a risk factor is a special type of correlate that requires documentation of precedence.[1] This is a crucial point, because concomitants or consequences of outcomes are likely to be much more highly correlated with the outcomes than are risk factors. It is easy to overlook the true risk factors and focus on the symptoms and scars of the disorder, in which case, the results of risk estimation might be misleading to risk evaluation or risk management.

In **Figure 2**, we continue this process by proposing a schematic representation of the steps necessary to document risk-factor status for a single characterization in a population. The first step is to establish that the factor is a correlate that precedes the outcome. This justifies use of the term risk factor. If precedence cannot be demonstrated, we suggest use of whichever of the terms *concomitant* or *consequence* is appropriate. If no effort has been made to determine precedence, the appropriate term is correlate.

A risk factor that can be demonstrated to change spontaneously within a subject (eg, age or weight) or to be changed within a subject by intervention (such as by administration of a drug or psychotherapy), we propose to call a *variable* risk factor. A risk factor that cannot be demonstrated to change we propose to call a *fixed marker* (eg, race, gender, or year of birth). If there is no empirical evidence documenting the stability or variability of a risk factor within subjects, the appropriate term is risk factor.

A variable risk factor that can be shown to be manipulable and, when manipulated, can be shown to change the risk of the outcome we term a *causal* risk factor. A variable risk factor that cannot be shown to be manipulable, or, if manipulated, cannot be shown to change the risk of the outcome we call a *variable* marker. If the manipulability or the efficacy or effectiveness of manipulation of a variable risk factor has not been tested, the appropriate term is variable risk factor.

The scientific term that is appropriate depends on what has been demonstrated to be true of a factor. At the moment, genes may be fixed markers, but not causal factors. Gene products, however, may be causal factors, because some are manipulable. If, at some future time, methods are devised to do "gene surgery," the gene that is currently a fixed marker may become manipulable. If gene surgery also could be shown to change the risk of the outcome, then the gene itself would be appropriately termed a causal risk factor. In short, the label that we propose to apply to any factor reflects the current state of scientific knowledge about that factor.

We use the term causal risk factor, not the term *the cause*. The latter use suggests a necessary and sufficient condition for the disorder, a single cause, an implication that often is inappropriate. The notion of cause has multiple meanings based on recognition of the direct and indirect ways in which a particular influence can operate, the dependence of one causal influence on the presence, level, and timing of other conditions for the outcome to emerge, the effect of multiple causes on and the multiple paths leading to an outcome, and the probabilistic nature of the outcome.[12] The present discussion of causal risk factor denotes that empirical research has shown that the factor is implicated in producing an outcome insofar as alteration of the factor alters the outcome. The term, as used here, allows for the diverse ways in which this relation may be evident, in keeping with the multiple meanings of cause. For example, causal risk factors for acquired immunodeficiency syndrome (AIDS) include unprotected sexual activity and sharing of needles. The cause of AIDS, however, seems to be the human immunodeficiency virus, in absence of which unprotected sex and sharing of needles would have no influence on risk of AIDS. When causal risk factors are identified for an outcome, questions may still remain about the mechanism or process by which those causal risk factors operate, ideally stimulating the additional work that would bring us closer to a full understanding of the cause and course of the disorder. Thus, if we yet knew nothing of the human immunodeficiency virus, knowledge of various fixed markers (hemophilia or Haitian origin) and of various causal risk factors (drug abuse, sharing of needles, unprotected sex, or use of blood products) might provide inspiration about where to look for the cause.

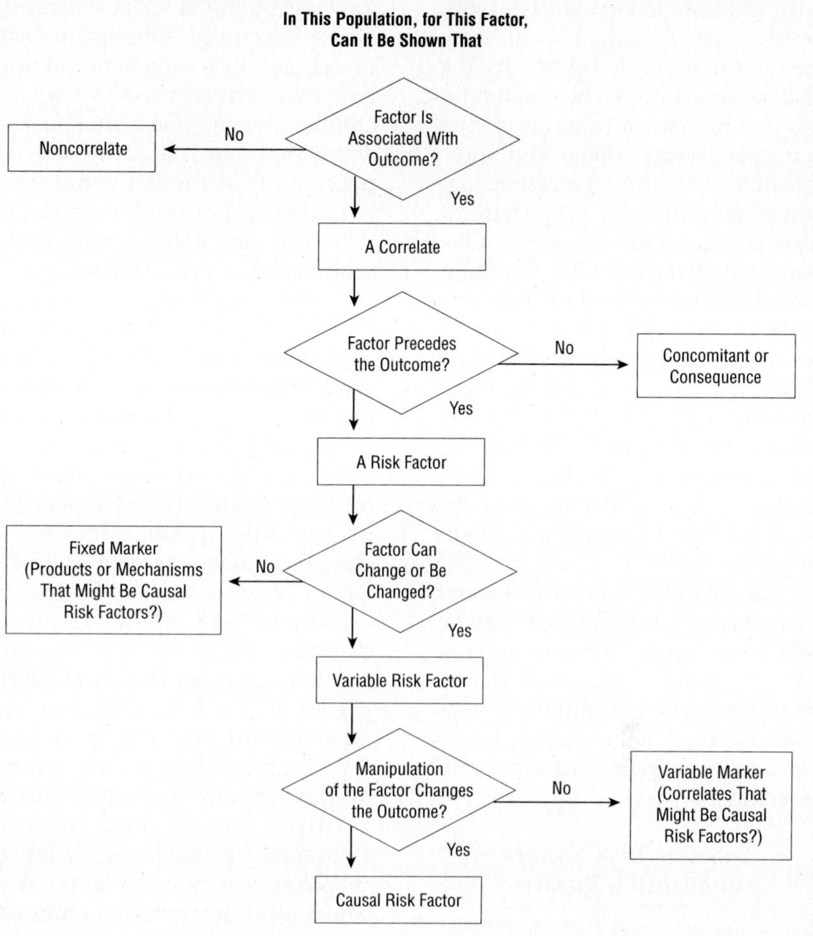

Figure 2. *The process of elucidation of risk-factor status for a factor in a population for a particular outcome.*

RISK FACTORS: APPLICATIONS

Time-Varying Risk Factors

In the typology shown in Figure 2, a crucial juncture is that in identifying a factor as variable or not. A factor that is fixed and nonvarying (a trait) over the lifetime of a subject (eg, race, sex, year of birth, or genotype) precedes any outcome during the lifetime of that subject. That removes the burden of demonstrating precedence. Such traits, consequently, are easily and validly assessed in retrospective or cross-sectional studies, which tend to be easier to do than prospective longitudinal studies. Moreover, when measuring such a trait at multiple occasions for a subject over a span of time, any variance among the multiple measures for a subject is error of measurement. Thus, a careful measurement any time during the lifetime of the subject suffices to define that characteristic of the subject for all time. All those advantages are counteracted by the fact that traits are at best fixed markers, which cannot be causal risk factors. The factors of greatest interest and importance are not fixed—they have time-varying (perhaps state) features to them.[13]

The emphasis in the risk-assessment literature, especially in psychiatry, has been on single-time point assessments, even for factors known to have substantial time variability within each subject. Because such time-varying factors are exactly the type of factors that might prove ultimately to be causal risk factors, such a focus on single-time point assessment is an impediment to searching for causal risk factors of psychiatric disorders.

Simultaneous Use of Multivariate Risk Factors

It is common to consider not 1 measure to define a possible risk factor but several to be used simultaneously (a multivariate risk factor), to identify the high- and low-risk subjects. A common way to deal with multiple factors is to develop a risk score, a mathematical function of the multiple factors, itself a risk factor. Although one could use any mathematical function of the multiple factors, linear and additive models (logistic regression, loglinear models, and discriminant analysis) generally are used.[14] One common example is the Framingham Risk Score.[15] An alternative way to deal with multiple factors is to develop a risk classification based on multiple factors to define the high- and low-risk groups.[3-16] For example, those who are below the poverty level and without strong family or social support might be the high-risk group for juvenile antisocial behavior.

Some of the individual factors in a multivariate risk factor may be potent risk factors, but some may not be. The joint use of several factors simultaneously generally increases potency, especially when risk factors act synergistically (risk-factor interactions).

Labeling Risk Factors in Research Reports

The quality of measurement (reliability, validity, and sensitivity) for risk factors and outcomes plays a major role in the ability to identify risk factors and measure their potency. The focus, however, is on issues concerning labeling in research reports, not on quality of measurement.

Because of the importance of time in risk-factor research, use of retrospective recall data to measure a factor or an outcome is problematic, not only because of the tendency of subjects to forget but also because of their tendency to reinterpret in light of subsequent experiences. Evidence suggests that retrospective information tends to be inaccurate and may be barely above chance level of accuracy when compared with the same information obtained prospectively.[17,18] This is particularly a problem with the retrospective measurement of possible risk factors.

When retrospective recall is obtained before an outcome, it may well be a risk factor for that outcome. For example, a retrospective report by an adult of childhood sexual abuse may be a risk factor for subsequent onset of depression in a general population. However, retrospective recall of childhood sexual abuse after onset of depression may reflect the subject's perception of the happenings reported as sexual abuse modified by the experience of the disorder, a consequence, not a risk factor.

More generally, maternal report of her child's characteristic may be a valuable risk factor for subsequent outcomes, but it is the maternal report of the characteristic and not the child's characteristic that is to be reported as the risk factor, eg, maternal report of child hyperactivity, not child hyperactivity itself. A clinician's assessment of the mental health status of a subject may be a valuable risk factor for subsequent outcomes, but it is the clinician's assessment that is to be reported as the risk factor, not the mental health status of the subject.

Such labeling issues, related to, but separate from, the issue of validity, are crucial to risk-assessment procedures. What researchers measure is what they study. Without precise communication of how risk factors were measured, rather than interpreted, the risk-outcome relation can be readily misinterpreted.

COMMENT

In the research literature on risk-factor estimation, terms such as *risk*, *marker*, and *cause* are used in various ways. The same term often is used for different constructs, and the same construct often is referred to by different terms. Thus, what we call a fixed marker, for example, may be called a vulnerability factor[1] or a susceptibility factor, and even a causal risk factor or cause. The terms *moderator* and *mediator*[19] may correspond to certain of these usages; the terms *necessary* and *sufficient* causes may correspond to others. The terms we have proposed are those that tend to carry no connotations beyond what is to be demonstrated to justify the application of the term.

Many factors labeled risk factors in the literature have not even been shown to precede the corresponding outcome. This is especially true because so many of the studies that provide the basis of such claims are cross-sectional, and many use retrospective reports. Many studies label risk factors based only on statistical significance, with no indication of potency. These factors may be risk factors by the present definition, but of negligible value in clinical, research, or policy application. Studies refer to high-risk subjects without specifying the outcome of which the subjects are at high risk.

We suggest that labeling a factor with the generic term risk factor with no further effort to delineate its role as a fixed marker, variable marker, or causal risk factor is a limited finding. Any causal risk factor for a disorder, any correlate of such a causal risk factor, and any correlate of a correlate of such a causal risk factor may be a risk factor. As one moves farther away from the causal risk factor, one might expect to see lower levels of potency, but this is not necessarily so. Causal risk factors may be difficult to measure reliably and noncausal risk factors relatively easy to measure. Because unreliability of measurement will attenuate apparent potency, the apparent potency of a causal risk factor may be lower than that of a marker. However, any disorder may have a myriad of risk factors, some of which play only a peripheral role in the development of the disorder or its course, and many of which will not be causal. An important purpose of the typology in Figure 2 is to encourage researchers not only to be very precise and specific about what is reported as a risk factor, but also to exert every possible effort to document its role as a fixed marker, a variable marker, or a causal risk factor. Such an effort will lay the basis for more productive future risk assessments. In psychiatric applications, there is a great deal of research evidence for correlates and fixed markers for onset of psychiatric disorders and other psychiatric outcomes of interest, but less evidence dealing with variable risk factors (specifically from longitudinal population studies) or distinguishing variable markers from causal risk factors (specifically, from randomized clinical trials of prevention programs).

Although the urgency for precise terminology in reporting risk research primarily relates to needs for clarity and consistency in risk estimation,[20] the typology of risk factors proposed herein also is intentionally closely tied to, and guided by, major social, clinical, and policy concerns. As a consequence of this decision, what emerges in terms of the relevance of risk factor to risk management is clear. If one had to choose a limited population to target for a prevention program, one would choose a population high on fixed markers. However, in structuring a prevention program to be used in that population, one needs to target causal risk factors. Fixed markers, by definition, cannot be changed, and changing variable markers, by definition, will have no influence on prevention.

The proposed typology of risk factors also is important to clinical decision-making. Markers and causal risk factors related to onset, duration, or relapse identify patients for whom a clinician might want to be particularly alert to forestall unwelcome medical outcomes. All 3 types of risk factors may serve as the basis of screening procedures. Generally, fixed markers (gender, race, or year of birth) are easiest to measure and, often, variable markers (eg, age) are easier to measure than causal risk factors. Moreover, markers are typically recognized long before causal risk factors are. For that reason, markers play a very important and special role in developing cost-effective screening procedures for use in clinical and research programs. However, as already discussed for prevention programs, structuring effective treatment programs requires a focus on causal risk factors, not markers.

Moving toward the complete understanding of the cause and course of any disease, our ultimate goal requires a deliberate and focused search for causal risk factors. Identification of markers is important in this process to the degree that such risk factors stimulate and motivate theoretical considerations about what correlated causal risk factors they might suggest for future study. Miscommunication about what are correlates but not risk factors, what are markers but not causal risk factors may be even more troubling, because imprecise reports can impede the search for such understanding of the cause and course of any disease and also may be a basis of inadequate medical intervention. The issues in risk-assessment research are much too important to tolerate less than precise terminology or the less than rigorous research reporting that results from imprecise and inconsistent terminology.

Accepted for publication July 31, 1996.

This work was supported by the John D. and Catherine T. MacArthur Foundation Research Network on Psychopathology and Development; Public Health Service grant SR01HL39770 from the National Heart, Lung and Blood Institute, Bethesda, Md; Public Health Service grant R01HD24240 from the National Institute for Child Health and Development, Bethesda; a Research Scientist award (MH00353) and grant MH35408 from the National Institute of Mental Health, Rockville, Md (Dr Kazdin); a National Health Scientist award from Health Canada, Ottawa, Ontario (Dr Offord); a Research Scientist award (K05-MH00507) (Dr Kessler) and grant MH30915 (Dr Kupfer) from the National Institute of Mental Health.

The opinions and assertions contained in this article are the private views of the authors and do not reflect the views of the Department of Health and Human Services of the National Institute of Mental Health.

We are grateful to the other members of the core group of the MacArthur Network on Psychopathology and Development, and to the Epidemiology Division of the Department of Health Research and Policy at Stanford University, Stanford, Calif, for critical, stimulating, and enlightening discussions of these issues; to John Richters, PhD, of the National Institute of Mental Health for his insights and his suggestion for the title of this article; and to the Stanford Center for Research in Disease Prevention for its input and for allowing free access to data from its library of risk estimation studies, completed or in progress, and permission to use an illustration from these studies.

Reprint requests to David J. Kupfer, MD, Western Psychiatric Institute and Clinic, Room 210, 3811 O'Hara St, Pittsburgh, PA 15213.

REFERENCES

1. Mrazek PJ, Haggerty RJ. *Reducing Risks for Mental Disorders: Frontiers for Prevention Intervention Research.* Washington, DC: National Academy Press; 1994.
2. Kraemer HC, Thiemann S. *How Many Subjects? Statistical Power Analysis in Research.* Beverly Hills, Calif: Sage Publications Inc; 1987.
3. Kraemer HC. *Evaluating Medical Tests: Objective and Quantitative Guidelines.* Beverly Hills, Calif: Sage Publications Inc; 1992.
4. Tanner JM. *Growth at Adolescence.* Cambridge, Mass: Blackwell Publishers; 1962.
5. Wilson DM, Killen JD, Hayward CH, Robinson TN, Hammer LD, Kraemer HC, Varady A, Taylor CB. Timing and rate of sexual maturation and the onset of cigarette and alcohol use among teenage girls. *Arch Pediatr Adolesc Med.* 1994; 148:789-795.
6. Miller RGJ. *Survival Analysis.* New York, NY: John Wiley & Sons Inc; 1981.
7. Frank E, Prien RF, Jarrett RB, Keller MB, Kupfer DJ, Lavari PW, Rush AJ, Weissman MM. Conceptualization and rationale for consensus definitions of terms in major depressive disorder: remission, recovery, relapse, and recurrence. *Arch Gen Psychiatry.* 1991;48:851-855.
8. Bancroft J, Skrimshire A, Reynolds F, Simkin S, Smith J. Self-poisoning and self-injury in the Oxford area: epidemiological aspects 1969-73. *Br J Prev Soc Med.* 1975;29:170-175.
9. Hawton K. *Suicide and Attempted Suicide Among Children and Adolescents.* Beverly Hills, Calif: Sage Publications Inc; 1986.
10. Kreitman N, Schreiber M. Parasuicide in young Edinburgh women, 1968-1975. *Psychol Med.* 1979;9:469-479.
11. Wetzel JW. *Clinical Handbook of Depression.* New York, NY: Gardner Press; 1984.
12. Haynes SN. *Models of Causality in Psychopathology: Toward Dynamic, Synthetic, and Nonlinear Models of Behavior Disorders.* Boston, Mass: Allyn & Bacon Inc; 1992.
13. Kraemer HC, Gullion CM, Rush AJ, Frank E, Kupfer DJ. Can state and trait variables be disentangled? a methodological framework for psychiatric disorders. *Psychiatry Res.* 1994;52:55-69.
14. Cox DR. *Analysis of Binary Data.* New York, NY: Chapman & Hall; 1970.
15. Truett J, Cornfield J, Kannel WA. A multivariate analysis of the risk of coronary heart disease in Framingham. *J Chron Dis.* 1967;20:511-524.
16. Breiman L, Friedman JH, Olshen RA, Stone CJ. *Classification and Regression Trees.* Belmont, Calif: Wadsworth Publishing Co; 1984.
17. Henry B, Moffitt TE, Caspi A, Langle J, Silva PA. On the 'remembrance of things past': a longitudinal evaluation of the retrospective method. *Psychol Assess.* 1994;6:92-101.
18. Robins LN, Schoenberg SP, Holmes SF, Ratcliff KS, Benham A, Works J. Early home environment and retrospective recall. *Am J Orthopsychiatry.* 1985;55:27-41.
19. Baron RM, Kenny DA. The moderator-mediator variable distinction in social psychological research: conceptual, strategic, and statistical considerations. *J Pers Soc Psychol.* 1986;51:1173-1182.
20. Finney DJ. On biometric language and its abuses. *Biometric Bull.* 1994;11:2-4.

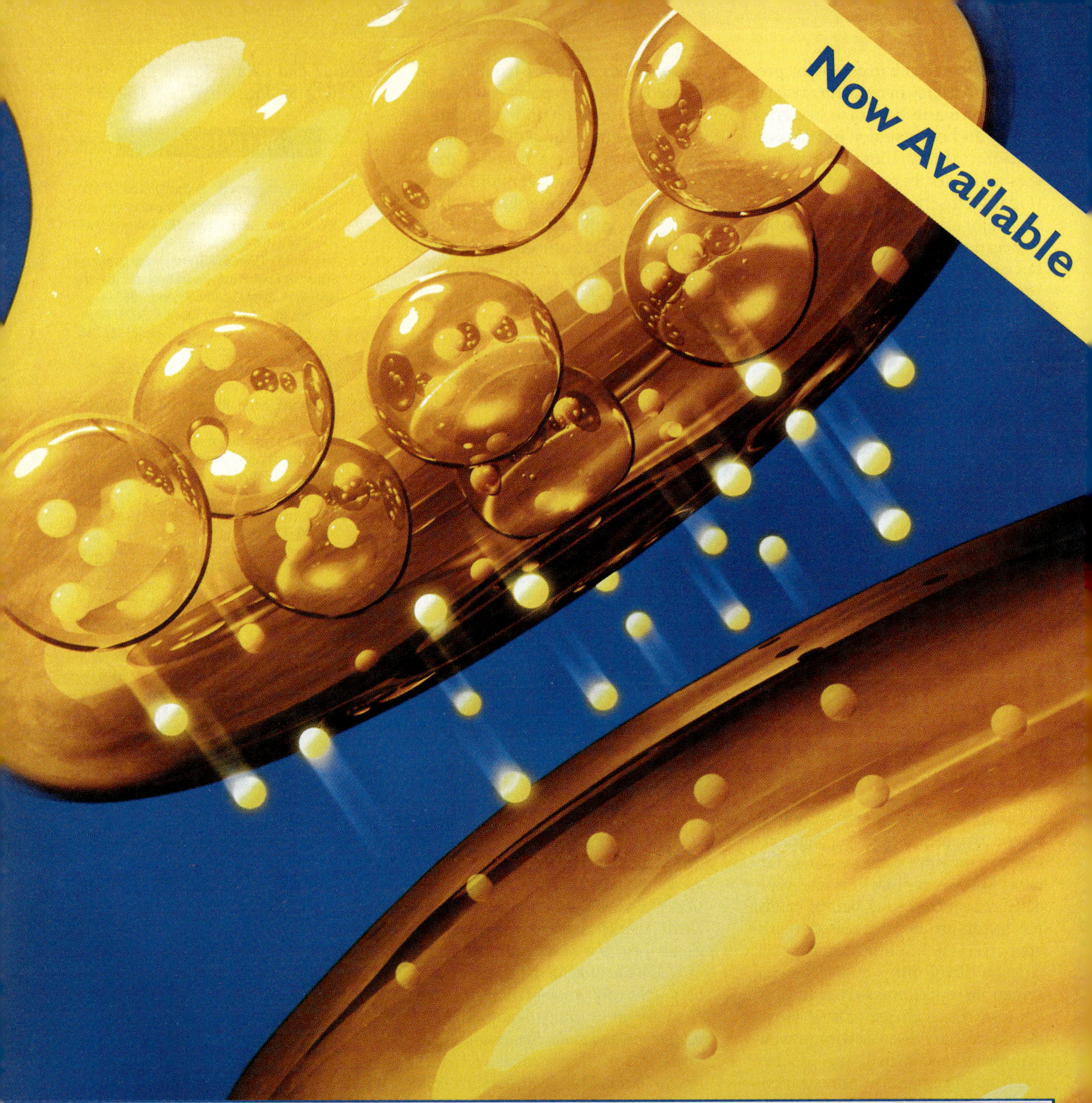
Now Available

ORIGINAL ARTICLE

Detecting Personality Disorders in a Nonclinical Population

Application of a 2-Stage Procedure for Case Identification

Mark F. Lenzenweger, PhD; Armand W. Loranger, PhD; Lauren Korfine, AM; Cynthia Neff, PhD

Background: There is no epidemiology of personality disorders (PDs) comparable with that currently available for most other mental disorders. One reason for this is that an Axis II diagnosis usually requires considerable clinical sophistication and it is expensive to deploy clinicians rather than trained laypersons to examine large community samples. This study explores the feasibility of using a 2-stage method in which only subjects who were screened as positive for PD would be interviewed by clinicians.

Methods: University students were screened with a self-administered Axis II inventory and subsequently interviewed by clinicians with the use of the International Personality Disorder Examination.

Results: The screen detected all individuals who subsequently received a definite diagnosis on the interview, and a specificity rate of detection was 61%. The point-prevalence estimate for diagnosable PD in this nonclinical population was 11.01% (95% confidence interval, 7.57%-14.52%).

Conclusion: If these results can be replicated in a more representative community sample, this 2-stage method might substantially reduce the number of persons who needed to be interviewed in a major epidemiological study of PDs, with little or no loss in diagnostic accuracy, while presumably lowering the cost of such an investigation.

Arch Gen Psychiatry. 1997;54:345-351

THE APPEARANCE of the multiaxial *DSM* classification systems,[1-3] with their explicit and detailed diagnostic criteria, has stimulated an unprecedented interest in the personality disorders (PDs).[4] Nevertheless, we still lack an epidemiology of PDs comparable with what is available for most mental disorders from the recently completed National Comorbidity Survey.[5] That study of a national probability sample of 8098 US residents provided information about the prevalence of 13 Axis I disorders, as determined by the *Composite International Diagnostic Interview*.[6]

The World Health Organization (WHO) (Geneva, Switzerland) and the National Institutes of Health (NIH) (Bethesda, Md) have had a long-term program of activities aimed at developing a battery of standardized diagnostic assessment instruments for use in clinical and epidemiological research worldwide.[7] The *Composite International Diagnostic Interview* is a major component of the WHO-NIH instrumentation package. It is highly structured, computer scored, and designed for use by trained lay interviewers in community surveys. When the *Composite International Diagnostic Interview* was first conceived, the state of the art of standardized interviews for PDs was in its infancy and considerably behind that of the clinical assessment of other mental disorders. Expert opinion within the WHO-NIH project favored the view that the complexity of the diagnostic criteria and level of inference and clinical sophistication required to make PD diagnoses, especially in those with other mental disorders, required an interview designed for experienced clinicians, ie, those capable of making independent psychiatric diagnoses. As a consequence of that decision, the Axis II coverage of the *Composite International Diagnostic Interview* was limited to antisocial disorder.

One of the principal deterrents to employing experienced clinicians in large-scale epidemiologic studies is its cost compared with that of employing the lay interviewers.[8] One way to curtail this expense might be to use a 2-stage design in which clinicians would only interview subjects with positive results from a screen-

From the Laboratory of Experimental Psychopathology, Cornell University (Dr Lenzenweger), Ithaca, NY; the Department of Psychiatry, Cornell University Medical College (Drs Lenzenweger and Loranger), New York, NY; the Department of Psychology, Harvard University, Cambridge, Mass (Ms Korfine); and Department of Psychology, University of Illinois at Champaign (Dr Neff).

SUBJECTS AND METHODS

SUBJECTS

Selection

The initial sample consisted of 2000 first-year, 18- to 19-year-old undergraduate students enrolled at Cornell University. They were selected from the complete roster of approximately 3000 incoming students during a recent fall semester using a stratified random sampling procedure, with simple random sampling (without replacement) within each of 15 strata. The 15 strata were identified a priori and coincided with established residence halls on the Cornell University campus. The students' participation was solicited by a team of 15 trained research assistants who used a door-to-door, face-to-face epidemiological-style survey distribution and collection method and made exhaustive efforts to personally approach each student. The project was described to the students as an National Institute of Mental Health–sponsored study of "Young Adult Development," and they were assured of the confidentiality of the information they provided. They were informed that their participation would involve the completion of a personality inventory, using the International Personality Disorder Examination (IPDE *DSM-III-R* Screen [IPDE-S]), for which they would be paid $5, and that they might also be asked to volunteer for additional assessments, for which they would be paid $50. Of the 2000 students who were invited to participate, 1684 accepted the offer. Thirty-five (2.1%) of those who accepted were excluded because they obtained scores greater than 3 on the Infrequency Scale. An additional 3 students were excluded because of incomplete responding. The sex profile of the sample was 48.7% male and 51.3% female participants. The response rate of 84.2% is an indication that the sample was reasonably representative of incoming Cornell University undergraduates. Moreover, by way of comparison with other epidemiological efforts, we note that our response rate is similar to that achieved in the National Comorbidity Survey (ie, 82.6%).[5]

Sampling

Based on the IPDE-S, the subject pool of 1646 students was divided into 2 groups: a PPD group and an NPD group. There were 708 subjects (43%) who exceeded the threshold for a PPD and 938 subjects (57%) who were below the threshold and presumed to have NPD. Smaller samples from these 2 groups were then selected, using simple random selection (without replacement), for participation in the second-stage of the project. Only 2 of those selected refused further participation. This yielded a second-stage pool of 121 male (47%) and 137 female (53%) subjects; 134 drawn from the PPD group and 124 from the NPD group. Prior to participation in the second-stage assessment procedure, all subjects gave voluntary written informed consent. These 258 subjects were interviewed with the IPDE and Structured Clinical Interview for *DSM-III-R:* Nonpatient Version (SCID-NP), and they are the focus of the present report.

Demographic Characteristics

The demographic characteristics of the initial-stage sample (N=1684) are given in **Table 1**. They are very similar to those of the entire entering class at Cornell University. Compared with the US population, the sample somewhat overrepresents Asians and underrepresents those of Hispanic, African American, and blue-collar origins. The ethnic-racial backgrounds of the second-stage subjects were as follows: Native American (n=1,0.4%), Asian–Pacific Islander (n=44, 17.0%), African American (n=10, (3.9%), Latin-Hispanic (n=10, 3.9%), white (n=188, 72.9%); and other (n=5, 1.9%). This distribution is comparable with that seen in the first-stage sample.

METHODS

Study Design

A 2-stage procedure for case identification[9] involves, first, an administration of a test or other procedure for the presumptive identification of possible, although not necessarily diagnosable, psychopathology in a defined population sample (in this instance, PD). The purpose of the initial screening is to differentiate broadly between those members of a population that might have a clinically significant psychiatric disorder from those who do not.[9] The initial screening is *not* meant to provide definitive diagnoses for the presumptive cases of disorder, but rather it merely identifies them, and such cases are then examined more thoroughly during the second-stage of the case identification process. During the second stage, actual diagnostic interview procedures and/or more detailed examination is carried out on the presumptive cases to verify the presence or absence of clinically significant psychopathologic features. It has been argued[9] that the first-stage screening procedure should be economical and characterized by ease of use (eg, administration by nonclinicians) and, therefore, reliable and valid self-report measures of psychopathology might be ideally suited for this task. The second stage in this approach should capitalize on the skills, talents, and abilities of more highly trained (and more expensive) diagnosticians.

ing and a random sample of subjects with negative results.[9] Because PDs do not occur in most of the population, this would result in a large savings, because most of the sample would never be interviewed. To be valid, the method would require a screen of high sensitivity (ie, low false-negative rate). The economic gain, however, would depend in part on the screen's specificity.

The initial screening and selection phase of the Longitudinal Study of Personality Disorders (LSPD) provided a unique opportunity to investigate the potential utility of the 2-stage procedure for detecting personality pathology in a nonclinical population. The LSPD is a large-scale, prospective, multiwave, longitudinal study of normal personality, temperament, PDs, and psychopathology under way at Cornell University, New York City, under the direction of one of us (M.F.L.). Its design required the identification of 2 large cohorts of subjects for long-term longitudinal

Assessment Instruments

IPDE-S. This is a 250-item self-administered true-false inventory developed and piloted by one of us (A.W.L.) to determine its potential value as a screen for the presence of the *DSM-III-R* Axis II disorders. The IPDE-S requires about 45 minutes for completion. The number of items measuring each criterion varies with the complexity of the criterion, and an algorithm determines whether the subject has met the criterion. The threshold for the presumptive diagnosis of a particular disorder is determined by the number of criteria stipulated in the *DSM-III-R*. A preliminary test of the reliability of the screen was conducted in a sample of 114 psychiatric patients, who were the subject of another investigation.[10] This reliability analysis focused on the internal consistency of the 3 major *DSM-III-R* PD clusters and employed the coefficient α[11] statistic. Analysis of the IPDE-S items used to operationalize the diagnostic criteria for the PDs in each of the 3 *DSM-III-R* PD clusters yielded the following α values: 0.88 for cluster A, 0.93 for cluster B, and 0.88 for cluster C.

IPDE. This is a semistructured interview developed in the WHO-NIH program and designed for use by experienced clinicians.[12,13] It surveys the behavior and life experiences relevant to the more than 150 criteria used in making PD diagnoses in the *DSM-III-R* and *International Classification of Diseases, 10th Revision*[14] classification systems. A *DSM-IV* version is also available.[15] In the present study, only the *DSM-III-R* criteria were assessed and the IPDE portion of the assessments required anywhere from 45 minutes to 4 hours (average, 1.5 hours) to complete. The IPDE was given by 2 PhD clinical psychologists, who were trained by the developer of the instrument (A.W.L.), and supervised throughout the project by the first author (M.F.L.), to monitor reliability. Prior to conducting study interviews with the subjects, the 2 clinical psychologists each conducted several joint practice interviews under direct supervision of the first author. The interviewers then jointly examined a series of subjects, and their reliability for IPDE assessments across all Axis II disorders was evaluated using the intraclass correlation coefficient (ICC). The interviewers attained a high degree of reliability in the use of the IPDE (median ICC across all Axis II PDs was 0.92 [dimensional criteria]). Interviewer reliability was reassessed midway through the data collection to ensure against criterion drift, and it was found to be excellent (median ICC across all Axis II PDs was 0.93). The interviewers were blind to the results of the screening and putative PD status of the subjects whom they interviewed.

SCID-NP. This is a semistructured *DSM-III-R* Axis I clinical interview for use with nonpatients.[16] It was administered prior to the IPDE by the same clinicians who administered the IPDE. They had completed the SCID-101 videocassette instructional series distributed by Robert L. Spitzer, MD, and had also conducted several practice interviews under the supervision of one of us (M.F.L.).

Personality Research Form–Infrequency Scale. This is a 14-item self-administered measure of extremely deviant, reckless, and/or random responding and was used as an indicator of invalid test-taking attitudes.[17]

Data Analyses

The internal consistency reliability of the IPDE-S was determined through the calculation of Cronbach's α [α; KR-20 formula].[11] The ICC was used to assess interrater reliability of the interviewers for the IPDE assessments.

Mean levels of PD features in the IPDE-S–assigned PPD and NPD groups on the IPDE were examined using the *t* test. Given the purpose of a general PD screen is to identify *any* likely diagnosable PD, we chose to examine our second-stage interview data using "any PD" on the IPDE as our unit of analysis. Thus, we collapsed individual diagnoses on the IPDE to yield the "any PD" variable, which was scored present or absent. The diagnostic efficiency of the IPDE-S in identifying any diagnosable personality pathology on the IPDE was evaluated using the well-known diagnostic efficiency indexes of sensitivity, specificity, positive predictive value, and negative predictive value. The χ^2 test was also used to contrast proportions of Axis I and Axis II diagnoses for the PPD vs NPD groups in the second-stage sample.

The point-prevalence estimates for personality pathology in this population, the SEs of these estimates, and the corresponding 95% confidence intervals (CIs) were calculated as shown by Shrout et al.[18,19] As noted earlier, in the 2-stage design, a sample of subjects is drawn from the general population and invited to participate in the screening phase. Those agreeing to participate complete the screen (stage 1) leading to assignment to group 1 (screened positive) or group 2 (screened negative). Samples from each of the 2 groups were selected and given the IPDE and SCID-NP as noted previously (stage 2). Define: *N* indicates the number of subjects who validly completed the *IPDE-S*; π_i, the proportion of the population in group *i*; λ_i, the prevalence rate in group *i*; f_i, the proportion of the group *i* sample referred for stage 2 assessment.

The population prevalence of the disorder is:

$$p = \lambda_1 \pi_1 + \lambda_2 \pi_2$$

and the large sample variance of the estimate *p* is (as per Newman et al[19(p192)]):

$$V = \frac{1}{N}\left[\frac{(\pi_1\sigma_1^2)}{f_1} + \frac{(\pi_2\sigma_2^2)}{f_2} + \beta^2\right],$$

where

$$\sigma^2_1 = \lambda_i (1-\lambda_i);\ i = 1, 2, \text{ and } \beta^2 = \pi_1 \pi_2 (\lambda_1 - \lambda_2)^2.$$

study: one cohort with a possible PD (PPD) and the other with no PD (NPD). All subjects for the LSPD were selected on the basis of an initial screening for PDs and subsequently interviewed by experienced clinicians. Information from the study about the performance of the screen in relation to the interview could be helpful in deciding whether it might be feasible to apply a similar 2-stage method in large-scale epidemiological studies of PDs in the general population.

RESULTS

RELIABILITY OF THE IPDE-S IN INITIAL-STAGE SAMPLE

As indicated, the reliability (internal consistency or α) of the IPDE-S had been previously established as satisfactory in a sample of 114 psychiatric patients. To determine whether this was also true of a nonpatient popu-

Table 1. Demographic Characteristics of Initial-Stage Screened Sample of 1684 University Students

Demographic Characteristics of Parents	Father, %	Mother, %
Educational level, y		
1-8	1.6	1.7
9-11	2.4	3.1
12	8.5	13.8
13-15	15.8	20.4
16+	70.6	60.4
Not available	1.1	0.6
Occupation		
Laborer/service	2.4	3.0
Operatives (machine)	1.6	0.7
Craftsman/foreman	4.5	1.6
Clerical/sales	4.2	15.4
Management/official	26.6	12.6
Professional/technical	52.0	42.0
Homemaker or not available	8.7	24.7
Ethnicity		
African American	4.2	
Latin-Hispanic	5.9	
White	66.8	
Asian-Pacific Islander	20.0	
Native American	0.3	
Other	2.5	
Not available	0.4	

Table 2. Lifetime *DSM-III-R* Axis I SCID-NP Diagnoses, Definite and Probable, of Those Screened Positive and Negative for PDs in Second-Stage Sample of 258 Subjects*

Disorder	Subjects, No.† (%) PPD (n=134)	NPD (n=124)	χ^2	*P*‡
Major depression	24 (17.9)	4 (3.2)	14.35	.001
Bipolar/bipolar NOS	5 (3.7)	0 (0)	4.72	.03
Dysthymia (current only)	11 (8.2)	3 (2.4)	4.21	.04
Other affective disorder	14 (10.4)	4 (3.2)	5.17	.02
Alcohol abuse	3 (2.2)	0 (0)	2.81	.09
Alcohol dependence	5 (3.7)	0 (0)	4.72	.03
Other drug dependence	1 (0.7)	0 (0)	0.93	.34
Social phobia	17 (12.7)	2 (1.6)	11.58	.001
Simple phobia	9 (6.7)	5 (4.0)	0.9	.34
Obsessive-compulsive	2 (1.5)	2 (1.6)	0.01	.94
Anorexia	3 (2.2)	1 (0.8)	0.87	.35
Bulimia	4 (3.0)	0 (0)	3.76	.05
Any Axis I diagnosis	57 (42.5)	16 (12.9)	27.87	.001

**SCID-NP indicates Structured Clinical Interview for* DSM-III-R*: Nonpatient Version; PPD, possible personality disorder (PD); NPD, no PD; and NOS, not otherwise specified.*

†*Values are the number of cases and percentages per diagnostic category observed in the 2 subject groups. Cases consist of both definite and probable Axis I diagnoses combined; some subjects have more than 1 Axis I diagnosis.*

‡*Significance based on Pearson χ^2 test (2-tailed),* df=*1.*

lation, we measured its reliability in the present sample (N=1646). The values of α coefficient, based on the IPDE-S items relevant to the PDs in each of the *DSM-III-R* PD clusters, were as follows: 0.84 for cluster A disorders, 0.91 for cluster B disorders, and 0.84 for cluster C disorders.

AXIS I CHARACTERISTICS OF SECOND-STAGE SAMPLE

The lifetime *DSM-III-R* Axis I diagnoses of the second-stage sample, as determined with the SCID-NP, are given in **Table 2**. Fifty-seven (42.5%) of those in the PPD group received an Axis I diagnosis compared with only 16 (12.9%) in the NPD group (χ^2=27.87, *df*=1, *P*<.001). The diagnoses were mostly mood and anxiety disorders; particularly common were major depression and social phobia. The SCID-NP inquires about any prior treatment for a mental disorder, and 22 (16.4%) in the PPD group and 12 (9.7%) in the NPD group reported a history of such treatment (χ^2=2.56, *df*=1, *P*=.14).

PD SYMPTOM LEVELS AND DISTRIBUTION OF DISORDERS

The mean (±SD) number of PD criteria met, as assessed by IPDE, in the entire sample (PPD and NPD combined; n=258) was 2.78±4.95, with a minimum of 0.00 and a maximum of 40.00. The average (±SD) total number of symptoms in the PPD subjects (4.62±6.13) exceeded that seen in the NPD subjects (0.79±1.73) (*t*=6.92, *df*=256, *P*<.001).

DSM-III-R provides a residual category (not otherwise specified) for those judged to have a PD that does not meet the requirements for any of the specific types. There are no diagnostic rules in the *DSM-III-R* for identifying PD not otherwise specified cases; therefore, we adopted an arbitrary conservative standard. The IPDE assigns a not otherwise specified diagnosis to those who do not meet the requirements for a specific disorder but nevertheless accumulate 10 or more criteria from the various disorders. The interview also assigns the designation "probable" to those who are 1 criterion short of the required number for a particular diagnosis. **Table 3** contains the *DSM-III-R* IPDE diagnoses of the second-stage sample. Twenty-one subjects (8.1%) had a definite PD, and 33 (12.8%) had either a definite or probable PD. With the exception of self-defeating, at least 1 case of each type of Axis II disorder appeared in this sample. The most common diagnoses were narcissistic and histrionic. Of those with either a definite or probable diagnosis, 19 (57.6%) received 1 diagnosis, 8 (24.7%) received 2 diagnoses, 4 (12.1%) received 3 diagnoses, 1 (3.0%) received 4 diagnoses, and 1 (3.0%) received 8 diagnoses; 42.4% of the subjects receiving PD diagnoses had more than 1 type of Axis II PD diagnosis.

PD DIAGNOSES IN THE SECOND-STAGE SAMPLE IN RELATION TO IPDE-S

Table 4 shows the performance of the IPDE-S in predicting the diagnosis of a PD on the IPDE interview. *All* 21 subjects who met criteria for a *definite* PD on the interview, had positive results on the screen. Of the 237 subjects with no PD on the interview, 113 had positive results on the screen. These data were used to calculate the diagnostic efficiency indexes, taking into account the 2-stage study design.[18,19] The sensitivity for the screen was

Table 3. *DSM-III-R* Axis II IPDE Diagnoses in Second-Stage Sample of 258 Subjects*

	Diagnosis, No.†	
Disorder	Definite	Probable
Paranoid	1	2
Schizoid	1	2
Schizotypal	0	4
Narcissistic	3	5
Antisocial	2	0
Borderline	0	4
Histrionic	5	4
Obsessive-compulsive	0	4
Dependent	1	1
Passive aggressive	0	2
Avoidant	1	2
Sadistic	0	1
Self-defeating	0	0
NOS	11	3

*IPDE indicates International Personality Disorder Examination; NOS, not otherwise specified.

†Values are the number of cases per disorder. Subjects who met criteria for a definite specific personality disorder (PD) could not receive a definite NOS PD diagnosis; subjects who met criteria for a probable specific PD could not receive a probable NOS PD diagnosis. Some individuals had multiple PD diagnoses; the distribution of the PD diagnoses (definite and probable combined) was: 1 diagnosis, 19 subjects; 2 diagnoses, 8 subjects; 3 diagnoses, 4 subjects; 4 diagnoses, 1 subject; and 8 diagnoses, 1 subject.

Table 4. Performance of PD Screening Inventory, IPDE Screen, in Predicting Diagnosis of a PD (Definite) Based on Clinician-Administered Semistructured Interview, IPDE, in 258 Subjects*

IPDE Screen	IPDE Interview, No. of Subjects: Definite PD†	NPD	Total
PPD	21	113	**134**
NPD	0	124	**124**
Total	**21**	**237**	**258**

*PD indicates personality disorder; PPD, possible PD; NPD, no PD; IPDE, International Personality Disorder Examination; and NOS, not otherwise specified.

†Subjects met criteria for a definite specific or NOS PD diagnosis on IPDE interview. χ^2 Test (2-tailed) (df=1) =21.15, P<.001.

Table 5. Performance of PD Screening Inventory, IPDE Screen in Predicting Diagnosis of a PD (Definite or Probable) Based on Clinician-Administered Semistructured Interview, IPDE, in 258 Subjects*

IPDE Screen	IPDE Interview, No. of Subjects: Definite or Probable PD†	NPD	Total
PPD	30	104	**134**
NPD	3	121	**124**
Total	**33**	**225**	**258**

*PD indicates personality disorder; IPDE, International Personality Disorder Examination; PPD, possible PD; NPD, no PD; and NOS, not otherwise specified.

†Subjects met criteria for a definite or probable specific or NOS PD diagnosis on IPDE interview. χ^2 Test (2-tailed) (df=1) =23.02, P<.001.

1.00 and the specificity was 0.61 for the definite PD diagnoses. The negative predictive value of the screen for a definite diagnosis on the interview was 1.00, and the positive predictive value was 0.16. The difference in the rates of definite PD in the PPD vs NPD groups in the second-stage sample was significant (χ^2=21.15, *df*=1, *P*<.001). An additional 12 subjects met criteria for a probable disorder, and **Table 5** combines the definite *and* probable cases. All but 3 of the 33 subjects in the combined group had positive results on the screen. Of the remaining 225 subjects with neither a definite nor a probable diagnosis on the interview, 104 had positive results on the screen. Diagnostic efficiency index calculations, which took into account the 2-stage study design, yielded a sensitivity of 0.87 and a specificity of 0.63. The negative predictive value of the screen for a definite or probable diagnosis on the IPDE was 0.98 and the positive predictive value was 0.22. The difference in the rates of definite or PPD in the PPD vs NPD groups in the second-stage sample was significant (χ^2=23.02, *df*=1, *P*<.001).

POINT-PREVALENCE ESTIMATES FOR PD

To estimate the point prevalence for any PD in this sample of university students, we used the prevalence estimation procedures for 2-staged screening applications described by Newman et al.[19] This takes into account the proportions of the first-stage population (N=1646) screened positive (PPD) (43%) and negative (NPD) (57%), in relation to the prevalence of PDs in the second-stage assessment, and provides an estimate of the point prevalence in the entire population that was screened. The estimates (±SE) provided by this method were 6.74%±1.36% (95% (CI, 4.07%-9.41%) for a definite PD and 11.01%±1.75% (95% CI, 7.57%-14.52%) for a definite PD or PPD. In this context, we note that width of the CIs around such prevalence estimates reflects 1 of the costs of a 2-stage design. The smaller the number of diagnostic interviews that are done at the second stage, the wider the CIs (Patrick Shrout, PhD, oral communication, April 3, 1996).

COMMENT

To our knowledge, there are no published studies demonstrating the applicability of a 2-stage procedure in determining the prevalence of PDs in the general population. The ongoing study of this large university population provided an opportunity to gauge the feasibility of implementing this cost-saving method. For each type of PD, item-based algorithms from a self-administered inventory were used to predict the presence or absence of each criterion for each type of disorder, and the *DSM-III-R* diagnostic rules were used to set the threshold for a diagnosis. If the present screening inventory should demonstrate a similar performance in other nonpatient populations, it would reduce the number of subjects requiring an interview by approximately half. This would represent a considerable decrease in the expense required to conduct a large-scale epidemiological study. It would be accomplished with a loss to the study of very few actual cases of PD. In fact, in the present sample, the screen failed to miss anyone who was found to have a definite PD, when examined by experienced clinicians with a reliable semistructured interview with extensive worldwide usage. Efforts to reduce the number of false-positive cases by raising the screening threshold resulted in a significant increase in the number of false-negative results, an undesirable feature of any screening device intended for epidemiological use.

Caseness was also redefined to designate those who were 1 criterion short of a diagnosis (probable). The screen missed 9% of those who were included in the combined definite or probable category. Use of the broader designation was associated with little reduction in the number of false-positive cases; therefore, one might argue in favor of dispensing with it. However, compared with clinicians, the IPDE generally tends to be especially conservative in making a diagnosis. For example, it requires that criterion behavior last at least 5 years, and that there be some manifestation of the disorder prior to age 25 years. Because of this strict interpretation of the *DSM-III-R* definition of a PD, some might prefer to retain the "probable" category, despite its adverse effect on sensitivity. The present screen may not have performed the same with each of the 14 *DSM-III-R* Axis II diagnoses taken individually. There were far too few subjects with the individual types of disorders, to permit any meaningful determination of its sensitivity and specificity with each of them. Future research using considerably larger initial and second-stage sample sizes might profitably explore the sensitivity and specificity of this, or another, screen in detecting individual types of PD on both initial screening and second-stage assessment.

The estimated point prevalence of a PD in the present sample of 18- to 19-year-old university students was 6.74% for a definite disorder and 11.01% for a definite or probable disorder. Currently available estimates for the general population are marred by sampling defects or dubious methods of case ascertainment. However, typical findings appear to be in the range of 5% to 15%,[20-22] with 1 of the studies actually using the IPDE[22] and reporting an unadjusted prevalence of 14.8%. Although at least some of the behavior indicative of a PD must have its onset by late adolescence or early adulthood,[1-3] the present estimates do not reflect the fact that 18- to 19-year-olds have yet to complete the period of risk for the development of all of the Axis II criteria and associated disorders. The 5-year requirement on the IPDE also extends the timeframe back to the middle of adolescence, where some of the adult-oriented criteria may be less relevant and, therefore, could not be assessed. Furthermore, 1 of the hallmarks of a PD is impaired social and occupational functioning. But one would expect that the high academic achievement of the present group reflects some censoring for mental health and personality adjustment. However, we also note that, although selection for university admission (ie, academic achievement) may mitigate against poor school and/or social functioning, academic ability does not preclude the presence or development of PD and other forms of psychopathology in this sample. Clearly, the prospective study of these particular subjects, currently under way through the LSPD, will shed light on their long-term social and occupational functioning and their mental health. All things considered, the prevalence of PD in this university sample approximates what might have been expected based on the information that is currently available in the literature.

One focus of our future work with the IPDE-S is to further increase the cost-effectiveness of the screen. As noted in some studies,[18,19] in light of available information on the accuracy of a screen, the utility of a 2-stage procedure depends on the relative cost of the screening to the diagnostic assessments. One method to further enhance the efficiency of the IPDE-S would be to accurately determine the optimal proportions of putative positive vs negative cases to be selected from the screened population for second-stage diagnostic workups.[18,19] Other changes in the IPDE-S or study design could also be considered. For example, efforts might be directed at continued refinement of the precision of the IPDE-S in its current form to reduce false-positive rates, substantial reduction in the length of the IPDE-S (hopefully with continued low false-negative rates) to reduce screening costs, and/or determining whether the actual IPDE interviews might be conducted in a valid fashion via telephone to reduce costs associated with second-stage assessments. In our view, telephone administration of the IPDE, however, must not be attempted without first carefully studying the impact this mode of administration might have on validity (eg, cluster A symptoms). We are considering all these options as we continue our efforts in this area.

Compared with the US population at large, the present sample is not only more homogeneous in age and educational achievement but also, to some extent, in social class and ethnicity. Moreover, our subjects displayed a high degree of cooperation with the second-stage assessments, higher than what one might anticipate in a community sample. Nevertheless, any screening procedure that can filter out at least half the cases, and still maintain perfect or near-perfect sensitivity, deserves a trial and cross-validation in larger and more representative community populations. If this or a similar screen should prove equally effective in the general population, it could remove the economic barrier to establishing an epidemiology of PDs, which is comparable with that already existing for most other mental disorders. Therefore, the present findings would seem to justify further exploration of the applicability of this 2-stage method of case identification in the pursuit of an epidemiology of PDs.

Accepted for publication June 18, 1997.

This research was supported in part by grant MH-45448 from the National Institute of Mental Health, Washington, DC (Dr Lenzenweger).

Preliminary results of this study were presented at the Third Meeting of the International Congress on the Disorders of Personality, International Society for the Study of Personality Disorders, Harvard University, Cambridge, Mass, September, 10, 1993.

We thank Patrick E. Shrout, PhD, for a helpful statistical consultation and Linda Foltz, PhD, for her assistance with second-stage assessments.

Reprints: Mark F. Lenzenweger, PhD, Laboratory of Experimental Psychopathology, Cornell University, Van Rensselaer Hall, Ithaca, NY 14853-4401.

REFERENCES

1. American Psychiatric Association. *Diagnostic and Statistical Manual of Mental Disorders, Third Edition.* Washington, DC: American Psychiatric Association; 1980
2. American Psychiatric Association. *Diagnostic and Statistical Manual of Mental Disorders, Third Edition, Revised.* Washington, DC: American Psychiatric Association; 1987.
3. American Psychiatric Association. *Diagnostic and Statistical Manual of Mental Disorders, Fourth Edition.* Washington, DC: American Psychiatric Association; 1994.
4. Loranger AW. The impact of *DSM-III* on diagnostic practice in a university hospital: a comparison of *DSM-II* and *DSM-III* in 10 914 patients. *Arch Gen Psychiatry.* 1990;47:672-675.
5. Kessler RC, NcGonagle KA, Zhao S, Nelson CB, Hughes M, Eshelman S, Wittchen H-U, Kendler KS. Lifetime and 12-month prevalence of *DSM-III-R* psychiatric disorders in the United States: results from the National Comorbidity Survey. *Arch Gen Psychiatry.* 1994;51:8-19.
6. World Health Organization. *Composite International Diagnostic Interview (CIDI), Version 1.0.* Geneva, Switzerland: World Health Organization; 1990.
7. Jablensky A, Sartorius N, Hirschfeld, R, Pardes H. Diagnosis and classification of mental disorders and alcohol- and drug-related problems: a research agenda for the 1980s. *Psychol Med.* 1983;13:907-921.
8. Loranger AW. Are current self-report and interview measures adequate for epidemiological studies of personality disorders? *J Pers Disord.* 1992;6:313-325.
9. Dohrenwend BP, Shrout PE. Toward the development of a two-stage procedure for case identification and classification in psychiatric epidemiology. *Res Commun Mental Health.* 1981;2:295-323.
10. Loranger AW, Lenzenweger MF, Gartner AF, Lehmann Susman V, Herzig J, Zammit GK, Gartner JD, Abrams RC, Young RC. Trait-state artifacts and the diagnosis of personality disorders. *Arch Gen Psychiatry.* 1991;48:720-728.
11. Cronbach LJ. Coefficient alpha and the internal structure of tests. *Psychometrika.* 1951;16:297-334.
12. Loranger AW, Sartorius N, Andreoli, A, Berger P, Buchheim P, Channabasavanna SM, Coid B, Dahl, A, Diekstra RFW, Ferguson B, Jacobsberg LB, Mombour W, Pull C, Ono Y, Regier D. The International Personality Disorder Examination (IPDE): the World Health Organization/Alcohol, Drug Abuse, and Mental Health Administration International Pilot Study of Personality Disorders. *Arch Gen Psychiatry.* 1994;51:215-224.
13. Loranger AW, Sartorius N, Janca A, eds. *Assessment and Diagnosis of Personality Disorders: The International Personality Disorder Examination (IPDE).* New York, NY: Cambridge University Press, 1996.
14. World Health Organization. *ICD-10 Chapter V: Mental and Behavioural Disorders (Including Disorders of Psychological Development): Diagnostic Criteria for Research: Draft for Field Trials.* Geneva, Switzerland: World Health Organization; 1990.
15. World Health Organization. *The International Personality Disorder Examination (IPDE): DSM-IV Module.* Washington, DC: American Psychiatric Association; 1995.
16. Spitzer RL, Williams JBW, Gibbon, M, First M. *User's Guide for the Structured Clinical Interview for DSM-III-R.* Washington, DC: American Psychiatric Press; 1990.
17. Jackson DN. *Manual for the Personality Research Form.* 3rd ed. Port Huron, Mich: Research Psychologists Press; 1984.
18. Shrout, PE, Newman, SC. Design of two-phase prevalence surveys of rare disorders. *Biometrics.* 1989;45:549-555.
19. Newman SC, Shrout PE, Bland RC. The efficiency of two-phase designs in prevalence surveys of mental disorders. *Psychol Med.* 1990;20:183-193.
20. Weissman M. The epidemiology of personality disorders: a 1990 update. *J Pers Disord.* 1993;7(suppl):44-62.
21. Samuels JF, Nestadt G, Romanoski AJ, Folstein M, McHugh PR. *DSM-III* personality disorders in the community. *Am J Psychiatry.* 1994;151:1055-1062.
22. Klein DN, Riso LP, Donaldson SK, Schwartz JE, Anderson RL, Ouimette PC, Lizardi H, Aronson TA. Family study of early-onset dysthymia: mood and personality disorders in relatives of outpatients with dysthymia and episodic major depression and normal controls. *Arch Gen Psychiatry.* 1995;52:487-496.

ORIGINAL ARTICLE

Multisomatoform Disorder

An Alternative to Undifferentiated Somatoform Disorder for the Somatizing Patient in Primary Care

Kurt Kroenke, MD; Robert L. Spitzer, MD; Frank V. deGruy III, MD; Steven R. Hahn, MD; Mark Linzer, MD; Janet B. W. Williams, DSW; David Brody, MD; Mark Davies, MS

Background: For clinical or research use in primary care, the *DSM-IV* diagnostic criteria for somatization disorder are too restrictive, while the criteria for undifferentiated somatoform disorder are overly inclusive. In this article, we examine the validity of multisomatoform disorder, defined as 3 or more medically unexplained, currently bothersome physical symptoms plus a long (≥2 years) history of somatization.

Methods: Data from the Primary Care Evaluation of Mental Disorders Study of 1000 patients from 4 primary care sites were analyzed. The outcomes assessed were 6 domains of health-related quality of life, using the 20-item Short-Form General Health Survey; self-reported disability days and health care use; satisfaction with care; and physician-rated difficulty of the encounter.

Results: Multisomatoform disorder was diagnosed in 82 (8.2%) of the 1000 patients who were enrolled in the Primary Care Evaluation of Mental Disorders Study. Compared with mood and anxiety disorders, multisomatoform disorder was associated with comparable impairment in health-related quality of life, more self-reported disability days and clinic visits, and greater clinician-perceived patient difficulty.

Conclusions: Multisomatoform disorder may be a valid diagnosis and potentially more useful than the *DSM-IV* diagnosis of undifferentiated somatoform disorder. Also, because multisomatoform disorder has a large and independent effect on impairment, its diagnosis should not be precluded simply because of a coexisting mood or anxiety disorder.

Arch Gen Psychiatry. 1997;54:352-358

From the Department of Medicine, Uniformed Services University of the Health Sciences, Bethesda, Md (Dr Kroenke); Biometrics Research Department, New York State Psychiatric Institute and Department of Psychiatry, Columbia University, New York (Drs Spitzer and Williams and Mr Davies); Department of Family Practice, University of South Alabama College of Medicine, Mobile (Dr deGruy); and Departments of Medicine, Albert Einstein College of Medicine of Yeshiva University, Bronx, NY (Dr Hahn), University of Wisconsin Medical School, Madison (Dr Linzer), and Medical College of Pennsylvania and Hahnemann University, Philadephia (Dr Brody).

MORE THAN half of all outpatient encounters in the United States are precipitated by physical symptoms,[1] of which at least one quarter to one third are somatoform (ie, lacking an adequate physical explanation even after a reasonable workup).[2-4] Multiple or poorly explained symptoms cause substantial patient disability,[2,5-7] excess health care use,[5-7] physician frustration,[6,8] and therapeutic disappointment.[9]

Somatization disorder, which first appeared in *DSM-III*, is a well-validated construct particularly useful in classifying some of the patients with somatoform symptoms who are seen by mental health specialists. However, it defines the extreme end of the spectrum of somatoform disorders, and most patients with unexplained symptoms undergoing treatment in the primary care setting do not meet the high symptom threshold.[6,10] Also, the diagnosis of somatization disorder involves lifetime symptom counts, and detailed inquiry about lifetime symptom experiences is typically not feasible in a busy primary care setting. Recognizing these limitations of somatization disorder for diagnosing many somatizing patients in primary care, an additional somatoform diagnosis was added to *DSM-III-R*—undifferentiated somatoform disorder—that requires only a single unexplained symptom persisting for 6 or more months. However, there is a common perception that undifferentiated somatoform disorder has been inconsistently applied and not well adopted in clinical practice[11,12]; we are unaware of any published data on its validity.

In the Primary Care Evaluation of Mental Disorders (PRIME-MD) 1000 Study of 1000 patients,[13] we developed criteria for a new somatoform disorder called *multisomatoform disorder*, defined as 3 or more current somatoform symptoms reported from a 15-symptom checklist along with at least a 2-year history of somatoform symptoms (**Table 1**). Alternative criteria sets were tested during an 8-month development phase that included 450 patients at 7 primary care sites. The final

PATIENTS AND METHODS

Details of the PRIME-MD Study, including patient sampling procedures, have been previously reported.[13] Briefly, the study population consisted of 1000 patients presenting for medical care at 4 primary care clinics. The mean age of the patients was 55 years (range, 18-91 years); 60% of the patients were women; 58%, white; and 28%, college graduates. The most common medical disorders in these patients were hypertension, 48%; arthritis, 23%; diabetes, 17%; and heart disease, 15%. The study protocol was approved by the institutional review boards at each site, and all patients gave signed, informed consent.

PSYCHIATRIC ASSESSMENT

All subjects were evaluated with PRIME-MD, a validated diagnostic interview that consists of a 26-item, self-administered patient questionnaire (PQ) and an accompanying clinician evaluation guide.[13] Criteria-based *DSM-III-R* diagnoses were made in 5 categories: mood, anxiety, somatoform, alcohol, and eating. (With minor modifications, the revised PRIME-MD makes *DSM-IV* diagnoses.) The average physician time required to complete the interview is less than 10 minutes, with an overall diagnostic accuracy and interobserver agreement comparable with other structured psychiatric interviews administered by mental health specialists.

The 15 physical symptoms on the somatoform section of the PQ are prefaced in the PQ by the query: "During the *past month*, have you *often* been bothered by . . . (1) stomach pain? (2) back pain? . . . " The clinician reviews the PQ and enters the somatoform module in the clinician evaluation guide only if the patient has endorsed 3 or more physical symptoms on the PQ. For each symptom endorsed on the PQ, patients are again asked: "Has (symptom) bothered you a *lot* in the past month?" If the patient replies yes, the clinician evaluation guide instructs the clinician to decide: "Based on your clinical judgment, does the symptom have a physical explanation that is adequate to explain its severity and associated disability?" Only if the clinician answers no is the symptom classified as somatoform. An important exception is that if the patient meets criteria for a mood or anxiety disorder, symptoms explicitly part of the diagnostic criteria for that disorder (eg, fatigue or insomnia for a mood disorder and cardiopulmonary or gastrointestinal tract symptoms for panic disorder) are not counted as somatoform. In short, a symptom endorsed on the PQ has to be verified by the patient as recently bothersome and be judged by the clinician as physically unexplained before it is classified as somatoform. A patient who meets all criteria for multisomatoform disorder, except for chronicity (criterion D, Table 1), is diagnosed as having somatoform disorder, not otherwise specified (NOS). Two other somatoform disorders were diagnosable by PRIME-MD in this study: chronic pain disorder (ie, a somatoform pain symptom that has interfered with the patient's activities for at least 6 months) and hypochondriasis (ie, unrealistic preoccupation with having a serious disease despite reassurance). Chronic pain disorder was not diagnosed if sufficient criteria were met for either multisomatoform disorder or somatoform disorder NOS.

OTHER MEASURES

Subjects also completed the 20-item Short-Form General Health Survey (SF-20), a validated instrument that measures HRQL in 6 domains: physical, mental, social, role, pain, and general health perceptions.[16] As an additional measure of functional status, disability days were estimated by asking patients how many days in the past 3 months they

Continued on next page

criteria set for the disorder accounted for prevalence, feasibility of diagnosis in the busy primary care setting, and the clinician's sense that the diagnosis would be useful in patient management. The 15 physical symptoms on PRIME-MD were chosen because they account for more than 90% of outpatient visits attributable to physical complaints (excluding symptoms related to upper respiratory infections).[1,9] Although listed in the new *DSM-IV-PC*[14] as a subtype of undifferentiated somatoform disorder, multisomatoform disorder is not included in *DSM-IV* and evidence regarding its validity, to our knowledge, has not previously been published.

With the use of data from the PRIME-MD Study of 1000 patients,[13] we examined the validity of this new somatoform disorder by addressing the following questions:

1. How does multisomatoform disorder compare with the mood and anxiety disorders commonly seen in the primary care setting in its effects on patient functional status and well-being, hereafter referred to as health-related quality of life (HRQL)?[15]

2. How does multisomatoform disorder compare with other disorders in its association with several secondary validators, namely, increased health care use, decreased satisfaction with care, and increased difficulty in the physician-patient relationship?

3. Is the threshold of 3 or more unexplained symptoms that is used in diagnosing multisomatoform disorder justified, or is the process of somatization a continuum for which no particular diagnostic cut point is defensible?

RESULTS

One hundred thirty-nine (14%) of the patients had a PRIME-MD somatoform diagnosis, including multisomatoform disorder in 82, somatoform disorder NOS in 42, hypochondriasis in 22, and chronic pain disorder in 8. Compared with patients without a somatoform disorder, patients with a somatoform disorder were younger (50 vs 56 years, $P<.001$), more likely to be women (75% vs 57%, $P<.001$), and less likely to be college graduates (17% vs 30%, $P<.001$). Psychiatric comorbidity was substantial: 61% of patients with a somatoform diagnosis had a coexisting mood disorder, and 50% had an anxiety disorder.

HEALTH-RELATED QUALITY OF LIFE

Table 2 shows the unique effects of common mood, anxiety, and somatoform disorders on HRQL. On 2 of the 6 SF-20 scales (ie, general health perceptions and bodily pain), were unable to pursue their usual activities because of not feeling well. Finally, subjects answered several questions regarding recent health care use and satisfaction with care.

After the visit, physicians completed the 10-item Difficult Doctor-Patient Relationship Questionnaire, a validated measure of physician-perceived difficulty of the patient encounter.[8,17] The Difficult Doctor-Patient Relationship Questionnaire was not administered until partway through the study, so this questionnaire was completed by 628 subjects who did not differ in demographic characteristics, medical comorbidity, and psychiatric diagnoses from the sample as a whole.

DATA ANALYSIS

One-way analysis of variance and a χ^2 analysis were used for univariate comparisons of continuous and categorical variables, respectively. Our primary dependent variables were HRQL (as measured by the 6 SF-20 scales), disability days, and health care use. For these continuous variables, we determined the unique effects of the 9 most common mood, anxiety, and somatoform disorders using a multivariate analysis of variance, adjusting for age, sex, number of general medical disorders, and each of the other 8 mental disorders. Indicator (dummy) variables were used for each of the mental disorders. This method of adjusting for psychiatric comorbidity identifies the independent association between each specific mental disorder and HRQL, disability days, and health care use.

For each SF-20 scale, total scores were estimated if information was available for more than 60% of the scale items; this resulted in missing data for 7% to 12% of the subjects for the different scales. There were missing data for 10% of the subjects for disability days, for 8% for health care use, and for 14% for satisfaction with care. Subjects with missing data on the SF-20 did not seem to be more or less healthy than subjects whose SF-20 forms were complete in that the mean number of disability days in the 2 groups was not notably different. For certain analyses involving SF-20 scores, we calculated an *effect size*, which is the difference between groups in scores on a particular scale, divided by the SD of the scale in the total sample. Effect sizes of 0.20, 0.50, and 0.80 or more are considered by some to represent small, moderate, and large differences, respectively.[18,19]

Two secondary outcomes assessed were patient satisfaction with care and physician-experienced difficulty of the encounter. For these categorical variables, patients with each disorder were compared with all patients without that disorder using logistic regression analysis, adjusting for age, sex, education, and number of general medical disorders. A second analysis was conducted, also adjusting for each of the other mental disorders to determine the unique effects of a specific disorder on satisfaction and difficulty. Satisfaction was dichotomized by combining patients who rated their care as very good or excellent; difficulty was dichotomized by using a Difficult Doctor-Patient Relationship Questionnaire cut point of 30 or more.

Finally, we assessed the relationship between number of somatoform and depressive symptoms and HRQL. The reference groups for these 2 analyses were the 659 subjects with no somatoform symptoms and the 719 subjects with no depressive symptoms, respectively. The impairment associated with increasing numbers of somatoform or depressive symptoms is the difference from the reference group expressed as the decrement in mean effect size for the 6 SF-20 scales (ie, the mean across all 6 domains), adjusted for age, sex, education, and number of general medical disorders. For logistic regression analysis, odds ratios with 95% confidence intervals are reported, while for all other tests of statistical significance, exact *P* values are calculated.

multisomatoform disorder exhibited the most severe impairment of any of the 9 disorders, and on 2 other scales (ie, social and role functioning), its impairment was among the most severe. On the physical functioning scale, only mood disorders were associated with at least moderate impairment (ie, effect size ≥0.50), while anxiety and somatoform disorders had only small effects. On the mental health scale, mood and anxiety disorders produced substantial decrements, while somatoform disorders produced little to no impairment; this is not surprising given that the 5 items on the SF-20 mental health scale inquire primarily about mood and anxiety symptoms.

DISABILITY DAYS AND HEALTH CARE USE

Table 3 shows the unique effects of specific mental disorders on disability days and health care use. Multisomatoform disorder was associated with more disability days than any other disorder; indeed, major depression was the only other disorder uniquely associated with an excess number of disability days. Multisomatoform disorder was also the only disorder associated with a notable increase in the number of clinic visits, as well as only 1 of 2 disorders to produce an excess number of emergency department visits.

PATIENT SATISFACTION AND DIFFICULTY

The proportion of patients in the entire sample who rated their care as very good or excellent was 76%, a level comparable with that generally reported in a large group practice or managed care setting.[20] After adjusting for age, sex, education, and number of general medical disorders, only 4 mental disorders were associated with decreased satisfaction (ie, rating care as less than very good or excellent): generalized anxiety disorder (odds ratio [OR], 3.1; 95% confidence interval [CI], 1.8-5.3), dysthymia (OR, 3.0; 95% CI, 1.8-5.2), major depression (OR, 2.3; 95% CI, 1.5-3.7), and multisomatoform disorder (OR, 1.7; 95% CI, 1.0-2.8). However, when further adjusting for psychiatric comorbidity, only generalized anxiety disorder remained uniquely associated with patient satisfaction (OR, 2.1; 95% CI, 1.0-4.3).

Mental disorders had a substantial effect on the physician's satisfaction with the encounter. As shown in **Table 4**, the presence of any of the mental disorders, with the exception of minor depression and anxiety disorder NOS, increased the likelihood of the patient's being considered difficult. When controlling for psychiatric comorbidity, only multisomatoform disorder, somatoform disorder NOS, and panic disorder were uniquely associated with patient difficulty. In particular, patients with multisomatoform disorder were more than 10 times as likely to be considered difficult.

WHAT IS THE APPROPRIATE SYMPTOM THRESHOLD FOR DIAGNOSING A DISORDER IN PATIENTS WITH MULTIPLE SOMATOFORM SYMPTOMS?

The **Figure** shows the relationship between HRQL and the number of somatoform and depressive symptoms. For somatoform and depressive symptoms, there is generally a dose-response relationship between increasing symptom counts and HRQL impairment. The linear relationship was significant at $P<.001$. An effect size of 0.50 or greater, which is often considered moderate, was approximated at a somatoform symptom count of 3 (effect size, 0.49; 95% CI, 0.26-0.71) and was exceeded at a depressive symptom count of 2 (effect size, 0.65; 95% CI, 0.46-0.84). The former finding further validates the 3-symptom threshold for PRIME-MD somatoform diagnoses, and the latter finding adds support to the 2-symptom threshold proposed for minor depressive disorder in *DSM-IV-PC*.[14] (Although there is a single departure from linear decline for somatoform symptoms and depressive symptoms, it is most likely due to the small sample size. There were 22 patients with 5 somatoform symptoms and 36 patients with 4 depressive symptoms.)

Table 1. Diagnostic Criteria for Multisomatoform Disorder*

A. Three or more somatoform symptoms currently present (ie, within the past month).
B. A somatoform symptom meets either criterion 1 or 2:
   1. After appropriate investigation, the symptom cannot be fully explained by a known general medical condition or the direct effects of a substance (eg, a drug of abuse or a medication).
   2. When there is a related general medical condition, the physical complaint or resulting social or occupational impairment is in excess of what would be expected from the history, physical examination, or laboratory findings.
C. The symptoms cause clinically significant distress or impairment in social, occupational, or other important areas of functioning.
D. Although specific symptoms may come and go, the person has had one or more somatoform symptoms, for more days than not, for at least 2 years.
E. Criteria for somatization disorder are not met nor are the symptoms part of the diagnostic criteria for a mental disorder that is currently present (eg, fatigue or insomnia in a patient with a depressive disorder or chest pain and dizziness that only occur during a panic attack in a patient with panic disorder).
F. The symptoms are not intentionally produced or feigned (as in factitious disorder or malingering).

**In the Primary Care Evaluation of Mental Disorders Study, the checklist included 15 symptoms or symptom groups: stomach pain, back pain, headache, chest pain, dizziness, fainting, palpitations, shortness of breath, bowel complaints (ie, constipation or diarrhea), dyspeptic complaints (ie, nausea, gas, or indigestion), fatigue, trouble sleeping, pain in joints or limbs, menstrual pain or problems, and pain or problems during sexual intercourse.*

COMMENT

Our study supports multisomatoform disorder as an alternative to the rather vague and unvalidated *DSM-IV* category of undifferentiated somatoform disorder. Characterized by 3 or more unexplained and currently bothersome symptoms along with a chronic history of somatization, multisomatoform disorder is associated with impairment in HRQL comparable with mood and anxiety disorders, a greater number of disability days and physician visits, and the highest level of provider frustration.

In examining an optimal symptom threshold for somatoform disorders in primary care, what justifies a 3-symptom cut point? First and most importantly, multisomatoform disorder was associated with impairment in multiple domains of HRQL as well as excess health care use, 2 outcomes increasingly salient in health care delivery and research.[15,21] At a somatoform symptom count of 3, the decline in HRQL approximated an effect size often judged to be clinically important, while disability days and clinic visits exceeded that of any mood or anxiety disorder. Because our estimates of effect size had wide

Table. 2 Unique Effects of Common Mood, Anxiety, and Somatoform Disorders on Health-Related Quality of Life

		Average Decrement (Effect Size) in SF-20 Health Status Scores*					
Mental Disorder	**No. of Patients**	**Physical Function**	**Bodily Pain**	**Role Function**	**General Health Perceptions**	**Social Function**	**Mental Health**
Multisomatoform disorder	82	−6.9 (0.25)	−18.0 (0.64)†	−18.6 (0.45)†	−21.4 (0.79)†	−13.0 (0.46)†	−2.5 (0.13)
Somatoform disorder, not otherwise specified	42	−7.9 (0.29)	−9.8 (0.35)	−18.1 (0.44)‡	−16.1 (0.60)†	−4.3 (0.15)	+3.6 (0.18)
Major depression	115	−13.6 (0.50)†	−11.0 (0.39)‡	−25.2 (0.61)†	−14.4 (0.53)†	−16.0 (0.67)†	−21.5 (1.10)†
Dysthymia	78	−6.8 (0.25)	+1.0 (0.03)	−17.4 (0.42)‡	−8.4 (0.31)	−12.5 (0.44)‡	−9.3 (0.47)†
Minor depression	64	−14.1 (0.52)†	−14.2 (0.51)†	−16.9 (0.41)†	−17.1 (0.63)†	−11.3 (0.40)†	−15.6 (0.78)†
Partial remission or recurrence of major depression	63	−12.2 (0.45)†	−9.0 (0.32)	−22.5 (0.55)†	−14.6 (0.54)†	−8.6 (0.30)	−15.7 (0.79)†
Anxiety disorder, not otherwise specified	90	−5.5 (0.20)	−9.8 (0.35)‡	−4.1 (0.10)	−6.1 (0.23)	−14.3 (0.35)†	−11.5 (0.58)†
Generalized anxiety disorder	70	−2.9 (0.11)	−9.0 (0.32)	−3.9 (0.09)	+0.2 (0.01)	−3.1 (0.11)	−12.2 (0.61)†
Panic disorder	36	−7.5 (0.28)	−0.6 (0.02)	−7.1 (0.17)	−4.9 (0.18)	−7.3 (0.26)	−8.7 (0.44)‡

**Patients with a specific disorder compared with all patients without that disorder, with scores adjusted for age, sex, education, number of physical disorders, and each of the other mental disorders. The effect size (in parentheses) is the average decrement divided by the SD for the entire sample. SF-20 indicates the 20-item Short-Form General Health Survey scale.*

†$P<.001$.

‡$P<.01$.

CIs because of the relatively few patients with any given somatoform symptom count, additional studies are needed to further validate the 3-symptom threshold.

Second, there is an epidemiological argument of reasonable prevalence: how much of a given population is defined as having a disorder when the defining variable is continuous? For example, using cut points of 1, 2, 3, 4, and 5 somatoform symptoms, the proportion of patients in our PRIME-MD Study that would qualify for a somatoform disorder would be 29%, 21%, 14%, 11%, and 7%, respectively. Adding the chronicity criterion (ie, several or more years of unexplained symptoms) to the 3-symptom threshold defines multisomatoform disorder, which has a reasonable prevalence of 8% in our primary care clinics.

A third and parallel argument relevant to separating diseased from normal individuals is the concept of reasonable risk.[22,23] At low levels of a risk factor (eg, mild hypertension or mild hyperlipidemia), the population prevalence is high (range, 25%-40%) but the morbidity for most patients exceeding a minimalistic threshold is fairly low. However, as the severity of a risk factor increases, there is a decrease in prevalence with a corresponding increase in morbidity. Thresholds arrived at by consensus abound in medicine and psychiatry: a diastolic blood pressure of 90 mm Hg, a serum cholesterol level exceeding 5.17 mmol/L (200 mg/dL), 4 of 11 criteria for systemic lupus erythematosus, 1 mm or more of ST segment depression on a cardiac stress test, 5 of 9 criteria for major depression, and 4 or more symptoms for a panic attack, to name a few. Fourth, thresholds for defining a disorder can be established at the point at which therapy has proven to be beneficial.[22,23] Management techniques effective for somatization disorder[24] have recently been shown to be useful in patients with lesser degrees of somatization as well.[25]

Why did we examine difficulty of the physician-patient encounter in our study? Difficulty experienced in caring for patients with somatoform symptoms may be important for several reasons: (1) physical (rather than psychological) symptoms are the most common presentation of psychopathologic features in medical patients,[12,26] (2) many physical symptoms remain poorly explained after diagnostic testing aimed at detecting simply physical causes,[2,27] and (3) such somatoform symptoms frustrate primary care physicians.[6,8,17] Our data suggest that, after adjusting for psychiatric comorbidity, much of the difficulty experienced by primary care physicians in caring for patients with mood and anxiety disorders may be attributable to coexisting somatoform disorders. Patients who have somatic manifestations of psychological distress may be more reluctant, at least ini-

Table 3. Unique Effects of Common Mood, Anxiety, and Somatoform Disorders on Sick Days and Health Care Visits During the Past 3 Months*

Mental Disorder	No. of Sick Days	No. of Clinic Visits	No. of Emergency Department Visits
Multisomatoform disorder	7.28†	1.24†	0.35‡
Major depression	7.05†	0.49	0.32‡
Partial remission or recurrence of major depression	4.93	0.41	−0.04
Panic disorder	4.52	−0.75	0.13
Dysthymia	2.73	0.75	0.11
Somatoform disorder, not otherwise specified	2.38	0.88	−0.08
Anxiety disorder, not otherwise specified	1.74	−0.07	0.03
Minor depression	1.61	0.14	0.18
Generalized anxiety disorder	−0.22	−0.04	−0.13
Mean, entire sample§	4.92	1.68	0.28

**Patients with each disorder are compared with patients without that disorder, adjusted for age, sex, education, number of physical disorders, and each of the other psychiatric disorders. For example, patients with major depression have 7.05 excess sick days compared with patients without major depression, while those with a generalized anxiety disorder have 0.22 fewer sick days than those without a generalized anxiety disorder.*

†*P*<.001.

‡*P*<.01.

§*These are simply mean values (ie, no comparison group) for all patients who provided information on sick days (n=832), clinic visits (n=846), and emergency department visits (n=868).*

Table 4. Unique Effects of Common Mood, Anxiety, and Somatoform Disorders on the Likelihood of Patients' Being Described as Difficult*

Mental Disorder	Patients Described as Difficult by Physician, %	Adjusted Odds Ratio (95% Confidence Interval)†	Adjusted Odds Ratio, Including Psychiatric Comorbidity (95% Confidence Interval)‡
Multisomatoform disorder	54	11.4 (5.9-22.2)	10.5 (4.9-22.5)
Panic disorder	56	8.2 (3.4-19.8)	4.7 (1.5-14.5)
Dysthymia	40	4.3 (2.2-8.3)	1.2 (0.4-3.2)
Generalized anxiety disorder	36	3.9 (2.0-7.6)	1.1 (0.4-2.8)
Major depression	31	3.1 (1.7-5.6)	1.6 (0.6-4.0)
Somatoform disorder, not otherwise specified	29	2.5 (1.0-6.2)	3.7 (1.4-9.9)
Partial remission or recurrence of major depression	30	2.3 (1.0-5.2)	1.5 (0.6-4.4)
Minor depression	19	1.3 (0.6-2.9)	1.6 (0.6-3.9)
Anxiety disorder, not otherwise specified	19	1.2 (0.6-2.3)	0.7 (0.3-1.6)

**There were 628 subjects for whom difficulty data were available.*

†*Odds ratio (with 95% confidence interval) of patients with a specific disorder being rated as difficult by their physician compared with patients without that disorder, adjusted for age, sex, education, and number of physical disorders.*

‡*Odds ratio adjusted for the variables mentioned in the previous footnote plus each of the other 8 mental disorders, thus showing the unique effect of a specific disorder on the likelihood of a patient being rated as difficult.*

tially, to explore emotional factors contributing to their symptoms, and the clinician may have to spend more time and extra visits so that the patient can undergo a gradual process of reattribution.

The 3 ways in which multisomatoform disorder differs from undifferentiated somatoform disorder are its higher symptom threshold (ie, 3 instead of 1), longer duration (ie, 2 years instead of 6 months), and fewer exclusionary psychiatric diagnoses (ie, its hierarchical rule). The 3-symptom threshold has already been discussed. The requirement for at least a 2-year history of unexplained symptoms recognizes the often chronic course of somatization and is analogous to the duration requirement for the chronic mood disorder, dysthymia. Also, compared with somatoform disorder NOS (ie, ≥3 unexplained symptoms but no chronicity criterion as defined in our study), multisomatoform disorder is associated with greater impairment in several domains of HRQL, more sick days, and a higher amount of health care use.

The criteria for multisomatoform disorder do not contain the hierarchical rule of undifferentiated somatoform disorder, which is not diagnosed if unexplained physical symptoms are better accounted for by another mental disorder, particularly a mood or anxiety disorder. Hierarchical rules can pose problems for diagnostic reliability because attributing headache, abdominal pain, or dizziness to a current mood or anxiety disorder involves considerable clinician judgment and even uncertainty or bias. Physical symptoms do not count toward a diagnosis of multisomatoform disorder when they are actually part of the diagnostic criteria for a current mood or anxiety disorder (criterion E, Table 1). However, there is no reason to exclude symptoms such as fatigue or insomnia from a somatoform diagnosis in patients with multiple other unexplained physical complaints who do not have a concurrent mood or anxiety disorder, particularly because there is evidence that it is not the specific type of somatoform symptom but rather the number of symptoms that determines the severity of functional impairment as well as psychiatric comorbidity.[2]

Abridged somatization disorder, consisting of 6 lifetime medically unexplained symptoms in women and 4 in men, is another less restrictive somatoform disorder that, like multisomatoform disorder, has been shown to be associated with excess functional impairment and health care use.[5,6,10,25,28] Abridged somatization disorder is not recognized in *DSM-IV*. A more important limitation is that the clinician must inquire about a patient's lifetime experiences with a long list of 37 symptoms. Typically, this is impractical in a busy primary care setting. While it is likely that there will be substantial overlap between abridged somatization disorder and multisomatoform disorder, this should be investigated in future studies.

Some might argue that somatoform disorders should remain a diagnosis of exclusion so that the clinician is not lulled into a false sense of security, quickly attributing unexplained physical complaints to a somatoform disorder while overlooking underlying and potentially treatable mental or general medical disorders. However, comorbidity is increasingly being established as the rule rather than the exception in patients with mental disorders.[13,29] For example, major depression frequently develops in patients with alcohol disorders and panic disorder may develop in those with schizophrenia. There is little evidence that important medical diagnoses are missed in patients with multiple somatoform symptoms, yet it is clear that such patients are exhaustively tested to exclude many rare physical causes before somatization is even considered.[10,12,26,27,30-32]

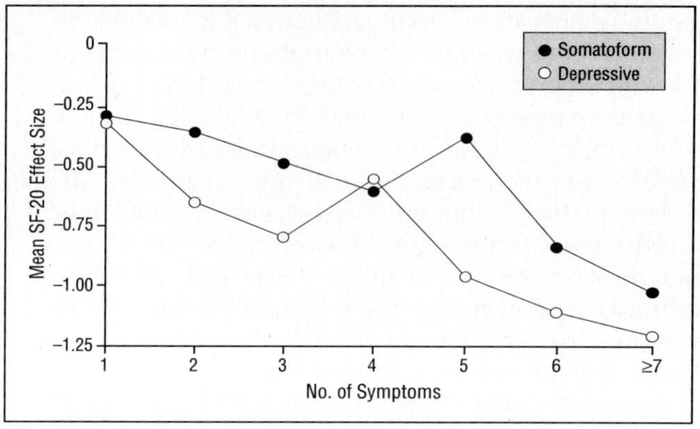

Decrement in health-related quality of life associated with a particular number of somatoform or depressive symptoms, using the 659 patients with no somatoform symptoms and the 719 patients with no depressive symptoms as the respective reference groups. Decrement is expressed as the mean effect size for the six 20-item Short-Form General Health Survey (SF-20) scales, adjusted for age, sex, education, and number of general medical disorders.

Our study has several limitations. First, the design was cross-sectional, and somatoform disorders more than many other Axis I disorders represent cumulative diagnoses, the certainty of which increases with longitudinal follow-up. Second, establishing the validity of criteria for somatoform disorders is one of the more challenging tasks in psychiatric nosology. "Hard" validators of mental disorders include genetic markers, family studies, natural history of the disorder, and treatment responsiveness, particularly to pharmacotherapy.[33] Family studies and natural history studies validating full somatization disorder are needed for lower threshold somatoform disorders. While there is no effective medication for somatoform disorders per se, nonpharmacological treatment strategies have shown some benefit for full and abridged somatization disorder.[24,25] Third, the measures of validity we were able to measure (ie, HRQL impairment, disability days, increased health care use, and satisfaction with care) are nonspecific in that many major mental or general medical disorders would be expected to affect these outcomes. While the evidence we provide to support the "caseness" of multisomatoform disorder is stronger than any published data available for undifferentiated somatoform disorder, prospective studies involving longitudinal follow-up of patients in primary care settings are certainly needed to further validate multisomatoform disorder.

In addition to the question of symptom thresholds, it is important to be aware of other problems regarding the definition of somatoform disorders, particularly in primary care. (1) There can be considerable physician or mental health professional bias in judging whether a symptom is somatoform, posing potential problems regarding diagnostic reliability. Criterion B is particularly susceptible to interclinician variability: what constitutes an "appropriate investigation" to exclude a physical basis for a patient's symptoms? Because other *DSM-IV* somatoform diagnoses (ie, somatization disorder, conversion disorder, and undifferentiated somatoform disorder) also include this criterion, we have retained it for multisomatoform disorder. However, particular caution must be exercised in an era of managed care not to overdiagnose somatoform disorders simply because of cost pressures to restrict the number of laboratory tests or referrals that are ordered. (2) Somatoform diagnoses depend on cumulative symptom counts, so that diagnostic confidence may be less at the onset of the clinician-patient relationship and increase with longitudinal follow-up. (3) Does somatoform mean only lacking an adequate physical explanation, or lack of a physical explanation plus the presence of a probable underlying psychological factor that is causing or aggravating the patient's symptom? While the first definition requires one to exclude potential physical suspects (a difficult enough task), the second requires sufficient positive evidence to justify psychological attribution. This raises problems of masking or denial of psychological factors, as well as physician bias in interpreting such factors even when they are present. (4) There is a high prevalence of individual symptoms in the general population[3] and in medical patients.[9] Also, symptom syndromes (eg, irritable bowel syndrome, fibromyalgia, premenstrual syndrome, and chronic fatigue syndrome), which currently lack either a satisfactory physical or psychiatric explanation, are among the most common disorders seen in primary care.[10,12,22,30] These factors pose particular challenges and must be recognized when diagnosing somatoform disorders in primary care.

In summary, multisomatoform disorder produces impairment at least as great as many Axis I disorders and should be given serious consideration as an alternative to undifferentiated somatoform disorder. Also, because somatoform disorders have a large and independent effect on impairment, their diagnosis should not be precluded simply because of a coexisting mood, anxiety, or other nonsomatoform mental disorder. We believe that changing the name as well as the criteria is warranted because undifferentiated somatoform disorder was never a formal diagnosis until it was included in *DSM-III-R* and has never been validated. On the other hand, the term *multisomatoform disorder* more accurately signifies that a higher symptom threshold (ie, 3 or more somatoform symptoms) may better define caseness for clinical and research purposes.

Accepted for publication August 20, 1996.

The development of the Primary Care Evaluation of Mental Disorders was underwritten by an unrestricted educational grant from the Roerig and Pratt Pharmaceuticals division of Pfizer Inc, New York, NY.

Corresponding author: Kurt Kroenke, MD, Department of Medicine, Uniformed Services University of the Health Sciences, 4301 Jones Bridge Rd, Bethesda, MD 20814.

REFERENCES

1. Schappert SM. National Ambulatory Medical Care Survey: 1989 summary. *Vital Health Stat 13.* 1992;110:2-11.
2. Kroenke K, Spitzer RL, Williams JBW, Linzer M, Hahn SR, deGruy FV III, Brody D. Physical symptoms in primary care: predictors of psychiatric disorders and functional impairment. *Arch Fam Med.* 1994;3:774-779.
3. Kroenke K, Price RK. Symptoms in the community: prevalence, classification, and psychiatric comorbidity. *Arch Intern Med.* 1993;153:2474-2480.
4. Kellner R. Functional somatic symptoms and hypochondriasis: a survey of empirical studies. *Arch Gen Psychiatry.* 1985;42:821-833.
5. Escobar JI, Rubio-Stipec M, Canino G, Karno M. Somatic Symptom Index (SSI): a new and abridged somatization construct: prevalence and epidemiological correlates in two large community samples. *J Nerv Ment Dis.* 1989;177:140-146.
6. Katon W, Lin E, Von Korff M, Russo J, Lipscomb P, Bush T. Somatization: a spectrum of severity. *Am J Psychiatry.* 1991;148:34-40.
7. Smith GR, Monson RA, Ray DC. Patients with multiple unexplained symptoms: their characteristics, functional health, and health care utilization. *Arch Intern Med.* 1986;146:69-72.
8. Hahn SR, Thompson KS, Wills TA, Stern V, Budner NS. The difficult doctor-patient relationship: somatization, personality and psychopathology. *J Clin Epidemiol.* 1994;47:647-657.
9. Kroenke K, Arrington ME, Mangelsdorff AD. The prevalence of symptoms in medical outpatients and the adequacy of therapy. *Arch Intern Med.* 1990;150:1685-1689.
10. Kirmayer LJ, Robbins JM, eds. *Current Concepts of Somatization: Research and Clinical Perspectives.* Washington, DC: American Psychiatric Press; 1991.
11. Martin RL, Yutzy SH. Somatoform disorders. In: Hales RE, Yudofsky SC, Talbott JA, eds. *The American Psychiatric Press Textbook of Psychiatry.* Washington, DC: American Psychiatric Press; 1994:591-622.
12. Bass CM, ed. *Somatization: Physical Symptoms and Psychological Illness.* Boston, Mass: Blackwell Scientific Publications; 1990.
13. Spitzer RL, Williams JBW, Kroenke K, Linzer M, deGruy FV III, Hahn SR, Brody D, Johnson JG. Utility of a new procedure for diagnosing mental disorders in primary care: the PRIME-MD 1000 Study. *JAMA.* 1994;272:1749-1756.
14. American Psychiatric Association. *Diagnostic and Statistical Manual of Mental Disorders, Fourth Edition: Primary Care Version (DSM-IV-PC).* Washington, DC: American Psychiatric Association; 1995.
15. Wilson IB, Cleary PD. Linking clinical variables with health-related quality of life. *JAMA.* 1995;273:59-65.
16. Stewart AL, Hays RD, Ware JE. The MOS Short-Form General Health Survey: reliability and validity in a patient population. *Med Care.* 1988;26:724-732.
17. Hahn SR, Kroenke K, Spitzer RL, Brody D, Williams JBW, Linzer M, deGruy FV. The difficult patient in primary care: prevalence, psychopathology and impairment. *J Gen Intern Med.* 1996;11:1-8.
18. Kazis LE, Anderson JJ, Meenan RF. Effect sizes for interpreting changes in health status. *Med Care.* 1989;27:S178-S189.
19. Light RJ, Pillemer DB. *Summing Up: The Science of Reviewing Research.* Cambridge, Mass: Harvard University Press; 1984.
20. Rubin HR, Gandek B, Rogers WH, Kosinski M, McHorney CA, Ware JE. Patients' ratings of outpatient visits in different practice settings: results from the Medical Outcomes Study. *JAMA.* 1993;270:835-840.
21. Franks P, Nutting PA, Clancy CM. Health care reform, primary care, and the need for research. *JAMA.* 1993;270:1449-1453.
22. Fletcher RH, Fletcher SW, Wagner EH. *Clinical Epidemiology: The Essentials.* Baltimore, Md: Williams & Wilkins; 1988.
23. Sackett DL, Haynes RB, Tugwell P. *Clinical Epidemiology: A Basic Science for Clinical Medicine.* Boston, Mass: Little Brown & Co Inc; 1985.
24. Smith GR, Monson RA, Ray DC. Psychiatric consultation in somatization disorder: a randomized, controlled study. *N Engl J Med.* 1986;314:1407-1413.
25. Smith GR, Rost K, Kashner TM. A trial of the effect of a standardized psychiatric consultation on health outcomes and costs in somatizing patients. *Arch Gen Psychiatry.* 1995;52:238-243.
26. Katon W, Kleinman A, Rosen G. Depression and somatization: a review: part I. *Am J Med.* 1982;72:127-135.
27. Kroenke K, Mangelsdorff AD. Common symptoms in ambulatory care: incidence, evaluation, therapy, and outcome. *Am J Med.* 1989;86:262-266.
28. Swartz M, Landerman R, George LK, Blazer DG, Escobar JI. Somatization disorder. In: Robins LN, Regier DA, eds. *Psychiatric Disorders in America.* New York, NY: Free Press; 1991:220-257.
29. Ormel J, Von Korff M, Ustun TB, Pini S, Korton A, Oldehinkel T. Common mental disorders and disability across cultures: results from the WHO Collaborative Study on Psychological Problems in General Health Care. *JAMA.* 1994;272:1741-1748.
30. Kellner R. *Psychosomatic Syndromes and Somatic Symptoms.* Washington, DC: American Psychiatric Press; 1991.
31. Goldberg DP, Bridges K. Somatic presentations of psychiatric illness in primary care setting. *J Psychosom Res.* 1988;32:137-144.
32. Barbour AB. *Caring for Patients: A Critique of the Medical Model.* Stanford, Calif: Stanford University Press; 1995.
33. Williams JBW. Psychiatric classification. In: Hales RE, Yudofsky SC, Talbott JA, eds. *The American Psychiatric Press Textbook of Psychiatry.* Washington, DC: American Psychiatric Press; 1994:221-246.

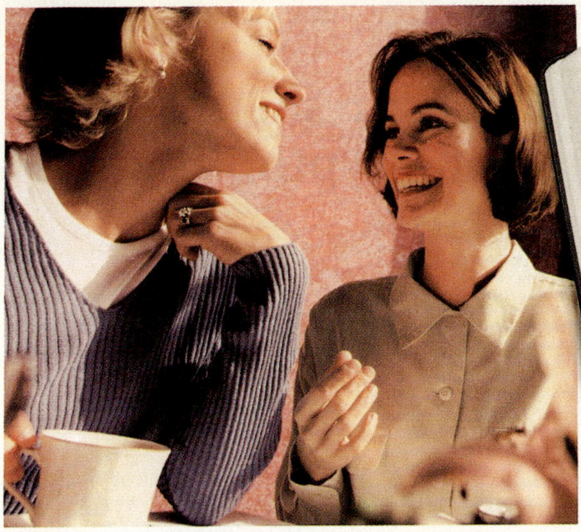

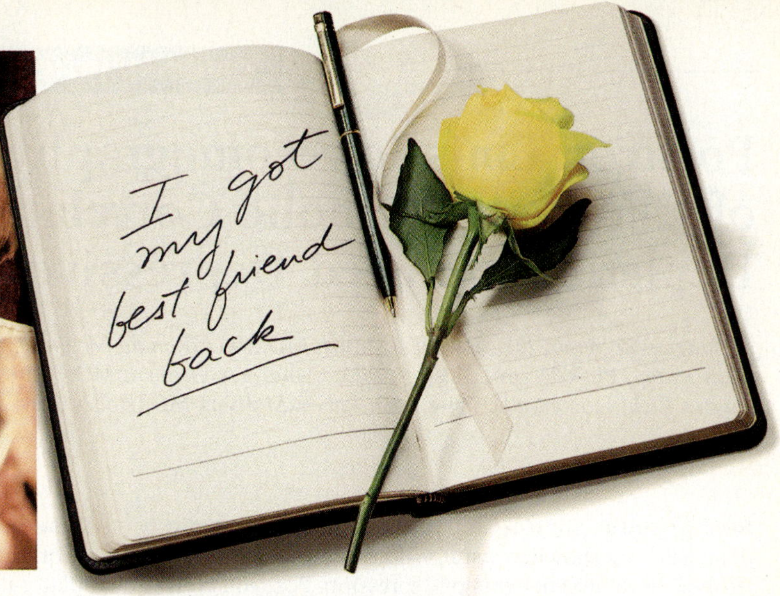

- Efficacy clearly demonstrated in depressed outpatients[6]
- Effective treatment in hospitalized depressed patients with major depressive disorder and melancholia meeting DSM-III-R™ criteria[7]

EFFEXOR is contraindicated in patients taking monoamine oxidase inhibitors (MAOIs). EFFEXOR should not be used in combination with an MAOI or within at least 14 days of discontinuing treatment with an MAOI because of potential for serious adverse reactions. Based on the half-life of EFFEXOR, at least 7 days should be allowed after stopping EFFEXOR before starting an MAOI.

Treatment with EFFEXOR is associated with sustained increases in blood pressure (BP) in some patients. The incidence was seen at >5% at dosages above 200 mg/day and appears to be dose dependent. It is recommended that patients have regular BP monitoring. For patients experiencing a sustained increase in BP, dose reduction or treatment discontinuation should be considered.

Low potential exists for interaction in patients taking lithium, diazepam, or cimetidine.[4]

—In combination with cimetidine, EFFEXOR should be used with caution in patients with preexisting hypertension, or in elderly patients, or in patients with hepatic dysfunction, as the interaction between the two drugs in these patients is not known and could be more pronounced.[6]

EFFEXOR at steady state increased the AUC of a single dose of haloperidol by 70%. The mechanism explaining this finding is unknown.

EFFEXOR is a relatively weak inhibitor of cytochrome P450 2D6.[4]

—Weak inhibition of cytochrome P450 2D6 is an important characteristic when considering other drugs metabolized by this enzyme.[4]

—Potential exists for a drug interaction between EFFEXOR and drugs that inhibit cytochrome P450 2D6 metabolism.[4]

The most common adverse events reported in EFFEXOR clinical trials (incidence >10% and ≥2× that of placebo) were nausea, somnolence, dry mouth, dizziness, constipation, nervousness, sweating, asthenia, abnormal ejaculation/orgasm, and anorexia.

EFFEXOR has not demonstrated any clinically significant impairment of psychomotor, cognitive, or complex behavior performance in healthy volunteers. However, as with any psychotropic drug, EFFEXOR may impair judgment, thinking, or motor skills; patients should be advised to exercise caution until they have adapted to therapy.

Please see brief summary of Prescribing Information on previous page of this advertisement.

Tablets: 25 mg, 37.5 mg, 50 mg, 75 mg, and 100 mg

VENLAFAXINE HCl

EFFEXOR® MEANS EFFECTIVE

Positron Emission Tomography Measurement of Cerebral Metabolic Correlates of Tryptophan Depletion–Induced Depressive Relapse

J. Douglas Bremner, MD; Robert B. Innis, MD, PhD; Ronald M. Salomon, MD; Lawrence H. Staib, PhD; Chin K. Ng, PhD; Helen L. Miller, MD; Richard A. Bronen, MD; John H. Krystal, MD; James Duncan, PhD; Dayton Rich; Lawrence H. Price, MD; Robert Malison, MD; Holley Dey, MD; Robert Soufer, MD; Dennis S. Charney, MD

Background: Short-term depletion of plasma tryptophan has been shown to result in depressive relapse in patients with remission of major depression. Positron emission tomography and single photon emission computed tomography studies implicated the dorsolateral prefrontal cortex, orbitofrontal cortex, thalamus, and caudate nucleus in the pathogenesis of depression. The purpose of this study was to measure cerebral metabolic correlates of tryptophan depletion–induced depressive relapse.

Methods: Patients diagnosed as having major depression (N=21) who clinically improved with serotonin reuptake inhibitors underwent 2 test days involving tryptophan depletion or placebo, followed 6 hours later by positron emission tomography scanning with fludeoxyglucose F18. Brain metabolism was compared in patients with (n=7) and without (n=14) a tryptophan depletion–induced depressive relapse.

Results: Tryptophan depletion resulted in a decrease in brain metabolism in the middle frontal gyrus (dorsolateral prefrontal cortex), thalamus, and orbitofrontal cortex in patients with a depletion-induced depressive relapse (but not in patients without depletion-induced relapse). Decreased brain metabolism in these regions correlated with increased depressive symptoms. Baseline metabolism was increased in prefrontal and limbic regions in relapse-prone patients.

Conclusion: Specific brain regions, including the middle frontal gyrus, thalamus, and orbitofrontal cortex, may mediate the symptoms of patients with major depression.

Arch Gen Psychiatry. 1997;54:364-374

From the Departments of Psychiatry (Drs Bremner, Innis, Salomon, Miller, Krystal, Price, Malison, and Charney) and Diagnostic Radiology (Nuclear Medicine [Drs Bremner, Staib, Ng, Duncan, Dey, and Soufer] and Neuroradiology [Dr Bronen]), Yale University School of Medicine, New Haven, Conn; and the National Center for Posttraumatic Stress Disorder (Drs Bremner, Innis, Krystal, and Charney), West Haven Veterans Affairs Medical Center (Drs Bremner, Innis, Salomon, Ng, Miller, Krystal, Dey, Soufer, and Charney and Mr Rich), and the Yale/Veterans Affairs Positron Emission Tomography Center (Drs Ng, Dey, and Soufer and Mr Rich), West Haven, Conn.

A WIDE range of evidence supports the hypothesis that alterations in central serotonergic function are involved in the pathogenesis of depression,[1-4] with specific findings often characterizing subgroups of patients with major depression.[5] Depression or suicidal behavior, or both, was associated with decreased cerebrospinal fluid levels of the serotonin metabolite 5-hydroxyindoleacetic acid,[6,7] decreased serotonin concentrations in platelets,[8] increased 5-hydroxytryptamine receptor binding in frontal cortex in some studies,[9-12] but not in others,[13] and reduction of prolactin response to the serotonin-releasing agent fenfluramine[14] and the serotonin precursor L-tryptophan.[15,16] Plasma L-tryptophan competes with other competing amino acids (CAAs) for uptake into the brain and is affected by factors that influence L-tryptophan plasma protein binding, such as levels of albumin or insulin.[17] Some studies,[18,19] but not others,[20-22] found a decrease in plasma tryptophan, or the ratio of tryptophan to CAAs in some studies,[18,23-26] but not in others,[20,27] in patients with major depression. Lower tryptophan availability was related to specific depressive symptoms (but not core depressive symptoms),[28] and it predicted treatment response to amitriptyline in some studies,[23] but not in others.[17] Dietary tryptophan depletion,[29-38] which was shown in animals to be associated with a decrease in brain levels of tryptophan, serotonin,[31,32] and 5-hydroxyindoleacetic acid,[33] was associated with depressive relapse in patients with major depression who were in remission with serotonin reuptake inhibitors,[29,37] but not in untreated patients with major depression.[30] Although these studies suggested that reduced serotonin availability in the brain is associated with depressive relapse, they did not provide information about specific brain mechanisms involved in depletion-induced depressive relapse.

Studies using positron emission tomography (PET) and single photon emission computed tomography have

SUBJECTS AND METHODS

SUBJECTS

The patient group comprised 21 patients between the ages of 18 and 65 years with clinically improved major depression who gave informed consent for participation. Patients were recruited by newspaper advertisement or clinician referral and were receiving treatment with outpatient clinicians at the time of the study. Nineteen of the patients were treated with fluoxetine hydrochloride and 2 with paroxetine. Patients were included who met the criteria for major depression based on the Structured Clinical Interview for *DSM-III-R*.[70] Patients were excluded if they had a history of meningitis, traumatic brain injury, loss of consciousness for more than 10 minutes, neurologic disorder, current alcohol or substance abuse or dependence, or schizophrenia based on the Structured Clinical Interview for *DSM-III-R*. Patients had not received benzodiazepines or sedatives for at least 4 weeks before the study. None of the patients had a history of loss of consciousness within the last year. Patients also were excluded if they had a history of foreign bodies that would preclude magnetic resonance imaging (MRI) scanning. Patients with risk factors for human immunodeficiency virus (HIV) infection were screened for HIV; HIV-positive patients were excluded. The patients (10 women and 11 men) had a mean±SD age of 40±7 years. Patients had been in remission and receiving a serotonin reuptake inhibitor from 1 to 335 weeks, with a mean±SD of 44.8±47.9 weeks of remission before participation in the study. Previous depressive events ranged from 0 to more than 10, with a mean±SD of 1.86±1.31 events. Eighteen of 21 patients had at least 1 previous episode of depression. Inpatient hospitalizations for depression ranged from 0 to 10 (mean±SD, 1.86±2.38).

Patients were evaluated with the Structured Clinical Interview for *DSM-III-R* for comorbid psychiatric diagnoses. All patients met criteria for a lifetime history of major depression. Eighteen (86%) of 21 patients had recurrent depression. Four (19%) of 21 patients met criteria for a lifetime history of panic disorder without agoraphobia, 1 (5%) for social phobia, 1 (5%) for simple phobia, 1 (5%) for anorexia, and 1 (5%) for bulimia. No patients had lifetime or current posttraumatic stress, generalized anxiety, obsessive-compulsive, bipolar, somatization, somatic pain, or undifferentiated somatization disorders; schizophrenia; dysthymia; or hypochondriasis. Three (14%) of 21 patients met criteria for a lifetime history of alcohol abuse, 4 (19%) of 21 for a lifetime history of alcohol dependence, 3 (14%) of 21 for polysubstance abuse, and 1 (5%) of 21 for polysubstance dependence. None of the patients met criteria for current alcohol or substance abuse, or for lifetime or current cannabis, sedative, hypnotic, anxiolytic, stimulant, opiate, cocaine, hallucinogen, or phencyclidine hydrochloride dependence or abuse.

PROCEDURES

Patients underwent 2 PET scanning days separated by 1 week, 1 following tryptophan depletion and the other following placebo. Tryptophan depletion and placebo were administered in a double-blind, placebo-controlled fashion, with randomized order of assignment. The tryptophan depletion day consisted of a 24-hour, 160 mg/d tryptophan diet (day 1) with blue placebo capsules taken 3 times daily, followed the next morning by a tryptophan-free, 15–amino acid drink (day 2). The amino acids consumed were L-alanine, 5.5 g; L-arginine, 4.9 g; L-cysteine, 2.7 g; L-glycine, 3.2 g; L-histidine, 3.2 g; L-isoleucine, 8.0 g; L-leucine, 13.5 g; L-lysine monohydrochloride, 11.0 g; L-methionine, 3.0 g; L-phenylalanine, 5.7 g; L-proline, 12.2 g; L-serine, 6.9 g; L-threonine, 6.9 g; L-tyrosine, 6.9 g; and L-valine, 8.9 g. Control testing consisted of a 24-hour, 160-mg/d tryptophan diet supplemented with blue capsules containing 500 mg of L-tryptophan taken 3 times daily, followed the next morning by a 16–amino acid drink containing L-tryptophan, 2.3 g, in addition to the aforementioned 15 amino acids.[71]

Patients underwent behavioral ratings, and plasma for free and total tryptophan levels was obtained at 9 AM before starting the diet (test day 1), 15 minutes before, and 5 and 7 hours after the drink (test day 2). Ratings were obtained again between 11 AM and 1 PM after each amino acid drink (the day after testing). Ratings were obtained by 1 of us (R.M.S.) or by a trained nurse-clinician. Raters had established reliability on the rating instruments used (interrater reliability for Hamilton Depression Scale (Ham-D) ranged from 88% to 95%) and were blinded to the sequence of placebo or active tryptophan supplementation.

Behavioral rating scales consisted of the Ham-D, the Hamilton Anxiety Scale, and the Symptom Checklist. A depressive relapse was defined as a 50% and a 9-point increase from baseline on the Ham-D. Seven patients met criteria for a depressive relapse with depletion, and 14 patients did not meet criteria. One patient had a depressive relapse with placebo.

BIOCHEMICAL METHODS

Total plasma tryptophan concentration was assayed by high-performance liquid chromatography with fluorometric detection as previously described.[21] Free plasma tryptophan concentration was assayed by obtaining the ultrafiltrate of plasma through a commercially available anisotropic, hydrophilic ultrafiltration membrane system (Amicon Inc, Beverly, Mass.) centrifuged (1000*g*) at room temperature and subjecting the ultrafiltrate to the high-performance liquid chromatography with fluorometric detection method. Plasma tryptophan levels were unavailable in 4 patients (1 with a tryptophan depletion–induced depressive relapse, and 3 without).

PET SCANNING METHODS

All subjects underwent 2 days of testing as described. The PET scans took place 6 hours after administration of the tryptophan-depleting low amino acid drink or placebo. Subjects were placed in the positron camera (Posicam 6.5, Positron Corp, Houston, Tex, at the Yale Veterans Affairs Positron Emission Tomography Center, West Haven, Conn), with the head positioned along the canthomeatal line and immobilized with head and chin straps. The Posicam 6.5 is a 21-slice camera with 5.125-mm interslice distance. The inherent resolution of the camera in-plane is 5.8 mm and 11.9 mm in the z-axis.[72] After application of the Butterworth filter, the in-plane resolution of the camera,

Continued on next page

measured as full-width half-maximum, is 7.5 mm. The sensitivity of the camera, measured in a 20-cm diameter cylinder phantom, can be expressed as the system sensitivity (165 kcounts/s per microcurie per cubic centimeter); slice sensitivity (9.5 kcounts/s per microcurie per cubic centimeter); or the sensitivity/axial cm (8.0 kcounts/μCi per cubic centimeter per axial centimeter).[72]

An intravenous line was inserted in the hand and warmed with heating pads for measurement of arterialized venous blood samples. This method has been shown to yield equivalent values of metabolism to arterial line placement.[73] A 10-minute ^{67}Ga/^{68}Ge rod transmission scan was performed for attenuation correction. Subjects then received an injection of 185 MBq of fludeoxyglucose F18 in a single intravenous bolus and were scanned for 60 minutes with eyes open in a dimly lit room. Arterialized venous blood samples were obtained at 23 time points after injection and spun down for measurement of radioactivity in plasma, which was used in the measurement of the plasma time-activity curve. A PET image was reconstructed 30 to 50 minutes after injection to determine brain tissue activity. Brain and tissue time-activity curves were then combined for measurement of cerebral glucose metabolic rate in milligrams per minute per 100 mL using the fixed rate constant approach of Sokoloff et al.[74] Separate kinetic rate constants were used for gray and white matter.[75]

PET IMAGE PROCESSING

Images were attenuation-corrected based on the transmission scan and reconstructed using a spatially varying convolution scatter subtraction technique and a Butterworth filter. A 20-cm cylindrical, fluid-filled phantom was scanned on the same day as each study to obtain a calibration factor for each of the 21 slices obtained with the PET camera for conversion of radioactivity in the PET image into units of microcuries per milliliter.

Magnetic resonance imaging scans were obtained in all subjects for coregistration with PET and determination of regions of interest (ROIs) from MRI scans subsequently resliced to correspond to the PET. The head was positioned with the canthomeatal line aligned with the laser light for reproducibility of data acquisition and to create MRI scans in the same plane as the PET images. Magnetic resonance imaging scans of 3-mm contiguous slices were obtained with a 1.5-T scanner (Signa, General Electric, Milwaukee, Wis). Axial images were acquired with a spoiled gradient recall acquisition in the steady state sequence with repetition time=25 milliseconds, echo time=5 milliseconds, number of excitations=2, matrix 256×256, and field of view=24 cm. The PET and MRI scans were transferred using a computer network to a SUN Sparc10 Workstation (SUN Microsystems, Mountain View, Calif). A surface-matching algorithm running under Analyze[76] was used for coregistration of PET and MRI scans. In this method, the surface of the brain is first identified in the PET image and in the corresponding MRI scan. A distance transform is calculated from the MRI scan using a Chamfer algorithm. The distance transform of an image is an image in which the value at each pixel is equal to the distance to the nearest surface point in the original image. The distance image values can then be summed at each point on the other transformed surface (or set of points) to give the total distance between the surfaces. The best transformation is then determined by minimizing the total distance using local gradient descent.[77] The MRI was then resliced to obtain 21 MRI slices, each of which corresponded to 1 of the 21 PET slices. Studies from our group using this surface-matching method and brain phantom data have had a registration error of 2.2 pixels (2.86 mm).[78]

MEASUREMENT OF ROIs

Measurements of ROIs on MRI were performed using specific criteria developed in conjunction with a

implicated specific brain regions in the pathogenesis of depression.[39-66] Some PET and SPECT studies,[41-44] but not others,[45,61] showed decreased global brain metabolism and blood flow in untreated unipolar depressives at baseline. Multiple PET and SPECT studies found decreased metabolism or blood flow, or both, in left[41,45,48,57] and bilateral[46,47,53,56,60] dorsolateral prefrontal cortex. Other PET and SPECT studies in patients with unipolar depression showed decreased metabolism or blood flow, or both, in caudate,[44,47,50,53,54] thalamus,[47] temporal,[47,50,53,55] cingulate,[48,53] parietal cortex,[47,50,60] and left putamen regions,[47] but orbitofrontal metabolism was increased[60] or unchanged.[66] Positron emission tomography studies in patients with Huntington[40] or Parkinson disease[49,65] and comorbid depression also showed decreased metabolism or blood flow, or both, in the prefrontal cortex,[40,49,65] orbitofrontal cortex,[40,49] and anterior cingulate region.[65] Treatment of depression was associated with a reversal of these metabolism and blood flow deficits.[64] Antidepressants increased metabolism or blood flow, or both, in the left prefrontal cortex in some studies,[41,45] but not in others,[50,56] and increased blood flow in anterior cingulate, right putamen, and right thalamus regions.[59] Sleep deprivation–induced improvement in depression was associated with increased baseline metabolism or blood flow, or both, in anterior cingulate,[61] amygdala,[57,61,63] orbitofrontal,[57,63] hippocampus,[57,63] and infratemporal regions,[57,63] but sleep deprivation in sleep responders resulted in a decrease in cingulate metabolism.[61] Treatment response to electroconvulsive therapy also was correlated with blood flow changes in cingulate cortex[58] and anterior frontal cortex.[62]

These findings led to the hypothesis that dysfunction of a circuit involving these regions mediates the symptoms of depression.[39,50] One PET study, however, found increased blood flow in unipolar depressives in left prefrontal cortex, left amygdala, and bilateral thalamus.[50] The authors hypothesized that rumination on depressive themes may have contributed to the increased blood flow. Consistent with this idea, active rumination on depressive themes in healthy subjects was associated with increased blood flow in prefrontal[51,52] and orbitofrontal cortex, caudate nucleus, putamen, and thalamus.[51] The use of a within-subjects design, in which subjects undergo scanning at baseline and after the experimental induction of depression with a technique such as tryptophan neuroradiologist (R.A.B.). These criteria were developed for reproducibility of measurements between observers and to have criteria based on an anatomical atlas that allows for the use of a common terminology and that is available to general access.[79] The criteria for ROIs use anatomical landmarks located on the individual subject's MRI to allow for decision-making in the measurement of ROIs that follow specific guidelines and are therefore reproducible. Regions of interest were drawn on the resliced MRI using a mouse-driven cursor by an operator blinded to subject identity and diagnosis. Templates for ROIs drawn on the MRI were transferred to the PET. Multiple brain regions were selected for analysis (**Table 1**). When a specific region was present in multiple slices as determined by these criteria, the mean of activity measured in each of these slices was determined. Global brain metabolism was calculated by obtaining the mean of brain tissue activity in all slices of the brain. Brain tissue activity determined from the coregistered scan was used in the determination of regional cerebral glucose metabolic rate. Normalization for global metabolic rate was performed by dividing metabolism in an individual region by global metabolism. We have recently tested these ROI criteria with 3 raters performing measurements on 11 fludeoxyglucose F18 scans coregistered with MRI. There was a high level of agreement between raters, with intraclass correlation coefficients ranging from 0.63 to 0.98. Intraclass correlation values for 3 of the hypothesized regions in this study were middle frontal gyrus (r=0.95), thalamus (r=0.85), and orbital cortex (r=0.78) (J.D.B., Gabriel De Erasquin, MD, Eric Vermetten, MD, et al, unpublished data, January 10, 1996, available on request).

DATA ANALYSIS

Specific ROIs were selected a priori as regions that were expected to change based on aforementioned neuroimaging and preclinical studies. The rationale was to include regions forwhich there were clinical and preclinical (increased metabolism with serotonergic stimulation) findings to support their role in depression. The primary region that was hypothesized to change was middle frontal gyrus, based on convergent evidence from aforementioned multiple sources, supporting a role for this region in depression. Other regions that were hypothesized to change were orbitofrontal cortex (studies showed decreased metabolism at baseline and a correlation with Ham-D score in secondary depression) and thalamus (decreased activity at baseline and increased metabolism with serotonergic stimulation in preclinical studies[67,68]). Two or more PET studies have found a decrease in caudate metabolism at baseline, although preclinical studies have shown no change in caudate metabolism with stimulation of serotonergic neurons.[67,68] Other regions given in Table 1 were examined because clinical evidence existed for their involvement in depression, for theoretical reasons to suggest their involvement, for purposes of comparison, or for exploratory purposes.

Data were analyzed for regional brain metabolic rates following administration of placebo or tryptophan depletion using a repeated measures analysis of variance (ANOVA) with depletion (tryptophan depletion vs placebo) as the repeated factor, and relapse status (patients with a relapse on the depletion day vs patients without a relapse on the depletion day) and hemisphere (left vs right) as factors in the analysis. Bonferroni corrections (dividing P value of .05 by the number of repeated measures comparisons, in this case P=.05/20=.003) were used to correct for multiple comparisons. Spearman rank order correlations were used to examine the relation between score on the Ham-D and brain metabolic response to tryptophan depletion. Normalization of regional metabolism for global metabolism was obtained by dividing regional metabolism by global metabolism.

depletion, would help resolve some of these state-related questions in a way that is impossible by scanning only at baseline.

The purpose of the present study was to examine brain metabolic correlates of tryptophan depletion–induced depressive relapse in patients with major depression who were in remission and receiving antidepressants. Studies in animals showed that electrical stimulation of the serotonergic system (rostral raphe nuclei) results in an increase in brain metabolism in thalamus,[67] the extrapyramidal system,[67,68] and other regions,[68] but PET fludeoxyglucose F18 studies showed increased brain metabolism with fenfluramine in prefrontal cortex in healthy human subjects.[69] Based on these findings and those already discussed, we hypothesized that tryptophan depletion–induced depressive relapse would be associated with decreases in metabolism in middle frontal gyrus (dorsolateral prefrontal cortex), orbitofrontal cortex, thalamus, and caudate nucleus regions. We also hypothesized that changes in regional brain metabolism would distinguish patients with depletion-induced depressive relapse from patients without depletion-induced depressive relapse.

RESULTS

EFFECTS OF TRYPTOPHAN DEPLETION ON REGIONAL CEREBRAL METABOLISM

Metabolism was decreased or unchanged with tryptophan depletion in all 7 of the patients with depletion-induced relapse (but not in patients without depletion-induced relapse) in thalamus (**Figure 1**) and middle frontal gyrus (**Figure 2**). Tryptophan depletion also reduced orbitofrontal cortex metabolism in the patients who experienced relapse (Table 1). Repeated measures ANOVA showed a significant interaction after correction for multiple comparisons between depletion status (depletion vs placebo) and relapse status (relapsers vs nonrelapsers) in these regions for absolute (Figures 1 and 2) and globally normalized (**Figure 3** and **Figure 4**) metabolism (P<.003). A significant correlation was seen between decrease in absolute and normalized metabolism and increase in depressive symptoms in these regions (**Figure 5** and **Figure 6**).

Tryptophan depletion had a tendency to decrease metabolism in a number of nonhypothesized regions in

Table 1. Metabolic Rates in Patients With and Without a Depletion-Induced Relapse*

	Patients						Depletion-Relapse Interaction	
	With Relapse (n=7)			Without Relapse (n=14)				
Brain Region	Placebo	Tryptophan Depletion	% Change	Placebo	Tryptophan Depletion	% Change	F	*P*
Brain Regions Hypothesized to Change With Tryptophan Depletion								
Thalamus	8.04 (3.07)	5.01 (0.98)	−37.69	5.39 (1.59)	6.53 (2.28)	21.15	23.39	<.001†
Middle frontal cortex	10.54 (3.19)	7.36 (1.43)	−30.17	7.59 (1.82)	9.54 (3.25)	25.69	16.06	<.001‡
Orbital cortex	7.77 (3.75)	4.92 (1.43)	−36.68	4.94 (1.93)	6.51 (3.30)	31.78	29.31	<.001†‡§
Caudate	10.01 (3.75)	6.47 (1.91)	−35.36	7.22 (1.90)	8.78 (3.14)	21.61	11.79	<.001
Normalized to Whole-Brain Metabolism								
Thalamus	1.26 (0.28)	0.95 (0.21)	−24.60	0.99 (0.20)	1.00 (0.20)	1.01	15.53	<.001†
Middle frontal cortex	1.71 (0.37)	1.41 (0.37)	−17.54	1.40 (0.19)	1.46 (0.29)	4.29	17.66	<.001†
Orbital cortex	1.19 (0.49)	0.81 (0.21)	−31.93	0.86 (0.20)	0.97 (0.30)	12.79	11.65	<.002
Caudate	1.60 (0.45)	1.25 (0.43)	−21.88	1.33 (0.23)	1.34 (0.25)	0.75	8.72	.005
Brain Regions Not Hypothesized to Change With Tryptophan Depletion								
Occipital cortex	8.31 (3.40)	6.87 (1.15)	−17.33	7.02 (1.45)	8.71 (2.90)	24.07	9.23	.004
Temporal cortex	9.23 (3.17)	7.00 (0.88)	−24.16	7.30 (1.77)	8.68 (2.75)	18.90	10.56	.002
Parietal cortex	9.74 (3.70)	7.43 (1.57)	−23.72	7.61 (1.43)	9.55 (2.95)	25.49	13.75	<.001
Postcentral gyrus	9.60 (3.82)	7.25 (1.26)	−24.48	6.81 (1.38)	8.53 (2.69)	25.26	16.11	<.001
Anteromedial frontal cortex	9.76 (3.98)	6.95 (0.96)	−28.79	6.81 (1.66)	8.35 (2.86)	22.61	13.50	<.001
Inferior frontal gyrus	10.10 (3.38)	7.48 (1.94)	−25.94	7.76 (2.10)	9.15 (2.95)	17.91	8.50	.006
Cingulate	8.74 (3.88)	7.06 (1.88)	−19.22	6.72 (1.49)	8.58 (2.93)	27.68	10.21	<.003
Globus pallidus	6.07 (2.78)	4.92 (1.86)	−18.95	4.52 (2.48)	5.63 (2.48)	24.56	5.32	.03
Putamen	11.63 (3.43)	7.89 (1.91)	−32.16	8.49 (2.26)	10.22 (3.35)	20.38	16.01	<.001
Parahippocampal gyrus	6.99 (2.44)	5.38 (1.13)	−23.03	4.67 (1.62)	5.39 (2.25)	15.42	7.07	.01
Hippocampus	6.56 (2.09)	4.83 (1.43)	−26.37	4.67 (1.69)	5.15 (2.35)	10.28	5.56	.02†‡
Amygdala	5.75 (2.40)	4.10 (0.84)	−28.70	3.98 (1.50)	4.35 (2.01)	9.30	5.72	.02
Pons	4.62 (1.92)	3.55 (1.31)	−23.16	2.85 (1.03)	3.79 (1.97)	32.98	7.92	.01‡
Midbrain	5.25 (2.30)	3.86 (1.15)	−26.48	3.32 (1.06)	3.92 (2.02)	18.07	7.10	.01
Cerebellum	7.84 (2.62)	6.20 (1.10)	−20.92	5.89 (1.66)	6.92 (2.31)	17.49	8.68	.005
White matter	5.26 (1.59)	4.12 (0.93)	−21.67	4.62 (1.55)	5.34 (2.74)	15.58	3.61	.06
Global	8.70 (2.59)	7.08 (0.85)	−18.62	7.46 (1.88)	8.65 (2.73)	15.95	3.86	.06
Normalized to Whole-Brain Metabolism								
Occipital cortex	1.28 (0.19)	1.30 (0.23)	1.56	1.30 (0.12)	1.34 (0.22)	3.08	0.13	.72
Temporal cortex	1.47 (0.30)	1.32 (0.21)	−10.20	1.34 (0.16)	1.33 (0.21)	−0.75	3.66	.06
Parietal cortex	1.51 (0.20)	1.39 (0.18)	−7.95	1.42 (0.16)	1.48 (0.18)	4.23	10.11	.003
Postcentral gyrus	1.49 (0.27)	1.36 (0.17)	−8.72	1.26 (0.15)	1.31 (0.20)	3.97	4.81	.03
Anteromedial frontal cortex	1.51 (0.20)	1.32 (0.26)	−12.58	1.26 (0.14)	1.26 (0.22)	0.00	7.27	.01†‡
Inferior frontal gyrus	1.62 (0.34)	1.45 (0.49)	−10.49	1.43 (0.26)	1.41 (0.27)	−1.40	2.02	.16
Cingulate	1.34 (0.34)	1.31 (0.25)	−2.24	1.25 (0.18)	1.33 (0.23)	6.40	1.64	.21
Globus pallidus	0.95 (0.26)	0.93 (0.34)	−2.11	0.84 (0.23)	0.82 (0.26)	−2.38	0.16	.69
Putamen	1.87 (0.36)	1.49 (0.35)	−20.32	1.57 (0.25)	1.57 (0.23)	0.00	14.82	<.001†
Parahippocampal gyrus	1.11 (0.22)	1.02 (0.25)	−8.11	0.84 (0.29)	0.85 (0.20)	1.19	0.57	.45†
Hippocampus	1.05 (0.23)	0.92 (0.29)	−12.38	0.78 (0.25)	0.85 (0.19)	8.97	0.47	.50
Amygdala	0.90 (0.20)	0.78 (0.19)	−13.33	0.68 (0.23)	0.72 (0.15)	5.88	0.72	.40‡
Pons	0.76 (0.37)	0.67 (0.21)	−11.84	0.52 (0.13)	0.57 (0.20)	9.62	2.01	.16
Midbrain	0.80 (0.14)	0.72 (0.18)	−10.00	0.61 (0.12)	0.59 (0.23)	−3.28	1.00	.32‡
Cerebellum	1.24 (0.21)	1.17 (0.17)	−5.65	1.07 (0.12)	1.07 (0.17)	0.00	1.91	.18
White matter	0.85 (0.22)	0.77 (0.15)	−9.41	0.85 (0.25)	0.81 (0.30)	−4.71	0.15	.70

*Metabolic rates are given as mean (±SD) milligrams of glucose per minute per 100 mL.
†Patients who experienced relapse had a decrease in metabolism with depletion compared with placebo (P<.003).
‡Patients who experienced relapse had higher metabolic rates at baseline (placebo day) compared with patients who did not (P<.003).
§Patients who did not experience relapse had an increase in metabolism with depletion compared with placebo (P<.003).

the patients who experienced relapse (Table 1). The effect of depletion on metabolism normalized to global metabolism is therefore an important variable to examine. Of the nonhypothesized regions, there was a significant effect after correction for multiple comparisons only for putamen. However, middle frontal gyrus, thalamus, and orbitofrontal cortex were the only regions that showed a reduction after correction for multiple comparisons and a correlation with change in depressive symptoms for absolute and normalized metabolism (putamen did not show a significant correlation with changes in depressive symptoms).

An unexpected finding was an increase in baseline metabolism (placebo day) in patients with depletion-induced relapse compared with patients without a depletion-induced relapse. This finding was significant for absolute

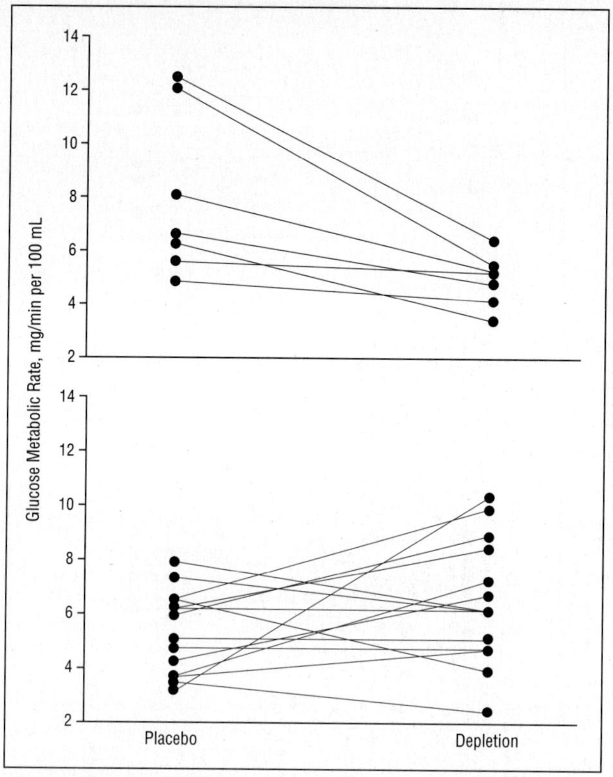

Figure 1. *Regional metabolism in the thalamus in patients with tryptophan depletion–induced depressive relapse (top) and without depressive relapse (bottom). Tryptophan depletion resulted in a decrease in brain metabolism in the thalamus for the patients with relapse compared with patients without relapse.*

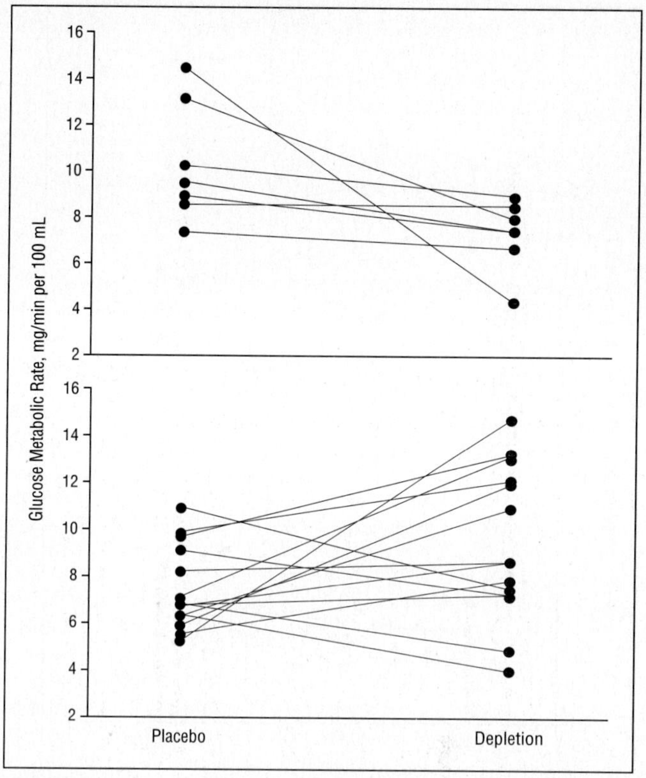

Figure 2. *Regional metabolism in the middle frontal gyrus in patients with tryptophan depletion–induced depressive relapse (top) and without depressive relapse (bottom). Tryptophan depletion resulted in a decrease in brain metabolism in the middle frontal gyrus for the patients with relapse compared with patients without relapse.*

metabolism in middle frontal gyrus, orbitofrontal cortex, hippocampus, and pons, and for globally normalized metabolism in amygdala, parahippocampal gyrus, anteromedial frontal cortex, and midbrain ($P<.003$).

ASSOCIATIONS BETWEEN VARIABLES

Ham-D Scores and Brain Metabolic Response to Tryptophan Depletion

Hamilton Depression Scale scores for patients with and without depletion-induced relapse are given in **Table 2**. Change in Ham-D score with tryptophan depletion was associated with changes in brain metabolism. We examined the relation between change from baseline in Ham-D score on the depletion day (minus the change from baseline on the placebo day) and placebo-subtracted metabolism on the depletion day. Increased baseline-subtracted scores on the Ham-D on the depletion day relative to the placebo day were associated with decreased brain metabolism on the depletion day relative to the placebo day in thalamus ($r=-0.66$, $df=20$; $P=.001$) (Figure 5), middle frontal gyrus ($r=-0.53$, $df=20$; $P=.01$) (Figure 6), and orbitofrontal cortex ($r=-0.55$, $df=20$; $P=.01$). Significant correlations were seen for these brain regions for left and right sides. Correlations between Ham-D scores and regional metabolism normalized for whole brain metabolism were found for thalamus ($r=-0.75$, $df=20$; $P<.001$), middle frontal gyrus ($r=-0.58$, $df=20$; $P=.006$), and orbitofrontal cortex ($r=-0.48$, $df=20$; $P=.02$), but not for any of the other regions measured in this study.

Plasma Tryptophan Levels With Tryptophan Depletion, Behavior, and Regional Brain Metabolism

Tryptophan depletion resulted in a marked reduction of plasma tryptophan levels in all patients. No difference was seen in free or total tryptophan levels between patients with and without a tryptophan depletion–induced depressive relapse at any time point on the placebo or the tryptophan depletion day (**Table 3**). The magnitude of reduction of free or total plasma tryptophan levels also was not different between patients with or without a depletion-induced depressive relapse. We did not find a correlation between change in brain metabolism (in any brain region) with depletion and magnitude of reduction of plasma free or total tryptophan.

Clinical Variables, Relapse Status, and Regional Brain Metabolism

No difference was seen in age between patients with a depletion-induced depressive relapse (mean±SD, 39±7 years) and patients without a depletion-induced depressive relapse (41±6 years). Two (20%) of the 10 women and 5 (45%) of the 11 men had a depressive relapse. Six (33%) of 18 patients with recurrent depression had a depressive relapse and 1 (33%) of 3 patients with first-time depression had a depressive relapse. One (14%) of

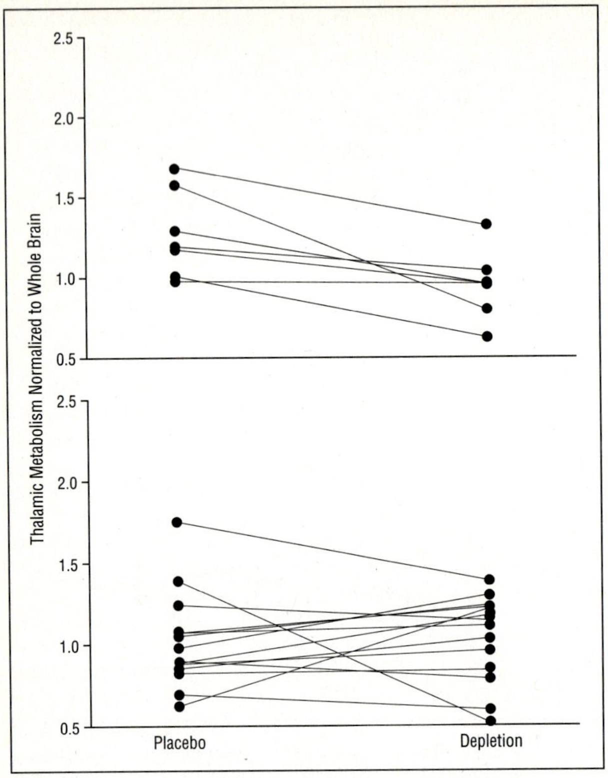

Figure 3. *Regional metabolism in the thalamus normalized to global metabolism in patients with tryptophan depletion–induced depressive relapse (top) and without depressive relapse (bottom). Tryptophan depletion resulted in a decrease in normalized brain metabolism in the thalamus for the patients with relapse compared with patients without relapse.*

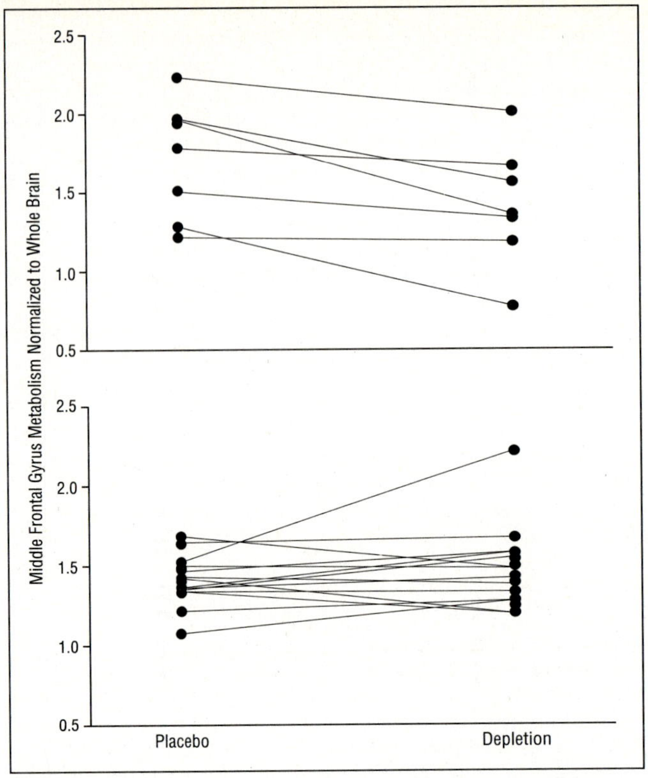

Figure 4. *Regional metabolism in the middle frontal gyrus normalized to global brain metabolism in patients with tryptophan depletion–induced depressive relapse (top) and without depressive relapse (bottom). Tryptophan depletion resulted in a decrease in globally normalized brain metabolism in the middle frontal gyrus for the patients with relapse compared with patients without relapse.*

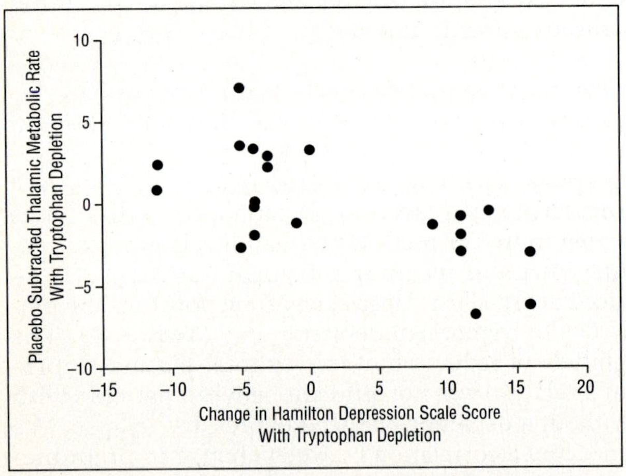

Figure 5. *Relation between change in Hamilton Depression Scale score and change in brain metabolism in the thalamus. Increases in baseline-subtracted Hamilton Depression Scale score were correlated with decreases in thalamic brain metabolism with tryptophan depletion* ($r = -0.66$, $df = 20$; $P = .001$).

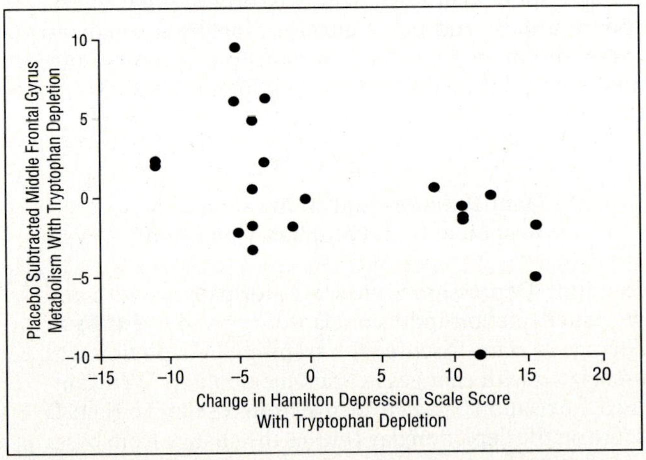

Figure 6. *Relation between change in Hamilton Depression Scale score and change in brain metabolism in the middle frontal gyrus. Increases in baseline-subtracted Hamilton Depression Scale score were correlated with decreases in middle frontal gyrus brain metabolism with tryptophan depletion* ($r = -0.53$, $df = 20$; $P = .01$).

7 patients with a lifetime history of alcohol abuse or dependence had a depressive relapse and 6 (43%) of 14 patients without a lifetime history of alcohol abuse or dependence had a depressive relapse. We did not find a difference in brain metabolic response to tryptophan depletion between men and women. We did not find a correlation between brain metabolic response to tryptophan depletion and number of weeks the patient had been in remission (clinically improved) from depression, number of previous episodes of depression, or number of hospitalizations for depression. Nine of the patients had tryptophan depletion on day 1; 11 had placebo on day 1. There was no difference in brain metabolic response to tryptophan depletion between patients who had depletion on the first or second day (ie, no order effect).

COMMENT

Tryptophan depletion was associated with a decrease in absolute and globally normalized brain metabolism in thalamus, middle frontal gyrus, and orbitofrontal cortex in patients with a tryptophan depletion–induced depressive relapse, but not in patients without a tryptophan depletion–induced depressive relapse. These regions were hypothesized to change based on previous studies. Tryptophan depletion had a tendency to decrease metabolism in several regions in the patients who experienced relapse, but the only nonhypothesized region in which this reached statistical significance was for putamen. Decreases in normalized brain metabolism were correlated with increases in Ham-D score for thalamus, middle frontal gyrus, and orbitofrontal cortex (but not putamen or other regions). In addition, increased baseline metabolism was seen in patients prone to depletion-induced relapse, which made a substantial contribution to the difference between patients who experienced relapse and those who did not. The variation in metabolism in these regions on the placebo day vs the tryptophan depletion day (33%) was greater in magnitude than the normal variation found in test-retest within subjects for PET fludeoxyglucose F18 (7%).[80,81]

Previous studies showed alterations in function as measured by brain metabolism and blood flow primarily in middle frontal gyrus (dorsolateral prefrontal cortex),[39,82] but also in limbic (orbitofrontal cortex, cingulate, thalamus, and amygdala) and striatal (caudate and putamen) regions. Normal subjects showed an activation during states of sadness, although most studies showed that depressed patients have decreased function in these regions when they are actively depressed, and our current findings show a reduction with depletion-induced relapse compared with baseline. This discrepancy may be explainable by the hypothesis that essential differences exist in brain function between normal subjects and patients with depression. Prefrontal cortex-limbic-striatal regions[83,84] comprise a functional circuit that may mediate normal dysphoria. This circuit may function abnormally in patients with depression (as previously hypothesized[39,50]), and this dysfunction may play a role in the pathogenesis of depression. Fundamental differences also may exist between induced sadness in normal subjects, which involves active rumination on sad themes, and symptoms of depression in the pathological states, which is essentially a passive process. In the single study of depressed patients that showed an increase in blood flow in prefrontal and limbic regions, the authors speculated that active rumination on depressive themes in their patients may have accounted for their discrepant findings.[50] A fundamental difference in base line brain function between normal subjects and patients with depression also may explain increased me-

Table 2. Hamilton Depression Scale Scores With Tryptophan Depletion and Placebo in Patients With and Without a Depletion-Induced Relapse*

	Patients			
	With Relapse (n=7)		Without Relapse (n=14)	
Test Time	Placebo	Tryptophan Depletion	Placebo	Tryptophan Depletion
Day				
1: 8 AM baseline	4.71 (2.98)	5.00 (4.20)	5.71 (4.79)	6.28 (4.95)
2: 8 AM baseline	7.00 (5.45)	6.86 (4.98)	6.21 (4.69)	4.79 (3.45)
2: 6 h postdrink	6.71 (6.07)	15.57 (6.92)†	9.21 (5.99)	6.36 (4.25)§
3: 8 AM	7.86 (6.61)	12.29 (7.39)‡	6.07 (4.55)	4.64 (2.59)‖

*Values are given as mean (±SD) score.

†Within patients with relapse only on the tryptophan-depletion day; significant increase from baseline: $t=3.45$, $df=12$; $P<.05$.

‡Within patients with relapse only on the tryptophan-depletion day; significant increase from baseline: $t=2.27$, $df=12$; $P=.04$.

§Difference between patients with and without relapse on the tryptophan-depletion day: $t=3.7$, $df=19$; $P<.01$.

‖Difference between patients with and without relapse on the tryptophan-depletion day: $t=2.75$, $df=19$; $P=.03$.

Table 3. Plasma Free and Total Tryptophan Levels With Tryptophan Depletion*

	Patients			
	With Relapse (n=7)		Without Relapse (n=14)	
Test Time	Placebo	Tryptophan Depletion	Placebo	Tryptophan Depletion
Plasma free tryptophan				
Day				
1: 8 AM baseline	1.85 (0.43)	1.70 (0.52)	2.05 (0.58)	1.99 (0.50)
2: 8 AM baseline	2.10 (0.50)	1.63 (0.51)	2.46 (0.81)	1.88 (0.51)
2: 6 h postdrink	4.56 (1.06)	0.36 (0.23)†	3.72 (2.18)	0.80 (1.00)†
3: 8 AM	1.96 (0.27)	1.76 (0.24)	2.02 (1.10)	1.88 (0.38)
Total tryptophan				
Day				
1: 8 AM baseline	11.23 (1.48)	11.33 (2.31)	10.63 (2.68)	10.17 (2.07)
2: 8 AM baseline	11.16 (1.50)	10.10 (2.93)	11.49 (2.03)	9.65 (2.13)
2: 6 h postdrink	16.88 (4.23)	1.61 (1.17)†	11.98 (5.35)	2.30 (2.87)†
3: 8 AM	11.20 (1.09)	10.35 (3.16)	9.52 (2.06)	9.44 (1.91)

*Values are given as mean (±SD) micrograms per milliliter of tryptophan.

†Significant decrease compared with baseline ($P\leq.05$).

tabolism at baseline in prefrontal and limbic regions in certain subgroups of patients with depression, including patients who have improvement in symptoms with sleep deprivation and patients vulnerable to tryptophan depletion–induced depressive relapse. In the case of the tryptophan-depletion findings, patients with depression who are in the "compensated" nonsymptomatic state have increased function, indicating that although they are not actively depressed, their brain function is different from normal, perhaps due to adaptive changes. Challenge to the system with tryptophan depletion leads to a decompensation, with a reduction in metabolism toward the level seen in patients with baseline depression, and an associated increase in depressive symptoms. Patients who respond to sleep deprivation have increased baseline function in orbitofrontal cortex, cingulate, and other limbic regions, with a reduction in cingulate function as their symptoms improve. These discrepant findings do not support the idea that all states of sadness or depression are associated with reduced prefrontal and limbic function from baseline. Rather, diversions from the normal pattern in these regions at baseline and during affective changes seem to be characteristic of patients with depression, even in the compensated nonsymptomatic state for at least a subgroup of patients.

Our study has several limitations. Our rates of depressive relapse were lower than those previously reported. Our method of normalization for global metabolism involved whole brain slice measurements, which include areas such as the ventricles, which have no functional brain tissue. The use of a conservative Bonferroni correction for multiple comparisons creates the possibility that regions that showed true changes after correction for global changes may not have been identified as statistically significant. This limits our ability to conclude that depletion-induced relapse results in specific decreases in thalamus, middle frontal gyrus, and orbitofrontal cortex. In fact, several nonhypothesized regions showed substantial reductions with depletion.

We did not find a relation between free or total L-tryptophan levels in the plasma and brain metabolism. In addition, plasma free and total L-tryptophan levels were reduced to an equal extent in patients with and without a depletion-induced depressive relapse. We did not, however, measure CAAs, which compete with L-tryptophan for uptake into the brain, or proteins such as albumin, which affect L-tryptophan binding. In addition, loading with CAAs and lowering L-tryptophan levels will induce changes in hormones such as insulin and glucagon (not measured in the present study) that will affect L-tryptophan uptake and possibly have behavioral or metabolic effects of their own. These factors limit the formation of definite conclusions about the relation among plasma L-tryptophan level, depressed mood, and brain metabolism. If plasma free L-tryptophan is related to brain serotonin in the current study, however, and if our findings are not confounded by the aforementioned factors, this suggests that decreased brain metabolism (with associated depressed mood) in the patients who experience relapse is not a function of brain serotonin levels, but rather is related to a postsynaptic effect of serotonin on brain function. According to this model, instead of a deficiency in serotonin, a dysfunction of specific brain regions that are vulnerable to a reduction below critical levels in various modulators, including serotonin and norepinephrine, taking the form of a change in postsynaptic receptor binding or affinity or other postreceptor mechanisms, leads to depressive relapse. This raises the question of why some brain regions are more vulnerable than others to the effect of a decrease in brain serotonin levels. Finding the answer to this question may help us to understand the pathogenesis of depression.

Accepted for publication August 20, 1996.

This work was supported by a Veterans Administration Career Development Award (Dr Bremner) and a Veterans Administration Merit Review Grant (Dr Charney).

We thank Melissa Giunti, Cathy Colonese, RN, Pat Barry, RN, and Angie Genovese, RN, for indispensable assistance in execution of the scanning studies; Hedy Sarofin, for acquisition of magnetic resonance images; Samuel M. Mazza, PhD, for preparation of fludeoxyglucose F18; and George Aghajanian, MD, and Helen Mayberg, MD, for useful and interesting discussions.

Reprints: J. Douglas Bremner, MD, West Haven Veterans Affairs Medical Center (116a), 950 Campbell Ave, West Haven, CT 06516.

REFERENCES

1. Mann JJ, Arango V, Marzuk PM, Theccanat S, Reis DJ. Evidence for the 5-HT hypothesis of suicide: a review of post-mortem studies. *Br J Psychiatry.* 1989; 155(suppl 8):7-14.
2. Risch SC, Nemeroff CB. Neurochemical alterations of serotonergic neuronal systems in depression. *J Clin Psychiatry.* 1992;53(suppl):3-7.
3. Maes M, Melzer HY. The serotonin hypothesis of major depression. In: Bloom FE, Kupfer DJ, eds. *Psychopharmacology: The Fourth Generation of Progress.* New York, NY: Raven Press; 1995:933-944.
4. Charney DS, Delgado PL, Price LH, Heninger GR. The receptor sensitivity hypothesis of antidepressant action: a review of antidepressant effects on serotonin function. In: Brown S-L, van Praag H, eds. *The Role of Serotonin in Psychiatric Disorders.* New York, NY: Brunner/Mazel Inc; 1991:29-56.
5. Asberg M, Bertilsson L, Martensson B, Scalia Tomba GP, Thoren P, Traskman-Bendz L. CSF monoamine metabolites in melancholia. *Acta Psychiatr Scand.* 1984;69:201-219.
6. Asberg M, Thoren P, Traskman L, Bertilsson L, Ringberger V. 'Serotonin depression': a biological subgroup within the affective disorders? *Science.* 1976; 191:478-480.
7. Jones JS, Stanley B, Mann JJ, Frances AJ, Guido JR, Traskman-Bendz L, Winchel R, Brown RP, Stanley M. CSF 5-HIAA and HVA concentrations in elderly depressed patients who attempted suicide. *Am J Psychiatry.* 1990;147:1225-1227.
8. Mann JJ, McBride A, Anderson GM, Mieczkowski TA. Platelet and whole blood serotonin content in depressed inpatients: correlations with acute and lifetime psychopathology. *Biol Psychiatry.* 1992;32:243-257.
9. Mann JJ, Stanley M, McBride A, McEwan BS. Increased serotonin$_2$ and β-adrenergic receptor binding in the frontal cortices of suicide victims. *Arch Gen Psychiatry.* 1986;43:954-959.
10. Stanley M, Mann JJ. Increased serotonin$_2$ binding sites in frontal cortex of suicide victims. *Lancet.* 1983;1:214-216.
11. Arango V, Ernsberger P, Marzuk PM, Chen J-S, Tierney H, Stanley M, Resi DJ, Mann JJ. Autoradiographic demonstration of increased serotonin 5-HT$_2$ and α-adrenergic receptor binding sites in the brain of suicide victims. *Arch Gen Psychiatry.* 1990;47:1038-1047.
12. Ferrier IN, McKeith IG, Cross AJ, Perry EK, Candy JM, Pemy RH. Postmortem neurochemical studies in depression. *Ann N Y Acad Sci.* 1986;487:128-142.
13. Lowther S, De Paermentier F, Crompton MR, Katona CLE, Horton RW. Brain 5-HT^2 receptors in suicide victims: violence of death, depression and effects of antidepressant medication. *Brain Res.* 1994;642:281-289.

14. Coccaro EF, Siever LJ, Klar HM, Maurer G, Cochrane K, Cooper TB, Mohs RC, Davis KL. Serotonergic studies in patients with affective and personality disorders. *Arch Gen Psychiatry.* 1989;46:587-599.
15. Heninger GR, Charney DS, Sternberg DE. Serotonergic function in depression: prolactin response to intravenous tryptophan in depressed patients and healthy subjects. *Arch Gen Psychiatry.* 1984;41:398-402.
16. Price LH, Charney DS, Delgado PL, Heninger GR. Serotonin function and depression: neuroendocrine and mood responses to intravenous L-tryptophan in depressed patients and healthy comparison subjects. *Arch Gen Psychiatry.* 1991; 148:1518-1526.
17. Baldessarini RJ. Treatment of depression by altering monoamine metabolism: precursors and metabolic inhibitors. *Psychopharmacol Bull.* 1984;2: 224-239.
18. Cowen PJEM, Charig EM, Fraser S, Elliott JM. Platelet 5-HT receptor binding during depressive illness and tricyclic antidepressant treatment. *J Affect Disord.* 1989;13:45-50.
19. Maes M, Vandewoude M, Schotte C, Martin M, D'Hondt P, Scharpe S, Blockx P. The decreased availability of L-tryptophan in depressed females: clinical and biological correlates. *Prog Neuropsychopharmacol Biol Psychiatry.* 1990;14: 903-919.
20. Meltzer HY. Role of serotonin in depression. *Ann N Y Acad Sci.* 1990;600: 486-499.
21. Moller SE, Kirk L, Fremming KH. Plasma amino acids as an index for subgroups in manic depressive psychosis: correlation to effect of tryptophan. *Psychopharmacology.* 1976;49:205-213.
22. Moller SE, Kirk L, Honore P. Relationship between plasma ratio of tryptophan to competing amino acids and the response to L-tryptophan treatment in endogenous depressed patients. *J Affect Disord.* 1980;2:47-59.
23. Moller SEP, Honore P, Larsen OB. Tryptophan and tyrosine ratios to neutral amino acids in endogenous depression: relation to antidepressant response to amitriptyline and lithium plus L-tryptophan. *J Affect Disord.* 1983;5:67-79.
24. De Meyer MK, Shea PA, Hendrie HC, Yoshimura NN. Plasma tryptophan and five other amino acids in depressed and normal subjects. *Arch Gen Psychiatry.* 1981;38:642-646.
25. Joseph M, Brewerton T, Reus V, Stebbins B. Plasma L-tryptophan/neutral amino acid ratio and dexamethasone suppression in depression. *Psychiatry Res.* 1984; 11:185-192.
26. Maes M, De Ruyter M, Claes R, Bosma G, Suy E. The cortisol responses to 5-hydroxytryptophan, orally, in depressive inpatients. *J Affect Disord.* 1987; 13:23-30.
27. Moller SE, Odum K, Kirk L, Bjerre M, Fog-Moller F, Knudsen A. Plasma tyrosine/neutral amino acid ratio correlated with clinical response to nortriptyline in endogenously depressed patients. *J Affect Disord.* 1985;9:223-229.
28. Maes M, Maes L, Suy E. Symptom profiles of biological markers in depression: a multivariate study. *Psychoneuroendocrinology.* 1990;15:29-37.
29. Delgado PL, Charney DS, Price LH, Aghajanian GK, Landis H, Heninger GR. Serotonin function and the mechanism of antidepressant action: reversal of antidepressant-induced remission by rapid depletion of plasma tryptophan. *Arch Gen Psychiatry.* 1990;47:411-418.
30. Delgado PL, Price LH, Miller HL, Salomon RM, Aghajanian GK, Heninger GR, Charney DS. Serotonin and the neurobiology of depression: effects of tryptophan depletion in drug-free depressed patients. *Arch Gen Psychiatry.* 1994; 51:865-874.
31. Biggio G, Fadda F, Fanni P, Tagliamonte A, Gesse GL. Rapid depletion of serum tryptophan, brain tryptophan, serotonin and 5-hydroxyindoleacetic acetic acid by a tryptophan-free diet. *Life Sci.* 1974;14:1321-1329.
32. Moja EA, Cipollo P, Castoldi D, Tofanetti O. Dose-response decrease in plasma tryptophan and in brain tryptophan and serotonin after tryptophan-free amino acid mixtures in rats. *Life Sci.* 1989;44:971-976.
33. Young SN, Ervin FR, Pihl RO, Finn P. Biochemical aspects of tryptophan depletion in primates. *Psychopharmacology (Berl).* 1989;98:508-511.
34. Young SN, Smith SE, Pihl RO, Ervin FR. Tryptophan depletion causes a rapid lowering of mood in normal males. *Psychopharmacology (Berl).* 1985;87:173-177.
35. Smith SE, Pihl RO, Young SN, Ervin FR. A test of possible cognitive and environmental influences on the mood lowering effect of tryptophan depletion in normal males. *Psychopharmacology (Berl).* 1987;91:451-457.
36. Delgado PL, Charney DS, Price LH, Landis H, Heninger GR. Neuroendocrine and behavioral effects of dietary tryptophan restriction in healthy subjects. *Life Sci.* 1989;45:2323-2332.
37. Heninger GR, Delgado PL, Charney DS, Price LH, Aghajanian GK. Tryptophan-deficient diet and amino acid drink deplete plasma tryptophan and induce a relapse of depression in susceptible patients. *J Chem Neuroanatomy.* 1992; 5:347-348.
38. Benkelfat C, Ellenbogen MA, Dean P, Palmour RM, Young SN. Mood-lowering effect of tryptophan depletion: enhanced susceptibility in young men at risk for major affective disorders. *Arch Gen Psychiatry.* 1994;51:687-697.
39. George MS, Ketter TA, Post RM. Prefrontal cortex dysfunction in clinical depression. *Depression.* 1994;2:59-72.
40. Mayberg HS, Starkstein SE, Peyser CE, Brandt J, Dannals RF, Folstein SE. Paralimbic frontal lobe hypometabolism in depression associated with Huntington's disease. *Neurology.* 1992;42:1791-1797.
41. Martinot J-L, Hardy P, Feline A, Huret J-D, Mazoyer B, Attar-Levy D, Pappata S, Syrota A. Left prefrontal glucose hypometabolism in the depressed state: a confirmation. *Am J Psychiatry.* 1990;147:1313-1317.
42. Sackeim HA, Prohovnik I, Moeller JR, Brown RP, Apter S, Prudic J, Devanand DP, Mukherjee S. Regional cerebral blood flow in mood disorders, I: comparison of major depressives and normal controls at rest. *Arch Gen Psychiatry.* 1990;47:60-70.
43. Sackeim HA, Prohovnik I, Moeller JR, Mayeux R, Stern Y, Devanand DP. Regional cerebral blood flow in mood disorders, II: comparison of major depression and Alzheimer's disease. *J Nucl Med.* 1993;34:1090-1101.
44. Baxter LR, Phelps ME, Mazziotta JC, Schwartz JM, Gerner RH, Selin CE, Sumida RM. Cerebral metabolic rates for glucose in mood disorders. *Arch Gen Psychiatry.* 1985;42:441-447.
45. Baxter LR, Schwartz JM, Phelps ME, Mazziotta JC, Guze BH, Selin CE, Gerner RH, Smida RM. Reduction of prefrontal cortex glucose metabolism common to three types of depression. *Arch Gen Psychiatry.* 1989;46:243-249.
46. Buchsbaum MS, DeLisi LE, Holcomb H, Cappelletti J, King AC, Johnson J, Hazlett E, Dowling-Zimmerman S, Post RM, Morihisa J, Carpenter W, Cohen R, Pickar D, Weinberger DR, Margolin R, Kessler RM. Anteroposterior gradients in cerebral glucose use in schizophrenia and affective disorders. *Arch Gen Psychiatry.* 1984;41:1159-1166.
47. Austin MP, Dougall N, Ross M, Murray C, O'Carroll RE, Moffoot A, Ebmeier KP, Goodwin GM. Single photon emission tomography with ^{99m}Tc-exametazime in major depression and the pattern of brain activity underlying the psychotic/neurotic continuum. *J Affect Disord.* 1992;26:31-43.
48. Bench CJ, Friston KJ, Brown RG, Scott LC, Frackowiak RSJ, Dolan RJ. The anatomy of melancholia: focal abnormalities of cerebral blood flow in major depression. *Psychol Med.* 1992;22:607-615.
49. Mayberg HS, Starkstein SE, Sadzot B, Preziosi T, Andrezejewski PL, Dannals RF, Wagner HN, Robinson RG. Selective hypometabolism in the inferior frontal lobe in depressed patients with Parkinson's disease. *Ann Neurol.* 1990;28:57-64.
50. Drevets WC, Raichle ME. Neuroanatomical circuits in depression: implications for treatment mechanisms. *Psychopharmacol Bull.* 1992;28:261-274.
51. Pardo JV, Pardo PJ, Raichle ME. Neural correlates of self-induced dysphoria. *Am J Psychiatry.* 1993;150:713-720.
52. George MS, Ketter TA, Parekh PI, Horwitz B, Herscovitch P, Post RM. Brain activity during transient sadness and happiness in healthy women. *Am J Psychiatry.* 1995;152:341-351.
53. Mayberg HS, Lewis PJ, Regenold W, Wagner HN. Paralimbic hypoperfusion in unipolar depression. *J Nucl Med.* 1994;35:929-934.
54. Buchsbaum MS, Wu J, DeLisi LE, Holcomb H, Kessler R, Johnson J, King AC, Hazlett E, Langston K, Post RM. Frontal cortex and basal ganglia metabolic rates assessed by positron emission tomography with [18F]2-deoxyglucose in affective illness. *J Affect Disord.* 1986;10:137-152.
55. Post RM, DeLisi LE, Holcomb HH, Uhde TW, Cohen R, Buchsbaum MS. Glucose utilization in the temporal cortex of affectively ill patients: positron emission tomography. *Biol Psychiatry.* 1987;22:545-553.
56. Hurwitz TA, Clark C, Murphy E, Klonoff H, Martin WRW, Pate BD. Regional cerebral glucose metabolism in major depressive disorder. *Can J Psychiatry.* 1990;35:684-688.
57. Ebert D, Feistel H, Barocka A. Effects of sleep deprivation on the limbic system and the frontal lobes in affective disorders: a study with Tc-99m-HMPAO SPECT. *Psychiatry Res Neuroimaging.* 1991;40:247-251.
58. Scott AIF, Dougall N, Ross M, O'Carroll RE, Riddle W, Ebmeier KP, Goodwin GM. Short-term effects of electroconvulsive treatment on the uptake of ^{99m}Tc-exametazime into brain in major depression shown with single photon emission tomography. *J Affect Disord.* 1994;30:27-34.
59. Goodwin GM, Austin MP, Dougall N, Ross M, Murray C, O'Carroll RE, Moffoot A, Prentice N, Ebmeier KP. State changes in brain activity shown by the uptake of ^{99m}Tc-exametazine with single photon emission tomography in major depression before and after treatment. *J Affect Disord.* 1993;29:245-255.
60. Biver F, Goldman S, Delvenne V, Luxen A, De Maertelaer V, Hubain P, Mendlewicz J, Lotstra F. Frontal and parietal metabolic disturbances in unipolar depression. *Biol Psychiatry.* 1994;36:381-388.
61. Wu JC, Gillin JC, Buchsbaum MS, Hershey T, Johnson JC, Bunney WE. Effect of sleep deprivation on brain metabolism of depressed patients. *Am J Psychiatry.* 1992;149:538-543.

62. Nobler MS, Sackeim HA, Prohovnik I, Moeller JR, Mukherjee S, Schnur DB, Prudic J, Devanand DP. Regional cerebral blood flow in mood disorders, III: treatment and clinical response. *Arch Gen Psychiatry.* 1994;51: 884-897.
63. Ebert D, Feistel H, Barocka A, Kaschka W. Increased limbic flow and total sleep deprivation in major depression with melancholia. *Psychol Res.* 1994;5:101-109.
64. Rubin E, Sackeim HA, Nobler MS, Moeller JR. Brain imaging studies of antidepressant treatments. *Psychiatry Ann.* 1994;24:653-658.
65. Ring RA, Bench CJ, Trimble MR, Brooks DJ, Frackowiak RSJ, Dolan RJ. Depression in Parkinson's disease: a positron emission study. *Br J Psychiatry.* 1994;165:333-339.
66. Baxter LR, Phelps ME, Mazziotta JC, Guze BH, Schwartz JM, Selin CE. Local cerebral glucose metabolic rates in obsessive-compulsive disorder: a comparison with rates in unipolar depression and normal controls. *Arch Gen Psychiatry.* 1987;44:211-218.
67. Cudennec A, Duverger D, Serrano A, Scatton B, MacKenzie ET. Influence of ascending serotonergic pathways on glucose use in the conscious rat brain, II; effects of electrical stimulation of the rostral raphe nuclei. *Brain Res.* 1988; 444:227-246.
68. Bonvento G, Lacombe P, MacKenzie ET, Seylaz J. Effects of dorsal raphe stimulation on cerebral glucose utilization in the anesthetized rat. *Brain Res.* 1991; 567:325-327.
69. Kapur S, Meyer J, Wilson AA, Houle S, Brown GM. Modulation of cortical neuronal activity by a serotonergic agent: a PET study in humans. *Brain Res.* 1994; 646:292-294.
70. Spitzer RL, Williams JBW, Gibbon M. *Structured Clinical Interview for DSM-III-R.* New York: New York State Psychiatric Institute, Biometrics Research Department; 1987.
71. Delgado PL, Price LH, Miller HL, Salomon RM, Licinio J, Krystal JH, Heninger GR, Charney DS. Rapid serotonin depletion as a provocative challenge test for patients with major depression: relevance to antidepressant action and the neurobiology of depression. *Psychopharmacol Bull.* 1991;27: 321-330.
72. Mulaney NA, Gould LK, Hartz RK, Hitchens RE, Wong WH, Bristow D, Adler S, Philippe EA, Bendrien B, Sanders M, Gibbs B. Design and performance of Posicam 6.5 BGO Positron camera. *J Nucl Med.* 1990;31:610-616.
73. Brownell GL, Kearfott KJ, Kairento A-L, Elmaleh DR, Alpert NM, Correia JA, Wechsler L, Ackerman RH. Quantitation of regional cerebral glucose metabolism. *J Comput Assist Tomagr.* 1983;7:919-924.
74. Sokoloff L, Reivich M, Kennedy C, Des Rosiers MH, Patlak CS, Pettigrew KD, Sakurada O, Shinohara M. The [14]deoxyglucose method for the measurement of local cerebral glucose utilization: theory, procedure, and normal values in the conscious and anesthetized albino rat. *J Neurochem.* 1977;28:897-916.
75. Huang S, Phelps ME, Hoffman EF, Kuhl DE. Error sensitivity of fluorodeoxyglucose method for measurement of cerebral rate of glucose. *J Cereb Blood Flow Metab.* 1981;1:391-401.
76. Robb RA, Hanson DP, Karwoski RA, Larson AG, Workman EL, Stacy MC. Analyze: a comprehensive, operator-interactive software package for multidimensional medical image display and analysis. *Comput Med Imaging Graph.* 1989;13:433-454.
77. Jiang H, Robb RA, Holton KS. A new approach to 3-D registration of multimodality medical images by surface matching. In: Robb R, ed. *Proceedings of the Second Conference on Visual Biomedical Computing.* Bellingham, Wash: SPIE; 1992;1808:196-213.
78. Zubal IG, Zhang L, Tagare B, Duncan JS. 3-D registration of SPECT and MRI brain images. *J Nucl Med.* 1993;34:187.
79. Duvernoy H. *The Human Brain: Surface Three-Dimensional Anatomy and MRI.* New York, NY: Springer-Verlag NY Inc; 1991.
80. Camargo EE, Szabo Z, Links JM, Sostre S, Dannals RF, Wagner HN. The influence of biological and technical factors on the variability of global and regional brain metabolism of 2-[^{18}F]fluoro-2-deoxy-D-glucose. *J Cereb Blood Flow Metab.* 1992;12:281-290.
81. Bartlett EJ, Brodie JD, Wolf AP, Christman DR, Laska E, Meissner M. Reproducibility of cerebral glucose metabolic measurements in resting human subjects. *J Cereb Blood Flow Metab.* 1988;8:502-512.
82. Baxter LR. PET studies of cerebral function in major depression and obsessive-compulsive disorder: the emerging prefrontal cortex consensus. *Ann Clin Psychiatry.* 1991;3:103-109.
83. Alexander GE, DeLong MR, Strick PL. Parallel organization of functionally segregated circuits linking basal ganglia and cortex. *Annu Rev Neurosci.* 1986;9: 357-381.
84. Clark CM, Klonoff H, Tyhurst JS, Ruth T, Adam M, Rogers J, Harrop R, Martin W, Pate B. Regional cerebral glucose metabolism in identical twins. *Neuropsychologia.* 1988;26:615-621.

Effects of *Meta*-chlorophenylpiperazine Infusions in Patients With Seasonal Affective Disorder and Healthy Control Subjects

Diurnal Responses and Nocturnal Regulatory Mechanisms

Paul J. Schwartz, MD; Dennis L. Murphy, MD; Thomas A. Wehr, MD; Diego Garcia-Borreguero, MD; Dan A. Oren, MD; Douglas E. Moul, MD, MPH; Norio Ozaki, MD; Alisa J. Snelbaker, MA; Norman E. Rosenthal, MD

Background: Multiple lines of evidence suggest that brain serotonergic systems may be disturbed in seasonal affective disorder (SAD). Previously, we found that the serotonergic agent *meta*-chlorophenylpiperazine (m-CPP) produced increases in activation and euphoria in depressed patients with SAD, but not in patients with SAD following light treatment or in the summer, nor in healthy control subjects in any condition. In the present study, we attempted to replicate and extend this finding using better methods.

Methods: Seventeen outpatients with SAD and 15 control subjects underwent successive 3-week periods of bright light treatment and light avoidance in a randomized order. During the third week of each condition, on 2 different occasions, subjects were admitted to the hospital for a night of sleep (core temperatures were recorded), followed by infusions of m-CPP (0.08 mg/kg) or placebo the next morning. Dependent measures included the 24-item National Institute of Mental Health Self-Rating Scale, plasma corticotropin, cortisol, prolactin, growth hormone, and norepinephrine concentrations, and core temperatures.

Results: *Meta*-chlorophenylpiperazine produced (1) significant increases in "activation-euphoria" ratings only in depressed patients with SAD in the untreated condition and (2) blunted corticotropin and norepinephrine responses in patients with SAD compared with controls across both light treatment conditions. In both groups, light treatment was associated with significant reductions in nocturnal core temperatures, which were correlated with similarly significant reductions in mean diurnal growth hormone concentrations. In patients with SAD, (1) the reductions in nocturnal core temperatures also were correlated with the reductions in baseline depression ratings and (2) the reductions in mean growth hormone concentrations were significantly smaller compared with controls.

Conclusions: The abnormal m-CPP–induced activation-euphoria responses represent a replicated state marker of winter depression in patients with SAD. The blunted m-CPP–induced responsiveness of the hypothalamic-pituitary-adrenal axis and the sympathetic nervous system may represent traitlike abnormalities. The improvements in mood following light treatment in patients with SAD seem to be associated with the lowering of nocturnal core temperatures. The findings, although not easily explained based on a uniform abnormality of serotonin receptors, are nonetheless compatible with the notion that selected regions of the central nervous system are deficient in serotonin transmission during winter depression.

Arch Gen Psychiatry. 1997;54:375-385

From the Clinical Psychobiology Branch (Drs Schwartz, Wehr, Garcia-Borreguero, Oren, Ozaki, and Rosenthal and Ms Snelbaker) and the Laboratory of Clinical Science (Dr Murphy), National Institute of Mental Health, Bethesda, Md; and the Epidemiology and Psychopathology Research Branch, National Institute of Mental Health, Rockville, Md (Dr Moul).

WINTER seasonal affective disorder (SAD) is a condition characterized by recurrent fall and winter depressions alternating with remissions or hypomanic episodes in the spring and summer.[1] Although there is a consensus that the winter depressions in SAD respond to light therapy,[2,3] the pathogenesis of the depressive episodes and the mechanism of action of light therapy are not well understood.

We and others have pursued the hypothesis that brain serotonergic systems are disturbed in SAD.[1] Indeed, many of the "atypical" vegetative symptoms of SAD (eg, hypersomnia, increased appetite, and carbohydrate craving) reflect disturbances in functions regulated, in part, by hypothalamic serotonin (5-HT),[4,5] which varies seasonally[6] and is regulated by environmental light.[7] Some clinical evidence supports the notion that the winter depressions in SAD are characterized by diminished brain 5-HT transmission. First, carbohydrate-rich meals, which increase brain 5-HT content,[5,8] energize patients with SAD but sedate control subjects.[9] Second, drugs that enhance neuronal 5-HT transmission (fenfluramine hydrochloride and fluoxetine hydrochloride) are effective in treating

SUBJECTS AND METHODS

SUBJECTS

Seventeen patients with SAD and 15 controls were recruited through the local media. Patients were required to (1) meet the criteria for SAD of Rosenthal et al[1]; (2) score at least 14 points on the 21-item Hamilton Depression Rating Scale (HDRS)[33] or score at least 12 on the HDRS with a total of 20 on the Structured Interview Guide for the HDRS-SAD Version (SIGH-SAD)[34]; and (3) be physically healthy on physical examination and routine laboratory testing. Patients (n=4) with histories of second Axis I conditions were permitted into the study provided these second conditions were in remission for at least a year before the study and did not confound the diagnosis of SAD. Exclusion criteria were (1) the use of any medications affecting the central nervous system within the 4 weeks before the study, (2) a history of migraine headaches,[35] and (3) pregnancy. The only medications permitted during the study were birth control pills (2 patients) and oral estrogens (3 patients).

Age- and sex-matched controls were required to (1) have no personal or family history of any *DSM-III-R*[36] Axis I psychiatric condition and (2) be physically healthy. There were no significant differences between groups in ages (mean ±SD age, patients with SAD, 36.0±9.5 years; controls, 36.4±10.2 years). There were 3 men in each group. Female patients and controls were matched for use of oral contraceptives or estrogens.

The study was conducted in the winter (December through March) at the National Institutes of Health Clinical Center, Bethesda, Md. Participants were fully informed about the nature, purpose, and procedures of the study. Informed consent was obtained before entry into the protocol, which was approved by the NIMH Institutional Review Board. Controls were paid for their participation.

STUDY DESIGN

All subjects underwent as outpatients a period of 3 weeks of light therapy (light-treated condition) and 3 weeks without light therapy (untreated condition). The order of light condition was randomized. We attempted to standardize ambient light exposures in the 2 light treatment conditions; all subjects wore dark goggles (3% transmittance) while outdoors on sunny days during the untreated condition; in the light-treated condition, all subjects received a 10 000-lux bright white light treatment[3] for 45 minutes twice a day, between 6 and 9 AM and between 6 and 9 PM. During the third week of each respective condition, all subjects underwent 1 m-CPP (0.08 mg/kg) and 1 placebo infusion on separate occasions, 3 to 5 days apart. The order of administration of m-CPP or placebo was assigned by balanced randomization.

Logistical difficulties did not permit us to control for phase of the menstrual cycle. Subjects adhered to their own self-selected sleep-wake schedules as outpatients, knowing their sleep times would be from 11 PM to 7 AM the nights before the infusions. Diet was not controlled as outpatients. Subjects were informed that (1) we were interested in measuring their emotional and physiological responses to m-CPP because of previous work suggesting the involvement of 5-HT in SAD; (2) m-CPP is not itself an antidepressant and is not intended to be a treatment for SAD; (3) m-CPP might cause temporary effects such as hot or cold sensations, dry mouth, nausea, headache, or mild nervousness; and (4) they could receive m-CPP or placebo on any given infusion day.

PROCEDURES

Subjects arrived on the research ward by 7 PM before their infusions. In the light-treated condition only, they completed a 10 000-lux bright light treatment from 8 to 9 PM. Subjects ingested nothing by mouth from 9 PM through 11 AM. Subjects wore hospital pajamas throughout the experiments. Sleep was permitted only after the lights were turned off (<1 lux) at 11 PM. Rectal temperatures were recorded every 3 minutes overnight and every minute in the morning with an indwelling probe (Mallinckrodt Medical Inc, St Louis, Mo) connected to an electronic temperature monitor (Isothermex, Columbus Instruments, Columbus, Ohio), accuracy of 0.1°C, resolution of 0.015°C. No restrictions were placed on the number of blankets used by the subjects overnight.

Subjects were awakened at 6:50 AM and the dim (30-lux) room lights were turned on. After voiding, subjects returned to bed, where they remained recumbent, without covers, with the head of the bed elevated to 45° for the remainder of the morning. Two antecubital intravenous catheters were inserted by 7:30 AM. Subjects did not read, watch television, or perform desk work. At 8 AM in the light-treated condition only, subjects received a 1-hour 10 000-lux light treatment. A SIGH-SAD rating was obtained between 9:10 and 9:30 AM by an experienced rater who was unaware of the light treatment condition.

SAD.[10,11] Third, rapid tryptophan depletion, which decreases brain 5-HT synthesis, antagonizes the antidepressant effects of light therapy in remitted patients with SAD.[12,13]

Meta-chlorophenylpiperazine (m-CPP) is a widely used and potentially informative probe of central 5-HT function,[14,15] having affinity for a number of different 5-HT receptors, in the following order of dissociation constants: 5-HT_{2C} greater than 5-HT_3 greater than 5-HT_{2A} greater than 5-HT_{1B} greater than 5-HT_{1A} greater than 5-HT_{1D}.[16] In addition, m-CPP has moderate affinity for α_2-adrenergic receptors and considerably lower affinity at other adrenergic and dopamine receptors and the human 5-HT transporter.[14-17] *Meta*-chlorophenylpiperazine consistently induces hormonal changes—including corticotropin (ACTH), cortisol, prolactin (PRL), growth hormone (GH), and norepinephrine (NE) release—and hyperthermia in humans,[18-21] nonhuman primates,[22] and rodents.[23,24] The behavioral effects of m-CPP in humans seem variable.[14,15]

We previously investigated the behavioral and hormonal effects of intravenous infusions of m-CPP in patients with SAD and controls before and after light treatment in the winter[25] and in the summer.[26] *Meta*-chlorophenylpiperazine consistently produced significant increases in "dysphoria" (a subscale of the 24-item

At 9:30 AM, a 20-mL solution of m-CPP (0.08 mg/kg) (Aldrich Chemical Co, Milwaukee, Wis) or saline placebo was administered intravenously for 90 seconds. Blood specimens were drawn through the intravenous line in the contralateral arm to avoid contamination of the plasma levels of m-CPP by residual drug in the intravenous apparatus used for the infusion. Specimens for m-CPP plasma levels were obtained at baseline and at 10, 30, 60, and 90 minutes after the infusions.

Subjects completed the 24-item NIMH Self-Rating Scale and a 24-item physical symptoms scale (assessing physical effects following the infusions) at 9:15 AM (considered baseline) and at 15, 30, 45, and 75 minutes after the infusions. Six subscale scores were compiled from the 24-item NIMH Self-Rating Scale: activation-euphoria, "depression," "anxiety," "altered self-reality," "functional deficit," and dysphoria.[27,28]

HORMONAL ASSAYS

Blood specimens for measurement of plasma concentrations of ACTH, cortisol, PRL, and GH were drawn at baseline and at 10, 20, 30, 40, 50, 60, and 90 minutes after the administration of m-CPP. Plasma NE concentrations were sampled only at baseline and at 10, 30, and 60 minutes after the infusions. Samples for ACTH and NE assays were collected in edetic acid tubes and stored at −70°C; those for PRL, cortisol, and GH were collected in heparinized tubes and stored at −30°C. The ACTH assay[37] had a detection limit of 0.3 pmol/L, with intra-assay coefficients of variation of 2.5% and 5.5% and interassay coefficients of variation of 23.4% and 17.0% for means of 5.0 and 28.2 pmol/L, respectively. The cortisol radioimmunoassay had a detection limit of 11.0 nmol/L with intra-assay coefficients of variation of 5.2% and 5.8% and interassay coefficients of variation of 16.1% and 14.0% for means of 182.1 and 364.2 nmol/L.[38] The PRL radioimmunoassay[39] had a detection limit of 2 μg/L, with intra-assay coefficients of variation of 11.0% and 7.2% and interassay coefficients of variation of 22.8% and 8.7% for means of 7.5 and 26.3 μg/L, respectively. The GH assay[40] had a detection limit of 0.1 μg/L, with intra-assay coefficients of variation of 5.8% and 7.4% and interassay coefficients of variation of 13.1% and 16.3% for means of 6.5 and 2.6 μg/L, respectively. Details of the NE collection and assay techniques are published elsewhere.[41]

STATISTICAL ANALYSIS

Two patients with SAD had severe physiological reactions following their first m-CPP infusion and were excluded from all postinfusion analyses, except the baseline analysis (ie, before the infusions). The first, whose 10-minute plasma m-CPP concentration was the highest of any subject throughout the study, had nausea, vomiting, and diarrhea. The second, whose blood pressure level dropped to 86/43 mm Hg, had a syncopal episode with a brief loss of consciousness. Three subjects were dropped from the ACTH analysis; 1 control had an m-CPP-induced ACTH response that was greater than 5 SDs above the mean of all other subjects; 1 patient and 1 control each had a missing ACTH data point at 10 minutes after m-CPP infusion that could not be reasonably interpolated.

Overnight temperatures were analyzed every 30 minutes by analysis of variance (ANOVA), with 2 grouping factors (diagnosis and order of light condition) and 3 repeated measures (light condition, night, and time). The morning baseline values for the behavioral, hormonal, and thermoregulatory measures were analyzed by means of ANOVAs with 2 grouping factors (diagnosis and order of light condition) and 2 repeated measures (drug and light condition). Effects of m-CPP on behavior, hormones, and temperatures were assessed with baseline-corrected ANOVAs, with 2 grouping factors (diagnosis and order of light condition) and 3 repeated measures (light condition, drug, and time). Where significant baseline differences were observed, the ANOVAs were checked by performing analysis of covariances (ANCOVAs), using baseline values as the covariates. These results are not shown because they did not alter any of the findings. Post hoc comparisons of the activation-euphoria data within each light condition separately were evaluated with (1) ANOVAs without light condition as a repeated measure and (2) nonparametric Mann-Whitney rank sum tests.

Values reported in the text are mean±SD unless otherwise specified. All tests were 2-tailed, and significance level was set at $P<.05$. Greenhouse-Geisser corrections were included for all repeated measures analyses. Because of previous studies showing a relation between changes in GH and PRL secretion and changes in core body temperature,[42-45] we had an a priori reason to look for correlations between the changes observed in these variables. Statistical analysis and data representation were performed using SuperANOVA (Abacus Concepts, Berkeley, Calif) and KaleidaGraph (Synergy Software, Reading, Pa).

There were no significant differences between groups or light treatment conditions in ambient room temperatures (mean±SD for all experiments, 22.5°C±1.5°C) or in the number of infusions conducted while women were in the follicular vs luteal phase of their menstrual cycles (χ^2, $P>.40$).

National Institute of Mental Health [NIMH] Self-Rating Scale[27,28]) in both groups and in all 3 conditions. By contrast, m-CPP produced significant increases in "activation-euphoria" (a subscale comprised of 4 items: "I feel energetic," "I feel elated," "I feel talkative," and "I have racing thoughts") only in depressed patients with SAD in the winter. As such, the abnormal m-CPP–induced activation-euphoria responses in patients with SAD might be regarded as a state-marker of winter depression,[25,26] and could disclose state-specific information about the nature of serotonergic dysfunction in SAD.

Certain experimental design issues limited the conclusions that could be drawn from our earlier studies; notably, the lack of a placebo control condition and the lack of a randomized order of presentation of the light treatment condition. In addition, depressed patients with SAD had exaggerated cortisol responses to m-CPP infusions compared with controls, which seemed to be at odds with our previous study suggesting that hypothalamic-pituitary-adrenal (HPA) axis tone and responsiveness is diminished in patients with SAD in the winter compared with controls.[29] We undertook the present study to address several limitations of our earlier studies and to clarify the nature of HPA axis activity in SAD. Specifically, we (1) used a placebo control, (2) randomly ordered the light treatment conditions, (3) studied a larger number of subjects, (4) used a lower dose of m-CPP (0.08 vs 0.1 mg/kg) in an attempt to reduce the likelihood of side effects, and (5) measured plasma ACTH and NE in addition to cortisol concentrations. We also wanted to extend our previous work concerning the effects of light therapy on the thermoregulatory and 5-HT systems.[30,31] Thus, we also measured nocturnal and diurnal core temperatures, and diurnal GH and PRL concentrations, because these variables are all regulated, in part, by 5-HT transmission, and modified by antidepressant treatments.[15,32] This study thus constitutes an attempted replication and extension of our earlier studies with improved methods.

RESULTS

BEFORE THE INFUSIONS

Behavioral

Patients with SAD were significantly more depressed in the untreated than in the treated condition (HDRS scores, 22.7±6.8 vs 9.7±5.8), and than controls in either condition (untreated, 2.6±4.1; light-treated, 2.9±3.6; group×light condition, $F_{(1,28)}$=38.56; *P*<.001). On the NIMH Self-Rating Scale, ANOVA showed a significant main effect for group on all 6 subscales (patients had higher scores than controls). There were also significant group×light condition interactions on the NIMH subscales depression, anxiety, dysphoria, and functional deficit, reflecting the reduction in these scores in patients with SAD, but not in controls, following light treatment. On the physical symptoms scale at baseline, patients scored significantly higher than controls on several items that reflected their depressed state: decreased sexual thoughts or feelings, dry mouth, itching, increased appetite, stiffness, tiredness, and weakness (all statistical analyses available on request).

Hormonal

Corticotropin. Analysis of variance showed no significant main effects or interactions involving group or light condition (untreated: SAD, 5.0±2.0 pmol/L; controls, 5.0±2.2 pmol/L; treated: SAD, 4.8±2.4 pmol/L; controls, 5.0±2.2 pmol/L).

Growth hormone. Analysis of variance showed no significant main effects or interactions involving group or light condition (group, *P*>.90; light condition, *P*>.40; group×light condition, *P*>.90).

Prolactin. Analysis of variance showed a significant main effect of light condition (means: untreated, 15.5±8.7 μg/L; treated, 13.7±6.5 μg/L; $F_{(1,28)}$=5.17; *P*<.05).

Norepinephrine. Untreated patients with SAD tended to have low baseline NE concentrations compared with untreated controls, and compared with themselves in the treated condition (SAD: untreated, 2.3±1.0 nmol/L; treated, 2.6±1.3 nmol/L; controls: untreated, 3.2±1.6 nmol/L; treated, 2.8±1.2 nmol/L; group×light condition: $F_{(1,24)}$=3.67; *P*=.07, 4 subjects with missing data).

Cortisol. Untreated patients with SAD tended to have high baseline plasma cortisol concentrations compared with untreated controls, and compared with themselves in the light-treated condition (SAD: untreated, 579.4±289.7 nmol/L; treated, 477.3±270.4 nmol/L; controls: untreated, 411.1±209.7 nmol/L; treated, 427.6±289.7 nmol/L; group×light condition: $F_{(1,28)}$=2.82; *P*=.10).

The effects of light and group on mean baseline PRL, NE, and cortisol concentrations also were present in the corresponding (time-averaged) means in the ANOVAs of the raw data from 9:30 to 11 AM (*P*=.002, *P*=.01, and *P*=.09, respectively).

Thermoregulatory (9:25-9:30 AM)

Analysis of variance showed no significant main effects or interactions involving group or light condition for core temperature (group, *P*>.70; light condition, *P*>.50; group×light condition, *P*>.40).

AFTER THE INFUSIONS

Behavioral

On the NIMH Self-Rating Scale, across groups and light treatment conditions, m-CPP produced significant increases in dysphoria (drug×time: $F_{(3,78)}$=5.10; *P*<.01), altered self-reality ($F_{(3,78)}$=16.37; *P*<.001), and functional deficit ($F_{(3,78)}$=8.63; *P*<.001) compared with placebo. Significant interactions involving group and/or light treatment were observed on only 2 subscales: activation-euphoria and anxiety (**Figure 1**).

Following m-CPP, patients with SAD showed significant increases in activation-euphoria in the untreated condition, but no such increases in the light-treated condition; controls showed no significant increases in either condition (group×light condition×drug×time; $F_{(3,78)}$=5.04; *P*<.01). The differences between patients with SAD and controls in m-CPP–induced activation-euphoria were significant in the untreated condition (post hoc ANOVA: drug×group×time; $F_{(3,78)}$=5.74; *P*<.005; Mann-Whitney *Z*=2.42; *P*=.02), but not in the light-treated condition (ANOVA: $F_{(3,78)}$; *P*>.40; Mann-Whitney *Z*=1.54; *P*>.10).

There was also a significant light condition×drug×group interaction in anxiety ($F_{(1,26)}$=6.91; *P*<.05). Increases in m-CPP–induced anxiety were absent in patients with SAD in the untreated condition, but they were present in patients with SAD in the light-treated condition and controls in both light treatment conditions.

On the physical symptoms scale, compared with placebo, m-CPP was associated with significant increases in many symptoms that did not differ between groups. *Meta-chlorophenylpiperazine*–induced "tremor," which was reported to a significantly greater degree in patients with SAD across light treatment conditions, was the only symptom that differed between groups.

Hormonal

Corticotropin. Patients with SAD showed blunted ACTH responses to m-CPP compared with controls across both light conditions (drug×time×group: $F_{(6,138)}$=6.39; *P*<.005; 3 subjects excluded) (**Figure 2**).

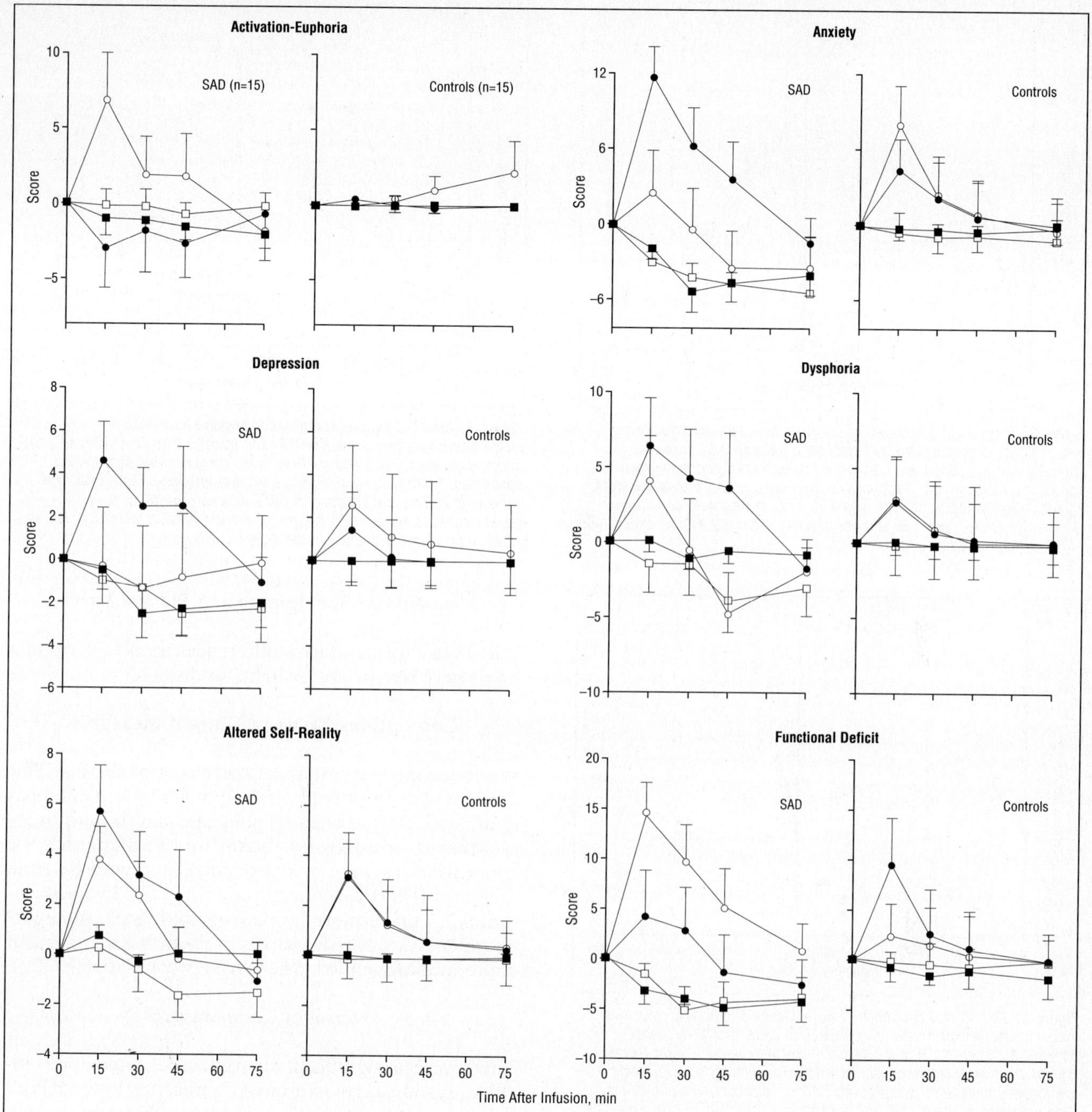

Figure 1. *Baseline-corrected scores on the National Institute of Mental Health Self-Rating Scale of patients with seasonal affective disorder (SAD) and controls following* meta-*chlorophenylpiperazine and placebo infusions in the untreated and light-treated conditions. Data are given as mean±SE. Open circles indicate the untreated condition,* meta-*chlorophenylpiperazine; open squares, the untreated condition, placebo; solid circles, light-treated condition,* meta-*chlorophenylpiperazine; and solid squares, light-treated condition, placebo.*

Norepinephrine. Patients with SAD showed blunted NE responses to m-CPP compared with controls across both light conditions (drug×group: $F_{(1,21)}=4.74$; $P<.05$, 5 subjects with missing data) (**Figure 3**).

Cortisol. *Meta*-chlorophenylpiperazine produced significant increases with no differences between groups or light conditions (drug×time: $F_{(6,144)}=25.98$; $P<.001$, 2 subjects with missing data; mean baseline corrected m-CPP–induced areas under the curve: SAD, 15 588±17 216; controls, 13 767±9443) ($P>.60$).

Prolactin. *Meta*-chlorophenylpiperazine produced significant increases with no differences between groups or light conditions (drug×time: $F_{(6,156)}=8.50$; $P<.001$).

Growth hormone. *Meta*-chlorophenylpiperazine produced significant increases with no differences between groups or light conditions (drug×time: $F_{(6,144)}=3.88$; $P<.05$, 2 subjects with missing data) (**Figure 4**). In addition, before baseline corrections, ANOVA on the raw data showed a main effect of light

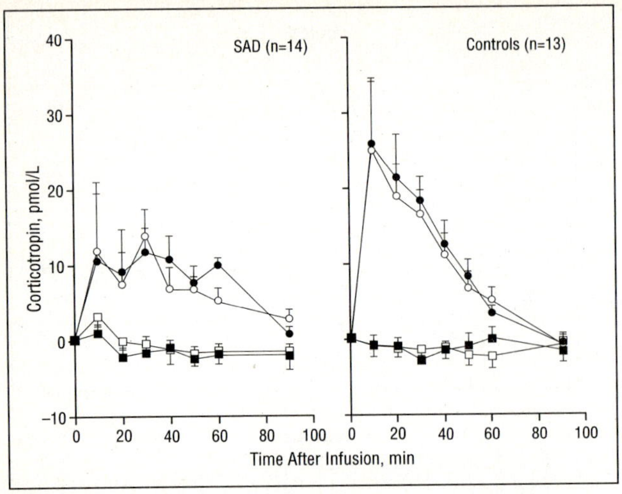

Figure 2. *Plasma concentrations of corticotropin following infusions of* meta-*chlorophenylpiperazine and placebo in patients with seasonal affective disorder (SAD) and controls in the untreated and light-treated conditions. Corticotropin responses to* meta-*chlorophenylpiperazine were significantly blunted in patients with SAD in both treatment conditions. Data are given as mean±SE and are baseline corrected. For an explanation of the symbols, see the legend to Figure 1.*

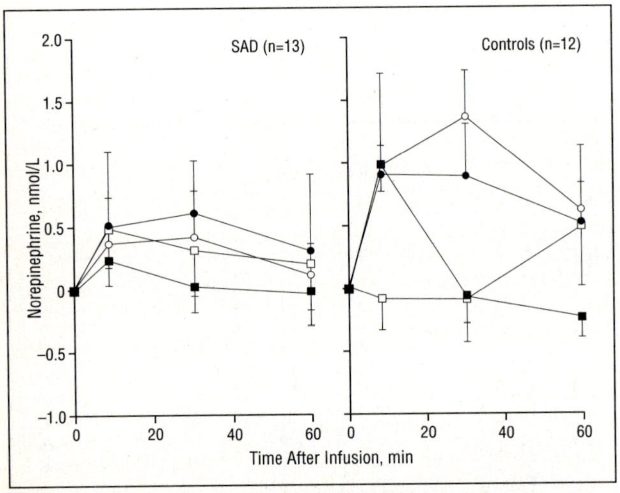

Figure 3. *Plasma concentrations of norepinephrine following infusions of* meta-*chlorophenylpiperazine and placebo in patients with seasonal affective disorder (SAD) and controls in the untreated and light-treated conditions. Norepinephrine responses to* meta-*chlorophenylpiperazine were significantly blunted in patients with SAD in both treatment conditions. Data are given as mean±SE and are baseline corrected. For an explanation of the symbols, see the legend to Figure 1.*

condition (means: untreated, 2.7±4.9 μg/L; treated, 1.7±3.6 μg/L; $F_{(1,24)}$=4.54; $P<.05$, 4 subjects with missing data).

Thermoregulatory

Meta-chlorophenylpiperazine caused significant biphasic changes in rectal temperature compared with placebo (drug×time: $F_{(11,253)}$=85.81; $P<.001$, 3 subjects with missing data, analyzed every 8 minutes) (**Figure 5**) with no differences between groups or light conditions (group, $P>.10$; light condition, $P>.80$; group×light condition, $P>.30$).

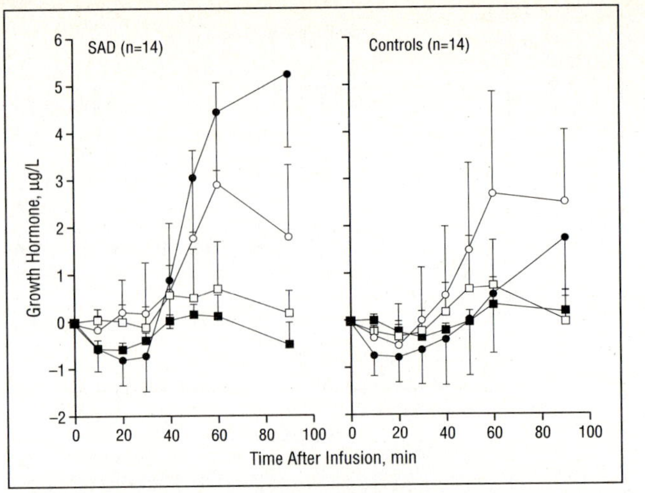

Figure 4. *Growth hormone responses following infusions of* meta-*chlorophenylpiperazine (m-CPP) and placebo in patients with seasonal affective disorder (SAD) and controls in the untreated and light-treated conditions. There were no differences between groups or light treatment conditions in baseline corrected m-CPP–induced growth hormone responses. Data are given as mean±SE and are baseline corrected. For an explanation of the symbols, see the legend to Figure 1.*

Meta-chlorophenylpiperazine Plasma Levels

There were no significant differences in m-CPP plasma levels between groups or light conditions.

Correlations Between Diurnal Measures

We found no physiological correlates of the m-CPP–induced activation-euphoria responses in untreated patients with SAD. Across all subjects, and in both light-treatment conditions, baseline (and mean) NE concentrations were inversely correlated with baseline (and mean) cortisol concentrations ($P<.05$ in both conditions). Furthermore, in patients with SAD, the light-treatment–associated changes in mean NE and cortisol concentrations tended to be inversely correlated (P=.09).

Overnight Temperatures

There were no significant main effects or interactions involving group. Light treatment significantly lowered both the absolute minimum ($F_{(1,23)}$=4.30; $P<.05$; 5 subjects with missing data from 1 night) and the mean level ($F_{(1,23)}$ =5.03; $P<.05$) of overnight rectal temperature (means for temperature minimum[T_{min}]—SAD: untreated, 36.65°C±0.31°C; treated, 36.48°C±0.26°C; controls: untreated, 36.52°C±0.42°C; treated, 36.44°C±0.34°C) (**Figure 6**). The mean±SD time to T_{min} after 11:00 PM lights out was not affected by group or light treatment condition (SAD: untreated, 303±223 minutes; light-treated, 303±189 minutes; controls: untreated, 370±184 minutes; light-treated, 269±201 minutes).

Correlations Between Nocturnal and Diurnal Measures

We found consistent negative correlations between the m-CPP–induced core temperature maximum change from

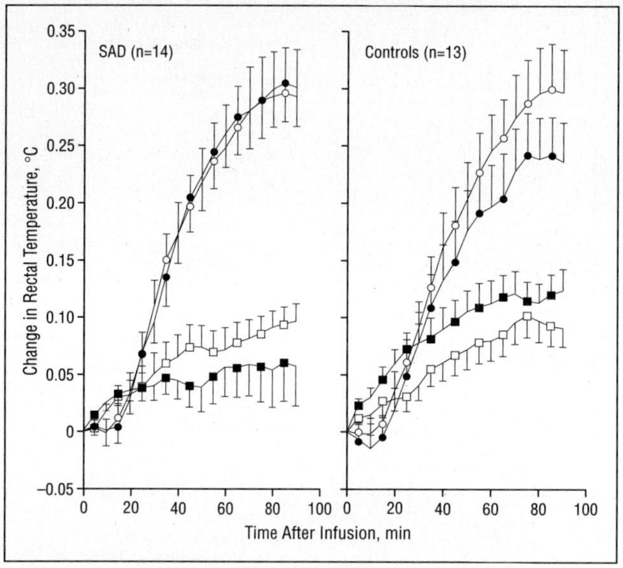

Figure 5. *Core temperature responses following infusions of meta-chlorophenylpiperazine (m-CPP) and placebo in patients with seasonal affective disorder (SAD) and controls in the untreated and light-treated conditions. There were no differences between groups or light treatment conditions in baseline-corrected m-CPP–induced core temperature responses. Data are given as mean±SE and are baseline corrected. For an explanation of the symbols, see the legend to Figure 1.*

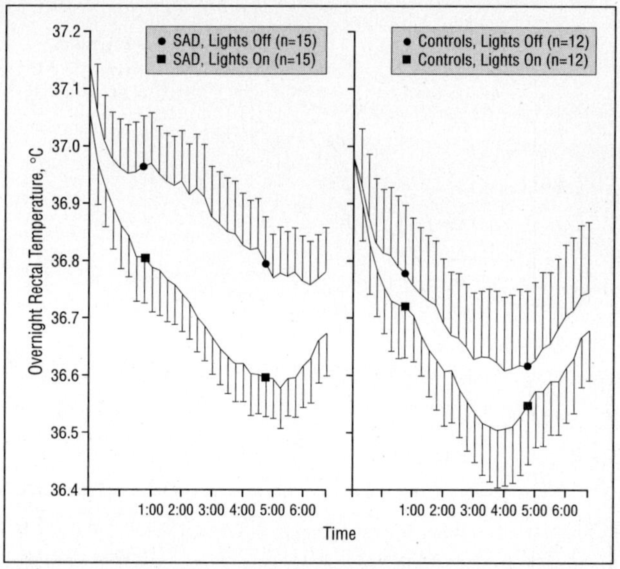

Figure 6. *Overnight core rectal temperature in patients with seasonal affective disorder (SAD) and controls in the untreated and the light-treated conditions. Two to 3 weeks of twice-daily light treatment significantly lowered the mean and minimum rectal temperature in both groups. Error bars represent SE.*

baseline (Max Δ) and T_{min} of the previous night within each of the 4 experimental blocks (**Figure 7**). By contrast, the Max Δ following the placebo infusions were uncorrelated with the T_{min} of the previous night. Repeated measures multivariate comparison of slopes[46] disclosed no significant effects of group or light condition on the slopes of these regression lines.

There were positive correlations between the light-treatment–associated changes in T_{min} and mean GH concentrations in patients with SAD ($F=10.03$; $r=0.68$; slope=3.41; $P=.008$) and controls ($F=12.66$; $r=0.72$; slope=3.55; $P=.004$; these slopes were not statistically different). Therefore, to further investigate whether patients with SAD and controls differed in their light-treatment–associated reductions in GH concentrations (main effect of light in raw ANOVA), an ANCOVA was performed (with Δ mean GH as the dependent variable and ΔT_{min} as the covariate). This ANCOVA yielded a significant main effect of group, such that the light-treatment–associated reductions in mean GH concentrations were greater in controls than in patients with SAD (Δ mean GH concentrations: controls, 1.7±2.6 μg/L; SAD, 0.2±1.9 μg/L; $F_{(1,24)}=11.52$, $P<.005$). ΔT_{min} also tended to be correlated with Δ mean PRL concentrations ($P=.06$).

We found a significant positive correlation ($r=0.61$; $P<.05$) between the percent reduction in total HDRS scores following light treatment and the degree of lowering of the nocturnal T_{min} (**Figure 8**) [$\%\Delta\text{Hamilton}=100\times(\text{HDRS}_{\text{untreated average}}-\text{HDRS}_{\text{treated average}})/(\text{HDRS}_{\text{untreated average}})$, and $\Delta T_{min}=(T_{\text{min treated average}}-T_{\text{min untreated average}})$].

COMMENT

The main findings of the present study are that (1) m-CPP produced significant increases in activation-euphoria ratings in untreated patients with SAD that were not seen in the light-treated condition or in controls in either condition; (2) m-CPP–induced ACTH and NE responses were significantly blunted in patients with SAD compared with controls across both light treatment conditions; (3) twice-daily bright light treatment was associated with reductions in mean nocturnal rectal temperatures and mean morning PRL and GH concentrations in both groups; (4) following light treatment, the degree to which depressed patients with SAD improved was correlated with the degree to which their nocturnal temperatures were lowered; (5) following light treatment, the changes in mean GH concentrations were correlated with the changes in the level of T_{min} in both groups; and (6) relative to the reductions in their T_{min}, patients with SAD had significantly smaller reductions in GH concentrations following light treatment compared with controls. We will discuss each of these findings in turn.

We suggest that the abnormal m-CPP–induced activation-euphoria responses of untreated patients with SAD reflect certain specific central nervous system abnormalities that are associated with their winter depressions. That is, these abnormal responses were not likely "merely psychological" reactions attributable to (1) patients' beliefs about the effects of m-CPP, (2) the nonspecific effects of infusions, or (3) abnormal physical effects produced by m-CPP in depressed patients with SAD, for the following reasons: First, patients were not led to believe that m-CPP would make them feel better, activated, or euphoric. Second, the abnormal activation-euphoria responses to m-CPP infusions were specific (there were no such group differences in 4 of the other 5 subscales), and the responses to placebo infusions were negligible. Finally, the physical effects of m-CPP—unlike the activation-euphoria effects—were similar across light conditions and groups. Furthermore, in a more re-

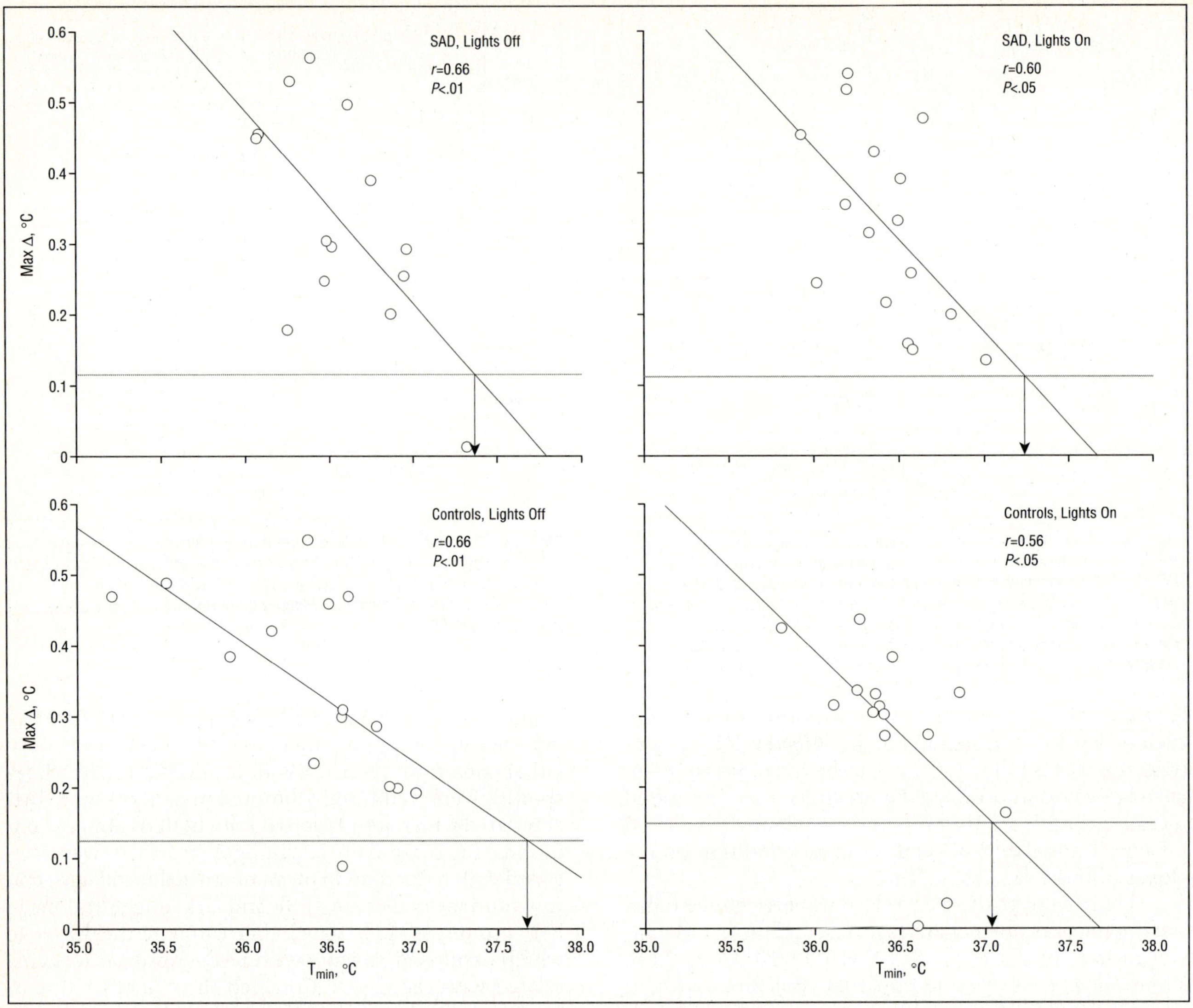

Figure 7. *The degree of hyperthermia following* meta-*chlorophenylpiperazine infusion (Max Δ) is negatively correlated with the level of the temperature minimum from the previous night in patients with seasonal affective disorder (SAD) and controls in both light treatment conditions. The horizontal lines represent the mean Max Δs following placebo infusions within each condition, ie, the mean intrinsic rise in core temperature from 9:30 to 11 AM. The projection onto the temperature axis of the intersection of each horizontal line with its corresponding regression line represents the location of the "set point" of the proportional controller. Thus, when the nocturnal temperature minimum is higher than the set point,* meta-*chlorophenylpiperazine results in no thermogenic reaction. The slope of each regression line represents the "gain" of the controller.*

cent study (N.E.R.; D.G.-B.; Erick H. Turner, MD; Rina G. Vetticad; Jan Sedway; P.J.S.; D.L.M., unpublished data, 1993-1994), administration of another physically and psychologically active serotonergic agent (ipsapirone hydrochloride) produced no abnormal behavioral responses in patients with SAD compared with controls. The reversal of these abnormal m-CPP–induced responses in the present study can be attributed safely to the preceding 2 weeks of light treatment—and not to the confounding effects of the acute light treatment on the mornings of the m-CPP infusions—because, in our previous m-CPP study,[25] comparable light-treatment–associated reductions in m-CPP–induced activation-euphoria were observed in patients with SAD, and light treatment was not administered on the mornings of the m-CPP infusions. In summary, these specific and abnormal behavioral responses to m-CPP seem to be a replicated state marker of winter depression in SAD because they are reversed following light therapy[25] and are absent in the summer.[26]

With regard to the blunted m-CPP–induced ACTH responses, in rats, m-CPP–induced ACTH release seems to be mediated by $5\text{-}HT_{2C}$ receptors in the paraventricular nucleus (PVN) of the hypothalamus,[47-49] which, when stimulated, result in CRH release. Although there are several subtypes of 5-HT receptors on the pituitary gland itself,[50] they do not seem to be involved in the mechanism of m-CPP–induced ACTH release.[48] Blunted ACTH responses also have been observed in patients with SAD in response to intravenous ovine corticotropin-releasing hormone (CRH) infusions.[29] Conceivably, the blunted ACTH responses seen in the previous CRH study and the present m-CPP study reflect diminished 5-HT function in the PVN, resulting in reduced CRH transmission and down-regulation of pituitary responsiveness to CRH.[29] In addition, it also remains possible that pituitary corticotroph function may be restrained in part due to intermittent stress-induced elevations in plasma cortisol concentrations.[51,52] However, because 5-HT modulates not only hypothalamic CRH release[48] but also pituitary ACTH[48] and brainstem NE release[53] (which, in turn, modulates ACTH release[54]), serotonergic lesions in any of several regions could account for the altered responsiveness of the HPA axis in SAD. In this regard, reciprocal circuits connect the brainstem locus caeruleus with the PVN, and agents which activate the PVN-HPA axis also tend to activate the locus caeruleus–sympathoadrenomedullary axis, and vice versa.[55-57] Thus, the blunted m-CPP–induced NE responses in patients with SAD are in keeping with the similarly blunted m-CPP–induced ACTH responses, and suggest a common restraining factor for the diminished responsiveness of these interconnected systems.

From another perspective, the balance between the basal tone of these 2 systems—reflected by the inverse correlations between baseline NE and cortisol concentrations[58]—seemed to be altered in depressed patients with SAD. Specifically, light treatment was accompanied by increases in mean plasma NE concentrations toward normal levels and decreases in mean cortisol concentrations toward normal levels in patients with SAD. Increased plasma NE concentrations[59] and increased whole body NE turnover[60] in response to light treatment have been reported in patients with SAD. Together, the results suggest that the underaroused state that characterizes winter depression is accompanied by reduced basal sympathetic tone,[61] and that the improvement with light treatment may be related in part to enhancing this tone.

We also have replicated our previous finding that twice-daily light treatment preferentially lowers nocturnal, as opposed to diurnal, core temperatures in depressed patients with SAD.[30] In addition, the observed correlation between the post–light-treatment reductions in the nocturnal core T_{min} and the levels of depression, similar to that observed in patients with nonseasonal depression following antidepressant medications,[62] is consistent with the hypotheses (1) that nocturnal core temperatures in patients with SAD are elevated during depression compared with during remission (as they are in patients with nonseasonal depression[62-66]) and (2) the antidepressant effects of light are associated with its nocturnal core temperature–lowering properties.[30,67] Consistent with these hypotheses, we have recently confirmed that nocturnal core temperatures in depressed patients with SAD in the winter become significantly lower during remission in the summer.[68] Whether these elevations in nocturnal core temperatures in patients with SAD might in some way contribute to the development of their recurrent depressions, or whether such elevations reflect epiphenomena of their depressive symptoms (eg, of decreased sleep efficiency) is unknown.

We have previously argued that, in healthy volunteers, the negative correlations observed between the m-CPP–induced Max Δs and the corresponding previous night T_{min} reflect the operation of a nocturnally sensitive proportional thermoregulatory controller that regulates basal metabolism and rest-phase temperature.[41] Briefly, in this model, both the intraindividual and interindividual variability in T_{min} depend on and correlate respectively with the intraindividual and interindividual variability in basal metabolism.[69-73] In the present context, we have $\text{Max}\,\Delta=\alpha(T_{min}-T_{set})$, where m-CPP augments a mode of metabolic thermogenesis (reflected in the increases in core temperature Max Δs) in proportion (α) to the difference between the level of rest-phase temperature (T_{min}) and the set point for metabolic thermogenesis (T_{set}). Insofar as these parameters were not different between groups or light treatment conditions, the results suggest that (1) α is not significantly affected by winter depression or by 2 weeks of twice-daily light treatment and (2) the reduction of T_{min} by light could be associated with a lowering of T_{set}.

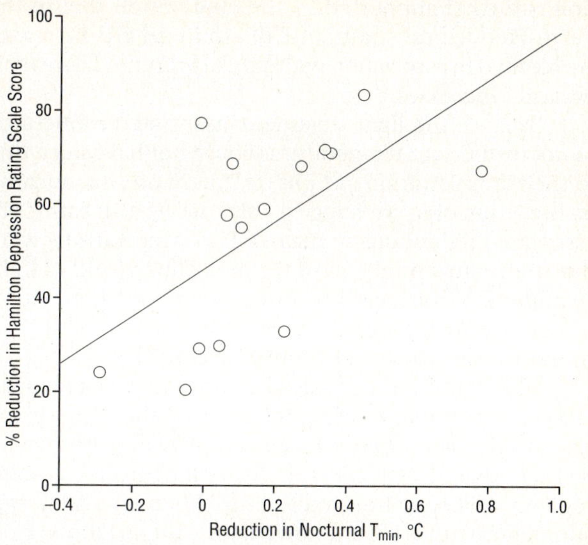

Figure 8. *In patients with seasonal affective disorder, the degree of clinical improvement (% reduction in Hamilton Depression Rating Scale score) following light treatment is correlated with the degree to which the nocturnal temperature minimum was lowered following light treatment.*

Several lines of reasoning suggest that the light-treatment–associated reductions in mean diurnal plasma GH (and possibly PRL) concentrations may also have been mediated, in part, by the mechanisms which govern the nocturnal core temperature-lowering effect of light. First, the delayed rise in GH concentrations following m-CPP suggests that m-CPP may affect GH secretion by an indirect mechanism. Second, the similarity in form between the m-CPP–induced profiles of GH and core temperature suggests that this indirect mechanism may involve the thermoregulatory system. Third, core temperature increases have been associated with increases in GH (and PRL) concentrations in animals and humans.[42-45] Fourth, the light-treatment–associated reductions in rest-phase temperatures were correlated with the corresponding reductions in mean GH (and PRL) concentrations. Given that PVN neurons, which mediate GH and PRL secretion,[74] are known to change their firing rate following thermal stimulation of the preoptic area/anterior hypothalamus (POAH),[75] it is possible that the action of light on these hormones is by modulation of thermally sensitive neuronal signals from the POAH to the PVN. These observations are consistent with the notion that 5-HT_{2C} receptors indirectly modulate GH release by their direct effect on core temperature. This notion is further supported by the observation that in the Fawn-Hooded rat strain, m-CPP–induced GH increases are blunted in association with similarly blunted core temperature increases.[24,76,77]

Because the light treatment–associated reductions in nocturnal core temperatures could not have been due to the administration of light treatment on the morning of the infusions, we suggest that the light-treatment–associated reductions in mean GH concentrations were due to the chronic effects of the preceding weeks of light treatment. With regard to PRL, an independent action of light on hypothalamic dopamine systems, which inhibit PRL secretion,[78] also must be considered.

The light-treatment–associated reductions in mean GH concentrations were significantly smaller (for a given reduction in nocturnal core temperature) in patients with SAD compared with controls. Several neuronal systems regulate GH secretion, including (1) an α_2-adrenergic stimulatory input (of unknown neural origin) to the PVN that causes the release of GH-releasing hormone,[79] (2) an ascending α_1-adrenergic inhibitory input to the PVN that arises from the locus caeruleus and seems to cause the release of GH releasing-inhibiting factor,[80] and (3) a descending influence from the POAH, which causes the release of GH-releasing hormone.[81] Given a role of GH in thermoregulation,[82] and the disturbances of thermoregulation and energy in patients with mood disorder,[83] the present GH findings may be of some interest.

A prominent theory about the pathogenesis of SAD posits an internal phase angle abnormality between the sleep-wake rhythm and other physiological rhythms.[84] Although we did not find a significant phase delay in the core rectal temperatures of patients with SAD compared with controls, our temperature data were "masked" by sleep, which, strictly speaking, precludes the determination of this internal phase angle.[67,84]

CONCLUSION

The significant m-CPP–induced activation-euphoria responses represent a replicated state marker of winter depression in SAD, and the blunted m-CPP–induced HPA and sympathoadrenomedullary axis responses seem more like trait abnormalities. In patients with SAD, the reduction in nocturnal core temperatures following light treatment may represent an important accompaniment of mood improvement. The GH abnormality in patients with SAD may be related to their disturbances in energy regulation. These abnormal findings in patients with SAD, although hard to explain based on a uniform 5-HT receptor abnormality, are not incompatible with the hypothesis that selected areas of the central nervous system are deficient in 5-HT transmission during winter depression.

Accepted for publication June 6, 1996.

We thank Charlotte Brown, PhD, Pamela Madden, PhD, and Fran Myers, RN, for their help with recruitment and Hamilton Depression Rating Scores; the nursing staff of 4-West, Bldg 10, National Institutes of Health, Bethesda, Md, for their assistance with patient care and data collection; and Philip W. Gold, MD, for his input into the manuscript.

Reprints: Paul J. Schwartz, MD, Clinical Psychobiology Branch, National Institute of Mental Health, Bldg 10, Room 4S-239, 10 Center Dr, MSC 1390, Bethesda, MD 20892-1390.

REFERENCES

1. Rosenthal NE, Sack DA, Gillin JC, Lewy AJ, Goodwin FK, Davenport Y, Mueller PS, Newsome DA, Wehr TA. Seasonal affective disorder: a description of the syndrome and preliminary findings with light therapy. *Arch Gen Psychiatry.* 1984;41:72-80.
2. Rosenthal NE, Sack DA, Skwerer RG, Jacobsen FM, Wehr TA. Phototherapy for seasonal affective disorder. *J Biol Rhythms.* 1988;3:101-120.
3. Terman M, Terman JS, Quitkin FM, McGrath PJ, Stewart JW, Rafferty B. Light therapy for seasonal affective disorder: a review of efficacy. *Neuropsychopharmacology.* 1989;2:1-22.
4. Jouvet M. Biogenic amines and the states of sleep. *Science.* 1969;163:32-41.
5. Fernstrom JD, Wurtman RJ. Brain serotonin content: increase following ingestion of a carbohydrate diet. *Science.* 1972;174:1023-1025.
6. Carlsson P, Svennerholm L, Winblad B. Seasonal and circadian monoamine variations in human brains examined post-mortem. *Acta Psychiatr Scand.* 1980; 61(suppl 280):75-82.
7. Cagampang FR, Inouye ST. Diurnal and circadian changes of serotonin in the suprachiasmatic nuclei: regulation by light and an endogenous pacemaker. *Brain Res.* 1994;639:175-179.
8. Wurtman RJ, Wurtman JJ. Carbohydrates and depression. *Sci Am.* 1989;260: 68-75.
9. Rosenthal N, Genhart M, Caballero B, Jacobsen F, Skwerer R, Coursey R, Rogers S, Spring B. Psychobiological effects of carbohydrate- and protein-rich meals in patients with seasonal affective disorder and normal controls. *Biol Psychiatry.* 1989;25:1029-1040.
10. O'Rourke D, Wurtman JJ, Wurtman RJ, Chebli R, Gleason R. Treatment of seasonal depression with *d*-fenfluramine. *J Clin Psychiatry.* 1989;50:343-347.
11. Lam RW, Gorman C, Michalon M, Steiner M, Levitt AJ. A multicentre, placebo-controlled study of fluoxetine in seasonal affective disorder. In: Program and abstracts of the annual meeting of the Society for Light Treatment and Biological Rhythms; June 1994:5; Bethesda, Md.
12. Neumeister A, Rieder N, Hesselmann B, Rao M-L, Gluck J, Kasper S. Serotonin function and mechanism of action of light therapy. In: Program and abstracts of the annual meeting of the Society for Light Treatment and Biological Rhythms; June 1995:7; Frankfort, Ky.
13. Lam RW, Zis AP, Grewal AK, Delgado PG, Charney DS, Krystal JH. Effects of rapid tryptophan depletion in patients with seasonal affective disorder in remission after light therapy. *Arch Gen Psychiatry.* 1996;53:41-44.
14. Kahn RS, Wetzler S. m-chlorophenylpiperazine as a probe of serotonin function. *Biol Psychiatry.* 1991;30:1139-1166.
15. Murphy DL, Lesch KP, Aulakh CS, Pigott TA. Serotonin-selective arylpiperazines with neuroendocrine, behavioral, temperature, and cardiovascular effects in humans. *Pharmacol Rev.* 1991;43:527-552.
16. Hoyer D, Clarke DE, Fozard JR, Hartig PR, Martin GR, Mylecharane EJ, Saxena PR, Humphrey PP. International union of pharmacology classification of receptors for 5-hydroxytryptamine (serotonin). *Pharmacological Rev.* 1994;46: 157-203.
17. Hamik A, Peroutka SJ. 1-(m-chlorophenyl)piperazine (mCPP) interactions with neurotransmitter receptors in the human brain. *Biol Psychiatry.* 1989;25:569-575.
18. Mueller EA, Sunderland T, Murphy DL. Neuroendocrine effects of m-CPP, a serotonin agonist, in humans. *J Clin Endocrinol Metab.* 1985;61:1179-1184.
19. Mueller EA, Murphy DL, Sunderland T. Further studies of the putative serotonin agonist, m-CPP: evidence for a serotonin receptor mediated mechanism of action in humans. *Psychopharmacology.* 1986;89:388-391.
20. Zohar J, Mueller EA, Insel TR, Zohar-Kadouich RC, Murphy DL. Serotonergic responsivity in obsessive-compulsive disorder: comparison of patients and healthy controls. *Arch Gen Psychiatry.* 1987;44:946-951.
21. Lawlor BA, Sunderland T, Mellow AM, Hill JL, Newhouse PA, Murphy DL. A preliminary study of the effects of intravenous m-chlorophenylpiperazine, a serotonin agonist, in elderly subjects. *Biol Psychiatry.* 1989;25:679-686.
22. Aloi JA, Insel TR, Mueller EA, Murphy DL. Neuroendocrine and behavioral effects of m-chlorophenylpiperazine administration in rhesus monkeys. *Life Sci.* 1984;34:1325-1331.
23. Maj J, Lewandowska A. Central serotoninmimetic action of phenylpiperazine. *Pol J Pharmacol.* 1980;32:495-504.
24. Mazzola-Pomietto P, Aulakh CS, Wozniak KM, Murphy DL. Evidence that m-CPP–induced hyperthermia in rats is mediated by stimulation of 5-HT2C receptors. *Psychopharmacology.* 1996;123:333-339.
25. Jacobsen FM, Mueller EA, Rosenthal NE, Rogers S, Hill JL, Murphy DL. Behavioral responses to intravenous *meta*-chlorophenylpiperazine in patients with seasonal affective disorder and control subjects before and after phototherapy. *Psychiatry Res.* 1994;52:181-197.
26. Joseph-Vanderpool JR, Jacobsen F, Murphy DL, Hill JL, Rosenthal NE. Seasonal variation in behavioral responses to m-CPP in patients with seasonal affective disorder and controls. *Biol Psychiatry.* 1993;33:496-504.

27. van Kammen DP, Murphy DL. Attenuation of the euphoriant and activation effects of *d*- and *l*-amphetamine by lithium carbonate treatment. *Psychopharmacologia.* 1975;44:215-244.
28. Murphy DL, Mueller EA, Hill JL, Tolliver TJ, Jacobsen FM. Comparative anxiogenic, neuroendocrine, and other physiologic effects of m-chlorophenylpiperazine given intravenously or orally to healthy volunteers. *Psychopharmacology.* 1989;98:275-282.
29. Joseph-Vanderpool JR, Rosenthal NE, Chrousos GP, Wehr TA, Skwerer R, Kasper S, Gold P. Abnormal pituitary-adrenal responses to corticotropin-releasing hormone in patients with seasonal affective disorder: clinical and pathophysiological implications. *J Clin Endocrinol Metab.* 1991;72:1382-1387.
30. Rosenthal NE, Levendosky AA, Skwerer RG, Joseph-Vanderpool JR, Kelly KA, Hardin T, Kasper S, DellaBella P, Wehr TA. Effects of light treatment on core body temperature in seasonal affective disorder. *Biol Psychiatry.* 1990;27:39-50.
31. Jacobsen FM, Murphy DL, Rosenthal NE. The role of serotonin in seasonal affective disorder and the antidepressant response to phototherapy. In: Rosenthal NE, Blehar MC, eds. *Seasonal Affective Disorders and Phototherapy.* New York, NY: Guilford Press; 1989.
32. Duncan WC, Johnson KA, Wehr TA. Antidepressant drug-induced hypothalamic cooling in Syrian hamsters. *Neuropsychopharmacology.* 1995;12:17-37.
33. Hamilton M. A rating scale for depression. *J Neurol Neurosurg Psychiatry.* 1960;12:56-62.
34. Williams JBW, Link MJ, Rosenthal NE, Terman M. Structured Interview Guide for the Hamilton Depression Rating Scale-Seasonal Affective Disorders Version (SIGH-SAD). New York, NY: New York State Psychiatric Institute; 1988.
35. Brewerton TD, Murphy DL, Mueller EA, Jimerson DC. Induction of migraine-like headaches by the serotonin agonist m-CPP. *Clin Pharmacol Ther.* 1988;43:605-609.
36. Spitzer RL, Williams JBW, Gibbon M, First MB. Structured clinical interview for DSM-III-R patient edition (SCID-P, 9/1/89 version). New York, NY: Biometrics Research Department, New York State Psychiatric Institute; 1989.
37. White A, Smith H, Hoadley M, Dobson SH, Ratcliffe JG. Clinical evaluation of a two-site immunoradiometric assay for adrenocorticotropin in unextracted human plasma using monoclonal antibodies. *Clin Endocrinol (Oxf).* 1987;26:41-51.
38. Abraham GE, Buster JE, Teller RC. Radioimmunoassay of plasma cortisol. *Anal Lett.* 1972;5:757-766.
39. Sinha YN, Selby FW, Lewis UJ, Vanderlaan WP. A homologous radioimmunoassay for prolactin. *J Clin Endocrinol Metab.* 1973;36:509-516.
40. Odell WD, Rayford PL, Ross GT. Simple partially automated method for radioimmunoassay of human thyroid stimulating, growth, luteinizing and follicle stimulating hormones. *J Lab Clin Med.* 1967;70:973-980.
41. Schwartz PJ, Wehr TA, Rosenthal NE, Bartko JJ, Oren DA, Luetke C, Murphy DL. Serotonin and thermoregulation: physiologic and pharmacologic aspects of control revealed by intravenous m-CPP in normal human subjects. *Neuropsychopharmacology.* 1995;13:105-115.
42. Christensen SE, Jorgensen O, Moller J, Moller N, Orskov H. Characterization of growth hormone release in response to external heating: comparison to exercise-induced release. *Acta Endocrinol.* 1984;107:295-301.
43. Christensen SE, Jorgensen O, Moller J, Moller N, Orskov H. Body temperature elevation, exercise and serum prolactin concentrations. *Acta Endocrinol.* 1985;109:458-462.
44. Brisson GR, Audet A, Ledoux M, Matton P, Pellerin-Massicotte J, Peronnet F. Exercise-induced blood prolactin variations in trained adult males: a thermic stress more than an osmotic stress. *Horm Res.* 1986;23:200-206.
45. Saini J, Brandenberger G, Libert JP, Follenius M. Nocturnal pituitary hormone and renin profiles during chronic heat exposure. *J Appl Physiol.* 1993;75:294-300.
46. Press SJ. Generalized multivariate regression. In: Overall JE, Klett CJ, eds. *Applied Multivariate Analysis.* New York, NY: Holt, Rinehart, and Winston; 1972:219-227.
47. Calogero AE, Gallucci WT, Chrousos GP, Gold PW. Effect of the catecholamines upon rat hypothalamic corticotropin releasing hormone secretion in vitro: clinical implications. *J Clin Invest.* 1988;82:839-846.
48. Calogero AE, Bagdy G, Szemeredi K, Tartaglia ME, Gold PW, Chrousos GP. Mechanisms of serotonin receptor agonist–induced activation of the hypothalamic-pituitary-adrenal axis in the rat. *Endocrinology.* 1990;126:1888-1894.
49. Calogero AE, Bagdy G, Moncada ML, D'Agata R. Effect of selective serotonin agonists on basal, corticotropin-releasing hormone- and vasopressin-induced ACTH release in vitro from rat pituitary cells. *J Endocrinol.* 1993;136:381-387.
50. Fuller RW. The involvement of serotonin in regulation of pituitary-adrenocortical function. *Front Neuroendocrinol.* 1992;13:250-270.
51. Jacobsen F, Sack D, Wehr T, Rogers S, Rosenthal N. Neuroendocrine response to 5-hydroxytryptophan in seasonal affective disorder. *Arch Gen Psychiatry.* 1987;44:1086-1091.
52. Garcia-Borreguero D, Jacobsen FM, Murphy DL, Joseph-Vanderpool JR, Chiara A, Rosenthal NE. Hormonal responses to the administration of m-CPP in patients with seasonal affective disorder and controls. *Biol Psychiatry.* 1995;37:740-749.
53. Segal M. Serotonergic innervation of the locus coeruleus from the dorsal raphe and its action on responses to noxious stimuli. *J Physiol (Lond).* 1979;286:401-405.
54. al-Damluji S. Adrenergic mechanisms in the control of corticotropin secretion. *J Endocrinol.* 1988;119:5-14.
55. Bagdy G, Szemeredi K, Hill JK, Murphy DL. The serotonin agonist, m-CPP, markedly increases levels of plasma catecholamines in the conscious rat. *Neuropharmacology.* 1988;27:975-980.
56. Chrousos GP, Gold PW. The concepts of stress and stress system disorders: overview of physical and behavioral homeostasis. *JAMA.* 1992;267:1244-1252.
57. Swanson LW, Sawchenko PE. Paraventricular nucleus: a site for the integration of neuroendocrine and autonomic mechanisms. *Neuroendocrinology.* 1980;31:410-417.
58. Sotsky SM, Lake CR, Goodwin FK. Adrenocortical function and plasma norepinephrine in normal human subjects. *Biol Psychiatry.* 1981;16:643-651.
59. Skwerer RG, Jacobsen FM, Duncan CC, Kelly KA, Sack DA, Tamarkin L, Gaist PA, Rosenthal NE. Neurobiology of seasonal affective disorder and phototherapy. In: Rosenthal N, Blehar M, eds. *Seasonal Affective Disorders and Phototherapy.* New York, NY: Guilford Press; 1989:135-154.
60. Anderson JL, Vasile RG, Mooney JJ, Bloomingdale KL, Samson JA, Schildkraut JJ. Changes in norepinephrine output following light therapy for fall/winter seasonal depression. *Biol Psychiatry.* 1992;32:700-704.
61. Rudorfer MV, Skwerer RG, Rosenthal NE. Biogenic amines in seasonal affective disorder: effects of light therapy. *Psychiatry Res.* 1993;46:19-28.
62. Souetre E, Salvati E, Wehr TA, Sack DA, Krebs B, Darcourt G. Twenty-four hour profiles of body temperature and plasma TSH in bipolar patients during depression and during remission and in normal control subjects. *Am J Psychiatry.* 1988;145:1133-1137.
63. Avery DH, Wildschiodtz G, Rafaelsen OJ. Nocturnal temperature in affective disorder. *J Affect Disord.* 1982;4:61-71.
64. Smallwood RG, Avery DH, Pascualy RA, Prinz PN. Circadian temperature rhythms in primary depression. *Sleep Res.* 1983;12:215.
65. Lund R, Kammerloher A, Dirlich G. Body temperature in endogenously depressed patients during depression and remission. In: Wehr TA, Goodwin FK, eds. *Circadian Rhythms in Psychiatry.* Pacific Grove, Calif: Boxwood Press; 1983:77-88.
66. Von Zerssen D, Barthelmes H, Dirlich G, Doerr P, Emrich HM, Von Lindern L, Lund R, Pirke KM. Circadian rhythms in endogenous depression. *Psychiatry Res.* 1985;16:51-63.
67. Czeisler CA, Kronauer RE, Mooney JJ, Anderson JL, Allan JS. Biologic rhythm disorders, depression, and phototherapy. *Psychiatr Clin North Am.* 1987:687-709.
68. Schwartz PJ, Rosenthal NE, Turner ET, Drake CD, Wehr TA. Abnormal seasonal variation in core temperature during sleep in patients with winter-seasonal affective disorder (SAD). *Biol Psychiatry.* In press.
69. Hammel HT. Temperature regulation and hibernation. In: Fisher KC, ed. *Mammalian Hibernation.* London, England: Oliver and Boyd; 1967:86-94.
70. Aschoff J, Pohl H. Rhythmic variations in energy metabolism. *Federation Proc.* 1970;29:1541-1552.
71. Heller HC, Colliver GW. CNS regulation of body temperature during hibernation. *Am J Physiol.* 1974;227:583-589.
72. Berger RJ, Phillips NH. Comparative aspects of energy metabolism, body temperature and sleep. *Acta Physiol Scand.* 1988;133:21-27.
73. Daan S, Masman D, Strijkstra A, Verhulst S. Intraspecific allometry of basal metabolic rate: relations with body size, temperature, composition, and circadian phase in the Kestrel, *Falco tinnunculus. J Biol Rhythms.* 1989;4:267-283.
74. Sawchenko PE, Swanson LW, Steinbusch HWM, Verhofstad AAJ. The distribution and cells of origin of serotonergic inputs to the paraventricular and supraoptic nuclei of the rat. *Brain Res.* 1983;277:355-360.
75. Matsumura K, Nakayama T, Ishikawa Y. Effects of preoptic thermal stimulation on electrical activities of neurosecretory cells in paraventricular and periventricular nuclei of the hypothalamus. *Brain Res.* 1983;289:330-333.
76. Aulakh CS, Hill JL, Lesch P, Murphy DL. Functional subsensitivity of 5-HT1c or α_2-adrenergic heteroreceptors mediating clonidine-induced growth hormone release in the Fawn-hooded rat strain relative to the Wistar rat strain. *J Pharmacol Exp Ther.* 1992;262:1038-1043.
77. Aulakh CS, Tolliver T, Wozniak KM, Hill JL, Murphy DL. Functional and biochemical evidence for altered serotonergic function in the fawn-hooded rat strain. *Pharmacol Biochem Behav.* 1994;49:615-620.
78. Ben-Jonathan N, Arbogast LA, Hyde JF. Neuroendocrine regulation of prolactin release. *Prog Neurobiol.* 1989;33:399-447.
79. Martin JB, Millard WJ. Brain regulation of growth hormone secretion. *J Anim Sci.* 1986;63(suppl 2):11.
80. Mounier F, Bluet-Pajot MT, Durand D, Kordon C, Epelbaum J. Alpha-1-noradrenergic inhibition of growth hormone secretion is mediated through the paraventricular hypothalamic nucleus in male rats. *Neuroendocrinology.* 1994;59:29-34.
81. Sawchenko PE, Swanson LW, Rivier J, Vale WW. The distribution of growth-hormone-releasing factor (GRF) immunoreactivity in the central nervous system of the rat: an immunohistochemical study using antisera directed against rat hypothalamic GRF. *J Comp Neurol.* 1985;237:100-115.
82. Juul A, Main K, Nielsen B, Skakkebaek NE. Decreased sweating in growth hormone deficiency: does it play a role in thermoregulation? *J Pediatr Endocrinol.* 1993;6:39-44.
83. Wehr TA, Rosenthal NE. Seasonality and affective illness. *Am J Psychiatry.* 1989;146:829-840.
84. Lewy AJ, Sack RL, Miller LS, Hoban TM. Antidepressant and circadian phase-shifting effects of light. *Science.* 1987;235:352-354.

The Motherhood Constellation: A Unified View of Parent-Infant Psychotherapy

by Daniel N. Stern, MD, 229 pp, ISBN 0-465-02602-8, New York, NY, Basic Books Inc Publishers, 1995.

Although the title of the new book, *The Motherhood Constellation: A Unified View of Parent-Infant Psychotherapy*, by Daniel Stern may suggest a selective audience of readers, the book, in fact, has broad appeal. The book is about an exciting, new area of interdisciplinary research, the mind sciences, which embrace emotion, motivation, and values as they affect behavior. The book also is relevant for those in the fields of developmental psychopathology, an area of research that examines individual development in interaction with specific environments, and mental health prevention.

This book represents the logical next step in Stern's persistent pursuit to understand the early development of the human infant's mind, before verbal speech. The book is about theory and practice and is grounded in the principles of development. The book is laced with Stern's creative and intuitive insights gained from his years of experience as a "baby watcher"; he is able to express complex phenomena in clinically relevant language. The book has many notable contributions. First, the research of the author and of other developmental psychologists, cognitive scientists, psycholinguists, and ethologists is summarized in the book; this research demonstrates conclusively that the human infant is an active, information-seeking organism with functional perceptual mechanisms available to signal and receive nonverbal communications. The infant's mind actively develops as the brain rapidly grows. Also, caregivers are biologically and experientially prepared to communicate with their infants.

Second, heuristic, theoretical models, which are derived from cognitive psychology, are presented about how mental representations are structured, activated, and enacted in the parent and the infant. Based on narrative memory and artificial intelligence research, Stern's notions of the "emerging moment," "schemas-of-being-with," and "protonarrative envelopes" provide testable models for scientists to better understand these cognitive, perceptual, and affective neural systems. His microanalytic observation and interview methods provide tools to study them.

Third, Stern's description of a special state in the life of a childbearing woman, the "motherhood constellation," addresses therapy. Stern's ability to integrate concepts from psychoanalysis, developmental psychology, cognitive neuroscience, and ethology is remarkable.

Part 1 of the book deals theoretically with the parents' and infants' representational worlds, taking into account the infant's immature cognitive system. After describing the richness of the representational world of the parent, Stern describes how a particular representation might be activated at any given moment-of-being-with and how, further, activated representations become enacted in interaction. The issue for Stern is how to conceive of the continuity of meaning in the passage from a mother's mental representation to her overt interactive behavior and then from the infant's experience of that overt behavior to his or her construction of his or her own mental representation.

From his method of microanalytic observation, Stern described regular occurrences of behavioral interaction sequences sometimes in synchrony and sometimes not. Now Stern focuses on the activation of specific maternal representations that guide a specific behavioral interaction using an analogous technique, the microanalytic interview. Pilot work, using the interview, suggests that mothers interacting with their infants activate many schemas-of-being-with during an interaction; few mother-infant behaviors occur without guidance from activated maternal schemas-of-being-with.

Stern provides a theory and model to explain the nature and formation of infant mental representations. Stern borrows heavily from memory researchers who have elucidated the construct of narrative event representations. Stern's contributions to event representation theory include (1) a model for incorporating affect and (2) the suggestion that affects serve as the mechanism for representing the whole experience as a meaningful happening. He develops the construct of a protonarrative envelope, which represents a discrete, brief epoch in which a feeling state can begin, crescendo, and diminish. The feeling shape within a particular temporal envelope, composed of intensity and duration, provides meaning to the experience.

The protonarrative envelope contains schemas of perceptions, concepts, sensory motor events, event sequences, and affects. Each of these schemas form simultaneously, in parallel; each exists independently, but they remain connected. Protonarrative envelopes represent meaningful interactive experiences that constitute the preverbal memories of infancy. Stern's speculations borrow from parallel distributed processing models of the brain that have emerged from computer simulations in the cognitive neurosciences and from Freud and Darwin who emphasized motives and goals as determining behavior. Stern suggests that protonarrative envelopes are representations based on developmentally relevant goal-directed motives, such as attempts to reestablish a state of equilibrium or physiological need satisfaction and states of object relatedness, affect sharing, safety, and self-esteem.

The therapeutic approaches of parent-infant psychotherapy are evaluated in part 2 of the book. Psychotherapies focused on changing parental representations are contrasted with approaches that attempt to alter behavioral interaction. Based on his own research with a group of interdisciplinary colleagues, Stern concludes that, irrespective of the theoretical focus of treatment or the hoped for target of change, if therapy alters any 1 element of the dyadic system, it will have an effect on all of the elements because of the dynamic interdependence of interaction and representation. Stern delineates some theoretical and applied differences between parent-infant and adult psychotherapies. He suggests that an immunization model of repeated serial, brief treatments, called "booster" sessions, may be more appropriate for parent-infant therapies, and he argues that rules guiding adult psychotherapy need to be revised for the mother-infant situation. Stern argues persuasively for maintaining a positive therapeutic alliance and transference relationship to enhance future booster treatments. He urges a family support model focused on the strengths of the parent-infant-therapist relationship.

In the final part of the book, Stern provides a synthesis. He describes the motherhood constellation as 4 themes that are awakened after the birth of the baby. The life growth theme focuses on the mother's attention to whether she, as a mother, can maintain her infant's life and sustain her infant's growth. The primary relatedness theme focuses on whether the mother can emotionally engage with her baby in her own authentic manner. The supportive matrix theme focuses on how the mother can create and permit a necessary support system to fulfill the other themes. Finally, the identity reorganization theme focuses on how the mother will function as a mother and transform her self-identity to permit and facilitate these functions. The activation of these themes, as the motherhood constellation, brings forth a further stage-specific set of preoccupations: the mother's discourse with her own mother, with herself as a mother, and with her baby. These discourses are defined as the motherhood "trilogy," which is constantly in interaction with the motherhood constellation as a mother's sense of herself as a mother for her baby shifts repeatedly during time and in different contexts. The motherhood constellation has features of a psychic organizational structure, features of a specific life-span phase, and features of an activated motivational system.

Stern has tackled 3 overlapping objectives. First, he has reviewed scientific data, including his own research, that provide a scaffold for the establishment of a theory regarding the development of the preverbal infant's mind in the context of the mother-infant relationship. Second, he has attempted to construct the scaffold. He has built a theory of mind based on the dynamic transformation of information from maternal internal mental representations to external interactional behavior to infant mental representation, and he has created models that can be used to test the theory. Third, he has reviewed the therapeutic approaches common among infant mental health clinicians, and he suggests specific recommendations about treatment. Dealing with any 1 of the 3 objectives (ie, data, theory, or treatment) would be formidable. Stern has risen to the challenge of all 3. Because of rapidly changing family constellations and parenting styles in our society, a theory of infant mental development and new approaches to early intervention are certainly important at this time.

What advice to give Dr Stern? Stern's contributions have affected primarily developmental psychoanalytic theory and clinicians who treat mothers and infants. His attention now needs to be set on neuroscientists to convince them that human infants and their experiences are worthy of systematic study. Nonhuman primate models, neurophysiological recording, functional neuroimaging, and computer simulation are methods that can be applied to the developmental model of the mind suggested by the ethological, adaptive approach of Daniel Stern.

Thomas F. Anders, MD
Department of Psychiatry
University of California, Davis
4430 V St
Sacramento, CA 95817

An Unquiet Mind

by Kay Redfield Jamison, 224 pp, $22, ISBN 0-679-44373-6, New York, NY, Knopf, 1995.

Kay Jamison provides unique insights for psychiatrists in this captivating autobiographical memoir. She writes prose eloquently, has lived as a person with manic-depression for 30 years, has treated and cared for bipolar patients as a clinical psychologist, and has performed and published thoughtful clinical research on this disorder. From these many perspectives, Jamison gives an informative autobiographical account of the symptoms and phases of manic-depressive illness, which is enriched by her masterful analysis of the broader implications, not only for the life she has lived, but also for illnesses occurring in clinicians and physicians involved in patient care. She also delves into deep philosophical issues raised by modern medical treatments and genetic discoveries. Jamison demonstrates a wonderful ability to shift from a deeply emotional subjective experience to an objective vantage of analysis, classification, and empiricism. From my perspective as a research psychiatrist having a special interest in bipolar illness, I found the personal aspects of her tale compelling. I also was stimulated by the insights provided for their clinical relevance and possible future research implications.

One of the author's most seminal contributions from the research standpoint has been her work on "noncompliance" with lithium carbonate therapy.[1] The current narrative elaborates the troublesome side effects of lithium as well as the psychological effect of the diagnosis and its treatment on the author/patient. She gives an illuminating description of the intoxicating and addictive quality of the manic states. She relates her unwillingness to relinquish them despite her knowledge about the potential destructiveness of the episodes and the likelihood of effective treatment. Clinical researchers seeking effective therapeutic interventions for noncompliance might benefit from reflection on these descriptions. Clinical psychopathological research could also investigate the implied link between premorbid personality and attitudes toward bipolar episodes and mood stabilizers. Neurobiologists seeking clues to underlying biochemical disturbances might exploit the analogy to addictive states and explore neurotransmitter systems not traditionally linked to bipolar illness.

Jamison gives a brilliant discussion of the cognitive changes associated with the depressed and manic phases. As is true for many professionals and creative individuals, the functioning of her brain mattered to her. She was aware of the heightened productivity, creativity, and alacrity of thought during the hypomania. Depression was a crush of low energy, slowing and deadening dullness. Brain circuits involved in these psychomotor oscillations in patients with bipolar disorder deserve greater in vivo illumination by modern neuroimaging methods. Sophisticated neuropsychological challenges will need to be administered to elaborate the functional neuroanatomy of memory, verbal associations, and creativity.

Rich description is given to potentially important nuances of symptom constellations during bipolar episodes. On page 82 Jamison states, "I felt infinitely worse, more dangerously depressed, during this first manic episode than when in the midst of my worst depressions." One wonders about biological differences that might distinguish pure or "white" mania from the excruciating mixed states, vs states of depression. This is an area of research that has received some, albeit insufficient, attention.[2,3] Her account also suggests a potentially definable biochemical switch triggering a psychotic mania in a patient whose episodes often did not achieve that level.

The search for the genetic bases for manic depression is at a critical stage and has the potential to provide major advances in the understanding and treatment of the disorder. Jamison raises vexing ethical and philosophical questions related to genetic research. Will people having the illness choose not to propagate? If the condition of a fetus can be diagnosed, will parents elect to abort? Can bipolar disorder be conceptualized as an evolutionary advance gone awry? Are mental disorders an important or necessary aspect of cultural evolution? What would become of societies lacking "mad" risk-taking behavior?

An Unquiet Mind is a courageous and helpful book. To paraphrase Paul McHugh, MD, chairman of the department of psychiatry, The Johns Hopkins University, Baltimore, Md, the field of psychiatry would be boring without Kay Jamison.

James Kocsis, MD
Department of Psychiatry
Cornell University Medical Center
525 E 68th St, Box 171
New York, NY 10021

1. Jamison KR, Gerner RH, Goodwin FK. Patient and physician attitudes toward lithium. *Arch Gen Psychiatry*. 1979;36:866-869.
2. Hudson JI, Lipinski JF, Keck PE, Aizley HG, Lukas SE, Rothschild AJ, Waternaux CM, Kupfer DJ. Polysomnographic characteristics of young manic patients: comparison with unipolar depressed patients and normal control subjects. *Arch Gen Psychiatry*. 1992;49:378-383.
3. Swann AC, Stokes PE, Secunda SK, Maas JW, Bowden CL. Depressive mania vs agitated depression: biogenic amine and hypothalamic-pituitary-adrenocortical function. *Biol Psychiatry*. 1994;35:803-813.

Professional Opportunities

Physician Recruitment

Psychiatry
Multiple Specialties/Group Practice
Locum Tenens Wanted
Graduate Training/Residencies/Fellowships
Chiefs/Department Heads/Directors
Academic/Faculty
CME Corner
Courses/Symposia/Seminars
Practices For Sale
Notices

1997 Professional Opportunity Rates

Regular	1x	1.15/wd	*3x	1.05/wd
Bold	1x	1.30/wd	*3x	1.20/wd

*In order to receive the 3-time frequency price, the request must be made upon initial placement. The minimum charge is 20 words. A word consists of one or more letters with space on each side.

For information on display advertising and our network buys contact an account representative.

Policy

Orders for classified advertising must be submitted in writing. Although the American Medical Association believes the classified advertisements in these pages to be from reputable sources, the Association does not investigate the offers made and assumes no liability concerning them. Acceptance of advertising is restricted to professional opportunities, practices for sale, and medical office space available. The Association reserves the right to decline, withdraw, or edit advertisements at its discretion. Every care is taken to avoid mistakes but responsibility cannot be accepted by the Association for clerical or printer's errors.

Reply Box Service

Confidential box numbers are available for an additional $20 per issue, plus the words: Box ________, c/o GNP.

When responding to a box number, please send to Archives of General Psychiatry, Box ________, c/o GNP, 515 N State St, Chicago, IL 60610.

Cancellations/Changes

Cancellations/changes must be received in writing at least 25 days prior to the date of the issue. In order to expedite, please fax to 312-464-5909 to the attention of your account representative.

General Information

To contact a Physician Recruitment Advertising account representative, call 312-464-2475/2490/2491/4485 or **800-AMA-2260**. Or fax your insertion order to **312-464-5909**. Mail your materials to **AMA Physician Recruitment Advertising, 12th Floor, 515 N State St, Chicago, IL 60610.**

STAFF PSYCHIATRISTS

Manatee Glens Corporation, a JCAHO-accredited, not-for-profit provider of psychiatric and substance abuse services located on Florida's captivating Central Gulf Coast, offers a flexible schedule and private practice opportunities.

We are now seeking Staff Psychiatrists (MDs or DOs) to work primarily with children in inpatient, outpatient, and partial hospitalization-managed care settings. Current Florida license and ability to be board certified in Child or Adolescent Psychiatry required.

A participant in the National Health Services Corporation and eligible for its programs, Manatee Glens offers a competitive compensation package and excellent benefits. Send resume to:

Director of Human Resources
P.O. Box 9478
391 6th Avenue W.
Bradenton, FL 34206
FAX: (941) 741-3112

Pre-employment drug testing is required. EOE

MANATEE GLENS

Psychiatry

GERIATRIC PSYCHIATRIST: with ABPN qualifications is sought by The University of Chicago for a full-time position with clinical and teaching responsibilities. A demonstrated record of scholarly productivity is required. Academic appointment and salary commensurate with experience. Reply to Neil H. Pliskin, PhD, Department of Psychiatry, The University of Chicago, 5841 South Maryland Ave, MC3077, Chicago, IL 60637. EOE.

TEXAS, the SOUTHEAST, and the SUNBELT STATES. There are Excellent Private Practice Opportunities Available in Psychiatry. Major Cities and Rural Communities Are Available.

Call 1-800-284-4560/Houston 281-493-2797
Or send CV to:
P.O. Box 42314
Houston, TX 77242-2314
FAX 281-493-2234

Reuben Bronstein & Associates

Chiefs/Department Heads/Directors

CHIEF OF PSYCHIATRY: Looking for experienced, energetic, and innovative medical staff leader for the Behavioral Health Services program at Samaritan Hospital as well as the expansion of programs throughout the entire Northeast Health system—an integrated delivery system including residential, community-based and homecare services. Samaritan's dynamic inpatient and outpatient programs offer innovative management and interventional strategies to meet the needs of specific patient populations. Expectations include the ongoing development of new dual diagnosis and geropsych inpatient services. Psychiatrist candidates must have previous administrative experience, be board certified, NYS license eligible. Send CV to Medical Director, 2212 Burdett Avenue, Troy, NY 12180. Fax 518-273-3307. EOE.

Locum Tenens Wanted

HKA LOCUM TENENS is looking for quality general psychiatry physicians to do Locum Tenens. We have opportunities coast-to-coast. We furnish Occurrence Malpractice Insurance (no tail necessary). Please call **HKA LOCUM TENENS at (800) 226-6347, Extension AM7.1.**

@ 1995 MAILSTAR

CALL 800 AMA-2260
for rate and deadline information

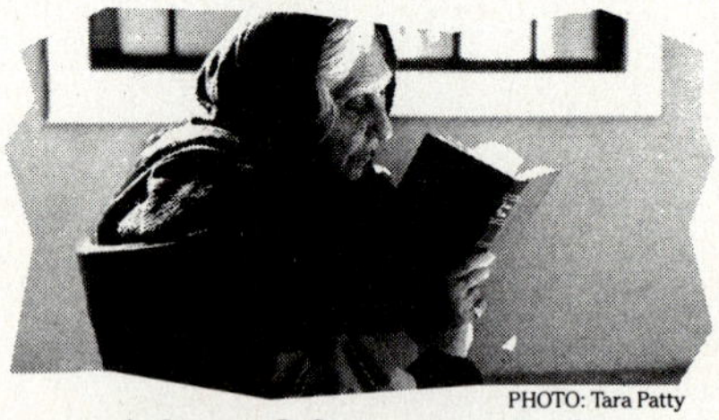

PHOTO: Tara Patty

After 80 years of good vision, we helped this lady see.

We combine adult reading programs with God's Word. That way we teach people to read and help open their eyes and hearts in the process. If this is the type of work you support, we would appreciate your donations.

THE SALVATION ARMY
Changing the World One Life at a Time.

Announcement

Volunteers Needed for Disaster Relief

Established in 1988, International Relief Teams is a nonprofit organization that mobilizes medical and nonmedical volunteers for short-term service (3 days to 2 weeks) to aid victims of disaster and severe poverty worldwide. The organization recently responded to Hurricane Fran in North Carolina, the refugee crisis in Lebanon, Hurricane Opal on the US Gulf Coast, the earthquake in Kobe, Japan, and the Rwanda refugee crisis. Ongoing medical projects are currently being conducted in Armenia, Ecuador, Latvia, and Romania.

For more information, call (619) 284-7979; or write International Relief Teams, 3547 Camino del Rio S, Suite C, San Diego, CA 92108; fax (619) 284-7938.

R E A C H

27,600 physicians monthly with *Archives of General Psychiatry.*

THIS MONTH IN

ARCHIVES OF GENERAL PSYCHIATRY

There is substantial public and professional controversy regarding the ethics of medication-free research in schizophrenia. To advance knowledge of the pathophysiology and treatment of this disease, off-drug protocols are often required, but the safety of the patient and the quality of informed consent have been questioned. **Carpenter et al** (page 401), however, found that data support the contention that medication-free research can be conducted safely. They propose guidelines to minimize risk, enhance benefit, and ensure adequacy of informed consent for patients who choose to participate in these studies. Two Commentaries about this article—by Henn et al and Fins et al—are also included in this issue.

Deficits in smooth pursuit eye tracking have been proposed as a genetic marker for schizophrenia. In a study of monozygotic twins discordant for schizophrenia, **Litman et al** (page 417) found that unaffected twins had significantly less eye tracking deficit compared with their affected counterparts and performed in the range of that of normal control twins. Their results suggest that eye tracking deficits may not be as useful as once thought for identifying unaffected gene carriers in genetic linkage studies. A Commentary about this article—by Holzman et al—is also included in this issue.

The human brain is bilaterally asymmetrical, and it has been suggested that schizophrenia may represent a disorder of cerebral laterality. **Reite and colleagues** (page 433) used magnetic source imaging to estimate neuronal sources of early auditory processing in left and right hemispheres of males and females with schizophrenia compared with nonschizophrenic controls. They found sex-specific anomalous asymmetry in the groups with schizophrenia; males with schizophrenia were less lateralized than controls, but females were more lateralized than controls. Males with schizophrenia also had smaller superior temporal gyri, whereas females did not.

Life-threatening water intoxication often occurs during psychotic exacerbations in schizophrenic patients with preexisting mild overhydration. While assessing factors known to influence water balance, **Goldman et al** (page 443) demonstrated that induced psychotic exacerbations lead to unexplained increases in plasma antidiuretic hormone in these patients, but not in schizophrenic controls. Antidiuretic hormone levels are a precisely regulated index of brain activity and are influenced by structures implicated in severe mental illness. The findings suggest a plausible mechanism for the potentially fatal water imbalance and a probe for exploring the pathophysiology of psychosis in a subset of patients with schizophrenia.

Maintenance treatment in schizophrenia requires medication and psychosocial interventions, but the relationship of these treatments has received scant research attention. **Schooler et al** (page 453) studied 3 dosing strategies using fluphenazine decanoate in patients who also received 1 of 2 family management strategies. They found that dosage reduction increased the use of rescue medication and relapse, but that rehospitalization increased only if a targeted treatment approach was used. There were no differences between family strategies. The value of antipsychotic medication for prevention of relapse and rehospitalization was supported. The absence of family treatment differences may be because both conditions engaged families.

Schizophrenic patients experience problems in relatively basic perceptual processes that could reflect either underlying predisposition to the disorder or the disruptive influence of psychiatric symptoms. **Green et al** (page 465) compared unaffected siblings of schizophrenic patients to normal controls on backward masking, a measure of early visual processing. The unaffected siblings showed poorer performance than controls and the differences were particularly prominent for the earliest phase. Early aspects of visual processing seem closely associated with vulnerability to schizophrenia and may be part of a phenotypic expression of schizophrenia that is separate from symptoms of the illness.

Kinney et al (page 475) systematically measured thought disorder in schizophrenia using an adoption research design to disentangle genetic and environmental sources of familial resemblance. Mean thought disorder was significantly higher in schizophrenic adoptees than in controls; thought disorder was also significantly elevated in biological, but not in adoptive, relatives of schizophrenic adoptees. Results suggest that elevated rates of thought disorder in schizophrenics' relatives primarily reflect genetic, rather than environmental, factors shared with the adoptees.

Cohen et al (page 481) compared the effects of clozapine, an atypical antipsychotic, with fluphenazine hydrochloride, a typical antipsychotic, on regional brain metabolism in patients with schizophrenia optimally treated with each agent. Both drugs led to a shift in the balance of limbic and frontal cortical activity, but differed in their effects on inferior prefrontal cortical and subcortical regions. Neither drug reversed low frontal metabolism seen in these and other patients with schizophrenia, suggesting that antipsychotics, typical and atypical, lead to "compensation" and "adaptation," rather than a "normalization" of brain activity in patients with schizophrenia.

Abnormal brain membrane metabolism may contribute to the symptoms of schizophrenia. A possible mechanism underlying the membrane disturbances is the increased activity of the phospholipid metabolizing enzyme phospholipase A_2, which regulates the rates of membrane renewal and the production of second messengers, such as prostaglandins, in the brain. **Ross et al** (page 487) reported that the activity of a specific subtype of phospholipase A_2 is increased in the blood of patients with the disorder. This change, if also present in the brain, may adversely affect neurotransmission, leading to the altered behavior observed.

The Rationale and Ethics of Medication-Free Research in Schizophrenia

William T. Carpenter, Jr, MD; Nina R. Schooler, PhD; John M. Kane, MD

Schizophrenia research is receiving intense scrutiny from an ethical perspective. Medication-free protocols present a most vexing dilemma in that they greatly enhance the opportunity for advancing knowledge but also raise the prospect of withholding known effective treatment. In this article, we discuss the purpose of medication-free protocols in new drug development and in nontreatment research. Potential benefits and risks associated with drug discontinuation are evaluated, and methods for minimizing risk and increasing benefits are proposed as guidelines for the protection of individual subjects. The complex problem of informed consent also is addressed. Medication-free research in schizophrenia is difficult, but it can be conducted relatively safely with freely consenting, competent subjects. Assurance that studies meet this standard is required. We believe that such investigations can meet high standards of ethics and subject protection, and that a radical revision of procedures for research review and implementation is not indicated.

Arch Gen Psychiatry. 1997;54:401-407

What is the scientific necessity, clinical wisdom, and ethics of research protocols that specify a treatment procedure for a cohort of patients rather than using the physician's best judgment for each individual? How is this addressed in serious diseases with known effective treatments? In schizophrenia, wherein research data and prevailing clinical opinion support continuous medication as a cornerstone of treatment for most patients, how can placebo-controlled clinical trials and medication delay or withdrawal for research purposes be justified? If a research protocol is justified as generating new knowledge, how is the participation of any given patient justified?

These issues are receiving intense scrutiny by investigators, ethicists, and laypersons concerned with the conduct of schizophrenia research. This follows extensive media coverage of allegations that a study conducted at the University of California, Los Angeles (UCLA), was unethical in its design, delinquent in its clinical responsibilities, and inadequate in informing participants of risks (*Time.* August 30, 1993:40-42; *The New York Times.* March 10, 1994, and May 24, 1994). However, an investigation by the National Institutes of Health Office of Protection From Research Risks found the scientific design of the UCLA study to be ethical and the standard of clinical care appropriate. Modifications were required in the consent form to ensure a thorough understanding by participants of the risks involved.[1] The widespread attention given to this case and public concern with human rights and safety in research fueled by recent revelations of the post–World War II radiation experiments makes it timely to reexamine these issues.

See also pages 412 and 415

We review the scientific questions in schizophrenia research that require medication-free periods and discuss the rationale for such studies. We then discuss the potential risks and benefits of con-

From the Department of Psychiatry, University of Maryland School of Medicine and Maryland Psychiatric Research Center, Baltimore (Dr Carpenter); University of Pittsburgh School of Medicine, Psychosis Research Program, Western Psychiatric Institute and Clinic, Pittsburgh, Pa (Dr Schooler); and Albert Einstein College of Medicine, Department of Psychiatry, Long Island Jewish Medical Center, Hillside Hospital, Glen Oaks, NY (Dr Kane).

trolled medication discontinuation under careful observation and suggest safeguards for study participants.

MEDICATION-FREE RESEARCH

There are 2 common types of studies that can require drug-free periods: those that study the development of new treatments and those used for the study of variables that might be confounded by medication effects. The latter studies are particularly important to advancing knowledge with regard to etiology and pathophysiology, and are the critical steps in ultimately finding a cure or prevention.

Development of New Pharmacological Treatments

Significant advances have been made in the short- and long-term pharmacological treatment of schizophrenia. Antipsychotic medications have been shown to be effective for a substantial proportion of patients in alleviating or reducing positive symptoms of schizophrenia and reducing the risk or delaying the recurrence of psychotic exacerbation. In the context of this antipsychotic effect, a broad range of symptom and functional attributes improve. However, available drugs are inadequate. Most patients respond only partially. Primary negative symptoms (ie, the deficit syndrome) are largely refractory to available treatments. Many patients relapse despite continuous medication treatment. Available compounds are associated with adverse effects that can be subjectively distressing, can interfere with psychosocial and vocational adjustment, are associated with poor medication compliance, and, in cases such as severe tardive dyskinesia or tardive dystonia, can be disabling.

There is now an unprecedented effort to develop better medications, reflecting both the dissatisfaction alluded to above and encouraging progress associated with newly marketed compounds.[2-4] It is essential that patients, their families, investigators, institutions, and society pursue the opportunities that these new and potentially more effective and safer medications represent with a consensus regarding the ethics of this research.

Why is medication-free research necessary in new drug development? The first reason is to provide an initial drug withdrawal period designed to minimize the risk for adverse drug-drug interaction as an experimental compound is introduced. Second is to prevent carry-forward effects of prestudy medication from confounding clinical response evaluation of the experimental treatment. Third is to establish a medication-free baseline against which therapeutic and adverse effects are measured. Fourth is to compare new compounds with placebo to establish that they are effective antipsychotic agents. Placebo controls are also necessary to determine an adverse effects profile of an experimental compound.[4] Depending on the stage of development, such studies also may incorporate comparison to standard antipsychotic agents or comparison of different doses or dose ranges of the experimental and/or standard drugs.

Because the goal of this research effort is to find medications that are safer and more effective than currently available treatments, it can be argued that the appropriate comparison should be between an experimental drug and a currently available medication, avoiding placebo altogether. A critical problem is the interpretation of study results. Consider a study in which the clinical effects of an experimental medication are not statistically different from those produced by a drug with established efficacy, but there is no placebo comparison group. Two interpretations are possible: one is that the treatments are equally effective; the other is that neither is effective because the particular patient sample studied is not treatment responsive. The second interpretation is plausible if the sample includes many patients who have received medication prior to study assignment, are poor neuroleptic responders, or are in a maintenance phase of treatment. These are common circumstances in clinical trials of new antipsychotic medications, and the inability to base efficacy conclusions on such designs has been demonstrated.[5,6] That poor response to known effective drugs is often observed has been verified in drug development studies in which haloperidol was an active control.[7] Using a criterion of at least 30% improvement on total Brief Psychiatric Rating Scale scores, the proportion of patients responding to haloperidol varied from 12% to 45%.[7]

The alternative design incorporates a placebo control. If the experimental drug and the standard medication are not distinguishable but both are better than placebo, then we conclude that they are both effective. If neither is better than placebo, we conclude that the study was insensitive to previously known effects and no conclusion is reached regarding effectiveness of the experimental drug. The placebo-controlled study is more informative scientifically, as well as potentially more sparing of risk. The effectiveness of an experimental drug that proves to be approximately as effective as standard treatment can be documented with adequate statistical power in a relatively small number of subjects participating in a placebo-controlled study. Failure to reject the null hypothesis that an experimental and a standard treatment are not different is not the same as finding them equivalent, and, if a study is conducted with inadequate power, the treatments may not differ statistically in their effect despite inferiority of the experimental drug.

A common misconception that placebo response rates in schizophrenia are minimal, consistent, and predictable leads to a misunderstanding of the need for placebo controls. In fact, placebo response rates vary substantially in both short- and long-term treatment trials, eg, ranging from 3% to 26% in the proportion of patients responding in one review of short-term trials.[7] In a recently published report from a large multicenter trial[4] comparing risperidone, haloperidol, and placebo, haloperidol was not significantly superior to placebo on a major outcome measure. Gilbert et al[8] reviewed 29 controlled trials involving neuroleptic withdrawal and found that relapse rates among patients withdrawn from medication ranged from 0% to 100% after follow-up intervals ranging from 0.5 to 24 months (mean, 9.7 months). It is not scientifically valid to substitute "historical" placebo response data for concurrent placebo control. A striking example of this problem occurred when hemodialysis was reported as remarkably superior to historical data,[9] only to be found no different from sham dialysis in controlled studies.[10-12]

In schizophrenia, treatment effects must be assessed in multiple outcome domains. Evaluating a treatment that is effective but is associated with an adverse effect profile causing low patient compliance requires several measures to describe the benefit-to-risk ratio. As an example, consider the prevalence (20%-25% in long-term treated patients) of tardive dyskinesia with antipsychotic drug treatment.[13] If a new medication were associated with little risk for tardive dyskinesia, but was also less effective than standard treatment in preventing relapse, could a decision be made regarding its use without proof that it was in fact superior to placebo?

It has been proposed[14] that once an effective treatment is available, new treatments should be introduced only if superior efficacy is expected. The hypothesis of superior efficacy to standard treatment can be tested without placebo control. This was the case when a superior efficacy hypothesis was tested for clozapine in comparison to chlorpromazine[2] and haloperidol.[15] But, clozapine's antipsychotic efficacy had been previously established.[16] New drug development in schizophrenia seeks advantages in motor side effects, sedation, negative symptoms, long-term cognitive functioning, patient acceptability, and other considerations. In all these instances, it is crucial to determine whether the new drug is an effective antipsychotic.

Nontreatment Studies

There are other research questions that require medication-free protocols and usually involve fewer subjects than are required in drug development programs. Of fundamental importance are studies designed to advance our knowledge of etiology and pathophysiology. Because of the wide range of effects of neuroleptic medication in the central nervous system, such treatment could either cause or confound the experimental results. For example, a positron emission tomographic scan study testing a dopamine receptor hypothesis cannot be conducted on subjects receiving neuroleptic medication because the drugs can alter receptor characteristics. Findings from most studies using dependent variables relating to pathophysiology may be confounded by neuroleptic drugs. These basic studies are necessary to gain sufficient understanding of the disease, which, in turn, provides a new basis for developing therapeutics and prevention. This type of study, in contrast to clinical trials, does not offer participants the possibility of specific benefits from the protocol, although the patient may benefit indirectly (through enhanced diagnosis and more intensive clinical care and therapeutics that are characteristic of settings conducting research with medication-free periods). However, study subjects may ultimately benefit if the research leads to new treatments in their lifetime. Subjects in the initial neuroleptic studies may not have benefited directly if receiving placebo, but their treatment for the years afterward has been enhanced by the new knowledge gained in these investigations.

A final class of studies involves medication-free periods to address specific clinical questions. Does early detection of dyskinesia reduce the risk of developing irreversible tardive dyskinesia? One early detection tool involves the observation of drug withdrawal dyskinesia requiring medication discontinuation,[13,17] another the provocation of dyskinesias by the administration of a dopamine agonist.[18] Does an increase in symptoms associated with initial drug withdrawal identify a subgroup of patients at heightened risk for relapse? Can this change distinguish patients who require substantial continuous medication from those who may be candidates for a medication reduction strategy? Gilbert et al,[8] who reviewed an extensive literature on neuroleptic withdrawal, concluded that discontinuation can usually be done safely with return to baseline levels of psychopathologic symptoms after about 3 weeks of retreatment if symptom exacerbation occurs. Considerable comment pro and con ensued,[19-26] but it is the case that in ordinary clinical care, drug withdrawal may be indicated in a number of circumstances.[19] These include (1) stable patients who refuse medication; (2) patients with emerging dyskinesia, dystonia, neuroleptic malignant syndrome, water intoxication, or severe cardiac effect; (3) aging patients whose psychosis is reduced and drug risks are increased; (4) stable, first-episode patients who may not have a recurrent psychotic illness; (5) pregnancy; and (6) a new approach to treatment that requires a drug washout for safety and/or observation of treatment response.

POTENTIAL BENEFITS AND RISKS OF DRUG DISCONTINUATION

Research protocols without apparent direct patient benefit provoke heated debate.[27] Should subjects be allowed to volunteer for such experiments, and, if so, at what risk or discomfort? We do not engage in this debate here, but rather provide a perspective on the clinical and research questions in medication-free protocols that must be understood if the debate is to be informed.

Potential benefits of drug withdrawal protocols include the ability to assess patients in a drug-free state and better characterize the nature of the illness, to have baseline assessments to more accurately assess treatment effects, to disentangle behavioral adverse effects of medication from manifestations of the disease, to identify early signs of tardive dyskinesia that may be masked by antipsychotic drugs, and to identify patients who may sustain remission without medication. The risks associated with medication-free periods include the prolongation or the reemergence of psychosis. If careful supervision is not in effect, or if severe exacerbations are not treated appropriately, subjects may be at risk for loss of judgment and insight, personal harm or harm to others, job or housing loss, increased burden to family or other caregivers, or other complications of psychosis. These risks are known and current studies must include safeguards to reduce such serious risks.

The question of long-term risk also has been raised. Are medication-free periods associated with substantial adverse effect on long-term course? In an illness that is often severe and persistent despite standard treatment, it is difficult to address this question decisively. Wyatt[28] reviewed the literature and argued that the longer a person is ill before initial treatment, and the more prolonged the psychotic experience is after initial treatment, the worse the ultimate treatment response and the poorer the long-term outcome. He speculates that psychosis is neurotoxic but cites no supportive evidence. On the other hand, animal studies have suggested that the administration of neuroleptic drugs might be capable of inducing neuronal pathologic effects in specific brain regions.[29-32] The interpretation of Wyatt's suggestions is complicated both in terms of the methods used and alternative explanations. First, long-term data that specifically address this issue are scarce. The study by May et al[33,34] involved random assignment of patients to 1 of 5 different conditions for 6 months. Those who did not receive medication during the 6-month trial had a poorer outcome during the next 5 years even though they ultimately received medication. Current drug withdrawal or medication-free research designs do not involve a 6-month "no drug treatment approach" for those experiencing a psychotic episode. The data that are available from trials of substantial dosage reduction or intermittent treatment[35-39] have not found differences in outcome on measures of psychopathology or psychosocial adjustment, even though patients in the medication reduction or withdrawal groups experienced significantly more symptomatic exacerbations. In fact, in one study,[40] patients receiving a very low dose were rated by their families as better on some psychosocial measures despite a 56% relapse rate in contrast to a control group with a 14% relapse rate.

These studies lasted 2 years at most and more data are needed regarding long-term outcome, but the hypothesis that drug-free periods have a long-term toxic effect is not yet substantiated. This view is reinforced by a 7-year follow-up study reported by Curson et al[41] of patients who were treated for 1 year with continuous medication or placebo (relapse rates of 8% and 67%, respectively). No difference in outcome was observed on any of the 11 psychopathology measures.

Although medication benefits are not doubted, it is important to recognize that medication does not cure or halt the progression of the disease. Medications diminish symptom expression and reduce relapse rates. For this reason, we agree with Wyatt concerning the desirability of early detection and initiation of drug therapy. However, this does not guarantee remission or prevention of relapse and may not alter long-term disability. Medication noncompliance is, perhaps, the principal source of lengthy off-medication periods, and dissatisfaction with current treatments is a contributing factor. The evidence from random assignment, controlled trials suggests that it is not the brief, closely monitored protocol-based, medication-free periods that contribute significantly to the adverse clinical course with which Wyatt is concerned. In addition, the potential long-term toxic effects of neuroleptic medication cannot be ignored in any discussion of medication-free research intended to develop safer and more effective treatments.

CONSIDERATIONS FOR INDIVIDUAL PROTECTION

Gaining new knowledge of schizophrenia has a clear scientific and societal benefit, but the issues of an individual's participation as a research subject must be addressed in the context of risk minimization, potential associated benefits, informed consent, and the individual's right to make an altruistic contribution.

If a study design increases risk for symptom exacerbation, how can maximum protection for individual participants be provided? The following points represent basic elements of guidelines to assure the ethical and prudent conduct of studies with schizophrenia patients.

Subject Selection

First, document that subjects understand the research information provided in informed consent. Second, exclude patients with known histories of rapid deterioration associated with substantial clinical management problems. Third, exclude patients who are at greatest risk for severe adverse effects. Fourth, include patients who are expected to have an excellent response to medication only if the following additional criteria are met: (1) the study tests a hypothesis regarding *superiority* of treatment to current medications in either efficacy or side effects or tests a major hypothesis relevant to etiology or pathophysiology that requires robust responders; (2) the placebo period is brief; (3) the protocol has clear criteria for withdrawing patients if response is inadequate or at early signs of clinical deterioration; and (4) if treatment research is involved, the protocol offers treatment advantages to the individual such as open-label treatment with the new drug being studied following research participation or the individual appreciates the absence of treatment advantages and exercises the right to participate to help others.

Enhanced Therapeutics and Clinical Care Monitoring

Several psychosocial treatments for schizophrenia have the potential to partially offset risks associated with medication-free research periods.[42] The protection of medication-free subjects should be enhanced by including a high-quality, broad-based clinical treatment program. In studies where symptom improvement or relapse prevention is the outcome variable of interest, effective psychosocial treatment may reduce power and, therefore, more time and/or subjects may be needed to answer the treatment question. However, if the psychosocial treatment program improves the ability to detect symptom change and rapid intervention is built into the protocol, such programs may enhance care while allowing the use of symptom change rather than full relapse as outcome criteria. Nontreatment studies requiring medication-free periods will similarly be enhanced by effective psychosocial treatment. These procedures facilitate close monitoring and emergency availability in the context of personal continuity of care.[43] Such procedures have proved safe and effective in outpatient research.[8,35-39,44] Any given patient's time in the medication-free component of a protocol may be brief compared with the overall length of care, and benefits from enhanced care can accumulate over time, while protocol restrictions affect only one aspect of treatment for a limited time.

Early Intervention

Early detection of symptom exacerbation and rapid treatment intervention has proved effective in targeted or intermittent drug treatment research in outpatient clinics. One study of maintenance treatment compared medication-free intervals coupled with rapid medication intervention and an enriched psychosocial treatment program with community standard treatment with continuous medication. These treatment approaches did not differ in overall effectiveness, and the treatment that incorporated medication-free intervals was associated with substantial reduction in drug administration.[36] Another study has shown that an early drug intervention strategy is better than crisis intervention in preventing serious relapse in medication-free patients.[44] Several studies have shown that continuous medication supplemented by psychosocial treatments in research settings is superior to low-dose continuous medication or to targeted medication in relapse prevention, but these same studies reveal advantages to the low-dose strategies in adverse drug effects and in the treatment of negative symptoms.[39,45]

Duration of Risk Period

Investigators should be explicit regarding the central study hypothesis. Design of acute treatment studies should incorporate the shortest medication-free period compatible with testing an efficacy hypothesis. Relapse prevention studies do not require severe symptomatic episodes as end points but can test prophylactic hypotheses with mild-to-moderate exacerbation compatible with rapid and effective intervention in most cases. Placebo-controlled studies testing experimental drug effect in actively psychotic patients may be informative in 2 to 6 weeks rather than the 4- to 10-week periods that are characteristic of most current designs. The potential weakness of less change in the shorter period can be compensated in many studies by adding more case subjects to increase statistical power.

Benefits to Participants

In studies evaluating an experimental treatment, providing all participants the opportunity to receive the treatment after study participation is highly desirable. This addresses the problem of patients participating in a study involving increased risk without potential advantage. When this is not possible, the investigator must ensure that the participant understands that the placebo assignment involves risks without the potential benefit of the experimental drug.

The material discussed above supports the propositions that medication-free research can be conducted while continuing other aspects of treatment, that rapid drug intervention can be an effective alternative to continuous medication during symptom exacerbation, that subject selection criteria can reduce risk, and that certain benefits may accrue to research participants. The question of treatment vs no treatment does not accurately address the key issue in most protocol-influenced treatment. Rather, the question is the relative risks and benefits of protocol-based clinical care vs standard care.

INFORMED CONSENT

It has been suggested that persons with schizophrenia be declared a vulnerable population meriting special protection, including requiring a guardianship to authorize research participation.[46-48] This proposal assumes that *all* persons with a diagnosis of schizophrenia are unable to participate in receiving and understanding information and making rational personal decisions regarding participation in research. This argument is not offered as a basis for incompetency and guardianship in all stroke victims, all panic disordered patients with irrational fears, all obsessive patients with irrational beliefs, all depressed patients with affect-distorted reasoning, or even cardiac patients whose apprehension may make them unduly reliant on the perceived wishes of their physician. The determination of competency simply on the basis of the diagnosis of schizophrenia is highly stigmatizing and would strip a large population of their civil rights because *some* schizophrenic individuals, at *some* points in their lives, are not competent to process information and reach informed decisions. Recent research suggests that approximately 75% of patients with schizophrenia incorporate information and make decisions similar to comparison groups when dealing with consent issues.[49]

There are special circumstances when an individual with schizophrenia is not able to participate adequately in informed consent. Investigators must avoid attempting to obtain informed consent when a patient is unable to interact in the receiving of information and determining his or her wishes. At a minimum, the patient should be able to explain what participation entails, identify significant risks and benefits, and know how to withdraw from the study. The signing of the informed consent document is essential for research participation, but the process of informing and assuring adequate patient participation in consent should involve ongoing discussion.[50-52] It is the research field's responsibility to develop documentation procedures to ensure that patient participation is based on an adequate process for informed consent and evidence that the prospective subject has competently processed the relevant information.

Informed consent is also essential for treatment in nonresearch clinical care, although procedures for obtaining and verifying consent are less formal. Clinical procedures have risks and benefits, and patients are entitled to this information and personal autonomy in making choices regarding their treatment (except in highly specified emergency situations or where legal incompetency and guardianship have been established). A written document is not routinely used, but this does not alter the informed consent obligation. There is no unique basis for depriving this entire class of patients of this right in favor of incompetency and guardianship, nor is it conceivable that all clinical care and study of persons with this diagnosis could be effectively conducted under guardianship conditions. What is needed is emphasis on full disclosure, assuring continuing discussion, and encouragement of family involvement.

CONCLUSIONS

Are human subjects participating in medication-free research adequately protected with current procedure? One answer to this question is provided by the observation that there are thousands of patients who have participated in such research and there have been few allegations of significant or long-lasting adverse consequences associated with their research participation. When adverse consequences are alleged, as in the recent UCLA case, the circumstances parallel those associated with difficulties in implementing effective care for schizophrenic patients that are often encountered in clinical settings. The risk that must be considered in medication-free studies is the extent to which such circumstances are *more* likely to occur and what protections are provided. Ultimately, patient welfare depends on the maintenance of effective clinical care and includes a capacity to rapidly and effectively intervene when the course of illness becomes complicated, including adverse consequences of medication-free periods. We know of no evidence that research participation leads to inferior treatment and a worse course of illness in the long term. In fact, many patients and their families anticipate a high level of expertise, a more extensive diagnostic evaluation, a more intensive (and often less expensive) clinical care effort, better follow-up, and perhaps an advantageous experimental treatment when selecting care in a research setting. Evidence supporting this view has been presented.[53-57]

Even when protocols require medication-free periods, cumulative days without antipsychotic drugs may be fewer and clinical supervision may be better than that which occurs in ordinary care settings. Patients often prefer to be without medication despite the risks, creating the very substantial problem of medication noncompliance in clinical care. Finally, all approaches to schizophrenia therapeutics have risks. Continuous medication is better for psychosis reduction and relapse prevention but worse for tardive dyskinesia, sedation, weight gain, a range of parkinsonian symptoms, and other adverse effects. Antipsychotic drug treatment is the cornerstone of modern therapeutics of schizophrenia, but this does not imply that continuous use in all cases is the only safe or effective approach. Nor is the risk-benefit analysis as straightforward as in treating diabetes with insulin. We acknowledge risk associated with medication-free research but we argue that the ethics and wisdom of such designs be viewed in the overall context of clinical care of a chronic illness. The high risk of prolonged off-drug status with infrequent monitoring, allowing severe relapse without intervention, is not the relevant comparison for time-limited, carefully monitored, multimodality clinical care with the capacity for a rapid intervention research design that is now common and that may represent the new standard for medication-free research.

We do not think that current approaches to medication-free research are associated with widespread problems of inadequate informed consent or adverse consequences to patients, nor do we believe that research-based clinical care is inferior. But, new data permitting more explicit examination of these issues are needed, and this is a propitious time to examine procedures and assure patients, society, and the research community that approaches are optimal and that the field is committed to developing better procedures whenever shortcomings are evident. We call for renewed emphasis on added protection. The first consideration is protocol design that ensures that the research questions are of high merit and that effective clinical interventions are in place to reduce risk during medication-free periods. The second has to do with ensuring that participants are competent and that they understand the risks and how to terminate research participation. Assessment of potential subjects in this regard is practical and can provide documentation that consent procedures are adequate and that patients can exercise choice.[58] The third is maximizing offsetting factors such as assuring enhanced psychosocial treatment and clinical monitoring and enabling all participants to have an opportunity to participate in any treatment hypothesized to be superior whenever practical. Ensuring that studies are well designed is the responsibility of investigators, the sponsors of research such as the pharmaceutical industry and the National Institutes of Health, and the established institutional review boards. Assuring the adequacy of protection to individuals who are potential participants in research is the responsibility of individual investigators and the clinical care systems that support the research. Ultimately, the hope of patients with schizophrenia and their families to benefit from further advances in treatment, as well as eventual prevention or cure, will hinge on how well we meet this challenge.

In this article, we described the most common conditions of research participation in medication-free protocols to increase the information used in public discussion of the ethics of this work. We are concerned that statements (*The New York Times.* March 10, 1994) comparing medication-free research in schizophrenia with withholding insulin from diabetic patients or giving placebo instead of immunosuppressant drugs during organ transplant surgery represents an astonishing unfamiliarity with the realities of schizophrenia therapeutics. We also remind the reader that no evidence of any widespread ethical problem in schizophrenia research has been presented and no indication that research participants have an adverse long-term course of illness has been forthcoming.

Based on the above considerations, we do not believe this is a time for radical reform of schizophrenia research procedures. Guardianships for research participants, external clinical monitors, new review boards, and regulations excluding placebo-controlled studies and medication-free research would, in our opinion, stigmatize patients, waste precious research funds, and deprive persons with this illness of the new knowledge on which better therapeutics and prevention will be based. Rather, we believe it is time for a careful assessment of current procedures to ensure their adequacy and to make any necessary modifications. Toward this end, we have identified some relevant strategies to ensure protection in protocol design and individual participation. It must be recognized that informed consent for research is problematic throughout medicine, and illness afflicting the brain presents particular problems in some patients. The general guidelines outlined in this article may apply in most situations but exceptions may have merit. If such guidelines defined the usual conduct of medication-free research in schizophrenia, investigators and review groups would know when an exceptional protocol is proposed and provide special scrutiny of novel provisions to make sure that the work, if undertaken, is conducted with due consideration to the protection of human subjects.

Accepted for publication March 26, 1996.

Supported in part by grants MH40279, MH35996, MH45156, and MH46672 from the National Institute of Mental Health, Rockville, Md.

Corresponding author: William T. Carpenter, Jr, MD, Maryland Psychiatric Research Center, PO Box 21247, Baltimore, MD 21228.

REFERENCES

1. Office for Protection From Research Risks, Division of Human Subject Protections. *Evaluation of Human Subject Protections in Schizophrenia Research.* Los Angeles: University of California, Los Angeles; May 11, 1994.
2. Kane J, Honigfeld G, Singer J, Meltzer H. Clozapine for the treatment-resistant schizophrenic: a double-blind comparison with chlorpromazine. *Arch Gen Psychiatry.* 1988;45:789-796.
3. Meltzer HY. Treatment of the neuroleptic nonresponsive schizophrenic patient. *Schizophr Bull.* 1992;18:515-542.
4. Marder SR, Meibach RC. Risperidone in the treatment of schizophrenia. *Am J Psychiatry.* 1994; 151:825-835.
5. Leber P. Is there an alternative to the randomized controlled trial? *Psychopharmacol Bull.* 1991; 27:3-8.
6. Temple R. Special study designs: early escape, enrichment, studies in non-responders. *Community Stat Theory Meth.* 1994;23:499-531.
7. Kane JM, Borenstein M. The use of placebo controls in psychiatric research. Presented at the First National Conference on Ethics in Neurobiologic Research With Human Subjects; January 7, 1995; Baltimore, Md.
8. Gilbert PL, Harris J, McAdams LA, Jeste DV. Neuroleptic withdrawal in schizophrenic patients: a review of the literature. *Arch Gen Psychiatry.* 1995; 52:173-188.
9. Wagemaker H Jr, Cade R. The use of hemodialysis in chronic schizophrenia. *Am J Psychiatry.* 1977; 134:684-685.
10. Schulz SC, van Kammen DP, Balow JE, Flye MW, Bunney WE Jr. Dialysis in schizophrenia: a double-blind evaluation. *Science.* 1981;211:1066-1068.
11. Carpenter WT, Sadler JH, Light PD, Hanlon TE, Kurland AA, Penna MW, Reed WP, Wilkinson EH, Bartko JJ. The therapeutic efficacy of hemodialysis in schizophrenia. *N Engl J Med.* 1983;308: 669-675.
12. Wagemaker H, Rogers JL, Cade R. Schizophrenia, hemodialysis, and the placebo effect: results and issues. *Arch Gen Psychiatry.* 1984;41:805-810.
13. Kane J, Jeste DV, Barnes TRE, Casey DE, Cole JO, Davis JM, Gualtieri CT, Schooler NR, Sprague RL, Wettstein RM. *American Psychiatric Association Task Force Report on Tardive Dyskinesia.* Washington, DC: American Psychiatric Press; 1992.
14. Rothman KJ, Michels KB. The continuing unethical use of placebo controls. *N Engl J Med.* 1994; 331:394-398.
15. Breier A, Buchanan RW, Kirkpatrick B, Davis OR, Irish D, Summerfelt A, Carpenter WT. Effects of clozapine on positive and negative symptoms in outpatients with schizophrenia. *Am J Psychiatry.* 1994;151:20-26.
16. Umbricht DSG, Lieberman JA, Kane JM. The clinical efficacy of clozapine in the treatment of schizophrenia. *Rev Contemp Pharmacother.* 1995;6: 165-186.
17. Carpenter WT, Rey AC, Stephens JM. Further remarks on covert dyskinesia in ambulatory schizophrenia. *Lancet.* June 19, 1982:1421.
18. Lieberman JA, Lesser M, John C, Pollack S, Saltz B, Kane J. Pharmacologic studies of tardive dyskinesia. *J Clin Psychopharmacol.* 1988;8(suppl 4): 57-63.
19. Carpenter WT, Tamminga CA. Why neuroleptic withdrawal in schizophrenia? *Arch Gen Psychiatry.* 1995;52:192-193.
20. Caldwell AE. *Origins of Psychopharmacology: From CPZ to LSD.* Springfield, Ill: Charles C Thomas Publisher; 1970.
21. Baldessarini RJ, Viguera AC. Neuroleptic withdrawal in schizophrenic patients. *Arch Gen Psychiatry.* 1995;52:189-192.
22. Greden JF, Tandon R. Long-term treatment for lifetime disorders? *Arch Gen Psychiatry.* 1995; 52:197-200.
23. Meltzer HY. Neuroleptic withdrawal in schizophrenic patients. *Arch Gen Psychiatry.* 1995;52: 200-202.
24. Nuechterlein KH, Gitlin MJ, Subotnik KL. The early course of schizophrenia and long-term maintenance neuroleptic therapy. *Arch Gen Psychiatry.* 1995;52:203-205.
25. Wyatt RJ. The risks of withdrawing antipsychotic medications. *Arch Gen Psychiatry.* 1995;52:205-208.
26. Jeste DV, Gilbert PL, McAdams LA, Harris MJ. Considering neuroleptic maintenance and taper on a continuum. *Arch Gen Psychiatry.* 1995;52:209-212.
27. *Proceedings From the First National Conference on Ethics in Neurobiological Research With Human Subjects.* Baltimore Marriott Inner Harbor, January 7-9, 1995; Baltimore, Md. Discussions.
28. Wyatt RJ. Neuroleptics and the natural course of schizophrenia. *Schizophr Bull.* 1991;17:235-280.
29. Gariano RF, Young SJ, Jeste DV, Segal DS, Groves PM. Effects of long-term administration of haloperidol on electrophysiologic properties of rat mesencephalic neurons. *J Pharmacol Exp Ther.* 1990; 255:108-113.
30. Benes FM, Paskevich PA, Domesick VB. Haloperidol-induced plasticity of axon terminals in rat substantia nigra. *Science.* 1983;221:969-971.
31. Meshul CK, Casey DE. Regional, reversible ultrastructural changes in rat brain with chronic neuroleptic treatment. *Brain Res.* 1989;489:338-346.
32. Roberts RC, Gaither LA, Gao XM, Kashyap SM, Tamminga CA. Ultrastructural correlates of haloperidol-induced oral dyskinesias in rat striatum. *Synapse.* 1995;20:234-243.
33. May PRA. *Treatment of Schizophrenia: A Comparative Study of Five Treatment Methods.* New York, NY: Science House; 1968.
34. May PRA, Tuma AH, Dixon WJ. Schizophrenia: a follow-up study of results of five forms of treatment. *Arch Gen Psychiatry.* 1981;38:776-784.
35. Herz MI, Glazer WM, Mostert MA, Sheard MA, Szymanski HV, Havez H, Mirza M, Vana J. Intermittent vs maintenance medication in schizophrenia: two-year results. *Arch Gen Psychiatry.* 1991; 48:333-339.
36. Carpenter WT Jr, Heinrichs DW, Hanlon TE. A comparative trial of pharmacologic strategies in schizophrenia. *Am J Psychiatry.* 1987;144:1466-1470.
37. Carpenter WT Jr, Hanlon TE, Heinrichs DW, Summerfelt AT, Kirkpatrick B, Levine J, Buchanan RW. Continuous versus targeted medication in schizophrenic outpatients: outcome results. *Am J Psychiatry.* 1990;147:1138-1148.
38. Schooler NR. Maintenance medication for schizophrenia: strategies for dose reduction. *Schizophr Bull.* 1991;17:311-324.
39. Schooler NR, Keith SJ, Severe JB, Matthews SM. Treatment strategies in schizophrenia: effects of dosage reduction and family management on outcome. *Schizophr Res.* 1993;9:260. Abstract.
40. Kreisman D, Blumenthal R, Borenstein M, Woerner M, Kane JM, Rifkin A, Reardon G. Family attitudes and patient social adjustment in a longitudinal study of outpatient schizophrenics receiving low-dose neuroleptics: the family's view. *Psychiatry.* 1988;51:3-13.
41. Curson DA, Hirsch SR, Platt SD, Bamber RW, Barnes TRE. Does short term placebo treatment of chronic schizophrenia produce long term harm? *BMJ.* 1986;293:726-728.
42. Bellack AS, Mueser KT. Psychosocial treatment for schizophrenia. *Schizophr Bull.* 1993;19:317-336.
43. Carpenter WT, Heinrichs DW. Early intervention, time-limited targeted pharmacotherapy in schizophrenia. *Schizophr Bull.* 1983;9:533-542.
44. Pietzcker A, Gaebel W, Kopcke W, Linden M, Muller P, Muller-Spahn F, Tegeler J. Intermittent versus maintenance neuroleptic long-term treatment in schizophrenia: 2 year results of a German multicenter study. *J Psychiatr Res.* 1993;27:321-339.
45. Kane JM, Marder SR. Psychopharmacologic treatment of schizophrenia. *Schizophr Bull.* 1993;19: 287-302.
46. Appelbaum P, Lidz C, Meisel A. *Informed Consent—Legal Theory and Clinical Practise.* Oxford, England: Oxford University Press; 1987.
47. National Commission for the Protection of Human Subjects of Biomedical and Behavioral Research. *The Belmont Report.* Washington, DC: Dept of Health, Education, and Welfare; 1978.
48. President's Commission for the Study of Ethical Problems in Medicine and Biomedical and Behavioral Research. *Summing Up.* Washington, DC: Government Printing Office; 1983.
49. Grisso T, Applebaum PS. The MacArthur Treatment Competence Study, III: abilities of patients to consent to psychiatric and medical treatments. *Law Human Behav.* 1995;19:149-174.
50. Carpenter WT. A new setting for informed consent. *Lancet.* March 23, 1974:500-501.
51. Katz J. Human experimentation and human rights. *St Louis University Law J.* 1993;38:7-54.
52. Katz J. Respecting autonomy. In: *The Silent World of Doctor and Patient.* New York, NY: Free Press; 1984:130-164.
53. Cardon PV, Dommel FW, Trumble RR. Injuries to research subjects: a survey of investigators. *N Engl J Med.* 1976;95:650-654.
54. Carroll RS, Miller A, Ross B, Simpson GM. Research as an impetus to improved treatment. *Arch Gen Psychiatry.* 1980;37:377-380.
55. Giller E, Strauss J. Clinical research: a key to clinical training. *Am J Psychiatry.* 1984;141:1075-1077.
56. Kalman TP, Talon NS, Frances A, Kocsis JH. A controlled study of satisfaction among psychobiology research patients. *Am J Psychiatry.* 1982; 139:344-347.
57. Kocsis JH, Frances A, Kalman TP, Shear MK. The effect of psychobiological research on treatment outcome: a controlled study. *Arch Gen Psychiatry.* 1981;38:511-515.
58. Love R, Conley RR. Obtaining informed consent from psychiatrically impaired subjects. *Psychiatr Serv.* In press.

Metabolic: Hyperammonemia (see **PRECAUTIONS**), hyponatremia, and inappropriate ADH secretion.

There have been rare reports of Fanconi's syndrome occurring chiefly in children.

Decreased carnitine concentrations have been reported although the clinical relevance is undetermined.

Hyperglycinemia has occurred and was associated with a fatal outcome in a patient with preexistent nonketotic hyperglycinemia.

Genitourinary: Enuresis and urinary tract infection.

Special Senses: Hearing loss, either reversible or irreversible, has been reported; however, a cause and effect relationship has not been established. Ear pain has also been reported.

Other: Edema of the extremities, lupus erythematosus, bone pain, cough increased, pneumonia, otitis media, bradycardia, cutaneous vasculitis, and fever.

OVERDOSAGE

Overdosage with valproate may result in somnolence, heart block, and deep coma. Fatalities have been reported; however patients have recovered from valproate levels as high as 2120 µg/mL.

In overdose situations, the fraction of drug not bound to protein is high and hemodialysis or tandem hemodialysis plus hemoperfusion may result in significant removal of drug. The benefit of gastric lavage or emesis will vary with the time since ingestion. General supportive measures should be applied with particular attention to the maintenance of adequate urinary output.

Naloxone has been reported to reverse the CNS depressant effects of valproate overdosage. Because naloxone could theoretically also reverse the antiepileptic effects of valproate, it should be used with caution in patients with epilepsy.

Ref. 03-4668-R3-Revised: June, 1996 (Bipolar)

ABBOTT LABORATORIES
NORTH CHICAGO, IL 60064, U.S.A. 609-731-7231A **MASTER**

PRINTED IN U.S.A.

Medication-Free Research With Schizophrenic Patients

A European Perspective

THE ARTICLE by Carpenter et al[1] in this issue of the ARCHIVES presents a clear evaluation of the role of medication-free research in schizophrenia and discusses the ethical implications of such research. The authors argue that medication-free research offers distinct advantages in treatment trials and that the risks for relapse can be limited through careful patient selection, close clinical monitoring, and psychosocial treatments. They further discuss the role of medication-free research in probing questions concerning etiology and provide some assessment of the issues in determining the risk-to-benefit ratio in these cases. They also suggest some relevant guidelines for patient selection in carrying out medication-free research. Finally, they provide some thoughtful insights on the issue of informed consent. They conclude that medication-free research in schizophrenia is clearly worthwhile and even necessary in treatment evaluations and in studies aimed at understanding etiology and that reasonable guidelines should be established by the profession for such research.

The arguments that delaying or withdrawing medication is unethical speak to the deep distrust of the research establishment by some who fear that patient rights may be infringed on in the name of scientific inquiry. That these fears have been realized in modern European history suggests that a European perspective on these issues may be useful. The sensitivity to the misuse of science plays itself out in the conduct of clinical trials. In schizophrenia research, no placebo-controlled trials are taking place in Germany. The standard for the government and industry is effectiveness of the new medication at least equal to standard treatment, which is almost always a comparison with haloperidol. We agree that only superiority can be demonstrated using this design but believe that in view of the limitations of standard therapy, one should only look for drugs with specific advantages over standard treatment. One suggestion for not missing drugs with markedly better side-effect profiles but equal efficacy is to attempt to establish superiority through comparison trials without placebo. If this shows equivalent efficacy and suggests a lower side-effect profile, consider a small placebo trial to establish efficacy unequivocally. This would result in the exposure of fewer patients to treatment with placebo.

See also pages 401 and 415

We believe that with detailed clinical monitoring and good psychosocial support, placebo-controlled treatment studies are ethical and ideal and should involve more intensive clinical care. This means extensive involvement of the primary caregiver in both consent procedures and clinical monitoring. Three dangers of placebo-controlled trials may require further discussion. First, care must be taken to avoid bias in patient selection toward either stable patients or rapidly responding noncompliant patients. Patient selection also occurs as a natural consequence of the detailed informed consent procedures that are recommended and necessary.[2] In general, as patients are given more detailed information for informed consent, fewer agree to participate in trials.[3] This limits the general applicability of the studies. Second, since the rapid withdrawal from medication appears to enhance the risk for relapse,[4,5] patients enrolled in placebo trials should either be in full relapse or already medication free, as study time deadlines mitigate against slow medication withdrawal. Finally, in view of the suggestion that relapses may worsen prognosis,[6-8] one should consider limiting placebo control patients to those who have experienced no relapses as a result of medication trials. This would mitigate against a pool of study patients being used repeatedly in industry-sponsored trials. Because in Great Britain and Germany, health care is considered a right, with mandatory universal insurance coverage, one must wonder about the coercive role of free clinical trials in a society such as the United States in which a substantial minority have no mental health care coverage.

Finally, in considering the role of medication-free research when studying etiological issues, several points must be kept in mind. In these studies it is not clear that any direct benefit will occur for the proband. Thus, every effort must be made to minimize risk. This would include a slow medication withdrawal for patients who were receiving medication, intensive clinical monitoring, and the initiation of pharmacological intervention at the first sign of prodromal symptoms. It is also necessary to attain a true drug-free state, which would mean a period of at least 6 weeks if depot medication is not a factor. Under these conditions, the welfare of the patients can be maximized even in studies that offer no immediate benefit to the patients.

Fritz A. Henn, PhD, MD
University of Heidelberg
Central Institute of Mental Health
Postfach 12 21 20
68072 Mannheim, Germany

Malcolm Lader, OBE, DSc, PhD, FRCPsych
London, England

Hanfried Helmchen, MD
Berlin, Germany

REFERENCES

1. Carpenter WT Jr, Schooler NR, Kane JM. The rationale and ethics of medication-free research in schizophrenia. *Arch Gen Psychiatry.* 1997;54:401-407.
2. Helmchen H, Lauter H. Ethische Probleme bei der biomedizinischen Forschung mit kognitiv beeinträchtigten älteren Menschen. *Nervenarzt.* 1995;66:231-238.
3. Grisso T, Appelbaum PS. Comparison of standards for assessing patients' capacities to make treatment decisions. *Am J Psychiatry.* 1995;152:1033-1037.
4. Green AI, Faraone SV, Brown WA, Gutterez J, Tsuang MT. Neuroleptic dose reduction studies: clinical and neuroendocrine effects. Presented at the 31st annual meeting of the American College of Neuropsychopharmacology; December 15, 1992; San Juan, Puerto Rico.
5. Baldessarini RJ, Viguera AC. Neuroleptic withdrawal in schizophrenic patients. *Arch Gen Psychiatry.* 1995;52:189-192.
6. Gilbert PI, Harris MJ, McAdams LA, Jeste DV. Neuroleptic withdrawal in schizophrenic patients: review of the literature. *Arch Gen Psychiatry.* 1995;52:173-188.
7. Wyatt KJ. Neuroleptics and the natural course of schizophrenia. *Schizophr Bull.* 1991;17:325-351.
8. Crow TJ, Macmillan JF, Johnson AL, Johnstone EC. A randomized controlled trial of prophylactic neuroleptic treatment. *Br J Psychiatry.* 1981;148:120-127.

ARCHIVES Circulation

The ARCHIVES is available by request to nonfederal physicians in the United States (50 states and Washington, DC) whose official American Medical Association masterfile record shows a primary specialty of psychiatry or child psychiatry in an office- or hospital-based practice as a staff physician, resident in training beyond the first year, or clinical fellow.

If you meet the above qualification criteria and are not currently receiving the ARCHIVES and would like to receive it each month, you must complete a free subscription request card. To receive a request card, please write to Kathryn Osten, American Medical Association, Circulation Processing Department, 515 N State St, Chicago, IL 60610 (fax 312-464-5831). A subscription request card will be sent to you in response. If you are a resident or fellow, please include verification of your training program and a complete mailing address.

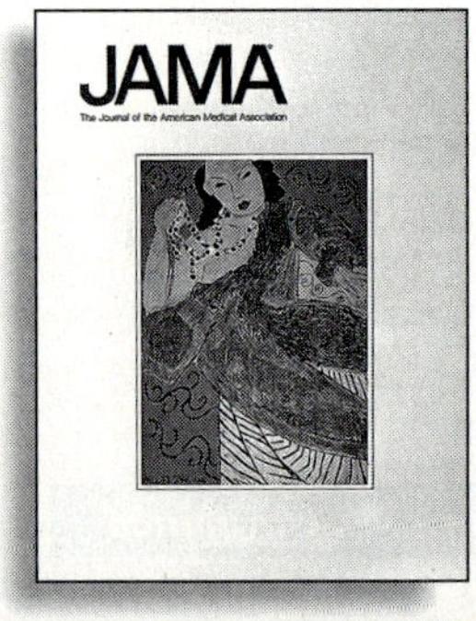
JAMA
The Journal of the American Medical Association

The Call of the Sirens

Navigating the Ethics of Medication-Free Research in Schizophrenia

IN THE *Odyssey*, Odysseus directs his men to tie him to their ship's mast as they approach the mind-altering call of the Sirens.[1] He forbids his crew to unlash him lest they all be destroyed and never reach their beloved Ithaca. Translated into a modern idiom, Odysseus outlines an advance directive for when he is decisionally incapacitated by the Sirens' seductions. He gives consent to his crew to bind and restrain him though he might ask for release.

See also pages 401 and 412

Addressing the ethics of medication-free research in schizophrenia, we can consider informed consent and protection of human subjects in light of this classical tale. Does the consent of a competent schizophrenic subject extend into a period of psychosis resulting from the agreed-upon drug-free interval? If consent is a process to be maintained over time,[2] then how is ongoing voluntariness[3] assured when the research subject loses insight necessary to judge research risks? Like the crew member who must decide whether to follow Odysseus' instructions, the psychiatric investigator must consider the quality of the subject's informed consent to determine the legitimacy of drug-free research. Moreover, the Siren call of future therapeutic advances may divert the attention of investigators from the ethical mandate to respect the rights of subjects and protect their welfare.

In this issue of the ARCHIVES, Carpenter et al[4] correctly note that schizophrenia—in and of itself—does not preclude the ability to consent to therapy or research.[5] Nonetheless, the authors are overly optimistic about the decision-making capacity of persons with schizophrenia. Appelbaum's observation that "hospitalized schizophrenics as a group are at elevated risk of having their capacities to consent impaired"[6] warrants a more nuanced assessment of the subject's ability to consent.

We suggest that psychiatric investigators adopt a "sliding scale" approach for consent to research to parallel ethical guidelines used for determining decision-making capacity in clinical practice.[7-9] Using this approach, the rigor of the capacity determination should vary depending on the risk-benefit profile of the study. Studies with greater risk, especially nontherapeutic experiments posing more than minimal risk, should have more exacting criteria for assessment and documentation of capacity.

An accurate appraisal of the subject's ability to participate in the decision-making process is critical because of our limited knowledge of the motivations and experiences of those participating in drug-free research. We do not know why these subjects volunteer, why they are prepared to accept periods without medication, and what their experiences have been. These questions warrant future systematic study and dictate procedural caution.

The conflict of interest that occurs when a psychiatric researcher assesses capacity and obtains consent also merits additional safeguards in some types of psychiatric research. Institutional review boards should consider independent capacity assessments in drug-free schizophrenia research because incapacity can result from the study intervention. We endorse the recommendation of Dresser that independent consent auditors and clinical monitors be employed in protocols that involve greater than minimal risk with no prospect of benefit.[10] We also second Appelbaum's suggestion that durable powers of attorney be used to direct health care decisions and authorize research when capacity is lost.[6]

Subjects who are deemed capable of consent need to appreciate the difference between research and clinical practice as well as the available therapeutic alternatives should they decline study enrollment. Justifying study participation, as the authors do, by analogizing the schizophrenic patient's right to consent to therapeutic interventions risks conflating clinical practice with research. In the former, the practitioner's intention is therapeutic. In the latter, direct patient benefit is not the primary goal and may be entirely absent.

The authors seem to appreciate that drug-free research imposes some additional responsibilities such as the provision of "enhanced therapeutics and clinical care monitoring" that offsets study risk. These protections should explicitly articulate safeguards for outpatient drug-free studies that pose greater monitoring challenges. Investigators should demonstrate that there is adequate and frequent monitoring to ensure subject safety in the outpatient setting.

Carpenter and his colleagues assert that medication-free research is ethically acceptable and that "this is not the time for radical reform of schizophrenia research procedures." We acknowledge the authors' cogent assessment of the risks and benefits of this research and agree that it should not be proscribed or burdened by excessive regulation. We believe that additional safeguards are indicated to ensure the adequacy of informed consent and subject protection, thereby promoting public acceptance of this worthy research. Only then can we navigate the currents of this complex research and avoid the treacherous shoals of the Sirens.

Joseph J. Fins, MD
Box 297
The New York Hospital–Cornell Medical Center
525 E 68th St
New York, NY 10021

Franklin G. Miller, PhD
Charlottesville, Va

Supported in part by a grant from the Emily Davie and Joseph S. Kornfeld Foundation, New York, NY.

REFERENCES

1. Homer. *The Odyssey.*
2. Lidz CW, Appelbaum PS, Meisel A. Two models of implementing informed consent. *Arch Intern Med.* 1988;148:1385-1389.
3. Nuremberg Code. Reprinted in Levine RJ. *Ethics and Regulation of Clinical Research.* 2nd ed. New Haven, Conn: Yale University Press; 1988.
4. Carpenter WT Jr, Schooler NR, Kane JM. The rationale and ethics of medication-free research in schizophrenia. *Arch Gen Psychiatry.* 1997;54:401-407.
5. Office for Protection From Research Risks. *Protecting Human Research Subjects: Institutional Review Board Guidebook.* Washington, DC: US Government Printing Office; 1993:6-29-30.
6. Appelbaum PS. Drug-free research in schizophrenia: an overview of the controversy. *IRB.* 1996;18(1):1-5.
7. Roth LH, Meisel A, Lidz CW. Tests of competency to consent to treatment. *Am J Psychiatry.* 1997;134:279-284.
8. Drane JF. Competency to give an informed consent: a model for making clinical assessments. *JAMA.* 1984;252:925-927.
9. Buchanan AE, Brock DW. Competence and incompetence. In: *Deciding for Others: The Ethics of Surrogate Decision Making.* New York, NY: Cambridge University Press; 1990:51-57.
10. Dresser R. Mentally disabled research subjects: the enduring policy issues. *JAMA.* 1996;276:67-72.

A Quantitative Analysis of Smooth Pursuit Eye Tracking in Monozygotic Twins Discordant for Schizophrenia

Robert E. Litman, MD; E. Fuller Torrey, MD; Daniel W. Hommer, MD; Allan R. Radant, MD; David Pickar, MD; Daniel R. Weinberger, MD

Background: Previous studies of discordant monozygotic (MZ) twins have suggested that abnormal smooth pursuit eye tracking is an indicator of genetic liability for schizophrenia. We attempted to replicate this in a different sample of twins.

Methods: Probands from 12 sets of MZ twins discordant for schizophrenia who met *DSM-III-R* criteria for schizophrenia or schizoaffective disorder and their co-twins without psychiatric diagnosis (except 2 with a history of substance abuse) and 12 sets of normal control MZ twins. Psychiatric diagnosis was based on Structured Clinical Interview; monozygosity was based on analysis of 19 red blood cell antigens. Smooth pursuit eye movement gain (equal to the ratio of eye-target velocity) and numbers, amplitudes, and subtypes of saccadic eye movements were compared. Measures were derived from computer analysis of digitized infrared oculographic recordings of constant velocity (16.67° per second) smooth pursuit eye tracking.

Results: Quantitative measures of eye tracking for the affected twin were inferior to those of the unaffected co-twin, with affected twins showing significant decreases in gain and significant increases in numbers and amplitudes of total and intrusive saccades. Moreover, whereas means for the group of affected twins differed significantly from those of normal controls on measures of gain and total saccades, means for the group of unaffected co-twins were well within the normal range.

Conclusions: These data are consistent with the hypothesis that abnormal eye tracking is associated with the expression of illness, or phenotype, in schizophrenia, at least in this twin sample. The data raise questions regarding the use of eye tracking measurement for identifying putative gene carriers among at-risk relatives in genetic linkage studies of schizophrenia.

Arch Gen Psychiatry. 1997;54:417-426

Recent success using molecular genetic techniques and linkage analysis to identify major genetic loci underlying hereditary illnesses such as Huntington disease[1,2] and other neurologic disorders has heightened expectations that such efforts will identify major genes for schizophrenia, a neuropsychiatric disorder for which evidence suggests a genetic liability.[3] To date, however, linkage studies in schizophrenic pedigrees have not yielded consistent, replicable results.[4-8] This lack of success may, in part, be due to the highly variable phenotypic expression of the putative gene(s) for schizophrenia, which makes it difficult to accurately determine, using established symptom or clinical criteria, which members of a pedigree possess the abnormal gene. Thus, classifying as unaffected pedigree members who are asymptomatic but nonetheless possess the abnormal gene(s) would distort the computation of linkage between a DNA marker for the gene and the disease.[9] One solution to this problem would be the use of objectively measured, biological markers for schizophrenia in conjunction with clinical assessments in linkage studies. Ideally, the marker would be linked to the presence of the gene, ie, it would occur not only in probands and family members who express symptoms of the illness but also in asymptomatic relatives who possess the gene.[10,11]

See also page 429

One marker for schizophrenia that shows promise in this regard is abnormal smooth pursuit eye tracking.[12] This abnormality is found in a high proportion of patients with schizophrenia; it involves an impairment in their ability to pursue a moving target visually. Studies of smooth pursuit tracking in schizophrenia suggest that the abnormality is a trait characteristic of schizophrenia, ie, the presence of the abnormality does not vary with experimental conditions, drug treatment, or clinical state.[13] Of significance for genetic studies, however, is the observation by Holzman et

From the Experimental Therapeutics Branch (Drs Litman and Pickar) and the Clinical Brain Disorders Branch (Drs Torrey and Weinberger), National Institute of Mental Health, and the Laboratory of Clinical Studies, National Institute on Alcohol Abuse and Alcoholism, National Institutes of Health, Bethesda, Md (Dr Hommer); and the Veterans Affairs Medical Center, Seattle, Wash (Dr Radant).

SUBJECTS AND METHODS

SUBJECTS

The recruitment, selection, and characterization of MZ twins in this study was performed according to methods previously described.[59] Twelve sets of MZ twins discordant for schizophrenia (9 male pairs and 3 female pairs) and 12 sets of normal controls (8 male pairs and 4 female pairs) gave written informed consent to participate in this study. Monozygosity for all twins was determined on the basis of physical similarity and analysis of 19 red blood cell antigens. All MZ twins discordant for schizophrenia underwent videotaped Structured Clinical Interview for *DSM-III-R* (SCID)[60] to establish *DSM-III-R* diagnoses, which were based on the consensus of 2 research psychiatrists.[61] Of the 12 affected twins or probands, 6 had chronic schizophrenia, undifferentiated type; 3 had chronic schizophrenia, paranoid type; 2 had schizoaffective disorder, depressed type; and 1 had chronic schizophrenia, disorganized type. Ten of the 12 unaffected co-twins received no psychiatric diagnosis, including no diagnoses of schizophrenia-spectrum disorders; 2 had a history of substance abuse. None of the discordant twins had tardive dyskinesia (on neurologic examination and by history), neurologic illness, or a history of chronic substance abuse. Discordant twins were recruited through the network of the National Alliance for the Mentally Ill; they are a subset of a larger sample of 26 discordant twins with schizophrenia available as part of a multidimensional study of MZ twins with schizophrenia.[59]

Eleven of the affected twins were receiving typical neuroleptic medication at the time of testing; 5 of these were receiving antiparkinsonian medication (either benztropine mesylate or trihexyphenidyl hydrochloride). Six were receiving nonneuroleptic psychotropic medication and 1 was receiving no medication. None of the affected twins were receiving lithium, benzodiazepines, clozapine,[48,62] or any other medication that might affect eye tracking performance.

Family histories were obtained from the mothers of twins via questionnaire and interview. Four sets of MZ twins had a family history of schizophrenia, 1 set with a definite diagnosis of schizophrenia in a first-degree relative and 3 sets with a diagnosis of probable schizophrenia in a second-degree relative.[59]

Two of the affected twins sustained possible brain trauma. One had a presumptive diagnosis of meningitis or encephalitis, according to the parent (medical records were unavailable). The other sustained severe head trauma from a vehicular crash resulting in loss of conciousness, seizures, and hospitalization for 3 weeks, although this twin also had a positive family history for schizophrenia and other predisposing factors for schizophrenia occurring before the head injury (eg, minor physical anomalies, lower birth weight, possible dyslexia). In both twins, the onset of symptoms of schizophrenia occurred more than 10 years after the episode of brain trauma.[59]

Affected twins had a mean±SD duration of illness of 10.1±5.6 years (range, 4-20 years) and had been hospitalized an average of 6.7 times. The minimum duration of illness for affected twins was long enough (>4 years) to make it unlikely that any twin pairs would become concordant for schizophrenia.[63]

Normal controls, recruited by word of mouth, underwent careful screening for absence of psychiatric disorders, history of neurologic illness or head trauma, and history of psychiatric illness in family members. Diagnostic screening was performed using the SCID (4 sets of normal controls) or the Schedule for Affective Disorders and Schizophrenia—Lifetime Version structured clinical interview (9 sets of normal controls).[64] (One set of normal controls underwent a second screening.)

The mean±SD age of discordant MZ twins was 29.6±7.8 years (range, 17-42 years); mean±SD age for normal controls was 30.7±10.8 years (range, 19-54 years). The 2 groups did not differ significantly in age (2-tailed $t=-0.40$; $P<.70$).

EYE MOVEMENT TESTING PROCEDURE AND SMOOTH PURSUIT TASK

Eye movements were recorded in a quiet, darkened room using an infrared limbus detection eye tracking device (Eye Trac Model 210, Applied Sciences Laboratories, Waltham, Mass). This device has a response time constant of 4 milliseconds, an accuracy of better than 0.25° of visual angle, and a range of 15° to the left and to the right of center. The subjects were seated 43 cm in front of a video monitor on which a small, bright square video target was displayed against a dark background. The target subtended a visual angle of less than 0.25°. The subject's head was secured by a bite bar and head restraint. Analog output of the infrared tracking device was sampled at 1000 Hz using an 8-bit analog to digital converter and was stored for subsequent analysis. Before each run of data collection, the system was electronically calibrated. This was done by asking the subject to look at the center of the screen and 15° to the left and to the right of center. Data were collected only from the eye from which the most rapid and accurate calibration was obtained.

Smooth pursuit eye tracking was recorded during a task where the target moved at a constant velocity of 16.67° per second horizontally across the screen, 15° to the left and to the right of center. Subjects performed the task for 1 full minute per trial. Subjects were instructed to keep their eyes on the target and follow it as accurately as they could. Data collection began 15 seconds into the task, and 30 seconds of smooth pursuit tracking data were subsequently collected. Symptom ratings from the Brief Psychiatric Rating Scale[65] and the Schedule for Assessment of Negative Symptoms[66] were collected on the day of or 1 to 2 days preceding the eye tracking procedure from all affected discordant twins.

EYE MOVEMENT DATA ANALYSIS

Eye movement data were analyzed using pattern recognition computer software developed by 2 of us (A.R.R. and D.W.H.) with methods as described previously.[48] Briefly,

al[14] that abnormal smooth pursuit tracking is found in the asymptomatic relatives of schizophrenic patients. Abnormal smooth pursuit tracking is present in 30% to 50% of the first-degree relatives of schizophrenic probands, but is only found in approximately 8% of first-degree relatives of patients with other psychiatric disorders, which is similar to its frequency in the general population.[15-17] This finding raises the possibility that abnormal smooth the raw data consisted of eye- and target-position values for each millisecond of recorded tracking, and they could be displayed on a computer screen as a plot of eye position vs time (**Figure 1**). Since the target moved horizontally at constant velocity, a triangular curve of target and eye motion was generated by the computer. Since the initiation of smooth pursuit is quite different from its maintenance,[67] we excluded the 250 milliseconds preceding or following changes in target direction from the analysis. Sequential manipulations were performed on the remaining data to isolate saccades from true pursuit and artifacts. First, the velocity for each millisecond of the tracking was calculated by subtracting the position value 5 milliseconds before the given point from the position value 5 milliseconds after the given point and dividing the result by 10 milliseconds. The next step in dissecting a subject's eye movement tracing was to identify all intervals with a peak velocity of greater than 35° per second. The beginning and end of these high-velocity intervals were extended to the point where the velocity dropped below 30° per second. High-velocity intervals with a simple uniphasic pattern were considered saccades. Saccade amplitude was derived as the length in degrees of visual arc of each interval deemed a saccade. Presaccadic and postsaccadic position errors were determined 5 milliseconds before the beginning and 5 milliseconds after the end of a saccade, respectively. High-velocity intervals with a peak velocity of greater than 850° per second or that were followed immediately by another high-velocity interval in the opposite direction were discarded as artifact. Both phases of any biphasic pattern were discarded, since preliminary studies (in which subjects purposely blinked) indicated that this pattern represents eye blinks. Inspection of all high-velocity intervals using interactive computer software was done by 1 of us (R.E.L) unaware of subject diagnosis to ensure that all intervals classified as saccades met these criteria and were not artifacts, as previously described.[48] All intervals of eye tracking not meeting the above criteria for being a high-velocity interval or artifact were considered to be SPEM. Since we were interested in measuring SPEM performance only when actively pursued targets were properly visualized by the fovea, we excluded from analysis intervals in which SPEM velocity was less than 5° per second or SPEM position error (eye position subtracted from target position) was greater than 2.5°, which is the radius of the fovea in humans.[48]

QUANTITATIVE EYE MOVEMENT VARIABLES AND SACCADE CLASSIFICATION CRITERIA

Quantitative variables were defined as follows. Gain of SPEM was defined as the mean (weighted for time) of the gain of each separate SPEM interval, across all such intervals. Total saccades were obtained by tabulating the number of all intervals considered to be saccades according to the criteria stated above (ie, high-velocity intervals with simple uniphasic pattern), per 30 seconds of smooth pursuit tracking. In addition, saccades were subclassified by their direction (in relation to target motion), and presaccadic and postsaccadic position errors were defined as the following 4 mutually exclusive subtypes: backup saccades, catch-up saccades, intrusive saccades, and intermediate saccades. All saccades in a direction opposite to target motion were defined as backup saccades. Saccades in the direction of target motion ending behind the target were classified as catch-up saccades. Saccades in the direction of target motion starting and ending ahead of the target were classified as intrusive saccades. Some saccades in the direction of target motion straddled the target, ie, started behind the target and ended ahead of it. These saccades were classified as catch-up saccades if at least two thirds of their saccadic amplitude moved gaze toward the target; if at least two thirds of the saccadic amplitude moved gaze ahead of the target, they were categorized as intrusive saccades; and if the saccades failed to meet either of these criteria, they were defined as intermediate saccades.

Saccades were also classified according to criteria proposed by Abel and Ziegler.[32] Saccades in the direction of target motion that ended ahead of the target and that were followed by a 50-millisecond interval of eye velocity of less than 5° per second were classified as anticipatory saccades. Complexes of 2 saccades (of roughly similar size), in opposite directions, separated by an interval (50-500 milliseconds) of smooth pursuit, were classified as square wave jerks (Figure 1).

STATISTICAL ANALYSIS

All data are expressed as mean±SD. Eye tracking variables (SPEM gain, numbers of total saccades and saccade subtypes, and mean amplitudes of total saccades and saccade subtypes) were compared by matched-pair *t* tests (2-tailed) in the discordant twins. This analysis is based on the difference in scores between members of a twin pair. Matched-pair *t* tests were also performed between members of normal control MZ twin pairs arbitrarily divided in 2 groups for this purpose. In addition, since normal controls could be divided in 2 groups in many (2^{12}) different ways for statistical analysis, the probability of obtaining significant difference scores for SPEM gain and numbers and amplitudes of total saccades was computed for 1000 randomly generated groupings using a resampling statistical software package (version 3.14, Resampling Stats Inc, Arlington, Va) for the normal control data. To assess the degree of similarity or concordance for eye tracking variables, intraclass correlation coefficients (ICCs) were computed for SPEM gain and numbers of total saccades in both the discordant and normal control MZ twins samples. Tracking variables of the group of affected discordant twins and the group of unaffected discordant co-twins were compared with those of normal controls using *t* tests for independent samples; to reduce type I error for this analysis, eye movement measures were averaged within normal control twin pairs. Data distributions for all variables were tested for normality using χ^2 and Kolmogorov-Smirnov tests before using parametric statistics. Rank-ordered (Spearman) correlations between eye tracking variables and psychiatric ratings, medication dosage, and duration of illness were performed for affected discordant twins.

pursuit tracking might be a specific, biological trait marker of genetic predisposition toward schizophrenia.[13,18,19]

Further support for this idea was suggested by studies of eye tracking conducted by Holzman and colleagues[20-22] in a sample of Norwegian monozygotic (MZ) and dizygotic twins characterized by Kringlen.[23] Using qualitative ratings (normal vs impaired tracking), these studies showed that concordance for eye tracking im-

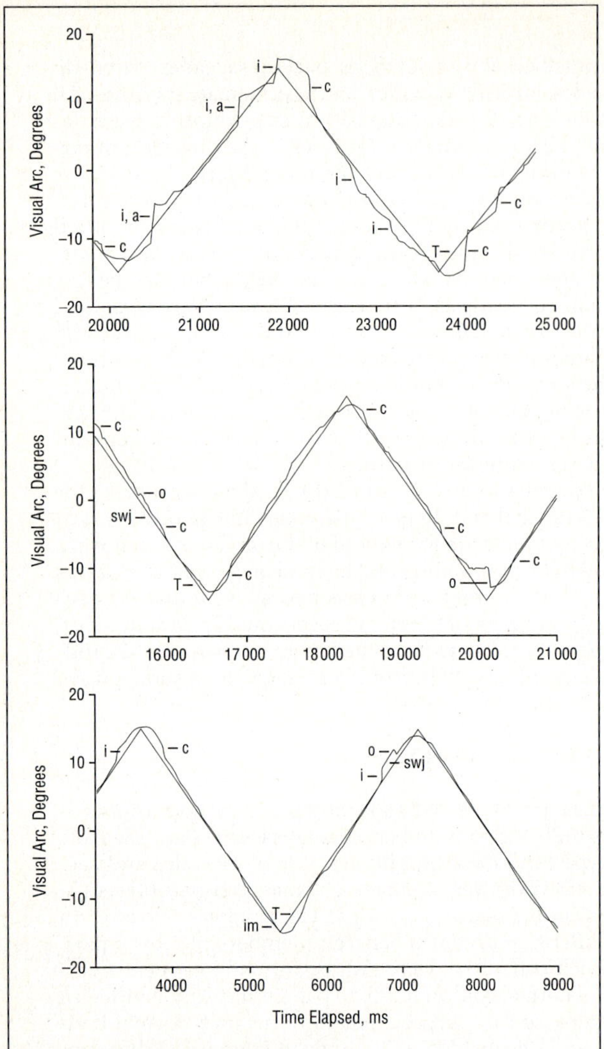

Figure 1. *Samples of smooth pursuit eye tracking recorded in an affected monozygotic twin with schizophrenia (top), her unaffected co-twin (middle), and an age- and sex-matched normal control twin (bottom). a indicates anticipatory saccade; c, catch-up saccade; i, intrusive saccade; im, intermediate saccade; swj, square wave jerk; and T, target motion. Criteria used to classify saccade subtypes are described in the "Quantitative Eye Movement Variables and Saccade Classification Criteria" subsection of the "Subjects and Methods" section of the text. Saccades occurring within 250 milliseconds preceding or following a change in target direction were excluded from data analysis.*

pairment was significantly greater than concordance for the clinical diagnosis of schizophrenia, ie, twins in their sample who were discordant for schizophrenia were highly concordant for abnormal eye tracking. Moreover, a global, quantitative measure of eye tracking performance (the natural logarithm of the signal-noise ratio) was significantly correlated within pairs. Concordance rates for qualitative eye tracking ratings and the natural logarithm of the signal-noise ratio correlations in MZ twins were twice those in dizygotic twins, suggesting that abnormal eye tracking was under strong genetic control. Studies in normal MZ twins have similarly found eye tracking performance to be highly correlated within twin pairs.[24,25]

Based on the results of the twin studies, Holzman[12,26,27] concluded that abnormal eye tracking was linked to the presence of the gene(s) for schizophrenia and proposed that abnormal eye tracking may be an indicator of genetic liability for schizophrenia in at-risk individuals without illness. Moreover, based on the frequency of abnormal eye tracking in the twins' offspring and in families, he proposed that abnormal eye tracking and/or schizophrenia could be accounted for by a single, underlying latent trait transmitted by an autosomal dominant gene. The latent trait model accounted for the curious observation in both twin and family data that abnormal eye tracking could be found in the asymptomatic relatives of schizophrenic probands who showed normal eye tracking. The model provides that, in a given individual, the latent trait can express the eye tracking abnormality, schizophrenic illness, or both.[28-30]

Two types of eye movement occur during smooth pursuit tracking: low-velocity smooth pursuit eye movements (SPEM), which hold the image of the target on the fovea by matching eye velocity to target velocity, and high-velocity saccadic eye movements (saccades), which reposition targets on the fovea if they become displaced. These eye movements are controlled by different central nervous system circuits that act in coordinated fashion to ensure accurate smooth pursuit tracking.[31] Although studies using qualitative ratings and global, quantitative assessments of eye tracking performance (like those used in previous twin studies) have been instrumental in documenting the eye tracking abnormality in patients with schizophrenia, several groups now advocate the use of neuro-ophthalmologically informed, quantitative measures of saccades and SPEM in eye tracking studies to better define the tracking deficit and its relationship to schizophrenia.[32-34] The majority of such quantitative studies suggest that the eye tracking abnormality in schizophrenia consists of reduced SPEM gain (a measure of smooth pursuit performance equal to eye velocity and target velocity)[35-48] and increased numbers of saccades produced during tracking.[36,40,42,43,45-54] A set of studies investigating the frequency of various saccade subtypes (eg, catch-up saccades, intrusive saccades, anticipatory saccades, and square wave jerks) and their relationship to reduced SPEM gain during smooth pursuit tracking in schizophrenia suggest that dysfunction in both the SPEM and saccadic central nervous system circuits occurs in schizophrenia. The former is indicated by observations of reduced gain and compensatory increases in catch-up saccade frequency and amplitude in patients with schizophrenia[44-47]; the latter, by patients' inability to suppress intrusive and anticipatory saccades during smooth pursuit tracking.[46-48,54]

Consistent with findings in previous family studies, several quantitative eye tracking studies have reported abnormal SPEM gain in first-degree relatives of schizophrenic probands[55-57]; 1 study found increases in anticipatory saccades but no impairment of gain in a small number of first-degree relatives.[58] In our study, we attempt to replicate previous eye tracking findings in twins with schizophrenia by quantifying SPEM and saccades in the eye tracking of MZ twins discordant for schizophrenia and in normal control MZ twins, according to methods previously described.[46,48] We hypothesized that if abnormal eye tracking was a genetic indicator for susceptibility to disease (as suggested by previous twin studies), quantitative characteristics of SPEM and saccades

Table 1. SPEM Gain and Saccades During Smooth Pursuit Eye Tracking in 12 Sets of MZ Twins Discordant for Schizophrenia and in 12 Pairs of Normal Control Twins*

	Mean±SD					
	Affected Twins (n=12)	Unaffected Co-twins (n=12)	Normal Controls (n=24)	*t* (*P*)†	*t* (*P*)‡	*t* (*P*)§
SPEM/gain	0.85±0.12	0.93±0.07	0.96±0.07	3.92 (**.002**)	−0.77 (.45)	−2.57 (**.02**)
Total saccades						
No.	47.3±14.5	36.8±15.8	32.3±15.8	−3.54 (**.005**)	0.79 (.44)	2.75 (**.01**)
Amplitude‖	1.98±0.82	1.53±0.44	1.69±0.58	−2.55 (**.03**)	−0.82 (.42)	1.21 (.23)

*SPEM indicates smooth pursuit eye movement; SPEM gain, ratio of eye velocity to target velocity; and MZ, monozygotic.
†Matched-pair t test, 2-tailed, discordant unaffected co-twins vs discordant affected twins. Boldface type indicates significant difference.
‡Independent sample t test, normal controls vs discordant unaffected co-twins.
§Independent sample t test, normal controls vs discordant affected twins. Boldface type indicates significant difference.
‖Given in degrees of visual arc.

would be similar for the affected and unaffected twins within a clinically discordant MZ pair, and would differ from values for normal controls.

RESULTS

Mean and individual values for SPEM gain and total saccades are displayed for all subjects in **Table 1** and **Figure 2**. Matched-pair analyses indicate that affected twins with schizophrenia have significantly decreased SPEM gain ($P<.003$) and significantly increased numbers ($P<.005$) and amplitudes ($P<.03$) of total saccades when compared with the unaffected twins (Table 1). This is further illustrated in Figure 2, which shows that 11 of 12 affected twins had lower SPEM gain and 10 of 12 affected twins had greater numbers of saccades than their unaffected co-twins; all 12 affected twins were inferior in comparison with their co-twins on at least 1 of these measures. Thus, when quantified in terms of SPEM gain and numbers of saccades, eye tracking performance differed between affected and unaffected members within MZ twins discordant for schizophrenia, with the performance of the affected twin almost always inferior to that of the unaffected co-twin. This is not the case for normal controls, where matched-pair analysis between arbitrarily divided members showed no significant differences (**Table 2**). Also, resampling normal control data revealed that different scores for SPEM gain and total saccades based on our arbitrarily divided groups will occur with a probability of 96% or greater (2-tailed).

Independent-sample *t* tests show that in the group of affected twins, mean SPEM gain is significantly reduced, and mean numbers of total saccades are significantly increased in comparison with these values in normal controls. By contrast, mean values for these variables in the group of unaffected co-twins do not differ from those in normal controls (Table 1).

The ICCs for SPEM gain and total saccades in discordant and normal control twin samples are as follows: for SPEM gain in discordant twins, 0.52 ($F=3.13$; $P=.03$); for SPEM gain in normal controls, 0.60 ($F=4.03$; $P<.01$); for total saccades in discordant twins, 0.59 ($F=3.85$; $P<.01$); and for total saccades in normal controls, 0.68 ($F=5.32$; $P<.004$).

Analyses were also performed on numbers and amplitudes of saccade subtypes, the mean values for which are displayed in **Table 3**. Numbers of intrusive saccades and amplitude of catch-up saccades were significantly higher ($P<.01$) in affected twins compared with unaffected co-twins. The amplitude and numbers of intermediate saccades (saccades that could not be categorized as intrusive or catch-up) were also increased in affected twins and unaffected co-twins ($P<.02$ and $P<.07$, respectively). Numbers of catch-up saccades, numbers and amplitudes of backup and anticipatory saccades, and numbers of square wave jerks did not differ between affected twins and unaffected co-twins. Numbers and amplitudes of saccade subtypes for both the affected and unaffected groups did not differ from those for normal controls, with the following exceptions: affected twins produced significantly more intermediate saccades than normal controls ($P<.02$), and both affected and unaffected twins produced slightly greater numbers of catch-up saccades than normal controls, although these differences did not reach statistical significance ($P<.14$ and $P<.16$, respectively).

Rank-ordered correlations between eye tracking variables and symptoms, duration of illness, and medication dosage for affected twins are listed in **Table 4**. Total saccades were significantly correlated with age and length of illness. Psychiatric symptoms were, in general, not correlated with eye tracking variables. In addition, neither lifetime neuroleptic dosage nor neuroleptic dosage at time of testing was significantly correlated with eye tracking variables.

Reanalysis of the data with the exclusion of discordant twins in whom there is a history of brain trauma does not substantiatively change within-pair differences observed on the matched-pair analysis (for SPEM gain in unaffected co-twins, ICC=0.93; for SPEM gain in affected twins, ICC=0.83 [$t=-3.00$; $P<.02$]; for total saccades in unaffected co-twins, ICC=32.3; and for total saccades in affected twins, ICC=43.7 [$t=3.27$; $P<.01$]) or group differences when comparing affected twins with normal controls (for SPEM gain, $t=1.75$, $P<.09$; for saccades, $t=-2.00$, $P<.05$). However, ICCs are further reduced for discordant twins (for SPEM gain, ICC=0.41 [$F=2.36$; $P=.10$]; for total saccades, ICC=0.38 [$F=2.23$; $P=.11$]).

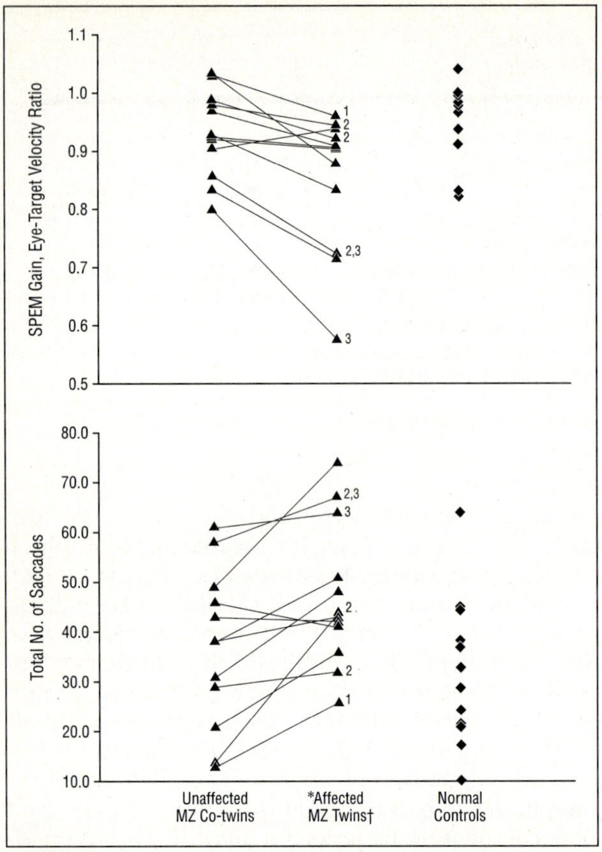

Figure 2. *Individual values for smooth pursuit eye movement (SPEM) gain and total saccades in 12 pairs of monozygotic (MZ) twins discordant for schizophrenia and 12 pairs of normal control MZ twins. 1 indicates twin set with history of a definite diagnosis of schizophrenia in a first-degree relative; 2, twin sets with history of a probable diagnosis of schizophrenia in a second-degree relative; 3, affected twins with history of brain trauma; asterisk, matched-pair analysis (affected twins vs unaffected co-twins) for SPEM gain (t=3.92; P<.002) and for saccades (t=−3.54; P<.005); and dagger, independent sample analysis (unaffected twins vs normal controls) for SPEM gain (t=−2.57; P<.02) and for saccades (t=2.75; P<.01).*

Table 2. SPEM Gain and Total Saccades During Smooth Pursuit Eye Tracking in 12 Sets of Normal Control MZ Twins*

	Mean±SD		
	Group 1 (n=12)	Group 2 (n=12)	*t* (*P*)†
SPEM gain	0.95±0.08	0.96±0.08	0.45 (.66)
Total No. of saccades	32.3±15.9	32.4±16.5	0.04 (.97)
Total saccades, amplitude‡	1.66±0.55	1.72±0.63	0.43 (.68)

**SPEM indicates smooth pursuit eye movement; SPEM gain, ratio of eye velocity to target velocity; and MZ, monozygotic. Twins were arbitrarily divided into paired groups 1 and 2.*
†Matched-pair t test, 2-tailed, group 1 vs group 2.
‡Given in degrees of visual arc.

COMMENT

In our study, we examined quantitative measures of smooth pursuit eye tracking in MZ twins discordant for schizophrenia and in normal control MZ twins. We found that, in virtually all discordant MZ twins, quantitative measures of eye tracking performance for the affected twin were inferior to those for the unaffected co-twin, with affected MZ twins showing significant decreases of SPEM gain and significant increases in numbers and amplitudes of total saccades. Moreover, whereas mean values for affected twins differed significantly from mean values for normal controls on these measures, values for virtually all unaffected co-twins were well within the normal range.

Our data showing significant differences in quantitative measures of eye tracking performance within discordant MZ twins are consistent with the hypothesis that, at least in our cohort, abnormal eye tracking is associated with the expression of illness, or phenotype, not genotype. By comparing affected and unaffected MZ twins reared together, we were able to control for both genetic and environmental determinants of eye tracking ability, thereby isolating for study the influence of the illness on the development of eye tracking impairment. Since members of an MZ twin pair should be endowed with the same innate eye tracking ability (as suggested by studies of normal MZ twins that show eye tracking ability to be under strong genetic control[24,25]), and to the extent that the eye tracking performance of the unaffected co-twin is the best available measure of what the affected twin's performance would have been if schizophrenia had not developed, we would conclude that the worsening in SPEM gain and numbers of saccades we observe in the group of affected twins is, most parsimoniously, a consequence of the expression of schizophrenic illness. Moreover, we would suggest that the difference or worsening observed in the affected twins relative to the unaffected co-twins constitutes the actual extent to which eye tracking is impaired by illness, relative to its intact, premorbid state, measured in the unaffected co-twins.

Based on observations in the Norwegian twin sample that qualitatively assessed eye tracking impairment was the same within a significant proportion (approximately 40%) of clinically discordant MZ pairs, and, moreover, that the concordance for abnormal eye tracking was significantly greater than concordance for clinical schizophrenia in MZ twins, Holzman and colleagues[20-22] concluded that abnormal eye tracking was linked to the presence of the gene(s) for schizophrenia and could be regarded as a genetic indicator of predisposition toward schizophrenia in at-risk individuals. Our data showing consistent within-pair differences in discordant MZ twins, with worsening of quantitative eye tracking measures found exclusively in the affected twins and a lack of concordance for eye tracking function among discordant twins, do not support these conclusions. Furthermore, our results do not support the notion that abnormal eye tracking may be an indicator of genetic predisposition for schizophrenia, at least not in this sample; if this were the case, one would expect a more substantial number of unaffected co-twins (who are presumably at highest genetic risk for schizophrenia) to have eye tracking abnormalities analogous to those found in affected twins, or at least to differ from normal subjects as a group. However, the overwhelming majority (11 of 12) of unaffected co-twins performed within the range of values of normal controls for quantitative eye tracking measures,

Table 3. Characteristics of Saccade Subtypes in the Smooth Pursuit Eye Tracking of 12 Sets of MZ Twins Discordant for Schizophrenia and 12 Pairs of Normal Control Twins*

Subtypes of Saccades	Mean±SD: Affected Twins (n=12)	Unaffected Co-twins (n=12)	Normal Controls (n=24)	*t* (*P*)†	*t* (*P*)‡	*t* (*P*)§
Catch-up						
No.	15.8±8.6	15.3±8.1	11.1±6.5	−0.14 (.88)	1.68 (.10)	1.83 (.08)
Amplitude‖	2.20±0.98	1.47±0.31	1.81±0.75	−3.12 (**.01**)	−1.48 (.15)	1.36 (.18)
Intrusive						
No.	18.8±13.4	12.5±10.5	13.2±8.6	−3.10 (**.01**)	0.22 (.83)	1.53 (.13)
Amplitude‖	2.66±1.74	2.82±2.58	2.76±1.88	−0.02 (.99)	0.07 (.94)	−0.16 (.88)
Backup						
No.	4.7±5.1	3.8±5.1	3.9±5.1	−0.66 (.53)	0.09 (.93)	0.42 (.68)
Amplitude‖	2.66±2.74	3.75±5.10	3.92±5.07	−0.90 (.40)	−0.03 (.97)	−0.10 (.92)
Intermediate						
No.	8.1±4.7	5.3±3.3	4.1±2.9	−2.05 (.07)	1.04 (.31)	3.11 (**.004**)
Amplitude‖	3.26±2.09	1.96±0.86	2.36±1.27	−2.79 (**.02**)	−0.97 (.34)	1.58 (.12)
Anticipatory						
No.	3.9±7.6	1.4±2.2	1.4±2.3	−1.12 (.29)	0.00 (.99)	1.51 (.14)
Amplitude‖	4.61±2.59	5.88±3.60	3.78±2.82	−0.33 (.76)	1.27 (.23)	0.59 (.56)
Square wave jerks, No.	1.9±4.1	1.5±1.9	1.0±2.3	−0.39 (.70)	0.59 (.56)	0.83 (.42)

**MZ indicates monozygotic. Subtypes of saccades are described in the "Quantitative Eye Movement Variables and Saccade Classification Criteria" subsection of the "Subjects and Methods" section of the text.*

†Matched-pair t test, 2-tailed, discordant unaffected twins vs discordant affected twins. Boldface type indicates significance difference.

‡Independent sample t test, normal controls vs discordant unaffected co-twins.

§Independent sample t test, normal controls vs discordant affected twins. Boldface type indicates significance difference.

‖Given in degrees of visual arc.

Table 4. Rank-Ordered Correlations Between Eye Tracking Variables and Clinical Measures in Affected Discordant MZ Twins With Schizophrenia*

	Age	BPRS Score	SANS Score	Neuroleptic Dosage, Current	Neuroleptic Dosage, Lifetime	Duration of Illness
SPEM gain	0.30	−0.14	0.00	−0.16	0.16	0.19
Total No. of saccades	0.60†	−0.36	−0.25	0.07	−0.35	0.61†
Total saccades, amplitude‡	−0.13	0.19	−0.08	−0.04	−0.22	−0.04

**MZ indicates monozygotic; BPRS, Brief Psychiatric Rating Scale; SANS, Schedule for the Assessment of Negative Symptoms; SPEM, smooth pursuit eye movement; and SPEM gain, ratio of eye velocity to target velocity.*

†P<.05.

‡Given in degrees of visual arc.

as well as within the range of values belonging to a large normal control sample previously undergoing the same testing methods in our laboratory.[48] This includes the 4 individuals with a family history of schizophrenia, who presumably have additional evidence of genetic risk.

Several methodologic factors, including sample size and selection and the small number of normal controls in our study, may account for our inability to confirm the results of previous studies. Perhaps the most significant factor is the use by previous twin studies of qualitative ratings to measure eye tracking impairment; these are dichotomous (normal vs impaired), subjective ratings performed by comparing subject eye tracking with target motion. Unlike the quantitative measures we used, qualitative ratings provide a global assessment of a subject's eye tracking performance without necessarily providing information regarding component eye movements during tracking (SPEM and saccades).[32-34] Interestingly, given the degree of overlap with normal control values in our data (Figure 2), it is possible to understand how high concordance rates for eye tracking performance may be obtained using dichotomous, qualitative ratings of the type used in previous studies. Other investigations of the heritability of eye tracking impairment have noted that the use of qualitative ratings may result in variable and/or overdetection of abnormal eye tracking in probands, family members, and normal controls.[57] Moreover, the insensitivity of qualitative ratings to the type and magnitude of dysfunction in SPEM and saccadic eye movements in the tracking of patients with schizophrenia has been the subject of several recent reviews.[32-34]

We suggest that, in contrast to global measures of eye tracking accuracy, the use of neuro-ophthalmologically informed, quantitative, continuous measures of SPEM and saccades (eg, SPEM gain, total saccades, and saccade subtypes) that have been previously shown to be abnormal in schizophrenia in a large number of studies[35-48] are better able to distinguish the eye tracking impairment associated with schizophrenia from genetically endowed eye tracking ability in discordant MZ twins.[24,25] The matched-pair analysis of quantitative eye tracking measures demonstrates that clinically discordant twin pairs maintain a parallel discordance for eye tracking, ie, all affected twins with schizophrenia experience some decrement or downward shift in eye tracking measures in comparison with their ideal control (the genetically identical, asymptomatic, unaffected co-twin). This occurs despite the fact that most affected twins perform within the range of normal controls. Thus, these data suggest that some disturbance in eye tracking function is almost always associated with having schizophrenia, even when a significant proportion of individuals with schizophrenia have values for eye tracking measures within the normal range. Moreover, they illustrate that dichotomous ratings may fail to detect dysfunction in certain individuals with schizophrenia, relative to their baseline genetic endowment. Similar distributions of data have been observed for neuroanatomical,[68] neurophysiological,[69] and neuropsychological[70] parameters in this discordant twin sample.

While the matched-pair analysis reveals significant within-pair differences in eye tracking performance for discordant twins, the ICCs for SPEM gain and total saccades suggest that discordant twins still retain some similarity for these measures. Since discordant MZ twins should share the same genetic endowment for eye tracking ability, a significant correlation in their abilities would be expected, given previous evidence for strong genetic control of eye tracking function in normal MZ twins.[24,25] However, it is also clear that ICCs in discordant twins are lower in magnitude than those in normal controls; indeed, the ICCs for eye tracking variables in the discordant twins decrease further in magnitude and become nonsignificant with the exclusion of the 2 pairs with histories of brain trauma. These data suggest that discordant MZ twins are less concordant for eye tracking measures than normal controls, which is consistent with the notion that illness expression in the affected twin impairs premorbid eye movement ability.

As noted above, other factors related to the selection and diagnosis of discordant MZ twins might also account for the lack of agreement between twin studies. Because we recruited twins through family advocacy groups, our sample may have been subject to greater selection bias (eg, higher socioeconomic status, and more severe, chronic illness) than the Norwegian sample, which was broadly recruited from a national twin registry. However, a significant proportion of the Norwegian MZ twins were older and further atypical in that they were much more fecund than one would expect for typical subjects with schizophrenia.[71] We obtained consensus diagnoses of schizophrenia in affected twins and excluded psychiatric illness in unaffected co-twins from videotaped SCIDs and extensive psychiatric histories.[59] However, less rigorous assessment was performed for the Norwegian twin sample,[22] resulting in uncertainty regarding the diagnosis of schizophrenia in probands and the absence of psychosis in co-twins in many of those MZ pairs. Thus, it is possible that the failure to find within-pair differences for abnormal eye tracking in previous studies is related to questionable diagnosis of schizophrenia in the proband or concordance for schizophrenia in the Norwegian MZ twins; preliminary data (not shown) from a small number of diagnostically concordant twins with schizophrenia show no within-pair differences for SPEM gain and saccades.

It is also possible that factors associated with illness, such as symptom acuity or the sedating effects of neuroleptic medication, might have caused the subtle worsening of eye tracking performance that we observed in the affected twins. However, we did not find psychiatric symptoms (including total, positive, and negative symptoms measured on the Brief Psychiatric Rating Scale and the Scale for Assessment of Negative Symptoms) or current or lifetime neuroleptic dosage to correlate with eye tracking performance in affected twins. These findings are consistent with previous studies in patients with schizophrenia, which show no relationship of eye tracking performance to symptom severity[13,26] and no effects of typical neuroleptic medications on quantitative measures of eye tracking.[48]

Limitations in our recording technique and sample size may have contributed to a high rate of false-negative findings (type II error), particularly among the unaffected co-twins. For example, within-pair differences we observed in MZ twins could be due to an underdetection of eye tracking abnormalities, especially saccades, in the unaffected co-twins in our study. One possible source for this error is the low-resolution, 8-bit eye movement recording we used, which cannot detect very small amplitude ($<0.5°$) saccades during tracking. However, it is unlikely that this limitation would apply only to unaffected co-twins and not to other groups in our study. Also, affected twins (but not unaffected co-twins) tended to have increased numbers of intrusive and anticipatory saccades, as well as greater numbers of high-amplitude, catch-up saccades in response to reduced SPEM gain, consistent with results of recent quantitative eye tracking studies that subtype saccades.[44-48,54] Moreover, 8-bit resolution is more than adequate for accurate measurement of SPEM gain, for which robust within-pair differences were observed. It is also conceivable that a more difficult tracking task might have elicited more errors in the tracking of unaffected co-twins[38,41]; however, given previous evidence that eye tracking dysfunction in schizophrenia is not altered by changes in task conditions,[13,26] there is no reason to suspect that differences between affected and unaffected twins would be abolished by a more difficult tracking task. The small numbers of discordant and normal control twins increase the likelihood of type II error in unaffected co-twins, although their values were well within the range of mean values we obtained in a much larger number of normal control subjects using similar methods.[48] In general, the fact that analogous data are found for neuroanatomical, neurophysiological, and neuropsychological parameters in this sample argues against the possibility that these findings are artifacts of our eye tracking method or sample size.[68-70]

Quantitative data on eye tracking function in our sample of discordant MZ twins do not support a genetic liability hypothesis for eye tracking dysfunction in schizophrenia. However, these data are not dispositive for the thesis, especially in view of the methodologic limitations noted above. These limitations could have prevented us from identifying abnormalities in unaffected twins, especially those performing in the low range of normal. In addition, increases in catch-up saccades, which have been found to be increased in several,[44-47] although not all,[38,39,48] eye tracking studies in schizophrenia, where one variable shown to be concordant among discordant twins (although their numbers were not significantly increased in comparison with those of normal controls in our data).

Perhaps the most significant evidence arguing against our interpretation of these data, however, are findings in family studies of eye tracking in schizophrenia that report eye tracking dysfunction in the asymptomatic first-degree relatives of schizophrenic probands,[14-17] including more recent quantitative studies of eye movements that found reduced SPEM gain and increased anticipatory saccades among first-degree relatives of probands with schizophrenia.[55-58] This body of evidence dictates that it would be premature to conclude that eye tracking impairment is not associated with the genetic liability for schizophrenia on the basis of our study alone. However, there are other plausible factors that may account for the apparent discrepancy between our results and the findings of family studies. For example, the use of qualitative ratings (or empirically derived cutoff scores in quantitative family studies) to dichotomize eye tracking dysfunction in family studies may imperfectly assess the presence of dysfunction in probands and relatives,[57] as they do in our data. Thus, the use of the cutoff score may explain why, in family data, some probands appear to have normal eye tracking, even when the eye tracking of their relatives is categorized as impaired.[57] It is also possible that another factor, heretofore unidentified, which is shared by family members but not linked to schizophrenia per se (eg, cigarette smoking)[72] accounts for similarities in eye tracking observed between probands and their first-degree relatives. Interestingly, one quantitative family study[55] shows reductions in SPEM gain to be significantly greater in relatives with symptoms of schizophrenia-spectrum disorders than in relatives with nonspectrum disorders, a finding consistent with the hypothesis that eye tracking dysfunction occurs as a consequence of schizophrenic illness. Moreover, 2 recent family studies find a significant proportion of families in whom eye tracking dysfunction occurred only in the proband, and not their asymptomatic relatives.[57,73] The possibility, suggested by these studies,[57,73] that schizophrenia is genetically heterogeneous (ie, genetic or familial forms of the illness in which eye tracking dysfunction is found among at-risk relatives, and nongenetic or sporadic forms in which relatives exhibit no eye tracking dysfunction) may also explain discrepancies in eye tracking results among twin and family samples with schizophrenia.[56] Thus, the lack of agreement between our study and previous studies in the Norwegian twins may be due to our sample being inherently less genetic (ie, containing more sporadic cases), a factor that may be endemic to discordant twin samples. Even this explanation is less than satisfactory, however, since one third of our twin pairs had first- or second-degree relatives with schizophrenia, a frequency that is greater than what would be expected in the general population.

In summary, our findings do not support previous hypotheses that abnormal eye tracking and schizophrenia are independent phenomena that are genetically linked; rather, they are more consistent with the notion that the eye tracking abnormality is associated with the expression of schizophrenic illness. However, in view of the small sample size, the potential for error in the detection of eye tracking abnormalities in our methods, possible bias in subject sampling, and the strong evidence from family studies, our study cannot definitively rule out an association between the genetic potential for schizophrenia and abnormal eye tracking. Given the importance of accurate phenotypic and genotypic characterization in schizophrenia pedigrees for linkage analysis, further attempts to replicate these findings in a larger sample of twins and their first-degree relatives, using more sensitive recording and measurement, are warranted.

Accepted for publication June 18, 1996.

We thank Philip Holzman, PhD, and Deborah Levy, PhD, for their willingness to review our oculographic records; Dr Holzman for his thoughtful review of our manuscript and his many suggestions; John J. Bartko, PhD, for statistical review of the manuscript; and Brett A. Clementz, PhD, Irving R. Gottesman, PhD, and John Hsiao, MD, for their general comments on the manuscript.

Reprints: Daniel R. Weinberger, MD, Clinical Brain Disorders Branch, National Institue of Mental Health Neuroscience Center at St Elizabeth's Hospital, 2700 Martin Luther King Ave SE, Washington, DC 20032.

REFERENCES

1. Gusella JF, Wexler NS, Connealy PM, Naylor SL, Anderson MA, Tanzi RE, Watkins PC, Ottina K, Wallace MR, Sakaguchi AY. A polymorphic DNA marker genetically linked to Huntington's disease. *Nature.* 1983;306:234-238.
2. Morrel V. Huntington's gene finally found. *Science.* 1993;260:28-30.
3. Gottesman II, Shields J, Hanson D. *Schizophrenia: The Epigenetic Puzzle.* New York, NY: Cambridge University Press; 1982.
4. Sherrington R, Brynjolfsson J, Petursson H, Potter M, Dudleston K, Barraclough B, Wasmuth J, Dobbs M, Gurling H. Localization of susceptibility locus for schizophrenia on chromosome 5. *Nature.* 1988;336:164-167.
5. Kennedy JL, Giuffra LA, Moises HW, Cavalli-Sforza LL, Pakstis AJ, Kidd JR, Castiglione CM, Sjogren B, Wetterberg L, Kidd KK. Evidence against linkage of schizophrenia to markers on chromosome 5 in a northern Swedish pedigree. *Nature.* 1988;336:167-170.
6. St Clair D, Blackwood D, Muir W, Baillie D, Hubbard S, Wright A, Evans HJ. No linkage of chromosome 5q11-q13 markers to schizophrenia in Scottish families. *Nature.* 1989;339:305-309.
7. Detera-Wadleigh SD, Goldin LR, Sherrington R, Encio I, de Miguel C, Berretini W, Gurling H, Gershon ES. Exclusion of linkage 5q11-q13 in families with schizophrenia and other disorders. *Nature.* 1989;340:391-393.
8. Aschauer HN, Aschauer-Treiber G, Isenberg KE, Todd RC, Knesevich MA, Garver DL, Reich T, Cloninger RC. No evidence for linkage between chromosome 5 markers and schizophrenia. *Hum Hered.* 1990;40:109-115.
9. Levinson DF, Mowry BJ. Defining the schizophrenia spectrum: issues for genetic linkage studies. *Schizophr Bull.* 1991;17:491-514.
10. Keefe RSE, Silverman JM, Siever LJ, Cornblatt BA. Refining phenotype characterization in genetic linkage studies in schizophrenia. *Soc Biol.* 1991;38:197-218.
11. Blackwood D, St Clair D, Muir W. DNA markers and biological vulnerability markers in families multiply affected with schizophrenia. *Eur Arch Psychiatry Clin Neurosci.* 1991;240:191-196.
12. Holzman PS. Behavioral markers of schizophrenia useful for genetic studies. *J Psychiatry Res.* 1992;26:427-445.
13. Holzman PS. Recent studies of psychophysiology in schizophrenia. *Schizophr Bull.* 1987;13:49-75.
14. Holzman PS, Proctor LR, Levy DL, Yassilo NJ, Meltzer HY, Hurt SW. Eye tracking dysfunctions in schizophrenic patients and their relatives. *Arch Gen Psychiatry.* 1974;31:141-151.
15. Holzman PS, Solomon CM, Levin S, Waternaux CS. Pursuit eye movement dysfunctions in schizophrenia: family evidence for specificity. *Arch Gen Psychiatry.* 1984;41:136-139.
16. Levy DL, Yassilo NJ, Jacniak PG, Gaviria M, Davis JM. Relative of unipolar and bipolar patients have normal pursuit. *Psychiatry Res.* 1983;10:285-293.
17. Siegel LJ, Waldo M, Miznor G, Adler LE, Freedman R. Deficits in sensory gating in schizophrenic patients and their relatives. *Arch Gen Psychiatry.* 1984;41:607-612.

18. Iacono WG. Psychophysiology and genetics: a key to psychopathology research. *Psychophysiology.* 1983;20:371-383.
19. Iacono WG. Eye tracking abnormalities in schizophrenic and affective disorders. In: Johnston CW, Pirozollo FJ, eds. *The Neuropsychology of Eye Movements.* Hillsdale, NJ: Lawrence Erlbaum Associates Inc; 1988:115-146.
20. Holzman PS, Kringlen E, Levy DL, Proctor LR, Haberman S, Yassilo NJ. Abnormal pursuit eye movements in schizophrenia: evidence for a genetic indicator. *Arch Gen Psychiatry.* 1977;34:802-805.
21. Holzman PS, Kringlen E, Levy DL, Proctor LR, Haberman S. Smooth pursuit eye movement in twins discordant for schizophrenia. *J Psychiatr Res.* 1978; 14:111-120.
22. Holzman PS, Kringlen E, Levy DL, Haberman S. Deviant eye tracking in twins discordant for psychosis: a replication. *Arch Gen Psychiatry.* 1980;37:627-631.
23. Kringlen E. *Heredity and Environment in the Functional Psychoses.* London, England: Heinemann Medical Books Ltd; 1968.
24. Iacono WG, Lykken DT. Eye tracking and psychopathology: new procedures applied to a sample of normal monozygotic twins. *Arch Gen Psychiatry.* 1979; 36:1361-1369.
25. Iacono WG. Eye tracking in normal twins. *Behav Genet.* 1982;12:517-526.
26. Holzman PS. Eye movement dysfunctions and psychosis. *Int Rev Neurobiol.* 1985;27:179-205.
27. Holzman PS. The use of eye movement dysfunctions in exploring the genetic transmission of schizophrenia. *Eur Arch Neurol Sci.* 1989;239:43-48.
28. Matthysse S, Holzman PS, Lange K. The genetic transmission of schizophrenia: application of mendelian latent structure analysis to eye tracking dysfunctions in schizophrenia and affective disorder. *J Psychiatr Res.* 1986;20:57-67.
29. Holzman PS. Genetic latent structure models: implication for research on schizophrenia? *Psychol Med.* 1987;17:271-274.
30. Holzman PS, Kringlen E, Matthysse S, Flanagan SD, Lipton RB, Cramer G, Levin S, Lange K, Levy DL. A single dominant gene can account for eye tracking dysfunctions and schizophrenia in offspring of discordant twins. *Arch Gen Psychiatry.* 1988;45:641-647.
31. Leigh RJ, Zee DS. *The Neurology of Eye Movements.* Philadelphia, Pa: FA Davis Co Publishers; 1990.
32. Abel LA, Ziegler AS. Smooth pursuit eye movements in schizophrenics: what constitutes quantitative assessment? *Biol Psychiatry.* 1988;24:747-762.
33. Clementz BA, Sweeney JA. Is eye movement dysfunction a biological marker for schizophrenia? a methodologic review. *Psychol Bull.* 1990;108:77-92.
34. Abel LA, Levin S, Holzman PS. Abnormalities of smooth pursuit and saccadic control in schizophrenia: a minireview. *Vision Res.* 1992;32:1009-1014.
35. Schmid-Burgk W, Becker W, Diekmann V, Jurgens R, Kornhuber HH. Disturbed smooth pursuit and saccadic eye movements in schizophrenia. *Arch Psychiatr Nervenkrankheiten.* 1982;232:381-389.
36. Mather JA, Putchat C. Motor control of schizophrenics, I: oculomotor control of schizophrenics: a deficit in sensory processing, not strictly in motor control. *J Psychiatr Res.* 1982-83;17:343-360.
37. Yee RD, Balogh RW, Marder SR, Levy DL, Sakala SM, Honrubia V. Eye movements in schizophrenia. *Invest Ophthalmol Vis Sci.* 1987;28:366-374.
38. Levin S, Luebke A, Zee DS, Hain TC, Robinson DA, Holzman PS. Smooth pursuit eye movements in schizophrenics: quantitative measurements with the search-coil technique. *J Psychiatry Res.* 1988;22:195-208.
39. Ross DE, Ochs AL, Hill MR, Goldberg SC, Pandurangi AK, Winfrey CJ. Erratic eye tracking in schizophrenic patients as revealed by high-resolution techniques. *Biol Psychiatry.* 1988;24:675-688.
40. Litman RE, Hommer DW, Clem T, Rapaport M, Pato CN, Pickar D. Smooth pursuit eye movements in schizophrenia: effects of neuroleptics and caffeine. *Psychopharmacol Bull.* 1989;25:473-477.
41. Allen JS, Matsunaga K, Hacisalihzade S, Stark L. Smooth pursuit eye movements of normal and schizophrenic subjects tracking an unpredictable target. *Biol Psychiatry.* 1990;28:705-720.
42. Moser A, Kompf D, Arolt V, Resch T. Quantitative analysis of eye movements in schizophrenia. *Neuro-ophthalmology.* 1990;10:73-80.
43. Oepen G, Thoden U, Warmke C. Association of tardive dyskinesia with increased frequency of eye movement disturbances in chronic schizophrenic patients. *Eur Arch Psychiatry Neurol Sci.* 1990;239:241-245.
44. Abel LA, Friedman L, Jesberger J, Malki A, Meltzer HY. Quantitative assessment of smooth pursuit gain and catch-up saccades in schizophrenia and affective disorders. *Biol Psychiatry.* 1991;29:1063-1072.
45. Friedman L, Jesberger JA, Meltzer HY. A model of smooth pursuit performance illustrates the relationship between gain, catch-up saccade rate and catch-up saccade amplitude in normal controls and patients with schizophrenia. *Biol Psychiatry.* 1991;30:537-556.
46. Radant A, Hommer DW. A quantitative analysis of saccades and smooth pursuit during visual pursuit tracking: a comparison of schizophrenics with normals and substance abusing controls. *Schizophr Res.* 1992;6:225-235.
47. Sweeney JA, Haas GL, Shuhua L. Neuropsychological and eye movement abnormalities in first-episode and chronic schizophrenia. *Schizophr Bull.* 1992; 18:283-294.
48. Litman RE, Hommer DW, Radant AR, Clem T, Pickar D. Quantitative effects of typical and atypical neuroleptics on smooth pursuit eye tracking in schizophrenia. *Schizophr Res.* 1994;12:107-112.
49. Mialet JP, Pichot P. Eye tracking patterns in schizophrenia: an analysis based on the incidence of saccades. *Arch Gen Psychiatry.* 1981;38:183-186.
50. Cegalis JA, Hafez H, Wong PS. What is deviant about deviant smooth pursuit eye movements in schizophrenia? *Psychiatry Res.* 1983;10:47-58.
51. Levin S, Jones AR, Stark L, Merrin EL, Holzman PS. Identification of abnormal patterns in eye movements of schizophrenic patients. *Arch Gen Psychiatry.* 1982;39:1125-1130.
52. Levin S, Jones A, Stark L, Merrin EL, Holzman PS. Saccadic eye movements of schizophrenic patients measured by reflected light technique. *Biol Psychiatry.* 1982;17:1277-1287.
53. Matsue Y, Okuma T, Saito H, Aneha S, Ueno T, Chiba H, Matsuoka H. Saccadic eye movements in tracking, fixation, and rest in schizophrenic and normal subjects. *Biol Psychiatry.* 1986;21:382-389.
54. Friedman L, Abel LA, Jesberger JA, Malki A, Meltzer HY. Saccadic intrusions into smooth pursuit in patients with schizophrenia or affective disorder and normal controls. *Biol Psychiatry.* 1992;31:1110-1118.
55. Clementz BA, Sweeney JA, Hirt M, Haas G. Pursuit gain and saccadic intrusions in the first-degree relatives of probands with schizophrenia. *J Abnorm Psychol.* 1991;99:327-335.
56. Grove WM, Lebow BS, Clementz BA, Cerri A, Medus C, Iacono WG. Familial prevalence and co-aggregation of schizotypy factors: a multitrait study. *J Abnorm Psychol.* 1991;100:115-121.
57. Clementz BA, Grove WM, Iacono WG, Sweeney JA. Smooth pursuit eye movement dysfunction and liability for schizophrenia: implications for genetic modeling. *J Abnorm Psychol.* 1992;101:117-129.
58. Whicker L, Abel LA, Dell'Osso LF. Smooth pursuit eye movements in the parents of schizophrenics. *Neuro-ophthalmology.* 1985;5:1-8.
59. Torrey EF, Bowler AE, Taylor EH, Gottesman II. *Schizophrenia and Manic Depressive Disorder: The Biological Roots of Mental Illness as Revealed by a Landmark Study of Identical Twins.* New York, NY: Basic Books Inc Publishers; 1994.
60. Spitzer RL, Williams JB, Gibbon M, First MB. *Structured Clinical Interview for the DSM-III-R.* New York: Biometrics Research Division, New York State Psychiatric Institute; 1988.
61. American Psychiatric Association. *Diagnostic and Statistical Manual of Mental Disorders, Third Edition, Revised.* Washington, DC: American Psychiatric Association; 1987.
62. Abel LA, Hertle RW. Effects of psychoactive drugs on ocular motor behavior. In: Johnston CW, Pirozzolo FJ, eds. *Neuropsychology of Eye Movements.* Hillsdale, NJ: Lawrence Erlbaum Associates Inc; 1988:81-114.
63. Belmaker R, Polin W, Wyatt RJ, Cohen S. A follow-up of monozygotic twins discordant for schizophrenia. *Arch Gen Psychiatry.* 1974;30:219-222.
64. Spitzer RL, Endicott J. *Schedule for Affective Disorders and Schizophrenia—Lifetime Version.* New York: Biometrics Research Division, New York State Psychiatric Institute; 1975.
65. Overall JE, Gorham DE. The Brief Psychiatric Rating Scale. *Psychol Rep.* 1961; 10:799-812.
66. Andreason NC. *The Scale for Assessment of Negative Symptoms (SANS).* Iowa City: University of Iowa; 1981.
67. Lisberger SG, Pavelko TA. Topographic and directional organization of visual motion inputs for initiation of horizontal and vertical smooth pursuit eye movements in monkeys. *J Neurophysiol.* 1989;61:173-185.
68. Suddath RL, Christison GW, Torrey EF, Weinberger DR. Cerebral anatomical abnormalities in monozygotic twins discordant for schizophrenia. *N Engl J Med.* 1990;322:789-794.
69. Berman KF, Torrey EF, Daniel DG, Weinberger DR. Regional cerebral blood flow in monozygotic twins discordant and concordant for schizophrenia. *Arch Gen Psychiatry.* 1992;49:927-934.
70. Goldberg TE, Ragland D, Torrey EF, Gold JH, Bigelow LB, Weinberger DR. Neuropsychological assessment of monozygotic twins discordant for schizophrenia. *Arch Gen Psychiatry.* 1990;47:1066-1072.
71. Kringlen E, Cramer G. Offspring of monozygotic twins discordant for schizophrenia. *Arch Gen Psychiatry.* 1989;46:873-877.
72. Thaker GK, Elsberry R, Moran M, Lahti A, Tamminga C. Tobacco smoking increases square wave jerks during pursuit eye movements. *Biol Psychiatry.* 1991; 29:82-88.
73. Iacono WG, Moreau M, Beiser M, Fleming JAE, Lin T. Smooth-pursuit eye tracking in first-episode psychotic patients and their relatives. *J Abnorm Psychol.* 1992;101:104-116.

COMMENTARY

Smooth Pursuit Eye Tracking in Twins

A Critical Commentary

LITMAN ET al[1] conducted a study of smooth pursuit eye movements in monozygotic (MZ) twins discordant for schizophrenia. Although their data show a high concordance for eye tracking among pairs of clinically discordant twins with schizophrenia, confirming previous twin studies of eye tracking,[2,3] they conclude that eye tracking dysfunction (ETD) is an outcome of having schizophrenia but does not represent a potential genetic indicator. We believe that this is an unwarranted conclusion and address this issue and other serious flaws in their design and interpretation.

SAMPLE AND SAMPLE SIZE

Litman et al compared 12 pairs of MZ twins discordant for schizophrenia with 12 pairs of MZ "normal" twins. Small samples permit nonrandom errors to exert a distorting effect on the data and, as we shall demonstrate, such distorting effects did occur in this particular study.

Included in the group of twins discordant for schizophrenia are 2 probands who had a brain disease that impairs pursuit eye movement[4] and, therefore, should have been excluded from the sample.

It is unusual, as occurs in this group of normal controls, to find gain scores less than 0.85[4] in young, normal subjects pursuing a 16.67° per second–target. What accounts for such poor performance in 2 of the normal twins?

As a consequence of the small sizes of all 3 groups, the poor performance of a few members of the normal group and the presence of brain disease in 2 members of the affected twin group contaminate the comparisons between groups. What happens is the 2 probands with a brain disease (16.67% of that group) are among the 3 people with the lowest gain scores, artificially inflating the rate of bad tracking and of low gain scores in the group of twins with schizophrenia. Including them, therefore, increases the likelihood of detecting differences between probands and other groups who do not have members with known brain disease, such as the unaffected co-twins and the normal controls. The presence of the 2 deviant control subjects, on the other hand, decreases the likelihood of detecting differences between controls and other groups, such as the unaffected co-twins. Thus, the inclusion of these 4 subjects in this study does 2 things: it produces a large overlap in scores between controls and unaffected co-twins, resulting in no differences between these groups, and it exaggerates differences between probands and their co-twins. The authors state that they reanalyzed their data excluding the 2 twin pairs with brain disease with no change in results. They report that after exclusion of the 2 twins with brain disease, who had 2 of the 3 lowest gain scores, the mean gain score of the affected twin group was 0.83, which must be an error since the gain score was 0.85 before they were excluded. Our estimation from their graph is a mean of 0.89.

See also page 417

For the overlap between the control twins and the unaffected co-twins in gain and saccade scores, the authors write "... all unaffected co-twins are well within the normal range." They conclude from this observation that the performance of the co-twins is not deviant and that ETD occurs only as a result of having schizophrenia, not as an indication of genetic predisposition. The error in this assertion is that if one excludes the 2 twins with schizophrenia who have brain disease from the analyses, as one should, then 9 of the remaining 10 twins with schizophrenia have gain scores and saccade counts that are also within the range of the normal control group. In other words, 90% of the twins with schizophrenia show the same overlap with the normal twins that the unaffected co-twins of subjects with schizophrenia show. Although this overlap is eventually acknowledged later in the article ("[the] majority of affected co-twins perform within the range of normal control twins"), neither the magnitude of the overlap nor its implications are addressed. Indeed, that overlap warrants the conclusion that, in this sample, ETD is not even associated with clinical schizophrenia. This finding contradicts the results of more than 80 studies, including another study by the authors of the article under discussion,[5] showing that subjects with schizophrenia have a significantly higher prevalence of ETD than the normal population, with no failure to replicate. A comprehensive review of those findings was published in 1993.[6]

REPLICATION ATTEMPT

The rationale of the authors is to "replicate previous eye tracking findings in twins with schizophrenia." Litman and colleagues asked one of us (P.S.H.) to assign qualitative scores to their data, as we had done in past twin studies,[2,3] and 2 of us (P.S.H. and D.L.L.) scored the data set independently of each other so that reliable ratings could be forwarded to the St Elizabeth's group. Twenty-six eye movement records were received and scored for the presence or absence of ETD. The researchers did the scoring without knowledge of group membership and acknowledgment for this effort appears at the end of their article. After the eye movement records had been scored and returned to Litman's group, they informed us that 16 of the 26 tracings were eye movement records of 8 pairs of discordant MZ twins and 10 were from 5 MZ pairs belonging to the control group. It is instructive to note that the qualitative scores we blindly assigned showed 100% concordance for eye tracking in the discordant twin group. Of the 8 sets of discordant twins, we identified ETD in both members of 3 and, in 5 sets of twins, we rated both members as having normal eye tracking. That is, each affected twin in whom we detected ETD had an unaffected co-twin who also had ETD.

These data are not included in the article by Litman et al. The results, nevertheless, are a strong replication of the Norwegian studies[2,3] in several respects. First, in the previous 2 studies, concordance for ETD in discordant MZ twins was 71%[2] and 100%.[3] In the Litman et al study, the concordance for ETD was 100%. Second, as in the Norwegian studies, the prevalence of ETD in the affected twins was 48%; in the Litman et al sample (considering only the 8 probands presented to us for evaluation), it is 37.5%. Third, the rate of ETD in 8 unaffected co-twins with MZ was 37.5% in the combined Norwegian studies and it was also 37.5% in the present study.

One finding is not replicated: the high rate of ETD (30%-40% [3 to 4 of 10 records]) in the normal twin pairs group. Among the twins in the normal group, we identified ETD in both members of a single twin pair, and ETD and borderline ETD in a second set of co-twins. Such a distribution of ETD is highly unlikely in the normal population, where the prevalence of ETD is about 8% or less[6-8] and most likely represents the nonrandom error that can plague small samples.

QUANTITATIVE SCORES USED

The claim is advanced that quantitative measures of gain and frequency of saccades provide a more superior indicator of eye tracking integrity than does the qualitative assessment. The computation and application of these 2 measures, however, raise questions about the usefulness of the data in assessing eye tracking integrity in this study. Because moderate-speed saccades are included as smooth pursuit, the gain scores in this study are inflated and saccade frequencies are underestimated. To understand the implications of our assertion for interpreting the data, it is important to note that gain is calculated as the ratio of eye velocity to target velocity during smooth pursuit only; the lower the gain score, the poorer the match. A gain score of 1.0 indicates a perfect match between eye velocity and target velocity. All events that are not smooth pursuit must be excluded from this calculation (ie, saccadic eye movements and blinks) or the velocities of these fast eye movements would be included in the calculation of eye velocity during pursuit, and artificially inflate the gain score. The authors set a criterion for identifying saccades as peak eye speed of at least 35° per second and returning to speeds of 30° per second and below. Eye movements as high as 29° per second would, therefore, be scored as smooth pursuit, with a gain of 1.74 (29° per second/16.67), an extraordinarily high gain. Since the target moved at a constant velocity of 16.67° per second, saccades that did not fall above the 30° per second criterion for identifying saccades will have been included as pursuit. The criterion for saccade detection set for this study, therefore, will fail to detect most moderate-speed saccades and instead will count them as fast pursuit, which, when averaged into calculations of pursuit velocity, will artificially inflate the gain scores. Furthermore, because these moderate-speed saccades are treated as pursuit, they are not included in the saccade counts, which results in an underestimation of the number of saccades. The influence of these events will be greater in poor trackers who make more saccades than good trackers, but the scores of all subjects will be distorted to some extent.

The saccade classification scheme is idiosyncratic and does not conform to any standard scheme for categorizing these fast eye movements. For example, catch-up saccades should end on the target, not behind it. It is also unclear why intrusive saccades would begin and end ahead of the target but go in the same direction as the target since such intrusions include square wave jerks, macro square wave jerks, saccadic pulses, and anticipatory saccades, all of which do not necessarily go in the direction of the target or begin or end ahead of the target. The category of intermediate saccades is particularly unclear; are these catch-up saccades occurring during a poorly calibrated portion of the recording, or anticipatory saccades, or something else? If they are the former, the rate of catch-up saccades would be further underestimated because intermediate saccades were considered as a separate category of saccades.

MISINTERPRETATION OF DATA

All of the correlations in the twin groups are positive and are within the range reported by other investigators who have studied eye tracking in twins, whether normal twins[9,10] or twins with schizophrenia.[2,3] The authors report an intraclass correlation for gain of 0.52 in the discordant twins and 0.60 in the normal group; for total saccades, the intraclass correlations are 0.59 in the discordant twins and 0.68 in the normal group. The authors interpret these differences in magnitude as if they were statistically significant by concluding "... the [intraclass correlations] in discordant twins are lower in magnitude than those for normal control twins.... These data suggest that discordant MZ twins are less concordant for eye tracking measures than normal twins." No confidence limits are included. According to our calculations, however, the 95% confidence limits of these correlations range from near 0 to greater than 0.84, indicating that these intraclass correlations do not differ from each other statistically.

What has this study shown? We believe that a more objective interpretation of these data, even granting the flaws in the measurement, would acknowledge the following. (1) Data based on blind qualitative ratings of the tracking in this MZ discordant twin sample replicate the original studies,[2,3] showing that in twins discordant for clinical schizophrenia, there is a high concordance in ETD. (2) There is a significant positive correlation in gain and saccade counts between MZ twins discordant for schizophrenia. (3) Data based on gain and saccade frequency fail to distinguish either subjects with schizophrenia or their unaffected co-twins from a normal comparison group. (4) Among the discordant twins, the affected twin seems to have lower gain, more saccades than the unaffected twin, or both. A similar result, using a global quantitative score (natural logarithm of the signal-noise ratio) was reported in earlier twin studies.[2,3] Such regularity suggests that there is some effect of the illness on eye tracking performance and calls for discussion and investigation, but does not mitigate the conclusion that clinically discordant twins have highly concordant eye tracking scores, using qualitative and quantitative measures. There is no reason why the affected twin should not show worse tracking than the clinically unaffected twin, since schizophrenia could be expected to affect behavior the same as other genetically transmitted traits influence susceptibility to disease: the outbreak of the disease may have an affect on the trait itself. For example, mild hypertension represents a liability trait for atherogenesis. With the outbreak of the disease, there is an effect of the disease itself on the severity of the trait, leading to a progressive accumulation of lipids in the smooth muscle cells and, hence, to an increase in blood pressure above that of the initial predisease elevation. An affected twin would, therefore, have a higher blood pressure than the well twin, who also has the genetic trait but not the disease and whose onset may be influenced by many other factors.[11]

The final proof of whether ETD represents a genetic factor in the transmission of schizophrenia rests on the discovery of chromosomal linkage with ETD. One such study has been published and awaits replication. Arolt and colleagues[8] recently reported linkage between a locus on chromosome 6 and ETD (measured qualitatively and using gain and saccade counts) in 63 members of 8 families with schizophrenia.

Given the errors of method and interpretation that we have described, the Litman et al study cannot, in our opinion, disprove the hypothesis that ETD is a genetically transmitted trait associated with schizophrenia.

Philip S. Holzman, PhD
Department of Psychology
Harvard University
33 Kirkland St
Cambridge, MA 02138

Deborah L. Levy, PhD
Steven W. Matthysse, PhD
Department of Psychiatry
Harvard Medical School
McLean Hospital
Belmont, Mass

Larry A. Abel, PhD
School of Orthoptics
Latrobe University
Bundoora, Victoria, Australia

REFERENCES

1. Litman RE, Torrey EF, Hommer DW, Radant AR, Pickar D, Weinberger DR. A quantitative analysis of smooth pursuit eye tracking in monozygotic twins discordant for schizophrenia. *Arch Gen Psychiatry.* 1997;54:417-428.
2. Holzman PS, Kringlen E, Levy DL, Proctor LR, Haberman S, Yasillo NJ. Abnormal-pursuit eye movements in schizophrenia: evidence for a genetic indicator. *Arch Gen Psychiatry.* 1977;34:802-805.
3. Holzman PS, Kringlen E, Levy DL, Haberman SJ. Deviant eye tracking in twins discordant for psychosis: a replication. *Arch Gen Psychiatry.* 1980;37:627-631.
4. Leigh RJ, Zee DS. *The Neurology of Eye Movements.* 2nd ed. Philadelphia, Pa: FA Davis Co Publishers; 1991:561.
5. Litman RE, Hommer DW, Clem T, Rapaport MH, Pato CN, Pickar D. Smooth pursuit eye movements in schizophrenia: effects of neuroleptic treatment and caffeine. *Psychopharmacol Bull.* 1989;25:473-478.
6. Levy DL, Holzman PS, Matthysse S, Mendell NR. Eye tracking and schizophrenia: a critical perspective. *Schizophr Bull.* 1993;19:461-536.
7. Arolt V, Lencer R, Nolte A, Pinnow M, Schwinger E. Eye tracking dysfunction in families with multiple cases of schizophrenia. *Eur Arch Psychiatry Clin Neurosci.* 1996;246:175-181.
8. Arolt V, Lencer R, Nolte A, Müller-Myhsok, Purmann S, Schürmann M, Leutelt J, Pinnow M, Schwinger E. Eye tracking dysfunction is a putative phenotypic susceptibility marker of schizophrenia and maps to a locus on chromosome 6p in families with multiple occurrence of the disease. *Am J Med Genet.* 1996;67:564-579.
9. Iacono WG, Lykken DT. Eye tracking and psychopathology: new procedures applied to a sample of normal monozygotic twins. *Arch Gen Psychiatry.* 1979;36:1361-1369.
10. Bell BB, Abel LA, Li W, Christian JC, Yee RD. Concordance of smooth pursuit and saccadic measures in normal monozygotic twin pairs. *Biol Psychiatry.* 1994;36:522-526.
11. Matthysse S, Holzman PS. Formal thought disorder in schizophrenics and their twins. *J Abnorm Psychol.* 1988;96:105-107.

ORIGINAL ARTICLE

Magnetic Source Imaging Evidence of Sex Differences in Cerebral Lateralization in Schizophrenia

Martin Reite, MD; Jeanelle Sheeder; Peter Teale, MSEE; Matthew Adams; Douglas Richardson; Jack Simon, MD, PhD; Richard H. Jones, PhD; Donald C. Rojas, PhD

Background: It has been postulated that schizophrenia represents a disorder of anomalous cerebral lateralization. This study is a replication of earlier preliminary findings using a multichannel neuromagnetometer, suggesting altered lateralization in schizophrenia in male subjects, with an extension of the findings to female subjects.

Methods: We used magnetoencephalography-based magnetic source imaging to estimate the intracranial location of the 100-millisecond latency auditory-evoked field component (M100) in both left and right hemispheres of 20 patients with paranoid schizophrenia and 20 controls without schizophrenia. Neuroanatomical data were obtained by means of magnetic resonance imaging, from which we segmented and computed volumes of both total brain and left and right superior temporal gyri.

Results: Locations of M100 source were compatible with neuronal generators located in the transverse gyri of Heschl on the superior temporal gyri in both study groups; M100 sources were asymmetric in all the control subjects. The male patient subgroup exhibited significantly less asymmetry than the control group, while the female patient subgroup actually showed significantly more asymmetry. The male patient subgroup generally had smaller superior temporal gyri than the control group. No evidence of total brain volume differences was observed.

Conclusions: Our findings support previous magnetoencephalography-based studies suggesting anomalous cerebral lateralization in schizophrenia. Further, in extending our studies to female patients, our data suggest that the nature of this anomaly is sex specific, a finding that, to our knowledge, has not previously been reported.

Arch Gen Psychiatry. 1997;54:433-440

THE BRAIN is not bilaterally symmetrical.[1-3] The hemispheres differ in size,[4] regional volumes,[5] androgen receptors,[6] electrical activity,[7] amine concentration,[8] metabolic activity,[9] and location of magnetic source imaging (MSI)–based auditory-evoked field (AEF) components.[10] Relatively few of these left-right hemisphere differences have been examined as a function of sex, which may be an important mediating factor. Kulynych et al[11] have found that female subjects do not exhibit temporal planum asymmetry to the same degree as do male subjects. Another example is the relative anteroposterior location of MSI-based locations of the 100-millisecond latency AEF component (M100). This component demonstrates greater asymmetry in male subjects (sources more anterior in the right hemisphere than in the left) than in female subjects.[10]

Schizophrenia has been postulated to represent a disorder of cerebral laterality. Crow[12] suggests that schizophrenia may be a genetic encephalopathy based on aberrant development of brain asymmetry, perhaps especially involving temporal lobes. Evidence for this hypothesis exists at both structural and functional levels. Hoff et al[13] and Falkai et al[14] found evidence of decreased asymmetry of lateral sulci in groups with schizophrenia, although Bartley and colleagues[15] could not confirm these findings.

Rubin et al,[16] in their computed-tomography–based study of 49 patients with newly diagnosed schizophrenia or schizophreniform disorder, found in the patient group a significant increase in size of the left sylvian fissures compared with those in 24 controls, with a similar, but statistically nonsignificant trend on the right side. In a recent study, Zipursky et al[17] found evidence of bilateral gray-matter deficits in patients with schizophrenia, but they did not support a major left-hemisphere emphasis, whereas Bilder and colleagues[18] found that regional cerebral volumes based on magnetic resonance imaging (MRI) were

From the Departments of Psychiatry (Drs Reite and Rojas and Ms Sheeder and Mssrs Teale, Adams, and Richardson), Radiology (Dr Simon), and Preventive Medicine and Biometrics (Dr Jones), University of Colorado Health Sciences Center; and Psychiatry Service, Denver Veterans Affairs Medical Center (Dr Reite), Denver.

SUBJECTS AND METHODS

SUBJECTS

We studied a total of 40 subjects, including 20 patients with schizophrenia (11 males and 9 females) and 20 normal controls (10 males and 10 females). Patients were recruited as volunteer participants from outpatient clinics in the Denver (Colo) metropolitan area. All were actively psychotic, all had a history of medication, and 16 were taking medication at the time of the recording. Two patients had a history of previous electroconvulsive treatment. Control subjects were normal healthy adults, recruited by advertisement from the Denver metropolitan area; they were never mentally ill by the Research Diagnostic Criteria.[39]

Diagnoses in the patient group were determined by criteria based on the Structured Clinical Interview for *DSM-III-R*-Patient Edition[40] in addition to review of all available medical records. Handedness was based on the Annett[41] handedness scale, on which handedness is a continuous variable ranging from 1.0 (purely right-handed) to −1.0 (purely left-handed). All study participants had normal hearing by audiometry. The research protocol was approved by the Colorado Multiple Institutional Review Board, and all patients and controls signed informed consent. A summary of subject information is provided in the **Table**.[42]

METHODS

Subject Positioning and Environment and Magnetoencephalographic Recordings

Magnetoencephalographic (MEG) recordings were made using a 7-channel, second-order biomagnetometer (BTI Model 607, Biomagnetic Technologies, Inc, San Diego, Calif), with 1.8-cm coil diameter and 4.0-cm baseline, and obtained inside a magnetically shielded room providing 34-dB attenuation at 0 Hz, and 55-dB attenuation at 60 Hz,[43] with subjects positioned in a nonmagnetic chair.

A sonic digitizer with customized software was used for absolute determination of the subject's fiduciary points (left and right preauricular points and nasion) and each dewar position. The relative location and orientation of each gradiometer coil in the 3-dimensional space defined by the fiduciary points were specified in terms of Cartesian coordinates *x*, *y*, and *z*. The x-axis is determined by the line connecting the preauricular points (positive *x* is out the right ear). The y-axis is the line normal to the x-axis at the midpoint (the origin), exiting through the front of the head, and contained in the plane defined by the x-axis and the nasion. The z-axis is normal to *x* and *y* at the midpoint and exits the top of the head (positive *z* is above the origin). Details of the method of localization with the sonic digitizer can be found in Reite et al.[44]

Stimuli

Stimuli were computer generated, 25 milliseconds long, 1-kHz tone pips, with 3-millisecond rise and fall times, at 90-dB sound pressure level, with random interstimulus intervals within a window of 1.2 to 1.8 seconds, delivered by a nonmagnetic piezoelectric earphone placed over the ear opposite the hemisphere from which magnetic recordings were being made. Subjects were instructed to ignore the auditory stimuli and to watch a 4-m distant video monitor on which a silent movie was being shown. Subjects were visually monitored on a closed circuit television system. Recordings were made from a sufficient number of locations (nominally 5-6) to encompass both ingoing and outgoing extrema of the component of interest over each hemisphere.

Data Processing

Magnetic recordings were wide band (0.1-300 Hz). Signals were amplified and digitized at a rate of 3 kHz, with a dynamic range of 3200 femtotesla peak to peak. Data were collected using a computer software package (SCAN, Neuroscan Inc, Herndon, Va) and raw data were retained. Recordings included a 100-millisecond prestimulus baseline and 250-millisecond poststimulus delivery. Averaging of responses to 100 stimuli provided averaged AEF responses. Averages were filtered with a phase invariant 24 dB per octave digital filter with a low pass of 20 Hz. All MEG channels were written out on paper for inspection of raw magnetic data and to facilitate elimination of eye movement, blink, subject movement, or extraneous magnetic artifact-contaminated trials.

The M100 component for each gradiometer position was computer selected, based on the largest absolute amplitude within the time window that contained the ingoing and outgoing extrema values (60- to 110-millisecond poststimulus). This ensemble of amplitude values was used as input for a customized software program (MEGEEG, Crazy Horse Software, Boulder, Colo), which provided inverse solution source location estimates. The MEGEEG software program performs inverse solutions for both multichannel magnetic and electric data, using an algorithm based on a globally convergent modification of the Newton method. It incorporates rectangular coordinates for positional encoding and reporting of results, provides 95% confidence intervals, includes corrections for tangential components (coil orientation with respect to a best-fit sphere is used to calculate both radial and tangential B-field components in the forward solution),[45] and models the effects of the areas and baselines of the coil arrays.[46] Studies using plastic sphere and skull phantoms demonstrate that MEGEEG localizes magnetic sources to an accuracy of within ±1.0 mm and it uses a single current dipole in a spherical model for source estimation. The local curvature of each subject's head over the nominal source location was used to establish the centerpoint and radius of the best-fit sphere.

significantly asymmetric in 51 control subjects, but 70 patients with first episode failed to exhibit the same degree of cerebral asymmetry. Petty and colleagues[19] have recently described a reversal of expected (left greater than right) asymmetry of the surface area of the temporal planum in schizophrenia.

Two previous reports[20,21] have suggested that male patients with paranoid schizophrenia may have altered cerebral lateralization based on MSI. In 1988, we[20,21] reported that the 50-millisecond latency AEF component (M50) failed to exhibit the same asymmetry in 6 subjects with schizophrenia compared with 6 male controls. Sub-

Source parameter estimates included 3-dimensional position (*x*, *y*, and *z*, defined earlier, with their respective 95% confidence intervals), orientation (θ in degrees counterclockwise from the vertex), current dipole strength (Q, in nanoampere meters), and fit, a measure of normalized error of the fit between measured and modeled field. Confidence intervals are estimated by analyzing the fit of the data to the model without using independent estimates of the measurement noise. They are generated by computing the difference between the residual error function associated with any given dipole and that associated with the optimum (least squares), divided by the optimum, and solving the resulting expression for all parameter values for which it is less than or equal to a statistical criterion derived from the Snedecor F distribution, as described in Reite et al.[44] Based on previous data, our primary interests were in the measures of anteroposterior location (the y value). We examined both absolute y values in left and right hemispheres and also computed a laterality score (Δy), by subtracting the left from the right y value.

An important issue in studies such as these is the reliability and replicability of MEG-determined source location. We have discussed this in some detail in a related article,[47] wherein we describe studies in which we have estimated the repeatability of M100 source location estimates using a 7-channel neuromagnetometer. We found, in independent recordings performed at least 1 week apart, root mean square differences in *x*, *y*, and *z* locations were approximately 0.7 cm on the 2 occasions; strength and orientation differences were 18 nanoampere meters and 11°, respectively. Although greater accuracy can generally be obtained in auditory source localization using a 37-channel instrument,[48] these values compare favorably with the repeatability of somatosensory-evoked field localizations using a large array biomagnetometer.[49]

MRI and Image Reconstruction

Magnetic resonance images of the head, including the fiduciary reference points (established with the sonic digitizer and marked with high proton density vitamin A capsules), were acquired with a standard head coil using a 1.5-Tesla system (GE Signa, General Electric Medical Systems, Inc, Waukesha, Wis). The spoiled-gradient echo acquisition resulted in 1.7-mm thick, T_1-weighted images with a repetition time per echo time of 40/5 milliseconds and a 40° flip angle, encompassed within a 256×256 matrix. These acquisition parameters resulted in 0.94 mm × 0.94 mm × 1.7 mm voxels. The entire head was imaged with 124 slices. Magnetic resonance images were transferred through an Ethernet link to a SUN SPARC station (Sun Microsystems Inc, Mountain View, Calif), compressed, and stored on optical disk. With the aid of 3-dimensional image rendering software (SunVision 1.2, Sun Microsystems Inc) and an image-processing software (Interactive Data Language 3.1.1, Research Systems Inc, Boulder), the entire brain was segmented, using a combination of automated computer thresholding and manual segmentation, and the total brain volume (TBV) was calculated. The volume computation algorithm was tested on irregular phantoms of known volume and was found to be accurate to ±1%. Additionally, the STG were manually segmented by one of us (M.R.), who was blind to subject, and reconstructed into 3-dimensional volumes whose surfaces were then tessellated and rendered as images. Details of the segmentation procedures can be obtained from the authors.

Herein, we report the constrained STG volumes, including those slices from the most anterior slice containing the temporal stem to the most posterior slice containing the fornix (inclusive) after the methods of Shenton et al.[50] All STG volumes are reported as a percentage of TBV.

Colocation of MEG-Determined Sources on MRI

The MRI fiduciary points were selected in a manner that most closely simulates the sonically digitized fiduciary points. These methods, accurate to 1 slice thickness, are detailed in Reite et al.[44] An example of M100 source locations placed on the reconstructed and surface-imaged STG of 1 of our normal control subjects, a 23-year-old man, is shown in **Figure 1**.

STATISTICAL ANALYSES

The Statistical Package for the Social Sciences (SPSS version 4.0, SPSS Inc, Chicago, Ill) was used for all the statistical analyses in this study. First, the laterality variable Δy (absolute right *y* location minus absolute left *y* location) was tested by a 2 × 2 between-subjects analysis of variance (ANOVA) (sex × diagnosis). Second, the relative STG volumes were evaluated by a 2 × 2 × 2 mixed-design ANOVA (sex × hemisphere × diagnosis), with hemisphere treated as a within-subjects factor. Third, possible differences in TBV were ascertained by 2 × 2 ANOVA (sex × diagnosis). All 3 designs were evaluated for significance at the .05 level, and in each case the within-cell sums-of-squares error was used to test effects. In each of the designs weighted means were used to account for differences in the number of subjects per cell. Because all main effects and interaction terms had only 1 *df* in the numerator, no post hoc analyses were needed, or performed, on the data. Power analyses were also conducted at the .05 α level and are discussed as applicable within the "Results" section.

Independent Student *t* tests (α=.05) were conducted between controls and patients (collapsed across sex) to determine whether our groups differed along the demographic variables (age, education, and handedness). To ascertain whether differences between our subject groups on demographic variables (ie, education [Table]) could explain some of the M100 and/or MRI results, Pearson *r* correlation coefficients were computed between the MEG and MRI variables and education. Each correlation was evaluated for significance at the .05 α level.

sequently, we[22] reported that the somewhat later M100 was also located asymmetrically in left and right hemispheres in 6 normal male subjects, with source locations further anterior in the right than the left hemisphere, whereas 6 male subjects with schizophrenia failed to exhibit this asymmetry. This was attributed primarily to M100 sources located more anterior in the left hemisphere in the patient group. We have also reported preliminary findings[23] suggesting that MSI of the M100 AEF component may also be different in female compared with male subjects with schizophrenia, but suggestive of predominantly right (rather than left) hemisphere differences.

Demographic Characteristics of Subjects*

Variable	Male Subjects: Controls	Male Subjects: Patients With Schizophrenia	Female Subjects: Controls	Female Subjects: Patients With Schizophrenia	*t* Value
Age, y	38.2±9.3	37.1±4.7	37.1±6.5	38.2±5.6	−0.07
Education, y	15.3±1.9	13.3±1.8	15.0±1.9	13.8±2.4	2.98†
Handedness‡	0.4±0.9	0.8±0.8	1.0±0.0	0.9±0.2	0.09
Chlorpromazine equivalent, mg/d§	...	248.0±306.2	...	864.0±786.8	...
Global Assessment of Functioning Scale score‖	...	46.4±11.6	...	46.3±11.9	...
Age of onset, y	...	19.3±2.4	...	21.9±6.3	...

**Values represent means (±SDs) for demographic characteristics of subjects. Ellipses indicate not applicable.*
†Indicates significant difference at .05 level between control and patient groups (independent t *tests), collapsed across sex.*
‡Handedness according to the Annett scale,[41] ranging from +1.0 (purely right-handed) to −1.0 (purely left-handed).
§After Davis.[42]
*‖Global Assessment of Functioning Scale (*DSM-III-R*, Axis V).*

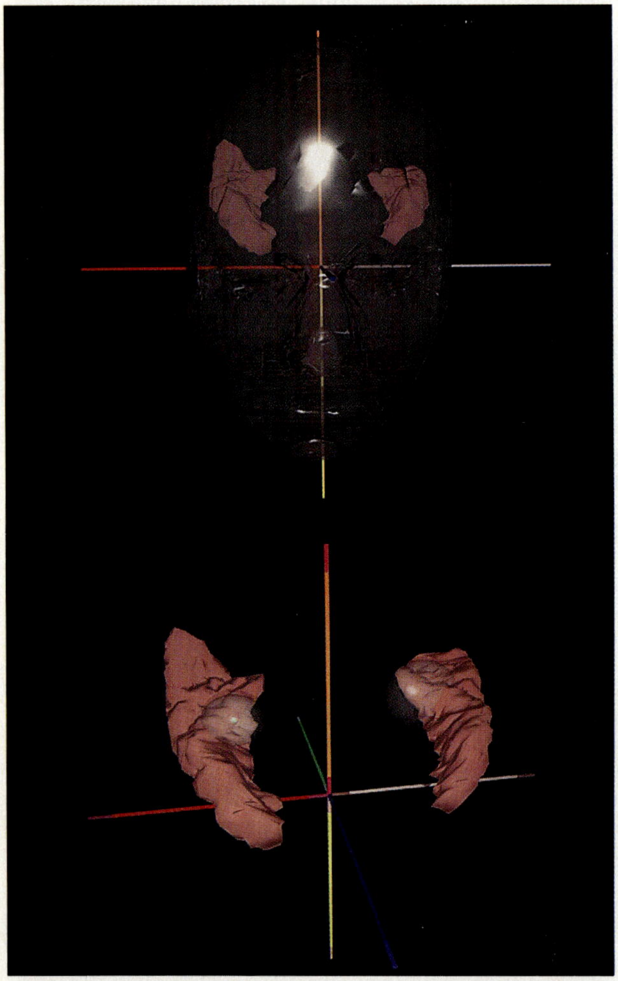

Figure 1. *Top, Magnetic resonance image reconstruction of the surface of the head (semitransparent) in a 23-year-old male control with right and left superior temporal gyri located at their true sites within the head. Magnetoencephalographic x-, y-, and z-axes indicated by the colored lines. Bottom, Reconstructed superior temporal gyri removed from the head and placed in actual position with respect to x- (mediolateral, connecting left and right preauricular points), y- (anteroposterior), and z- (vertical) axes (colored lines). Bright white dots indicate M100 source locations; translucent ellipsoids, source location confidence regions.*

The possible sex-related differences in laterality are interesting in light of the considerable evidence that the schizophrenic disorders are sexually dimorphic. In women, schizophrenia has been reported as having a later onset,[24-28] being clinically less severe,[29] having greater affective symptoms,[30,31] being more responsive to treatment, and having a better outcome.[32,33] There have also been reports that apparent structural deficits found in male subjects with schizophrenia may not be as prominent, or appear at all, in affected female subjects.[34-38]

The early MSI-based observations from our laboratory, while compatible with abnormalities in hemispheric lateralization in schizophrenia, were compromised by the fact that a single-channel gradiometer was used as the measuring instrument, limiting the accuracy of the MSI. We designed the present study to more accurately test the 2 hypotheses: that M100 sources exhibit altered interhemispheric asymmetry in patients with schizophrenia and that the lack of asymmetry seen in male subjects would not be present in female subjects. We also used MRI and image reconstruction to determine whether associated anatomical abnormalities in the superior temporal gyri (STG) might be correlated with the MSI-based auditory source location findings.

RESULTS

MEG-BASED M100 SOURCE LOCATION DIFFERENCES

A significant 2-way interaction was obtained from the first ANOVA on the Δy variable ($F[1,36]=5.11$; $P<.05$), indicating that the mean (±SD) variable Δy was smaller in male patients with schizophrenia ($\Delta y=0.48\pm1.06$ cm) than in male controls ($\Delta y=1.26\pm.95$ cm), whereas it was larger in the female patients with schizophrenia ($\Delta y=1.52\pm0.35$ cm) than in the female controls ($\Delta y=1.16\pm0.55$ cm). Because there were significant differences between the patient and control groups in education (Table), a correlation coefficient was computed between Δy and education and was found to be nonsignificant ($r=0.18$; $P>.05$), suggesting no linear relationship between those variables.

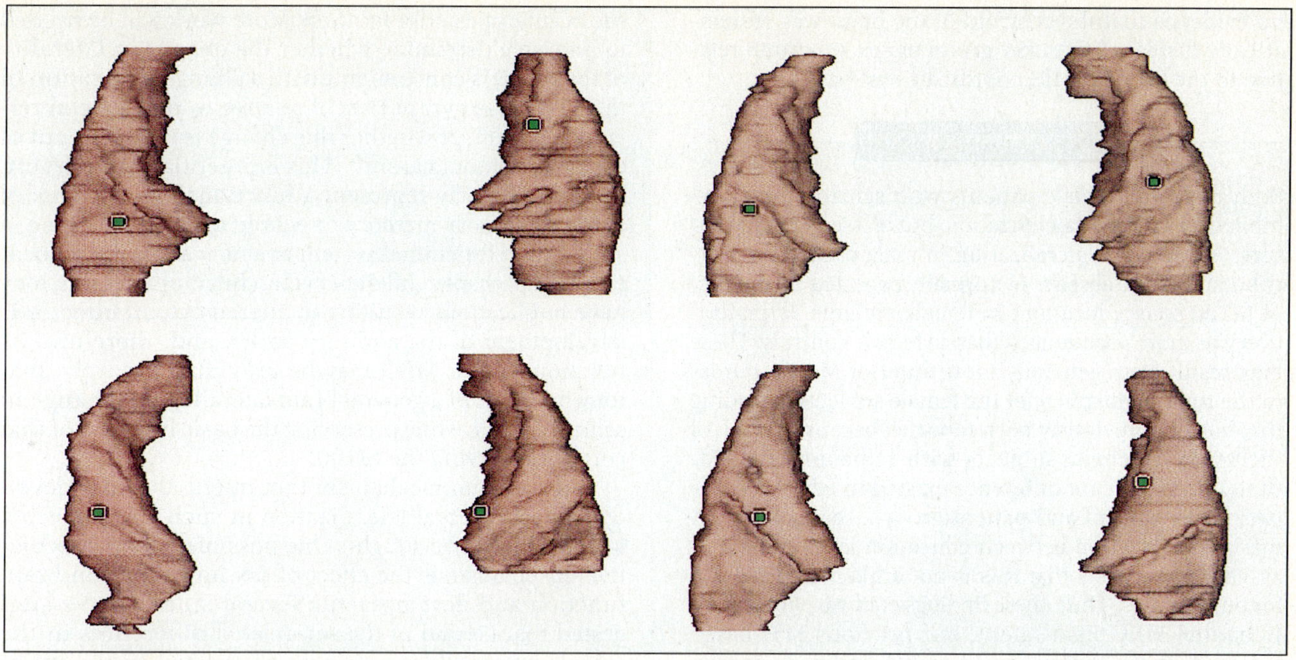

Figure 2. *Reconstructed top views of the left and right superior temporal gyri (STG) in 4 representative subjects: a male control (top left) and patient with schizophrenia (bottom left), and a female control (top right) and patient with schizophrenia (bottom right). Left and right STG are represented in their in vivo orientation with respect to each other in anteroposterior position. Locations of M100 (100-millisecond latency auditory-evoked field component) source are projected on to the surface of the STG (green squares). Because these are 2-dimensional representations of 3-dimensional reconstructions, the apparent length of the STG may be foreshortened as a function of the orientation and slope of the sylvian fissure (which defines the top surface of the STG) in each head and hemisphere, and as a result of differences in head placement in the magnetic resonance imaging head coil. Calibration lines are, therefore, omitted because they would be misleading. (Data regarding the absolute dimensions of these structures are available from the authors.)*

ABSOLUTE LOCATION OF M100 SOURCES ON THE STG OF SUBJECTS

When M100 source locations were plotted on the reconstructed STG, source location confidence intervals included the transverse gyri of Heschl for both patient and control groups. **Figure 2** illustrates representative M100 source locations (green squares) plotted on the reconstructed STG of 4 representative subjects, a male and female control, and a male and female patient with schizophrenia. These subjects were chosen on the basis of their individual y (anteroposterior) locations value being representative of the means for their group.

STRUCTURAL MRI

The second ANOVA on relative STG volume revealed no significant 3-way interaction (F[1,36]=0.83; *P*>.05. A significant hemisphere main effect was obtained (F[1,36]=12.27; *P*<.05), but the group × hemisphere and sex × hemisphere interactions were nonsignificant (F[1,36]=0.96; *P*>.05 and F[1,36]=0.00; *P*>.05, respectively), indicating that the mean (±SD) left STG volume is slightly smaller (1.08% ± 0.15%) than the right STG (1.20% ± 0.18%) across all subjects in our sample, when corrected for TBV. The sex main effect was significant (F[1,36]=4.87; *P*<.05), and the sex × diagnosis interaction approached significance at the .05 level (F[1,36]=3.20; *P*=.08), indicating a general trend for the mean (±SD) female relative STG volumes (1.18%±0.17%) to be higher than male STG volumes (1.09%±0.13%), but that this was most likely due to the lower STG volumes in the male patients with schizophrenia (0.95%±0.13%), rather than in the male controls (1.15%±.15%). Educational level did not correlate significantly with either left (*r*=0.03) or right (*r*=0.20) relative STG volume (*P*>.05).

The third ANOVA revealed that the mean (±SD) TBVs were smaller in females (1236 ± 115 mL) than in males (1398 ± 101 mL) (F[1,36]=22.46; *P*<.05). The sex × diagnosis interaction was nonsignificant (F[1,36]=2.65; *P*=.11); TBV did not correlate significantly with education (*r*=0.15; *P*>.05).

Caution should be used in interpreting any of the nonsignificant findings pertaining to the MRI data as evidence of lack of effect, given the relatively poor power of some of the interaction tests (eg, 0.35 for the sex × diagnosis interaction on the TBVs). It is possible that with a larger sample, results that approached significance at the .05 level would have reached statistically significant levels.

THE COORDINATE SYSTEM

Because all MEG and MRI spatial references are based on a skeletal reference system (preauricular points and nasion), it is important to consider whether the control and populations with schizophrenia might exhibit systematic alterations in these reference points. We examined absolute lengths of the lines from nasion to left and right preauricular points in both groups and their sex subgroups and found no significant difference. We also noted no evidence that the centroid of the brain was systematically displaced in either group or sex subgroup relative to the MEG or MRI coordinate systems.

COMMENT

Both male and female patients with schizophrenia exhibited anomalous lateralization, but of a sex-specific nature. Anomalous lateralization in male patients was attributable to the absence of normally expected asymmetry of M100 source location; in female patients, lateralization was more pronounced than in female controls. These may result from generally more anterior M100 sources in the right hemisphere of the female subjects, a finding that has not previously been reported because of lack of inclusion of female subjects with schizophrenia. Although a significant difference existed in education between our control and patient groups, the lack of significant correlation between education level and M100 assymetry suggests that this is not a likely explanation for our findings. Thus, these findings confirm, with a multichannel MEG instrument, our previous MSI-based (using a single-channel instrument) findings suggesting anomalous lateralization in the schizophrenic brain and also suggest that the direction of the anomaly is sex specific.

One trend within the anatomical data emerged. Male patients had smaller STGs than male controls. This finding is in essential agreement with those of Shenton et al,[50] who also found smaller STG volumes in male patients with schizophrenia. However, Shenton and colleagues found volumetric reductions specific to the left hemisphere STG and although they did not report STG data about female subjects, we saw no evidence of a difference in volume of the STG in this sample of female subjects with schizophrenia.

Our finding that TBVs did not differ between control and patient groups was consonant with earlier findings by Nasrallah et al[51] in male subjects with schizophrenia, but it contradicts the findings of Rubin et al[16] and Gur et al,[52] who found smaller brain volumes in both male and female subjects with schizophrenia. However, this measure is likely very sensitive to the method used to estimate brain volume, and that may account for the differences between these studies. Another recent study[53] reported smaller total volumes of heteromodal association cortex (STG, dorsolateral prefrontal cortex, and inferior parietal lobule) in patients compared with those in controls, with the effect mainly accounted for by the female schizophrenic group. More studies using larger numbers of male and female subjects will need to be conducted before this issue is resolved.

In this group of subjects, M100 source locations were again compatible with generators in, or immediately contiguous to, the transverse gyri of Heschl, as has been previously described in nonschizophrenic subjects.[44] However, as described elsewhere,[54] uncertainty about the precise anatomical delimiters of the transverse gyri of Heschl complicates interpretation of this issue. The recent article by Petty and colleagues[19] found no evidence of altered surface area of the transverse gyrus of Heschl in schizophrenia, but this study did not address the issue of anteroposterior location. More work will be needed to precisely determine whether the change in laterality of the M100 is concomitant with a change in location of the transverse gyri of Heschl relative to the skeletal reference system, or whether this change is independent of a general anatomical shift. This is potentially important, as the M100 may represent a functional MEG index of auditory sensory memory or echoic memory.[55,56] If so, a shift of that functional system to a new anatomical location, and perhaps a different cytoarchitectural region, may have implications resulting in altered cytoarchitectonic development of the auditory cortex and, therefore, its function. If not, MEG may be providing a purely anatomical index of a general brain lateralization change in schizophrenia, while preserving the basic function of that cortex subserving the M100.

A common mechanism that might alter the development of cerebral lateralization in such a sex-specific fashion should be sought. One possible, albeit speculative, mechanism is the effect of sex hormones on brain function and development. Several studies have suggested that certain of the sex-related differences in the schizophrenic illness are possibly related to the influence of sex hormones. Seeman and Lang[57] have recently reviewed proposed roles of the organizational and activational effects of estrogens in accounting for sex differences in schizophrenia, and some evidence suggests estrogens that may exert a protective effect in women prone to schizophrenia,[58] possibly mediated by modulation of dopamine systems.[59-62] Substantial data exist, primarily from nonprimate animals, supporting the important role of prenatal sex-hormone exposure on brain development in the fetus.[63] Several investigators have hypothesized that the lateralization of the brain is accomplished in utero, and that sex hormones are important in this process.[2,64] The possibility of schizophrenia being associated with a fundamental abnormality of the development of tonotopic organization within the auditory cortex should be considered, as well as the potential influence of sex hormones on this cytoarchitectural organization. The first of these issues can be directly addressed by MSI methods.[65,66]

The receptive fields of neurons within the auditory cortex are generally spatially organized by both frequency (tonotopic organization) and amplitude (amplitopic organization) of the sound stimuli. It seems likely that the M100 component would be restricted to an ensemble of neurons in primary auditory cortex whose position should be fixed early in development in a tonotopic[65] and amplitopic[67,68] lattice. Intuitively, it would seem unlikely that this location would shift appreciably in response to a later developing schizophrenic process, although longitudinal developmental studies will be required to substantiate this. The implication of such a hypothesis is that the schizophrenic process is operative at the earliest developmental stages.

It is not yet known whether such changes are present at the onset of the disorder, in which case they may suggest a neurodevelopmental vulnerability. We also cannot yet discount the schizophrenic process, or its treatment, as being a causative element in changes of this nature. The recent findings of DeLisi and colleagues[69] suggest that subtle cortical atrophy may continue after first symptom onset in patients with schizophrenia, although STG volume change in the subjects with schizophrenia during 4 years was not different from that of controls.

Another consideration is whether schizophrenic symptoms per se could be related to findings of the type we have described. Magnetic source imaging has revealed that the cortical representation for the digits of the left hand is increased in violin players, suggesting that cortical reorganization in adult humans reflects functional demands.[70] Thus, we cannot exclude the possibility that the psychotic hallucinatory experiences of our subjects, presumably reflecting in part the activity of the auditory cortex, may have resulted in a cortical reorganization, reflected in a change in M100 dipole source location on the STG. This explanation is supported by preliminary data from Tiihonen and colleagues,[71] who found an increase in M100 latency and poorer fit to a simple dipole model (a single dipole within a spherical homogeneous volume conductor) in a single subject with schizophrenia studied while actively hallucinating. Such an explanation would seemingly not account for sex differences, since all of our patients were hallucinating.

In summary, these findings strongly support the notion of anomalous lateralization of the brain in the schizophrenic disorders. They should not be cause to unduly emphasize the role of such changes in schizophrenic pathology, because evidence of altered brain structure and function in schizophrenia is widespread, including, but probably not limited to, temporal limbic regions,[72,73] basal ganglia,[36,74] frontal and parietal lobes[75,76] and thalamus.[77] Rather, they are but 1 more piece of a complex puzzle of which all pieces are not yet known. Furthermore, these findings are based on a small and relatively homogeneous sample of patients with schizophrenia. They will clearly need to be independently verified in nonparanoid subtypes of schizophrenia and extended to include other forms of psychotic illness and the influence of pharmacological and other treatments. We do believe that the findings are of sufficient interest to merit continuation of this avenue of research.

Accepted for publication March 26, 1996.

This research was supported by grant MH47476 from the National Institute of Mental Health, Rockville, Md. Dr Reite was supported in part by Research Scientist Award grant MH46335 from the National Institute of Mental Health.

We thank Julie Worlein, PhD, for her critical review of the manuscript. We also gratefully acknowledge Bernhard Geiger from Institut National de Recherche en Informatique et en Automatique, Rocquencourt, France, for his MRI contour triangulation software package NUAGES 4.0 (e-mail: ftp://betelgeuse.inria.fr/pub/Nuages/NUAGES—SUN4.tar.Z).

Reprints: Martin Reite, MD, Department of Psychiatry, Box C268-68, University of Colorado Health Sciences Center, 4200 E Ninth Ave, Denver, CO 80262.

REFERENCES

1. Galaburda AM, Lemay M, Kemper TL, Geschwind N. Right-left asymmetries in the brain. *Science.* 1978;199:852-856.
2. Galaburda AM. Anatomic basis of cerebral dominance. In: RJ Davidson, K Hugdahl, eds. *Brain Asymmetry.* Cambridge, Mass: The MIT Press; 1995:51-73.
3. Geschwind N, Galaburda AM. Cerebral lateralization: biological mechanisms, associations, and pathology, I: a hypothesis and a program for research. *Arch Neurol.* 1985;42:428-458.
4. Willerman L, Schultz R, Rutledge JN, Bigler ED. Hemisphere size asymmetry predicts relative verbal and nonverbal intelligence differently in the sexes: an MRI study of structure-function relations. *Intelligence.* 1992;16: 315-328.
5. Weinberger D, Luchins D, Morihisa J, Wyatt R. Asymmetrical volumes of the right and left frontal and occipital regions of the human brain. *Ann Neurol.* 1982;11:97-100.
6. Sholl SA, Kim KL. Androgen receptors are differentially distributed between right and left cerebral hemispheres of the fetal male rhesus monkey. *Brain Res.* 1990;516:122-126.
7. Gevins AS, Schaffer RE, Doyle JC, Cutillo BA, Tannehill RS, Bressler SL. Shadows of thought: shifting lateralization of human brain electrical patterns during brief visuomotor task. *Science.* 1983;220:97-99.
8. Oke A, Keller R, Mefford I, Adams RN. Lateralization of norepinephrine in human thalamus. *Science.* 1978;200:1411-1413.
9. Gur RE, Mozley PD, Resnick SM, Harper-Mozley L, Shtasel DL, Gallacher F, Arnold SE, Karp JS, Alavi A, Reivich M, Gur RC. Resting cerebral glucose metabolism in first-episode and previously treated patients with schizophrenia relates to clinical features. *Arch Gen Psychiatry.* 1995;52:657-667.
10. Reite M, Sheeder J, Teale P, Richardson D, Adams M, Simon J. MEG based brain laterality: sex differences in normal adults. *Neuropsychologia.* 1995;33: 1607-1616.
11. Kulynych JJ, Vladar K, Jones DW, Weinberger DR. Gender differences in the normal lateralization of the supratemporal cortex: MRI surface-rendering morphometry of Heschl's gyrus and the planum temporale. *Cereb Cortex.* 1994; 4:107-118.
12. Crow TJ. Temporal lobe asymmetries as the key to the etiology of schizophrenia. *Schizophr Bull.* 1990;16:433-443.
13. Hoff AL, Riordan H, O'Donnell D, Stitzke P, Neale C, Boccio A, Anand AK, DeLisi LE. Anomalous lateral sulcus asymmetry and cognitive function in first-episode schizophrenia. *Schizophr Bull.* 1992;18:257-270.
14. Falkai P, Bogerts B, Greve B, Pfeiffer U, Machus B, Folsch-Reetz B, Majtenyi C, Ovary I. Loss of sylvian fissure asymmetry in schizophrenia: a quantitative postmortem study. *Schizophr Res.* 1992;7:23-32.
15. Bartley AJ, Jones DW, Torrey EF, Zigun JR, Weinberger DR. Sylvian fissure asymmetries in monozygotic twins: a test of laterality in schizophrenia. *Biol Psychiatry.* 1993;34:853-863.
16. Rubin P, Karle A, Moller-Madsen S, Hertel C, Povlsen UJ, Noring U, Hemmingsen R. Computerised tomography in newly diagnosed schizophrenia and schizophreniform disorder: a controlled blind study. *Br J Psychiatry.* 1993; 163:604-612.
17. Zipursky RB, Marsh L, Lim KO, DeMent S, Shear PK, Sullivan EV, Murphy GM, Csernansky JG, Pfefferbaum A. Volumetric MRI assesment of temporal lobe structures in schizophrenia. *Biol Psychiatry.* 1994;35:501-616.
18. Bilder RM, Wu H, Bogerts B, Degreef G, Ashtari M, Alvir JMJ, Snyder PJ, Lieberman JA. Absence of regional hemispheric volume asymmetries in first-episode schizophrenia. *Am J Psychiatry.* 1994;151:1437-1447.
19. Petty RG, Barta PE, Pearlson GD, McGilchrist IK, Lewis RW, Tien AY, Pulver A, Vaughn DD, Casanova MF, Powers RE. Reversal of aymmetry of the planum temporale in schizophrenia. *Am J Psychiatry.* 1995;152:715-721.
20. Reite M, Teale P, Zimmerman JE, Davis K, Whalen J. Source location of a 50-msec latency auditory-evoked field component. *Electroencephalogr Clin Neurophysiol.* 1988;70:490-498.
21. Reite M, Teale P, Zimmerman JE, Davis K, Whalen J, Edrich J. Source origin of a 50-msec latency auditory-evoked field component in young schizophrenic men. *Biol Psychiatry.* 1988;24:495-506.
22. Reite M, Teale P, Goldstein L, Whalen J, Linnville S. Late auditory sources may differ in the left hemisphere of schizophrenic patients: a preliminary report. *Arch Gen Psychiatry.* 1989;46:565-572.
23. Scheuneman D, Teale PT, Linnville S, Goldstein L, Reite M. Magnetic auditory M100 source location in normal females. *Brain Res Bull.* 1991;26:747-751.
24. Forrest A, Hay A. Sex differences and the schizophrenia experience. *Acta Psychiatr Scand.* 1971;47:137-149.
25. Loranger A: Sex differences in age of onset of schizophrenia. *Arch Gen Psychiatry.* 1984;41:157-161.
26. Flor-Henry P. Influence of gender in schizophrenia as related to other psychopathological syndromes. *Schizophr Bull.* 1990;16:211-227.
27. Hafner H, Maurer K, Loffler W, Reicher-Rossler A. The influence of age and sex on the onset and early course of schizophrenia. *Br J Psychiatry.* 1993; 162:80-86.

28. Hafner H, Reicher-Rossler A, An Der Heiden W, Maurer K, Fatkenheuer B, Loffler W. Generating and testing a causal explanation of the gender difference in age at first onset of schizophrenia. *Psychol Med.* 1993;23:925-940.
29. Goldstein JM, Link BG. Gender and the expression of schizophrenia. *J Psychiatry Res.* 1988;22:141-155.
30. Goldstein JM. Gender differences in the course of schizophrenia. *Am J Psychiatry.* 1988;145:684-689.
31. Goldstein J, Santangelo S, Simpson J, Tsuang M. The role of gender in identifying subtypes of schizophrenia: a latent class analytic approach. *Schizophr Bull.* 1990;16:263-275.
32. Angermeyer MC, Kuhn L, Goldstein JM: Gender and the course of schizophrenia: differences in treated outcomes. *Schizophr Bull.* 1990;16:293-307.
33. Szymanski S, Lieberman JA, Alvir JM, Mayerhoff D, Loebel A, Geisler S, Chakos M, Koreen A, Jody D, Kane J, Woerner M, Cooper T. Gender differences in onset of illness, treatment response, course, and biologic indexes in first-episode schizophrenic patients. *Am J Psychiatry.* 1995;152:698-703.
34. Flaum M, Arndt S, Andreasen NC. The role of gender in studies of ventricle enlargement in schizophrenia: a predominantly male effect. *Am J Psychiatry.* 1990;147:1327-1332.
35. Andreasen NC, Ehrhardt JC, Swayze VW, Alliger RJ, Yuh WTC, Cohen G, Ziebell S. Magnetic resonance imaging of the brain in schizophrenia: the pathophysiological significance of structural abnormalities. *Arch Gen Psychiatry.* 1990; 47:35-44.
36. Swayze VW, Andreasen NC, Alliger RJ, Yuh WT, Erhardt JC. Subcortical and temporal structures in affective disorder and schizophrenia: a magnetic resonance imaging study. *Biol Psychiatry.* 1992;31:221-240.
37. Waddington JL. Schizophrenia: developmental neuroscience and pathobiology. *Lancet.* 1993;341:531-536.
38. Waddington JL. Neurodynamics of abnormalities in cerebral metabolism and structure in schizophrenia. *Schizophr Bull.* 1993;19:55-69.
39. Spitzer RL, Endicott J, Robins E. Research Diagnostic Criteria: rationale and reliability. *Arch Gen Psychiatry.* 1978;35:773-782.
40. Spitzer RL, Williams JB, Gibbon M, First MB. *Structured Clinical Interview for DSM-III-R-Patient Edition (SCID-P, Version 1).* Washington, DC: American Psychiatric Press; 1990.
41. Annett M. *Left, Right, Hand and Brain: The Right Shift Theory.* Hillsdale, NJ: Lawrence A Erlbaum Associates; 1985.
42. Davis J. Dose equivalent of the antipsychotic drugs. *J Psychiatr Res.* 1974; 11:65-69.
43. Edrich J, Teale P, Reite M, Zimmerman J. Doorless and economic shield for clinical magnetoencephalography. In: Book of Abstracts from the Proceedings of the Ninth International Conference on Biomagnetism: Advances in Biomagnetism; Vienna, Austria; August 14-20, 1993.
44. Reite M, Adams M, Simon J, Teale P, Sheeder J, Richardson D, Grabbe R. Auditory M100 component 1: relationship to Heschl's gyri. *Cogn Brain Res.* 1994;2:13-20.
45. Sarvas J. Basic mathematical and electromagnetic concepts of the biomagnetic inverse problem. *Physiol Med Biol.* 1987;32:11-22.
46. Goldstein L, Teale P, Reite M. Monte Carlo study of confidence region accuracy for MEG dipole inverse solutions. In: Williamson SJ, Hoke M, Stroink G, Kotani M, eds. *Advances in Biomagnetism.* New York, NY: Plenum Press; 1989:555-558.
47. Teale P, Goldstein L, Reite M, Sheeder J, Richardson D, Edrich J, Zimmerman JE. Reproducibility of MEG auditory-evoked field source localizations in normal human subjects using a 7-channel gradiometer. *IEEE Trans Biomed Eng.* 1996;43:967-969.
48. Gallen C, Pantev C, Hampson S, Buchanan DS, Sobel D. Reliability and validity of auditory neuromagnetic source localization using a large array biomagnetometer. In: Hoke M, Erne SN, Okada YC, Romani GL, eds. *Biomagnetism: Clinical Aspects.* Amsterdam, the Netherlands: Elsevier Science Publishers; 1992: 171-175.
49. Gallen CC, Schwartz B, Rieke K, Pantev C, Sobel D, Hirschkoff E, Bloom FE. Intrasubject reliability and validity of somatosensory source localization using a large array biomagnetometer. *Electroencephalogr Clin Neurophysiol.* 1994; 90:145-156.
50. Shenton M, Kikinis R, Jolsz FA, Pollak SD, Lemay M, Wible CG, Hokama H, Martin J, Metcalf D, Coleman M, McCarley R. Abnormalities of the left temporal lobe and thought disorder in schizophrenia: a quantative magnetic resonance imaging study. *N Engl J Med.* 1992;327:604-612.
51. Nasrallah HA, Schwarzkopf SB, Olson SC, Coffman JA. Gender differences in schizophrenia on MRI brain scans. *Schizophr Bull.* 1990;16:205-210.
52. Gur RE, Mozley D, Shtasel DL, Cannon TD, Gallacher F, Turetsky B, Grossman R, Gur RC. Clinical subtypes of schizophrenia: differences in brain and CSF volume. *Am J Psychiatry.* 1994;151:343-350.
53. Schlaepfer TE, Harris GJ, Tien AY, Penn LW, Lee S, Chase GA, Barta PE, Pearlson GD. Decreased regional cortical gray matter volume in schizophrenia. *Am J Psychiatry.* 1994;151:842-848.
54. Reite M, Sheeder J, Teale P, Richardson D, Adams M, Simon J. MEG based brain laterality: sex differences in normal adults. *Neuropsychologia.* 1995;33: 1607-1616.
55. Lu Z-L, Williamson SJ, Kaufman L. Human auditory primary and association cortex have differing lifetimes for activation traces. *Brain Res.* 1992;572:236-241.
56. Lu Z-L, Williamson SJ, Kaufman L. Behavioral lifetime of human auditory sensory memory predicted by physiological measures. *Science.* 1992;258:1668-1670.
57. Seeman MV, Lang M. The role of estrogens in schizophrenia gender differences. *Schizophr Bull.* 1990;16:184-194.
58. Oades RD, Schepker T. Serum gonadal steroid hormones in young schizophrenic patients. *Psychoneuroendocrinology.* 1994;19:373-385.
59. DiPaolo T: Modulation of brain dopamine transmission by sex steroids. *Rev Neurosci.* 1994;5:27-41.
60. Gattaz WF, Vogel P, Riecher-Rossler A, Soddu G. Influence of the menstrual cycle phase on the therapeutic response in schizophrenia. *Biol Psychiatry.* 1994; 36:137-139.
61. Riecher-Rossler A, Hafner H, Dutsch-Strobel A, Oster M, Stumbaum M, van Gulick-Bailer M, Loffler W. Further evidence for a specific role of estradiol in schizophrenia? *Biol Psychiatry.* 1994;36:492-495.
62. Riecher-Rossler A, Hafner H, Stumbaum M, Maurer K, Schmidt R. Can estradiol modulate schizophrenic symptomatology? *Schizophr Bull.* 1994;20:203-214.
63. Breedlove SM: Sexual differentiation of the human nervous system. In: Porter LW, Rosenzweig MR, eds. *Annual Review of Psychology.* Palo Alto, Calif: Annual Reviews Inc; 1994:389-418.
64. Lewis DW, Diamond MC. The influence of gonadal steriods on the asymmetry of the cerebral cortex. In: Davidson RJ, Hugdahl K. *Brain Asymmetry.* Cambridge, Mass: The MIT Press; 1995:31-50.
65. Romani GL, Williamson SJ, Kaufman L. Tonotopic organization of the human auditory cortex. *Science.* 1982;216:1339-1340.
66. Pantev C, Hoke M, Lehnertz K, Lutkenhoner B, Anogianakis G, Wittkowski W. Tonotopic organization of the human auditory cortex revealed by transient auditory evoked magnetic fields. *Electroencephalogr Clin Neurophysiol.* 1988;69: 160-170.
67. Tunturi AR. A difference in the representation of auditory signals for the left and right ears in the iso-frequency contours of the right middle ectosylvian auditory cortex of the dog. *Am J Physiol.* 1952;168:712-727.
68. Merzenich MM, Brugge JF. Representation of the cochlear partition on the superior temporal plane of the macaque monkey. *Brain Res.* 1973;50:275-296.
69. DeLisi LE, Tew W, Shu-Hong X, Hoff AL, Sakuma M, Kushner M, Lee G, Shedlack K, Smith AM, Grimson R. A perspective follow-up study of brain morphology and cognition in first-episode schizophrenic patients: preliminary findings. *Biol Psychiatry.* 1995;38:349-360.
70. Elbert T, Pantev C, Wienbruch C, Rockstroh B, Taub E. Increased cortical representation of the fingers of the left hand in string players. *Science.* 1995;270: 305-307.
71. Tiihonen J, Hari R, Naukkarinen H, Rimon R, Jousmaki V, Kajola M. Modified activity of the human auditory cortex during auditory hallucinations. *Am J Psychiatry.* 1992;149:255-257.
72. Conrad AJ, Abebe R, Austin R, Forsythe S, Scheibel AB. Hippocampal pyramidal cell disarray in schizophrenia as a bilateral phenomenon. *Arch Gen Psychiatry.* 1991;48:413-417.
73. Breier A, Buchanan RW, Elkashef A, Munson RC, Kirkpatrick B, Gellad F. Brain morphology and schizophrenia: a magnetic resonance imaging study of limbic, prefrontal cortex, and caudate structures. *Arch Gen Psychiatry.* 1992;49: 921-926.
74. Bogerts B, Meertz E, Schonfeldt-Bausch R. Basal ganglia and limbic system pathology in schizophrenia. *Arch Gen Psychiatry.* 1985;42:784-791.
75. Deicken RF, Calabrese G, Merrin EL, Meyerhoff DJ, Dillon WP, Weiner MW, Fein G. ^{31}Phosphorus magnetic resonance spectroscopy of the frontal and parietal lobes in chronic schizophrenia. *Biol Psychiatry.* 1994;36:503-510.
76. Harvey SA, Nelson E, Haller JW, Early TS. Lateralized attentional abnormality in schizophrenia is correlated with severity of symptoms. *Biol Psychiatry.* 1993; 33:93-99.
77. Andreasen NC, Arndt S, Swayze V, Cizadlo T, Flaum M, O'Leary D, Erhardt JC, Yuh WT. Thalamic abnormalities in schizophrenia visualized through magnetic resonance image averaging. *Science.* 1994;266:294-298.

ORIGINAL ARTICLE

Psychotic Exacerbations and Enhanced Vasopressin Secretion in Schizophrenic Patients With Hyponatremia and Polydipsia

Morris B. Goldman, MD; Gary L. Robertson, MD; Daniel J. Luchins, MD; Donald Hedeker, PhD; Ghanshyam N. Pandey, PhD

Background: For unclear reasons, life-threatening water intoxication often coincides with acute psychosis in polydipsic schizophrenic patients with chronic hyponatremia. In contrast, most polydipsic schizophrenic patients are normonatremic and never manifest hyponatremia. To explore whether the effect of acute psychosis on water balance differs in these 2 schizophrenic subgroups, we compared their responses to drug-induced psychotic exacerbations.

Methods: Matched polydipsic schizophrenic patients with (n=6) and without (n=8) hyponatremia were identified based on past and current indexes of fluid intake and hydration. A transient psychotic exacerbation was induced with an infusion of the psychotomimetic methylphenidate hydrochloride (0.5 mg/kg of body weight over a 60-second period). Antidiuretic hormone levels, subjective desire for water, and factors known to influence water balance were measured at 15-minute intervals for 2 hours.

Results: Except for the expected differences in plasma osmolality and sodium, basal measures were similar in the 2 groups. Following methylphenidate administration, antidiuretic hormone levels increased more in the hyponatremic patients ($P<.02$), despite their consistently lower plasma osmolality ($P<.007$). No known or putative antidiuretic hormone stimulus could account for this finding. Only basal positive psychotic symptoms ($P<.09$) and plasma sodium ($P<.18$) were even marginally associated with the peak antidiuretic hormone responses, but neither factor could explain the difference in the response by the 2 groups.

Conclusion: Psychotic exacerbations are associated with enhanced antidiuretic hormone secretion, for unknown reasons, in schizophrenic patients with hyponatremia and polydipsia, thereby placing them at increased risk of life-threatening water intoxication.

Arch Gen Psychiatry. 1997;54:443-449

From the Department of Psychiatry, University of Chicago Pritzker School of Medicine, Chicago, Ill (Drs Goldman and Luchins); the Psychiatric Institute, University of Illinois at Chicago in affiliation with the University of Chicago (Drs Goldman, Luchins, and Pandey); the Department of Medicine, Northwestern University School of Medicine, Chicago (Dr Robertson); and the Division of Epidemiology and Biostatistics, School of Public Health (Dr Hedeker) and the Department of Psychiatry, College of Medicine (Dr Pandey), University of Illinois at Chicago.

THREE PERCENT to 5% of patients with chronic schizophrenia are hyponatremic and experience episodes of life-threatening water intoxication.[1] Their basal hyponatremia compromises neuropsychological functioning,[2] and water intoxication can cause seizures, delirium, irreversible neurologic deficits,[3] and death.[1] These patients show increased water intake and impaired water excretion. The enhanced intake manifests as a defect in osmotic and oropharyngeal regulation of the subjective desire for water,[4-6] and usually is not associated with increased thirst or hydrophilic delusions.[7] The impaired excretion is a consequence of increased release and perhaps action of the antidiuretic hormone arginine vasopressin (AVP).[4,6,8,9] The aforementioned defects can account for these patients' chronic mild hyponatremia, but not for the profound hyponatremia associated with water intoxication, for which an additional factor must be invoked.[4,6,8]

Water intoxication often coincides with exacerbations of schizophrenia, but the significance of the association is unclear.[9] Some contend that the aggravated water imbalance is a consequence of psychotic exacerbations,[10-13] others have come to the opposite conclusion,[14] and a third group argues that the 2 events are indirectly related.[15-17] Those who favor the first interpretation point out that transient elevations of plasma AVP during acute psychosis have been observed in hyponatremic[6,18] and some normonatremic schizophrenic patients.[19,20] Within this group of investigators, some argue that the increased AVP levels are fundamentally related to the psychotic exacerbation, and others believe that recognized or putative AVP stimuli are responsible (eg, hypotension, stress, adaptation to polydipsia, and long-term treatment with neuroleptic medication).[9] Those who con-

MATERIALS AND METHODS

Subjects were recruited from among the 2000 beds of acute- and extended-treatment units of Illinois state psychiatric facilities. We reviewed the medical charts of patients who were diagnosed as having schizophrenia or schizoaffective disorder who were competent and voluntarily admitted to the hospital, between 21 and 55 years of age, and without factors known to affect water balance.

Serum sodium concentrations and urine specific gravities from current and previous laboratory records were then inspected in qualifying patients who had been identified by the clinical staff as having polydipsia. Potential subjects were initially classified as follows: those with multiple morning spot urine samples of a specific gravity of less than 1.008 and serum sodium concentrations of less than 125 mmol/L and at least 1 serum sodium sample of less than 120 mmol/L were classified as potentially having hyponatremic polydipsia; those with equally severe hyposthenuria but no current or previous serum sodium values of less than 133 mmol/L were classified as potentially having normonatremic polydipsia. We attempted to balance groups for age, sex, duration of psychiatric illness, and current neuroleptic dose (chlorpromazine hydrochloride equivalents). We initially recruited subjects from both sexes, but later limited patients to men because of the recommendation of a funding agency.

Subjects who met this first stage of selection were transferred to the Psychiatric Institute, University of Illinois at Chicago. Definitive psychiatric diagnosis (based on criteria in the *DSM-III-R*)[21] was determined in a multidisciplinary diagnostic conference. To provide further validity to the grouping process, we measured morning plasma osmolality and afternoon urine osmolality 3 times each week for 2 weeks.[22] Based on these findings, final group assignment was as follows: hyponatremic patients (n=6; 1 woman) had mean morning plasma osmolalities of less than 280 mmol/kg and mean afternoon urine osmolalities of less than 150 mmol/kg; and normonatremic patients (n=8; all men) had mean plasma osmolalities of more than 285 mmol/kg and mean urine osmolalities of less than 150 mmol/kg. Duration of polydipsia was estimated by determining when hyposthenuria (urine specific gravity <1.008) consistently occurred in the laboratory record.

Because (1) methylphenidate hydrochloride reliably induces transient psychotic exacerbations in schizophrenic patients even when they are receiving neuroleptic medication,[23,24] (2) the effects of exacerbated psychosis should be most apparent when baseline psychosis is minimal, (3) neuroleptic medications block stimulant-induced nausea and emesis (which independently stimulate AVP release),[25] (4) neuroleptic washout has been linked to water intoxication[17] and does not eliminate defects in AVP secretion in hyponatremic patients,[26] (5) water intoxication occurs in schizophrenic patients never treated with neuroleptic medications and in those who have not received the drug for a prolonged period,[9-11] and (6) neuroleptic medications do not seem to alter AVP secretion in the absence of recognized stimuli,[20] we continued neuroleptic medication. The subject was switched, on admission to the hospital, from his or her previous neuroleptic medication to an equivalent dose of fluphenazine hydrochloride, which was then adjusted during 1 to 2 weeks by the attending psychiatrist to optimize clinical response. The subject was then maintained at this dose for 2 weeks before the study.

Patients who participated provided informed, written consent. Consent was obtained before transfer to the research unit in the presence of a staff member who was unaffiliated with the research. Family members were asked to participate in the consent process. Patients and family members were told that methylphenidate could temporarily worsen the patient's clinical condition.

PROCEDURE

Methylphenidate was chosen over other psychotomimetics because it seems to have a lower incidence of hypotension and nausea,[23,27] both of which independently stimulate AVP release.[25] Smoking, food, and water were restricted

tend that exacerbated psychosis is a consequence of water intoxication point out that many schizophrenic patients with polydipsia remain normonatremic during psychotic exacerbations,[1] that profound hyponatremia may aggravate psychosis, and that water intoxication–induced seizures or hyponatremia may stimulate AVP release.[13,14] Finally, those who believe the 2 events are indirectly related observe that the introduction of recognized or putative AVP stimuli (eg, increased smoking and adjustment of neuroleptic dose) often coincide with psychotic exacerbations.[12,14]

To clarify if, and how, acute psychosis contributes to water intoxication, we pharmacologically induced psychotic exacerbations in polydipsic schizophrenic patients with and without hyponatremia. We chose polydipsic schizophrenic patients without a history of hyponatremia as controls, because this group resembles the hyponatremic patients but their history suggests that their water balance is unaffected by acute psychosis.

RESULTS

DEMOGRAPHIC, PRESTUDY, AND BASELINE MEASURES

Demographic and prestudy measures were similar in the 2 groups except for mean morning plasma osmolality, which was, as expected, lower in the hyponatremic patients (**Table 1**). On the day of the infusion, total BPRS scores were almost identical in the 2 groups (**Table 2**). Plasma AVP, subjective desire for water, and other factors implicated in water-balance regulation were stable during the 3 baseline time points and similar across groups, except for the expected differences in plasma osmolality and sodium (**Table 3**). Plasma growth hormone and cortisol fell slightly during the 3 baseline time points but also were similar across groups.

from the night before the study until its completion (total time=12 hours). Smoking was restricted because it stimulates AVP release; food and water because they affect plasma osmolality, the main physiological stimulus for AVP. Compliance with the smoking restriction was assessed by measuring expired-air carbon monoxide, from which carboxyhemoglobin content can be determined with a carboxyhemoglobin analyzer (Ecolyzer 211, National Draeger, Inc, Pittsburgh, Pa).[28] Throughout the study, subjects remained supine (except for the measuring of upright vital signs immediately following the 30-minute sample) to minimize the influence of postural change on AVP.[29]

At 8 AM, a cuff was attached over the brachial artery, and blood pressure and pulse were recorded every 15 minutes for the duration of the study. Continuous monitoring of cardiac rhythm was performed with an electrocardiogram. An intravenous catheter was inserted into an arm vein, and, starting 30 minutes later, 3 baseline blood samples were obtained at 15-minute intervals. Methylphenidate hydrochloride (Ritalin, IND 27083, Ciba-Geigy Corp, Summit, NJ), 0.5 mg/kg, was then infused over a 60-second period. Blood samples were drawn, and abdominal discomfort, nausea, and desire for water were assessed every 15 minutes for the next 2 hours by the research nurse. Abdominal discomfort and nausea were assessed by direct inquiry; desire for water was estimated by asking the subject, while displaying a 250-mL cup, how many cups of water he or she would like to drink.[4,5] Thirty minutes before and after the methylphenidate infusion, 2 unblinded trained raters completed the Brief Psychiatric Rating Scale (BPRS) (16 items, 0=absent to 6=extremely severe)[30] and the Dyskinesia Identification System Condensed User Scale (individual score ≥5 suggests tardive dyskinesia).[31] Ad lib water intake was measured for 10 minutes at the end of the study.

LABORATORY STUDIES

Blood was placed in chilled heparin-treated tubes, and spun down (1800 g for 10 minutes at 4°C) within 1 hour. Plasma and urine osmolality were determined by freezing-point depression (model 2D, Advanced Instruments, Needham, Mass). Other chemistries were determined at the University of Chicago Clinical Research Center core lab (ASTRA IV autoanalyzer, Beckman Instruments Inc, Palo Alto, Calif). Plasma samples were stored at −20°C before measuring AVP (intra-assay coefficient of variation at 2.6 pg/mL=6.2%; interassay coefficient of variation at 2.7 pg/mL=13.0%, at 0.8 pg/mL=26%),[32] human growth hormone (hGH RIA kit, INCSTAR Corporation, Stillwater, Minn), and cortisol (Coat-a-count, Diagnostic Products Corporation, Los Angeles, Calif) by radioimmunoassay, and plasma homovanillic acid (HVA) by high-performance liquid chromatography with electrochemical detection[33] (assayed only on 0-, 30-, and 120-minute samples). Growth hormone and plasma HVA were measured because they reflect central dopaminergic activity, which has been posited to be enhanced in some schizophrenic patients.[24,34,35] Cortisol was measured because its release seems to be closely tied to that of AVP[36,37] and also may be enhanced in schizophrenic patients with water imbalance.[38]

STATISTICAL ANALYSIS

For the analysis of recurrent measures, if the 3 baseline values did not vary within groups, they were averaged; otherwise all time points were included in the analysis. We relied on univariate or multivariate analysis of variance for repeated measures, depending on whether the compound symmetry assumption (ie, equal variances and covariances across time) was met. Reported F values are from the univariate procedure unless otherwise noted. In either approach, if the time effect or group X time interaction was significant, the response was more precisely characterized by examining only the linear, quadratic, and cubic components of the polynomial time contrast. Results are expressed as mean±SD unless otherwise noted. Two-tailed probability tests (α=.05) are reported throughout.

BEHAVIORAL AND CARDIOVASCULAR RESPONSES TO METHYLPHENIDATE

Behavioral response to methylphenidate peaked within 30 minutes and rapidly dissipated during the next half hour. Total BPRS scores tended to increase more in the hyponatremic patients (Table 2). Positive psychotic symptoms increased in both groups and tended to be consistently higher in the hyponatremic patients, but negative psychotic symptoms decreased and anxiety and depression tended to increase to a similar extent in the 2 groups. Ratings of tardive dyskinesia increased to a slight, but significantly greater, extent in normonatremics.

Mean arterial pressure rose sharply and then fell slowly to a similar extent in both groups (**Figure**) (time effect, F[3,36]=2.89, $P<.05$; cubic trend, F[1,36]=10.35, $P<.05$; group X time interaction, F[3,36]=1.35, $P<.30$). Heart rate showed a similar response (data not shown). On standing 30 minutes after methylphenidate administration, mean arterial pressure increased to the same extent that it had at baseline, and the response was similar in the 2 groups (data not shown).

RESPONSE OF PLASMA AVP, DESIRE FOR WATER, AND OTHER RELATED VARIABLES

After methylphenidate administration, AVP rose sharply and rapidly returned to baseline in the hyponatremic patients; the response in the normonatremic patients was blunted (Figure). Statistical analysis confirmed the impressions that the overall (group X time interaction, multivariate F[3,10]=5.52; $P<.02$) and the peak responses (hyponatremic, 1.9±0.7 pg/mL; normonatremic, 1.0±0.7 pg/mL; independent t test=2.37; $P<.05$, 95% confidence interval for difference, 0.1-1.4 pg/mL) were greater in the hyponatremic patients. These comparisons remained significant when the single female hyponatremic subject was excluded.

Desire for water seemed to increase similarly in both groups (Figure), but due to considerable individual variation, the response did not achieve statistical significance (time effect, F[3,36]=2.35, $P<.10$; group X time interaction, F[3,36]=0.69, $P<.60$). Plasma osmolality fell slightly and to a similar extent in both groups (Figure) (time effect, F[3,36]=4.43, $P<.02$; linear trend, F[1,36]=8.7, $P<.02$; group X time interaction, F[3,36]=0.82, $P<.35$), and values remained consistently lower in the hyponatremic patients (group effect, F[1,12]=11.83; $P<.007$). Plasma sodium showed a similar response (data not shown). Plasma potassium, glucose, urea, and creatinine levels and hematocrit were unchanged and remained similar across the groups (data not shown). All subjects denied nausea and abdominal discomfort. Ad libitum water consumption after the study was similar (hyponatremic patients, 1.5±1.01; normonatremics, 1.3±0.8; $P<.65$).

Because no recognized factors could account for the enhanced AVP response in the hyponatremic patients, the demographic, physiological, and behavioral variables (Tables 1 through 3), and the mean responses to methylphenidate were added individually as covariates into an analysis of covariance (ANCOVA) comparing the peak AVP response in the 2 groups. Only the addition of basal plasma sodium (t=1.47; $P<.18$) and basal positive psychotic symptoms approached statistical significance (t=1.92; $P<.09$), but neither factor accounted for the different response in the 2 groups (ANCOVA with sodium, group F[1,11]=8.32, $P<.02$; ANCOVA with basal psychotic symptoms, group F[1,11]=5.28, $P<.05$).

Table 1. Demographic and Prestudy Measures*

Measure	Subjects: Hyponatremic (n=6)	Subjects: Normonatremic (n=8)
Age, y	36.2 (±6.7)	33.6 (±4.5)
Sex, M/F	5/1	8/0
Smoker/nonsmoker	6/0	6/2
Schizophrenia/schizoaffective	5/1	7/1
Age at onset, y	16.8 (±3.2)	17.7 (±3.1)
Duration of polydipsia, y	8.6 (±4.5)	6.9 (±3.8)
Fluphenazine dose, mg/d	28.3 (±20.4)	29.0 (±18.5)
PM urine osmolality, mmol/kg	122.5 (±65.7)	112.4 (±57.5)
24-hour urine volume, L†		
Measured	7.8 (±4.3)	11.1 (±3.6)
Estimated	6.5 (±2.0)	7.1 (±1.9)
AM plasma osmolality, mmol/kg‡	276.2 (±3.3)	287.9 (±1.5)
Serum thyroxine, nmol/L	108 (±24)	114 (±27)
Time on unit before infusion, d	25.7 (±11.9)	33.1 (±17.1)

*Values are given as mean (±SD) unless otherwise indicated. Measures were compared by 2-tailed Student t test or χ^2 test for categorical data.
†Measured urine volume is from a single 24-hour complete collection; estimated volume is calculated from spot morning and afternoon urine creatinine concentrations obtained on multiple occasions.
‡$P<.05$.

RESPONSES OF OTHER HORMONES AND HVA

Plasma cortisol levels seemed to increase slightly with methylphenidate administration but varied considerably within individuals, so the response was not statistically significant and values remained similar across groups (data not shown). Growth hormone levels rose, peaked at 45 minutes, and slowly returned to baseline and remained similar throughout in the 2 groups. Plasma HVA levels did not change, and remained similar in the 2 groups.

COMMENT

We found that psychotic exacerbations are associated with enhanced release of the antidiuretic hormone in poly-

Table 2. Behavioral Profile 30 Minutes Before and After Methylphenidate Administration*

Test	Hyponatremic	Normonatremic	Time Effect F	Time Effect P	Group X Time Effect F	Group X Time Effect P
Total (BPRS)†						
Before	20.8 (±7.2)	19.8 (±9.2)	20.7	<.001	3.1	<.07
After	36.6 (±4.8)	26.1 (±10.3)				
BPRS positive psychotic symptom factor (hallucinations, delusions, thought disorder)‡						
Before	6.0 (±4.4)	4.7 (±4.5)	12.5	<.005	1.5	<.25
After	12.5 (±2.0)	7.9 (±2.8)				
BPRS negative psychotic symptom factor (blunted affect, emotional withdrawal, motor retardation)						
Before	4.8 (±5.1)	4.3 (±3.2)	5.1	<.05	1.2	<.30
After	3.6 (±2.6)	1.0 (±1.2)				
BPRS anxious/depressed factor (anxiety, depression, guilt)						
Before	1.3 (±1.6)	3.9 (±3.2)	3.4	<.10	1.2	<.30
After	3.8 (±3.6)	4.5 (±3.8)				
Dyskinesia identification system condensed user scale						
Before	0.3 (±0.5)	0.3 (±0.5)	7.9	<.02	7.7	<.02
After	0.0 (±0.0)	2.5 (±2.1)				

*Values are given as mean (±SD) unless otherwise indicated. BPRS indicates Brief Psychiatric Rating Scale.
†Score increased in all but 1 control.
‡Group effect marginally significant (F [1,12]=4.34; $P<.06$). Factor score increased by 4 points in all but 2 controls.

Table 3. Baseline Measures of Water Balance and Related Variables*

Variable	Hyponatremic	Normonatremic
Plasma		
Vasopressin, pg/mL	0.6 (±0.2)	0.6 (±0.2)
Osmolality, mmol/kg†	278.6 (±6.2)	288.2 (±5.4)
Sodium, mmol/L‡	134.7 (±6.0)	140.3 (±3.2)
Glucose, mmol/L (mg/dL)	4.9 (±1.0) (88.6 [±18.4])	4.9 (±0.3) (88.4 [±4.9])
Potassium, mmol/L	4.5 (±0.5)	4.4 (±0.3)
Creatinine, μmol/L (mg/dL)	70.7 (±8.8) (0.8 [±0.1])	80.0 (±10.0) (0.9 [±0.1])
Total calcium, mmol/L	2.2 (±0.1)	2.1 (±0.1)
Growth hormone, μg/L	1.5 (±0.3)	1.6 (±0.5)
Cortisol, nmol/L	340.2 (±85.5)	289.0 (±298.6)
Homovanillic acid, μmol/mL	.031 (±.022)	.035 (±.018)
Urine osmolality, mmol/kg	304.2 (±154.3)	402.5 (±262.1)
Hematocrit, %	43.0 (±2.0)	45.5 (±1.4)
Pulse, beats per min	68.3 (±13.7)	77.8 (±16.1)
Mean arterial pressure, mm Hg	84.8 (±12.7)	95.9 (±18.5)
Upright-supine mean arterial pressure, mm Hg	12.4 (±3.7)	10.1 (±9.2)
Desire for water, cups	1.0 (±0.7)	2.5 (±3.5)
Expired-air carbon monoxide, ppm	9.0 (±5.6)	11.7 (±9.0)

**Values are for time=0 minutes, except for urine osmolality, change in mean arterial pressure on arising, and expired air carbon monoxide, which were obtained at −60 minutes. All measures, except the aforementioned 3, were also obtained at −30 and −15 minutes and were included in the statistical analysis. Values are given as mean (±SD).*

†*P*<.05.

‡*P*<.10.

dipsic schizophrenic patients with chronic hyponatremia. The data also support the interpretation that exacerbated psychosis is responsible for the enhanced AVP release, rather than the reverse, or that the events are only indirectly related. These conclusions are based on the observation that a pharmacologically induced psychotic exacerbation elevated antidiuretic hormone levels in a sample of these patients. If levels remained even slightly elevated as plasma osmolality continued to fall, life-threatening water intoxication would soon ensue.[29] The conclusions are tempered by the small sample size and by our limited knowledge of the extent to which methylphenidate replicates naturally occurring psychotic exacerbations.[23,24] Still, the finding is consistent with a considerable literature showing that water excretory capacity diminishes in this subgroup of schizophrenic patients during psychotic relapses.[9-13,18]

In contrast to the hyponatremic subjects, AVP levels rose little, if at all, in a closely matched group of normonatremic polydipsic schizophrenic patients. This blunted response in the normonatremic patients is in keeping with the observation that they never manifest hyponatremia and is especially striking because their higher plasma osmolality might be expected to enhance their response.[25,39] Although many others have observed that psychotic exacerbations are associated with enhanced plasma AVP in some schizophrenic patients,[9,11-13,18-20] in this study, we varied the severity of psychotic symptoms and assessed recognized and putative AVP stimuli in 2 closely matched groups of polydipsic schizophrenic patients, 1 with, and 1 without, a history of im-

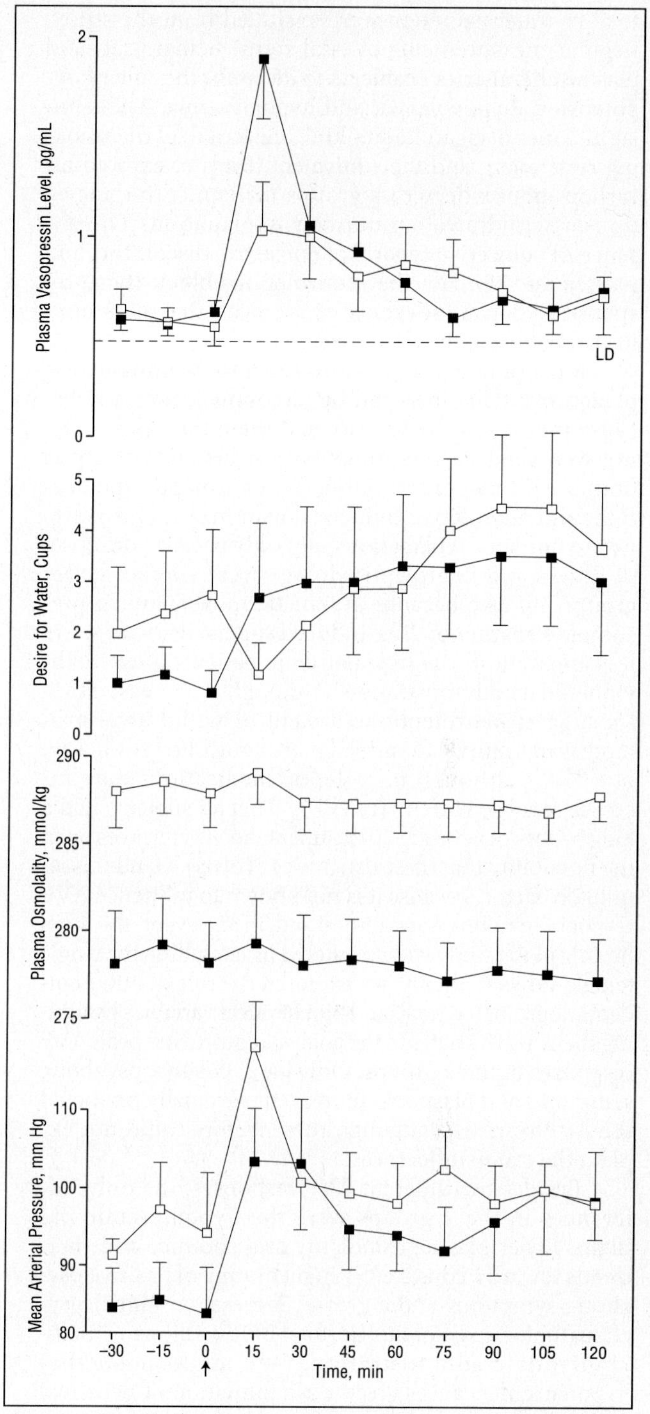

Effects of methylphenidate hydrochloride (0.5-mg/kg intravenous push) (arrow) on plasma vasopressin levels and related variables (mean± SEM) in polydipsic schizophrenic patients with (solid squares) and without (open squares) hyponatremia. LD indicates limit of detection of the vasopressin assay.

paired water excretion. Thus, this controlled demonstration of a difference in the AVP response to psychotic exacerbations provides a unique opportunity to explore the cause of the finding.

The difference in the AVP response in the 2 groups cannot be accounted for by recognized AVP stimuli, although we admittedly have weak power to eliminate them from consideration. Thus, patients with factors known to alter water excretion were excluded from the study. Regular measurements of vital signs, hematocrit, and plasma chemistries enable us to discount the role of hypotension, hypovolemia, and hypoglycemia. The similar histories of cigarette smoking, the length of the smoking restriction, and the equivalent levels of expired-air carbon monoxide across groups make nicotine ingestion or withdrawal an unlikely explanation. The absence of subjective reports of epigastric discomfort and nausea and the fact that neuroleptics block these responses to dopamine agonists[25,40] indicate that this stimulus probably can be dismissed.

Most putative factors also seem to be unlikely explanations. Polydipsia can be discounted, not only because indexes of the severity and the duration of polyuria were similar across groups but also because polydipsia blunts AVP responses. Similarly, neuroleptic medications and neuroleptic-induced dopamine supersensitivity are unlikely explanations, not only because duration of illness and neuroleptic dosage were similar across groups but also because dyskinetic movements, a presumptive marker of drug-induced supersensitivity, were less apparent in the hyponatremic patients after methylphenidate administration. Although a few case studies suggest neuroleptic treatment or withdrawal promote water intoxication,[9,15,17] more controlled studies do not[1,9,41,42] (although neuroleptic medications may increase renal sensitivity to AVP).[6] That all subjects had a long history of neuroleptic treatment, however, leaves open the possibility that these drugs are involved. Gender is an unlikely factor, because it is not known to influence AVP response to nonosmotic stimuli and, in any event, the main finding of the study was not altered by excluding the single female subject. Finally, we explored the role of other epidemiologic, behavioral, and biochemical variables by adding them as covariates to the analysis comparing peak AVP responses in the 2 groups. Only basal positive psychotic symptoms and plasma sodium even marginally predicted the AVP response, although these factors could not explain the group differences.

Besides the different AVP responses, the only differences in the 2 groups were the hyponatremic patients' lower plasma osmolality and sodium, and their trends toward a consistently higher rating of positive psychotic symptoms and a greater increase in global psychopathologic symptoms (ie, total BPRS) following methylphenidate administration. One might posit that hyponatremia causes greater accumulation of neuronal AVP, which in turn is released by methylphenidate.[43] Such an explanation, however, is inconsistent with studies in chronically hyponatremic animals,[39] the responses of hyponatremic schizophrenic patients to other AVP stimuli,[6] and the almost significant positive correlation between plasma sodium and peak AVP in this study. Alternatively, one might attribute the enhanced AVP response to greater stress, because hyponatremic patients seemed to display more intense positive psychotic symptoms and an exaggerated behavioral response to methylphenidate. Stress (ie, a factor that enhances measures of arousal and threatens the well-being of the organism), however, does not increase, and probably diminishes, AVP release in the absence of recognized AVP stimuli.[44-47]

The difference in the AVP response of the 2 groups may be more fundamentally related to differences in the nature or severity of their psychiatric illnesses. Some propose that dopaminergic hyperactivity accounts for the association between exacerbated psychosis and enhanced AVP release,[9,20,43] although the similarity of plasma HVA and growth hormone levels in our 2 groups, their equally poor clinical response to dopaminergic antagonists, and the unclear role of the dopaminergic system in schizophrenia or AVP release cast doubt on this interpretation. Medial temporal lobe dysfunction is implicated in schizophrenia, and this region seems to be smaller (and associated cognitive functions may be more impaired)[48,49] in hyponatremic patients compared with the normonatremic schizophrenic patients.[50,51] Furthermore, this region may normally restrain behavioral and neuroendocrine (including AVP)[52-55] responses to psychological stress.[56,57] Because peripheral AVP is precisely regulated[29] and these regulatory influences are well-characterized,[58] our findings may provide an ideal opportunity to explore the mechanisms underlying neuroendocrine and psychiatric illnesses.

The clinical implication of our finding is that hyponatremic patients should be closely monitored for signs and symptoms of latent water intoxication (eg, lethargy, confusion, nausea, ataxia, coarse tremor, and large diurnal weight gain)[1] during periods of incipient psychosis or when neuroleptic dosage is reduced. Clinicians also may want to consider a trial of clozapine in appropriate patients, because it seems to correct the hyponatremia and may prevent water intoxication.[59]

Accepted for publication May 15, 1996.

Supported in part by the Brain Research Foundation, an affiliate of the University of Chicago, Chicago, Ill, the Scottish Rite Program for Schizophrenia Research, Lexington, Mass, and a Clinical Research Center grant (RR-00055) and a First Award (MH43618) from the National Institute of Mental Health, Bethesda, Md.

Presented at the Society for Neuroscience, Miami, Fla, November 17, 1994.

We thank Robert C. Marks, MD, Lesley Blake, MD, Miljana Petkovic, BS, John Savaglio, RN, Annette Miller, RN, Jackie Imperial, RN, Javaid Javaid, PhD, John Davis, MD, Rajiv Sharma, MD, Barbara Brown, MS, Nijole Grazulis, MS, the staffs of the Clinical Research Center at the University of Chicago, the Psychiatric Research Unit at the Psychiatric Institute, the University of Illinois at Chicago, and the Elgin (Ill) Mental Health Center; and the Department of Mental Health and Developmental Disabilities, State of Illinois, for their assistance.

Reprints: Morris B. Goldman, MD, Department of Psychiatry, MC 3077, University of Chicago Medical Center, 5841 S Maryland Ave, Chicago, IL 60637.

REFERENCES

1. de Leon J, Verghese C, Tracy JI, Josiassen RC, Simpson GM. Polydipsia and water intoxication in psychiatric patients: a review of the epidemiological literature. *Biol Psychiatry.* 1994;35:519-530.
2. Shutty MS, Briscoe L, Sautter S, Leadbetter RA. Neuropsychological manifestations of hyponatremia in chronic schizophrenic patients with the syndrome of psychosis, intermittent hyponatremia and polydipsia. *Schizophr Res.* 1993;10:125-130.

3. Tanneau RS, Henry A, Rouhart F, Bourbigot B, Garo B, Mocquard Y, Goas J. High incidence of neurological complications following rapid correction of severe hyponatremia in polydipsic patients. *J Clin Psychiatry.* 1994;55:349-354.
4. Goldman MB, Luchins DJ, Robertson GL. Mechanisms of altered water metabolism in psychotic patients with polydipsia and hyponatremia. *N Engl J Med.* 1988;318:397-403.
5. Goldman MB, Robertson GL, Hedeker D. Oropharyngeal regulation of water balance in polydipsic schizophrenics. *Clin Endocrinol (Oxf).* 1996;44:31-37.
6. Goldman MB, Robertson GL, Luchins DJ, Hedeker D. The influence of polydipsia on water excretion in hyponatremic, polydipsic schizophrenic patients. *J Clin Endocrinol Metab.* 1996;81:1465-1470.
7. Millson RC, Koczapski AB, Cook MI, Daskiewicz M. A survey of patient attitudes toward self-induced water intoxication. *Can J Psychiatry.* 1992;37:46-47.
8. Berl T. Psychosis and water balance. *N Engl J Med.* 1988;318:441-443.
9. Riggs AT, Dysken MW, Kim WS, Opsahl JA. A review of disorders of water homeostasis in psychiatric patients. *Psychosomatics.* 1991;32:133-148.
10. Dubovsky SL, Grabon S, Berl T, Schrier R. Syndrome of inappropriate secretion of antidiuretic hormone with exacerbated psychosis. *Ann Intern Med.* 1974; 79:551-554.
11. Suzuki M, Takeuchi O, Mori I, Takegoshi K, Kurachi M. Syndrome of inappropriate secretion of antidiuretic hormone associated with schizophrenia. *Biol Psychiatry.* 1992;31:1057-1061.
12. Raskind MA, Orenstein H, Christopher TG. Acute psychosis, increased water ingestion and inappropriate antidiuretic hormone secretion. *Am J Psychiatry.* 1975;132:907-910.
13. Hariprasad MK, Eisinger RP, Nadler IM, Padmanabhan CS, Nidus BD. Hyponatremia in psychogenic polydipsia. *Arch Intern Med.* 1980;140:1639-1642.
14. Inoue K, Tadai T, Kamura H, Miki H, Hashimoto H, Nakajima T. The syndrome of self-induced water intoxication in psychiatric patients. *Folia Psychiat Neurol Jpn.* 1985;39:121-128.
15. Ajlouni K, Kern MW, Tures JF, Theil GB, Hagen TC. Thiothixene-induced hyponatremia. *Arch Intern Med.* 1974;134:1103-1105.
16. Allon M, Allen HM, Deck LV. Role of cigarette use in hyponatremia in schizophrenic patients. *Am J Psychiatry.* 1990;47:1075-1077.
17. Shen WW, Sata LS. Hypothalamic dopamine receptor supersensitivity? a pilot study of self-induced water intoxication. *Psychiatr J Univ Ottawa.* 1983;8:154-158.
18. Ragavan V, Verbalis J, Wood M, Randels P, French G, Robinson A. Psychogenic polydipsia and hyponatremia: evidence for a reset osmostat. *Excerpta Med.* 1984;652:1182. Abstract.
19. Emsley R, Potgieter A, Taljaard F, Joubert G, Gledhill R. Water excretion and plasma vasopressin in psychotic disorders. *Am J Psychiatry.* 1989;146:250-253.
20. Raskind MA, Courtney N, Murburg MM, Backus FI, Bokan JA, Ries RK. Antipsychotic drugs and plasma vasopressin in normals and acute schizophrenic patients. *Biol Psychiatry.* 1987;22:453-462.
21. American Psychiatric Association. *Diagnostic and Statistical Manual of Mental Disorders, Third Edition, Revised.* Washington, DC: American Psychiatric Association; 1987.
22. Goldman MB, Marks RC, Blake L, Petkovic M, Hedeker D, Luchins DJ. Estimating daily urine volume in psychiatric patients: empiric confirmation. *Biol Psychiatry.* 1992;31:1228-1231.
23. Lieberman JA, Kane JM, Alvir J. Provocative tests with psychostimulant drugs in schizophrenia. *Psychopharmacology.* 1987;91:415-433.
24. Lieberman JA, Kane JM, Sarantakos S, Gadaleta D, Woerner M, Alvir J, Ramos-Lorenzi J. Prediction of relapse in schizophrenia. *Arch Gen Psychiatry.* 1987; 44:597-603.
25. Rowe JW, Shelton RL, Helderman JH, Vestal RE, Robertson GL. Influence of the emetic reflex on vasopressin release in man. *Kidney Int.* 1979;16:729-735.
26. Lawson WB, Williams I, Inagami T, Kirch DG, Robertson GL, Iager A. Response to osmotic challenges in schizophrenia. American Psychiatric Association Annual Meeting, Washington, DC; May 5, 1992; Symposium 49B. Abstract.
27. Sharma RP, Javaid JL, Pandey GN, Janicak PG, Davis JM. Behavioral and biochemical effects of methylphenidate in schizophrenic and nonschizophrenic patients. *Biol Psychiatry.* 1991;30:459-466.
28. Gori GB, Benowitz NL, Lynch CJ. Mouth versus deep airways absorption of nicotine in cigarette smokers. *Pharmacol Biochem Behav.* 1986;25:1181-1184.
29. Robertson GL. Physiology of ADH secretion. *Kidney Int.* 1987;32(suppl 21): 20-26.
30. Overall JE, Gorham DR. The brief psychiatric rating scale. *Psychol Rep.* 1962; 10:799-812.
31. Kalachnik JE, Sprague RL. The dyskinesia identification system condensed user scale: reliability, validity, and a total score cut-off for mentally ill and mentally retarded populations. *J Clin Psychol.* 1993;49:177-188.
32. Davison JM, Gilmore EA, Durr J, Robertson GL, Lindheimer MD. Altered osmotic thresholds for vasopressin secretion and thirst in human pregnancy. *Am J Physiol.* 1984;246(Renal Fluid Electrolyte Physiol 15):F105-F109.
33. Javaid JI, Liu TS, Mass JW, Davis JM. Measurement of 3-methoxy-4-hydroxyphenylacetic acid (HVA) in plasma by high-performance liquid chromatography with electrochemical detector (HPLC-EC). *Anal Biochem.* 1983; 135:326-331.
34. Kane JM. Efficacy, mechanisms, and side effects of typical and atypical neuroleptics. In: Andreasen NC, ed. *Schizophrenia: From Mind to Molecule.* Washington, DC: American Psychiatric Press; 1994:173-188.
35. Lieberman JA, Jody D, Alvir JMJ, Ashtari M, Levy DL, Bogerts B, Degreef G, Mayerhoff DI, Cooper T. Brain morphology, dopamine, and eye-tracking abnormalities in first-episode schizophrenia. *Arch Gen Psychiatry.* 1993;50:357-368.
36. Yamada K, Yasushi T, Yoshida S. Effect of administration of corticotropin-releasing hormone and glucocorticoid on arginine vasopressin response to osmotic stimulation in normal subjects and patients with hypocorticotropinism without overt diabetes insipidus. *J Clin Endocrinol Metab.* 1989;69:396-401.
37. Rittmaster RS, Cutler GB, Gold PW, Brandon DD, Thomas T, Loriaux DL, Chrousos GP. The relationship of saline-induced changes in vasopressin secretion to basal and corticotropin-releasing hormone-stimulated adrenocorticotropin and cortisol secretion in man. *J Clin Endocrinol Metab.* 1987;64:371-376.
38. Goldman MB, Blake L, Marks RC, Hedeker D, Luchins DJ. Association of nonsuppression of cortisol on the DST with primary polydipsia in chronic schizophrenia. *Am J Psychiatry.* 1993;150:653-655.
39. Verbalis JG. Osmotic inhibition of neurohypophysial secretion. In: North WG, Moses AM, Share L, eds. *The Neurohypophysis: A Window on Brain Function.* New York, NY: Annals of the New York Academy of Sciences; 1993;689:146-160.
40. Miaskiewicz SL, Stricker EM, Verbalis JG. Neurohypophysial secretion in response to cholecystokinin but not meal-induced gastric distention in humans. *J Clin Endocrinol Metab.* 1989;68:837-843.
41. Canuso CM, Goldman MB. Does minimizing neuroleptic dosage influence hyponatremia? *Psychiatry Res.* 1996;63:227-229.
42. Umbricht DS, Saltz B, Pollack S, Woerner M, Kane JM, Lieberman JA. Polydipsia and tardive dyskinesia in chronic psychiatric patients-related disorders? *Am J Psychiatry.* 1993;150:1536-1538.
43. Sladek CD, Armstrong WE. Effect of neurotransmitters and neuropeptides on vasopressin release. In: Gash DM, Boer GJ, eds. *Vasopressin: Principles and Properties.* New York, NY: Plenum Publishing Corp; 1987:275-333.
44. Raskind MA, Weitzman RE, Orenstein H, Fisher DA, Courtney N. Is antidiuretic hormone elevated in psychosis? a pilot study. *Biol Psychiatry.* 1978;13:385-390.
45. Dohanics J, Hoffman GE, Verbalis JG. Hyponatremia-induced inhibition of magnocellular neurons causes stressor-selective impairment of stimulated adrenocorticotropin secretion in rats. *Endocrinology.* 1991;128:331-340.
46. Yagi K, Onaka T. Stress and nociceptive inputs to VP neurons. In: Jard S, Jamison R, eds. *Vasopressin.* London, England: Colloque INSERM/John Libbey Eurotext; 1991;208:245-255.
47. Edelson JT, Robertson GL. The effect of the cold pressor test on vasopressin secretion in man. *Psychoneuroendocrinology.* 1986;11:307-316.
48. Illowsky BP, Kirch DG. Polydipsia and hyponatremia in psychiatric patients. *Am J Psychiatry.* 1988;145:675-683.
49. Emsley RA, Spangenberg JJ, Roberts MC. Disordered water homeostasis and cognitive impairment in schizophrenia. *Biol Psychiatry.* 1993;34:630-633.
50. Luchins DJ, Nettles KW, Goldman MB. Anterior medial temporal lobe volume in polydipsic schizophrenic patients with and without hypoosmolemia: a pilot study. *Biol Psychiatry.* In press.
51. Elkashef AM, Leadbetter RA, Kirch DG. Structural brain imaging in patients with schizophrenia and polydipsia-hyponatremia syndrome. In: Schnor DB, Kirch DG, eds. *Water Balance in Schizophrenia.* Washington, DC: American Psychiatric Association Press; 1996:125-136.
52. Umbricht D. Polydipsia and hippocampal pathology. *Biol Psychiatry.* 1994;36: 709-710.
53. Renaud LP, Jhamandas JH, Randle JCR. Electrophysiology of rostral afferents to supraoptic nucleus neurosecretory neurons. In: Cowley AW, Liard JF, Ausiello DA, eds. *Vasopressin: Cellular and Integrative Functions.* New York, NY: Raven Press; 1988:335-340.
54. Morris JF, Chapman DB, Sokol HW. Anatomy and function of the classic vasopressin-secreting hypothalamus-neurohypophysial systems. In: Gash DM, Boer GJ, eds. *Vasopressin: Principles and Properties.* New York, NY: Plenum Publishing Corp; 1987:91-117.
55. Goldman MB, Nettles KW. Influence of the hippocampus subiculum on antidiuretic hormone levels during stress. *Psychoneurol Endocrinol.* In press.
56. Jacobsen L, Sapolsky R. The role of the hippocampus in feedback regulation of the hypothalamic-pituitary-adrenocortical axis. *Endocr Rev.* 1991;12:118-134.
57. Plotsky PM, Thrivikraman KV, Meaney MJ. Central and feedback regulation of hypothalamic corticotropin-releasing factor secretion. In: *Corticotropin Releasing Factor.* New York, NY: John Wiley & Sons Inc; 1993:59-84.
58. Cunningham ET, Sawchenko PE. Reflex control of magnocellular vasopressin and oxytocin secretion. *Trends Neurosci.* 1991;14:406-411.
59. de Leon J, Verghese C, Stanilla JK, Lawrence T, Simpson GM. Treatment of polydipsia and hyponatremia in psychiatric patients: can clozapine be a new option? *Neuropsychopharmacology.* 1995;12:133-138.

ESTABLISHED THERAPY FOR OCD

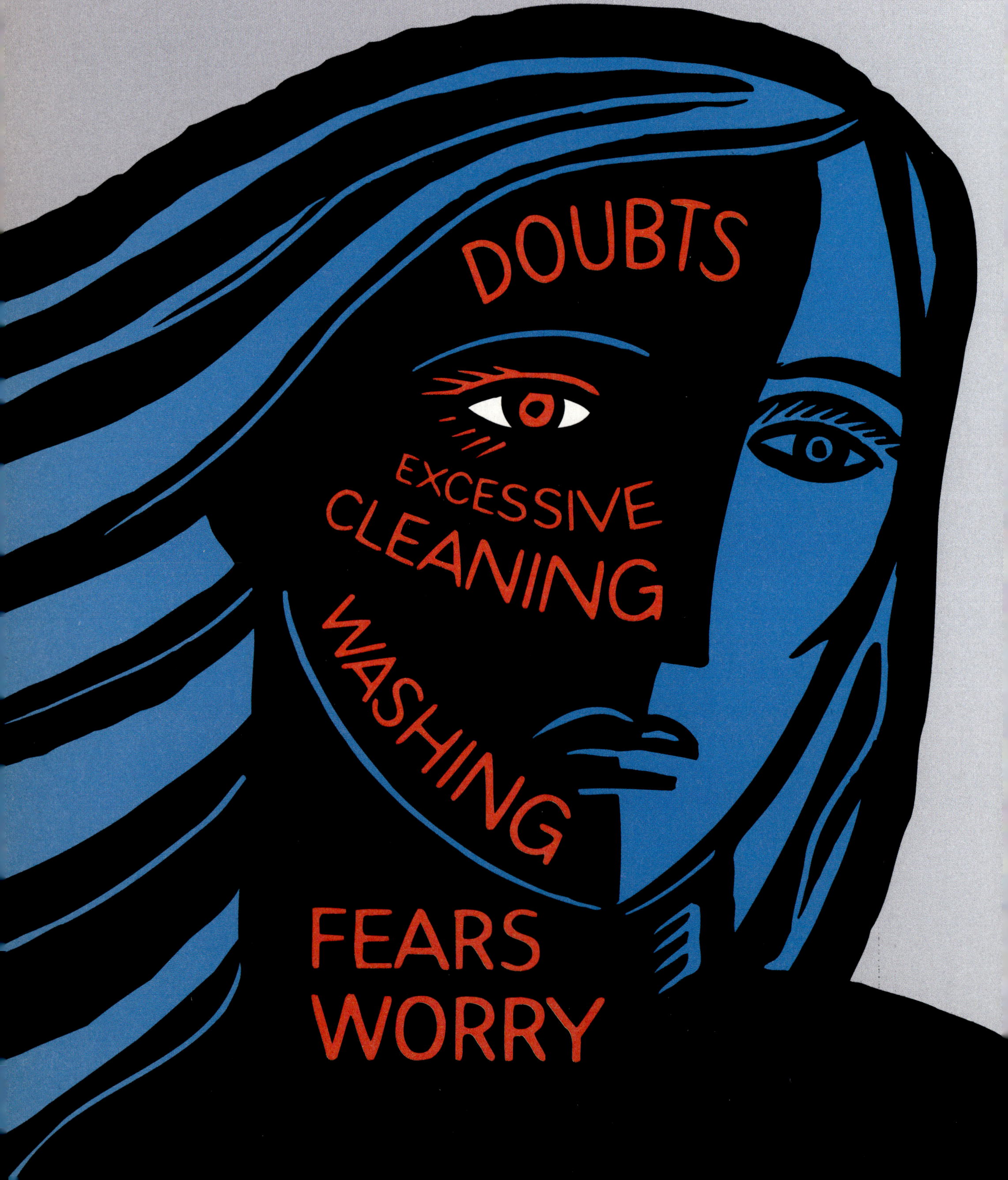

Relapse and Rehospitalization During Maintenance Treatment of Schizophrenia

The Effects of Dose Reduction and Family Treatment

Nina R. Schooler, PhD; Samuel J. Keith, MD; Joanne B. Severe, MS; Susan M. Matthews; Alan S. Bellack, PhD; Ira D. Glick, MD; William A. Hargreaves, PhD; John M. Kane, MD; Philip T. Ninan, MD; Allen Frances, MD; Marc Jacobs, MD; Jeffrey A. Lieberman, MD; Rosalind Mance, MD; George M. Simpson, MD; Margaret G. Woerner, PhD

Background: Previous studies have examined dose reduction and family treatment in schizophrenia, but none has examined their interaction. This study assessed the impact of dose reduction of antipsychotic medication and family treatment on relapse and rehospitalization during maintenance treatment.

Methods: Subjects were 313 male and female outpatients at 5 centers with a *DSM-III-R* diagnosis of schizophrenia or schizoaffective disorder. In a 3×2 design, subjects were randomized to 1 of 3 medication strategies using fluphenazine decanoate under double-blind conditions: continuous moderate dose (standard) (12.5-50 mg every 2 weeks); continuous low dose (2.5-10 mg every 2 weeks); or targeted, early intervention (fluphenazine only when symptomatic). Subjects also were randomized to 1 of 2 family treatment strategies (supportive or applied). Supportive family management involved monthly group meetings. The more intensive applied family management involved monthly group meetings and home visits where communication and problem-solving skills were taught. Patients and families were treated and assessed for 2 years.

Results: Both continuous low-dose and targeted treatment increased use of rescue medication and relapse; only targeted treatment increased rehospitalization. This pattern was consistent across both family treatments; there were no differences between family treatments.

Conclusions: These findings reaffirm the value of antipsychotic medication in preventing relapse and rehospitalization. The absence of family treatment differences may be because both conditions engaged families.

Arch Gen Psychiatry. 1997;54:453-463

As a chronic illness, schizophrenia requires a range of treatments and services for successful community tenure. Determining treatment efficacy requires specification and experimental control. Such evaluation, using clinical trial methods, is standard for pharmacologic treatments of schizophrenia,[1] but experimental assessment of psychosocial treatments has been limited and there has been little work on the interaction of specific medications and psychosocial treatments. Investigations of family treatments that include treatment specification and controls represent a notable exception and have yielded impressive results. The National Institute of Mental Health Treatment Strategies in Schizophrenia Study, a multicenter study of dose-reduction strategies and specified family treatment methods, is the first long-term maintenance study to examine both the main effects and interaction of these modalities.

The efficacy of antipsychotic medication in the maintenance treatment of schizophrenia is well established.[2] Primary goals are to sustain symptom remission and forestall relapse. Secondary goals are to improve functioning beyond psychopathologic symptoms such as social adjustment. Dose-reduction strategies aim to reduce the amount of medication received while forestalling relapse and reducing the risk of tardive dyskinesia, neuroleptic-induced negative symptoms, and other neuroleptic side effects. Further, patients freed of some neuroleptic side effects might increase social and instrumental activities, be less burdensome to their families, and more treatment compliant. Two dose-reduction strategies have been studied extensively: continuous "low-dose" and targeted or intermittent treatment.[3,4] Both treatments require ongoing monitoring to detect signs or symptoms that may signal impending relapse or psychotic exacerbation but differ in assumptions regarding medication's role during maintenance treatment.

The affiliations of the authors appear in the acknowledgment section at the end of the article.

SUBJECTS AND METHODS

CENTERS

Five centers, selected by competitive review from 27 that responded to a Request for Applications from the National Institute of Mental Health, participated in the trial. All were affiliated with academic departments of psychiatry, but represented a range of clinical settings where schizophrenic patients receive treatment in the United States. Grady Memorial Hospital, Atlanta, Ga, and San Francisco (Calif) General Hospital are general public hospitals with psychiatric units. Hillside Hospital, New Hyde Park, NY, is a private psychiatric hospital in a medical center. Payne Whitney Clinic, New York, NY, is a university hospital. Eastern Pennsylvania Psychiatric Institute, Philadelphia, is a public psychiatric hospital in a medical center. Patients were admitted from the community, and length of hospital stay varied from an average of 9 days at San Francisco General Hospital to 30 days at Hillside Hospital.

SUBJECTS

Five hundred twenty-eight acutely ill patients were recruited between 1985 and 1990. Inclusion criteria were (1) a *DSM-III-R*[38] diagnosis of schizophrenia (any subtype), schizoaffective disorder, or schizophreniform disorder as determined by the Structured Clinical Interview for *DSM-III-R* (SCID-Psychotic Disorders), which makes these diagnoses as well as diagnosis of major depressive disorder, bipolar disorder, brief reactive psychosis, delusional disorder, and psychotic disorder not otherwise specified; (2) age between 18 and 55 years; (3) living with, or having more than superficial contact with, family of origin defined as a minimum of 4 hours of regular face-to-face contact per week; (4) living close enough to the clinic to permit home visits; and (5) informed consent from the patient and at least 1 family member to participate in both medication and family treatment. Exclusion criteria were (1) unequivocal liver damage; (2) acute or chronic organic brain syndrome; (3) *DSM-III-R* diagnosis of psychoactive substance dependence and, additionally, for patients with schizophreniform disorder, *DSM-III-R* diagnosis of psychoactive substance abuse; and (4) pregnancy.

Ninety-three percent of subjects were recruited during hospitalization; the remainder were outpatients experiencing acute exacerbations.

PROCEDURES

Following consent, subjects entered a 16- to 24-week stabilization phase defined by hospital admission date or by study entry for outpatients. They were randomly assigned to AFM or SFM and those treatments began. They were discharged, with the goal of stabilization, to receive assigned family management and injectable fluphenazine decanoate only. A priori stabilization criteria included the following: stable dosage of 12.5 to 50 mg of fluphenazine decanoate every 2 weeks for 4 weeks without the use of other antipsychotic or psychotropic medications (eg, lithium, antidepressants); stable psychotic symptoms as assessed by the Brief Psychiatric Rating Scale (BPRS)[39,40] for 4 weeks; no psychotic symptom (conceptual disorganization, grandiosity, hallucinatory behavior, and unusual thought content) greater than moderate. Successfully stabilized patients entered the maintenance phase at which time they were randomized to 1 of the 3 medication conditions. Treatment with the combination of medication condition and family management continued for 24 months.

The flowchart in **Figure 1** presents the 2-stage randomization and the numbers of subjects in the 2×3 factorial design.

TREATMENT

Family Management

Family members were invited to a psychoeducational workshop modeled on the survival skills workshop developed by Anderson and coworkers[41] and received 3 study-specific booklets: "What is Schizophrenia?" "Medication for Schizophrenia," and "The Role of the Family." The workshop emphasized a vulnerability/stress model of schizophrenia and its treatment using medication and family participation. Following the workshop, patients and families were assigned to a family management clinician and randomized to SFM or to the more intensive AFM. The family management clinicians were trained in AFM by Ian R. H. Falloon, MD, and Christine W. McGill, PhD, and assigned cases in both conditions. They were almost exclusively women and had social work, psychology, or nursing backgrounds, with a mean of 7.4 years of clinical experience, but only 28% had experience with behavioral methods.[42]

The SFM participants were invited to monthly family group meetings that continued throughout the stabilization and maintenance phases. Meetings were led by a family management clinician, lasted approximately 1½ hours, and included presentations consonant with the treatment model and discussion of issues raised by participants. In addition, family management clinicians answered questions and provided case management and consultation regarding problems. Families were relied on to initiate contacts unless the treatment team decided that a problem or crisis required family intervention.

The AFM subjects had individual meetings scheduled in the home to assess functional status and knowledge of schizophrenia. Home sessions that included the patient followed individual assessments. Sessions, following a detailed treatment manual,[43] were held weekly for 13 weeks, biweekly for 13 visits, and monthly until the end of the first year of the maintenance phase, for a maximum of 32 sessions. Presentation of educational materials and training in communication skills preceded teaching and practice of problem-solving techniques. Separate monthly

Continuous low-dose treatment assumes that dosage can be reduced substantially following remission to less than was required to treat psychotic symptoms. Published comparisons[5-13] of low-dose treatment to a "standard" dosage in outpatients have used injectable medication to ensure that covert noncompliance did not compromise the dosage differences and, with the exception of the 6-week study of Goldstein et al,[5] were meetings for AFM participants paralleled the SFM groups. Case management was also available to AFM families.

Maintenance Phase

Two hundred fifteen subjects (41%) did not enter the maintenance phase: 105 could not be stabilized according to study criteria; 21 were stable, but only with treatment above the study dose range (50 mg of fluphenazine decanoate every 2 weeks); 80 withdrew consent; and 9 were withdrawn for administrative reasons.

As shown in Figure 1, 313 patients (58% of the 272 patients randomized to AFM and 61% of the 256 patients randomized to SFM) were further randomized to 1 of 3 medication conditions: standard dose (StanD), fluphenazine decanoate, 12.5 to 50 mg every 2 weeks; low dose (LowD), fluphenazine decanoate, 2.5 to 10 mg every 2 weeks; and targeted dose (TargD), an injection of the sesame oil or miglioil vehicle every 2 weeks. Benztropine mesylate was the preferred antiparkinsonian medication and temazepam or lorazepam was used for sleep. Subjects either met the a priori stabilization criteria or, if BPRS symptom levels exceeded the stabilization criteria, they could enter the maintenance phase by meeting a "clinical" criterion of being symptomatic, but stable and suitable for dosage reduction. The blind was maintained by administering the same volume of medication to all groups with a 20% dilution for the LowD group and the vehicle only in the TargD group. An adaptive randomization algorithm[44,45] was used in an attempt to maximize equality of randomization using the following parameters: family management assignment; gender; Abnormal Involuntary Movements Scale score at the end of stabilization (mild or greater in any body area vs less than mild); diagnosis (*DSM-III-R* schizophrenia vs schizoaffective disorder vs schizophreniform disorder); length of stabilization phase (16 weeks vs >16 weeks).

If subjects showed prodromal signs of relapse, open-label rescue medication was added—either oral fluphenazine or fluphenazine decanoate, if compliance was a concern. Once patients were restabilized, as defined by the same criteria as for initial stabilization, rescue medication was discontinued. Patients who required rescue medication for a cumulative total of more than 140 days (20 weeks) were discontinued from receiving double-blind medication and were treated openly. They continued with their assigned family management condition and received study assessments for the full 2-year maintenance phase.

ASSESSMENTS

Clinical and social functioning assessments were completed at points determined by study design and patients' clinical course. Psychopathologic symptoms were rated by psychiatrists using the Hillside anchored version of the BPRS,[40] a modification of the Scale for Assessment of Negative Symptoms,[46,47] and the severity and improvement items of the Clinical Global Impressions.[48] Extrapyramidal side effects were rated by psychiatrists using the Neurological Rating Scale, which is a modification of the Simpson-Angus Scale for Extrapyramidal Side Effects.[49] Prodromal signs were monitored by nurses using a modified Early Signs Questionnaire[50] and a summary of idiosyncratic signs tailored for each patient following interviews with the patient and a family member regarding prior episodes.

Psychiatric assessments using the BPRS and Clinical Global Impressions were completed monthly. In addition, during periods that subjects received rescue medication, assessments were completed weekly. Nursing evaluations were completed at biweekly injection visits. Detailed assessments of psychopathologic symptoms, side effects, and social functioning were completed at 6, 12, 18, and 24 months during the maintenance phase, and after 20 weeks of rescue medication, if that occurred.

DATA ANALYSIS

We addressed 3 major areas of the clinical trial: (1) To determine whether there were differences among groups in the 3×2 factorial design at the start of the maintenance phase despite randomization, we used analysis of variance (ANOVA) to compare demographic characteristics, treatment history, and symptoms. (2) To assess treatment implementation, we used ANOVA to compare the total biweekly medication dosage received for 6-month study intervals by treatment group; we compared the treatment groups' attendance at the psychoeducational workshop and the monthly support group meetings during the stabilization phase and at 6-month intervals of the maintenance phase; and we compared the number of family home sessions for those randomized to AFM by medication group. (3) To assess treatment outcome, we examined 5 dependent variables for survival time using a Cox proportional hazards model[51] with 3 medication conditions, 2 family management conditions, and their interaction as covariates. Dependent variables were the times to first use of rescue medication, 20 weeks of rescue medication, psychotic relapse, and first rehospitalization, during the period that patients were in the full medication × family management design and for the 2-year maintenance phase regardless of whether they were still receiving double-blind medication. Psychotic relapse was defined by a rating of "moderate" or greater, representing an increase of at least 2 scale points on any 1 of 5 psychosis items of the BPRS (conceptual disorganization, grandiosity, suspiciousness, hallucinatory behavior, and unusual thought content) that persisted for 2 monthly ratings or a monthly rating and a rating at rescue medication start. We also used log linear analysis to evaluate the proportions of patients in each treatment group who were rehospitalized, comparing AFM with SFM under each medication condition. To assess site differences, we repeated the Cox proportional hazards analysis separately by site for 1 measure, time to 20 weeks of rescue medication. To control for the influence of baseline psychopathologic status on outcome, we repeated the Cox proportional hazards analysis for time to 20 weeks of rescue medication with the addition of severity of illness at the start of the maintenance phase to the model. Two-tailed tests and an alpha level of .05 were used to define significance.

at least 1 year long. Low-dose treatment increases the risk for relapse under some circumstances. The dose level, patients' stage of illness, how minor exacerbations are treated, and the length of time that the strategy is used all influence relapse risk. On balance, dose reduction is feasible as long as extremely low doses are not involved and patients are not in an acute phase of their illness. Most studies report some clinical advantages to

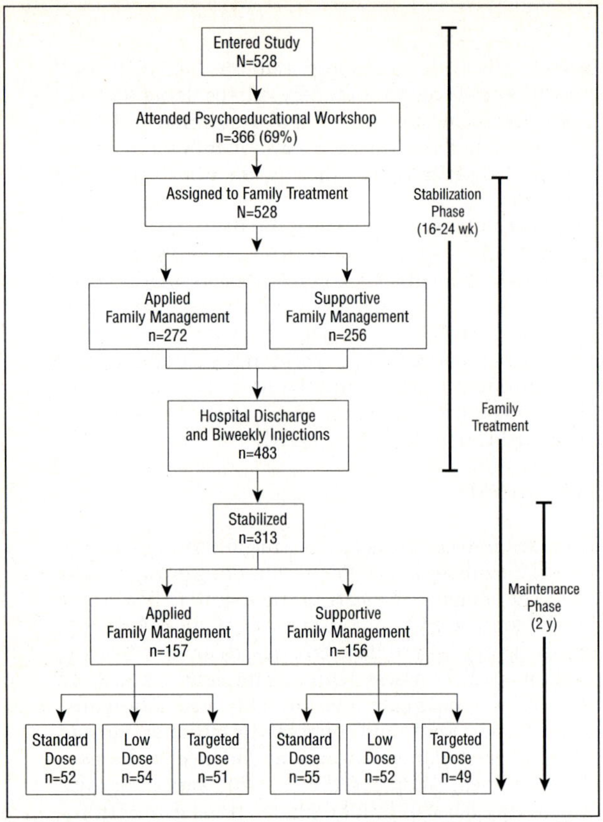

Figure 1. *Study flowchart of 2-stage randomization to family treatment and medication treatment.*

low-dose treatment such as side-effect reduction, improvement of negative symptoms, and reduction of family burden.

Targeted treatment assumes that stable patients require neuroleptic medication only when they experience prodromal signs or psychotic symptoms. Compared with continuous medication, patients receiving targeted treatment receive less medication and experience fewer side effects, particularly extrapyramidal symptoms.[14-20] In one study that included a third condition, "neuroleptic crisis intervention," medication was given only at relapse, directly testing the hypothesis that delaying treatment until a full episode develops is inferior to treating prodromal symptoms. There was a higher relapse rate in the crisis intervention group than in the early intervention group.[20] Although an early intervention or targeted strategy is feasible and may be superior to delaying intervention until relapse, the risk for relapse is significantly increased compared with a continuous medication strategy and the gains in social functioning and side effects do not compensate.

There are several reported controlled comparisons of the effects of psychoeducational family treatment of schizophrenia.[21-23] When family treatment was compared with either routine treatment or other psychosocial interventions, statistically significant and clinically substantial differences in relapse or rehospitalization were seen.[24-30] In contrast, there were no significant overall differences among family treatments.[31-36] Tarrier and his colleagues[34,35] compared 4 groups: 2 family treatments, education, and routine treatment. They found no differences between family treatments, but substantial differences between family treatment and the other conditions after 9 months. In tacit acceptance of the hypothesis that the distinction between family treatment and routine care is the critical one, subsequent comparisons merged the family treatment groups.[34,35] Two studies by Leff et al[28,29] provide a similar pattern of results. One compared family treatment with routine care and found relapse differences. The second attempted to deconstruct the family social intervention, but did not include a routine care group and found no difference; however, post hoc comparison of the family treatment groups from both studies vs routine care suggested that family treatment enhanced outcome.[31,32]

One study examined the interaction of family treatment vs usual care and moderate vs low dose of injectable medication. In this brief, 6-week trial, the 2 treatments had an additive effect: relapse was lowest when patients received both moderate dose and family treatment and highest if they received the low dose and usual care.[5]

The Treatment Strategies in Schizophrenia Study was designed to address gaps in knowledge regarding medication and family treatment. Specifically, the study directly compared targeted, early intervention with continuous low-dose drug treatment, as well as the interaction of family treatment with controlled medication treatment, in long-term maintenance. The medication factor of the design compared a moderate dose, a continuous low-dose, and the targeted early intervention approach under double-blind conditions over a period of 2 years. All 3 conditions allowed the addition of open-label rescue medication if prodromal signs or symptom exacerbation occurred so that the value of the medication strategies including a rescue protocol could be tested. The family treatment factor of the design compared 2 well-specified forms of family psychoeducation–supportive family management (SFM) and applied family management (AFM). Their common elements included an initial psychoeducational workshop for families and monthly support group meetings for 2 years for patients and families. The AFM added individual family sessions conducted in the home modeled on behavioral family treatment developed by Falloon and his colleagues.[37] These families received individualized psychoeducation and were coached in communication and problem-solving skills. To test the maintenance effects of the strategy, the added treatment component of AFM ended after the first year.

We examined the effects on temporal measures of efficacy: need for rescue medication, relapse, and rehospitalization. We hypothesized that targeted treatment would require more added medication and result in higher relapse rates and more rehospitalization than low-dose treatment, which in turn would require more added medication and result in higher relapse rates and more rehospitalization than the standard dose. We also hypothesized that AFM would be more effective than SFM. Further, we hypothesized that medication effects would be attenuated by AFM; differences among medication conditions would be smaller for subjects who received AFM, the more intensive family treatment.

Table 1. Demographic Characteristics and Treatment History (n=313)*

SCID-PD† diagnosis, %	
Schizophrenia	79.6
Schizoaffective disorder	13.1
Schizophreniform disorder	7.4
Sex, % male	66.1
Race, % white	39.6
Marital status, % ever married	18.2
Mean (SD) age, y	
At study admission	29.6 (7.4)
At first hospitalization	23.8 (5.8)
At first illness	21.1 (5.7)
Prior hospitalizations, % ever	73.2
Mean (SD) No. of months hospitalized, if ever (n=229)	7.6 (13.8)
Hospitalized prior 24 mo, %	43
Mean (SD) No. of months hospitalized, if during 24 mo	2.1 (2.6)
Neuroleptic medication received, % ever	76.3
Mean (SD) length of stabilization, wk	23.2 (4.3)

*All variables were examined for differences by analysis of variance for 3 medication × 2 family management conditions. Trends and significant effects are as follows: age at admission, applied family management (30.3 y) vs supportive family management (28.8 y) ($P>.05<.10$); age at first illness, standard-dose (21.6 y) vs low-dose (20.0 y) vs targeted-dose (21.7 y) treatment ($P<.05$).

†Structured Clinical Interview for DSM-III-R–Psychotic Disorders.

Table 2. Psychopathologic Symptoms at Start of Maintenance Phase*

Brief Psychiatric Rating Scale (BPRS) (n=313)	
Anxious depression	1.8 (0.8)
Anergia	1.8 (0.7)
Thought disturbance	1.5 (0.8)
Activation	1.4 (0.6)
Hostility	1.5 (0.6)
Total score	29.4 (7.6)
Scale for Assessment of Negative Symptoms (SANS) global ratings (n=290)	
Affective flattening	2.2 (1.0)
Alogia	1.7 (0.9)
Avolition/Apathy	2.4 (1.1)
Anhedonia/asociality	2.5 (1.2)
Attention	1.9 (0.9)
Physician Severity of Illness Rating (n=313)	3.0 (1.0)

*Data are given as mean (SD) scores. All variables were examined for differences by analysis of variance for 3 medication × 2 family management conditions. Significant effects are as follows: BPRS, anxious depression, applied family management (AFM) (1.7) vs supportive family management (SFM) (1.9) ($P<.05$); SANS attention, family management × medication interaction: standard dose, AFM (2.0); standard dose, SFM (1.9); low dose, AFM (1.6); low dose, SFM (2.1); targeted dose, AFM (2.0); targeted dose, SFM (1.9); $P<.05$.

RESULTS

SUBJECT CHARACTERISTICS

Demographic characteristics and treatment history are presented in **Table 1**. Differences among treatment groups are identified in this table. Sixty-six percent of the sample was male; 79% met *DSM-III-R* criteria for schizophrenia at study entry. By the start of the maintenance phase, all subjects initially diagnosed as having schizophreniform disorder met criteria for schizophrenia.

Psychopathologic symptoms at the maintenance phase baseline are shown in **Table 2**. Again, treatment group differences are noted. Psychopathologic symptoms were in the minimal to mild range for virtually all of the measures examined, including negative symptoms assessed on the Scale for the Assessment of Negative Symptoms. Eighty-eight percent of patients met a priori stabilization criteria. Seventy percent met a more stringent criterion for remission: no BPRS psychotic symptom worse than mild.

TREATMENT IMPLEMENTATION

Medication

Dosage includes double-blind and rescue medication. Oral fluphenazine dose is converted to fluphenazine decanoate based on the following formula: 15-mg/d oral fluphenazine hydrochloride = 25-mg fluphenazine decanoate every 2 weeks. **Table 3** presents dosage for 2-week intervals by treatment group by 6-month period, but only for patients who were receiving blind medication during each period. There were no significant differences between AFM and SFM, no interactions of family management and medication conditions, and no site differences. During all 4 periods, subjects in the StanD group received significantly more medication than subjects in the LowD and TargD groups. During the first 6 months, the difference between LowD and TargD mirrored the randomized condition. During subsequent periods, dosage did not differ significantly between LowD and TargD groups. During the last period, the dose for the few patients in the TargD group did not differ from either StanD or LowD. For the TargD group, dose increases over time.

Fluphenazine decanoate was used as rescue medication if compliance was a concern. There were no differences among the medication conditions in its use. The proportion of subjects who received fluphenazine decanoate as rescue medication was as follows: StanD, 64%; LowD, 77%; and TargD, 71% ($\chi^2=2.61$, $P>.05$).

Family Management

There were no differences between SFM and AFM in attendance at the initial workshop (AFM, 75.2%; SFM, 79.2%) or monthly meetings (AFM, 53.5%; SFM, 60.3%) during the stabilization phase. As shown in **Table 4**, the percentage of families who attended monthly meetings during each 6-month period of the maintenance phase ranged from 71% to 30%. For families who attended at least once during a period, the mean number of meetings attended ranged from 3.0 to 3.8 (maximum of 6). There were no significant differences among sites, medication condition, family management condition, or their interactions. For patients randomized to AFM, there were no differences among the 3 medication groups in number of home sessions.

Table 3. Treatment Implementation: Medication Dosage by Treatment Group and 6-Month Study Interval*

Period	Standard Dose (StanD) AFM	Standard Dose (StanD) SFM	Low Dose (LowD) AFM	Low Dose (LowD) SFM	Targeted Dose (TargD) AFM	Targeted Dose (TargD) SFM	Significant Effects†
0-6 mo							
n	51	54	54	52	51	49	F=66.77 (*df*=2/305); all pairwise comparisons significant
2-wk dose	33.2 (21.3)	28.8 (18.8)	13.0 (11.9)	13.7 (13.7)	7.9 (9.6)	6.8 (10.3)	
7-12 mo							
n	43	50	46	42	40	41	F=15.91 (*df*=2/256); StanD differs from LowD and TargD
2-wk dose	31.3 (20.0)	27.6 (19.4)	16.6 (20.9)	17.2 (15.4)	15.0 (13.6)	15.6 (18.1)	
13-18 mo							
n	37	37	30	29	16	24	F=16.26 (*df*=2/167); StanD differs from LowD and TargD
2-wk dose	29.4 (23.8)	26.6 (20.0)	8.4 (5.5)	11.9 (11.7)	18.5 (34.5)	10.5 (11.5)	
19-24 mo							
n	23	29	23	21	3	9	F=12.93 (*df*=2/102); StanD differs from LowD
2-wk dose	25.1 (20.4)	25.9 (19.4)	8.3 (8.1)	9.7 (8.1)	19.9 (13.8)	15.6 (19.5)	

**Dosage is reported as mean (SD) milligrams of fluphenazine decanoate every 2 weeks. Dosage includes both double-blind fluphenazine decanoate and open-label fluphenazine decanoate and fluphenazine hydrochloride. Fluphenazine hydrochloride is converted to fluphenazine decanoate dosage using the following formula: 15-mg fluphenazine hydrochloride per day = 25-mg fluphenazine decanoate every 2 weeks. AFM indicates applied family management; SFM, supportive family management.*

†*P*<.*001.*

Table 4. Treatment Implementation: Family Management Parameters by Treatment Group and Study Interval During Maintenance Phase

	Applied Family Management: Standard Dose (n=52)	Applied Family Management: Low Dose (n=54)	Applied Family Management: Targeted Dose (n=51)	Supportive Family Management: Standard Dose (n=54)	Supportive Family Management: Low Dose (n=52)	Supportive Family Management: Targeted Dose (n=49)
Monthly support group meetings						
Months 1-6						
% Attended	63	63	55	61	67	71
No. attended*	3.6 (1.8)	3.3 (1.8)	3.5 (1.9)	3.6 (2.1)	3.1 (1.4)	3.0 (1.7)
Months 7-12						
% Attended	56	57	37	48	50	55
No. attended*	3.7 (1.6)	3.1 (1.9)	3.8 (1.4)	3.2 (1.8)	3.3 (1.7)	3.1 (1.6)
Months 13-18						
% Attended	44	42	43	39	46	49
No. attended*	3.7 (2.0)	3.3 (1.7)	3.8 (1.7)	3.7 (1.9)	3.4 (1.9)	3.2 (1.8)
Months 19-24						
% Attended	40	39	39	30	35	35
No. attended*	3.7 (2.1)	3.0 (1.7)	3.8 (1.6)	3.2 (1.8)	3.6 (1.8)	3.4 (1.9)
No. of home visits†	24.7 (5.8)	23.4 (7.1)	23.8 (6.9)	...	...	...

**Only for those who attended; data are mean (SD).*

†*Only applicable to applied family management condition; data are mean (SD).*

Treatment Effects on Rescue Medication, Relapse, and Rehospitalization

Figure 2 presents Kaplan-Meier survival curves for the 6 treatment groups for time to 20 weeks of rescue fluphenazine to illustrate findings of the Cox regression analyses. The statistical tests for differences among the 6 survival curves show highly significant effects whether treatment failures are equally weighted (Savage test) or early failures are more heavily weighted (Wilcoxon test). Within each medication condition, curves for the 2 family management groups are virtually identical. Curves for the medication groups are more easily distinguished after 6 months of maintenance treatment.

Table 5 presents the results of the Cox regression analyses for the 5 outcomes. Time to 20 weeks of rescue medication is also presented separately for the 5 sites and for the model that included baseline clinical severity of illness rating. In these regression models, covariates represent the treatment factors in the design and their interactions. For family management (AFM vs SFM), 1 covariate estimates the effect. For the medication condition (StanD vs LowD vs TargD), 2 covariates are required to define the model. Significant contrasts for main effects are identified: AFM vs SFM; StanD vs LowD; StanD vs TargD; and LowD vs TargD. Because no interactions of family management and medication conditions were significant, interactions are not included in the table. Table 5 also presents mean survival times for each level of family management and medication condition.

The model for time to first rescue medication was highly significant. All medication contrasts are significant. Time to first rescue was shortest in the TargD group and longest in the StanD group. There was no significant difference between AFM and SFM. The model for time to 20 weeks of rescue medication was also highly significant and showed the same pattern (Figure 2). The test of that model was significant for 4 of the 5 centers and the pattern of effects is consistent with the analysis of combined centers. When baseline severity of illness was added to the model, it had a significant effect, but did not change the findings for the treatments.

The model for psychotic symptom relapse was significant ($P<.01$), but only the contrast between StanD and TargD approached significance ($P>.05<.10$). The mean time to psychotic relapse was 431 days in the TargD group and 609 days in the StanD group.

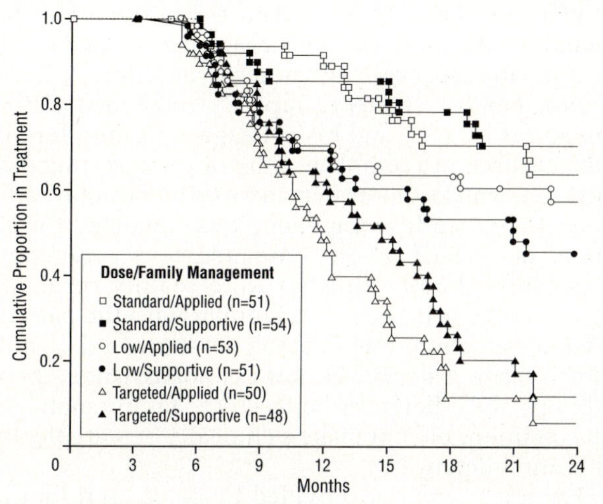

Figure 2. *Survival times for 6 treatment groups for 20 weeks of rescue medication. Savage test (treatment failures equally weighted)* χ^2, $P<.001$; *Wilcoxon test (early treatment failures more heavily weighted)* χ^2, $P<.001$.

Time to rehospitalization was examined for the period that subjects participated in the full 3×2 factorial design (before 20 weeks of rescue medication) and for the 2-year maintenance phase. There is a significant effect of medication on rehospitalization during the period that subjects received double-blind medication ($P<.05$). Time to rehospitalization was shorter for the TargD group (456 days) than for the LowD group (579 days). In the analysis that examined rehospitalization during the entire maintenance phase, the overall model shows a trend toward significance ($P>.05<.10$) as do the contrasts between TargD and both StanD and LowD. Time to rehospitalization is longest for the StanD condition (554 days) and shortest for the TargD condition (420 days).

The proportion of subjects rehospitalized over the 2-year period, by medication and family management conditions, is given in **Table 6**. **Table 7** presents log linear analysis of rehospitalization during the maintenance phase. The effects labeled medication, family management, and medication × family management represent the study design and nonsignificant χ^2 values indicate successful randomization. The significant χ^2 associated with rehospitalization indicates that the difference between rehospitalized and not rehospitalized differed from chance. Interaction effects (medication × rehospitalization, family management × rehospitalization, and medication × family management × rehospitalization) test differences in rehospitalization by treatment. Only the medication × rehospitalization interaction is significant. Twenty-five percent of subjects in the StanD and LowD groups were rehospitalized, compared with 46% of TargD group subjects.

Table 5. Effects of Family Management and Medication on Longitudinal Measures of Outcome: Mean Times by Family Management and Medication Condition*

	Model	Significance of Contrasts†			Mean Time, d				
					Family Management		Medication		
Variable	χ^2 (*P*)	StanD vs LowD	StanD vs TargD	LowD vs TargD	AFM	SFM	StanD	LowD	TargD
Time to first rescue medication	55.69 (.001)	.01	.001	.01	323	351	495	346	187
Time to 20 wk of rescue medication									
All sites‡	58.94 (.001)	.01	.001	.05	518	527	618	532	406
Hillside Hospital	10.29 (.10)	...	.10	...	510	575	667	565	411
Eastern Pennsylvania Psychiatric Institute	29.08 (.001)	...	.10	.05	555	525	595	663	362
Payne Whitney Clinic	6.77 (NS)	...	...	...	487	533	574	510	438
San Francisco General Hospital	19.09 (.01)	.01	.05	...	479	409	592	384	338
Grady Memorial Hospital	12.23 (.05)	.10	.05	...	546	571	663	516	469
Time to psychotic relapse§	15.46 (.01)	...	.10	...	524	544	609	520	431
Time to rehospitalization, full medication condition	17.85 (.01)	...	...	.05	557	545	601	579	456
Time to rehospitalization, full 2-y study period	9.06 (.10)	...	.10	.10	515	504	554	532	420

**StanD indicates standard dose; LowD, low dose; TargD, targeted dose; AFM, applied family management; SFM, supportive family management; and NS, not significant.*

†*No contrasts of AFM to SFM or interactions of medication and family management were significant.*

‡*The all sites analysis was repeated including physician's rating of Global Severity of Illness at start of maintenance phase as a covariate.* χ^2 *for the model=58.28 (6 df) ($P<.001$), Global Severity of Illness ($P<.01$); significance of other contrasts remains as shown in the table.*

§*Defined by a rating of "moderate" or greater that represents an increase of at least 2 scale points on any 1 of 5 psychotic items of the Brief Psychiatric Rating Scale (conceptual disorganization, grandiosity, suspiciousness, hallucinatory behavior, and unusual thought content) that is sustained for 2 assessments.*

Table 6. Percentage of Subjects Rehospitalized Over 2-Year Period by Medication and Family Management Conditions

Family Management	Standard Dose	Low Dose	Targeted Dose	Total
Applied	19	26	43	29
Supportive	31	25	49	35
Total	25	25	46	32

Table 7. Log Linear Analysis of Rehospitalization During the Maintenance Phase (n=313)

Effect	*df*	χ^2	*P*
Medication	2	0.28	.87
Family management	1	0.00	.95
Medication × family management	2	0.30	.86
Rehospitalization	1	41.73	<.001
Medication × rehospitalization	2	13.14	.001
Family management × rehospitalization	1	1.16	.28
Medication × family management × rehospitalization	2	1.15	.56

COMMENT

Our findings extend the understanding of the role of dose reduction and specified family treatments in the maintenance treatment of schizophrenia. The study is definitive because of the treatment duration, the large sample size, and the generalization to 5 centers. The outcomes reported—amount of medication required, relapse rates, and rehospitalization rates—address major study questions and are key for clinicians treating patients with schizophrenia.

MEDICATION

Treatment with LowD and TargD medication had not been compared directly before. Our findings are consistent with earlier studies. Both strategies were successfully implemented, but both required use of rescue medication that limit their clinical use. This was especially true for TargD: almost all subjects in this condition required rescue medication, 60% within 6 months. In contrast, 45% of subjects in the StanD group required some rescue medication within 2 years. The direct comparison of LowD and TargD reveals clinically meaningful differences. On average, a patient receiving LowD first received rescue medication 159 days later than a patient receiving TargD and reached 20 weeks of rescue medication 126 days later. Further, patients in the LowD group were first rehospitalized on average 123 days later than those receiving TargD and did not differ significantly from patients receiving StanD in either time to or risk for rehospitalization.

Medication differences were seen despite close monitoring for prodromal signs and cannot be attributed to use of depot medication for rescue, which was used in the majority of patients in all of the groups.

FAMILY TREATMENT

We found no differential effects of AFM and SFM in measures sensitive to effects of medication, but not necessarily to psychosocial interventions. Earlier studies comparing family interventions to usual treatment or psychosocial treatment that did not involve families reported effects on these measures and influenced our study design. The Treatment Strategies in Schizophrenia Study offered support and therapeutic intervention to all families. Psychoeducational workshop attendance predicted continuation into the maintenance phase, suggesting that family engagement is valuable.[52] Rehospitalization rates for AFM and SFM in combination with StanD or LowD treatment are similar to those reported in the literature for family treatments (25% over a 2-year period) and lower than those for usual care and other treatments.

Does family treatment simply increase medication compliance? Hogarty and his colleagues[27] found family treatment effects in a compliant subgroup, suggesting that family treatment does more than increase medication compliance. In our study, compliance was enhanced for all subjects: depot medication eliminated covert noncompliance; missed appointments were readily rescheduled; a research team member, familiar with the patient and family situation, was available 24 hours a day; and treatment teams had relatively low case loads. Under these conditions, the differences between the family management conditions did not make a clinically or statistically significant difference.

Treatment was not provided by behavioral family therapy originators, although Drs Falloon and McGill collaborated in the study and trained and supervised the family management clinicians.[42] Family management clinician certification, based on review of videotaped sessions demonstrating proficiency in each specific component of AFM, was required before clinicians could treat study subjects, and not all trainees were certified. Ongoing competency was monitored through review of audiotaped sessions and supervisory telephone calls. The Behavioral Family Therapy Competency Scale was used to assess adherence to specific components and skills of AFM. The family management clinicians in our study maintained competency that ranged from adequate to outstanding (Laporta et al, written communication, 1994). There was consistent exposure to monthly meetings, no differences between family management conditions in attendance at the initial psychoeducational workshop, and no differences in the number of AFM sessions among the medication conditions.

LIMITATIONS

Only patients in frequent contact with families of origin were included. Thus, older and married patients were less likely to be included. A review of the 6012 patients screened for the study found that 2374 met "tentative" inclusion or exclusion criteria; 528 (9% of the screened sample and 22% of potentially eligible subjects) entered the trial.[53] These rates are not unusually low, but limit generalizablity to the broad population of schizophrenic patients. The 528 subjects in the stabilization phase were further reduced to 313 subjects in the maintenance phase. We have reported on characteristics that predict successful stabilization.[54-56] There were no differences between AFM and SFM in likelihood of stabilization, but 20% of subjects did not meet stabilization criteria. Thus, our findings may not apply to more persistently and severely ill schizophrenic patients.

A reviewer suggested that eliminating subjects who did not successfully stabilize limited our ability to show family treatment effects. Two prior studies that showed effects support that view. Subjects in the study of Goldstein et al[5] were all acutely symptomatic. McFarlane and colleagues[33] found no overall effect of single vs multiple family groups, but found differences among more symptomatic patients. The design constraints required to study dose-reduction strategies (clinical stability and minimal psychotic symptoms) may not be optimal for detecting psychosocial treatment effects. Alternatively, it can be argued that clinical stability is required in order to profit from psychosocial treatments. The present study and its subjects balance these constraints. The most severely and persistently symptomatic patients were excluded, but patients were clinically stable for less than 6 months.

The study sites were not randomly chosen from treatment facilities for schizophrenia in the United States but span a range of settings where patients are treated: psychiatric units in public general hospitals, public psychiatric clinics, and private psychiatric clinics. We examined site effects for one major outcome—time to use of rescue medication for 20 weeks—and found that the Cox regression model was significant at 4 of the 5 sites despite reduced power. Although fewer contrasts were significant, the pattern mirrored the effects seen in the full sample.

CLINICAL RECOMMENDATIONS

There is no added benefit of the more intensive AFM in patients' need for rescue medication, delay of relapse, or rehospitalization. However, the 2-year rehospitalization rates in both the StanD and LowD groups in our study are lower than those reported for the usual care condition of studies in which family treatment was compared with usual care. Thus, our findings, in conjunction with earlier research, support the engagement of families within a psychoeducational framework and the development of family support groups. Our study lends no support to the provision of an intervention involving home visits or training in communication and problem-solving skills.

The benefits of medication are clear. Relapse or need for additional medication may not occur for weeks or months after dosage reduction or medication discontinuation, particularly for stable patients treated with depot medication. Since there is no immediate response against which to judge success, dose reduction in clinically stable patients is problematic. Our study suggests that relatively low dosage can be sustained for 2 years in about 50% of patients. Dosage increases avert relapse in some patients and rehospitalization rates are no higher with low doses than with the moderate dose we studied.

The use of medication only when symptoms emerge carries higher risks for relapse and rehospitalization. This strategy should be reserved for patients who refuse medication but accept clinical monitoring. Such patients are better served by remaining in treatment rather than being discharged as uncooperative. For most patients with schizophrenia, a moderate dose of medication appears to be the best clinical recommendation.

FUTURE RESEARCH

This report focused on a limited number of outcomes. Other important questions will be addressed in future reports. These include clinical outcome of subjects who required 20 weeks of rescue medication; efficacy of family treatment for families who participated fully; the course of psychopathologic symptoms and social functioning; risk for tardive dyskinesia and other extrapyramidal symptoms; and the influence on outcome of patient and family characteristics such as gender, race, education, chronicity of illness, nature of family constellation, symptom pattern, and initial response to treatment.

The treatment of schizophrenia stands at a juncture as significant as that represented by the introduction of antipsychotic agents in the 1950s. New antipsychotic agents, not restricted in use like clozapine, are available or on the horizon.[57,58] We have little information regarding their efficacy in maintenance treatment. New psychosocial treatments for schizophrenia are being developed, including primary prevention strategies. Ideally, new medications and psychosocial treatments will prompt a generation of studies to investigate their additive and interactive effects.

Accepted for publication July 10, 1996.

From the Western Psychiatric Institute and Clinic, Department of Psychiatry, University of Pittsburgh School of Medicine, Pittsburgh, Pa (Dr Schooler); the National Institute of Mental Health Division of Clinical and Treatment Research, Rockville, Md (Dr Keith and Mss Severe and Matthews); and the Departments of Psychiatry, Eastern Pennsylvania Psychiatric Institute, Medical College of Pennsylvania, Philadelphia (Drs Bellack and Simpson), Payne Whitney Clinic–Cornell Medical Center, New York, NY (Drs Glick and Frances), San Francisco General Hospital, University of California, San Francisco (Drs Hargreaves and Jacobs), Hillside Hospital–Long Island Jewish Medical Center, New Hyde Park, NY (Drs Kane, Lieberman, and Woerner), and Grady Memorial Hospital, Emory University, Atlanta, Ga (Drs Ninan and Mance). Now with the Departments of Psychiatry at the following institutions are Dr Keith, University of New Mexico, Albuquerque; Dr Bellack, University of Maryland, Baltimore; and Dr Frances, Duke University Medical Center, Durham, NC; and now with the Departments of Psychiatry and Behavioral Sciences are Dr Lieberman, University of North Carolina, Chapel Hill; and Dr Simpson, University of Southern California, Los Angeles.

All double-blind medication supplies as well as open-label fluphenazine decanoate and fluphenazine hydrochloride were provided courtesy of Bristol-Myers Squibb Company, Princeton, NJ.

The Treatment Strategies in Schizophrenia Cooperative Agreement Program was a multicenter clinical trial carried out by 5 research teams in collaboration with the Division of Clinical and Treatment Research of the National Institute of Mental Health (NIMH). The NIMH principal collaborators are Nina R. Schooler, PhD; Samuel J. Keith, MD; Joanne B. Severe, MS; and Susan M. Matthews. The NIMH principal collaborators for the Adjunctive Lithium Trial are S. Charles Schulz, MD, and Carol L. Odbert. The principal investigators and coprincipal investigators at the 5 sites are as follows: John M. Kane, MD, Jeffrey A. Lieberman, MD, and Margaret Woerner, PhD (Albert Einstein School of Medicine and Hillside Hospital–Long Island Jewish Medical Center [UO1 MH39992]); Alan S. Bellack, PhD, and George M. Simpson, MD (Medical College of Pennsylvania and Eastern Pennsylvania Psychiatric Institute [UO1 MH39998]); Ira D. Glick, MD, and Allen J. Frances, MD (Cornell University Medical College and Payne Whitney Clinic [UO1 MH40007]); William A. Hargreaves, PhD, and Marc Jacobs, MD (University of California at San Francisco and San Francisco General Hospital [UO1 MH40042]); and Philip T. Ninan, MD, and Rosalind M. Mance, MD (Emory University and Grady Memorial Hospital [UO1 MH40597]). Consultants for applied family management are Ian R. H. Falloon, MD, Department of Psychiatry, University of New Zealand, Aukland, and Christine W. McGill, PhD, Palo Alto, Calif. We thank Franz Kulhanek, MD, Bristol-Myers Squibb GMBH, Munich, Germany, for his assistance in securing medication supplies.

Reprints: Nina R. Schooler, PhD, Western Psychiatric Institute and Clinic, 3811 O'Hara St, Pittsburgh, PA 15213.

REFERENCES

1. Kane J, Schooler NR, Marder SR, Simpson GM, Casey DE. Methods for clinical evaluation of pharmacologic treatments of schizophrenia. In: Prien RF, Robinson DS, eds. *Clinical Evaluation of Psychotropic Drugs.* New York, NY: Raven Press; 1994:345-372.
2. Davis JM. Overview: maintenance therapy in psychiatry, I: schizophrenia. *Am J Psychiatry.* 1975;132:1237-1245.
3. Schooler NR. Maintenance medication for schizophrenia: strategies for dose reduction. *Schizophr Bull.* 1991;17:311-324.
4. Kane JM, Marder SR. Psychopharmacologic treatment of schizophrenia. *Schizophr Bull.* 1993;19:287-302.
5. Goldstein MJ, Rodnick EH, Evans JR, May PRA, Steinberg MR. Drug and family therapy in the aftercare of acute schizophrenics. *Arch Gen Psychiatry.* 1978; 35:1169-1177.
6. Kane JM, Rifkin A, Woerner M, Reardon G, Sarantakos S, Schiebel D, Ramos-Lorenzi J. Low-dose neuroleptic treatment of outpatient schizophrenics. *Arch Gen Psychiatry.* 1983;40:893-896.
7. Kane JM, Rifkin A, Woerner M, Reardon G, Kreisman D, Blumenthal R, Borenstein M. High dose vs low dose strategies in the treatment of schizophrenia. *Psychopharmacol Bull.* 1985;21:533-537.
8. Kane JM, Woerner M, Sarantakos S. Depot neuroleptics: a comparative review of standard, intermediate, and low dose regimens. *J Clin Psychiatry.* 1986;47 (suppl):30-33.
9. Marder SR, Van Putten T, Mintz J, McKenzie J, Lebell M, Faltico G, May PRA. Costs and benefits of two doses of fluphenazine. *Arch Gen Psychiatry.* 1984; 41:1025-1029.
10. Marder SR, Van Putten T, Mintz J, Lebell M, McKenzie J, May PR. Low and conventional dose maintenance therapy with fluphenazine decanoate: two-year outcome. *Arch Gen Psychiatry.* 1987;44:518-521.
11. Johnson DAW, Ludlow JM, Street K, Taylor RDW. Double-blind comparison of half-dose and standard flupenthixol decanoate in the maintenance treatment of stabilized out-patients with schizophrenia. *Br J Psychiatry.* 1987;151:634-638.
12. Hogarty GE, McEvoy JP, Munetz M, DiBarry AL, Bartone P, Cather R, Cooley SJ, Ulrich RJ, Carter M, Madonia JM, Environmental/Personal Indicators in the Course of Schizophrenia Research Group. Dose of fluphenazine, familial expressed emotion, and outcome in schizophrenia. *Arch Gen Psychiatry.* 1988; 45:797-805.
13. Kane JM, Davis JM, Schooler NR, Marder SR, Brauzer B, Casey DE. A one-year comparison of four dosages of haloperidol decanoate. *Schizophr Res.* 1993;9:239-240.
14. Herz MI, Szymanski HV, Simon JC. Intermittent medication for stable schizophrenic outpatients: an alternative to maintenance medication. *Am J Psychiatry.* 1982;139:918-922.
15. Herz MI, Glazer WM, Mostert MA, Sheard MH, Szymanski HV, Hafez H, Mirza M, Vaha J. Intermittent vs maintenance medication in schizophrenia. *Arch Gen Psychiatry.* 1991;48:333-339.
16. Carpenter WT Jr, Hanlon TE, Heinrichs DW, Kirkpatrick B, Levine J, Buchanan RW. Continuous vs targeted medication in schizophrenic outpatients: outcome results. *Am J Psychiatry.* 1990;147:1138-1148.
17. Jolley AG, Hirsch SR, McRink A, Manchanda R. Trial of brief intermittent prophylaxis for selected schizophrenic outpatients: clinical outcome at one year. *BMJ.* 1989;298:985-990.
18. Jolley AG, Hirsch SR, Morrison E, McRink A. Trial of brief intermittent neuroleptic prophylaxis for selected schizophrenic outpatients: clinical and social outcome at two years. *BMJ.* 1990;301:837-842.
19. Pietzcker A, Gaebel W, Kopcke W. A German multi-center study on the neuroleptic long-term therapy of schizophrenic patients: preliminary report. *Pharmacopsychiatry.* 1986;19:161-166.
20. Pietzcker A, Gaebel W, Kopcke W, Linden M, Müller P, Müller-Spahn S, Tiegler J. Intermittent versus maintenance neuroleptic long-term treatment in schizophrenia: 2 year results of a German multicenter study. *J Psychiatr Res.* 1993; 27:321-339.
21. Keith SJ, Schooler NR. Psychosocial and psychotherapeutic strategies for long-term treatment of schizophrenia. In: Costa e Silva JA, Nadelson CC, eds. *International Review of Psychiatry.* Washington, DC: American Psychiatric Press Inc; 1993:229-262.
22. Bellack AS, Mueser KT. Psychosocial treatment for schizophrenia. *Schizophr Res.* 1993;19:317-336.
23. Schooler NR, Keith SJ, Severe JB, Matthews SM. Maintenance treatment of schizophrenia: a review of dose reduction and family management strategies. *Psychiatr Q.* 1995;66:279-292.
24. Falloon IRH, Boyd JL, McGill CW, Razani J, Moss HB, Gilderman AM. Family management in the prevention of exacerbations of schizophrenia. *N Engl J Med.* 1982;306:1437-1440.
25. Falloon IRH, Boyd J, McGill C, Williamson M, Razani J, Moss HG, Gilderman AM, Simpson GM. Family management in the prevention of morbidity of schizophrenia: clinical outcome of a two-year longitudinal study. *Arch Gen Psychiatry.* 1985;42:887-896.
26. Hogarty GE, Anderson CM, Reiss DJ, Kornblith SJ, Greenwald DP, Javna CD, Madonia MJ. Family psychoeducation, social skills training, and maintenance chemotherapy in the aftercare treatment of schizophrenia, I: one-year effects of a controlled study on relapse and expressed emotion. *Arch Gen Psychiatry.* 1986;43:633-642.
27. Hogarty GE, Anderson CM, Reiss DJ, Kornblith SJ, Greenwald DP, Ulrich RJ, Carter M, the Environmental-Personal Indicators in the Course of Schizophrenia (EPICS) Research Group. Family psychoeducation, social skills training, and maintenance chemotherapy in the aftercare treatment of schizophrenia, II: two-year effects of a controlled study on relapse and adjustment. *Arch Gen Psychiatry.* 1991;48:340-347.
28. Leff J, Kuipers L, Berkowitz R, Eberlein-Vries R, Sturgeon D. A controlled trial of social intervention in the families of schizophrenic patients. *Br J Psychiatry.* 1982;141:121-134.
29. Leff J, Kuipers L, Berkowitz R, Sturgeon D. A controlled trial of social intervention in the families of schizophrenic patients: two year follow-up. *Br J Psychiatry.* 1985;146:594-600.
30. Randolph ET, Eth S, Glynn S, Paz GB, Leong GB, Shaner AL, Strachan A, Van Vort W, Escobar J, Liberman RP. Behavioural family management in schizophrenia: outcome from a clinic-based intervention. *Br J Psychiatry.* 1994;144: 501-506.
31. Leff JP, Berkowitz R, Shavit N, Strachan A, Glass I, Vaughn C. A trial of family therapy versus a relatives' group for schizophrenia. *Br J Psychiatry.* 1989;154:58-66.
32. Leff J, Berkowitz R, Shavit N, Strachan A, Glass I, Vaughn C. A trial of family

therapy versus a relatives' group for schizophrenia: two-year follow-up. *Br J Psychiatry.* 1990;157:571-577.
33. McFarlane WR, Lukens E, Link B, Dushay R, Deakins SA, Dunne EJ, Horen B, Newmark M, Toran J. The multiple family group, psychoeducation, and maintenance medication in the treatment of schizophrenia. *Arch Gen Psychiatry.* 1995;52:679-687.
34. Tarrier N, Barrowclough C, Vaughn C, Bamrah JS, Porceddu K, Watts D, Freeman H. The community management of schizophrenia: a controlled trial of a behavioural intervention with families to reduce relapse. *Br J Psychiatry.* 1988; 153:532-542.
35. Tarrier N, Barrowclough C, Vaughn C, Bamrah JS, Porceddu K, Watts D, Freeman H. Community management of schizophrenia: a two-year follow-up of a behavioural intervention with families. *Br J Psychiatry.* 1989;154:625-628.
36. Zastowny TR, Lehman AF, Cole RE, Kane C. Family management of schizophrenia: a comparison of behavioral and supportive family treatment. *Psychiatr Q.* 1992;63:159-186.
37. Falloon IRH, Boyd JL, McGill CW. *Family Care for Schizophrenia: A Problem-Solving Approach to Mental Illness.* New York, NY: Guilford Press; 1984.
38. American Psychiatric Association. *Diagnostic and Statistical Manual of Mental Disorders, Third Edition, Revised.* Washington, DC: American Psychiatric Association; 1987.
39. Overall JE, Gorham DR. The Brief Psychiatric Rating Scale (BPRS). *Psychol Rep.* 1962;10:799-812.
40. Woerner MG, Mannuza S, Kane JM. Anchoring the BPRS: an aid to improved reliability. *Psychopharmacol Bull.* 1988;24:112-117.
41. Anderson CM, Reiss DJ, Hogarty G. *Schizophrenia in the Family.* New York, NY: Guilford Press; 1986.
42. Falloon IRH, McGill CW, Matthews SM, Keith SJ, Schooler NR. Family treatment for schizophrenia: the design and research application of therapist training models. *J Psychother Prac Res.* 1996;5:45-56.
43. Falloon I, Mueser K, Gingerich S, Rappaport S, McGill C, Hole V. *Behavioural Family Therapy: A Workbook.* Buckingham, England: Buckingham Mental Health Services; 1988.
44. Pocock SJ, Simon R. Sequential treatment assignment with balancing for prognostic factors in the controlled clinical trial. *Biometrics.* 1975;31:103-115.
45. White SJ, Freedman LS. Allocation of patients to treatment groups in a controlled clinical study. *Br J Cancer.* 1978;37:849-857.
46. Andreasen NC. *The Scale for the Assessment of Negative Symptoms (SANS).* Iowa City, Iowa: University of Iowa; 1983.
47. Mueser KT, Sayers SL, Schooler NR, Mance R, Haas GL. A multi-site investigation of the reliability of the Scale for the Assessment of Negative Symptoms. *Am J Psychiatry.* 1994;151:1453-1462.
48. Guy W. *EDCEU Assessment Manual for Psychopharmacology.* Rockville, Md: Dept of Health, Education and Welfare, National Institute of Mental Health; 1976. Publication (ADM)76-338.
49. Simpson GM, Angus JWS. Drug-induced extrapyramidal disorders. *Acta Psychiatr Scand.* 1970;212(suppl):17-19.
50. Herz MI, Melville C. Relapse in schizophrenia. *Am J Psychiatry.* 1980;137:801-805.
51. Cox DR, Oakes D. *Analysis of Survival Data.* London, England: Chapman & Hall; 1984.
52. Keith SJ, Bellack A, Frances A, Mance R, Matthews S, the Treatment Strategies in Schizophrenia Collaborative Study Group. The influence of diagnosis and family treatment on acute treatment response and short term outcome in schizophrenia. *Psychopharmacol Bull.* 1989;25:336-339.
53. Robinson D, Woerner M, Pollack S, Lerner G. Subject selection biases in clinical trials: data from a multicenter schizophrenia treatment study. *J Clin Psychopharmacol.* 1996;16:170-176.
54. Schooler NR, Keith SJ, Severe JB, Matthews S, the Treatment Strategies in Schizophrenia Collaborative Study Group. Acute treatment response and short term outcome in schizophrenia: first results of the NIMH Treatment Strategies in Schizophrenia Study. *Psychopharmacol Bull.* 1989;25:331-335.
55. Hargreaves WA, Kane JM, Ninan PT, Severe JB, Woerner M, the Treatment Strategies in Schizophrenia Collaborative Study Group. Demographic characteristics, treatment history, presenting psychopathology and early course in schizophrenia. *Psychopharmacol Bull.* 1989;25:340-343.
56. Glick ID, Jacobs M, Lieberman J, Simpson G, Schooler NR, the Treatment Strategies in Schizophrenia Collaborative Study Group. Prediction of short term outcome in schizophrenia: depressive symptoms, negative symptoms, and extrapyramidal signs. *Psychopharmacol Bull.* 1989;25:344-347.
57. Kane JM. Risperidone. *Am J Psychiatry.* 1994;151:802-803.
58. Marder SR, Meibach RC. Risperidone in the treatment of schizophrenia. *Am J Psychiatry.* 1994;151:825-835.

ORIGINAL ARTICLE

Backward Masking Performance in Unaffected Siblings of Schizophrenic Patients

Evidence for a Vulnerability Indicator

Michael F. Green, PhD; Keith H. Nuechterlein, PhD; Bruno Breitmeyer, PhD

Background: Visual masking is a procedure that is used to assess the earliest components of visual processing. In backward masking, the identification of an initial stimulus (the target) is disrupted by a later stimulus (the mask). The masking function can be divided into an early component (eg, up to about 60 ms) that reflects the involvement of sensory-perceptual processes, and a later component that reflects susceptibility to attentional disengagement as the mask diverts processing away from the representation of the target. Schizophrenic patients show anomalies on both masking components. It is not known whether backward masking deficits reflect enduring genetic vulnerability to schizophrenia.

Methods: We assessed 32 unaffected siblings of schizophrenic patients and 52 normal control subjects on the early and late components of 4 masking conditions. The conditions differentially involved the sustained and transient visual pathways.

Results: The unaffected siblings showed poorer overall performance than control subjects on the masking procedures. More specifically, siblings showed anomalies on the early, sensory-perceptual component, but not on the later, attentional disengagement component.

Conclusions: The backward masking performance deficits that have been observed in schizophrenic patients appear to reflect enduring vulnerability to the disorder rather than only the symptoms of the illness. This vulnerability appears to be associated with early, sensory-perceptual processes.

Arch Gen Psychiatry. 1997;54:465-472

SCHIZOPHRENIC patients experience difficulties in a broad range of neurocognitive domains, including relatively basic perceptual processes. The origins of these problems are rarely obvious; some may reflect underlying predisposition to the disorder whereas others may reflect the disruptive influence of psychiatric symptoms. Deciphering the origins of the deficits requires specialized designs and procedures.

The backward masking procedure is used to assess the earliest components of visual processing. In backward masking, a brief visual stimulus (the *target*) is followed in very rapid succession by a second stimulus (the *mask*). The interval between target offset and mask onset is called the *interstimulus interval* (ISI). Subjects are able to detect the target accurately when it is presented by itself. However, the additional presentation of the mask makes it harder to identify the target. Because the mask appears to work backward in time, the procedure is called "backward" masking.

Everyone experiences masking effects, but schizophrenic patients require a longer interval between target and mask (ie, a longer ISI) to identify the target.[1-6] This masking performance deficit does not seem to result from neuroleptic medication,[1] which appears to improve performance. Nor is poor performance strictly related to psychotic symptoms because deficits are found among nonpsychotic individuals who are hypothesized to be in the schizophrenia spectrum based on mild clinical symptoms or psychometric test results.[7-10]

Although masking performance is not related to psychotic symptoms, several studies have reported associations with negative symptoms.[2,11,12] Similarly, Braff[13] reported that patients with negative symptoms required a longer stimulus duration to detect the target compared with patients with predominantly psychotic symptoms. Even with this longer target duration, the patients with negative symptoms tended to have larger masking performance deficits than patients with predominantly psychotic symptoms. Besides nega-

From the Department of Psychiatry and Biobehavioral Sciences, University of California, Los Angeles (Drs Green and Nuechterlein); West Los Angeles Veterans Affairs Medical Center (Dr Green); the Department of Psychology, University of California, Los Angeles (Dr Nuechterlein); and the Department of Psychology, University of Houston, Houston, Tex (Dr Breitmeyer).

SUBJECTS AND METHODS

Written informed consent was obtained from all study participants. Forty-two siblings of schizophrenic patients participated in this project. A description of the patients and their masking data are presented elsewhere.[22,23] Siblings within a 128-km (80-mile) radius of the hospital were invited to participate. All siblings shared both biological parents with a proband. If more than 1 sibling was available, the one closest in age to the proband was invited to participate regardless of psychiatric history. Siblings received an expanded version of the Present State Examination[24] supplemented with sections of the Structured Clinical Interview for *DSM-III-R*[25] (SCID) and the Schedule for Schizophrenia and Affective Disorders.[26] The expanded Present State Examination assessed both current and lifetime conditions. In addition, the siblings received the sections on schizotypal and paranoid personality disorder from the SCID-II.[27]

We used 2 definitions of unaffected sibling because a key aim of this study was to determine whether backward masking deficits are indicators of genetic vulnerability to schizophrenia that are sometimes present even in the absence of any clinical psychiatric disorder. The first group excluded siblings who were considered to be in the schizophrenia spectrum because of a diagnosis of schizophrenia (n=2) or schizotypal or paranoid personality disorder (n=2). Recent studies of spectrum disorder in the families of probands have emphasized *DSM-III* and *DSM-III-R* schizotypal and paranoid personality disorder.[28] Second, to test the possibility that observed group differences were due to the presence of other psychiatric disorders among the siblings, we conducted an additional analysis with stricter selection criteria that excluded any sibling who would have been excluded from the control group. For this sample, we omitted siblings with a history of bipolar disorder (n=2) or substance dependence (n=4). These exclusions resulted in sample sizes of 38 and 32, respectively, for unaffected siblings. The latter group, selected with the stricter criteria, was 37.5% male; the mean (SD) age was 33.5 (7.1) years (range, 17-46 years) and the mean education level was 14.2 years.

The control subjects (n=52; 44% male) were drawn from the psychiatric technician training program at Camarillo State Hospital, Camarillo, Calif. They received the expanded Present State Examination and the sections of the SCID-II on schizotypal, paranoid, and borderline personality disorder. Their mean (SD) age was 33.0 (10.3) years (range, 20-55 years) and the mean education level was 13.8 years. Potential control subjects were excluded if they (1) had a history of drug or alcohol dependence, (2) had an acquired neurological disorder, (3) had a history of a seizure disorder, (4) met criteria for any of the personality disorders that were probed, or (5) had a history of any psychotic disorder, bipolar disorder, or more than 1 major depressive episode. In addition, to make the control subjects distinct from the siblings in genetic relationship to a person with schizophrenia, potential control subjects were excluded if they had a first-degree relative with a history of a psychotic disorder.

MASKING PROCEDURES

The subjects were tested on a 3-channel projection tachistoscope (model G1176, Gerbrand Corporation, Arlington, Mass). Subjects sat 1 m from a rear-projection screen and were presented with 1 of 4 letters (S, C, O, Q), which could appear at any 1 of 4 locations that were 2.2° of visual angle away from fixation (top, right, bottom, or left). Target letters subtended 0.3° of visual angle. The mask consisted of overlapping Xs and covered all of the possible target locations. The tester sat on the other side of the rear-projection screen and could ensure that the subject was looking at the screen during each trial. Luminance was determined with a light meter (Gossen Luna Pro, Gossen, Woodside, NY) held 1 m from the screen at eye level. Subjects were tested in a lighted room with ambient light at approximately 111 candelas per square meter (with a light diffuser). The target and mask displays (stimuli and background) were both presented at a luminance of approximately 732 cd/m^2 (without light diffuser) and the luminance of the stimuli alone was approximately 9.5 cd/m^2. The presentations (letters and locations) were randomized. A fixation point was presented for 400 ms and it ended 200 ms prior to the target presentation.

During practice, the target was presented without the mask at a duration of 10 ms. Subjects were required to identify the target on at least 8 of 10 trials, which was generally easy for them. Next, subjects practiced with both target and mask at an ISI of 100 ms, the longest interval within our masking functions, and an interval for which we did not expect much masking based on prior studies.[2] To ensure that the masking function was essentially complete at an ISI of 100 ms, subjects were required to correctly identify at least 4 of 5 targets at this ISI before proceeding with the test. If the subjects could not identify the target at criterion levels, the duration of the target was increased by 4-ms increments until subjects met the criterion. For the few subjects who required adjustment (2 siblings and 1 control), the duration of the mask was adjusted in the experimental conditions to maintain a constant target-mask ratio across subjects.

tive symptoms, poor masking performance has been associated with poor premorbid functioning,[14] poor prognosis,[3] and greater chronicity.[6]

Although the deficits in masking performance have been well documented in schizophrenic patients, fundamental questions remain unanswered. While masking performance deficits have been hypothesized to be indicators of vulnerability to schizophrenia,[15] empirical support for this view is limited. Two types of designs are typically used to provide evidence for vulnerability indicators: studies of first-degree relatives of patients and studies of patients' performance when they are in symptomatic remission. We are aware of only one study of masking performance in remitted schizophrenic patients.[15] In that study, 10 remitted patients showed deficits compared with 10 matched control subjects, suggesting that masking performance might be an indicator of vulnerability to schizophrenia. However, the degree of remission was unclear because the remitted patients were medicated and exhibiting poor social functioning.

To our knowledge, there have been no published studies of masking in first-degree relatives of schizophrenic patients. If a masking anomaly is truly an indicator of genetic vulnerability to schizophrenia, a disproportionate

Four masking conditions used in our previous studies of schizophrenic patients[19,20] were administered in a counterbalanced order across subjects. The masking functions differentially emphasize the sustained or transient visual channels. For the 3 target identification conditions, the ISIs were set at 5, 10, 20, 40, 70, and 100 ms. The ISIs for the target location condition, which has a compressed masking function, were set at 5, 10, 15, 20, 30, and 50 ms. Twelve targets were presented at each ISI. Both the targets and the ISIs were presented in a block-randomized fashion with the constraint that the same ISI could not be presented twice in succession. This constraint eliminated the possibility that any performance differences were due to redundancy-associated deficits.[29] The conditions included:

1. *Target identification with a high-energy mask.* This condition requires the identification of a clearly focused target that involves high spatial frequency information and, consequently, relies on sustained channels. The energy of the mask in this condition is greater than the energy of the target. The term "energy" in this context refers to the light intensity × the duration of a stimulus. A high-energy mask typically generates a masking function in which the masking effect gradually decreases (ie, performance gradually increases) as the ISIs become longer. In this condition, the energy of the mask was twice the energy of the target (20 ms for a 10-ms target).

2. *Target identification with a low-energy mask.* This condition also involves the identification of a clearly focused target and relies on sustained channels. It was designed to generate a masking function in which performance does not regularly increase as the ISIs become longer (eg, U-shaped). A U-shaped function indicates that maximal masking occurred when the transient channels of the mask inhibited the sustained channels of the target. In this condition, the energy of the mask was one half the energy of the target (eg, 5 ms for a 10-ms target).

3. *Target identification of blurred target.* This condition used an identification task in which the target was blurred. Sustained visual pathways are sensitive to high spatial frequencies; blurring the target reduces high spatial frequency information and consequently reduces reliance on sustained channels while increasing reliance on transient channels. The target was blurred to a standardized degree by changing the lens-to-screen distance from 95 cm to 107.5 cm (which defocuses the stimuli), and then refocusing the mask but not the target. As a by-product of blurring, the visual discrimination became more difficult. To obtain performance comparable to the low-energy condition and to prevent floor effects, the duration of the target was doubled (eg, from 10-20 ms) and the duration of the mask was one fourth the duration of the target (eg, 5 ms for a 20-ms target).

4. *Target location.* For this condition, subjects stated the location of a focused target (up, down, left, right), but did not need to identify it. To reduce any confusion, a response card was placed in front of the subject, displaying the 4 possible responses in their respective spatial locations. For briefly presented stimuli, such as those in this study, transient channels convey information about the location of objects. Hence, this task was intended to rely largely on transient channels. Locating is generally easier than identifying a target. To prevent a ceiling effect, the target-mask ratio was 1:1 (eg, 10 ms for both target and mask). The transient channels have a shorter latency than sustained channels, so the sampling of ISIs was compressed and included 5, 10, 15, 20, 30, and 50 ms (12 targets at each ISI).

STATISTICAL ANALYSIS

Data from the 4 masking conditions were analyzed in a 2 (group) by 4 (condition) by 6 (ISI) (2×4×6) multivariate analysis of variance. The primary question was whether the unaffected siblings would show abnormalities in masking performance as evidenced by a main effect for group. In addition, we considered 2 more specific questions. The first question was whether the groups showed differential performance on the early vs later aspects of the masking function. For this, a separate analysis was conducted across conditions to test for a group by temporal position interaction in which the first 4 ISIs (early) were contrasted with the last 2 ISIs (late). Second, we considered whether the groups would be differentially affected by the manipulations of the relative activity in transient and sustained visual channels. The groups were compared on the 2 conditions that relied on sustained channels (identification of focused targets with high- and low-energy masks) vs the 2 conditions that restricted the role of sustained visual channels (blurred target and location). For all tests, the significance level was set at .05, 2 tailed.

Two sets of analyses with unaffected siblings were conducted, one with only the schizophrenia spectrum siblings excluded, and one that also excluded siblings with disorders that would have led to exclusion from the control group. A parallel set of analyses with all siblings was done as a cross-check to determine whether the results would be changed by the inclusion of siblings who may be genetically prone and also affected. Because the results for the 3 sets of analyses were essentially the same, we report the findings from the most strictly defined unaffected group.

number of the first-degree relatives of patients would be expected to show performance deficits compared with control subjects, even without any signs of illness. This prediction is based on the fact that first-degree relatives are more likely to carry a genetic predisposition to the disorder than the general population. However, only a minority of vulnerable individuals actually develop the disorder, depending on the degree of vulnerability, psychological coping mechanisms, and compensatory biological and neurodevelopmental processes.[16-18]

Masking procedures are well suited for isolating rather specific visual processes. Masking performance includes 2 primary components, early and late. The early part of the masking function (ie, ISIs roughly less than 60 ms) reflects *sensory-perceptual* processes.[19,20] Masking performance at these short ISIs is determined primarily by the interaction of sustained and transient visual pathways. In contrast, the later part of the masking function (roughly greater than 70 ms) does not rely primarily on the interactions of sensory pathways. It reflects a susceptibility to *attentional disengagement.* The masking effect at these later intervals indicates that the mask has diverted attention away from the representation of the target.[20,21] **Figure 1** illustrates a model of the masking

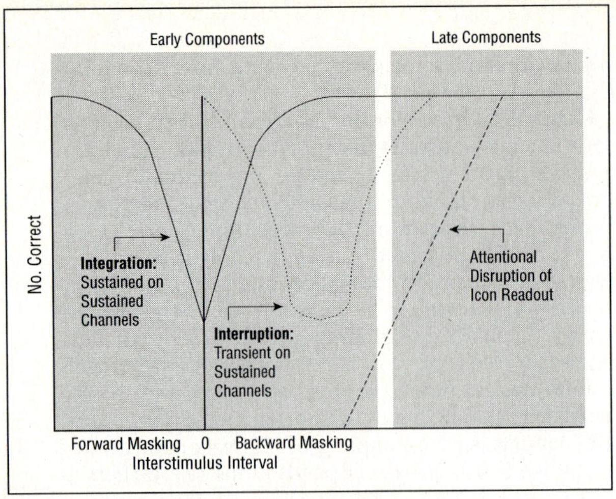

Figure 1. *Model of the components of a backward masking function. The figure shows hypothetical processes that underlie backward masking functions. The early masking processes (integration and interruption) are sensory-perceptual components and rely on the interactions of transient and sustained visual channels. The later component does not rely directly on the interactions of sensory pathways. It reflects an attentional disengage component in which attention is diverted away from the target by the mask. Adapted with permission from Michaels and Turvey.*[21]

components adapted from Michaels and Turvey.[21] Such a fine-grained analysis of specific processes that underlie masking performance may allow isolation of the specific neurocognitive abnormalities that indicate vulnerability to schizophrenia.[14]

Schizophrenic patients show anomalies on both the early and the later components of the masking function. We hypothesized, based on work from our laboratory and from others, that deficits on the early, sensory-perceptual aspects of masking may reflect overactive transient channels.[22,23] The anomalies on the later component may indicate that patients either are unusually susceptible to disengagement from the target or have unusual difficulty in re-engaging target processing after presentation of the mask.

The present study examined whether unaffected full siblings of schizophrenic patients differ from normal control subjects in backward masking performance. In addition, the current study considered whether the unaffected siblings of patients show masking abnormalities in one or both of the masking components. Finally, we tested the possibility that siblings are differentially affected by the masking conditions that minimize sustained channel activity and maximize transient channel activity. This study explored these questions with 4 masking conditions used in our previous studies with schizophrenic patients.[22,23]

RESULTS

The main effect for group was significant ($F[1,81]=6.92$, $P=.01$), indicating that the unaffected siblings of schizophrenic patients showed performance deficits across conditions compared with control subjects. The main effects of condition ($F[3,79]=38.37$, $P<.001$) and ISI ($F[5,77]=367.51$, $P<.001$) were also significant. The group × ISI interaction was significant ($F[5,77]=2.84$, $P=.02$), indicating that the groups showed nonparallel masking functions across conditions. The results for all 4 masking conditions are displayed in **Figure 2** through **Figure 5**.

A contrast was conducted to compare the 2 groups on early vs late masking components across conditions. This analysis revealed a significant group × temporal position (early vs late) interaction ($F[1,81]=7.29$, $P<.01$). Examination of the figures indicates that the siblings departed from the control subjects in the early, sensory-perceptual parts of the masking function, but the 2 groups converged at the later component of the function. This pattern appeared in each of the masking conditions, although the group contrasts were not significant for the low-energy mask condition.

Figure 6 through **Figure 8** show the frequency distributions of scores for the early masking component from the 3 masking conditions in which the groups differed significantly. A normal curve was fit to the data from the control subjects and the unaffected siblings. Data for the affected siblings were included, but were too sparse to fit with a normal curve. In general, the distribution for the siblings appears to be shifted to the left, with no obvious bimodality.

Next, we contrasted the 2 conditions that relied on high-spatial-frequency-sustained channels (high- and low-energy mask) to those that limited the role of sustained channels and increased the role of transient channels (blurred target and location). The group × condition interaction showed a directional tendency, but did not reach significance ($F=2.39[1,81]$, $P<.15$). The siblings tended to show a larger difference from control subjects in the 2 conditions that restricted sustained (and emphasized transient) visual channels. The 3-way interaction for group × ISI (early vs late) × type of condition (emphasizing vs deemphasizing sustained channels) was nonsignificant.

The finding that the groups differed at the early, but not the late, components of the masking function is intriguing, but could be due to an artifact. If the trials with longer ISIs were too easy for the subjects, a ceiling effect could obscure group differences at these ISIs. The nonlinear shapes of the masking functions argue against, but do not rule out, such an interpretation. We tested this possibility more directly by selecting points (1 early and 1 late) at which the performance of control subjects was comparable in terms of mean level and internal consistency (coefficient α). If the groups differ on 1 ISI and not the other, it cannot be easily explained by a ceiling effect. For the high-energy mask condition, control subjects performed comparably at the 20- and 70-ms ISIs (means, 10.2 and 11.0; coefficient α, 0.62 and 0.60 for the 20- and 70-ms ISIs, respectively). The groups differed substantially at the early ($P=.001$) but not the later ($P=.35$) ISI. For the location condition, control subjects performed comparably at ISIs of 20 and 50 ms (means, 11.2 and 11.6; coefficient α, 0.60 and 0.68 for 20- and 50-ms ISIs, respectively). Again, the groups differed at the early ($P=.01$) but not the later ($P=.23$) ISI. These results, although not definitive, suggest that the findings of significant group differences for early, but not late, components of the masking function are not simply due to psychometric artifact.

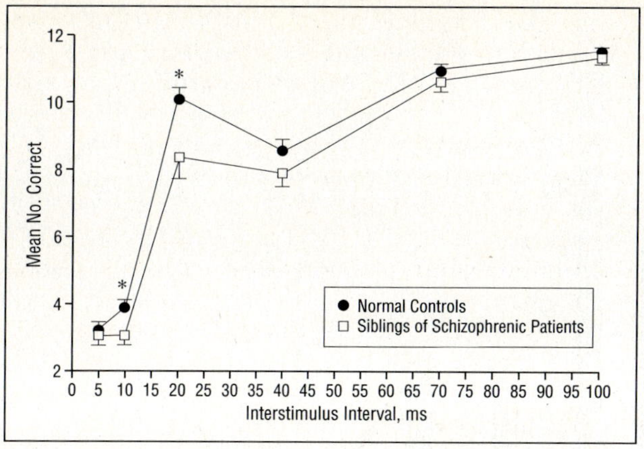

Figure 2. *Results for unaffected siblings of schizophrenic patients and control subjects on an identification masking task with a high-energy mask. The energy of the mask was twice that of the target. Asterisk indicates* P<.025.

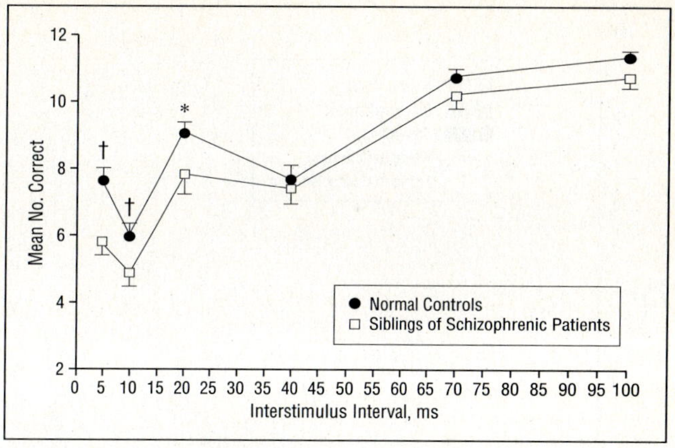

Figure 4. *Results for unaffected siblings of schizophrenic patients and control subjects on an identification masking task with a blurred target. The energy of the mask was one fourth that of the target. Asterisk indicates* P<.05; *dagger,* P<.025.

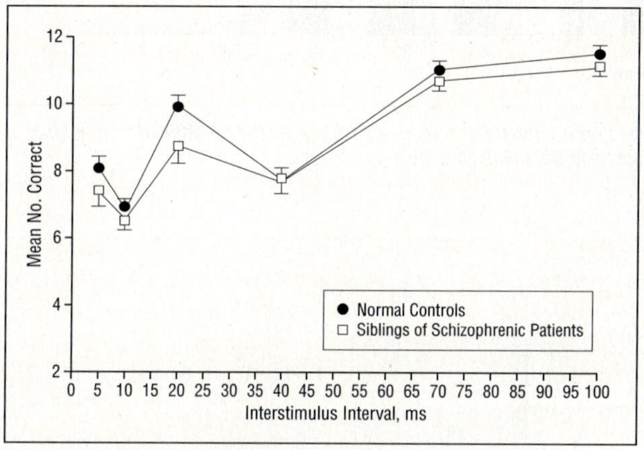

Figure 3. *Results for unaffected siblings of schizophrenic patients and control subjects on an identification masking task with a low-energy mask. The energy of the mask was one half that of the target.*

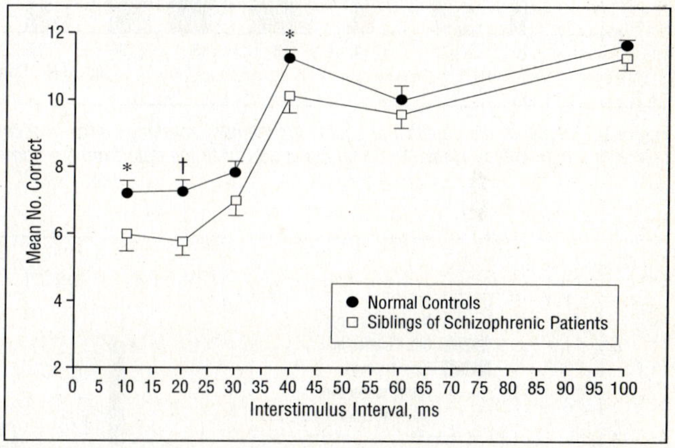

Figure 5. *Results for unaffected siblings of schizophrenic patients and control subjects on a location masking task with a focused target. The energy of the mask was equal to that of the target. Asterisk indicates* P<.05; *dagger,* P<.025.

COMMENT

These results suggest that certain anomalies of visual masking in schizophrenia reflect vulnerability to the disorder as opposed to the symptoms of the illness. To our knowledge, this is the first study to demonstrate visual masking deficits in biological relatives of schizophrenic probands. Our results indicate that unaffected siblings of schizophrenic patients have deficits, in comparison with control subjects, on the early component of the masking function, suggesting that altered sensory-perceptual processes may be relevant to genetic vulnerability to schizophrenia. In contrast, sibling performance appears intact on the later component of the masking function, which has been hypothesized to involve disengagement of attention from the target. Analyses with and without affected siblings produced essentially the same results. Although the similarity in results may be attributable to the relatively small number of affected siblings, it is also consistent with the hypothesized pattern for a stable vulnerability indicator,[17] which remains constant across clinical states.

The actual rate of schizophrenia in the sibling group (4.8%) is entirely consistent with the rates of morbid risk (age corrected) for schizophrenia in first-degree relatives reported in other studies (1.4%-6.5%[28]). The rate of spectrum personality disorders (also 4.8%) is at the low end of a range for studies that have assessed paranoid and schizotypal personality disorder in first-degree relatives (2.8%-30.0%; median, 8.2%[28]).

The finding that the later, attentional disengagement mechanism, was not associated with vulnerability to schizophrenia might at first glance appear inconsistent with other studies that have documented attentional deficits in the first-degree relatives of schizophrenic patients.[30,31] Performance on this component depends on how well subjects resist disengaging from the target, or how easily they reengage the target. This type of attentional process differs from other types of attention, such as vigilance, which have been the primary focus of studies with first-degree relatives.

Vigilance (or sustained focused attention) is often measured by tests such as the continuous performance test (CPT) that assess the subject's ability to respond

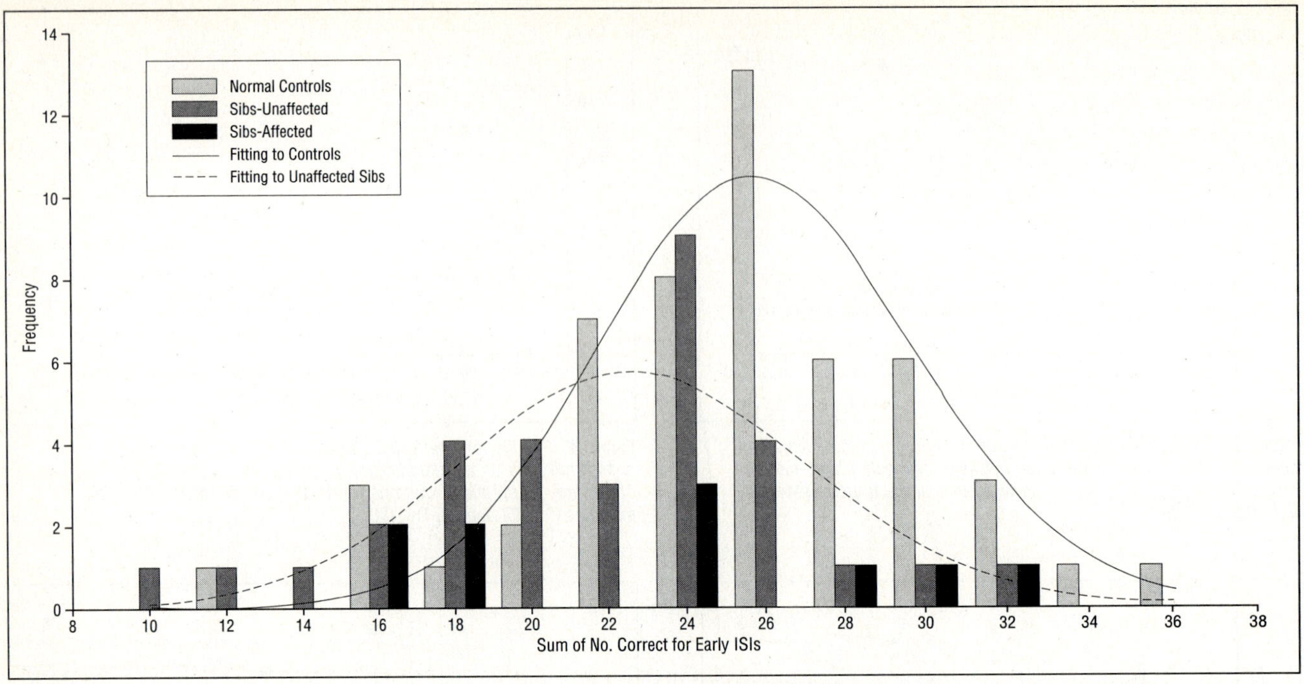

Figure 6. *Frequency distributions of scores for the early masking component (sum of the first 4 interstimulus intervals [ISIs]) on the identification masking task with a high-energy mask. A normal curve was fit to the data from the control subjects and the unaffected siblings.*

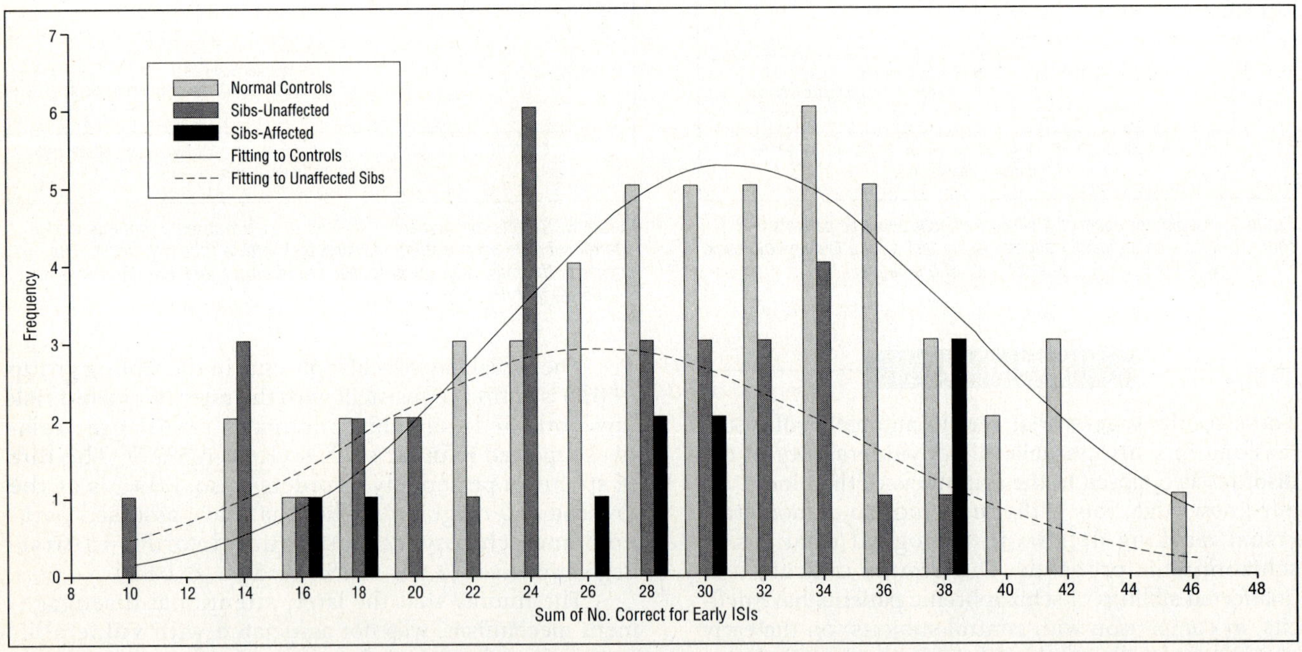

Figure 7. *Frequency distributions of scores for the early masking component (sum of the first 4 interstimulus intervals [ISIs]) on the identification masking task with a blurred target. A normal curve was fit to the data from the control subjects and the unaffected siblings.*

to targets over time. Deficits in the CPT have been found among first-degree relatives of schizophrenic patients[30-33] and among patients who are in remission.[34] Findings with the CPT have sometimes been interpreted to mean that sustained attention deficits reflect vulnerability to schizophrenia. An alternative possibility, noted by Nuechterlein et al,[35] is that at least some CPT deficits may involve early perceptual processes. The CPT stimuli are presented tachistoscopically and involve relatively poor perceptual images, a quality further emphasized with degraded stimuli.[32] Perhaps one vulnerability factor for schizophrenia revealed by the CPT is not sustained attention per se, but instead a sensory-perceptual process that is also relevant to backward masking.

Indirect evidence from family studies supports such a reformulation. First-degree relatives do not generally show abnormalities in their performance

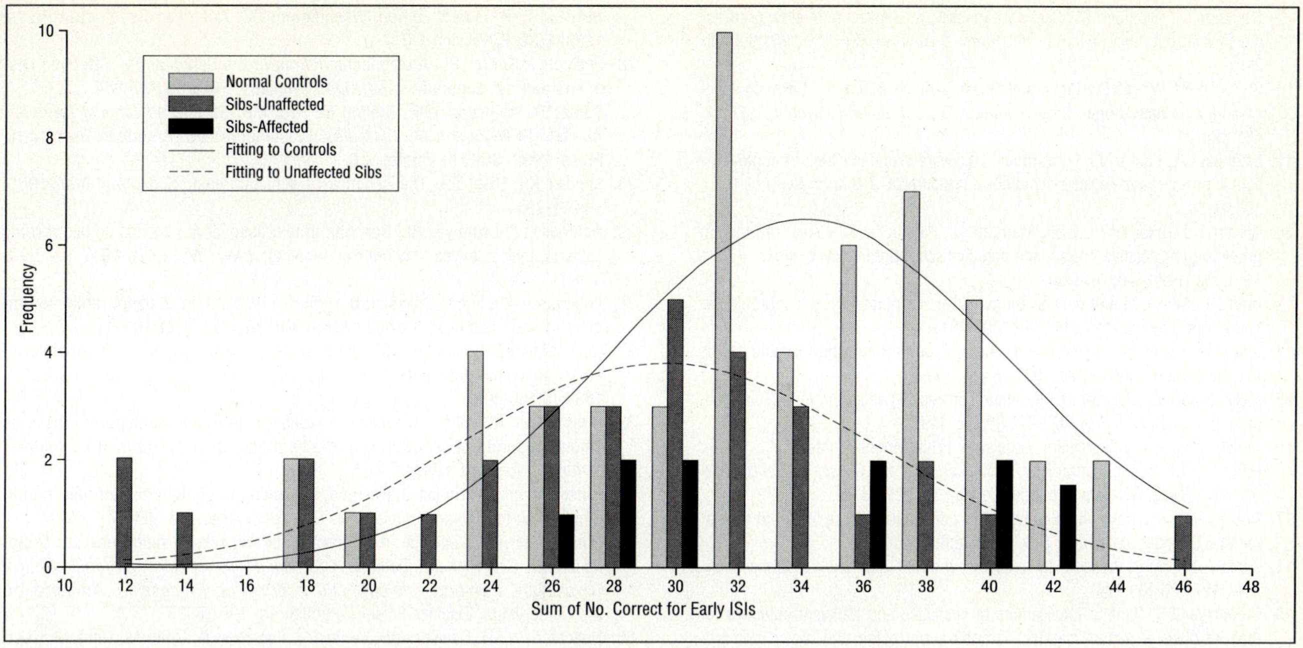

Figure 8. *Frequency distributions of scores for the early masking component (sum of the first 4 interstimulus intervals [ISIs]) on the location masking task with a focused target. A normal curve was fit to the data from the control subjects and the unaffected siblings.*

decrement from beginning to end of a vigilance task. Instead, they differ from controls in their ability to separate signal stimuli from noise stimuli throughout the task, which involves sensory-perceptual processes in tachistoscopic tasks.[36]

An underlying problem in dopamine dysregulation at the level of the retina might provide a neurochemical explanation for abnormalities in the early components of visual processing[37] because there is dopaminergic activation of the retinal amacrine cells.[38] Although such a retinal process is unlikely to last as long as 60 to 70 ms after stimulus presentation, retinal dopaminergic cells might contribute to an initial disruption of visual processing.

The 2 major conclusions from this study are that (1) backward masking holds promise as an indicator of vulnerability to schizophrenia and (2) the early, sensory-perceptual component of visual masking is most closely associated with vulnerability. Other neurocognitive measures have previously been linked to vulnerability, but masking procedures have an advantage in that they help to isolate particular subcomponents of neurocognitive processes associated with vulnerability. Masking procedures lend themselves to a program of experimental reductivism that attempts to identify the smallest meaningful units that make up a more complex behavior.[39] By parsing neurocognition in this way, we can develop more precise models of the nature of vulnerability to schizophrenia and also develop a more complete picture of the phenotypic expression of schizophrenia that is separate from the symptoms of the illness.

Accepted for publication July 10, 1996.

Funding for this project came from grant MH-43292 from the National Institute of Mental Health, Rockville, Md (Dr Green).

The authors thank Maryam Aslani, David Chavez, Cynthia Christenson, Donna Gaier, Daniel Gutkind, Robert Kern, PhD, David King, PhD, Susan G. Hellman, Sharon Mitchell, MA, Chad Nelson, Julie Van Sickle, MA, and Jennifer Smith for their help in subject recruitment and data collection. Kimmy Kee, PhD, and Mary Jane Robertson, MS, helped with the preparation of the manuscript. The statistical analyses were conducted by Sun Hwang, MS, MPH, of the Methodology and Statistical Support Unit of the UCLA Clinical Research Center for the Study of Schizophrenia. The patients were obtained through the excellent cooperation of the staff and administration of Camarillo State Hospital.

Reprints: Michael F. Green, PhD, UCLA Neuropsychiatric Institute, 760 Westwood Plaza, C9-420, Los Angeles, CA 90024-1759.

REFERENCES

1. Braff DL, Saccuzzo DP. Effect of antipsychotic medication on speed of information processing in schizophrenic patients. *Am J Psychiatry.* 1982;139:1117-1130.
2. Green M, Walker E. Symptom correlates of vulnerability to backward masking in schizophrenia. *Am J Psychiatry.* 1986;143:181-186.
3. Saccuzzo DP, Braff DL. Early information processing deficit in schizophrenia. *Arch Gen Psychiatry.* 1981;38:175-179.
4. Saccuzzo DP, Braff DL. Information-processing abnormalities. *Schizophr Bull.* 1986;12:447-459.
5. Schwartz BD, Winstead DK, Adinoff B. Temporal integration deficit in visual information processing by chronic schizophrenics. *Biol Psychiatry.* 1983;18:1311-1320.
6. Rund BR. Backward-masking performance in chronic and nonchronic schizophrenics, affectively disturbed patients, and normal control subjects. *J Abnorm Psychol.* 1993;102:74-81.
7. Braff DL. Impaired speed of information processing in non-medicated schizotypal patients. *Schizophr Bull.* 1981;7:499-508.
8. Merritt RD, Balogh DW. The use of a backward masking paradigm to assess information-processing deficits among schizotypics: a re-evaluation of Steronko and Woods. *J Nerv Ment Dis.* 1984;172:216-224.

9. Saccuzzo DP, Schubert DL. Backward masking as a measure of slow processing in schizophrenia spectrum disorders. *J Abnorm Psychol.* 1981;90:305-312.
10. Steronko RJ, Woods DJ. Impairment in early stages of visual information processing in nonpsychotic schizotypic individuals. *J Abnorm Psychol.* 1978;87:481-490.
11. Slaghuis WL, Bakker VJ. Forward and backward visual masking of contour by light in positive- and negative-symptom schizophrenia. *J Abnorm Psychol.* 1995;104:41-54.
12. Weiner RU, Opler LA, Kay SR, Merriam AE, Papouchis N. Visual information processing in positive, mixed, and negative schizophrenic syndromes. *J Nerv Ment Dis.* 1990;178:616-626.
13. Braff DL. Sensory input deficits and negative symptoms in schizophrenic patients. *Am J Psychiatry.* 1989;146:1006-1011.
14. Knight R. Specifying cognitive deficiencies in premorbid schizophrenics. *Prog Exp Pers Psychopathol Res.* 1992;15:252-289.
15. Miller S, Saccuzzo D, Braff D. Information processing deficits in remitted schizophrenics. *J Abnorm Psychol.* 1979;88:446-449.
16. Nuechterlein KH. Vulnerability models for schizophrenia: state of the art. In: Hafner H, Gattaz WF, Janzarik W, eds. *Search for the Causes of Schizophrenia.* Heidelberg, Germany: Springer-Verlag; 1987:297-316.
17. Nuechterlein KH, Dawson ME. A heuristic vulnerability/stress model of schizophrenic episodes. *Schizophr Bull.* 1984;10:300-312.
18. Zubin J, Spring B. Vulnerability: a new view of schizophrenia. *J Abnorm Psychol.* 1977;86:103-126.
19. Breitmeyer BG, Ganz L. Implications of sustained and transient channels for theories of visual pattern masking, saccadic suppression, and information processing. *Psychol Rev.* 1976;83:1-36.
20. Breitmeyer BG. *Visual Masking: An Integrative Approach.* New York, NY: Oxford University Press; 1984.
21. Michaels CF, Turvey MT. Central sources of visual masking: indexing structures supporting seeing at a single, brief glance. *Psychol Res.* 1979;41:1-61.
22. Green MF, Nuechterlein KH, Mintz J. Backward masking in schizophrenia and mania, I: specifying a mechanism. *Arch Gen Psychiatry.* 1994;51:939-944.
23. Green MF, Nuechterlein KH, Mintz J. Backward masking in schizophrenia and mania, II: specifying the visual channels. *Arch Gen Psychiatry.* 1994;51:945-951.
24. Wing JK, Cooper JE, Sartorius N. *The Measurement and Classification of Psychiatric Symptoms.* London, England: Cambridge University Press; 1974.
25. Spitzer RL, Williams JBW, Gibbon M, First MB. *Structured Clinical Interview for* DSM-III-R*–Patient Edition.* Washington, DC: American Psychiatric Press; 1990. SCID-P, Version 1.0.
26. Endicott J, Spitzer RL. A diagnostic interview: the Schedule for Affective Disorders and Schizophrenia. *Arch Gen Psychiatry.* 1978;35:837-844.
27. Spitzer RL, Williams JBW, Gibbon M, First MB. *Structured Clinical Interview for* DSM-III-R*–Personality Disorders.* Washington, DC: American Psychiatric Press; 1990. SCID-II, Version 1.0.
28. Kendler KS, Diehl SR. The genetics of schizophrenia. *Schizophr Bull.* 1993;19:261-285.
29. DeAmicis LA, Cromwell RL. Reaction time crossover in process schizophrenic patients, their relatives, and control subjects. *J Nerv Ment Dis.* 1977;167:593-600.
30. Erlenmeyer-Kimling L, Cornblatt B. High risk research in schizophrenia: a summary of what has been learned. *J Psychiatr Res.* 1987;21:401-411.
31. Nuechterlein KH, Dawson ME. Information processing and attentional functioning in the developmental course of schizophrenic disorders. *Schizophr Bull.* 1984;10:160-203.
32. Nuechterlein KH. Signal detection in vigilance tasks and behavioral attributes among offspring of schizophrenic mothers and among hyperactive children. *J Abnorm Psychol.* 1983;92:4-28.
33. Rutschmann J, Cornblatt B, Erlenmeyer-Kimling L. Sustained attention in children at risk for schizophrenia. *Arch Gen Psychiatry.* 1977;34:571-575.
34. Nuechterlein KH. Vigilance in schizophrenia and related disorders. In: Steinhauer SR, Gruzelier JH, Zubin J, eds. *Handbook of Schizophrenia: Neuropsychology, Psychophysiology, and Information Processing.* Amsterdam, the Netherlands: Elsevier Science Publishers; 1991;5.
35. Nuechterlein KH, Dawson ME, Ventura J, Fogelson D, Gitlin M, Mintz J. Testing vulnerability models: stability of potential vulnerability indicators across clinical state. In: Hafner H, Gattaz WF, eds. *Search for the Causes of Schizophrenia.* Heidelberg, Germany: Springer-Verlag; 1991;2:177-191.
36. Nuechterlein KH, Dawson ME, Green MF. Information-processing abnormalities as neuropsychological vulnerability indicators for schizophrenia. *Acta Psychiatr Scand.* 1994;90:71-79.
37. Maguire G, Hamasaki DI. The retinal dopamine network alters the adaptational properties of retinal ganglion cells in the cat. *J Neurophysiol.* 1994;72:730-741.
38. Schwartz BD, Evans WJ, Pena JM, Winstead DK. Visible persistence decay rates for schizophrenics and substance abusers. *Biol Psychiatry.* 1994;36:662-669.
39. Holzman PS. Parsing cognition: the power of psychology paradigms. *Arch Gen Psychiatry.* 1994;51:952-954.

ORIGINAL ARTICLE

Thought Disorder in Schizophrenic and Control Adoptees and Their Relatives

Dennis K. Kinney, PhD; Philip S. Holzman, PhD; Bjørn Jacobsen, MD; Lennart Jansson, MD; Britta Faber, MD; Wera Hildebrand, PhD; Eva Kasell; Morris E. Zimbalist

Background: Previous research showed significantly elevated levels of thought disorder in the relatives of persons with schizophrenia, as well as in the persons with schizophrenia themselves. Comparisons of schizophrenic and control adoptees and their respective relatives provide a method for minimizing the confounding of genetic and environmental sources of familial resemblance and for elucidating whether the elevated levels of thought disorder in persons with schizophrenia and their relatives reflect the influence of shared genetic factors, shared environmental factors, or both. The present study provides the first such adoption-sample data on an operationally defined measure of thought disorder.

Methods: Speech samples elicited by standard interview questions from schizophrenic and control adoptees and their respective biological and adoptive relatives were tape-recorded. Verbatim transcripts of these speech samples were scored, while unaware of the personal or family diagnoses of the subjects, using the Thought Disorder Index (TDI).

Results: The mean TDI scores were significantly higher in schizophrenic than in control adoptees and in biological relatives of the schizophrenic adoptees than in the biological relatives of the control adoptees, whereas the respective groups of adoptive relatives did not differ significantly. The differences were most marked for the samples of biological sibs and half sibs, which were larger and more representative than the samples of parents.

Conclusion: Results suggest that the elevated TDI scores in the relatives of persons with schizophrenia that have been found in other studies reflect the operation of genes increasing the liability for schizophrenia, rather than the rearing experiences that were shared in common with schizophrenic probands.

Arch Gen Psychiatry. 1997;54:475-479

THOUGHT DISORDER has long been considered a cardinal feature of schizophrenia. Kraepelin,[1] for example, described disordered thought processes in persons with schizophrenia as "derailments." Bleuler[2,3] deemed "loosening of associations" a key feature of schizophrenic thinking—and also a pathologic feature of a latent form of schizophrenia often found in the biological relatives of persons with schizophrenia. Meehl[4,5] suggested that mild thought disorder, or "cognitive slippage," was a core form of psychiatric dysfunction found in "schizotypic" individuals who, although not schizophrenic, carried genetic liability for schizophrenia.

Numerous subsequent studies have reported elevated rates of disordered thinking in persons with schizophrenia, as well as in patients with other disorders, such as organic brain diseases and affective psychoses.[6-16] Evidence from these studies confirming the importance of thought disorder in schizophrenia has prompted the development of objective scales for measuring thought disorder, including the Scale for the Assessment of Thought, Language, and Communication developed by Andreasen,[17,18] a scale developed by Harrow and Quinlan[19] and Marengo et al,[20] and the Thought Disorder Index, or TDI.[13,16,21,22]

The TDI offers a number of advantages for studying thought disorder in persons with schizophrenia and their families. The TDI provides a standard method for scoring thought disorder, with multiple indications of reliability and validity. It was designed to assess a broad range of deficits and dysfunction in various aspects of thinking. It provides clear operational definitions and scoring guidelines, with examples of 4 different levels of severity on each of 23 different categories of thought disturbance (eg, incoherent or confused thinking, neologisms, and pe-

From the Department of Psychiatry, Harvard Medical School, Boston, Mass (Drs Kinney and Holzman); the Laboratories for Psychiatric Research (Drs Kinney and Hildebrand, Ms Kasell, and Mr Zimbalist) and the Psychology Research Laboratory (Dr Holzman), McLean Hospital, Belmont, Mass; the Department of Psychology, Harvard University, Cambridge, Mass (Dr Holzman); and the Institute of Preventive Medicine, Copenhagen Hospital Corporation, Copenhagen, Denmark (Drs Jacobsen, Jansson, and Faber).

SUBJECTS AND METHODS

SUBJECTS

Subjects were drawn from a large comprehensive sample of adopted persons with schizophrenia (the *index probands*) and adopted control probands, along with their respective adoptive and biological relatives, who were all previously ascertained by Kety et al.[27,31-33] This systematic sample consisted of all persons with schizophrenia born in Denmark between 1924 and 1947 and subsequently adopted at an early age by parents to whom they were not biologically related. For each index proband, a *control proband* with no record of psychiatric hospitalization was selected and matched with the index proband for age, sex, socioeconomic status of the adoptive home, and age at placement with adoptive parents. Most probands were separated from their biological parents shortly after birth and had little or no subsequent contact with the biological relatives. Subjects in the study are from the "provincial" subsample, consisting of probands adopted through courts outside greater Copenhagen, along with their respective biological and adoptive parents, sibs, and half sibs. All probands and relatives 18 years old or older and residing in Scandinavia were invited to participate; more than 88% agreed to be interviewed.

Subjects were first interviewed by 1 of 2 Danish psychiatrists, using a standard schedule that included the Schedule for Affective Disorders and Schizophrenia—Lifetime Version of Spitzer and Endicott.[34] Subjects were then asked to answer 4 standard questions, and their responses were recorded with a high-fidelity audiotape recorder. The first question followed the standard procedure used by Gottschalk and Gleser[35] (which asks subjects to talk about an interesting or dramatic life experience) to elicit speech samples for content analysis. Three other questions, selected after pilot testing, asked subjects for their views on various topics affecting Danish society. Most subjects were tape-recorded the day they were interviewed, and all were taped within several months of being interviewed. All subjects were white. The mean±SD ages of the schizophrenic (44.2±6.4 years) and control (43.3±5.3 years) probands with valid speech samples were similar. The Pearson product-moment correlation of the ages of the subjects with TDI scores was not statistically significant for the probands (r=0.08) or for any other subject groups (r=0.09 for biological relatives; 0.17 for adoptive relatives).

SPEECH SAMPLES

Several steps were used to keep those who obtained, transcribed, and scored the interviews and speech samples unaware of the index or control group status of the subjects. For example, scheduling of subjects was arranged so that the relatives of the probands were typically interviewed by investigators different from those who interviewed the proband.

The tape-recorded responses of the subjects were transcribed verbatim in Danish by a native Dane who was fluent in English and Danish. The typed transcript was then proofread by a second bilingual Dane who compared the tape and transcript for accuracy and deleted any potentially biasing information. Photocopies of this edited transcript were then distributed to the raters.

SCORING OF THOUGHT DISORDER

Before rating the Danish transcripts, the raters (W.H. and E.K.) were trained by 1 of the other authors (P.S.H.) until they were proficient in scoring the TDI with English samples. Both raters were native Danes fluent in English and Danish and had graduate training in linguistic analysis. The principal rater (W.H.), moreover, had experience as a Danish-English translator and a PhD in Scandinavian languages. Thus, speech samples were collected, transcribed, and scored in Danish by native Danes. Once use of the TDI was mastered, scoring of the transcripts from the present study began. Questions about scoring difficult cases were discussed with 1 of us (P.S.H.), while all were still unaware of the status of the subjects. Coders were knowledgeable about Danish dialects, so that colloquial differences in language usage are unlikely to have been misconstrued as instances of thought disorder. Speech samples likely to contain artifacts or invalid data (eg, because of noisy tape

culiar verbalizations). Interscorer reliability is high.[22] Several studies have found that TDI scores are significantly higher in persons with schizophrenia than in healthy controls or patients with most other psychiatric disorders.[13,16,21] The TDI has also been used to detect thought disorder in subjects with schizotypal and borderline personality disorders.[23]

Of particular interest for the present study, the nonschizophrenic *relatives* of persons with schizophrenia also show elevated TDI scores.[13,24] In the nonpsychotic relatives of persons with schizophrenia, scores on the TDI are a rather stable, traitlike, variable. Moreover, the TDI scores of relatives are not lowered by antipsychotic medications, as they are in patients.[25,26] These results suggest that high (ie, deviant) TDI scores tend to characterize not only persons with schizophrenia, but also persons without schizophrenia who carry genes for the illness, just as persons without schizophrenia who are likely to carry a gene for schizophrenia seem to have elevated rates of *other* types of milder symptomatology, such as schizotypal personality disorder.[27,28]

Thought disorder in the relatives of persons with schizophrenia might also, however, reflect the influence of *environmental* factors in the rearing families of the persons with schizophrenia, such as patterns of disordered thinking or deviant communication in the rearing parents that may contribute to the development of schizophrenic pathology in the offspring, as suggested, for example, by the work of Wynne et al[29] and Tienari et al.[30] Interpretation of previous studies of thought disorder in the families of schizophrenics is thus clouded by the confounding of genetic and environmental factors that can occur in nonadoptive samples.

Comparisons of schizophrenic and control *adoptees,* and of their respective relatives, provide a method for minimizing such potential confounding. The present study provides the first such adoption-sample data on an operationally defined measure of thought disorrecordings, very brief speech samples, or organic brain disorders, such as senile dementia or aphasia secondary to strokes) were excluded from data analyses. So that conditions for eliciting speech samples would be comparable across subjects, subjects were not included in analyses unless they provided valid speech samples for at least 3 of the 4 questions.

The transcripts for all subjects were scored by the main coder (W.H.), whose scores were used for data analyses, so that between-coder differences in applying coding guidelines were not another source of variance. However, a check was done on a representative subsample of 30 subjects, which indicated high interrater reliability ($r=0.90$, $P<.001$). To help avoid possible halo effects in scoring, responses to the 4 questions by a given subject were rated at different times.

DIAGNOSTIC EVALUATIONS

Two sets of consensus psychiatric diagnoses were available on the subjects, each set representing the consensus reached by a pair of experienced psychiatric diagnosticians who reviewed English transcripts of the psychiatric interviews of subjects while unaware of the TDI scores and the index or control group status of the subjects. The first set of diagnoses, made by Seymour Kety, MD, and Paul Wender, MD,[27] were also based on a review, while still unaware of the TDI scores and index or control status of the subjects, of abstracts of medical records for subjects who had been hospitalized for psychiatric conditions. An independent set of consensus diagnoses, made by Kenneth Kendler, MD, and Alan Gruenberg, MD,[28] applied *DSM-III*[36] criteria and were also based on a review of medical record abstracts for the index probands. The major findings of Kety et al[27] were that schizophrenia-spectrum disorders (chronic and latent schizophrenia) were each significantly more prevalent in the biological relatives of index probands with schizophrenia-spectrum diagnoses than of control probands, whereas no significant difference was found between respective groups of adoptive relatives. Parallel results were found by Kendler et al[28] when they defined the schizophrenia spectrum to include diagnoses, based on *DSM-III*[36] criteria, of schizophrenia, schizotypal personality disorder, or schizoaffective disorder, mainly schizophrenic subtype. Details of the procedures and results of these diagnostic studies in the provincial sample are reported elsewhere.[27,28] The diagnostic agreement between the 2 groups of diagnosticians was high, but not perfect. For the analyses of TDI, therefore, we used the 29 index and 25 control families in which both diagnostic groups agreed that probands were appropriately classified as to index vs control group status. All 29 index probands were given a schizophrenia-spectrum diagnosis by both diagnostic groups, and all but 2 were given a diagnosis of schizophrenia by 1 or both groups.

STATISTICAL ANALYSES

For our key analyses, we followed the procedures outlined in the TDI manual[13]: the algebraic sum of all thought-disordered responses that fell within the various TDI categories was obtained, so that summary scores considered the number and severity of all instances of thought disorder. To control for verbal productivity, a subject's algebraic sum score (the number of thought-disordered responses multiplied by the severity level) was divided by an index of the number of words spoken by the subject (the number of lines of typed transcript, averaging 7 words per line) and multiplied by 100, to yield the score used for statistical analyses. The Student *t* test was used to test for group differences in thought-disorder scores, with 1-tailed tests used where the direction of group differences had been hypothesized. Computer-based software (Statistical Analysis System, SAS Inc, Cary, NC) was used to perform the statistical procedures. If a test for heterogeneity of variance indicated that sample variances differed significantly, we used the alternative *t* test that generates a *t* statistic and degrees of freedom appropriate for the case of unequal variances that was developed by the statisticians, Welch and Satterthwaite.[37-39] As a supplementary nonparametric test, we studied whether the proportions of subjects with extremely high scores differed between groups. As a cutoff for extreme scores, we chose the score that was higher than that for any of the subjects in our largest and most representative subsample of control subjects, which was composed of the biological sibs and half sibs of the control adoptees.

der, the TDI. Although it was also of interest whether, in a Danish sample, TDI scores would differentiate persons with schizophrenia from control subjects, the *primary* aim of the study was to investigate whether high TDI scores are significantly higher in the *biological* relatives of persons with schizophrenia than in the biological relatives of control subjects, supporting a genetic hypothesis, or in the *adoptive* relatives of persons with schizophrenia than in the adoptive relatives of control subjects, as would be expected if the rearing environment contributed significantly to the familial resemblance for TDI scores.

Our general hypothesis was that thought disorder is a behavioral indicator of increased genetic liability for schizophrenia. Specific key corollary hypotheses were that thought disorder scores would be significantly worse in schizophrenic than in control adoptees and would be significantly worse in the *biological* relatives of adoptees with schizophrenia than in the biological relatives of control adoptees, but in the respective *adoptive* relatives of schizophrenic and control probands, the scores would *not* differ significantly.

RESULTS

The mean TDI score for the index probands was significantly higher than for the control probands, as shown in the **Table**, which gives the means and SD of TDI scores for the index and control probands and for the main analyses comparing their respective biological and adoptive relatives. The mean TDI score was also significantly greater for the *biological* relatives of the index probands than for the biological relatives of the control probands. Group differences were particularly striking for the sample of biological *sibs* and *half sibs*, which was larger and more representative than the sample of biological parents. (A majority of the parents was deceased or, because of great age or disability, unable to provide valid speech samples.)

Mean Thought-Disorder Scores for Schizophrenic and Control Adoptees and Their Relatives

	Mean (SD) Score on Thought Disorder Index	P*
Adoptee probands		
Control probands (n=16)	1.15 (1.23)	.01
Schizophrenic probands (n=9)	4.82 (4.01)	
All biological relatives of		
Control probands (n=53)	0.99 (0.99)	<.05
Schizophrenic probands (n=80)	1.37 (1.65)	
Biological sibs and half sibs of		
Control probands (n=39)	0.82 (0.74)	.006
Schizophrenic probands (n=69)	1.44 (1.74)	
Adoptive relatives of		
Control probands (n=13)	1.31 (1.07)	.56
Schizophrenic probands (n=17)	1.11 (0.81)	

**Student* t *test of significance of difference in means.*

Thus, although the samples of biological parents did not differ significantly on TDI scores, the TDI scores were significantly higher for the index than the control biological sibs and half sibs.

Of these 69 index biological sibs and half sibs, both diagnostic teams agreed that 6 had diagnoses within the schizophrenia spectrum (3 had schizophrenia, and 3 had borderline schizophrenia or schizotypal personality disorder); by contrast, none of the 39 control biological sibs and half sibs was determined to have a spectrum diagnosis. The 6 index sibs and half sibs with spectrum diagnoses had higher TDI scores (mean, 3.76; SD, 3.68) than did the 63 index sibs and half sibs without a spectrum diagnosis (mean, 1.22; SD, 1.28), although the difference was not quite significant (t=1.68; P=.08). When the 6 spectrum cases were removed from the analysis, however, the mean TDI score for the remaining 63 sibs and half sibs without a spectrum diagnosis was still significantly higher than that for control sibs and half sibs (t=1.97; P=.026).

By contrast, the mean TDI score for *adoptive* relatives of the index probands, as is also shown in the Table, was low and not significantly different from the adoptive relatives of the control probands. Indeed, the mean for control adoptive relatives was somewhat *higher*.

Parallel results were obtained for proportions of the index vs control groups with extremely high scores. Thus, the proportion of the index probands with a high score (ie, above the cutoff) was 67% (6/9), vs 12% (2/16) for the control probands (P<.01). The proportions of subjects with high scores were also significantly greater for all index than all control biological relatives (11/80 vs 2/53; P=.05) and for the index than the control biological sibs and half sibs (11/69 vs 0/39; P=.005). No significant differences in proportions of high scores were found for index vs control biological parents (0/11 vs 2/14) or for index vs control adoptive relatives (0/17 vs 2/13).

COMMENT

The overall pattern of results supported our key hypotheses. The index probands had significantly higher thought-disorder scores than did control probands. The elevated mean score for subjects with a diagnosis of schizophrenia is consistent with previous studies,[13,16,21] but provides the first such data on *adopted* schizophrenic and control subjects and on *Danish* schizophrenic and control samples. More important, significantly higher TDI scores were found in the *biological* relatives of the index probands than in the biological relatives of control probands.

That the evidence for increased rates of disordered thinking was stronger for the biological *sibs and half sibs* of the index probands than for their *parents* is consistent with the diagnostic finding in these same samples that schizophrenia-spectrum disorders were significantly more prevalent, compared with controls, in the biological sibs and half sibs of the index probands than in their biological parents.[27,28] Kety et al[27] have noted that this higher prevalence of spectrum disorders in the sibs and half sibs of adoptees with schizophrenia is not surprising, because Danish social authorities had, at the time the adoptions were made, discouraged adoption if the biological *parents* of potential adoptees were known to have schizophrenia. These adoption placement policies should thus have worked against our finding significantly elevated rates of thought disorder among the biological *parents* of the index probands (but not among the biological sibs and half sibs of the index probands).

The results of the present study complement extensive previous research[6,12,13,17,20,21] that points to thought disorder as a central feature of schizophrenic pathology. More important, the significantly elevated rates of thought disorder in the biological sibs and half sibs of the index probands, who did not share the same rearing environment with the index probands, suggests that other, probably genetic, factors are important in mediating familial resemblance for thought disorder. Moreover, while TDI scores were most highly elevated among the subjects with schizophrenia-spectrum disorders, the mean score was *also* significantly elevated even among the index probands' biological sibs and half sibs *without* spectrum disorders. This latter finding suggests that subtle forms of thought disorder may represent a subclinical indicator of individuals who carry increased genetic liability for schizophrenia, as suggested by keen clinical observers such as Bleuler[2,3] and Meehl.[4,5]

The absence of a significant difference between the index and control *adoptive* relatives suggests that the elevated levels of thought disorder found among the relatives of persons with schizophrenia in earlier studies were primarily the result of shared genes rather than shared factors in the postnatal environment. The data in the present study do not seem to offer support for hypotheses that deviant patterns of thinking in the rearing family are causal contributors to schizophrenia (or, for that matter, that having a child or sibling with schizophrenia is an environmental stressor contributing to thought disorder in the relatives of the person with schizophrenia). Although caution is warranted for the interpretation of this study's findings on the adoptive relatives, given the modest sample size for adoptive relatives, it is noteworthy that there was not even a trend for thought-disorder scores to be elevated among the adoptive relatives of the index probands. The overall pattern of results of this study provides some of the strongest evidence available indicating that the significantly elevated prevalence of thought disorder in the relatives of persons with schizophrenia reflects to a significant degree their increased genetic liability for schizophrenia.

Accepted for publication June 21, 1996.

This research was supported in part by grants MH31154, MH31340, MH41582, MH01021, and MH36088 from the Public Health Service, grant 81-171 from the MacArthur Foundation, a grant from the Foundations Fund For Research in Psychiatry, and grant RR 0584 from the National Institutes of Health Biomedical Research Support Program, Bethesda, Md.

We thank Seymour Kety, MD, David Rosenthal, MD, Fini Schulsinger, MD, and Paul Wender, MD, for making the adoption study sample available for participation; Seymour Kety, Paul Wender, Kenneth Kendler, and Alan Gruenberg for use of their diagnostic data; Jean Endicott, PhD, for consultation on the Schedule for Affective Disorders and Schizophrenia—Lifetime Version; Seymour Kety, MD, and Steven Matthysse, PhD, for their helpful advice; and Anne Beardsley, Hanne Beck, Sandra M. Cole, MA, Annete Ganz, Lisa Muchnicki, and Sharon Tramer for research assistance.

Reprints: Dennis K. Kinney, PhD, Laboratories for Psychiatric Research, McLean Hospital, NB-G-28, 115 Mill St, Belmont, MA 02178.

REFERENCES

1. Kraepelin E; Barclay RM, trans. In Robertson GM, ed. *Dementia Praecox and Paraphrenia.* Edinburgh, Scotland: Livingstone; 1919.
2. Bleuler E; Brill AA, trans. *Textbook of Psychiatry.* New York, NY: Macmillan Publishing Co Inc; 1924.
3. Bleuler E; Zinkin J, trans. *Dementia Praecox or the Group of Schizophrenias.* Madison, Conn: International Universities Press; 1950.
4. Meehl P. Schizotaxia, schizotypy, schizophrenia. *Am Psychol.* 1962;17:827-838.
5. Meehl P. Schizotaxia revisited. *Arch Gen Psychiatry.* 1989;46:935-944.
6. Andreasen NC, Powers PS. Overinclusive thinking in mania and schizophrenia. *Br J Psychiatry.* 1974;125:452-456.
7. Cameron N. Experimental analysis of schizophrenic thinking. In: Kasanin JS, ed. *Language and Thought in Schizophrenia.* Berkeley, Calif: University of California Press; 1946;50-64.
8. Carlson GA, Goodwin FK. The stages of mania: a longitudinal analysis of the manic episode. *Arch Gen Psychiatry.* 1973;28:221-228.
9. Clayton PJ, Pitts FN, Winokur G. Affective disorder, IV: mania. *Compr Psychiatry.* 1965;6:313-322.
10. Gershon SN, Benson DF, Frazier SH. Diagnosis: schizophrenia versus posterior aphasia. *Am J Psychiatry.* 1974;134:966-969.
11. Goldstein K. Methodological approach to the study of schizophrenic thought disorder. In: Kasanin JS, ed. *Language and Thought in Schizophrenia.* Berkeley, Calif: University of California Press; 1946;17-40.
12. Harrow M, Quinlan D. Is disordered thinking unique to schizophrenia? *Arch Gen Psychiatry.* 1977;34:15-21.
13. Johnston MH, Holzman PS. *Assessing Schizophrenic Thinking.* San Francisco, Calif: Jossey-Bass Publishers Inc; 1979.
14. O'Connell M, Cooper S, Perry JC, Hoke L. The relationship between thought disorder and psychotic symptoms in borderline personality disorder. *J Nerv Ment Dis.* 1989;177:273-278.
15. Shenton ME, Solovay MR, Holzman PS. Comparative studies of thought disorder, II: schizoaffective disorder. *Arch Gen Psychiatry.* 1987;44:21-30.
16. Solovay MS, Shenton ME, Holzman PS. Comparative studies of thought disorder, I: mania and schizophrenia. *Arch Gen Psychiatry.* 1987;44:13-20.
17. Andreasen NC. Thought, language, and communication disorders, I: clinical assessment, definition of terms, and evaluation of their reliability. *Arch Gen Psychiatry.* 1979;36:1315-1321.
18. Andreasen NC. Scale for the Assessment of Thought, Language, and Communication (TLC). *Schizophr Bull.* 1986;12:473-482.
19. Harrow M, Quinlan D. *Disordered Thinking and Schizophrenic Psychopathology.* New York, NY: Gardner Press; 1985.
20. Marengo JT, Harrow M, Lanin-Kettering I, Wilson A. Evaluating bizarre-idiosyncratic thinking. *Schizophr Bull.* 1986;12:497-509.
21. Holzman PS, Solovay MR, Shenton ME. Thought disorder specificity in functional psychoses. In: Alpert M, ed. *Controversies in Schizophrenia: Changes and Constancies.* New York, NY: Guilford Press; 1985:228-245.
22. Coleman MJ, Carpenter JT, Waternaux C, Levy DL, Shenton ME, Perry J, Medoff D, Wong H, Monach D, Meyer P, O'Brian C, Valentino C, Robinson D, Smith M, Makowski D, Holzman PS. The thought disorder index: a reliability study. *Psychol Assess.* 1993;5:336-342.
23. Edell WS. Role of structure in disordered thinking in borderline and schizophrenic disorders. *J Pers Assess.* 1987;51:23-41.
24. Shenton ME, Solovay MR, Holzman PS, Coleman M, Gale HJ. Thought disorder in the relatives of psychotic patients. *Arch Gen Psychiatry.* 1989;46:897-901.
25. Hurt SS, Holzman PS, Davis JM. Thought disorder: the measurement of its changes. *Arch Gen Psychiatry.* 1983;40:1281-1285.
26. Spohn H, Coyne L, Larson J, Mittleman F, Spray J, Hayes K. Episodic and residual thought pathology in chronic schizophrenics. *Schizophr Bull.* 1986; 12:394-407.
27. Kety SS, Wender PH, Jacobsen B, Ingraham LJ, Jansson L, Faber B, Kinney DK. Mental illness in the biological and adoptive relatives of schizophrenic adoptees, II: replication of the Copenhagen Study in the rest of Denmark. *Arch Gen Psychiatry.* 1994;51:442-455.
28. Kendler SS, Gruenberg AM, Kinney DK. Independent diagnoses of adoptees and relatives, using *DSM-III* criteria, in the provincial and national samples of the Danish Adoption Study of Schizophrenia. *Arch Gen Psychiatry.* 1994;51: 456-468.
29. Wynne LC, Singer MT, Toohey M. Communication of the adoptive parents of schizophrenics. In: Jorstad J, Ugelstad E, eds. *Schizophrenia 75: Psychotherapy, Family Studies, Research.* Oslo, Norway: University of Oslo Press; 1976:413-451.
30. Tienari P, Wynne LC, Moring J, Lahti I, Naarala M, Sorri A, Wahlberg K-E, Saarento O, Seitamaa M, Kaleva M, Laksy K. The Finnish adoptive family study of schizophrenia: implications for family research. *Br J Psychiatry.* 1994;164 (suppl 23):20-26.
31. Kety SS, Rosenthal D, Wender PH, Schulsinger F. The types and prevalence of mental illness in the biological and adoptive families of adopted schizophrenics. In: Rosenthal D, Kety S, eds. *The Transmission of Schizophrenia.* Elmsford, NY: Pergamon Press Inc; 1968:345-362.
32. Kety SS, Rosenthal D, Wender PH, Schulsinger F, Jacobsen B. The biological and adoptive families of adopted individuals who became schizophrenic: prevalence of mental illness and other characteristics. In: Wynne L, Cromwell R, Matthysse S, eds. *The Nature of Schizophrenia: New Approaches to Research and Treatment.* New York, NY: John Wiley & Sons Inc; 1978:25-37.
33. Kety SS. Mental illness in the biological and adoptive relatives of schizophrenic adoptees: findings relevant to genetic and environmental factors in etiology. *Am J Psychiatry.* 1983;140:720-727.
34. Spitzer RI, Endicott J. *Schedule for Affective Disorders and Schizophrenia: Lifetime Version.* New York, NY: Biometrics Research Division, New York State Psychiatric Institute; 1976.
35. Gottschalk LA, Gleser GC. *The Measurement of Psychological States Through the Content Analysis of Verbal Behavior.* Berkeley, Calif: University of California Press; 1969.
36. American Psychiatric Association. *Diagnostic and Statistical Manual of Mental Disorders, Third Edition.* Washington, DC: American Psychiatric Association; 1980.
37. SAS Institute. *SAS/STAT User's Guide,* Volume 2, Version 6, 4th Edition. Cary, NC: SAS Institute Inc; 1990.
38. Satterthwaite FW. An approximate distribution of estimates of variance components. *Biometrics Bull.* 1946;2:100-144.
39. Howell DC. *Statistical Methods for Psychology.* 3rd ed. Belmont, Calif: Duxbury Press; 1992.

ORIGINAL ARTICLE

The Brain Metabolic Patterns of Clozapine- and Fluphenazine-Treated Patients With Schizophrenia During a Continuous Performance Task

Robert M. Cohen, PhD, MD; Thomas E. Nordahl, PhD, MD; William E. Semple, PhD; Paul Andreason, MD; Robert E. Litman, MD; David Pickar, MD

Background: The comparison of the effects of 2 classes of neuroleptic drugs on regional brain functional activities may reveal common mechanisms of antipsychotic drug efficacy.

Methods: The regional cerebral glucose metabolic rates of patients with schizophrenia who were and were not receiving neuroleptic drugs and normal control subjects were obtained by positron emission tomography using fludeoxyglucose F 18 as the tracer.

Results: Compared with normal controls and patients not receiving medication, fluphenazine hydrochloride–and clozapine-treated patients had lower global gray matter absolute metabolic rates throughout the cortex. When normalized regional glucose metabolic rates were examined, both medications lowered rates in the superior prefrontal cortex and increased rates in the limbic cortex. Fluphenazine, but not clozapine, increased metabolic rates in the subcortical and lateral temporal lobes, whereas clozapine, but not fluphenazine, decreased inferior prefrontal cortex activity.

Conclusions: These changes are consistent with the idea that neuroleptic drugs lead to "compensation" and "adaptation" rather than "normalization" of the functional activities of brain structures in schizophrenia. The overall similarity of their global and regional metabolic effects suggests that both classes of antipsychotic drugs share some common mechanisms of action. One possibility is that of inducing a shift in the balance of cortical to limbic cortex activity. Differential effects in the inferior prefrontal cortex and the basal ganglia might underlie differences in the therapeutic efficacy and side effect profile of clozapine and fluphenazine.

Arch Gen Psychiatry. 1997;54:481-486

FOR MORE than 30 years, neuroleptic drugs have remained the focal point of the pharmacologic treatment of schizophrenia. Although it is likely that the dopamine system is the target of these drugs, how the blockade of dopamine receptors leads to antipsychotic drug efficacy is unknown. The most direct hypotheses posit that neuroleptic drugs halt an overactive dopamine system. However, despite considerable efforts, the evidence of an aberrant dopamine system in patients with schizophrenia remains weak.[1,2] Alternatively, it has been proposed that the dopamine system, although not the cause of schizophrenia, permits the development and/or maintenance of the psychotic state.

In prior studies, we evaluated both hypotheses by examining the positron emission tomography (PET)–determined brain metabolic patterns of patients with schizophrenia who had been withdrawn from their medication or who were receiving neuroleptic drugs at the time of scan.[3-5] Those metabolic deficits of the midprefrontal cortex that were present in medication-withdrawn patients with schizophrenia were also present in patients treated with classical neuroleptic drugs; there were additional brain areas that discriminated the treated patient group from the medication-withdrawn patients and normal control subjects, ie, a further decrease in metabolic rates of the normalized frontal cortex and abnormally high metabolic rates of the temporal lobe and subcortex.

Thus, our data did not support the hypothesis that neuroleptic drugs act directly to normalize the abnormalities of schizophrenia, but supported the hypothesis that neuroleptic drugs induce compensatory or adaptive changes in brain function that alter the course of psychosis. It remained possible, however, that our findings resulted from an inability to delineate the significant abnormalities of schizophrenia because of the heterogene-

From the Section on Clinical Brain Imaging, Laboratory of Cerebral Metabolism, National Institute of Mental Health and Experimental Therapeutics Branch, National Institute of Mental Health, Bethesda, Md. Dr Nordahl is now affiliated with the Department of Psychiatry, University of California Medical Center, Davis. Dr Semple is now affiliated with the Cleveland Veterans Administration Medical Center and the Department of Psychiatry, Case Western Reserve Medical School, Cleveland, Ohio. Dr Andreason is now with the Food and Drug Administration, Bethesda.

ity of the patients and/or the intrinsic or extant capabilities of our PET methods. For example, the metabolic abnormalities induced by neuroleptic drugs could reflect the side effect profile of these drugs, not their efficacy.

Herein, we report on the data acquired from 2 different approaches embodied in 2 independent studies used to discriminate between these possibilities. Study 1 of medication-withdrawn patients (DF1 group), patients receiving fluphenazine hydrochloride (FLU1 group), and normal control subjects (NC1) incorporated significant improvements in experimental design and regional metabolic rate determination to lessen the likelihood that inadequate methods were responsible for the absence of PET findings supporting the hypothesis that neuroleptic drugs reverse the metabolic abnormalities of schizophrenia. Previous studies[6-17] evaluating the effects of neuroleptic drugs on regional metabolism frequently suffered from studying patients who were not receiving the same neuroleptic drug, and the absence of 1 or more of the following: the study of normal controls, medication-withdrawn patients and neuroleptic drug-treated patients undergoing scanning in parallel; the use of a controlled behavioral state during scanning; and calculations based on an arterial tracer input curve and an empirically determined attenuation correction.

Because of clozapine's enhanced clinical efficacy and favorable side effect profile compared with typical neuroleptic drugs,[18,19] study 2 of fluphenazine-treated patients (FLU2 group), clozapine-treated patients (CLOZ group), and normal controls (NC2 group) was expected to clarify those metabolic alterations associated with efficacy from those associated with the induction of side effects.

SUBJECTS AND METHODS

Unless otherwise indicated, data are given as mean±SD.

SUBJECTS

In study 1, 20 male subjects in the NC1 group (mean age, 32.5±9.6 years; range, 23-56 years), 12 male patients in the FLU1 group (mean age, 29.9±4.3 years; range, 23-37 years), and 10 male patients in the DF1 group (mean age, 29.9±4.8 years; range, 22-39 years) were studied using PET. In study 2, there were 21 male subjects in the NC2 group (mean age, 30.4±7.6 years; range, 19-46 years), 10 male patients in the FLU2 group (mean age, 34.1±7.5 years; range, 21-47 years), and 11 male patients in the CLOZ group (mean age, 34.3±6.2 years; range, 21-44 years).

The diagnosis of schizophrenia was made on the basis of the evaluation of 2 psychiatrists. All patients were given a modified Schizophrenic Affective Disorders Scale and met *DSM-III-R*[20] criteria. Patients were excluded if a significant medical or neurological problem was present. The medication-withdrawn patients had received no medications for at least 14 days (mean time, 17.3±3.7 days). During the scan week, the average dose of fluphenazine hydrochloride in study 1 was 25.4±12.5 mg/d. Average doses of fluphenazine hydrochloride and clozapine in study 2 were 22.5±11.6 mg/d and 431.2±200.9 mg/d, respectively. At the time of scan, the FLU1 group had received the drug for an average of 69.6±8.0 days (median, 29.5 days). The FLU2 group had received fluphenazine for an average of 473.8±121.7 days (median, 35 days), and the CLOZ group had received clozapine for an average of 91.5±76.4 days (median, 66 days). Patients did not receive any medication on the day of their scan. An optimal dose design strategy was used, as we were interested in determining those regional changes associated with neuroleptic drug efficacy.

Symptoms during the week of scan were measured using the Bunney-Hamburg Rating Scale for Psychosis (BHRS-P)[21] and the Brief Psychiatric Rating Scale (BPRS).[22] The average BHRS-P score was 6.21±1.53 for the FLU1 group and 5.75±1.82 and 5.72±1.71 for the FLU2 and CLOZ groups, respectively. The average BPRS score was 54.8±15.0 for the FLU1 group and 52.4±12.0 and 53.0±11.4 for the FLU2 and CLOZ groups, respectively. A detailed description of the patient populations and their clinical and biological responses to fluphenazine and clozapine treatment has been reported elsewhere.[23]

Each normal control subject was interviewed by a psychiatrist, received a medical examination, completed a Minnesota Multiphasic Personality Inventory, and submitted blood and urine samples for routine laboratory evaluation. On the basis of all the available information, control subjects were proscribed from participating if they had any serious medical illness, history of significant mental (*DSM-III-R* criteria) or neurological disorder, or first-degree relatives with histories consistent with *DSM-III-R* diagnoses of schizophrenia, major mood disorder, or alcohol abuse.

All patients were residing on a research unit at the National Institutes of Health, Bethesda, Md, at the time of scan. All patients and normal controls gave informed consent before their scans.

PET SCAN PROCEDURE

Subjects, with eyes patched, began their auditory discrimination task several minutes before the injection of 148 to 185 MBq of fludeoxyglucose F 18 and completed the task 30 minutes after injection. The auditory discrimination task in which subjects must identify 1 of 3 auditory tones has been described in detail elsewhere.[24] Scanning, beginning 30 minutes after isotope injection, was performed on a Scanditronix PET scanner (Scanditronix, Essex, Mass) with a 5- to 6-mm full-width-half-maximum in-plane resolution and a z-axis resolution of 11.8 mm. A transmission scan was used

RESULTS

ABSOLUTE METABOLIC RATES

The FLU1 group had lower global gray glucose metabolic rates than the NC1 and DF1 groups, whereas the NC1 and DF1 groups did not differ from each other (FLU1 rate, 46.8±7.2 μmol of glucose/100 g of tissue per minute; NC1 rate, 54.2±7.6 μmol of glucose/100 g of tissue per minute; P=.01; DF1 rate, 54.6±8.3 μmol of glucose/

to calculate attenuation, and the tracer input curve was calculated from blood samples obtained from the radial artery. Four sets of 7 planes were obtained for each subject, starting at 5 mm above the plane parallel to the canthomeatal (CM) line. The interslice interval was approximately 3.5 mm.

DATA ANALYSIS

Raw pixel values were converted to glucose metabolic rates in micromoles of glucose per 100 g of tissue per minute by means of previously reported kinetic constants.[25-27] To extract regional glucose metabolic rates, 60 rectangular boxes were located in 5 standard planes (plane A, 94 mm above the CM line; plane B, 81 mm above the CM line; plane C, 67 mm above the CM line; plane D, 53 mm above the CM line; and plane E, 40 mm above the CM line) chosen from one of the four 7-plane scan sets.[24,28,29] Anatomical structures were judged as contained within these regions according to Matsui and Hirano.[30]

TERMS USED

Metabolic rates are expressed as global gray glucose metabolic rate, an estimate of the average glucose metabolic rate of gray matter–rich areas determined by averaging the glucose metabolic rates obtained from all the gray matter–rich areas of the cortex sampled in planes B through E (an adequate match for plane A could not be found in a few subjects); absolute regional metabolic rate, the actual glucose metabolic rate for a region of interest (ROI); and normalized or relative glucose metabolic rate, the absolute regional metabolic rate divided by the global gray glucose metabolic rate.

STATISTICAL ANALYSIS

The significance of global absolute metabolic rate differences between 2 groups was evaluated by 1-way analyses of variance (ANOVAs) and Student t tests. Because regional absolute metabolic rates are highly correlated with the global glucose metabolic rate, normalized metabolic rates were used to examine the localized effects of neuroleptic drugs.[31,32]

Our prior studies with schizophrenic patients who were receiving neuroleptic drugs[3-5] generated the hypotheses that neuroleptic drugs induce a broad decrease in normalized frontal cortex metabolism and an increase in normalized temporal lobe and subcortical metabolism. In study 1, we tested these hypotheses by using the normalized regional metabolic rates of the FLU1 group in comparison with those of the NC1 and DF1 groups.

Study 2 was designed to specifically test any new hypotheses that might be generated from study 1 based on the improved methods of study 1 compared with those of our earlier work while generating a new set of hypotheses concerning regional differences in fluphenazine-treated patients compared with clozapine-treated patients. Thus, any new findings in study 1 not replicated in study 2 should and would be viewed with considerable skepticism and as likely being the result of type I error.

To avoid the likelihood of a type I error in the regional normalized metabolic rate comparisons, the original 60 ROIs were combined into the 6 larger regions of superior prefrontal cortex (planes B and C), inferior prefrontal cortex (planes D and E), parietal-occipital cortex, lateral temporal cortex, limbic cortex (cingulate and medial temporal cortex), and subcortex (thalamus and basal ganglia). This allowed for a single multivariate test, the Hotelling T^2, to evaluate whether there were significant localized differences between the various patient groups. Student t tests were then used to determine the location of the regionalized differences. Because we are reporting on only a single study with clozapine, any reported differences between the regional effects of clozapine compared with fluphenazine should still be considered exploratory in nature and thus requiring replication.

100 g of tissue per minute; P=.03). These findings were tested in study 2, in which the FLU2 group and the CLOZ group were compared with the NC2 group. Results of the 1-way ANOVA were significant (F[2,39]=3.69; P=.03). By the least significant difference method of comparison, the FLU2 and CLOZ groups differed significantly from the NC2 group (P=.02 and P=.05, respectively), but not from each other (NC2 rate, 52.3±8.5 μmol of glucose/100 g of tissue per minute; FLU2 rate, 44.3±10.2 μmol of glucose/100 g of tissue per minute; CLOZ rate, 45.6±7.3 μmol of glucose/100 g of tissue per minute).

NORMALIZED REGIONAL METABOLIC RATES

Fluphenazine-Treated Patients vs Normal Controls

To eliminate the effects of global gray glucose metabolic rates on tests of the localized, ie, regional, effects of neuroleptic drug treatment, while maximizing the power and reliability of these comparisons, multivariate analyses of variance (MANOVAs) were performed on normalized regional metabolic rates. The MANOVA for the 6 major regions examined in the comparison of the FLU1 and NC1 groups was significant (Hotelling T^2=54.5; F[6,25]=7.57; P<.001). As expected from our earlier study, the normalized metabolic rate of the superior prefrontal cortex was lower, whereas the normalized metabolic rates of the lateral temporal lobe, limbic cortex, and subcortex were higher in the FLU1 group than in the NC1 group (**Table 1**). These effects were highly reproducible (Table 1).

Clozapine-Treated Patients vs Normal Controls

The normalized metabolic rate pattern of the CLOZ group also differed from the NC2 group (**Table 2**) (Hotelling T^2=70.17; F[6,25]=9.75; P<.001). As was the case for the FLU2 group, the CLOZ group had lower normalized metabolic rates in the prefrontal cortex and higher normalized metabolic rates in the limbic cortex. In addition, higher metabolic rates were found for the parietal-occipital cortex, but not for the lateral temporal lobes and subcortex, where rates were found to be higher in the FLU2 group than in the NC2 group. Despite the ab-

Table 1. Normalized Metabolic Rates for Fluphenazine-Treated Patients Compared With Normal Control Subjects*

Brain Region	Study 1† Normalized Metabolic Rate: FLU1 Group (n=12)	NC1 Group (n=20)	FLU1-NC1 Rate, %	*P*
Superior prefrontal cortex	1.028 (0.048)	1.064 (0.021)	−3.4	.005
Inferior prefrontal cortex	0.998 (0.043)	1.013 (0.036)	−1.5	.30
Parietal-occipital cortex	1.013 (0.042)	0.995 (0.039)	1.8	.22
Lateral temporal cortex	0.990 (0.056)	0.955 (0.039)	3.7	.05
Limbic cortex	0.914 (0.065)	0.861 (0.042)	6.2	.008
Subcortex	1.165 (0.159)	0.981 (0.072)	18.7	<.001

Brain Region	Study 2‡ Normalized Metabolic Rate: FLU2 Group (n=10)	NC2 Group (n=21)	FLU2-NC2 Rate, %	*P*
Superior prefrontal cortex	1.014 (0.032)	1.063 (0.033)	−4.6	<.001
Inferior prefrontal cortex	0.981 (0.046)	1.001 (0.028)	−1.9	.15
Parietal-occipital cortex	1.034 (0.033)	1.002 (0.025)	3.3	.008
Lateral temporal cortex	0.991 (0.031)	0.962 (0.036)	3.0	.04
Limbic cortex	0.933 (0.067)	0.868 (0.046)	7.5	.004
Subcortex	1.171 (0.081)	0.999 (0.075)	17.2	<.001

*Unless otherwise indicated, data are given as mean (SD).

†FLU1 indicates patients receiving fluphenazine hydrochloride; NC1, normal control subjects. For all comparisons, Hotelling T^2 for the multivariate analysis of variance=54.5; F (6, 25)=7.57; and P<.001.

‡FLU2 indicates patients receiving fluphenazine; NC2, normal control subjects. Hotelling T^2 for the multivariate analysis of variance=53.9; F (6, 22)=7.32; and P<.001.

sence of a significant clozapine effect in the subcortex, a separate multivariate comparison of the 6 ROIs comprising the basal ganglia was performed. We elected to add this additional test of the effects of clozapine treatment because of the high metabolic rates in the basal ganglia of patients receiving typical neuroleptic drugs observed in prior studies as well as in studies 1 and 2 and because of the importance attributed to hypotheses relating changes in basal ganglia activity to behavioral changes. This additional test yielded a positive result (Hotelling T^2=27.15; F[6,25]=3.8; *P*=.008) with higher metabolic rates in the right anterior (15.8%; *P*=.002) and posterior (14%; *P*=.02; separate variances) putamen ROIs of the CLOZ group.

Clozapine-Treated Patients vs Fluphenazine-Treated Patients

To directly compare regional differences between the 2 drugs, we pooled the fluphenazine data from studies 1 and 2 to form a combined fluphenazine-treated patient group (FLU group). A significant difference was found between the FLU and CLOZ groups (Hotelling T^2=19.4; F[6,24]=2.67; *P*=.04), with fluphenazine showing a greater effect on increasing subcortical normalized metabolic rates, whereas clozapine had a greater effect on lowering the metabolic rate of the inferior prefrontal cortex. To be consistent with the earlier analysis of the clozapine data, an additional separate multivariate analysis of the 6 ROIs comprising the basal ganglia was performed, and results were consistent with the above subcortex finding in that the FLU group had higher basal ganglia rates than the CLOZ group (Hotelling T^2=17.6; F[6,26]=2.46; *P*=.05).

COMMENT

Because of concerns about the replicability of regional brain metabolic studies of antipsychotic drug treatment in schizophrenia,[33] our current studies were designed to demonstrate replicability while attempting to improve many of the quantitative aspects of the regional metabolic determination. We hoped that these results would provide a basis for the examination of hypotheses that typical and atypical antipsychotic drugs share a unified or differing antipsychotic mechanism. To this end, we have now examined 30 fluphenazine-treated patients with schizophrenia, 36 medication-withdrawn patients, and, in parallel, more than 60 normal controls in 3 independent studies.

In studies 1 and 2, fluphenazine-treated patients with schizophrenia had lower global and regional metabolic rates than normal controls and medication-withdrawn patients. Superimposed on this overall global effect were those of relatively increased temporal lobe, limbic cortex, and subcortical metabolism and decreased superior frontal cortex metabolism.

COMPARISON OF CLOZAPINE WITH FLUPHENAZINE

The overall similarity of the metabolic patterns found in the FLU2 and CLOZ groups is consistent with the 2 drugs sharing, at least, some common mechanisms of action. Of the regions effected in common by the 2 drugs, the prefrontal cortex and limbic cortex show the most robust responses, with the putamen showing a somewhat attenuated response with clozapine. Whether these are direct effects of neuroleptic drugs

Table 2. Normalized Metabolic Rates for Clozapine-Treated Patients Compared With Normal Control Subjects and Fluphenazine-Treated Patients*

	Study 2† Normalized Metabolic Rate			
Brain Region	CLOZ Group (n=11)	NC2 Group (n=21)	CLOZ-NC2 Rate, %	*P*
Superior prefrontal cortex	1.021 (0.039)	1.063 (0.033)	−4.0	.003
Inferior prefrontal cortex	0.957 (0.035)	1.001 (0.028)	−4.3	<.001
Parietal-occipital cortex	1.047 (0.049)	1.002 (0.025)	4.6	.002
Lateral temporal cortex	0.973 (0.043)	0.962 (0.036)	1.2	.42
Limbic cortex	0.927 (0.045)	0.868 (0.046)	6.8	.002
Subcortex	1.045 (0.094)	0.999 (0.075)	4.6	.14

	All Drug-Treated Patients‡ Normalized Metabolic Rate			
Brain Region	CLOZ Group (n=11)	FLU Group (n=22)	FLU-CLOZ Rate, %	*P*
Superior prefrontal cortex	1.021 (0.039)	1.022 (0.041)	−0.1	.96
Inferior prefrontal cortex	0.957 (0.035)	0.990 (0.044)	−3.3	.04
Parietal-occipital cortex	1.047 (0.049)	1.021 (0.039)	2.5	.12
Lateral temporal cortex	0.973 (0.043)	0.990 (0.046)	−1.7	.32
Limbic cortex	0.927 (0.045)	0.923 (0.065)	0.4	.86
Subcortex	1.045 (0.094)	1.168 (0.127)	−10.5	.008

**Unless otherwise indicated, data are given as mean (SD).*

†CLOZ indicates clozapine-treated patients; NC2, normal control subjects. Hotelling T^2 *for the multivariate analysis of variance=70.17;* $F_{(6, 25)}=9.75$*; and* $P<.001$.

‡CLOZ indicates clozapine-treated patients; FLU, all patients in studies 1 and 2 treated with fluphenazine hydrochloride. Hotelling T^2 *for the multivariate analysis of variance=19.38;* $F_{(6, 24)}=2.67$*; and* $P=.04$.

on all of these regions or indirect ones, eg, mediated through the parallel circuits linking the frontal and limbic, basal ganglia, and thalamus,[34] remains to be determined. In either case, however, the data suggest that alterations in the balance of limbic vs frontal cortical activity underlie the therapeutic effects of antipsychotic drugs.

Assuming that these common regional effects reflect the mechanism of action of the neuroleptic drugs, it is important to examine whether there is any evidence of preexisting abnormalities in these brain regions that neuroleptic drugs might be correcting. The evidence of abnormally high frontal cortex activity and abnormally low basal ganglia functional activity in medication-withdrawn patients is either weak or nonexistent.[3,4,35-41] Decreased limbic cortex activity (anterior cingulate and hippocampal and parahippocampal cortex) was reported by Tamminga et al[37] in a preliminary study of resting patients with schizophrenia that the authors stated required replication. We have not observed decreases in these areas in our studies, but because normal control subjects performing our task have lower limbic cortex (anterior cingulate and parahippocampal cortex) metabolic rates than resting subjects, it is possible that our task precluded this observation. To our knowledge, however, the findings by Tamminga et al have not been replicated, with a recent larger study failing to find any regional abnormalities in resting patients with schizophrenia.[41] Thus, the most parsimonious explanations of neuroleptic drug efficacy would seem to be those that hypothesize that neuroleptic drugs affect functional brain activities in ways that ultimately compensate for schizophrenia. This explanation is consistent with the correlations observed by Buchsbaum et al[16,17] of pretreatment basal ganglia metabolic rates and changes in basal ganglia metabolic rates in response to neuroleptic drug treatment with clinical response.

Areas where fluphenazine and clozapine differ in their metabolic effects may be regions that determine side effects or selective therapeutic efficacy. For example, fluphenazine's greater effects in the basal ganglia may be related to its capacity to induce extrapyramidal symptoms and tardive dyskinesia. The greater effect of clozapine on the functional activity of the inferior prefrontal cortex might indicate why treatment with clozapine has been associated with the induction and/or modulation of obsessive-compulsive symptoms,[42,43] as abnormal activity of the orbital frontal cortex has been observed in obsessive-compulsive disorder.[44,45]

To provide support for these hypotheses, it will be important to continue to evaluate the regional metabolic effects of antipsychotic drugs of different classes and, as in the studies of Buchsbaum et al,[16,17] to examine in our own within-subject data whether the higher relative basal ganglia and thalamic metabolic rates relate to clinical response. Ultimately, clarifying the importance of regionally specific effects of neuroleptic drugs as biological determinants of behavioral change should lead to a more rational basis for the drug treatment of schizophrenia.

Accepted for publication March 26, 1996.

We are grateful for the assistance of A. Catherine King, Susan Dowling, Garrett Bagley, Glinda Fitzgerald, and the PET technicians of the Department of Nuclear Medicine, National Institutes of Health Clinical Center, Bethesda.

Reprints: Robert M. Cohen, PhD, MD, Clinical Brain Imaging Section, Laboratory of Cerebral Metabolism, National Institute of Mental Health, Bldg 36, Room 1A05, 36 Convent Dr, MSC 4030, Bethesda, MD 20892-4030.

REFERENCES

1. Carlsson A. The current status of the dopamine hypothesis of schizophrenia. *Neuropsychopharmacology.* 1988;1:179-186.
2. Meltzer HY. The role of dopamine in schizophrenia. In: Lindenmayer J-P, Kay SR, eds. *New Biological Vistas on Schizophrenia.* New York, NY: Brunner/Mazel; 1992:131-157.
3. DeLisi LE, Holcomb HH, Cohen RM, Pickar D, Carpenter W, Morihisa JM, King AC, Kessler R, Buchsbaum MS. Positron emission tomography in schizophrenic patients with and without neuroleptic medication. *J Cereb Blood Flow Metab.* 1985;5:201-206.
4. Cohen RM, Semple WE, Gross M, Nordahl TE, DeLisi LE, Holcomb HH, King AC, Morihisa JM, Pickar D. Dysfunction in a prefrontal substrate of sustained attention in schizophrenia. *Life Sci.* 1987;40:2031-2039.
5. Cohen RM, Semple WE, Gross M, Nodahl TE, Holcomb HH, Dowling MS, Pickar D. The effect of neuroleptics on dysfunction in a prefrontal substrate of sustained attention in schizophrenia. *Life Sci.* 1988;43:1141-1150.
6. Buchsbaum MS, Wu JC, DeLisi LE, Holcomb HH, Hazlett E, Cooper-Langston K, Kessler R. Positron emission tomography studies of basal ganglia and somatosensory cortex neuroleptic drug effects: differences between normal controls and schizophrenic patients. *Biol Psychiatry.* 1987;22:479-494.
7. Wolkin A, Jaeger J, Brodie JD, Wolf AP, Fowler J, Retrosen J, Gomez-Mont F, Cancro R. Persistence of cerebral metabolic abnormalities in chronic schizophrenia as determined by positron emission tomography. *Am J Psychiatry.* 1985;142:564-571.
8. Volkow ND, Brodie JD, Wolf AP, Angrist B, Russell J, Cancro R. Brain metabolism in patients with schizophrenia before and after acute neuroleptic administration. *J Neurol Neurosurg Psychiatry.* 1986;49:1199-1202.
9. Volkow ND, Brodie JD, Wolf AP, Gomez-Mont F, Cancro R, van Gelder P, Russell JAG, Overall J. Brain organization in schizophrenia. *J Cereb Blood Flow Metab.* 1986;6:441-446.
10. Volkow ND, Levy A, Brodie JD, Wolf AP, Cancro R, van Gelder P, Henn F. Lower cerebellar metabolism in medicated patients with chronic schizophrenia. *Am J Psychiatry.* 1992;149:686-688.
11. Gur RE, Resnick SM, Gur RC, Alavi A, Caroff S, Kushner M, Reivich M. Regional brain function in schizophrenia, II: repeated evaluation with positron emission tomography. *Arch Gen Psychiatry.* 1987;44:126-129.
12. Resnick SM, Gur RE, Alavi A, Gur RC, Reivich M. Positron emission tomography and subcortical glucose metabolism in schizophrenia. *Psychiatry Res.* 1988;24:1-11.
13. Szechtman H, Nahmias C, Garnett S, Firnau G, Brown GM, Kaplan RD, Cleghorn JM. Effect of neuroleptics on altered cerebral glucose metabolism in schizophrenia. *Arch Gen Psychiatry.* 1988;45:523-532.
14. Wik G, Wiesel F-A, Sjogren I, Blomqvist G, Stone-Elander S. Effects of sulpiride and chlorpromazine on regional cerebral glucose metabolism in schizophrenic patients as determined by positron emission tomography. *Psychopharmacology.* 1989;97:309-318.
15. Bartlett EJ, Wolkin A, Brodie JD, Laska EM, Wolf AP, Sanfilipo M. Importance of pharmacologic control in PET studies: effects of thiothixene and haloperidol on cerebral glucose utilization in chronic schizophrenia. *Psychiatry Res Neuroimaging.* 1991;140:115-124.
16. Buchsbaum MS, Potkin SG, Marshall JF, Lottenberg S, Teng C, Heh CW, Tafalla R, Reynolds C, Abel L, Plon L, Bunney WE. Effects of clozapine and thiothixene on glucose metabolic rate in schizophrenia. *Neuropsychopharmacology.* 1992;6:155-163.
17. Buchsbaum MS, Potkin SG, Siegel BV Jr, Lohr J, Katz M, Gottschalk LA, Gulasekaram B, Marshall JF, Lottenberg S, Teng CY, Abel L, Plon L, Bunney WE Jr. Striatal metabolic rate and clinical response to neuroleptics in schizophrenia. *Arch Gen Psychiatry.* 1992;49:966-974.
18. Baldessarini RJ, Frankenburg FR. Clozapine: a novel antipsychotic agent. *N Engl J Med.* 1991;324:746-754.
19. Kane J, Honigfeld G, Singer J, Meltzer H. Clozapine for the treatment-resistant schizophrenic: a double blind comparison with chlorpromazine. *Arch Gen Psychiatry.* 1988;45:789-796.
20. American Psychiatric Association. *Diagnostic and Statistical Manual of Mental Disorders, Third Edition, Revised.* Washington, DC: American Psychiatric Press; 1987.
21. Bunney WE Jr, Hamburg DA. Methods for reliable longitudinal observation of behavior. *Arch Gen Psychiatry.* 1963;9:280-294.
22. Overall JE, Gorham DE. The Brief Psychiatric Rating Scale. *Psychol Res.* 1992;10:799-812.
23. Pickar D, Owen RR, Litman RE, Konicki PE, Gutierrez R, Rapaport MH. Clinical and biologic response to clozapine in patients with schizophrenia: crossover comparison with fluphenazine. *Arch Gen Psychiatry.* 1992;49:345-353.
24. Cohen RM, Semple WE, Gross M, Holcomb HH, Dowling MS, Nordahl TE. Functional localization of sustained attention: comparison to sensory stimulation in the absence of instruction. *Neuropsychiatry Neuropsychol Behav Neurol.* 1988;1:3-20.
25. Sokoloff L, Reivich M, Kennedy C, DesRosiers MH, Patlak CS, Pettigrew KD, Sakurada O, Shinohara M. The [^{14}C]deoxyglucose method for the determination of local cerebral glucose utilization: theory, procedure, and normal values in the conscious and anesthetized albino rat. *J Neurochem.* 1977;28:897-916.
26. Phelps ME, Huang S-C, Hoffman EJ, Selin C, Sokoloff L, Kuhl DE. Tomographic measurement of local cerebral glucose metabolic rate in humans with [F-18]1-fluoro-2-deoxy-D-glucose: validation of method. *Ann Neurol.* 1979;6:371-388.
27. Brooks R. Alternative formula for glucose utilization using labeled deoxyglucose. *J Nucl Med.* 1982;23:538-539.
28. Cohen RM, Semple WE, Gross M, King AC, Nordahl TE. The metabolic brain pattern of sustained auditory discrimination. *Exp Brain Res.* 1992;92:165-172.
29. Semple WE, Johnson JL, Cohen R. Reliability in positron emission tomography. In: London ED, ed. *Imaging Drug Action in the Brain.* Boca Raton, Fla: CRC Press Inc; 1993:297-316.
30. Matsui T, Hirano A. *An Atlas of the Human Brain for Computerized Tomography.* New York, NY: Igaku-Shoin Medical Publishers; 1978.
31. Metter EJ, Riege WH, Kuhl DE, Phelps ME. Cerebral metabolic relationships for selected brain regions in healthy adults. *J Cereb Blood Flow Metab.* 1984;4:1-7.
32. Clark C, Carson R, Kessler R, Margolin R, Buchsbaum M, DeLisi L, King C, Cohen R. Alternative statistical models for the examination of clinical positron emission tomography/fluorodeoxyglucose data. *J Cereb Blood Flow Metab.* 1985;5:142-150.
33. Sedvall G. The current status of PET scanning with respect to schizophrenia. *Neuropsychopharmacology.* 1992;7:41-54.
34. Alexander GE, DeLong MR, Strick PL. Parallel organization of functionally segregated circuits linking basal ganglia and cortex. *Annu Rev Neurosci.* 1986;9:357-381.
35. Kotrla KJ, Weinberger DR. Brain imaging in schizophrenia. *Annu Rev Med.* 1995;36:1275-1281.
36. Wolkin A, Sanfilipo M, Wolf AP, Angrist B, Brodie J, Rotrosen J. Negative symptoms and hypofrontality in chronic schizophrenia. *Arch Gen Psychiatry.* 1992;49:959-965.
37. Tamminga CA, Thaker GK, Buchanan R, Kirkpatrick B, Alphs LD, Chase TN, Carpenter WT. Limbic system abnormalities identified in schizophrenia using positron emission tomography with fluorodeoxyglucose and neocortical alterations with deficit syndrome. *Arch Gen Psychiatry.* 1992;49:522-530.
38. Buchsbaum MS, Nuechterlein KH, Haier RJ, Wu J, Sicotte N, Hazlett E, Asarnow R, Potkin S, Guich S. Glucose metabolic rate in normals and schizophrenics during the continuous performance task assessed by positron emission tomography. *Br J Psychiatry.* 1990;156:216-227.
39. Early TS, Reiman EM, Raichle ME, Spitznagel EL. Left globus pallidus abnormality in never-medicated patients with schizophrenia. *Proc Natl Acad Sci U S A.* 1987;84:561-563.
40. Sheppard G, Gruzelier J, Machanda R, Hirsch SR. ^{15}O positron emission tomographic scanning in predominantly never-treated acute schizophrenic patients. *Lancet.* 1983;2:1448-1452.
41. Gur RE, Mozley D, Resnick SM, Mozley L, Shtasel E, Gallacher R, Arnold SE, Karp JS, Alavi A, Reivich M, Gur RC. Resting cerebral glucose metabolism in first-episode and previously treated patients with schizophrenia. *Arch Gen Psychiatry.* 1995;52:657-667.
42. Dursun SM, Reveley MA. Obsessive-compulsive symptoms and clozapine. *Br J Psychiatry.* 1994;165:267-268.
43. Allen L, Tejera C. Treatment of clozapine-induced obsessive-compulsive symptoms with sertraline. *Am J Psychiatry.* 1994;151:1096-1097.
44. Baxter LR, Phelps ME, Mazziotta JC, Guze BH, Schwartz JM, Selin CE. Local cerebral glucose metabolic rates in obsessive-compulsive disorder: a comparison with rates in unipolar depression and normal controls. *Arch Gen Psychiatry.* 1987;44:211-218.
45. Nordahl TE, Benkelfat C, Semple WE, Gross M, King AC, Cohen RM. Cerebral glucose metabolic rates in obsessive compulsive disorder. *Neuropsychopharmacology.* 1989;2:23-28.

ORIGINAL ARTICLE

Increased Phospholipid Breakdown in Schizophrenia

Evidence for the Involvement of a Calcium-Independent Phospholipase A_2

Brian M. Ross, PhD; Craig Hudson, MD; Jeffrey Erlich; Jerry J. Warsh, MD, PhD; Stephen J. Kish, PhD

Background: Magnetic resonance spectroscopy studies have suggested above-normal turnover of membrane phospholipids in brains of patients with schizophrenia. One possible explanation for these findings is increased activity of the phospholipid-catabolizing enzyme phospholipase A_2 (PLA_2). However, attempts to demonstrate higher PLA_2 activity in the serum of subjects with schizophrenia have led to conflicting results. We hypothesized that this was due to serum PLA_2 activity consisting of a family of different enzymes, with each group of investigators measuring activity of different PLA_2 forms.

Design: Activity of PLA_2 in serum samples obtained from 24 individuals with schizophrenia was compared with serum obtained from 33 age- and sex-matched control subjects, using both fluorometric and radiometric assays with different substrates. Each method had previously yielded conflicting results concerning the status of the enzyme in schizophrenia.

Results: With the fluorometric assay, serum PLA_2 activity in individuals with schizophrenia was markedly increased by 49% compared with control subjects ($P<.001$). In contrast, radiometric assay of the same serum samples resulted in PLA_2 activity not significantly different between patients and control subjects. Further investigations demonstrated that, whereas the radiometric assay measured activity of a calcium-dependent enzyme, the fluorometric assay detected a calcium-insensitive enzyme possessing an acid-neutral pH optimum.

Conclusions: Increased calcium-independent PLA_2 activity was seen in the serum of patients with schizophrenia. This change, if present also in the brain, may well explain the increased levels of phosphodiesters observed using magnetic resonance spectroscopy and therefore may contribute to the pathophysiological features of the disorder.

Arch Gen Psychiatry. 1997;54:487-494

A SUBSTANTIAL body of data suggests that membrane phospholipid metabolism is altered in patients with schizophrenia.[1,2] For example, most investigators,[3-9] although not all,[10,11] observed decreased levels of 1 or both major membrane phospholipids, phosphatidylcholine and phosphatidylethanolamine (PE), in serum and fibroblasts of patients with schizophrenia. In addition, altered levels of specific fatty acids have been observed in erythrocytes of patients with schizophrenia,[12] whereas the turnover of platelet phosphatidylinositol[13] and arachidonic acid[14] is increased. Taken together, these findings suggest elevated phospholipid breakdown in schizophrenia.

Recently, direct evidence for perturbed phospholipid metabolism in the brain of subjects with schizophrenia was obtained using phosphorus 31 magnetic resonance spectroscopy, which allows the abundance of phosphorous-containing compounds to be measured in vivo. Several independent investigators have reported increased levels of membrane breakdown products (phosphodiesters) in the frontal and temporal cortices of drug-naive[15-17] and drug-treated[18,19] subjects with schizophrenia. Furthermore, the abundance of metabolites used in membrane synthesis (phosphomonoesters) is decreased consistently in the frontal cortex of drug-treated and drug-naive patients,[16,17,20-23] implying more rapid use of these compounds for membrane biosynthesis. Taken together, these data suggest that membrane turnover is accelerated in schizophrenia. The consequences of such a perturbation are unclear, but may include membrane breakdown and altered interneuronal communication, in particular the production of phospholipid-derived second messengers (eg, prostaglandins, leukotrienes, and inositol phosphates),[24-26] ul-

From the Clarke Institute of Psychiatry (Drs Ross, Hudson, Warsh, and Kish and Mr Erlich), the Departments of Psychiatry (Drs Ross, Warsh, and Kish) and Pharmacology (Drs Warsh and Kish), and the Institute of Medical Science (Drs Hudson, Warsh, and Kish), University of Toronto, Toronto, Ontario.

SUBJECTS AND METHODS

SUBJECTS

Subjects with schizophrenia were recruited by advertisement from the patient population of the Clarke Institute of Psychiatry, Toronto, Ontario. All received diagnoses according to *DSM-III-R* criteria[34] using the Structured Clinical Interview for *DSM-III-R* (SCID), and their psychopathological states were assessed using the Positive and Negative Syndrome Scale (PANSS). Control subjects had no history of mental illness as assessed during the SCID interview and were recruited by advertisement from the greater Toronto area. The sample consisted of 24 hospitalized individuals suffering from paranoid schizophrenia (15 male and 9 female patients; mean±SEM age, 40±2 years) as described in **Table 1** and 33 healthy control subjects (20 male and 13 female subjects; mean±SEM age, 38±2 years), all of whom had given written informed consent. There were no significant differences between the mean ages (P=.26, Student t test) or relative numbers of male and female subjects (P=.64, Pearson χ^2 goodness of fit) in each group. The subjects with schizophrenia were all receiving neuroleptic therapy at the time of blood withdrawal (397±75 chlorpromazine equivalents). Both control subjects and subjects with schizophrenia showed no signs of physical illness and had no recent history of alcohol or other drug abuse based on information collected during the SCID interview. In addition, subjects had not taken any anti-inflammatory medication for at least 2 weeks before blood withdrawal. Venous blood (10 mL) was withdrawn into Vacutainers without anticoagulant and allowed to clot for approximately 30 minutes at room temperature. Blood was centrifuged at $1500g_{average}$ for 20 minutes at room temperature, and the resulting serum samples were stored at −80°C until assay.

MATERIALS

The 1-octasanyl-2-(pyren-l-yl)-hexanoyl-*sn*-phosphatidylmethanol (C28-O-PHPM) was purchased from Oy Acadexim Ab, Helsinki, Finland. The 1-alk-1′-enyl-2-$[^{14}C]$-arachidonyl phosphatidylcholine (choline plasmalogen) was a gift from Ernest Do, PhD, New England Nuclear, Boston, Mass. All other radiochemicals were purchased from New England Nuclear, Toronto, Ontario. Porcine pancreatic PLA_2 ($pPLA_2$) was purchased from Sigma Chemical Company, St Louis, Mo, whereas secretory ($sPLA_2$) and cytosolic PLA_2 ($cPLA_2$) were a gift from Ruth Kramer, PhD, Lilly Research Laboratories, Indianapolis, Ind.

DETERMINATION OF PLA_2 ACTIVITY

Serum PLA_2 activity was assayed fluorometrically,[34] based on the procedure used by Gattaz et al[28,29] in their studies of serum and plasma PLA_2 in schizophrenia, and radiometrically, based on the procedure used by Albers et al[32] in their study of PLA_2 in the disorder. Assays were performed in duplicate, with the investigator unaware of the diagnosis.

The fluorometric assay measures the rate of hydrolysis of the pyrene-labeled phospholipid analogue, C28-O-PHPM. The *sn*-1 ether bond of this compound makes it resistant to hydrolysis by serum lipases.[35] Briefly, 40 μL serum was incubated in the presence of 30 μmol/L C28-0-PHPM and 14 mmol/L Tris(hydroxymethyl) aminomethane (Tris)/hydrogen chloride (pH, 7.4) (final assay volume, 200 μL) for 90 minutes at 37°C, and the released pyrenyl-hexanoic acid was extracted and quantified as described.[35] "Blank" reactions (to measure nonenzymatic hydrolysis) contained serum but were stopped at zero time. No difference in blank values was observed between control subjects and subjects with schizophrenia. Hydrolysis of the *sn*-1 ester bond by incubation in the presence of 1 mol/L hydrogen chloride did not lead to increased release of fluorescent product (data not shown). The assay was linear with respect to time for at least 2 hours, and with respect to volume of serum up to 70 μL. We were concerned that the low ionic strength of Tris in the assay buffer would be

timately leading to the behavioral abnormalities observed in the disorder.

It is therefore of great interest to discover the mechanisms that underlie the observed membrane abnormalities. We and others[22] suggest that a likely mechanism, which offers a simple explanation for the schizophrenia-associated increase in phosphodiester levels, is an increase in the activity of phospholipase A_2 (PLA_2), the rate-limiting enzyme of phospholipid breakdown.[27] However, whereas 2 groups of investigators have found that PLA_2 activity is increased in serum of subjects with schizophrenia,[28-31] another group did not.[32] These conflicting results may relate to the fact that PLA_2 is not a single protein species, but a family of different enzymes.[33] We hypothesized that different investigators, using various assay procedures, have detected different PLA_2 subtypes, and that a change in the activity of the enzyme is confined to a specific isoform. In an attempt to resolve this controversy, PLA_2 activity was assayed in the serum of control subjects and patients with schizophrenia using 2 different methods characterized with respect to the distinct PLA_2 isoforms that each detects.

RESULTS

Phospholipase A_2 activity, measured using the fluorometric assay (**Figure 1**, left), was significantly (P<.001) and markedly increased by 49% in the subjects with schizophrenia (41.1±2.2 pmol fatty acid per minute per milliliter of serum) compared with control subjects (27.6±1.5 pmol fatty acid per minute per milliliter of serum). To confirm the reproducibility of the assay, a subset of subjects (n=21) underwent reassay, with similar results (data not shown; r_s=0.94). Kinetic analysis (**Figure 2**) in 3 subjects with schizophrenia possessing high serum PLA_2 levels and in 3 randomly selected control subjects revealed that elevated activity was due to significantly increased maximal velocity (69.6±1.6 vs 32.6±3.6 pmol fatty acid per minute per milliliter of serum in subjects with schizophrenia and control subinsufficient to adequately buffer the incubation mix. However, measurement of the assay buffer pH following the addition of serum did not reveal any significant fluctuation from 7.4 (3 control subjects and 3 patients with schizophrenia).

The radiometric method used autoclaved *Escherichia coli* bacteria labeled with hydrogen 3–labeled arachidonic acid at the *sn*-2 position as substrate,[32] modified to make use of commercially available reagents. Specifically, 30 μL serum was incubated in the presence of approximately 60 000 disintegrations per minute of ^{3}H-arachidonyl–labeled *E coli* (specific activity, 407 MBq/mmol phosphate), 1 mmol/L calcium chloride, and 100 mmol/L N-[2-hydroxyethyl]piperazine-*N′*-2-ethanesulfonic acid/sodium hydroxide (pH, 7.4) (final assay volume, 75 μL) for 30 minutes at 37°C. The reaction was terminated by the addition of 75 μL ethanol containing 1% acetic acid and 100 μg/mL arachidonic acid, and the release of radiolabeled free fatty acid was quantitated using thin-layer chromatography and liquid scintillation spectroscopy.[36] Blank reactions contained serum but were stopped at zero time. The reaction was linear with respect to time up to 40 minutes and with respect to serum up to 60 μL. Since specific radioactivity of the *E coli* was given in terms of moles of phosphate, activities are described in terms of picomole (pmol) of phosphate equivalents of fatty acid. However, since almost all the radioactivity is associated with the fatty acid fraction, the specific radioactivity per mole of phosphate is very similar to that per mole of fatty acid. In experiments using synthetic radiolabeled phospholipids, substrates were dried by vacuum centrifugation and resuspended in ethanol. One hundred microliters serum was incubated with 10 mmol/L ethylenediaminetetraacetic acid (EDTA), 100 mmol Tris/hydrogen chloride (pH, 7.4), and 6.5 μmol/L phospholipid substrate (specific activity, approximately 1850 MBq/mmol) in 5 μL ethanol (final assay volume, 400 μL) at 37°C for 60 minutes. The reaction was terminated by the addition of 400 μL butanol, followed by vortexing and centrifugation at 13 000$g_{average}$ for 5 minutes.[37] An aliquot of the butanol phase was dried by vacuum centrifugation, the residue was resuspended in ethanol, and radiolabeled free fatty acid was quantitated as described above.

PURIFIED PLA_2 SUBTYPES

To determine the PLA_2 subtypes detected by each assay, purified enzymes were used. Each enzyme was diluted in 20 mmol/L Tris/hydrogen chloride (pH, 7.4) containing 1 mg/mL bovine serum albumin (essentially fatty acid free) immediately before use. In preliminary experiments, the linear range of fatty acid release with respect to protein concentration was determined, and concentrations were chosen that gave similar activities to those obtained using human serum. The protein concentrations used for the fluorometric assay were 130, 40, and 1000 ng protein per tube of $pPLA_2$, $sPLA_2$, and $cPLA_2$, respectively, and for the radiometric assay were 0.65, 200, and 1000 ng protein per tube of $pPLA_2$, $sPLA_2$, and $cPLA_2$, respectively.

STATISTICAL ANALYSIS

Data from the control subjects and subjects with schizophrenia were compared using a 2-tailed, unpaired, Student *t* test, after first confirming normality of the data using a Liliefors test. Interaction between subject group and assay type was investigated by 2-way analysis of variance (ANOVA). Spearman correlation coefficients were used throughout (r_s), as was an α level of .05.

DETERMINATION OF pH OPTIMUM

The buffers used at each pH were MES (2-[*N*-Morpholino]ethanesulfonic acid]), 5.0 to 6.5; HEPES (*N*-[2-hydroxyethyl]piperazine-*N′*-[2-ethanesulfonic acid]), 7.0 to 8.0; and borate, 8.5 to 10.0.

Data are given as mean±SEM.

jects, respectively; $P<.001$), whereas the substrate Michaelis constant was not significantly altered (6.9±2.0 μmol/L in subjects with schizophrenia vs 3.9±0.1 μmol/L in control subjects; $P=.21$). Fluorometrically assayed PLA_2 activity was significantly correlated with overall severity ($r_s=0.44$; $P=.03$) and positive symptom scores ($r_s=0.42$; $P=.04$) of the PANSS scale, but not with the negative symptom ($r_s=0.25$) or general psychopathology score ($r_s=0.33$) (**Figure 3**).

In contrast, no significant difference ($P>.99$) was apparent between control subjects and subjects with schizophrenia when PLA_2 activity was assayed radiometrically (Figure 1, right), using the same serum samples as for the fluorometric assay (mean activities, 91.4±7.4 vs 91.3±4.2 pmol phosphate equivalents of fatty acid per minute per milliliter of serum in subjects with schizophrenia and control subjects, respectively). The discordance between both methods was further revealed by the lack of correlation between the activity measured in each subject by the different assays ($r_s=0.091$; **Figure 4**), and the statistically significant ($P=.007$) interaction between assay type and subject group as assessed by 2-way ANOVA. In addition, no significant correlation was observed between radiometrically assayed PLA_2 activity and any PANSS scores ($-0.15<r_s<0.22$).

Measured PLA_2 activity was not significantly different in male and female subjects and was not correlated with age, treatment duration, or chlorpromazine equivalents of neuroleptic medication ($P>.25$ in all cases). Furthermore, the addition of 20 nmol/L haloperidol (a concentration typical of that found in serum of patients receiving neuroleptic therapy[38]) to each assay had no significant effect on activity (n=5 control subjects; data not shown).

The dissimilarity between the results of both PLA_2 assays was further investigated by an examination of the calcium ion requirements of the activity revealed by each method. As expected,[32,39] activity measured by the radiometric assay was almost completely abolished by the addition of the calcium ion chelator EDTA to the assay

Table 1. Clinical Details of Subjects With Schizophrenia

Subject No./ Sex/Age, y*	Duration of Treatment, y†	PANSS Scale Scores‡ Positive	Negative	General Psychopathology	Medication at Time of Blood Withdrawal
1/M/42	22	22	22	30	Fluphenazine hydrochloride; 50 mg/2 wk
2/M/42	21	20	11	27	Perphenazine; 80 mg/d
3/F/41	15	7	11	16	Flupenthixol; 60 mg/4 wk
4/M/38	20	7	7	17	Flupenthixol; 20 mg/3 wk
5/M/28	3	13	20	25	Fluphenazine; 5 mg/d
6/M/46	20	12	12	23	Trifluoperazine hydrochloride; 20 mg/d
7/M/36	14	15	12	25	Haloperidol; 100 mg/2 wk
8/M/42	22	10	14	27	Perphenazine; 12 mg/d
9/M/33	15	28	10	27	Fluspirilene; 4 mg/wk
10/M/33	15	35	24	50	Clozapine; 250 mg twice daily
11/F/25	6	15	16	29	Risperidone; 6 mg/d
12/F/65	41	7	14	22	Thioridazine hydrochloride; 100 mg twice daily
13/F/43	24	8	13	21	Fluphenazine; 13 mg/3 wk
14/F/40	23	16	11	ND	Pipotiazine palmitate; 100 mg/2 wk
15/M/43	25	16	10	ND	Flupenthixol; 50 mg/2 wk
16/F/46	28	18	18	31	Flupenthixol; 2 mg/2 wk
17/F/48	30	17	25	20	Pimozide; 6 mg/d
18/M/32	13	16	13	25	Pimozide; 4 mg/d
19/F/43	21	7	7	16	Haloperidol; 0.5 mg/d
20/F/43	25	8	8	24	Fluphenazine; 100 mg/4 wk
21/M/34	16	ND	ND	ND	Fluphenazine; 24 mg/d
22/M/30	6	8	11	21	Risperidone; 4 mg/d
23/M/31	15	19	8	28	Flupenthixol; 3 mg twice daily
24/M/49	30	29	29	42	Clozapine; 300 mg twice daily

**Mean±SEM age was 40±2 years.*

†Mean±SEM duration of treatment was 18±2 years.

‡PANSS indicates Positive and Negative Syndrome Scale; ND not determined. For positive symptoms, mean±SEM score was 15±2; for negative symptoms, 14±1; and for general psychopathology, 26±2.

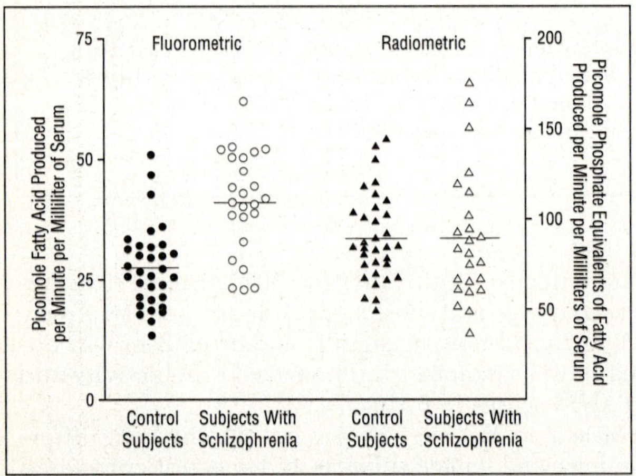

Figure 1. *Phospholipase A_2 (PLA_2) activity in the serum of subjects with schizophrenia (n=24) compared with that in control subjects (n=33). The PLA_2 activity was significantly (P<.001) increased in subjects with schizophrenia compared with control subjects when assayed fluorometrically (left) but unchanged (P>.99) when assayed radiometrically (right). Bars indicate the mean activity in each group.*

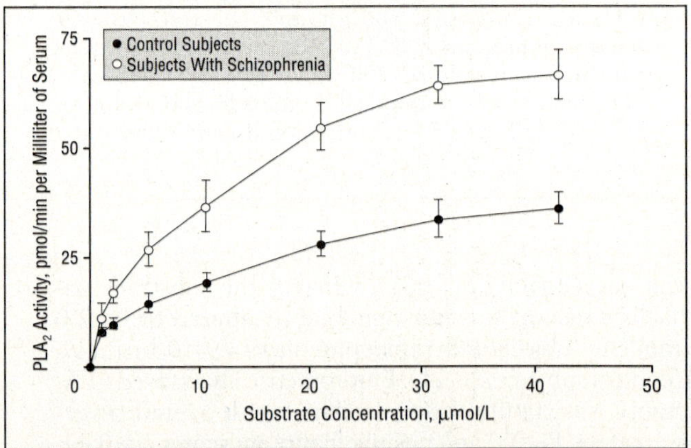

Figure 2. *Effect of substrate concentration on serum phospholipase A_2 (PLA_2) activity in control subjects and subjects with schizophrenia. The PLA_2 activity was measured fluorometrically under varying substrate concentrations in control subjects or subjects with schizophrenia. Each point represents the mean values of 3 subjects analyzed in separate experiments. Bars indicate the SEM.*

buffer, although activity in the presence of 1 mmol/L calcium chloride was not significantly different from that without added calcium, indicating that PLA_2 is fully activated by endogenous calcium ions (**Table 2**). In contrast, the inclusion of EDTA in the fluorometric assay did not significantly alter the rate of hydrolysis (Table 2). The EDTA-insensitive activity was investigated further and found to possess a slightly acidic pH optimum of 6.0 to 7.0 (**Figure 5**) and was moderately inhibited (by 29.1%±5.5% in 5 control subjects) by 5 mmol/L dithiothreitol.

We next compared the characteristics of 3 purified PLA_2s in each assay, ie, porcine $pPLA_2$, human low-molecular-weight $sPLA_2$, and human high-molecular-

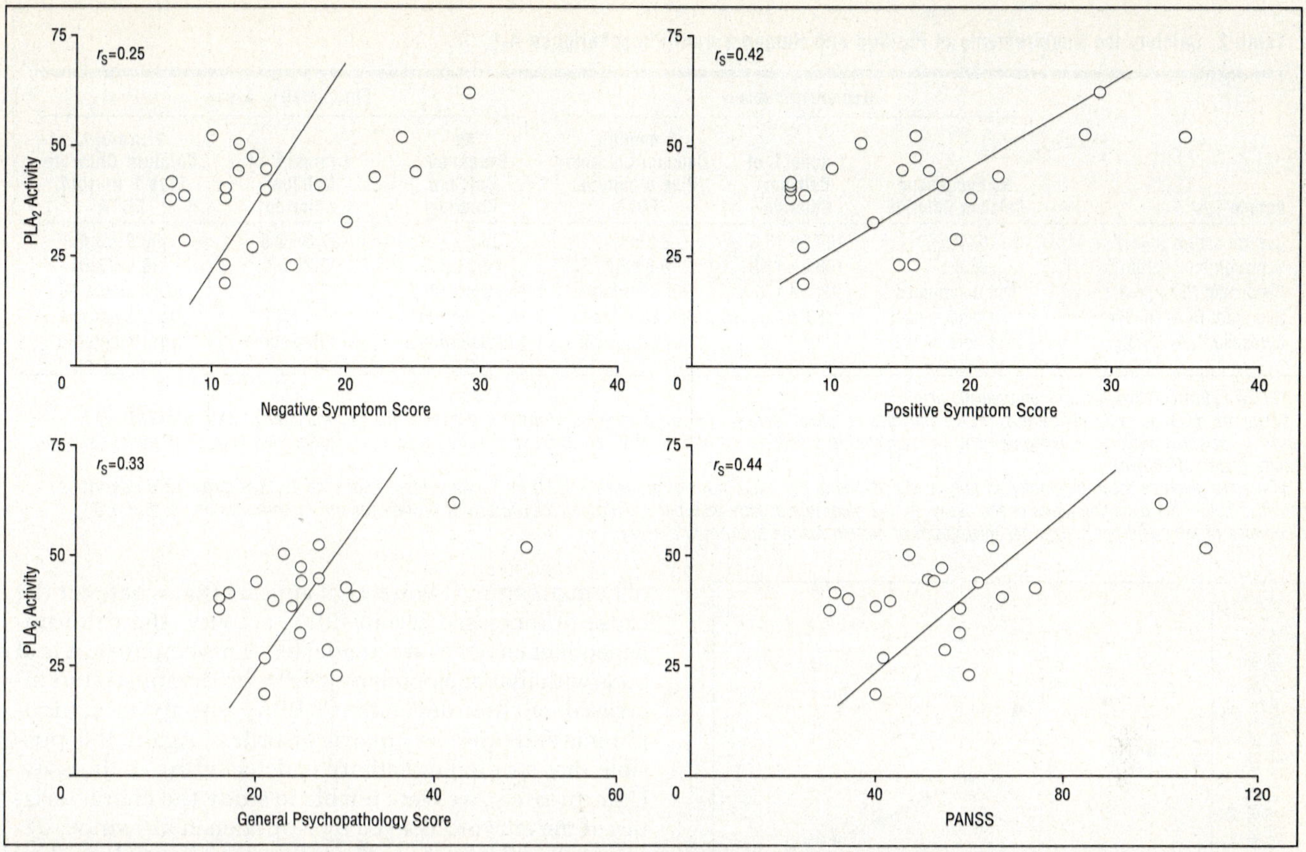

Figure 3. *Correlation between phospholipase A_2 (PLA_2) activity and Positive and Negative Syndrome Scale (PANSS) scores. Serum PLA_2 activity in subjects with schizophrenia measured fluorometrically was significantly correlated ($P<.05$) with positive symptom and overall PANSS scores but not with negative symptom or general psychopathology score. Each panel also shows the best-fit line and the Spearman regression coefficient (r_s).*

weight $cPLA_2$. In the radiometric assay, $pPLA_2$ was much more active than $sPLA_2$ or $cPLA_2$, while in the fluorometric assay $cPLA_2$ was completely inactive, the highest rate of hydrolysis being catalyzed by $sPLA_2$ followed by $pPLA_2$ (Table 2). Furthermore, irrespective of assay type, no hydrolysis was detected in the presence of EDTA. It is therefore unlikely that the enzymatic activity in human serum that catalyses the hydrolysis of C28-O-PHPM in the fluorometric assay derives from $cPLA_2$, $sPLA_2$, or $pPLA_2$.

Finally, we investigated whether human serum contained a calcium-insensitive PLA_2 able to hydrolyze phospholipid species normally found in the body, as opposed to the atypical phospholipid analogue C28-O-PHPM. No evidence was found for such an enzyme active against phosphatidylinositol or diacylphosphatidylcholine. However, PE was hydrolyzed in the presence of 10 mmol/L EDTA, with low rates of hydrolysis of 1-alk-1′-enyl-2-acyl phosphatidylcholine (choline plasmalogen) also being observed (**Table 3**). Furthermore, we also detected the presence of a lysophospholipase activity (the enzyme that hydrolyzes the lysophospholipid product of PLA_2 catalysis) in serum (Table 3).

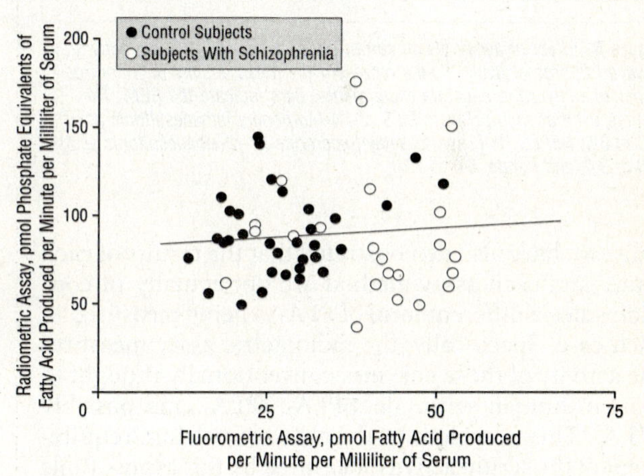

Figure 4. *Lack of correlation between phospholipase A_2 activity measured fluorometrically and radiometrically in control subjects and subjects with schizophrenia. The best-fit line through all points is shown.*

COMMENT

To our knowledge, this is the first investigation in which multiple forms of PLA_2 have been simultaneously assayed in the serum of patients with schizophrenia. Our major finding was that calcium-independent PLA_2 ($iPLA_2$) activity was increased in schizophrenia, whereas calcium-dependent activity was unaltered.

In agreement with Gattaz et al,[29] if serum PLA_2 is assayed by the fluorometric procedure, we found activity to be markedly elevated in patients with schizophrenia, whereas if the enzyme is assayed radiometrically we found, like Albers et al,[32] the activity to be unaltered. Criti-

Table 2. Calcium Ion Requirements of Purified and Human Serum Phospholipase A_2*

	Radiometric Assay			Fluorometric Assay		
Source	No Exogenous Calcium Chloride	1 mmol/L of Calcium Chloride	1 mmol/L Calcium Chloride Plus 5 mmol/L EDTA	No Exogenous Calcium Chloride	1 mmol/L of Calcium Chloride	1 mmol/L Calcium Chloride Plus 5 mmol/L EDTA
Control serum (n=5)†	103.2±7.1	104.2±13.9	8.8±4.0	26.2±4.1	27.3±2.5	30.0±3.4
Schizophrenic serum (n=5)†	96.8±7.4	108.3±11.2	8.8±2.2	40.3±3.7	42.2±5.0	38.9±3.0
Pancreatic PLA_2 (n=3)‡	Not determined	4225±126	Not detectable	Not determined	16.2±2.1	Not detectable
Secretory PLA_2 (n=3)‡	Not determined	18.2±2.6	Not detectable	Not determined	55.5±4.2	Not detectable
Cytosolic PLA_2 (n=3)‡	Not determined	4.1±0.8	Not detectable	Not determined	Not detectable	Not detectable

*EDTA indicates ethylenediaminetetraacetic acid.

†Data are given as phospholipase A_2 (PLA_2) activities of human serum in mean picomoles of fatty acid per minute per milliliter of serum (SEM) of 5 randomly selected subjects. This experiment was repeated in a second set of 5 control subjects and 5 subjects with schizophrenia, with qualitatively similar results (data not shown).

‡Data are given as mean picomoles of fatty acid per minute per microgram of protein (±SEM) in 3 independent experiments. Not detectable describes activities below the detection limits of the assay, ie, 0.2 picomole of fatty acid per minute per microgram of protein for the radiometric assay and 1.5 picomoles of fatty acid per minute per microgram of protein for the fluorometric assay.

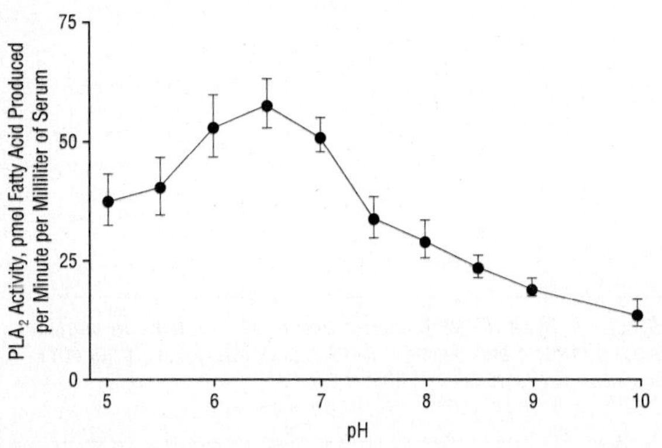

Figure 5. *Effect of assay pH on serum phospholipase A_2 (PLA_2) activity assayed fluorometrically. Points represent the mean activity of 3 control subjects analyzed in separate experiments. Bars indicate the SEM. The buffers used at each pH were MES (2-[N-Morpholino]ethanesulfonic acid]), 5.0 to 6.5; HEPES (N-[2-hydroxyethyl]piperazine-N′-[2-ethanesulfonic acid]), 7.0 to 8.0; and borate, 8.5 to 10.0.*

cally, we have also demonstrated that the results of each study and each assay method are not actually in conflict, since a different form of PLA_2 is being measured in each case. Specifically, the radiometric assay measures the activity of those enzymes conventionally thought to exist in human serum, ie, $pPLA_2$, $sPLA_2$, and possibly $cPLA_2$. This is evident by the absolute calcium requirement of the serum activity measured by this assay (Table 2). Thus, our data and those of Albers et al[32] strongly suggest that the activity of "classical" calcium-sensitive serum PLA_2 is unchanged in serum of subjects with schizophrenia. This finding firmly differentiates schizophrenia-associated alterations in serum PLA_2 activity from those observed in, for example, acute pancreatitis, rheumatoid arthritis, and multiple injuries, which are due to increased serum levels of $sPLA_2$ occurring as part of the acute-phase response in these diseases.[40] We suggest that enhanced PLA_2 activity in schizophrenia, assayed using the substrate C28-O-PHPM, may involve an $iPLA_2$ activity. Moreover, since no correlation was apparent between the calcium-dependent and calcium-independent activities of human serum (Figure 4), it appears that whatever the cause of increased serum $iPLA_2$ activity, the calcium-dependent enzymes are unaffected. This conclusion is at odds with that of Noponen et al,[31] who demonstrated increased calcium-dependent[39] PLA_2 activity in schizophrenia and other psychiatric disorders. Again, it is possible that a different activity is detected by each assay. Unfortunately, we were unable to study the characteristics of the enzyme assayed by Noponen et al[31] since, despite using identical assay conditions to those described in their report, no significant hydrolysis of the phospholipid substrate could be detected in 8 of 10 serum samples assayed.

Although purified $sPLA_2$ and $pPLA_2$ are capable of hydrolyzing C28-O-PHPM in a calcium-dependent manner, the lack of inhibition of serum activity by calcium chelators (EDTA) suggests that they do not contribute significantly to serum PLA_2 activity as measured fluorometrically (Table 2). This can be explained by reference to the levels of these enzymes present in normal human serum, approximately 4 ng/mL for $pPLA_2$ and 3 ng/mL for $sPLA_2$.[40] Based on the specific activities of the purified enzymes (Table 2), the enzyme levels in normal serum are below the detection limit of the assay. Admittedly, the activity of our $pPLA_2$ preparation was lower than that used in the original characterization of the fluorometric assay.[35] However, even using this higher specific activity (2 pmol of fatty acid per minute per nanogram of protein), the rate of fatty acid release would be only 8 pmol of fatty acid per minute per milliliter of serum (given that serum contains 4 ng/mL $pPLA_2$), which in our hands would be only slightly above blank values. Thus, the fluorometric assay is simply not sensitive enough to detect the low levels of $pPLA_2$ and $sPLA_2$ normally present in human serum.

The identity of the $iPLA_2$ we detected in serum is unclear. Blood is known to contain at least 4 calcium-independent lipases, ie, hepatic endothelial lipase,[41] lipoprotein lipase,[42] platelet activating factor acetylhydrolase,[43] and lecithin-cholesterol acyltransferase.[44] However, the characteristics of these enzymes are dissimilar to the $iPLA_2$ activity we have identified, suggesting that the en-

Table 3. Calcium-Independent Phospholipid Hydrolyzing Activities in Human Serum

Substrate	Activity*
1-Palmitoyl, 2-[^{14}C]-arachidonyl, phosphatidylethanolamine	1.21±0.21
1-Stearoyl, 2-[^{3}H]-arachidonyl, phosphatidylcholine	Not detectable
1-Alk-1′-enyl, 2-[^{14}C]-arachidonyl, phosphatidylcholine	0.20±0.02
1-Stearoyl, 2-[^{14}C]-arachidonyl, phosphatidylinositol	Not detectable
1-[^{14}C]-Palmitoyl, lysophosphatidylcholine	1.57±0.90

Activity was measured at a pH of 7.5 in the presence of 10 mmol/L of ethylenediaminetetraacetic acid. Values are given as mean picomoles of fatty acid released per minute per milliliter of serum (±SEM) of 6 control subjects analyzed in 3 separate experiments. Not detectable describes activities below 0.2 picomole of fatty acid produced per minute per milliliter of serum, the detection limits of the assay.

zyme described herein may be of a novel form. Interestingly, a phosphatidylmethanol hydrolyzing $iPLA_2$ activity has recently been detected in platelets.[45] A platelet source for serum $iPLA_2$ is also supported by the observation that platelet PLA_2 activity is increased, albeit marginally, in schizophrenia.[30]

Importantly, we have also demonstrated that the natural phospholipids PE and choline plasmalogen can be hydrolyzed in a calcium-independent manner by an enzyme present in human serum, suggesting that the actions of serum $iPLA_2$ are not limited to the hydrolysis of atypical phospholipids such as C28-O-PHPM (Table 3). This is of particular interest given that many,[3-6] although not all,[7,9,10] investigators have reported reduced platelet or erythrocyte PE levels in schizophrenia.

Our findings differ from those of Gattaz et al[28] with respect to the effect of neuroleptic medication on serum PLA_2 in schizophrenia, in that all of our patients were treated with neuroleptics and those observed by Gattaz et al with increased activity were not. Indeed, they found that PLA_2 activity was reduced after the commencement of neuroleptic therapy to the point where there was no longer a difference between the activities of patients with schizophrenia and control subjects.[28] However, whereas the duration of drug treatment of our subjects always exceeded 1 year, and in most cases was considerably longer, Gattaz et al[28] only monitored PLA_2 activity for 3 weeks after the commencement of therapy. Thus, the neuroleptic-associated reduction in serum PLA_2 activity described by Gattaz et al[28] may be a temporary effect reversed after more extended treatment. It is worth noting that addition of haloperidol to the assay at a concentration typical of that found in the serum of neuroleptic-treated patients with schizophrenia (20 nmol/L[38]) did not affect PLA_2 activity. Clearly, longer-term studies of the effect of neuroleptic treatment will be required to resolve this issue.

It is presently unclear the degree to which perturbed phospholipid metabolism is specific to schizophrenia. Gattaz et al[28-30] have consistently reported unaltered PLA_2 activity in subjects suffering from psychiatric disorders (primarily major depression) other than schizophrenia. However, recent reports have indicated that phospholipid metabolites in the brains of patients suffering from bipolar disorder are changed in a similar manner to those in schizophrenia.[46-48] To address this issue, we are currently investigating serum $iPLA_2$ activity in bipolar disorder, as well as other well-defined psychiatric and neurological conditions.

Interestingly, the increase in serum PLA_2 activity in schizophrenia was positively, although weakly, correlated with overall psychopathological severity, a finding due mainly to a correlation between the positive symptom component of the PANSS scale and PLA_2 activity (Figure 3). In contrast, negative symptom scores correlated poorly with PLA_2 activity. Thus, if increased PLA_2 activity is the basis for the elevated levels of brain phosphodiester observed during brain imaging, one would expect to find a correlation between phosphodiester levels and positive, but not negative, symptoms. Indeed, although increased brain phosphodiester levels are present in groups of patients possessing marked positive symptoms,[18] phosphodiester levels are unchanged in subjects with mainly negative symptoms.[22,23] Differences in degree of positive symptoms also may explain why some researchers report increased phosphodiester levels in individuals with schizophrenia receiving long-term neuroleptic treatment,[18,19] whereas others only detect a change in neuroleptic-naive patients,[16] although other interstudy variables, such as differing anatomical regions or stages of illness, may also account for the contrasting findings of individual studies. A causative role of $iPLA_2$ in increasing levels of brain phosphodiesters and in the pathophysiological features of the disorder is dependent on a serumlike $iPLA_2$ being present in the brain. To this end, our experiments have indicated that human brain contains $iPLA_2$ activities capable of hydrolyzing PE[49] and C28-O-PHPM (B.M.R., unpublished data, July 1995).

In summary, we have shown that the failure by some groups to detect increased PLA_2 activity in the serum of individuals with schizophrenia is due to methodological differences and that the affected activity is attributable, at least in part, to a calcium-independent enzyme. If a similar increase occurs in the brains of subjects with schizophrenia, this may explain why brain phosphodiester levels are increased, especially in those with pronounced positive symptoms. Currently, it is unknown whether increased PLA_2 activity represents a primary detrimental phenomena, eg, increased membrane breakdown and production of eicosanoids, or is a beneficial compensatory change in response to other biochemical abnormalities such as decreased prostaglandin synthesis.[2] Future experiments using PLA_2 inhibitors to reduce the rate of membrane turnover in patients with schizophrenia will likely resolve this issue.

Accepted for publication March 26, 1996.

Supported by the Ontario Mental Health Foundation (Drs Ross and Kish) and Physician Services Incorporated (Dr Hudson), Toronto, Ontario. Dr Ross is an Ontario Mental Health Foundation scientist.

Reprints: Brian M. Ross, PhD, Human Neurochemical Pathology Laboratory, Clarke Institute of Psychiatry, 250 College St, Toronto, Ontario, Canada M5T 1R8.

REFERENCES

1. Pettegrew JW, Keshavan MS, Minshew NJ. ^{31}P nuclear magnetic resonance spectroscopy: neurodevelopment and schizophrenia. *Schizophr Bull.* 1993;19:36-53.
2. Horrobin DF, Glen AIM, Vaddadi K. The membrane hypothesis of schizophrenia. *Schizophr Res.* 1994;13:195-207.
3. Stevens JD. The distribution of phospholipid fractions in the red cell membranes of schizophrenics. *Schizophr Bull.* 1972;6:60-61.
4. Sengupta N, Datta SC, Sengupta D. Platelet and erythrocyte membrane lipid and phospholipid patterns in different types of mental patients. *Biochem Med.* 1981;25:267-275.
5. Tolbert LC, Monti JA, O'Shields H, Walter-Ryan W, Meadows D, Smythies JR. Defects in transmethylation and membrane lipids in schizophrenia. *Psychopharmacol Bull.* 1993;19:594-599.
6. Keshavan MS, Mallinger AG, Pettegrew JW, Dippold C. Erythrocyte membrane phospholipids in psychotic patients. *J Psychiatr Res.* 1993;49:89-95.
7. Hitzemann R, Hirschowitz J, Garver D. Membrane abnormalities in the psychoses and affective disorders. *J Psychiatr Res.* 1984;18:319-326.
8. Hitzemann RJ, Mark C, Hirschowitz J, Garver DL. Characteristics of phospholipid methylation in human erythrocyte ghosts: relationship(s) to the psychoses and affective disorders. *Biol Psychiatry.* 1985;20:297-307.
9. Lautin A, Mandio CD, Segarnick DJ, Wod L, Mason MF, Rotrosen J. Red cell phospholipids in schizophrenia. *Life Sci.* 1982;31:3051-3056.
10. Pangerl AM, Steudle A, Jaroni HW, Rufer R, Gattaz WF. Increased platelet membrane lysophosphatidylcholine in schizophrenia. *Biol Psychiatry.* 1991;30:837-840.
11. Mahadik SP, Mukherjee S, Correnti EE, Kelkar HS, Wakade CG, Costa RM, Scheffer R. Plasma membrane phospholipid and cholesterol distribution of skin fibroblasts from drug-naive patients at the onset of psychosis. *Schizophr Res.* 1994;13:239-247.
12. Glen AI, Glen EMT, Horrobin DF, Vaddadi KS, Spellman M, Morse-Fisher N, Ells K, Skinner FK. A red cell membrane abnormality in a subgroup of schizophrenic patients: evidence for two diseases. *Schizophr Res.* 1994;12:53-61.
13. Yao JK, Yasaei P, van Kammen DP. Increased turnover of platelet phosphatidylinositol in schizophrenia. *Prostaglandins Leukot Essent Fatty Acids.* 1992; 46:39-46.
14. Demisch L, Gerbaldo H, Gebhart P, Georgi K, Bochnik HJ. Incorporation of ^{14}C-arachidonic acid into platelet phospholipids of untreated patients with schizophreniform or schizophrenic disorders. *Psychiatry Res.* 1987;22:275-282.
15. Keshavan MS, Sanders RD, Pettegrew JW, Dombrowsky SM, Panchalingam KS. Frontal lobe metabolism and cerebral morphology in schizophrenia: ^{31}P MRS and MRI studies. *Schizophr Res.* 1993;10:241-246.
16. Stanley JA, Williamson PC, Drost DJ, Carr TJ, Rylett J, Malla A, Thompson T. An in vivo study of the prefrontal cortex of schizophrenic patients at different stages of illness via phosphorous magnetic resonance spectroscopy. *Arch Gen Psychiatry.* 1995;52:399-406.
17. Pettegrew JW, Keshavan MS, Panchalingam K, Strychor S, Kaplan DB, Tretta MG, Allen M. Alterations in brain high energy phosphate metabolism in first episode drug naive schizophrenics. *Arch Gen Psychiatry.* 1991;48:563-568.
18. Fukazako H, Takeuchi K, Ueyama K, Fukazako T, Hokazono Y, Hirakawa K, Yamada K, Hashiguchi T, Takigawa M, Fujimoto T. ^{31}P magnetic resonance spectroscopy of the medial temporal lobe of schizophrenic patients with neuroleptic-resistant marked positive symptoms. *Eur Arch Psychiatry Clin Neurosci.* 1994; 244:236-240.
19. Fujimoto T, Nakano T, Hokazano Y, Asakura T, Tsuji T. Study of chronic schizophrenics using ^{31}P magnetic resonance chemical shift imaging. *Acta Psychiatr Scand.* 1992;86:455-462.
20. Kato T, Shiori T, Murashita J, Hamakawa H, Inubushi T, Takahashi S. Lateralized abnormality of high-energy phosphate and bilateral reduction of phosphomonoester measured by phosphorous-31 magnetic resonance spectroscopy of the frontal lobes in schizophrenia. *Psychiatry Res: Neuroimaging.* 1995;61:151-160.
21. Stanley JA, Williamson PC, Drost DJ, Carr TJ, Rylett RJ, Morrison-Stewart S, Thompson RT. Membrane phospholipid metabolism and schizophrenia: an in vivo ^{31}P-MR spectroscopy study. *Schizophr Res.* 1994;13:209-215.
22. Williamson P, Drost D, Stanley J, Carr T, Morrison S, Merskey H. Localized phosphorous-31 magnetic resonance spectroscopy in chronic schizophrenic patients and normal controls. *Arch Gen Psychiatry.* 1991;48:578.
23. Shiori T, Kato T, Inubushi T, Murashita J, Takahashi S. Correlations of phosphomonoesters measured by phosphorous-31 magnetic resonance spectroscopy in the frontal lobes and negative symptoms in schizophrenia. *Psychiatry Res.* 1995;55:223-235.
24. Agranoff BW, Hajra AK. Lipids. In: Siegel GJ, Agranoff BW, Albers RW, Molinoff PB, eds. *Basic Neurochemistry.* New York, NY: Raven Press; 1993:97-116.
25. Agranoff BW, Fisher SK. Phosphoinositides. In: Siegel GJ, Agranoff BW, Albers RW, Molinoff PB, eds. *Basic Neurochemistry.* New York, NY: Raven Press; 1993:417-428.
26. Wolfe LS, Horrocks LA. Eicosanoids. In: Siegel GJ, Agranoff BW, Albers RW, Molinoff PB, eds. *Basic Neurochemistry.* New York, NY: Raven Press; 1993: 475-490.
27. Dawson RMC. Enzymic pathways of phospholipid metabolism in the nervous system. In: Eichberg J, ed. *Phospholipids in Nervous Tissues.* New York, NY: John Wiley & Sons Inc; 1985:45-77.
28. Gattaz WF, Kollisch M, Thurn T, Virtanen JA, Kinnunen PKJ. Increased plasma phospholipase-A_2 activity in schizophrenic patients: reduction after neuroleptic therapy. *Biol Psychiatry.* 1987;22:421-426.
29. Gattaz WF, Hübner CK, Nevalainen TJ, Thuren T, Kinnunen PKJ. Increased serum phospholipase-A_2 activity in schizophrenia: a replication study. *Biol Psychiatry.* 1990;28:495-501.
30. Gattaz WF, Schmitt A, Maras Athanasios M. Increased platelet phospholipase A_2 activity in schizophrenia. *Schizophr Res.* 1995;16:1-6.
31. Noponen M, Sanfilipo M, Samanich K, Ryer H, Ko G, Angrist B, Wolkin A, Duncan E, Rotrosen J. Elevated PLA_2 activity in schizophrenics and other psychiatric disorders. *Biol Psychiatry.* 1993;34:641-649.
32. Albers M, Meurer H, Marki F, Klotz J. Phospholipase A_2 activity in serum of neuroleptic-naive psychiatric inpatients. *Pharmacopsychiatry.* 1993;26:94-98.
33. Mayer RJ, Marshall LA. New insights on mammalian phospholipase A_2(s): comparison of arachidonyl-selective and -nonselective enzymes. *FASEB J.* 1993; 7:339-348.
34. American Psychiatric Association. *Diagnostic and Statistical Manual of Mental Disorders, Third Edition, Revised.* Washington, DC: American Psychiatric Press; 1987.
35. Thuren T, Virtanen JA, Lalla M, Kinnunen PKJ. Fluorometric assay for phospholipase A_2 in serum. *Clin Chem.* 1985;31:714-717.
36. Ross BM, Kish SJ. Characterization of lysophospholipid metabolizing enzymes in human brain. *J Neurochem.* 1994;63:1839-1848.
37. Gross RW, Ramanadham S, Kruszka KK, Han X, Turk J. Rat and human pancreatic islet cells contain a calcium ion dependent phospholipase A_2 activity selective for hydrolysis of arachidonate which is stimulated by adenosine triphosphate and is specifically localized to islet β-cells. *Biochemistry.* 1993;32:327-336.
38. Seeman P. Brain dopamine receptors. *Pharmacol Rev.* 1981;32:229-313.
39. Schädlich HR, Büchler M, Beger HG. Improved method for the determination of phospholipase A_2 catalytic activity concentration in human serum and ascities. *J Clin Chem Clin Biochem.* 1987;25:505-509.
40. Nevalainen TJ. Serum phospholipases A_2 in inflammatory diseases. *Clin Chem.* 1993;39:2453-2459.
41. Ennholm C, Shaw W, Greten H, Brown WV. Purification from human plasma of a heparin-released lipase with activity against triglyceride and phospholipids. *J Biol Chem.* 1975;250:6756-6761.
42. Jackson RL, McLean LR. Human postheparin plasma lipoprotein lipase and hepatic triglyceride lipase. In: Dennis EA, ed. *Methods in Enzymology.* Orlando Fla: Academic Press Inc; 1991;197:339-345.
43. Stafforini DM, Prescott SM, McIntyre TM. Human plasma platelet-activating factor acetylhydrolase. *J Biol Chem.* 1987;262:4223-4230.
44. Aron L, Jones S, Fielding CJ. Human plasma lecithin-cholesterol acyltransferase. *J Biol Chem.* 1978;253:7220-7226.
45. Riendeau D, Guay J, Weech PK, Laliberte F, Yergey J, Li C, Desmarais S, Perrier H, Liu S, Nicoll-Griffith D, Street IP. Arachidonyl trifluoromethyl ketone, a potent inhibitor of 85-kDa phospholipase A_2, blocks production of arachidonate and 12-hydroxyeicosatetraenoic acid by calcium ionophore-challenged platelets. *J Biol Chem.* 1994;269:15,619-15,624.
46. Kato T, Shiori T, Murashita J, Hamakawa H, Inubushi T, Takahashi S. Phosphorous-31 magnetic resonance spectroscopy and ventricular enlargement in bipolar disorder. *Psychiatry Res Neuroimaging.* 1994;55:41-50.
47. Deicken RF, Weiner MW, Fein G. Decreased temporal lobe phosphomonoesters in bipolar disorder. *J Affect Disord.* 1995;33:195-199.
48. Deicken RF, Fein G, Weiner MW. Abnormal frontal lobe phosphorous metabolism in bipolar disorder. *Am J Psychiatry.* 1995;152:915-918.
49. Ross BM, Kim DK, Bonventre J, Kish SJ. Characterization of a novel phospholipase A_2 activity in human brain. *J Neurochem.* 1995;64:2213-2221.

Interference with Cognitive and Motor Performance: Because of initial sedation, CLOZARIL® (clozapine) may impair mental and/or physical abilities, especially during the first few days of therapy. The recommendations for gradual dose escalation should be carefully adhered to, and patients cautioned about activities requiring alertness.

Use in Patients with Concomitant Illness: Clinical experience with CLOZARIL® (clozapine) in patients with concomitant systemic diseases is limited. Nevertheless, caution is advisable in using CLOZARIL® (clozapine) in patients with renal or cardiac disease.

Use in Patients Undergoing General Anesthesia: Caution is advised in patients being administered general anesthesia because of the CNS effects of CLOZARIL® (clozapine). Check with the anesthesiologist regarding continuation of CLOZARIL® (clozapine) therapy in a patient scheduled for surgery.

Information for Patients: Physicians are advised to discuss the following issues with patients for whom they prescribe CLOZARIL® (clozapine):

– Patients who are to receive CLOZARIL® (clozapine) should be warned about the significant risk of developing agranulocytosis.They should be informed that weekly blood tests are required to monitor for the occurrence of agranulocytosis, and that CLOZARIL® (clozapine) tablets will be made available only through a special program designed to ensure the required blood monitoring. Patients should be advised to report immediately the appearance of lethargy, weakness, fever, sore throat, malaise, mucous membrane ulceration or other possible signs of infection. Particular attention should be paid to any flu-like complaints or other symptoms that might suggest infection.

– Patients should be informed of the significant risk of seizure during CLOZARIL® (clozapine) treatment, and they should be advised to avoid driving and any other potentially hazardous activity while taking CLOZARIL® (clozapine).

– Patients should be advised of the risk of orthostatic hypotension, especially during the period of initial dose titration.

– Patients should be informed that if they stop taking CLOZARIL® (clozapine) for more than 2 days, they should not restart their medication at the same dosage, but should contact their physician for dosing instructions.

– Patients should notify their physician if they are taking, or plan to take, any prescription or over-the-counter drugs or alcohol.

– Patients should notify their physician if they become pregnant or intend to become pregnant during therapy.

– Patients should not breast feed an infant if they are taking CLOZARIL® (clozapine).

Drug Interactions: The risks of using CLOZARIL® (clozapine) in combination with other drugs have not been systematically evaluated.

The mechanism of CLOZARIL® (clozapine) induced agranulocytosis is unknown; nonetheless, the possibility that causative factors may interact synergistically to increase the risk and/or severity of bone marrow suppression warrants consideration. Therefore, CLOZARIL® (clozapine) should not be used with other agents having a well-known potential to suppress bone marrow function.

Given the primary CNS effects of CLOZARIL® (clozapine), caution is advised in using it concomitantly with other CNS-active drugs or alcohol.

Orthostatic hypotension in patients taking clozapine can, in rare cases (approximately 1 case per 3,000 patients), be accompanied by profound collapse and respiratory and/or cardiac arrest. Some of the cases of collapse/respiratory arrest/cardiac arrest during initial treatment occurred in patients who were being administered benzodiazepines; similar events have been reported in patients taking other psychotropic drugs or even CLOZARIL® (clozapine) by itself. Although it has not been established that there is an interaction between CLOZARIL® (clozapine) and benzodiazepines or other psychotropics, caution is advised when clozapine is initiated in patients taking a benzodiazepine or any other psychotropic drug.

Because CLOZARIL® (clozapine) is highly bound to serum protein, the administration of CLOZARIL® (clozapine) to a patient taking another drug which is highly bound to protein (e.g., warfarin, digitoxin) may cause an increase in plasma concentrations of these drugs, potentially resulting in adverse effects. Conversely, adverse effects may result from displacement of protein-bound CLOZARIL® (clozapine) by other highly bound drugs.

Cimetidine and erythromycin may both increase plasma levels of CLOZARIL® (clozapine), potentially resulting in adverse effects. Although concomitant use of CLOZARIL® (clozapine) and carbamazepine is not recommended, it should be noted that discontinuation of concomitant carbamazepine administration may result in an increase in CLOZARIL® (clozapine) plasma levels. Phenytoin may decrease CLOZARIL® (clozapine) plasma levels, resulting in a decrease in effectiveness of a previously effective CLOZARIL® (clozapine) dose.

A subset (3%-10%) of the population has reduced activity of certain drug metabolizing enzymes such as the cytochrome P450 isozyme P450 2D6. Such individuals are referred to as "poor metabolizers" of drugs such as debrisoquin, dextromethorphan, the tricyclic antidepressants, and clozapine. These individuals may develop higher than expected plasma concentrations of clozapine when given usual doses. In addition, certain drugs that are metabolized by this isozyme, including many antidepressants (clozapine, selective serotonin reuptake inhibitors, and others), may inhibit the activity of this isozyme, and thus may make normal metabolizers resemble poor metabolizers with regard to concomitant therapy with other drugs metabolized by this enzyme system, leading to drug interaction.

Concomitant use of clozapine with other drugs metabolized by cytochrome P450 2D6 may require lower doses than usually prescribed for either clozapine or the other drug. Therefore, co-administration of clozapine with other drugs that are metabolized by this isozyme, including antidepressants, phenothiazines, carbamazepine, and Type 1C antiarrhythmics (e.g., propafenone, flecainide and encainide), or that inhibit this enzyme (e.g., quinidine), should be approached with caution.

CLOZARIL® (clozapine) may also potentiate the hypotensive effects of antihypertensive drugs and the anticholinergic effects of atropine-type drugs. The administration of epinephrine should be avoided in the treatment of drug induced hypotension because of a possible reverse epinephrine effect.

Carcinogenesis, Mutagenesis, Impairment of Fertility: No carcinogenic potential was demonstrated in long-term studies in mice and rats at doses approximately 7 times the typical human dose on a mg/kg basis. Fertility in male and female rats was not adversely affected by clozapine. Clozapine did not produce genotoxic or mutagenic effects when assayed in appropriate bacterial and mammalian tests.

Pregnancy Category B: Reproduction studies have been performed in rats and rabbits at doses of approximately 2-4 times the human dose and have revealed no evidence of impaired fertility or harm to the fetus due to clozapine. There are, however, no adequate and well-controlled studies in pregnant women. Because animal reproduction studies are not always predictive of human response, and in view of the desirability of keeping the administration of all drugs to a minimum during pregnancy, this drug should be used only if clearly needed.

Nursing Mothers: Animal studies suggest that clozapine may be excreted in breast milk and have an effect on the nursing infant. Therefore, women receiving CLOZARIL® (clozapine) should not breast feed.

Pediatric Use: Safety and effectiveness in pediatric patients have not been established.

ADVERSE REACTIONS

Associated with Discontinuation of Treatment: Sixteen percent of 1080 patients who received CLOZARIL® (clozapine) in premarketing clinical trials discontinued treatment due to an adverse event, including both those that could be reasonably attributed to CLOZARIL® (clozapine) treatment and those that might more appropriately be considered intercurrent illness. The more common events considered to be causes of discontinuation included: CNS, primarily drowsiness/sedation, seizures, dizziness/syncope; cardiovascular, primarily tachycardia, hypotension and ECG changes; gastrointestinal, primarily nausea/vomiting; hematologic, primarily leukopenia/granulocytopenia/agranulocytosis; and fever. None of the events enumerated accounts for more than 1.7% of all discontinuations attributed to adverse clinical events.

Commonly Observed: Adverse events observed in association with the use of CLOZARIL® (clozapine) in clinical trials at an incidence of greater than 5% were: central nervous system complaints, including drowsiness/sedation, dizziness/vertigo, headache and tremor; autonomic nervous system complaints, including salivation, sweating, dry mouth and visual disturbances; cardiovascular findings, including tachycardia, hypotension and syncope; and gastrointestinal complaints, including constipation and nausea; and fever. Complaints of drowsiness/sedation tend to subside with continued therapy or dose reduction. Salivation may be profuse, especially during sleep, but may be diminished with dose reduction.

Incidence in Clinical Trials: The following table enumerates adverse events that occurred at a frequency of 1% or greater among CLOZARIL® (clozapine) patients who participated in clinical trials. These rates are not adjusted for duration of exposure.

Treatment-Emergent Adverse Experience Incidence Among Patients Taking CLOZARIL® (clozapine) in Clinical Trials (N = 842) (Percentage of Patients Reporting)

Body System Adverse Event[a]	Percent
Central Nervous System	
Drowsiness/Sedation	39
Dizziness/Vertigo	19
Headache	7
Tremor	6
Syncope	6
Disturbed sleep/Nightmares	4
Restlessness	4
Hypokinesia/Akinesia	4
Agitation	4
Seizures (convulsions)	3[b]
Rigidity	3
Akathisia	3
Confusion	3
Fatigue	2
Insomnia	2
Hyperkinesia	1
Weakness	1
Lethargy	1
Ataxia	1
Slurred speech	1
Depression	1
Epileptiform movements/Myoclonic jerks	1
Anxiety	1
Cardiovascular	
Tachycardia	25[b]
Hypotension	9
Hypertension	4
Chest pain/Angina	1
ECG change/Cardiac abnormality	1
Gastrointestinal	
Constipation	14
Nausea	5
Abdominal discomfort/Heartburn	4
Nausea/Vomiting	3
Vomiting	3
Diarrhea	2
Liver test abnormality	1
Anorexia	1
Urogenital	
Urinary abnormalities	2
Incontinence	1
Abnormal ejaculation	1
Urinary urgency/frequency	1
Urinary retention	1
Autonomic Nervous System	
Salivation	31
Sweating	6
Dry mouth	6
Visual disturbances	5
Integumentary (Skin)	
Rash	2
Musculoskeletal	
Muscle weakness	1
Pain (back, neck, legs)	1
Muscle spasm	1
Muscle pain, ache	1
Respiratory	
Throat discomfort	1
Dyspnea, shortness of breath	1
Nasal congestion	1
Hemic/Lymphatic	
Leukopenia/Decreased WBC/Neutropenia	3
Agranulocytosis	1[b]
Eosinophilia	1
Miscellaneous	
Fever	5
Weight gain	4
Tongue numb/sore	1

[a]Events reported by at least 1% of CLOZARIL® (clozapine) patients are included.

[b]Rate based on population of approximately 1700 exposed during premarket clinical evaluation of CLOZARIL® (clozapine).

Other Events Observed During the Premarketing Evaluationof CLOZARIL® (clozapine): This section reports additional, less frequent adverse events which occurred among the patients taking CLOZARIL® (clozapine) in clinical trials. Various adverse events were reported as part of the total experience in these clinical studies; a causal relationship to CLOZARIL® (clozapine) treatment cannot be determined in the absence of appropriate controls in some of the studies. The table above enumerates adverse events that occurred at a frequency of at least 1% of patients treated with CLOZARIL® (clozapine). The list below includes all additional adverse experiences reported as being temporally associated with the use of the drug which occurred at a frequency less than 1%, enumerated by organ system.

Central Nervous System: loss of speech, amentia, tics, poor coordination, delusions/hallucinations, involuntary movement, stuttering, dysarthria, amnesia/memory loss, histrionic movements, libido increase or decrease, paranoia, shakiness, Parkinsonism, and irritability.

Cardiovascular System: edema, palpitations, phlebitis/thrombophlebitis, cyanosis, premature ventricular contraction, bradycardia, and nose bleed.

Gastrointestinal System: abdominal distention, gastroenteritis, rectal bleeding, nervous stomach, abnormal stools, hematemesis, gastric ulcer, bitter taste, and eructation.

Urogenital System: dysmenorrhea, impotence, breast pain/discomfort, and vaginal itch/infection.

Autonomic Nervous System: numbness, polydypsia, hot flashes, dry throat, and mydriasis.

Integumentary (Skin): pruritus, pallor, eczema, erythema, bruise, dermatitis, petechiae, and urticaria.

Musculoskeletal System: twitching and joint pain.

Respiratory System: coughing, pneumonia/pneumonia-like symptoms, rhinorrhea, hyperventilation, wheezing, bronchitis, laryngitis, and sneezing.

Hemic and Lymphatic System: anemia and leukocytosis.

Miscellaneous: chills/chills with fever, malaise, appetite increase, ear disorder, hypothermia, eyelid disorder, bloodshot eyes, and nystagmus.

Postmarketing Clinical Experience: Postmarketing experience has shown an adverse experience profile similar to that presented above. Voluntary reports of adverse events temporally associated with CLOZARIL® (clozapine) not mentioned above that have been received since market introduction and that may have no causal relationship with the drug include the following:

Central Nervous System: delirium; EEG abnormal; exacerbation of psychosis; myoclonus; overdose; paresthesia; possible mild cataplexy; and status epilepticus.

Cardiovascular System: atrial or ventricular fibrillation and periorbital edema.

Gastrointestinal System: acute pancreatitis; dysphagia; fecal impaction; intestinal obstruction/paralytic ileus; and salivary gland swelling.

Hepatobiliary System: cholestasis; hepatitis; jaundice.

Hepatic System: cholestasis.

Urogenital System: acute interstitial nephritis and priapism.

Integumentary (Skin): hypersensitivity reactions: photosensitivity, vasculitis, erythema multiforme, and Stevens-Johnson Syndrome.

Musculoskeletal System: myasthenic syndrome and rhabdomyolysis.

Respiratory System: aspiration and pleural effusion.

Hemic and Lymphatic System: deep vein thrombosis; elevated hemoglobin/hematocrit; ESR increased; pulmonary embolism; sepsis; thrombocytosis; and thrombocytopenia.

Miscellaneous: CPK elevation; hyperglycemia; hyperuricemia; hyponatremia; and weight loss.

DRUG ABUSE AND DEPENDENCE

Physical and psychological dependence have not been reported or observed in patients taking CLOZARIL® (clozapine).

OVERDOSAGE

Human Experience: The most commonly reported signs and symptoms associated with CLOZARIL® (clozapine) overdose are: altered states of consciousness, including drowsiness, delirium and coma; tachycardia; hypotension; respiratory depression or failure; hypersalivation. Aspiration pneumonia and cardiac arrhythmias have also been reported. Seizures have occurred in a minority of reported cases. Fatal overdoses have been reported with CLOZARIL® (clozapine), generally at doses above 2500 mg. There have also been reports of patients recovering from overdoses well in excess of 4 g.

Management of Overdose: Establish and maintain an airway; ensure adequate oxygenation and ventilation. Activated charcoal, which may be used with sorbitol, may be as or more effective than emesis or lavage, and should be considered in treating overdosage. Cardiac and vital signs monitoring is recommended along with general symptomatic and supportive measures. Additional surveillance should be continued for several days because of the risk of delayed effects. Avoid epinephrine and derivatives when treating hypotension, and quinidine and procainamide when treating cardiac arrhythmia.

There are no specific antidotes for CLOZARIL® (clozapine). Forced diuresis, dialysis, hemoperfusion and exchange transfusion are unlikely to be of benefit.

In managing overdosage, the physician should consider the possibility of multiple drug involvement.

Up-to-date information about the treatment of overdose can often be obtained from a certified Regional Poison Control Center. Telephone numbers of certified Poison Control Centers are listed in the Physicians' Desk Reference®.*

DOSAGE AND ADMINISTRATION

In order to minimize the risk of agranulocytosis, CLOZARIL® (clozapine) is available only through a distribution system that ensures weekly WBC testing prior to delivery of the next week's supply of medication. Upon initiation of CLOZARIL® (clozapine) therapy, up to a 1 week supply of additional CLOZARIL® (clozapine) tablets may be provided to the patient to be held for emergencies (e.g., weather, holidays).

Initial Treatment: It is recommended that treatment with CLOZARIL® (clozapine) begin with one-half of a 25 mg tablet (12.5 mg) once or twice daily and then be continued with daily dosage increments of 25-50 mg/day, if well-tolerated, to achieve a target dose of 300-450 mg/day by the end of 2 weeks. Subsequent dosage increments should be made no more than once or twice-weekly, in increments not to exceed 100 mg. Cautious titration and a divided dosage schedule are necessary to minimize the risks of hypotension, seizure, and sedation.

In the multicenter study that provides primary support for the effectiveness of CLOZARIL® (clozapine) in patients resistant to standard antipsychotic drug treatment, patients were titrated during the first 2 weeks up to a maximum dose of 500 mg/day, on a t.i.d. basis, and were then dosed in a total daily dose range of 100-900 mg/day, on a t.i.d. basis thereafter, with clinical response and adverse effects as guides to correct dosing.

Therapeutic Dose Adjustment: Daily dosing should continue on a divided basis as an effective and tolerable dose level is sought. While many patients may respond adequately at doses between 300-600 mg/day, it may be necessary to raise the dose to the 600-900 mg/day range to obtain an acceptable response. [Note: In the multicenter study providing the primary support for the superiority of CLOZARIL® (clozapine) in treatment resistant patients, the mean and median CLOZARIL® (clozapine) doses were both approximately 600 mg/day.]

Because of the possibility of increased adverse reactions at higher doses, particularly seizures, patients should ordinarily be given adequate time to respond to a given dose level before escalation to a higher dose is contemplated.

Dosing should not exceed 900 mg/day.

Because of the significant risk of agranulocytosis and seizure, events which both present a continuing risk over time, the extended treatment of patients failing to show an acceptable level of clinical response should ordinarily be avoided.

Maintenance Treatment: While the maintenance effectiveness of CLOZARIL® (clozapine) in schizophrenia is still under study, the effectiveness of maintenance treatment is well established for many other antipsychotic drugs. It is recommended that responding patients be continued on CLOZARIL® (clozapine), but at the lowest level needed to maintain remission. Because of the significant risk associated with the use of CLOZARIL® (clozapine), patients should be periodically reassessed to determine the need for maintenance treatment.

Discontinuation of Treatment: In the event of planned termination of CLOZARIL® (clozapine) therapy, gradual reduction in dose is recommended over a 1-2 week period. However, should a patient's medical condition require abrupt discontinuation (e.g., leukopenia), the patient should be carefully observed for the recurrence of psychotic symptoms.

Reinitiation of Treatment in Patients Previously Discontinued: When restarting patients who have had even a brief interval off CLOZARIL® (clozapine), i.e., 2 days or more since the last dose, it is recommended that treatment be reinitiated with one-half of a 25 mg tablet (12.5 mg) once or twice daily *(see WARNINGS)*. If that dose is well tolerated, it may be feasible to titrate patients back to a therapeutic dose more quickly than is recommended for initial treatment. However, any patient who has previously experienced respiratory or cardiac arrest with initial dosing, but was then able to be successfully titrated to a therapeutic dose, should be re-titrated with extreme caution after even 24 hours of discontinuation.

Certain additional precautions seem prudent when reinitiating treatment. The mechanisms underlying CLOZARIL® (clozapine) induced adverse reactions are unknown. It is conceivable, however, that re-exposure of a patient might enhance the risk of an untoward event's occurrence and increase its severity. Such phenomena, for example, occur when immune mediated mechanisms are responsible. Consequently, during the reinitiation of treatment, additional caution is advised. Patients discontinued for WBC counts below 2000/mm^3 or an ANC below 1000/mm^3 must *not* be restarted on CLOZARIL® (clozapine). *(See WARNINGS)*

HOW SUPPLIED

CLOZARIL® (clozapine) is available only through a distribution system that ensures weekly WBC testing prior to delivery of the next week's supply of medication.

CLOZARIL® (clozapine) is available as 25 mg and 100 mg round, pale-yellow, uncoated tablets with a facilitated score.

CLOZARIL® (clozapine) Tablets

25 mg: Engraved with "CLOZARIL" once on the periphery of one side. Engraved with a facilitated score and "25" once on the other side.

Bottle of 100 (NDC 0078-0126-05).

SandoPak® unit-dose packages of 100: 2 × 5 strips, 10 blisters per strip (NDC 0078-0126-06).

100 mg: Engraved with "CLOZARIL" once on the periphery of one side. Engraved with a facilitated score and "100" once on the other side.

Bottle of 100 (NDC 0078-0127-05).

SandoPak® unit-dose packages of 100: 2 × 5 strips, 10 blisters per strip (NDC 0078-0127-06).

Store and Dispense: Storage temperature should not exceed 86°F (30°C). Drug dispensing should not ordinarily exceed a weekly supply. Dispensing should be contingent upon the results of a WBC count.

*Trademark of Medical Economics Company, Inc.

Sandoz Pharmaceuticals Corporation
East Hanover, New Jersey 07936

REV: MARCH 1997 P30118906

ARCHIVES OF GENERAL PSYCHIATRY

In the first community-based study of the cause of bulimia nervosa, **Fairburn et al** (page 509) found that while many of the causative factors previously implicated were more common among women with bulimia nervosa than matched healthy control subjects, there were far fewer differences between those with bulimia nervosa and those with other psychiatric disorders. However, among women with bulimia nervosa, experiences that were likely to increase the risk of dieting were more common, as were childhood low self-esteem and certain parental problems. The findings suggest that bulimia nervosa is the result of exposure to general risk factors for psychiatric disorder and risk factors for dieting.

Evidence is strong that serotonin plays an important role in the regulation of feeding, mood, and impulse control, all of which are abnormal in bulimia nervosa (BN). **Levitan et al** (page 521) reported that patients with BN have markedly abnormal hormonal and mood responses to the serotonergic drug *meta*-chlorophenylpiperazine. These results suggest that patients with BN have a significant decrease in central serotonin activity and that several brain regions may be affected.

In bulimia nervosa, binge eating may be linked to impaired function in brain serotonin pathways that regulate food intake. **Jimerson et al** (page 529) found that serotonergic responsiveness was abnormally low in patients with bulimia nervosa based on the measurement of serum prolactin response following the administration of the serotonergic drug D,L-fenfluramine hydrochloride. Blunted neuroendocrine responses were most apparent in patients with a history of frequent binge eating. Additional study of serotonergic medications may lead to new treatment approaches for this disorder.

A Commentary by Katherine A. Halmi, MD, titled "Models to Conceptualize Risk Factors for Bulimia Nervosa," is also included in this issue.

Anorexia nervosa may have long-term consequences even after weight recovery. In a magnetic resonance imaging study, **Lambe et al** (page 537) showed that the brains of women who are weight-recovered have lower volumes of gray matter than the brains of control subjects. Such brain changes were formerly thought to be fully reversible. The identification of an irreversible component of the brain changes found in anorexia nervosa underscores the importance of early detection and treatment.

Little is known concerning the mediators of health-damaging effects of high strain jobs that impose high workload demands on the worker while allowing little control over how those demands are met. **Williams et al** (page 543) found that women in blue- and white-collar jobs who reported high job strain also reported less social support and were more depressed, anxious, and hostile than coworkers with low job strain. This clustering of psychosocial risk factors among women in high strain jobs may be a likely contributor to their increased health problems.

Quetiapine fumarate is a new atypical antipsychotic drug that shows promise in the treatment of schizophrenia. In an international, placebo-controlled, double-blind, randomized trial, **Small et al** (page 549) found that quetiapine fumarate, at doses greater than 250 mg/d, was consistently superior to placebo in reducing the positive symptoms of schizophrenia and, on one scale, the negative symptoms of schizophrenia. Quetiapine was well tolerated and did not induce extrapyramidal symptoms, sustained elevations of prolactin, or significant changes in hematological parameters after 6 weeks of treatment. Somnolence and headache were the most common nondisease-related adverse events.

Many of the structural abnormalities in the brains of subjects with schizophrenia consist of the disarray of the neuronal organization of the cerebral cortex. **Gabriel et al** (page 559) reasoned that this disorganization may be reflected in proteins in the cortices of schizophrenics. Compared with normal elderly controls, the concentration of these synaptic proteins, including synaptophysin, were increased in the cingulate cortex of schizophrenics. These findings show that the synaptic organization of a cortical region that is important to cognition and affect is altered in schizophrenia.

Given the greater potency of clozapine at D_4 dopamine receptors compared with D_2 receptors, it had been eagerly anticipated that selective D_4 antagonism might be a breakthrough therapy for schizophrenia. **Kramer et al** (page 567) reported that the pure D_4 dopamine receptor antagonist (L-745,870) given to schizophrenic inpatients for 4 weeks (at doses indirectly estimated to block >90% of D_4 receptors) was not an effective antipsychotic. Their results suggest that D_4 antagonism alone is not the unique factor that endows clozapine with improved efficacy and indicate that further work is necessary to solve the puzzle of clozapine.

COMMENTARY

Models to Conceptualize Risk Factors for Bulimia Nervosa

BULIMIA NERVOSA is a disorder identified by specific symptom constellations that most likely emerge from a complex integration of physiological, psychological, and environmental influences. In the search for risk factors from these influences for bulimia nervosa, the authors of the 3 articles about bulimia nervosa published in this issue have implicitly conceptualized a model of the development of bulimia nervosa. This model, which was initially proposed by Lucas[1] and later expanded by Ploog[2] and by myself,[3] proposes that bulimia nervosa develops after the stress of dieting. This dieting experience is influenced by antecedent conditions that include genetic and physiological vulnerability, psychological predispositions that are often affected by the family, and societal influences. It is notable to remember that the salient feature of bulimia nervosa is disturbed eating behavior.

See also pages 509, 521, and 529

Many years of comprehensive studies of the eating behaviors of animals have provided direction for human studies. Blundell and Hill[4] proposed that the final behavior of eating was the result of an interaction of "variables under the skin" and "variables beyond the skin." The former includes neurotransmitter hormones, peptide hormones, metabolic rate, gastrointestinal state, amount of storage tissue, metabolic formation, and sensory receptors. The variables beyond the skin have 2 categories. The first category is features of food, which include taste, familiarity, texture, nutritional composition, and variety. The second category is features of the environment, which include temperature, location (for humans it would be home, bar, or restaurant), current stresses (for humans it would be family, work, individual psychological stress, constraints on behavioral repertoire, and cultural and societal beliefs). Blundell and Hill[4] stated that the capacity to control nutrients to meet bodily needs requires special mechanisms to harmonize physiological information in the internal milieu with nutritional information in the external environment. Two essential features are necessary for this integration. First, perceptual capacities are necessary to identify the characteristics of food materials in the environment and second, a mechanism is needed to link the biochemical consequences of the ingested food with the characteristics of the consumed food.

Booth[5] developed the concept of nutritional hedonic conditioning to explain the integration mechanism linking physiological information of the internal milieu with external nutritional information. The selection of foods involves conditioned and unconditioned components in which satiation cues from the gastrointestinal tract (peptide hormones) and neurotransmitters are part of the conditioning process along with the sensory characteristics of foods and cognitive sets, which are culturally derived attitudes.

Many studies of laboratory animals have shown that central serotonin pathways modulate feeding. The administration of serotonin antagonists increases food intake and, consequently, weight gain; conversely, administration of serotonin agonists decreases food intake. Serotonin seems to increase postprandial satiety rather than to decrease appetite.[6] Thus, it is reasonable to hypothesize that an impaired serotonergic response may contribute to the blunted satiety and prolonged periods of rapid food ingestion present in bulimia nervosa.[7] The techniques by which we can study serotonin functioning in the human are limited. Levitan et al[8] and Jimmerson et al[9] used the pharmacological challenge test with *meta*-chlorophenylpiperazine and D,L-fenfluramine, respectively. A blunted prolactin response to these serotonin agonists was present in both studies. Previous work by McBride et al[10] has shown that the pituitary lactotroph is intact in patients with bulimia nervosa. Thus, the blunted prolactin response is likely to reflect dysfunction in the transmission of serotonin in the central nervous system. The studies presented in this issue confirm the results of previous studies[7,10,11] and suggest an abnormality of postsynaptic serotonergic neurons in patients with bulimia nervosa.

A hypofunctioning serotonergic neurotransmitter system provides the pharmacological rationale for treating patients with bulimia nervosa with serotonin-agonist medications. A large multicenter, placebo-controlled treatment study with fluoxetine showed that this serotonergic agonist was indeed effective in reducing binge behavior in patients with bulimia nervosa.[12]

This article is also available on our Web site: www.ama-assn.org/psych.

To ascertain more accurately the specifics of serotonin dysfunction in bulimia nervosa it will be necessary to move beyond pharmacological challenge tests. Perhaps functional neuroimaging with ligand studies will provide more specific information about the physiological mechanisms of binge eating.

Although dieting, which is the common stress factor that precipitates binge eating behavior, alters brain serotonin function more markedly in women than in men,[13] it does not provide a sufficient explanation for the development of bulimia nervosa. It is reasonable to hypothesize that some vulnerability exists in the overall functioning of the serotonergic neurotransmitter system and this creates a risk factor for developing bulimia nervosa.

Risk factors for bulimia nervosa were investigated by Fairburn et al[14] with a case-control study technique that compared the contents of interviews with patients with bulimia nervosa with those of controls (people in the general population who did not have eating disorders) and patients with other psychiatric disorders who did not have eating disorders. This design provided the opportunity to determine what risk factors may be unique to bulimia nervosa. Punitive risk factors were categorized a priori into 3 domains: personal vulnerability factors, environmental factors, and dieting vulnerability factors. Only factors in the dieting vulnerability and environmental domains distinguished bulimia nervosa cases from general psychiatric cases. Within these categories, only 2 factors—risk of obesity and parental problems—distinguished patients with bulimia nervosa from controls. In comparing the cases of bulimia nervosa with normal controls, premorbid psychiatric disorder was found to be a notable risk factor. A study by Braun et al[15] of psychiatric comorbidity in patients with eating disorders showed that only 33.3% of patients with bulimia nervosa developed their eating disorder as their first Axis I disorder. In this study, 37% of the patients with bulimia nervosa had an affective disorder first, 22.2% had an anxiety disorder first, and 7.4% had an alcohol or substance abuse disorder first.

Unfortunately, the ideal prospective risk factor study is probably prohibitive because of cost. The study by Fairburn et al[14] has definite limitations because the data were preponderantly retrospective information. Another problem with the method was that all information concerning the families, including psychiatric diagnoses, was obtained from the patient and not from personal interviews of family members. It is possible to interview first-degree relatives of patients with bulimia nervosa as demonstrated in previous studies.[16-19] Another methodological problem in the risk factor study by Fairburn et al is a potential bias introduced by the fact that the risk factor interviewer was not blind to the case status of the subject or to the hypothesis of the study.

The study by Fairburn et al has provided a preliminary glimpse at risk factors in bulimia nervosa and hopefully an impetus for the development of prospective studies. Developing preventive interventions and assessing their effectiveness in dieters who are at risk for obesity and psychiatric disorder in general to prevent the development of bulimia nervosa is, indeed, an awesome challenge not only to researchers, but also to those who control the financial structure of our society.

Katherine A. Halmi, MD
Department of Psychiatry
Cornell University Medical College
The New York Hospital—Westchester Division
21 Bloomingdale Rd
White Plains, NY 10605

This Commentary was supported by a fund established in The New York Community Trust by DeWitt Wallace, New York.

REFERENCES

1. Lucas AR. Towards the understanding of anorexia nervosa as a disease entity. *Mayo Clin Proc.* 1981;56:254-264.
2. Ploog D. The importance of physiologic, metabolic and endocrine studies for the understanding of anorexia nervosa. In: Pirke KM, Ploog D, eds. *The Psychobiology of Anorexia Nervosa.* Berlin, Germany: Springer-Verlag; 1989:chap 1.
3. Halmi KA. A multi-modal model for understanding and treating eating disorders. *J Women's Health.* 1994;3:487-493.
4. Blundell JE, Hill A. Nutrition, serotonin and appetite: case study in the evolution of scientific idea. *Appetite.* 1987;8:183-194.
5. Booth DA. How should questions about satiation be asked? *Appetite.* 1981;2:237-244.
6. Blundell JE, Rogers PJ. Effects of anorectic drugs on food intake, food selection and preferences, hunger motivation and subjective experiences. *Appetite.* 1980;1:151-165.
7. Brewerton TD, Brandt HA, Lessen MD. Serotonin in eating disorders. In: Coccaro EF, Murphy DL, eds. *Serotonin in Major Psychiatric Disorders.* Washington, DC: American Psychiatric Press; 1990:153-184.
8. Levitan RD, Kaplan AS, Joffe RT, Levitt AJ, Brown GM. Hormonal and subjective responses to intravenous *meta*-chlorophenylpiperazine in bulimia nervosa. *Arch Gen Psychiatry.*1997;54:521-527.
9. Jimerson DC, Wolfe BE, Metzger ED, Finkelstein DM, Cooper TB, Levine JM. Decreased serotonin function in bulimia nervosa. *Arch Gen Psychiatry.* 1997;54:529-534.
10. McBride PA, Anderson GM, Halmi KA. Serotonergic responsiveness in eating disorders. *Psychopharmacol Bull.* 1991;27:365-372.
11. Halmi KA, McBride PA, Sunday SR. Serotonin responsivity and hunger and satiety in eating disorders. *Adv Biosc.* 1993;90:123-131.
12. Fluoxetine Bulimia Nervosa Collaborative Study Group. Fluoxetine in the treatment of bulimia nervosa: a multicenter, placebo-controlled, double-blind trial. *Arch Gen Psychiatry.* 1992;49:139-147.
13. Goodwin GM, Fairburn CG, Cowen PJ. Dieting changes serotonergic function in women not men: implications for the etiology of anorexia nervosa? *Psychol Med.* 1987;17:839-842.
14. Fairburn CG, Welch SL, Doll HA, Davies BA, O'Connor ME. Risk factors for bulimia nervosa: a community-based case-control study. 1997; 54:509-517.
15. Braun DL, Sunday SR, Halmi KA. Psychiatric comorbidity in patients with eating disorders. *Psychol Med.* 1994;24:859-867.
16. Kendler K, MacLean C, Neal M. The genetic epidemiology of bulimia nervosa. *Am J Psychiatry.* 1991;148:1627-1637.
17. Strober M, Lampert C, Morrell W. A controlled study of anorexia nervosa: evidence of familial aggregation and lack of shared transmission with affective disorders. *Int J Eat Disord.* 1990;9:239-253.
18. Halmi KA, Eckert E, Marchi P, Sampugnaro V, Apple R, Cohen J. Comorbidity of psychiatric diagnoses in anorexia nervosa. *Arch Gen Psychiatry.* 1991;48:712-718.
19. Gershon ES, Schreiber J, Hamovit. Clinical findings in patients with anorexia nervosa and affective illness in their relatives. *Am J Psychiatry.* 1984;141:1419-1422.

ORIGINAL ARTICLE

Risk Factors for Bulimia Nervosa

A Community-Based Case-Control Study

Christopher G. Fairburn, DM, MPhil, FRCPsych; Sarah L. Welch, DPhil, MRCPsych; Helen A. Doll, MSc; Beverley A. Davies; Marianne E. O'Connor

Background: Many apparently disparate risk factors have been implicated as causes of eating disorders. This study was designed to test the hypothesis that 2 broad classes of risk factors exist for bulimia nervosa: those that increase the risk for development of a psychiatric disorder in general and those that increase the risk of dieting. It was predicted that the latter are especially common among persons with bulimia nervosa.

Methods: A case-control design was used involving 2 integrated comparisons. First, 102 subjects with bulimia nervosa were compared with 204 healthy control subjects without an eating disorder. Second, the same 102 subjects with bulimia nervosa were compared with 102 subjects with other psychiatric disorders. To reduce sampling bias, the subjects were recruited directly from the community. A broad range of putative risk factors was assessed.

Results: The subjects with bulimia nervosa and the healthy control subjects differed in their rates of exposure to most of the putative risk factors. Far fewer differences were evident between the subjects with bulimia nervosa and the control subjects with other psychiatric disorders, although exposure to factors that were likely to increase the risk of dieting and to negative self-evaluation and certain parental problems (including alcohol use disorder) were substantially more common among those with bulimia nervosa.

Conclusions: The findings support the hypothesis that bulimia nervosa is the result of exposure to general risk factors for psychiatric disorder and risk factors for dieting. An unexpected finding was the particularly high rates of premorbid negative self-evaluation and certain parental problems among those with bulimia nervosa.

Arch Gen Psychiatry. 1997;54:509-517

THE RESEARCH on the cause of eating disorders has implicated many apparently disparate risk factors. These include a family history of an eating disorder,[1-6] affective disorder,[3,7-12] substance abuse,[3,8,10,11,13] and obesity[14-16]; a history of exposure to adverse events and circumstances,[17] including sexual and physical abuse[18-20]; and the presence of certain traits such as perfectionism, excessive compliance, and low self-esteem.[21,22] This research has had certain limitations. First, most of the work has focused on anorexia nervosa, whereas bulimia nervosa and the "atypical eating disorders"[23] (in *DSM-IV* terms, eating disorders not otherwise specified[24]) have been relatively neglected despite being substantially more common.[25-27] Second, samples representative of all those with eating disorders have not been studied except in the study by Rastam and Gillberg.[28] Almost all the research has used patient samples, yet evidence shows that many of those with eating disorders do not seek medical attention.[29-33] The research findings may therefore be distorted by sampling bias.[34] Third, most studies have had a narrow perspective and have investigated a limited number of putative causes. As a result, almost nothing is known about the relative contributions of different classes of factors and whether they interact. Once again, the study by Rastam and Gillberg[28] is an exception. Fourth, because few studies have included general psychiatric control groups, determining whether the causative factors implicated are particularly common among those with eating disorders or whether they are risk factors for psychiatric disorder in general has not been possible. Fifth, little attention has been paid to when the putative risk factors occurred; therefore, whether the risk factors could have operated before the onset of the eating disorder is not clear.

See also pages 507, 521, and 529

Our study was designed to overcome some of these limitations. We had 2 main aims. The first was to identify risk factors for the development of bulimia nervosa, and the second was to determine which of these risk factors are especially common among subjects with bulimia nervosa when com-

From the Department of Psychiatry, Oxford University, Warneford Hospital, Oxford, United Kingdom.

SUBJECTS AND METHODS

DESIGN

A matched case-control design was used with 2 related comparisons that corresponded with the 2 main aims. The first comparison (for aim 1) was between 102 subjects with bulimia nervosa recruited from a community sample of young women and 204 control subjects without an eating disorder who were recruited from the same community sample (healthy control subjects). The second comparison (for aim 2) was between the same 102 subjects with bulimia nervosa and 102 control subjects with other psychiatric disorders ("general psychiatric control subjects"), also recruited from the same community sample.

The 2 groups of control subjects were individually matched to the subjects with bulimia nervosa for 2 variables: age and parental social class. Subjects were matched within 1 year of age and within 3 parental social class bands using the customary classification scheme of the United Kingdom.[35] Briefly, the classification scheme includes 5 classes labeled I through V. Classes I and II are considered high, III is considered middle, and IV and V, low. Matching for age ensured that the length of recall required of the subjects with bulimia nervosa and control subjects was equivalent, and matching for parental social class removed an important potential confounding variable.

RECRUITMENT PROCEDURE

Practically all the British population is registered with a local general practitioner,[36] and these physicians keep lists of the patients registered with them. Therefore, these lists contain the names and addresses of the great majority of the local population. To obtain a study group from the local general population, we contacted the people on the lists of 23 general practices located in urban and rural parts of Oxfordshire, England.

All women and girls between 16 and 35 years old on these lists were sent 2 self-report questionnaires. One was the self-report version of the Eating Disorder Examination (EDE-Q), a questionnaire designed to detect cases of eating disorders in community samples.[37,38] The other was the 30-item General Health Questionnaire,[39] an instrument designed to detect cases of psychiatric disorders in community samples. Subjects who did not reply to the first mailing were sent a second set of questionnaires. Those whose responses on the EDE-Q suggested that they might have bulimia nervosa were invited for an interview to establish their true case status. Those who met diagnostic criteria for bulimia nervosa then underwent a more detailed interview to assess the presence of putative risk factors for the disorder.

Each time a subject with bulimia nervosa was recruited, 3 individually matched control subjects (2 healthy control subjects and 1 general psychiatric control subject) were sought from the same community sample. Potential healthy control subjects were identified from their responses on the EDE-Q. Potential psychiatric control subjects were identified from their scores on the General Health Questionnaire. As with the subjects with bulimia nervosa, the case status of these subjects was established by interview. Subjects who met the case or control criteria (see "Subject and Case Definitions") were assessed using the same risk-factor interview.

Identifying the response rate in a study that uses this recruitment method is difficult. The lists kept by general practitioners are invariably overinclusive because they include the names of people who have subsequently moved away from the area. Therefore, we cannot conclude that nonresponse is indicative of a decision not to participate in the study. For this reason, a detailed pilot study was undertaken using 2 general practice case registers. The pilot study involved attempting to trace all women and girls aged 16 to 35 years (N=583) to calculate the true response rate. Three of these subjects (0.5%) could not be traced, and 243 (42%) were found to have moved away. When the potential subjects who were unavailable to participate were eliminated from the study population, the response rate at interview was 83.6% (290/347).[40]

SUBJECT AND CASE DEFINITIONS

The subjects with bulimia nervosa met a strict operational definition of *DSM-IV* bulimia nervosa based on ratings on the Eating Disorder Examination.[41-43] The healthy control subjects were required to have no current or past eating disorder, established by interview. The general psychiatric control subjects were required to have the diagnosis of a current Axis I *DSM-III-R*[44] psychiatric disorder, confirmed by interview using the Structured Clinical Interview for *DSM-III-R*.[45,46] Potential general psychiatric control subjects with a current or past eating disorder were excluded. The selection criteria for the 2 control groups excluded subjects with eating disorders of clinical severity (as defined in *DSM-IV*) but not subjects with normative degrees of dieting or overeating or normative levels of concern about body shape or weight. The following exclusion criteria were applied to all 3 subject groups: current pregnancy or pregnancy within the preceding 4 months; a physical disorder or medication likely to influence eating or weight, such as diabetes or treatment with corticosteroids; and lack of fluency in English.

RISK FACTOR ASSESSMENT

Exposure to putative risk factors for bulimia nervosa was assessed by interviewing the subjects (usually in their own

pared with control subjects with other psychiatric disorders. The study was designed to test the hypothesis that 2 broad classes of risk factors exist for bulimia nervosa: those that increase the risk of development of psychiatric disorder in general and those that increase the risk of dieting. We predicted that a family history of obesity; family concerns about shape, weight, and eating; and childhood obesity would all be more common among those with bulimia nervosa than among persons with other psychiatric disorders.

RESULTS

CHARACTERISTICS OF THE 3 SUBJECT GROUPS

Subjects With Bulimia Nervosa

Their mean±SD age was 23.7±4.9 years, and their parental social class distribution was as follows[35]: social class I or II (high), 47 (46%); social class III homes). Other informants were not used because a characteristic feature of bulimia nervosa is that the person with the disorder tends to keep it secret.[29,47] Few subjects would have given us permission to contact other informants. Had we insisted on having an additional informant, our response rate would have been substantially reduced, thereby increasing sampling bias.

The risk-factor interview was designed for this study. It was intended to identify the biological, psychological, and social factors believed to place persons at risk for the development of eating disorders. The interview focused on the period *before* the onset of the eating disorder. "Onset" was conservatively defined as the age at which the first noteworthy and persistent behavioral characteristic of an eating disorder began (ie, sustained dieting, regular episodes of overeating, self-induced vomiting, or misuse of laxatives), rather than the age at which the subject first met full diagnostic criteria for bulimia nervosa. "Sustained dieting" was defined as a period, lasting at least 3 months, of *continuous* attempted restriction of food intake to control shape or weight. "Overeating" was defined using EDE concepts,[41-43] it being required that there be at least 12 objective bulimic episodes or episodes of objective overeating over a 3-month period. This conservative definition of onset was chosen to ensure that the exposure preceded the eating disorder and therefore could have contributed to its development. To match the subjects for the period considered, each healthy control subject was interviewed about the period up to the age at onset of their matched subjects with bulimia nervosa. The presence of 5 risk factors with a possible hereditary influence (ie, family history of depression, alcohol misuse, drug misuse, obesity, and eating disorders) was assessed before and after the onset of the eating disorder (as previously defined). These factors were analyzed in 2 forms: when present at any time, and when present before the age at onset. The subjects also completed the Parental Bonding Instrument.[48,49]

The risk-factor interview was designed to minimize the problems associated with retrospective reporting. Thus, it used clear behavioral definitions to reduce subjectivity and post-hoc rationalization. For example, "low parental contact" was defined as a sustained period when the participant regularly did not see a parent for a week or more because the parent was away from home or because the parent returned home late at night and left early in the morning. A further example is "physical abuse," which was defined as any deliberate physical contact resulting in injury such as bruising (including physical punishment by parents or teachers), whereas "severe physical abuse" included more severe injuries such as burns or fractures and any injury to the participant's head or face. The definition of sexual abuse has been described elsewhere.[18] An inescapable limitation of the study was that it was impossible to conduct the risk-factor interview using an assessor who was unaware of the case status of the participant because this would have required separate interviews with 2 different people, an arrangement that few of these community-based participants would have been willing to accept. To minimize the risk of biased assessment, interviewer bias was discussed repeatedly during the training and ongoing supervision of the assessors, and they were taught how to adopt a standard but flexible approach. An interrater reliability study (with the second rater unaware of the case status of the participant) obtained a high level of agreement across the risk factors (mean weighted κ, 0.66; SD, 0.17).

A large number of putative risk factors was assessed (**Table 1**). They were categorized a priori into 1 of 3 domains: factors in the individual or family that might increase the risk for development of psychiatric disorder in general (personal vulnerability factors); adverse circumstances (environmental factors); and factors that might heighten concerns about shape, weight, or eating, and thereby increase the risk of dieting (dieting vulnerability factors). Within each domain, a number of subdomains were distinguished a priori, reflecting certain types of exposure. Additional factors, which did not naturally belong to any 1 of the 3 domains, were age at onset of menstruation, a history of pregnancy or abortion, and parity.

DATA ANALYSIS

Two sets of case-control comparisons, corresponding to the 2 aims of the study, were made. Each involved using conditional logistic regression analyses appropriate for a case-control design with individual matching.[50] The relationships between individual putative risk factors and case status were assessed by univariate analysis. Each risk factor was considered as a single indicator variable and coded 0 for no and 1 for yes. Statistical significance was assessed using the χ^2 likelihood ratio statistic. Because of the number of comparisons performed, $P<.001$ was considered statistically significant. To assess the relative importance of different types of exposure, the relationships between case status and exposure in each subdomain and domain were first assessed by univariate analysis and then in multivariate stepwise regression analyses. An overall measure of exposure to risk in each subdomain and domain was obtained by summing the numbers of component risk factors to which each participant had been exposed, and the scores were grouped in categories of as equal size as possible. To test for the significance of any apparent linear trend, the categorized scores (each assigned a value of average exposure) were entered in the regression analyses in factored and unfactored forms. Statistical significance for these analyses was assessed using the χ^2 likelihood ratio statistic, set at $P<.05$.

(middle), 46 (45%); and social class IV or V (low), 9 (9%). The mean±SD age at which the first established feature of an eating disorder began was 15.5±3.9 years, and the mean±SD age at onset of bulimia nervosa was 19.0±4.0 years. Eighty-nine percent (85/95 [95 is the subset of those who provided this information]) were not undergoing treatment; of these, 18% (15/85) had previously undergone treatment for an eating disorder.

Healthy and General Psychiatric Control Subjects

Because the control subjects were individually matched to the subjects with bulimia nervosa for age and parental social class, the distribution of these characteristics in the groups was very similar. The diagnoses of the general psychiatric control subjects belonged to the following principal categories: major depressive disorder, 83 (81%); bipolar disorder,

Table 1. Distribution of Putative Risk Factors in the 3 Subject Groups and the Results of Matched Univariate Conditional Regression Analyses*

Factors	Group, No (%)			Bulimia Nervosa Subjects vs					
				Healthy Control Subjects			General Psychiatric Control Subjects		
	Bulimia Nervosa Subjects	Healthy Control Subjects	General Psychiatric Control Subjects	*P*	Odds Ratio	95% CI	*P*	Odds Ratio	95% CI
Personal vulnerability domain									
Subdomain 1 (childhood characteristics)									
Negative self-evaluation	55 (54)	27 (13)	31 (30)	<.001	7.4†	(3.9-14.0)	<.001	2.8†	(1.5-5.4)
Shyness	41 (40)	35 (17)	45 (44)	<.001	3.8†	(2.1-6.8)	.56	0.8	(0.5-1.5)
Perfectionism	42 (42)	49 (24)	26 (26)	<.001	2.6‡	(1.5-4.6)	.01	2.3§	(1.2-4.6)
Extreme compliance	29 (29)	42 (21)	27 (27)	.13	1.5	(0.9-2.6)	.76	1.1	(0.6-2.0)
No close friends	18 (18)	10 (5)	10 (10)	<.001	4.2†	(1.8-9.6)	.11	1.9	(0.8-4.2)
School absence through anxiety	8 (8)	4 (2)	4 (4)	<.02	4.0§	(1.2-13.3)	.24	2.0	(0.6-6.6)
Subdomain 2 (premorbid psychiatric disorder)									
Major depression	30 (29)	9 (4)	17 (17)	<.001	17.4†	(5.3-57.3)	.02	2.3§	(1.1-4.8)
Drug abuse	3 (3)	1 (<1)	3 (3)	.09	6.0	(0.1-6.0)	>.99	1.0	(0.2-5.0)
Alcohol abuse	13 (14)	19 (10)	14 (14)	.31	1.6	(0.6-3.9)	.81	0.9	(0.3-2.3)
Subdomain 3 (behavioral problems)									
Marked conduct problems	16 (16)	4 (2)	7 (7)	<.001	10.2†	(3.0-35.1)	.04	3.0	(1.0-9.3)
School absence (truancy)	16 (16)	7 (3)	7 (7)	<.001	4.6†	(1.9-11.1)	.04	2.8§	(1.0-7.8)
Deliberate self-harm	13 (13)	2 (1)	9 (9)	<.001	24.5‡	(3.2-188.0)	.34	1.6	(0.6-4.1)
Subdomain 4 (parental psychiatric disorder [ever])									
Parental depression	23 (23)	10 (5)	20 (20)	<.001	6.7†	(2.7-16.7)	.62	1.2	(0.6-2.2)
Parental alcoholism	24 (24)	8 (4)	7 (7)	<.001	6.7†	(2.9-15.5)	<.001	4.4‡	(1.7-11.6)
Parental drug abuse	9 (9)	1 (<1)	3 (3)	<.001	18.0‡	(2.3-142.1)	.08	3.0	(0.8-11.1)
Environmental domain									
Subdomain 1 (parental problems)									
Low parental contact	34 (34)	36 (18)	14 (14)	.003	2.3‡	(1.3-4.1)	<.001	3.2‡	(1.5-6.8)
Separation from parents	13 (14)	9 (5)	10 (10)	.01	3.2§	(1.3-8.2)	.25	1.7	(0.7-4.4)
Parental									
Arguments	58 (57)	52 (26)	36 (36)	<.001	4.8†	(2.6-8.6)	.003	2.2‡	(1.3-3.9)
Criticism	34 (33)	11 (5)	17 (17)	<.001	7.2†	(3.5-15.1)	.01	2.2§	(1.2-4.2)
High expectations	51 (51)	43 (21)	25 (25)	<.001	3.7†	(2.2-6.3)	<.001	3.4†	(1.7-6.6)
Overinvolvement	15 (15)	6 (3)	7 (7)	<.001	5.7†	(2.1-15.8)	.08	2.1	(0.9-5.3)
Underinvolvement	59 (58)	70 (34)	43 (42)	<.001	2.7†	(1.6-4.5)	.02	1.9§	(1.1-3.5)
Minimal affection	41 (40)	17 (8)	28 (28)	<.001	8.7†	(4.0-18.6)	.06	1.7	(1.0-3.1)
PBI (low care and high overprotection)									
Maternal	55 (63)	44 (22)	39 (46)	<.001	7.2†	(3.5-14.8)	.07	1.8	(0.9-3.6)
Paternal	44 (52)	54 (26)	41 (49)	<.001	2.7†	(1.6-4.5)	.63	1.2	(0.6-2.2)
Subdomain 2 (disruptive events)									
Parental death	2 (2)	3 (2)	5 (5)	.76	1.3	(0.2-8.0)	.25	0.4	(0.1-2.1)
Change of parent figure	18 (18)	23 (11)	20 (20)	.12	1.7	(0.9-3.5)	.72	0.9	(0.4-1.8)
Parental chronic illness	28 (28)	40 (20)	36 (35)	.14	1.5	(0.9-2.6)	.24	0.7	(0.4-1.3)
Frequent house moves	22 (22)	25 (12)	19 (19)	.04	1.9§	(1.0-3.6)	.56	1.3	(0.6-2.7)
Severe personal health problems	12 (12)	7 (3)	14 (14)	.003	5.0‡	(1.6-15.7)	.68	0.8	(0.4-1.9)
Subdomain 3 (parental psychiatric disorder)									
Parental depression	19 (19)	6 (3)	9 (9)	<.001	8.8†	(3.0-26.0)	.05	2.3	(1.0-5.2)
Parental alcoholism	20 (20)	5 (3)	6 (6)	<.001	9.6†	(3.3-28.3)	.002	4.5‡	(1.5-13.3)
Parental drug abuse	9 (9)	1 (<1)	2 (2)	<.001	18.0‡	(2.3-142.1)	.03	4.5	(1.0-20.8)
Subdomain 4 (teasing and bullying)									
Teasing (not about shape, weight, eating, or appearance)	15 (15)	25 (12)	12 (12)	.59	1.2	(0.6-2.4)	.56	1.3	(0.6-2.7)
Bullying	11 (11)	9 (4)	13 (13)	.04	2.6§	(1.0-6.5)	.67	0.8	(0.4-1.9)

Table 1. Distribution of Putative Risk Factors in the 3 Subject Groups and the Results of Matched Univariate Conditional Regression Analyses (cont)*

	Group, No (%)			Bulimia Nervosa Subjects vs					
				Healthy Control Subjects			General Psychiatric Control Subjects		
Factors	Bulimia Nervosa Subjects	Healthy Control Subjects	General Psychiatric Control Subjects	*P*	Odds Ratio	95% CI	*P*	Odds Ratio	95% CI
Subdomain 5 (sexual or physical abuse)									
Sexual abuse	36 (35)	22 (11)	26 (26)	<.001	4.4†	(2.3-8.2)	.13	1.6	(0.9-2.9)
Repeated severe sexual abuse	9 (9)	1 (<1)	3 (3)	<.001	18.0‡	(2.3-142.1)	.02	7.0	(0.9-56.9)
Physical abuse	33 (32)	18 (9)	30 (29)	<.001	6.0†	(2.8-12.6)	.64	1.2	(0.6-2.1)
Repeated severe physical abuse	8 (8)	1 (<1)	10 (10)	<.001	16.0‡	(2.0-127.9)	.62	0.8	(0.3-2.1)
Repeated severe physical or severe sexual abuse	12 (12)	2 (2)	12 (12)	<.001	12.0‡	(2.7-53.6)	>.99	1.0	(0.4-2.5)
Dieting vulnerability domain									
Subdomain 1 (dieting risk)									
Family member dieting									
For any reason	64 (63)	74 (36)	44 (43)	<.001	2.8†	(1.7-4.7)	.005	2.3‡	(1.2-4.1)
For shape or weight	50 (49)	54 (27)	37 (36)	<.001	2.6†	(1.6-4.2)	.07	1.7	(0.9-2.9)
Critical comments by family about shape, weight, or eating	66 (65)	51 (25)	32 (31)	<.001	6.3†	(3.4-11.6)	<.001	5.9†	(2.6-13.1)
Repeated comments by others about shape or weight	34 (33)	28 (14)	23 (23)	<.001	3.0†	(1.7-5.3)	.08	1.7	(0.9-3.3)
Teasing about shape, weight, eating, or appearance	50 (50)	57 (28)	43 (42)	<.001	2.5†	(1.5-4.1)	.28	1.3	(0.8-2.3)
Parental obesity	34 (34)	23 (11)	20 (20)	<.001	4.3†	(2.2-8.2)	.02	2.4§	(1.1-5.0)
Childhood obesity	41 (40)	31 (15)	13 (13)	<.001	3.2†	(1.9-5.6)	<.001	4.5†	(2.1-9.7)
Parental history of anorexia nervosa or bulimia nervosa	5 (5)	0 (0)	1 (1)	...	...	...	.09	5.0	(0.6-42.8)
Subdomain 2 (obesity risk)									
Childhood obesity	41 (40)	31 (15)	13 (13)	<.001	3.2†	(1.9-5.6)	<.001	4.5†	(2.1-9.7)
Parental obesity (ever)	44 (44)	31 (15)	29 (29)	<.001	4.6†	(2.5-8.6)	<.001	2.4§	(1.2-4.8)
Subdomain 3 (parental eating disorder)									
Parental history of anorexia nervosa or bulimia nervosa (ever)	6 (6)	1 (<1)	2 (2)	.004	12.0§	(1.4-99.7)	.15	3.0	(0.6-14.9)
Additional risk factors									
Age at menarche, y									
14-18	19 (19)	60 (30)	30 (30)	<.001	1.00	...	.007	1.00	
13	28 (28)	70 (35)	35 (35)	...	1.20	(0.6-2.5)	...	1.20	(0.6-2.5)
12	23 (23)	46 (23)	23 (23)	...	1.47	(0.7-3.1)	...	1.66	(0.7-3.9)
9-11	31 (31)	22 (11)	13 (13)	...	5.01†	(2.2-11.4)	...	4.39‡	(1.7-11.4)
Pregnancy	13 (13)	4 (2)	7 (7)	<.001	8.2‡	(2.3-28.9)	.02	7.00	(0.9-56.9)
Parity, No. of children									
1	7 (7)	4 (2)	3 (3)	...	...	...	...	...	...
2-4	6 (6)	0 (0)	4 (4)	...	...	...	...	...	...
Abortion	5 (5)	2 (1)	5 (5)	.04	5.0	(1.0-25.8)	>.99	1.00	(0.3-4.0)

**The significance of the exposure (likelihood ratio statistic, χ^2) and odds ratios with their significance levels and 95% confidence intervals (CI) are given for each factor. All exposures, except those labeled (ever), predate the onset of the eating disorder. PBI indicates Parental Bonding Instrument.*

†$P<.001$.

‡$P<.01$.

§$P<.05$.

1 (1%); and anxiety disorder, 18 (18%). Thus, depressive disorder was overrepresented, possibly because chronic cases of anxiety disorder were missed by the General Health Questionnaire.[51] Of the general psychiatric control subjects, 70 (69%) were not receiving treatment.

COMPARISON WITH THE HEALTHY CONTROL SUBJECTS (AIM 1)

Individual Risk Factors

In comparison with the healthy subjects, the bulimia nervosa subjects reported significantly greater levels of expo-

Table 2. Number of Factors in Each Domain to Which the Subjects Were Exposed and the Results of Matched Univariate Conditional Regression Analyses*

	Group, No (%)			Bulimia Nervosa Subjects vs					
				Healthy Control Subjects			General Psychiatric Control Subjects		
Domain/ No. of Factors	Bulimia Nervosa Subjects	Healthy Control Subjects	General Psychiatric Control Subjects	*P*	Odds Ratio	95% CI	*P*	Odds Ratio	95% CI
Personal vulnerability domain									
0	5 (5)	76 (37)	19 (19)	<.001	1.00	...	<.001	1.00	...
1	16 (16)	70 (34)	27 (27)		2.64	(0.9-7.8)		2.82	(0.8-10.6)
2	15 (15)	31 (15)	13 (13)		6.75†	(2.1-22.0)		6.06‡	(1.3-28.1)
3-9	66 (65)	27 (13)	43 (43)		35.30§	(11.5-108.1)		9.11†	(2.4-34.3)
Environmental domain									
0-1	8 (8)	73 (36)	20 (20)	<.001	1.00	...	<.001	1.00	...
2-3	8 (8)	74 (36)	21 (21)		1.50	(0.5-4.9)		0.84	(0.2-3.0)
4-5	25 (25)	35 (17)	24 (24)		9.80§	(3.0-31.8)		2.79	(1.0-8.0)
6-18	61 (60)	22 (11)	37 (36)		42.48§	(12.3-146.7)		4.77†	(1.7-13.4)
Dieting vulnerability domain									
0	4 (4)	59 (29)	16 (16)	<.001	1.00	...	<.001	1.00	...
1-2	36 (35)	107 (52)	58 (57)		3.88‡	(1.3-11.6)		2.02	(0.5-8.0)
3	20 (20)	25 (12)	13 (13)		9.99§	(2.9-34.3)		4.14‡	(1.1-16.1)
4-8	42 (41)	13 (6)	15 (15)		30.80§	(9.2-102.8)		11.41†	(2.7-49.0)

*The significance of the exposure (likelihood ratio statistic χ^2) and odds ratios with their significance levels and 95% confidence intervals (CI) are given for each domain.
†P<.01.
‡P<.05.
§P<.001.

sure (*P*<.001) to all except 4 of the personal vulnerability factors, most of the environmental factors, and all but 1 of the dieting vulnerability factors (Table 1). They were also younger at menarche and more likely to have been pregnant. The younger the subject at menarche, the higher the risk that bulimia nervosa would subsequently develop.

Overall Level of Exposure in Each Subdomain

The bulimia nervosa subjects reported a significantly greater level of exposure than did the healthy control subjects to all except 1 of the 12 subdomains (teasing and bullying); the greater the degree of exposure within each subdomain, the greater the risk of developing bulimia nervosa. On multivariate analysis across the subdomains, 5 subdomains entered the regression model: parental problems (χ^2=85.1; *df*=3; *P*<.001); obesity risk (χ^2=23.6; *df*=2; *P*<.001); parental psychiatric disorder (χ^2=15.9; *df*=2; *P*<.001); sexual or physical abuse (χ^2=21.2; *df*=3; *P*<.001); and premorbid psychiatric disorder (χ^2=6.7; *df*=2; *P*=.03).

Overall Level of Exposure in Each Domain

Univariate analysis showed that the bulimia nervosa subjects had a significantly greater level of exposure than did the healthy control subjects to all 3 domains (*P*<.001) (**Table 2**). The odds ratios increased, in a linear fashion, from the subjects exposed to the smallest number of factors, to those exposed to the largest.

On multivariate analysis across the 3 domains, all three entered the logistic regression model (**Table 3**). Exposure in the environmental domain entered first (χ^2=100.8; *df*=3; *P*<.001), followed by exposure in the personal vulnerability domain (χ^2=26.4; *df*=3; *P*<.001), and then by exposure in the dieting vulnerability domain (χ^2=9.2; *df*=3; *P*=.03). The resulting odds ratios for each domain were lower than on univariate analysis, indicating a degree of confounding among the domains. However, no statistically significant interactions were found among the domains, suggesting that the effect of exposure in any 1 domain did not depend on the degree of exposure in any other and that the effect of combined exposures was additive.

COMPARISON WITH THE GENERAL PSYCHIATRIC CONTROL SUBJECTS (AIM 2)

Individual Risk Factors

Although the bulimia nervosa subjects reported a significantly greater level of exposure than the healthy control subjects to most of the personal vulnerability and environmental risk factors, few significant differences (at *P*<.001) were found between the bulimia nervosa subjects and their general psychiatric control subjects (Table 1). The 4 factors on which they did differ were negative self-evaluation, parental alcoholism (ever), low parental contact, and parental high expectations; in each case the level of exposure was higher in the subjects with bulimia nervosa. The 2 groups differed significantly with respect to 3 dieting vulnerability factors: critical comments by family about shape, weight, or eating; childhood obesity; and parental obesity (ever). Again, the level

Table 3. Results of Matched Stepwise Conditional Regression Analyses*

	Bulimia Nervosa Subjects vs					
	Healthy Control Subjects			General Psychiatric Control Subjects		
Domain/No. of Factors	***P***	**Odds Ratio**	**95% CI**	***P***	**Odds Ratio**	**95% CI**
Personal vulnerability domain						
0	<.001	1.00	...	...	...	...
1		1.86	(0.5-7.1)		...	...
2		2.39	(0.5-10.7)		...	...
3-9		8.65†	(2.3-33.1)		...	...
Environmental domain						
0-1	<.001	1.00	...	<.05	1.00	...
2-3		1.06	(0.2-4.6)		0.51	(0.1-2.0)
4-5		4.82‡	(1.1-21.1)		1.45	(0.5-4.7)
6-18		14.90§	(3.0-73.6)		2.31	(0.7-7.5)
Dieting vulnerability domain						
0	<.05	1.00	...	<.001	1.00	...
1-2		2.83	(0.7-11.9)		1.63	(0.4-7.0)
3		2.12	(0.4-12.6)		2.66	(0.6-11.6)
4-8		7.92‡	(1.6-39.3)		8.19†	(1.7-39.2)

**The significance of the exposure (likelihood ratio statistic, χ^2) and odds ratios with their significance levels and 95% confidence intervals (CI) are given for each domain that had an independent relationship with case status.*

†$P<.01$.

‡$P<.05$.

§$P<.001$.

of exposure was higher in the subjects with bulimia nervosa. The 2 groups did not differ significantly with respect to the additional risk factors.

Overall Level of Exposure to Each Subdomain

The bulimia nervosa subjects reported a significantly greater level of exposure than did the general psychiatric control subjects to all except 3 of the 12 subdomains, slightly fewer than in the comparison of the bulimia subjects with the healthy control subjects. The exceptions were teasing and bullying, childhood characteristics, and sexual and physical abuse. As in the previous case-control comparison, the greater the degree of exposure within each subdomain, the greater the risk of developing bulimia nervosa. The subjects with bulimia nervosa had been exposed to a greater extent than had the general psychiatric control subjects to each of the 3 dieting vulnerability subdomains.

On multivariate analysis across the subdomains, 2 entered the regression model, 1 from the environmental domain (parental problems, χ^2=26.8; *df*=3; $P<.001$) and 1 from the dieting vulnerability domain (obesity risk, χ^2=18.3; *df*=2; $P<.001$). This contrasts with the comparison of the subjects with bulimia nervosa with the healthy control subjects in which exposure to 3 other subdomains also had an independent relationship with case status.

Overall Level of Exposure to Each Domain

On univariate analysis, the bulimia nervosa subjects had a significantly greater level of exposure than did the general psychiatric control subjects to all 3 domains ($P<.001$) (Table 2). The odds ratios increased, in a linear fashion, from the subjects exposed to the smallest number of factors, to those exposed to the largest.

On multivariate analysis across the 3 domains, exposure in the dieting vulnerability domain entered the model first (χ^2=26.6; *df*=3; $P<.001$) followed by exposure in the environmental domain (χ^2=8.6; *df*=3; P=.03) (Table 3). After adjusting for exposure in these 2 domains, exposure in the personal vulnerability domain was no longer significantly related to case status (χ^2=3.5; *df*=3; P=.32). This contrasts with the comparison of the subjects with bulimia nervosa with the healthy control subjects in which exposure to all 3 domains had an independent relationship with case status. No significant statistical interaction was found between the dieting vulnerability domain and the environmental domain.

COMMENT

The findings from the first of the case-control comparisons, between the bulimia nervosa subjects and the healthy control subjects, generally supported earlier studies of individual risk factors. They showed that the great majority of the previously implicated risk factors were indeed risk factors for bulimia nervosa. Multivariate analysis of the 3 domains indicated that all 3 were independently related to case status; and a dose-response effect was evident. The higher the degree of exposure, the higher the risk of developing bulimia nervosa. Within the domains, 5 subdomains were most strongly associated with case status: parental problems, obesity risk, parental psychiatric disorder, sexual or physical abuse, and premorbid psychiatric disorder. These findings are consistent with our hypothesis that factors that are likely to increase the risk for dieting and those likely to increase the risk for development of psychiatric disorder in general contribute to the etiology of bulimia nervosa.

As expected, only a few of the risk factors identified in the first case-control comparison were significantly more common among the subjects with bulimia nervosa than among the general psychiatric control subjects. Independent exposure to factors in the dieting vulnerability and environmental domains, but not the personal vulnerability domain, distinguished these 2 groups. On multivariate analysis across the subdomains, just 2 entered the regression model: obesity risk and parental problems. The overall results of the second case-control comparison, that between the subjects with bulimia nervosa and the general psychiatric control subjects, support our hypothesis that factors that increase concerns about shape, weight, or eating, and thereby increase the risk of dieting (including intrafamilial factors), are especially common among persons with bulimia nervosa. They also support and extend the striking finding from the multivariate genetic analysis by Kendler et al[52] that family environmental factors are especially important in the development of bulimia nervosa.

We did not predict that certain parental problems (low contact and high expectations), parental alcohol use disorder (ever), and negative self-evaluation would be more common among the subjects with bulimia nervosa than among the general psychiatric control subjects. The parental problems do, however, resemble descriptions of the parents of *patients* with bulimia nervosa.[53] The association with parental alcohol use disorder is intriguing and warrants further examination. Negative self-evaluation might encourage dieting by distorting the views of girls on their appearance.[54] That menarche occurred earlier in the subjects with bulimia nervosa than in the general psychiatric control subjects ($P<.01$) is noteworthy. Early menarche has been implicated in the development of anorexia nervosa,[55] and it may be a risk factor for dieting because it involves early exposure to the changes in body shape associated with puberty.[56]

The findings of this study confirm that there are many risk factors for bulimia nervosa, and, for the first time, data are provided on their relative contributions. How these risk factors operate, however, is not clear. The study needs to be repeated using another sample of subjects with bulimia nervosa because limited inferences can be drawn from a single investigation. It would be desirable in any replication for the general psychiatric control group to be more heterogeneous than that in our study, in which most subjects had a diagnosis of major depressive disorder. There is also a need for prospective studies of the onset of the disorder to illuminate the causal processes that are likely to be involved, because a shift in research emphasis is required away from risk factors and toward risk mechanisms. Prospective studies would also have the advantage of recruiting incident cases, whereas in our study the cases were well established.

From the perspective of prevention, we are impressed by the uniformly negative results of attempts to reduce the prevalence of dieting among young girls.[57-62] Indeed, it is possible that school-based interventions of this type may do more harm than good.[63] We believe that focusing on particular subgroups of dieters, rather than on dieting in general, might be more fruitful. If this strategy were adopted, knowledge of which dieters are at particular risk for the development of bulimia nervosa would be important because this would assist in the targeting of preventive interventions. Our findings suggest that bulimia nervosa is most likely to develop in dieters who are at risk of obesity and psychiatric disorder in general.

Accepted for publication June 21, 1996.

This study was funded by program grant 18157 from the Wellcome Trust, London, United Kingdom. Professor Fairburn holds a Wellcome Principal Research Fellowship (046386); Dr Welch and Ms Doll were supported by grants 030583 and 13123 from the Wellcome Trust.

We thank Professor George Brown, (Bedford College, London) and Dr Emily Simonoff (Institute of Psychiatry, London) for their advice on the design of the risk-factor interview. Dr David Jones (Park Hospital, Oxford, United Kingdom) advised on the assessment of sexual abuse. We also thank the participating general practitioners, and Faith Barbour, Jenny Burton, Jan Francis, Phillipa Hay, and Patricia Norman, for their work as interviewers. Dr Hay conducted the reliability study.

The operational definitions used for the EDE ratings and a copy of the interview schedule may be obtained by writing to Professor Fairburn. A charge will be made to cover the cost of postage and photocopying.

Corresponding author: Christopher G. Fairburn, DM, MPhil, FRCPsych, Department of Psychiatry, Oxford University, Warneford Hospital, Oxford OX3 7JX, United Kingdom.

REFERENCES

1. Holland AJ, Hall A, Murray R, Russell GFM, Crisp AH. Anorexia nervosa: a study of 34 twin pairs and one set of triplets. *Br J Psychiatry.* 1984;145:414-419.
2. Holland AJ, Sicotte N, Treasure JL. Anorexia nervosa: evidence for a genetic basis. *J Psychosom Res.* 1988;32:561-571.
3. Kassett JA, Gershon ES, Maxwell ME, Guroff JJ, Kazuba DM, Smith AL, Brandt HA, Jimerson DC. Psychiatric disorders in the first-degree relatives of probands with bulimia nervosa. *Am J Psychiatry.* 1989;146:1468-1471.
4. Hsu LKG, Chesler BE, Santhouse R. Bulimia nervosa in eleven sets of twins: a clinical report. *Int J Eat Disord.* 1990;9:275-282.
5. Strober M, Lampert C, Morrell W, Burroughs J, Jacobs C. A controlled family study of anorexia nervosa: evidence of familial aggregation and lack of shared transmission with affective disorders. *Int J Eat Disord.* 1990;9:239-253.
6. Kendler KS, MacLean C, Neale M, Kessler R, Heath A, Eaves L. The genetic epidemiology of bulimia nervosa. *Am J Psychiatry.* 1991;148:1627-1637.
7. Winokur A, March V, Mendels J. Primary affective disorder in relatives of patients with anorexia nervosa. *Am J Psychiatry.* 1980;137:695-698.
8. Hudson JI, Pope HG, Jonas JM, Yurgelun-Todd D. Family history study of anorexia nervosa and bulimia. *Br J Psychiatry.* 1983;142:133-138.
9. Gershon ES, Schreiber JL, Hamovit JR, Dibble ED, Kaye W, Nurnberger JI, Andersen AE, Ebert M. Clinical findings in patients with anorexia nervosa and affective illness in their relatives. *Am J Psychiatry.* 1984;141:1419-1422.
10. Rivinus TM, Biederman J, Herzog DB, Kemper K, Harper GP, Harmatz JS, Houseworth S. Anorexia nervosa and affective disorders: a controlled family history study. *Am J Psychiatry.* 1984;141:1414-1418.
11. Hudson JI, Pope HG, Jonas JM, Yurgelun-Todd D, Frankenburg FR. A controlled family history study of bulimia. *Psychol Med.* 1987;17:883-890.
12. Logue CM, Crowe RR, Bean JA. A family study of anorexia nervosa and bulimia. *Compr Psychiatry.* 1989;30:179-188.
13. Bulik CM. Drug and alcohol abuse by bulimic women and their families. *Am J Psychiatry.* 1987;144:1604-1606.

14. Garfinkel PE, Moldofsky H, Garner DM. The heterogeneity of anorexia nervosa: bulimia as a distinct subgroup. *Arch Gen Psychiatry.* 1980;37:1036-1040.
15. Strober M. The significance of bulimia in juvenile anorexia nervosa: an exploration of possible aetiological factors. *Int J Eat Disord.* 1981;1:28-43.
16. Fairburn CG, Cooper PJ. The clinical features of bulimia nervosa. *Br J Psychiatry.* 1984;144:238-246.
17. Schmidt U, Tiller J, Treasure J. Setting the scene for eating disorders: childhood care, classification and course of illness. *Psychol Med.* 1993;23:663-672.
18. Welch SL, Fairburn CG. Sexual abuse and bulimia nervosa: three integrated case-control comparisons. *Am J Psychiatry.* 1994;151:402-407.
19. Everill JT, Waller G. Reported sexual abuse and eating psychopathology: a review of the evidence for a causal link. *Int J Eat Disord.* 1995;18:1-11.
20. Welch SL, Fairburn CG. Childhood sexual and physical abuse as risk factors for the development of bulimia nervosa. *Child Abuse Negl.* 1996;20:633-642.
21. Garfinkel PE, Garner DM. *Anorexia Nervosa: A Multidimensional Perspective.* New York, NY: Brunner-Mazel Publications; 1982.
22. Johnson CL, Connors ME. *The Etiology and Treatment of Bulimia Nervosa. A Biopsychosocial Perspective.* New York, NY: Basic Books Inc Publishers; 1987.
23. Fairburn CG, Walsh BT. Atypical eating disorders. In: Brownell KD, Fairburn CG, eds. *Eating Disorders and Obesity: A Comprehensive Handbook.* New York, NY: Guilford Press; 1995:135-140.
24. American Psychiatric Association. *Diagnostic and Statistical Manual of Mental Disorders, Fourth Edition.* Washington, DC: American Psychiatric Association; 1994.
25. Fairburn CG, Beglin SJ. Studies of the epidemiology of bulimia nervosa. *Am J Psychiatry.* 1990;147:401-408.
26. Clinton DN, Glant R. The eating disorders spectrum of *DSM-III-R*: clinical features and psychosocial concomitants of 86 consecutive cases from a Swedish urban catchment area. *J Nerv Ment Dis.* 1992;180:244-250.
27. Mitrany E. Atypical eating disorders. *J Adolesc Health.* 1992;13:400-402.
28. Rastam M, Gillberg C. Background factors in anorexia nervosa. *Eur Child Adolesc Psychiatry.* 1992;1:54-65.
29. Fairburn CG, Cooper PJ. Self-induced vomiting and bulimia nervosa: an undetected problem. *BMJ.* 1982;284:1153-1155.
30. Fairburn CG, Cooper PJ. Binge-eating, self-induced vomiting and laxative abuse: a community study. *Psychol Med.* 1984;14:401-410.
31. King MB. *Eating Disorders in a General Practice Population: Prevalence, Characteristics and Follow-up at 12 to 18 Months.* New York, NY: Cambridge University Press; 1989:14. Psychological Medicine Monograph.
32. Whitaker A, Davies M, Shaffer D, Johnson J, Abrams S, Walsh BT, Kalikow K. The struggle to be thin: a survey of anorexic and bulimic symptoms in a non-referred adolescent population. *Psychol Med.* 1989;19:143-163.
33. Whitehouse AM, Cooper PJ, Vize CV, Hill C, Vogel L. Prevalence of eating disorders in three Cambridge general practices: hidden and conspicuous morbidity. *Br J Gen Pract.* 1992;42:57-60.
34. Fairburn CG, Welch SL, Norman PA, O'Connor ME, Doll HA. Bias and bulimia nervosa: how typical are clinic cases? *Am J Psychiatry.* 1996;153:386-391.
35. Office of Population Censuses and Surveys. *Classification of Occupations.* London, England: HMSO; 1980.
36. Office of Health Economics. *Compendium of Health Statistics.* London, England: Office of Health Economics; 1987.
37. Beglin SJ, Fairburn CG. Evaluation of a new instrument for the detection of eating disorders in community samples. *Psychiatry Res.* 1992;44:191-201.
38. Fairburn CG, Beglin SJ. Assessment of eating disorders: interview or self-report questionnaire? *Int J Eat Disord.* 1994;16:363-370.
39. Goldberg D, Williams P. *A User's Guide to the General Health Questionnaire.* Windsor, UK: NFER Publishing Company; 1988.
40. Beglin SJ. *Eating Disorders in Young Adult Women.* Oxford, UK: University of Oxford; 1990. Thesis.
41. Cooper Z, Fairburn CG. The Eating Disorder Examination: A semi-structured interview for the assessment of the specific psychopathology of eating disorders. *Int J Eat Disord.* 1987;6:1-8.
42. Cooper Z, Cooper PJ, Fairburn CG. The validity of the Eating Disorder Examination and its subscales. *Br J Psychiatry.* 1989;154:807-812.
43. Fairburn CG, Cooper Z. The Eating Disorder Examination (12th edition). In: Fairburn CG, Wilson GT, eds. *Binge Eating: Nature, Assessment and Treatment.* New York, NY: Guilford Press; 1993:317-360.
44. American Psychiatric Association. *Diagnostic and Statistical Manual of Mental Disorders, Third Edition, Revised.* Washington, DC: American Psychiatric Association; 1987.
45. Spitzer RL, Williams JBW, Gibbon M, First MB. The Structured Clinical Interview for *DSM-III-R* (SCID), I: history, rationale and description. *Arch Gen Psychiatry.* 1992;49:624-629.
46. Williams JBW, Gibbon M, First MB, Spitzer RL, Davis M, Borus J, Howes MJ, Kane J, Pope HG, Rounsaville B, Wittchen HU. The Structured Clinical Interview for *DSM-III-R* (SCID), II: multisite test-retest reliability. *Arch Gen Psychiatry.* 1992;49:630-636.
47. Herzog DB. Bulimia: the secretive syndrome. *Psychosomatics.* 1982;23:481-484.
48. Parker G, Tupling H, Brown LB. A Parental Bonding Instrument. *Br J Med Psychol.* 1979;52:1-10.
49. Parker G. The Parental Bonding Instrument: psychometric properties reviewed. *Psychiatr Dev.* 1989;4:317-335.
50. Breslow NE, Day NE. *Statistical Methods in Cancer Research. Volume 1: The Analysis of Case-Control Studies.* Lyon, France: International Agency for Research on Cancer; 1980.
51. Koeter M, Van den Brink W, Ormel J. Chronic psychiatric complaints and the General Health Questionnaire. *Br J Psychiatry.* 1989;155:186-190.
52. Kendler KS, Walters EE, Neale MC, Kessler RC, Heath AC, Eaves LJ. The structure of the genetic and environmental risk factors for six major psychiatric disorders in women. *Arch Gen Psychiatry.* 1995;52:374-383.
53. Vandereycken W, Kog E, Vanderlinden J. *The Family Approach to Eating Disorders.* Costa Mesa, Calif: PMA Publishing Corporation; 1989.
54. Fairburn CG. Eating disorders. In: Clark DM, Fairburn CG, eds. *Science and Practice of Cognitive Behaviour Therapy.* New York, NY: Oxford University Press; 1997:209-241.
55. Crisp AH. Reported birth weights and growth rates in a group of patients with primary anorexia nervosa (weight phobia). *J Psychosom Res.* 1970;14:23-50.
56. Striegel-Moore RH. Etiology of binge eating: a developmental perspective. In: Fairburn CG, Wilson GT, eds. *Binge Eating: Nature, Assessment and Treatment.* New York, NY: Guilford Press; 1993:144-172.
57. Shisslak CM, Crago M, Neal ME. Prevention of eating disorders among adolescents. *Am J Health Promotion.* 1990;5:100-106.
58. Rosen JC. Prevention of eating disorders. *Natl Anorexic Aid Soc Newsletter.* 1989;12:1-3.
59. Moriarty D, Shore R, Maxim N. Evaluation of an eating disorder curriculum. *Eval Program Plann.* 1990;13:407-413.
60. Moreno AB, Thelen MH. A preliminary prevention program for eating disorders in a junior high school population. *J Youth Adolescence.* 1993;22:109-124.
61. Paxton SJ. A prevention program for disturbed eating and body dissatisfaction in adolescent girls: a 1 year follow-up. *Health Educ Res.* 1993;8:43-51.
62. Killen JD, Barr Taylor C, Hammer LD, Litt I, Wilson DM, Rich T, Hayward C, Simmonds B, Kraemer H, Varady A. An attempt to modify unhealthful eating attitudes and weight regulation practices of young adolescent girls. *Int J Eat Disord.* 1993;13:369-384.
63. Carter JC, Stewart DA, Dunn VJ, Fairburn CG. Primary prevention of eating disorders: might it do more harm than good? *Int J Eat Disord.* In press.

EFFECTIVE SSRI THERAPY WITH LOW

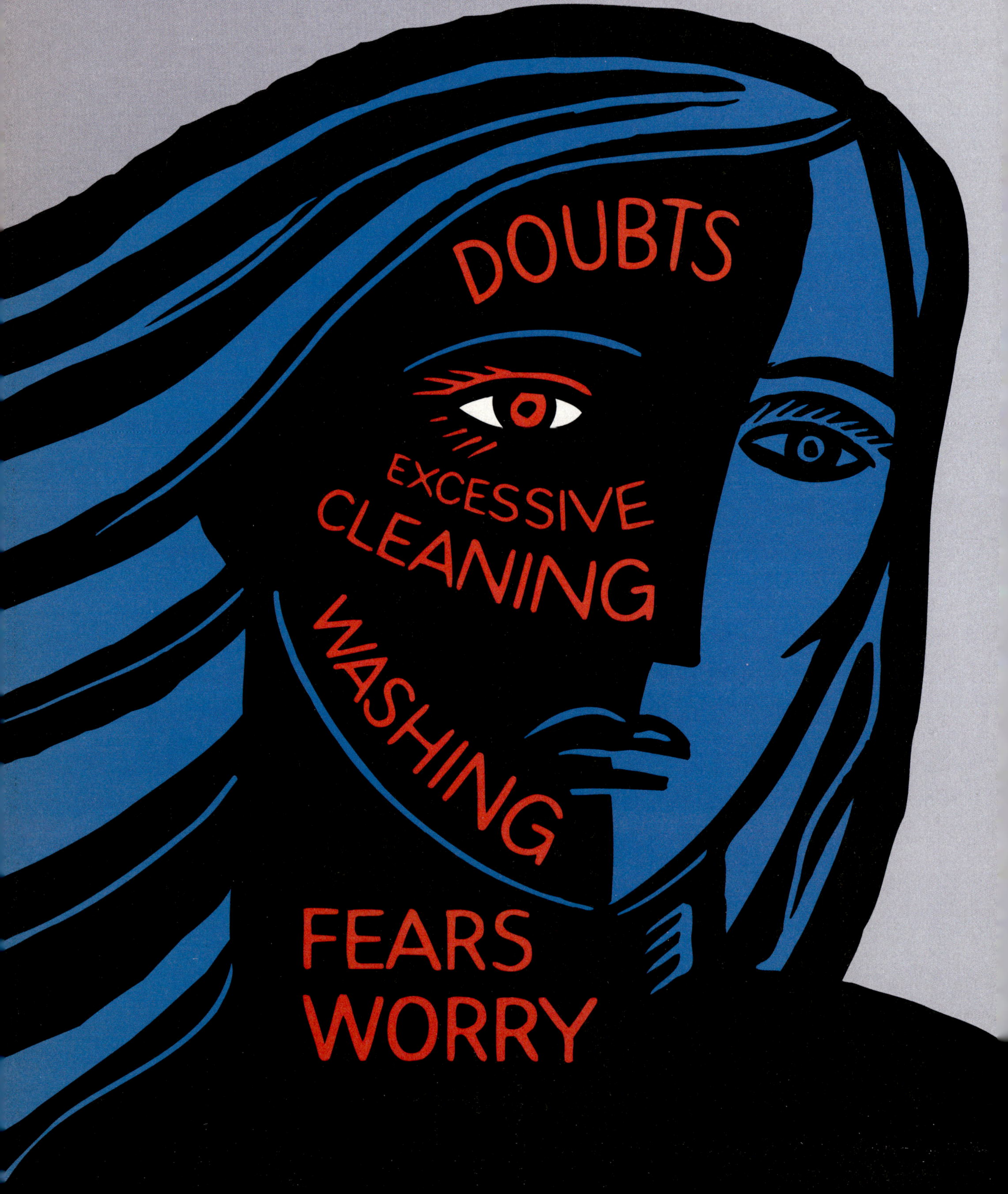

ORIGINAL ARTICLE

Hormonal and Subjective Responses to Intravenous *meta*-Chlorophenylpiperazine in Bulimia Nervosa

Robert D. Levitan, MD; Allan S. Kaplan, MD; Russell T. Joffe, MD; Anthony J. Levitt, MD; Gregory M. Brown, MD

Background: Several lines of evidence point to serotonergic abnormalities in patients with bulimia nervosa (BN). Our goal was to further examine central serotonergic function in bulimic patients using neuroendocrine and subjective responses to the postsynaptic serotonin receptor agonist *meta*-chlorophenylpiperazine (mCPP).

Method: Using a double-blind, randomized, placebo-controlled design, we assessed neuroendocrine and subjective responses to intravenous mCPP (0.1 mg/kg) and placebo in 16 patients with BN, free of medication, and 14 normal control subjects. Plasma prolactin and cortisol levels were used as neuroendocrine measures, whereas subjective responses were measured using a visual analog scale of 10 different mood states.

Results: Compared with controls, the BN group exhibited blunted prolactin and net cortisol responses following mCPP challenge. Subjective responses, while preliminary, also differed between groups on items related to anxiety, calmness, and altered self-awareness.

Conclusion: Evidence of dysfunction at or downstream of central serotonergic receptors in BN confirms and extends findings of prior research.

Arch Gen Psychiatry. 1997;54:521-527

Bulimia nervosa (BN) is a complex, relatively poorly understood disorder with numerous factors playing a role in its cause and pathophysiological features. One factor that may contribute to several clinical features of BN and that may also be a reasonable target therapeutically is the neurotransmitter serotonin (5-HT). In addition to playing a key role in satiety mechanisms,[1-5] 5-HT has been implicated in depression,[6-16] anxiety,[17-22] and impulsive behaviors,[23-33] all of which are common in subjects with BN.[34-36]

A number of studies have found alterations in 5-HT function in BN. An initial report found that in weight-recovered anorexic patients, those with continuing bulimic symptoms had lower probenecid-induced 5-hydroxyindoleacetic acid (5-HIAA) accumulation in cerebrospinal fluid, suggesting a relationship between bingeing and reduced brain 5-HT metabolism.[37] Later studies of normal-weight bulimic patients have found normal cerebrospinal fluid levels of 5-HIAA relative to those of controls,[38,39] although patients who binge at least twice daily may have lower levels of this metabolite.[39] This may be consistent with decreased release of 5-HT in bulimic patients with high binge frequency.

Other studies have looked at peripheral measures of 5-HT activity as an indirect means of assessing central 5-HT function. High platelet 5-HT uptake, which may reflect increased 5-HT uptake at central nervous system synapses,[40] and decreased platelet imipramine binding[41] have been reported

See also pages 507, 509, and 529

in BN. The plasma ratio of tryptophan to large neutral amino acid (TRP/LNAA) has been used as a peripheral indicator of central 5-HT precursor availability in BN.[42,43] A study of baseline measures found no difference in the TRP/LNAA ratio between patients with BN and normal control subjects[42]; however, patients who fail to exhibit an increase in the TRP/LNAA ratio during bingeing may experience prolongation of the binge-purge cycle.[43] This suggests that, notwithstanding normal baseline levels of tryptophan, an inability to increase the synthesis or turnover of brain 5-HT may play a role in abnormal satiety mechanisms in some bulimic individuals.

Preliminary evidence exists for abnormal neuroendocrine responses to both presynaptic and postsynaptic serotonergic

From the Eating Disorders Center, The Toronto Hospital (Drs Levitan and Kaplan), and the Clarke Institute of Psychiatry (Drs Joffe, Levitt, and Brown), Department of Psychiatry University of Toronto, Toronto, Ontario. Dr Levitan is now at the Mood Disorders Clinic, Clarke Institute of Psychiatry, Toronto. Dr Joffe is now with the Department of Psychiatry, McMaster University, Hamilton, Ontario. Dr Levitt is now at the Mood Disorders Clinic, Sunnybrook Hospital, Department of Psychiatry, University of Toronto.

PATIENTS AND METHODS

DEMOGRAPHICS AND CLINICAL CHARACTERISTICS

The BN group included consecutive female outpatients who presented for an initial eating disorder consultation or were awaiting admission to an eating disorder day hospital program. They ranged in age from 18 to 45 years, were greater than 85% of the matched population mean weight (MPMW), and met *DSM-III-R*[56] criteria for current BN based on the eating disorder section of the Structured Clinical Interview for *DSM-III*.[57] Patients were excluded from the study if they were acutely suicidal or current substance abusers, but were not excluded if they had comorbid depression. All subjects in the BN group were actively bingeing and purging and had been free of psychiatric medication for at least 8 weeks at entry to the study.

Normal controls included 14 healthy volunteer female subjects, ranging in age from 18 to 45 years, with greater than 85% MPMW, and with no history of psychiatric illness or substance abuse based on a semistructured screening interview. Controls were recruited through posters and announcements distributed at the University of Toronto and The Toronto Hospital, Toronto, Ontario.

No subject was pregnant, had significant medical illnesses, and or had irregular menstrual cycles during the 3 months before the study date. Menstrual phase was documented by self-report, defined as menstrual days 0 to 5, follicular days 5 to 14, and luteal days 14 to menses. All subjects underwent testing during the follicular phase to control for possible effects of menstrual cycle on serotonergic function. Each subject underwent a routine physical examination and laboratory tests, including electrocardiography and blood work. Each subject was given an oral and written summary of the purposes, procedures, and potential risks of the project and gave informed consent.

PREPARATION OF mCPP

Fifteen hundred milligrams of dry mCPP-dihydrochloride powder (Research Biochemicals, Natick, Mass) was diluted with 500 mL of normal saline solution to create a 3-mg/mL solution (based on the salt with molecular weight 269.7). Sodium hydroxide solution was added to bring the final pH to 5.15. Under sterile conditions, the solution was passed through a 0.22-μm polymer filter. A portion was obtained for pyrogen and sterility testing, and the remainder was packaged in sterile 10-mL vials in 5-mL aliquots.

mCPP TEST PROCEDURE

All subjects were admitted to the clinical investigation unit of The Toronto Hospital in the evening before the first challenge and allowed nothing by mouth except for clear fluids after 8 PM. On the evening of admission, patients completed the Beck Depression Inventory[58] and were administered the Hamilton Depression Rating Scale (HAM-12)[59] and a modified version of the Eating Disorders Examination[60] by one of us (R.D.L.).

At 7 AM the next morning, an indwelling venous catheter was inserted in a forearm vein and kept patent with normal saline solution. At 8 AM, vital signs were taken and, using a double-blind procedure, an injection of 0.1 mg/kg of mCPP or normal saline solution was administered for 10 minutes. On each day, the test solution was diluted in 50 mL of normal saline solution for intravenous administration. Blood samples were taken 15 minutes before, at the same time as, and at 30, 60, 90, 120, and 180 minutes after placebo or drug challenge to measure prolactin and cortisol levels. Samples were kept on ice and centrifuged, and plasma was divided into aliquots and frozen until subsequent radioimmunoassay. At the same time that blood samples were drawn, each subject completed subjective mood ratings using visual analog scales consisting of 10 parallel 100-mm lines. Each line had a left border marked "not at all" and a right border marked "most ever." The following 10 different mood variables were assessed: happy, sad, anxious, drowsy, nervous, energetic, calm, fearful, high, and mellow.[61]

Following completion of the first challenge, subjects were given a day pass and returned to the unit in the evening. Following the same protocol as described above, subjects completed a second challenge the next morning with the agent not used in the first test. The investigator who administered the challenge tests (R.D.L.) was unaware of which substance was injected; however, a coinvestigator (A.S.K.) was aware of the placebo-mCPP condition.

DATA ANALYSIS

All data were tested for normal distribution and met criteria for normality. For hormonal variables, comparisons between groups were analyzed using a repeated measures analysis of variance (RANOVA) with baseline hormone levels as a single covariate. Post hoc analysis of group differences was performed using simple effects. For mood variables, insufficient degrees of freedom were available for a single multivariate ANOVA, and the 10 mood items were analyzed separately using a RANOVA. Pearson correlation coefficients were used to evaluate relationships among neuroendocrine responses, subjective responses, and key clinical variables. For all results, the α level of significance was set at .05.

agents in BN. Blunted prolactin responses to the 5-HT precursor 5-hydroxytryptophan,[44] the 5-HT–releasing drug fenfluramine hydrochloride,[45] and the postsynaptic 5-HT receptor agonist *meta*-chlorophenylpiperazine (mCPP)[46] have been reported. Notwithstanding the consistency of these findings, their interpretation is open to debate. A blunted response to a 5-HT precursor or releaser may be due to a variety of presynaptic or postsynaptic defects, including mechanisms not directly related to 5-HT.[47] Two of the studies[45,46] used oral as opposed to intravenous challenges, introducing the possible confound of variable gastrointestinal absorption patterns across subjects,[48] a particular concern in bulimic subjects.[49]

Given these potential limitations of prior research, we decided to examine central serotonergic function in bulimic patients (BN group) using neuroendocrine and subjective responses to intravenous mCPP. An active metabolite of the antidepressant trazodone hydrochloride, mCPP is a postsynaptic 5-HT receptor agonist known to reliably stimulate release of prolactin and cortisol in normal human subjects in a safe manner.[50] It binds with highest affinity to 5-HT_{2c} receptors, but it also binds to 5-HT_{1a}, 5-HT_{1b} (not in human brain), and 5-HT_2 and moderately to α_2-noradrenergic receptors.[51,52] Studies with mCPP in humans indicate that its hormonal and behavioral effects (eg, anxiety production) are serotonergically mediated.[50,53,54]

It was decided to use mCPP based on the working hypothesis that, due to postsynaptic 5-HT dysfunction in patients with BN, blunted hormonal and subjective responses to serotonergic challenge would occur in this group. Intravenous mCPP was chosen based on previous work indicating less variability in blood levels in comparison with oral administration.[48,55] A 0.1-mg/kg dose was used based on previous studies showing robust hormonal and subjective responses in normal controls in this dose range.[54]

RESULTS

DEMOGRAPHICS

All error terms are SDs. There were no significant differences between the BN group and controls in age (23.7±4.8 vs 23.8±2.9 years), weight (55.7±10.9 vs 63.7±16.6 kg), or MPMW (99.9±19.1 vs 106.6±26.9 kg). The BN group had a mean HAM-21 score of 14.7±7.7 (range, 2-27) and a mean Beck Depression Inventory score of 18.6±8.4 (range, 8-39). Binge and vomiting frequencies for the BN group were 8.1±8.7 and 9.1±11.8 per week, respectively.

NEUROENDOCRINE MEASURES

Prolactin

Baseline Measures. For the mCPP and placebo challenges, both prechallenge plasma prolactin levels (ie, 15 minutes before and at baseline) were found to be highly correlated (r=0.89, P<.001, for mCPP challenge; r=0.97, P<.001, for placebo challenge) across all subjects. Based on these results, baseline prolactin level was defined as the average of the 2 prechallenge prolactin levels on a given test day.

For each subject, a mean baseline prolactin level was calculated by averaging the baseline prolactin levels for both study days. The BN group had significantly lower mean baseline prolactin levels than controls (11.1±3.9 vs 18.0±5.5 μg/L, respectively; P<.001, unpaired t test). The correlation between mean baseline prolactin level and MPMW was insignificant within each group and for the total group of subjects. Within the BN group, there was no significant correlation between baseline prolactin levels and clinical measures, including current monthly binge frequency, current monthly vomiting frequency, and Beck Depression Inventory and HAM-21 scores.

Response to mCPP and Placebo. Prolactin responses to mCPP and placebo in controls and the BN group are graphed in **Figure 1**. The RANOVA indicated a significant group by drug by time interaction (F=2.86; df=5, 24; P=.04) and a significant group by drug interaction

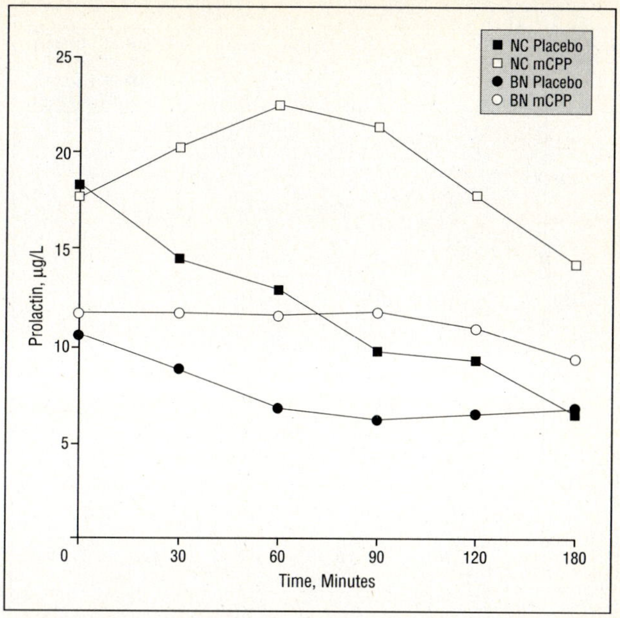

Figure 1. *Prolactin responses to* meta-*chlorophenylpiperazine (mCPP) and placebo in patients with bulimia nervosa (BN) and normal control subjects (NC).*

(F=6.13; df=1, 28; P=.02). The main effects of drug (F=73.33; df=1, 28; P<.001) and time (F=12.09; df=5, 24; P<.001) were significant. The main effect of group was not significant.

Post hoc analysis indicated that the peak prolactin level following mCPP challenge, defined as the maximum increase in prolactin level from baseline, was significantly greater in controls than in the BN group (6.6±5.5 vs 1.9±4.3 μg/L, respectively; P=.02, unpaired t test). Within the BN group, no significant correlations were found between peak prolactin levels and clinical variables, including age, weight, MPMW, binge and vomiting frequency, or HAM-21 scores.

To further investigate the effect of the drug relative to placebo, prolactin change scores were calculated by subtracting baseline prolactin levels from each post-challenge data point. Net change scores, defined as the difference in prolactin change scores on the mCPP and placebo challenge days, were then calculated. A RANOVA using these net change scores revealed significant main effects of group (F=12.01; df=1, 28; P=.002) and time (F=15.375; df=4, 25; P<.001). Simple effects tests on these net change scores at each time revealed significant differences between controls and the BN group at 30 minutes (F=4.58; df=1, 28; P=.04), 60 minutes (F=8.41; df=1, 28; P=.007), 90 minutes (F=13.54; df=1, 28; P=.001), and 120 minutes (F=10.15; df=1, 28; P=.004) after challenge.

To control for possible order effects, a RANOVA with group and day of mCPP challenge as between-group factors was completed on the prolactin scores. The group by mCPP day and group by mCPP day by drug interactions and the main effect of mCPP challenge day were all nonsignificant. The group by drug interaction remained significant (F=5.13; df=1, 26; P=.03), and there was a trend for a group by drug by time interaction using this model (F=2.29; df=5, 22; P=.08).

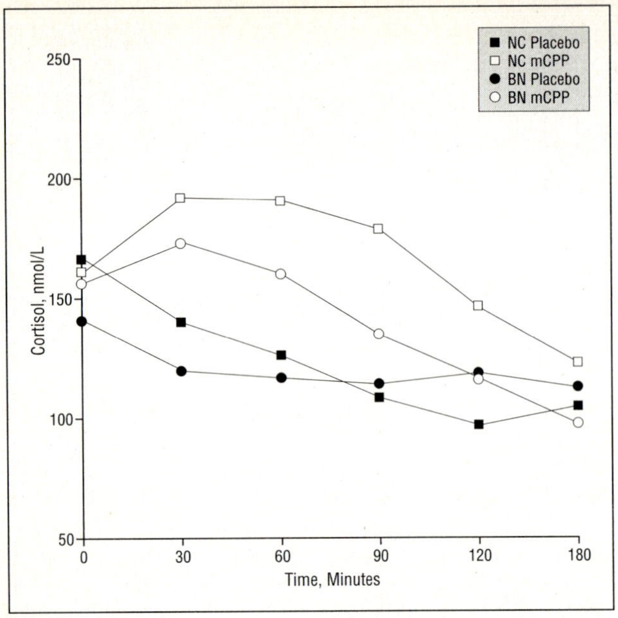

Figure 2. *Cortisol responses to* meta-*chlorophenylpiperazine (mCPP) and placebo in patients with bulimia nervosa (BN) and normal control subjects (NC).*

Cortisol

Baseline Measures. For the mCPP and placebo challenges, both prechallenge plasma cortisol levels were found to be highly correlated (r=0.65, P<.001, for mCPP challenge; r=0.67, P<.001, for placebo challenge) across all subjects. Based on these findings, mean baseline cortisol level was defined as the average of both prechallenge cortisol levels on a given test day.

For each subject, a mean baseline cortisol level was calculated by averaging the baseline cortisol levels for both study days. There was no statistical difference in mean baseline cortisol level between controls and the BN group (162.1±42.0 vs 147.5±58.1 nmol/L, respectively; P=.44, unpaired t test). The correlation between mean baseline cortisol level and MPMW was insignificant within each group and for the total group of subjects. Within the BN group, there was no significant correlation between baseline cortisol levels and clinical measures, including current monthly binge and vomiting frequency and Beck Depression Inventory and HAM-21 scores.

Response to mCPP and Placebo. Cortisol responses to mCPP and placebo in controls and the BN group are graphed in **Figure 2**. The RANOVA indicated no significant interaction or main effect related to group. There were significant main effects of drug (F=14.06; df=1, 28; P=.001) and time (F=15.85; df=5, 24; P<.001).

The peak cortisol level following mCPP challenge, defined as the maximum increase in cortisol level from baseline, was not significantly different between controls and the BN group (66.9±98.4 vs 26.9±54.6 nmol/L; P=.17, unpaired t test).

Cortisol net change scores, defined as the difference in cortisol change scores on days of mCPP and placebo challenges, were then calculated for each time. A RANOVA on these change scores revealed a significant main effect of group (F=5.04; df=1, 28; P=.03) and time (F=5.98; df=4, 25; P=.002). Calculation of simple effects at each time revealed significant differences between groups at 90 minutes (F=4.38; df=1, 28; P=.05), 120 minutes (F=4.73; df=1, 28; P=.04), and 180 minutes (F=6.23; df=1, 28; P=.02) following challenge.

To control for possible order effects, a RANOVA with group and day of mCPP challenge as between-group factors was completed on the cortisol net change scores. The group by mCPP day interaction and the main effect of mCPP challenge day were nonsignificant. The main effect of group continued to be significant (F=5.00; df=1, 26; P=.03).

SUBJECTIVE RESPONSES

Subjective responses were available for 29 of the 30 subjects participating in the study (not performed by 1 subject in the BN group). To capture only acute subjective responses likely to be attributable to the placebo or drug, only baseline values and the first 3 postchallenge times (ie, 30, 60, and 90 minutes) were included in this analysis.

Baseline Scores

For each of the 10 mood variables on a given day, baseline was defined as the average of both prechallenge ratings on that day. For a given mood state of each subject, a mean baseline rating was calculated by averaging the baseline levels for both study days. Unpaired t tests revealed no significant difference in mean baseline ratings between groups on any of the 10 mood states.

Subjective Responses to mCPP and Placebo

Raw data for subjective responses to mCPP and placebo (baseline and the first 2 postchallenge times) are summarized in the **Table**. Significant group by drug by time interactions were found for ratings of fearful (F=3.46; df=3, 25; P=.03) and high (F=3.00; df=3, 25; P=.05). Significant group by drug interactions were found for ratings of anxious (F=4.35; df=1, 27; P=.05), calm (F=5.33; df=1, 27; P=.03), and mellow (F=9.87; df=1, 27; P=.004).

Examination of the raw data suggests that group by drug interactions on ratings of mellow and high may have been largely attributable to baseline differences and responses to placebo, and not to responses to mCPP per se, although the decrease in mellow ratings following mCPP challenge appeared to last longer (60 minutes) in the BN group. Differential response to the mCPP challenge in the BN group and controls is more apparent on ratings of anxiety and fearful. Overall, these results should be considered preliminary and subject to further study with a larger sample.

COMMENT

Our study is the first to use an intravenously administered postsynaptic challenge agent in BN and the first to find blunted neuroendocrine and altered subjective re-

Subjective Responses to *meta*-Chlorophenylpiperazine and Placebo in Patients With Bulimia Nervosa and Normal Control Subjects*

	mCPP Responses			Placebo Responses		
Mood Item	At Baseline	After 30 Minutes	After 60 Minutes	At Baseline	After 30 Minutes	After 60 Minutes
Anxious						
Controls	21.4±21.4	33.1±28.3	22.4±20.4	16.4±17.8	14.5±20.0	12.4±17.8
BN Group	27.9±23.4	29.5±16.0	22.9±14.9	27.6±22.3	26.5±22.1	26.9±24.9
Nervous						
Controls	20.4±21.9	27.4±28.3	19.0±20.0	16.0±18.3	14.1±19.9	12.4±17.3
BN Group	25.1±22.1	22.9±20.8	16.1±15.5	21.5±18.9	16.6±19.3	17.8±17.8
Fearful						
Controls	16.7±19.9	23.9±23.6	15.7±17.7	18.3±19.9	16.2±19.2	15.6±20.3
BN Group	15.3±18.2	14.3±16.3	10.1±16.4	11.3±12.5	10.8±11.2	9.8±13.0
Calm						
Controls	51.8±18.2	43.9±22.3	50.7±17.2	53.0±18.3	49.6±20.3	51.3±18.3
BN Group	52.3±18.5	38.1±24.7	44.6±18.8	55.4±13.3	58.4±18.1	55.4±24.1
Mellow						
Controls	45.7±22.6	37.0±25.3	47.7±22.7	39.4±22.6	36.9±23.8	34.1±24.3
BN Group	47.3±15.5	33.7±23.0	39.1±23.7	51.4±17.1	46.9±23.8	51.7±21.5
High						
Controls	13.9±17.2	35.3±31.0	23.8±22.1	13.8±16.1	13.9±16.9	13.8±19.6
BN Group	21.3±21.5	43.9±31.2	27.8±24.1	18.0±21.1	26.7±27.7	22.5±25.3
Happy						
Controls	46.8±11.1	43.4±11.3	46.1±8.7	43.7±12.1	47.1±10.1	47.7±8.3
BN Group	47.2±16.4	53.2±17.6	52.2±16.1	48.3±15.1	49.8±20.0	53.3±18.1
Sad						
Controls	17.8±20.0	18.7±20.6	17.6±19.6	14.8±17.7	11.9±14.6	13.1±17.4
BN Group	22.6±26.1	24.8±27.2	20.8±23.6	26.2±26.6	25.7±26.6	24.4±23.0
Drowsy						
Controls	30.2±26.9	35.7±28.0	17.9±17.7	27.0±21.6	17.6±23.5	18.4±22.1
BN Group	33.2±28.5	28.5±25.8	28.8±26.4	36.8±25.9	29.0±23.9	27.9±24.9
Energetic						
Controls	29.5±20.2	32.6±21.1	30.0±19.9	20.5±13.9	24.6±14.0	30.3±14.2
BN Group	28.5±14.2	37.4±25.4	31.6±17.6	30.1±13.7	40.0±19.4	38.1±16.1

**Scoring is described in the "Subjective Responses" subsection of the "Results" section of the text. mCCP indicates* meta*-chlorophenylpiperazine; BN, bulimia nervosa.*

sponses to serotonergic challenge in this population. These results may be consistent with decreased activity at or downstream of central 5-HT receptors in BN and confirm and extend prior research.

In a previous study using oral mCPP challenges in BN, bulimic patients had low baseline prolactin levels, blunted prolactin responses, and no difference in cortisol responses to mCPP compared with controls[46]; most patients had abstained from bingeing and purging for 1 month at the time of the challenge. Our results are generally consistent with those of this prior study, with the major difference being our finding of blunted cortisol net change scores in the BN group. This discrepancy may have been due to the higher dose of mCPP used in the prior study; evidence supports an early ceiling effect for cortisol release with serotonergic stimulation.[62] Alternatively, the difference in studies may have been due in some way to the greater degree of active bingeing and purging in our BN group.

The finding of low baseline prolactin levels in BN is consistent with prior research[46,63]; however, it is unclear to what extent altered 5-HT activity contributes to this. Several[64-66] but not all[67] studies have shown that depletion of 5-HT stores or destruction of 5-HT nerve terminals decreases basal as well as stimulated prolactin release in rats. A defect in prolactin secretion beyond the serotonergic influence, such as a primary defect in pituitary lactotroph cells and/or overactivity of tuberoinfundibular dopaminergic neurons (which tonically inhibit prolactin secretion), could also account for lower baseline and blunted prolactin responses. The fact that patients with BN exhibit normal prolactin responses to thyrotropin-releasing hormone, which acts directly on the pituitary lactotroph,[63,68] makes these mechanisms less likely to account for our results. Furthermore, the BN group exhibited blunted net cortisol responses to mCPP in our study with normal baseline cortisol levels, suggesting serotonergic dysfunction at sites other than the pituitary lactotroph.

A different pattern of acute subjective responses to mCPP and placebo on mood ratings related to anxiety, calmness, and altered self-awareness was found in the BN group relative to controls. It is difficult to determine to what extent the observed differences were due to mCPP effects as opposed to baseline differences and responses to placebo, although, for anxiety ratings, the BN group appeared to have blunted responses to mCPP relative to controls. It is also not clear whether these data reflect true group differences in 5-HT receptor activity or simply discrepancies in reporting of moods; patients with BN have difficulty in labeling emotions.[69] While no firm conclusions can be drawn regarding subjective responses to mCPP in our BN group, our data suggest that further study in a larger sample of bulimic patients is merited.

MECHANISM OF SEROTONERGIC DYSFUNCTION IN BN

Why do patients with BN exhibit altered 5-HT activity? A number of mechanisms, acting alone or in combination, may play a role. It is possible that abnormal 5-HT function exists premorbidly, perhaps due to inherited abnormalities at or beyond the 5-HT receptor. Not mutually exclusive to this is the possibility that changes in 5-HT function are at least in part state related, with several potential factors involved.

Short-term starvation up-regulates rather than down-regulates hypothalamic 5-HT receptors[70] and cannot account for our findings. On the other hand, women with anorexia nervosa exhibit reduced rather than increased prolactin responses to L-trypotophan and mCPP,[71] suggesting that longer-term starvation may lead to down-regulation of the 5-HT system in time. This being the case, blunted 5-HT activity in BN may be related to long-term intermittent starvation.

Binge eating and/or vomiting may increase central 5-HT synthesis and lead to a compensatory down-regulation of postsynaptic 5-HT receptors.[43] This may prevent the compensatory increase in postsynaptic receptor sensitivity associated with shorter-term starvation.[39] Assessment of 5-HT function in nonpurging vs purging bulimic patients and in chronic vomiters who do not binge may be necessary to address this further.

Interactions between the 5-HT system and circulating hormones may contribute to altered 5-HT activity. Endogenous corticosteroid secretion has been shown to enhance activity of midbrain tryptophan hydroxylase, the rate-limiting enzyme in the biosynthesis of 5-HT from tryptophan.[72] In animals, long-term treatment with cortisol produces blunted prolactin responses to mCPP.[62] This may be due to enhanced 5-HT release and receptor down-regulation in time. An inverse relationship between baseline cortisol and peak prolactin levels in response to mCPP has been described previously in bulimic subjects.[46] This suggests that, in at least some bulimic patients, long-term stress or other factors raising cortisol levels in time may play a role in altering central 5-HT receptor sensitivity.

LIMITATIONS AND FINAL CONCLUSIONS

It is difficult to sort out to what extent intermittent starvation, bingeing, and purging may have contributed to our results. The fact that our findings were similar to those in patients who were abstinent from bingeing and purging for several weeks[46] suggests that serotonergic dysfunction in BN may not be state dependent. On the other hand, it may take several months for biological systems and receptors to recover once disrupted. Further research in bulimic patients with long-term abstinence from symptoms is required to sort out this state vs trait issue.

The general lack of specificity of mCPP makes it difficult to ascertain which particular 5-HT receptor subtypes might be abnormal in BN, although a parsimonious explanation for our findings might be dysfunction at or beyond the central $5\text{-}HT_{2c}$ receptors in particular. These receptors have been implicated in prolactin and cortisol secretion,[22,73] anxiety production,[21,22] and the mediation of satiety.[74-77] Further assessment of this possibility awaits the development of more specific 5-HT agonists and antagonists suitable for use in the human population.

Notwithstanding these potential limitations, the combination of hormonal and subjective rating abnormalities strongly supports a model of central serotonergic dysfunction in BN. Whereas the hormonal results are most consistent with dysfunction of hypothalamic serotonergic receptors, it is possible that subjective results reflect serotonergic dysfunction at other brain sites, particularly those involved in modulation of anxiety such as the amygdala, thalamus, hippocampus, and/or neocortex.

Accepted for publication July 10, 1996.

Supported by the Ontario Mental Health Foundation, Toronto.

Sidney Kennedy, MD, Franco Vaccarino, PhD, and Dennis Murphy, MD, provided valuable assistance at various stages of this project. Ongoing technical assistance was provided by staff of The Toronto Hospital, Clinical Investigation Unit. Statistical consultation was provided by David Streiner, PhD, and Cathy Spegg, MBA.

Reprints: Robert D. Levitan, MD, Clarke Institute of Psychiatry, Room 1135, 250 College St, Toronto, Ontario, Canada M5T 1R8.

REFERENCES

1. Goudie A, Thornton E, Wheeler T. Effects of Lilly 110 140, a specific inhibitor of 5-hydroxytryptamine uptake, on food intake and on 5-hydroxytryptophan-induced anorexia: evidence for serotonergic inhibition of feeding. *J Pharm Pharmacol.* 1976;28:318-320.
2. Blundell JE. Is there a role for serotonin in feeding? *Int J Obesity.* 1977;1:15-42.
3. Wurtman JJ, Wurtman RJ. Drugs that enhance central serotonergic transmission diminish selective carbohydrate consumption by rats. *Life Sci.* 1979;24:895-904.
4. Blundell J. Serotonin and appetite. *Neuropharmacology.* 1984;23:1537-1551.
5. Leibowitz S, Shor-Posner G. Brain serotonin and eating behavior. *Appetite.* 1986;7:1-14.
6. Meltzer HY, Aurora RC, Baber R, Tricou BJ. Serotonin uptake in blood platelets of psychiatric patients. *Arch Gen Psychiatry.* 1981;38:1322-1326.
7. DeMeyer MK, Shea PA, Hendrie HC, Yoshimura NN. Plasma tryptophan and five other amino acids in depressed and normal subjects. *Arch Gen Psychiatry.* 1981;38:642-646.
8. Moller SE, Kirk L, Brandrup E, Ortmann J, Elley J. Plasma tryptophan in depression. *Biol Psychiatry.* 1983;10:30-46.
9. Heninger GR, Charney DS, Sternberg DE. Serotonergic function in depression. *Arch Gen Psychiatry.* 1984;41:398-402.
10. Briley M. Imipramine binding: its relationship with serotonin. In: Green AR, ed. *Neuropharmacology of Serotonin.* New York, NY: Oxford University Press Inc; 1985:50-78.
11. Young SN, Smith SE, Pihl R, Ervin FR. Tryptophan depletion causes a rapid lowering of mood in normal males. *Psychopharmacology (Berl).* 1985;87:173-177.
12. Koyama T, Meltzer HY. A biochemical and neuroendocrine study of the serotonergic system in depression. In: Hippius H, Klerman GL, Matussek N, eds. *New Results in Depression Research.* New York, NY: Springer-Verlag NY Inc; 1986:169-188.
13. Cowen PJ, Charig EM. Neuroendocrine responses to intravenous tryptophan in major depression. *Arch Gen Psychiatry.* 1987;44:958-966.
14. Delgado PL, Charney DS, Price LH, Aghajanian GK, Landis H, Heninger GR. Serotonin function and the mechanism of antidepressant action: reversal of antidepressant-induced remission by rapid depletion of plasma tryptophan. *Arch Gen Psychiatry.* 1990;47:411-418.
15. Price LH, Charney DS, Delgado PL, Heninger GR. Serotonin function and depression: neuroendocrine and mood responses to intravenous L-tryptophan in depressed patients and healthy comparison subjects. *Am J Psychiatry.* 1991; 148:1515-1525.

16. Benkelfat C, Ellenbogen MA, Dean P, Palmour RM, Young SN. Mood-lowering effect of tryptophan depletion: enhanced sensitivity in young men at genetic risk for major affective disorders. *Arch Gen Psychiatry.* 1994;51:687-697.
17. Zohar J, Mueller EA, Insel TR, Zohar-Kadouch RC. Serotonergic responsivity in obsessive-compulsive disorder: comparison of patients and healthy controls. *Arch Gen Psychiatry.* 1987;44:946-951.
18. Glennon R. Central serotonin receptors as targets for drug research. *J Med Chem.* 1987;30:1-12.
19. Kahn RS, Wetzler S, van Praag HM, Asnls GM, Strauman T. Behavioral indications for serotonin receptor hypersensitivity in panic disorder. *Psychiatry Res.* 1988;25:101-104.
20. Charney DS, Woods SW, Krystal JH, Nagy LM, Heninger GR. Hypotheses relating serotonergic dysfunction to the etiology and treatment of panic and generalized anxiety disorders. In: Coccaro EF, Murphy DL, eds. *Serotonin in Major Psychiatric Disorders.* Washington, DC: American Psychiatric Press; 1990:71-97.
21. Germine M, Goddard AW, Woods SW, Charney DS, Heninger GR. Anger and anxiety responses to m-chlorophenylpiperazine in generalized anxiety disorder. *Biol Psychiatry.* 1992;32:457-461.
22. Seibyl JP, Krystal JH, Price LH, Woods SW, D'Amico C, Heninger GR, Charney DS. Effects of ritanserin on the behavioral, neuroendocrine, and cardiovascular responses to *meta*-chlorophenylpiperazine in healthy human subjects. *Psychiatry Res.* 1991;38:227-236.
23. Valzelli L. Aggressive behavior induced by isolation. In: Garattini S, Sigg E, eds. *Excerpta Medica.* Belle Meade, NJ: Excerpta Medica-Princeton; 1969:70-76.
24. Asberg M, Traskman L, Thoren P. 5-HIAA in the cerebrospinal fluid: a biochemical suicide predictor? *Arch Gen Psychiatry.* 1976;33:1193-1197.
25. Brown GL, Ballenger JC, Minchiello MD, Goodwin FK. Human aggression and its relationship to cerebrospinal fluid 5-hydroxyindolacetic acid, 3-methoxy-4-hydroxyphenolglycol and homovanillic acid. In: Sandler M, ed. *Psychopharmacology of Aggression.* New York, NY: Raven Press; 1979:131-148.
26. Ballenger JC, Goodwin FK, Major LF, Brown GL. Alcohol and central serotonin metabolism in man. *Arch Gen Psychiatry.* 1979;36:224-227.
27. Kantak K, Hegstrand L, Eichelman B. Facilitation of shock-induced fighting following intraventricular 5,7-dihydroxytryptamine and 6-hydroxy DOPA. *Psychopharmacololgy (Berl).* 1981;74:157-160.
28. Brown GL, Ebert MH, Goyer PF, Jimerson D, Klein WJ, Bunney WE, Goodwin FK. Aggression, suicide and serotonin: relationship to CSF amine metabolites. *Am J Psychiatry.* 1982;139:741-746.
29. Linnoila M, Virkunnen M, Scheinin M, Nuutila A, Rimon R, Goodwin FK. Low cerebrospinal fluid 5-hydroxy-indolacetic acid concentration differentiates impulsive from nonimpulsive violent behavior. *Life Sci.* 1983;33:2609-2614.
30. Molina V, Gobaille S, Mandel P. Effects of serotonin-mimetic drugs on mouse-killing behavior. *Aggressive Behav.* 1986;12:201-211.
31. Soubrie P. Reconciling the role of central serotonin neurons in human and animal behavior. *Behav Brain Sci.* 1986;9:319-364.
32. Virkkunen M, Nuutila A, Goodwin FK, Linnoila M. Cerebrospinal fluid monoamine metabolite levels in male arsonists. *Arch Gen Psychiatry.* 1987;44:241-247.
33. Hollander E, Stein DJ, Decaria CM, Cohen L, Saoud JB, Skodol AE, Kellman D, Rosnick L, Oldham JM. Serotonergic sensitivity in borderline personality disorder: preliminary findings. *Am J Psychiatry.* 1994;151:277-280.
34. Hatsukami D, Eckert E, Mitchell J, Pyle RL. Affective disorders and substance abuse in women with bulimia. *Psychol Med.* 1984;14:701-704.
35. Mitchell J, Hatsukami D, Eckert E, Pyle RL. Characteristics of 275 patients with bulimia. *Am J Psychiatry.* 1985;142:482-485.
36. Laessle R, Wittchen H, Fichter M, Pirke KM. The significance of subgroups of bulimia and anorexia nervosa: lifetime frequency of psychiatric disorders. *Int J Eat Disord.* 1989;8:569-574.
37. Kaye WH, Ebert MH, Gwirtsman HE, Weiss SR. Differences in brain serotonergic metabolism between nonbulimic and bulimic patients with anorexia nervosa. *Am J Psychiatry.* 1984;141:1598-1601.
38. Kaye WH, Ballenger JC, Lydiard RB, Stuart GW, Laraia RN, O'Neil P, Fossey MD, Stevens V, Lesser S, Hsu G. CSF monoamine levels in normal-weight bulimia: evidence for abnormal noradrenergic activity. *Am J Psychiatry.* 1990;147:225-229.
39. Jimerson DC, Lesem MD, Kaye WH, Brewerton TD. Low serotonin and dopamine metabolite concentrations in cerebrospinal fluid from bulimic patients with frequent binge episodes. *Arch Gen Psychiatry.* 1992;49:132-138.
40. Goldbloom DS, Hicks L, Garfinkel PE. Platelet serotonin uptake in bulimia nervosa. *Biol Psychiatry.* 1990;28:644-647.
41. Marazziti D, Macchi E, Rotondo A, Placidi GF, Cassano GB. Involvement of the serotonin system in bulimia. *Life Sci.* 1988;43:2123-2126.
42. Lydiard RB, Brady KT, O'Neil PM, Schleisier-Carter B, Hamilton S, Rogers Q, Ballenger GC. Precursor amino acid concentrations in normal weight bulimics and normal controls. *Prog Neuropsychopharmacol Biol Psychiatry.* 1988;12:893-898.
43. Kayef WH, Gwirtsman HE, Brewerton TD, George DT, Wurtman RJ. Bingeing behavior and plasma amino acids: a possible involvement of brain serotonin in bulimia nervosa. *Psychiatry Res.* 1988;23:31-43.
44. Goldbloom DS, Garfinkel PE, Katz R, Brown G. The hormonal response to intravenous 5-hydroxytryptophan in bulimia nervosa. *Psychosom Med.* 1990; 52:225-226.
45. Jimerson DC, Wolfe BE, Metzger ED, Levine JM. Serotonin function in bulimia nervosa. Presented at the 147th Annual Meeting of the American Psychiatric Association; May 26, 1994; Philadelphia, Pa.
46. Brewerton TD, Mueller E, Lesem MD, Brandt HA, Quearry B, George DT, Murphy DL, Jimerson DC. Neuroendocrine responses to m-chlorophenylpiperazine and L-tryptophan in bulimia. *Arch Gen Psychiatry.* 1992;49:852-861.
47. Kahn RS, Wetzler S. m-Chlorophenylpiperazine as a probe of serotonin function. *Biol Psychiatry.* 1991;30:1139-1166.
48. Kahn RS, Wetzler S, Asnis GM, Kling MA, Suckow RF, van Praag HM. Effects of m-chlorophenylpiperazine in normal subjects: a dose-response study. *Psychopharmacology (Berl).* 1990;100:339-344.
49. Walsh BT, Lo ES, Cooper T, Lindy DC, Roose SP, Gladis M, Glassman AH. Dexamethasone suppression test and plasma dexamethasone levels in bulimia. *Arch Gen Psychiatry.* 1987;44:797-803.
50. Mueller EA, Murphy DL, Sunderland T. Neuroendocrine effects of m-chlorophenylpiperazine, a serotonergic agonist, in humans. *J Clin Endocrinol Metab.* 1985;61:1179-1184.
51. Hamik A, Petrouka SJ. 1-(m-chlorophenylpiperazine) interactions with neurotransmitter receptors in the human brain. *Biol Psychiatry.* 1989;25:569-575.
52. Hoyer D. Functional correlates of serotonin 5-HT-1 recognition sites. *J Recept Signal Transduct Res.* 1988;8:59-81.
53. Mueller EA, Murphy DL, Sunderland T. Further studies of the putative serotonin agonist m-chlorophenylpiperazine: evidence for a serotonin receptor mediated mechanism of action in humans. *Psychopharmacology (Berl).* 1986;89:388-391.
54. Murphy DL, Mueller EA, Hill JL, Tolliver TJ, Jacobsen FM. Comparative anxiogenic, neuroendocrine, and other physiological effects of m-chlorophenylpiperazine given intravenously to healthy volunteers. *Psychopharmacology (Berl).* 1989;98:275-282.
55. Kalus O, Wetzler S, Kahn RS, Asnis GM, van Praag HM. A dose-response study of m-chlorophenylpiperazine in normal subjects. *Psychopharmacology (Berl).* 1992;106:388-390.
56. American Psychiatric Association. *Diagnostic and Statistical Manual of Mental Disorders, Third Edition, Revised.* Washington, DC: American Psychiatric Association; 1987.
57. Spitzer RL, Williams JBW. *Structured Clinical Interview for* DSM-III. New York: New York State Psychiatric Institute, Biometrics Research; 1982.
58. Beck AT, Ward CH, Mendelson M, Mock J, Erbaugh J. An inventory for measuring depression. *Arch Gen Psychiatry.* 1961;4:561-571.
59. Hamilton M. A rating scale for depression. *J Neurol Neurosurg Psychiatry.* 1960;6:278-296.
60. Johnson C. Initial consultation for patients with bulimia and anorexia nervosa. In: Garner DM, Garfinkel PE, eds. *Handbook of Psychotherapy for Anorexia Nervosa and Bulimia.* New York, NY: Guilford Press; 1985:34-49.
61. Charney DS, Goodman WK, Price LH, Woods SW, Rasmussen SA, Heninger GR. Serotonin function in obsessive-compulsive disorder: a comparison of the effects of tryptophan and m-CPP in patients and healthy subjects. *Arch Gen Psychiatry.* 1988;45:177-185.
62. Bagdy G, Calogero AE, Murphy DL, Szemeredi K. Serotonin agonists cause parallel activation of the sympathoadrenomedullary system and the hypothalamo-pituitary-adrenocortical axis in conscious rats. *Endocrinology.* 1989;125:2664-2669.
63. Levy AB, Dixon KN, Malarkey WB. Pituitary response to TRH in bulimia. *Biol Psychiatry.* 1988;23:476-484.
64. Gil-Ad I, Zambotti F, Carruba MO, Vicentini L, Muller EE. Stimulatory role for brain serotonergic system on prolactin secretion in male rat. *Proc Soc Exp Biol Med.* 1976;151:512-518.
65. Advis JP, Simpkins JW, Bennett J, Meites J. Serotonergic control of prolactin release in male rats. *Life Sci.* 1979;24:359-366.
66. Schettini G, Quattrone A, Di Renzo G, Preziosi P. Serotonergic involvement in neuroendocrine function. *Pharmacol Res.* 1980;12:249-254.
67. Willoughby JO, Menadue M, Jervois P. Function of serotonin in physiological secretion of growth hormone and prolactin: action of 5,7-dihydroxytryptamine, fenfluramine and p-chlorophenylalanine. *Brain Res.* 1982;249:291-299.
68. Kaplan AS, Garfinkel PE, Brown GM. The DST and TRH test in bulimia nervosa. *Br J Psychiatry.* 1989;154:86-92.
69. deGroot J, Rodin G, Olmstead M. Alexithymia, depression and treatment outcome in bulimia nervosa. *Comp Psychiatry.* 1995;36:1-9.
70. Goodwin GM, Fairburn CG, Cowen PJ. The effects of dieting and weight loss on neuroendocrine responses to tryptophan, clonidine, and apomorphine in volunteers: important implications for neuroendocrine investigations in depression. *Arch Gen Psychiatry.* 1987;44:952-957.
71. Brewerton TD, Brandt HA, Lesem MD, Murphy DL, Jimerson DC. Serotonin in eating disorders. In: Coccaro EF, Murphy DL, eds. *Serotonin in Major Psychiatric Disorders.* Washington, DC: American Psychiatric Press; 1990:153-184.
72. Azmitia EC, McEwen BE. Adrenal-cortical influence on rat brain tryptophan hydroxylase activity. *Brain Res.* 1974;78:291-302.
73. Rittenhouse PA, Levy AD, Bethea CL, Van de Kar LD. Neurons in the hypothalamic paraventricular nucleus mediate the serotonergic stimulation of prolactin secretion via 5-HT1c/2 receptors. *Endocrinology.* 1993;133:661-667.
74. Leibowitz S, Weiss G, Suh J. Medial hypothalamic nuclei mediate serotonin's inhibitory effect on feeding behavior. *Pharmacol Biochem Behav.* 1990;37:735-742.
75. Kennett GA, Curzon G. Evidence that mCPP may have behavioral effects mediated by central 5-HT1c receptors. *Br J Pharmacol.* 1988;94:137-147.
76. Kennett GA, Curzon G. Potencies of antagonists indicate that 5-HT1c receptors mediate 1-3 (chlorophenyl) piperazine-induced hypophagia. *Br J Pharmacol.* 1991;103:2016-2020.
77. Dourish C, Clark M, Fletcher A, Iversen S. Evidence that blockade of post-synaptic 5-HT-1 receptors elicits feeding in satiated rats. *Psychopharmacology (Berl).* 1989;97:54-58.

ORIGINAL ARTICLE

Decreased Serotonin Function in Bulimia Nervosa

David C. Jimerson, MD; Barbara E. Wolfe, RN, PhD; Eran D. Metzger, MD; Dianne M. Finkelstein, PhD; Thomas B. Cooper, MA; Jeffrey M. Levine, MD

Background: Evidence that serotonin-active antidepressant medications decrease binge eating in patients with bulimia nervosa has fueled interest in the hypothesis that abnormal serotonergic neurotransmitter function contributes to symptoms of the disorder. To evaluate this hypothesis, we employed pharmacological challenge testing to compare serotonin function in patients with bulimia nervosa and healthy controls.

Methods: Neuroendocrine response patterns were compared for 15 nonhospitalized, medication-free, normal-weight women with bulimia nervosa and 14 age-matched healthy female controls. Behavioral assessment included ratings of eating disorder symptoms, depression, and anxiety. Serotonergic response patterns were assessed by measuring the increase in serum prolactin concentration during 5 hours following single-dose, oral administration of 60 mg of d,l-fenfluramine hydrochloride (Pondimin).

Results: For patients with bulimia nervosa, the fenfluramine-stimulated increase in serum prolactin concentration was significantly less than for controls. Within the patient group, the frequency of binge eating episodes during the 4 weeks prior to the study exhibited a significant inverse correlation with serotonin-stimulated prolactin secretion.

Conclusion: Our study provides new evidence that impaired central nervous system serotonergic responsiveness may contribute to the onset or maintenance of abnormal eating patterns in patients with bulimia nervosa.

Arch Gen Psychiatry. 1997;54:529-534

From the Department of Psychiatry, Beth Israel Deaconess Medical Center and Harvard Medical School (Drs Jimerson, Wolfe, Metzger, and Levine), and the Department of Biostatistics, Harvard School of Public Health (Dr Finkelstein), Boston, Mass; and the Nathan Kline Institute for Psychiatric Research, Orangeburg, and the New York State Psychiatric Institute, College of Physicians & Surgeons, Columbia University, New York (Mr Cooper). Dr Levine is now with the Department of Psychiatry, St Mary's Hospital, Waterbury, and Yale University School of Medicine, New Haven, Conn.

INDIRECT EVIDENCE suggests that biological predisposition, acting in concert with recurrent dieting behavior and psychosocial stressors, contributes to the pathophysiology of bulimia nervosa.[1,2] The central nervous system (CNS) neurotransmitter serotonin has attracted particular attention in this regard.[3] Brain hypothalamic serotonin pathways participate in postingestive satiety, and premeal administration of serotonin-agonist drugs decreases food intake.[4-8] In comparison with healthy controls, patients with bulimia nervosa demonstrate diminished postingestive satiety responses.[9,10] The efficacy of serotonin-active antidepressants in patients with bulimia nervosa may be related to serotonergic effects on eating behavior.[11-13]

In a previous challenge study, medication-free, hospitalized patients with severe symptoms of bulimia nervosa demonstrated significantly blunted prolactin responses following the administration of the serotonin receptor agonist *m*-chlorophenylpiperazine.[14] To follow up on this result, we assessed serotonin-stimulated prolactin secretion following the administration of the serotonergic drug fenfluramine hydrochloride in nonhospitalized patients with bulimia nervosa. Because the presence of comorbid depression in some patients with bulimia nervosa may have contributed to previous evidence for altered serotonin function,[15] we excluded subjects with current major depressive disorder. Moreover, although serotonin-stimulated prolactin secretion in women varies with menstrual cycle phase,[16,17] it has been impractical to control for this variable in previous investigations with hospitalized patients. In our study with nonhospitalized patients, challenge procedures were scheduled during the follicular phase of the subjects' menstrual cycles. Baseline blood samples were obtained to assess related hormone, neurotransmitter, and metabolic measurements, including estradiol, progesterone, and tryptophan concentrations. Thyroid

See also pages 507, 509, and 521

This article is also available on our Web site: ama-assn.org/psych.

SUBJECTS AND METHODS

SUBJECT SELECTION

Nonhospitalized women with bulimia nervosa were recruited from university-affiliated eating disorder programs and from the community by media announcements. Patients met *DSM-III-R* criteria for bulimia nervosa,[18] with the additional requirement that the frequency of binge eating and purging (through self-induced vomiting or laxative abuse) had averaged at least 3 times per week for the preceding 6 months. Patients were free of psychotropic medication at least 6 weeks prior to the study. Based on diagnostic assessment by a trained interviewer (B.E.W.) using the Schedule for Affective Disorders and Schizophrenia-Life Version,[19] patients with bulimia nervosa were free of major depression, substance abuse disorder, and other major psychiatric disorders for at least 6 months prior to the study, and they had no history of psychotic disorder. Healthy female volunteers (controls), recruited from the community, were free of current or past major psychiatric disorder. Controls were additionally screened to exclude individuals who reported a history of major psychiatric disorder, including eating disorders and obesity, in first-degree relatives.

Subject enrollment criteria included age between 18 and 45 years; normal body weight (85%-115% age-adjusted, height-adjusted US population average body weight)[20]; stable body weight (±5%) during the month prior to the study; and good medical health, as assessed by findings from medical history, physical examination, electrocardiogram, and routine laboratory studies. Subjects agreed to abstain from alcohol use for the week prior to the study. Pregnancy and toxicology screening tests were obtained prior to the study. Skinfold measurements for calculation of percentage lean body mass were obtained by the research dietitian of the General Clinical Research Center at Beth Israel Deaconess Medical Center, Boston, Mass. Subjects gave written informed consent prior to study participation.

STUDY PROTOCOL

Subjects were admitted to a general clinical research center for an overnight stay prior to pharmacological challenge studies. Studies were conducted using a fixed sequence, placebo-first, single-blind design to avoid possible medication carryover effects.[21] Study days were consecutive for all subjects with the exception of 2 controls who had 2 intervening days between studies. Studies were scheduled during the first 14 days of the subjects' menstrual cycles. One patient had secondary amenorrhea and, because of scheduling conflicts, 2 patients were studied at a later time (day 15 and day 21) in their menstrual cycles.

Subjects remained at bed rest, with brief bathroom privileges, and abstained from food and fluids other than water, from the preceding midnight until completion of procedures at 2 PM. An intravenous catheter was placed in a forearm vein between 7:30 and 8 AM, and baseline blood samples were drawn between 8:40 and 8:55 AM. At 9 AM, the subjects received matching tablets containing placebo or 60 mg of d,l-fenfluramine hydrochloride (Pondimin).

Blood samples for the measurement of prolactin response were obtained at baseline and at 60-minute intervals during the next 5 hours following the administration of the drug or placebo. Plasma concentrations of fenfluramine and its major metabolite, norfenfluramine, were measured at 5 hourly time points following the administration of the active drug. Additional laboratory measurements obtained from baseline blood samples on the morning of the active study day included values for cortisol, estradiol, progesterone, thyroid hormones, β-hydroxybutyrate, tryptophan, large neutral amino acids (valine, methionine, isoleucine, leucine, tyrosine, and phenylalanine), and homovanillic acid.

Patients were interviewed to assess the average frequency of binge eating and self-induced vomiting during the 4 weeks preceding admission to the general clinical research center. Baseline ratings obtained on the morning of the active study day included the Hamilton Depression Scale,[22] the Eating Attitudes Test,[23] and the state anxiety scale of the State-Trait Anxiety Inventory.[24] Using a 5-point Likert scale, subjects rated side-effect symptoms at baseline, 2 hours, and 5 hours following the administration of the drug or placebo. Items on the scale included "tiredness," "nausea," "stomachache," "headache," and "decreased appetite."

hormones and β-hydroxybutyrate were measured in baseline blood samples as indirect indexes of nutritional status.

RESULTS

As summarized in the **Table**, the 15 patients and 14 controls were similar in mean age, body weight, and percentage of lean body mass. The studies of response to active fenfluramine coincided with menstrual cycle day 9.6±4.5 for patients (excluding 1 amenorrheic patient) and 7.6±2.8 for controls. Seasonal distribution of study procedures was not significantly different for patients and controls (χ^2=1.2, *df*=3, *P*>.1). For the 4 weeks prior to the study, patients reported an average of 6.4±2.6 binge eating episodes per week. Fourteen of the 15 patients reported regular use of self-induced vomiting, with an average of 6.8±3.2 episodes per week. Patients had significantly higher ratings than controls on the Eating Attitudes Test (*P*<.001), the Hamilton Depression Scale (*P*<.001), and the state anxiety scale of the State-Trait Anxiety Inventory (*P*<.001) (Table).

Baseline serum prolactin values were significantly lower for patients than for controls (5.5±1.9 vs 8.2±2.2 μg/L, *t*=3.85, *df*=27, *P*<.001). For the patient group, the baseline prolactin level was not significantly correlated with frequency of binge eating; frequency of self-induced vomiting; body mass index (the weight in kilograms divided by the height in meters squared); or scores on the Eating Attitudes Test, Hamilton Depression Scale, or the state anxiety scale of the State-Trait Anxiety Inventory.

The time course of the serum prolactin response to the administration of fenfluramine is shown in **Figure 1**. Prolactin response on the active study day was not significantly correlated with the baseline prolactin concentration for patients (*r*=−0.03, *df*=13, *P*=.91) or for controls (*r*=−0.28, *df*=12, *P*=.33).

LABORATORY METHODS

Serum and plasma samples were stored at −70°C until assayed. Serum prolactin level was measured by dissociation-enhanced fluoroimmunoassay (DELFIA kit, Wallac Inc, Gaithersberg, Md). Plasma fenfluramine and norfenfluramine levels were measured by gas chromatography.[25] Serum estradiol and progesterone levels were measured by radioimmunoassay following extraction and, for estrogen, celite column chromatography (Hazleton Laboratories, Vienna, Va). Serum cortisol, thyrotropin, triiodothyronine, free thyroxine, and reverse triiodothyronine concentrations were measured by radioimmunoassay. Plasma β-hydroxybutyrate concentration was measured by an enzymatic method (Metpath, Teterboro, NJ); plasma tryptophan was measured by a fluorometric method[26]; and plasma large neutral amino acids and plasma homovanillic acid[27] levels were measured by high-pressure liquid chromatography.

STATISTICAL METHODS

Statistical analyses were performed using Statistical Package for Social Sciences software (SPSS for Windows, SPSS, Chicago, Ill).[28] Two-sided significance levels are reported, with statistical significance indicating $P<.05$. Group values for outcome measurements are reported as mean±SD. Variables not normally distributed (as indicated by the Kolmogorov-Smirnov test) were log-transformed and retested for normality prior to analysis by parametric methods. Transformed variables included baseline concentrations of prolactin, estradiol, thyrotropin, reverse triiodothyronine and homovanillic acid, and prolactin response. Review of baseline hormone levels revealed that the original group of 16 patients included 1 patient thought to be studied on menstrual cycle day 9 who had an estradiol level of more than 6 SDs higher than the mean value for other patients. To avoid potential confounding influence of an elevated estradiol level on prolactin response, results for this patient were excluded from data analysis. Demographic data and baseline laboratory measurements for the remaining 15 patients and the 14 controls were compared by Student *t* test or, for baseline behavioral ratings, by Wilcoxon *W* test. Comparability of seasonal distribution of studies for patients and controls was assessed by χ^2 test.

Placebo-controlled prolactin response to fenfluramine for patients and controls was compared by analysis of variance. The placebo-adjusted value for serum prolactin concentration at each postdrug time point on the active medication day was calculated by subtracting the change from baseline at the corresponding time point on the placebo day. Prolactin response was evaluated based on area-under-the-curve (AUC) increase over baseline in placebo-adjusted serum prolactin concentration during the 5 hours following the administration of fenfluramine, calculated using the trapezoidal rule. A secondary outcome measure was the maximal prolactin increase over baseline value based on individual placebo-adjusted postdrug time points. The primary and secondary indexes of placebo-adjusted prolactin response were computed using nontransformed measurements of serum prolactin concentration. Because prolactin response data were not normally distributed for the controls, values for AUC response and maximal prolactin response for both subject groups were log-transformed prior to comparison by analysis of variance.

To control for possible influence of intersubject variations in plasma fenfluramine concentration, prolactin response for patients and controls was compared by analysis of covariance, using fenfluramine concentration as a continuous covariate. Fenfluramine concentration for each subject was evaluated using AUC for concentration over time, using the sum of plasma fenfluramine plus norfenfluramine concentrations at the 5 hourly postdrug time points. For the patient group, Pearson product moment correlation coefficients were calculated between prolactin response, covarying for plasma fenfluramine concentration and frequency of binge eating, frequency of self-induced vomiting, and scores on the symptom rating scales.

Side-effect ratings, measured as the difference from baseline to the 2-hour and 5-hour time points, were compared for active and placebo days by Wilcoxon matched-pairs signed-rank test.

Placebo-controlled prolactin response to fenfluramine, based on AUC increase over baseline concentration, was significantly smaller for patients (1545±767 μg/L·minute) than for controls (2879±2246 μg/L·minute) (t=2.43, df=27, P=.02). Expressed as the mean increase over baseline (averaged across the 180-, 240-, and 300-minute time points), the prolactin response was 8.6±4.2 μg/L for patients and 15.5±9.2 μg/L for controls. A secondary analysis based on peak prolactin level increase over baseline demonstrated a similar significant difference between patients (11.2±4.8 μg/L) and controls (20.2±12.3 μg/L) (t=2.79, df=27, $P<.001$).

Plasma fenfluramine concentration was not significantly different for patients (80.3±32.6 μmol/L·minute) and controls (87.9±21.4 μmol/L·minute) (t=.73, df=27, P=.47). Placebo-controlled prolactin AUC response was significantly correlated with fenfluramine concentration for the patient group (r=0.57, df=13, P=.03) and for the combined subject group (r=0.41, df=27, P=.03), although not for controls taken separately (r=0.19, df=12, P=.51). Comparison of serum prolactin AUC response for patient and control groups by analysis of covariance revealed a significant effect for diagnostic group ($F_{1,26}$=5.13, P=.03) after adjusting for plasma fenfluramine concentration ($F_{1,26}$=4.70, P=.04). A similar result was obtained for the secondary outcome measure prolactin peak response. When these analyses were repeated excluding the 2 patients studied on menstrual cycle days 15 and 21, significant differences between patients and controls continued to be present for prolactin AUC response (P=.04) and prolactin peak response (P=.03).

For the patient group, frequency of binge eating during the 4 weeks prior to the study was inversely correlated with prolactin response after adjusting for fenfluramine concentration (r=−0.59, df=12, P=.03) (**Figure 2**). There was a similar trend toward an in-

Descriptive Characteristics of Study Sample*

Characteristics	Patients With Bulimia Nervosa (n=15)	Healthy Controls (n=14)	Significance†
Age, y	22.5±2.0	22.5±3.2	t=.06, P>.1
Weight, kg	60.0±7.5	58.0±6.8	t=.72, P>.1
Weight (% adjusted US average)	98.7±10.0	99.8±9.7	t=.32, P>.1
Lean body mass, %	74.5±5.6	71.7±5.4	t=1.36, P>.1
Eating Attitudes Test score	34.4±7.2 (35)	2.2±2.6 (2)	w=105.0, P<.001
Hamilton Depression Scale score	5.3±5.1 (4)	0.4±0.5 (0)	w=136.0, P<.001
State anxiety scale score	39.5±11.0 (39)	25.9±4.9 (26)	w=127.5, P<.001

*Values expressed as mean±SD. Median values for rating scale scores are in parentheses.

†W indicates Wilcoxon W statistic.

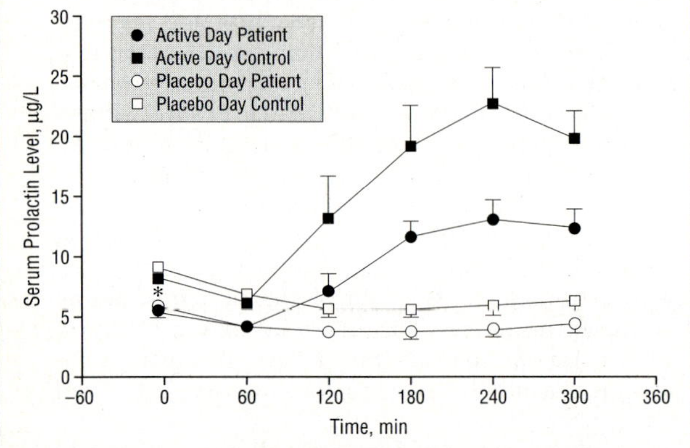

Figure 1. *Time course of serum prolactin response (mean±SEM) following administration of 60 mg of d,l-fenfluramine hydrochloride or placebo.*

verse relationship between frequency of vomiting behavior and prolactin response (r=−0.47, df=12, P=.09). Scores on the Eating Attitudes Test, the Hamilton Depression Scale, and the state anxiety scale of the State-Trait Anxiety Inventory were not significantly correlated with prolactin response (P>.1). Prolactin response did not differ significantly between the 4 patients who met criteria for a past episode of major depression and the other 11 patients.

In comparison with controls, patients had lower baseline concentrations of serum triiodothyronine (t=2.01, df=27, P=.06), free thyroxine (t=4.03, df=27, P<.001), thyrotropin (t=2.49, df=27, P<.02), and reverse triiodothyronine (t=3.35, df=27, P<.001) (all thyrotropin values were within the normal reference range for the assay). Patients and controls did not differ significantly on baseline concentrations of serum estradiol (146±130 vs 157±76 pmol/L), progesterone (1.49±0.89 vs 1.34±0.64 nmol/L), β-hydroxybutyrate (0.38±0.16 vs 0.29±0.12 mmol/L), or other baseline laboratory test results (including cortisol, homovanillic acid, plasma total tryptophan, or ratio of tryptophan to sum of large neutral amino acids).

Correlational analysis for the patient group revealed no significant relationships between baseline pro-

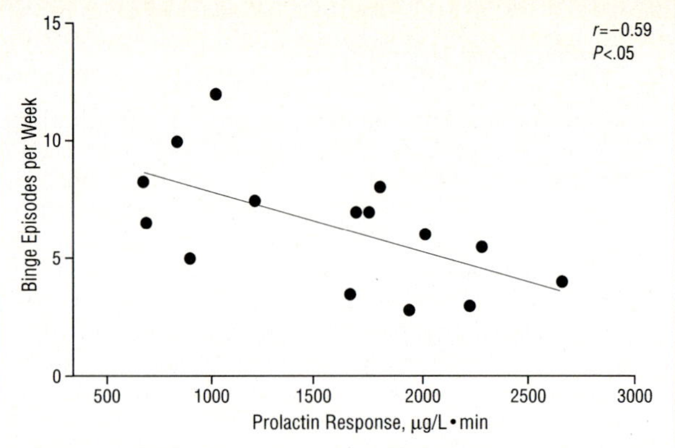

Figure 2. *Relationship between placebo-controlled prolactin response (adjusted for plasma fenfluramine level) and average frequency of binge eating episodes in patients with bulimia nervosa.*

lactin concentration or prolactin response to fenfluramine and other baseline laboratory measurements. Prolactin response was not significantly correlated with baseline concentration of plasma tryptophan or the ratio of tryptophan to the sum of large neutral amino acids for either patient or control groups. For the controls, there was a positive correlation between prolactin response to fenfluramine and baseline concentrations of plasma β-hydroxybutyrate (r=0.70, df=13, P<.001). Analysis of covariance comparing prolactin response for patients and controls revealed a significant effect for diagnostic group ($F_{1,25}$=8.65, P<.001) after adjusting for plasma levels of fenfluramine and β-hydroxybutyrate.

Changes in side-effect ratings from baseline to values at 2 hours and 5 hours following the administration of medication were not significantly different on active study and placebo days for patients or for controls.

COMMENT

In our study, bulimia nervosa was associated with decreased responsiveness in CNS serotonergic pathways, consistent with a model implicating impaired postingestive serotonergic satiety signals in this disorder. Based on our results, it seems that outpatients with moderate levels of symptom severity have serotonergic abnormalities similar to those previously found in highly symptomatic hospitalized patients.[14,29] Diminished serotonergic prolactin response in patients with bulimia nervosa has been observed in several additional preliminary reports.[30-32]

The observation that serotonergic responses were inversely correlated with the frequency of binge eating episodes points toward specificity of an association between serotonergic alterations and symptoms of bulimia nervosa. It is possible that patients with the highest frequency of binge eating may also have had the shortest interval between preadmission binge episodes and pharmacological challenge testing. The finding of diminished neuroendocrine response to fenfluramine and other serotonin-agonist drugs is not unique to bulimia nervosa.[33-36] Thus, altered central serotonin function may reflect a shared neurobiological diathesis across several psychiatric disorders. Given that controlled trials in patients with bulimia nervosa have demonstrated therapeutic responses to antidepressant medications thought to preferentially affect serotonergic function (eg, fluoxetine) or noradrenergic function (eg, desipramine), it is possible that altered regulation in several neurotransmitter systems may contribute to the disorder.[37]

Based on the current cross-sectional investigation, it is uncertain whether apparent abnormalities in CNS serotonergic function predate the appearance of eating disorder symptoms. Preliminary data from a companion investigation suggest that fenfluramine-stimulated prolactin secretion in individuals who have maintained long-term recovery from bulimia nervosa does not differ significantly from control values.[38]

In healthy female volunteers, dieting can result in increased neuroendocrine responses to serotonergic pharmacological challenge testing. This increased responsiveness is thought to reflect a counterregulatory response to diet-induced decreases in CNS serotonin synthesis.[39-41] The significant positive correlation between plasma β-hydroxybutyrate concentration, an indirect index of metabolic state, and prolactin response to fenfluramine in the control group may reflect an influence of restrained eating in some of the volunteers. Although the sample size in this study is limited, a significant relationship between β-hydroxybutyrate concentration and prolactin response was not observed in the patient group.

Reduced levels of serum thyroid hormones in patients with bulimia nervosa have been noted previously and are likely to be reflective of impaired nutritional status.[42-44] The finding that baseline serum prolactin concentrations were significantly lower in patients with bulimia nervosa than in healthy controls is also consistent with other investigations.[14,45,46] This finding may reflect nutritional factors, although experimental dieting in healthy volunteers seems to have little effect on the baseline concentration of serum prolactin.[40] Prolactin secretion following neuroendocrine challenge testing with the nonserotonergic secretogogue protirelin has previously been found to be normal or increased in patients with bulimia nervosa,[45,47] indicating that response at the level of the pituitary lactotroph is not diminished. Low baseline concentration of serum prolactin could reflect an increase in the tonic inhibitory influence of CNS dopamine.[48] Plasma levels of the dopamine metabolite homovanillic acid were not, however, significantly different for patients and controls.

The increase in the serum prolactin concentrations following the administration of fenfluramine is thought to provide a relatively specific probe of CNS serotonergic responsiveness.[33,49-53] Neuroendocrine responses to racemic d,l-fenfluramine could be influenced by interactions of the l-fenfluramine isomer with CNS dopamine pathways.[54] In healthy volunteers, however, prolactin responses to d,l-fenfluramine were highly correlated with prolactin responses to d-fenfluramine.[55] Moreover, although prolactin responses to d,l-fenfluramine are most likely to reflect serotonergic regulation in hypothalamic pathways modulating pituitary hormone secretion, prolactin responses are significantly correlated with cerebrospinal fluid concentrations of 5-hydroxyindoleacetic acid in clinical studies.[52]

Severe weight loss and associated changes in the hypothalamic-pituitary-gonadal axis are thought to contribute to diminished prolactin responses in serotonergic challenge testing in patients with anorexia nervosa.[48,56,57] Abnormalities in menstrual cycle hormone patterns have also been noted in patients with bulimia nervosa.[58] In our study, patients and controls were matched for body weight, and baseline estradiol and progesterone levels were not significantly different for the 2 subject groups.

CONCLUSION

Results of our study, in concert with previous investigations, indicate an association between decreased CNS serotonergic responsiveness and abnormal eating patterns in patients with bulimia nervosa. Additional investigations are needed to clarify the extent to which the apparent serotonergic alterations may contribute to the onset, persistence, or recurrence of symptoms in bulimia nervosa. In conjunction with controlled trials of psychotherapeutic interventions, research on serotonin-active antidepressant medications and related serotonergic drugs may contribute to the development of new treatment approaches for bulimia nervosa.

Accepted for publication October 8, 1996.

Supported by grants R01 MH45466 (Dr Jimerson) and K07 MH00965 (Dr Wolfe) from the National Institute of Mental Health, Rockville, Md, and grant RR01032 (the General Clinical Research Center at Beth Israel Deaconess Medical Center) from the National Center for Research Resources, National Institutes of Health, Bethesda, Md.

We thank Debra Franko, PhD, Beth Israel Hospital, and David Herzog, MD, Massachusetts General Hospital, for their assistance in patient recruitment, and Joseph Mortola, MD, for his assistance in the evaluation of menstrual cycle–related hormone data. We also gratefully acknowledge the technical assistance of Karin Nauth and Lisa Beyer; and the nursing, nutritionist, and laboratory staff of the general clinical research center at Beth Israel Deaconess Medical Center.

Matching d,l-fenfluramine hydrochloride (Pondimin) and placebo tablets were provided by A. H. Robbins Co Inc, Richmond, Va, and Wyeth-Ayerst Laboratories, Philadelphia, Pa.

Corresponding author: David C. Jimerson, MD, Department of Psychiatry, Beth Israel Deaconess Medical Center, 330 Brookline Ave, Boston, MA 02215.

REFERENCES

1. Kassett JA, Gershon ES, Maxwell ME, Guroff JJ, Kazuba DM, Smith AL, Brandt HA, Jimerson DC. Psychiatric disorders in the first-degree relatives of probands with bulimia nervosa. *Am J Psychiatry.* 1989;146:1468-1471.
2. Kendler KS, MacLean C, Neale M, Kessler R, Heath A, Eaves L. The genetic epidemiology of bulimia nervosa. *Am J Psychiatry.* 1991;148:1627-1637.
3. Jimerson DC, Lesem MD, Hegg AP, Brewerton TD. Serotonin in human eating disorders. *Ann N Y Acad Sci.* 1990;600:532-544.
4. Leibowitz SF, Weiss GF, Suh JS. Medial hypothalamic nuclei mediate serotonin's inhibitory effect on feeding behavior. *Pharmacol Biochem Behav.* 1990; 37:735-742.
5. Blundell JE. Serotonin and appetite. *Neuropharmacology.* 1984;23:1537-1551.

6. Kitchener SJ, Dourish CT. An examination of the behavioural specificity of hypophagia induced by $5\text{-}HT_{1b}$, $5\text{-}HT_{1c}$ and $5\text{-}HT_2$ receptor agonists using the postprandial satiety sequence in rats. *Psychopharmacology.* 1994;113:369-377.
7. Aulakh CS, Mazzola-Pomietto P, Wozniak KM, Hill JL, Murphy DL. Evidence that 1-(2,5-dimethoxy-4-methylphenyl)-2-aminopropane-induced hypophagia and hyperthermia in rats is mediated by serotonin-2A receptors. *J Pharmacol Exp Ther.* 1994;270:127-132.
8. Brewerton TD, Murphy DL, Jimerson DC. Testmeal responses following *m*-chlorophenylpiperazine and L-tryptophan in bulimics and controls. *Neuropsychopharmacology.* 1994;11:63-74.
9. Chiodo J, Latimer PR. Hunger perceptions and satiety responses among normal-weight bulimics and normals to a high-calorie, carbohydrate-rich food. *Psychol Med.* 1986;16:343-349.
10. LaChaussee JL, Kissileff HR, Walsh BT, Hadigan CM. The single-item meal as a measure of binge-eating behavior in patients with bulimia nervosa. *Physiol Behav.* 1992;51:593-600.
11. Chaput Y, Demontigny C, Blier P. Presynaptic and postsynaptic modifications of the serotonin system by long-term administration of antidepressant treatments: an in vivo electrophysiologic study in the rat. *Neuropsychopharmacology.* 1991;5:219-229.
12. Fluoxetine Bulimia Nervosa Collaborative Study Group. Fluoxetine in the treatment of bulimia nervosa: a multicenter, placebo-controlled, double-blind trial. *Arch Gen Psychiatry.* 1992;49:139-147.
13. Jimerson DC, Herzog DB, Brotman AW. Pharmacological approaches in the treatment of eating disorders. *Harvard Rev Psychiatry.* 1993;1:82-93.
14. Brewerton TD, Mueller EA, Lesem MD, Brandt HA, Quearry B, George DT, Murphy DL, Jimerson DC. Neuroendocrine responses to *m*-chlorophenylpiperazine and L-tryptophan in bulimia. *Arch Gen Psychiatry.* 1992;49:852-861.
15. Price LH, Charney DS, Delgado PL, Heninger GR. Serotonin function and depression: neuroendocrine and mood responses to intravenous L-tryptophan in depressed patients and healthy comparison subjects. *Am J Psychiatry.* 1991;148:1518-1525.
16. O'Keane V, O'Hanlon M, Webb M, Dinan T. d-fenfluramine prolactin response throughout the menstrual cycle: evidence for an oestrogen-induced alteration. *Clin Endocrinol (Oxf).* 1991;34:289-292.
17. Dannies PS. Control of prolactin production by estrogen. In: Litwack G, ed. *Biochemical Actions of Hormones.* Orlando, Fla: Academic Press Inc; 1985:289-307.
18. American Psychiatric Association. *Diagnostic and Statistical Manual of Mental Disorders, Third Edition, Revised.* Washington DC: American Psychiatric Press; 1987.
19. Endicott J, Spitzer RL. A diagnostic interview: the Schedule for Affective Disorders and Schizophrenia. *Arch Gen Psychiatry.* 1978;35:837-844.
20. Society of Actuaries, Association of Life Insurance Medical Directors of America. *Build Study, 1979.* Chicago, Ill: Society of Actuaries; 1980.
21. Gilmore JH, Ruegg RG, Ekstrom RD, Knight B, Carson SW, Mason GA, Golden RN. Altered prolactin response to clomipramine rechallenge in healthy subjects. *Biol Psychiatry.* 1993;34:885-888.
22. Hamilton M. A rating scale for depression. *J Neurol Neurosurg Psychiatry.* 1960;23:56-62.
23. Garner DM, Olmsted MP, Bohr Y, Garfinkel PE. The Eating Attitudes Test: psychometric features and clinical correlates. *Psychol Med.* 1982;12:871-878.
24. Spielberger CD. *Manual for the State-Trait Anxiety Inventory (STAI-Form-Y).* Palo Alto, Calif: Consulting Psychologist Press; 1983.
25. Krebs HA, Cheng LK, Wright GJ. Determination of fenfluramine and norfenfluramine in plasma using a nitrogen-sensitive detector. *J Chromatogr.* 1984;310:412-417.
26. Denckla WD, Dewey HK. The determination of tryptophan in plasma, liver, and urine. *J Lab Clin Med.* 1967;69:160-169.
27. Salzman C, Jimerson D, Vasile R, Watsky E, Gerber J. Response to SSRI antidepressants correlates with reduction in plasma HVA: pilot study. *Biol Psychiatry.* 1993;34:569-571.
28. Norusis MJ. *SPSS for Windows: Base System User's Guide, Release 6.0.* Chicago, Ill: SPSS Inc; 1993.
29. Jimerson DC, Lesem MD, Kaye WH, Brewerton TD. Low serotonin and dopamine metabolite concentrations in cerebrospinal fluid from bulimic patients with frequent binge episodes. *Arch Gen Psychiatry.* 1992;49:132-138.
30. Goldbloom D, Garfinkel P, Katz R, Brown G. The hormonal response to intravenous 5-hydroxytryptophan in bulimia nervosa. *Psychosom Med.* 1990;52:225-226. Abstract.
31. McBride PA, Anderson GM, Khait VD, Sunday SR, Halmi KA. Serotonergic responsivity in eating disorders. *Psychopharmacol Bull.* 1991;27:365-372.
32. Levitan RD, Kaplan AS, Levitt AJ, Joffe RT. Hormonal and subjective responses to intravenous *m*-chlorophenylpiperazine (*m*-CPP) in bulimia nervosa and normal controls. *Proc Int Conference Eating Disord.* 1994;6:104. Abstract.
33. Siever LJ, Murphy DL, Slater S, de la Vega E, Lipper S. Plasma prolactin changes following fenfluramine in depressed patients compared to controls: an evaluation of central serotonergic responsivity in depression. *Life Sci.* 1984;34:1029-1039.
34. O'Keane V, Dinan TG. Prolactin and cortisol responses to d-fenfluramine in major depression: evidence for diminished responsivity of central serotonergic function. *Am J Psychiatry.* 1991;148:1009-1015.
35. Coccaro EF, Siever LJ, Owen K, Davis KL. Serotonin in mood and personality disorders. In: Coccaro EF, Murphy DL, eds. *Serotonin In Major Psychiatric Disorders.* Washington DC: American Psychiatric Press; 1990:69-97.
36. McBride PA, Anderson GM, Hertzig ME, Sweeney JA, Kream J, Cohen DJ, Mann JJ. Serotonergic responsivity in male young adults with autistic disorder: results of a pilot study. *Arch Gen Psychiatry.* 1989;46:213-221.
37. Miller HL, Delgado PL, Salomon RM, Berman R, Krystal JH, Heninger GR, Charney DS. Clinical and biochemical effects of catecholamine depletion on antidepressant-induced remission of depression. *Arch Gen Psychiatry.* 1996;53:117-128.
38. Wolfe BE, Jimerson DC, Metzger ED, Levine JM. Serotonergic challenge responses in women with a history of bulimia nervosa. *Biol Psychiatry.* 1994;35:736-737. Abstract.
39. Delgado PL, Charney DS, Price LH, Landis H, Heninger GR. Neuroendocrine and behavioral effects of dietary tryptophan restriction in healthy subjects. *Life Sci.* 1989;45:2323-2332.
40. Anderson IM, Parry-Billings M, Newsholme EA, Fairburn CG, Cowen PJ. Dieting reduces plasma tryptophan and alters brain 5-HT function in women. *Psychol Med.* 1990;20:785-791.
41. Walsh AES, Oldman AD, Franklin M, Fairburn CG, Cowen PJ. Dieting decreases plasma tryptophan and increases the prolactin response to d-fenfluramine in women but not men. *J Affect Disord.* 1995;33:89-97.
42. Serog P, Apfelbaum M, Autissier N, Baights F, Brigant L, Ktorza A. Effects of slimming and composition of diets on $\dot{V}O_2$ and thyroid hormones in healthy subjects. *Am J Clin Nutr.* 1982;35:24-35.
43. Pirke KM, Pahl J, Schweiger U, Warnhoff M. Metabolic and endocrine indices of starvation in bulimia: a comparison with anorexia nervosa. *Psychiatry Res.* 1985;15:33-39.
44. Obarzanek E, Lesem MD, Goldstein DS, Jimerson DC. Reduced resting metabolic rate in patients with bulimia nervosa. *Arch Gen Psychiatry.* 1991;48:456-462.
45. Levy AB, Dixon KN, Malarkey WB. Pituitary response to TRH in bulimia. *Biol Psychiatry.* 1988;23:476-484.
46. Weltzin TE, McConaha C, McKee M, Hsu LKG, Perel J, Kaye WH. Circadian patterns of cortisol, prolactin, and growth hormone secretion during binging and vomiting in normal weight bulimic patients. *Biol Psychiatry.* 1991;30:37-48.
47. Kaplan AS, Garfinkel PE, Brown GM. The DST and TRH test in bulimia nervosa. *Br J Psychiatry.* 1989;154:86-92.
48. Ben-Jonathan N. Regulation of prolactin secretion. In: Imura H, ed. *The Pituitary Gland.* 2nd ed. New York, NY: Raven Press; 1994:261-283.
49. Garattini S, Mennini T, Bendotti C, Invernizzi R, Samanin R. Neurochemical mechanism of action of drugs which modify feeding via the serotoninergic system. *Appetite.* 1986;7(suppl):15-38.
50. Murphy DL. Peripheral indices of central serotonin function in humans. *Ann N Y Acad Sci.* 1990;600:282-295.
51. Van de Kar LD. Neuroendocrine pharmacology of serotonergic (5-HT) neurons. *Annu Rev Pharmacol Toxicol.* 1991;31:289-320.
52. Mann JJ, McBride PA, Brown RP, Linnoila M, Leon AC, DeMeo M, Mieczkowski T, Myers JE, Stanley M. Relationship between central and peripheral serotonin indexes in depressed and suicidal psychiatric inpatients. *Arch Gen Psychiatry.* 1992;49:442-446.
53. Cowen PJ. Serotonin receptor subtypes in depression: evidence from studies in neuroendocrine regulation. *Clin Neuropharmacol.* 1993;16(suppl 3):S6-S18.
54. Invernizzi R, Bertorelli R, Consolo S, Garattini S, Samanin R. Effects of the l-isomer of fenfluramine on dopamine mechanisms in the rat brain: further studies. *Eur J Pharmacol.* 1989;164:241-248.
55. Coccaro EF, Kavoussi RJ, Hauger R. PRL and HVA responses to d- and d,l-fenfluramine in humans. *Biol Psychiatry.* 1994;35:644. Abstract.
56. Brewerton TD, Brandt HA, Lesem MD, Murphy DL, Jimerson DC. Serotonin in eating disorders. In: Coccaro EF, Murphy DL, eds. *Serotonin in Major Psychiatric Disorders.* Washington DC: American Psychiatric Press; 1990:153-184.
57. Hadigan CM, Walsh BT, Buttinger C, Hollander E. Behavioral and neuroendocrine responses to *meta*CPP in anorexia nervosa. *Biol Psychiatry.* 1995;37:504-511.
58. Schweiger U, Pirke KM, Laessle RG, Fichter MM. Gonadotropin secretion in bulimia nervosa. *J Clin Endocrinol Metab.* 1992;74:1122-1127.

Cerebral Gray Matter Volume Deficits After Weight Recovery From Anorexia Nervosa

Evelyn K. Lambe, MSc; Debra K. Katzman, MD; David J. Mikulis, MD; Sidney H. Kennedy, MD; Robert B. Zipursky, MD

Background: Structural changes have been observed in the brains of low-weight patients with anorexia nervosa (AN), including increased cerebrospinal fluid (CSF) volumes and decreased gray matter and white matter volumes. We hypothesized that subjects who are weight-recovered from AN would show elevated CSF volumes and reduced gray matter volumes compared with controls.

Methods: We used magnetic resonance imaging to compare the brains of 12 subjects who are weight-recovered from AN (time since weight recovery, 1-23 years) with those of 18 healthy control subjects and 13 low-weight patients with AN. Axial, dual-echo scans of the whole brain were segmented into gray matter, white matter, and CSF compartments by means of a computerized volumetric approach. Brain measures were corrected for the significant effects of intracranial volume and age, based on regression analysis of a larger group of 30 healthy female controls.

Results: *t* Tests showed that the weight-recovered group had significantly greater CSF volumes and smaller gray matter volumes than the control group. By comparison with low-weight patients, the weight-recovered subjects had significantly smaller CSF volumes and significantly larger gray matter and white matter volumes. In the weight-recovered group, neither the CSF elevations nor gray matter deficits were correlated with the length of time since weight recovery.

Conclusions: The persistent gray matter volume deficits in subjects who are weight-recovered from AN suggest that there may be an irreversible component to the brain changes associated with the illness. The neuropathological features of this irreversible component have yet to be characterized.

Arch Gen Psychiatry. 1997;54:537-542

Computed tomography and magnetic resonance imaging (MRI) studies[1-3] have consistently shown that young women with anorexia nervosa (AN) have structural brain abnormalities. During the past 2 decades, many studies of AN[2-10] have found that the brains of low-weight patients have significantly enlarged cerebrospinal fluid (CSF) spaces. Furthermore, when compared with healthy controls,[1] these patients have significant reductions in both gray matter and white matter volumes.

In our previous MRI study[1] of adolescents with AN, gray matter volumes in the patient group were positively correlated with lowest body mass index (BMI) (expressed as the weight, in kilograms, divided by the height, in meters, squared) and negatively correlated with 24-hour urinary free cortisol levels. These findings are consistent with previously reported associations between brain abnormalities and degree of starvation.[3,6] The high cortisol levels seen in patients with AN[11] may have lasting effects on the brain. In animals, high physiological levels of cortisol have been shown to make neurons more vulnerable to stressors such as hypoglycemia or dehydration.[12]

Structural brain abnormalities have been well documented in AN and may result in cognitive impairment during and after the illness. A comprehensive study by Kingston et al[13] reported cognitive deficits in a large group of patients with AN both before and after treatment. Deficits on memory tasks and on flexibility and inhibition tasks persisted despite substantial weight recovery. Performance on these tasks was correlated with BMI on admission to the hospital and ventricular size on MRI at admission.[13] It is also conceivable that alterations in brain structure caused by starvation may play a role in perpetuating the illness or in determining a person's vulnerability to relapse.

To quantify the long-term consequences of AN on total CSF, gray matter, and white matter volumes, we studied former patients with AN who had been weight-recovered for at least 1 year.[14] Although several longitudinal studies[2,3,6] have reported partial or full normalization of ventricular CSF volumes within months after recovery, these studies did not quantify total CSF or total gray and white matter volumes. Furthermore, previous studies[2,3,6] focused on patients with AN who had been weight-recovered for a relatively brief time.

From the Institute of Medical Science (Ms Lambe) and the Departments of Pediatrics (Dr Katzman), Medical Imaging (Dr Mikulis), and Psychiatry (Drs Kennedy and Zipursky), University of Toronto School of Medicine, Toronto, Ontario. Ms Lambe is now with the Interdepartmental Neuroscience Program, Yale University, New Haven, Conn.

SUBJECTS AND METHODS

SUBJECTS

This study involved 4 subject groups: (1) a group of healthy subjects who are weight-recovered from AN, (2) a large control group used to calculate the correction factors for the significant effects of intracranial volume (ICV) and age, (3) a subset of this large control group selected as an age-matched comparison group for the weight-recovered subjects, and (4) a group of low-weight patients with AN included as a second comparison group for the healthy weight-recovered subjects.

The weight-recovered subjects were recruited through 2 university research and teaching hospitals in Toronto, Ontario—The Hospital for Sick Children and the Clarke Institute of Psychiatry. Staff physicians at both institutions were asked to suggest former patients known to have successfully recovered from AN and to have agreed to participate in research. These former patients were contacted by telephone to describe the study and to screen interested subjects using the exclusion criteria described below. Twelve healthy female subjects were included in the study: 11 were former patients of the Eating Disorder Program at The Hospital for Sick Children and 1 was a former patient of the Clarke Institute of Psychiatry. All subjects had *DSM-III-R*–verified[15] past diagnoses of AN, restricting type; all were free of current *DSM-III-R* eating disorders. The mean±SD age of the subjects who were weight-recovered from AN was 18.9±6.9 years (range, 11.7-37.6 years). The minimum BMI for inclusion as a weight-recovered subject was 18 kg/m^2.[16,17] All of the subjects were right-handed and all were white. Physical and clinical characteristics of the weight-recovered subjects are further described in **Table 1**. Six had been hospitalized more than once for the treatment of AN, 3 had been hospitalized once, and 3 had received outpatient treatment only. Exclusion criteria included past or current chronic medical illness, substance abuse, psychotic illness, major depressive episode(s) not concurrent with AN, corticosteroid treatment, intellectual impairment, seizures or head injuries, as well as current claustrophobia, metallic implants, or pregnancy.

Although 13 weight-recovered subjects were originally recruited and underwent MRI, 1 weight-recovered subject was omitted from the analysis after her scan was read by a radiologist (D.J.M.) as abnormal because of possible communicating hydrocephalus. Including this subject in the analysis would have unduly biased the study toward finding a significant effect.

Because of the large age range of the weight-recovered subjects, it seemed most conservative to correct all brain measures for age by regression analysis using a large, evenly age-distributed control group before comparing the weight-recovered subjects with the smaller, age-matched group of controls.

Data from a group of 30 healthy female subjects were used to calculate the correction factors for the effects of ICV and age on the brain measures. These adults and adolescents had been recruited from the community as healthy control subjects for concurrent studies that involved an MRI scan. In addition, 1 control subject was recruited specifically as a match for the youngest weight-recovered subject. The mean±SD age of this large control group was 24.6±8.7 years (range, 12.0-41.3 years). Although the large control group was older on average than the group of AN subjects, previous work has demonstrated that the relationship between age and the brain measures is approximately linear over the age range used in this study.[18] All of the controls were white; 29 were right-handed and 1 was left-handed. A history of a *DSM-III-R* eating disorder (assessed by the Structured Clinical Interview for *DSM-III-R*—Nonpatient Version [SCID-NP]) was added to the exclusion criteria described above.

From this larger control group, 18 healthy females were selected to form a comparison group, similar in mean age and age range, to the weight-recovered subjects. This matching was accomplished by omitting the 10 controls between the ages of 26 and 35 years and the 2 controls older than 37 years. The mean±SD age of the comparison group was 19.9±7.1 years (range, 12.0-37.1 years). All of the controls in this age-matched comparison group were right-handed. The age-matched control group is further described in Table 1.

A previously published data set[1] of 13 low-weight patients with AN was also used as a comparison group. At the time of MRI scan, these adolescents were receiving inpatient treatment for AN, restricting type, at The Hospital for Sick Children. Physical and clinical characteristics of these subjects are further described in Table 1 as well as in the article by Katzman et al.[1]

All subjects and controls were given extensive structured interviews about their past and current medical and psychological health. This interview included the SCID-Patient or SCID-Nonpatient versions.[15] The interview also assessed the frequency of specific disturbed behaviors such as self-induced vomiting, laxative abuse, diuretic abuse, and binge eating. The Beck Depression Inventory (BDI)[19] and the Eating Attitudes Test (EAT-26)[20] were used to measure depression and abnormal eating attitudes in the weight-recovered subjects. The weight-recovered subjects had blood samples taken the week of the MRI scan to measure electrolyte, serum urea nitrogen, total protein, and serum cortisol levels.

The study protocols were approved by the Research Ethics Committees at The Hospital for Sick Children and the Department of Psychiatry at the University of Toronto. Before participation in the study, informed written consent was provided by subjects 16 years and older. For subjects younger than 16 years, informed written consent was provided by a parent, and verbal assent was given by the subject.

The subjects in the weight-recovered group had been within a normal weight range for 1 year or more as assessed by self-report. This group had a mean±SD BMI of 20.5±2.3 (range, 18.1-25.6). Menstruation had started or returned in 10 of the 12 subjects: 7 had regular menses, 3 had irregular menses, a 22-year-old had primary amenorrhea, and a 12-year-old subject had not yet reached menarche. Two subjects were taking the oral contraceptive pill; however, both were above the BMI at which they previously had regular menses. At the time of the MRI scan, all subjects had normal electrolyte, serum urea nitrogen, and total protein measures. Three of the young women had above-average serum cortisol levels for the time of day that they were tested.[21] The weight-recovered group obtained significantly lower scores on the BDI than the low-weight comparison group (7±6 vs 21±9; $t[22]=-4.6$, $P<.001$) and on the EAT-26 (15±12 vs 35±11; $t[22]=-4.1$, $P<.001$). The weight-recovered group had BDI and EAT-26 mean scores that were comparable to those obtained in previous studies of the general population (BDI, adolescents: 8.47±8.03[22]; BDI, adults: 6.18±6.82[23]; EAT-26, female college students: 15.6±9.3[20]). Based on the SCID interview, 1 subject received a *DSM-III-R* diagnosis of past bulimia nervosa for a 6-month period years before involvement in this study. No subject reported inducing vomiting for the purpose of weight control within the 3 months prior to scanning. As illustrated in Table 1, the weight-recovered subjects and the patients with AN had comparable lowest BMIs and durations of illness.

MRI SCAN ACQUISITION

All patients and controls were scanned (GE Signa 1.5-T MRI scanner) at The Toronto Hospital—Western Division. A 17-minute conventional spin-echo sequence was used to acquire contiguous axial images of 3-mm thickness from the base of the pons to the vertex of the brain (TR, 5000-5500 milliseconds; field of view, 20 cm; matrix size, 256×192 pixels; TE, 30/90 milliseconds; interleaved images). The images were oriented perpendicularly to the sagittal plane and parallel to a plane passing through both the anterior and posterior commissures. The MRI sequence was selected to facilitate image processing with Brain Image software (Behavioral Genetics and Neuroimaging Research Center, Kennedy Krieger Institute, Baltimore, Md).[24]

MRI ANALYSIS

The images were processed and segmented into gray matter, white matter, and CSF compartments by 2 trained research assistants who were unaware of subject identity and diagnosis. The procedures involved in image preparation are described in detail by Katzman et al.[1] The present analysis included all sections with nonpartially volumed white matter from the inferior surface of the temporal lobes to the vertex of the brain. The mean±SD number of slices included were 32.5±1.5 per weight-recovered subject and 31.9±1.8 per control subject.

Interrater and intrarater reliabilities were calculated for all procedures by using intraclass correlations to measure agreement. The reliability tests were performed on 3 randomly selected brains. Interrater and intrarater (for raters 1 and 2) interclass coefficients for all brain measures were as follows: 1.00, 1.00, and 1.00 for outer CSF; 0.97, 0.99, and 0.98 for outer gray matter; 0.94, 0.98, and 0.95 for outer white matter; 0.99, 0.99, and 0.99 for inner CSF; 1.00, 1.00, and 1.00 for inner gray matter; 1.00, 1.00, and 1.00 for inner white matter; 1.00, 1.00, and 1.00 for measurement of ventricular CSF; and 0.99, 0.99, and 0.99 for removal of the cerebellum and brain stem.

STATISTICAL ANALYSIS

Data from the large control group (n=30) were used to correct the brain measures from all subjects for the significant effects of ICV and age.[25] First, linear regressions were used to calculate ICV-corrected residuals for all brain measures. Then linear regressions were used to calculate age-corrected residuals from the ICV-corrected residuals. The Pearson coefficients and *P* values for the ICV and age relationships are given in **Table 2**. The mean brain measures for the weight-recovered subjects and age-matched controls are shown in **Table 3**. The regressions were based on the brain measures from only the large control group. The ICV- and age-corrected *z* scores were used in all subsequent analyses.

Student *t* tests were used to measure significance when the *z* scores for total CSF, total gray matter, and total white matter volumes were compared between the weight-recovered group (n=12) and the age-matched control group (n=18). The differences in sulcal and ventricular CSF volumes between the weight-recovered subjects and the age-matched controls were also assessed.

Effect sizes were calculated from the division of the difference between the mean *z* scores for the weight-recovered group and the large control group by the SD for the large control group to obtain the most accurate estimate of normal variance.

Within the weight-recovered group, associations were explored between the brain measures and time since recovery, lowest BMI, current BMI, serum cortisol level at MRI, and duration of illness. The first set of correlations was performed with and without the oldest subject who was an outlier on time since recovery.

The CSF and gray matter volumes for the weight-recovered subjects and age-matched controls were compared using *t* tests a second time after omitting from the analysis the weight-recovered subjects with above-average serum cortisol levels, and then after omitting the weight-recovered subjects who had BMIs less than 20 kg/m^2 at the time of the MRI scan.

The final set of analyses compared the weight-recovered group with the low-weight reference group. Student *t* tests were used to compare total CSF, gray matter, and white matter *z* scores from the weight-recovered group (n=12) with those from a group of previously described[1] low-weight adolescents with AN (n=13). For the purpose of this analysis, however, corrections for the effects of ICV and age were based on the large control group (n=30) described above. Effect sizes were calculated for the low-weight group in the same manner as described above for the weight-recovered group.

All *P* values have been adjusted for the number of comparisons using the Holm sequentially rejective step-down correction.[26,27] Because the sample size is small, all significant comparisons have been confirmed using the Mann-Whitney nonparametric test.

Table 1. Physical and Clinical Characteristics of Subject Groups*

Characteristic	Control Group (n=18)	Weight-Recovered Group (n=12)	Low-Weight Group (n=13)
Age at MRI, y	19.9±7.1 (12.0-37.1)	18.9±6.9 (11.7-37.6)	15.2±1.2 (13.3-17.0)
BMI at MRI	21.9±3.4† (15.1-27.3)	20.5±2.3 (18.1-25.6)	15.6±1.7‡ (12.7-17.8)
Lowest BMI, kg/m²	NA	13.7±1.9 (11.3-16.4)	14.3±1.7 (10.5-17.2)
Age at AN onset, y	NA	13±2 (9-16)	14±1 (12-16)
Duration of AN, mo	NA	14±10 (4-36)	11±6 (3-24)

*Data are presented as mean±SD (range). MRI indicates magnetic resonance imaging; BMI, body mass index (expressed as the weight, in kilograms, divided by the height, in meters, squared); AN, anorexia nervosa; and NA, not applicable.
†n=16.
‡P<.001, low-weight vs weight-recovered group and low-weight vs control group.

Table 2. Pearson Correlation Coefficients for the Effects of Intracranial Volume and Age in the Large Control Group (n=30)

Brain Measure	Intracranial Volume	Age*
Total cerebrospinal fluid	0.05	0.47†
Sulcal cerebrospinal fluid	−0.04	0.47†
Ventricles	0.11	0.30
Total gray matter	0.82‡	−0.81‡
Cortical gray matter	0.79‡	−0.72‡
Central gray matter	0.75‡	−0.63‡
Total white matter	0.72‡	0.71‡

*After correction for intracranial volume.
†P<.01.
‡P<.001.

RESULTS

WEIGHT-RECOVERED SUBJECTS VS CONTROLS

The weight-recovered group had significantly smaller total gray matter volumes ($t[28]=-3.3$, $P=.02$) and significantly greater total CSF volumes ($t[28]=2.8$, $P=.04$) when compared with the age-matched controls. The weight-recovered group did not differ significantly from the control group on total white matter volumes ($t[28]=0.2$, $P=.80$). Replacement of the linear age regression by a quadratic age regression did not affect the white matter z scores. Further analysis of CSF volumes showed that weight-recovered subjects had significantly larger sulcal CSF volumes ($t[28]=2.7$, $P=.02$) but not significantly larger ventricles ($t[28]=1.8$, $P=.20$), compared with the age-matched control group. **Figure 1** and **Figure 2** show that the weight-recovered group had greater CSF volumes and smaller gray matter volumes compared with the large control group. The effect sizes for all brain measures are reported in **Table 4**.

There were no significant correlations between any of the brain measures and time since recovery, lowest BMI, current BMI, or duration of illness within the weight-recovered group.

The differences between the weight-recovered group and the age-matched control group were robust. The weight-recovered group still had significantly lower gray matter ($t[22]=-3.0$, $P=.01$) and higher CSF volumes ($t[22]=3.0$, $P=.02$) than the age-matched controls after the weight-recovered subjects who had BMIs below 20 kg/m² at the time of the MRI scan were omitted from analysis. Likewise, the weight-recovered group had significantly lower gray matter volumes ($t[25]=-3.0$, $P=.02$) and higher CSF volumes ($t[25]=2.5$, $P=.02$) than the age-matched controls after the weight-recovered subjects with above-average serum cortisol levels at the time of the MRI scan were omitted from the analysis.

WEIGHT-RECOVERED SUBJECTS VS LOW-WEIGHT SUBJECTS

The gray matter and CSF volumes for the weight-recovered group were intermediate between those of the low-weight group and those of the large control group, as described in Figure 1 and Figure 2. Compared with the low-weight group, the weight-recovered group had significantly smaller CSF volumes ($t[23]=-3.6$, $P=.003$) and significantly larger white matter ($t[23]=2.7$, $P=.02$) and gray matter volumes ($t[23]=2.3$, $P=.03$). Table 4 shows the effect sizes for the low-weight group compared with the large control group. Because the brain measures reported by Katzman et al[1] were corrected with regressions based on 8 controls and 13 low-weight subjects, the magnitude (but not the direction) of the results are different from those previously reported.[1,28]

COMMENT

This study suggests that structural brain abnormalities may remain after long-term weight recovery from AN. Compared with age-matched controls, healthy weight-recovered subjects have significantly lower gray matter volumes and significantly higher CSF volumes. Neither the CSF elevations nor gray matter deficits were significantly correlated with length of time since weight recovery. These findings suggest that AN may have long-lasting and global effects on the brain.

To our knowledge, this is the first study to examine gray matter and white matter tissue volumes in subjects who are weight-recovered from AN. The finding of long-term volume deficits in gray matter but not white matter supports the hypothesis that brain changes in AN have both irreversible and reversible components. In comparison with a group of low-weight patients with AN, the weight-recovered subjects had significantly higher white matter volumes and lower CSF volumes. Although these findings need to be replicated in a longitudinal study, we believe that the gray matter volume deficits and CSF elevations seen in long-term weight-

Table 3. Brain Measures for the Weight-Recovered Anorectic and Age-Matched Control Subjects Before and After Correction for Intracranial Volume (ICV) and Age

Brain Measure	Mean±SD Voxels: Control Group (n=18)	Mean±SD Voxels: Weight-Recovered Group (n=12)	Mean±SD Age- and ICV-Corrected Voxels: Control Group (n=18)	Mean±SD Age- and ICV-Corrected Voxels: Weight-Recovered Group (n=12)
ICV	568 171±47 075	592 638±48 110	...	...
Total cerebrospinal fluid	47 300±8421	58 414±16 641	−1980±8300	9381±13 842*
Sulcal cerebrospinal fluid	34 630±4536	59 038±10 943	−1315±9321	7807±11 988*
Ventricles	6245±2048	8271±3742	−492±2224	1440±3573
Total gray matter	307 383±33 849	312 305±27 033	1705±9998	−10 508±9882*
Cortical gray matter	228 520±22 387	233 188±20 897	1131±9321	−5354±7557
Central gray matter	78 863±13 607	79 117±8784	574±6502	−5154±7727
Total white matter	213 488±22 018	221 919±20 394	275±10 422	1126±7312

*P≤.01.

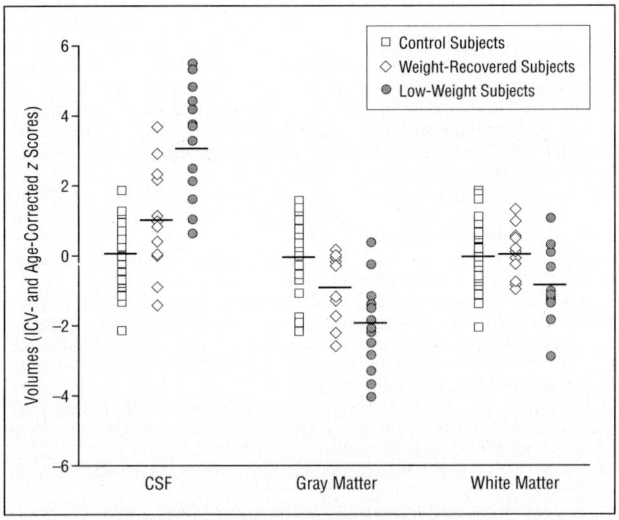

Figure 1. *Intracranial (ICV)- and age-corrected volumes of total cerebrospinal fluid (CSF), gray matter, and white matter in control subjects and weight-recovered subjects and low-weight patients with anorexia nervosa.*

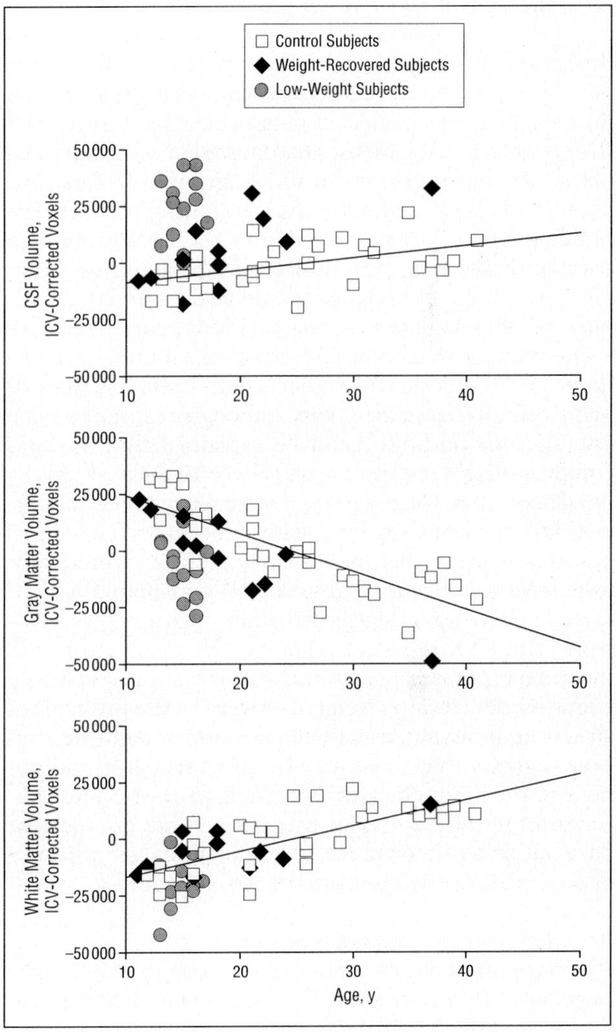

Figure 2. *Intracranial (ICV)-corrected brain measures vs age. Linear regression is based on the data from the large control group. For CSF, r=0.47, P=.009 (29 df); gray matter, r=−0.81, P<.001 (29 df); and white matter, r=0.71, P<.001 (29 df).*

recovered subjects in the present study most likely represent an irreversible component of brain changes that occurs during starvation.

By focusing on a reasonably homogeneous group, this study has narrowed the range of possible explanations for the gray matter volume deficits. The study included only subjects who had an early onset of AN, a relatively brief duration of illness, and minimal comorbidity. They had been weight-recovered for a relatively long time compared with subjects studied previously and, as a group, reported normal eating attitudes and behavior at the time of MRI.

As suggested by Katzman et al,[1] the gray matter deficits may result from prolonged exposure to the high physiological levels of cortisol present in AN.[11] Katzman et al[1] reported a correlation between cortisol levels and brain measures in female adolescents who had relatively short durations of illness. Tumors in the hypothalamic-pituitary axis, as well as administration of exogenous steroids, can result in elevated cortisol levels, and both have been linked to brain changes such as tissue atrophy and fluid space enlargement.[12,29-31]

The differences between the brains of the weight-recovered subjects and those of the age-matched controls do not appear to be related to differences in the current descriptive or clinical characteristics of the 2 groups. Based on the literature, one might speculate that the weight-recovered subjects who had high cortisol levels would have more serious CSF elevations or gray matter volume deficits. However, there were no significant correlations between the brain measures and serum cortisol levels at the time of the MRI scan. Furthermore, removing the weight-

Table 4. Effect Sizes for All Brain Measures for the Weight-Recovered and Low-Weight Anorectic Groups*

Brain Measure	Weight-Recovered Group (n=12)	Low-Weight Group (n=13)
Total cerebrospinal fluid	1.1	3.4
Sulcal cerebrospinal fluid	1.1	3.3
Ventricles	0.5	1.4
Total gray matter	−1.0	−2.1
Cortical gray matter	−0.6	−1.0
Central gray matter	−0.8	−1.9
Total white matter	0.1	−0.8

*Compared with the large control group (n=30).

recovered subjects with above-average serum cortisol levels at the time of scan did not change the results.

Given the evidence for persisting brain differences in this sample, it is important to reexamine whether this group of subjects can be considered "weight-recovered." At the time this study was conducted, none of the subjects met *DSM-III-R* criteria for AN. Menses had started or returned in 10 of the 12 subjects. The mean and range for BMI were consistent with those reported in the literature for other groups of subjects who have recovered from AN.[16,17] We found no correlation between current BMI and the abnormal brain measures; such a correlation would be expected if incomplete weight recovery were responsible for continued gray matter volume deficits or CSF elevations. Finally, removing from the analysis the subjects with BMIs less than 20 kg/m^2 did not change the results. Although it cannot be ruled out that our findings could be explained by less-than-complete weight restoration, we believe for the reasons outlined above that the differences most likely reflect significant structural abnormalities in a weight-recovered sample.

The finding that long-term weight-recovered subjects have significantly reduced total gray matter and elevated CSF volumes suggests that the apparent reversibility of the CSF measures reported in prior studies is incomplete. This is consistent with reports of persisting cognitive deficits after weight recovery.[13] The presence of structural brain abnormalities years after weight restoration suggests that there may be an irreversible component to the brain changes associated with AN. The neuropathological features of this irreversible component have yet to be characterized; the functional significance of these deficits requires further investigation.

Accepted for publication December 18, 1996.

Supported by the Associates Fund of the Clarke Institute of Psychiatry, the Ontario Mental Health Foundation, and the Medical Research Council of Canada.

Presented in part at the Society for Neuroscience Meeting, Washington, DC, November 19, 1996.

We thank Shitij Kapur, MD, PhD, for permitting us to include control subjects from the PET Centre at the Clarke Institute of Psychiatry, and Corey Jones for helping us to obtain the MRI scans. We also acknowledge David Streiner, PhD, for his help as a statistical consultant, and Paul Garfinkel, MD, and Allan Kaplan, MD, for helping to recruit subjects. Edmond Chong and Brigit Swenson gave assistance in all aspects of image processing.

This article is based on a thesis submitted to fulfill in part the requirements for the degree of Master of Science at the University of Toronto (Ms Lambe).

Reprints: Robert B. Zipursky, MD, Clarke Institute of Psychiatry, 250 College St, Toronto, Ontario, Canada M5T 1R8 (e-mail: rz@sig.clarke-inst.on.ca).

REFERENCES

1. Katzman DK, Lambe EK, Mikulis DJ, Ridgely JN, Goldbloom DS, Zipursky RB. Cerebral gray matter and white matter volume deficits in adolescent females with anorexia nervosa. *J Pediatr.* 1996;129:794-803.
2. Dolan RJ, Mitchell J, Wakeling A. Structural brain changes in patients with anorexia nervosa. *Psychol Med.* 1988;18:349-353.
3. Krieg JC, Pirke KM, Lauer C, Backmund H. Endocrine, metabolic, and cranial computed tomographic findings in anorexia nervosa. *Biol Psychiatry.* 1988;23:377-387.
4. Artmann H, Grau H, Adelmann M, Schleiffer R. Reversible and non-reversible enlargement of cerebrospinal fluid spaces in anorexia nervosa. *Neuroradiology.* 1985;27:304-312.
5. Datlof S, Coleman PD, Forbes GB, Kreipe RE. Ventricular dilation on CT scans of patients with anorexia nervosa. *Am J Psychiatry.* 1986;143:96-98.
6. Golden NH, Ashtari M, Kohn MR, Patel M, Jacobson MS, Fletcher A, Shenker IR. Reversibility of cerebral ventricular enlargement in anorexia nervosa, demonstrated by quantitative magnetic resonance imaging. *J Pediatr.* 1996;128:296-301.
7. Hoffman GWJ, Ellinwood EHJ, Rockwell WJ, Herfkens RJ, Nishita JK, Guthrie LF. Cerebral atrophy in anorexia nervosa: a pilot study. *Biol Psychiatry.* 1989;26:321-324.
8. Kohlmeyer K, Lehmkuhl G, Poutska F. Computed tomography of anorexia nervosa. *AJNR Am J Neuroradiol.* 1983;4:437-438.
9. Kornreich L, Shapira A, Horev G, Danziger Y, Tyano S, Mimouni M. CT and MR evaluation of the brain in patients with anorexia nervosa. *AJNR Am J Neuroradiol.* 1991;12:1213-1216.
10. Nussbaum M, Shenker IR, Marc J, Klein M. Cerebral atrophy in anorexia nervosa. *J Pediatr.* 1980;96:876-869.
11. Gold PW, Gwirtsman H, Avgerinos PC, Nieman LK, Gallucci WT, Kaye W, Jimerson D, Ebert M, Rittmaster R, Loriaux DL, Chorousos GP. Abnormal hypothalamic-pituitary-adrenal function in anorexia nervosa. *N Engl J Med.* 1986;314:1335-1342.
12. Sapolsky RM. *Stress, the Aging Brain, and the Mechanisms of Neuron Death.* Cambridge, Mass: MIT Press; 1992.
13. Kingston K, Szmukler G, Andrewes D, Tress B, Desmond P. Neuropsychological and structural brain changes in anorexia nervosa before and after refeeding. *Psychol Med.* 1996;26:15-28.
14. Lambe EK. *Gray-Matter Volume Deficits in Weight-Recovered Anorexics.* Toronto, Ontario: University of Toronto; 1996. Thesis.
15. American Psychiatric Association. *Diagnostic and Statistical Manual of Mental Disorders, Third Edition, Revised.* Washington, DC: American Psychiatric Association; 1987.
16. Bachrach LK, Katzman DK, Litt IF, Guido D, Marcus R. Recovery from osteopenia in adolescent girls with anorexia nervosa. *J Clin Endocrinol Metab.* 1991;72:602-606.
17. Eckert ED, Halmi KA, Marchi P, Grove W, Crosby R. Ten-year follow-up of anorexia nervosa: clinical course and outcome. *Psychol Med.* 1995;25:143-156.
18. Pfefferbaum A, Mathalon DH, Sullivan EV, Rawles JM, Zipursky RB, Lim KO. A quantitative MRI study of changes in brain morphology from infancy to late adulthood. *Arch Neurol.* 1994;51:874-887.
19. Beck A, Ward C, Mendelson M, Mock J, Erbaugh J. An inventory for measuring depression. *Arch Gen Psychiatry.* 1961;4:561-571.
20. Garner DM, Garfinkel PE. The Eating Attitudes Test: an index of the symptoms of anorexia nervosa. *Psychol Med.* 1979;9:273-279.
21. Mt Sinai Hospital Clinical Laboratories. *Lab User's Handbook.* Toronto, Ontario: Mt Sinai Hospital; 1992:175.
22. Teri L. The use of the Beck Depression Inventory with adolescents. *J Abnorm Child Psychol.* 1982;10:277-284.
23. Oliver JM, Simmons ME. Affective disorders and depression as measured by the Diagnostic Interview Schedule and the Beck Depression Inventory in an unselected adult population. *J Clin Psychol.* 1985;41:469-477.
24. Reiss AL, Hennessey J, Subramanium B, Rubin M, Beach L. *Brain Image.* Baltimore, Md: Behavioral Genetics and Neuroimaging Research Center, Kennedy Krieger Institute; 1994.
25. Zipursky RB, Lim KO, Sullivan EV, Brown BW, Pfefferbaum A. Widespread cerebral gray matter volume deficits in schizophrenia. *Arch Gen Psychiatry.* 1992;49:195-205.
26. Holm S. A simple sequentially rejective multiple test procedure. *Scand J Statistics.* 1979;6:65-70.
27. Wright SP. Adjusted P-values for simultaneous inference. *Biometrics.* 1992;48:1005-1013.
28. Zipursky RB, Lambe EK, Goldbloom D, Ridgely J, Mikulis DJ, Katzman DK. Gray matter and white matter volume loss in anorexia nervosa. *Biol Psychiatry.* 1996;39:603. Abstract.
29. Momose KJ, Kjellberg RN, Kliman B. High incidence of cortical atrophy of the cerebral and cerebellar hemispheres in Cushing's disease. *Radiology.* 1971;99:341-348.
30. Okuno T, Ito M, Konishi Y, Yoshioka M, Nakano Y. Cerebral atrophy following ACTH therapy. *J Comput Assist Tomogr.* 1980;4:20-23.
31. Bentson J, Reza M, Winter J, Wilson G. Steroids and apparent cerebral atrophy on computed tomography scans. *J Comput Assist Tomogr.* 1978;2:16-23.

Psychosocial Correlates of Job Strain in a Sample of Working Women

Redford B. Williams, MD; John C. Barefoot, PhD; James A. Blumenthal, PhD; Michael J. Helms, MS; Linda Luecken, MA; Carl F. Pieper, DPH; Ilene C. Siegler, PhD, MPH; Edward C. Suarez, PhD

Background: This study identifies potential mediators of job strain effects on health by determining whether psychosocial factors known to predict an increased risk of cardiovascular disease and all-cause mortality are higher among women who report high levels of job strain.

Methods: Measures of job strain and other psychosocial risk factors were obtained in a sample of 152 female employees of a local corporation. Canonical correlation and analyses of covariance were used to assess relationships between job demands and decision latitude and other psychosocial risk factors.

Results: A significant (P=.002) solution to the canonical correlation analysis showed that high job demands and low decision latitude were correlated with a pattern of psychosocial factors consisting of (1) increased levels of negative emotions like anxiety, anger, depression, and hostility; (2) reduced levels of social support; and (3) a preponderance of negative compared with positive feelings in dealings with coworkers and supervisors. This pattern was confirmed by analyses of covariance that adjusted for demographic and specific job characteristics.

Conclusions: The canonical correlation analysis results provide empirical support for the job strain construct. The most important finding is that health-damaging psychosocial factors like job strain, depression, hostility, anxiety, and social isolation tend to cluster in certain individuals.

Arch Gen Psychiatry. 1997;54:543-548

A CONSIDERABLE amount of recent behavioral medicine research has focused on the role of occupational stress in physical health and disease. The most widely used conceptualization of occupational stress in this research has been the job strain model promulgated by Karasek and Theorell.[1] According to this model, the most stressful jobs are those characterized by the combination of high psychological workload demands and low decision latitude. A job with high workload demands is one that requires workers to work fast and hard to accomplish an excessive amount of work in too short a time. A job with low decision latitude is one that does not allow workers to make decisions on their own, does not involve learning new skills or developing special abilities, and does involve a lot of repetitive work.

In a recent comprehensive review of the research on job strain and health, Schnall and coworkers[2] concluded that of 37 articles about job strain published between 1981 and 1993, almost all found a notable positive association between increased job strain and increased risk of cardiovascular disease (CVD), all-cause mortality, or CVD risk factors like hypertension. The job strain effect size was similar in cross-sectional and prospective designs, in blue- and white-collar workers, and in men and women, although more research is needed in female working groups.[2]

Although few of the reviewed studies evaluated potential modifiers of the effect of job strain on risk,[2] there is some indication that other psychosocial factors can moderate the health-damaging effects of job strain. Thus, the effect of high job strain on increased CVD risk was stronger in workers with a low socioeconomic status (SES) in Sweden[3-5] and the United States.[6] Studies of Swedish working groups[3,7,8] reported a larger increase in all-cause mortality and CVD prevalence as a function of high job strain when there was also a low level of social support.

In contrast with the positive evidence that social factors like SES and social support moderate the effect of job strain on health, Schnall and coworkers[2] note that there is a paucity of studies on

From the Departments of Psychiatry (Drs Williams, Barefoot, Blumenthal, Siegler, and Suarez, Mr Helms, and Ms Luecken) and Community and Family Medicine (Dr Pieper), Behavioral Medicine Research Center, Duke University Medical Center, Durham, NC.

SUBJECTS AND METHODS

SUBJECTS

The subjects were 152 female employees who worked in 2 departments of a large local corporation. In 1 department (ie, customer services), the job involves talking on the telephone with potentially irate customers all day. In the other department (ie, paperwork processing), the workers spend their day processing paperwork in a more or less assembly line arrangement. The sample included 94 women from customer services and 58 from paperwork processing. The mean (±SD) age of the women was 32±9 years, and their mean (±SD) length of employment was 76±70 months. The racial composition of the sample was white, 53%; African American, 41%; and other, 6%. Data from men working in the 2 departments were not evaluated because they constituted less than 10% of the workers.

The data on which this report is based were collected during the preliminary phase of a large-scale intervention trial to evaluate the effect of stress management training on the psychobiological concomitants of workplace stress among employees in this local corporation. All employees in the 2 departments were invited to attend orientation sessions in which the overall study plan would be described. At the end of these sessions, those attending were asked to complete several questionnaires that measure job stress factors and psychological factors that may be affected by job stress. There was no coercion to participate in this testing, and all employees were informed that their responses to the questionnaires would be kept in confidence and that no individual would be identified to management. There was no compensation for this phase of the study. Informed consent was obtained using a form approved by the Institutional Review Board of Duke University Medical Center, Durham, NC.

PSYCHOSOCIAL MEASURES

The job demands and decision latitude dimensions that make up the job strain construct were measured using an abbreviated version of the job content instrument formulated by Karasek and coworkers,[10] which contains items assessing work pace and difficulty, time available to do the work, freedom to make decisions on one's own, repetitiveness of work, and variety of tasks. A short form of the NEO Personality Inventory, the NEO Five Factor Inventory,[11] was used to measure 5 personality dimensions: neuroticism, extroversion, openness, conscientiousness, and agreeableness. Depression was assessed using the Beck Depression Inventory.[12] Social desirability was assessed with the scale developed by Crowne and Marlow.[13] The State-Trait Personality Inventory developed by Spielberger and coworkers[14] was used to measure anxiety, anger, and curiosity. Hostility was measured using the Cook and Medley[15] Hostility scale. The Interpersonal Support Evaluation List[16] was used to measure 4 dimensions of social support. The perceived adequacy of social contacts in meeting a person's needs is assessed by the appraisal subscale. The number of social contacts making up a person's social network is assessed by the belonging subscale. The availability of help from others to meet specific needs (eg, child care) is assessed by the tangible subscale. And a person's sense of self-worth derived from contacts with others is assessed by the self-esteem subscale.

To provide a measure of the overall tone of their interactions with coworkers and supervisors, we asked the employees participating in this preliminary phase of the study to rate the degree (ie, from not at all to extremely)

the question of whether personality factors modify the effect of job strain. Citing one study[9] that failed to find an association between trait anxiety and either job strain or blood pressure levels while at work among employed men, they conclude that "it is unlikely that personality variables account for the association between job strain and hypertension or CVD."[2] However, they acknowledge the need for more research to "develop a theory that specifies possible interactions between environmental stressors [like job strain] and personality characteristics, and to improve the methodology of such studies."[2]

This study addresses this need by examining the association between job strain and a range of psychosocial factors that have been found in other research to be health damaging. By studying these associations in a large sample of working blue- and white-collar women, the study also addresses the need for expanded research on the effect of job strain among women workers.

RESULTS

The canonical correlation analysis found that the first "Job Characteristics" canonical variable explained 55% of the variance for job demands and decision latitude and was positively weighted for job demands and negatively weighted for decision latitude. It was correlated (Wilks $\lambda=0.62$, $P=.002$) with the first "Psychosocial Factors" canonical variable that explained 24% of the variance in the psychosocial measures. The psychosocial measure weightings reflected a general trend toward increased psychosocial distress.

As shown in **Table 1**, the first canonical variable characterized by high demands and low decision latitude is associated with a psychosocial profile indicating (1) higher levels of negative emotions and related traits (eg, depression, anxiety, anger, neuroticism, and hostility), (2) reduced levels of social support, and (3) a preponderance of negative compared with positive feelings associated with dealings with coworkers and supervisors. By finding a first canonical variable positively weighted for demands and negatively weighted for decision latitude, the results of this analysis are consistent with the job strain construct as originally described by Karasek and Theorell.[1] The results also suggest that high job strain is associated with a potentially harmful pattern of other psychosocial factors.

To provide a replication of the findings of the canonical correlation analysis and to gain a more complete and detailed impression of the psychosocial profile associated with reports of high job strain, we performed a series of ANCOVAs—controlling for the de-to which they had experienced various positive (eg, happy, glad, and contented) and negative (eg, angry, sad, and frustrated) feelings "during the past week, including today" with coworkers and supervisors. With the use of these ratings, we created 2 summary variables, coworkers-moods and supervisors-moods, combining the total of ratings for positive moods with the reverse of negative moods ("reverse" means that on a 1-5 scale, a 1 becomes a 5, a 2 becomes a 4, and so on). These variables enabled us to index the overall tone of moods aroused by workers' interactions with other workers and supervisors, with a high score indicating a relative preponderance of positive moods compared with negative moods.

STATISTICAL ANALYSIS

Prior research on job strain[2] has used various approaches to define high strain, such as (1) those above the median on demands and below the median on decision latitude, (2) use of the quotient of demands divided by decision latitude to create a continuous strain variable, and (3) use of a threshold level (eg, top 20%) above which high strain is considered to be present. Rather than impose any of these arbitrary definitions, we chose as our first step an empirical multivariable approach employing canonical correlation to determine whether there is an optimal combination of the demand and decision latitude measures that relates to a particular and meaningful pattern of the other psychosocial factors. Finding a canonical variable weighted positively for demands and negatively for decision latitude that correlates with a specific pattern of the other psychosocial factors would provide empirical support for the job strain construct and help identify other psychosocial factors that cluster in women who report high job strain.

Various demographic factors (eg, age, race, marital status, and various job-related characteristics) could confound any relationships between job strain and the other psychosocial factors. Therefore, we conducted a series of analyses of covariance (ANCOVAs) to evaluate relationships between the independent variable job strain—using a more traditional "strain" variable defined as the sum of demands and the reverse of decision latitude—and the dependent psychosocial factor variables with potential demographic (ie, race and age) and objective job characteristic (ie, department and length of employment) confounders as covariates. In addition to controlling for possible confounders, these separate ANCOVAs also provide a series of univariate replications of the multivariable analysis previously described using canonical correlation but with a priori specification of the job strain construct.

To gain an impression of demographic and psychosocial profiles, we used analyses of variance to compare workers in the 2 departments for demographic characteristics and the psychosocial variables being studied. With the exception of the demands and decision latitude variables, workers in the 2 departments were remarkably similar on all variables tested. Workers in the customer services department had significantly higher ($P \leq .001$) demands and decision latitude than those in paperwork processing. However, because demands and decision latitude were higher, customer service employees did not differ from those in paperwork processing on the strain measure. Thus, it seemed warranted to collapse subjects from the 2 departments into a single sample in the analyses to evaluate clustering of psychosocial risk factors in this sample. Even so, the previously described ANCOVAs would control for any unmeasured departmental effects.

An $\alpha = .05$ was used to establish statistical significance for all analyses.

partment in which they work, race, age, and months employed at the corporation—that compared levels of the psychosocial factors among workers scoring in each quartile on the job strain variable (ie, sum of demands and reverse of decision latitude). Independently of department, race, age, and length of employment, those workers reporting higher levels of job strain differ significantly (**Table 2**) from workers reporting lower strain for several psychosocial characteristics. These results remained essentially unchanged in further ANCOVAs that included—in addition to department, race, age, and months of employment—marital status, presence of children living in the home, specific job title (ie, a rough measure of job differences within the 2 departments), and supervisor as covariates.

An inspection of Table 2 reveals a consistently adverse psychosocial profile among workers reporting higher levels of job strain. Psychologically, they are more depressed, anxious, angry, neurotic, and hostile than their counterparts reporting lower levels of job strain. They also show reduced levels of a positive trait, curiosity. From the social perspective, their scores on the Interpersonal Support Evaluation List scales suggest that persons reporting high job strain appraise their sources of social support as less adequate in meeting their emotional needs or enhancing their self-esteem. Workers with a high level of job strain also reported less of a sense of belonging, and they had a preponderance of negative compared with positive dealings with coworkers and supervisors encountered at this particular work site.

A comparison of the results depicted in Tables 1 and 2 shows that all of those psychosocial variables that differed significantly across the job strain quartiles in Table 2 had loading coefficients on the "Psychosocial Factors" canonical variable at the 0.40 level or higher. In contrast, all of those psychosocial factors that were not significant in the ANCOVAs reported in Table 2 had loading coefficients lower than 0.40. Thus, the 2 analyses, one empirical and one based on an a priori definition of job strain, produced essentially similar results.

With the exception of Hostility scale scores, the results shown in Table 2 describe a similar pattern of increase in negative, or decrease in positive, psychosocial factor scores going from lower to higher job strain quartiles. Thus, those in the 2 lowest quartiles were similar to each other, with those in the third quartile showing a moderate and those in the fourth quartile a marked deterioration in score. It was not until relatively high levels of job strain were reported that the other psychosocial factors showed adverse (ie, increased depression and decreased social support) effects.

Table 1. Canonical Correlation Analysis Relating Demands and Latitude Variables to the Set of Psychosocial Variables Collected in This Sample*

Variables	*r* With First Canonical Variable
First Job Characteristics Canonical Variable	
Demands	+0.64
Decision latitude	−0.83
First Psychosocial Factors Canonical Variable	
Crowne-Marlowe scale	−0.30
Hostility scale	+0.43
Neuroticism	+0.60
Extroversion	−0.32
Openness	−0.13
Conscientiousness	−0.09
Agreeableness	−0.18
Beck Depression Inventory	+0.70
STPI	
Anxiety	+0.70
Anger	+0.42
Curiosity	−0.61
ISEL	
Appraisal	−0.44
Belonging	−0.65
Tangible	−0.33
Self-esteem	−0.74
Coworkers-moods	−0.55
Supervisors-moods	−0.48

**STPI Indicates State-Trait Personality Inventory; ISEL, Interpersonal Support Evaluation List. The coeffictients shown in the table are correlations of each individual variable with the canonical variable on its side of the equation; these coefficients can be interpreted as "loadings" of each variable on a single combined variable.*

COMMENT

The most important finding of this study is that health-damaging psychosocial factors like job strain, depression, hostility, and social isolation are not randomly distributed as independent entities among the working women we studied. Instead, these factors seem to cluster in certain individuals. Those who fall within the highest high job strain quartile are characterized by a pattern of adverse psychosocial characteristics: (1) increased depression, anxiety, neuroticism, hostility, and anger; (2) decreased social support and a preponderance of negative compared with positive feelings in their dealings with coworkers and supervisors; and (3) decreased curiosity.

Hostility,[17] depression,[18] anxiety,[19] and low levels of social support or social isolation[20] have each been found, when considered singly, to increase the risk for various adverse health outcomes, including coronary heart disease, all-cause mortality, and mortality after heart attacks. Research during the past 5 years indicates that a combination of 2 or more of these psychosocial factors is even more damaging to health than a single factor acting alone. Thus, the combination of type A behavior and low social support predicts a higher mortality from coronary heart disease[21] and correlates more strongly with coronary artery disease severity[22] than either factor alone.

The health consequences are compounded even more when 3 psychosocial risk factors are present. Kaplan[23] found, for example, that all-cause mortality was increased far more by the combination of depression and social isolation in residents with a low SES than those with a high SES in Alameda County, California. He also reports a similar compounding of mortality risk among participants in the Kuopio, Finland, study who are cynically hostile, poor, and socially isolated. Barefoot and coworkers[24] found a similar compounding of all-cause mortality among residents of Glostrup, Denmark, who are hostile and depressed and who have a lower SES.

The clustering of increased depression, anxiety, anger, hostility, and social isolation found among the working women reporting high job strain in this study suggests, therefore, that women who perceive their jobs as high in strain will be at particularly high risk for a range of health problems. Indeed, the Beck Depression Inventory score of 14.8 among women in the highest quartile of job strain (Table 2) is itself already in the range in which depression is considered to be clinically significant.[12] The present findings contrast with those found in a study of men that did not find anxiety associated with job strain,[9] suggesting the possibility that high job strain may have a greater adverse effect on women than men. A more extensive evaluation of the associations between job strain and psychosocial risk factors in men will be required before firm conclusions regarding sex differences in the psychosocial correlates of job strain can be drawn. Women in professional and executive positions should be studied to see if the links between job strain and psychosocial distress we found in this study are also present among women in higher-status jobs.

Because psychosocial risk factors tend to cluster in the same individuals or groups where their health-damaging effects are compounded, it will be important in future psychosocial risk factor research to assess the complete array of psychosocial risk factors. Such an approach will facilitate the identification of the pathways responsible for the increased mortality rates and shorter life expectancy found among persons in high-strain jobs, as well as other groups exposed to environmental stressors, like low SES, that also predispose[25-28] to increased morbidity and mortality.

The available data from this cross-sectional study do not permit us to conclude which comes first, high job strain or the adverse array of psychosocial characteristics. There is some evidence from prior research suggesting that individual differences can influence the perception of job characteristics. Kristensen[29] found, for example, that even among slaughterhouse workers with objectively identical job descriptions there is a range in levels of job strain using self-report instruments. Spector[30] found that only 10% to 20% of the variability in self-reports of job strain is due to objective characteristics of the job. This study found that associations between job strain and psychological distress and social isolation were not diminished when we controlled for such objective characteristics of the job as the department worked in, specific job title, and even supervisor. These results suggest that high levels of psychosocial distress may themselves contribute to individual differences in self-reports of job strain.

Whatever the direction of causality for associations between job strain and other psychosocial risk fac-

Table 2. Psychosocial Characteristics of Workers in the 4 Quartiles of Job Strain

	Job Strain Quartiles†				
Psychosocial Factors*	First	Second	Third	Fourth	P‡
Crowne-Marlowe scale	21.6 (0.9)	19.5 (0.9)	19.2 (0.9)	19.0 (1.0)	≥.10
Hostility scale	12.3 (0.7)	14.8 (0.7)	14.2 (0.7)	14.7 (0.8)	.04
Neuroticism	32.5 (1.2)	32.0 (1.2)	35.2 (1.2)	37.7 (1.4)	.008
Extroversion	39.7 (0.9)	41.7 (0.9)	40.4 (0.9)	38.0 (1.1)	≥.10
Openness	36.4 (0.9)	37.2 (0.8)	36.5 (0.9)	37.0 (1.0)	≥.10
Conscientiousness	46.8 (0.9)	46.8 (0.9)	46.2 (0.9)	46.3 (1.0)	≥.10
Agreeableness	45.9 (0.9)	45.0 (0.9)	45.8 (0.9)	44.3 (1.1)	≥.10
Beck Depression Inventory	7.7 (1.0)	8.3 (1.0)	10.1 (1.0)	14.8 (1.1)	<.001
STPI					
Anxiety	19.7 (0.8)	19.5 (0.8)	21.2 (0.8)	25.1 (0.9)	<.001
Anger	18.7 (0.9)	20.3 (0.9)	20.9 (0.9)	22.1 (1.0)	.09
Curiosity	26.5 (0.8)	27.4 (0.8)	26.3 (0.8)	23.2 (0.9)	.007
ISEL					
Appraisal	23.7 (0.9)	23.9 (0.9)	21.6 (0.9)	19.7 (1.1)	.01
Belonging	22.6 (0.8)	24.0 (0.8)	21.8 (0.8)	19.4 (0.9)	.003
Tangible	25.8 (0.8)	25.4 (0.8)	24.1 (0.9)	23.1 (0.9)	≥.10
Self-esteem	21.4 (0.7)	21.6 (0.7)	19.6 (0.7)	18.1 (0.8)	.004
Coworkers-moods	63.7 (2.7)	63.5 (2.6)	62.8 (2.2)	54.8 (3.2)	.05
Supervisors-moods	61.6 (2.7)	59.0 (2.7)	52.4 (2.2)	53.3 (3.0)	.005

**STPI indicates State-Trait Personality Inventory; ISEL, Interpersonal Support Evaluation List.*
†All data are given as the mean (±SEM). Number in each quartile: first, 39; second, 40; third, 39; and fourth, 32.
‡Based on analyses of covariance with department, race, age, and length of employment entered first as covariates. The means and SEMs shown are adjusted for the covariates; analysis with unadjusted values yielded essentially the same results.

tors, their compounded pathogenic potential would remain the same. Moreover, it seems that self-reports of job strain are stronger predictors of health outcomes than objective indexes of job stress. Self-reports of job strain identify persons at a higher risk of myocardial infarction than do objective measures of job characteristics.[4,31] Thus, the effect of psychosocial factors on individual differences in how the job is perceived (and hence, perhaps, on the psychosocial distress experienced) may be critical in determining the health consequences of job strain.

The profile of psychosocial characteristics found among the women in our study reporting high job strain suggests various pathways whereby job strain can affect health. From a biological perspective, the negative affects and social isolation that cluster in women reporting high job strain have been found in prior research[2,3,32-34] to be associated with biological characteristics that are plausible contributors to pathogenesis: increased sympathetic nervous system activation, decreased parasympathetic activation, increased cortisol secretion, and decreased immune function. Similarly from a behavioral perspective, such risk behaviors as smoking, overeating, increased alcohol consumption, and failure to adhere to prescribed medical regimens have all been found among persons exhibiting the same psychosocial profile as the women reporting high job strain in this study.[2,3,32-34] However, prospective studies will be required to document the precise biobehavioral mechanisms whereby job strain and other psychosocial factors contribute to health problems.

We already know that psychosocial distress in the absence of objective medical illness is responsible for many patient visits to primary care physicians.[35] Therefore, any intervention that can reduce the distress associated with high job strain has the potential for immediate benefits in reduced use of costly medical services. Even more important, there is reason to expect that interventions effective in reducing this psychosocial distress will also lead to a reduced incidence of debilitating medical problems during the long-term. Controlled clinical trials are already showing that psychosocial interventions aimed at reducing psychological distress improve prognosis in patients with coronary heart disease[36,37] and cancer.[38,39] If reducing health-damaging psychosocial distress in patients who already have a life-threatening medical disorder can improve prognosis, it is likely that similar approaches can ameliorate health risks associated with high job strain.

This study of women employed in blue- and white-collar jobs found that job strain and other health-damaging characteristics tend to co-occur in the same individuals. Because the disease risks are compounded when psychosocial risk factors co-occur, the present findings make it likely that the health-damaging effects of job strain that have been reported among men will be at least as severe among women workers. This tendency of health-damaging psychosocial characteristics to cluster in the same individuals and groups should compel us in future research to obtain measures of the entire known array of psychosocial risk factors to help understand pathogenic mechanisms and to guide the development of interventions to promote health and prevent disease.

Accepted for publication April 22, 1996.

This study was supported by grants HL36587 from the National Heart, Lung, and Blood Institute, MH70482 from the National Institute of Mental Health, and

AG11268 and AG12085 from the National Institute on Aging, Bethesda, Md.

Reprints: Redford B. Williams, MD, Box 3926, Department of Psychiatry, Duke University Medical Center, Durham, NC 27710.

REFERENCES

1. Karasek RA, Theorell T. *Healthy Work: Stress, Productivity, and the Reconstruction of Working Life.* New York, NY: Basic Books Inc Publishers; 1990.
2. Schnall PL, Landsbergis PA, Schwartz JE, Warren K, Pickering TG. Job strain and cardiovascular disease. *Annu Rev Public Health.* 1994;15:381-411.
3. Johnson JV, Hall EM. Job strain, work place social support, and cardiovascular disease: a cross-sectional study of a random sample of the Swedish working population. *Am J Public Health.* 1988;78:1336-1342.
4. Johnson JV, Hall EM, Theorell T. Combined effects of job strain and social isolation on cardiovascular disease morbidity and mortality in a random sample of the Swedish male working population. *Scand J Work Environ Health.* 1989; 15:271-279.
5. Karasek RA, Baker D, Marxer F, Ahlbon A, Theorell T. Job decision latitude, job demands, and cardiovascular disease: a prospective study of Swedish men. *Am J Public Health.* 1981;71:694-705.
6. LaCroix AZ. *High Demand/Low Control Work and the Incidence of CHD in the Framingham Cohort.* Chapel Hill: University of North Carolina; 1984. Thesis.
7. Falk A, Hanson BS, Isacsson S-O, Ostergren P-O. Job strain and mortality in elderly men: social network, support, and influence as buffers. *Am J Public Health.* 1992;82:1136-1139.
8. Astrand NE, Hanson BS, Isacson SO. Job demands, job decision latitude, job support, and social network factors as predictors of mortality in a Swedish pulp and paper company. *Br J Ind Med.* 1989;46:334-340.
9. Landsbergis PA, Schnall PL, Dietz D, Friedman R, Pickering TG. The patterning of psychological attributes and distress by job strain and social support in a sample of working men. *J Behav Med.* 1992;15:379-405.
10. Karasek RA, Pieper C, Schwartz J, Fry L, Schrier D. *Job Content Instrument Questionnaire and User's Guide.* New York, NY: Columbia University Job/Heart Project; 1985.
11. Costa PT, McCrae RR. *NEO Five Factor Inventory.* Odessa, Fla: Psychological Assessment Resources; 1989.
12. Beck AT, Steer RA. *Beck Depression Inventory Manual.* San Antonio, Tex: The Psychological Corporation, Harcourt Brace Jovanovich; 1987.
13. Crowne DP, Marlow D. A new scale of social desirability independent of psychopathology. *J Consult Psychol.* 1960;24:349-354.
14. Spielberger CD, Gorsuch RL, Lushene R, Vagg PR, Jacobs GA. *Manual for the State-Trait Anxiety Inventory (Form Y ['Self-Evaluation Questionnaire']).* Palo Alto, Calif: Consulting Psychologists' Press; 1983.
15. Cook W, Medley D. Proposed hostility and phariasaic-virtue scales for the MMPI. *J Appl Psychol.* 1954;38:414-418.
16. Cohen S, Mermelstein R, Kamarck T, Hoberman H. Measuring the functional components of social support. In: Sarason IG, Sarason BR, eds. *Social Support: Theory, Research and Applications.* The Hague, Holland: Martinus Nijhoff Publishers; 1983.
17. Smith TW. Hostility and health: current status of a psychosomatic hypothesis. *Health Psychol.* 1992;11:139-150.
18. Frasure-Smith N, Lesperance F, Talajic M. Depression following myocardial infarction: impact on 6-month survival. *JAMA.* 1993;270:1819-1825.
19. Kawachi I, Sparrow D, Vokonas PS, Weiss ST. Symptoms of anxiety and risk of coronary heart disease. *Circulation.* 1994;90:2225-2229.
20. House JS, Landis KR, Umberson D. Social relationships and health. *Science.* 1988;241:540-545.
21. Orth-Gomer K, Unden A-L. Type A behavior, social support, and coronary risk: interaction and significance for mortality in cardiac patients. *Psychosom Med.* 1990;52:59-72.
22. Blumenthal JA, Burg MM, Williams RB, Barefoot JC, Haney T, Zimet G. Social support, type A behavior, and coronary artery disease. *Psychosom Med.* 1987; 49:331-340.
23. Kaplan GA. Where do shared pathways lead? some reflections on a research agenda. *Psychosom Med.* 1995;57:208-212.
24. Barefoot JC, Williams RB, Siegler IC, Schroll M. Depressive affect, hostility and socioeconomic status (SES): interrelationships and joint effects on health. Presented at the Annual Meeting of the American Psychosomatic Society; March 3, 1995; New Orleans, La.
25. Adler NE, Boyce T, Chesney MA, Folkman S, Syme SL. Socioeconomic inequalities in health: no easy solution. *JAMA.* 1993;269:3140-3145.
26. Kaplan GA, Kiel JE. Socioeconomic factors and cardiovascular disease: a review of the literature. *Circulation.* 1993;88:1973-1993.
27. Pincus T, Callahen LF. What explains the association between socioeconomic status and health: primarily access to medical care or mid-body variables? *Advances.* 1995;11:4-36.
28. Marmot MG, Rose G, Shipley M, et al. Employment grade and coronary heart disease in British civil servants. *J Epidemiol Community Health.* 1978;3:244-249.
29. Kristensen T. Information bias in measurement of psychosocial work environment factors. Presented at the APA Conference on Work, Stress, and Health; September 18, 1995; Washington, DC.
30. Spector PE. A consideration of the validity and meaning of self-report measures of job conditions. In: Cooper CL, Robertson IT, eds. *International Review of Industrial and Organizational Psychology.* New York, NY: John Wiley & Sons Inc; 1992;7:123-151.
31. Hammar N, Alfredsen L, Theorell T. Job characteristics and the incidence of myocardial infarction. *Int J Epidemiol.* 1994;23:277-284.
32. Suarez EC, Luecken LJ, Kuhn CM, Schanberg SM, Siegler IC, Stallone L, Swoap RA, Zimmerman E, Williams RB. Mommy, are you stressed? the effect of marital status and children on excretion rates of urinary neuroendocrines in working women. Presented at the Annual Meeting of the Society of Behavioral Medicine; April 16, 1994; Boston, Mass.
33. Williams RB, Barefoot JC, Califf RM, Haney TL, Saunders WB, Pryor DB, Hlatky MA, Siegler IC, Mark DB. Prognostic importance of social and economic resources among medically treated patients with angiographically documented coronary artery disease. *JAMA.* 1992;267:520-524.
34. Williams RB. Somatic consequences of stress. In: Friedman MJ, Charney DS, Deutch A, eds. *Neurobiological and Clinical Consequences of Stress: From Normal Adaptation to PTSD.* New York, NY: Raven Press; 1995:403-412.
35. Keita G, Sauter S, eds. *Work and Well-Being.* Washington, DC: American Psychological Association; 1992.
36. Friedman M, Thoresen CE, Gill JJ. Alteration of type A behavior and its effect on cardiac recurrences in post myocardial infarctions patients: summary results of the Recurrent Coronary Prevention Project. *Am Heart J.* 1986;112: 653-665.
37. Frasure-Smith N, Prince R. The Ischemic Heart Disease Life Stress Monitoring Program: impact on mortality. *Psychosom Med.* 1985;47:431-445.
38. Spiegel D, Bloom JR, Kraemer HC, Gottheil E. Effect of psychosocial treatment on survival of patients with metastatic breast cancer. *Lancet.* 1989;2:888-891.
39. Fawzy FI, Fawzy NW, Hyun CS, Elashoff R, Guthrie D, Fahey JL, Morton DL. Malignant melanoma: effects of an early structured psychiatric intervention, coping, and affective state on recurrence and survival 6 years later. *Arch Gen Psychiatry.* 1993;50:681-689.

Quetiapine in Patients With Schizophrenia

A High- and Low-Dose Double-blind Comparison With Placebo

Joyce G. Small, MD; Steven R. Hirsch, MPhil, MD, FRCP, FRCPPsych; Lisa A. Arvanitis, MD; Barbara G. Miller, MS; Christopher G. G. Link, MB, ChB, MPhil, MRCPsych, Dip Pharm Med, MFPM; and the Seroquel Study Group

Background: Quetiapine fumarate (Seroquel [ICI 204,636]) is an atypical dibenzothiazepine antipsychotic with a greater affinity for 5-hydroxytryptamine$_2$ (5-HT_2) receptors than for D_2 dopamine receptors; its efficacy in patients with schizophrenia was shown in early phase 2 trials (maximum dose, 750 mg/d).

Methods: In this multicenter, double-blind, placebo-controlled trial, 286 patients hospitalized with chronic or subchronic schizophrenia (*DSM-III-R*) were randomized to 6 weeks of treatment with high-dose quetiapine fumarate (≤750 mg/d), n=96; low-dose quetiapine fumarate (≤250 mg/d), n=94; or placebo, n=96. The Brief Psychiatric Rating Scale (BPRS) and Clinical Global Impression Severity of Illness item scores were the primary efficacy variables. Secondary efficacy variables included the BPRS positive-symptom cluster score, the Modified Scale for the Assessment of Negative Symptoms summary score (United States only), and the total score from the negative scale of the Positive and Negative Syndrome Scale (Europe only). Scores were analyzed using an analysis of covariance for change from baseline at end point with last observations carried forward. The model included baseline score (covariate), center, and treatment. Extrapyramidal symptoms were assessed using the Simpson-Angus Scale and the Barnes Akathisia Scale; abnormal involuntary movements were assessed using the Abnormal Involuntary Movement Scale. Frequency distributions of grouped change-from-baseline scores were analyzed using χ^2 tests.

Results: Of 280 patients in whom the efficacy of quetiapine was evaluated, 159 (42% of those receiving high-dose treatment; 57%, low-dose treatment; and 59%, placebo) withdrew before trial completion, primarily because of treatment failure. Significant ($P<.001$, BPRS; $P=.003$, Clinical Global Impression Severity of Illness item; and $P=.003$, BPRS positive-symptom cluster) differences were identified between patients receiving high-dose quetiapine and placebo for both primary efficacy variables, with end point differences in the BPRS positive-symptom cluster score showing quetiapine's consistency in reducing positive symptoms. The reduction of negative symptoms was less consistent; high-dose quetiapine was superior on the Modified Scale for the Assessment of Negative Symptoms but not on the negative scale of the Positive and Negative Syndrome Scale. Quetiapine was well tolerated and did not induce extrapyramidal symptoms, sustained elevations of prolactin, or clinically significant changes in hematologic parameters.

Conclusions: Quetiapine is an effective antipsychotic with a favorable safety profile. The optimum dose is probably greater than 250 mg/d.

Arch Gen Psychiatry. 1997;54:549-557

From the Division of Mental Health, Larue D. Carter Memorial Hospital, Indianapolis, Ind (Dr Small); Departments of Psychiatry, Charing Cross Hospital, London, England (Dr Hirsch); Clinical and Medical Affairs, Zeneca Pharmaceuticals, Wilmington, Del (Dr Arvanitis and Ms Miller); and Medical Affairs, Zeneca Pharmaceuticals, Macclesfield, England (Dr Link). A complete list of the members of the Seroquel Study Group appears in the box on page 552.

ALTHOUGH palliative, pharmacotherapy plays an important role in the treatment of schizophrenia. The benefits of standard antipsychotic agents are well established (eg, reduced hallucinations and delusions, reduced hospitalizations, and increased patient self-reliance and productivity). Equally established are their limitations (eg, treatment-related adverse events and partial effectiveness). The commonality of these effects has been attributed to presynaptic or postsynaptic blockade of central dopamine receptors, primarily D_2 dopamine receptors,[1] giving credence to the dopamine hypothesis of schizophrenia. While standard agents differ in dosage and tolerability, comparatively, none have represented a therapeutic advance. In contrast, research prompted by the clozapine experience has produced notable advance, not merely in developing compounds that closely reproduce clozapine's atypical pharmacological features but by stimulating interest to further characterize receptor activity and possibly the disease, beyond activity at D_2 dopamine and 5-hydroxytryptamine$_2$ (5-HT_2) receptors.[2]

Quetiapine fumarate (Seroquel [ICI 204,636], Zeneca Pharmaceuticals, Wilmington, Del) is a new atypical dibenzothiazepine antipsychotic with an affinity for multiple receptors. Like clozapine, quetiapine is characterized by a greater affinity for $5HT_2$ receptors than for D_2 dopamine receptors (IC_{50} [inhibitory

PATIENTS AND METHODS

The efficacy and tolerability of 2 dose ranges of quetiapine were compared with the effects of placebo in a 6-week randomized, multicenter, double-blind, parallel-group clinical trial. Patients were recruited from 37 centers in the United States (18) and Europe (19) and provided written, informed consent before enrollment in the trial. The trial was conducted in accordance with the Declaration of Helsinki, and institutional review board or ethics committee approval was granted for each center. To ensure the reliability of data, staff at each center were trained on protocol requirements and trial procedures. Principal investigators or designated subinvestigators, all experienced in clinical interviewing and the application of *DSM-III-R* diagnostic criteria, were responsible for recorded diagnoses.

PATIENTS

Hospitalized men and women, aged 18 through 65 years, were eligible for enrollment in the trial if, based on current and historical findings, they met the *DSM-III-R* criteria[11] for chronic or subchronic schizophrenia with acute exacerbation. Other key enrollment criteria included a total score of at least 27 on the Brief Psychiatric Rating Scale[12] (BPRS) (scoring, 0-6) and scores of 3 (moderate) or greater for at least 2 of the 4 items in the BPRS positive-symptom cluster: conceptual disorganization, suspiciousness, hallucinatory behavior, and unusual thought content. A Clinical Global Impression[13] (CGI) Severity of Illness item score of at least 4 (moderately ill) was also required for enrollment.

Reasons for exclusion included any other *DSM-III-R* Axis I diagnosis; serious suicidal threats or behavior within a year of trial enrollment; mental retardation; history of convulsive disorders, severe head trauma, or organic brain disease; and risk of pregnancy. Other exclusionary criteria included use of injectable long-acting antipsychotic agents within 4 weeks of trial participation.

PROCEDURES

Screening procedures included demographic and diagnostic assessments, physical examination, review of medical history, clinical laboratory tests, and electrocardiography. Psychotropic medications were discontinued for all patients who met the enrollment criteria. In Europe, patients were drug free for at least 24 hours; in the United States, patients received placebo for a minimum of 2 days. Patients were then randomized to 1 of 3 treatments for 42 days: high-dose quetiapine fumarate (maximum daily dose, 750 mg), low-dose quetiapine fumarate (maximum daily dose, 250 mg), or placebo. Randomization was based on computer-generated randomization schemes produced per center, with patient numbers allocated in balanced blocks in a 1:1:1 ratio. Trial tablets were packaged according to randomization schedules, and patients received treatment according to sequentially assigned patient numbers. The daily dose was escalated within the dose range designated per treatment group, until an adequate therapeutic effect was achieved. Dose adjustments were permitted in response to side effects, such as sedation and postural hypotension. In the high-dose group, the maximum daily dose of 750 mg was limited to 14 days; after that, reductions to 500 mg or less were required. (This limitation was based on toxicologic data available at the time of the trial.)

Limited use of drugs for minor complaints (eg, headache, indigestion, and constipation) was permitted. Chloral hydrate, 500 to 1000 mg, was permitted orally for acute agitation or insomnia, up to 2000 mg/d. In the United States, lorazepam, 1 to 2 mg, was permitted orally or intramuscularly for severe agitation or insomnia unresponsive to chloral hydrate or dose escalation of quetiapine. In Europe, other benzodiazepines were permitted within protocol-specific guidelines for frequency of use and maximum dose. Neither chloral hydrate nor lorazepam use was permitted within 6 and 24 hours, respectively, of psychiatric or neurologic assessments. When present for at least 24 hours, EPS rated as moderate, according to the Simpson-Angus Scale for EPS,[14] were treated orally with 50 mg of diphenhydramine hydrochloride or up to 4 mg of benztropine mesylate (2 mg if given parenterally) for up to 3 days per episode. In Europe, alternate treatments for EPS were prescribed according to local practices.

ASSESSMENTS

Psychiatric symptomatology was assessed using the BPRS and CGI and the Modified Scale for the Assessment of Negative Symptoms[15] (SANS) in the United States or the negative scale of the Positive and Negative Syndrome Scale[16] (PANSS[N]) in Europe. Assessments were completed before randomization (day 0) and weekly thereafter for 6 weeks (on days 7, 14, 21, 28, 35, and 42) by personnel trained in the use of these scales (typically the investigator or designated subinvestigator).

In the United States, blood samples were collected weekly for the determination of drug plasma concentrations and were sent to the sponsor for analysis. A capillary gas chromatographic method with mass selective detection, developed and validated for the measurement of quetiapine, was used.

All adverse events were assessed for severity and relationship to treatment. On day 0 and weekly thereafter, EPS were assessed using the Simpson-Angus Scale and the 4 items on the Barnes Akathisia Scale[17]: observable restlessness, subjective awareness of restlessness, related distress, and global severity. Abnormal involuntary movements were assessed using the Abnormal Involuntary Movement Scale.[18] Other measures of safety included weekly clinical laboratory testing and urinalysis (United States only); weekly weight monitoring and daily vital signs assessments in the United States and daily assessments through day 14, then weekly, in Europe; an electrocardiographic examination on days 21 and 42; determination of plasma prolactin levels on days 21 and 42 in the United States and weekly in Europe; and a physical examination on day 42. If treatment was discontinued before day 42, patients

concentration, ie, the concentration needed to displace 50% of a given ligand from the receptor] = 148 and 329 nmol/L, respectively).[3] Although quetiapine's affinity at the D_2 dopamine receptor is considered modest in rat models, models used to predict antipsychotic activity provide considerable evidence of quetiapine's antipsychotic effects.[4] In primates, quetiapine blocks conditioned avoidance responses, reverses blinking induced underwent all efficacy and safety assessments at the time of withdrawal.

STATISTICAL METHODS

Power calculations were based on the ability to detect a minimum difference of 9 units for mean changes from baseline in BPRS total scores between the high-dose and placebo treatment groups. An SD of 14, obtained earlier in a noncomparative trial with quetiapine (data on file), was used to estimate the expected degree of patient variability. As a result, an estimated 50 patients per treatment group would provide a power of at least 0.90 to detect this difference with a 2-sided $\alpha=.05$.

Efficacy

The primary efficacy variables were the BPRS total score and the CGI Severity of Illness item score. Secondary efficacy variables included response rate, BPRS positive-symptom cluster score, the CGI Global Improvement score, and the SANS summary score (ie, the total of global ratings for affective blunting, alogia, avolition-apathy, anhedonia-asociality, and attention) or the PANSS(N) total score. Response to treatment was defined as a reduction of at least 30% from baseline in BPRS total score at any time during the randomized treatment phase.

The population for the analysis of efficacy included all patients who were randomized to treatment and had efficacy data for at least one time point after day 0. The primary end point for the analysis of efficacy was day 42, the last day of randomized treatment. However, patients who withdrew before day 42 were included in end point analyses using data carried forward from final evaluations. Data corresponding to other designated evaluation days were also analyzed with the last observations carried forward.

The proportions of patients who withdrew per treatment group, along with reasons for withdrawal, were tabulated. Baseline characteristics were compared between treatment groups using an analysis of variance (ANOVA) for continuous variables and a Cochran-Mantel-Haenszel χ^2 test for categorical measures. The ANOVA models included treatment and center. Except for CGI Global Improvement data, efficacy data were analyzed using an analysis of covariance (ANCOVA) (PROC GLM procedure, SAS Institute, Cary, NC) for change from baseline. The model included baseline score (covariate), center, and treatment. Adjusted means from the ANCOVA were compared, the pairwise differences were calculated, and 95% confidence intervals were constructed for these differences. Clinical Global Impression Global Improvement scores were analyzed using an ANOVA model. In addition to pairwise comparisons, a formal assessment of the linear relationship between dose group and response was conducted using an ANCOVA (PROC GLM procedure).

Residuals from all final ANCOVA models were evaluated for deviation from normality using the Shapiro-Wilk test. The assumption of equal variances among treatment groups was evaluated using the F test for equality of variances. The assumption of parallelism (ie, no significant baseline-by-treatment interaction, $P>.05$) and possible treatment-by-center interactions were investigated by including these interaction terms in the final model. A stratified Wilcoxon rank-sum test (a nonparametric method) was used to corroborate the findings when (in a few instances) the assumptions of the ANCOVA were untenable.

Fourteen centers (4 in the United States and 10 in Europe) did not recruit the number of patients needed (2 per treatment group) to estimate treatment effects within the center; therefore, for all efficacy analyses, data from the 4 US centers were pooled for analysis and data from the 10 European centers were pooled for a separate analysis. Overall, no treatment-by-center interactions were identified.

All statistical tests were conducted using a 2-sided $\alpha=.05$. Unless otherwise indicated, all mean changes refer to adjusted mean changes.

In the analysis of trough plasma concentrations, scatterplots of median plasma levels (calculated per patient) vs change from baseline for BPRS total, BPRS positive-symptom cluster, and CGI Severity of Illness item scores were generated for each treatment group by trial day. Linear dose-response relationships were then investigated by fitting a simple linear regression model for each treatment group, predicting median plasma level based on change from baseline for the efficacy variable.

Tolerability

All randomized patients were included in analyses of safety. Adverse events were classified using preferred terms from the Food and Drug Administration's COSTART (coding symbols for thesaurus of adverse reaction terms) dictionary. Crude incidence rates and numbers of events and their severity were tabulated by body system and preferred term for each treatment group. Vital signs and weight were summarized using descriptive statistics for actual values as well as for changes from baseline.

The distributions of Simpson-Angus Scale total scores and Abnormal Involuntary Movement Scale total scores at baseline were extremely skewed, with most patients having minimum total scores for each scale. Therefore, frequency distributions of grouped total scores and grouped change-from-baseline scores were calculated; changes less than 0 denoted improvement, changes equal to 0 denoted no change, and changes greater than 0 denoted worsening. Because a large proportion of patients also had normal responses on the Barnes Akathisia Scale, data were similarly categorized for each Barnes Akathisia Scale item. The analyses of the change from baseline for Simpson-Angus Scale and Abnormal Involuntary Movement Scale total scores and Barnes Akathisia Scale scores were based on χ^2 tests, using Cochran-Mantel-Haenszel methods to control for center effects.

An ANCOVA was also used to compare changes from baseline in laboratory data (with baseline values as covariates) and changes from baseline in electrocardiographic parameters (with baseline, center, and treatment included in the model).

by apomorphine (a dopamine agonist),[5] fully substitutes for clozapine in drug discrimination tests,[6] and, in a model valid for negative symptoms, reverses social isolation induced by amphetamine.[7] In models predictive of dystonic or dyskinetic liability, quetiapine produces few, if any, weak and variable reactions in haloperidol-sensitized and drug-naive monkeys[5] and produces only weak cataleptic responses (comparable with clozapine)

The Seroquel Study Group

Clinical Centers and Principal Investigators in the United States

Audie L. Murphy Veterans Memorial Hospital, San Antonio, Tex: C. L. Bowden, MD. *Veterans Affairs Medical Center, Philadelphia, Pa:* C. P. O'Brien, MD, PhD. *Jackson Memorial Medical Center, Miami, Fla:* R. M. Steinbook, MD. *Institute of Mental Health, Cranston, RI:* R. L. Wagner, MD. *University of Mississippi Medical Center, Jackson:* W. M. Pitts, Jr, MD. *Veterans Affairs Medical Center, Jackson, Miss:* Brian Crabtree, PharmD. *Dorothea Dix Hospital, Raleigh, NC:* M. H. N. Corrigan, MD. *Veterans Affairs Medical Center, San Diego, Calif:* J. B. Lohr, MD. *University of Texas Health Science Center at San Antonio:* A. L. Miller, MD. *San Antonio State Hospital, San Antonio, Tex:* L. Ereshefsky, PharmD. *Clinical Pharmacy Programs, San Antonio, Tex:* C. B. Anderson, PharmD. *Terrell State Hospital, Terrell, Tex:* M. A. Knesevich, MD. *New York Veterans Affairs Medical Center, New York:* J. Rotrosen, MD. *Veterans Affairs Medical Center, Little Rock, Ark:* R. R. Owen, Jr, MD. *Arkansas State Hospital, Little Rock:* C. N. Karson, MD. *Schizophrenic Research Unit, Bronx, NY:* J. P. Lindenmayer, MD. *Stanford/Veterans Affairs Mental Health Clinical Research Center, Palo Alto, Calif:* A. Pfefferbaum, MD; W. O. Faustman, PhD. *University of Cincinnati College of Medicine, Cincinnati, Ohio:* P. E. Keck, Jr, MD. *Birmingham Research Group, Hillcrest Hospital, Birmingham, Ala:* W. M. Patterson, MD. *DeKalb Medical Center, Decatur, Ga:* R. A. Riesenberg, MD; M. B. Gladson, MD. *Sand Lake Hospital, Orlando, Fla:* I. S. Kolin, MD.

Clinical Centers and Principal Investigators in Europe

Horton Hospital, Surrey, England: T. R. E. Barnes, MD, MB, BS. *West Middlesex Hospital, Middlesex, England:* T. Sensky, MB, BS, PhD. *St Mary Abbot Hospital, London, England:* M. Riccio. *Gordon Hospital, London:* S. Franks, MD, MB, BS. *Ealing Hospital, Middlesex, England:* A. Jolley, MD. *Charing Cross Hospital, London:* C. Hallstrom, MD, MB, ChB. *Levernadale Hospital, Glasgow, Scotland:* E. Bennie, MB, ChB. *Clinique de Psychiatrie et de Psycologie Hospital Pasteur, Nice, France:* G. Darcourt, MD. *Clinique Psychiatre, Strasbourg, France:* M. Patris, MD. *Heatherwood Hospital, Berkshire, England:* M. DeSilva, MB, BS. *Fairfield Hospital, Hertfordshire, England:* A. G. Patel, MB, BS. *Innsbruck University Clinic, Innsbruck, Austria:* W. W. Fleischhacker, MD. *Psychiatric University Clinic, Vienna, Austria:* M. Dietzel, Dr Med. *Psychiatric Research Institute, Prague, Czechoslovakia:* D. Seifertova, MD, CSc, PhD. *Psychiatric Hospital, Prague:* O. Vinar, Dr Med. *Charles University, Prague:* F. Faltus, DrSc. *Semmelweis Orvostudomanyi Egyetem, Budapest, Hungary:* I. Bitter, MD, PhD. *Unversity Medical School of Pecs, Pecs, Hungary:* K. Ozsvath, MD, PhD. *Stanley Road Hospital, West Yorkshire, England:* S. H. Shaw, MB, ChB. *The General Hospital, Hartlepool, England:* S. N. Mahapatra, MB, BS. *Bassetlaw District General Hospital, Nottingham, England:* T. K. Szulecka, MD. *Halifax General Hospital, West Yorkshire, England:* K. Sundararajan, MB, BS. *St Mary's Psychiatric Hospital, Caslebar, County Mayo, Ireland:* F. Creaven, MB, BCh. *St Luke's Hospital, Clonmel, County Tipperary, Ireland:* J. Lynch, LRCPI. *Psychiatrische Klinik, Düsseldorf, Germany:* E. Klieser, Dr Med. *The Queen's University of Belfast, Belfast, Northern Ireland:* S. J. Cooper, MD. *University Clinic of Vienna, Vienna:* H. Aschauer, MD.

in monkeys trained in movement control.[6] These preclinical findings—all consistent with an atypical profile—proved applicable in predicting efficacy and the liability of extrapyramidal symptoms (EPS) in humans. In early phase 2 placebo-controlled trials,[8,9] quetiapine was superior to placebo in treating positive and negative symptoms, with tolerability comparable with placebo. In the first active-controlled trial,[10] quetiapine was comparable with chlorpromazine in efficacy and it was well tolerated. In the last in a series of 5 phase 2 trials, 2 dose ranges of quetiapine (ie, high and low) were compared with placebo. The results are provided in this article.

RESULTS

PATIENTS

A total of 286 patients (169 from the United States and 117 from Europe) were randomized to treatment: 96 to high-dose quetiapine, 94 to low-dose quetiapine, and 96 to placebo. None of the 37 centers (18 in the United States and 19 in Europe) recruited more than 12% of all randomized patients.

Generally, treatment groups were well balanced for demographic and baseline characteristics. The typical patient was a 77-kg man, aged 37 years, with a diagnosis of acute exacerbation of either chronic paranoid schizophrenia or chronic undifferentiated schizophrenia (**Table 1**).

Forty-eight patients in the high-dose group, 54 in the low-dose group, and 57 in the placebo-treated group withdrew before they completed 6 weeks of treatment for reasons shown in Table 1. Most withdrawals (25 in the high-dose group, 34 in the low-dose group, and 42 in the placebo group) were attributed to treatment failure.

CLINICAL EFFICACY

A total of 280 patients (94 in the high-dose group, 92 in the low-dose group, and 94 in the placebo group) were included in BPRS analyses, with one additional patient (in the high-dose group) included in CGI analyses.

At baseline, mean BPRS total scores were comparable between both groups who received quetiapine and between the groups who received low-dose quetiapine and placebo. A statistically significant (P=.05) 3-point difference in mean scores between the high-dose group (score, 41) and the placebo group (score, 38) was adjusted by the inclusion of the baseline score as a covariate. The mean change from baseline in BPRS total score was significantly greater at end point (**Table 2**) for the high-dose group (change, −8.7) compared with mean changes in the low-dose (change, −4.2) and placebo (change, −1.0) groups ($2.24>t>1.96$, df=184, P=.04 and

Table 1. Demographics, Psychiatric History, and Reasons for Withdrawal

	Patients Who Received*		
Characteristic	High-Dose Quetiapine Fumarate (n=96)	Low-Dose Quetiapine Fumarate (n=94)	Placebo (n=96)
Patients			
M	66 (69)	73 (78)	64 (67)
F	30 (31)	21 (22)	32 (33)
Mean age (SD) [range], y	36 (9)[20-61]	37 (9)[19-63]	38 (10)[21-63]
Race			
White	66 (69)	63 (67)	73 (76)
Black	19 (20)	20 (21)	16 (17)
Other	11 (11)	11 (12)	7 (7)
DSM-III-R diagnosis: schizophrenia with acute exacerbation			
Paranoid	50 (52)	57 (60)	50 (52)
Undifferentiated	32 (33)	24 (25)	29 (30)
Disorganized	14 (15)	10 (11)	12 (12)
Other	0	3 (3)	5 (5)
Mean age at first treatment (US patients only) (SD) [range], y	22 (6)[9-42]	23 (6)[4-44]	22 (6)[4-39]
Previous hospitalizations (US patients only)			
≤8	31 (58)	24 (48)	25 (51)
>8	22 (42)	26 (52)	24 (49)
Unknown	4	5	8
Withdrawals, total	48 (50)	54 (57)	57 (59)
Treatment failure†	25 (52)	34 (63)	42 (74)
Withdrawn consent†	10 (21)	4 (7)	8 (14)
Adverse event†	7 (15)	7 (13)	3 (5)
Intercurrent medical event†	1 (2)	1 (2)	0
Protocol violation†	1 (2)	1 (2)	0
Other†	4 (8)	7 (13)	4 (7)

All data are given as the number (percentage) of patients unless otherwise specified.
†*The number (percentage of total) patients is given.*

$t>3.29$, $df=186$, $P<.001$, respectively). From day 14 onward, differences between mean changes in the high-dose and placebo groups were significant ($P\leq.01$, BPRS total scores) (**Figure 1**). For each evaluation made before end point, mean decreases from baseline in BPRS total score for the high-dose group were larger than mean decreases in the low-dose group, which were larger than those in the placebo group. The test for a linear dose-response relationship was significant ($P\leq.05$) from day 14 onward. Across treatment groups, more patients responded to quetiapine (high dose, 53%; low dose, 50%) than placebo (37%). The difference in the distribution of responders among treatment groups was significant (χ^2 [adjusted for center]=6.002, $df=2$, $P=.05$).

A significant ($P=.003$) end point difference between the high-dose and placebo groups was also achieved for change from baseline in the BPRS positive-symptom cluster score (Table 2), which showed quetiapine's consistency of effect in reducing positive symptoms.

Mean CGI Severity of Illness item scores were comparable among treatment groups at baseline. Differences between the high-dose and placebo groups were significant at end point ($P=.003$) (Table 2) and from day 21 onward ($P\leq.02$) (**Figure 2**). Mean changes indicated improvement in patients treated with quetiapine, with greater decreases in the high-dose group than in the low-dose group; changes in the placebo group were negligible. A dose-response relationship was shown with significance ($P\leq.05$) achieved from day 21 onward.

Mean CGI Global Improvement scores at end point were significantly better (lower) in the high-dose group (score, 3.4) than in either the low-dose group (score, 4.0; $P\leq.03$) or the placebo group (score, 4.1; $P=.006$) (Table 2). Differences between the high-dose and placebo groups were significant ($P\leq.02$) from day 14 onward. Differences between high-dose and low-dose groups were marginally significant on days 21 and 35 ($P=.08$ for both days), with lower (better) scores in the high-dose group.

Mean SANS summary scores for patients treated with high-dose quetiapine (n=55) steadily improved (ie, decreased) through day 42. For patients treated with low-dose quetiapine (n=51), small mean decreases were seen through day 28 before scores increased toward those at baseline. Scores for placebo-treated patients (n=56) increased from day 21 onward, indicating deterioration. Differences between the high-dose group and both the low-dose and placebo groups were significant at end point ($2.63>t>2.28$, $df=104$, $P=.02$ and $3.39>t>2.87$, $df=109$, $P=.004$, respectively) (Table 2) as well as from day 28 onward. Mean changes from baseline for subscale global item scores indicated improvement in all 5 items for patients treated with high-dose quetiapine.

Differences among treatment groups in PANSS(N) scores were not significant ($P\geq.10$) at end point (Table 2) or throughout the trial with one exception (day 14, high-dose vs placebo group, $P=.04$ favoring the high-dose group).

Table 2. Assessments of Efficacy: Pairwise Comparisons at End Point for Change From Baseline*

Scale	Treatment	No. of Patients	Baseline, Mean±SD	End Point, Mean±SD	Change From Baseline, Mean±SE†	P‡ (ANCOVA)
Primary measures						
BPRS total score	Quetiapine (H)	92	41.0±9.6	31.2±15.4	−8.7±1.64	<.001 vs P
	Quetiapine (L)	94	38.9±9.8	34.4±16.0	−4.2±1.62	.04 vs H
	P	92	38.4±9.7	37.1±18.8	−1.0±1.61	.15 vs L
CGI Severity of Illness item score	Quetiapine (H)	95	5.1±0.8	4.4±1.3	−0.6±0.13	.003 vs P
	Quetiapine (L)	92	5.1±0.8	4.7±1.4	−0.3±0.13	.08 vs H
	P	94	4.9±0.7	4.9±1.3	−0.1±0.13	.23 vs L
Secondary measures						
BPRS positive-symptom cluster score	Quetiapine (H)	92	3.5±0.8	2.7±1.4	−0.9±0.13	.003 vs P
	Quetiapine (L)	94	3.6±0.9	3.0±1.5	−0.6±0.13	.11 vs H
	P	92	3.6±1.0	3.2±1.5	−0.4±0.13	.17 vs L
CGI Global Improvement	Quetiapine (H)	95	NA	3.4±1.7§	NA	.006 vs P
	Quetiapine (L)	94	NA	4.0±1.7§	NA	.03 vs H
	P	92	NA	4.1±1.8§	NA	.55 vs L
SANS summary score	Quetiapine (H)	55	15.8±3.6	14.0±3.6	−1.7±0.47	.02 vs P
	Quetiapine (L)	51	15.8±3.9	15.9±4.6	0.3±0.48	.004 vs H
	P	56	14.5±3.6	14.8±4.3	−0.1±0.46	.54 vs L
PANSS(N) total score	Quetiapine (H)	38	27.5±9.4	22.4±8.6	−4.4±1.2	.10 vs P
	Quetiapine (L)	38	25.5±8.7	22.5±9.2	−2.9±1.1	.32 vs H
	P	37	24.4±6.6	22.7±8.9	−1.9±1.1	.52 vs L

**ANCOVA indicates analysis of covariance; BPRS, Brief Psychiatric Rating Scale; CGI, Clinical Global Impression; H, high-dose group; L, low-dose group; NA, not applicable; P, placebo group; PANSS(N), negative scale of the Positive and Negative Syndrome Scale; and SANS, Modified Scale for the Assessment of Negative Symptoms.*

†Adjusted mean from ANCOVA.

‡All values are from pairwise t tests of adjusted means from ANCOVA models including baseline score, center, and treatment.

§Adjusted mean from analysis of variance.

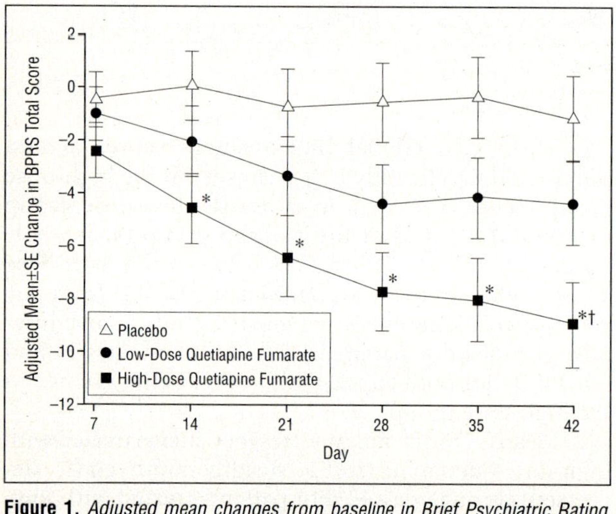

Figure 1. *Adjusted mean changes from baseline in Brief Psychiatric Rating Scale (BPRS) total score for each treatment group by day. The asterisks indicate P≤.05 for the high-dose group vs the placebo group; dagger, P≤.05 for the high-dose group vs the low-dose group.*

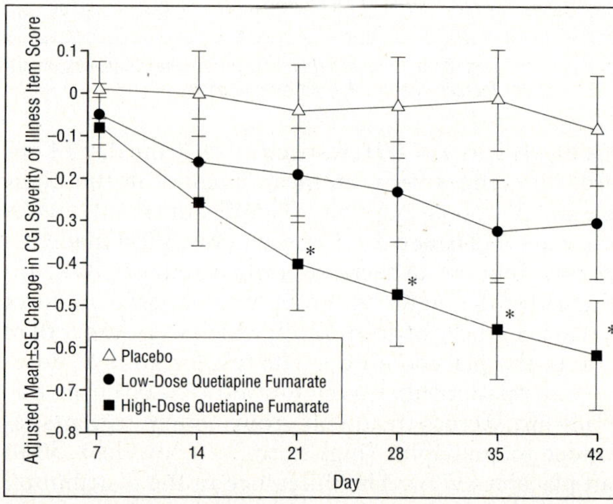

Figure 2. *Adjusted mean changes from baseline in the Clinical Global Impression (CGI) Severity of Illness item score for each treatment group by day. The asterisks indicate P≤.05 for the high-dose group vs the placebo group.*

At end point, trough plasma concentrations of quetiapine ranged from 21.5 to 169.0 ng/mL (mean, 67.8 ng/mL) in the high-dose group and from 17.3 to 90.4 ng/mL (mean, 41.5 ng/mL) in the low-dose group. No statistically significant relationships were found at end point between the efficacy variables tested and plasma concentrations of quetiapine.

TOLERABILITY

The mean daily dose of quetiapine fumarate was 360 mg in the high-dose group (range, 50-566 mg) and 209 mg in the low-dose group (range, 50-267 mg) (one patient erroneously received one 750-mg dose); for patients who completed the trial, the mean daily dose increased to 488 and 248 mg/d, respectively. The mean duration of treatment was 29, 28, and 26 days for patients in the high-dose (median, 38 days), low-dose (median, 28 days), and placebo (median, 26 days) groups, respectively. Approximately 50% of the patients in each treatment group received chloral hydrate, on average, for 9 to 10 days. One hundred twenty-two patients—36 (38%) in the high-dose group, 48 (51%) in the low-dose group, and 38 (40%) in the placebo group—received lorazepam or some other

Table 3. Most Frequent Adverse Events by Treatment Group*

Adverse Event	High-Dose Quetiapine Fumarate (n=96)	Low-Dose Quetiapine Fumarate (n=94)	Placebo (n=96)
	No. (%) of Patients Who Received		
Agitation†	26 (27)	26 (28)	19 (20)
Somnolence	24 (25)	18 (19)	14 (15)
Headache	18 (19)	11 (12)	11 (11)
Dizziness	11 (11)	10 (11)	1 (1)
Constipation	11 (11)	6 (6)	3 (3)
Insomnia	10 (10)	12 (13)	18 (19)
Tachycardia	7 (7)	5 (5)	5 (5)
Pain	7 (7)	3 (3)	5 (5)
Pharyngitis	7 (7)	2 (2)	4 (4)
Rash	7 (7)	0	3 (3)
Alanine aminotransferase level increased	6 (6)	11 (12)	1 (1)
Dry mouth	6 (6)	4 (4)	1 (1)
Dyspepsia	6 (6)	3 (3)	4 (4)
Nausea	6 (6)	3 (3)	4 (4)
Asthenia	5 (5)	3 (3)	1 (1)
Vomiting	1 (1)	5 (5)	7 (7)

**Those with an incidence of greater than 5% in any treatment group.*

†Agitation accounted for 60% of all adverse events rated as severe: in 13% of patients in the high-dose group, 16% in the low-dose group, and 10% in the placebo group. All other adverse events reported as severe (ie, insomnia, psychosis, hostility, and somnolence) occurred in 2 or fewer patients per treatment group, with the exception of somnolence (3 patients in the high-dose group). Most severe adverse events were representative of the illness.

benzodiazepine, on average, for 3 to 6 days. Medications indicated for the treatment of EPS were prescribed infrequently and for fewer patients (3) in the low-dose group than in either the high-dose group (7) or the placebo group (10).

Most adverse events were rated mild or moderate; those events that occurred in more than 5% of patients (in any treatment group) appear in **Table 3**. Agitation was the most frequently reported adverse event in each treatment group and was likely associated with the underlying illness. Somnolence, not unexpected with antipsychotic medications, occurred in both groups who received quetiapine (25% in the high-dose group and 19% in the low-dose group) as well as in the placebo group (15%). Motor system adverse events were limited, with similar incidences seen across treatment groups, and may have reflected worsening of symptoms after anticholinergic medications were discontinued at trial enrollment. The incidence of akathisia ranged from 1% in the placebo group to 4% in the high-dose group. Conversely, tremor occurred in 5% of placebo-treated patients but not in patients treated with quetiapine.

Seventeen patients (7 in the high-dose group, 7 in the low-dose group, and 3 in the placebo group) withdrew because of adverse events. Events at the high dose included postural hypotension, dizziness, and somnolence (singularly and in combination); hypotension; agitation; and a decreased white blood cell count (which remained within normal limits). Events at the low dose included hypotension with tachycardia; postural hypotension; peripheral edema with maculopapular rash;

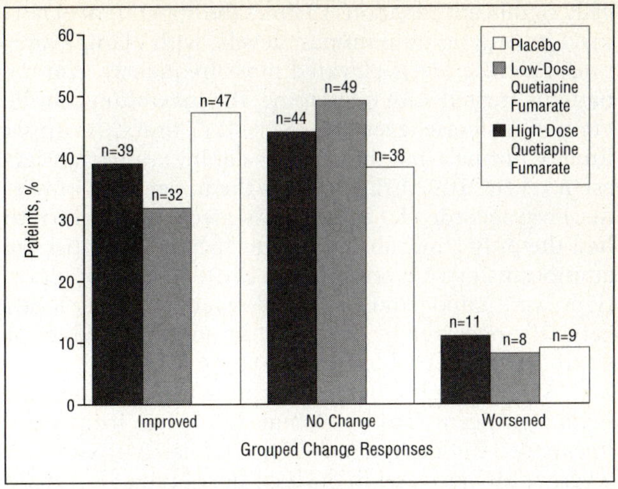

Figure 3. *Simpson-Angus Scale total score: grouped change responses for extrapyramidal symptoms at end point. Improved indicates a change of less than 0; no change, a change of 0; and worsened, a change greater than 0.*

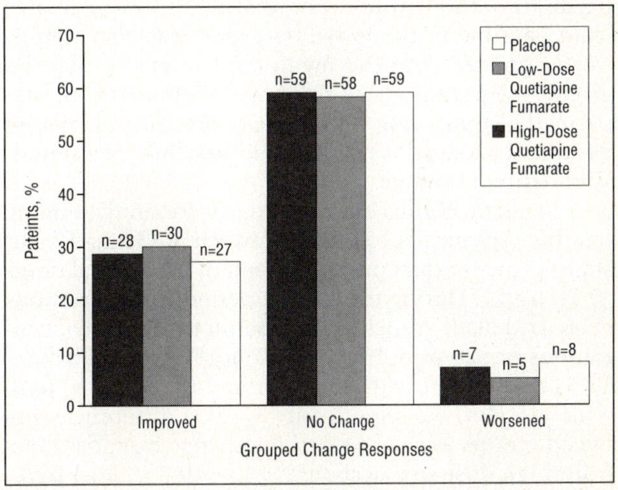

Figure 4. *Barnes Akathisia Scale score: grouped change responses for global clinical assessment of akathisia at end point. Improved indicates a change of less than 0; no change, a change of 0; and worsened, a change greater than 0.*

sinus bradycardia; increased concentrations of alanine aminotransferase, aspartate aminotransferase, and γ-glutamyltransferase; depression; and anorexia with somnolence, speech disorder, and hypokinesia. In the placebo group, tachycardia, nausea and vomiting, and rash with flatulence, pain, and peripheral edema led to withdrawal. No patients died.

No statistically significant differences were identified at end point for any pairwise comparison of change from baseline in Simpson-Angus Scale total scores (**Figure 3**), Barnes Akathisia Scale scores for any item, including global clinical assessment of akathisia (**Figure 4**), or Abnormal Involuntary Movement Scale total scores.

Quetiapine had no clinically important effects on hematologic parameters when administered for up to 6 weeks.

Fourteen patients (5 in the high-dose group, 8 in the low-dose group, and 1 in the placebo group) had clinically significant elevations (3 times the upper limit of normal) in hepatic transaminase levels, with alanine aminotransferase levels elevated most frequently. Among patients treated with quetiapine, the maximum alanine aminotransferase level was 387 U/L (7 times the upper limit of normal), but the greatest alanine aminotransferase level (ie, 1092 U/L, 18 times the upper limit of normal) was recorded for a placebo-treated patient who also had the only clinically significant increase in aspartate aminotransferase levels (to 402 U/L). Generally, elevations were minor, transient, and reversible; peak levels generally occurred by day 14 or 21 and returned to, or approached, pretrial levels during the trial.

At end point, differences among treatment groups were significant ($P \leq .05$) for mean change from baseline in total triiodothyronine (T_3) and total thyroxine (T_4) levels; mean decreases in the high-dose group (T_3, −0.13 nmol/L; T_4, −25 nmol/L [1.9 μg/dL]) were significantly greater than mean changes in the low-dose (T_3, −0.01 nmol/L, $P=.05$; T_4, −13 nmol/L [1.0 μg/dL], $P<.001$) and placebo (T_3, 0.08 nmol/L, $P<.001$; T_4, −1 nmol/L [−0.08 μg/dL], $P<.001$) groups. For total T_4, the mean change from baseline in the low-dose group was also significantly greater than the mean change in the placebo group, suggesting a dose-response relationship. No statistically significant differences were found among treatment groups for change from baseline for thyroid-stimulating hormone.

Mean prolactin concentrations were similar among treatment groups at baseline (between 30-37 μg/L) and slightly greater than the upper limit of the normal range (0-20 μg/L). During the 6-week period, concentrations decreased in all groups. At end point, the mean concentrations (±SD) were 13.3 (±11.3) μg/L at the high dose, 12.5 (±14.6) μg/L at the low dose, and 18.3 (±20.4) μg/L with placebo. No significant ($P>.05$) differences between groups were identified for change from baseline: from high dose to placebo (±SE), −19.0 (±1.9) μg/L, −19.9 (±1.8) μg/L, and −14.9 (±1.9) μg/L.

Quetiapine had no clinically important effects on electrocardiographic parameters. Small increases (7-8 beats per minute) in atrial and ventricular rates were observed at end point in patients treated with quetiapine. Although differences between quetiapine and placebo were significant (high dose, $2.58>t>2.24$, $df=153$, $P=.01$; low dose, $3.29>t>2.81$, $df=152$, $P=.003$), increased heart rates as identified by electrocardiogram were not corroborated by pulse rates. No statistically significant differences were identified between treatment groups for change in QTc intervals.

Treatment with quetiapine was associated with clinically significant weight gain (an increase of ≥7% from baseline weight) in 25% of the patients in the high-dose group compared with 16% in the low-dose group and 5% in the placebo group.

COMMENT

The results of this placebo-controlled multicenter trial showed that, at daily doses greater than 250 mg, quetiapine fumarate was effective for the treatment of acute exacerbation of chronic or subchronic schizophrenia, evident in the consistency of treatment effects across all primary and most secondary efficacy variables. Statistically significant differences were identified primarily between high-dose quetiapine fumarate (≤750 mg/d) and placebo with significant ($P \leq .05$) dose-response relationships identified among the 3 treatment groups for both of the primary efficacy variables (ie, BPRS total score and CGI Severity of Illness item score). Daily treatment with low-dose quetiapine was never statistically superior to placebo, thereby suggesting that the optimum daily dose of quetiapine fumarate is probably greater than 250 mg.

The consistency of effect in reducing positive symptoms was supported by a statistically significant end point difference between high-dose quetiapine and placebo for change from baseline in BPRS positive-symptom cluster scores.

The effect of quetiapine on negative symptoms was less consistent. Clinically and statistically significant differences between treatment groups were demonstrated based on SANS summary scores (US patients) but not PANSS(N) scores (European patients). Regardless of the scale used, severity of baseline negative symptoms seemed to be similar among patients when ratings for subscale global items or PANSS(N) items were reviewed. Differences in the way in which negative symptoms were conceptualized or defined between the 2 scales may have accounted for some of the discrepancy in results.

Overall, quetiapine was well tolerated. Adverse events were generally not alarming and fell into 2 categories: those known to occur with antipsychotic agents, including sedation and somnolence, and those related to the underlying illness, such as agitation and insomnia. The use of concomitant sedatives was similar among treatment groups; therefore, somnolence was considered a mild treatment effect in patients treated with quetiapine even though it was reported for placebo-treated patients as well.

Analysis of Simpson-Angus Scale total scores and Barnes Akathisia Scale scores, similar incidences of motor system adverse events across quetiapine and placebo treatment groups, and the limited need for anticholinergic medications suggest a minimal liability of EPS with quetiapine. These results and those from other phase 2 quetiapine trials[8-10] suggest that patients may better tolerate quetiapine and thereby gain maximum benefit from treatment.

Although the decreases in total T_3 and T_4 concentrations seen in this trial are not typically seen with other antipsychotic agents, the implications of these changes, given the relative lack of change in thyroid-stimulating hormone, cannot be fully understood without evaluating other measures of thyroid function, namely, free T_4, free T_3, and thyroid-binding globulin. Notably, clinical hypothyroidism was not seen.

Mean decreases in prolactin levels at end point in the groups receiving quetiapine were similar to those in the placebo group. The lack of sustained serum prolactin elevations in this trial, and in other phase 2 trials, further distinguishes quetiapine from standard antipsychotic medications and suggests that treatment will not be compromised by effects typically seen when prolactin is elevated (eg, impotence, amenorrhea, and galactorrhea).

Patients treated with quetiapine had a mean weight gain of 2 kg, compared with 0.1 kg for patients in the placebo group; however, weight gain did not necessitate withdrawal of treatment for any patient and may or may not have been clinically important during the 6-week period. Often weight gain in patients treated for acute psychosis seems more a function of a return to preexacerbation status and other aspects of well-being associated with improvement in psychosis rather than of treatment.

This trial was limited by several design factors. A fixed, rather than a flexible, dosing schedule may have provided a better comparison between the targeted 250-mg low dose and 750-mg high dose. Additionally, while findings at 6 weeks provide a good indication of treatment effect, effects of longer-term exposure, currently under investigation, are unclear. Other limitations, such as lack of structured diagnostic interview assessments, in all likelihood did not adversely affect clinical judgments of improvement or worsening. The dropout rate was not ideal but neither was it unexpected nor inconsistent with findings from other placebo-controlled trials of currently accepted antipsychotic medications.[19,20]

Results from this trial strengthen and corroborate results from previous phase 2 trials in which quetiapine was effective in the treatment of acute exacerbation of schizophrenia, with consistency of effects seen across all primary efficacy variables. In 2 other placebo-controlled trials and 1 active-controlled trial, quetiapine was superior to placebo and comparable with chlorpromazine, respectively, in reducing positive symptoms. Efficacy in reducing negative symptoms has been consistent to date based on SANS data.

With statistically significant differences seen primarily between the group that received high-dose quetiapine and the placebo group, the optimal total daily dose of quetiapine fumarate is most likely greater than 250 mg. Clearly additional trials using fixed doses are needed to determine quetiapine's ideal therapeutic dose range; its comparability with haloperidol and newer antipsychotic medications, such as risperidone; and its efficacy in treatment-resistant patients. Until such research is complete, quetiapine's pharmacological features may still offer considerable insight about the drug's potential. In certain animal models, quetiapine, unlike risperidone, is indistinguishable from clozapine. Should these findings equate with clinical significance, especially in treatment-resistant patients, quetiapine will play an important role in the treatment of schizophrenia and our understanding of the disease.

Accepted for publication November 6, 1996.

This study was supported by a grant from Zeneca Pharmaceuticals, Macclesfield, England, and Wilmington, Del.

We thank Suzanne Bristow-Marcalus for medical writing support; Jean Fennimore, RN, and Alison Smith, MSc, for trial organization and management support; Gary Cooper, MS, Jacqueline Fiore, Lesley Farrow, and Barney Horne for trial monitoring support; and Kathleen Jelliffe, Denise Redkar-Brown, Joy Russo, and Thais Womack for data management support.

Reprints: Lisa A. Arvanitis, MD, CNS Clinical Research, Clinical and Medical Affairs, Zeneca Pharmaceuticals, Office Wing 2 (OW-2), 1800 Concord Pike, Wilmington, DE 19850.

REFERENCES

1. Peroutka SJ, Snyder SH. Relationship of neuroleptic drug effects at brain dopamine, serotonin, alpha-adrenergic, and histamine receptors to clinical potency. *Am J Psychiatry.* 1980;137:1518-1522.
2. Kane JM, Freeman HL. Towards more effective antipsychotic treatment. *Br J Psychiatry.* 1994;165:22-31.
3. Saller CF, Salama AI. Seroquel: biochemical profile of a potential atypical antipsychotic. *Psychopharmacology.* 1993;112:285-292.
4. Goldstein JM. Pre-clinical pharmacology of new atypical antipsychotics in late stage development. *Expert Opinion Invest Drugs.* 1995;4:291-298.
5. Migler BM, Litwin LC, Sutton EB, Malick JB. Seroquel: behavioral effects in conventional and novel tests for atypical antipsychotic drug. *Psychopharmacology.* 1993;112:293-307.
6. Carey G, Bergman J. Discriminative stimulus effects of proposed atypical antipsychotics in clozapine-trained squirrel monkeys. *Behav Pharmacol.* 1994;5 (suppl 1):114.
7. Ellenbroek BA, Lubbers LJ, Cools AR. The activity of 'Seroquel' (ICI 204,636) in animal models for atypical properties of antipsychotics: a comparison with clozapine. *Neuropsychopharmacology.* In press.
8. Fabre LF, Arvanitis LA, Pultz J, Jones VM, Malick JB, Slotnick VB. ICI 204,636, a novel atypical antipsychotic: early indication of safety and efficacy in patients with chronic and subchronic schizophrenia. *Clin Ther.* 1995;17:366-378.
9. Borison RL, Arvanitis LA, Miller BG, and the US Seroquel Study Group. ICI 204,636, an atypical antipsychotic: efficacy and safety in a multicenter, placebo-controlled trial in patients with schizophrenia. *J Clin Psychopharmacol.* 1996; 16:158-169.
10. Goldstein JM, Arvanitis LA. ICI 204,636 (Seroquel): a dibenzothiazepine atypical antipsychotic: review of preclinical pharmacology and highlights of phase II clinical trials. *CNS Drug Rev.* 1995;1:50-73.
11. American Psychiatric Association. *Diagnostic and Statistical Manual of Mental Disorders, Third Edition, Revised.* Washington, DC: American Psychiatric Association; 1987.
12. Overall JE, Gorham DR. The Brief Psychiatric Rating Scale. *Psychol Rep.* 1962; 10:799-812.
13. *CGI Clinical Global Impressions: ECDEU Assessment Manual for Psychopharmacology (Revised Edition).* Rockville, Md: US Dept of Health, Education, and Welfare; 1976:218-222.
14. Simpson GM, Angus JW. A rating scale for extrapyramidal side effects. *Acta Psychiatr Scand.* 1970;212:11-19.
15. Andreasen N. *Modified Scale for the Assessment of Negative Symptoms.* Rockville, Md: Dept of Health and Human Services, Public Health Administration; 1984. National Institutes of Mental Health publication ADM 9-102.
16. Kay SR, Opler LA, Lindenmayer J-P. The positive and negative syndrome scale (PANSS): rationale and standardisation. *Br J Psychiatry.* 1989;155:59-65.
17. Barnes TRE. A rating scale for drug-induced akathisia. *Br J Psychiatry.* 1989; 154:672-676.
18. *AIMS: ECDEU Assessment Manual for Psychopharmacology (Revised Edition).* Rockville, Md: US Dept of Health, Education, and Welfare; 1976:534-535. US Dept of Health, Education, and Welfare publication ADM 76-338.
19. Marder SR, Meibach RC. Risperidone in the treatment of schizophrenia. *Am J Psychiatry.* 1994;151:825-835.
20. Chouinard G, Jones B, Remington G, Bloom D, Addington D, MacEwan GW, Labelle A, Beuclair L, Arnott W. A Canadian multicenter placebo-controlled study of fixed doses of riperidone and haloperidol in the treatment of chronic schizophrenic patients. *J Clin Psychopharmacol.* 1993;13:25-40.

ORIGINAL ARTICLE

Increased Concentrations of Presynaptic Proteins in the Cingulate Cortex of Subjects With Schizophrenia

Steven M. Gabriel, PhD; Vahram Haroutunian, PhD; Peter Powchik, MD; William G. Honer, MD, FRCPC; Michael Davidson, MD; Peter Davies, PhD; Kenneth L. Davis, MD

Background: Cytoarchitectural and neurochemical studies demonstrate disorganization in the cerebral cortex in schizophrenia, which perhaps underlies the severe behavioral disturbances of the disease. This neuronal disarray should be accompanied by synaptic abnormalities. As such, presynaptic proteins have proved valuable indexes of synaptic density and their concentrations have correlated markedly with synaptic loss. Our study sought to determine whether abnormalities exist in the concentrations of presynaptic proteins in the postmortem cerebral cortex of subjects with schizophrenia.

Methods: Presynaptic protein immunoreactivities were assessed in 4 different cerebrocortical regions derived from 16 elderly controls, 19 elderly subjects with schizophrenia, and 24 subjects with Alzheimer's disease. Tissues were assayed with the monoclonal antibodies EP10 and SP4, which recognize synaptophysin, and the monoclonal antibodies SP6 and SP14, which detect syntaxin and synaptosomal–associated protein-25-kd immunoreactivities, respectively.

Results: In subjects with schizophrenia relative to controls, presynaptic proteins were increased in the cingulate cortex, but were unchanged in the temporal, frontal, and parietal cortices. In contrast, when cases with Alzheimer's disease were compared with controls, presynaptic proteins were decreased in the frontal, temporal, and parietal samples.

Conclusions: These findings reveal changes in the synaptic organization of the cingulate cortex in schizophrenia relative to other areas examined. These changes are distinct from the deficits in presynaptic proteins observed in Alzheimer's disease.

Arch Gen Psychiatry. 1997;54:559-566

Studies consistently report changes in the postmortem cingulate and prefrontal cortices in schizophrenia.[1,2] Reports of decreased γ-amino butyric acid (GABA) neurotransmission in the cortex and hippocampus[3-5] are complemented by findings of increased numbers of $GABA_A$ receptors and ascending vertical axons.[6,7] These changes do not seem to result from prolonged neuroleptic exposure, postmortem interval (PMI), sex, or age.[6,8,9] We investigated whether neuropathologic alterations in schizophrenia are accompanied by changes in a fundamental neuronal element like the synapse.

Synaptic neurotransmission, like all forms of exocytosis, requires an array of proteins. These proteins have varying ion and guanine nucleotide sensitivities and possess intricate functional and biochemical kinships. The key links in this interaction are the soluble *N*-ethylmaleimide–sensitive fusion proteins, which, together with the soluble *N*-ethylmaleimide–sensitive fusion attachment proteins, bind to cellular membranes throughout the body in many species.[10-12] The soluble *N*-ethylmaleimide–sensitive fusion attachment proteins attach to soluble *N*-ethylmaleimide–sensitive fusion attachment protein receptors embedded in membranes. Synaptosomal–associated protein-25 kd (SNAP-25) and syntaxins are localized to the presynaptic membrane and are considered target soluble N-ethylmaleimide–sensitive fusion attachment protein receptors.[10] In mature neurons, these target receptors are complemented by vesicular proteins that include synaptotagamin and vesicle-associated membrane protein/synaptobrevin.[10-12] These complex interactions enable vesicles to be docked and ready for neurotransmitter release. The 38-d molecular weight protein, synaptophysin, may exist as a hexamer and enter the exocytotic process by forming a gap junction or fusion pore.[12,13]

From the Departments of Psychiatry, Mount Sinai School of Medicine, New York, NY (Drs Gabriel, Haroutunian, Powchik, Davidson, and Davis); the Bronx Veterans Affairs Medical Center (Drs Gabriel, Haroutunian, Powchik, Davidson, and Davis); and the Department of Pathology, Albert Einstein College of Medicine, (Dr Davies), Bronx NY; and the Department of Psychiatry, University of British Columbia, Vancouver (Dr Honer).

SUBJECTS, MATERIALS, AND METHODS

SUBJECTS

The subjects with schizophrenia were inpatients that met *DSM-III-R* criteria based on a retrospective review of medical records (n=13) or antemortem assessment with a review of medical records (n=6).[27] They did not meet criteria for AD.[28,29] Their average length of hospitalization was 45 years, ranging from 21 to 66 years. The cases with AD were nursing home residents who satisfied the criteria for AD [28,29] and had no history of additional psychiatric illness. The elderly control group contained nursing home residents who were cognitively and histopathologically normal subjects (n=13) or subjects with multi-infarct dementia based on a review of medical records with findings of cerebrovascular disease and multiple infarcts sufficient to account for a dementia (n=3). These cases of multi-infarct dementia had infarcts distal to the regions sampled, had no neurochemical abnormalities based on earlier studies,[30,31] and the exclusion of their data did not affect the outcome of any of the significance tests described herein. Cognitive impairment was assessed with the clinical dementia rating scale.[32]

MATERIALS AND METHODS

Specimen Preparation

Four left hemispheric samples were excised in single gyri. Cytoarchitectural verifications of Brodmann areas (Br) were not performed. The areas were the anterior cingulate gyrus at the level of the corpus callosum approximating Br 24, the superior frontal gyrus at the level of the corpus callosum approximating Br 8, the inferior temporal gyrus caudal to the amygdala approximating Br 20, and the inferior parietal lobule rostral to the parietal-occipital sulcus approximating Br 7. Samples were not available for all cases in all regions. No more than a 1-mm, white-matter border and no visible infarcts were included. Samples were processed blind for diagnosis. Specimens weighing approximately 25 mg were homogenized in 1 mL of TRIS-buffered saline (10 mm of TRIS chloride, and 150 mm of sodium chloride, with a 7.4 pH). Aliquots were prepared for protein analysis[33] or frozen at −85°C before the assay. Immunoreactivity measurements in a single aliquot were stable to 3 freeze-thaw cycles. The right hemisphere was used for neuropathologic studies.[27] Cases were assigned ratings for plaques in the medial frontal, superior temporal, inferior parietal, and occipital visual cortices.[29] Ratings were modified (0, none; 1, sparse; 2, moderate; rather than 3; 3, severe; rather than 5) to obtain a mean plaque rating.

Immunoassays

Presynaptic proteins were quantified by immunoassay using monoclonal antisera generated against human synaptic isolates. The EP10 and SP4 antibodies detect synaptophysin-like immunoreactivity as determined by Western blot analysis and immunoprecipitation.[24,25] Comparisons between species, and with the SY38 antisera (Boehringer Manheim, Indianapolis, Ind), suggest that the 2 antisera detect different epitopes on synaptophysin.[24,25] Based on analyses with fusion proteins, the SP6 antibody detects an epitope on the 34- to 36-kd molecular weight syntaxin molecule.[12,25,26] The SP14 antibody recognizes SNAP-25 immunoreactivity based on comparison with previously characterized SNAP-25 antisera and in studies with fusion proteins.[26]

The abundance of these integral presynaptic proteins has contributed to the isolation and elucidation of their properties.[12,14-16] In addition to regulating vesicle docking and exocytosis,[10,11] presynaptic proteins seem to be crucial for neuronal development in embryogenesis.[17-20] Further, under some experimental conditions, presynaptic proteins may change in concert with one another.[21] Being localized to the synapse, concentrations of synaptophysin correlate with direct, and more laborious, electronmicrographic measures of synapse numbers and, in Alzheimer's disease (AD), correlate strongly with the severity of cognitive impairment.[22] This would attest to the utility of quantifying presynaptic proteins as markers for synaptic connectivity and, potentially, for symptoms of schizophrenia.

It was hypothesized that altered concentrations of presynaptic proteins would be found in the cerebral cortex of subjects with schizophrenia. The anterior cingulate, superior frontal, and inferior temporal gyri plus the inferior parietal lobule were sampled from postmortem tissues collected from subjects with schizophrenia and elderly controls. Tissues from a cohort of subjects with AD were also included. These cortical regions were selected based on their reported involvement in schizophrenia or AD. Four monoclonal antibodies were employed to strengthen the possibility of detecting changes related to a general alteration in presynaptic structures and not to idiosyncratic changes in any particular antigen. These monoclonal antibodies were generated against crude synaptic membrane preparations from brain tissue from subjects with AD or schizophrenia and the identities of the proteins detected by these reagents were determined after their selection based on reactivity to human brain tissues. Two of these antibodies, EP10 and SP4, detect synaptophysin immunoreactivity.[23-25] The SP6 antibody detects syntaxin immunoreactivity and the SP14 antibody recognizes SNAP-25 immunoreactivity.[25,26] These 2 proteins are distinct from synaptophysin, but are associated with the presynaptic membrane, vesicle docking, and neurotransmitter release.[10-12]

RESULTS

SUBJECT GROUPS

As summarized in **Table 1**, PMI was greater in the subjects with schizophrenia compared with the control and AD groups ($F_{2,56}$=14.06 [$P>.001$]). Age was nominally greater in the controls compared with the groups with schizophrenia and AD ($F_{2,56}$=2.23 [$P>.1$]). These 2 variables, along with sex, were included as covariables in all statistical procedures. The group with schizophrenia and the group severely impaired with AD had greater clinical dementia rating scale scores compared with controls

Tissue homogenates were diluted with water (60-μg/mL protein). A 6-μg/100 μL aliquot was transferred to microplate wells (F96, Nunc MaxiSorp, VWR Scientific, Bridgeport, NJ) and serially diluted 7 times (1:1) with water. Therefore, total protein amount ranged from 3 to 0.024 μg. Tissues were adhered to the microplate well by rotary evaporation. More sample mass (3 μg) can be adhered to rather than absorbed in the polystyrene matrix (100 ng) of a microplate, making this method more appropriate for detecting antigens contained in membrane fractions. Substantial sample detachment does not occur in the range of plate washing. Dried wells were incubated with 5% powdered milk in TRIS–buffered saline for 1 hour at room temperature, then incubated overnight at 4°C with primary antibody diluted (1:10) in TRIS–buffered saline–treated milk. The next day, the plates were washed in TRIS–buffered saline containing 0.1% Tween-20, incubated for 1 hour at room temperature with an anti–mouse IgG-horseradish peroxidase conjugate diluted (1:1000) (PI-2000, Vector Laboratories, Burlingame, Calif) in TRIS–buffered saline–treated milk, washed again, and developed with substrate (3,3′,5,5′-tetramethylbenzidine peroxidase [TMB], BioRad, Hercules, Calif).

These assays detect epitopes from molecules for which synthetic or purified standards are unavailable. Therefore, each plate contained a pool of human cerebral cortex homogenate diluted identically to the samples that served as a standard curve with values corresponding to the total protein content added to each well. Relative optical densities were read at 655 nm (3550, BioRad). Calculations were performed using the BioRad Microplate Manager (BioRad) and the Statistical Analysis System (SAS, Cary, NC). Immunoreactivity in unknowns that read in the linear portion of the standard curve were multiplied by the appropriate dilution factor (1:128). Values represent the mean of 2 to 4 dilutions in duplicate and are expressed as relative optical density per microgram of protein.

Concentrations of neuron-specific enolase (NSE) were determined by antibody capture enzyme-linked immunosorbent assay using antisera (rabbit antihuman NSE) (17437, Polysciences Inc, Warrington, Pa) and antigen 17436 (Polysciences Inc). Buffers, blocking conditions, and incubations were as described earlier. Controls, standards (500-3.9 ng), and homogenized cerebral cortical samples (3, 1.5, and 0.75 μg) were adhered by rotary evaporation. After an overnight primary antibody incubation (1:5000 final), the plates were washed and incubated with goat anti–rabbit IgG-horseradish peroxidase conjugate (1:500 final) (4010-05, Southern Biotechnology, Birmingham, Ala) followed by substrate development. The relative optical density$_{1.0}$ for this assay was 143 ng; the (twice background) sensitivity was 6.3 ng.

STATISTICAL ANALYSIS

Data were analyzed using analysis of variance. Because the immunoreactivities are intimately associated with presynaptic elements,[10-12] they were treated as repeated measures, with the regions analyzed separately. Comparisons between subject groups were performed using the Tukey test ($P<.05$). Correlation coefficients were calculated for different immunoreactivities assessed in identical samples using pooled in-group regressions. For comparisons among the 4 presynaptic protein measures, the significance was $P<.004$ ($P<.05$ corrected for 12 comparisons). For comparisons between NSE and the 4 presynaptic protein measures, the significance was $P<.001$ ($P<.05$ corrected for 16 comparisons).

($F_{2,50}$ =22.01 [$P<.001$]). Mean plaque ratings varied by diagnosis ($F_{2,55}$=110.2 [$P<.001$]), with the group with AD being higher compared with either the control group or the group with schizophrenia ($P<.001$). Mean plaque ratings did not differ between the control group and the group with schizophrenia. Similarly, in a subset of cases in which actual plaque counts were obtained, subjects with AD had greater plaque counts compared with the controls and the subjects with schizophrenia ($F_{2,30}$=49.53 [$P<.001$]).

PRESYNAPTIC PROTEIN CONCENTRATIONS IN THE SUBJECT GROUPS

Figure 1 through **Figure 4** show presynaptic protein immunoreactivities detected by 4 monoclonal antibodies for subjects with schizophrenia, controls, and subjects with AD. On each histogram, the first 2 antibodies, EP10 and SP4, detect synaptophysin immunoreactivity; the third antibody, SP6, detects syntaxin immunoreactivity; and the fourth antibody, SP14, detects SNAP-25 immunoreactivity. In the anterior cingulate gyrus, a significant subject group effect (Figure 1) ($F_{2,51}$=5.07 [$P<.005$]) was reflected by increased presynaptic protein immunoreactivities for subjects with schizophrenia relative to the control and cases with AD ($P<.02$). These data contrast with the 3 other cortical regions, in which presynaptic protein concentrations in subjects with schizophrenia were not different from controls. Significant effects were found for subject groups in the superior frontal gyrus (Figure 2) ($F_{2,40}$=10.78 [$P<.001$]), the inferior temporal gyrus (Figure 3) ($F_{2,49}$=9.15 [$P<.004$]), and the inferior parietal lobule (Figure 4) ($F_{2,30}$=3.30 [$P<.05$]). In the temporal gyrus, a significant interaction of subject group with presynaptic protein measure was found ($F_{6,156}$=2.03 [$P<.012$]). These effects reflected decreases in all 4 presynaptic proteins for the group with AD relative to the control and schizophrenia cohorts in the superior frontal ($P<.004$) and inferior ($P<.04$) temporal gyri. In the inferior parietal lobule, the 4 presynaptic protein concentrations were significantly decreased in the group with AD compared with the elderly control group ($P<.003$).

EFFECTS OF PMI AND NEUROLEPTIC TREATMENT

Regression analyses performed on the combined subject groups revealed no significant correlations between individual immunoreactivity measures and PMI (16 analyses of 4 immunoreactivities with 4 regions) ($-0.09<r<0.159$, $.19<P<.77$). Similarly, when the analyses were restricted to the subjects with schizophrenia, none of the analyses were significant ($0.02<r<0.569$,

Table 1. Demographic Characteristics of the Study Groups

Feature*	Elderly Subjects in Control Group	Subjects With Alzheimer's Disease	Subjects With Schizophrenia
No. of subjects	16	24	19
Age, y			
Mean±SD	81.4±11.9	73.6±11.5	74.1±12.0
Range	55-99	58-97	52-95
PMI, h			
Mean±SD	5.87±2.83	6.62±3.97	32.7±30.1†
Range	2.67-10.4	1.75-15.3	3.53-88.2
Sex			
Ratio, male-female	6:10	16:8	11:8
CDR‡			
Mean±SD	1.2±2.0	4.2±0.9§	2.0±1.3§
Range	0-5	0-5	0-4
Plaque rating			
Mean±SD	0.15±0.32	2.53±0.47†	0.59±0.96
Plaque count‖			
Mean±SD	0.0±0.0	20.8±9.0†	2.2±3.0
No.	8	6	19
Cardiac medications¶			
Ratio, yes:no:missing	8:6:2	2:8:14	2:17:0
Anti-inflammatory medications¶			
Ratio, yes:no:missing	2:12:2	1:9:14	2:17:0
Alcoholism¶			
Ratio, yes:no:missing	1:13:2	0:10:14	0:2:17

**PMI indicates postmortem interval; CDR, clinical dementia rating.*
†Significantly different from the elderly subjects in the control group (P<.001).
‡The CDR scores were not obtained on 1 control and 4 cases of Alzheimer's disease.
§Significantly different from the elderly control group (P<.05).
‖The numbers associated with the plaque count represent the subset of cases for that measure only.
¶Ratios for the use of cardiac or anti-inflammatory medications at the time of death and histopathologic or other evidence of alcoholism are based on evidence from the review of the medical records of the subjects. There was no evidence of the use of elicit drugs in any of the subjects.

.067<*P*<.936). Given the range of PMI (3.53-88.2) and the size of the schizophrenia cohort (n=19), these data do not suggest that PMI influences the immunoreactivity measures in the subjects with schizophrenia or the entire cohort. Lack of variation in PMI in the control group and the group with AD negated separate regression analyses.

Despite the lack of correlation in the schizophrenia cohort, an additional repeated measures analysis of variance was performed on a subset of cases with schizophrenia with the 9 lowest PMI matched to an equal number of controls to within 100 minutes (control=393±180 min; subjects with schizophrenia=441±206 min [mean±SD]). For the anterior cingulate gyrus, a significant effect of subject group ($F_{1,11}$=7.52 [*P*<.019]) was evidenced as an increase in all 4 presynaptic proteins in subjects with schizophrenia compared with controls (*P*<.012). In this smaller subset of cases, a significant effect of subject group ($F_{1,11}$=11.42 [*P*<.006]) also was found for the inferior temporal gyrus, with all 4 presynaptic protein concentrations being greater in the subjects with schizophrenia relative to the controls (*P*<.006). No differences were found for similar analyses in the superior frontal gyrus or the inferior parietal lobule (data not shown).

An additional factor that might affect the cerebral cortical presynaptic concentrations in the group with schizophrenia relative to the control group and the group with AD was exposure to neuroleptics. Seven of the 17 cases with schizophrenia, for which presynaptic protein concentrations were determined in the anterior cingulate gyrus, were judged to be free of neuroleptic medication more than 1 year prior to death (**Table 2**). In that region, none of the 4 presynaptic protein immunoreactivities differed between the group treated with vs the group not treated with neuroleptic drugs. In the superior frontal gyrus, inferior temporal gyrus, and inferior parietal lobule, presynaptic protein concentrations also did not differ between the group with schizophrenia treated with vs the group with schizophrenia not treated with neuroleptic drugs (data not shown).

CORRELATIONS BETWEEN PRESYNAPTIC PROTEIN IMMUNOREACTIVITIES

Because these monoclonal antibodies detect antigens common to the synapse, correlation coefficients were calculated for immunoreactivities determined in identical analytes. In any particular region, pairs of immunoreactivity measures were highly correlated with *r*, ranging from 0.63 to 0.94 (all *P*<.002). Only 2 correlations, EP10 vs SP4 in the inferior parietal lobule and SP4 vs SP6 in the inferior temporal gyrus, failed to reach significance. Correlation coefficients were not calculated for individual presynaptic proteins vs clinical dementia rating because of the limited number of cases in each subject group and the lack of range in the clinical dementia rating in each subject group (Table 1).

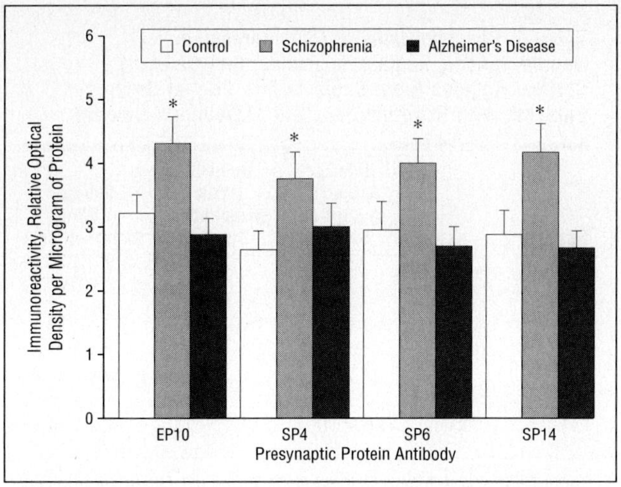

Figure 1. *Presynaptic protein immunoreactivities detected by 4 monoclonal antibodies in the anterior cingulate gyrus approximating Brodmann area 24 from elderly controls (n=15), subjects with schizophrenia (n=17), and subjects with Alzheimer's disease (n=24). The EP10 and SP4 antibodies recognize synaptophysin, SP6 detects syntaxin, and SP14 identifies synaptosomal–associated protein-25 kd. Error bars indicate uncorrected mean±SEM; asterisk, significantly different from elderly controls and subjects with Alzheimer's disease (P<.02).*

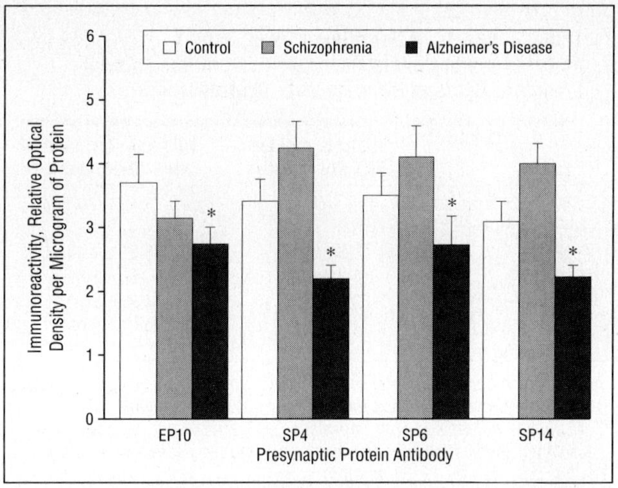

Figure 3. *Presynaptic protein immunoreactivities detected by 4 monoclonal antibodies in the inferior temporal gyrus approximating Brodmann area 20 from elderly controls (n=12), subjects with schizophrenia (n=19), and subjects with Alzheimer's disease (n=22). The EP10 and SP4 antibodies recognize synaptophysin, SP6 detects syntaxin, and SP14 identifies synaptosomal–associated protein-25 kd. Error bars indicate uncorrected mean±SEM; asterisk, significantly different from elderly controls and subjects with schizophrenia (P<.04).*

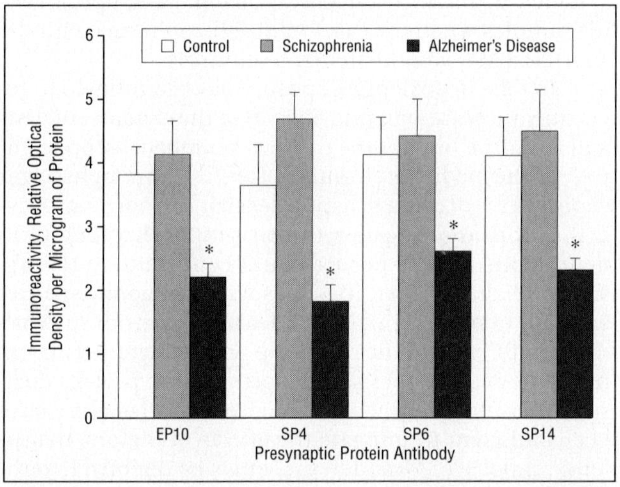

Figure 2. *Presynaptic protein immunoreactivities detected by 4 monoclonal antibodies in the superior frontal gyrus approximating Brodmann area 8 from elderly controls (n=13), subjects with schizophrenia (n=10), and subjects with Alzheimer's disease (n=22). The EP10 and SP4 antibodies recognize synaptophysin, SP6 detects syntaxin, and SP14 identifies synaptosomal–associated protein-25 kd. Error bars indicate uncorrected mean±SEM; asterisk, significantly different from elderly controls and subjects with schizophrenia (P<.004).*

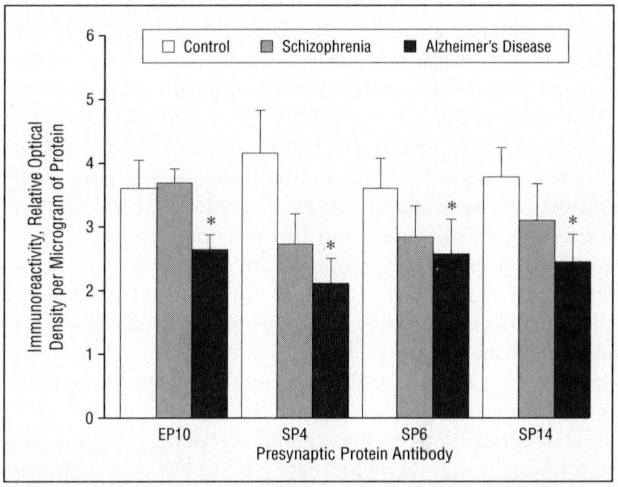

Figure 4. *Presynaptic protein immunoreactivities detected by 4 monoclonal antibodies in the inferior parietal lobule approximating Brodmann area 7 from elderly controls (n=12), subjects with schizophrenia (n=8), and subjects with Alzheimer's disease (n=15). The EP10 and SP4 antibodies recognize synaptophysin, SP6 detects syntaxin, and SP14 identifies synaptosomal–associated protein-25 kd. Error bars indicate uncorrected mean±SEM; asterisk, significantly different from elderly controls (P<.003).*

NSE CONCENTRATIONS IN THE SUBJECT GROUPS

To evaluate the specificity of the increased presynaptic protein concentrations observed in schizophrenia, concentrations of NSE, an enzyme not exclusively confined to presynaptic terminals, were determined (**Table 3**). This enzyme did not differ among the 3 subject groups in the 4 areas. In the anterior cingulate gyrus, regression analyses revealed that synaptophysin (EP10) (r=0.511, P<.001) and syntaxin (SP6) (r=0.498, P<.002) correlated with NSE. In the inferior temporal gyrus, synaptophysin (EP10) (r=0.587, P<.001) and syntaxin (SP6) (r=0.552, P<.002) correlated with NSE.

COMMENT

Our study demonstrates increased concentrations of presynaptic proteins in the postmortem cingulate cortex of subjects with schizophrenia. That these presynaptic proteins change in concert and are correlated with one another supports the contention that these changes reflect a common neuronal element, namely, the synapse. Indeed, electron microscopy of the anterior limbic cortex

Table 2. Effects of Neuroleptic Treatment on Presynaptic Protein Concentrations in the Anterior Cingulate Gyrus of Patients With Schizophrenia*

Features	Subjects Treated With Neuroleptics	Subjects Not Treated With Neuroleptics†
No. of subjects	10	7
Synaptophysin		
SP4‡	3.81±1.99	3.81±1.40
EP10	3.60±1.06	4.54±1.83
Syntaxin (SP6)	3.65±2.12	4.37±1.72
SNAP-25§ (SP14)	4.10±1.97	4.07±2.08

*Concentrations are expressed in relative optical density units (ROD/μg of protein). Unless otherwise indicated, all values are mean±SD.

†Subjects not treated with neuroleptic drugs were not exposed to any neuroleptic medications for at least 1 year prior to death (44.3±39.0 [mean±SD]; range, 12-20 months).

‡Codes indicate the particular monoclonal antibody used to detect that immunoreactivity.

§SNAP-25 indicates synaptosomal–associated protein-25 kd.

Table 3. Concentrations of Immunoreactive Neuron-Specific Enolase in Postmortem Cerebral Cortical Regions From Subjects in a Control Group and Subjects With Schizophrenia and Alzheimer's Disease*

Feature	Elderly Subjects in Control Group	Subjects With Alzheimer's Disease	Subjects With Schizophrenia
No. of subjects	15	24	17
Gyrus			
Anterior cingulate	159.7±32.8	153.2±36.9	152.1±29.1
Superior frontal	112.0±23.1	113.4±45.7	95.8±27.5
Inferior temporal	70.4±19.6	67.4±21.3	66.6±20.6
Labule			
Inferior parietal	48.0±15.4	44.1±11.3	40.5±14.4

*Concentrations are expressed as micrograms per milligram of protein. All values represent mean±SD.

indicates increased synaptic density in the postmortem brains of subjects with schizophrenia.[34] Cortical presynaptic protein concentrations were also increased in a small study of subjects with schizophrenia.[23] Another brief article found decreased synapsin I concentrations in the hippocampus of subjects with schizophrenia, but synaptophysin concentrations were unchanged and the cingulate cortex was not evaluated.[35] If the alterations in the synapse implied by our data reflect increases in the neuronal population relative to the total brain volume, other neuronal proteins such as the cytosolic enzyme, NSE, might be expected to increase. While NSE concentrations did not differ among the subjects groups, in 2 instances, presynaptic protein concentrations did correlate with NSE concentrations. Because disturbances in the numbers of small neurons, as well as individual neuronal elements, have been described in schizophrenia,[5,7,36] our data may also reflect alterations in intrinsic cortical neurons.

Decreases in nonneuronal elements, such a glia, could result in relative increases in neuronal density and, therefore, neuronal proteins. Changes in glial populations might also indicate postnatal nerve damage. Glia generally have not been found to be altered in schizophrenia, although the quantitation of this cell population is problematic.[37] A recent preliminary study describes increased astrocytosis in subjects with demented schizophrenia.[38] Unfortunately, glial fibrillary acidic protein was undetectable in the homogenates used in our study (data not shown).

The subject groups we studied differed to varying degrees in age, sex, PMI, cognitive functioning, neuroleptic exposure, and hospitalization. Postmortem interval is always a concern in neurochemical studies. Postmortem degradation may have increased or revealed antigens normally embedded in membranes or not otherwise detected by the antibodies. Additionally, postmortem detritus may interfere nonspecifically with binding to increase the apparent sample blank and read as a false immunoreactivity increase. Still, regression analyses failed to reveal any relationship between PMI and immunoreactivity in the schizophrenia cohort. The limitation of changes noted for the schizophrenia cohort to 1 cortical area argues against this possibility. A more likely consequence of postmortem degradation (ie, immunoreactivity loss) is suggested by the significant increase in presynaptic protein concentrations in the temporal lobule samples when the cases with schizophrenia with the shortest PMIs were matched to controls.

In rats, neuroleptic exposure has been shown to reversibly increase synaptic density in the caudate nucleus and striatum, but not the nucleus acumbens, hippocampus, or the medial prefrontal cortex,[39-41] although longer exposure may reduce synaptic density.[42] In our study, several factors argue against the possibility that long-term neuroleptic drug exposure could contribute to the observed changes. First, the cases with schizophrenia not exposed to neuroleptics for at least 1 year prior to death did not differ from the subgroup with schizophrenia exposed to neuroleptics for any presynaptic protein measure. Admittedly, the neuroleptic-free period may not have been sufficient to mitigate the effects of lifelong neuroleptic exposure. Although there may be regional heterogeneity in responses to prolonged neuroleptic treatment, it is difficult to contend that neuroleptic exposure would preferentially effect presynaptic proteins in the cingulate cortex and not the superior frontal gyrus, which receives dense dopaminergic innervation.

Finally, recent findings of increased $GABA_A$ receptor binding[6] and decreased dopaminergic activity[9] in the postmortem anterior cingulate cortex from subjects with schizophrenia do not seem to be influenced by exposure to neuroleptic drugs.

A final between-group factor that could have influenced the findings is chronic institutionalization among the cohort with schizophrenia that averaged 45 years. This potential confound in any postmortem examination of a population of subjects with schizophrenia is difficult to replicate in comparison subjects. However, the most parsimonious explanation regarding the influence of possible environmental impoverishment would posit a decrease in the concentration of presynaptic proteins and synaptic number[43] rather than the increase observed here.

Our observation of decreased presynaptic proteins in AD concurs with previous studies that link decreased synaptophysin to diminished synaptic contacts.[22,44,45] The 50% decrease in synaptophysin noted by Masliah and coworkers[44] compares with that seen in our study. Additional validation of our observations in the cohort with schizophrenia is provided by the simultaneous immunoassay of identically handled specimens. The subjects with schizophrenia were cognitively impaired, although not as profoundly as the subjects with AD. Although synaptophysin immunoreactivity has been found to correlate with cognitive dysfunction in subjects with AD,[22] only nominal decreases in presynaptic proteins were noted for the group with schizophrenia in the inferior parietal lobule. It is unclear whether a group of subjects with schizophrenia that have more severe cognitive impairment would also have reduced presynaptic proteins in this region implicated in cognition. Thus, present data indicate a discordance in an index of synaptic density known to correlate with cognitive impairment in the brains of subjects with AD relative to subjects with schizophrenia.

Synaptophysin, SNAP-25, and the syntaxins regulate synaptic vesicle traffic in mature neurons and have additional roles in the migration of axonal growth cones during development.[10,13,17-20] At first glance, the dual roles of these proteins seem to prevent distinguishing between their involvement in a developmental vs maturational component of schizophrenia. On the contrary, these proteins may be uniquely suited to inducing the double defect of a neurodevelopmental insult compounded by disturbances manifest during adolescence and continuing through early adulthood.[1,2,46] This intimate link of presynaptic proteins to neuronal growth, neurotransmission, and vesicular traffic suggests a biological basis for abnormal information processing in a region of the brain that has been implicated in affect, emotion, and schizophrenia.[47,48]

Despite the devastating consequences for behavior, this and previous postmortem depictions of the brain in schizophrenia are not as dramatic as the plaques and dystrophic neurons described for AD. The weight of evidence that implicates a disruption of GABA-containing neurons in the cingulate and prefrontal cortex of subjects with schizophrenia includes small interneuron loss, increased $GABA_A$-receptor numbers, increased ascending apical fiber staining, and pervasive deficits in intrinsic neuropeptides.[3,4,6,7,31,36,49,50] Dysfunction in this major inhibitory component in the prefrontal cerebral cortex of subjects with schizophrenia is also indicated by descriptions of a decrease in glutamate amino decarboxylase gene expression.[5] A synaptic analogue complements these cytological and neurochemical alterations in the cingulate cortex of a subject with schizophrenia and could reflect increased synaptic numbers or increased activity in a constant number of synapses. While the cingulate cortex is implicated, the pathophysiology of schizophrenia and its constellation of symptoms certainly involves the interactions of many brain regions. Indeed, time-honored and more recent observations of schizophrenia involve neurotransmitter systems efferent to the cerebral cortex (ie, dopamine and serotonin).[51] The relatively small and homogenous area occupied by the anterior cingulate cortex, the cytoarchitectonics of the associated Br 24 with its prominent layer 5 pyramidal neurons,[48] together with its connectivity to prefrontal and subcortical structures, may have contributed to the demonstration of defects that are present, but less readily revealed, in the brains of people with schizophrenia.

Accepted for publication June 4, 1996.

This research was supported by grant VA5118 from the Department of Veterans Affairs, Washington, DC, (Dr Davidson); grants MH46436 (Dr Haroutunian), AG02219, AG5138, MH45212, and VA4125 (Dr Davis) from the Department of Health and Human Services, Washington, DC; the Stanley Foundation (Dr Homer); and the Medical Research Council of Canada (Dr Homer).

These data were presented in preliminary form at the Society for Neuroscience Meeting, Miami, Fla, November 13-18, 1994, and the American College of Neuropsychopharmacology Meeting, San Juan, Puerto Rico, December 11-16, 1994.

We thank Debra Lazarus, Nancy Ruiz, and W. Ahmed, MD, for their technical assistance. We also thank James Schmeidler, PhD, for his comments on the statistical analysis and D. P. Perl, MD, and D. P. Purohit, MD, for their neuropathologic characterization of the cases studied.

Corresponding author: Vahram Haroutunian, PhD, Department of Psychiatry, Bronx Veterans Affairs Medical Center, 130 W Kingsbridge Rd, Bronx, NY 10468.

REFERENCES

1. Carpenter WT Jr, Buchanan RW, Kirkpatrick B, Tamminga C, Wood F. Strong inference, theory testing, and the neuroanatomy of schizophrenia. *Arch Gen Psychiatry.* 1993;50:825-831.
2. Weinberger DR. Neurodevelopmental prespectives in schizophrenia. In: Bloom FE, Kupfer DJ, eds. *Psychopharmacology: The Fourth Generation of Progress.* New York, NY: Raven Press; 1995:1171-1184.
3. Kutay FZ, Pogun S, Hariri NI, Peker G, Erlacin S. Free amino acid level determinations in normal and schizophrenic brain. *Prog Neuropsychopharmacol Biol Psychiatry.* 1989;13:119-126.
4. Reynolds GP, Czudek C, Andrews HB. Deficit and hemispheric asymmetry of GABA uptake sites in the hippocampus in schizophrenia. *Biol Psychiatry.* 1990; 27:1038-1044.
5. Akbarian S, Kim JJ, Potkin SG, Hagman JO, Tafazzoli A, Bunney WE Jr, Jones EG. Gene expression for glutamic acid decarboxylase is reduced without loss of neurons in prefrontal cortex of schizophrenics. *Arch Gen Psychiatry.* 1995; 52:258-266; discussion 267-278.
6. Benes FM, Vincent SL, Alsterberg G, Bird ED, SanGiovanni JP. Increased $GABA_A$ receptor binding in superficial layers of cingulate cortex in schizophrenics. *J Neurosci.* 1992;12:924-929.
7. Benes FM, Sorensen I, Vincent SL, Bird ED, Sathi M. Increased density of glutamate-immunoreactive vertical processes in superficial laminae in cingulate cortex of schizophrenic brain. *Cereb Cortex.* 1992;2:503-512.
8. Ruano D, Machado A, Vitorica J. Absence of modifications of the pharmacological properties of the $GABA_A$ receptor complex during aging, as assessed in 3- and 24-month-old rat cerebral cortex. *Eur J Pharmacol.* 1993;246:81-87.
9. Wyatt RJ, Karoum F, Casanova MF. Decreased DOPAC in the anterior cingulate cortex of individuals with schizophrenia. *Biol Psychiatry.* 1995;38:4-12.
10. Sollner T, Whiteheart SW, Brunner M, Erdjument-Bromage H, Geromanos S, Tempst P, Rothman JE. SNAP receptors implicated in vesicle targeting and fusion. *Nature.* 1993;362:318-324.
11. Littleton JT, Bellen HJ. Synaptotagmin controls and modulates synaptic-vesicle fusion in a Ca^{2+}-dependent manner. *Trends Neurosci.* 1995;18:177-183.

12. Bajjalieh SM, Scheller RH. The biochemistry of neurotransmitter secretion. *J Biol Chem.* 1995;270:1971-1974.
13. Edelmann L, Hanson PI, Chapman ER, Jahn R. Synaptobrevin binding to synaptophysin: a potential mechanism for controlling the exocytotic fusion machine. *EMBO J.* 1995;14:224-231.
14. Oyler GA, Higgins GA, Hart RA, Battenberg E, Billingsley M, Bloom FE, Wilson MC. The identification of a novel synaptosomal-associated protein, SNAP-25, differentially expressed by neuronal subpopulations. *J Cell Biol.* 1989;109: 3039-3052.
15. Bennett MK, Calakos N, Scheller RH. Syntaxin: a synaptic protein implicated in docking of synaptic vesicles at presynaptic active zones. *Science.* 1992;257: 255-259.
16. Jahn R, Schiebler W, Ouimet C, Greengard P. A 38,000-dalton membrane protein (p38) present in synaptic vesicles. *Proc Natl Acad Sci U S A.* 1985;82: 4137-4141.
17. Oyler GA, Polli JW, Wilson MC, Billingsley ML. Developmental expression of the 25-kDa synaptosomal-associated protein (SNAP-25) in rat brain. *Proc Natl Acad Sci U S A.* 1991;88:5247-5251.
18. Osen-Sand A, Catsicas M, Staple JK, Jones KA, Ayala G, Knowles J, Grenningloh G, Catsicas S. Inhibition of axonal growth by SNAP-25 antisense oligonucleotides in vitro and in vivo. *Nature.* 1993;364:445-448.
19. Fletcher TL, Cameron P, De Camilli P, Banker G. The distribution of synapsin I and synaptophysin in hippocampal neurons developing in culture. *J Neurosci.* 1991;11:1617-1626.
20. Leclerc N, Beesley PW, Brown I, Colonnier M, Gurd JW, Paladino T, Hawkes R. Synaptophysin expression during synaptogenesis in the rat cerebellar cortex. *J Comp Neurol.* 1989;280:197-212.
21. Ferreira A, Kosik KS, Greengard P, Han HQ. Aberrant neurites and synaptic vesicle protein deficiency in synapsin II–depleted neurons. *Science.* 1994;264: 977-979.
22. Terry RD, Masliah E, Salmon DP, Butters N, DeTeresa R, Hill R, Hansen LA, Katzman R. Physical basis of cognitive alterations in Alzheimer's disease: synapse loss is the major correlate of cognitive impairment. *Ann Neurol.* 1991; 30:572-580.
23. Honer WG, Kaufmann CA, Kleinman JE, Casanova MF, Davies P. Monoclonal antibodies to study the brain in schizophrenia. *Brain Res.* 1989;500:379-383.
24. Honer WG, Kaufmann CA, Davies P. Characterization of a synaptic antigen of interest in neuropsychiatric illness. *Biol Psychiatry.* 1992;31:147-158.
25. Honer WG, Hu L, Davies P. Human synaptic proteins with a heterogeneous distribution in cerebellum and visual cortex. *Brain Res.* 1993;609:9-20.
26. Honer WG, Falkai P, Young C, Wang T, Xie J, Bonner J, Hu L, Boulianne GL, Lu Z, Trimble WS. Cingulate cortex synaptic terminal proteins and neural cell adhesion molecule in schizophrenia. 1997. In press.
27. Purohit DP, Davidson M, Perl DP, Powchik P, Haroutunian V, Bierer LM, McCrystal J, Losonczy M, Davis KL. Severe cognitive impairment in elderly schizophrenic patients: a clinicopathological study. *Biol Psychiatry.* 1993;33: 255-260.
28. Khachaturian ZS. Diagnosis of Alzheimer's disease. *Arch Neurol.* 1985;42: 1097-1105.
29. Mirra SS, Heyman A, McKeel D, Suni SM, Crain BJ, Brownlee LM, Vogel FS, Hughes JP, van Belle G, Berg L. The consortium to establish a registry for Alzheimer's disease (CERAD), part II: standardization of the neuropathologic assessment of Alzheimer's disease. *Neurology.* 1991;41:479-486.
30. Gabriel SM, Bierer LM, Harotunian V, Purohit DP, Perl DP, Davis KL. Widespread deficits in somatostatin but not neuropeptide Y concentrations in Alzheimer's disease cerebral cortex. *Neurosci Lett.* 1993;155:116-120.
31. Gabriel SM, Davidson M, Haroutunian V, Powchik P, Bierer LM, Purohit DP, Perl DP, Davis KL. Neuropeptide deficits in schizophrenia versus Alzheimer's disease cerebral cortex. *Biol Psychiatry.* 1996;39:82-91.
32. Hughes CP, Berg L, Danziger WL, Coben LA, Martin RL. A new clinical scale for the staging of dementia. *Br J Psychiatry.* 1982;140:566-572.
33. Lowry OH, Rorebrough NJ, Farr AL, Randall RJ. Protein measurement with folin reagent. *J Biol Chem.* 1951;193:265-272.
34. Aganova EA, Uranova NA. Morphometric analysis of synaptic contacts in the anterior limbic cortex in the endogenous psychoses. *Neurosci Behav Physiol.* 1992;22:59-65.
35. Browning MD, Dudek EM, Rapier JL, Leonard S, Freedman R. Significant reductions in synapsin but not synaptophysin specific activity in the brains of some schizophrenics. *Biol Psychiatry.* 1993;34:529-535.
36. Benes FM, McSparren J, Bird ED, SanGiovanni JP, Vincent SL. Deficits in small interneurons in prefrontal and cingulate cortices of schizophrenic and schizoaffective patients. *Arch Gen Psychiatry.* 1991;48:996-1001.
37. Casanova MF, Stevens JR, Kleinman JE. The neuropathology of schizophrenia: old and new findings. In: Lindenmayer JP, Kay SR, eds. *New Biological Vistas in Schizophrenia.* New York, NY: Brunner-Mazel; 1992:82-109.
38. Arnold SE, Franz BR, Moberg PJ, Martinoli M, Gur RE, Trojanowski JQ. Molecular markers of neural injury and neurodegeneration in elderly patients with schizophrenia. Presented at the American College of Neuropsychopharmacology; December 11-15, 1995; San Juan, Puerto Rico.
39. Meshul CK, Janowsky A, Casey DE, Stallbaumer RK, Taylor B. Effect of haloperidol and clozapine on the density of perforated synapses in caudate, nucleus accumbens, and medial prefrontal cortex. *Psychopharmacology (Berl).* 1992; 106:45-52.
40. Uranova NA, Orlovskaya DD, Apel K, Klintsova AJ, Haselhorst U, Schenk H. Morphometric study of synaptic patterns in the rat caudate nucleus and hippocampus under haloperidol treatment. *Synapse.* 1991;7:253-259.
41. Meshul CK, Casey DE. Regional, reversible ultrastructural changes in rat brain with chronic neuroleptic treatment. *Brain Res.* 1989;489:338-346.
42. Roberts RC, Gaither LA, Gao XM, Kashyap SM, Tamminga CA. Ultrastructural correlates of haloperidol-induced oral dyskinesias in rat striatum. *Synapse.* 1995; 20:234-243.
43. Greenough WT, Anderson BJ. Cerebellar synaptic plasticity: relation to learning versus neural activity. *Ann N Y Acad Sci.* 1991;627:231-247.
44. Masliah E, Terry RD, Alford M, DeTeresa R, Hansen LA. Cortical and subcortical patterns of synaptophysinlike immunoreactivity in Alzheimer's disease. *Am J Pathol.* 1991;138:235-246.
45. Hamos JE, DeGennaro LJ, Drachman DA. Synaptic loss in Alzheimer's disease and other dementias. *Neurology.* 1989;39:355-361.
46. Stevens JR. Abnormal reinnervation as a basis for schizophrenia: a hypothesis. *Arch Gen Psychiatry.* 1992;49:238-243.
47. Siegel BV Jr, Buchsbaum MS, Bunney WE Jr, Gottschalk LA, Haier RJ, Lohr JB, Lottenberg S, Najafi A, Nuechterlein KH, Potkin SG, Wu JC. Cortical-striatal–thalamic circuits and brain glucose metabolic activity in 70 unmedicated male schizophrenic patients. *Am J Psychiatry.* 1993;150:1325-1336.
48. Devinsky O, Morrell MJ, Vogt BA. Contributions of the anterior cingulate cortex to behavior. *Brain.* 1995;118:279-306.
49. Manberg PJ, Nemeroff CB, Bissette G, Widerlov E, Youngblood WW, Kizer JS, Prange AJ Jr. Neuropeptides in CSF and postmortem brain tissue of normal controls, schizophrenics and Huntington's choreics. *Prog Neuropsychopharmacol Biol Psychiatry.* 1985;9:97-108.
50. Roberts GW, Ferrier IN, Lee Y, Crow TJ, Johnstone EC, Owens DG, Bacarese-Hamilton AJ, McGregor G, O'Shaughnessey D, Polak JM, et al. Peptides, the limbic lobe and schizophrenia. *Brain Res.* 1983;288:199-211.
51. Roth BL, Meltzer HY. The role of serotonin in schizophrenia. In: Bloom FE, Kupfer DJ, eds. *Psychopharamacology: The Fourth Generation of Progress.* New York, NY: Raven Press; 1995:1215-1227.

ORIGINAL ARTICLE

The Effects of a Selective D_4 Dopamine Receptor Antagonist (L-745,870) in Acutely Psychotic Inpatients With Schizophrenia

Mark S. Kramer, MD, PhD; Barbara Last; Albert Getson, PhD; Scott A. Reines, MD, PhD; and the D_4 Dopamine Antagonist Group

Background: Based mainly on the selective antagonism of clozapine at D_4 compared with D_2 dopamine receptors, hopes have run high that a selective D_4 dopamine receptor antagonist might improve the pharmacological treatment of patients with schizophrenia. We report, to our knowledge, the first multicenter study of the antipsychotic potential of a highly specific D_4 dopamine receptor antagonist (ie, L-745,870) in patients with acute schizophrenia.

Methods: Thirty-eight acutely psychotic and neuroleptic responsive (by history) newly admitted inpatients with schizophrenia were randomized to 4 weeks of double-blind treatment (2:1) with either L-745,870 (n=26), 15 mg/d, or placebo (n=12) after a 3- to 5-day placebo run-in period.

Results: Overall, a greater percentage of patients receiving L-745,870 compared with patients receiving placebo discontinued the study for insufficient therapeutic response (32% vs 16%). At the end of 4 weeks by last observation carried forward analysis, the mean change from baseline to week 4 on the total Brief Psychiatric Rating Scale favored placebo (ie, −8 points [−15% change from baseline] vs −1 point [−2% change from baseline] for placebo vs L-745,870, P=.09). Similar differences in favor of placebo in changes from baseline mean scores were observed for the not carried forward analysis on the total Brief Psychiatric Rating Scale (P<.03), for not carried forward and last observation carried forward analyses on the sum of selected positive symptom items of the Brief Psychiatric Rating Scale, and for the Clinical Global Impression analysis (P=.03, last observation carried forward). A greater percentage of patients receiving L-745,870 had scores indicative of some level of worsening (compared with baseline) on the total Brief Psychiatric Rating Scale and the Clinical Global Impressions' Severity of Illness Scale as well as positive symptoms compared with those receiving placebo.

Conclusion: The selective D_4 dopamine receptor antagonist L-745,870 was ineffective as an antipsychotic for the treatment of neuroleptic responsive inpatients with acute schizophrenia.

Arch Gen Psychiatry. 1997;54:567-572

IN THE LATE 1980s, it became widely appreciated through a landmark study[1] that some patients, previously refractory to standard antipsychotic medications, were symptomatically and functionally improved with clozapine treatment. The enhanced efficacy and safety (ie, fewer extrapyramidal events) of clozapine suggest that, somewhere within its heterogeneous biochemical pharmacological features, clozapine holds the clue(s) for the discovery of new, improved treatments for patients with schizophrenia. Lower than expected numbers of D_2 dopamine receptors are occupied in patients receiving therapeutic doses of clozapine.[2] This suggested that the efficacy of clozapine is either not due to blockade of D_2 dopamine receptors at all or to low D_2 dopamine receptor blockade that is then functionally augmented by some other aspect(s) of its pharmacological features. Of the known dopamine receptor affinities of clozapine, its affinity for D_4 dopamine receptors is approximately an order of magnitude greater than for D_2 dopamine receptors,[3] and this may contribute to its unusual antipsychotic profile. In addition, some reports[4-9] suggest, albeit arguably,[10] that the number of D_4 dopamine receptors might be elevated in the postmortem brains of patients with schizophrenia compared with normal control subjects. Hence, it seemed reasonable that D_4 dopamine receptor antagonism might underlie the therapeutic benefits of clozapine.

To test the hypothesis clinically, the D_4 dopamine receptor antagonist L-745,870 (3-{[4-(4-chlorophenyl) piperazin-1-yl]methyl}-1H-pyrrolo[2,3-b] pyridine) was chosen because of its high selectivity as an antagonist at D_4 dopamine receptors and because of its advantageous pharmacokinetic profile (half-life≈15 hours in humans). L-745,870 displaced the specific binding of

From the Departments of Clinical Neuroscience (Drs Kramer and Reines and Ms Last) and Clinical Biostatistics (Dr Getson), Merck & Co Inc, West Point, Pa; and Psychiatry and Human Behavior, Thomas Jefferson Medical College, Philadelphia, Pa (Dr Kramer). A complete list of the members of the D_4 Dopamine Antagonist Group appears in the box on page 570.

PATIENTS AND METHODS

PATIENTS

Eligible inpatients were aged 18 to 60 years, men or women, and in need of treatment with an antipsychotic medication. This double-blind, randomized study was begun in men and surgically sterilized women; when developmental and reproduction toxicologic studies became available, women with childbearing potential were also included. For their present episode of psychosis, patients should not have been hospitalized for longer than 3 weeks.

DIAGNOSTIC ASSESSMENT AND SEVERITY OF ILLNESS AT BASELINE

Investigators determined that study patients met *DSM-IV* criteria for the diagnosis of schizophrenia,[13] episodic or continuous, except those with the residual type, single episode in full remission, schizophreniform disorder, or schizoaffective disorder. In addition, the patients were required to have a Brief Psychiatric Rating Scale (BPRS) total score[14,15] for items 1 to 18 of greater than 38 (scale, 1-7); a Clinical Global Impressions (CGI) Severity of Illness Scale score at the end of the placebo run-in of 4 (moderately) to 6 (severely ill); and a score of at least 4 (moderate) on 2 of the following 4 BPRS items: conceptual disorganization, suspiciousness, hallucinatory behavior, and unusual thought content. All ratings were done by research psychiatrists, often with other skilled research personnel. By protocol, the investigators only included patients who were judged by history to have been responsive to antipsychotic medication or who had never received antipsychotic medication. Refractory patients were defined as those who had failed to respond in their most recent episode to at least 2 or more antipsychotic medications, each given consecutively for at least 6 weeks, at daily doses at least equivalent to 600 mg of chlorpromazine hydrochloride.

OTHER ENROLLMENT CRITERIA

Patients were excluded from the study if they presently or in the past had a clinically significant systemic disease; a concurrent or past history of a psychiatric or neurologic diagnosis; treatment with depot neuroleptics within 2 months of screening; clinically significant abnormalities in electrocardiographic findings, blood chemistries, or other laboratory parameters; a positive screening for substance abuse, excluding benzodiazepines; or evidence of tardive dyskinesia and scoring greater than 2 on any item of the Simpson-Angus Scale[16] or similarly anchored items for akathisia and akinesia. To provide a safe framework for the trial, patients were not enrolled if, in the opinion of the investigator on screening, they were dangerous to themselves, dangerous to others, or unusually uncooperative so as to interfere with the evaluation process.

General Design

Before initiation of the study, the study protocol was reviewed and approved by the Investigational Review Board at each of the investigative sites. Furthermore, the investigators discussed with patients the nature of the study and its requirements and restrictions and obtained their written, informed consent.

A complete physical examination, an electrocardiographic examination, and a psychiatric diagnostic examination were performed within 1 week before the onset of a 3- to 5-day placebo run-in period; fasting blood and urine samples for laboratory evaluations were also obtained before this run-in period. All prior regimens of antidepressants, antipsychotics, mood stabilizers (eg, lithium, valproic acid, and carbamazepine), anticholinergics, amantadine, and diphenhydramine were gradually discontinued before the placebo run-in period at clinically determined rates, which minimized the effect of withdrawing the medication(s) too rapidly. On the day after the last dose of previous psychotropic medications was received, patients received 3 placebo tablets, once daily, for 3 to 5 days. Patients in whom extrapyramidal symptoms developed during the placebo run-in period were excluded from double-blind treatment. The electrocardiographic examination, laboratory evaluations, and physical examination were performed again before randomization; vital signs and weight were also obtained again before randomization.

After this run-in period, patients were randomized in a 2:1 ratio to L-745,870, 15 mg (3 tablets of 5 mg) or placebo (3 identically appearing tablets) once daily for 4 weeks.

Medications

All study medications were taken once daily, in the presence of a nurse, in the morning after blood samplings or other study measurements. Patients who required rescue with standard antipsychotic medications or other interventions at any time during the study were withdrawn. Antidepressants, antipsychotics, or mood stabilizers were prescribed. However, chloral hydrate, 500 to 1000 mg daily, could be prescribed sparingly for insomnia. Extrapyramidal symptoms could be treated (not prophylactically) with anticholinergic medications as indicated per the label, if necessary. Acute agitation was treated sparingly with single parenteral or oral doses (no standing orders were allowed) of lorazepam (Ativan, Wyeth-Ayerst Laboratories, Philadelphia, Pa) at doses consistent with

0.2-nmol/L [^{3}H]spiperone to cloned human D_4 dopamine receptors (K_i [negative log of inhibitory concentration] = 0.43 nmol/L); L-745,870 exhibited greater than 2000-fold selectivity for the D_4 dopamine receptor compared with other dopamine receptor subtypes, with affinities (IC_{50} [inhibitory concentration that causes a 50% reduction in in vivo response] ≥400 nmol/L) for serotonin type 2 and ς- and α-adrenergic receptors. In vitro, L-745,870 (0.1-1.0 μmol/L) exhibited D_4 dopamine receptor antagonist activity, reversing dopamine (1 μmol/L) mediated inhibition of adenylate cyclase in hD_4HEK and hD_4CHO cells, stimulation of [^{35}S]GTPγS [sulfur 35 guanosine triphosphate-γ–sulfur] binding, and stimulation of the extracellular acidification rate, but without any notable intrinsic activity in these assays.

Because in vivo neurochemical or behavioral responses were not observed with L-745,870 alone at doses in excess of those required for the blockade of D_4 dopamine receptors, D_4 dopamine receptor occupancy of L-745,870 was indirectly determined through (1) inhibition of in vivo [^{3}H]SKF10047 binding in mice, (2) inhibition of mescaline-induced head twitches in mice, and labeling. Any patient who required lorazepam for agitation was to be reassessed by the investigator to determine if the patient should remain in the study. Alcohol consumption was not permitted during the study. Otherwise, there were no dietary or other restrictions.

Assessments

All assessments were made by skilled research psychiatrists. Patients were assessed on the BPRS before the study, at the end of the placebo run-in period (to serve as a baseline for subsequent comparisons), and on the last day of each treatment week. The 18-item version, which designates 1 (not present) to 7 (very severe) as the anchor points, was used. Items 3, 4, 6, 7, 13, 14, 16, 17, and 18 were rated on the basis of observations made during the interview. The remaining items were rated on the basis of reported (ie, subjective) information pertaining to the week before the evaluation. The response of positive and negative symptoms was assessed through subsequent analysis of positive symptoms[17] of the BPRS (ie, conceptual disorganization, grandiosity, hostility, suspiciousness, hallucinatory behavior, and excitement) and the withdrawal-retardation factor (ie, the anergy factor minus disorientation [ie, emotional withdrawal, blunted affect, and motor retardation items]) subscale of the BPRS, respectively. The CGI[18] Severity of Illness Scale was completed before the study, at the end of the placebo run-in period (to serve as a baseline for subsequent comparisons), and on the last day of each treatment week. The ratings were from 1 (normal) to 7 (among the most extremely ill patients). Safety observations included physical examination, weight, laboratory evaluations, vital signs, and electrocardiographic examination at specified intervals and adverse experience reporting, including extrapyramidal signs and symptoms.

Plasma Samples for Drug Levels

Blood samples for drug levels were obtained on the last day of each treatment week before the morning dose of medication. To obtain an estimate of exposure of patients to L-745,870, plasma levels of 10 patients receiving L-745,870 were analyzed at random; average (±SD) trough plasma levels of 12±7 ng/mL were observed throughout the study. These levels were consistent with those observed in human volunteers; based on preclinical data described in the introduction of this article, such levels are estimated to yield a D_4 dopamine receptor central occupancy of greater than 90%.

Logistics

Up to 10 experienced investigators were to have enrolled a total of 75 patients, 50 to receive L-745,870 and 25 to receive placebo. Based on the results of a sampling of other studies of hospitalized patients, it was estimated that approximately 72% (n=54) of the patients would complete 4 weeks of study. Patients who discontinued treatment for any reason were not replaced. All patients who discontinued the study for adverse effects remained under medical supervision and received appropriate care for as long as clinically indicated.

As the study was exploratory, data from the study were reviewed by 2 of us (M.S.K. and A.G.) after approximately half of the patients (n=38) had reached a valid end point. Investigators remained blinded. Given the unanticipated results of that analysis, as reported below, a decision was made to discontinue the study.

STATISTICAL ANALYSES

The database and automated graphing and tabulation systems (Microsoft EXCEL 5.0, Microsoft Corporation, Redmond, Wash) were developed and all analyses (Statistica, Statsoft, Tulsa, Okla) were done using mainstream software packages. The study was powered at 90% ($P<.05$, 2-tailed Student t test) to detect a week 4 change from baseline in total BPRS score (last observation carried forward [LOCF]) between L-745,870 and placebo of approximately 10 points on total BPRS.

Approximately midway through the study, an unplanned interim analysis was performed. All 38 patients (ie, 26 patients receiving L-745,870 and 12 receiving placebo) reached a valid end point. For the primary outcome, an analysis of LOCF data of a week 4 change from baseline in total BPRS score for placebo vs L-745,870 was performed as a Student t test for independent samples. Secondary analyses included the following: not carried forward (NCF) analysis for total BPRS score, LOCF analysis, and NCF analysis for positive symptoms, negative symptoms, and CGI score. To justify post hoc significance testing, repeated measures analysis of variance (ANOVA) tests—by times (baseline and weeks 1, 2, 3, and 4) and groups (placebo and L-745,870)—were done for total BPRS, CGI, and positive or negative symptoms (from the BPRS); their effects and interactions were noted. As the group by time interactions were significant ($P<.02$), exploratory post hoc testing was performed for each outcome measure. The results seemed to be consistent across multicenter sites.

In addition, the cumulative distributions of the percentage of patients who achieved a particular week 4 change from baseline scores are included. Finally, an exploratory analysis of week 4 change from baseline LOCF data was done for each individual item score of the BPRS.

(3) induction of mild parkinsonianlike symptoms in squirrel monkeys (ie, via its weak affinity for ς, serotonin type 2, and D_2 dopamine receptors, respectively). The median effective dose values obtained for L-745,870 in these in vivo surrogate marker studies were extrapolated to estimate the doses of L-745,870 required to occupy D_4 dopamine receptors, using the relative ratios between the binding affinity of L-745,870 at the D_4 dopamine receptor and the respective surrogate marker. These estimations of D_4 dopamine receptor blockade were closely correlated. In addition, the doses of haloperidol and clozapine estimated through these assays to stimulate dopamine metabolism, reverse amphetamine-induced hyperactivity in mice, and block apomorphine-induced stereotypy were correlated better with those required to occupy D_2 compared with D_4 dopamine receptors.[11,12] Based on ratios of preclinical in vivo exposure levels in appropriate species compared with those observed in humans, a clinical dose of L-745,870, 15 mg/d, was predicted to occupy greater than 90% of central D_4 dopamine receptors at all times throughout the dosing interval.

The D_4 Dopamine Antagonist Group

Clinical Centers and Investigators

Loma Linda University Behavioral Medical Center, Redlands, Calif: Dan Zimbroff, MD. *Charter Brookside Hospital, Nashua, NH:* Hisham Hafez, MD. *New York Veterans Administration Medical Center, New York:* Murray Alpert, PhD; John Rotrosen, MD. *John Umstead Hospital, Butner, NC:* Joseph McEvoy, MD. *Hillside Hospital and Long Island Jewish Medical Center, Glen Oaks, NY:* John Kane, MD; Michael Kronig, MD. *Affiliated Research Institute, San Diego, Calif:* Charles Merideth, MD. *University of Texas Health Sciences Center, San Antonio:* Larry Ereshefsky, PharmD, FCCP. *West Los Angeles Veterans Administration Medical Center and University of California, Los Angeles:* Stephen Marder, MD; Donna Ames, MD.

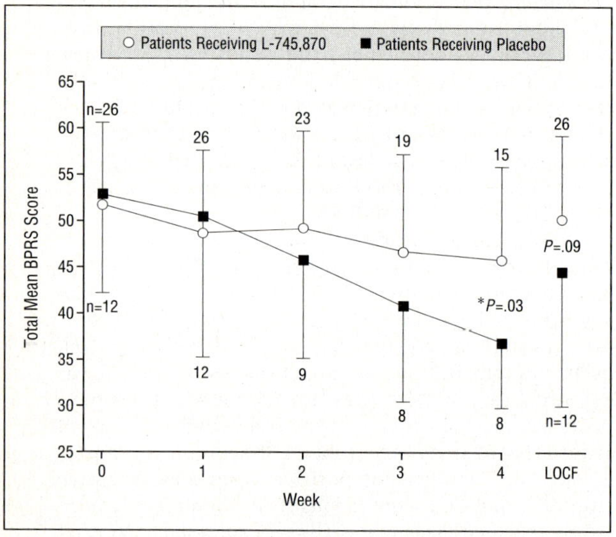

Figure 1. *Effect of L-745,870 or placebo on total mean Brief Psychiatric Rating Scale (BPRS) scores. LOCF indicates last observation carried forward; asterisk, a significant difference.*

This article describes the results of a placebo-controlled, double-blind study in which 38 acutely psychotic patients with schizophrenia were treated with L-745,870, 15 mg/d, for up to 4 weeks.

RESULTS

DEMOGRAPHICS AND PATIENT ACCOUNTING

The mean (±SD) age for patients randomized to L-745,870 or placebo was 38 (±8) years (n=26) and 42 (±6) years (n=12), respectively. Three of the 26 patients receiving L-745,870 were women compared with 1 of the 12 patients receiving placebo. At baseline, the mean severity of illness as measured by the total BPRS (**Figure 1**) or CGI (**Figure 2**) score was almost identical for patients randomized to L-745,870 or placebo. Of the patients receiving L-745,870, 14 (54%) completed all 4 weeks of the study compared with 8 (67%) of the patients receiving placebo. Of the patients receiving L-745,870, 9 (35%) were withdrawn from the study early because of lack of efficacy compared with 2 (17%) of patients receiving placebo.

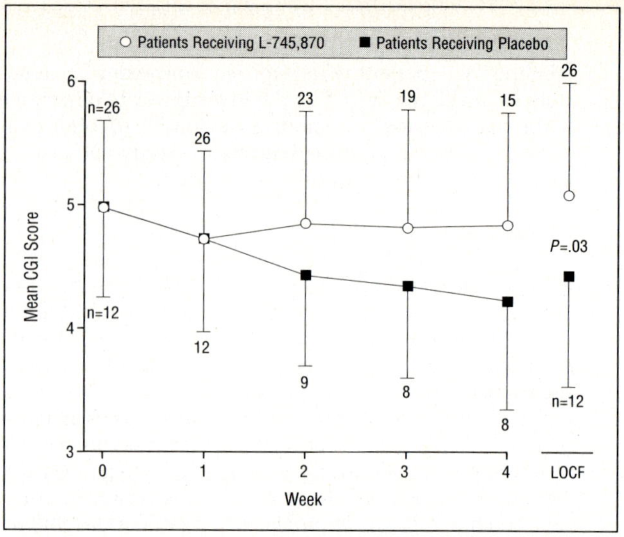

Figure 2. *Effect of L-745,870 on mean Clinical Global Impressions (CGI) scores. LOCF indicates last observation carried forward.*

EFFICACY RESULTS

Total BPRS

Figure 1 shows the mean change from baseline to week 4 on the LOCF total BPRS and the estimate of the NCF mean score at each time point. On LOCF analyses, the difference in mean week 4 change from baseline between L-745,870 and placebo, although numerically in favor of placebo, only tended toward statistical significance (2-tailed Student *t* test=−1.71, *P*=.09). A gradual but definite reduction of mean total BPRS scores was observed over time in patients receiving placebo, whereas little change from baseline was observed for patients receiving L-745,870 (NCF group by time interaction, F[4,84]=2.71, *P*=.03; LOCF group by time interaction, F[4,144]=2.28, *P*=.06). The difference in mean week 4 change from baseline L-745,870 and placebo on the NCF analysis was statistically significant in favor of placebo (2-tailed Student *t* test=−2.30, *P*=.03).

Clinical Global Impressions

Figure 2 shows the CGI score (LOCF, change from baseline to week 4) plus the NCF estimate at each time point and the change from baseline to week 4 NCF analysis. The results of the CGI analysis are consistent with those of the total BPRS (ie, a gradual but definite reduction of mean CGI scores was observed in patients receiving placebo compared with little change from baseline in patients receiving L-745,870). The difference in mean week 4 change from baseline between L-745,870 and placebo on the LOCF analysis was statistically significant in favor of placebo (group by time interaction F[4,144]=.03; 2-tailed Student *t* test=−2.19, *P*=.03). No significant differences between the groups were detected on the NCF repeated measures ANOVA or change from baseline to week 4 (group by time interaction F[4,84]=1.58, *P*=.19; 2-tailed Student *t* test=−1.67, *P*=.11).

As seen in **Figure 3**, a greater percentage of patients receiving L-745,870 compared with those receiving placebo had worse scores on the CGI analysis at week 4 compared with baseline. Similar cumulative distributions were observed for total BPRS analysis and positive symptoms.

Positive and Negative Symptom Scores

As shown in **Figure 4**, the differences between patients receiving L-745,870 and those receiving placebo in mean positive symptom score changes from baseline were similar in direction and magnitude with those observed for mean total BPRS scores and mean CGI scores but were not statistically significant either on the NCF (2-tailed Student *t* test=−0.96, *P*=.34) or LOCF (2-tailed Student *t* test=−1.06, *P*=.29) analyses. No significant differences (*P*=.82) in mean negative symptom scores were observed for patients receiving L-745,870 compared with those receiving placebo.

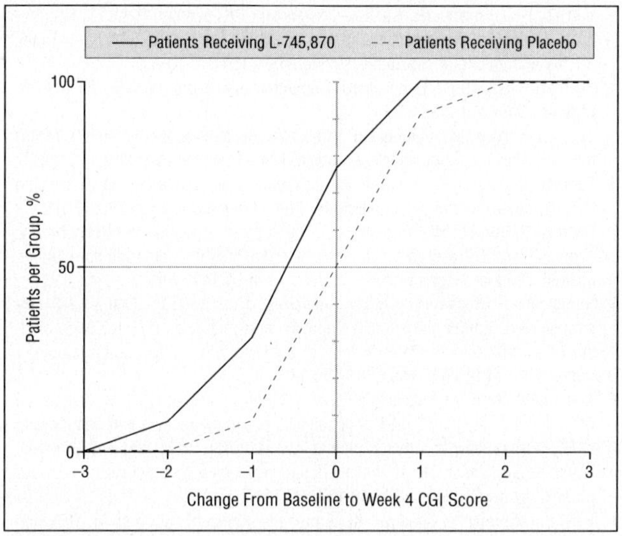

Figure 3. *Cumulative percentage of patients per group at or below a given Clinical Global Impressions (CGI) change from baseline at week 4 (last observation carried forward analysis).*

Item Scores of the BPRS

An exploratory analysis of BPRS individual item scores was undertaken to discern which aspects of behavior might be contributing to the differences that were observed on the total BPRS and CGI measures. There were modest trends between the groups in favor of placebo on hostility (2-tailed Student *t* test=−1.71, *P*=.06) and unusual thought content (2-tailed Student *t* test=−1.71, *P*=.05). Although this exploratory analysis was not adjusted for multiplicity of comparisons, consistent trends were observed in favor of placebo treatment for most items. On average, patients receiving L-745,870 were more uncooperative, excited, hostile, and tense at week 4 (LOCF) compared with baseline, whereas patients receiving placebo were more cooperative, less tense, and less conceptually disorganized at week 4 (LOCF) than at baseline.

ADJUNCTIVE USE OF LORAZEPAM OR CHLORAL HYDRATE

Lorazepam was prescribed adjunctively for patients receiving L-745,870 and placebo for a comparable (23% and 22%, respectively) number of days that the patients were in the study. Chloral hydrate was prescribed on significantly more treatment days for patients receiving L-745,870 (157 of 584 days [27%]) than those receiving placebo (25 of 286 days [9%]) (χ^2=27, *df*=890, *P*<.001).

SAFETY RESULTS

In general, L-745,870 and placebo were well tolerated in this study. There were few reports of clinical, laboratory, or other adverse experiences. No treatment emergent extrapyramidal symptoms were observed in this study in patients receiving either L-745,870 or placebo. A total of 5 adverse experiences was reported by 3 of 12 patients receiving placebo compared with 17 reports by 7 of 26 patients receiving L-745,870. Most of the adverse experiences that were reported by patients receiving L-745,870 were related to worsening of psychiatric sta-

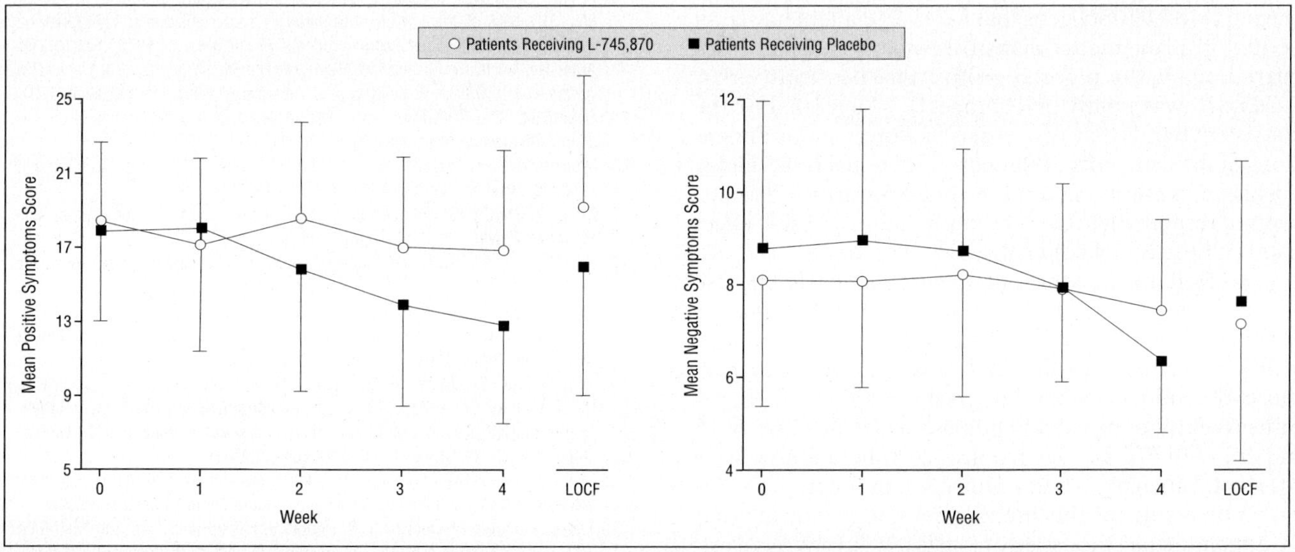

Figure 4. *Effect of L-745,870 on positive and negative symptoms of the Brief Psychiatric Rating Scale. LOCF indicates last observation carried forward.*

tus (eg, bizarre behavior, agitation, hallucinations, suspiciousness, and hostility). There were no adverse experiences related to psychiatric worsening for patients receiving placebo.

COMMENT

This preliminary study suggests that L-745,870 at a dose of 15 mg/d for 4 weeks, indirectly estimated to have occupied greater than 90% of D_4 dopamine receptors, was not therapeutically efficacious in this sample of inpatients with schizophrenia. As L-745,870 is markedly selective for the human D_4 dopamine receptor (K_i=0.43 nmol/L [eg, ~2000-fold more specific for D_4 than D_2 dopamine receptors]),[19] within the limitations of this initial study, these results suggest that D_4 dopamine receptor antagonism alone is apparently not the beneficial element within the complex pharmacological features of clozapine that endows it with uniquely enhanced efficacy and few extrapyramidal symptoms.

The role, if any, of D_4 dopamine receptors[20] in the human brain, therefore, remains obscure. L-745,870 exhibited no behavioral effects in animals, except at high doses at which D_4 dopamine receptor selectivity was lost, so there was no indication from preclinical study as to the function of the D_4 dopamine receptor. In this study, the only finding was a possible mild worsening of the symptoms of acute schizophrenia in patients with schizophrenia who were receiving L-745,870 compared with those receiving placebo. This finding was due to improvement of many patients receiving placebo and a mild worsening of patients receiving L-745,870 after 4 weeks of therapy. Because of the relatively small sample size, this may have been a chance finding.

In this study, the 30% change on total BPRS score in baseline mean to week 4 mean in the patients receiving placebo is within the historical range of expected results,[21] but it is clearly at the high end. This is probably because these patients, who were preselected for past responsiveness to neuroleptics or who were naive to treatment, particularly benefited from nonspecific nonpharmacological factors (eg, placebo washout, hospitalization, and milieu therapy). On the other hand, the minimal responsiveness of patients receiving L-745,870 suggests that L-745,870 might have prevented improvements that otherwise would have occurred, as in the placebo group. The possibility that L-745,870 was mildly psychotogenic is suggested by the consistent trends that were observed along various dimensions of the data: total BPRS score, individual BPRS items, positive symptoms, CGI score, and cumulative distributions of response patterns, discontinuation and side effect data, and the use of adjunctive chloral hydrate.

Overall our data must be viewed cautiously because the study was small; it is also unknown whether higher or lower doses of L-745,870 would have been associated with a different clinical profile than was observed. Furthermore, the indirect estimate of greater than 90% D_4 dopamine receptor occupancy in humans receiving doses of 15 mg of L-745,870 per day requires corroboration by neuroreceptor imaging studies, which are in progress.

The results of this initial experiment indicate that D_4 dopamine receptor antagonism is not effective as a primary treatment for patients with schizophrenia.

Accepted for publication December 18, 1996.

We acknowledge the additional contributions of J. Arturo Silva, MD, Audie Murphy Veterans Administration Medical Center, San Antonio, Tex; William Wirshing, MD, West Los Angeles Veterans Administration Medical Center, Los Angeles, Calif; Robert Conley, MD, University of Maryland, Baltimore; Edward Allan, MD, Franklin D. Roosevelt Veterans Administration Medical Center, Montrose, NY; and Haiyung Cheng, PhD, and Cynthia Chavez-Eng, Merck Research Laboratories, West Point, Pa.

Reprints not available from the authors.

REFERENCES

1. Kane JM, Honigfeld G, Singer J, Meltzer H, and the Clozaril Collaborative Study Group. Clozapine for the treatment-resistant schizophrenic: a double-blind comparison with chlorpromazine. *Arch Gen Psychiatry.* 1988;45:789-796.
2. Farde L, Nordström A-L, Wiesel F-A, Pauli S, Halldin C, Sedvall G. Positron emission tomographic analysis of central D_1 and D_2 dopamine receptor occupancy in patients treated with classical neuroleptics and clozapine: relation to extrapyramidal side effects. *Arch Gen Psychiatry.* 1992;49:538-544.
3. Van Tol HH, Bunzow JR, Guan H-C, Sunahara RK, Seeman P, Niznik HB, Civelli O. Cloning of the gene for a human dopamine D_4 receptor with high affinity for the antipsychotic clozapine. *Nature.* 1991;350:610-614.
4. Seeman P, Guan H-C, Van Tol HH. Dopamine D_4 receptors elevated in schizophrenia. *Nature.* 1993;365:441-445.
5. Seeman P, Guan H-C, Van Tol HH, Niznik HB. Low density of dopamine D_4 receptors in Parkinson's, schizophrenia, and control brain striata. *Synapse.* 1993;14:247-253.
6. Seeman P, Guan H-C, Van Tol HH. Elevation of dopamine D_4-like sites using [^{3}H]nemonapride and [^{125}I]epidepride. *Eur J Pharmacol.* 1995;286:R3-R5.
7. Seeman P, Van Tol HH. Dopamine D_4-like receptor elevation in schizophrenia: cloned D_2 and D_4 receptors cannot be discriminated by raclopride competition against [^{3}H]nemonapride. *J Neurochem.* 1995;64:1413-1415.
8. Sumiyoshi T, Stockmeier CA, Overholser JC, Thompson PA, Meltzer HY. Dopamine D_4 receptors and effects of guanine nucleotides on [^{3}H]raclopride binding in postmortem caudate nucleus of subjects with schizophrenia or major depression. *Brain Res.* 1995;681:109-116.
9. Murray AM, Hyde TM, Knable MB, Herman MM, Bigelow LB, Carter JM, Weinberger DR, Kleinman JE. Distribution of putative D_4 dopamine receptors in postmortem striatum from patients with schizophrenia. *J Neurosci.* 1995;15(pt 2):2186-2191.
10. Reynolds GP, Mason SL. Are striatal dopamine D_4 receptors increased in schizophrenia? *J Neurochem.* 1994;63:1576-1577.
11. Patel S, Freedman S, Chapman KL, Emms F, Fletcher AE, Knowles M, Marwood R, McAllister G, Myers J, Patel SH, Curtis N, Kulagowski J, Leeson PD, Ridgill M, Graham M, Matheson S, Rathbone D, Watt AP, Bristow LJ, Rupniak NMJ, Baskin E, Lynch JJ, Ragan CI. Biological profile of L-745,870, a selective antagonist with high affinity for the dopamine D_4 receptor. *J Pharmacol Exp Ther.* In press.
12. Bristow LI, Saywell KL, Cook GP, Kulagowski JJ, Leeson PD, Ragan CI, Tricklebank MD. Lack of effect of the dopamine D_4 receptor antagonist, L-745,870, on amphetamine-induced behaviors in rodents. *Br J Pharmacol.* 1996;119:210-212.
13. American Psychiatric Association. *Diagnostic and Statistical Manual of Mental Disorders, Fourth Edition.* Washington, DC: American Psychiatric Association; 1994.
14. Overall JE. The Brief Psychiatric Rating Scale in psychopharmacology research. *Pharmacopsychiatry.* 1974;7:67-78.
15. Woerner MG, Mannuzza S, Kane JM. Anchoring the BPRS: an aid to improved reliability. *Psychopharmacol Bull.* 1988;24:112-114.
16. Simpson GM, Angus JSW. A rating scale for extrapyramidal side effects. *Acta Psychiatr Scand.* 1970;212(suppl):11-19.
17. Opler LA, Kay SR, Rosado V, Lindenmayer JP. Positive and negative syndromes in chronic schizophrenic inpatients. *J Nerv Ment Dis.* 1984;172:317-325.
18. Guy W. *Early Clinical Drug Evaluation Unit (ECDEU) Assessment Manual.* Rockville, Md: US Dept of Health and Human Services; 1976:218-222. US Dept of Health and Human Services publication (ADM) 91-338.
19. Patel S, Patel SH, Marwood R, Fletcher AE, Kulagowski J, Ragan CI, Leeson PD, Freedman SB. L-745,870 (3-{[4-(4-chlorophenyl)piperazin-1-yl]methyl}-1H-pyrrolo[2,3-b]pyridine): a high affinity and selective dopamine D_4 receptor antagonist. *Br J Pharmacol.* 1996;119(suppl):29P.
20. Lahti RA, Roberts RC, Tamminga CA. D_2-family receptor distribution in human postmortum tissue: an autoiradiographic study. *Neuroreport.* 1995;6:2505-2512.
21. Kane J. Conduct of studies: II. Presented at a Food and Drug Administration Advisory Committee Meeting on the Development of Antipsychotic Medications; July 25, 1995; Gaithersburg, Md.

Electronic *DSM-IV*

American Psychiatric Association, $89.95, ISBN 0-88048-736-4, Washington, DC, American Psychiatric Press Inc, 1994. (Electronic System Requirements: Diskette (3.5 in) with 7-page user manual. Windows: 386 or later IBM personal computer or IBM-compatible computer, DOS 5.0 or higher, at least 7-MB available hard disk space, 4-MB RAM, and Windows version 3.0 or higher. Macintosh: at least 7-MB available hard disk space, 2-MB RAM, and system version 6.0.7 or later.

The *DSM-IV* and the *International Classification of Diseases, Tenth Revision,* have established themselves as the main diagnostic references for mental health disorders worldwide. The full text of *DSM-IV,* like other major medical textbooks, has recently become available in searchable computerized format. This technological advance offers superior searching capability with fast retrieval times, compact storage, and text printing and pasting capabilities. For some mental health professionals, this software may be their first encounter with electronic media.

For research as well as clinical settings, the main advantage of the electronic version of the *DSM-IV* is the ability to search for a combination of subjects or key words. For example, a search for "anxiety" found 296 hits and a search for "sexual," 194 hits; a search for a crossmatch of both items yielded 50 hits. Studying each and every hit would be a Sisyphean job. To overcome this difficulty, the search utility of the *Electronic DSM-IV* offers 2 convenient tools.

The Precision Bar determines the distance allowed in the text for these search terms to be apart and still qualify as a match. In our example, searching for "anxiety" and "sexual" with the bar set on the option of "all search terms must occur in the text" retrieved 50 matches. Changing the precision bar setting to "search terms must occur within 10 words of each other" resulted in 7 matches. When we refined our search by setting the bar to "search terms must be adjacent to each other," we had a single match about sexual dysfunction, which we considered as fulfilling the aims of the search.

With the Smart Match option, the software presents a relative relevance score for each match and ranks the top 20 matches in descending order.

The *Electronic DSM-IV* has many useful advantages, such as the ability to search by *DSM-IV* numeric codes, by disorder, or by phrase. Moreover, when a search term is misspelled, an alphabetical list of all possible textbook terms is displayed, opened to the appropriate alphabetic position. Another practical tool is the ability to attach multiple electronic bookmarks and sticky notes. These can be placed at specific locations and notes can be added for future reference.

The software is easy to use; opening a new window places it over the previous one, enabling the user to switch between them. It is also possible to view the complete list of open windows and jump directly to any one of them. An important feature of this electronic version is the ability to print paragraphs of the text from *DSM-IV.* This utility is useful as a teaching aid and for inclusion in patient files.

We found the software to be an important addition to the electronic library of those wishing access to the *DSM-IV.* It performs well on a 486-equipped IBM or IBM-compatible computer. The software is supported for IBM, IBM-compatible, and Macintosh computers.

A minor drawback of the software is the missing decision trees for differential diagnosis appearing in "Appendix A" of the printed version. Another drawback may be the questionable convenience of reading large sections of text from a computer screen.

Considering *DSM-IV* as undoubtedly a reference source rather than a textbook, we think that for most users, this electronic version may entirely replace the printed version of the manual.

Daniel Mimouni, MD
Beilinson Medical Center
Petah-Tiqva, 49100 Israel
Yuval Bloch, MD
Shalvata Mental Health Center
Hod-Hasharon, 45100 Israel

George Winokur, MD, 1925-1996

George Winokur, MD, was born on February 10, 1925, and died on October 12, 1996. He was a truly remarkable member of the academic psychiatric community. His commitment to systematic, controlled psychiatric research was never in question. His entire career was spent trying to learn more about our diagnostic system, the differential diagnosis of psychiatric disorders, the course and long-term outcome of such disorders, and the nature of the familiality of psychiatric illness. He was a prolific writer, having published approximately 400 articles and individual chapters as well as a dozen textbooks and monographs. His work was known and respected all over the world, evidenced by his many invitations to participate in international meetings and to deliver lectures at leading medical schools throughout the world.

Dr Winokur was born in Philadelphia, Pa, but moved early in life to Baltimore, Md, where he graduated from the Johns Hopkins University in 1944 with a bachelor of arts degree. He then attended the University of Maryland School of Medicine, Baltimore, receiving his doctor of medicine degree in 1947. He completed a rotating internship at the Church Home and Hospital, Baltimore, in 1948 and served for 2 years as an assistant resident in psychiatry at the Seton Institute, also in Baltimore, finishing in the summer of 1950. He completed his residency training at Barnes Hospital and Washington University, St Louis, Mo, in 1951. Dr Winokur joined the faculty at Washington University in 1951 and rose through the academic ranks, being appointed professor of psychiatry in 1966. He served in this capacity for 5 years before moving to the University of Iowa College of Medicine, Iowa City, in 1971 where he became the Paul W. Penningroth professor and head of the Department of Psychiatry.

He served in that capacity until 1990 when he stepped down. Dr Winokur was certified by the American Board of Psychiatry and Neurology in 1953. He was a member of all of the distinguished research societies in psychiatry and served on 18 different editorial boards including those of the *Journal of Affective Disorders, Neuropsychobiology, Archives of General Psychiatry, Comprehensive Psychiatry, Journal of Clinical Psychiatry, Journal of Nervous and Mental Disease,* and *Biological Psychiatry,* to name a few.

Dr Winokur received many awards and honors including the Hofheimer Prize for Research from the American Psychiatric Association, Washington, DC; the Anna-Monika First Prize Award for Research in Affective Disorders; the Samuel W. Hamilton Award from the

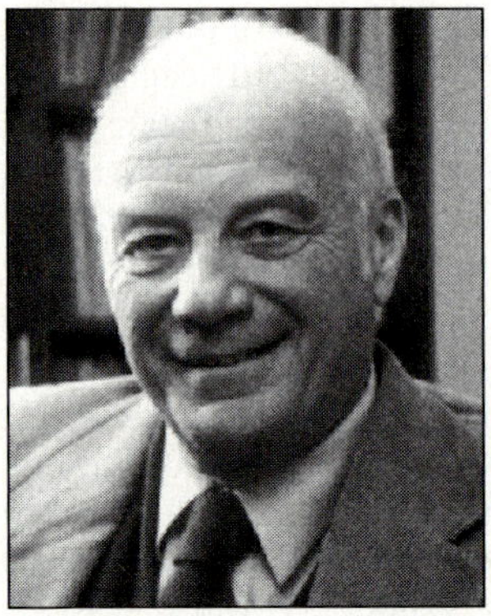
George Winokur, MD

American Psychopathological Association; the Leonard Cammer Memorial Award from Columbia College of Physicians and Surgeons, New York, NY; the Paul Hoch Award from the American Psychopathological Association; the Gold Medal Award from the Society of Biological Psychiatry; the Lifetime Research Award from the National Depressive and Manic Depressive Association, New York; the Joseph Zubin Award from the American Psychopathological Association; the Lifetime Achievement Award from the International Society of Psychiatric Genetics; and an Honorary Fellowship from the Royal College of Psychiatrists in Great Britain.

Dr Winokur married his wife Betty, a social worker, in 1951. They had 3 children: 2 sons and 1 daughter. One of their sons became a pathologist and is on the faculty of the University of Alabama, Birmingham. Their daughter is an internist interested in infectious diseases and she is on the faculty at the University of Iowa. Their other son is a musician and works all over the country. The Winokurs have 2 grandsons. Even though George Winokur occasionally feigned a certain aloofness about his family, he was a devoted husband, father, and grandfather.

At the University of Iowa, Dr Winokur developed an outstanding group of young investigators, some recruited from elsewhere and many trained within the department. One of George Winokur's most outstanding characteristics was his ability to attract people into research and to encourage them to pursue their careers in this area. He was very informal in his dealings with his faculty, dropping in on them regularly for informal chats and discussions. In this way, he kept himself informed about their progress and problems, had an opportunity to make suggestions and to offer encouragement, and, more importantly, to be sure that they appreciated the importance of what they were doing. He was highly respected by his colleagues within and without the Department of Psychiatry. In addition to his professional work and research, he had a very highly developed interest in literature. Here, as in his professional work, he impressed everyone by his phenomenal memory. It seemed he never forgot any experience. He remembered details from his reading as well as details from the life histories of his colleagues and friends. He loved to bring up episodes from the past, partly to impress people but also to look for humorous implications. Very few individuals could get away with being as candid and open as George Winokur. Somehow, people recognized that he was not mean, but that he was always looking for the interesting, the odd, or the unanticipated phenomenon or experience.

His professional accomplishments were truly outstanding. There are few, if any, individuals in his generation who have made more important or greater contributions to the advancement of psychiatry than did George Winokur. He never waivered in his determination to make this the core activity of his life and to stimulate his students, residents, and colleagues to do likewise. He was truly an outstanding, internationally recognized leader in the field. He was also an unusual individual and colleague with a wonderful sense of humor and varied interests in literature, politics, and art.

Samuel B. Guze, MD
St Louis, Mo

Ray W. Fuller, PhD, 1936-1996

Ray W. Fuller, PhD, noted neuropsychopharmacologist, died in his home in August 1996 after a 10-year struggle with chronic lymphocytic leukemia. Ray was a deeply private individual and most of his friends and associates were unaware of his long battle with this disease.

Ray's contributions to neuropsychopharmacology included seminal studies on the central monoamines, serotonin, norepinephrine, and dopamine. Ray's interest in biogenic amines, coupled with his commitment to finding better treatments for neuropsychiatric disorders, contributed immensely to the discovery and development by him and his Eli Lilly and Co colleagues of several important psychotropic medications, including fluoxetine (Prozac), a well-established selective serotonin reuptake inhibitor for the treatment of depression; pergolide (Permax), a long-acting dopamine receptor agonist for Parkinson disease; and olanzapine (Zyprexa), a novel antipsychotic agent recently introduced into clinical practice.

Ray was born and raised in southern Illinois on a farm, in the rural town of Dongola, without electricity, telephones, indoor plumbing, or school buses. Many years later, Ray noted in an invited address to the commencement class from his alma mater, Southern Illinois University, Carbondale, that his elementary schooling occurred in a 1-room school house and that he never expected to attend high school. However, because of his tenacity and the wisdom of his parents, Ray's family moved to Anna, Ill, so that he and his brother could attend high school. From there, Ray matriculated at Southern Illinois University, earning a bachelor of arts degree in chemistry and, several years later, a master's degree in microbiology.

During his years at Southern Illinois University, Ray worked as a ward attendant in a state mental hospital, then called the Anna State Hospital, during weekends and summers to help pay for his education. It was during this time that Ray developed his intense interest in the brain and realized that a better understanding of normal brain function and dysfunction might lead to new treatments for the mentally ill. At Anna State Hospital, Ray assisted in administering electroconvulsive shock therapy to patients with severe depression, an effective, albeit frightening, treatment in those days. These early experiences helped Ray to formulate his lifelong interest and commitment to alternative and better therapies for treating mental disorders.

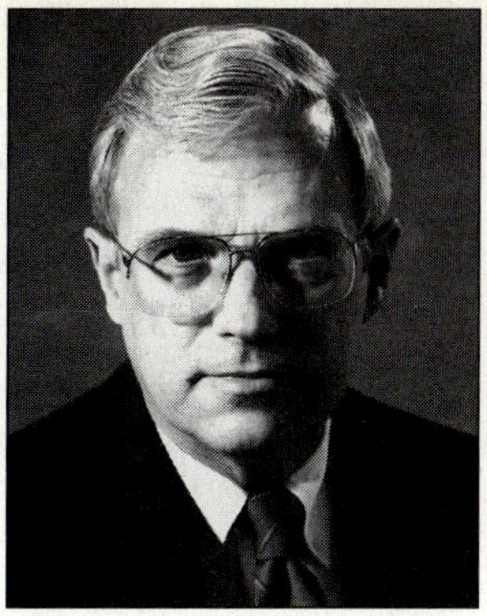
Ray W. Fuller, PhD

With these ideas shaping in young Fuller, he enrolled at Purdue University, Lafayette, Ind, receiving his doctor of philosophy degree in biochemistry, followed by a brief position as director of the biochemistry research laboratory at Fort Wayne State Hospital, Fort Wayne, Ind. During this time, Ray published 2 articles in *Science* on his studies of Down syndrome (1962;137:868-869; 1963;141:535). In 1963, Dr Irwin Slater, director of research for Lilly Research Laboratories, met young Fuller and, impressed with his potential abilities, convinced Ray to join the Lilly Research Laboratories. These 2 gentlemen developed an enormous respect for each other and, ultimately, a friendship that encouraged and permitted Ray to grow and develop as a scientist and discoverer of novel drugs for the treatment of psychiatric disorders. Ray began his early studies at Lilly with a focus on the role of serotonin in brain function. During the mid-1960s, Ray published several important papers on the metabolism of tryptophan and serotonin. In fact, Ray's interest in the treatment of depression was expressed as early as 1965 in a letter to *Lancet* (1965;2:640) where he expanded on theories regarding the potential importance of biogenic amine neurotransmitters in the biochemical basis of depression. Ray was also interested in the interactions of phenylethylamines and amphetamines with monoamine oxidase and serotonergic and noradrenergic receptor mechanisms in the brain.

In 1989, after several promotions and a mercifully brief foray in administration, Ray was promoted to Lilly research fellow. During this time, Ray held adjunct faculty positions at the Indiana University School of Medicine, Indianapolis, and the Southern Illinois School of Medicine. He was also a visiting lecturer at Massachusetts Institute of Technology, Cambridge. Until his death, Ray served on the editorial board of 14 major scientific journals. Ray was a member of many professional societies and served as a reviewer for the many National Institutes of Health, Bethesda, Md, and other study sections.

As a scientist, Ray exhibited remarkable insight and clarity of thought. In part, this resulted from his conviction that scientific writing was a fundamental responsibility and requirement for all scientists. Ray believed that "doing good experiments is not enough; the results have to be communicated acceptably to the right people." He wrote, "writing is a valuable tool for clear thinking, necessary for the accurate transmission of ideas and information" and that "the quality of writing gives the reader an impression of the scientist" (*The Pharmacologist*. 1992; 34:248-251). During his career, Ray contributed more than 500 scientific articles in the areas of neuropharmacology and neurochemistry. The example that Ray provided affirmed his contention that the best scientists in the industry not only discover drugs, but also publish their data in the best scientific journals available. Ray's prowess and expertise in discovering drugs and communicating his scientific observations were enhanced by his legendary typing and shorthand skills. For some time within the Lilly Research Laboratories, Ray served as secretary at research management meetings, since his scientific prowess, coupled with his secretarial skills, permitted minutes to be distributed rapidly from each of these meetings. Ray was also an advocate of precise and specific grammar in scientific writing and he was the owner of several reference sources on scientific writing that were used by virtually all Lilly scientists at one time or another. Scientists often used Ray's expertise in providing the most expeditious and precise syntax for a given idea.

During the course of his career, Ray received many honors for which he was humble and proud. These included 2 honorary doctorate degrees from Southern Illinois University and Purdue University, Lafayette, Ind. In addition, he received the Outstanding Professional Achievement and Alumni Achievement Awards from Southern Illinois University. Most notably, in 1993, Ray was the co-recipient (with David Wong and Bryan Molloy) of the coveted Pharmaceutical Manufacturer's Association Discoverer's Award for his work on fluoxetine. This award, one of the most prestigious for scientists in the pharmaceutical industry, has been awarded to some of the most distinguished scientists in biomedical research, such as Sir James Black, Gertrude Elion, George Hitchings, Max Tischler, and Paul Janssen.

In addition to his scientific work, Ray enjoyed fishing and bird watching. He was also an aficionado of country music and a connoisseur of gourmet food. Ray's scientific, professional, and personal standards were impeccable. He had a well-defined and established sense of integrity and fairness. These qualities were exhibited in many ways. In 1970, for instance, Ray wrote a letter (*Science*. 1970;167:1562) indicating that he "felt obliged to provide the name of a supplier and the lot numbers of erroneously labeled catecholamines, epinephrine, and norepinephrine" that had been provided to him in bottles bearing the opposite labels! When discussing data or the design of experiments, Ray was always able to provide an impartial and objective perspective and to ask the fairest and most appropriate critical questions. For all of these qualities, Ray earned the profound respect of his colleagues around the world.

Ray had a marvelous work ethic, believing strongly that every activity in life should be accomplished to the absolute best of one's ability. During a commencement address he delivered at his beloved alma mater, Southern Illinois University, he closed with 3 points of advice. "First, be yourself, nobody can do that. Second, don't let the fear of making mistakes keep you from finding out what you can accomplish and, third, keep learning—continue your education—throughout your life."

Ray was fond of collecting "quotes" on topics of personal importance to him. In fact, in 1992 Ray distributed a copy of "Some Philosophies I Have Tried To Use In My Own Life" to Lilly neuroscientists. The quotes covered topics on *wisdom* (Know your ignorance if you are to be wise. Be curious. Wisdom is the ability to ask good questions and see the total picture.), *independence* (Be an independent thinker. Don't be afraid to rock the boat. Don't be afraid to get into trouble if it is the right thing to do.), *openness* (This is very important and rare; be open to new points of view and new ideas. If data don't fit the theory, don't get rid of the data. Search out individuals who will disagree with you, and in that way you may learn.), *courage* (Have the fortitude to face difficulty. Say what you believe.), *ability to reason* (Reason works by logic, not by force. Reason is the joining of knowledge and intuition.), *communication* (Listen. The objective of dialogue is to understand, searching and questioning in pursuit of truth.), *learning* (Commit yourself to lifelong learning.), *responsibility* (Be accountable for your actions; do not try to shift the blame to someone else.), and *authenticity* (Your thoughts, words, and actions should be congruent; others will trust you then.). Ray deeply believed in these principles, and he spent the latter part of his career instilling similar principles in others with whom he came in contact. Although Ray was a man of few words, when he spoke, his words were always highly influential.

Despite his many honors and awards and his exceptional character, Ray was a modest, humble, and unassuming person. In fact, his most prized "award" was a plastic gumball machine filled with Lifesaver's that he had received from a Phoenix television anchor who was a Prozac user who had used the Lifesaver's logo as a way to thank Ray for "saving my life." Ray's collection of quotes consisted of one that he particularly liked; a quote that we believe captures the essence of his career and life. This quote is from Leo Rosten and reads:

> I can't believe the purpose of life is to be happy. I think the purpose of life is to be useful, to be responsible, to be compassionate. It is above all to matter, to count, to stand for something, to have made some difference that you lived at all.

Ray is survived by his wife Sue, son Ray W. Fuller II, and daughter Angela L. Shock, as well as his mother, brother, and 5 grandchildren. In addition, through his mentoring and his science, Ray will influence generations of psychopharmacologists to come.

Marlene L. Cohen, PhD
David L. Nelson, PhD
Steven M. Paul, MD
Indianapolis, Ind

Schizophrenia After Prenatal Famine

If an event like the Dutch Hunger Winter caused a unique and dramatic decline in population fertility that differentially affected the social classes, confounding by socioeconomic status must be ruled out before conclusions can be drawn about a possible association between prenatal nutritional deficiency and later schizophrenia, as suggested by Susser et al.[1] The exposed (EX2) cohort was marked by a 50% decline in fertility. This decrease was associated with socioeconomic status, because it particularly affected the class of manual occupations.[2] The authors state that "no relation has been found in the Netherlands between schizophrenia and low social class of origin." The question, however, is whether the outcome under investigation (discharge from a psychiatric hospital with a diagnosis of schizophrenia in the Netherlands) is possibly associated with higher socioeconomic status of origin, because only this would lead to a spurious association. In fact, the well-known Dutch study[3] on social class and schizophrenia referred to by Susser et al[1] reported findings to this effect. For example, 39% of the fathers of a randomly selected Dutch control sample performed skilled or unskilled manual labor, compared with only 15% of the fathers of patients with schizophrenia as classified by the *International Classification of Diseases (ICD)* (relative risk, 2.7; 95% confidence interval, 1.2-6.1; $P<.01$; our calculations from the data provided). Patients and patients' fathers were also better educated than their control sample counterparts. The Dutch study is by no means the only one to report such associations. The recent British 1946 Birth Cohort Study[4] to which Susser et al[1] also refer reports an association at the 10% significance level between cumulative risk of schizophrenia and higher social class. Whether the association between higher socioeconomic status and schizophrenia in these studies is real or an artifact of, for example, filters operating at the level of hospital admission or diagnosis, is not at issue; what matters is the likely confounding mechanism.

If the results for schizophrenia were confounded by social class because both the famine exposure and the schizophrenia outcome were associated with higher socioeconomic status, one would expect the opposite, namely, a "protective," effect of the famine exposure, on a disorder that is associated with lower social class. Because there is evidence that lower social status is associated with an increased risk of affective disorder,[5] one would expect such a protective effect of the famine exposure on the cumulative risk of admission to a psychiatric hospital for affective disorder. For a previous study,[6] we had obtained from the Dutch National Psychiatric Case Register a list of all 143 316 individuals discharged from the hospital with an *ICD-8* or *ICD-9* discharge diagnosis of functional psychosis (295.0-298.9) for the first time from 1970 through 1992. The diagnostic distribution among these individuals with functional psychosis who were born in the 6 cities in the famine region was markedly different in the EX2 cohort as compared with the unexposed cohort (as defined by Susser et al[1]). There was an excess of "narrow" schizophrenia (as defined by Susser et al[1]) in the EX2 cohort [EX2 cohort, 25% (9/36); unexposed cohort, 14% (138/987); χ^2, 3.4; *df*, 1, $P=.06$], but a deficit of affective (*ICD* 296.0-296.9) psychosis cases [EX2, 11% (4/36); unexposed cohort, 28% (273/987); χ^2, 4.8; *df*, 1; $P=.03$]. Relating these figures to the source population provided by Susser et al[1] yielded a similar picture. The EX2 cohort was at an increased risk of developing schizophrenia (relative risk, 2.1; 95% confidence interval, 1.1-4.2; $P=.03$), but at a decreased risk of developing affective psychosis (relative risk, 0.5; 95% confidence interval, 0.2-1.3; $P=.13$). Although this latter association failed to reach the conventional statistical significance level, it was large and in the predicted direction.

Another issue is the role of numerator/denominator discrepancy. Since 1945, Dutch cities have undergone substantial boundary changes, to the effect that many smaller municipalities have merged with the larger cities. The Dutch National Psychiatric Case Register codes place of birth according to the most recent boundary changes, whereas the figures used in the denominator refer to the city boundaries of 1944 and 1945. Therefore, subjects born during the Hunger Winter in the nearly 50 smaller municipalities[7] that were later added to the 6 large cities in the study were included in the numerator, whereas their corresponding birth cohorts were excluded from the denominator. While this is unlikely to have led to spurious results, it may have led to spurious precision. The likely effect of this discrepancy should therefore be quantified.

Jim van Os, MSc, PhD
Department of Psychiatry and Neuropsychology
Maastricht University
PO Box 616
6200 MD Maastricht
the Netherlands

1. Susser E, Neugebauer R, Hoek HW, Brown AS, Lin S, Labovitz D, Gorman JM. Schizophrenia after prenatal famine: further evidence. *Arch Gen Psychiatry.* 1995;53:25-31.
2. Stein Z, Susser M, Saenger G, Marolla F, eds. *Famine and Human Development: The Dutch Hunger Winter of 1944-45.* New York, NY: Oxford University Press Inc; 1975:80-81.
3. Wiersma D, Giel R, De Jong A, Slooff CJ. Social class and schizophrenia in a Dutch cohort. *Psychol Med.* 1983;13:141-150.

4. Jones P, Rodgers B, Murray R, Marmot M. Child developmental risk factors for adult schizophrenia in the British 1946 birth cohort. *Lancet.* 1994;344:1398-1402.
5. Dohrenwend BP, Dohrenwend BS. *Social Status and Psychological Disorder: A Causal Inquiry.* New York, NY: John Wiley & Sons Inc; 1969:113-127.
6. van Os J, Howard N, Takei N, Murray R. Increasing age is a risk factor for psychosis in the elderly. *Soc Psychiatry Psychiatr Epidemiol.* 1995;30:161-165.
7. *Historisch Gemeenteregister versie 1994* [computer program]. Code CBS29D. Voorburg, the Netherlands: Centraal Bureau voor de Statistiek; 1994.

In reply

We thank Dr van Os for his thoughtful comments and careful reading of our work. In addition, his letter provides us with a welcome opportunity to demonstrate that social class confounding cannot account for our result from the Dutch famine study.[1]

First, if there were confounding due to social class of origin, it would most likely have diminished the association between prenatal exposure to famine and the risk of hospitalization for schizophrenia. As Dr van Os rightly indicates, the lower class was underrepresented in the exposed cohorts. Most studies suggest that individuals in the lower class are at an increased risk of hospitalization for schizophrenia; therefore, the effect would be to reduce the observed risk in the exposed cohort and to reduce the relative risk of hospitalization for schizophrenia. The result of the Dutch study[2] *to which Dr van Os refers was atypical. That study included only a small number of patients with schizophrenia (N=34) and was conducted in a university town; the authors noted these limitations and did not infer from their results that individuals in the upper class in Holland were at a higher risk for schizophrenia.*

Second, in the unlikely circumstance that upper social class were associated with schizophrenia, the confounding would have been minimal. To see this, consider an example. Assume that we have 5000 exposed and 100 000 unexposed individuals and that the risk of schizophrenia is the same in the exposed and unexposed groups within a given social class (ie, there is no effect of exposure on risk). Next assume that the risk of schizophrenia is twice as high in the upper class (0.5%) than in the lower class (0.25%). Allow the ratio of upper to lower class births to be 3:2 in the exposed group and 1:1 in the unexposed group, as it actually was in the data of our study.[1] *The risk of schizophrenia in the exposed group can be computed as a weighted average of the risk in the upper and lower class, ie, [(0.5% × 3000)+(0.25% × 2000)]/5000=4/1000, and the risk of schizophrenia in the unexposed group can be computed in the same way to be 3.75/1000. The relative risk is 4/3.75=1.07. This example shows that, while being born into the upper class is assumed to have a strong effect on schizophrenia, even if prenatal famine exposure is assumed to have no effect on schizophrenia, the artifactual relative risk due to social class confounding is barely detectable and cannot account for a relative risk of the magnitude that we observed.*

Third, a subsequent study has provided empirical evidence that social class was not a confounding factor.[3] *This study examined the related outcome of schizophrenia spectrum personality disorder in men aged 18 years in the same exposed and unexposed birth cohorts. Unlike the schizophrenia study, that study included data about the social class of origin of the subjects. The effect was found to be the same among individuals in the upper and lower classes. Finally, we were unable to verify the decrease in ICD-9 affective psychoses in the exposed birth cohort that is noted by Dr van Os. It seems that he has made some errors in the data analysis (eg, by the omission of female cases). Nevertheless, it should be underscored that had this decrease in affective psychoses been real, it would not by any means indicate that the result we have reported for schizophrenia was due to social class confounding.*

In summary, social class confounding does not explain the increased risk of schizophrenia after early prenatal exposure to famine.

Ezra S. Susser, MD, DrPH
Division of Epidemiology and Community Psychiatry
Department of Psychobiology
New York State Psychiatric Institute
College of Physicians and Surgeons of Columbia University
722 W 168th St, Box 24
New York, NY 10023
Richard Neugebauer, PhD
Hans W. Hoek, MD
Alan S. Brown, MD
Shang P. Lin, PhD
Daniel Labovitz, MD
Jack M. Gorman, MD
New York

1. Susser E, Neugebauer R, Hoek HW, Brown AS, Lin S, Labovitz D, Gorman JM. Schizophrenia after prenatal famine: further evidence. *Arch Gen Psychiatry.* 1996;53:25-31.
2. Wiersma D, Giel R, DeJong A, Slooff CJ. Social class and schizophrenia in a Dutch cohort. *Psychol Med.* 1983;13:141-150.
3. Hoek HW, Susser E, Buck KA, Lumey LH, Lin SP, Gorman JM. Schizoid personality disorder after prenatal exposure to famine. *Am J Psychiatry.* 1996: 153;1637-1639.

N-Methyl-D-Aspartate Receptor Hypofunction in Schizophrenia Could Arise From Reduced Cortical Connectivity Rather Than Receptor Dysfunction

An article by Olney and Farber[1] outlines an intriguing theory of schizophrenia based on studies of the glutamate *N*-methyl-D-aspartate (NMDA) receptor. Their model relies on the observation that NMDA antagonists such as phencyclidine hydrochloride can induce psychoticlike symptoms in human subjects and has demonstrated neurotoxic reactions in animals. The latter could provide an explanation for the downhill course of many patients with schizophrenia. Their model also notes that dopamine is known to inhibit glutamate release, an observation that suggests a possible therapeutic action, namely, disinhibition of glutamate release, of dopamine-blocking antipsychotic drugs. The authors postulate that NMDA receptor dysfunction underlies the pathology of schizophrenia.

Other recent studies suggest that NMDA receptor hypofunction in schizophrenia may derive not from receptor dysfunction per se, but from altered cortical connectivity. N-Methyl-D-aspartate receptors are widespread in the cerebral cortex[2,3] and mediate neuronal plasticity associated with development and learning.[4-6] Selemon et al[7] demonstrated reduced neuropil volume (ie, gray matter tissue surrounding neuronal cell bodies) in the cerebral cortex of patients with schizophrenia. These data suggest a reduction in the dendritic-axonal matrix that enwraps neurons. Two independently conducted Golgi stain studies of prefrontal layer IV pyramidal neurons in postmortem brain samples of cases with schizophrenia have also been reported recently.[8,9] Marked reductions in dendritic spine density relative to control brain samples were found in both studies. Dendritic spines provide anatomic loci for synaptic contacts between axons and dendrites.

These studies suggest that NMDA receptor hypofunction in schizophrenia could be due to the loss of microanatomic structures that incorporate these receptors rather than a disturbance of the receptor itself. Phencyclidinelike drugs could mimic this neuroanatomic condition by "functionally pruning" cortical circuits. Recent data suggest that NMDA receptors modulate corticocortical connections rather than thalamocortical connections.[10] We have described computer models of memory retrieval and perception using simulated neural networks that receive information from outside sources. These networks produced analogs of psychotic symptoms when interneuron connections were pruned away.[11,12] One of these models demonstrated marked curtailment of these "symptoms" when dopamine blockade was simulated.[12]

Postulating a primary disturbance of the NMDA receptor in schizophrenia allowed Olney and Farber[1] to invoke the neurotoxic effects of phencyclidinelike drugs to account for the downward course of this disorder. However, the doses of phencyclidine hydrochloride used to induce these effects in animals were much larger (ranging from 0.5 mg/kg to 50 mg/kg[13]) than the dose ranges of phencyclidine hydrochloride used to induce experimentally psychotic symptoms in humans (generally ranging from 0.05 mg/kg to 0.1 mg/kg).[14] Moreover, we are not aware of any evidence indicating that phencyclidine-induced neuropathological changes described by the authors are present in the brains of patients with schizophrenia. The absence of gliosis in the brains of patients with schizophrenia is also evidence against a neurodegenerative process in these disorders.[15]

Olney and Farber[1] report that the pharmacologic blockade of NMDA receptors by phencyclidinelike drugs does not have the same psychotogenic effect in preadolescence. They did not provide an explanation for this interesting observation. Normally there is an overelaboration of frontal synapses during this time; excessive synapses are later reduced during adolescence to relatively stable adult levels.[16] Perhaps preadolescent overelaboration of frontal synapses could compensate for reduced interneuron communication caused by NMDA receptor blockade by phencyclidinelike drugs.

The distinction between an NMDA receptor dysfunction model vs a synaptic elimination model of schizophrenia is not trivial. The former model predicts that molecular study of the expression and the nature of the NMDA receptor itself will be key to solving the riddle of schizophrenia. The latter model views schizophrenia as a neurodevelopmental disorder best approached by studying the regulation of synaptic pruning during adolescence and early adulthood.[17,18]

Ralph E. Hoffman, MD
Thomas H. McGlashan, MD
Yale Psychiatric Institute
PO Box 208038
New Haven, CT 06520-8038

1. Olney JW, Farber NB. Glutamate receptor dysfunction and schizophrenia. *Arch Gen Psychiatry.* 1995;52:998-1007.
2. Young AB, Dauth GW, Hollingsworth Z, Penney JB, Katz K, Gilman S. Quisqualate- and NMDA-sensitive [^{3}H] glutamate binding in primate brain. *J Neurosci Res.* 1990;27:512-521.
3. Conti F, Minelli A, Molnar M, Brecha NC. Cellular localization and laminar distribution of NMDAAR1 mRNA in the rat cerebral cortex. *J Comp Neurol.* 1994;343:554-565.
4. Hofer M, Constantine-Paton M. Regulation of N-methyl-D-aspartate (NMDA) receptor function during the rearrangement of developing neuronal connections. *Prog Brain Res.* 1994;102:277-285.
5. Keller EA, Borghese CM, Carrer HF, Ramirez OA. The learning capacity of high and low performance rats is related to hippocampus NMDA receptors. *Brain Res.* 1992;576:162-164.
6. Huang YY, Colino A, Selig DK, Malenka RC. The influence of prior synaptic activity on the induction of long-term potentiation. *Science.* 1992;255:730-733.
7. Selemon LD, Rajkowska G, Goldman-Rakic PS. Abnormally high neuronal density in the schizophrenic cortex: a morphometric analysis of prefrontal area 9 and occipital area 17. *Arch Gen Psychiatry.* 1995;52:805-818.
8. Garey LJ, Ong WY, Patel TS, Kanani M, Davis A, Hornstein C, Bauer M. Reduction in dendritic spine number on cortical pyramidal neurons in schizophrenia. *Soc Neurosci.* 1995;21:237. Abstract.
9. Glantz LA, Lewis DA. Assessment of spine density on layer III pyramidal cells in the prefrontal cortex of schizophrenic subjects. *Soc Neurosci.* 1995; 21:239. Abstract.
10. Salt TE, Meier CL, Seno N, Krucker T, Herrling PL. Thalamocortical and corticocortical excitatory postsynaptic potentials mediated by excitatory amino acid receptors in the cat motor cortex in vivo. *Neuroscience.* 1995;64:433-442.
11. Hoffman RE, Dobscha SK. Cortical pruning and the development of schizophrenia: a computer model. *Schizophr Bull.* 1989;15:477-490.
12. Hoffman RE, Rapaport J, Ameli R, McGlashan TH, Harcherik D, Servan-Schreiber D. A neural network simulation of hallucinated 'voices' and associated speech perception impairments in schizophrenic patients. *J Cognitive Neurosci.* 1995;7:479-496.
13. Olney JW, Labruyere J, Price MT. Pathological changes induced in cerebrocortical neurons by phencyclidine and related drugs. *Science.* 1989;244: 1360-1362.
14. Javitt DC, Zukin SR. Recent advances in the phencyclidine model of schizophrenia. *Am J Psychiatry.* 1991;148:1301-1308.
15. Bogerts B. Recent advances in the neuropathology of schizophrenia. *Schizophr Bull.* 1993;19:431-445.
16. Huttenlocher PR. Synaptic density in the human frontal cortex: developmental changes and effects of aging. *Brain Res.* 1979;163:195-205.
17. Feinberg I. Schizophrenia: caused by a fault in programmed synaptic elimination during adolescence? *J Psychiatry Res.* 1982/1983;17(4):319-334.
18. Hoffman RE, McGlashan T. Parallel, distributed processing and the emergence of schizophrenic symptoms. *Schizophr Bull.* 1993;19:119-140.

In reply

Hoffman and McGlashan are generally accepting of our NMDA receptor hypofunction (NRH) hypothesis of schizophrenia, but they argue that NRH could arise from reduced cortical connectivity rather than receptor dysfunction per se, and in their closing paragraphs they introduce a neurodevelopmental twist (faulty synaptic pruning) that they would like to see emphasized in an alternate framing of our hypothesis.

Implicit in their letter is the suggestion that reduced cortical connectivity, faulty synaptic pruning, and a neu-

rodevelopmental twist are novel ideas that did not occur to us. However, we included all of this thinking in our article and the accompanying commentary. We emphasized that our hypothesis was not limited to NMDA receptor dysfunction per se or to pathological processes originating in adulthood. Rather, a unique aspect of our hypothesis is that it rests on a neurodevelopmental foundation. We specifically postulated that during early development a pathologic event occurs that deletes NMDA receptors or the GABAergic neurons on which they synapse. We stressed that loss of GABAergic neurons would be an NRH "equivalent" and it is obvious that loss of either NMDA receptors or GABAergic neurons would set the stage for altered cortical connectivity in adulthood. In addition, we cited the work of Lewis et al[1] pertaining to synaptic pruning in adolescence and suggested that what would otherwise be normal pruning could become abnormal in schizophrenia because of the prior loss of NMDA receptors or the neural network to which they are attached and through which their functions are expressed. Specifically, we stated that "a GABAergic system that is already impaired due to a pathological event in utero might be further weakened beyond a critical threshold by the synaptic pruning process." Thus we would not agree with Hoffman and McGlashan that our model fails to consider neurodevelopment or synaptic pruning. Our model postulates that a neurodevelopmental anomaly and subsequent synaptic pruning may play key roles in the pathophysiology of schizophrenia.

In the commentary accompanying our article, Crow[2] characterized our hypothesis as flawed because it did not emphasize defects in cortical connectivity as the primary basis for psychopathology in schizophrenia. Our response was that our hypothesis does, in fact, rest solidly on the assumption that defective cortical connectivity plays an important role in schizophrenia. Crow did not recognize the connectionistic implications of our hypothesis because we did not shroud the hypothesis in the kind of "connectionistic" terminology with which he is familiar. Hoffman and McGlashan also seem to have failed to recognize the connectionistic implications of our hypothesis, perhaps because they may not have read the accompanying commentary where connectionistic aspects were highlighted.

Hoffman and McGlashan raise the issue that the dose of NMDA antagonists used in rats to produce the neurotoxic effects is greater than that needed to produce psychotic symptoms in humans. To evaluate this criticism, it would be necessary to know how rodents and humans compare in the rate at which they metabolize these drugs. It is well known that for many, if not most, drugs, rodents metabolize at a much higher rate, so that usually a dose 5 to 10 times higher is required to produce a given effect in the rodent compared with the human.

As an apparent criticism of our hypothesis. the authors assert that there is no evidence for "phencyclidine-induced neuropathological changes . . . in the brains of patients with schizophrenia." To the best of our knowledge, nobody has studied in schizophrenic brains the specific regions (posterior cingulate and retrosplenial cortices) that are most sensitive to damage from phencyclidine. However, it is a misunderstanding of our hypothesis to assume that we are postulating a role for phencyclidine in schizophrenia. If a patient with schizophrenia is an abuser of phencyclidine, and if the brain of that patient becomes available for autopsy evaluation, it would certainly be of interest to look for neuropathological changes that might be attributable to phencyclidine. However, most patients with idiopathic schizophrenia have never been exposed to phencyclidine, so one would not expect to find phencyclidine-induced neuropathological changes in their brains. Apparently Hoffman and McGlashan are erroneously assuming that we consider phencyclidine exposure or phencyclidine-induced neuropathology a prerequisite to the development of schizophrenia, which is not at all what we are proposing. We regard phencyclidine as a tool for studying the receptor mechanisms and circuitry in the animal brain that underlie phencyclidine-induced neurotoxic effects on cerebrocortical neurons, which we propose may be related to psychotic symptom formation in the psychotic syndrome triggered by phencyclidine and in schizophrenia, by virtue of these psychotic processes and phencyclidine neurotoxic effects having the same underlying mechanism (NRH). By deciphering the receptor systems and circuitry underlying the neurotoxic effects of phencyclidine, we hope to gain insight into mechanisms that give rise to psychotic symptom formation in schizophrenia and hopefully develop these insights in directions that will provide improved therapeutic treatment of schizophrenia. A major feature of our hypothesis is that the NRH mechanism, by a disinhibition principle, can trigger psychotic symptom formation without inducing permanent brain damage. However, if the disinhibitory state is particularly severe and long lasting, it could result eventually in neurodegenerative changes.

To further buttress their argument that NRH degeneration does not occur in schizophrenia, Hoffman and McGlashan cite the lack of gliosis in the brains of patients with schizophrenia. We would disagree with their statement because, as we discussed at length in our article and accompanying commentary, NRH produces only a very mild and transient glial response that easily could be missed in autopsy studies.

John W. Olney, MD
Nuri B. Farber, MD
Department of Psychiatry
Washington University School of Medicine
4940 Children's Place
St Louis, MO 63110

1. Lewis DA, Anderson SA, Rosenberg DR, Lund JS, Conde F. Postnatal refinements of prefrontal cortical circuitry and schizophrenia. *Schizophrenia Res.* 1995;15:29-30.
2. Crow TJ. Constraints on concepts of pathogenesis: language and the speciation process as the key to the etiology of schizophrenia. *Arch Gen Psychiatry.* 1995;52:1011-1014.

Information for Patients: Physicians are advised to discuss the following issues with patients for whom they prescribe CLOZARIL® (clozapine):

– Patients who are to receive CLOZARIL® (clozapine) should be warned about the significant risk of developing agranulocytosis. They should be informed that weekly blood tests are required to monitor for the occurrence of agranulocytosis, and that CLOZARIL® (clozapine) tablets will be made available only through a special program designed to ensure the required blood monitoring. Patients should be advised to report immediately the appearance of lethargy, weakness, fever, sore throat, malaise, mucous membrane ulceration or other possible signs of infection. Particular attention should be paid to any flu-like complaints or other symptoms that might suggest infection.

– Patients should be informed of the significant risk of seizure during CLOZARIL® (clozapine) treatment, and they should be advised to avoid driving and any other potentially hazardous activity while taking CLOZARIL® (clozapine).

– Patients should be advised of the risk of orthostatic hypotension, especially during the period of initial dose titration.

– Patients should be informed that if they stop taking CLOZARIL® (clozapine) for more than 2 days, they should not restart their medication at the same dosage, but should contact their physician for dosing instructions.

– Patients should notify their physician if they are taking, or plan to take, any prescription or over-the-counter drugs or alcohol.

– Patients should notify their physician if they become pregnant or intend to become pregnant during therapy.

– Patients should not breast feed an infant if they are taking CLOZARIL® (clozapine).

Drug Interactions: The risks of using CLOZARIL® (clozapine) in combination with other drugs have not been systematically evaluated.

The mechanism of CLOZARIL® (clozapine) induced agranulocytosis is unknown; nonetheless, the possibility that causative factors may interact synergistically to increase the risk and/or severity of bone marrow suppression warrants consideration. Therefore, CLOZARIL® (clozapine) should not be used with other agents having a well-known potential to suppress bone marrow function.

Given the primary CNS effects of CLOZARIL® (clozapine), caution is advised in using it concomitantly with other CNS-active drugs or alcohol.

Orthostatic hypotension in patients taking clozapine can, in rare cases (approximately 1 case per 3,000 patients), be accompanied by profound collapse and respiratory and/or cardiac arrest. Some of the cases of collapse/respiratory arrest/cardiac arrest during initial treatment occurred in patients who were being administered benzodiazepines; similar events have been reported in patients taking other psychotropic drugs or even CLOZARIL® (clozapine) by itself. Although it has not been established that there is an interaction between CLOZARIL® (clozapine) and benzodiazepines or other psychotropics, caution is advised when clozapine is initiated in patients taking a benzodiazepine or any other psychotropic drug.

Because CLOZARIL® (clozapine) is highly bound to serum protein, the administration of CLOZARIL® (clozapine) to a patient taking another drug which is highly bound to protein (e.g., warfarin, digitoxin) may cause an increase in plasma concentrations of these drugs, potentially resulting in adverse effects. Conversely, adverse effects may result from displacement of protein-bound CLOZARIL® (clozapine) by other highly bound drugs.

Cimetidine and erythromycin may both increase plasma levels of CLOZARIL® (clozapine), potentially resulting in adverse effects. Although concomitant use of CLOZARIL® (clozapine) and carbamazepine is not recommended, it should be noted that discontinuation of concomitant carbamazepine administration may result in an increase in CLOZARIL® (clozapine) plasma levels. Phenytoin may decrease CLOZARIL® (clozapine) plasma levels, resulting in a decrease in effectiveness of a previously effective CLOZARIL® (clozapine) dose.

A subset (3%-10%) of the population has reduced activity of certain drug metabolizing enzymes such as the cytochrome P450 isozyme P450 2D6. Such individuals are referred to as "poor metabolizers" of drugs such as debrisoquin, dextromethorphan, the tricyclic antidepressants, and clozapine. These individuals may develop higher than expected plasma concentrations of clozapine when given usual doses. In addition, certain drugs that are metabolized by this isozyme, including many antidepressants (clozapine, selective serotonin reuptake inhibitors, and others), may inhibit the activity of this isozyme, and thus may make normal metabolizers resemble poor metabolizers with regard to concomitant therapy with other drugs metabolized by this enzyme system, leading to drug interaction.

Concomitant use of clozapine with other drugs metabolized by cytochrome P450 2D6 may require lower doses than usually prescribed for either clozapine or the other drug. Therefore, co-administration of clozapine with other drugs that are metabolized by this isozyme, including antidepressants, phenothiazines, carbamazepine, and Type 1C antiarrhythmics (e.g., propafenone, flecainide and encainide), or that inhibit this enzyme (e.g., quinidine), should be approached with caution.

CLOZARIL® (clozapine) may also potentiate the hypotensive effects of antihypertensive drugs and the anticholinergic effects of atropine-type drugs. The administration of epinephrine should be avoided in the treatment of drug induced hypotension because of a possible reverse epinephrine effect.

Carcinogenesis, Mutagenesis, Impairment of Fertility: No carcinogenic potential was demonstrated in long-term studies in mice and rats at doses approximately 7 times the typical human dose on a mg/kg basis. Fertility in male and female rats was not adversely affected by clozapine. Clozapine did not produce genotoxic or mutagenic effects when assayed in appropriate bacterial and mammalian tests.

Pregnancy Category B: Reproduction studies have been performed in rats and rabbits at doses of approximately 2-4 times the human dose and have revealed no evidence of impaired fertility or harm to the fetus due to clozapine. There are, however, no adequate and well-controlled studies in pregnant women. Because animal reproduction studies are not always predictive of human response, and in view of the desirability of keeping the administration of all drugs to a minimum during pregnancy, this drug should be used only if clearly needed.

Nursing Mothers: Animal studies suggest that clozapine may be excreted in breast milk and have an effect on the nursing infant. Therefore, women receiving CLOZARIL® (clozapine) should not breast feed.

Pediatric Use: Safety and effectiveness in pediatric patients have not been established.

ADVERSE REACTIONS: Associated with Discontinuation of Treatment: Sixteen percent of 1080 patients who received CLOZARIL® (clozapine) in premarketing clinical trials discontinued treatment due to an adverse event, including both those that could be reasonably attributed to CLOZARIL® (clozapine) treatment and those that might more appropriately be considered intercurrent illness. The more common events considered to be causes of discontinuation included: CNS, primarily drowsiness/sedation, seizures, dizziness/syncope; cardiovascular, primarily tachycardia, hypotension and ECG changes; gastrointestinal, primarily nausea/vomiting; hematologic, primarily leukopenia/granulocytopenia/agranulocytosis; and fever. None of the events enumerated accounts for more than 1.7% of all discontinuations attributed to adverse clinical events.

Commonly Observed: Adverse events observed in association with the use of CLOZARIL® (clozapine) in clinical trials at an incidence of greater than 5% were: central nervous system complaints, including drowsiness/sedation, dizziness/vertigo, headache and tremor; autonomic nervous system complaints, including salivation, sweating, dry mouth and visual disturbances; cardiovascular findings, including tachycardia, hypotension and syncope; and gastrointestinal complaints, including constipation and nausea; and fever. Complaints of drowsiness/sedation tend to subside with continued therapy or dose reduction. Salivation may be profuse, especially during sleep, but may be diminished with dose reduction.

Incidence in Clinical Trials: The following table enumerates adverse events that occurred at a frequency of 1% or greater among CLOZARIL® (clozapine) patients who participated in clinical trials. These rates are not adjusted for duration of exposure.

Treatment-Emergent Adverse Experience Incidence
Among Patients Taking CLOZARIL® (clozapine) in Clinical Trials
(N = 842)
(Percentage of Patients Reporting)

Body System / Adverse Event[a]	Percent
Central Nervous System	
Drowsiness/Sedation	39
Dizziness/Vertigo	19
Headache	7
Tremor	6
Syncope	6
Disturbed sleep/Nightmares	4
Restlessness	4
Hypokinesia/Akinesia	4
Agitation	4
Seizures (convulsions)	3[b]
Rigidity	3
Akathisia	3
Confusion	3
Fatigue	2
Insomnia	2
Hyperkinesia	1
Weakness	1
Lethargy	1
Ataxia	1
Slurred speech	1
Depression	1
Epileptiform movements/Myoclonic jerks	1
Anxiety	1
Cardiovascular	
Tachycardia	25[b]
Hypotension	9
Hypertension	4
Chest pain/Angina	1
ECG change/Cardiac abnormality	1

(Continued)

Treatment-Emergent Adverse Experience Incidence
Among Patients Taking CLOZARIL® (clozapine) in Clinical Trials
(N = 842)
(Percentage of Patients Reporting)

Body System / Adverse Event[a]	Percent
Gastrointestinal	
Constipation	14
Nausea	5
Abdominal discomfort/Heartburn	4
Nausea/Vomiting	3
Vomiting	3
Diarrhea	2
Liver test abnormality	1
Anorexia	1
Urogenital	
Urinary abnormalities	2
Incontinence	1
Abnormal ejaculation	1
Urinary urgency/frequency	1
Urinary retention	1
Autonomic Nervous System	
Salivation	31
Sweating	6
Dry mouth	6
Visual disturbances	5
Integumentary (Skin)	
Rash	2
Musculoskeletal	
Muscle weakness	1
Pain (back, neck, legs)	1
Muscle spasm	1
Muscle pain, ache	1
Respiratory	
Throat discomfort	1
Dyspnea, shortness of breath	1
Nasal congestion	1
Hemic/Lymphatic	
Leukopenia/Decreased WBC/Neutropenia	3
Agranulocytosis	1[b]
Eosinophilia	1
Miscellaneous	
Fever	5
Weight gain	4
Tongue numb/sore	1

[a]Events reported by at least 1% of CLOZARIL® (clozapine) patients are included.

[b]Rate based on population of approximately 1700 exposed during premarket clinical evaluation of CLOZARIL® (clozapine).

Other Events Observed During the Premarketing Evaluation of CLOZARIL® (clozapine): This section reports additional, less frequent adverse events which occurred among the patients taking CLOZARIL® (clozapine) in clinical studies. Various adverse events were reported as part of the total experience in these clinical studies; a causal relationship to CLOZARIL® (clozapine) treatment cannot be determined in the absence of appropriate controls in some of the studies. The table above enumerates adverse events that occurred at a frequency of at least 1% of patients treated with CLOZARIL® (clozapine). The list below includes all additional adverse experiences reported as being temporally associated with the use of the drug which occurred at a frequency less than 1%, enumerated by organ system.

Central Nervous System: loss of speech, amentia, tics, poor coordination, delusions/hallucinations, involuntary movement, stuttering, dysarthria, amnesia/memory loss, histrionic movements, libido increase or decrease, paranoia, shakiness, Parkinsonism, and irritability.

Cardiovascular System: edema, palpitations, phlebitis/thrombophlebitis, cyanosis, premature ventricular contraction, bradycardia, and nose bleed.

Gastrointestinal System: abdominal distention, gastroenteritis, rectal bleeding, nervous stomach, abnormal stools, hematemesis, gastric ulcer, bitter taste, and eructation.

Urogenital System: dysmenorrhea, impotence, breast pain/discomfort, and vaginal itch/infection.

Autonomic Nervous System: numbness, polydypsia, hot flashes, dry throat, and mydriasis.

Integumentary (Skin): pruritus, pallor, eczema, erythema, bruise, dermatitis, petechiae, and urticaria.

Musculoskeletal System: twitching and joint pain.

Respiratory System: coughing, pneumonia/pneumonia-like symptoms, rhinorrhea, hyperventilation, wheezing, bronchitis, laryngitis, and sneezing.

Hemic and Lymphatic System: anemia and leukocytosis.

Miscellaneous: chills/chills with fever, malaise, appetite increase, ear disorder, hypothermia, eyelid disorder, bloodshot eyes, and nystagmus.

Postmarketing Clinical Experience: Postmarketing experience has shown an adverse experience profile similar to that presented above. Voluntary reports of adverse events temporally associated with CLOZARIL® (clozapine) not mentioned above that have been received since market introduction and that may have no causal relationship with the drug include the following:

Central Nervous System: delirium; EEG abnormal; exacerbation of psychosis; myoclonus; overdose; paresthesia; possible mild cataplexy; and status epilepticus.

Cardiovascular System: atrial or ventricular fibrillation and periorbital edema.

Gastrointestinal System: acute pancreatitis; dysphagia; fecal impaction; intestinal obstruction/paralytic ileus; and salivary gland swelling.

Hepatobiliary System: cholestasis; hepatitis; jaundice.

Hepatic System: cholestasis.

Urogenital System: acute interstitial nephritis and priapism.

Integumentary (Skin): hypersensitivity reactions: photosensitivity, vasculitis, erythema multiforme, and Stevens-Johnson Syndrome.

Musculoskeletal System: myasthenic syndrome and rhabdomyolysis.

Respiratory System: aspiration and pleural effusion.

Hemic and Lymphatic System: deep vein thrombosis; elevated hemoglobin/hematocrit; ESR increased; pulmonary embolism; sepsis; thrombocytosis; and thrombocytopenia.

Miscellaneous: CPK elevation; hyperglycemia; hyperuricemia; hyponatremia; and weight loss.

DRUG ABUSE AND DEPENDENCE: Physical and psychological dependence have not been reported or observed in patients taking CLOZARIL® (clozapine).

Store and Dispense: Storage temperature should not exceed 86°F (30°C). Drug dispensing should not ordinarily exceed a weekly supply. Dispensing should be contingent upon the results of a WBC count.

*Trademark of Medical Economics Company, Inc.

Sandoz Pharmaceuticals Corporation, East Hanover, New Jersey 07936

REV: MARCH 1997   P30118906

THIS MONTH IN ARCHIVES OF GENERAL PSYCHIATRY

Recent advances in molecular and cellular neurobiology have led to new hypotheses concerning the pathophysiology and treatment of depression. The hypothesis presented by **Duman et al** (page 597) states that certain forms of depression may result from the injury and loss of function of specific groups of neurons in the brain, and that antidepressant treatments may repair or protect these neurons from further damage by increasing levels of neurotrophic factors. These factors are critical to the survival of neurons and to the maintenance of normal synaptic activity. This article discusses the mechanisms by which antidepressant treatments increase these factors in certain target brain regions and suggests new strategies for the development of novel therapeutic agents. *A Commentary about this article by Post is also included in this issue.*

Does depression run in the families of school-age patients with affective disorder? **Kovacs et al** (page 613) found that such families are 5 times as likely to have a member with depression as families of youngsters with other psychiatric disorders. First-degree relatives of depressed youths were most likely to have been depressed. Mothers of these children were particularly likely to have had their first depressive episode at a young age.

The study of the early seeds of affective disorder has largely focused on the role of childhood psychosocial adversity. Recent meta-analytic studies have shown that patients with affective disorder display cerebral ventricular enlargement and sulcal prominence, indicating a possible neurodevelopmental pathway to adult mood disorder. **van Os et al** (page 625) analyzed prospective data from a national general population birth cohort and found that early cognitive and motor development differentiated children destined to develop affective disorder. These findings suggest that part of the vulnerability to mood disorder can be explained by aberrant neurodevelopment.

Women are more likely to have a first episode of major depression than are men; however, it is unclear whether the subsequent course of depression differs between the sexes. **Simpson et al** (page 633) used prospective data to examine male and female subjects with 1 major depressive episode. There was no significant sex difference in the time to recovery, the time to recurrence, or the number and severity of recurrences during up to 15 years of follow-up. These findings influence theories advanced to explain why women are more likely to have depression than are men.

The efficacy of selective serotonin reuptake inhibitors (SSRIs) in panic disorder (PD) raises the possibility that enhancement of serotonin neurotransmission may stabilize the noradrenergic system. **Coplan et al** (page 643) describe a novel clonidine method assessing noradrenergic dysregulation, whereby untreated patients with PD are strongly differentiated from healthy volunteers. Using this method, noradrenergic dysregulation declined significantly following the effective treatment of patients with PD with the SSRI fluoxetine hydrochloride. Confirming serotonin's critical role in panic disorder, SSRI-induced treatment response was paralleled by the normalization of noradrenergic dysregulation.

The actions of antipsychotics are probably mediated by the blockade of D_2 dopaminelike receptors, but the location of these effects remains uncertain. **Goldsmith et al** (page 649) found that schizophrenic subjects exhibited significantly disrupted patterns of D_2 receptors in the perirhinal, superior, and inferior temporal cortices, including that of modular D_2 receptor bands, without alterations in the hippocampus. Blockade of the regionally specific, aberrant pattern of D_2 receptors in auditory and auditory-visual association cortices may provide a mechanism for the clinical efficacy of D_2 antagonists in reducing hallucinations.

Many of the cognitive functions mediated by the prefrontal cortex are disturbed in schizophrenia. **Glantz and Lewis** (page 660) assessed the integrity of synaptic circuitry in postmortem brain specimens from subjects with schizophrenia, nonschizophrenic psychiatric case subjects, and controls. Compared with the control groups, immunoreactivity for synaptophysin, a marker of the synaptic vesicles involved in neurotransmitter release, was decreased in the prefrontal cortex of the subjects with schizophrenia. Although several different pathological mechanisms may produce these findings, each is consistent with a disturbance in synaptic transmission in the prefrontal cortex of subjects with schizophrenia.

Despite the high social and economic costs of conduct disorder (CD), few preventable risk factors have been identified. **Wakschlag et al** (page 670) found that pregnant mothers who smoked more than a half a pack of cigarettes daily were significantly more likely to have sons with CD than were nonsmokers, even with associated risk factors controlled. Although this study cannot establish causality, it provides strong evidence that smoking is an independent risk factor for CD.

A Molecular and Cellular Theory of Depression

Ronald S. Duman, PhD; George R. Heninger, MD; Eric J. Nestler, MD, PhD

Recent studies have begun to characterize the actions of stress and antidepressant treatments beyond the neurotransmitter and receptor level. This work has demonstrated that long-term antidepressant treatments result in the sustained activation of the cyclic adenosine 3′, 5′-monophosphate system in specific brain regions, including the increased function and expression of the transcription factor cyclic adenosine monophosphate response element-binding protein. The activated cyclic adenosine 3′, 5′-monophosphate system leads to the regulation of specific target genes, including the increased expression of brain-derived neurotrophic factor in certain populations of neurons in the hippocampus and cerebral cortex. The importance of these changes is highlighted by the discovery that stress can decrease the expression of brain-derived neurotrophic factor and lead to atrophy of these same populations of stress-vulnerable hippocampal neurons. The possibility that the decreased size and impaired function of these neurons may be involved in depression is supported by recent clinical imaging studies, which demonstrate a decreased volume of certain brain structures. These findings constitute the framework for an updated molecular and cellular hypothesis of depression, which posits that stress-induced vulnerability and the therapeutic action of antidepressant treatments occur via intracellular mechanisms that decrease or increase, respectively, neurotrophic factors necessary for the survival and function of particular neurons. This hypothesis also explains how stress and other types of neuronal insult can lead to depression in vulnerable individuals and it outlines novel targets for the rational design of fundamentally new therapeutic agents.

Arch Gen Psychiatry. 1997;54:597-606

Depression is thought to be a heterogenous illness that can result from the dysfunction of several neurotransmitter or metabolic systems. Basic and clinical studies have provided evidence that the serotonin and norepinephrine (NE) neurotransmitter systems are involved in the treatment of depression. These studies have led to a series of hypotheses concerning the mechanism of the action of antidepressant treatments, as well as the pathophysiology of depression, that have focused on alterations in levels of these monoamines or their receptors. Although these models have guided research efforts in the field for 3 decades, they have not generated a compelling model of antidepressant action or the pathophysiology of depression. For example, studies to date have failed to identify a common action of antidepressant treatments at the level of monoamines or their receptors. This is not surprising given that different types of antidepressant treatments exert widely dif-

For editorial comment see page 607

From the Laboratory of Molecular Psychiatry, Departments of Psychiatry and Pharmacology, Yale University School of Medicine, Connecticut Mental Health Center, New Haven.

This article is also available on our Web site: ama-assn.org/psych.

ferent effects on the serotonin and NE systems. It is also possible that there is more than a single mechanism by which antidepressant treatments exert their therapeutic actions.

An updated hypothesis that builds on previous work suggests that the long-term, therapeutic action of antidepressant treatments is mediated by postreceptor intracellular targets. Advances in molecular and cellular biology have elucidated the intracellular machinery through which monoamines ultimately act to control the functioning of neurons. These advances have made it possible to begin the process of delineating the specific signal transduction pathways that mediate the short-term effects of different types of antidepressant treatments and that underlie the adaptations in neuronal function responsible for the long-term effects of these treatments.

We present a brief review of the basic and clinical work about the role of serotonin and NE systems in the treatment of depression. We also discuss, in greater detail, recent advances that demonstrate a role for intracellular signal transduction pathways and the regulation of specific target genes in antidepressant treatments. Specifically, we describe recent findings that demonstrate that the transcription factor cyclic adenosine 3′, 5′-monophosphate (cAMP) response element-binding protein (CREB) is one intracellular target of long-term antidepressant treatment and that brain-derived neurotrophic factor (BDNF) is one target gene of CREB. These studies support an emerging hypothesis of the mechanisms by which stress and other environmental insults may damage specific populations of neurons and, thereby, contribute to the pathophysiology of depression in vulnerable individuals. This provides a framework for future studies needed to test this potentially unifying hypothesis for antidepressant action and the pathophysiology of at least certain forms of depression.

MONOAMINES AND DEPRESSION

Early studies indicated that agents that deplete monoamines, such as reserpine, could lead to depression in a small percentage of individuals. This led to the theory that reduced availability of monoamine neurotransmitters, particularly NE and serotonin, could play a role in the formation of depression.[1-3] This hypothesis was supported by the discovery that prototypical antidepressant treatments, the tricyclics and monoamine oxidase inhibitors, cause a short-term increase in synaptic levels of monoamines. However, despite extensive research, it remains unclear whether long-term antidepressant treatments result in the increased or decreased function of the many monoamine pathways located throughout the brain.

The role of monoamines in depression has been further examined with the use of serotonin and NE depletion paradigms in normal and drug-remitted individuals with depression.[4-6] The results of these studies demonstrate that although the depletion of serotonin or NE does not lead to depressive symptoms in normal individuals, patients who experienced remission on either serotonin or NE selective reuptake inhibitors are vulnerable to relapse on depletion of the corresponding monoamine. This indicates that serotonin and NE are somehow involved in the maintenance of an antidepressant response, but cannot alone explain either the mechanism of action of antidepressant treatments or the pathophysiology of depression. This conclusion is also supported by the time required for the therapeutic action of antidepressant treatments (several weeks), even though levels of monoamines are increased rapidly by these treatments. Together, the results suggest that additional factors contribute to antidepressant responses and the onset of depression.

MONOAMINE RECEPTORS AND DEPRESSION

A consequence of antidepressant treatment and elevated levels of serotonin or NE is the activation of monoamine receptors. One possibility is that persistent activation of these receptors would lead to adaptations in the receptors that would then contribute to the delayed therapeutic action of antidepressant treatments.[7-9] Indeed, early studies demonstrated that long-term antidepressant treatments down-regulate the density of receptor sites for serotonin and NE. The best-characterized example is that the long-term, but not short-term, administration of many types of antidepressant treatments decreases levels of β-adrenergic receptor (βAR) ligand–binding sites in limbic brain regions, such as the cerebral cortex and the hippocampus.[10,11] The ability of βARs to stimulate the formation of cAMP is similarly decreased in these regions by long-term antidepressant treatments. Serotonin$_2$-receptor–binding sites were also found to be down-regulated by many antidepressant treatments.[12] These and other receptor studies led to various receptor sensitivity hypotheses—for example, that the action of antidepressant treatments is dependent on the down-regulation of βAR or serotonin$_2$ receptors and that enhanced sensitivity of these receptors may lead to depression.[7,8]

However, there are many problems with these hypotheses. First, not all antidepressant treatments effectively regulate the levels of βAR or serotonin$_2$-receptor sites.[9] This could mean that the action of different antidepressant treatments is mediated by different receptors or that other sites are more relevant. Second, the time course for down-regulation of βAR and serotonin$_2$ receptor–binding sites is more rapid than the therapeutic onset of these treatments.[9,13,14] Third, levels of serotonin$_2$ receptors are increased, not decreased, by long-term electroshock seizure treatment, one of the most effective therapies for depression.[9,14] Fourth, the reduction of βAR function by the administration of selective βAR receptor antagonists is not an effective treatment for depression and actually produces depression in some individuals.[15,16] In fact, the activation or facilitation of βAR function by the administration of thyroid hormone or a specific receptor agonist can have antidepressant efficacy in some patients.[17]

A serotonin$_{1A}$ receptor sensitivity hypothesis has also been put forth by Blier and de Montigny.[18] This hypothesis states that long-term antidepressant treatments increase the function of postsynaptic serotonin$_{1A}$ receptors in the hippocampus. Depending on the type of antidepressant treatment, they propose that this could occur by either the increased sensitivity of postsynaptic serotonin$_{1A}$ receptors or the desensitization of serotonin autoreceptors. One problem with this hypothesis is that direct-acting serotonin$_{1A}$ receptor agonists are not clearly effective antidepressant treatments, although the serotonin$_{1A}$ agonists tested (buspirone hydrochloride and gepirone) are thought to be partial agonists at postsynaptic serotonin$_{1A}$ receptors and may not adequately test the hypothesis. Another possibility is that increased serotonin$_{1A}$ neurotransmission is necessary, but insufficient, for antidepressant efficacy and that the activation of additional factors is required.

Several other monoamine receptor subtypes are reported to be regulated by antidepressant treatments.[8,9] However, as with the βAR, serotonin$_2$, and serotonin$_{1A}$ receptors, regulation of these other monoamine receptors alone cannot account for the mechanism of action of antidepressant treatments. Rather, alterations in the levels of these receptors or in their functional sensitivity probably represent adaptations to increased levels of monoamines. In fact, it can be argued that the observed receptor down-regulations are indicative of continued receptor activation secondary to continued elevations in monoamine levels after long-term antidepressant treatments. Indeed, levels of these receptors are decreased, and not completely eliminated, by long-term antidepressant treatments, raising the possibility that there could be sufficient levels of receptor remaining to respond to the elevated levels of serotonin and NE (**Figure 1**). If this is the case, the functional output of the monoamine receptors would be increased, not decreased, by long-term treatments, a possibility that was entertained in an early review.[19] This would suggest that long-term antidepressant treatments result in the sustained activation of the intracellular signal transduction cascades that mediate the actions of monoamine receptors. Such intracellular factors represent potential common targets for many different types of antidepressant treatments because they could be regulated by the activation of either the serotonin or NE receptor systems. This could include the activation of serotonin and NE receptor subtypes that are not themselves regulated by antidepressant treatments. It will be important in future studies to determine which serotonin and NE receptor subtypes mediate the relevant therapeutic actions of antidepressant treatments, although identification of the critical intracellular targets will likely facilitate this process.

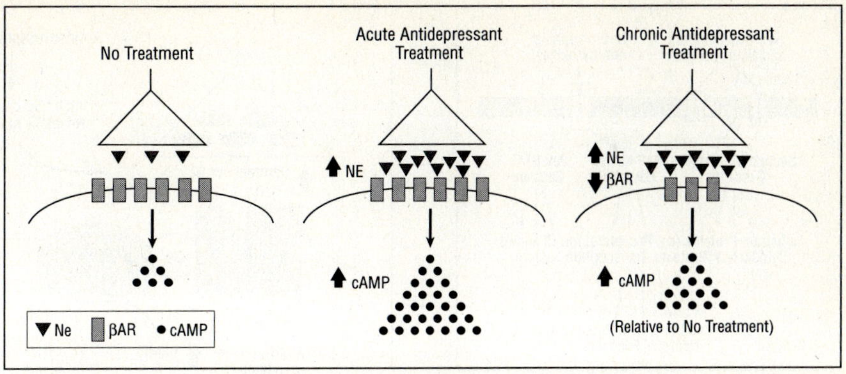

Figure 1. *A model demonstrating antidepressant regulation of the β-adrenergic receptor (βAR)–coupled cyclic adenosine 3′, 5′-monophosphate (cAMP) system. When there is no treatment, basal levels of norepinephrine (NE) stimulate the βAR–coupled cAMP system. Short-term administration of certain types of antidepressants elevates levels of NE, increasing levels of βAR–stimulated cAMP formation. Long-term administration of many types of antidepressants causes down-regulation of the number of βAR-binding sites available to stimulate cAMP production. This in turn leads to a decrease in the maximal level of βAR–stimulated cAMP formation. However, with synaptic levels of NE still elevated as a result of continued antidepressant treatment, the level of cAMP formed remains elevated relative to the no-treatment condition. This possibility requires further testing to determine if levels of βAR–stimulated cAMP formation are indeed elevated. However, this model provides a mechanism to explain how long-term antidepressant treatments activate the cAMP pathway even though levels of βAR are decreased.*

INTRACELLULAR MESSENGERS, NEUROTROPHIC FACTORS, AND DEPRESSION

Advances in molecular and cellular biology have paved the way for studies to determine how antidepressant treatments ultimately regulate the function of target neurons in the brain. There are many comprehensive reviews on intracellular signal transduction pathways,[20-25] and this information will not be discussed in detail herein except as it pertains to antidepressant treatments. In general, these pathways can be divided into 2 broad categories. The first category includes those pathways that are controlled by receptor-coupled second messengers (eg, cAMP, inositol triphosphate, Ca^{2+}, and nitric oxide) and are usually regulated by classic neurotransmitters, such as the monoamines, amino acids, and neuropeptides (**Figure 2**). The second category includes those pathways that are controlled by receptors that contain, or interact with, protein tyrosine kinases and are usually regulated by neurotrophic factors and cytokines; activation of these receptors leads to the regulation of other intracellular cascades, such as the mitogen-activated protein kinase pathway (Figure 2). As the protein kinases and phosphatases, phosphoproteins, transcription factors, and target genes that make up these pathways are increasingly identified and characterized, it is becoming possible to examine how adaptations of these complex pathways are involved in the long-term actions of antidepressant treatments and other psychotropic drugs.

The ability to study these adaptations is a critical advance because these pathways control all aspects of neuronal function and ultimately underlie the ability of the brain to adapt and respond to pharmacological and environmental inputs. The functional consequences of such molecular adaptations can be determined at the cellular level by analysis of the electrophysiological and morpho-

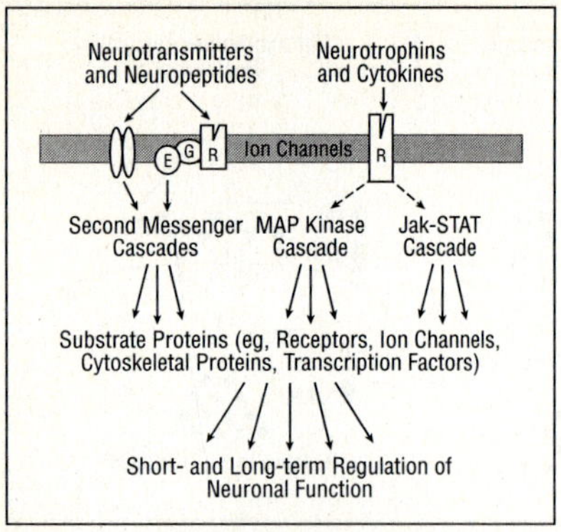

Figure 2. *A general model of receptor-coupled intracellular signal transduction pathways. Intracellular pathways can be subdivided into 2 general categories. Intracellular pathways in the first general category are the second messenger-regulated signaling cascades. These pathways are activated by neurotransmitter or neuropeptide receptors that couple to effector (E) proteins via G proteins. Examples of second messenger cascades include cyclic adenosine monophosphate, cyclic guanosine monophosphate, Ca^{2+}, inositol triphosphate, and nitric oxide. Neurotransmitter regulation of ion channels can also result in regulation of second messenger-dependent pathways. These second messengers lead to the regulation of second messenger-dependent protein serine–threonine kinases. Intracellular pathways in the second general category are the tyrosine kinase–mediated cascades. These pathways are regulated by neurotrophins and cytokines via the activation of receptors (R) that have intrinsic tyrosine kinase activity on the intracellular aspect of the receptors (eg, trkB) or interact with cytoplasmic tyrosine kinases. Activation of these kinases leads to association with other proteins that subsequently activate the mitogen-activated protein (MAP) kinase and Jak-STAT cascades. Regulation of these and the second messenger-dependent protein kinase cascades results in the short- and long-term regulation of neuronal function via the phosphorylation of specific substrate proteins.*

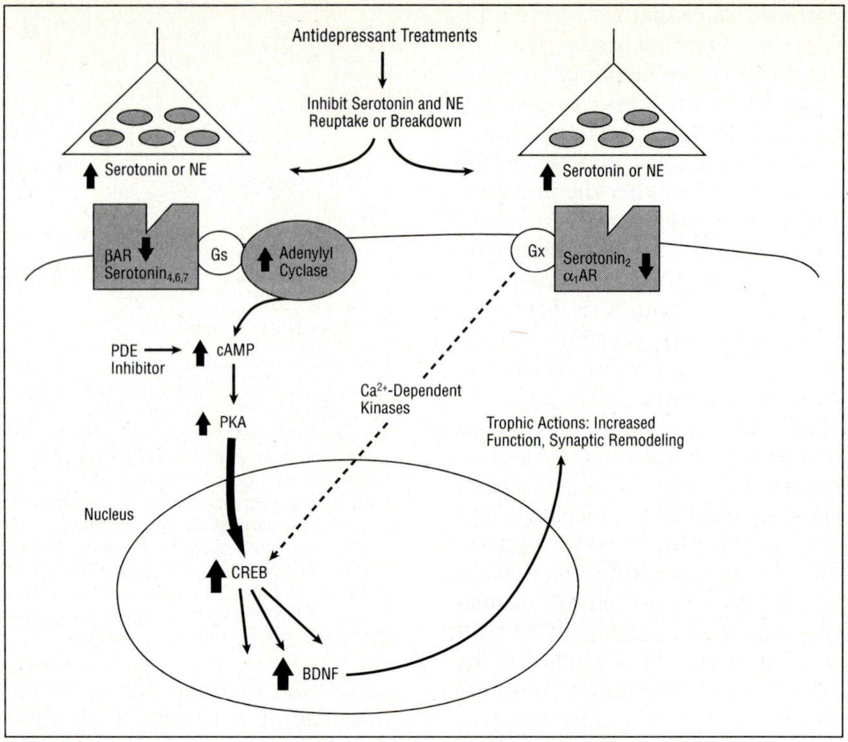

Figure 3. *A model for the molecular mechanism of action of long-term antidepressant treatments. Antidepressants cause a short-term increase in levels of serotonin and noreprinephrine (NE) by inhibiting the reuptake or breakdown of these monoamines. Long-term antidepressant administration decreases the function and expression of certain serotonin and NE receptors (eg, β-adrenergic receptor [βAR] and serotonin$_2$), but the cyclic adenosine 3', 5'-monophosphate (cAMP) signal transduction pathway is increased by long-term antidepressant treatments, including increased levels of adenylyl cyclase and cAMP-dependent protein kinase (PKA), as well as the translocation of PKA to the cell nucleus. Moreover, recent studies demonstrate that expression and function of the transcription factor cAMP response element–binding protein (CREB) is increased by different types of antidepressant treatments, suggesting that CREB is a common postreceptor target for antidepressants. Cyclic adenosine monophosphate response element–binding protein could be regulated by monoamine receptors that couple to the cAMP-PKA cascade (serotonin$_{4,6,7}$ and βAR) or via receptors that lead to the activation of Ca^{2+}-dependent kinases (eg, serotonin$_2$ and α_1-adrenergic receptor [α_1AR]). Increased activity of the cAMP signal transduction cascade indicates that the functional output of serotonin and NE are up-regulated at least in some brain regions, even though levels of certain serotonin and NE receptors are partially down-regulated. This conclusion is further supported by the finding that expression of brain-derived neurotrophic factor (BDNF) and trkB, 2 potential targets of CREB, is also increased by long-term antidepressant treatment. Up-regulation of BDNF and trkB could influence the function of hippocampal neurons or the neurons innervating this brain region, such as serotonin and NE neurons. This could include increased neuronal survival, function, and remodeling of synaptic or cellular architecture.*

logical properties of neurons. Examples of these types of adaptations are the enhanced or diminished synaptic efficacy that is observed in cellular models of learning and memory.[26-29] Morphological changes include atrophy or the sprouting of neurons in response to damaging or growth-promoting stimuli.[30-32]

These types of responses can be viewed as prototypical ways in which the brain adapts to repeated perturbations. Our hypothesis is that similar types of molecular and cellular adaptations occur in response to antidepressant treatments and are involved in the pathophysiology of depression. These types of adaptations are complicated and, in many cases, are difficult to identify, but recognition of their potential importance has stimulated studies that have investigated the role of intracellular pathways and their cellular adaptations in antidepressant action and in depression. Characterization of such adaptations is at a relatively early stage, but has already led to notable conceptual advances in the field.

ANTIDEPRESSANT TREATMENTS ACTIVATE THE cAMP SIGNAL TRANSDUCTION PATHWAY

There are many potential intracellular pathways that could mediate the action of antidepressant treatments. One such pathway that is regulated by the serotonin and NE systems is the cAMP signal transduction cascade (**Figure 3**). Receptor activation leads to the formation of cAMP by coupling to adenylyl cyclase via the stimulatory G protein subtype, Gs. Certain forms of adenylyl cyclase can be activated independent of Gs in response to elevated cellular Ca^{2+} levels.[24] The effects of cAMP are then mediated by the activation of cAMP-dependent protein kinase, which, in turn, leads to the regulation of cellular function by the phosphorylation of specific proteins. One of these is the transcription factor CREB, which mediates many of the actions of the cAMP system on gene expression.[33,34] In addition to its regula-

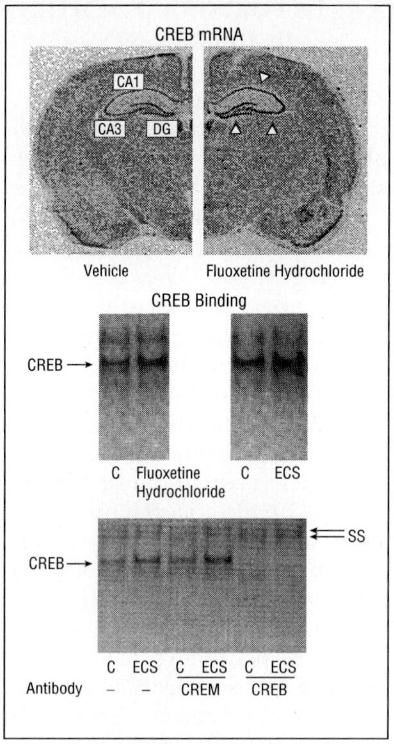

Figure 4. *Long-term antidepressant treatments increase levels of cyclic adenosine 3′, 5′-monophosphate (cAMP) response element–binding protein (CREB) messenger RNA (mRNA) and binding in the hippocampus. The finding that long-term antidepressant treatments increase the expression and function of CREB in the hippocampus is illustrated. The influence of long-term (21 days) fluoxetine hydrochloride administration on levels of CREB messenger RNA was determined by in situ hybridization analysis. Levels of CREB messenger RNA were increased in the major subfields of the hippocampus, including CA3 and CA1 pyramidal and dentate gyrus granule cell layers. Levels of CREB binding were also increased by long-term fluoxetine treatment, as well as electroshock seizures (ECS) (10 days). For this assay, homogenates of the hippocampus are incubated with a radiolabeled, synthetic fragment of DNA that contains a consensus cAMP response element. Binding of CREB shifts the migration of the radiolabeled DNA through the gel. The identity of CREB is confirmed in several ways. First, the CREB binding is reduced by competition with unlabeled DNA containing the cAMP response element, but not with DNA containing a mutated cAMP response element sequence (not shown). Second, supershift (SS) studies (bottom) demonstrate that a specific antibody to CREB, but not CREM (cAMP response element modulatory protein), alters the cAMP response element–binding band. For ss analysis, the homogenate is preincubated with antibody before the radiolabeled DNA is added. If the specific antibody binds to the protein-DNA complex, it either disrupts the complex or supershifts the migration of the complex through the gel.*[44]

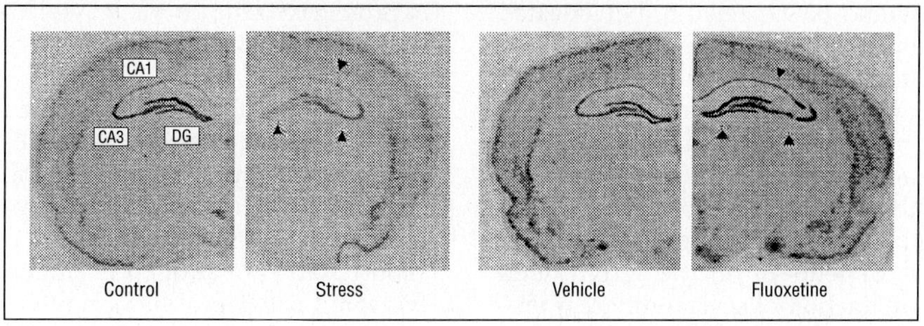

Figure 5. *Stress decreases and antidepressant treatments increase the expression of brain-derived neurotrophic factor in the hippocampus. The influence of acute restraint stress (90 minutes) or long-term fluoxetine hydrochloride administration (21 days) on levels of brain-derived neurotrophic factor messenger RNA were determined by in situ hybridization analysis. The CA3 and CA1 pyramidal and dentate gyrus granule cell layers of the hippocampus are indicated. Pretreatment with fluoxetine or other antidepressants also blocks the down-regulation of brain-derived neurotrophic factor in response to stress.*[52]

tion by phosphorylation, recent studies have demonstrated that expression of the total amount of CREB is another mechanism by which the function of CREB can be regulated.[35-37] The cAMP system is a potential common target for serotonin and NE because there are receptor subtypes for both monoamines that stimulate the formation of this second messenger (Figure 3). In addition to the βAR, there are 3 serotonin receptor subtypes that stimulate the cAMP system (serotonin$_{4,6,7}$), and one of these (serotonin$_7$) is reported to be regulated by long-term antidepressant treatments.[38] Moreover, CREB may represent a common intracellular target for antidepressant treatments because other serotonin or NE receptors (eg, serotonin$_{2A,C}$ and α_1-adrenergic receptors) could also activate CREB via the stimulation of Ca^{2+}-dependent protein kinases (**Figure 4**).[33,34]

Several studies have demonstrated that the postreceptor components of the cAMP system are regulated by long-term antidepressant treatments (Figure 3). Levels of guanine nucleotide–stimulated adenylyl cyclase and cAMP–dependent protein kinase enzyme activity are reported to be increased by long-term antidepressant treatments.[39-43] In addition, we have found that the levels of CREB messenger RNA and protein in the hippocampus are increased by long-term antidepressant treatments, including serotonin and NE selective reuptake inhibitors (Figure 4 and **Figure 5**).[44] The time course for the induction of CREB is consistent with that for the therapeutic actions of antidepressant treatments (ie, 10-21 days of treatment). To further test the hypothesis that CREB is involved in antidepressant actions, it will be important to determine whether the time course for the reversal of these effects is consistent with the offset of therapeutic actions. Increased expression of CREB could be mediated by the up-regulation of cAMP function discussed previously because CREB expression can be induced in cultured cells by the activation of the cAMP cascade.[35] These findings contrast to those of a recent study of CREB function in PC12 cells, an adrenal chromafin cell line.[45] However, in the latter study, the short-term incubation of PC12 cells with antidepressant treatments inhibited depolarization-induced activation of CREB, an effect owing to the blockade of Ca^{2+} channels. To our knowledge, such inhibition of CREB has not been demonstrated in vivo.

Increased function and expression of CREB provides direct support for the proposal that the cAMP signal transduction system is increased in the hippocampus by long-term antidepressant treatments. Induction of the intracellular components of the cAMP cascade may also explain the requirement for long-term antidepressant treatments, even though levels of cAMP may be elevated by short-term antidepressant treatments (Figure 1 and Figure 3). Our results also indicate the types of specific gene elements likely to be regulated by long-term antidepressant treatments; that is, those with functional cAMP response elements. However, not all genes with a cAMP response element would be expected to be activated by antidepressant treatments. First, up-regulation of the cAMP system and CREB is not observed in all brain regions (there is evidence for down-regulation of the cAMP system in the locus coeruleus[46]). Second, regulation of gene expression is dependent on the activity and interaction of several different promoter elements and transcription factors. Thus, activation of the cAMP system and CREB may lead to the regulation of a specific set of genes in the hippocampus that are involved in the action of antidepressant treatments. One goal of current studies is to identify these genes and to determine their relevance to the clinical responses to antidepressant treatments. Recent studies have identified BDNF and its receptor, trkB, as 2 potential target genes of interest.

ANTIDEPRESSANT TREATMENTS REGULATE NEUROTROPHINS

Brain-derived neurotrophic factor is a member of the nerve growth factor family, which also includes the prototype nerve growth factor as well as neurotrophin-3 and neurotrophin-4. These growth factors are involved in the differentiation and growth of many types of neurons in the developing brain as well as the maintenance and survival of neurons in the mature brain.[30-32,47] For example, the survival and growth of serotonin neurons in the adult brain is increased by BDNF and, to a lesser degree, by neurotrophin-3, but not by the nerve growth factor.[48] Also, neurotrophins can rapidly influence the function of neurons, as demonstrated by the finding that short-term exposure of hippocampal slices to BDNF increases the strength of certain synaptic connections.[28,29] These types of findings, along with an increasing appreciation of the neurotrophic actions of the monoamines,[49,50] highlight the large overlap between the roles played by neurotrophins and monoamines in the regulation of brain function. The actions of neurotrophins are mediated by binding to specific receptors, referred to as trkB receptors, which lead to the activation of protein tyrosine kinase activity located on the intracellular domain of the receptors.

Recent studies have provided support for the notion that neurotrophins and neuronal plasticity and survival may be involved in the treatment of depression. First, BDNF is reported to have antidepressant effects in 2 behavioral models of depression, the forced swim and learned helplessness paradigms.[51] Second, long-term, but not short-term, antidepressant administration, including serotonin and NE selective reuptake inhibitors, a monoamine oxidase inhibitor, an atypical antidepressant, as well as electroshock seizures, increases the expression of BDNF and trkB in the hippocampus (Figure 3 and Figure 5).[44,52] Third, BDNF is reported to enhance the growth of serotonin and NE neurons, as well as to protect these neurons from neurotoxic damage.[48,53] While these findings support a role for BDNF in the actions of antidepressant treatments, studies of additional antidepressant and nonantidepressant agents are required to further test this hypothesis. In addition, the role of other neurotrophic factors (eg, nerve growth factor, neurotrophin-3, and neurotrophin-4) should be examined.

The possibility that increased expression of BDNF results from the activation of CREB is supported by several lines of evidence. First, the time course for the up-regulation of CREB is similar to that of BDNF. Second, the regulation of CREB and BDNF is observed in the same populations of neurons in the hippocampus (Figure 4 and Figure 5). Third, studies in primary neuronal cultures have demonstrated that the stimulation of cAMP- or Ca^{2+}-activated protein kinases increases the expression of BDNF.[54,55] Finally, the reduction of CREB levels in the hippocampus by the administration of antisense oligonucleotides to CREB messenger RNA decreases basal levels of BDNF and blocks the induction of BDNF by antidepressant treatments.[49] Additional in vitro and in vivo studies are needed to demonstrate a direct link between CREB and the expression of BDNF.

A ROLE FOR NEUROTROPHINS IN DEPRESSION

There is also evidence of a neurotrophic element in the pathophysiology of certain forms of depression. First, immobilization stress causes a dramatic reduction in BDNF expression in the hippocampus of rats (Figure 5).[56] The relevance of this finding requires further examination. For example, do other types of stress (eg, psychosocial), which can precipitate or exacerbate depression, also decrease the expression of BDNF? Second, chronic stress of several types (ie, restraint or psychosocial) or glucocorticoid treatments are reported to cause atrophy, or even death, of vulnerable neurons in the hippocampus in rats and nonhuman primates.[57-63] The CA3 pyramidal neurons seem to be most vulnerable to stress, although other populations of neurons seem to be sensitive to stress, glucocorticoids, cytokines, and other types of neuronal insult, such as hypoxia-ischemia or hypoglycemia.[64] Third, the ability of the hippocampus to inhibit the hypothalamic–pituitary–adrenal axis is reduced in certain patients with depression, consistent with a deficit of hippocampal function in these individuals.[65] Fourth, there is a small decrease in hippocampal volume as determined by magnetic resonance imaging in patients with depression or posttraumatic stress disorder.[66-68] In addition, a recent review of the literature provides evidence to suggest that there may be a decrease in the size of certain brain structures in depression.[69] Down-regulation of BDNF may contribute to the atrophy of neurons in the hippocampus in response to stress. However, not all episodes of depression are associated with stress, and the model presented may be limited to certain subtypes of depression. Postmortem studies to demonstrate atrophy or neuronal death directly in the hippocampus of patients with depression are required to further test this hypothesis.

These studies form the basis of a molecular and cellular model of depression and antidepressant action (**Figure 6**). Depression, particularly stress-associated cases, may result from the atrophy or death of vulnerable pyramidal neurons in the CA3 region of the hippocampus. This could be a consequence, at least in part, of the decreased levels of BDNF available to these neurons. Elevated levels of glucocorticoids are also known to play a notable role in stress-induced damage of CA3 neurons.[57-63] Antidepressant treatments could reverse this atrophy by increasing BDNF expression and function. In fact, we have found that long-term antidepressant pretreatment blocks the down-regulation of BDNF in response to stress.[52] Normalization of glucocorticoid levels by antidepressant treatments in some individuals could be an additional mechanism for the prevention of further neuronal damage.[70] Further studies are required to determine whether antidepressant treatments have direct neuroprotective effects or neurotrophic actions on hippocampal neurons as suggested by early studies.[71,72] Recent studies are encouraging. We have found that long-term electroshock treatment causes sprouting of granule neurons in the hippocampus.[73] Unlike the sprouting observed in response to kindling or excitotoxin treatment, there was no obvious cell damage after long-term electroshock treatment. In addition, electroshock-induced sprouting was markedly attenuated in mutant knockout mice that express reduced levels of BDNF. These results indicate that electroshock induces sprouting of certain hippocampal neurons and that the response is mediated by the increased expression of BDNF in these neurons. The observation that antidepressant treatments can lead to the reinstatement of hippocampal control of the hypothalamic–pituitary–adrenal axis in some patients further supports the possibility that the function of these neurons, indeed, can be improved.[65]

One challenge in depression research is the difficulty of identifying specific anatomical substrates involved in the disorder. The hippocampus is involved in the control of emotion, learning and memory, and the regulation of the hypothalamic–pituitary–adrenal axis, as well as other vegetative processes. Changes in the structure or function of hippocampal neurons could be involved in the affective, neuroendocrine, cognitive, and vegetative abnormalities observed in depression. However, these abnormalities are also likely to be influenced by several other limbic brain structures and it is possible that stress alters the structure and function of neurons in these brain regions as well.

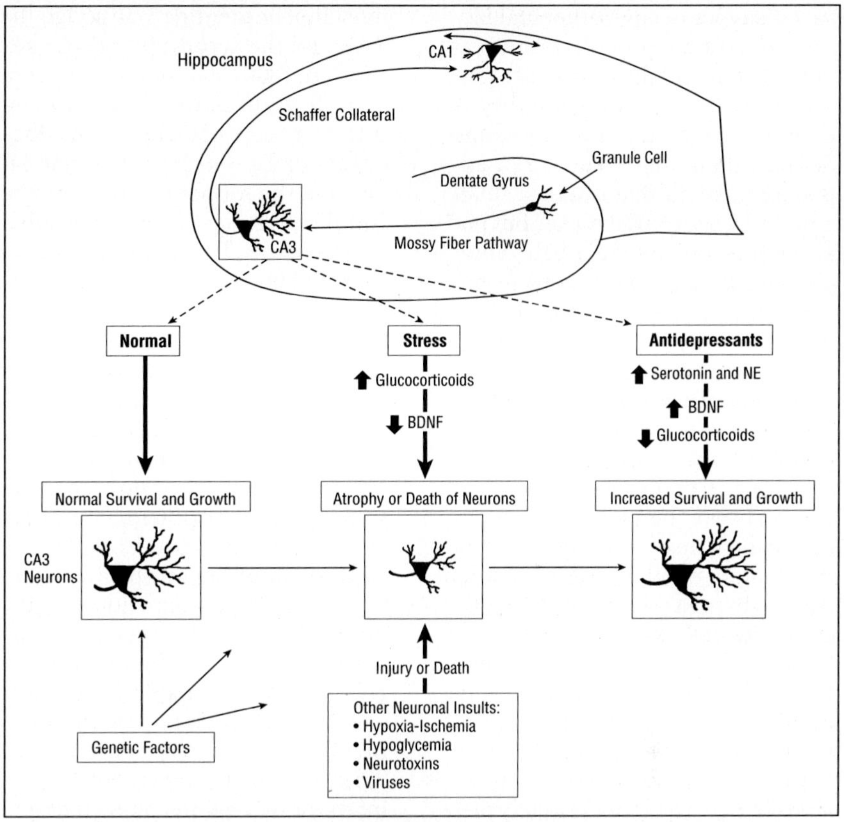

Figure 6. *A molecular and cellular model for the action of antidepressant treatments and the pathophysiology of stress-related disorders. This model of the hippocampus shows the major cell types in the hippocampus and how stress and antidepressant treatments may influence CA3 pyramidal cells. The 3 major subfields of the hippocampus (CA3 and CA1 pyramidal cells and dentate gyrus granule cells) are connected by the mossy fiber and Schaffer collateral pathways. Recent studies demonstrate that chronic stress decreases the expression of brain-derived neurotrophic factor (BDNF) in the hippocampus. This could contribute to the atrophy or death of neurons in the CA3 pyramidal cell layer of the hippocampus. Long-term elevation of glucocorticoid levels is also known to decrease the survival of these neurons. Other types of neuronal insult such as hypoxia-ischemia, hypoglycemia, neurotoxins, and viral infections could also cause atrophy or damage of neurons and could, thereby, make an individual vulnerable to subsequent insults. These types of interactions could underlie the observations of decreased function and volume of hippocampus in patients with affective disorders and could explain the selective vulnerability of certain individuals to become depressed. Long-term antidepressant treatments increase the expression of BDNF, as well as trkB, and prevent the down-regulation of BDNF elicited by stress. This could increase the growth or survival of neurons, or help repair or protect neurons from further damage. Increased expression of BDNF and trkB seems to be mediated by the sustained elevation of the serotonin and norepinephrine (NE) systems and the cyclic adenosine monophosphate cascade. Normalization of glucocorticoid levels by long-term antidepressant treatments could also contribute to the recovery of CA3 neurons.*

A HYPOTHESIS FOR GENETIC AND ENVIRONMENTAL VULNERABILITIES

It is widely believed that depression results from a combination of genetic and environmental factors. Yet, virtually nothing is known about the specific genes that may predispose certain individuals to depression and render others relatively resistant. Studies of the cAMP pathway, CREB, and BDNF, discussed previously, demonstrate the enormous number of genes that could be involved. Indeed, these studies highlight the naivete of candidate gene strategies to identify depression vulnerability genes, which remain focused on monoamine metabolic enzymes, receptors, and reuptake proteins. These studies indicate the need for more open-ended investigations of the genetic factors involved in depression.

However, it could be immediately informative to examine how

various types of environmental factors may predispose certain individuals to mood disorders based on our hypothesis. One possibility is that many individuals who become depressed may have had a prior exposure to stress that causes a small amount of neuronal damage, but not enough to precipitate a behavioral change. If additional damage occurs, either as a result of normal aging or further stressful stimuli, these effects may then be manifested in the symptoms of a mood disorder. These types of events could explain the decreased volume of specific brain structures in depression. This model could also explain how other types of neuronal insult predispose an individual to mood disorders. Insults such as hypoxia-ischemia, hypoglycemia, neurotoxins, or viral infections could cause direct neuronal damage or render neurons more vulnerable to psychosocial stress (Figure 6). Such changes could lead to depression at later times or, if severe enough, could immediately precipitate a depressive episode. For example, a high incidence of depression is well documented in patients who have had a stroke.[74-76] The possible involvement of myriad environmental factors implicates many additional sets of genes that could conceivably alter an individual's inherent responses to stress and establish a diathesis for depression. The possible role of a subtle neurodegenerative contribution to the pathophysiology of depression should be directly examined by analysis of postmortem tissue, as discussed previously.

RATIONAL DESIGN OF NOVEL THERAPEUTIC AGENTS

New information indicating a role for the cAMP pathway and CREB in the actions of antidepressant treatments suggests novel approaches to develop faster-acting and more effective agents. The development and testing of such agents will also help to further test our hypothesis. First, receptor agonists could be targeted at the specific serotonin or NE receptors that stimulate cAMP- or Ca^{2+}-activated protein kinases and mediate the antidepressant induction of BDNF. These receptor sites must first be identified, although the βAR and the $serotonin_{4,6,7}$ receptor sites are likely candidates. Second, identification of other neurotransmitter receptors that stimulate cAMP- or Ca^{2+}-activated protein kinases in the hippocampus could be additional targets. Third, agents that directly stimulate cAMP- or Ca^{2+}-activated kinases, or that directly activate CREB, could be developed. Fourth, the inhibition of cAMP breakdown would enhance the function of CREB and increase BDNF expression. Fifth, agents that activate the BDNF-trkB signaling pathway may be of some use. The first 2 possibilities have the potential for regulating the function of CREB and the expression of BDNF specifically in the hippocampus, depending on the distribution of the receptors targeted, but may not be much more effective than available treatments. Conversely, the last 3 possibilities may be less specific because they would be expected to influence many brain regions as well as peripheral tissues that express these intracellular targets, but may be more effective. There has been legitimate concern regarding the specificity and safety of such agents. However, it is impossible to predict the effects of such agents until prototypical compounds are available for evaluation. Moreover, some agents, such as lithium and nonsteroidal anti-inflammatory agents (which affect arachidonic acid metabolism), are enormously effective for their respective indications despite their generalized actions.

The possibility that the inhibition of cAMP breakdown increases BDNF expression has been examined. Long-term administration of inhibitors of phosphodiesterases, the enzymes that metabolize cAMP, increases the expression of CREB and BDNF in the hippocampus of rats.[44] Moreover, coadministration of a phosphodiesterase inhibitor with a tricyclic antidepressant results in a more rapid induction of CREB and BDNF.[44] These findings provide additional support for the hypothesis that the cAMP system regulates the expression of BDNF and suggest that the inhibition of cAMP metabolism may provide a mechanism for a more rapid treatment of depression. The notion that the inhibition of cAMP metabolism may have antidepressant effects was raised several years ago[77] and was supported by preliminary clinical studies with rolipram, a potent phosphodiesterase inhibitor.[78] The lack of further progress on the therapeutic potential of phosphodiesterase inhibitors raises questions about the efficacy of these agents in the treatment of depression. However, given the recent observations, it may be time to reevaluate the therapeutic potential of phosphodiesterase inhibitors. One potential application that has not been investigated is the use of phosphodiesterase inhibitors as augmenting agents with other antidepressant treatments that block the reuptake or metabolism of monoamines. This approach could allow the cAMP system to be augmented in specific brain regions that contain the appropriate serotonin and NE receptors.

COMMENT

Although the regulation of CREB and BDNF may be important in the actions of antidepressant treatments, it would be preliminary and naive to suggest that these are the sole targets of these treatments. There are many genes that are known to be regulated by the cAMP system and certain antidepressant treatments.[70,79-86] In addition, the cAMP cascade is just one of many intracellular pathways that could be regulated by serotonin and NE and could be important to the action of antidepressant treatments. One example is the regulation of the phosphatidylinositol system and protein kinase C by lithium.[87-91]

The findings discussed herein indicate that antidepressant action is not mediated by the simple up- or down-regulation of monoamines and their receptors. Elucidation of the role of the cAMP system and BDNF in the response to antidepressant treatments provides fundamentally new leads in understanding antidepressant action and the pathophysiology of depression. Although the studies discussed provide a framework for a unifying hypothesis, it requires further testing of its several components. However, the model incorporates the important role of the monoamines in these phenomena and begins to elaborate the many molecular and cellular mechanisms influenced by the monoamines that are more proximal to the complex adaptations in brain function that underlie depression and its treatment.

Accepted for publication June 18, 1996.

This study was supported by grants MH45481, MH53199, and 2 PO1 MH25642 from the National Institute of Mental Health, National Institutes of Health, Bethesda, Md; a Veterans Administration National Center Grant, Veterans Affairs Medical Center, West Haven, Conn; and the Abraham Ribicoff Research Facilities of the Connecticut Mental Health Center, State of Connecticut Department of Mental Health and Addiction Services, New Haven.

Corresponding author: Ronald S. Duman, PhD, Connecticut Mental Health Center, 34 Park St, New Haven, CT 06508.

REFERENCES

1. Schildkaut JJ. The catecholamine hypothesis of affective disorders: a review of supporting evidence. *Am J Psychiatry.* 1965;122:509-522.
2. Bunney WE, Davis J. Norepinephrine in depressive reactions: a review. *Arch Gen Psychiatry.* 1965;13:483-494.
3. Coppen A. The biochemistry of affective disorders. *Br J Psychiatry.* 1967;113:1237-1264.
4. Shopsin B, Gershon S, Goldstein M, Friedman E, Wilk S. Use of synthesis inhibitors in defining a role for biogenic amines during imipramine treatment in depressed patients. *Psychopharmacol Commun.* 1975;1:239-249.
5. Delgado PL, Price LH, Miller HL, Salomon RM, Aghajanian G, Heniner GR, Charney D. Serotonin and the neurobiology of depression. *Arch Gen Psychiatry.* 1994;51:865-874.
6. Miller HL, Delgado PL, Salomon RM, Berman R, Krystal JH, Heninger GR, Charney DS. Clinical and biochemical effects of catecholamine depletion on antidepressant-induced remission of depression. *Arch Gen Psychiatry.* 1996;53:117-128.
7. Sulser F, Vetulani J, Mobley P. Mode of action of antidepressant drugs. *Biochem Pharmacol.* 1978; 27:257-261.
8. Charney DS, Menkes DB, Heninger GR. Receptor sensitivity and the mechanism of action of antidepressant treatment: implications for the etiology and therapy of depression. *Arch Gen Psychiatry.* 1981;38:1160-1180.
9. Heninger GR, Charney DS. Mechanisms of action of antidepressant treatments: implications for the etiology and treatment of depressive disorders. In: Meltzer HY, ed. *Psychopharmacology: The Third Generation of Progress.* New York, NY: Raven Press; 1987:535-544.
10. Vetulani J, Sulser F. Action of various antidepressant treatments reduces reactivity of noradrenergic cAMP-generating system in limbic forebrain. *Nature.* 1975;257:495-496.
11. Banerjee SP, Kung LS, Riggi SJ, Chanda SK. Development of β-adrenergic receptor subsensitivity by antidepressants. *Nature.* 1977;268:455-456.
12. Peroutka SL, Snyder SH. Long-term antidepressant treatment decreases spiroperidol-labeled serotonin receptor binding. *Science.* 1980;210:88-90.
13. Riva MA, Creese I. Re-evaluation of the regulation of β-adrenergic receptor binding by desipramine treatment. *Mol Pharmacol.* 1989;36:211-218.
14. Butler MO, Morinobu S, Duman RS. Chronic electroconvulsive seizures increase the expression of serotonin$_2$ receptor mRNA in rat frontal cortex. *J Neurochem.* 1993;61:1270-1276.
15. Paykel ES, Fleminger R, Watson JP. Psychiatric side effects of antihypertensive drugs other than reserpine. *J Clin Psychopharmacol.* 1982;2:14-39.
16. Avorn J, Everitt DE, Weiss S. Increased antidepressant use in patients prescribed β-blockers. *JAMA.* 1986;255:357-360.
17. Goodwin FK, Prange AJ, Post RM, Muscettola G, Lipton MA. Potentiation of antidepressant effect by triiodothyronine in tricyclic nonresponders. *Am J Psychiatry.* 1982;139:34-38.
18. Blier P, de Montigny C. Current advances and trends in the treatment of depression. *Trends Pharmacol Sci.* 1994;15:220-226.
19. Stone EA. Problems with the current hypotheses of antidepressant agents: speculations leading to a new hypothesis. *Behav Brain Sci.* 1983;6:535-577.
20. Berridge MJ. Inositol triphosphate and calcium signaling. *Nature.* 1993;361:315-325.
21. Blenis J. Signal transduction via the MAP kinases: proceed at your own RSK. *Proc Natl Acad Sci U S A.* 1993;90:5889-5892.
22. Hudson CJ, Young LT, Li PP, Warsh JJ. CNS signal transduction in the pathophysiology and pharmacotherapy of affective disorders and schizophrenia. *Synapse.* 1993;13:278-293.
23. Darnell JE, Kerr IM, Stark GR. Jak-STAT pathways and transcriptional activation in response to IFNs and other extracellular signaling proteins. *Science.* 1994;264:1415-1421.
24. Nestler EJ, Duman RS. G proteins and cyclic nucleotides in the nervous system. In: Siegel G, Agranoff B, Albers RW, Molinoff P, eds. *Basic Neurochemistry.* 5th ed. New York, NY: Raven Press; 1994:429-448.
25. Duman RS, Nestler EJ. Signal transduction pathways for catecholamine receptors. In: Meltzer H, ed. *Psychopharmacology: The Fourth Generation of Progress.* New York, NY: Raven Press; 1995:303-320.
26. Madison DV, Malenka RC, Nicoll RA. Mechanisms underlying long-term potentiation of synaptic transmission. *Ann Rev Neurosci.* 1991;14: 379-397.
27. Bliss TVP, Collingridge G. A synaptic model of memory: long-term potentiation in the hippocampus. *Nature.* 1993;361:31-39.
28. Kang H, Schuman EM. Long-lasting neurotrophin-induced enhancement of synaptic transmission in the adult hippocampus. *Science.* 1995;267:1658-1662.
29. Levine ES, Dreyfus CF, Black IB, Plummer MR. Brain-derived neurotrophic factor rapidly enhances transmission in hippocampal neurons via postsynaptic tyrosine kinase receptors. *Proc Natl Acad Sci U S A.* 1995;92:8074-8077.
30. Lindsay RM, Wiegand SJ, Altar CA, Di Stefano PS. Neurotrophic factors: from molecule to man. *Trends Neurosci.* 1994;17:182-190.
31. Lindvall O, Kokaia Z, Bengzon J, Elmer E, Kokaia M. Neurotrophins and brain insults. *Trends Neurosci.* 1994;17:490-496.
32. Thoenen H. Neurotrophins and neuronal plasticity. *Science.* 1995;270:593-598.
33. Meyer TE, Habener JF. Cyclic adenosine 3′,5′-monophosphate response element-binding protein (CREB) and related transcription-activating deoxyribonucleic acid-binding proteins. *Endocr Rev.* 1993;14:269-290.
34. Ghosh A, Greenberg ME. Calcium signaling in neurons: molecular mechanisms and cellular consequences. *Science.* 1995;268:239-247.
35. Walker WH, Fucci L, Habener JF. Expression of the gene encoding transcription factor cyclic adenosine 3′,5′-monophosphate (cAMP) response element-binding protein (CREB): regulation by follicle-stimulating hormone-induced cAMP signalling in primary rat Sertoli cells. *Endocrinology.* 1995; 136:3534-3545.
36. Widnell KL, Russell DS, Nestler EJ. Regulation of expression of cAMP response element-binding protein in the locus coeruleus in vivo and in a locus coeruleus-like cell line in vitro. *Proc Natl Acad Sci U S A.* 1994;91:10947-10951.
37. Widnell KL, Self DW, Lane SB, Russell DS, Vaidya VA, Miserendino MJD, Rubin CR, Duman RS, Nestler EJ. Regulation of CREB expression: in vivo evidence for a functional role in morphine action in the nucleus accumbens. *J Pharmacol Exp Ther.* 1996;276:306-315.
38. Sleight AJ, Carolo C, Petit N, Zwingelstein C, Bourson A. Identification of 5-hydroxytryptamine$_7$ receptor binding sites in rat hypothalamus: sensitivity to chronic antidepressant treatments. *Mol Pharmacol.* 1995;47:99-103.
39. Menkes DB, Rasenick MM, Wheeler MA, Bitensky MW. Guanosine triphosphate activation of brain adenylate cyclase: enhancement by long-term antidepressant treatment. *Science.* 1983; 129:65-67.
40. Ozawa H, Rasenick MM. Chronic electroconvulsive treatment augments coupling of the GTP-binding protein Gs to the catalytic moiety of adenylyl cyclase in a manner similar to that seen with chronic antidepressant drugs. *J Neurochem.* 1991; 56:330-338.
41. Colin SF, Chang HC, Mollner S, Pfeuffer T, Reed RR, Duman RS, Nestler EJ. Chronic lithium regulates the expression of adenylate cyclase and Gi-protein alpha in rat cerebral cortex. *Proc Natl Acad Sci U S A.* 1991;88:10634-10637.
42. Nestler EJ, Terwilliger RZ, Duman RS. Chronic antidepressant administration alters the subcellular distribution of cyclic AMP-dependent protein kinase in rat frontal cortex. *J Neurochem.* 1989; 53:1644-1647.
43. Perez J, Tinelli D, Brunello N, Racagni G. cAMP-dependent phosphorylation of soluble and crude microtubule fractions of rat cerebral cortex after prolonged desmethylimipramine treatment. *Eur J Pharmacol.* 1989;172:305-316.
44. Nibuya M, Nestler EJ, Duman RS. Chronic antidepressant administration increases the expression of cAMP response element-binding protein (CREB) in rat hippocampus. *J Neurosci.* 1996;16: 2365-2372.
45. Schwaninger M, Schoel C, Blume R, Rossig L, Knepel W. Inhibition by antidepressant drugs of cyclic AMP response element-binding protein/cyclic AMP response element-directed gene transcription. *Mol Pharmacol.* 1995;47:1112-1118.

46. Melia KR, Rasmussen K, Haycock J, Terwilliger RZ, Nestler EJ, Duman RS. Coordinate regulation of firing rate, tyrosine hydroxylase, and the cyclic AMP system in rat locus coeruleus: effects of chronic stress and norepinephrine depleting agents. *J Neurochem.* 1992;58:494-502.
47. Lo DC. Neurotrophic factors and synaptic plasticity. *Neuron.* 1995;15:979-981.
48. Mamounas LA, Blue ME, Siuciak JA, Altar CA. BDNF promotes the survival and sprouting of serotonergic axons in the rat brain. *J Neurosci.* 1995; 15:7929-7939.
49. Duman RS, Vaidya VA, Nibuya M, Morinobu S, Rydelek-Fitzgerald L. Stress, antidepressant treatments, and neurotrophic factors: molecular and cellular mechanisms. *Neuroscientist.* 1995;1:351-360.
50. Azmitia EC, Rubenstein VJ, Strafaci JA, Rios JC, Whitaker-Azmitia PM. 5-HT_{1A} agonist and dexamethasone reversal of para-chloroamphetamine-induced loss of MAP-2 and synaptophysin immunoreactivity in adult rat brain. *Brain Res.* 1995; 677:181-192.
51. Siuciak JA, Lewis D, Wiegand SJ, Lindsay RM. Antidepressant-like effect of brain-derived neurotrophic factor. *Pharmacol Biochem Behav.* 1996; 56:131-137.
52. Nibuya M, Morinobu S, Duman RS. Regulation of BDNF and trkB mRNA in rat brain by chronic electroconvulsive seizure and antidepressant drug treatments. *J Neurosci.* 1995;15:7539-7547.
53. Sklair-Tavron L, Nestler EJ. Opposing effects of morphine and the neurotrophins NT-3, NT-4, and BDNF, on locus coeruleus neurons in vitro. *Brain Res.* 1995;702:117-125.
54. Ghosh A, Carnahan J, Greenberg ME. Requirement for BDNF in activity-dependent survival of cortical neurons. *Science.* 1994;263:1618-1623.
55. Condorelli DF, Dell'Albani P, Mudo G, Timmusk T, Belluardo N. Expression of neurotrophins and their receptors in primary astroglial cultures: induction by cAMP-elevating agents. *J Neurochem.* 1994;63:509-516.
56. Smith MA, Makino S, Kvetnansky R, Post RM. Stress alters the expression of brain-derived neurotrophic factor and neurotrophin-3 mRNAs in the hippocampus. *J Neurosci.* 1995;15:1768-1777.
57. Sapolsky RM, Krey LC, McEwen BS. Prolonged glucocorticoid exposure reduces hippocampal neuron number: implications for aging. *J Neurosci.* 1985;5:1222-1227.
58. Uno H, Tarara R, Else JG, Suleman MA, Sapolsky RM. Hippocampal damage associated with prolonged and fatal stress in primates. *J Neurosci.* 1989;9:1705-1711.
59. Sapolsky RM, Uno H, Robert CS, Finsh CE. Hippocampal damage associated with prolonged glucocorticoid exposure in primates. *J Neurosci.* 1990;10:2897-2902.
60. Wooley CS, Gould E, McEwen BS. Exposure to excess glucocorticoids alters dendritic morphology of adult hippocampal pyramidal neurons. *Brain Res.* 1990;531:225-231.
61. Watanabe Y, Gould E, McEwen BS. Stress induces atrophy of apical dendrites of hippocampal CA3 pyramidal neurons. *Brain Res.* 1982;588: 341-345.
62. Stein-Behrens B, Mattson MP, Chang I, Yeh M, Sapolsky R. Stress exacerbates neuron loss and cytoskeletal pathology in the hippocampus. *J Neurosci.* 1994;14:5373-5380.
63. Magarinos AM, McEwen BS, Flugge G, Fuchs E. Chronic psychosocial stress causes apical dendritic atrophy of hippocampal CA3 pyramidal neurons in subordinate tree shrews. *J Neurosci.* 1996; 16:3534-3540.
64. Sapolsky R. Glucocorticoids, hippocampus, and the glutamatergic synapse. *Prog Brain Res.* 1990; 86:13-23.
65. Young EA, Haskett RF, Murphy-Weinberg V, Watson SJ, Akil H. Loss of glucocorticoid fast feedback in depression. *Arch Gen Psychiatry.* 1991; 48:693-699.
66. Sheline YI, Wany P, Gado MH, Csernansky JG, Vannier MW. Hippocampal atrophy in recurrent major depression. *Proc Natl Acad Sci U S A.* 1996; 93:3908-3913.
67. Sapolsky RM. Glucocorticoids and atrophy of the human hippocampus. *Science.* 1996;273:749-775.
68. Bremner JD, Randall P, Scott TM, Bronen RA, Seibyl JP, Southwick SM, Delaney RC, McCarthy G, Charney DS, Innis RB. MRI-based measurement of hippocampal volume in patients with combat-related posttraumatic stress disorder. *Am J Psychiatry.* 1995;152:973-981.
69. Elkis H, Friedman L, Wise A, Meltzer HY. Meta-analysis of studies of ventricular enlargement and cortical sulcal prominence in mood disorders. *Arch Gen Psychiatry.* 1995;52:735-746.
70. Barden N, Reul JMH, Holsboer F. Do antidepressants stabilize mood through actions on the hypothalamic-pituitary-adrenocortical system? *Trends Neurosci.* 1995;18:6-11.
71. Nakamura S. Antidepressants induce regeneration of catecholaminergic axon terminals in the rat cerebral cortex. *Neurosci Lett.* 1990;111:64-68.
72. Watanabe Y, Gould E, Daniels DC, Cameron H, McEwen BS. Tianeptine attenuates stress-induced morphological changes in the hippocampus. *Eur J Pharmacol.* 1992;222:157-162.
73. Vaidya VA, Duman RS. Chronic ECS induces mossy fiber sprouting. *Soc Neurosci.* 1996;22: 181.
74. Reding MJ, Orto LA, Winter SW, Firtuna IM, Di Ponte P, McDowell FH. Antidepressant therapy after stroke: a double-blind trial. *Arch Neurol.* 1986; 43:763-765.
75. Stern RA, Bachmann DL. Depressive symptoms following stroke. *Am J Psychiatry.* 1991;148:351-356.
76. Fedoroff J, Starkstein S, Forrester A, et al. Depression in patients with acute traumatic brain injury. *Am J Psychiatry.* 1992;149:918-923.
77. Wachtel H. Potential antidepressant activity of rolipram and other selective cyclic adenosine 3',5'-monophosphate phosphodiesterase inhibitors. *Neuropharmacology.* 1983;22:267-272.
78. Horowski R, Sastre-Y-Hernandez M. Clinical effects of the neurotrophic selective cAMP phosphodiesterase inhibitor rolipram in depressed patients: global evaluation of the preliminary reports. *Curr Ther Res.* 1985;38:23-29.
79. Duman RS, Heninger GR, Nestler EJ. Adaptations of receptor-coupled signal transduction pathways underlying stress- and drug-induced neural plasticity. *J Nerv Ment Disease.* 1994;182:692-700.
80. Hosoda K, Duman RS. Regulation of β-adrenergic receptor mRNA and ligand binding by antidepressant treatments and norepinepnrine depletion in rat frontal cortex. *J Neurochem.* 1993;60: 1335-1343.
81. Hosoda K, Feussner GK, Rydelek-Fitzgerald L, Fishman PH, Duman RS. Agonist and cyclic AMP-mediated regulation of β_1-adrenergic receptor mRNA and gene transcription in rat C6 glioma cells. *J Neurochem.* 1994;63:1635-1645.
82. Li PP, Tam YK, Young T, Warsh JJ. Lithium decreases Gs, Gi-1 and Gi-2α-subunit mRNA levels in rat cortex. *Eur J Pharm.* 1991;206:165-166.
83. Winston SM, Hayward MD, Nestler EJ, Duman RS. Chronic electroconvulsive seizures down-regulate expression of the immediate-early genes c-fos and c-jun proto-oncogenes in rat cerebral cortex. *J Neurochem.* 1990;54:1920-1925.
84. Duncan GE, Johnson KB, Breese GR. Topographic patterns of brain activity in response to swim stress: assessment by 2-deoxyglucose uptake and expression of fos-like immunoreactivlty. *J Neurosci.* 1993;13:3932-3934.
85. Hope BT, Kelz M, Duman RS, Nestler EJ. Chronic electroconvulsive seizure (ECS) treatment results in expression of a long-lasting AP-1 complex in brain with altered composition and characteristics. *J Neurosci.* 1994;14:4318-4328.
86. Morinobu S, Nibuya M, Duman RS. Chronic antidepressant treatment down-regulates the induction of c-fos mRNA in response to acute stress in rat frontal cortex. *Neuropsychopharmacology.* 1995;12:221-228.
87. Casebolt TL, Jope RS. Effects of chronic lithium treatment on protein kinase C and cyclic AMP-dependent protein phosphorylation. *Biol Psychiatry.* 1991;29:233-243.
88. Lenox RH, Watson DG, Patel J, Ellis J. Chronic lithium administration alters a prominent PKC substrate in rat hippocampus. *Brain Res.* 1992;570: 333-340.
89. Li PP, Sibony D, Green MA, Warsh JJ. Lithium modulation of phosphoinositide signaling system in rat cortex: selective effect on phorbol ester binding. *J Neurochem.* 1993;61:1722-1730.
90. Manji HK, Etcheberrigaray R, Chen G, Olds JL. Lithium decreases membrane-associated protein kinase C in hippocampus: selectivity for the a isozyme. *J Neurochem.* 1993;61:2303-2310.
91. Manji HK, Potter WZ, Lenox RH. Signal transduction pathways: molecular targets for lithium's actions. *Arch Gen Psychiatry.* 1995;52:531-543.

Molecular Biology of Behavior

Targets for Therapeutics

IN THIS ISSUE of the ARCHIVES, the article by Duman and colleagues[1] helps clarify the next layer of understanding of the neurobiology of depression and, ultimately, brings to light more powerful and selective treatment interventions. As in the catecholamine and indoleamine hypotheses of the 1960s, Duman et al appropriately rely heavily on a pharmacological bridge to better understand potential alterations in depression based on the effects of antidepressant medications. In addition, microstructural alterations in the brains of patients with depression have begun to be reported, with initial reports of increased expression of corticotropin-releasing hormone in the brains of suicide victims who had depression; increased size of the pituitary and adrenal glands; and a variety of findings concerning receptor, peptide, and structural alterations in the hippocampus, including preliminary findings of decreased hippocampal size as a function of duration of prior depressions.[2] It is against this background that tracing the effects of stress and antidepressant treatments through second messenger systems to immediate early genes, neurotrophins, and, potentially, late-effector genes becomes so exciting.

Recently, Bolwig and colleagues (personal communication, 1996) reported that of 21 600 patients studied, the best predictor of incidence and latency to rehospitalization for depression was the number of prior hospitalizations for depression. Thus, considering the pathophysiology of depression at the level of neurotrophic factors and gene expression provides candidate mechanisms by which stresses and episodes themselves could leave behind developmental lesions and additional vulnerabilities to new episode recurrence.[3] Recent work of Zhang and associates (unpublished data, 1996) revealed that a single day of maternal deprivation in the neonatal rodent can lead to marked decrements in hippocampal brain-derived neurotrophic factor associated with an increased number of "apo-tagged" cells (likely indicative of apoptosis or preprogrammed cell death). With these types of acute effects and the studies of repeated separation stress leading to a lifelong resetting of the hypothalamic-pituitary-adrenal axis by Plotsky et al,[4] there is no reason to believe that the same types of developmental vulnerabilities that Hubel and Wiesel[5] demonstrated in the visual system will not be readily discernible in neural systems related to the neurobiology of emotion regulation and social affiliation.

See also page 597

Given these types of models and the use of antidepressants in either the prevention of some of the neurobiological alterations or their amelioration once they have occurred,[1,4,6] some of the major remaining stigmas of psychiatric illness and its treatment should diminish further. New data on the neuroplasticity of the brain at the level of gene expression in response to environmental stimuli, pharmacologic agents, psychosocial stresses, and antidepressants raise some persisting elements of psychiatric stigma to an absurd level. One can readily ask why an as yet untreatable degenerative neuropsychiatric illness such as Huntington chorea is somehow more worthy of respect and more eligible for medical reimbursement than the more malleable neuropsychiatric illnesses of depression and bipolar illness—for which many effective treatments already exist, with more on the horizon.

Thus, the synthesis of the article by Duman and colleagues brings us to a fundamental new level of understanding, which should have wide ramifications for the conceptualization of depressive illnesses and their treatment. While Duman and colleagues allude to many possibilities in their article, perhaps several should be made more explicit. For many decades, the field has searched for rapid-acting antidepressants without success. If the neurotrophic factors or other late-effector gene, neuropeptide, or receptor system candidates (ie, the trkB receptor for brain-derived neurotrophic factor), which may be dysregulated in depression, are appropriately targeted pharmacologically, perhaps a rapid onset of antidepressant response can be achieved.

In addition to pharmacotherapeutic approaches, one might also wonder about the ultimate possibilities of affecting some of these neurotrophic factor and late-effector gene systems with repeated transcranial magnetic stimulation of the brain.[7,8] Some of the effects of repeated transcranial magnetic stimulation are

This article is also available on our Web site: www.ama-assn.org/psych.

likely to be frequency dependent, with higher frequencies enhancing neural excitability and glucose utilization and lower frequencies producing decrements in these parameters and quenchinglike effects via effects on transcriptional activity and neurotrophic factor gene expression.[9]

Not only does the molecular neurobiology revolution give us a new fundamental understanding of potential mechanisms of depression and its therapeutics, but, as noted by the investigators previously mentioned as well as others,[10] it also provides an equally compelling structure for understanding the short- and long-term consequences of psychologically relevant variables that can only be studied in a behavioral context.[1,10] As such, this beginning probe of the neurobiology of depression at the level of alterations in gene expression will ultimately lead to a better combination of modern biological psychiatry with its earlier roots in development, learning and memory, neuropsychology, and behavior.

Robert M. Post, MD
Biological Psychiatry Branch
National Institute of Mental Health
National Institutes of Health
9000 Rockville Pike
Bethesda, MD 20892

REFERENCES

1. Duman RS, Heninger GR, Nestler EJ. A molecular and cellular theory of depression. *Arch Gen Psychiatry.* 1997;54:597-606.
2. Sapolsky RM. Why stress is bad for your brain. *Science.* 1996;273:749-750.
3. Post RM. Transduction of psychosocial stress into the neurobiology of recurrent affective disorder. *Am J Psychiatry.* 1992;149:999-1010.
4. Plotsky PM, Eisler JA, Anand KJS. Long-term consequences of neonatal stress. *J Eur Coll Neuropsychopharmacol.* 1996;6(suppl 3):217. Abstract.
5. Hubel DH, Wiesel TN. Brain mechanisms of vision. *Sci Am.* 1979;241:150-162.
6. Smith MA, Makino S, Kvetnansky R, Post RM. Stress and glucocorticoids affect the expression of brain-derived neurotropic factor and neurotrophin-3 mRNAs in the hippocampus. *J Neurosci.* 1995;15:1768-1777.
7. George MS, Wassermann EM, Williams WA, Callahan A, Ketter TA, Basser P, Hallett M, Post RM. Daily repetitive transcranial magnetic stimulation (rTMS) improves mood in depression. *Neuroreport.* 1995;6:1853-1856.
8. Pascual-Leone A, Rubio B, Pallardo F, Catala MD. Rapid-rate transcranial magnetic stimulation of left dorsolateral prefrontal cortex in drug-resistant depression. *Lancet.* 1996;348:233-237.
9. Post RM, Kimbrell T, Frye M, George M, McCann U, Little J, Dunn R, Li H, Weiss SRB. Implications of kindling and quenching for the possible frequency dependence of rTMS. *CNS Spectrums.* 1997;2:54-60.
10. Smith MA. Hippocampal vulnerability to stress and aging: possible role of neurotrophic factors. *Behav Brain Res.* 1996;78:25-36.

A Controlled Family History Study of Childhood-Onset Depressive Disorder

Maria Kovacs, PhD; Bernie Devlin, PhD; Myrna Pollock, MSW; Cheryl Richards, MBA; Protap Mukerji, MS

Background: We studied the family psychiatric history of 125 youths with childhood-onset depressive disorder (a portion of whom developed bipolar disorder) and 55 psychiatric controls with nonaffective disorder.

Methods: Probands were classified according to prospectively observed clinical course in childhood. Family psychiatric history was determined by interviewers blind to probands' diagnoses, with mothers typically informing about themselves and about remaining first- and all second-degree adult relatives.

Results: Families of affectively ill juveniles had 5-fold greater odds of lifetime depressive disorder and 2-fold greater odds of recurrent unipolar depressive disorder than did families of psychiatric controls. The higher risk of depression was most evident in first-degree and female relatives. Mothers of affectively ill youths were younger at onset of depression than were mothers of controls. Alcoholism and substance use disorders were more prevalent in relatives of affectively ill probands than in controls and cosegregated with familial depression. However, other covariates were more important at predicting patterns of familial depression. Familial illness patterns also varied somewhat with proband characteristics.

Conclusions: Child probands with affective disorder identify families enriched with affective disorder (even compared with families of psychiatric controls), suggesting that juvenile- and adult-onset forms of this condition share the same diathesis. Rates of affective illness in the families of depressed youngsters also are notably higher than population-based estimates. The findings therefore indicate that very-early-onset affective disorder is familial and that pedigrees ascertained through affectively ill children are good candidates for family and genetic studies.

Arch Gen Psychiatry. 1997;54:613-623

Depressive disorders diagnosed by *DSM-III*[1] and *DSM-III-R*[2] have been identified in psychiatrically referred youths, nonreferred children at risk for affective disorders, and juveniles in school- or community-based samples.[3-13] It also has been shown that major depressive and *DSM-III* dysthymic disorders in youngsters are associated with high rates of recovery but subsequent episodes of affective illness.[5,6,14-19] In general, rates of remission, recurrence, and comorbidity in depressed juvenile and adult patients are strikingly similar,[20] suggesting that childhood-onset and later-onset depressions are variants of the same condition.

Patterns of familial psychiatric illness should shed further light on the nature of very-early-onset affective disorder and its relationship to later-onset depression. However, only 4 controlled studies exist of family psychiatric history of school-age, depressed, clinically referred probands who had been assessed with structured interviews and diagnosed by accepted operational criteria, and whose relatives were evaluated by interviewers kept blind to the probands' identity.[21-24] Two studies included 6- to 12-year-old patient probands,[21,22] 1 included 7- to 17-year-old patient probands,[23] and 1 had only adolescent probands.[24] Psychiatric as well as normal controls served as comparisons.

According to the results,[21-24] clinically referred youths with depressive disorder have consistently and significantly higher rates of depression in their families than do normal control youths. Furthermore, familial depression appears to be more prevalent among depressed children than depressed adolescents. But rates of affective illness in families of depressed youngsters vs youngsters with

From the Department of Psychiatry, University of Pittsburgh School of Medicine, and Western Psychiatric Institute and Clinic (Drs Kovacs and Devlin, Mss Pollock, and Richards, and Mr Mukerji); and Carnegie Mellon University (Dr Devlin), Pittsburgh, Pa.

SUBJECTS AND METHODS

DESIGN

We review relevant aspects of our methods; more details are provided elsewhere.[5,6,14] Subjects for the main longitudinal investigation were recruited primarily from among sequential referrals to the child psychiatry outpatient service, University of Pittsburgh, Pittsburgh, Pa, and the general medical clinic, Children's Hospital of Pittsburgh (83% and 15%, respectively, of all depressed subjects in the present article); the remaining cases were obtained through other avenues. Subjects were screened by us irrespective of referral reason or the service provider's diagnosis. Children had to meet the following study entry criteria: 8 to 13 years old; not mentally retarded; no major systemic medical illness; ambulatory status; and living with parent or guardian within commuting distance of greater Pittsburgh. Signed consents were obtained for a repeated-assessment 5-year follow-up and then for further optional follow-up periods. Families received monetary reimbursement at each assessment.

PSYCHIATRIC DIAGNOSIS OF PROBANDS

At each assessment, the parent and child were interviewed separately by the same research clinician with the use of the semistructured Interview Schedule for Children and Adolescents and its diagnostic addenda, which have satisfactory reliability.[25,26] Interviewers were experienced and specifically trained mental health professionals (MSW and PhD level). Subsequent to each interview, clinical history and Interview Schedule for Children and Adolescents symptom ratings were used to assign diagnoses by *DSM-III*[1,5] and by additional operational rules, namely (1) a protracted, partially remitted major depressive disorder (MDD) was never diagnosed as dysthymic disorder (DD), (2) *DSM-III* criteria for hypomania[1(p220)] with at least 1-week duration served to diagnose "bipolar II" disorder, and (3) specific criteria were defined for adjustment disorder.[27] Interviewers knew the outcomes of a child's previous assessments. Final *DSM-III* diagnoses were assigned by consensus among the research clinicians and subsequently verified by 1 of us (M.K.).

Shortly after entry into the main study, patients were classified by "index diagnosis" (*DSM-III*[1]): MDD (n=60); DD (n=32); MDD superimposed on DD (MDD/DD; n=23); adjustment disorder with depressed mood (ADDM; n=19); bipolar disorder (BP; n=8); and nonaffective or control psychiatric disorder (n=49). The diagnoses (either primary or secondary) of control cases included behavior (attention and/or conduct) disorder (59%), developmental disorder, enuresis (10%), only adjustment disorder and/or V-code (24%), and other disorders (6%). All diagnostic groups had high rates of initial psychiatric comorbidity, from 68% to 83% among children with affective problems, and 63% among the controls.

CLASSIFICATION OF CASENESS OF PROBANDS

Three groups were identified on the basis of clinical outcome during the follow-up: 99 probands with early-onset depressive disorder (group 1), 26 with early-onset BP (group 2), and 55 psychiatric controls free of early-onset depressive or BP disorder (group 3). Early-onset depressive disorder refers to MDD and/or DD by 14 years of age, corresponding to the upper age limit at study entry. Early-onset BP refers to bipolar I or II forms of this condition by 17 years of age.

Our groupings are based on 3 observations: some youths with an initial nonaffective diagnosis developed affective disorder on follow-up,[27] childhood-onset MDD and DD are variants of the same illness,[6,28] and most children with bipolar II convert to bipolar I disorder.[29] In group 1, 95 cases originally had MDD/DD, 1 had ADDM, and 3 were controls; in group 2, 8 originally had BP, 16 had MDD/DD, 1 had ADDM, and 1 was a control; and in group 3, 42 were originally controls and 13 had ADDM. Of the original sample, 5 children were adopted and were not included in the present data set; no pedigree information was available on 6 further children.

The proband groups differed on several demographic variables and rates of comorbid diagnoses by late adolescence

nonaffective psychiatric disorder have not consistently differed, raising questions of specificity. Also, it has been unclear whether alcoholism and substance use disorders cosegregate in the pedigrees of youths and affect rates of depression. Finally, it has not been resolved whether proband characteristics, such as absence of comorbid "externalizing" disorders, can identify more homogeneous phenotypes of familial depression.

To address these issues, we report on a controlled, blind, family psychiatric history study of first- and second-degree adult relatives of 8- to 13-year-old clinically referred patients with a research diagnosis of affective disorder. Determination of familial psychiatric illness was one component of a larger longitudinal investigation of depressive disorders. The working hypothesis was that probands with childhood-onset depression have significantly higher familial rates of affective illness than do controls with childhood-onset nonaffective psychiatric disorder. Mothers of probands were generally assessed directly. Information on most other relatives was gathered through the family history method. Therefore, our findings should be regarded as preliminary but necessary for future attempts at direct family study of childhood-onset affective disorders.

RESULTS

LIFETIME PSYCHIATRIC DIAGNOSES FOR FAMILIES

A family was considered to be affected with a specific disorder if at least 1 member had that diagnosis (**Table 2**). Families of probands with affective disorder had significantly greater odds of major depression and recurrent unipolar depression than did control families. Furthermore, families of bipolar probands had a significantly higher rate of mania than did families of probands with

(**Table 1**). However, probands with early-onset depressive disorder and those with BP had their first depressive episode at comparable ages (10.0 and 11.4 years, on average, respectively). Two controls became depressed at the mean age of 17.8 years, which disqualified them from being in group 1.

FAMILY PSYCHIATRIC HISTORY

Family psychiatric history was obtained by trained master's level mental health professionals, who were not otherwise affiliated with the project and who were kept blind to probands' psychiatric diagnoses. Across the 180 families, informants were 150 mothers, 17 fathers, 9 grandmothers, and 6 other relatives, with 2 informants each for 13 probands. For 11 other families, partial information from parents was supplemented by data from medical records. Information was gathered on 1727 adults aged 18 years or older at the time of the assessments: parents, probands' siblings, and second-degree relatives on whom the informant could report. The extent of information varied, with limited data on some fathers and many paternal relatives. For close to 350 relatives, only nondiagnostic indexes of potential caseness were available, which are not included in this article.

Pedigree sizes and average ages of relatives were nearly identical across the proband groups. Specifically, the mean numbers of relatives for groups 1, 2, and 3 were 9.8±5.5, 9.7±4.7, and 9.2±4.3, respectively. Mean ages of mothers were 35.9±5.9, 35.8±4.3, and 37.1±5.5 years. Fathers' mean ages were 38.6±7.4, 38.8±6.1, and 40.4±9.7 years. Grandparents' mean ages were 60.5±9.1, 62.0±10.3, and 62.2±9.2 years; ages of aunts and uncles for the 3 proband groups were 35.4±9.6, 35.6±10.7, and 35.8±9.8 years.

Mothers were generally assessed directly via the Schedule for Affective Disorders and Schizophrenia–Lifetime Version[30] and diagnosed by Research Diagnostic Criteria (RDC).[31] Almost all fathers, older siblings of probands, and second-degree relatives were diagnosed by family history RDC (FH-RDC)[32,33] with mothers generally serving as informants. All assessments were tape-recorded.

Altogether, 28 randomly selected Schedule for Affective Disorders and Schizophrenia–Lifetime Version/RDC and 90 FH-RDC taped assessments were rated blindly by a second interviewer. Diagnostic agreement, computed as the κ coefficient,[34] was satisfactory. For RDC diagnoses in this article, the κ statistics were 1.00 each for major depression, recurrent unipolar depression, and mania. Owing to low variability, percentage agreements were computed for other diagnoses, yielding concordance rates of 100% each for alcoholism, substance abuse, and antisocial personality. For FH-RDC, κ values were between 1.00 and 0.90 for major depression, alcoholism, and substance abuse, and between 0.71 and 0.79 for recurrent unipolar depression, mania, and antisocial personality.

DATA ANALYSES

The expected age-at-onset distribution of psychiatric illness in families of probands with childhood-onset affective disorders is not known. Because the age distributions were similar for all 3 groups, we report morbidity risks uncorrected for age at assessment, namely, the number of relatives with a specific diagnosis divided by the number of relatives surveyed. Diagnostic rates were compared across groups by odds ratios (ORs)[35] and associated statistics by unconditional maximum likelihood (2-sided tests of significance). Given the assumption that probands with early-onset affective illness differ in family histories from probands who had nonaffective disorders, groups 1 and 2 were combined and contrasted with group 3. If the 2 early-onset affective disorder groups differed on an outcome variable, then ORs were computed separately for group 1 vs group 3 and group 2 vs group 3.

Because the Schedule for Affective Disorders and Schizophrenia–Lifetime Version (administered to mothers) elicits age at onset of disorders, selected maternal diagnoses also were modeled by the Kaplan-Meier method,[36] providing sample-specific, age-corrected estimates. Finally, to examine the impact of familial nonaffective disorders and selected proband characteristics on the likelihood of depression in relatives, the data were modeled by means of stepwise logistic regression techniques.[35]

early-onset depression (OR, 3.08; *P*=.03; 95% CI, 1.10-8.63) or controls (OR, 3.14; *P*=.05; 95% CI, 0.98-10.07).

LIFETIME PSYCHIATRIC DIAGNOSES FOR FIRST-DEGREE RELATIVES

Affective Disorders

Major depression (**Table 3**) was more common in group 2 than group 1 first-degree relatives (OR, 2.09; *P*=.03; 95% CI, 1.05-4.15). Additionally, the odds of major depression were significantly greater in group 2 than group 3 relatives (OR, 3.06; *P*=.003; 95% CI, 1.48-6.32), but only somewhat elevated in group 1 vs group 3 relatives (OR, 1.45; *P*=.12; 95% CI, 0.92-2.34). Likewise, the rate of recurrent unipolar depression for relatives was highest in group 2 and lowest in group 3.

Mothers had particularly high rates of major depression (72.5% in group 1 and 76.0% in group 2, vs 54.0% in group 3; OR, 2.34; *P*=.02; 95% CI, 1.17-4.66) and recurrent unipolar depression (37.1% in group 1 and 47.8% in group 2, vs 20.8% in group 3; OR, 2.46; *P*=.03; 95% CI, 1.11-5.43). Rates of major depression and recurrent unipolar depression did not significantly differ for fathers of the proband groups.

Nonaffective Disorders

The increased rate of alcoholism in first-degree relatives of probands with affective disorder (Table 3) reflects the combined contribution of maternal (17.4% in group 1 and 12.5% in group 2, vs 6.4% in group 3) and paternal (48.1% in group 1 and 28.6% in group 2, vs 31.9% in group 3) histories. There also was a trend of a higher rate of familial substance abuse among children with affective disorder as compared with controls.

Table 1. Characteristics of Juvenile Probands

Variable	Group 1: Depressive Disorder (n=99)	Group 2: Bipolar Disorder (n=26)	Group 3: Nonaffective Disorder (n=55)	Significant Contrasts*
Demographics at Study Entry				
Female, %	57	35	29	a, b
White, %	67	65	58	None
Socioeconomic status, %†				a
High (I)	1	2	7	
Middle (II, III, IV)	72	58	73	
Low (V)	28	31	20	
Intact family of origin, %	26	38	33	None
Two-parent household, %	50	65	51	None
Age, y				
Mean±SD	11.3±1.6	11.4±1.6	10.5±1.5	b, c
Range	8-13	8-13	8-13	
Clinical Characteristics by Age 18 y	**Group 1:**	**Group 2:**	**Group 3:**	**Significant Contrasts**
Age at first major disorder, y (mean±SD)‡	8.4±2.5	8.6±3.2	8.8±4.1	None
Age at first depression, y (mean±SD)	10.0±2.1	11.4±3.5	17.8§	b, c
Behavior disorder, %‖	47	69	60	a
Anxiety disorder, %	56	46	13	b, c
Suicide attempt, %	31	31	7	b, c

*By χ^2 ($P<.05$) or *t* tests ($P<.025$): a indicates group 1 vs group 2; b, group 1 vs group 3; and c, group 2 vs group 3.
†Hollingshead index.
‡Not including adjustment disorder, enuresis/encopresis, V-codes.
§Two cases developed depression after age 14 years.
‖Attention deficit, conduct, or substance use/abuse disorder.

Table 2. Rates of Lifetime Psychiatric Diagnoses for Families of Probands*

Variable	Group 1: Depressive Disorder (n=95†)	Group 2: Bipolar Disorder (n=26†)	Group 3: Nonaffective Disorder (n=52†)	Odds Ratio‡ (95% CI)	*P*
Major depression	0.937	1.000	0.788	5.1 (1.77-14.67)	.003
Recurrent unipolar depression	0.602	0.625	0.451	1.88 (0.97-3.65)	.06
Mania	0.140	0.333	0.137	. . .§	. . .
Alcoholism	0.753	0.667	0.680	1.31 (0.63-2.69)	.47
Substance abuse	0.495	0.435	0.408	1.35 (0.69-2.66)	.38
Antisocial personality	0.344	0.560	0.347	1.21 (0.60-2.43)	.59

*Rates are adjusted for missing data.
†Number of families.
‡Groups 1 and 2 vs group 3. CI indicates confidence interval.
§Group 2 differs from group 1. Separate odds ratios are reported in the text.

AGE-CORRECTED RISK OF DEPRESSION AND FIRST PSYCHIATRIC PROBLEM FOR MOTHERS

Mothers of the proband groups significantly differed in the cumulative probability of depression (**Figure 1**) and its median age at onset (Mantel Cox statistic=7.903, *df*=2, *P*=.02). Median age at first depression was 21.50 years for group 2 mothers, 27.00 years for group 1 mothers, and 36.06 years for control mothers. Categorizing maternal depression as having onset in childhood (up to age 14 years), adolescence (ages 15-19 years), or adulthood (age 20 years and later) showed no differences between group 1 and group 2 mothers (exact χ^2, *P*=.79). However, mothers of children with affective disorder were significantly more likely to have had childhood- or adolescent-onset depression than were control mothers (χ^2=6.6, *df*=2, *P*=.04). For example, 21% of depressed mothers of affectively ill probands, but none of the control mothers, had their first depression by age 14 years.

The groups of mothers also significantly differed in the cumulative probability of any first psychiatric problem (**Figure 2**, Mantel Cox statistic=6.161, *df*=2, *P*=.05). Median age at onset of first problem was 15 years for mothers of each of the 2 proband groups with affective disorder and 18.50 years for control mothers.

Table 3. Rates of Lifetime Psychiatric Diagnoses for First-Degree Relatives of Probands*

	Child Proband Group				
Variable	Group 1: Depressive Disorder (n=197†)	Group 2: Bipolar Disorder (n=49†)	Group 3: Nonaffective Disorder (n=116†)	Odds Ratio‡ (95% CI)	P
Major depression	0.537	0.708	0.442	. . .§	. . .
Recurrent unipolar depression	0.247	0.333	0.173	1.71 (0.97-3.06)	.07
Mania	0.048	0.065	0.063	0.81 (0.31-2.12)	.67
Alcoholism	0.298	0.196	0.177	1.98 (1.02-3.14)	.04
Substance abuse	0.178	0.111	0.091	1.80 (0.95-4.13)	.07
Antisocial personality	0.081	0.152	0.063	1.57 (0.65-3.80)	.32

*Rates are adjusted for missing data.
†Number of relatives.
‡Groups 1 and 2 vs group 3. CI indicates confidence interval.
§Group 2 differs from group 1. Separate odds ratios are reported in the text.

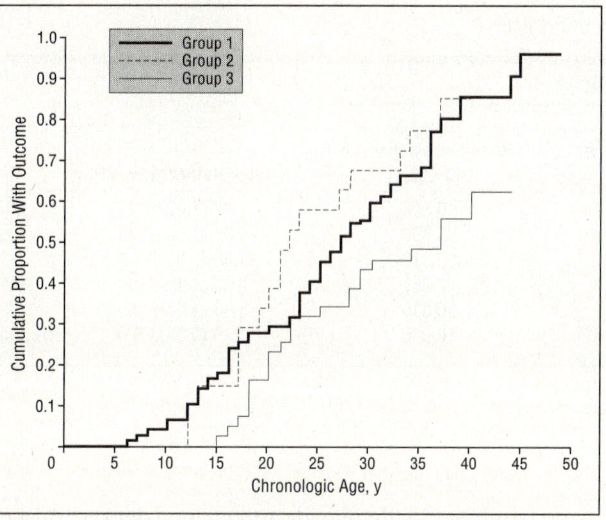

Figure 1. *Cumulative probability of first-episode depressive disorder for mothers in the 3 proband groups as a function of chronologic age of mothers (group 1, probands with depressive disorder; group 2, probands with bipolar disorder; group 3, probands with nonaffective disorder).*

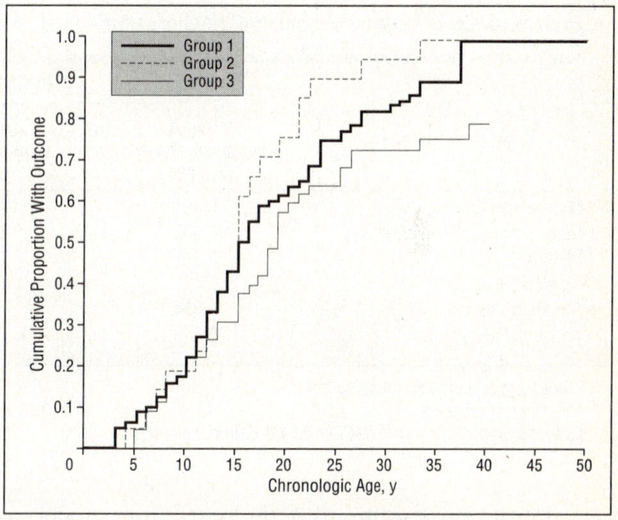

Figure 2. *Cumulative probability of any first psychiatric problem for mothers in the 3 proband groups as a function of chronologic age of mothers (group 1, probands with depressive disorder; group 2, probands with bipolar disorder; group 3, probands with nonaffective disorder).*

LIFETIME PSYCHIATRIC DIAGNOSES FOR SECOND-DEGREE RELATIVES

The odds of recurrent unipolar depression were approximately 2-fold higher in second-degree relatives (**Table 4**) of children with depressive disorder than in relatives of bipolar probands (OR, 2.13; P=.05; 95% CI, 1.00-4.57) or control probands (OR, 1.82; P=.03; 95% CI, 1.05-3.14). Alcoholism also was more likely in second-degree relatives of affectively ill probands than in controls.

LIFETIME PSYCHIATRIC DIAGNOSES BY SEX OF RELATIVE

The odds of depressive disorder, recurrent unipolar depression, alcoholism, and drug abuse were significantly higher in female relatives of affectively ill probands than in female control relatives (**Table 5**). Male relatives of affectively ill probands only had elevated rates of alcoholism and antisocial personality as compared with control male relatives (**Table 6**).

MODELING THE PROBABILITY OF DEPRESSIVE DISORDER IN RELATIVES

To clarify the relationship of depression to alcoholism and substance abuse in the pedigrees, we fit a logistic regression model with depression as the response and alcoholism or substance abuse as predictors. Groups 1, 2, and 3 were similar in their patterns. Both alcohol (OR, 1.36; P=.04; 95% CI, 1.02-1.82) and drug abuse (OR, 1.78; P=.004; 95% CI, 1.20-2.66) tended to cosegregate with depression in families.

We also explored a more complex model to explain depression in group 1 vs group 3 and group 2 vs group 3 families, in which the following variables were included: alcoholism (yes, no), drug abuse (yes, no), status of relative (mother, father, sibling, and second-degree maternal and paternal relatives or half-siblings), sex of relative, and proband group. Suicide attempt of relative (yes, no) also was included because of its documented association with depression and substance abuse. The full model (up to first-order interactions) was simplified by means of standard parsimony criteria.[35]

Table 4. Rates of Lifetime Psychiatric Diagnoses for Second-Degree Relatives of Probands*

Variable	Child Proband Group: Group 1: Depressive Disorder (n=574†)	Group 2: Bipolar Disorder (n=150†)	Group 3: Nonaffective Disorder (n=298†)	Odds Ratio‡ (95% CI)	*P*
Major depression	0.221	0.229	0.208	1.09 (0.78-1.54)	.61
Recurrent unipolar depression	0.114	0.057	0.066	. . .§	. . .
Mania	0.020	0.042	0.010	2.36 (0.67-12.66)	.22
Alcoholism	0.207	0.209	0.147	1.51 (1.05-2.19)	.03
Substance abuse	0.073	0.088	0.048	1.64 (0.90-3.01)	.11
Antisocial personality	0.083	0.090	0.059	1.46 (0.84-2.55)	.18

**Rates are adjusted for missing data.*
†*Number of relatives.*
‡*Groups 1 and 2 vs group 3. CI indicates confidence interval.*
§*Group 2 differs from group 1. Separate odds ratios are reported in the text.*

Table 5. Rates of Lifetime Psychiatric Diagnoses for Female Relatives of Probands*

Variable	Child Proband Group: Group 1: Depressive Disorder (n=402†)	Group 2: Bipolar Disorder (n=99†)	Group 3: Nonaffective Disorder (n=205†)	Odds Ratio‡ (95% CI)	*P*
Major depression	0.381	0.454	0.308	1.47 (1.03-2.10)	.03
Recurrent unipolar depression	0.207	0.185	0.099	2.31 (1.36-3.90)	<.01
Mania	0.018	0.031	0.015	1.38 (0.35-7.90)	.77
Alcoholism	0.131	0.124	0.065	2.15 (1.15-3.99)	.02
Substance abuse	0.064	0.073	0.020	3.45 (1.20-9.90)	.02
Antisocial personality	0.025	0.042	0.030	0.95 (0.33-3.05)	≅1.00

**Rates are adjusted for missing data.*
†*Number of relatives.*
‡*Groups 1 and 2 vs group 3. CI indicates confidence interval.*

For group 1 vs group 3, the best-fitting model included relative's sex (χ^2=4.17, *df*=1, *P*=.04), status (χ^2=79.15, *df*=5, *P*<.001), and attempted suicide (χ^2=65.96, *df*=1, *P*<.001). Female relatives were approximately twice as likely to be depressed as male relatives. Mothers and fathers were at greater risk than aunts and uncles, with siblings and half-siblings at intermediate risk (and not differing significantly from the family mean risk). Suicide attempt of a relative was strongly associated with depression (OR, 17.87; 95% CI, 9.53-33.49). Neither alcoholism nor drug abuse was significantly associated with depression, and none of the interactions with group was significant.

Because bipolar probands had few siblings, relative's status in group 2 vs group 3 analyses was coded as mother, father, or maternal and paternal second-degree relatives. The best-fitting model included group (χ^2=5.28, *df*=1, *P*=.02), sex (χ^2=10.52, *df*=1, *P*=.001), group-by-sex interaction (χ^2=3.94, *df*=1, *P*=.05), relative status (χ^2=55.10, *df*=3, *P*<.001), group-by–relative status interaction (χ^2=8.46, *df*=3, *P*=.04), suicide (χ^2=14.75, *df*=1, *P*<.001), and group-by-suicide interaction (χ^2=8.91, *df*=1, *P*=.003). The rate of depression was significantly higher for females than males in group 2, but it approached 50:50 for men and women in group 3. Mothers and fathers were at greater risk of depression than were second-degree relatives. The group-by–relative status interaction reflects a dearth of depressed maternal relatives in bipolar proband families. Finally, suicide attempt and depression were much more strongly associated in group 3 families (OR, 72.40; 95% CI, 9.62-544.90) than group 2 families (OR, 3.18; 95% CI, 1.15-8.81).

COMORBIDITY IN AFFECTIVELY ILL PROBANDS AND FAMILIAL DIAGNOSES

Among depressed youths, behavior disorders may affect long-term outcomes[37] and constitute frequent comorbid conditions.[38] Therefore, we examined the effects of comorbid behavior (attention deficit, conduct, substance use/abuse) disorder in the affectively ill probands on familial aggregation of selected conditions.

Youths with comorbid affective and behavior disorders had higher familial rates of alcoholism, substance abuse, and antisocial personality (but similar rates of depression and mania) than relatives of youths with affective illness but no behavior disorder. These trends approached significance in first-degree relatives (OR, 1.67; *P*=.08; 95% CI, 0.94-2.98 for alcoholism; OR, 1.88; *P*=.08; 95% CI, 0.92-3.83 for substance abuse; OR, 2.14; *P*=.11; 95% CI, 0.84-5.47 for antisocial personality), were significant in second-degree relatives (OR, 2.10; *P*<.001; 95% CI, 1.44-3.06 for alcoholism; OR, 1.81; *P*=.04; 95% CI, 1.02-3.24 for substance abuse; OR, 3.10; *P*<.001; 95% CI, 1.70-5.68 for antisocial personality), and were

Table 6. Rates of Lifetime Psychiatric Diagnoses for Male Relatives of Probands*

Variable	Child Proband Group: Group 1: Depressive Disorder (n=369†)	Group 2: Bipolar Disorder (n=100†)	Group 3: Nonaffective Disorder (n=209†)	Odds Ratio‡ (95% CI)	*P*
Major depression	0.215	0.242	0.244	0.88 (0.59-1.31)	.53
Recurrent unipolar depression	0.081	0.064	0.094	0.81 (0.44-1.47)	.49
Mania	0.037	0.065	0.035	1.21 (0.48-3.48)	.83
Alcoholism	0.338	0.289	0.244	1.51 (1.04-2.19)	.03
Substance abuse	0.137	0.113	0.098	1.40 (0.82-2.39)	.21
Antisocial personality	0.146	0.167	0.090	1.78 (1.03-3.07)	.04

**Rates are adjusted for missing data.*
†Number of relatives.
‡Groups 1 and 2 vs group 3. CI indicates confidence interval.

detectable in both female and male relatives compared with same-sex relatives of youths without comorbidity. However, the propensity for antisocial personality was evident only in male relatives of youths with comorbidity, compared with male relatives of youths without comorbidity (OR, 2.59; $P=.001$; 95% CI, 1.47-4.57).

POST HOC ANALYSES

To examine possible effects of socioeconomic status (SES) (Table 1) on familial patterns of depression, alcoholism, and/or substance abuse, we fit logistic regression models for groups 1 and 2 and for group 3. The dependent variables were major depression, alcoholism, or drug abuse (each yes/no) and the independent variables were group, SES, and their interaction. Last grade of formal education served as a surrogate for SES; it was trichotomized as follows: 1, less than high school; 2, high school degree; and 3, 1 or more years of college. Socioeconomic status was treated as a continuous or categorical variable in separate analyses.

Socioeconomic status had no significant effect on between- or within-group rates of depression. Socioeconomic status was inversely related to familial alcoholism and substance abuse, but there were no significant between-group differences. For simple logistic regression models in which SES was the only independent variable and all family members and groups were included, the slopes were −0.632 (SE=0.095) for alcoholism and −0.462 (SE=0.132) for substance abuse (both $P<.001$).

COMMENT

The main findings of the present study are that relatives of young patients with affective illness are at greater risk for major depression and recurrent unipolar depression than are relatives of psychiatric controls, and that mothers of depressed youths have an earlier age at onset of depression than do mothers of controls. In our pedigrees, familial rates of alcoholism and substance use disorder are higher for the target probands than for controls, tend to cosegregate with depression, but are not important explanatory variables after other covariates are accounted for. Furthermore, patterns of nonaffective familial psychiatric illness vary with certain proband characteristics. The results, however, have to be interpreted in the context of methodological constraints.

POTENTIAL LIMITATIONS OF THE PRESENT STUDY

Because of the methods of case ascertainment, our results and all extant information on familial psychiatric morbidity of affectively ill youths are generalizable only to clinical populations. Additionally, because we used a psychiatric control group, we cannot estimate the absolute magnitude of morbid risk to relatives of a depressed child as compared with a "normal" child. However, psychiatric comparisons can help to determine whether trends in familial psychopathology are specific to depressed probands and provide some control for comorbidity among them, as recently suggested.[39] A related issue is the relatively small sizes of our samples, just as in other family history studies of depressed youths,[21-24] reflecting the fact that subjects were clinically referred. Multisite designs may be needed to gather more juvenile probands and thereby increase the power to detect effects of interest.

Another limitation is our use of the family history method of psychiatric diagnosis for fathers and second-degree relatives. The FH-RDC can obscure the extent of familiality because it yields lower psychiatric morbidity rates, particularly for depression, than direct family study does. Nonetheless, the results do provide a gross indication of whether disorders are familial.[40] Using a single informant for most family data also may bias results because the informant may not be equally knowledgeable about all relatives. However, such a bias should be similar across proband groups.

Questions can also be raised about having combined, for most analyses, probands with depressive disorder and BP. This decision was based on 3 considerations. First, if we defined caseness of our probands by their initial diagnoses, which is the usual approach in family history studies, the vast majority of them would be depressive; the switch in polarity typically occurred during follow-up. Second, no differences have been found in familial rates of depressive disorders and BP among depressed children who did and those who did not develop bipolarity.[22] Third, age at onset of first disorder and first depression, which have been associated with differential familial histories of affective illness in youths[41] and adults,[42,43] were comparable in our depressed and bipolar probands.

Notwithstanding such methodological constraints, results of our study converge with other data on familial psychiatric illness in affectively ill youths. As we now discuss, the findings underscore the need for further research in this area.

AFFECTIVE DISORDERS IN RELATIVES

As reported previously,[21-24] familial morbid risk of depression is higher for depressed than for normal children. Our results and those from another blind family history study[39] indicate that the elevated rate of depression in the pedigrees of depressed children distinguish them from nondepressed psychiatric control children. Moreover, by all accounts, rates of familial depressive illness for depressed youths are higher than those for depressed adults,[42,44] whereas familial patterns appear to be the same. Namely, the higher rates of depression in first-degree than in second-degree relatives and in female as compared with male relatives that typify adult probands[42,45,46] also are evident in the families of affectively ill youths.

The excess affective morbidity in the pedigrees of juveniles could mean that childhood-onset depression is more familial than later-onset depression. Alternatively, it could be argued that methodological factors are at play. For example, the high rate of familial depression among young depressed patients has been thought to reflect that depressed parents are particularly inclined to bring their children for treatment.[47] It also could be argued that secular changes in rates and age at onset of depression[48-50] may explain the high prevalence of depression in relatives of depressed youths. However, despite secular trends, major depression has been found to be strongly familial in younger as well as older adult cohorts.[45]

It appears that from 34%[21] to 57% (present study) of first-degree relatives of depressed children have depressive disorder; in first-degree relatives of adolescents, a 25% rate was reported.[24] These figures represent about a 2-fold increase in rates of depression compared with rates in various juvenile control groups. The prevalence of maternal depression among depressed children is particularly high (from 56%[23] to 73% [present study]).

Compared with the above figures, and consistent with a putative genetic component to childhood-onset depression, there is a lower risk of the disorder in second-degree relatives. From 8%[21] to 25%[22] of such relatives of depressed children have depressive disorder; in second-degree relatives of adolescents, a 5% rate was reported.[24] The prevalence rates of depression in second-degree relatives represent anywhere from no increase to a 2-fold increase in risk depending on the comparison group, but are probably underestimates of true rates.[40]

To place our findings in a broader context, we compared the prevalence of parental depression with population rates of the National Comorbidity Survey.[51,52] Because the National Comorbidity Survey rates are higher than those from other epidemiological studies,[53] our contrasts are conservative. Nonetheless, it appears that an affectively ill child represents a notably increased risk of depression in parents as compared with the rate of depression among same-sex and similar-age community residents. Mothers of our affectively ill youths have a 3.8-fold higher rate of depression than do 25- to 34-year-old women in the general population (73.3% vs 19.4%) and a 3.1-fold increase as compared with 35- to 44-year-old women (73.3% vs 23.8%).[52] Fathers of our youths with affective disorder have a 3.3-fold higher rate of depression than do 25- to 34-year-old men in the general population (42.9% vs 13.1%) and a 2.9-fold increase as compared with 35- to 44-year-old men (42.9% vs 14.7%).[52]

Consistent with findings on children[18,22] and adults,[46] our youths with BP originate from pedigrees with high rates of depressive illness. There also was a significantly elevated familial rate of mania for bipolar children when the family was the unit of analysis. However, our sample sizes did not provide sufficient statistical power to detect proband-group differences in mania across specific classes of relatives.

NONAFFECTIVE DISORDERS IN RELATIVES

An excess of nonaffective psychiatric illness has been detected in the families of affectively ill youths both on blind[21,23,24] and on nonblind evaluation,[54] although there have been contrary reports as well.[39,55] The most consistent findings have been elevated rates of alcoholism and/or substance abuse among first-degree, particularly female, relatives[21,23] and/or second-degree relatives.[21,24] In adult probands and their families, affective illness and alcoholism also are often associated with one another.[56-60]

On cursory examination, our results support the cosegregation of depression and alcoholism in relatives. This finding may reflect some "familial clustering of social risk factors"[56,61] or, possibly, familial subtypes.[60] In our study, however, the cosegregation of depression and alcoholism is not compelling and is overshadowed by the relationship of depression and attempted suicide.

SEVERITY OF PSYCHIATRIC DISORDER IN RELATIVES

Relatives' age at onset of disorders and rates of suicidal behaviors have been examined as indicators of illness severity in families of young patients.[21-24] The findings suggest that depressed youngsters originate from more seriously ill families than do psychiatric control or normal youths, and that families of probands with childhood-onset affective disorder are more ill than families of adolescent-onset cases.

Considering either age at onset of first depression or of any first psychiatric disorder, mothers of our target probands were significantly younger when they became ill than were mothers of psychiatric controls. Relatives of depressed and bipolar children in other samples also have had earlier onset of depression and first psychiatric disorder than have relatives of normal probands,[22] although this trend was not evident in the relatives of depressed adolescents.[24] Furthermore, mothers of depressed children have their first depression significantly earlier than do mothers of depressed adolescents.[23] Additionally, female (but not male) relatives of our probands with affective disorder were twice as likely to have attempted suicide than were comparable relatives of controls, paralleling reports on other samples of youths.[21,23]

Recurrent unipolar depression (vs ever having had a depressive disorder) may also be considered an index of illness severity. We found that recurrent unipolar depression was more prevalent among all relatives of affectively ill youths than controls, with a particularly strong trend among first-degree and female relatives. In future studies, it would be useful to obtain more precise information on indexes of illness severity in grandparents. For example, our data suggest an 11% rate of recurrent unipolar depression in grandparents of our affectively ill youths, about 26% in first-degree adult relatives, and about 40% in the juvenile probands themselves.[6] Suicidal behavior, as an index of severity, shows a similar trend: about 15% of the adult first-degree relatives of our affectively ill juveniles have attempted suicide, whereas 31% of the probands themselves already had suicide attempts. Therefore, earlier onset of depression and its apparently increased severity in successive generations of pedigrees identified by a depressed child resemble genetic anticipation.[62]

COMORBID DISORDERS IN PROBANDS

Psychiatric comorbidity is common in depressed patients across the age span,[20] as well as in the offspring of depressed parents,[11,12,63] and has been used to define depression subtypes.[64] Comorbid conduct or behavior disorder has been of particular interest in studies of youths, presumably because it may identify a less familial form of childhood-onset depression.[21] However, whereas conduct disorder (vs its absence) in depressed children has been associated in 1 study with lower rates of major depression in all relatives and higher rates of alcoholism in second-degree relatives,[21] these results were not replicated in other studies.[23,24] Possibly reflecting a diagnostic subtype, comorbid conduct disorder in depressed youths prognosticated a low risk of depression on long-term follow-up,[37] although shorter observation intervals have yielded contrary conclusions.[38]

Our results do not support the assumption that comorbid behavior disorder identifies a less familial form of childhood-onset depression. Probands with affective and behavior disorders did not differ from the remainder of the affectively ill youths in rates of depression or mania in their families, although depressed probands with comorbidity had higher familial rates of alcoholism, substance use, and antisocial personality, particularly among second-degree relatives. Possibly, therefore, problems involving serious dysregulation of behavior may be familially transmitted in the pedigrees of depressed youths along with, but not strictly in association with, depressive illness.

AGE AT ONSET AND FAMILIALITY OF AFFECTIVE DISORDERS

Three lines of evidence suggest that proband's age at onset of depression may be an indicator of familial transmission of the disorder, namely, family histories of affectively ill youngsters, characteristics of the offspring of depressed parents, and the relationship of age at onset of depression in adults to rates of depression in their relatives. As already discussed, rates of familial depressive illness are higher for depressed youths than for depressed adult probands. Furthermore, in a series of influential articles, Weissman and associates[11,65-67] reported that, compared with the offspring of normal controls, children of depressed parents were at increased risk for major depressive and nonaffective disorders. Other investigators similarly found that depressive disorder was the most prevalent diagnosis in children of affectively ill parents.[9,10,12,63]

Finally, among depressed adults,[47,68-70] age at depression onset tends to be inversely related to rates of depression in relatives, although this association has not been uniformly confirmed.[45] Early-onset probands, originally defined as having developed depression before age 40 years, were found to have greater familial morbidity of depression, alcoholism, and sociopathy than did late-onset probands.[68] The cutoff for early age at onset eventually was reduced to 30 years[69] and then to 20 years,[47,70] yielding increasingly higher rates of familial morbidity for early-onset cases.

On the basis of these convergent lines of evidence regarding the association of age, depression, and morbid risk in relatives, the most familial variant of this condition should be childhood-onset depressive disorder. Although the available information strongly supports this supposition, the data are not conclusive because of the absence of direct family studies of depressed youngsters, the likelihood of informant bias, and the relatively small samples that have been examined. Nonetheless, it is now evident that direct assessment of family members of young depressed patients should be a research priority.

FINAL NOTE

As noted by Kendler,[61] the major psychiatric disorders tend to aggregate in families. One important question is the extent to which such phenomena reflect a common genetic diathesis within particular disorders as well as shared or nonshared environmental variables, including risk factors that may be familially transmitted.[61,71] On the basis of information concerning the hereditability of affective illness in adults,[42,44,72] it is reasonable to suppose that genetic factors are involved in the familial transmission of very-early-onset depressive illness as well. Although the exact mode of genetic-psychosocial transmission of depressive illness is yet to be identified, our data and the findings of others suggest that pedigrees that are ascertained through a depressed child would be good candidates for such studies.[22]

Accepted for publication August 28, 1996.

This study was supported by grant MH33990 from the National Institute of Mental Health, Health and Human Services Administration, Bethesda, Md.

Much appreciation is due to Phoebe L. Parrone for computer programming assistance.

Corresponding author: Maria Kovacs, PhD, Western Psychiatric Institute and Clinic, 3811 O'Hara St, Pittsburgh, PA 15213.

REFERENCES

1. American Psychiatric Association, Committee on Nomenclature and Statistics. *Diagnostic and Statistical Manual of Mental Disorders, Third Edition.* Washington, DC: American Psychiatric Association; 1980.
2. American Psychiatric Association, Committee on Nomenclature and Statistics. *Diagnostic and Statistical Manual of Mental Disorders, Revised Third Edition.* Washington, DC: American Psychiatric Association; 1987.
3. Mitchell J, McCauley E, Burke PM, Moss SJ. Phenomenology of depression in children and adolescents. *J Am Acad Child Adolesc Psychiatry.* 1988;27:12-20.
4. Ryan ND, Puig-Antich J, Ambrosini P, Rabinovich H, Robinson D, Nelson B, Iyengar S, Twomey J. The clinical picture of major depression in children and adolescents. *Arch Gen Psychiatry.* 1987;44:854-861.
5. Kovacs M, Feinberg TL, Crouse-Novak MA, Paulauskas SL, Finkelstein R. Depressive disorders in childhood, I: a longitudinal prospective study of characteristics and recovery. *Arch Gen Psychiatry.* 1984;41:229-237.
6. Kovacs M, Akiskal HS, Gatsonis C, Parrone PL. Childhood-onset dysthymic disorder: clinical features and prospective naturalistic outcome. *Arch Gen Psychiatry.* 1994;51:365-374.
7. Biederman J, Faraone S, Mick E, Lelon E. Psychiatric comorbidity among referred juveniles with major depression: fact or artifact? *J Am Acad Child Adolesc Psychiatry.* 1995;34:579-590.
8. Ferro T, Carlson GA, Grayson P, Klein DN. Depressive disorders: distinctions in children. *J Am Acad Child Adolesc Psychiatry.* 1994;33:664-670.
9. Keller MB, Beardslee WR, Dorer DJ, Lavori PW, Samuelson H, Klerman GR. Impact of severity and chronicity of parental affective illness on adaptive functioning and psychopathology in children. *Arch Gen Psychiatry.* 1986;43:930-937.
10. Hammen C, Burge D, Burney E, Adrian C. Longitudinal study of diagnoses in children of women with unipolar and bipolar affective disorder. *Arch Gen Psychiatry.* 1990;47:1112-1117.
11. Weissman MM, Gammon GD, John K, Merikangas KR, Warner V, Prusoff BA, Sholomskas D. Children of depressed parents. *Arch Gen Psychiatry.* 1987;44:847-853.
12. Orvaschel H. Early onset psychiatric disorder in high risk children and increased familial morbidity. *J Am Acad Child Adolesc Psychiatry.* 1990;29:184-188.
13. Fleming JE, Offord DR. Epidemiology of childhood depressive disorders: a critical review. *J Am Acad Child Adolesc Psychiatry.* 1990;29:571-580.
14. Kovacs M, Feinberg TL, Crouse-Novak M, Paulauskas SL, Pollock M, Finkelstein R. Depressive disorders in childhood, II: a longitudinal study of the risk for a subsequent major depression. *Arch Gen Psychiatry.* 1984;41:643-649.
15. McCauley E, Myers K, Mitchell J, Calderon R, Schloredt K, Treder R. Depression in young people: initial presentation and clinical course. *J Am Acad Child Adolesc Psychiatry.* 1993;32:714-722.
16. Harrington R, Fudge H, Rutter M, Pickles A, Hill J. Adult outcomes of childhood and adolescent depression, I: psychiatric status. *Arch Gen Psychiatry.* 1990;47:465-473.
17. Rao U, Ryan ND, Birmaher B, Dahl RE, Williamson DE, Kaufman J, Rao R, Nelson B. Unipolar depression in adolescents: clinical outcome in adulthood. *J Am Acad Child Adolesc Psychiatry.* 1995;34:566-578.
18. Strober M, Carlson G. Bipolar illness in adolescents with major depression. *Arch Gen Psychiatry.* 1982;39:549-555.
19. Hughes CW, Preskorn SH, Wrona M, Hassanein R, Tucker S. Follow-up of adolescents initially treated for prepubertal-onset major depressive disorder with imipramine. *Psychopharmacol Bull.* 1990;26:244-248.
20. Kovacs M. Presentation and course of major depressive disorder during childhood and later years of the life span. *J Am Acad Child Adolesc Psychiatry.* 1996;35:705-715.
21. Puig-Antich J, Goetz D, Davies M, Kaplan T, Davies S, Ostrow L, Asnis L, Twomey J, Iyengar S, Ryan ND. A controlled family history study of prepubertal major depressive disorder. *Arch Gen Psychiatry.* 1989;46:406-418.
22. Todd RD, Neuman R, Geller B, Fox LW, Hickok J. Genetic studies of affective disorders: should we be starting with childhood onset probands? *J Am Acad Child Adolesc Psychiatry.* 1993;32:1164-1171.
23. Mitchell J, McCauley E, Burke P, Calderon R, Schloredt K. Psychopathology in parents of depressed children and adolescents. *J Am Acad Child Adolesc Psychiatry.* 1989;28:352-357.
24. Williamson DE, Ryan ND, Birmaher B, Dahl RE, Kaufman J, Rao U, Puig-Antich J. A case-control family history study of depression in adolescents. *J Am Acad Child Adolesc Psychiatry.* 1995;34:1596-1607.
25. Kovacs M. The Interview Schedule for Children (ISC). *Psychopharmacol Bull.* 1985;21:991-994.
26. Last CG, Hersen M, Kazdin AE, Finkelstein R, Strauss CC. Comparison of *DSM-III* separation anxiety and overanxious disorders: demographic characteristics and patterns of comorbidity. *J Am Acad Child Adolesc Psychiatry.* 1987;26:527-531.
27. Kovacs M, Gatsonis C, Pollock M, Parrone PL. A controlled prospective study of *DSM-III* adjustment disorder in childhood: short-term prognosis and long-term predictive validity. *Arch Gen Psychiatry.* 1994;51:535-541.
28. Klein DN, Riso LP, Donaldson SK, Schwartz JE, Anderson RL, Ouimette PC, Lizardi H, Aaronson TA. Family study of early-onset dysthymia. *Arch Gen Psychiatry.* 1995;52:487-496.
29. Kovacs M, Pollock M. Bipolar disorder and comorbid conduct disorder in childhood and adolescence. *J Am Acad Child Adolesc Psychiatry.* 1995;34:715-723.
30. Endicott J, Spitzer RL. A diagnostic interview: the Schedule for Affective Disorders and Schizophrenia. *Arch Gen Psychiatry.* 1978;35:837-844.
31. Spitzer RL, Endicott J, Robins E. Research Diagnostic Criteria: rationale and reliability. *Arch Gen Psychiatry.* 1978;34:136-141.
32. Andreasen NC, Endicott J, Spitzer RL, Winokur G. The family history method using diagnostic criteria: reliability and validity. *Arch Gen Psychiatry.* 1977;34:1229-1235.
33. Zimmerman M, Coryell W, Pfohl B, Stangl D. The reliability of the family history method for psychiatric diagnoses. *Arch Gen Psychiatry.* 1988;45:320-322.
34. Bartko JJ, Carpenter WT. On the methods and theory of reliability. *J Nerv Ment Dis.* 1976;163:307-317.
35. Agresti A. *Categorical Data Analysis.* New York, NY: John Wiley & Sons Inc; 1990.
36. Kalbfleisch JD, Prentice RL. *The Statistical Analysis of Failure Time Data.* New York, NY: John Wiley & Sons Inc; 1980.
37. Harrington R, Fudge H, Rutter M, Pickles A, Hill J. Adult outcomes of childhood and adolescent depression, II: links with antisocial disorders. *J Am Acad Child Adolesc Psychiatry.* 1991;30:434-439.
38. Kovacs M, Paulauskas S, Gatsonis C, Richards C. Depressive disorders in childhood, III: a longitudinal study of comorbidity with and risk for conduct disorders. *J Affect Disord.* 1988;15:205-217.
39. Harrington RC, Fudge H, Rutter ML, Bredenkamp D, Groothues C, Pridham J. Child and adult depression: a test of continuities with data from a family study. *Br J Psychiatry.* 1993;162:627-633.
40. Andreasen NC, Rice J, Endicott J, Reich T, Coryell W. The family history approach to diagnosis. *Arch Gen Psychiatry.* 1986;43:421-429.
41. Strober M, Morrell W, Burroughs J, Lampert C, Danforth H, Freeman R. A family study of bipolar I disorder in adolescence: early onset of symptoms linked to increased familial loading and lithium resistance. *J Affect Disord.* 1988;15:255-268.
42. Moldin SO, Reich T, Rice JP. Current perspectives on the genetics of unipolar depression. *Behav Genet.* 1991;21:211-242.
43. McMahon FJ, Stine OC, Chase GA, Meyers DA, Simpson SG, DePaulo JR. Influence of clinical subtype, sex, and lineality on age at onset of major affective disorder in a family sample. *Am J Psychiatry.* 1994;151:210-215.
44. Gershon ES, Bunney WE, Leckman JF, Van Eerdewegh M, DeBauche BA. The inheritance of affective disorders: a review of data and of hypotheses. *Behav Genet.* 1976;6:227-261.
45. Reich T, Van Eerdewegh P, Rice J, Mullaney J, Endicott J, Klerman GL. The familial transmission of primary major depressive disorder. *J Psychiatr Res.* 1987;21:613-624.
46. Weissman MM, Gershon ES, Kidd KK, Prusoff BA, Leckman JF, Dibble E, Hamovit J, Thompson WD, Pauls DL, Guroff JJ. Psychiatric disorders in the relatives of probands with affective disorders. *Arch Gen Psychiatry.* 1984;41:13-21.
47. Weissman MM, Wickramaratne P, Merikangas KR, Leckman JF, Prusoff BA, Caruso KA, Kidd KK, Gammon D. Onset of major depression in early adulthood. *Arch Gen Psychiatry.* 1984;41:1136-1143.
48. Klerman GL, Lavori PW, Rice J, Reich T, Endicott J, Andreason NC, Keller MB, Hirschfeld RMA. Birth-cohort trends in rates of major depressive disorder among relatives of patients with affective disorder. *Arch Gen Psychiatry.* 1985;42:689-693.
49. Lavori PW, Klerman GL, Keller MB, Reich T, Rice J, Endicott J. Age-period-cohort analysis of secular trends in onset of major depression: findings in siblings of patients with major affective disorder. *J Psychiatr Res.* 1987;21:23-35.

50. Wickramaratne PJ, Weissman MM, Leaf PJ, Holford TR. Age, period and cohort effects on the risk of major depression: results from five United States communities. *J Clin Epidemiol.* 1989;42:333-343.
51. Kessler RC, McGonagle KA, Zhao S, Nelson CB, Hughes M, Eshleman S, Wittchen H-U, Kendler KS. Lifetime and 12-month prevalence of *DSM-III-R* psychiatric disorders in the United States. *Arch Gen Psychiatry.* 1994;51:8-19.
52. Blazer DG, Kessler RC, McGonagle KA, Swartz MS. The prevalence and distribution of major depression in a national community sample: the National Comorbidity Survey. *Am J Psychiatry.* 1994;151:979-986.
53. Robins LN, Regier DA, eds. *Psychiatric Disorders in America: The Epidemiologic Catchment Area Study.* New York, NY: Free Press; 1991.
54. Kutcher S, Marton P. Affective disorders in first-degree relatives of adolescent onset bipolars, unipolars, and normal controls. *J Am Acad Child Adolesc Psychiatry.* 1991;30:75-78.
55. Weller RA, Kapadia P, Weller EB, Fristad M, Lazaroff LB, Preskorn SH. Psychopathology in families of children with major depressive disorders. *J Affect Disord.* 1994;31:247-252.
56. Merikangas KR, Leckman JF, Prusoff BA, Pauls DL, Weissman MM. Familial transmission of depression and alcoholism. *Arch Gen Psychiatry.* 1985;42:367-372.
57. Kendler KS, Heath AC, Neale MC, Kessler RC, Eaves LJ. Alcoholism and major depression in women. *Arch Gen Psychiatry.* 1993;50:690-698.
58. Maier W, Lichtermann D, Minges J. The relationship between alcoholism and unipolar depression: a controlled family study. *J Psychiatr Res.* 1994;28:303-317.
59. Coryell W, Winokur G, Keller M, Scheftner W, Endicott J. Alcoholism and primary major depression: a family study approach to co-existing disorders. *J Affect Disord.* 1992;24:93-99.
60. Winokur G, Coryell W. Familial subtypes of unipolar depression: a prospective study of familial pure depressive disease compared to depression spectrum disease. *Biol Psychiatry.* 1992;32:1012-1018.
61. Kendler KS. Familial risk factors and the familial aggregation of psychiatric disorders. *Psychol Med.* 1990;20:311-319.
62. Petronis A, Kennedy JL. Unstable genes—unstable mind? *Am J Psychiatry.* 1995; 152:164-172.
63. Welner Z, Rice J. School-aged children of depressed parents: a blind and controlled study. *J Affect Disord.* 1988;15:291-302.
64. Weissman MM, Merikangas KR, Wickramaratne P, Kidd KK, Prusoff BA, Leckman JF, Pauls DL. Understanding the clinical heterogeneity of major depression using family data. *Arch Gen Psychiatry.* 1986;43:430-434.
65. Weissman MM, Prusoff BA, Gammon GD, Merikangas KR, Leckman JF, Kidd KK. Psychopathology in the children (ages 6-18) of depressed and normal parents. *J Am Acad Child Psychiatry.* 1984;23:78-84.
66. Weissman MM, Leckman JF, Merikangas KR, Gammon GD, Prusoff BA. Depression and anxiety disorders in parents and children. *Arch Gen Psychiatry.* 1984; 41:845-852.
67. Weissman MM, Warner V, Wickramaratne P, Prusoff BA. Early-onset major depression in parents and their children. *J Affect Disord.* 1988;15:269-277.
68. Mendlewicz J, Baron M. Morbidity risks in subtypes of unipolar depressive illness: differences between early and late onset forms. *Br J Psychiatry.* 1981;139: 463-466.
69. Price RA, Kidd KK, Weissman MM. Early onset (under age 30 years) and panic disorder as markers for etiologic homogeneity in major depression. *Arch Gen Psychiatry.* 1987;44:434-440.
70. Kupfer DJ, Frank E, Carpenter LL, Neiswanger K. Family history in recurrent depression. *J Affect Disord.* 1989;17:113-119.
71. Reiss D, Plomin R, Hetherington EM. Genetics and psychiatry: an unheralded window on the environment. *Am J Psychiatry.* 1991;148:283-291.
72. Kendler KS, Neale MC, Kessler RC, Heath AC, Eaves LJ. A population-based twin study of major depression in women. *Arch Gen Psychiatry.* 1992;49:257-266.

ORIGINAL ARTICLE

Developmental Precursors of Affective Illness in a General Population Birth Cohort

Jim van Os, MSc, PhD; Peter Jones, MSc; Glyn Lewis, MSc, PhD; Michael Wadsworth, MPhil, PhD; Robin Murray, DSc

Background: Recent evidence suggests that neurodevelopmental impairment may be a risk factor for later affective disorder.

Methods: Associations between childhood developmental characteristics and affective disorder were examined in a prospectively studied national British birth cohort of 5362 individuals born between March 3 and March 9, 1946. Mental state examinations by trained interviewers performed at ages 36 and 43 years identified 270 case subjects with adult affective disorder (AD). Teachers' questionnaires completed at age 13 and 15 years identified 195 case subjects who had shown evidence of childhood affective disturbance (CAD).

Results: Female gender and low educational test scores at ages 8, 11, and 15 years were a risk factor for AD, CAD, and AD without CAD. In addition, attainment of motor milestones was later in the CAD group (odds ratio [OR]=1.2; 95% confidence interval [CI], 1.1-1.3), followed by, and independent of, greater risk for speech defects between the ages of 6 and 15 years (OR=2.0; 95% CI, 1.3-3.0), decreased psychomotor alertness on medical examination between ages 4 and 11 years (OR=4.6; 95% CI, 2.2-9.7), and an excess of twitching and grimacing motor behaviors in adolescence (OR=3.9; 95% CI, 2.5-6.1). Persistent CAD was strongly associated with persistent AD (OR=7.8; 95% CI, 2.6-23.2).

Conclusion: The findings give credence to the suggestion that affective disorder, especially its early-onset form, is preceded by impaired neurodevelopment.

Arch Gen Psychiatry. 1997;54:625-631

From the Department of Psychiatry and Neuropsychology, University of Maastricht, European Graduate School of Neuroscience, Maastricht, the Netherlands (Dr van Os); the Department of Psychiatry, University of Nottingham, Nottingham, England (Dr Jones); the Department of Community and Epidemiological Psychiatry, Division of Psychological Medicine, University of Wales College of Medicine, Cardiff (Dr Lewis); MRC National Survey of Health and Development and the Department of Epidemiology and Public Health, University College London Medical School, London, England (Dr Wadsworth); and the Department of Psychological Medicine and Social, Genetic and Developmental Research Centre, Institute of Psychiatry, London (Dr Murray).

YOUTH IN general,[1] and adolescent development in particular,[2] is an important period of risk for the onset of affective disorder. The view that stressful experiences acquired in childhood or adolescence produce enduring and substantial effects on liability to affective disorder has been challenged.[3] Patients with (unipolar and bipolar) mood disorders display both cerebral ventricular enlargement and sulcal prominence,[4-6] suggesting that early neurodevelopmental processes increase the risk for later affective outcomes.

Developmentally compromised individuals who develop affective symptoms may also have poorer outcome. Poor childhood adjustment, impaired adolescent friendship patterns, low academic achievement, neurotic personality traits, and early-onset dysthymia have all been found to predict poor prognosis in unipolar, bipolar, and schizoaffective disorders.[7-15]

We wished to examine whether impaired childhood neurodevelopment is associated with the onset and persistence of affective disorder by using data from the 1946 British national birth cohort, which assessed subjects on 20 occasions over a period of 4 decades. Mental state assessments of survey members at various ages enabled us to identify a group of subjects who had had evidence of affective disturbance of varying persistence during adolescence and/or adulthood.

RESULTS

AD CASES

Female gender, lower scores on childhood cognitive tests, and presence of twitches and grimaces at age 15 years predicted later depression. Presence of speech defects was weakly associated with later AD (**Table 1**).

Within the AD sample, illness persistence (n=75) was predicted significantly only by behavioral apathy on the medical examination alertness rating between the ages of 6 and 11 years (Table 1).

SUBJECTS AND METHODS

The Medical Research Council National Survey of Health and Development (NSHD) is an ongoing longitudinal study of a stratified sample of 5362 subjects (52.5% male) born in Britain during the week of March 3 to 9, 1946. Data were collected on 11 occasions at intervals of 2 years until age 16 years, and on 9 occasions thereafter, with the most recent contact occurring in 1989 at the age of 43 years.[16,17]

CASE DEFINITION

Case definition involved 4 criteria as follows: (1) evidence of affective disorder in adulthood, (2) evidence of affective disturbance in childhood, (3) evidence of illness persistence, and (4) identification of schizophrenia cases.

AD Cases

The caseness criterion was defined conservatively as a score of 5 or higher on either (1) the index of definition scale of the Present State Examination (PSE), a short version of which was administered by trained lay interviewers in 1982,[18] and which included all PSE neurotic and affective features; or (2) the equivalent score on a similar instrument, the Psychiatric Symptom Frequency scale (PSF), administered in 1989 by trained nurses.[19] The PSF is a 19-item scale that rates symptoms of anxiety and depression for the 12 months preceding the interview. The reliability, validity, and internal consistency of the PSE and PSF in this investigation were found to be satisfactory.[18,19] The cutoff for the caseness criterion in the PSF score was placed at the same percentile (96.3%) as the median total PSE score of the risk set (defined below) in the PSE index of definition cutoff category of 5.

Childhood Affective Disturbance

The 16 items of teachers' questionnaires, completed when children were 13 and 15 years old (when teachers usually would have been different), had, independent of the current investigation, previously been grouped into 3 factors, one of which constituted an anxiety-depression factor (depression items included statements such as "persistently sad and gloomy," "unable to make friends," "tired and washed out," "fearful"[20,21]). Presence of CAD was defined as a score above the cutoff (a priori also set at the 96th percentile) on this anxiety-depression rating at either age 13 or 15 years.

Illness Persistence

Adult affective disorder (AD) cases met this criterion if subjects had reported, among a variety of questions on chronic health problems, in 1982 *and* in 1989 that they had experienced "nervous or emotional trouble or persistent depression" all or most of the time (1982) and that they had experienced recurrent "nervous or emotional trouble or depression" (1989). Individuals with CAD met the illness persistence criterion if they had had evidence of affective disturbance at ages 13 *and* 15 years.

Absence of Schizophrenia or Schizoaffective Disorder

Schizophrenia cases were defined by means of a 2-stage screen.[20,21] First, subjects for whom there was any evidence to suggest schizophrenia, severe mental illness, psychiatric hospital admission, or use of prescribed antipsychotic drugs were identified using (1) the 9 questionnaire and interview contacts obtained between 16 and 43 years of age that made inquiries into all hospital inpatient and outpatient contacts and general practice visits and that recorded subjects' own descriptions of their illnesses and antipsychotic drug use; (2) appearances in the Mental Health Inquiry (a national psychiatric hospital registration system); and (3) the short version of the PSE discussed above, which included probes for psychosis. In the second stage, *DSM-III-R*[22] criteria for schizophrenia and schizoaffective disorder were applied to all clinical information on subjects thus identified. Clinical data other than those from NSHD interviews were available from a variety of sources, including details of mental state during admissions that were supplied by hospitals in response to routine requests by the NSHD whenever a hospital admission had been identified. Subjects meeting *DSM-III-R* criteria, as well as those meeting positive *DSM-III-R* criteria for schizophrenia or schizoaffective disorder but for whom no statement of relevant exclusion criteria could be found, were not included as AD or CAD cases.

Adult affective disorder was defined as meeting case definition criteria 1 and 4 (n=270; 8.2%). Ninety-seven percent of these subjects had admitted to low mood at either the 1982 or the 1989 interview. Of the 270 AD cases, 75 (27.8%) met the AD illness persistence criterion. Childhood affective disturbance (CAD) was defined as meeting case definition criteria 3 and 4 (n=195; 5.9%). Of these, 27 (13.9%) met the CAD illness persistence criterion and 34 (17.4%) also met criteria for AD as adults. These latter cases will be referred to as CAD with adult continuity.

INDIVIDUALS AT RISK OF BEING IDENTIFIED AS DEPRESSED IN ADULTHOOD

Included in the analyses were all individuals at risk of being identified as having AD in 1982 (hereafter referred to as the risk set). These were the individuals who, in the 1982 interview, had answered the question on persistent depression and had had valid PSE interview results (n=3293). All noncases in the risk set, including schizophrenia cases, were included as control cases.

Developmental variables, particularly later motor milestone attainment, twitching and grimacing, cognitive test scores at ages 11 and 15 years, and behavioral apathy on the medical examination alertness rating at ages 6 to 11 years, discriminated between those who did and those who did not meet CAD criteria within the AD sample.

In the comparison between the AD group and control group, associations with gender and cognitive ability at ages

DEVELOPMENTAL VARIABLES

All of the variables included in the analyses (motor development, medical examinations, cognitive tests, teacher reports, etc) were collected specifically for the purpose of the NSHD. Individuals who collected data (teachers, nurses, health visitors, lay interviewers) received specific training. Therefore, all variables were specifically probed for at various times and identical information was collected in the same standardized way for each subject.[17]

To reduce spurious positive findings, and guided by existing literature on the relationship between early development and psychiatric outcomes, an a priori selection of a limited group of variables was made for the analyses from a total of 2000 available childhood variables. This choice was made independent of the current investigation, the variables having been selected first for the purposes of a previous analysis involving subjects with schizophrenia.[20,21] Thus, variables from the following developmental domains were included in the analyses.

Neurodevelopmental and Physical

This domain included data on the timing of language (saying words other than "mumma" or "dadda" as recalled by the mother at age 2 years); motor milestones (sitting, walking, and standing unaided); speech abnormalities observed during medical examinations at ages 6, 7, 11, and 15 years; and teachers' observations on presence of motor habits of twitching and grimaces at age 15 years.

Cognitive Ability

Cognitive ability was measured by nonverbal, verbal, and reading ability tests administered at ages 8, 11, and 15 years; vocabulary at ages 8 and 11 years; and arithmetic tests at ages 11 and 15 years.[23,24] Test scores of survey members had been normalized,[25] adjusting for sex and social class.

Sociobehavioral

At ages 6, 7, and 11 years, the examining physician rated the level of alertness of the child on a 3-point scale, where the highest score indicated "apathetic." At age 4 years, mothers were probed by the health visitor on children's preference for solitary play.

Other variables included social class, defined as the 1946 Registrar General's Classification of the father's occupation at birth.[26]

Given the possible confounding effect of early childhood environmental adversity on the association between developmental variables and AD,[27,28] the following variables were adjusted for: household crowding, health visitor's opinion on mother's understanding and management of the child and cleanliness of the child at age 4 years, history of seizures in the child, parental death or separation, teacher's opinion on whether schoolwork was adversely affected by factors outside the school, and teacher's impression of parental interest in school progress. An indication of parental history of psychiatric disorder was obtained from parents and subjects, defined as whether the parent had ever experienced "nervous trouble."

SAMPLE ATTRITION AND MISSING DATA

In 1989, 983 survey members (18.3%) were known to have died or left the country. Of the remaining 4379 subjects, 646 (14.8%) refused further participation, 276 (6.3%) were untraced, and 195 (4.5%) were not willing to be interviewed on that occasion. Thus, the response rate in 1989 was 74.5% of those subjects thought to be still living in Britain (n=3262).

Within the risk set, AD case subjects and control subjects did not differ in the proportion who had missing values on any of the developmental variables such as motor milestones (cases, 12.2%; controls, 10.3%), solitary play at age 4 years (cases, 4.4%; controls, 4.8%), medical examination alertness rating (cases, 4.4%; controls, 6.2%), speech defects (cases, 5.2%; controls, 5.7%), cognitive test score at age 8 years (cases, 9.6%; controls, 10.7%), cognitive test score at age 11 years (cases, 14.8%; controls, 13.7%), cognitive test score at age 15 years (cases, 15.2%; controls, 14.0%), and twitches and grimaces at age 15 years (cases, 14.8%; controls, 14.2%). Similarly, there was no evidence that results could have been biased by differential probability of missing data in the groups meeting CAD or illness persistence criteria.

ANALYSES

The main analyses used odds ratios (ORs) that, in view of the relative rarity of the outcome, estimated the desired incidence rate ratio. The ORs and 95% confidence intervals (CIs) were calculated using the logistic regression[29] procedure of the STATA computer program.[30]

Principal component analysis was used to reduce a larger number of correlated variables to a smaller number of transformed variables that accounted for most of the variation. For example, highly correlated measures of age at reaching motor milestones (sitting, standing, walking) yielded a general motor attainment measure, explaining 73% of the variance. Similarly, highly correlated educational test scores at ages 8, 11, and 15 years yielded a general measure of cognitive ability, explaining approximately 75% of the variance.

Analyses were performed to examine associations between developmental risk factors and both AD and CAD. Subsequently, we examined whether the same developmental variables discriminated, *within* the AD and CAD groups, (1) between persistent and nonpersistent cases; (2) within the group of AD cases, between childhood-onset (ie, also meeting CAD criteria) and adult-onset cases; and (3) within the group of CAD cases, between cases with adult continuity (ie, also meeting the criteria for AD as adults) and cases without adult continuity.

All analyses are presented after adjustment for gender and social class.

8, 11, and 15 years persisted after exclusion of AD case subjects who also met the criteria for CAD (ORs of 2.3, 1.4, 1.3, and 1.4, respectively; all $P<.01$). However, associations with twitches and grimaces and speech defects all but disappeared (OR=1.1 [$P=.68$] and OR=1.2 [$P=.27$], respectively). After exclusion of CAD cases, behavioral apathy continued to predict illness persistence within the AD group (no control subjects rated as such; $P=.02$).

Table 1. Childhood Developmental Variables and Risk for Adult Affective Disorder*

Developmental Variable	Adjusted OR (95% CI): Whole Sample: Subjects With AD (n=270) vs Controls	Within AD Sample: Persistent (n=75) vs Others	Within AD Sample: Childhood Onset† (n=34) vs Others
Female gender	2.4¶ (1.8-3.1)	1.2 (0.7-2.2)	1.8 (0.8-4.4)
Social class‡	1.1 (0.9-1.3)	1.3 (0.9-1.8)	1.3 (0.8-2.2)
Motor milestone attainment§	1.0 (0.9-1.1)	1.2 (0.9-1.4)	1.6¶ (1.2-2.1)
Age at first speech§	1.0 (0.8-1.3)	1.2 (0.7-1.9)	0.6 (0.3-1.3)
Speech defect between ages 6 and 15 y	1.5 (1-2.2)	1.8 (0.8-4.2)	2.1 (0.8-5.6)
Twitching/grimacing at age 15 y	1.7# (1.0-2.8)	1.6 (0.5-4.5)	6.1¶ (2.0-18.6)
Cognitive ability‖			
At age 8 y	1.4¶ (1.2-1.6)	1.0 (0.7-1.4)	1.4 (0.9-2.0)
At age 11 y	1.3¶ (1.1-1.6)	1.0 (0.7-1.3)	1.9¶ (1.2-2.8)
At age 15 y	1.5¶ (1.3-1.7)	1.0 (0.7-1.3)	1.8¶ (1.2-2.7)
Prefers to play alone at age 4 y	1.1 (0.8-1.4)	1.1 (0.6-2.3)	1.9 (0.8-4.6)
Behavioral apathy on medical examination alertness rating at ages 6-11 y	1.6 (0.6-4.1)	11.3# (1.2-106.0)	4.9 (0.8-31.1)

*OR indicates odds ratio; CI, confidence interval; and AD, adult affective disorder.
†Also meeting criteria for childhood affective disturbance.
‡Highest social class was used as the baseline.
§Higher values indicate later attainment of milestone.
‖Higher values indicate worse performance.
¶$P \leq .01$.
#$P \leq .05$.

CAD CASES

Most variables discriminated between case subjects and control subjects, including lower social class and later motor milestone attainment (**Table 2**). Presence of CAD predicted AD (OR=2.6; 95% CI, 1.6-3.5). Evidence of CAD at both ages 13 and 15 years also strongly predicted AD (OR=4.0; 95% CI, 1.7-9.5), especially AD meeting the additional illness persistence criterion (OR=7.8; 95% CI, 2.6-23.2).

Female gender and lower cognitive test scores also predicted persistence within the CAD group. These variables also tended to predict adult continuity of disorder within the CAD group (Table 2).

Adjustment for possible residual socioeconomic and other potential confounders did not change the pattern of results. For example, the association between CAD and cognitive test scores at ages 8, 11, and 15 years persisted after adjusting for, apart from gender and social class, household crowding, the teacher's opinion on whether schoolwork was adversely affected by factors outside the school, the teacher's impression of parental interest in school progress, and family history of "nervous trouble" (adjusted ORs of 1.7, 2.0, and 1.7, respectively; all $P<.001$). The association between AD and cognitive test scores also remained large and significant after adjustment for the same variables.

Similarly, the association with delayed motor milestones remained after additional adjustment for the health visitor's opinion on mother's understanding and management of the child and cleanliness of the child at age 4 years, crowding in the household, family history of nervous disorder, and history of seizures in the child (OR=1.3, $P<.001$). Further restriction of the CAD case subjects to those whose parents were alive and who had never been separated from their parents before the age of 5 years also did not affect the association (OR=1.3, $P<.01$).

INDEPENDENCE OF RISK FACTORS AND GENDER EFFECT MODIFICATION

Analyses were performed with all significant predictors entered jointly in the equation (of the 3 cognitive test scores, that obtained at age 11 years was entered). This revealed that all the risk factors were independent (**Table 3**).

There was no evidence that statistical interaction with gender occurred more often than would be expected by chance.

Repeating the analyses with log-transformed continuous developmental variables gave similar results, indicating that the findings were not the result of a subgroup with outlier values. Similarly, adding squared exposure terms to the model gave no indication of extralinear variation.

CLINICAL VALIDITY OF AD/CAD CONSTRUCTS AND PERSISTENCE CRITERION

Thirty-six percent of the AD case subjects vs 6% of control subjects had indicated in the 1982 interview that they had seen their general practitioner or a psychiatrist in the year before for their "nerves." For subjects meeting the AD illness persistence criterion, this percentage was 57%. For CAD subjects, the percentage with service contacts in 1982 was 12%, and was 26% for subjects meeting the CAD persistence criterion.

To examine the possibility that the cases labeled as persistent affective disorder were schizophrenia cases that had escaped the screening process, all available hospital

Table 2. Childhood Developmental Variables and Risk for Childhood Affective Disturbance*

Developmental Variable	Adjusted OR (95% CI): Whole Sample: Subjects With CAD (n=195) vs Controls	Within CAD Cases: Persistent (n=27) vs Others	Within CAD Cases: Adult Continuity† (n=34) vs Others
Female gender	1.6¶ (1.2-2.1)	2.6# (1.0-6.7)	3.0# (1.2-7.2)
Social class‡	1.5¶ (1.2-1.8)	1.1 (0.6-1.9)	0.9 (0.6-1.5)
Motor milestone attainment§	1.2¶ (1.1-1.3)	1.1 (0.9-1.3)	1.1 (0.9-1.4)
Age at first speech§	0.9 (0.6-1.1)	0.6 (0.3-1.4)	0.9 (0.5-1.8)
Speech defect between ages 6 and 15 y	2.0¶ (1.3-3.0)	0.7 (0.2-2.6)	1.4 (0.5-3.8)
Twitches/grimaces at age 15 y	3.9¶ (2.5-6.1)	1.1 (0.3-3.5)	1.8 (0.7-4.7)
Cognitive ability‖			
At age 8 y	1.7¶ (1.5-2.1)	1.8# (1.1-3.1)	1.1 (0.8-1.7)
At age 11 y	1.9¶ (1.6-2.3)	1.4 (0.9-2.2)	1.3 (0.9-1.9)
At age 15 y	1.8¶ (1.5-2.1)	1.7# (1.1-2.7)	1.5# (1.0-2.3)
Preference for playing alone at age 4 y	1.2 (0.9-1.8)	2.3 (0.9-5.6)	1.7 (0.7-4.2)
Behavioral apathy on medical examination alertness rating at ages 6-11 y	4.6¶ (2.2-9.7)	1.5 (0.3-7.5)	1.1 (0.2-5.6)

*OR indicates odds ratio; CI, confidence interval; and CAD, childhood affective disturbance.
†Also meeting the criteria for affective disorder as adults.
‡Highest social class was used as the baseline.
§Higher values indicate later attainment of milestone.
‖Higher values indicate worse performance.
¶$P \leq .01$.
#$P \leq .05$.

clinical details, which are collected systematically for all survey members as described above, were studied for the 75 AD case subjects who also met the illness persistence criterion. Details included clinical diagnosis, treatment, and clinical synopsis. Twenty-five (33%) of the 75 AD subjects were known to have had outpatient or inpatient contact with psychiatric services; 23 (92%) had a confirmed clinical diagnosis of affective disorder, with the majority being neurotic, reactive, or anxiety depression. Twenty-one (84%) of the 25 had been psychiatric inpatients; 3 patients had received lithium carbonate, 5 had received trifluoperazine hydrochloride, and 4 had been treated with electroconvulsive therapy.

COMMENT

LIMITATIONS

One quarter of the contactable survey members were not interviewed in 1989. In a separate investigation, however, it has been established that it is unlikely that any major bias due to differential attrition exists in the data.[31] Furthermore, such a bias would have occurred only if missing follow-up data were correlated with both affective disorder and each of the independent developmental risk factors separately, which is unlikely. Similarly, the likelihood of missing developmental data in the risk set was similar for case subjects and controls, which makes bias due to differential probability of missing data unlikely.

Adult affective disorder and CAD are not well-defined constructs. The following, however, attests to their validity. There were the expected gender and social class effects,[32] and there were the expected low numbers of case subjects in contact with services.[32] Subjects with persistent AD were nearly 10 times more likely to have sought professional help for mental disorder than control subjects, and among those who had been in contact with specialized psychiatric services, 92% received a diagnosis of depression. The validity of the childhood measure of af-

Table 3. Independence of Developmental Risk Factors for Affective Disorder*

Developmental Variable	Adjusted OR (95% CI): Subjects With CAD (n=195) vs Controls	Adjusted OR (95% CI): Subjects With AD (n=270) vs Controls
Female gender	2.1‖ (1.5-2.9)	2.6‖ (1.9-3.5)
Social class†	1.3 (1.0-1.6)	. . .
Motor milestone attainment‡	1.2‖ (1.1-1.4)	. . .
Age at first speech‡	. . .	. . .
Speech defect between ages 6 and 15 y	1.8¶ (1.1-2.9)	1.4 (0.9-2.1)
Twitches/grimaces at age 15 y	3.2‖ (1.9-3.2)	1.7¶ (1.0-2.9)
Cognitive ability§		
At age 8 y	. . .	. . .
At age 11 y	1.7‖ (1.4-2.0)	1.3‖ (1.1-1.6)
At age 15 y	. . .	. . .
Preference for playing alone at age 4 y	. . .	. . .
Behavioral apathy on medical examination alertness rating at ages 6-11 y	3.2‖ (1.3-8.3)	. . .

*OR indicates odds ratio; CI, confidence interval; CAD, childhood affective disturbance; and AD, adult affective disorder.
†Highest social class was used as the baseline.
‡Higher values indicate later attainment of milestone.
§Higher values indicate worse performance.
‖$P \leq .01$.
¶$P \leq .05$.

fective disturbance derived from teacher questionnaires was supported by (1) the expected[33,34] high risk for subsequent AD established through mental state interviews; (2) the fact that one quarter of case subjects with persistent CAD, so "diagnosed" at age 13 and 15 years, admitted to contact with services for mental disorder at the age of 36 years; and (3) the fact that teachers usually have a much lower threshold for reporting behavioral deviance than for reporting the appearance of sadness and anxiety,[35] which makes misclassification unlikely.

Persons with AD and CAD may comprise subgroups with medical conditions, alcohol misuse, or other depressogenic factors that might also be associated with developmental deviance. However, there was no evidence that risk for AD and CAD was confined to any subgroup with, for example, very low educational test scores or older age at motor attainment. The results indicated significant linear trends across continuous distributions. Furthermore, we examined the possibility of confounding by medical disorder by excluding those who had been separated from their mothers before the age of 6 years, thus effectively removing those with severe childhood illnesses needing hospital admission. Exclusion of these case subjects did not change the results.

Although we can be fairly certain that there were no cases of schizophrenia or schizoaffective disorder among the AD and CAD groups, it is likely that some subjects had experienced psychotic symptoms at some time during their illness (5 had received trifluoperazine). The conservative interpretation is that case subjects represented affective disorders at the severest end of the spectrum.

Some control subjects would have gone on to develop depression after the 1989 interview. Any resulting misclassification, however, would have served to obscure existing differences with control subjects rather than to produce spurious results.

THE FINDINGS

Low childhood cognitive ability predicted both childhood and adult affective disorder, the latter independent of the former. Previous prospective work established similar associations,[36] but case identification depended entirely on hospital admission before age 28 years. These and related findings,[37] however, strongly suggest that intellectual impairment is a risk factor for affective disorder.

Subjects with CAD but not AD had an additional excess risk for abnormal motor and speech development, and, within the AD group, the same variables discriminated between CAD cases and non-CAD cases. This suggests that children with disordered neurodevelopment are at increased risk for adolescent affective disorder, as reported in a recent prospective study.[38] The contrast in risk profile between subjects with AD and those with CAD may indicate that childhood-onset disorder is the more severe form, because it is associated with more pervasive developmental deficits. This notion corresponds with findings that, across the entire age spectrum, earlier onset of affective disturbance predicts more severe disease,[7,39-45] and higher morbid risk in the relatives.[46-48] Alternatively, CAD may be *qualitatively* different from AD. This, however, is unlikely, given the strong associations between CAD and later AD.

There was no evidence that neuromotor development was associated with persistence of AD. There was, however, a strong effect of behavioral apathy, consistent with previous work showing associations between abnormal psychosocial development and outcome in affective disorder.[7-15] Persistence of CAD, as well as adult continuity, was associated with low IQ. During the critical phase of adolescent development, intellectual impairment may render an individual more vulnerable to the disruptive effects of affective disturbance.[49]

Analyses of data from the US National Comorbidity Survey revealed that women do not have a higher risk for *chronic* depression than do men.[50] Our findings concur for AD. However, girls with CAD had greater risk for illness persistence and adult continuity, suggesting that female childhood-onset affective disorder runs a more deteriorated course. This conclusion disagrees with the results of a previous follow-up investigation,[34] which, however, lacked statistical power to examine this issue.

In conclusion, our findings complement a substantial body of evidence attesting to a possible neurodevelopmental origin of affective disorder. First, patients with (unipolar and bipolar) mood disorders display both cerebral ventricular enlargement and sulcal prominence.[4-6] Second, there is genetic overlap between affective disorder (especially depression) and disorders associated with neurodevelopmental deviance, such as schizophrenia[51,52] and attention-deficit disorder.[53] Third, the (as yet) unaffected children of parents with affective disorder have been shown to have lower IQs, poorer academic performance, and poorer social competence in childhood and adolescence.[54,55]

Accepted for publication October 8, 1996.

This study benefited from earlier work by Bryan Rodgers, PhD, and Sheila Mann, FRCPsych. We are also grateful to the technical and scientific staff of the Medical Research Council National Survey of Health and Development.

Reprints: Jim van Os, MSc, PhD, Department of Psychiatry and Neuropsychology, University of Maastricht, European Graduate School of Neuroscience, PO BOX 616, 6200 MD Maastricht, the Netherlands.

REFERENCES

1. Coryell W, Endicott J, Keller M. Major depression in a nonclinical sample. *Arch Gen Psychiatry.* 1992;49:117-125.
2. Burke KC, Burke JD, Regier DA, Rae DS. Age at onset of selected mental disorders in five community populations. *Arch Gen Psychiatry.* 1990;47:511-518.
3. Kendler KS, Neale MC, Kessler RC, Heath AC, Eaves LJ. A longitudinal twin study of 1-year prevalence of major depression in women. *Arch Gen Psychiatry.* 1993; 50:843-852.
4. Jeste DV, Lohr JB, Goodwin FK. Neuroanatomical studies of major affective disorders: a review and suggestions for further research. *Br J Psychiatry.* 1988; 153:444-459.
5. Elkis H, Friedman L, Wise A, Meltzer H. Meta-analyses of studies of ventricular enlargement and cortical sulcal prominence in mood disorders: comparisons with controls or patients with schizophrenia. *Arch Gen Psychiatry.* 1995;52:735-746.
6. Nasrallah HA, Coffman JA, Olson SC. Structural brain-imaging findings in affective disorders: an overview. *J Neuropsychiatry.* 1989;1:21-26.

7. Warner V, Weissman MM, Fendrich M, Wickramaratne P, Moreau D. The course of depression in the offspring of depressed patients: incidence, recurrence, and recovery. *Arch Gen Psychiatry.* 1992;49:795-801.
8. Deister A, Marneros A. Predicting the long-term outcome of affective disorders. *Acta Psychiatr Scand.* 1993;88:174-177.
9. Scott J, Eccleston D, Boys R. Can we predict the persistence of depression? *Br J Psychiatry.* 1992;161:633-637.
10. Harder D, Greenwald D, Ritzler B, Strauss J, Kokes R, Gift T. Prediction of outcome among adult psychiatric admissions. *J Clin Psychol.* 1990;46:119-129.
11. Duggan CF, Lee AS, Murray RM. Does personality predict long-term outcome in depression? *Br J Psychiatry.* 1990;157:19-24.
12. Coryell W, Endicott J, Keller M. Outcome of patients with chronic affective disorder: a five year follow-up. *Am J Psychiatry.* 1990;147:1627-1633.
13. Kovacs M, Feinberg TL, Crouse-Novak MA, Paulauskas SL, Pollock M, Finkelstein R. Depressive disorders in childhood, II: a longitudinal study of the risk for a subsequent major depression. *Arch Gen Psychiatry.* 1984;41:643-649.
14. van Os J, Takei N, Castle D, Wessely S, Der G, Murray RM. Premorbid abnormalities in mania, schizomania, acute schizophrenia and chronic schizophrenia. *Soc Psychiatry Psychiatr Epidemiol.* 1995;30:274-279.
15. Vocisano C, Klein DN, Keefe RSE, Dienst ER, Kincaid MM. Demographics, family history, premorbid functioning, developmental characteristics, and course of patients with deteriorated affective disorder. *Am J Psychiatry.* 1996;153:248-255.
16. Atkins E, Cherry N, Douglas JWB, Kiernan KE, Wadsworth MEJ. The 1946 birth cohort: an account of the origins, progress and results of the National Survey of Health and Development. In: Mednick SA, Baerts AE, eds. *Prospective Longitudinal Research: An Empirical Basis for the Primary Prevention of Psychosocial Disorders.* London, England: Oxford University Press; 1981:57-81.
17. Wadsworth MEJ. *The Imprint of Time: Childhood History and Adult Life.* Oxford, England: Clarendon Press; 1991.
18. Rodgers B, Mann SA. The reliability and validity of PSE assessments by lay interviewers: a national population survey. *Psychol Med.* 1986;16:689-700.
19. Rogers B. Reported parental behaviour and adult affective symptoms, 1: associations and moderating factors. *Psychol Med.* 1991;26:51-61.
20. Jones P, Rodgers B, Murray R, Marmot M. Child developmental risk factors for adult schizophrenia in the British 1946 birth cohort. *Lancet.* 1994;344:1398-402.
21. Jones P, Murray R, Rodgers B. Childhood risk factors for adult schizophrenia in a general population birth cohort at age 43 years. In: Mednick SA, Hollister JM, eds. *Neural Development in Schizophrenia: Theory and Research.* New York, NY: Plenum Press; 1996:151-176.
22. American Psychiatric Association. *Diagnostic and Statistical Manual of Mental Disorders, Third Edition, Revised.* Washington, DC: American Psychiatric Association; 1987.
23. Pidgeon DA. Tests used in the 1954 and 1957 surveys. In: Douglas JWB, ed. *The Home and the School.* London, England: MacGibbon & Kee; 1964:129-132.
24. Pidgeon DA. Details of the fifteen year tests. In: Douglas JWB, Ross JM, Simpson HR. *All Our Futures.* London, England: Peter Davies; 1968:194-197.
25. Andrews F, Morgan J, Sonquist J, Klein L. *Multiple Classification Analysis.* 2nd ed. Ann Arbor: University of Michigan; 1973.
26. Office of Population Census and Surveys. *Classification of Occupations.* London, England: Her Majesty's Stationery Office; 1970.
27. Kessler RC, Magee WJ. Childhood adversities and adult depression: basic patterns of association in a US national survey. *Psychol Med.* 1993;23:679-690.
28. Rogers B. Adult affective disorder and early environment. *Br J Psychiatry.* 1990; 157:539-550.
29. Breslow NE, Day NE. *Statistical Methods in Cancer Research.* Lyon, France: World Health Organization; 1987;2:192-246.
30. STATA Corporation. *STATA Statistical Software: Release 4.* College Station, Tex: STATA Corp; 1993.
31. Wadsworth MEJ, Mann SL, Rodgers B, Kuh DL, Hilder WS, Yusuf EJ. Loss and representativeness in a 43 year follow-up of a national birth cohort. *J Epidemiol Community Health.* 1992;46:300-304.
32. Kessler RC, McGonagle KA, Zhao S, Nelson CB, Hughes M, Eshleman S, Wittchen HU, Kendler KS. Lifetime and 12-month prevalence of *DSM-III-R* psychiatric disorders in the United States: results from the National Comorbidity Survey. *Arch Gen Psychiatry.* 1994;51:8-19.
33. Kovacs M, Akiskal HS, Gatsonis C, Parrone PL. Childhood-onset dysthymic disorder: clinical features and prospective naturalistic outcome. *Arch Gen Psychiatry.* 1994;51:365-374.
34. Harrington R, Fudge H, Rutter M, Pickles A, Hill J. Adult outcomes of childhood and adolescent depression, I: psychiatric status. *Arch Gen Psychiatry.* 1990;47: 465-473.
35. Watt NF. Patterns of childhood social development in adult schizophrenics. *Arch Gen Psychiatry.* 1978;35:160-165.
36. Done DJ, Sacker A, Crow TJ. Childhood antecedents of schizophrenia and affective illness: intellectual performance at ages 7 and 11. *Schizophr Res.* 1994; 11:96-97.
37. Sackeim HA, Freeman J, McElhiney M, Coleman E, Prudic J, Devanand DP. Effects of major depression on estimates of intelligence. *J Clin Exp Neuropsychol.* 1992;14:268-88.
38. Hellgren L, Gillberg IC, Bagenholm A, Gillberg C. Children with deficits in attention, motor control and perception almost grown up: psychiatric and personality disorders at age 16 years. *J Child Psychol Psychiatry.* 1994;35:1255-71.
39. Winokur G, Coryell W, Keller M, Endicott J, Akiskal H. A prospective follow-up study of patients with bipolar and primary unipolar affective disorder. *Arch Gen Psychiatry.* 1993;50:457-465.
40. Coryell W, Endicott J, Keller M. Major depressive disorder in a non-clinical sample: predictors of relapse. *Am J Psychiatry.* 1991;148:1353-1358.
41. Keitner GI, Ryan CE, Miller IW, Norman WH. Recovery and major depression: factors associated with twelve-month outcome. *Am J Psychiatry.* 1992;149:93-99.
42. Kovacs M, Feinberg TL, Crouse-Novak MA, Paulauskas SL, Finkelstein R. Depressive disorders in childhood, I: a longitudinal study of characteristics and recovery. *Arch Gen Psychiatry.* 1984;41:229-237.
43. Greenhouse JB, Kupfer DJ, Frank E, Jarrett DB, Rejman KA. Analysis of time to stabilization in the treatment of depression: biological and clinical correlates. *J Affect Disord.* 1987;13:259-266.
44. Giles DE, Jarret RB, Biggs MM, Guzick DS, Rush AJ. Clinical predictors of recurrence in depression. *Am J Psychiatry.* 1989;146:764-767.
45. Brodaty H, Harris L, Peters K, Wilhelm K, Hickie I, Boyce P, Mitchell P, Parker G, Eyers K. Prognosis of depression in the elderly: a comparison with younger patients. *Br J Psychiatry.* 1993;163:589-596.
46. James NM. Early- and late-onset bipolar affective disorder: a genetic study. *Arch Gen Psychiatry.* 1977;34:715-717.
47. Weissman MM, Wickramaratne P, Merikangas KR, Leckman JF, Prusoff BA, Caruso KA, Kidd KK, Gammon GD. Onset of major depression in early adulthood: increased familial loading and specificity. *Arch Gen Psychiatry.* 1984;41:1136-1143.
48. Rice J, Reich T, Andreasen NC, Endicott J, Van Eerdewegh M, Fishman R, Hirschfeld RM, Klerman GL. The familial transmission of bipolar illness. *Arch Gen Psychiatry.* 1987;44:441-447.
49. Kovacs M, Goldston D. Cognitive and social cognitive development of depressed children and adolescents. *J Am Acad Child Adolesc Psychiatry.* 1991; 30:388-392.
50. Kessler RC, McGonagle KA, Swartz M, Blazer DG, Nelson CB. Sex and depression in the National Comorbidity Survey, I: lifetime prevalence, chronicity and recurrence. *J Affect Disord.* 1993;29:85-96.
51. Taylor M. Are schizophrenia and affective disorder related? a selective literature review. *Am J Psychiatry.* 1992;149:22-32.
52. Maier W, Lichtermann D, Minges J, Hallmayer J, Heun R, Benkert O, Levinson DF. Continuity and discontinuity of affective disorders and schizophrenia: results of a controlled family study. *Arch Gen Psychiatry.* 1993;50:871-883.
53. Biederman J, Faraone SV, Keenan K, Tsuang MT. Evidence of familial association between attention deficit disorder and major affective disorders. *Arch Gen Psychiatry.* 1991;48:633-642.
54. Dworkin RH, Cornblatt BA, Friedmann LM, Kaplansky JA, Lewis AR, Shilliday C, Erlenmeyer-Kimling L. Childhood precursors of affective vs social deficits in adolescents at risk for schizophrenia. *Schizophr Bull.* 1993;19:563-577.
55. Anderson C, Hammen CL. Psychosocial outcomes of children of unipolar depressed, bipolar, medically ill, and normal women: a longitudinal study. *J Consult Clin Psychol.* 1993;61:448-454.

First-Episode Major Depression

Few Sex Differences in Course

H. Blair Simpson, MD, PhD; John C. Nee, PhD; Jean Endicott, PhD

Background: There is a sex difference in the prevalence of unipolar major depression. This study sought to determine whether there is a sex difference in its course.

Methods: The National Institute of Mental Health Collaborative Program on the Psychobiology of Depression–Clinical Studies provided data on 96 male and 101 female subjects who were diagnosed as having a first episode of unipolar major depressive disorder at intake and on whom prospective data were available. We looked for differences at intake in factors other than sex that might affect the course of illness: demographic factors, characteristic features of the first depressive episode, psychiatric history, and family history of depression. We then examined the course of depression of these subjects during the following 15 years.

Results: The subjects were similar at intake, enabling us to focus on sex when we looked for differences in the course. Most subjects recovered from their first episode of major depression, but the majority had at least 1 recurrence in the following 5 years. During the following 15 years, male and female subjects did not differ significantly in the time to recovery, the overall time to first recurrence, or the number or severity of recurrences of major depressive episodes. There was no evidence for a more chronic course of depression in women.

Conclusion: There were few significant sex differences in the course of major depressive disorder in this study population.

Arch Gen Psychiatry. 1997;54:633-639

WOMEN HAVE a reported higher lifetime prevalence of unipolar major depression than men,[1-5] with a relative risk reported to range from 1.7[6,7] to 2.4.[8] It is not clear whether there is a sex difference in the course of major depression, an important issue for several reasons. First, a sex difference in course (eg, a higher rate of recurrent episodes or of chronic depressive symptoms) could underlie a sex difference in observed prevalence.[9,10] Second, clinicians and researchers would need to take into account such a sex difference. Finally, a sex difference in course would be consistent with some, but not all, of the biological and social theories advanced to explain the sex difference in the prevalence of depression.[1,2,5,11]

Relatively few reports have focused on sex differences in the course of depression; moreover, the findings vary. Some studies report that women are significantly more likely to suffer recurrences[9,10,12,13]; others do not.[7,14] Some suggest that women are more likely not to recover or to recover more slowly[11,15]; others find no difference in the length or chronicity of depressive episodes.[7,9] Because the studies vary in their designs, sample sizes, and measures of depression, as well as their results, it is difficult to come to any clear conclusions about sex differences in the course of major depression.

Using data from the National Institute of Mental Health (NIMH) Collaborative Program on the Psychobiology of Depression–Clinical Studies, we examined whether there are sex differences in the course of major depressive disorder (MDD). The advantages of this data set are that (1) it is a prospective, naturalistic study; (2) it uses standardized diagnostic instruments; (3) it includes frequent follow-up evaluations; and (4) it has followed subjects after intake for up to 15 years. We focused on subjects who entered the study with a first episode of MDD as defined by the Research Diagnostic Criteria (RDC).[16] Because differences other than sex could lead to differences in course, male and female subjects were first compared at intake on demographic information, features of their first episode of

From the Department of Psychiatry, College of Physicians and Surgeons, Columbia University, New York, NY.

SUBJECTS AND METHODS

METHODS

Subjects for this study were probands of the NIMH Collaborative Program on the Psychobiology of Depression–Clinical Studies; the full protocol has been described.[17] At intake, subjects had to be experiencing a current episode that met RDC criteria for MDD, schizoaffective disorder, or manic disorder; be 17 years of age or older, white, and English-speaking; have an IQ greater than 70 and no evidence of an organic brain syndrome; and have knowledge of their biological parents. Subjects entered the study after hospital admission or within 2 months of the first outpatient visit for the intake episode. Treatment was not controlled for by the study protocol. At the time of this writing, subjects have been followed for up to 15 years.

At intake, all patients were evaluated with the Schedule for Affective Disorders and Schizophrenia (SADS).[18] Data from the SADS were used in combination with medical records and interviews with informants and physicians to determine current and lifetime diagnoses based on RDC criteria. Demographic data were gathered using the Personal History of Depressive Disorders[19]; family history was gathered from the subject and, in most instances, a family informant, using the Family History–RDC[20,21]; work, recreation, and interpersonal relationships were assessed by using the Longitudinal Interval Follow-up Evaluation Base.[22]

After intake, raters interviewed consenting subjects at 6-month intervals for the first 5 years, using the Longitudinal Interval Follow-up Evaluation,[23] and at yearly intervals after that, using the Streamlined Longitudinal Interval Continuation Evaluation. The weekly severity of depressive symptoms during follow-up was quantified by using the Psychiatric Status Ratings (PSR) scale, which ranges from 1 (no current symptoms) to 6 (definite and severe MDD).

Recovery was defined as the first week of 8 or more consecutive weeks of PSR ratings of 2 or less. Recurrence could only occur after recovery and was defined as the first week of 2 or more consecutive weeks of PSR ratings of 4 or greater. Somatic treatments received during the course of the study were also recorded weekly and converted into a measure called the "composite antidepressant" (CAD) level (ranging from 0 [no treatment] to 4 [eg, ≥300 mg of imipramine hydrochloride or the equivalent, or ≥900 mg of lithium carbonate, or 3 or more electroconvulsive treatments per week]).[24-26] At 2, 5, 10, and 15 years after intake, relevant material was reviewed by the current rater and updated RDC diagnoses were determined.

This report focused on subjects who, during the intake episode, met criteria for a first episode of definite MDD with no history of a prior manic, hypomanic, schizoaffective, or schizophrenic disorder and for whom prospective data are available. Of 955 subjects at intake, 96 male and 101 female subjects met these criteria. Subjects at intake would also have met criteria for a first episode of MDD as defined by *DSM-IV*.[27]

STATISTICAL ANALYSIS

For descriptive data, *t* tests were used for continuous data; χ^2 tests or odds ratios (OR) were used (with continuity correction) for categorical data. No adjustments for multiple tests were made because multiple domains of interest were tested. Survival analyses[28] were used to examine the time to the first recovery and time to the first recurrence. Subjects were censored 1 week after the last week data were available, if the event of interest was not observed. Survival curves were compared by means of the Wilcoxon χ^2 test. Kaplan-Meier estimates of the time to first recurrence were found to best fit a Weibull distribution, and thus permitted both univariate and covariate parametric analyses using life regression methods (SAS procedure of LIFEREG; SAS Institute Inc, Cary, NC). This method is equivalent to the Cox proportional hazards model with an acceleration parameter and was used because the hazard rate changed over time. Variables with skewed distributions were treated by logarithmic transformation (eg, duration of intake episode for the univariate and covariate analyses) or by arcsine transformation (eg, mean proportion of weeks during follow-up at PSR level of ≥5 for the *t* test). To compute group means for the PSR and CAD data, each subject's mean for all weeks of follow-up was first calculated; group means for male and female subjects were then determined. For all tests, significance was defined as a *P* value less than .05 (2 tailed). Confidence intervals (CIs), when given, are at the 95% level.

depression, psychiatric history, and family history of depression. Next, we examined the course of depression over the ensuing 15 years of follow-up, looking at the time to recovery, time to the first recurrence, number of recurrences, severity and chronicity of depressive episodes, and rate of death. This is the first article from the NIMH Collaborative Study to focus on the outcome of subjects with a first episode of MDD at intake.

RESULTS

INTAKE CHARACTERISTICS

Demographics at Intake

Demographic data for the male and female subjects at intake are presented in **Table 1**.

Characteristics of the Intake Episode and History of Mental Disorders

In many respects, the intake episode was similar for male and female subjects: most subjects met criteria for endogenous MDD (male=85.4%, female=88.1%); few met criteria for psychotic major depression (male=5.2%, female=12.9%); and about half had an external stressor prior to the onset of the major depressive episode (male=49.0%, female=58.4%). Neither the mean Extracted Hamilton Depression Rating Scale score (equivalent to a raw Hamilton score between 25 and 26 for each sex) nor the mean Global Assessment Scale score (equivalent to a raw Global Assessment Scale score of 39-40 for each sex) differed significantly. There also was no significant difference in the treatment that subjects received for the intake episode prior to admission to the study. Treatment included antidepressants (male=55.2%, female=60.4%), psychotherapy or counseling (male=49.0%, female=52.5%), "minor" tranquilizers (eg, diazepam) (male=40.6%, female=47.5%), "major" tranquilizers (eg, chlorpromazine) (male=19.8%, female=22.8%), electroconvulsive shock therapy (male=2.0%, female=7.9%), and lithium (male=3.0%, female=5.9%). There was no significant sex difference in the length of the first episode of major depression (mean [SD]: male=151 [192] weeks, female=114 [146] weeks; median: male=77 weeks, female=67 weeks).

There were only 2 RDC features of the intake episode that were significantly different: more female subjects met RDC criteria for primary depression (male=51.0%, female=68.3%), while more male subjects met criteria for secondary depression (male=50.0%, female=30.7%; χ^2=5.42, *df*=1, *P*=.02); and significantly more female subjects met criteria for simple depression, having no RDC nonaffective disorder for more than 1 year prior to the first episode (male=35.4%, female=53.5%; χ^2=5.78, *df*=1, *P*=.02). Of 12 SADS summary scale scores that reflect features of the intake episode, only 2 differed significantly between the sexes. Male subjects had a significantly greater SADS summary score for current alcohol or other drug abuse (*t*=2.37, *df*=195, *P*=.02), which was due to alcohol (*P*=.02) and not other drug abuse. Second, female subjects scored significantly higher than male subjects on the SADS anxiety summary score for the intake episode (*t*=2.26, *df*=195, *P*=.03). This difference was due to significantly more somatic anxiety (*P*<.001) and phobias (*P*=.02) reported by women; there were no significant differences in reports of panic attacks or of psychic anxiety, other single items that constitute the SADS anxiety summary score.

Subjects also were assessed for all other lifetime RDC mental disorders at intake, including minor and intermittent depressive disorder. There was only 1 significant difference: more male than female subjects had a lifetime diagnosis of alcoholism (male=43%, female=25%; χ^2=6.34, *df*=1, *P*=.02).

Finally, as assessed using the Longitudinal Interval Follow-up Evaluation Base questionnaire, male and female subjects did not differ significantly at intake or in the previous 5 years in their degree of work impairment (either outside or inside the home), level of functioning, interpersonal relationships, level of satisfaction with their life, or degree of involvement with recreational activities.

Family History of MDD

There was no significant sex difference in the rates of parental depression (mother depressed: male=15.3%, female=23.1%; father depressed: male=22.4%, female=18.3%; both father and mother depressed: male=4.1%, female=7.7%).

SUBSEQUENT COURSE

Length of Follow-up

Seventy-two men and 82 women were followed up for at least 5 years. There was no significant difference in the rate of subjects unavailable for follow-up in the first 5 years (OR=1.44; CI, 0.73-2.84). However, after 5 years, more male than female subjects were unavailable for follow-up. Thus, in the first 10 years after intake, there was a sex difference in the rate of subjects unavailable for follow-up (OR=2.37; CI, 1.32-4.28). During the total follow-up period of 15 years, female subjects were followed up longer than male subjects (mean [SD]: male=399.4 [214] weeks, female=474.0 [201] weeks; median: male and female=520 weeks). Because of this differential length of follow-up, there was more opportunity to observe recurrent episodes of depression in female subjects. Therefore, the outcome measures took into account the length of follow-up, as detailed below, and survival analysis was used to determine the time to recovery and the time to first recurrence.[29] Reasons for censorship during the total follow-up period were death or suicide (male=18, female=10), refusal (male=21, female=15), and unavailable data for other reasons (male=8, female=4).

Table 1. Demographic Characteristics at Intake

Characteristic	Males (n=94)*	Females (n=101)
Mean (SD) age, y	37 (15)	37 (14)
Marital status, No. (%)		
Never married†	39 (41.5)	23 (22.8)
Married or living together	42 (44.7)	56 (55.4)
Separated, divorced, widowed	13 (13.8)	22 (21.8)
Education, No. (%)		
Graduate school	15 (16.0)	10 (9.9)
College graduate	12 (12.8)	14 (13.9)
High school graduate or partial college	53 (56.4)	59 (58.4)
Partial high school or less	14 (14.9)	18 (17.8)
Residential description, No. (%)		
City‡	53 (56.4)	39 (38.6)
Town	14 (14.9)	17 (16.8)
Suburban	23 (24.5)	36 (35.6)
Rural	4 (4.3)	9 (8.9)
Current work status,§ No. (%)		
Full-time	58 (61.7)	38 (37.6)
Homemaker	0	32 (31.7)
Unemployed	17 (18.1)	6 (5.9)
Part-time, student, retired, other	19 (20.2)	25 (24.8)

*Two male subjects did not have demographic data.
†χ^2=7.03, df=1, P≤.008.
‡χ^2=5.48, df=1, P≤.02.
§Not statistically tested.

Diagnosis at Follow-up

At final follow-up, 38 of 96 men and 50 of 101 women met RDC criteria for recurrent unipolar MDD; 3 male subjects and 5 female subjects met criteria for bipolar I disorder; 7 men and 12 women met criteria for bipolar II disorder; and 3 men met criteria for schizoaffective disorder. The remaining subjects at follow-up continued to carry the diagnosis of unipolar MDD, single episode.

Table 2. Time to First Recovery

Week of Follow-up	No. (%) Recovered* Males (n=96)	Females (n=101)
13 (3 mo)	37 (39)	43 (43)
26 (6 mo)	53 (56)	57 (56)
52 (1 y)	62 (65)	72 (72)
260 (5 y)	83 (91)	87 (90)
520 (10 y)	86 (100)	90 (94)

**Ten men and 11 women were censored before recovering. Percentages are of those remaining subjects and were based on the Kaplan-Meier product limit estimate of the survival function.*

Table 3. Time to First Recurrence

Week Following Recovery	No. (%) With First Recurrence* Males (n=86)	Females (n=90)
13 (3 mo)	4 (5)	15 (17)
26 (6 mo)	10 (12)	20 (22)
52 (1 y)	17 (21)	28 (31)
260 (5 y)	44 (59)	54 (64)
520 (10 y)	48 (68)	62 (78)

**Thirty-eight men and 27 women were censored before their first recurrence. Percentages are of those remaining subjects and were based on the Kaplan-Meier product limit estimate of the survival function.*

Time to Recovery From the Intake Episode

Most subjects recovered in the following 10 years (**Table 2**). The majority recovered in the first 6 months after intake. Comparing survival curves, men and women did not differ in the time to first recovery (Wilcoxon χ^2=0.46, *df*=1, *P*=.50).

Time to First Recurrence

Of the male (n=86) and female (n=90) subjects who recovered, the majority had at least 1 more major depressive episode in the following 5 years (**Table 3**). The rate of first recurrence was highest in the early years of follow-up, but then diminished with time.

During the whole follow-up period of 15 years, the time to first recurrence was not significantly different between the sexes (Wilcoxon χ^2=2.23, *df*=1, *P*=.14). The average rate of first recurrence for men was 0.4% per week and for women was 0.5% per week. A univariate analysis using life regression methods showed there was no significant difference between male and female subjects either in the initial time to first recurrence (*z*=1.15, *df*=1, *P*>.25) or in the change in the time to first recurrence (*z*=1.14, *df*=1, *P*>.25).

Although the overall time to first recurrence and the initial time to first recurrence were not significantly different between the sexes, women tended to experience recurrence earlier than men; however, this difference decreased with time (**Figure**). The median time to first recurrence was 138 weeks for women and 170 weeks for men. A post hoc analysis restricted to the first 6 months after recovery revealed a significant sex difference in the time to first recurrence (Wilcoxon χ^2=4.78, *df*=1, *P*=.03), with the average recurrence rate in the first 6 months 0.4% for male subjects and 1% for female subjects. By 1 year after recovery, there no longer was a significant sex difference.

A covariate analysis using life regression methods showed that sex had no significant effect on the overall time to first recurrence when the following predictor variables were controlled for: age at intake, duration of the index episode, number of parents with major affective disorder, life history of some other affective disorder, life history of substance abuse, and life history of an anxiety disorder.

Number of Recurrences

To control for the length of follow-up, we compared the subset of 72 (of the 96) male subjects and 82 (of the 101) female subjects who were followed up for 5 years after intake. There was no significant difference in the rate of men (44%) and women (48%) who had at least 1 additional episode of major depression (OR=0.88; CI, 0.47-1.66). There was no significant difference between the sexes in the number of recurrent depressive episodes during this period (χ^2=0.27, *df*=3, *P*<.97).

Chronicity and Severity of Depressive Episodes

Male and female subjects did not differ in the chronicity of their depressive symptoms as measured in the following 2 ways. First, as noted above, men and women did not differ in the rate of recovery. Second, the PSR data enabled a calculation of the proportion of weeks of depressive symptoms at each severity level, thus taking into account the number of weeks of follow-up. There was no sex difference in the mean PSR level after intake (mean [SD]: male=2.10 [1.00], female=2.17 [1.17]; CI of the difference, −0.38 to 0.24). There also was no significant sex difference in the proportion of weeks subjects reported the most severe depressive symptoms (mean [SD] proportion of weeks with PSR of ≥5: male=0.13 [0.16], female=0.15 [0.21]; CI of the difference, −0.10 to 0.03).

Death and Suicide

Eighteen (18.8%) of 96 male subjects died during follow-up: 14 died of medical causes (5 from cardiovascular problems); 4 committed suicide. Ten (9.9%) of 101 female subjects died during follow-up: 8 died of medical causes (2 from cardiovascular problems); 2 committed suicide. To control for the length of follow-up, we compared the number of deaths among male and female subjects in the first 5 years of follow-up: there was no significant sex difference (9/[72+9] males=11%, 5/[82+5] females=6%; OR=1.97; CI, 0.66-5.88).

Treatment

There was no significant sex difference in the somatic treatments received during follow-up. This was determined by calculating the proportion of weeks at different CAD levels, taking into account the number of weeks of follow-up. The mean (SD) CAD level during follow-up was not significantly different between the sexes (male=0.48 [0.70], female=0.50 [0.65]). In fact, during the follow-up period, most subjects received no antidepressant treatment (mean [SD] proportion of weeks of follow-up with a CAD level of 0: male=0.80 [0.25], female=0.77 [0.27]).

We also looked at the mean CAD level for each of the 4 weeks prior to the first recurrence and for the week of recurrence in the 48 male and 63 female subjects who had a first recurrence. In all cases, the mean CAD level for both sexes was less than 1 (CAD level 1=imipramine hydrochloride up to 99 mg or the equivalent, or 1 electroconvulsive treatment), and thus of questionable clinical significance. Women did have a significantly lower mean CAD level 1 week prior to the first recurrence (mean [SD]: male=0.90 [1.36], female=0.41 [0.91]; $t=2.13$, $df=78$, $P<.04$).

COMMENT

In this sample of subjects suffering from their first episode of major depression, there were no significant sex differences in measures used to quantify the course of depression over the 15 years of follow-up. First, there was no sex difference in the duration of the intake episode, which is in agreement with the findings of others.[9] Second, there was no sex difference in the time to first recovery: almost all of the subjects recovered from their first episode, most within the first 6 months after intake, a finding consistent with other reports from the NIMH Collaborative Study using different samples.[26] Third, there was no significant sex difference in the time to first recurrence, even when controlling for variables known to affect the recurrence rate of major depression. Moreover, there also was no significant sex difference in the rate of subjects who had any recurrence or in the number of recurrences that subjects had in the first 5 years of follow-up. Fourth, there was no significant sex difference in the severity of depressive periods during follow-up. Finally, there was no evidence for a more chronic course of depression in women, as determined by the absence of a significant sex difference in both (1) the initial recovery rate and (2) the proportion of weeks of follow-up with depressive symptoms at varying levels of severity.

Others have reported that women have more recurrences than men; however, the difference has not always been statistically significant.[9,12-14,30-33] These studies are difficult to compare with each other and with ours for several reasons: the follow-up period varies, subjects with first episodes are often not separated from those with multiple episodes (despite the fact that a previous history of depression has been shown to increase the likelihood of another depressive

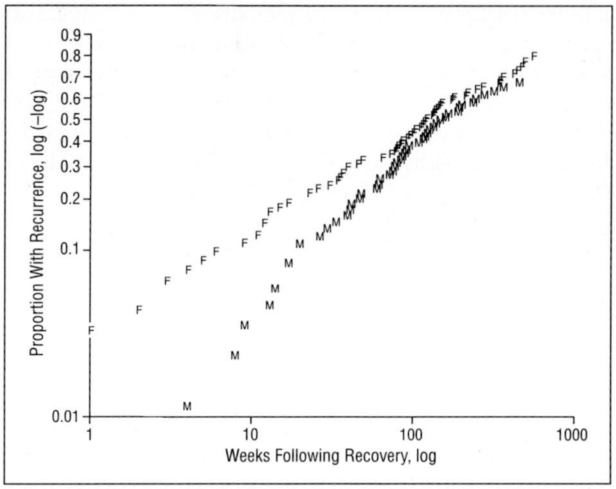

Time to first recurrence of major depressive disorder following first recovery. A plot of the survival function vs time, using log vs log (−log) scales to demonstrate the fit of the data to a Weibull function; the data plotted are the same as in Table 3. Each symbol (M, male; F, female) represents a recurrence. Women initially experienced recurrence earlier than men, but there was no significant sex difference in the overall time to first recurrence.

episode[14]), the studies include both retrospective and prospective designs, and some of the studies have long intervals in between evaluations, which may lead to the problem of bias due to differential recall. Finally, 2 studies that found a significant sex difference in recurrence rates[9,12] did not separate episodes of major depression from minor or intermittent episodes of depression when tabulating recurrence.

Our study suggests 2 additional sources of possible bias that could occur in other studies. First, if women are generally followed up longer than men, as they were in our study, then women could appear to have more recurrences if the length of follow-up was not taken into account. Second, we found that women initially tended to experience recurrences earlier than men. In fact, a post hoc analysis restricted to the first 6 months after intake revealed a significant difference. If it is generally true that women tend to have recurrence earlier than men, then women could be found to have more recurrences if the follow-up period of a study were short.

Our findings that, (1) with a 15-year follow-up, women do not significantly differ from men in the time to first recurrence and, (2) with a 5-year follow-up, women do not significantly differ from men in the number of recurrences they have, are supported by at least 3 other studies. One large retrospective study found no evidence for a sex difference in recurrence.[7] Using a sample different from ours, Coryell et al[14] also concluded that sex was not an important predictor of recurrence. Finally, in a prospective study with a 10-year follow-up, Ernst and Angst[10] found that milder depressive syndromes were more recurrent in women, but that if one used *DSM* criteria for major depression, the sex difference was not significant, which is in agreement with our findings.

Besides a sex difference in recurrence rate, some authors[10,11,15] have suggested that women have a more chronic course than men (eg, either because of slower recovery rates leading to longer major depressive episodes or because of persistent minor depressive symptoms after the resolution of an episode of major depression). As described earlier, we found no evidence for a more chronic course of depression in women, in agreement with a recent large retrospective study.[7]

Our study has several strengths. First, it is a prospective study that includes an intensive intake evaluation and frequent follow-up evaluations, uses standardized diagnostic instruments, and has followed up subjects for up to 15 years. Second, there was a low rate of change to a diagnosis other than MDD at follow-up, making us confident that we were studying a diagnostically stable population. Finally, male and female subjects were similar at intake in terms of demographics, features of their first depressive episode, psychiatric history, and family psychiatric history, which enabled us to focus on sex as we looked for differences in course.

Some aspects of this study limit the generalizability of the findings. First, to be in the study, subjects had to meet criteria for MDD as defined by the RDC and had to seek treatment; most were hospitalized at the time of intake. Second, we believe that subjects at intake were undergoing their first episode of MDD, but there is no guarantee of this. Third, the sample size was small, limiting our ability to find small differences statistically significant. However, we did have sufficient power (following the methods of Lachin[34]) to detect a clinically relevant sex difference, as defined by a 2-fold difference in risk, for all of the following outcome measures: time to recovery, time to first recurrence, and rate with any recurrence in the first 5 years. We also had sufficient power to detect a 1-point difference in mean PSR values.

Treatment received during follow-up was not controlled for in this study. Sex differences in treatment could obscure sex differences in course, since treatment can alter course.[35] As best as we can determine, there were no meaningful sex differences in the somatic treatment received during follow-up. In fact, what is striking is how little somatic treatment subjects received during the follow-up period, consistent with earlier reports from the NIMH Collaborative Study.[24-26]

Multiple factors have been reported to influence the recurrence of MDD: age, a history of previous episodes, a family history of depression, and certain comorbid psychiatric conditions, such as alcoholism and anxiety disorders.[14,30,33,36,37] When these factors were controlled for in our covariate analysis, sex had no significant effect on the time to recurrence. However, male and female subjects were not identical at intake, and we cannot exclude that some uncontrolled factor obscured our ability to detect a sex difference in course.

In summary, MDD is a debilitating illness. Although most of our subjects recovered from their first episode of depression, the majority had a recurrence within 5 years. During the 15 years of the study, there were no outcome measures that differed significantly by sex. Our results from this prospective study are in agreement with a recent large retrospective study[7] that also reported no significant sex differences in the course of MDD. It appears that women, at least during their reproductive years, are more likely to have a first episode of major depression than men,[7,32] but, after a first episode of *major* depression, the overall recurrence rate and the chronicity of depressive symptoms may not differ between the sexes. These results have implications for theories advanced to explain the sex difference in the lifetime prevalence of major depression.

Accepted for publication August 20, 1996.

This work was supported in part by the New York State Department of Mental Health and grants MH23864 and 30906 from the NIMH, Rockville, Md.

The NIMH Collaborative Program on the Psychobiology of Depression–Clinical Studies was conducted with the participation of the following investigators: M. B. Keller, MD, Providence, RI (chairperson); W. Coryell, MD, Iowa City, Iowa (cochairperson); H. S. Akiskal, MD, J. D. Maser, PhD, Washington, DC; P. W. Lavori, PhD, T. I. Mueller, MD, M. T. Shea, PhD, Providence; J. Fawcett, MD, W. A. Scheftner, MD, Chicago, Ill; G. Winokur, MD (deceased), J. Haley, Iowa City; J. Endicott, PhD, A. Leon, PhD, J. Loth, MSW, New York, NY; J. Rice, PhD, T. Reich, MD, St Louis, Mo. Other contributors include N. C. Andreasen, MD, PhD, P. J. Clayton, MD, J. Croughan, MD, G. L. Klerman, MD (deceased), R. M. A. Hirschfeld, MD, M. M. Katz, PhD, E. Robins, MD, R. W. Shapiro, MD (deceased), R. L. Spitzer, MD, and M. A. Young, PhD. The manuscript has been reviewed by the Publication Committee of the Collaborative Depression Study and has its endorsement.

We would like to thank A. Leon, PhD, R. O. Rieder, MD, D. Solomon, MD, D. S. Vicario, PhD, and S. Wolk, MD, for commenting on earlier versions of the manuscript.

Corresponding author: Jean Endicott, PhD, New York State Psychiatric Institute, Unit 123, 722 W 168th St, New York, NY 10032.

REFERENCES

1. Weissman MM, Klerman GL. Sex differences and the epidemiology of depression. *Arch Gen Psychiatry.* 1977;34:98-109.
2. Weissman MM, Klerman GL. Gender and depression. *Trends Neurosci.* 1985;8:416-420.
3. Smith AL, Weissman MM. Epidemiology. In: Paykel E, ed. *Handbook of Affective Disorders.* 2nd ed. London, England: Churchill Livingstone; 1992:111-129.
4. Leon AC, Klerman GL, Wickramaratne P. Continuing female predominance in depressive illness. *Am J Public Health.* 1993;83:754-757.
5. Wolk SI, Weissman MM. Women and depression: an update. In: Oldham JM, Riba MB, eds. *American Psychiatric Press Review of Psychiatry.* Washington, DC: American Psychiatric Press; 1995;14:227-259.
6. Young MA, Scheftner, WA, Fawcett J, Klerman GL. Gender differences in the clinical features of unipolar major depressive disorder. *J Nerv Mental Dis.* 1990;178:200-203.
7. Kessler RC, McGonagle KA, Swartz M, Blazer DG, Nelson CB. Sex and depression in the National Comorbidity Survey, I: lifetime prevalence, chronicity and recurrence. *J Affect Disord.* 1993;29:85-96.
8. Weissman MM, Bruce ML, Leaf PJ, Florio LP, Holzer C. Affective disorders. In: Robins LN, Regier DA, eds. *Psychiatric Disorders in America.* New York, NY: The Free Press; 1991:53-80.
9. Amenson CS, Lewinsohn PM. An investigation into the observed sex difference in prevalence of unipolar depression. *J Abnorm Psychol.* 1981;90:1-13.

10. Ernst C, Angst J. The Zurich Study XII: sex differences in depression: evidence from longitudinal epidemiological data. *Eur Arch Psychiatry Clin Neurosci.* 1992; 241:222-230.
11. Nolen-Hoeksema S. Sex differences in unipolar depression: evidence and theory. *Psychol Bull.* 1987;101:259-282.
12. Lewinsohn PM, Zeiss AM, Duncan EM. Probability of relapse after recovery from an episode of depression. *J Abnorm Psychol.* 1989;98:107-116.
13. Winokur G, Coryell W, Keller M, Endicott J, Akiskal H. A prospective follow-up of patients with bipolar and primary unipolar affective disorder. *Arch Gen Psychiatry.* 1993;50:457-465.
14. Coryell W, Endicott J, Keller MB. Predictors of relapse into major depressive disorder in a nonclinical population. *Am J Psychiatry.* 1991;148:1353-1358.
15. Frank E, Carpenter LL, Kupfer DJ. Sex differences in recurrent depression: are there any that are significant? *Am J Psychiatry.* 1988;145:41-45.
16. Spitzer RL, Endicott J, Robins E. Research Diagnostic Criteria: rational and reliability. *Arch Gen Psychiatry.* 1978;35:773-782.
17. Katz MM, Secunda SK, Hirschfeld RMA, Koslow SH. NIMH clinical research branch collaborative program on the psychobiology of depression. *Arch Gen Psychiatry.* 1979;36:765-771.
18. Endicott J, Spitzer RL. A diagnostic interview: the Schedule for Affective Disorders and Schizophrenia. *Arch Gen Psychiatry.* 1978;35:837-844.
19. Larkin BH, Hirschfeld RMA. *The Personal History of Depressive Disorders (PHDD).* Rockville, Md: National Institute of Mental Health, Clinical Research Branch; 1977.
20. Andreasen NC, Endicott J, Spitzer RL, Winokur G. The family history method using diagnostic criteria. *Arch Gen Psychiatry.* 1977;34:1229-1235.
21. Andreasen NC, Rice J, Endicott J, Reich T, Coryell W. The family history approach to diagnosis. *Arch Gen Psychiatry.* 1986;43:421-429.
22. Shapiro R, Keller M. *Longitudinal Interval Follow-up Evaluation Base (LIFE-Base).* Boston: Massachusetts General Hospital; 1979.
23. Keller MB, Lavori PW, Friedman B, Neilsen E, Endicott J, McDonald-Scott P, Andreasen N. The Longitudinal Interval Follow-up Evaluation. *Arch Gen Psychiatry.* 1987;44:540-548.
24. Keller MB, Klerman GL, Lavori PW, Fawcett JA, Coryell W, Endicott J. Treatment received by depressed patients. *JAMA.* 1982;248:1848-1855.
25. Keller M, Lavori PW, Klerman GL, Andreasen NC, Endicott J, Coryell W, Fawcett J, Rice JP, Hirschfeld RMA. Low levels and lack of predictors of somatotherapy and psychotherapy received by depressed patients. *Arch Gen Psychiatry.* 1986; 43:458-466.
26. Keller MB, Lavori PW, Mueller TI, Endicott J, Coryell W, Hirschfeld RMA, Shea T. Time to recovery, chronicity, and levels of psychopathology in major depression: a 5-year prospective follow-up of 431 subjects. *Arch Gen Psychiatry.* 1992; 49:809-816.
27. American Psychiatric Association. *Diagnostic and Statistical Manual of Mental Disorders, Fourth Edition.* Washington, DC: American Psychiatric Association; 1994.
28. Kalbfleisch JD, Prentice RL. *The Statistical Analysis of Failure Time Data.* New York, NY: John Wiley & Sons; 1980.
29. Leon AC, Friedman RA, Sweeney JA, Brown RP, Mann JJ. Statistical issues in the identification of risk factors for suicidal behavior: the application of survival analysis. *Psychiatry Res.* 1990;31:99-108.
30. Gonzales LR, Lewinsohn PM, Clarke GN. Longitudinal follow-up of unipolar depressives: an investigation of predictors of relapse. *J Consult Clin Psychol.* 1985; 53:461-469.
31. Perugi G, Musetti L, Simonini E, Piagentini F, Cassano GB, Akiskal HS. Gender-mediated clinical features of depressive illness: the importance of temperamental differences. *Br J Psychiatry.* 1990;157:835-841.
32. Coryell W, Endicott J, Keller M. Major depression in a nonclinical sample: demographic and clinical risk factors for first onset. *Arch Gen Psychiatry.* 1992; 49:117-125.
33. Merikangas KR, Wicki W, Angst J. Heterogeneity of depression: classification of depressive subtypes by longitudinal course. *Br J Psychiatry.* 1994;164:342-348.
34. Lachin JM. Introduction to sample size determination and power analysis for clinical trials. *Control Clin Trials.* 1981;2:93-113.
35. Frank E, Kupfer DJ, Perel JM, Cornes C, Jarrett DB, Mallinger AG, Thase ME, McEachran AB, Grochocinski VJ. Three-year outcomes for maintenance therapies in recurrent depression. *Arch Gen Psychiatry.* 1990;47:1093-1099.
36. Zis AP, Grof P, Webster M, Goodwin FK. Prediction of relapse in recurrent affective disorder. *Psychopharmacol Bull.* 1980;16:47-49.
37. Keller MB, Lavori PW, Lewis CE, Klerman G. Predictors of relapse in major depressive disorder. *JAMA.* 1983;250:3299-3304.

Break the debilitating cycle of

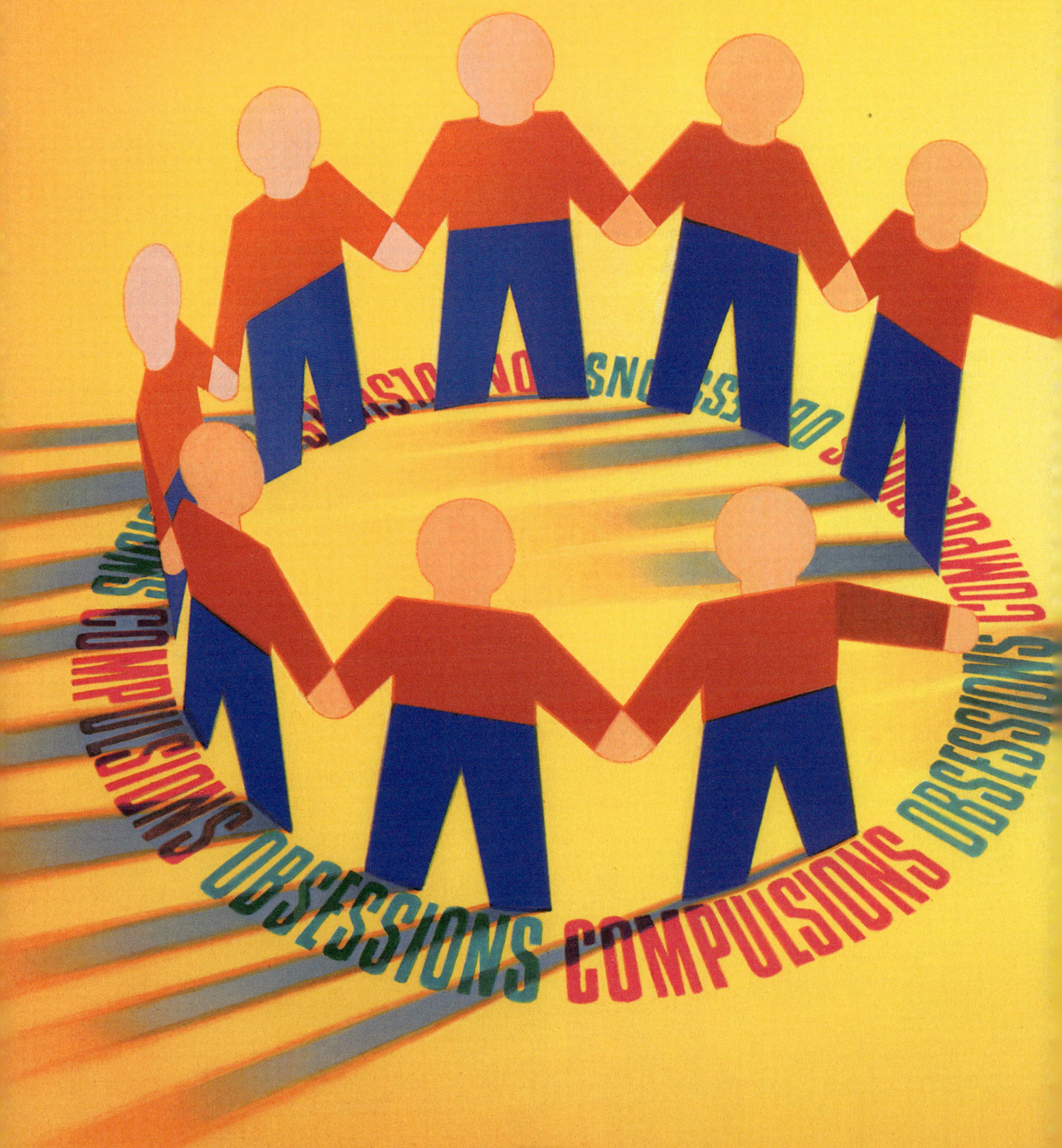

ORIGINAL ARTICLE

Clinical Improvement With Fluoxetine Therapy and Noradrenergic Function in Patients With Panic Disorder

Jeremy D. Coplan, MD; Laszlo A. Papp, MD; Daniel Pine, MD; Jose Martinez, MA; Thomas Cooper, MA; Leonard A. Rosenblum, PhD; Donald F. Klein, MD; Jack M. Gorman, MD

Background: Central noradrenergic (NA) dysregulation has provided a major theoretical framework for understanding the pathogenesis of panic disorder (PD). Using clonidine, an α_2-adrenergic receptor agonist, as a probe of NA function, we investigated the hypothesis that the antipanic efficacy of the selective serotonin reuptake inhibitors may be associated with normalization of a putatively dysregulated NA system.

Methods: We report further analyses on data from 17 subjects with PD and 16 healthy volunteers who underwent measurement of the plasma NA metabolite 3-methoxy-4-hydroxyphenylglycol (MHPG) immediately before and after oral clonidine administration. Thirteen patients with PD were rechallenged after 12 weeks during open fluoxetine hydrochloride treatment using the same clonidine paradigm; 13 healthy volunteers were rechallenged at 12 weeks, not having received treatment between challenges.

Results: Patients with PD, compared with healthy volunteers, have markedly elevated plasma MHPG volatility during the first clonidine challenge. Volatility describes the magnitude of within-subject plasma MHPG oscillatory activity as assessed by the root of the mean square successive difference. A greater degree of clinical global improvement was predicted by a greater magnitude of basal MHPG reduction with fluoxetine treatment. Antipanic response to fluoxetine was accompanied by a significant decrease of MHPG volatility to volunteer levels. Volunteer MHPG volatility remained unchanged from the first to second clonidine challenge.

Conclusions: Further evidence is provided for the hypothesis of NA dysregulation in PD as reflected by elevations of within-subject plasma MHPG volatility during clonidine challenge. Effective selective serotonin reuptake inhibitor–antipanic treatment in this clinical sample was paralleled by normalization of dysregulated NA function.

Arch Gen Psychiatry. 1997;54:643-648

From the College of Physicians and Surgeons of Columbia University, New York State Psychiatric Institute (Drs Coplan, Papp, Pine, Klein, and Gorman and Messrs Martinez and Cooper) and the Phobia and Stress Clinic, Hillside Hospital, Long Island Jewish Medical Center (Drs Coplan, Papp, and Gorman) New York, NY; and the Department of Psychiatry and Primate Behavior Laboratory, SUNY Health Sciences Center at Brooklyn, Brooklyn, NY (Dr Rosenblum).

THE SELECTIVE serotonin reuptake inhibitors (SSRIs) have been shown in open and controlled studies to be effective antipanic medications.[1,2] In this article, we address the influence of the SSRIs on noradrenergic (NA) function in patients with panic disorder (PD). Central NA function has been proposed to be prone to "dysregulation" in PD, based on enhanced responsivity to α_2-adrenergic autoreceptor agonists or antagonists (clonidine hydrochloride and yohimbine, respectively).[3,4] The question is therefore raised whether chronic serotonin reuptake blockade mediates antipanic effects through down-modulation of an abnormally "volatile" NA system. Noradrenergic volatility describes the magnitude of plasma 3-methoxy-4-hydroxyphenylglycol (MHPG) oscillatory activity as assessed by the root of the mean square successive difference (MSSD) statistic. The down-modulation of volatility may occur directly (through inhibitory serotonergic projections that arise from brainstem raphe nuclei and project to NA neurons located in the nucleus locus coeruleus[5]) and/or indirectly (through down-modulation of neurotransmitters that stimulate brain-stem NA activity, including corticotropin-releasing factor,[6,7] glutamate,[8] somatostatin,[9] and substance P[10]).

Our data indicating persistently reduced human growth hormone response and exaggerated cortisol decrements to clonidine in fluoxetine hydrochloride–improved patients with PD[11,12] were inconsistent with literature about rodents, in which at least 2 studies showed that fluoxetine modifies α_2-adrenoceptor sensitivity.[13,14]

We therefore reexamined, in greater detail, plasma MHPG, a peripheral NA metabolite,[15,16] which had been measured immediately before and during oral cloni-

SUBJECTS AND METHODS

SUBJECTS

Seventeen patients meeting *DSM-III-R* criteria for PD with or without agoraphobia as assessed by a structured clinical interview for *DSM-III-R* (Structured Clinical Interview)[17] were recruited by advertisement in local newspapers. Inclusion and exclusion criteria were discussed in detail previously.[11,12] Sixteen healthy subjects, as assessed by the Structured Clinical Interview,[17] served as a control group.

The routine baseline evaluation included physical examination, blood tests for liver profile and electrolyte function, complete blood cell count and thyroid function tests, electrocardiogram, pregnancy test, and urinalysis. Patients were medication-free for 4 weeks before the study but were permitted to take benzodiazepines as needed up to 3 days before the clonidine challenges. Five patients took benzodiazepines as needed up to 3 days before the first clonidine challenge and 2 of these, both subsequently assessed as being nonresponders, took benzodiazepines as needed up to 3 days before the second challenge. Persons who received benzodiazepines as needed were not permitted to exceed 1 mg alprazolam per day or its equivalent.

Before the first challenge, patients with PD were evaluated using the Hamilton Depression Scale, Hamilton Anxiety Scale, and Clinical Global Assessment Scale (CGAS)[18]; the number of panic attacks during the week before the evaluation were tallied. Overall improvement on all measures was seen in the patient group.[11,12] None of the patients experienced benzodiazepine withdrawal during either clonidine challenge. To obviate possible effects of menstrual phase on NA function, women were studied during the first half of the menstrual cycle. Thirteen of 17 patients with PD (4 treatment dropouts) and 13 of 16 volunteers repeated the clonidine challenge 12 weeks later.

There was no significant difference between groups for sex distribution (patients, 7 males and 10 females; controls, 8 males and 8 females, Pearsonian $\chi^2=.26$, $df=1$). There was a trend for the patients (n=17) to be older than the control subjects (n=16; mean±SD, 40.53±10.24 years vs 33.94±10.45 years, $t=1.83$; $df=31$; $P=.077$) (2-tailed). There was no weight difference between groups. Informed consent was obtained from all subjects.

CHALLENGE PROCEDURES

At 9 AM, an indwelling venous cannula was placed in an antecubital vein and kept open with heparinized solution. Subjects remained in a semireclining comfortable position. At 9:30 AM (0 time), clonidine (0.15 mg) was given by mouth. Blood samples were drawn at times 0, 60, 120, 180, and 240 minutes for plasma MHPG and cortisol. Clonidine blood levels were measured at 60, 120, and 180 minutes.

TREATMENT PHASE

Following the completion of the challenge study, patients were entered into an open flexible fluoxetine treatment phase. The mean±SD final daily dose of fluoxetine was 17.7±16.7 mg/d.[11,12]

BIOCHEMICAL ANALYSES

Clonidine blood levels were quantitated using gas chromatography mass spectrometry in the simultaneous ion-monitoring mode using methods developed in this laboratory (T.C., unpublished data, January 1995). Within-run and between-run relative SDs were 4.2% and 5.6%, respectively. The lower limit of detection is 100 pg/mL.

Plasma MHPG was measured by gas chromatography mass spectrometry operated in the simultaneous ion-monitoring mode using deuterated MHPG as an internal standard. The method is essentially the same as that of Jimerson et al.[19] Plasma cortisol levels were assayed as in previous reports.[20]

dine challenge in patients with PD and in healthy volunteers.[12] After the initial clonidine challenge, patients were treated openly with fluoxetine for 12 weeks and then rechallenged with clonidine while receiving treatment. Healthy volunteers received no treatment between equivalently spaced clonidine challenges. We posed the following questions: Can differences be detected between patients and controls for within-subject volatility of NA function, supporting the NA dysregulation hypothesis of panic disorder?[3,4] Can a significant influence of SSRI action on NA function be documented in PD through correlation of fluoxetine antipanic response with magnitude of normalization of plasma MHPG variables?

RESULTS

PRETREATMENT NA VOLATILITY FINDINGS

Untreated patients with PD showed markedly increased within-subject plasma MHPG volatility during clonidine challenge compared with healthy controls. Only a limited group overlap was observed (patients, mean±SD, 1.96±0.92 ng/mL per hour vs controls, 0.519±0.28 ng/mL per hour; Mann-Whitney *U* test, $z=-4.7$; $P<.001$; effect size, 2.18) (**Figure 1** and **Table**). The excessive plasma MHPG volatility can be visualized directly in **Figure 2**, which shows each subject's baseline and successive postclonidine plasma MHPG levels. A high degree of line "verticality" between time points, in strong contrast to the controls' "horizontal" plasma MHPG levels, indicates the large oscillations of NA function observed in patients with PD during clonidine challenge.

All 16 controls had values of plasma MHPG change per hour of less than 1.25 ng/mL per hour (100% specificity), but only 3 of 17 patients showed values below this post hoc cutoff (82% sensitivity) ($P<.001$, Fisher exact) (Figure 1).

Indicating volatility beyond that predicted by group differences of conventional variance alone, the ratio of MSSD to conventional variance was significantly greater in patients (n=17) vs controls (n=16) (mean±SD, 2.7±3.2 vs 0.7±0.9); Mann-Whitney *U* test, $z=-2.9$; $P<.003$).

DATA ANALYSIS

Because no significant group, challenge, or interactive effect for blood clonidine levels had been previously observed using an analysis of variance with repeated measures (ANOVAR),[11,12] these are not examined further in the current article.

Four missing plasma MHPG values of a total of 295 measures were replaced by substituting the adjacent plasma MHPG values. Plasma MHPG volatility was computed using the MSSD calculated from the 3 values derived from 4 postclonidine time points (120 minutes–60 minutes, 180 minutes–120 minutes, 240 minutes–180 minutes) for both clonidine challenges. Baseline values are excluded because clonidine was not yet pharmacologically active. Volatility can be determined by applying the formula of von Neumann et al:[21]

$$\delta^2 = \frac{\sum_{i=1}^{n-1} (x_i - x_i)^2}{n-1}$$

According to von Neumann et al,[21] δ^2 (MSSD) must differ significantly from s^2 (conventional variance, which is measured independently of the order of the observations).

$$s^2 = \frac{\sum_{i=1}^{n} (x_i - \bar{x})^2}{n}$$

We computed the ratio of the MSSD to conventional variance and then ascertained group differences. If larger in patients compared with controls, this ratio indicates that the magnitude of volatility is greater than that expected by group differences of conventional variance alone. Rifkin et al[22] have applied this statistical procedure to measure mood lability in emotionally unstable character disorder. To accurately reflect mean MHPG volatility levels, we took the square root of the computed MSSD value to fulfill the units of mean plasma MHPG change in nanograms per milliliter per hour during clonidine challenge. Because assumptions of normality may not be fulfilled by measures of variability, the groups were compared using nonparametric tests and also by application of a post hoc cutoff for sensitivity and specificity assessments.

We used an ANOVAR to analyze time and group by time effects of the raw plasma MHPG levels in response to clonidine challenge to ascertain if these were influencing the volatility computations. Correlations of pretreatment MHPG volatility and basal MHPG were performed.

To address the question of the influence of fluoxetine antipanic treatment on NA function, patients were designated by responder status. Eleven patients with PD were assessed as being treatment responders (moderate to marked response on the CGAS). Two patients who were assessed as being nonresponders to fluoxetine (minimal improvement and no improvement on the CGAS) were excluded from subsequent ANOVAR analyses. The ANOVAR tested whether the magnitude of between-visit reductions of MHPG variables was greater in fluoxetine-responsive patients than in healthy controls. We assessed 2 MHPG variables—basal levels (those obtained before clonidine administration) and the aforementioned MSSD-derived values. Significant group-by-visit interactions for both plasma MHPG measures would reflect normalization of basal and volatility-related NA function in patients treated for PD. Significant ANOVAR effects were followed up by paired and unpaired post hoc tests.

A final correlational analysis included all patients with PD who had completed both clonidine challenges (including nonresponders) (n=13). Clinical global improvement as assessed by administration of the CGAS was nonparametrically correlated with the plasma MHPG between-visit difference using the Spearman rank order correlation coefficient.

Identical analyses were applied to the cortisol data.

All results reported are 2-tailed, set at an α level of significance of $P<.05$.

A strong time effect ($F=8.22$; $df=4,124$; $P<.001$) was evident for subjects in general (group-by-time effect not significant [NS]), reflecting the decline of plasma MHPG following clonidine administration. However, when baseline measures are excluded from the ANOVAR analysis, there is no longer a significant time effect for plasma MHPG levels (60-240 minutes). Both groups undergo significant reductions of MHPG in the first hour following clonidine, but thereafter measures remain stable in both groups (group-by-time interaction NS), suggesting tonic NA presynaptic inhibition by clonidine during the period of increased volatility.

Conceivably, the group differences of intrasubject plasma MHPG volatility could be attributed to the artifact introduced by the general elevations of plasma MHPG levels in patients with PD during the clonidine challenge. Group comparisons using plasma MHPG levels from the 4 postclonidine time points indicated only a trend elevation in patients vs controls ($F=2.24$; $df=3,93$; $P=.09$). Nevertheless, to eliminate this potential source of bias, we reanalyzed the data assessing each subject's reconverted volatility measure as a percentage of his or her mean MHPG levels during clonidine administration. The results were essentially unchanged (patients, mean±SD, 38%±13% vs controls, 13%±6%; Mann-Whitney *U* test, $z=-4.6$; $P<.001$).

The 5 patients who were taking benzodiazepines as needed up to 72 hours before the first clonidine challenge may have differed from the other 12 patients with PD. Of the 5 patients who were taking benzodiazepines as needed, 2 were subsequent nonresponders (who have been separately grouped), 1 other patient dropped out, and the 2 remaining patients did not differ in any systematic fashion from patients who had not taken benzodiazepines as needed.

There was no significant correlation between age or sex and plasma MHPG volatility.

Basal plasma MHPG in patients correlated with pretreatment MHPG volatility during clonidine (Spearman $r=0.64$; $P=.006$) but this was not the case in controls (Spearman $r=0.28$; $P=.30$). The magnitude of the correlations, using the Fisher *r* to *z* transformation, did not differ between groups (NS). Correlations between basal plasma MHPG or plasma MHPG volatility during clonidine and the pretreatment Hamilton Anxiety Scale, clinical global improvement, or clinical global severity assessments were NS.

EFFECTS OF FLUOXETINE ON NA VARIABLES

In previous analyses of basal or preclonidine plasma MHPG,[12] a visit effect with equivalent declines in patients and controls from first to second measurement was observed. By excluding the 2 nonresponders from the analysis, the magnitude of the basal plasma MHPG decrease between visits is more marked in the patients than in controls (**Figure 3** and Table).

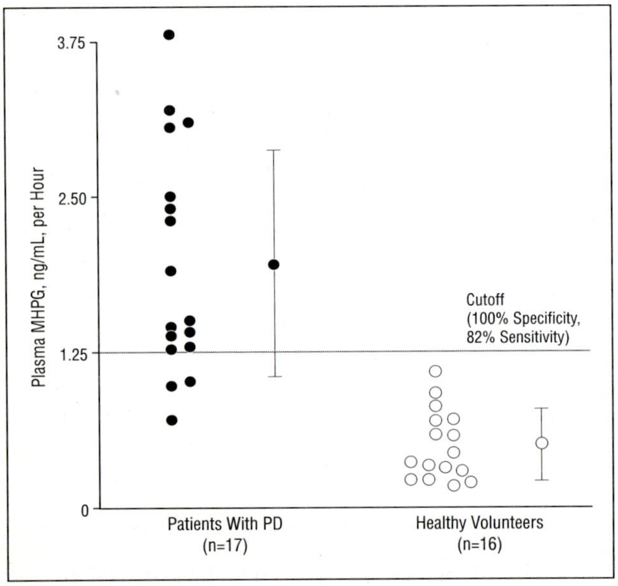

Figure 1. *Comparison of the means and SDs of within-subject plasma 3-methoxy-4-hydroxyphenylglycol (MHPG) volatility during clonidine challenge between untreated patients with panic disorder (PD) and healthy volunteers. The scatterplot depicting the individual values is on the left of the group mean and SD. Mann-Whitney* U *test,* $z=-4.7$; $P<.001$. *Application of cutoff is post hoc,* $P<.001$, *Fisher exact test.*

Because the 2 nonresponders showed a basal plasma MHPG pattern opposite to that of treatment responders, their inclusion in previous analyses obscured a significant group-by-visit interaction. The 2 nonresponders had numerically lower levels of pretreatment preclonidine MHPG than the mean of the patient responders or controls and exhibited an increase, rather than decrease, of between-visit basal plasma MHPG levels, which was observed in responders (Figure 3 and Table). The between-visit change of preclonidine plasma MHPG correlated inversely with clinical global improvement (Spearman $r=-0.55$; n=13; $P<.05$). Those patients with PD who were treated with fluoxetine and experienced the greatest between-visit reductions of basal plasma MHPG were more likely to show clinical improvement.

Fluoxetine treatment response was also associated with a significant reduction of MHPG volatility during clonidine administration (**Figure 4**). Posttreatment patient measures were indistinguishable from either control challenge. There was no statistically detectable difference from visit 1 to visit 2 for plasma MHPG volatility during clonidine for controls (Table). In patients with PD who had undergone both challenges (n=13), the magnitude of reduction by fluoxetine of intrasubject plasma MHPG volatility during clonidine challenge was not correlated with clinical global improvement.

PLASMA CORTISOL DATA

No group differences in pretreatment plasma cortisol volatility were observed. Basal and volatility measures of plasma cortisol were unchanged in both study groups when comparing the first with the second clonidine challenge. None of the cortisol variables examined disclosed significant correlations with clinical measures.

COMMENT

Our data support the view that markedly elevated levels of plasma MHPG volatility during clonidine challenge are observed in untreated patients with PD compared with

Basal Plasma MHPG and Plasma MHPG Volatility During Clonidine Administration in Patients With Panic Disorder and in Healthy Volunteers*

Group	Patients With PD (n=11)	Healthy Volunteers (n=13)	Nonresponders† (n=2)	ANOVAR Effect	F	*df*	*P*	Paired Testing	Test Used	Statistic Value	*P*
Preclonidine MHPG											
Visit											
1	6.65 (±2.74) a	4.37 (±1.03) b	3.50 (±0.70)	Group	5.9	1,22	<.03	a vs b	Unpaired *t*	$t=-2.8$	.01
				Visit	24.3	1,22	<.001	a vs c	Paired *t*	$t=3.3$	.007
2	4.45 (±1.67) c	3.67 (±0.96) d	4.45 (±1.34)	Group-by-visit	6.4	1,22	<.02	b vs d	Paired *t*	$t=3.7$	.004
MHPG volatility during clonidine administration											
Visit											
1	1.9 (±1.0) a	0.5 (±0.3) b	2.0 (±0.8)	Group	7.9	1,22	.01	a vs b	MW U	$z=-3.9$	<.001
				Visit	2.8	1,22	.10	a vs c	WMP	$z=2.8$	.006
2	0.9 (±0.8) c	0.9 (±0.8) d	1.3 (±0.6)	Group-by-visit	13.6	1,22	.001	...	...	...	...

**Patients were challenged before and after 12 weeks of fluoxetine treatment; controls were challenged 12 weeks apart with no treatment. MHPG indicates 3-methoxy-4-hydroxyphenylglycol; PD, panic disorder; and ANOVAR, analysis of variance with repeated measures; MW U, Mann-Whitney* U*; WMP, Wilcoxon matched pairs. MHPG values are given as mean (±SD).*

†*Two fluoxetine nonresponders not included in analyses.*

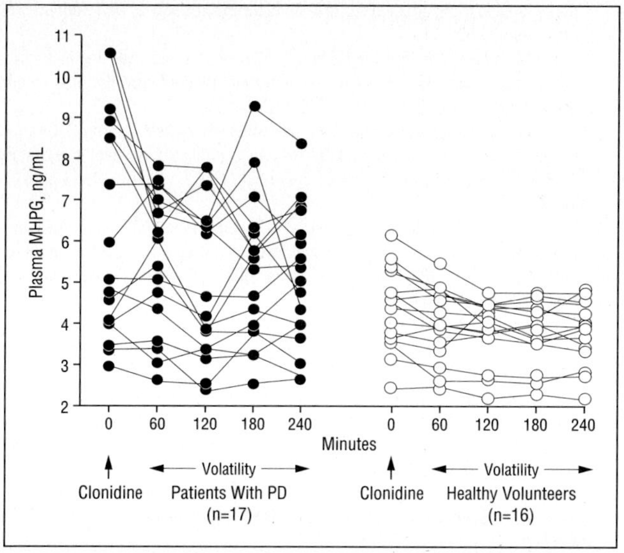

Figure 2. *Successive plasma 3-methoxy-4-hydroxyphenylglycol (MHPG) levels following administration of clonidine (indicated by "Clonidine" and arrow) in patients with panic disorder [PD] and in healthy volunteers). The mean group differences in patterns of plasma MHPG production are shown in Figure 1. Plasma MHPG volatility is determined using the root of the mean square successive difference[23] from the 4 postclonidine time points (indicated by "Volatility" and arrows).*

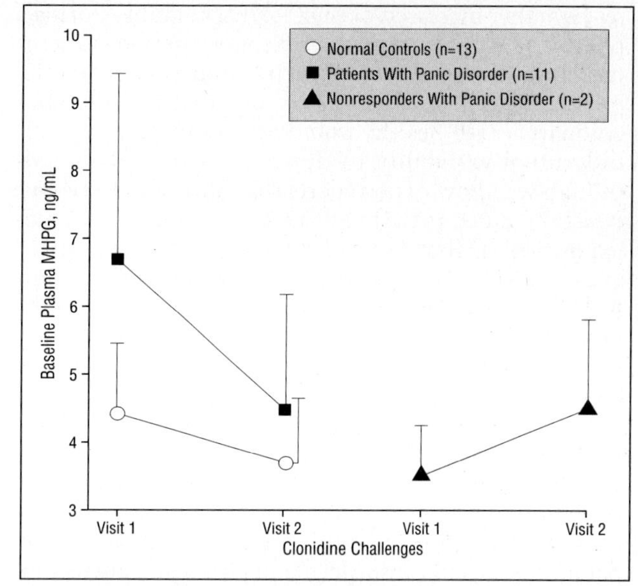

Figure 3. *Effects of antipanic fluoxetine treatment on preclonidine 3-methoxy-4-hydroxyphenylglycol (MHPG) levels. Visit 1=preclonidine plasma MHPG before the first clonidine challenge. Visit 2=preclonidine plasma MHPG before a second clonidine challenge following 12 weeks of open fluoxetine treatment for patients and no treatment for controls. Although all subjects show a reduction in basal plasma MHPG for visit 2, when the 2 nonresponders with panic disorder are excluded from the analysis, the effect is more marked in the patients than in the controls..*

healthy volunteers. The SSRIs appeared to have exerted an "NA stabilizing" role by reducing pretreatment MHPG volatility to levels equivalent to that seen in controls.

Supporting the view that normalization of the NA system occurred in parallel to treatment response, the magnitude of decrease in basal MHPG from the first to second visit correlated with clinical global improvement as assessed by the clinical CGAS. It is of interest, but requires an expanded study, that the 2 nonresponders had low pretreatment basal plasma MHPG and displayed increases rather than decreases of basal plasma MHPG following unsuccessful fluoxetine treatment.

The increased MHPG volatility in untreated subjects with PD during clonidine challenge supports the views proposed by Charney and Heninger[3] and Nutt[4] of "NA dysregulation" in PD. Noradrenergic dysregulation may be viewed as an inability of the neuronal system to maintain homeostasis of its neurotransmitter activity, due to a malfunction of a putative neurobiological "buffering capacity."[23] Loss of homeostatic control of NA function in PD may occur along cybernetic lines, a dysfunction in which a system is unable to contain bidirectional perturbations (increases and decreases).[24,25] That basal MHPG was significantly correlated with MHPG volatility in patients, but not in controls, suggests that rheostat (unidirectional) increases of NA function may relate to the putative cybernetic dysfunction of NA homeostasis in PD.

The normalizing effects of SSRIs on NA function in the present study contrast with previous observations in patients with PD. The reduced human growth hormone response[11] and the exaggerated decline of plasma cortisol[12] to clonidine, and the enhanced MHPG response to yohimbine,[26] persist despite SSRI-induced clinical improvement. Only the anxiogenic effects of yohimbine were attenuated by fluvoxamine in that study.[26]

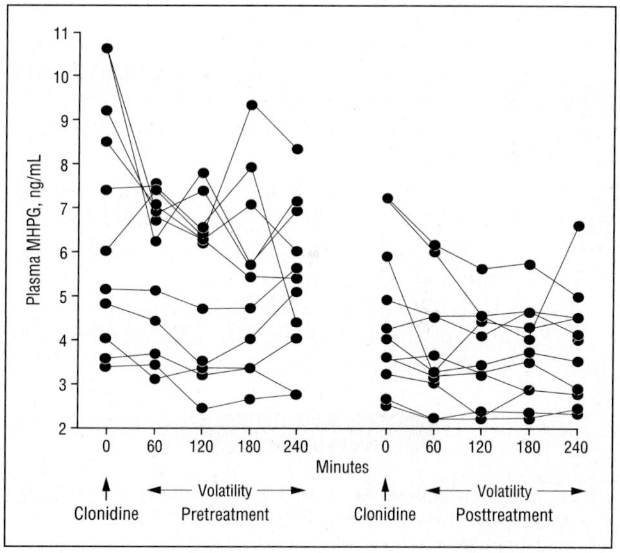

Figure 4. *Individual successive plasma 3-methoxy-4-hydroxyphenylglycol (MHPG) levels following clonidine administration before and after fluoxetine treatment in 11 responders with panic disorder. Fluoxetine response was associated with a significant reduction of plasma MHPG volatility.*

Several important limitations are evident. The validity of plasma MHPG levels as reflective of central NA activity has been questioned because of large peripheral contributions.[3,16] Nevertheless, adrenal medullary sympathetic activity is regulated by central NA structures, so detectable peripheral changes should parallel central NA activity. The lack of placebo-treated patients leaves open the possibility that the treatment response may be partially due to a placebo and not a fluoxetine response. Moreover, placebo-controlled clonidine challenges should test whether increased plasma MHPG volatility during a pharmacologically unperturbed control period is abnormal. In a diurnal neuroendocrine study of acutely depressed males, Trestman et al[27] reported no difference compared with healthy volunteers in the mean intra-individual variability of diurnal plasma MHPG, although we know of no reports that have addressed this question in PD. In the present study, women were studied during the first 2 weeks (14 days) of their menstrual cycle. Clonidine studies are probably best performed during the first 10 days of the menstrual cycle to avoid the periovulatory period. Levels of reproductive hormones, which affect human growth hormone secretion, also may affect NA function.

Documentation of increased within-subject NA volatility during clonidine challenge is in accordance with our group's work examining ventilatory function in PD. In those studies, an increased variance of tidal volume or chaotic breathing patterns are evident at baseline in patients with panic disorder.[28] Future studies are recommended in which simultaneous ventilatory, serotonergic, and NA measures may be integrated. In addition, the diagnostic specificity of elevated NA volatility needs to be determined. Noradrenergic volatility during clonidine challenge, like the human growth hormone response to clonidine, may be elevated in other anxiety and affective disorders and represent a nonspecific common dysregulation.

Accepted for publication September 27, 1996.

Supported in part by National Institute of Mental Health Clinical Research Center grant MH-30906, National Institute of Mental Health (NIMH) Research Scientist Award MH-00416 (Dr Gorman), NIMH Research Scientist Development Award MH-00858 (Dr Papp), and clinical training grant MH-18641 and NIMH Research Scientist Development Award MH-01039 (Dr Coplan), Bethesda, Md.

We thank Andrew Goddard, MBBCh, Yale University, New Haven, Conn, for his helpful input.

Reprints: Jeremy D. Coplan, MD, 722 W 168th St, PO Box 24, New York, NY 10032.

REFERENCES

1. Gorman JM, Liebowitz MR, Fyer AJ, et al. An open trial of fluoxetine in the treatment of panic attacks. *J Clin Psychopharmacol.* 1987;7:329-332.
2. Den Boer JA, Westenberg HG. Serotonin function in panic disorder: a double blind placebo controlled study with fluvoxamine and ritanserin. *Psychopharmacology (Berl).* 1990;102:85-94.
3. Charney DS, Heninger GR. Abnormal regulation of noradrenergic function in panic disorders: effects of clonidine in healthy subjects and patients with agoraphobia and panic disorder. *Arch Gen Psychiatry.* 1986;43:1042-1055.
4. Nutt DJ. Altered central alpha-2 sensitivity in panic disorder. *Arch Gen Psychiatry.* 1989;46:165-169.
5. Morgane JP, Jacobs MS. Raphe projections to the locus coeruleus in the rat. *Brain Res Bull.* 1979;4;519-534.
6. Reul JM, Labeur MS, Grigoriadis DE, De Souza EB, Holsboer F. Hypothalamic-pituitary-adrenocortical axis changes in the rat after long-term treatment with the reversible monoamine oxidase-A inhibitor moclobemide. *Neuroendocrinology.* 1994;60:509-519.
7. Butler PD, Weiss JM, Stout JC, Nemeroff CB. Corticotropin-releasing factor produces fear-enhancing and behavioral activating effects following infusion into the locus coeruleus. *J Neurosci.* 1990;10:176-183.
8. Charlety PJ, Chergui K, Akaoka H, Saunier CF, Buda M, Aston-Jones G, Chouvet G. Serotonin differentially modulates responses mediated by specific excitatory amino acid receptors in the locus coeruleus. *Eur J Neurosci.* 1993;5:1024-1028.
9. Lima L, Arce V, Tresguerres JA, Devesa J. Clonidine potentiates the growth hormone response in norepinephrine synthesis-inhibited rats: evidence for an α_2-adrenergic control of hypothalamic release of somatostatin. *Neuroendocrinology.* 1993;57:1155-1160.
10. Yeomans DC, Proudfit HK. Antinociception induced by microinjection of substance P into the A7 catecholamine cell group in the rat. *Neuroscience.* 1992; 49:681-691.
11. Coplan JD, Papp LA, Martinez J, Pine D, Rosenblum LA, Cooper T, Liebowitz MR, Gorman JM. Persistence of decreased human growth hormone (HGH) response to clonidine in fluoxetine-treated panic disorder patients. *Am J Psychiatry.* 1995;152:619-622.
12. Coplan JD, Pine D, Papp LA, Rosenblum LA, Cooper T, Gorman JM. Noradrenergic/HPA axis uncoupling in panic disorder. *Neuropsychopharmacology.* 1995;13: 65-73.
13. Aulakh CS, Hill JL, Murphy DL. Attenuation of clonidine-induced growth hormone release following chronic glucocorticoid and 5-hydroxytryptamine uptake-inhibiting antidepressant treatments. *Neuroendocrinology.* 1994;59: 35-41.
14. Pilc A. The role of α_2-adrenoceptors in the mechanism of action of antidepressant drugs. *Pol J Pharmacol.* 1987;39:691-713.
15. Uhde TW, Tancer ME, Rubinow DR, et al. Evidence for hypothalamo-growth hormone dysfunction in panic disorder: profile of growth hormone responses to clonidine, yohimbine, caffeine, glucose, GRF and TRH in panic disorder patients versus healthy volunteers. *Neuropsychopharmacology.* 1992;6:101-118.
16. Abelson JL, Glitz D, Cameron OG, Lee MA, Bronzo M, Curtis GC. Endocrine, cardiovascular and behavioral responses to clonidine in patients with panic disorder. *Biol Psychiatry.* 1992;32:18-25.
17. Spitzer RL, Williams JBW, Gibbon M, First M. *SCID: User's Guide for the Structured Clinical Interview for DSM-III-R.* Washington, DC: American Psychiatric Press; 1990.
18. Schneier FR, Liebowitz MR, Davies SO, et al. Fluoxetine in panic disorder. *J Clin Psychopharmacol.* 1990;10:119-121.
19. Jimerson DC, Markey SP, Oliver JA, et al. Simultaneous measurement of plasma 3-hydroxy-4-methoxyphenylglycol and 3, 4-dihydroxyphenylethylene glycol by gas chromatography mass spectrometry. *Biomed Mass Spectrom.* 1981;8:256-259.
20. Murphy BE. Some studies of the protein binding of steroids and their application to the micro and ultramicro measurement of various binding radio assay. *J Clin Neuroendocrinol Metab.* 1967;27:973-990.
21. von Neumann J, Kent RH, Bellinson HR, Hart BI. The mean square successive difference. *Ann Math Stat.* 1941;12:442-451.
22. Rifkin A, Quitkin F, Carrillo C, Blumberg A, Klein DF. Lithium carbonate in emotionally unstable character disorder. *Arch Gen Psychiatry.* 1972;27:519-523.
23. Siever LJ, Trestman RL, Coccaro EF, et al. The growth hormone response to clonidine in acute and remitted depressed male patients. *Neuropsychopharmacology.* 1992;6:165-177.
24. Klein DF. Cybernetics, activation and drug effects. *Acta Psychiatrica Scand.* 1988; 77:126-137.
25. Coplan JD, Gorman JM, Klein DF. Serotonin-related function in panic disorder: a critical overview. *Neuropsychopharmacology.* 1992;6:189-200.
26. Goddard AW, Woods SW, Sholomkas DE, Goodman WK, Charney DS, Heninger GR. Effects of the serotonin reuptake inhibitor fluvoxamine on yohimbine-induced anxiety in panic disorder. *Psychiatry Res.* 1993;48:119-133.
27. Trestman RL, Yehuda R, Coccaro E, Horvath T, Knott P, Gabriel S, Siever LJ. Diurnal neuroendocrine and autonomic function in acute and remitted depressed males. *Biol Psychiatry.* 1995;37:448-456.
28. Gorman JM, Papp LA, Coplan JD, Martinez JM, Lennon S, Goetz RR, Klein DF. Anxiogenic effects of carbon dioxide and hyperventilation in panic patients. *Am J Psychiatry.* 1994;151:547-553.

ORIGINAL ARTICLE

Disrupted Pattern of D_2 Dopamine Receptors in the Temporal Lobe in Schizophrenia

A Postmortem Study

Sara K. Goldsmith, PhD; Raymond M. Shapiro, MD, PhD; Jeffrey N. Joyce, PhD

Background: Anatomical substrates for the clinical efficacy of D_2 dopamine receptor antagonism in ameliorating positive symptoms, including auditory hallucinations, in schizophrenia are not fully known. We previously identified a modular organization of D_2 receptors unique to the temporal lobe. The dense bands of D_2 receptors showed highest frequency in auditory and speech association cortices (Brodmann areas 22, 39, and 42) and auditory-visual association areas (Brodmann areas 20 and 37) but were rarely found in somatosensory association regions (Brodmann area 21). Since the anatomical localization of these bands mirrors the presumed sites underlying hallucinations in schizophrenia, the modular and laminar distribution of D_2 receptors was studied in the temporal cortex in the brains of schizophrenic and control subjects.

Methods: Tissue obtained post mortem from 12 elderly schizophrenic subjects and 13 controls matched for age and postmortem interval was examined by quantitative receptor autoradiography for D_2 receptor binding with [^{125}I]epidepride. All regions of the temporal lobe were sampled in all cases.

Results: Schizophrenic cases exhibited significantly disrupted patterns of D_2 receptors in the perirhinal, superior, and inferior temporal cortices, including disrupted patterns in the modular D_2 receptor bands. The schizophrenic cases had reduced concentrations of D_2 receptors in the supragranular layers and elevated concentrations of D_2 receptors in the granular layer in isocortical regions of the temporal lobe. This disruption does not appear to be due to long-term treatment with antipsychotic drugs and is regionally specific as there were no differences between groups for concentrations or patterns of expression in the hippocampal complex.

Conclusions: Blockade of the disrupted distribution of D_2 receptors in auditory and auditory-visual association cortices is a likely mechanism for the clinical efficacy of D_2 antagonists in reducing hallucinations. The regionally specific, aberrant pattern of D_2 receptors may be a symptom of anomalous cortical development in these regions.

Arch Gen Psychiatry. 1997;54:649-658

From the Department of Psychiatry and the Center for Neurobiology and Behavior, University of Pennsylvania School of Medicine, Philadelphia. Dr Goldsmith is now a Science and Engineering Congressional Fellow, Washington, DC. Dr Shapiro is now with East Ridge Health Systems, Martinsburg, WVa, and Dr Joyce is now with the Christopher Center for Parkinson's Disease Research, Sun City, Ariz.

THE DOPAMINE (DA) hypothesis of schizophrenia has been based largely on pharmacological evidence that manipulations of DA systems either augment or depress the symptoms of schizophrenia.[1-4] The evidence that antipsychotic drugs have high affinity for members of the D_2 dopamine receptor family has focused on their involvement in the disorder. However, the anatomical localization of these antipsychotic effects via D_2 receptors remains undefined.

Studies in rats implicate both mesolimbic and/or nigrostriatal DA pathways in pharmacological actions of antipsychotic drugs.[5,6] This is supported by reports of elevations in D_2-like receptors in the postmortem schizophrenic brain.[7,8] There is limited evidence, however, that these changes in receptor number are directly involved in the production of psychotic symptoms. Increasing evidence including in vivo imaging studies favors limbic over striatal DA circuits in the production of positive psychotic symptoms.[9-12] In addition, there are anatomical abnormalities in limbic structures of the medial temporal lobe that suggest a neurodevelopmental disorder.[13] Neurons in these regions in schizophrenic individuals underexpress a number of markers of cell integrity, including microtubule-associated protein (MAP-2),[14] synapsin,[15] and the embryonic form of neural cell adhesion molecule.[16] In addition, various regions of the parahippocampus exhibit reduced cell number and altered laminar arrangement of neurons.[17-20]

We have identified a highly organized modular pattern of D_2 receptors in the medial temporal lobe of the normal postmortem brain,[21] including D_2 receptor–enriched and poor bands, which are unique to isocortical regions of the temporal lobe.[22] The D_2 bands appear to be another example of iterative cortical elements that play a role in feature extraction. Hence, this modular organization of D_2 receptors may

SUBJECTS AND METHODS

CASE MATERIAL

Brain tissue was obtained from each of 13 control subjects (10 males, 3 females) and 12 schizophrenic subjects (5 males, 7 females) (**Table**). Control case subjects had no known history of neurologic or psychiatric disease and died of natural causes. Schizophrenic brain tissue was derived post mortem from long-term, institutionalized patients.[25] These individuals met *DSM-III-R*[26] criteria for a primary diagnosis of schizophrenia for all of their adult lives, which was established by standardized chart review and caretaker interviews. Diagnostic gross and microscopic neuropathological examination, including visual inspection for neuron loss, gliosis, vascular accidents, and tumors, confirmed the absence of neuropathological abnormalities in the tissue.[27] Alzheimer disease pathology identified by senile plaque and neurofibrillary tangle density was strikingly absent in this group of schizophrenics. Notably, the hippocampus, which invariably shows the highest density of neurofibrillary tangles of any area of the brain in Alzheimer disease,[28] was virtually absent of such pathological characteristics in these schizophrenic cases. Antipsychotic drug treatment given in average daily chlorpromazine equivalents (milligrams)[29] was calculated as the range of doses determined at 3 time points: within 72 hours of death, 1 month prior to death, and 1 year prior to death.

Schizophrenic subjects were significantly older at death than control subjects (t=2.98, $P \leq .01$, 23 *df*). There were also significant age differences when male and female subjects were examined separately, although the direction differed across groups. Schizophrenic males were significantly older than control males (t=4.63, $P \leq .001$, 13 *df*), whereas schizophrenic females (mean±SD, 75.86±3.27 years) were significantly younger than control females (82.33±2.309 years) (t=3.46, $P \leq .01$, 8 *df*). There was no significant difference in postmortem interval between schizophrenic and control cases. With regard to brain weight, there was no significant effect of group, but there was a significant effect of gender (F=13.44, $P \leq .002$) and no significant interaction between group and gender (schizophrenic males, 1278.00±58.48 g [mean±SD]; schizophrenic females, 1128.57±63.10 g; control males, 1363.40±147.57 g; and control females, 1166.67±80.83 g).

Receptor Autoradiography

Each case was represented with tissue blocks from 3 to 7 rostral-caudal levels of the temporal lobe. D_2 receptors were labeled with [^{125}I]epidepride as previously published.[21,22,30] Tissue sections from all cases were processed simultaneously by incubating 20-μm-thick slide mounted tissue sections with [^{125}I]epidepride at a concentration approximately twice the K_D for the D_2 receptor (80-99 pmol/L, 2200 Ci/mmol) for 60 minutes at 30°C. Idazoxan (100 nmol/L) was included to block binding to α-adrenergic receptors. Previous studies have shown that under the conditions used, [^{125}I]epidepride is labeling a single population of D_2-like receptors within the temporal cortex. [^{125}I]epidepride binding to D_3 receptors is not detectable in the cortex of the human brain.[31] Our studies have established that the affinity of [^{125}I]epidepride to the human D_4 receptor is more than 100 times lower than that to D_2 or D_3 receptors (K_D of 5.4 nmol/L).[8] Thus, at the concentrations used, only binding to D_2 receptors was detected. Sections and high specific activity tritiated hydrogen-plastic standards (American Radiolabeled Chemicals, St Louis, Mo) were apposed to autoradiography film (Hyperfilm, Amersham Life Sciences, Arlington Heights, Ill) for 1 week. Films were developed in developer for 4 minutes at 15°C, stopped in distilled water,

provide a mechanism for functional regulation of compartments within these regions by DA. The D_2 bands have their greatest frequency in auditory association cortex, next highest frequency in auditory-visual areas, and very low incidence in somatosensory association areas. The anatomical distribution of these D_2 bands correlates with that of the locus for other markers of neural systems subserving hallucinatory activity in schizophrenia.[23,24] Since there have been several recent reports indicating that these same regions exhibit an altered laminar arrangement of neurons, we used receptor autoradiography to determine if there was a disrupted laminar pattern of D_2 receptors in the temporal cortex, including that within the D_2 bands, in postmortem schizophrenic tissue.

RESULTS

D_2 DA RECEPTOR–RICH CORTICAL BANDS

A detailed analysis of the D_2 receptor–enriched bands of the association regions of the superior and inferior cortices in normal humans is reported elsewhere.[22] D_2 receptor–enriched bands were defined by an almost 2-fold increase in concentrations of D_2 receptors as compared with the immediately adjacent region (F=113.47, $P \leq .001$) (Figure 1, **Figure 2**, A and C, and **Figure 3**, E). These D_2 receptor–enriched bands were restricted to the temporal lobe and were distributed heterogeneously across isocortical regions with the highest frequency of bands observed in higher-order auditory association areas 22 and 42 in the superior temporal gyrus. Adjacent Nissl-stained sections show that the bands exhibit a well-defined granular layer IV, with consistently lower concentrations of D_2 receptors over the granular layer (**Figure 4**).

D_2 DA receptor–enriched bands were found in schizophrenic tissue but differed on 2 characteristics—laminar pattern and band width. There was no main effect of diagnosis for concentrations of D_2 receptors in the bands when the analysis was collapsed across all laminae. There was a less distinct laminar differentiation in the bands in schizophrenic cases (in Figure 2, compare D with C). The interaction between diagnosis and laminae was significant (F=6.55, $P \leq .001$), with lower concentrations of D_2 receptors in laminae I-II of schizophrenic cases (**Figure 5**, A and C). In addition, in the superior temporal cortex there were higher concentrations of D_2 receptors in lamina IV of the D_2 receptor–enriched bands (Figure 2, D, and Figure 5, C). The altered laminar arrangement of receptors did not appear to reflect a poorly defined laminar arrangement of neurons as the schizophrenic cases did exhibit a well-defined granular layer (Figure 4, B). There was an al-fixed in fixer (Kodak GBX) and washed. All binding values are reported in femtomoles per milligram of protein.

Histological Stains

To aid in the identification of the regions, analyzed sections adjacent to those processed for receptor autoradiography were stained with cresyl violet acetate or Timm stain (for hippocampus only). Timm staining for heavy metals was performed on alternate sections to those used for autoradiography for identification of hippocampal subregions as described in detail elsewhere.[32] Slide-mounted sections alternate to those used for histochemistry and autoradiography were stained with 0.5% cresyl violet acetate for anatomical analysis of the adjacent autoradiograms.

STATISTICAL ANALYSES

Analysis of the generated autoradiograms was performed by digitizing the film image with a computer-based image analysis system.[21,22] The mean optical density of each brain region of interest was converted to a value of femtomoles per milligram of protein from a standard curve.[33] Sections from all cases were divided along the rostral-caudal axis of the temporal lobe into 4 levels that corresponded to plates 5 to 13, 13 to 25, 25 to 31, and 31 to 35 of the atlas of Roberts and Hanaway.[34] For each of the 4 rostral-caudal levels, a minimum of 4 samples (4 sections for total binding and 2 sections for nonspecific binding established 1 sample) were analyzed for each level of each case. The average specific binding was defined as total binding minus nonspecific binding for each region of interest within the temporal lobe. The regions of interest were identified a priori based on previous studies of the distribution of D_2 receptors in the hippocampus, parahippocampus, and temporal cortex complex.[21,22,30] The criteria for analysis of the hippocampus and parahippocampus are presented in those articles (5 regions: dentate gyrus, hilus, CA3, CA1, and subiculum). The parahippocampus was analyzed as 2 regions (entorhinal cortex, perirhinal cortex) and 6 laminae. The D_2 bands of the inferior, middle, and superior temporal cortices were analyzed similarly. The D_2 receptor–enriched bands of the temporal isocortex were identified and quantified as detailed elsewhere (**Figure 1**).[22] Laminar analysis of the concentration of D_2 receptors was made by examining the adjacent Nissl-stained slides overlaid by the autoradiographic film.

Main effects of diagnosis (control vs schizophrenia), region, laminar organization within each region, and laminar organization of D_2-enriched bands for concentrations of D_2 receptor binding were tested for significance by means of a repeated-measures analysis of variance. Effects of postmortem interval, age, and brain weight on D_2 receptor concentration were examined with regression analyses. The frequency of bands in each gyrus of the temporal lobe was estimated as the mean percent incidence of D_2 bands per gyrus (number of bands observed divided by number of rostral-caudal planes sampled for that area in each case). Differences across control and schizophrenic groups in mean percent incidence of D_2 bands across temporal gyri were tested with analysis of variance. Post hoc comparisons were tested for significant differences using the Scheffé F test at the 99% confidence level. Tests for significant differences in the frequency distribution of the widths of the D_2 receptor–enriched bands between groups were made by χ^2 analysis. Specific binding of [^{125}I]epidepride to D_2 receptors (total–nonspecific) in control tissues was 90.23%±7.89% (mean±SD), and was not different from the schizophrenic cases (85.67%±8.23%). In the present sample, there were no significant effects of age, hemisphere, postmortem interval, gender, or brain weight on concentration of D_2 receptors for control or schizophrenic cases in any region examined.

Cases Matched for Postmortem Interval (PMI)

Control Subjects*				Schizophrenic Subjects					
Case No./ Sex/Age, y	PMI, h	Hemisphere	Cause of Death	Case No./ Sex/Age, y	PMI, h	Hemisphere	Cause of Death	Age at Onset, y	Chlorpromazine Equivalents†
1/M/59	14.0	R	Pulmonary embolism	1/F/74	14.0	L	Pneumonia	18	600
2/M/56	12.0	R	Cardiac arrest	2/F/76	12.0	R	Perforated bowel	16	200-300
3/F/85	11.0	L	Pulmonary embolism	3/M/71	11.5	R	Septic shock	20	1350-1700
4/F/81	22.0	R	Cardiac arrest	4/F/79	22.0	R	Cardiac arrest	24	200
5/M/68	18.0	R	Pneumonia	5/M/78	18.0	R	Pneumonia	21	0
6/M/64	15.0	R	Cancer	6/F/72	15.0	R	Cardiac arrest	20	250-300
7/M/60	16.0	R	Cardiac arrest	7/M/74	14.0	L	Cardiac arrest	21	100
8/M/70	18.5	R	Multiple organ failure	8/F/73	14.5	L	Pneumonia	24	100-250
9/M/37	8.0	L	Renal failure	...	...	...	...	...	...
10/F/81	3.0	L	Cardiac arrest	10/F/82	7.0	R	Cardiac arrest	20	0-25
11/M/54	2.0	R	Cancer	11/M/79	7.0	L	Pneumonia	22	0-100
12/M/67	8.0	L	Cancer	12/M/83	7.0	L	Pneumonia	30	0
13/M/65	10.5	L	Cardiac arrest	13/F/75	10.0	R	Sepsis	33	300
Mean±SD 65.1±13.0	12.1±5.9			Mean±SD 76.3±14.0	12.8±4.6				

*Control case subjects had no known history of neurologic or psychiatric disease and died of natural causes.
†All values are the range of average daily chlorpromazine equivalents during year prior to death.

tered cortical distribution of the bands in schizophrenic cases, with a reduced incidence of bands in the superior and inferior temporal gyri (in Figure 2, compare B with A). The highest incidence of bands relative to all regions of temporal cortex in control and schizophrenic cases was found in the superior temporal gyrus (con-

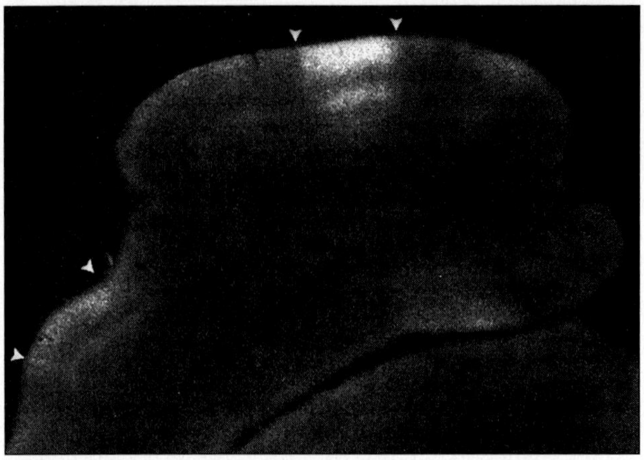

Figure 1. *Examples of 2 D_2 dopamine receptor bands (delimited by arrowheads) in a control case in auditory association cortices (Brodmann area 42 dorsally and area 52 medially). In dark-field photomicrographs, increasing densities of [^{125}I]epidepride binding to D_2 receptors appear as lighter areas. The D_2 bands unique to temporal isocortex appear as "columns" of dense binding of [^{125}I]epidepride to D_2 receptors in the coronal plane and were observed throughout the rostral-caudal extent of the temporal lobe. The bands were identified by the boundary between the column of dense concentrations of [^{125}I]epidepride binding to D_2 receptors and the immediately adjacent region of lower binding. These bands were often superimposed on the already existing laminar pattern of binding, but concentrations of [^{125}I]epidepride binding within the bands were 1.5 to 2.5 times higher than the immediately adjacent region and show a different laminar pattern, due to the higher concentration of [^{125}I]epidepride binding in layer III of the bands than in the immediately adjacent cortex. In addition, the columns were aligned in adjacent coronal sections, revealing their 3-dimensional modular structure extending at least 2500 μm in the anteroposterior plane.*[22]

trols vs schizophrenics, 138.30%±50.00% vs 100.80%±67.58%), followed by the lateral occipital (41.50%±52.90% vs 48.70%±50.20%), inferior (54.2%±45.50% vs 27.10%±40.27%), and middle (10.00%±30.00% vs 15.33%±26.15%) temporal gyri. Regression analyses for the control and schizophrenic groups revealed no significant effects of age, brain weight, or dementia in the schizophrenic cases on the number of D_2 bands or D_2 receptor concentrations. In 2 schizophrenic cases (cases 1 and 8), no bands could be identified. This was unlikely to be due to sampling error since 3 to 5 levels were sampled, and control cases with 3 to 5 levels sampled exhibited from 3 to 12 bands. In addition, all control cases exhibited bands. Schizophrenic cases exhibited a significantly different distribution of band widths (χ^2=39.45, $P\leq.02$). There was a shift toward increase in the percentage of wide bands and a decrease in the percentage of narrower bands.

PATTERN OF D_2 DA RECEPTOR DISTRIBUTION IN HIPPOCAMPUS AND TEMPORAL ISOCORTEX

The hippocampus of control and schizophrenic cases exhibited the same cytoarchitectonically defined pattern of D_2 receptors with significant differences across subregions for both groups (F=10.05, $P<.001$) (**Figure 6**). There was no main effect of diagnosis on concentrations of D_2 receptors in hippocampus. There were low levels of specific [^{125}I]epidepride binding to D_2 receptors in the entorhinal cortex of control cases (**Figure 7**, A, C, and E) and schizophrenic cases (Figure 7, B, D, and F). There were no differences between groups.

In control tissue, the concentrations of D_2 receptors were elevated at the border of the entorhinal cortex and the transentorhinal cortex coincident with the appearance of an internal granular layer IV. At this cytoarchitectonic juncture, a trilaminar pattern of D_2 receptors became evident (Figure 7, A, C, and E), was well developed in the perirhinal cortical regions 35 and 36, and continued throughout the other isocortical regions of the temporal lobe. In the control group, the highest concentrations of [^{125}I]epidepride were in perirhinal layers I-II, the lowest concentrations were in layers III-IV, and there were slightly increased values in layers V-VI (Figure 5, E). Post hoc tests revealed a significant difference between concentration of D_2 receptors in laminae I-II compared with lamina III, and/or lamina IV in control cases (I-II vs III: Scheffé F=2.76, $P\leq.04$; I-II vs IV: Scheffé F=2.75, $P\leq.04$). This pattern was significantly disrupted in schizophrenic cases (lamina × diagnosis interaction, F=9.87, $P<.001$). The concentration of D_2 receptors was significantly reduced in laminae I-II of the schizophrenic cases, apparent in the transentorhinal cortex (controls, 6.92±3.22; schizophrenics, 3.85±1.96, Scheffé F=7.06, $P\leq.02$), and throughout the perirhinal cortex (Figure 5, E, and Figure 7, B). Similarly, for other regions of temporal isocortex, the pattern of D_2 receptors was significantly disrupted in the schizophrenic group (lamina × diagnosis interaction: F=8.67, $P<.001$), with lower concentrations in laminae I-II, compared with the control group (Figure 5, B and D).

When individual schizophrenic cases were examined with control cases matched for postmortem interval (Table), there were 2 patterns of disruption evident. In 6 of the schizophrenic cases (cases 1, 5, 7, 8, 10, and 13), diminution of the laminar patterning was due to very low concentrations of D_2 receptors across all cortical laminae, as seen in the inferior temporal cortex (Figure 3, B), but normal concentrations of D_2 receptors in the hippocampus. In the other cases, however, there was an aberrantly high expression of D_2 receptors in the internal granule layer IV, as seen in photomicrographs of [^{125}I]epidepride binding in the inferior temporal gyrus of 2 matched cases (Figure 3, E and F). This was never observed in the control cases. Despite the altered laminar patterning of D_2 receptor, the identification of the internal granule layer was easily made in the adjacent Nissl-stained sections of all control and schizophrenic cases (Figure 4).

COMMENT

Our results demonstrate that the modular and laminar pattern of D_2 receptors in the temporal lobe, including the D_2 receptor–enriched bands, is disrupted in a group of elderly schizophrenic subjects without a similar disruption in the hippocampus. The tissue used for this study was derived from an aged and long-term institutionalized population, most of whom exhibited a severe illness and pronounced cognitive impairment. In addition, all schizophrenic subjects had long treatment histories that included long-term use of antipsychotics. Despite these limitations, it is unlikely that the observed differences are due to long-term drug treatment. Regression analyses revealed no significant relationship between drug dosages and D_2 receptor concentrations in any region or number of D_2 receptor–enriched bands. There was also no relationship

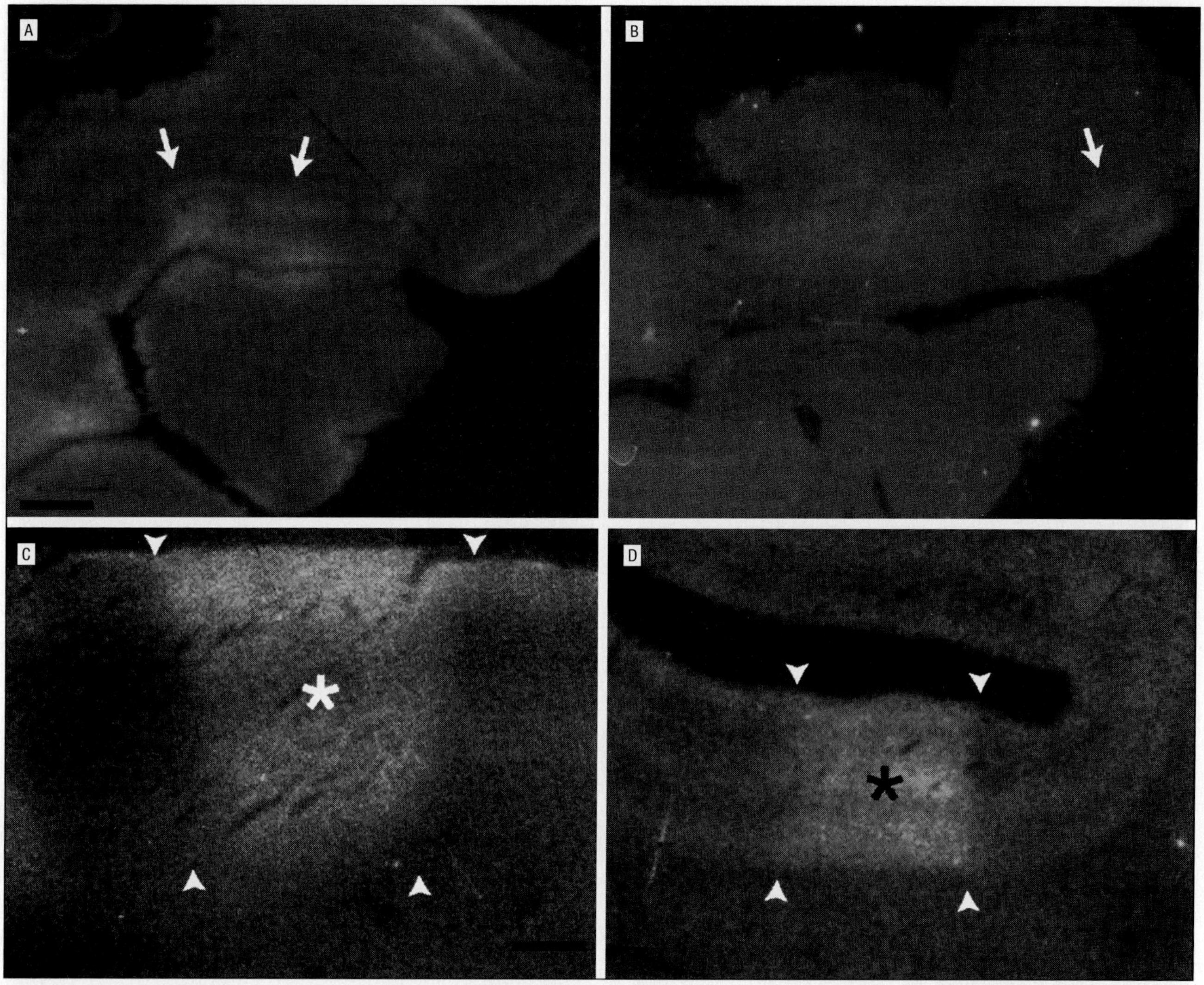

Figure 2. *Dark-field photomicrographs of [^{125}I]epidepride binding to D_2 dopamine receptors in the D_2 receptor–enriched bands in the multimodal association region of Brodmann area 42 of 2 control (A, C) and schizophrenic (B, D) cases matched for age and postmortem interval. In a coronal section, 2 such bands are marked with arrows in control case 11 (A), as compared with the single band of markedly lower contrast, of D_2 receptors within a band (arrow) in schizophrenic case 11 (B). The D_2 receptor–enriched bands, defined by an almost 2-fold increase in concentrations of D_2 receptors in the supragranular and infragranular layers vs the immediately adjacent region (C, arrowheads demarcate border), and a lower concentration of D_2 receptors over the granular layer (C, asterisk), were disrupted in schizophrenics. As depicted in photomicrograph D (case 4), some cases exhibited a less distinct laminar appearance due to the elevated concentrations of D_2 receptors over the granular layer (asterisk). A and B, bar=3.5 mm; C and D, 1.0 mm.*

between drug history and the degree of disruption of D_2 receptor patterns in the schizophrenic cases. The lack of difference between the schizophrenic and control groups in D_2 receptor concentrations in the hippocampus also helps rule out a general drug effect. Unlike observations in the striatum of schizophrenic patients who had received long-term treatment with antipsychotic drugs,[7] we did not find any evidence of elevated concentrations of D_2 receptors in the parahippocampus or temporal lobe. Our present results also differ from our observations for D_3 receptor concentrations in the striatum where antemortem drug history was the primary determinant of receptor levels.[8] D_3 receptors were elevated in drug-free schizophrenics as compared with controls or schizophrenics receiving antipsychotics near the time of death. This suggests the changes in D_2 receptor expression in the medial temporal lobe are not related to long-term treatment with antipsychotic drugs.

Alzheimer disease was ruled out in the present schizophrenic cases. Arnold and colleagues[27] found that Alzheimer disease pathology, measured by the number of neurofibrillary plaques and tangles, and anatomical distribution, was strikingly absent in this group of demented schizophrenics. Notably, the hippocampus, which invariably shows the highest density of neurofibrillary tangles of any area of the brain in Alzheimer disease,[28] was virtually absent of such pathology in these schizophrenic cases. In addition, neither the concentration nor anatomical distribution of D_2 receptors in the hippocampus differed between schizophrenics and controls. This stands in contrast to what is observed in Alzheimer disease, where there are significant losses of D_2 receptors in the hippocampus and all laminae of the parahippocampus and temporal lobe (Amanda Myers and J.N.J., unpublished results, December 1993).[30]

The present sample of schizophrenic subjects showed a significant reduction in whole brain weight. A loss in tissue volume alone, would, if anything, artificially *increase* measures of the apparent concentration of D_2 receptors. Hence, the evidence for a disrupted laminar patterning of

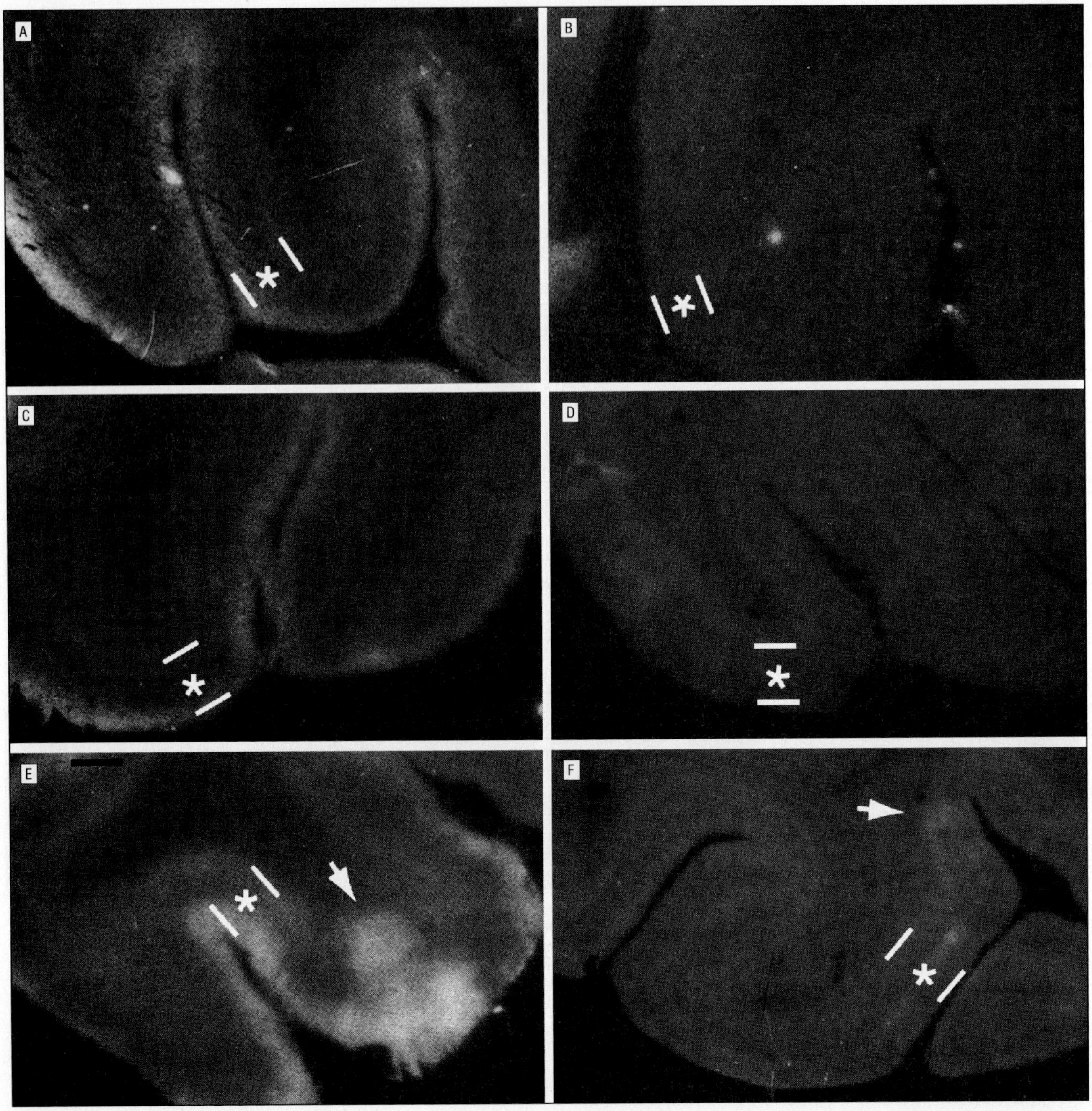

Figure 3. *Dark-field photomicrographs of [^{125}I]epidepride binding to D_2 dopamine receptors in inferior temporal cortex (Brodmann area 20) of 3 control (A, C, and E) and schizophrenic (B, D, and F) cases matched for age and postmortem interval. In control cases, there was a robust trilaminar pattern of D_2 receptors with highest levels in external laminae I-II, lowest in III-IV, and moderate levels in deep layers V-VI. An asterisk between parallel bars marks granule cell layer with lowest concentration of D_2 receptors in controls. The trilaminar pattern of D_2 receptors was disrupted in schizophrenics. In case 1 (A and B) and case 7 (C and D), the concentration of D_2 receptor is reduced in the external laminae of the schizophrenic cases. In case 4 (E and F), an elevated concentration of D_2 receptors is evident over the granule cell layer of the schizophrenic case (bar=5 mm). E and F, the shift from the diffuse laminar pattern of D_2 receptors to the modular organization is indicated by an arrow.*

D_2 receptors in the absence of an elevation in D_2 receptor concentrations makes it unlikely that our results are due to end-stage changes in the patient population.

DISEASE-SPECIFIC EFFECTS

The altered arrangement of D_2 receptors might reflect one of several potential deficits that have already been shown to occur in neurons of this region in schizophrenia. Akbarian and associates[35] demonstrated that persons with schizophrenia showed significantly reduced expression of glutamic acid decarboxylase messenger RNA (mRNA) in the dorsolateral prefrontal cortex. This occurred without a loss of neuronal number or reduction in another mRNA (CamIIK), indicative of failure of these cells to express particular mRNAs. Pyramidal neurons of these regions may also have reduced expression of D_2 mRNA, leading to reduced protein levels.[36] Alternatively, as Arnold and associates[14] have demonstrated, the schizophrenic cases used in this study exhibited a marked reduced expression of neuronal cytoskeletal proteins in neurons of the medial temporal lobe. This might lead to a failure to transport all pro-

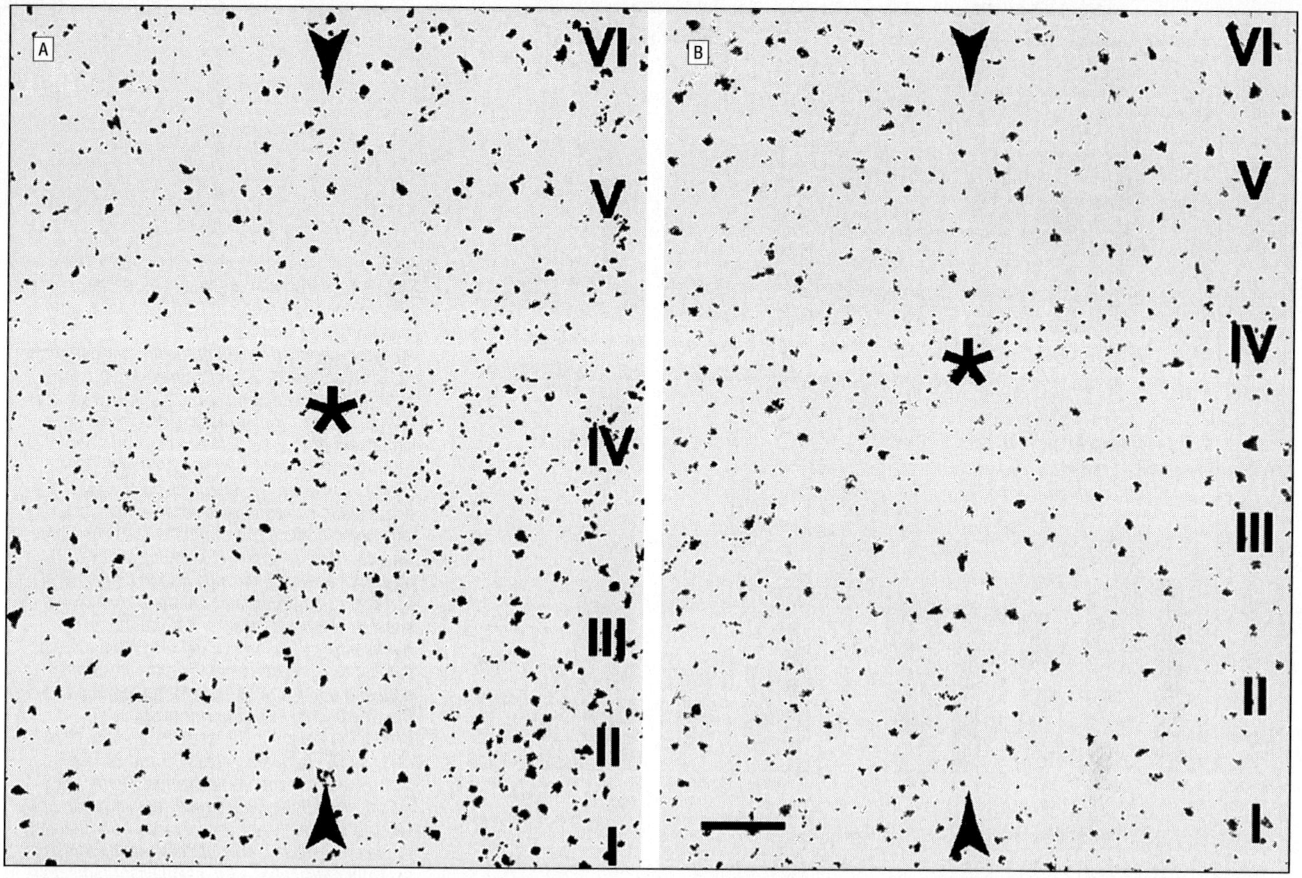

Figure 4. *Nissl-stained sections, adjacent to those used for autoradiography, to identify cytoarchitecture of the junction of the D_2 band and nonband adjacent cortex depicted in Figure 2, C and D (Brodmann area 42). A and B, The arrowheads coincide with the left border of the D_2 bands in Figure 2, C, and D, respectively. The Nissl-stained sections show that the bands exhibit a well-defined granular layer IV (asterisks). All bands occurred in temporal isocortex with a distinct granule layer, regardless of whether there was an decrease in D_2 receptors over layer IV as in all control bands, or an increase as was observed in some bands in schizophrenic tissue. Bar=240 μm.*

teins, including D_2 receptors, in apical dendrites of infragranular pyramidal neurons (eg, due to loss of MAP-2) and, consequently, a reduced concentration of D_2 receptors in the supragranular layers. Neither process would, however, explain the aberrant patterns observed in some schizophrenic cases where higher than normal concentrations of D_2 receptor were identified in the granular layer. It also should be pointed out that the subiculum is a region that was particularly affected in the loss of MAP-2 and this region does not show significant alterations in D_2 receptor number in our study. Thus, other explanations, such as an altered distribution of D_2 receptor–expressing neurons, seem more likely.

The altered laminar patterning of D_2 receptors identified in the temporal lobe might be the result of, or contribute to, abnormal brain development previously reported. Recent studies of Akbarian and associates[17] supported earlier results indicative of a disturbance in the migration of neurons into the cortical plate of the medial temporal lobe in schizophrenia.[18-20] This hypothesis, based on work in fetal monkey neocortex,[37] states that there is a disturbance in the migration of immature neurons of the ventricular wall to their final position in the cortical plate resulting in an inappropriate arrangement of neurons. The altered arrangement of D_2 receptors could be related to an underrepresentation of neurons expressing D_2 receptors in supragranular layers. Dopamine acting through D_2-like receptors plays a direct role in normal cellular differentiation and morphology of cortical neurons.[38,39] This appears to include axons' elongation and connectivity. Thus, the altered laminar arrangement and underexpression of D_2 receptors may lead to further alterations in brain development.

The DA hypothesis of schizophrenia in its classic formulation (DA hyperactivity in schizophrenia) is thought to be more relevant to the pathophysiology of positive rather than negative symptoms. However, negative symptoms can sometimes be improved by drugs that stimulate the DA system.[1,4] Therefore, several theories have been advanced to explain how schizophrenia could be associated with both an excess and a deficiency of dopaminergic activity. Several reformulations of the DA hypothesis of schizophrenia have been proposed, emphasizing a dysfunction between cortical and subcortical DA transmission.[5,6,40] The DA hypothesis of schizophrenia in its classic formulation is also difficult to reconcile with a neurodevelopmental model that is based on an increasing body of in vivo[41] and postmortem evidence.[17-20] Our results may provide a way to reconcile these disparate areas of research. Our study reveals that there are significant, regionally specific disturbances in the distribution and expression of D_2 receptors in temporal lobe regions (particularly of D_2 receptor–enriched bands) that have been linked with auditory hallucinations, reduced tissue volume, altered glucose metabolism, and altered auditory-evoked potentials.[9,11,23,24,42-44] Glucose metabolism in these same

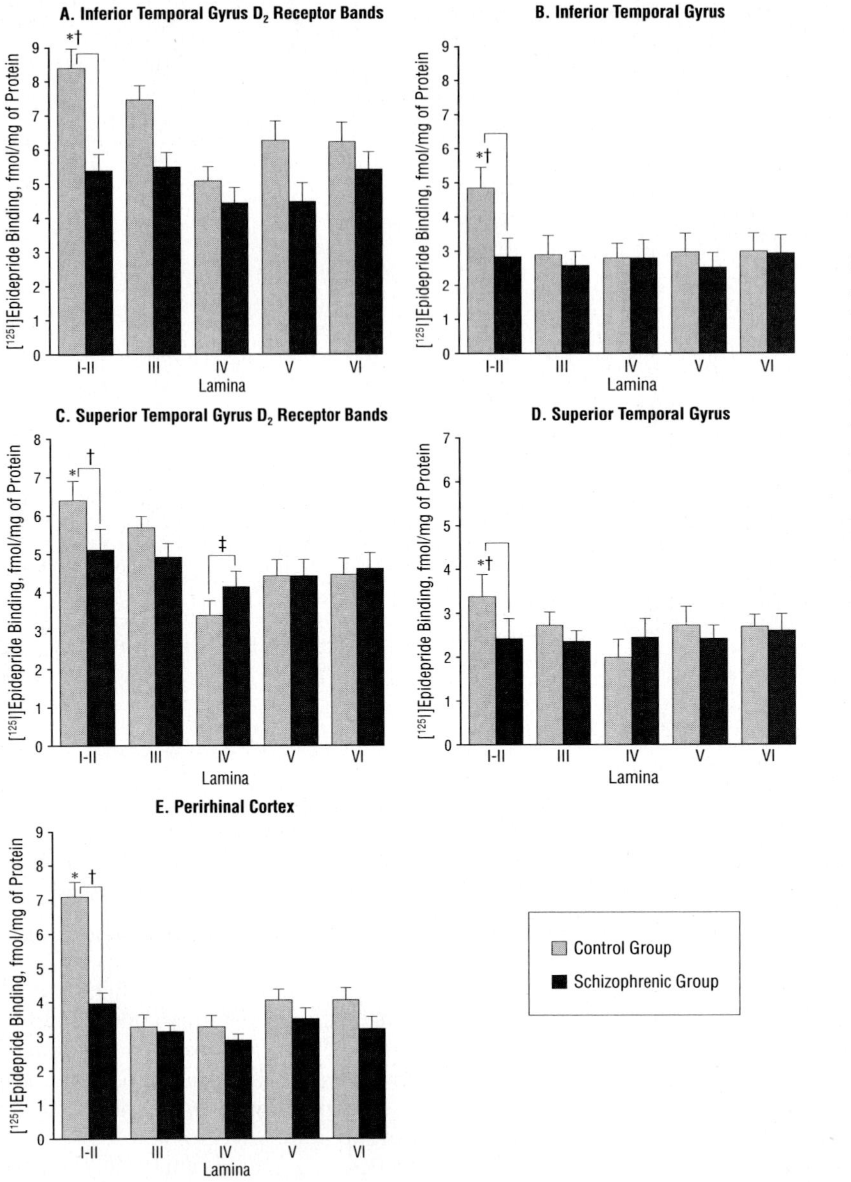

Figure 5. *Bar graphs of the mean±SEM for [125I]epidepride binding to D_2 dopamine receptors in the different laminae of the D_2 receptor–enriched bands of the inferior temporal (A, Brodmann area 21) and superior temporal cortices (C, Brodmann areas 22, 39, and 42) for control and schizophrenic groups. There was a significant difference between concentration of D_2 receptors in laminae I-II compared with III, and/or IV in control cases. This pattern was disrupted in schizophrenic cases with a significant reduction in laminae I-II as compared with controls. In addition, concentrations of D_2 receptors were significantly less in lamina IV of controls vs schizophrenics in the D_2 bands in the superior temporal regions. Bar graphs representing the mean±SEM for [125I]epidepride binding to D_2 receptors in the different laminae of nonband regions of the inferior temporal (B, Brodmann area 20), superior temporal (D, Brodmann areas 22, 39, and 42), and perirhinal cortices (E, Brodmann areas 35 and 36) for control and schizophrenic groups. There was a significant difference between concentration of D_2 receptors in laminae I-II compared with III and/or IV in control cases. This pattern was disrupted in schizophrenic cases with a significant reduction in laminae I-II compared with controls. Asterisk indicates* $P \leq .04$*; dagger,* $P < .001$*; and double dagger,* $P \leq .05$*.*

regions of schizophrenics respond to dopaminergic agents.[10-12] We hypothesize that normal functioning at the D_2 receptor–enriched bands, found only in higher-order auditory and multimodal association cortices of the temporal lobe, serves to normally inhibit hallucinatorylike experiences. The disturbed D_2 receptor distribution in these bands in persons with schizophrenia results in a breakdown of normal functioning at these multimodal circuits, resulting in hallucinations. Blockade of D_2 receptors at the point of altered synaptic organization might reduce the functional contribution of these regions (ie, have antipsychotic actions).[45] These regions, as well as their target structures in the basal ganglia,[8,46] could functionally respond to antipsychotic agents by modifying different clusters of symptoms associated with schizophrenia.

Accepted for publication August 22, 1996.

This research was supported by grants MH 56824, MH 43880, and AG 09215 from the Public Health Service, Washington, DC.

Brain tissue was obtained from the Hospital of the University of Pennsylvania, Philadelphia (John Trojanowski, MD, PhD), and Sun Health Research Institute and Graduate Hospital (Joseph Rogers, PhD).

[125I]epidepride was a gift of Kim Neve, MD, Oregon Health Sciences University, Portland.

Reprints: Jeffrey N. Joyce, PhD, Christopher Center for Parkinson's Disease Research, Sun Health Institute, Sun City, AZ 85351.

REFERENCES

1. Angrist B, Rotrosen J, Gershon S. Differential effects of amphetamine and neuroleptics on negative vs positive symptoms in schizophrenia. *Psychopharmacology.* 1980;72:17-19.
2. Bowers MB. The role of drugs in the production of schizophreniform psychoses and related disorders. In: Meltzer HV, ed. *Psychopharmacology: The Third Generation of Progress.* New York, NY: Raven Press; 1987:819-832.
3. Snyder SH. Catecholamines in the brain as mediator of amphetamine psychosis. *Arch Gen Psychiatry.* 1973;130:61-67.

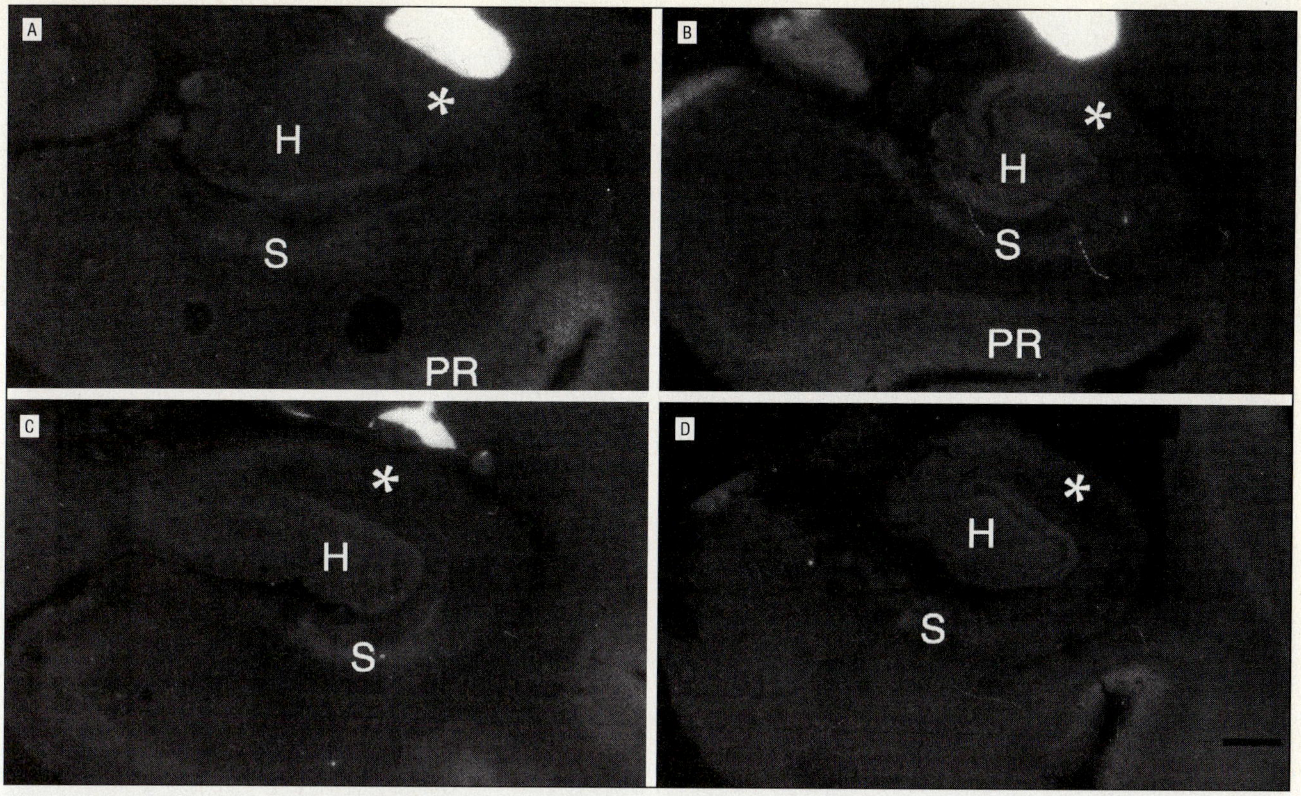

Figure 6. *Dark-field photomicrographs of [^{125}I]epidepride binding to D_2 dopamine receptors in hippocampus of 2 control (A and C) and 2 schizophrenic (B and D) cases matched for age and postmortem interval (control and schizophrenic cases 2 and 12). H indicates hilus of hippocampus; PR, perirhinal cortex; S, subiculum; asterisk, distal border of CA3 region of hippocampus; and bar, 2.1 mm. For the hippocampus, there was no evidence of a difference in concentration or pattern of D_2 receptors between groups.*

4. Tamminga CA, Schaffer MH, Smith RC, Davis JM. Schizophrenic symptoms improve with apomorphine. *Science.* 1978;200:567-568.
5. Davis KL, Kahn RS, Ko G, Davidson M. Dopamine in schizophrenia: a review and reconceptualization. *Am J Psychiatry.* 1991;148:1474-1486.
6. Grace AA. Cortical regulation of subcortical systems and its possible relevance to schizophrenia. *J Neural Transm.* 1993;91:111-134.
7. Seeman P, Bzowej NH, Guan HC, Bergeron C, Reynolds GP, Bird ED, Riederer P, Jellinger K, Tourtellote WW. Human brain D_1 and D_2 dopamine receptors in schizophrenia, Alzheimer's, Parkinson's and Huntington's disease. *Neuropsychopharmacology.* 1987;1:5-15.
8. Gurevich EV, Bordelon Y, Shapiro R, Arnold S, Gur R, Joyce JN. Mesolimbic dopamine D_3 receptors and use of antipsychotic drugs in patients with schizophrenia: a postmortem study. *Arch Gen Psychiatry.* 1997;54:225-232.
9. Gur RE, Jaggi JL, Shtasel DL, Ragland JD, Gur RC. Cerebral blood flow in schizophrenia. *Biol Psychiatry.* 1994;35:3-15.
10. Tamminga CA, Burrows GH, Chase TN, Alphs LD, Thaker GK. Dopamine neuronal tracts in schizophrenia. *Ann N Y Acad Sci.* 1988;537:443-450.
11. Tamminga CA, Thaker GK, Buchanan R, Kirkpatrick B, Alphs LD, Chase N, Carpenter WT. Limbic system abnormalities identified in schizophrenia using positron emission tomography with fluorodeoxyglucose and neocortical alterations with deficit syndrome. *Arch Gen Psychiatry.* 1992;49:522-530.
12. Wolkin A, Sanfilipo M, Angrist B, Duncan E, Wieland S, Wolf AP, Brodie JD, Copper TB, Laska E, Rostrosen JP. Acute d-amphetamine challenge in schizophrenia. *Biol Psychiatry.* 1994;36:317-332.
13. Shapiro RM. Regional neuropathology in schizophrenia: where are we? where are we going? *Schizophr Res.* 1993;10:187-239.
14. Arnold SE, Lee VM, Gur RE, Trojanowski JQ. Abnormal expression of two microtubule-associated proteins (MAP2 and MAP5) in specific subfields of the hippocampal formation in schizophrenia. *Proc Natl Acad Sci U S A.* 1991;88:10850-10854.
15. Browning MD, Dudek EM, Rapier JL, Leonard S, Freedman R. Significant reduction in synapsin but not synaptophysin specific activity in the brains of some schizophrenics. *Biol Psychiatry.* 1993;34:529-535.
16. Barbeau D, Liang JJ, Robitaille Y, Quiron R, Srivastava LK. Decreased expression of the embryonic form of the neural cell adhesion molecule in schizophrenic brains. *Proc Natl Acad Sci U S A.* 1995;92:2785-2789.
17. Akbarian S, Vinuela A, Kim JJ, Potkin SG, Bunney WE Jr, Jones EG. Distorted distribution of nicotinamide-adenine dinucleotide phosphate-diaphorase neurons in temporal lobe of schizophrenics implies anomalous cortical development. *Arch Gen Psychiatry.* 1993;50:178-187.
18. Arnold SE, Hyman BT, Van Hoesen GW, Damasio AR. Some cytoarchitectural abnormalities of the entorhinal cortex in schizophrenia. *Arch Gen Psychiatry.* 1991;48:625-632.
19. Jacob H, Beckmann H. Prenatal development disturbances in the limbic allocortex in schizophrenics. *J Neural Transm.* 1986;65:154-161.
20. Jakob H, Beckmann H. Gross and histological criteria for developmental disorders in brains of schizophrenics. *J R Soc Med.* 1989;82:466-469.
21. Goldsmith SK, Joyce JN. D_2 receptor expression in hippocampus and parahippocampal cortices of human, rat and cat in comparison with tyrosine hydroxylase immunoreactive fibers. *Hippocampus.* 1994;4:1-20.
22. Goldsmith S, Joyce JN. Dopamine D_2 receptors are organized in bands in normal human temporal cortex. *Neuroscience.* 1996;74:435-451.
23. Barta PE, Pearlson GD, Powers RE, Richards S, Tune LE. Auditory hallucinations and smaller superior temporal gyral volume in schizophrenia. *Am J Psychiatry.* 1990;147:1457-1462.
24. McGuire PK, Shah GMS, Murray RM. Increased blood flow in Broca's area during auditory hallucinations in schizophrenia. *Lancet.* 1993;342:703-706.
25. Arnold SE, Gur RE, Shapiro RM, Fisher KR, Moberg PJ, Gibney MR, Gur RC, Blackwell P, Trojanowski, JQ. Prospective clinicopathological studies of schizophrenia: accrual and assessment. *Am J Psychiatry.* 1995;152:731-737.
26. American Psychiatric Association. *Diagnostic and Statistical Manual of Mental Disorders, Third Edition, Revised.* Washington, DC: American Psychiatric Association; 1987.
27. Arnold SE, Franz BR, Trojanowski JQ. Elderly patients with schizophrenia exhibit infrequent neurodegenerative lesions. *Neurobiol Aging.* 1994;15:299-303.
28. Arnold SE, Hyman BT, Flory J, Damasio AR, Van Hoesen GW. The topographical and neuroanatomical distribution of neurofibrillary tangles and neuritic plaques in the cerebral cortex of patients with Alzheimer's disease. *Cereb Cortex.* 1991;1:103-116.
29. Kane JM. In: Kaplan HI, Sadock BJ, eds. *Comprehensive Textbook of Psychiatry.* Baltimore, Md: Williams & Wilkins; 1989:777-792.

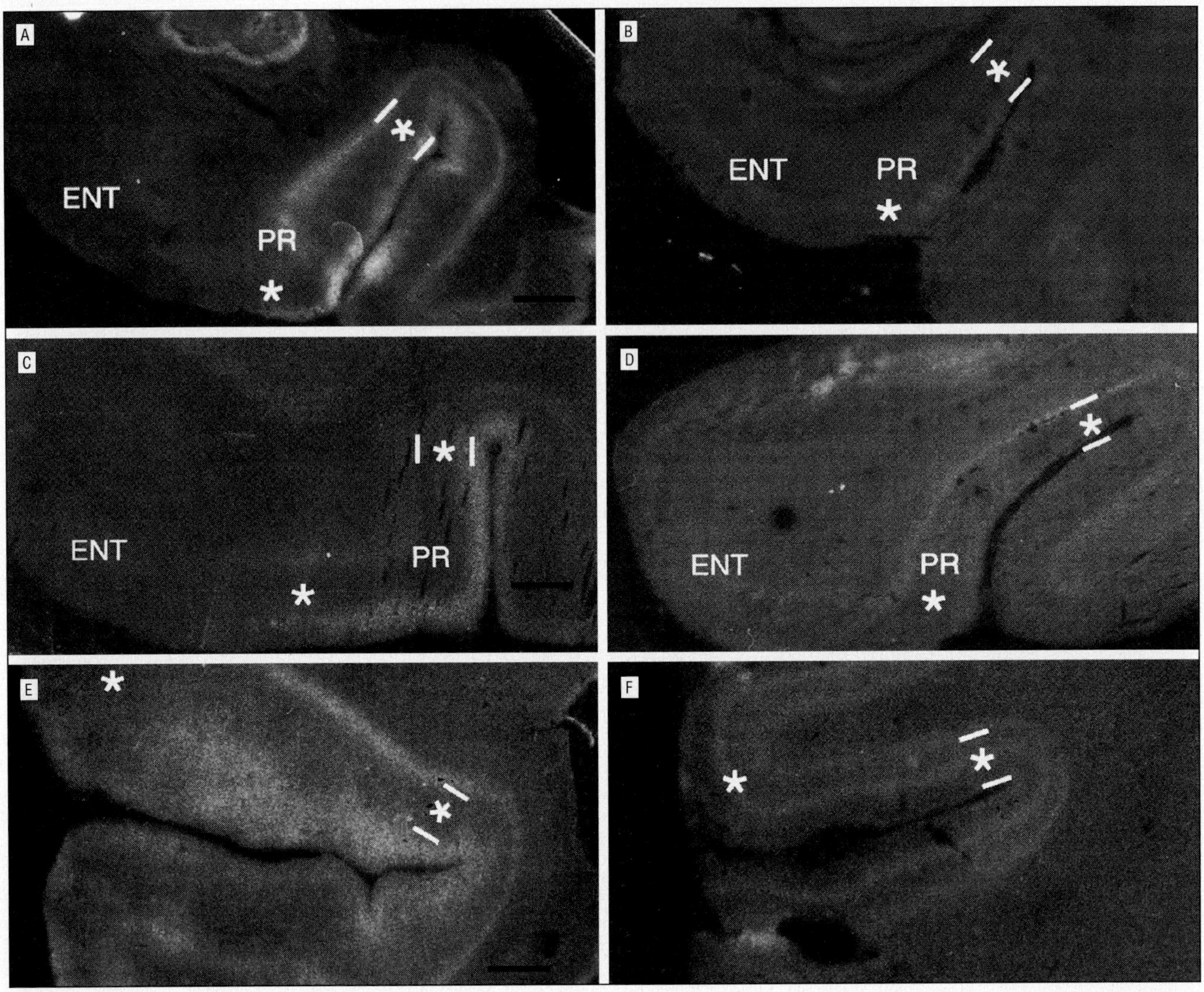

Figure 7. *Dark-field photomicrographs of [^{125}I]epidepride binding to D_2 dopamine receptors in parahippocampus (entorhinal [Brodmann area 28] and perirhinal [Brodmann areas 35 and 36] cortices) of 3 control (A, C, and E) and 3 schizophrenic (B, D, and F) cases matched for age and postmortem interval. ENT indicates entorhinal cortex; PR, perirhinal cortex; asterisks, the border of the ENT and the transentorhinal cortex coincident with the appearance of a trilaminar pattern of D_2 receptors; and asterisk between parallel bars, granule cell layer of perirhinal cortex. For the ENT, there was no evidence of a difference in concentration or pattern of D_2 receptors between groups. The trilaminar pattern of D_2 receptors in the PR was disrupted in schizophrenics. In case 6 (A and B) and case 13 (C and D), the concentration of D_2 receptor is reduced in the external laminae of the schizophrenic cases (bar=1.44 mm). In case 5 (E and F), an elevated concentration of D_2 receptors is evident over the granule cell layer of the PR (bar=1.9 mm). The section in F is cut at an oblique angle such that the PR is continuous with the piriform cortex rostral to the ENT.*

30. Ryoo H, Joyce JN. The loss of dopamine D_2 receptors varies along the rostrocaudal axis of the hippocampal complex in Alzheimer's disease. *J Comp Neurol.* 1994;348:94-110.
31. Murray AM, Ryoo H, Gurevich E, Joyce JN. Localization of dopamine D_3 receptors to mesolimbic and D_2 receptors to mesostriatal regions of human forebrain. *Proc Natl Acad Sci U S A.* 1994;91:11271-11275.
32. Goldsmith S, Joyce JN. Alterations in the hippocampal mossy fiber pathway in schizophrenia and Alzheimer's disease. *Biol Psychiatry.* 1995;37:122-126.
33. Artymyshyn R, Smith A, Wolfe BB. The use of ^{3}H standards in ^{125}I autoradiography. *J Neurosci Methods.* 1990;32:185-192.
34. Roberts SJ, Hanaway J. *Atlas of the Human Brain in Section.* Philadelphia, Pa: Lea & Febiger; 1971.
35. Akbarian S, Kim JJ, Potkin SG, Hagman JO, Tafazzoki A, Bunney WE Jr, Jones EG. Gene expression for glutamic acid decarboxylase is reduced without loss of neurons in prefrontal cortex of schizophrenics. *Arch Gen Psychiatry.* 1995;52:258-266.
36. Meador-Woodruff JH, Grandy DK, Van Tol HHM, Damask SP, Little KY, Civelli O, Watson SJ. Dopamine receptor gene expression in the human medial temporal lobe. *Neuropsychopharmacology.* 1994;10:239-248.
37. Rakic P. Mode of cell migration to the superficial layers of the fetal monkey neocortex. *J Comp Neurol.* 1972;145:61-84.
38. Reinoso BS, Undie AS, Levit P. Dopamine receptors mediate differential morphological effects on cerebral cortical neurons in vitro. *J Neurosci Res.* 1996;43:439-453.
39. Swarzenski BC, Tang L, Oh YJ, O'Malley KL, Todd RD. Morphogenic potentials of D_2, D_3, and D_4 dopamine receptors revealed in transfected neuronal cell lines. *Proc Natl Acad Sci U S A.* 1994;91:649-653.
40. Weinberger DR, Berman KF, Illowsky BP. Physiological dysfunction of dorsolateral prefrontal cortex in schizophrenia, III. *Arch Gen Psychiatry.* 1988;45:609-615.
41. Stabenau JR, Pollin W. Heredity and environment in schizophrenia, revisited: the contribution of twin and high-risk studies. *J Nerv Ment Dis.* 1993;181:290-297.
42. Shenton ME, Kikinis R, Jolesz FA, Pollak SD, Le May M, Wible CG, Hokama H, Martin J, Colemean M, McCarley RW. Abnormalities of the left temporal lobe and thought disorder in schizophrenia. *N Engl J Med.* 1992;327:604-612.
43. McCarley RW, Shenton ME, O'Donnell BF, Gaux SF, Kikinis R, Nestor G, Jolesz FA. Auditory 300 abnormalities and left superior temporal gyrus volume reduction in schizophrenia. *Arch Gen Psychiatry.* 1993;50:190-197.
44. Penfield W, Perot P. The brains record of auditory and visual experience. *Brain.* 1963;86:595-696.
45. Joyce JN. The dopamine hypothesis of schizophrenia: limbic interactions with serotonin and norepinephrine. *Psychopharmacology.* 1993;112(suppl):S16-S34.
46. Cleghorn JM, Franco S, Szechtman B, Kaplan RD, Szechtman H, Brown GM, Nahmias C, Garnett ES. Toward a brain map of auditory hallucinations. *Am J Psychiatry.* 1992;149:1062-1069.

COMING SOON

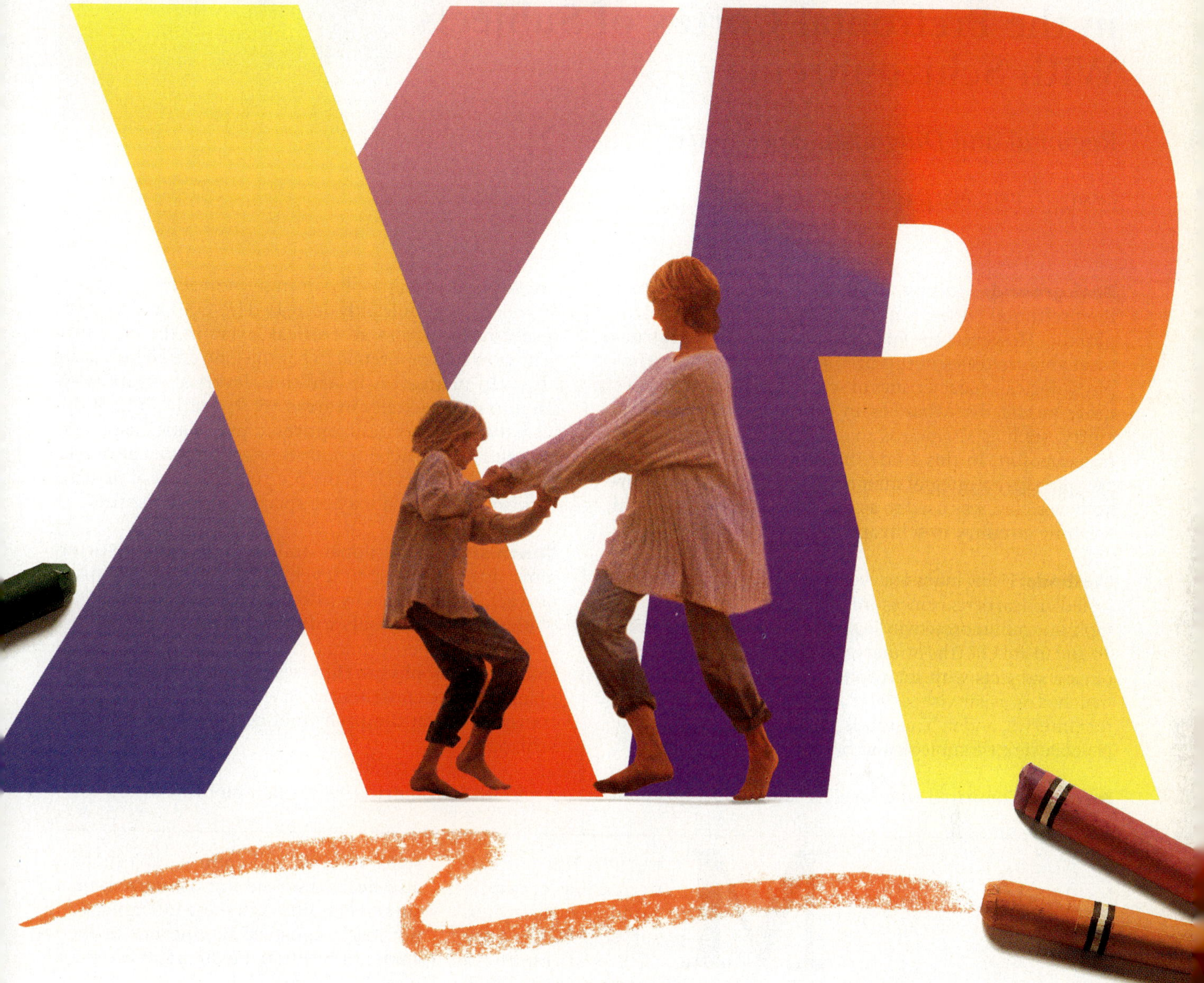

VENLAFAXINE HCl

EFFEXOR® XR EXTENDED RELEASE CAPSULES

67323-02

WYETH-AYERST LABORATORIES
Philadelphia, PA 19101

Reduction of Synaptophysin Immunoreactivity in the Prefrontal Cortex of Subjects With Schizophrenia

Regional and Diagnostic Specificity

Leisa A. Glantz, MS; David A. Lewis, MD

Background: Multiple lines of evidence indicate that the prefrontal cortex is a site of dysfunction in schizophrenia. However, the apparent absence of gross structural abnormalities in this area suggests that the pathophysiological characteristics of schizophrenia may involve more subtle disturbances in prefrontal cortical circuitry, such as alterations in synaptic connectivity and transmission. In this study, immunoreactivity for synaptophysin, an integral membrane protein of small synaptic vesicles, was used to assess the integrity of cortical synaptic circuitry in schizophrenia.

Methods: Using immunocytochemical techniques and adjusted optical density measurements, we examined synaptophysin immunoreactivity in prefrontal cortical areas 9 and 46 and in area 17 (the primary visual cortex) from 10 pairs of case subjects with schizophrenia and control subjects matched on a pairwise basis for age, sex, race, and postmortem interval, and in 5 matched pairs of nonschizophrenic psychiatric case subjects and normal control subjects.

Results: Compared with levels found in matched control subjects, synaptophysin immunoreactivity in areas 46 and 9 was significantly decreased ($P<.001$ and $P<.008$, respectively) across all cortical layers in the case subjects with schizophrenia. In contrast, no differences were observed in area 17. In addition, levels of synaptophysin immunoreactivity in areas 46, 9, and 17 did not differ between 5 nonschizophrenic psychiatric case subjects and their matched controls, suggesting that decreased synaptophysin levels in the prefrontal cortex of patients with schizophrenia may be specific to that disorder.

Conclusions: Additional studies are required to determine if the decrease in levels of synaptophysin immunoreactivity is caused by a decrease in the number or size of presynaptic terminals, a decrease in the number of synaptic vesicles per terminal, or a decrease in the expression of synaptophysin. However, all of these potential explanations are consistent with a disturbance in synaptic transmission in the prefrontal cortex of patients with schizophrenia.

Arch Gen Psychiatry. 1997;54:660-669

MULTIPLE lines of evidence have implicated the prefrontal cortex (PFC) as a site of dysfunction in schizophrenia. For example, many of the negative or deficit symptoms of schizophrenia are similar to those exhibited by patients with frontal lobe lesions.[1] In addition, a variety of functional neuroimaging and neuropsychological studies have identified abnormalities in the prefrontal cortex of subjects with schizophrenia.[2-8]

Attempts to identify the neuroanatomical basis for this dysfunction of the PFC have included both structural imaging and postmortem investigations. Many,[9-13] but not all,[14] structural imaging studies have revealed a decrease in PFC gray-matter volume in subjects with schizophrenia. Similar differences in the thickness or volume of the PFC[15-18] between subjects with schizophrenia and control subjects have also been observed in postmortem measurements, although these differences did not reach statistical significance in every study. In addition, postmortem investigations have revealed that the density,[18] but not the number,[15,17] of PFC neurons is increased in subjects with schizophrenia compared with control subjects, although some investigators have observed decreased numbers of certain populations of PFC neurons.[19,20] The combination of decreased PFC volume and increased cell packing density suggests that the amount of neuropil in this cortical region may be diminished in at least a subpopulation of subjects with schizophrenia. The cortical neuropil is composed of small dendrites, dendritic spines, and axon terminals,[21] critical elements in the structure of most cortical synapses. Consequently, a decrease in PFC neuropil volume in subjects with schizophrenia is

From the Departments of Neuroscience (Ms Glantz and Dr Lewis) and Psychiatry (Dr Lewis), University of Pittsburgh, Pittsburgh, Pa.

SUBJECTS AND METHODS

SUBJECTS

Specimens from 32 human brains were obtained during autopsies conducted at the Allegheny County Coroner's Office, Pittsburgh, Pa, or the University of Pittsburgh Medical Center. No neuropathological abnormalities were detected in any subjects except for 2 brains (Nos. 207 and 313) in which thioflavin S revealed a few senile plaques. The density of the plaques was insufficient to meet diagnostic criteria for Alzheimer disease,[30] and there was no clinical history of dementia in either subject. An independent committee of experienced clinicians made consensus *DSM-III-R* diagnoses for each subject using information obtained from clinical records, and, whenever possible (for 20 subjects), a structured interview with a surviving relative of the subject. All procedures were approved by the University of Pittsburgh's Institutional Review Board for Biomedical Research.

The first set of experiments (**Table 1**) used tissue specimens from 10 subjects with schizophrenia, 5 of whom also met diagnostic criteria for an alcohol-related disorder at some point during their life. This frequency of alcoholism is comparable with that observed in clinical studies of schizophrenia.[31] Eight subjects were receiving treatment with antipsychotic medications at the time of death. Case subject 207 had not taken antipsychotic medications for 10 years prior to death. Case subject 185 was known to be noncompliant with prescribed medications, and toxicology studies at autopsy failed to detect evidence of antipsychotic medications.

Each subject with schizophrenia was matched to 1 control subject on a pairwise basis for age, sex, race, and postmortem interval (PMI). Interviews with relatives confirmed that 8 control subjects had no history of any neurologic or psychiatric disorder. One subject (No. 230) had a history of alcohol dependence, and the other subject (No. 249) met diagnostic criteria for recurrent major depressive disorder with psychotic features. This individual had been treated intermittently for 25 years with antipsychotic medications.

The second study involved 5 case subjects in whom organic delusional disorder, major depressive disorder, or alcohol dependence or abuse had been diagnosed (**Table 2**). Case 217 was receiving antipsychotic treatment at the time of death, but the other 4 case subjects had no history of exposure to antipsychotic medications. These case subjects were matched with 5 control subjects who had no history of neurologic or psychiatric disease.

Finally, 1 additional pair of cases was studied. A 68-year-old white man (PMI, 16.8 hours) in whom major depression had been diagnosed and who had been receiving antipsychotic medications at the time of death, was matched with a 70-year-old white man (PMI, 16.5 hours) in whom major depression had been diagnosed, but who had never received antipsychotic medications.

PREPARATION OF TISSUE

The left hemisphere of each brain was cut into coronal blocks and immersed in a solution of 4% paraformaldehyde for 48 hours at 4°C.[32] Tissue blocks were then washed in a series of sucrose solutions in phosphate-buffered saline and stored in an antifreeze solution at -30°C. Mean (±SD) storage time did not differ between the case subjects with schizophrenia and their controls (29.3±14.0 and 29.5±12.3 months, respectively), or between the nonschizophrenic psychiatric case subjects and their controls (42.0±15.5 and 36.2±22.4 months, respectively). Previous studies have also shown that storage under these conditions does not affect immunoreactivity.[33] Sections (40 μm) were cut on a motor-driven cryostat to ensure maximal consistency in section thickness, and every 10th section was stained using the Nissl method.

AREAS EXAMINED

To assess the regional specificity of any changes in synaptophysin immunoreactivity, 3 areas with substantial differences in cytoarchitecture and afferent input were examined: PFC areas 9 and 46 and area 17, the primary visual cortex. These areas were identified using published cytoarchitectonic criteria.[32,34,35] Camera lucida drawings were made of Nissl-stained sections from each case subject, and the boundaries of each region were plotted to establish the appropriate zones for analysis on the sections labeled for synaptophysin immunoreactivity.

IMMUNOCYTOCHEMICAL PROCEDURES

Tissue sections from each pair of case and control subjects were pretreated in aqueous 1% hydrogen peroxide for 7½

Continued on next page

likely to involve alterations in the synaptic connectivity of this region.

One way to test the hypothesis that the synaptic connectivity of the PFC is disturbed in schizophrenia is to assess the integrity of specific proteins that are known to be essential for synaptic function. For example, synaptophysin, a 38-kd integral membrane protein of small synaptic vesicles,[22-24] seems to be critical for calcium-dependent synaptic transmission.[25,26] Synaptophysin is present in more than 95% of cortical synaptic terminals,[22,23] and levels of synaptophysin immunoreactivity have been shown to be reliable measures of synaptic density.[27-29] Consequently, we used immunocytochemical techniques and optical density measurements to address the following 3 questions: Is synaptophysin immunoreactivity decreased in the PFC of subjects with schizophrenia compared with matched control subjects? If so, is the decrease selective to this region? Is the decreased synaptophysin immunoreactivity specific to the disease process of schizophrenia?

RESULTS

QUALITATIVE COMPARISONS OF SYNAPTOPHYSIN IMMUNOREACTIVITY IN THE BRAINS OF SUBJECTS WITH SCHIZOPHRENIA AND MATCHED CONTROL SUBJECTS

Examination of the brains of subjects with schizophrenia and control subjects revealed a punctate pattern of minutes to remove endogenous peroxidase activity, washed, and then incubated at room temperature for 30 minutes in phosphate-buffered saline containing 0.3% Triton X-100 and 4.5% normal horse serum. Sections were incubated for 40 to 48 hours at 4°C in phosphate-buffered saline containing 0.3% Triton X-100, 0.05% bovine serum albumin, 3% normal horse serum, and 1 of 2 mouse monoclonal antibodies (Sigma, St Louis, Mo, diluted 1:1000 or Boehringer Mannheim, Indianapolis, Ind, diluted 1:100) that specifically recognize[24,36] synaptophysin. Sections were then processed using a standard kit (Vectastain ABC kit, Vector Laboratories, Burlingame, Calif) and diaminobenzidine.

Control experiments involved replacing each primary antibody with normal mouse serum and processing the tissue as usual. No immunoreactivity was observed in these experiments. Specificity of the labeling was further indicated by the identical regional and laminar patterns of immunoreactivity produced by both antibodies.

Using the synaptophysin antibody from Sigma, 5 separate immunocytochemical experiments were performed for each cortical area of the case subjects with schizophrenia and their matched control subjects. A total of 4 experiments were performed for each area for the nonschizophrenic psychiatric case subjects and their matched controls. For each experiment, sections from a matched pair of subjects were processed together throughout the entire immunocytochemical procedure. Thus, for each of the 3 regions of interest, a total of 100 sections were prepared for the schizophrenia case-control study, and a total of 40 sections were prepared for the nonschizophrenia psychiatric case-control study. All of these sections were used in the quantitative analyses described herein.

ANALYSIS

Slide-mounted sections from each pair were randomly coded and scanned together, and the images were imported into an image analysis software program (Bioscan Inc, Edmonds, Wash) to obtain light transmittance measurements of synaptophysin immunoreactivity. Within each cytoarchitectonic region, rectangles that extended for 5 to 10 mm across the cortical surface and from the pial surface into the subjacent white matter were drawn. Rectangles varied in size because measurements were restricted to those portions of the areas of interest that were cut perpendicular to the pial surface and that were free of any discontinuities in the tissue. The average light transmittance (ranging 0-255) was determined in 3 different rectangles for each area on each section. The values from each rectangle were then averaged to produce a mean cortical and a mean white matter light transmittance value from each section of each cortical area of each case. Because synaptophysin immunoreactivity was virtually absent in the white matter of all subjects, light transmittance measurements in the white matter were used to control for possible differences between case in nonspecific labeling. Adjusted optical density values were calculated from the mean light transmittance values according to the equation: adjusted optical density=log (light transmittance in white matter/light transmittance in cortex).[37] The adjusted optical density values were then used for comparisons between the matched pairs of subjects. Light transmittance values within the cortex were also divided into superficial and deep halves to determine adjusted optical density values for the supragranular and infragranular cortical layers.

Rescanning and remeasurement of the same coded sections produced mean adjusted optical density values that differed from the previous measurements by less than 1%. As an additional check on the reliability of these measurements, 5 neuroanatomists were asked to examine coded sections from 1 immunocytochemical experiment involving each of the subjects shown in Table 1, and to determine which section of a pair was more intensely immunoreactive, or if there was no discernible difference. In 49 of the resulting 50 comparisons, these ratings agreed with the findings of the quantitative comparisons (98% concordance).

STATISTICAL ANALYSES

For each of the 3 cortical regions, analysis of variance (ANOVA) was used to assess the significance (α=.05) of differences in adjusted optical density measurements between matched pairs of case subjects with schizophrenia and their control subjects, and between matched pairs of nonschizophrenic psychiatric case subjects and their control subjects. The ANOVA model factors were diagnostic group, matched pair, immunocytochemical experiment, and their second-order interactions. Diagnostic group effect, adjusting for pairing and immunocytochemical experiment, used F-statistics obtained from corresponding SAS Type III (SAS, Cary, NC) sums of squares. Linear regression analyses were used to evaluate the effects of age and PMI on adjusted optical density values.

synaptophysin immunoreactivity throughout the cortical neuropil (**Figure 1**). In contrast, cell bodies and the proximal portions of dendrites were not labeled. This pattern of immunoreactivity is consistent with the location of synaptophysin in small synaptic vesicles that aggregate in presynaptic axon terminals.

For each case subject, the laminar distribution of synaptophysin immunoreactivity differed consistently between the prefrontal and visual cortices. In areas 9 and 46, synaptophysin immunoreactivity was intense in layer 1, progressively decreased from the pial surface to the layer 6 white matter border (**Figure 2**, B), and then sharply declined to undetectable levels in the white matter. In contrast, a more complex laminar pattern of immunoreactivity was present in area 17, the primary visual cortex (Figure 2, D). These laminar changes were clearly reflected in adjusted optical density measurements of synaptophysin immunoreactivity in this region (**Figure 3**).

Within each region, similar laminar patterns of synaptophysin immunoreactivity were found in subjects with schizophrenia and control subjects. However, in areas 9 and 46, the intensity of immunoreactivity seemed to be decreased, especially in the superficial layers, in many of the case subjects with schizophrenia (Figure 2, A) compared with the matched controls (Figure 2, B). In contrast, no differences in the intensity of label were apparent between subjects with schizophrenia (Figure 2, C) and control subjects in area 17 (Figure 2, D).

Table 1. Characteristics of Matched Pairs of Subjects With Schizophrenia and Control Subjects*

	Subjects With Schizophrenia					Control Subjects			
Pair	Subject No.	*DSM-III-R* Diagnosis	Sex/Race/ Age, y	Postmortem Interval, h	Cause of Death	Subject No.	Sex/Race/ Age, y	Postmortem Interval, h	Cause of Death
1	131	Chronic undifferentiated schizophrenia†	M/B/62	3.9	Pneumonia	249	M/B/57	4.3	ASCVD‡
2	153	Chronic paranoid schizophrenia§	M/B/24	18.3	Suicide by drowning	230	M/W/33	18.2	ASCVD‡
3	185	Schizophrenia§	M/W/64	8.6	ASCVD‡	313	M/W/60	11.0	ASCVD‡
4	236	Residual schizophrenia	M/W/69	17.0	Thermal burns	321	M/W/71	14.0	Aortic aneurysm
5	317	Chronic undifferentiated schizophrenia	M/W/48	8.3	Bronchopneumonia	278	M/W/50	4.5	ASCVD‡
6	398	Schizoaffective disorder	F/W/41	10.3	Pulmonary embolus	247	F/W/38	6.8	Pulmonary embolus
7	207	Schizophrenia	M/W/72	3.8	Subdural hematoma	168	M/W/77	6.2	ASCVD‡
8	377	Chronic undifferentiated schizophrenia‖	M/W/52	10.0	Gastrointestinal tract bleeding	178	M/W/48	7.4	ASCVD‡
9	341	Chronic undifferentiated schizophrenia¶	F/W/47	14.5	Suicide by drug overdose	208	F/W/56	18.0	ASCVD‡
10	333	Chronic undifferentiated schizophrenia	F/W/66	17.9	ASCVD‡	420	F/B/67	19.5	Carbon monoxide interaction#
		Mean (±SE)	**54.5 (±15.0)**	**11.3 (±5.4)**		**Mean (±SE)**	**55.7 (±14.0)**	**10.9 (±6.0)**	

**Results of toxicology screening were available for all subjects, excluding subjects 131 and 207, and were negative except for prescription drugs or alcohol in some subjects.*

†Also met criteria for alcohol abuse, in remission at time of death.

‡ASCVD indicates atherosclerotic coronary vascular disease.

§Also met criteria for alcohol dependence, in remission at time of death.

‖Also met criteria for alcohol dependence, current at time of death.

¶Also met criteria for alcohol abuse, current at time of death.

#Accidental due to defective stove.

QUANTITATIVE COMPARISONS OF SYNAPTOPHYSIN IMMUNOREACTIVITY IN THE BRAINS OF SUBJECTS WITH SCHIZOPHRENIA AND MATCHED CONTROL SUBJECTS

The mean (±SE) adjusted optical density value of synaptophysin immunoreactivity in area 46 (**Figure 4**, A) of the brains of subjects with schizophrenia (0.169±0.018) was significantly decreased ($F_{1,19}$=23.0; $P<.001$) compared with those of control subjects (0.198±0.027). Levels of synaptophysin immunoreactivity were decreased by 15% to 30% in the brains of subjects with schizophrenia relative to those of the matched control subjects in 6 of the 10 pairs (Figure 4, B). Similarly, in area 9 (Figure 4, C), the mean adjusted optical density value was significantly decreased ($F_{1,19}$=8.78; $P<.008$) in the brains of subjects with schizophrenia (0.164±0.017) compared with those of control subjects (0.192±0.030). In 8 pairs, the brains of subjects with schizophrenia exhibited a reduction in the amount of synaptophysin immunoreactivity relative to those of the matched control, with the reduction ranging from 10% to 35% in 5 pairs (Figure 4, D).

The intense synaptophysin immunoreactivity present in layer 1, which might represent surface artifact staining, could confound comparisons across subjects. Exclusion of values from layer 1 resulted in lower mean adjusted optical density measurements for the brains of subjects with schizophrenia (area 9, 0.152±0.015; area 46, 0.159±0.017) and those of the control subjects (area 9, 0.180±0.029; area 46, 0.185±0.025). These differences in adjusted optical density measurements between the brains of subjects with schizophrenia and those of control subjects remained statistically significant ($P<.005$)and were identical in magnitude to those found with measurements of the entire cortical thickness.

In contrast with these differences in the PFC, no group differences in levels of synaptophysin immunoreactivity were observed in area 17 (Figure 4, E). Only 1 pair showed a decrease of more than 10% in the brain of the subject with schizophrenia (Figure 4, F).

In both prefrontal regions, neither age (area 46, r=−0.07; area 9, r=−0.38) nor PMI (area 46, r=−0.36; area 9, r=−0.06) was significantly correlated with the magnitude of the difference in synaptophysin immunoreactivity between subjects with schizophrenia and control subjects. In addition, there was no effect of sex on the group differences in synaptophysin immunoreactivity, although only 3 pairs of female subjects were available for this study.

Table 2. Characteristics of Matched Pairs of Nonschizophrenic Psychiatric Subjects and Normal Control Subjects*

	Nonschizophrenic Psychiatric Subjects					Control Subjects			
Pair	Subject No.	*DSM-III-R* Diagnosis	Sex/ Age, y	Postmortem Interval, h	Cause of Death	Subject No.	Sex/ Age, y	Postmortem Interval, h	Cause of Death
1	217	Organic delusional disorder†	M/29	9.0	Acute ethanol intoxication	187	M/32	7.6	Myocarditis
2	223	Major depression†	M/29	27.5	Suicide by drug overdose	457	M/25	17.0	Carbon monoxide intoxication‡
3	228	Major depression	F/66	5.4	Asphyxiation	365	M/68	10.0	ASCVD§
4	248	Major depression and somatization disorder	F/48	6.3	Suicide by hanging	250	F/47	5.3	ASCVD§
5	282	Alcohol abuse	M/58	11.5	Suicide by hanging	166	M/63	8.2	ASCVD§
		Mean (±SE)	**46.0 (±16.8)**	**11.9 (±9.0)**		**Mean (±SE)**	**47.0 (±18.7)**	**9.6 (±4.5)**	

**Results from toxicology screening were available for all subjects and were negative except for prescription drugs or alcohol in some subjects. All normal control subjects were white.*

†Also met criteria for alcohol dependence, current at time of death.

‡Accidental due to explosion.

§ASCVD indicates atherosclerotic coronary artery disease.

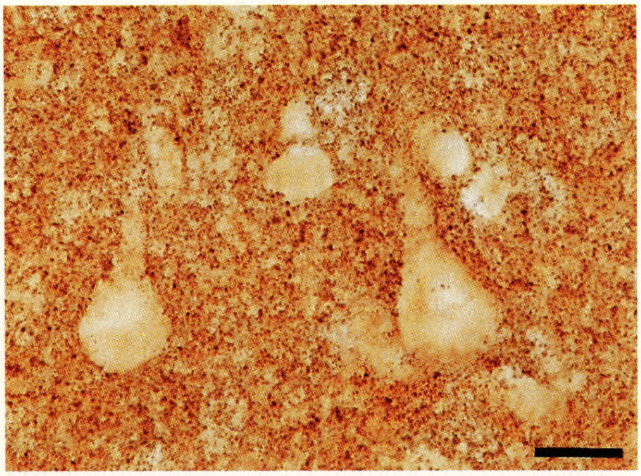

Figure 1. *Brightfield photomicrograph illustrating the typical appearance of synaptophysin immunoreactivity in area 46 of the prefrontal cortex of control subject 247. Synaptophysin immunoreactivity typically labels the neuropil in a punctate manner. Cell bodies and proximal dendrites are outlined by the terminal labeling. Calibration bar is equivalent to 20 μm.*

LAMINAR COMPARISONS OF SYNAPTOPHYSIN IMMUNOREACTIVITY IN THE BRAINS OF SUBJECTS WITH SCHIZOPHRENIA AND OF MATCHED CONTROL SUBJECTS

To determine if the decrease in synaptophysin immunoreactivity in the subjects with schizophrenia was greater in the superficial cortical layers (Figure 2), adjusted optial density values for the superficial half (approximately layers 1-3) and deep half (layers 4-6) of the prefrontal areas were analyzed. The 2 pairs of subjects (pairs 5 and 10) that showed an increase in synaptophysin immunoreactivity in the brain of the subject with schizophrenia were excluded from this analysis. The magnitude of the absolute differences in mean adjusted optical density values was greater in the superficial cortical layers than in the deep layers for both areas 46 and 9 (**Figure 5**, top). However, when expressed as a percentage of the matched control value, the superficial and deep layers of the brains of subjects with schizophrenia exhibited a 20% decrease in adjusted optical density values in both prefrontal regions (Figure 5, bottom). These findings suggest that synaptophysin immunoreactivity was decreased across all cortical layers in the brains of subjects with schizophrenia, and that the greater absolute difference in adjusted optical density levels in the superficial layers may reflect the relatively higher synaptic density in these cortical layers.[21]

SYNAPTOPHYSIN IMMUNOREACTIVITY IN THE BRAINS OF NONSCHIZOPHRENIC PSYCHIATRIC CASE SUBJECTS AND OF MATCHED NORMAL CONTROL SUBJECTS

Similar studies were conducted on the brains of nonschizophrenic psychiatric case subjects and of matched normal control subjects to determine the diagnostic specificity of the observations on the brains of subjects with schizophrenia. In contrast with the findings in the schizophrenia case-control studies, levels of synaptophysin immunoreactivity were not decreased in any region of the brains of nonschizophrenic psychiatric case subjects (**Figure 6**). In areas 9 and 46, the brains of all nonschizophrenic psychiatric case subjects exhibited either no difference or an increase in the levels of synaptophysin immunoreactivity compared with their control subjects. The only exception was area 9 of pair 4, where synaptophysin levels were 7% lower in the brain of the nonschizophrenic psychiatric subject. These findings suggest that the reduction in synaptophysin immunoreactivity is not a common characteristic of individuals with psychiatric disorders, raising the possibility that it may be specific to schizophrenia.

COMMENT

These findings demonstrate that synaptophysin immunoreactivity is decreased in at least 2 regions of the PFC in most subjects with schizophrenia compared with

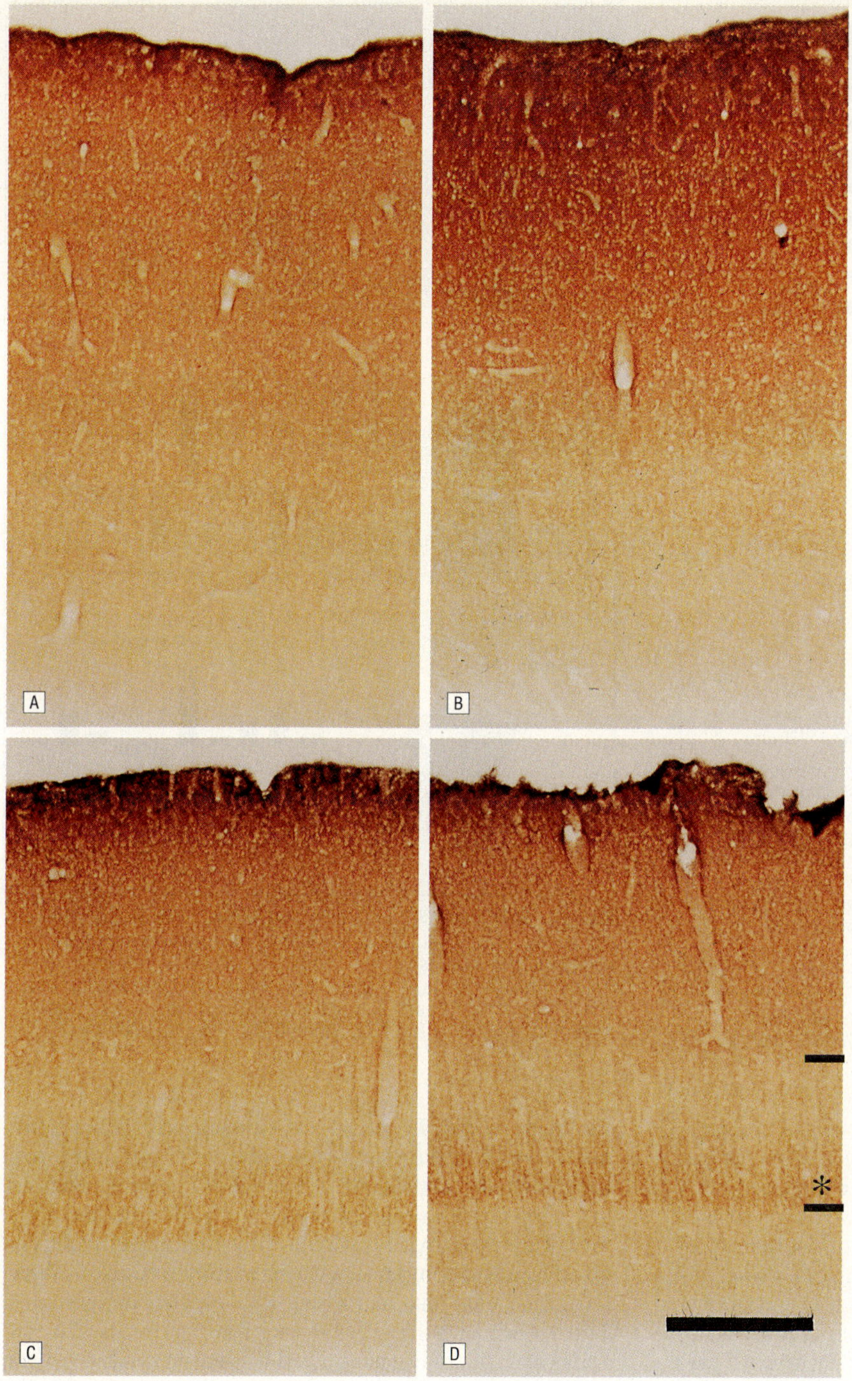

Figure 2. *Brightfield photomicrographs of synaptophysin immunoreactivity in areas 46 (A,B) and 17 (C,D) of a subject with schizophrenia (A and C) and the matched normal control subject (B and D; pair 1 in Table 1). Compared with the matched control subject, the intensity of synaptophysin immunoreactivity seems to be decreased in area 46, but not in area 17, of the subject with schizophrenia. Also apparent is the different laminar distribution of synaptophysin immunoreactivity in areas 46 and 17 in both subjects. D, Hash marks indicate the locations of the borders between layers 3 and 4 and layers 4 and 5, and the asterisk indicates the band of increased synaptophysin immunoreactivity located in layer 4cβ. Calibration bar is equivalent to 500 μm.*

matched control subjects, but is unchanged in the primary visual cortex. These results suggest that the reduction of synaptophysin immunoreactivity in schizophrenia is not a global cortical effect, but exhibits regional selectivity. Consistent with these observations, synaptophysin protein levels have been reported to be significantly decreased in the PFC and inferior temporal cortex, but not in the primary visual cortex, of subjects with schizophrenia.[38] Other investigators have also observed a decrease in synaptophysin immunoreactivity in the hippocampal formation of subjects with schizophrenia.[39,40] In contrast with these findings of regional specificity, both the PFC and the primary visual cortex of subjects with schizophrenia have been reported to exhibit similar alterations in neuronal density.[18]

Although synaptophysin immunoreactivity was decreased in the PFC of most of the subjects with schizophrenia, levels were clearly increased in 1 subject with schizophrenia (No. 317) compared with the matched control subject (No. 278) in all 3 areas. To determine whether this finding reflected heterogeneity across subjects with schizophrenia or abnormally low levels of synaptophysin immunoreactivity in the matched control, we measured synaptophysin immunoreactivity in control subject 278 and 4 other closely matched normal white men (age range, 45-50 years; PMI range, 5.1-7.8 hours). This comparison

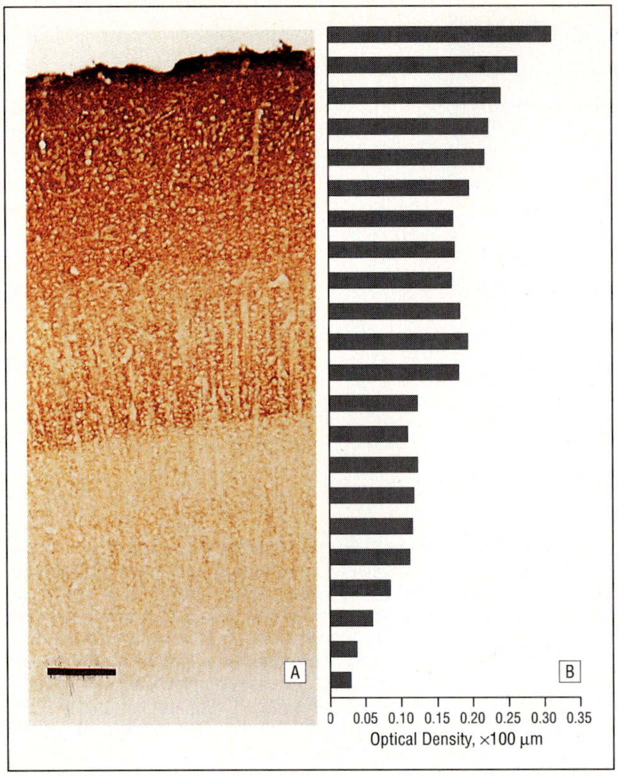

Figure 3. *A, Brightfield photomicrograph of synaptophysin immunoreactivity in area 17, the human primary visual cortex. Synaptophysin immunoreactivity progressively decreased from the pial surface through layer 3. At the border between layers 3 and 4, the intensity of immunoreactivity seemed to decrease stepwise, to remain relatively low in layers 4a and 4b, and then to increase again in layer 4c, with a particularly striking band in sublayer 4cβ. The border between sublayer 4cβ and layer 5 was defined by a sharp decline in immunoreactivity that continued throughout layer 5. The synaptophysin immunoreactivity then increased slightly in layer 6 before declining abruptly at the border between layer 6 and the white matter. Calibration bar on the left is equivalent to 200 µm. The distinctive laminar pattern of synaptophysin immunoreactivity in this region is reflected in the optical density values shown in the 100-µm-deep bins, right.*

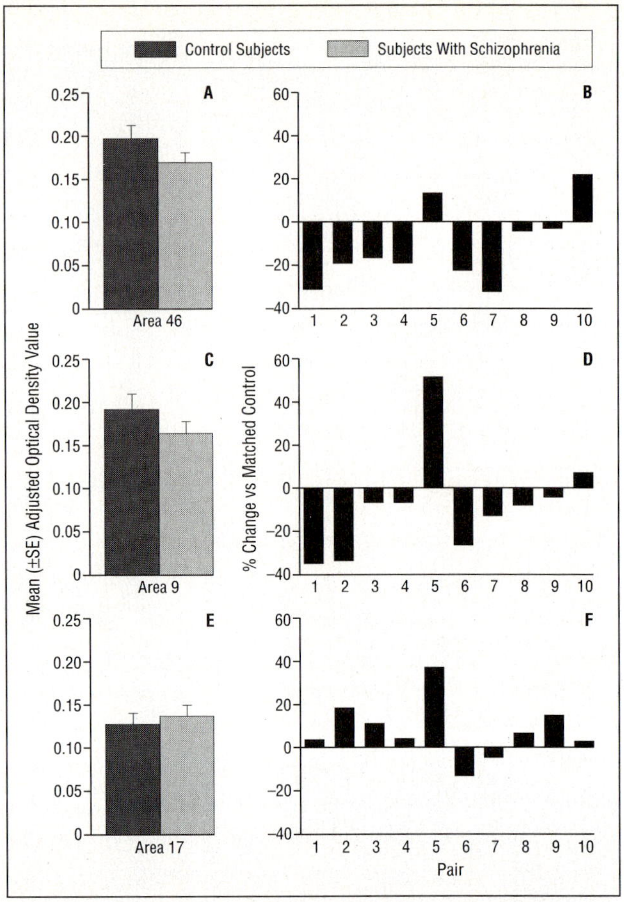

Figure 4. *The mean (± SE) adjusted optical density values of synaptophysin immunoreactivity for the 10 subjects with schizophrenia and matched control subjects in areas 46 (A; $F_{1,19}$=23.0; P<.001), 9 (C; $F_{1,19}$=8.78; P<.008), and 17 (E; $F_{1,23}$; P>.05). The percentage change in adjusted optical density of each subject with schizophrenia relative to the matched control subject for areas 46, 9, and 17 is shown in B, D, and F, respectively.*

suggested that adjusted optical density levels of synaptophysin immunoreactivity in control subject 278 were unusually low. For example, in area 9, mean adjusted optical density levels in control subject 278 were only 61% of the value for the matched case subject with schizophrenia, whereas in the other 4 matched controls, these values ranged from 88% to 95% of the levels for case subject 317. Thus, the apparent marked elevation (Figure 4) of adjusted optical density values in all 3 cortical areas of case subject 317 seems to have been an artifact of the matched control subject used in the initial study.

The decreased synaptophysin immunoreactivity in the PFC may be specific to schizophrenia, since no differences were observed between the brains of nonschizophrenic psychiatric case subjects and of matched normal control subjects. In addition, 2 of the control subjects (Nos. 230 and 249) used in the first study had a history of a psychiatric disorder, but levels of synaptophysin immunoreactivity were substantially reduced in both prefrontal regions of the case subjects with schizophrenia matched to these control subjects (pairs 1 and 2 of Figure 4, B and D). Several lines of evidence also indicate that the coexistence of a diagnosis of alcohol dependence or abuse in 5 schizophrenic subjects is unlikely to account for our findings. First, synaptophysin levels in the PFC of 2 of the subjects with schizophrenia who met criteria for alcohol abuse did not differ from the matched controls (pairs 8 and 9 of Figure 4). Second, in 1 subject with schizophrenia (No. 153) who had a history of alcoholism, PFC synaptophysin immunoreactivity was decreased compared with the matched control subject (No. 230) who also had a history of alcohol dependence. Third, none of the 5 subjects with schizophrenia who had a history of alcoholism showed decreased synaptophysin immunoreactivity in the primary visual cortex. Finally, the 3 nonschizophrenic psychiatric case subjects who met diagnostic criteria for alcohol dependence or abuse did not show decreased levels of synaptophysin immunoreactivity. Together, these findings strongly suggest that the decrease in synaptophysin immunoreactivity in schizophrenia may be specific to that disorder and not a general correlate of psychiatric illness or a consequence of alcoholism.

POSSIBLE CONFOUNDING VARIABLES

As indicated previously, multiple technical controls were used to minimize the potential pitfalls of quantitative immunocytochemical techniques.[41] Although we cannot completely exclude the influence of such potential con-

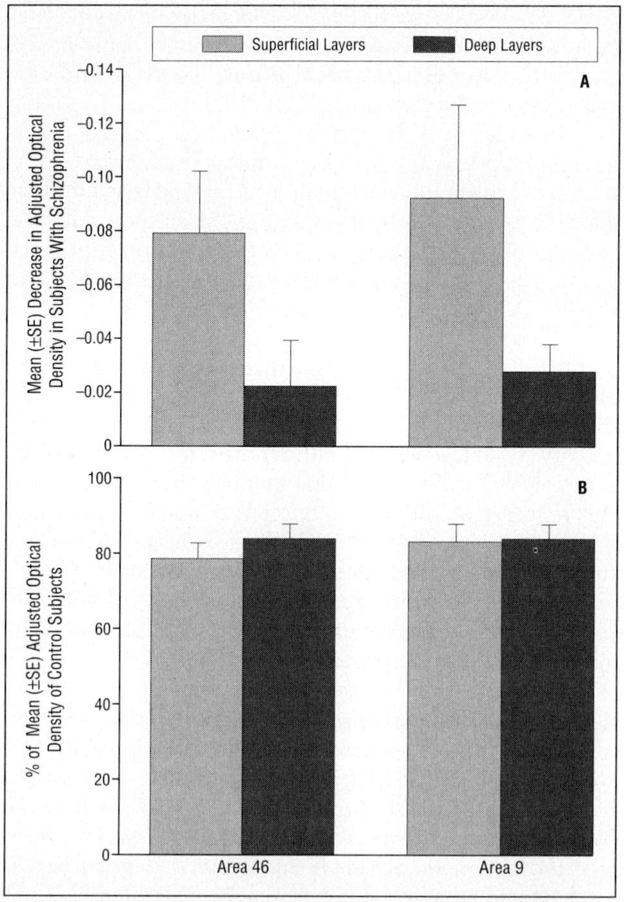

Figure 5. *Comparison of adjusted optical density values in the superficial and deep layers of areas 46 and 9 for 8 pairs of subjects with schizophrenia and their matched control subjects (see text). A, Mean (±SE) decrease in the adjusted optical density of the 8 subjects with schizophrenia relative to their matched control subjects. B, Mean (±SE) adjusted optical density of 8 subjects with schizophrenia as a percentage of the mean adjusted optical density of the 8 matched control subjects.*

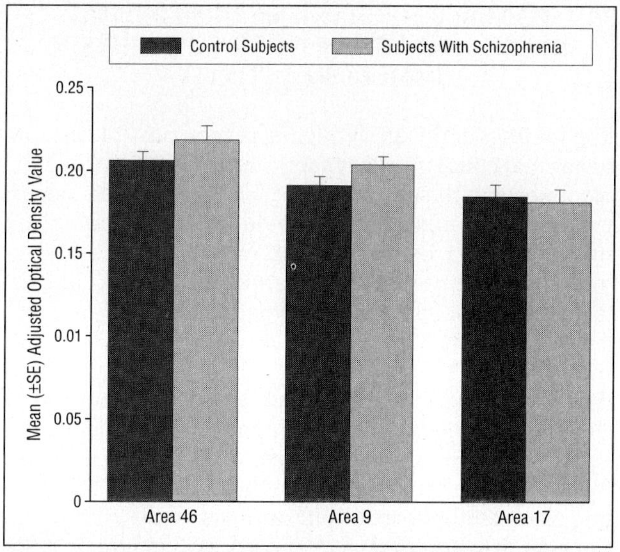

Figure 6. *The mean (±SE) adjusted optical density values of synaptophysin immunoreactivity for the nonschizophrenic psychiatric case subjects and matched normal control subjects for areas 46 (left), 9 (center), and 17 (right) (in each comparison,* P>*.05).*

founding variables, perhaps the best evidence for their absence is the confirmation of the findings of the present study by the use of complementary techniques.[38]

The observed decrease in adjusted optical density measurements could be a consequence of increased cortical vascularization in the subjects with schizophrenia. That is, an increase in the density of cortical blood vessels would result in fewer axon terminals per unit area of cortex and, consequently, decreased adjusted optical density measurements of synaptophysin immunoreactivity. However, 2 observations argue against this explanation for our findings. First, the primary visual cortex is more highly vascularized than the PFC in the human brain[42] and might be expected to exhibit an even larger difference between subjects with schizophrenia and control subjects than would the PFC. However, no differences in levels of synaptophysin immunoreactivity in the visual cortex were detected. Second, quantitative measurements were made of blood vessel cross-sectional area for the 5 pairs of case subjects in whom the greatest decrease in synaptophysin levels was found in area 46 (Figure 4, B). In these pairs, the mean (±SE) area (per 1.0 mm^2 of cortex) of blood vessels in the subjects with schizophrenia (0.017±0.002 mm^2) was actually smaller than that of the controls (0.022±0.004 mm^2). Thus, the observed decrease in adjusted optical density measurements of synaptophysin immunoreactivity does not seem to be attributable to increased vasculature in the PFC of subjects with schizophrenia.

Finally, several lines of evidence suggest that the findings of this study are not due to medication effects. First, in 2 case subjects with schizophrenia not receiving antipsychotic medications at the time of death (Nos. 207 and 185), levels of synaptophysin immunoreactivity were decreased in the PFC. Second, case subject 341 who committed suicide by taking an overdose of chlorpromazine did not show a decrease in synaptophysin levels. Third, adjusted optical density measurements of synaptophysin immunoreactivity were more than 30% lower in the PFC of case subject 131 than in the matched control (No. 249), a subject who did not have schizophrenia but who had received treatment with antipsychotic medications. Fourth, synaptophysin levels were not decreased in control subject 217, who did not have schizophrenia and who had also been treated for with antipsychotic medications. Fifth, in an additional pair of subjects (see "Subjects and Methods" section), in whom major depressive disorder had been diagnosed, synaptophysin levels in the PFC were not lower in the subject who had received treatment with antipsychotic medications. Sixth, administration of haloperidol for 2 weeks had no effect on synaptophysin protein levels in rodent cerebral cortex specimens.[40] Finally, although the decrease in synaptophysin immunoreactivity in schizophrenia could be due to a decrease in the number or size of axon terminals or in the density of synaptic vesicles per terminal, these types of changes are unlikely to be a consequence of antipsychotic medications. For example, although chronic treatment of rats with haloperidol or clozapine may cause a shift in the relative percentages of the types of postsynaptic membrane specializations, they do not change the total number or average size of cortical axon terminals or the density of synaptic vesicles per terminal.[43]

POSSIBLE MECHANISMS UNDERLYING DECREASED LEVELS OF SYNAPTOPHYSIN IMMUNOREACTIVITY

The findings of this study suggest several possible mechanisms that could impair synaptic transmission in the PFC of subjects with schizophrenia. First, decreased synaptophysin immunoreactivity could be due to a decrease in the number of presynaptic terminals, and consequently in the number of synapses, in the PFC of subjects with schizophrenia. Presynaptic terminals are major components of the cortical neuropil, and a variety of recent studies, though not all,[14,15,19,20] have produced findings consistent with a decreased amount of neuropil in the PFC of subjects with schizophrenia. First, both imaging and postmortem studies have revealed a decrease in PFC volume in subjects with schizophrenia.[9-13,16-18] Second, increased phospholipid turnover in the PFC of patients with schizophrenia observed with magnetic resonance spectroscopy[44-47] may also reflect a loss of neuropil.[45,46] Third, an increase in neuronal density[18] without a change in total cell number[15,17] has also been observed in the PFC of subjects with schizophrenia. Finally, the density of dendritic spines, the major sites of excitatory synapses on pyramidal neurons, is decreased in the PFC of subjects with schizophrenia.[48,49] These findings and those of the present study converge on the common hypothesis that the number of presynaptic terminals and synaptic contacts is decreased in the PFC of subjects with schizophrenica. This interpretation is consistent with previous suggestions that PFC dysfunction in schizophrenia is related to the elimination of cortical synapses during adolescence.[50-52]

Alternatively, a reduction in the number of synaptic vesicles per terminal could produce the observed decrease in synaptophysin immunoreactivity. Because the size of an axon terminal is directly correlated with the number of vesicles it contains,[53] a decrease in the number of synaptic vesicles per terminal in subjects with schizophrenia would be associated with a decrease in terminal size and a decrease in synaptophysin immunoreactivity. Such a decrease in axon terminal size might also contribute to a decrease in PFC neuropil and volume in schizophrenia.

Finally, the results of this study could be caused by a decrease in the expression of synaptophysin messenger RNA, as has been observed in the hippocampal formation of subjects with schizophrenia.[40] Although such changes might not produce structural alterations in the PFC, they would likely disrupt neurotransmission in this region, given the critical role of synaptophysin in exocytosis.[25]

What elements of PFC circuitry might contribute to the altered synaptophysin immunoreactivity in subjects with schizophrenia? The decreased synaptophysin immunoreactivity across all cortical layers suggests that the involved system or systems must have axon terminals distributed throughout the cortical gray matter. Thus, it seems unlikely that abnormalities in projections from the mediodorsal thalamic nucleus, which terminate in the middle layers of the PFC,[54] could, at least in isolation, account for these findings. However, abnormalities in these afferents could have secondary effects on synaptophysin levels across all cortical layers. Projections to the PFC from many other cortical regions terminate across all cortical layers.[55] Thus, decreased synaptophysin immunoreactivity could reflect alterations in corticocortical input, which would certainly impair the function of the PFC.

In addition, although they comprise a variety of different subtypes, as a group, PFC γ-aminobutyric acid (GABA) neurons provide axon terminals in all cortical layers.[56] Thus, alterations in GABA terminals might also account for the findings of the present study, an interpretation supported by studies demonstrating alterations in GABA systems in the PFC of subjects with schizophrenia.[15,57-59]

Clearly, it is impossible to determine from the results of this study exactly which neural system(s) are altered in the PFC of subjects with schizophrenia. In addition, although a decline in synaptophysin immunoreactivity could lead to altered function of the PFC in schizophrenia,[2-4,6-8] it is also possible that impaired activation of this region may induce a reduction in markers of synaptic transmission. However, whatever pathological mechanism(s) lead to these alterations, disturbances in the levels of synaptophysin, a critical component of synaptic transmission, are likely to have profound effects on PFC synaptic function in schizophrenia.

Accepted for publication June 21, 1996.

This work was supported in part by the Independent Scientist Award MH00519 (Dr Lewis) and the Center for the Neuroscience of Mental Disorders grant MH45156, from the National Institute of Mental Health (Dr Lewis), and by a grant from the Scottish Rite Schizophrenia Research Program, Northern Masonic Jurisdiction, Lexington, Ky (Ms Glantz).

Presented as a poster exhibit at the Society for Neuroscience Meeting, Miami, Fla, November 15, 1994.

We thank Mayada Akil, MD,and Larry Glanz, PhD, for their help in obtaining the clinical information on the subjects used in this study, and Gretchen Haas, PhD, Matcheri Keshavan, MD, and Nina Schooler, PhD, for their participation in the diagnostic conferences. We also thank Allan Sampson, PhD, and Kris Schmidt, MA, for statistical consultation, Mary Brady for photographic assistance, and Dr Akil and Michele Pucak, PhD, for helpful comments on the manuscript.

Corresponding author: David A. Lewis, MD, Western Psychiatric Institute and Clinic, W1651 BST, 3811 O'Hara St, Pittsburgh, PA 15213.

REFERENCES

1. Levin S. Frontal lobe dysfunctions in schizophrenia, II: impairments of psychological and brain functions. *J Psychiat Res.* 1984;18:57-72.
2. Berman KF, Torrey EF, Daniel DG, Weinberger DR. Regional cerebral blood flow in monozygotic twins discordant and concordant for schizophrenia. *Arch Gen Psychiatry.* 1992;49:927-934.
3. Buchsbaum MS, Haier RJ, Potkin SG, Neuchterlein K, Bracha HS, Katz M, Lohr J, Wu J, Lottenberg S, Jerabek PA, Trenary M, Tafalla R, Reynolds C, Bunney WE Jr. Frontostriatal disorder of cerebral metabolism in never-medicated schizophrenics. *Arch Gen Psychiatry.* 1992;49:935-942.
4. Ingvar DH, Franzen G. Abnormalities of cerebral blood flow distribution in patients with chronic schizophrenia. *Acta Psychiat Scand.* 1974;50:425-462.
5. Park S, Holzman PS. Schizophrenics show spatial working memory deficits. *Arch Gen Psychiatry.* 1992;49:975-982.
6. Rubin P, Holm S, Friberg L, Videbech P, Anderson HS, Bendsen BB, Stromso N, Larsen JK, Lassen NA, Hemmingsen R. Altered modulation of prefrontal and subcortical brain activity in newly diagnosed schizophrenia and schizophreniform

disorder: a regional cerebral blood flow study. *Arch Gen Psychiatry.* 1991;48:987-995.

7. Wolkin A, Sanfilipo M, Wolf AP, Angrist B, Brodie JD, Rotrosen J. Negative symptoms and hypofrontality in chronic schizophrenia. *Arch Gen Psychiatry.* 1992; 49:959-965.
8. Weinberger DR, Berman KF, Zec RF. Physiologic dysfunction of dorsolateral prefrontal cortex in schizophrenia, I: regional cerebral blood flow evidence. *Arch Gen Psychiatry.* 1986;43:114-124.
9. Andreasen NC, Flashman L, Flaum M, Arndt S, Swayze V II, O'Leary DS, Ehrhardt JC, Yuh WT. Regional brain abnormalities in schizophrenia measured with magnetic resonance imaging. *JAMA.* 1994;272:1763-1769.
10. Breier A, Buchanan RW, Elkashef A, Munson RC, Kirkpatrick B, Gellad F. Brain morphology and schizophrenia: a magnetic resonance imaging study of limbic, prefrontal cortex, and caudate structures. *Arch Gen Psychiatry.* 1992;49:921-926.
11. Schlaepfer TE, Harris GJ, Tien AY, Peng LW, Lee S, Federman EB, Chase GA, Barta PE, Pearlson GD. Decreased regional cortical gray matter volume in schizophrenia. *Am J Psychiatry.* 1994;151:842-848.
12. Shelton RC, Karson CN, Doran AR, Pickar D, Bigelow LB, Weinberger DR. Cerebral structural pathology in schizophrenia: evidence for a selective prefrontal cortical defect. *Am J Psychiatry.* 1988;145:154-163.
13. Zipursky RB, Lim KO, Sullivan EV, Brown BW, Pfefferbaum A. Widespread cerebral gray matter volume deficits in schizophrenia. *Arch Gen Psychiatry.* 1992; 49:195-205.
14. Wible CG, Shenton ME, Hokama H, Kikinis R, Jolesz FA, Metcalf D, McCarley RW. Prefrontal cortex and schizophrenia: a quantitative magnetic resonance imaging study. *Arch Gen Psychiatry.* 1995;52:279-288.
15. Akbarian S, Kim JJ, Potkin SG, Hagman JO, Tafazzoli A, Bunney WE Jr, Jones EG. Gene expression for glutamic acid decarboxylase is reduced without loss of neurons in prefrontal cortex of schizophrenics. *Arch Gen Psychiatry.* 1995;52:258-266.
16. Pakkenberg B. Post-mortem study of chronic schizophrenic brains. *Br J Psychiatry.* 1987;151:744-752.
17. Pakkenberg B. Total nerve cell number in neocortex in chronic schizophrenics and controls estimated using optical disectors. *Biol Psychiatry.* 1993;34:768-772.
18. Selemon LD, Rajkowska G, Goldman-Rakic PS. Abnormally high neuronal density in the schizophrenic cortex: a morphometric analysis of prefrontal area 9 and occipital area 17. *Arch Gen Psychiatry.* 1995;52:805-818.
19. Benes FM, Davidson J, Bird ED. Quantitative cytoarchitectural studies of the cerebral cortex of schizophrenics. *Arch Gen Psychiatry.* 1986;43:31-35.
20. Benes FM, McSparren J, Bird ED, SanGiovanni JP, Vincent SL. Deficits in small interneurons in prefrontal and cingulate cortices of schizophrenic and schizoaffective patients. *Arch Gen Psychiatry.* 1991;48:996-1001.
21. Bourgeois J-P, Goldman-Rakic PS, Rakic P. Synaptogenesis in the prefrontal cortex of rhesus monkeys. *Cereb Cortex.* 1994;4:78-96.
22. Jahn R, Schiebler W, Ouimet C, Greengard P. A 38,000-dalton membrane protein (p38) present in synaptic vesicles. *Proc Natl Acad Sci U S A.* 1985;82:4137-4141.
23. Navone F, Jahn R, DiGioia G, Stukenbrok H, Greengard P, DeCamilli P. Protein p38: an integral membrane protein specific for small vesicles of neurons and neuroendocrine cells. *J Cell Biol.* 1986;103:2511-2527.
24. Wiedenmann B, Franke WW. Identification and localization of synaptophysin, an integral membrane glycoprotein of M_r 38,000 characteristic of presynaptic vesicles. *Cell.* 1985;41:1017-1028.
25. Alder J, Lu B, Valtorta F, Greengard P, Poo M. Calcium-dependent transmitter secretion reconstituted in *Xenopus* oocytes: requirement for synaptophysin. *Science.* 1992;257:657-661.
26. Alder J, Kanki H, Valtorta F, Greengard P, Poo M. Overexpression of synaptophysin enhances neurotransmitter secretion at xenopus neuromuscular synapses. *J Neurosci.* 1995;15:511-519.
27. Hamos JE, DeGennaro LJ, Drachman DA. Synaptic loss in Alzheimer's disease and other dementias. *Neurology.* 1989;39:355-361.
28. Masliah E, Terry RD, Alford M, DeTeresa R. Quantitative immunohistochemistry of synaptophysin in human neocortex: an alternative method to estimate density of presynaptic terminals in paraffin sections. *J Histochem Cytochem.* 1990;38:837-844.
29. Masliah E, Terry RD, Alford M, DeTeresa R, Hansen LA. Cortical and subcortical patterns of synaptophysinlike immunoreactivity in Alzheimer's disease. *Am J Pathol.* 1991;138:235-246.
30. Khachaturian ZS. Diagnosis of Alzheimer's disease. *Arch Neurol.* 1985;42:1097-1105.
31. Dixon L, Haas G, Weiden PJ, Sweeney J, Frances AJ. Drug abuse in schizophrenic patients: clinical correlates and reasons for use. *Am J Psychiatry.* 1991;148:224-230.
32. Daviss SR, Lewis DA. Local circuit neurons of the prefrontal cortex in schizophrenia: selective increase in the density of calbindin-immunoreactive neurons. *Psychiatry Res.* 1995;59:81-96.
33. Rosenberg DR, Lewis DA. Postnatal maturation of the dopaminergic innervation of monkey prefrontal and motor cortices: a tyrosine hydroxylase immunohistochemical analysis. *J Comp Neurol.* 1995;358:383-400.
34. Lewis DA, Campbell MJ, Terry RD, Morrison JH. The laminar and regional distribution of neurofibrillary tangles and neuritic plaques in Alzheimer's disease: a quantitative study of visual and auditory cortices. *J Neurosci.* 1987;7:1799-1808.
35. Rajkowska G, Goldman-Rakic PS. Cytoarchitectonic definition of prefrontal areas in the normal human cortex, I: remapping of areas 9 and 46 using quantitative criteria. *Cereb Cortex.* 1995;5:307-322.
36. Devoto SH, Barnstable CJ. SVP38: a synaptic vesicle protein whose appearance correlates closely with synaptogenesis in the rat nervous system. *Ann N Y Acad Sci.* 1987;493:493-496.
37. Smolen AJ. Image analytic techniques for quantification of immunohistochemical staining in the nervous system. In: Conn PM, ed. *Quantitative and Qualitative Microscopy.* Orlando, Fla: Academic Press Inc; 1990:208-229.
38. Perrone-Bizzozero NI, Sower AC, Bird ED, Benowitz LI, Ivins KJ, Neve RL. Levels of the growth-associated protein GAP-43 are selectively increased in association cortices in schizophrenia. *Proc Natl Acad Sci U S A.* 1996;93:14182-14187.
39. Browning MD, Dudek EM, Rapier JL, Leonard S, Freedman R. Significant reductions in synapsin but not synaptophysin specific activity in the brains of some schizophrenics. *Biol Psychiatry.* 1993;34:529-535.
40. Eastwood SL, Harrison PJ. Decreased synaptophysin in the medial temporal lobe in schizophrenia demonstrated using immunoautoradiography. *Neuroscience.* 1995;69:339-343.
41. Peretti-Renucci R, Feuerstein C, Manier M, Lorimier P, Savasta M, Thibault J, Mons N, Geffard M. Quantitative image analysis with densitometry for immunohistochemistry and autoradiography of receptor binding sites—methodological considerations. *J Neurosci Res.* 1991;28:583-600.
42. Duvernoy H, Delon S, Vannson JL. Cortical blood vessels of the human brain. *Brain Res Bull.* 1981;7:519-579.
43. Vincent SL, McSparren J, Wang RY, Benes FM. Evidence for ultrastructural changes in cortical axodendritic synapses following long-term treatment with haloperidol or clozapine. *Neuropsychopharmacology.* 1991;5:147-155.
44. Deicken RF, Calabrese G, Merrin EL, Meyerhoff DJ, Dillon WP, Weiner MW, Fein G. ^{31}Phosphorus magnetic resonance spectroscopy of the frontal and parietal lobes in chronic schizophrenia. *Biol Psychiatry.* 1994;36:503-510.
45. Pettegrew JW, Keshavan MS, Panchalingam K, Strychor S, Kaplan DB, Tretta MG, Allen M. Alterations in brain high-energy phosphate and membrane phospholipid metabolism in first-episode, drug-naive schizophrenics: a pilot study of the dorsal prefrontal cortex by in vivo phosphorus 31 nuclear magnetic resonance imaging. *Arch Gen Psychiatry.* 1991;48:563-568.
46. Stanley JA, Williamson PC, Drost DJ, Carr TJ, Rylett RJ, Malla A, Thompson RT. An *in vivo* study of the prefrontal cortex of schizophrenic patients at different stages of illness via phosphorus magnetic resonance spectroscopy. *Arch Gen Psychiatry.* 1995;52:399-406.
47. Williamson P, Drost D, Stanley J, Carr T, Morrison S, Merskey H. Localized phosphorous 31 magnetic resonance spectroscopy in chronic schizophrenic patients and normal controls. *Arch Gen Psychiatry.* 1991;48:578.
48. Glantz LA, Lewis DA. Assessment of spine density on layer III pyramidal cells in the prefrontal cortex of schizophrenic subjects. *Soc Neurosci Abstr.* 1995;21:239.
49. Garey LJ, Ong WY, Patel TS, Kanani M, Davis A, Hornstein C, Bauer M. Reduction in dendritic spine number on cortical pyramidal neurons in schizophrenia. *Soc Neurosci Abstr.* 1995;21:237.
50. Feinberg I. Schizophrenia: caused by a fault in programmed synaptic elimination during adolescence? *J Psychiat Res.* 1982;17:319-334.
51. Hoffman RE, Dobscha SK. Cortical pruning and the development of schizophrenia: a computer model. *Schizophr Bull.* 1989;15:477-490.
52. Hoffman RE, McGlashan TH. Parallel distributed processing and the emergence of schizophrenic symptoms. *Schizophr Bull.* 1993;19:119-140.
53. Pierce JP, Lewin GR. An ultrastructural size principle. *Neuroscience.* 1994;58:441-446.
54. Giguere M, Goldman-Rakic PS. Mediodorsal nucleus: areal, laminar, and tangential distribution of afferents and efferents in the frontal lobe of rhesus monkeys. *J Comp Neurol.* 1988;277:195-213.
55. Goldman-Rakic PS, Schwartz ML. Interdigitation of contralateral and ipsilateral columnar projections to frontal association cortex in primates. *Science.* 1982; 216:755-757.
56. Lund JS, Lewis DA. Local circuit neurons of developing and mature macaque prefrontal cortex: golgi and immunocytochemical characteristics. *J Comp Neurol.* 1993;328:282-312.
57. Sherman AD, Davidson AT, Baruah S, Hegwood TS, Waziri R. Evidence of glutamatergic deficiency in schizophrenia. *Neurosci Lett.* 1991;121:77-80.
58. Benes FM, Vincent SL, Alsterberg G, Bird ED, SanGiovanni JP. Increased $GABA_A$ receptor binding in superficial layers of cingulate cortex in schizophrenics. *J Neurosci.* 1992;12:924-929.
59. Benes FM, Vincent SL, Marie A, Khan Y. Up-regulation of $GABA_A$ receptor binding on neurons of the prefrontal cortex in schizophrenic subjects. *Neuroscience.* 1996;75:1021-1031.

ORIGINAL ARTICLE

Maternal Smoking During Pregnancy and the Risk of Conduct Disorder in Boys

Lauren S. Wakschlag, PhD; Benjamin B. Lahey, PhD; Rolf Loeber, PhD; Stephanie M. Green, MS; Rachel A. Gordon, MA; Bennett L. Leventhal, MD

Background: Previous animal and human studies have indicated that prenatal exposure to nicotine is associated with adverse reproductive outcomes, including altered neural structure and functioning, cognitive deficits, and behavior problems in the offspring. Our study extends previous research on humans by controlling a broad range of correlates of maternal smoking during pregnancy to determine if smoking is associated with behavior problems in the offspring severe enough to qualify for *DSM-III-R* diagnoses.

Method: Subjects were 177 clinic-referred boys, ages 7 to 12 years at the time of the first assessment, who underwent longitudinal assessment for 6 years using annual structured diagnostic interviews. Correlates of maternal smoking during pregnancy and previously identified demographic, parental, perinatal, and family risk factors for the disruptive behavior disorders were controlled in logistic regression analyses.

Results: Mothers who smoked more than half a pack of cigarettes daily during pregnancy were significantly more likely to have a child with conduct disorder (odds ratio, 4.4; $P=.001$) than mothers who did not smoke during pregnancy. This association was statistically significant when controlling for socioeconomic status, maternal age, parental antisocial personality, substance abuse during pregnancy, and maladaptive parenting.

Conclusions: Maternal smoking during pregnancy appears to be a robust independent risk factor for conduct disorder in male offspring. Maternal smoking during pregnancy may have direct adverse effects on the developing fetus or be a marker for a heretofore unmeasured characteristic of mothers that is of etiologic significance for conduct disorder.

Arch Gen Psychiatry. 1997;54:670-676

YOUTH ARE said to exhibit conduct disorder (CD) if they frequently and persistently engage in a variety of serious antisocial behaviors. Conduct disorder differs from normal delinquent behavior in terms of the variety of antisocial behaviors manifested and the severity, persistence, and precocity of those antisocial behaviors. Because CD is a serious problem to the affected youths, their families, and society at large, and because it is usually refractive to treatment,[1] research on the cause and subsequent prevention of CD must be a high priority for society.

Our study explores the possibility that maternal cigarette smoking during pregnancy is a risk factor for CD in the offspring. At least 20% to 25% of pregnant women are estimated to smoke cigarettes, although smoking is associated with low birth weight, prematurity, and infant mortality.[2,3] Maternal smoking is believed to contribute to adverse reproductive outcomes through fetal hypoxia resulting from nicotine-mediated restriction of uteroplacental blood flow and increased carboxyhemoglobin in fetal blood, but there is evidence that nicotine is also a neurobehavioral teratogen. Nicotine crosses the human placenta and has direct effects on the developing fetus.[4-9] Preclinical studies suggest that maternal smoking during pregnancy produces changes in the offspring's neural functioning, including reductions in uptake of serotonin,[10] alterations in dopaminergic systems,[11,12] alterations in peripheral and central noradrenergic neurons,[13-15] inhibited cholinergic brain cell growth in rats (perhaps due to precocious stimulation of nicotinic receptors),[7,8,16] and changes in DNA and RNA synthesis in the brain.[17] Functional deficits following nicotine exposure persist well after effects on receptor binding have attenuated and occur even at levels not generally considered toxic.[14,15] Behavioral consequences of in utero nicotine exposure in animals include de-

From the Department of Psychiatry, University of Chicago, Chicago, Ill (Drs Wakschlag, Lahey, and Leventhal and Ms Gordon), and the Western Psychiatric Institute and Clinic, School of Medicine, University of Pittsburgh, Pittsburgh, Pa (Dr Loeber and Ms Green).

SUBJECTS AND METHODS

SUBJECTS

Data used in the present analyses are from the Developmental Trends Study, a longitudinal study of 177 boys referred to 1 of 2 university child psychiatry and child psychology outpatient clinics in Pennsylvania (n=96) and Georgia (n=81). Participation rate at the time of the first assessment (year 1) was 88.5%, and retention rate across the subsequent 5 years was high, averaging 98%. Additional details on this sample have been reported previously.[33,34] Four annual assessments were conducted, and a fifth assessment was conducted 2 years later, between October 1, 1987, and May 30, 1993. The use of repeated assessments of CD into adolescence was designed to minimize the false-negative classification of youth that is common in cross-sectional studies of risk-behavior relationships using a single time of measurement.

Subjects ranged from 7 to 12 years of age at the onset of the study and were 12 to 17 years of age in year 6. Seventy-one percent of the sample were non-Hispanic white, and 29% were African American. Family SES was distributed across all 5 levels of the Hollingshead 4-factor index.[36] Fifty-two percent of the mothers were married, 10% were cohabiting, and 38% were living alone in year 1.

ASSESSMENTS

Demographic, Perinatal, and Family Factors

Maternal smoking during pregnancy and all other pregnancy factors were assessed via a structured interview of the biological mother about her pregnancy history in year 1 (ie, 7-12 years following pregnancy). Maternal smoking status was based on maternal report in response to the question "Did you smoke cigarettes during your pregnancy?" with choices as follows: no, occasionally (less than daily), half a pack or less daily, more than half to 1 pack daily, and more than 1 pack daily. Due to low frequencies in several of the groups, these categories were then collapsed into the following 3 smoking groups: none (includes occasionally), half a pack or less daily, and more than half a pack daily. Data on smoking behavior in each trimester were not available, and data on paternal smoking behavior were not available.

Age of the mother at the birth of the study child was entered as a continuous variable (mean±SD, 25.0±5.1 years; range, 15-38 years). All other pregnancy and perinatal variables (prenatal alcohol and illicit drug use, pregnancy and birth complications, prematurity, and low birth weight) were treated dichotomously (0 indicates no; 1, yes). Pregnancy complications were defined as the occurrence of high blood pressure, bleeding, and/or infection during pregnancy. Birth complications were defined as the occurrence of delivery or perinatal complications such as severe jaundice or oxygen deprivation. Prematurity and low birth weight were defined by standard usage; ie, gestational age below 37 weeks and birth weight less than 2500 g.[37]

Family factors were also derived from this interview. The marital status of the biological parents in year 1 was treated dichotomously (0 indicates married; 1, not currently married), as was ethnicity (0 indicates non-Hispanic white; 1, African American). The number of siblings in the household in year 1 was entered as a continuous variable (mean±SD, 1.2±0.9 siblings; range, 0-5 siblings).

In addition, a series of parental self-report questionnaires was used to assess parenting in year 1. These questionnaires were adapted from the Parent-Adolescent Communication Scale[38] and from parenting measures developed and extensively validated in the Oregon Youth Study.[39] Parenting measures were constructed by extracting items representing dimensions of parenting identified in previous research as familial antecedents to CD,[40] ie, supervision, discipline, and communication. Supervision was assessed as the degree to which the parent actively monitored the child's daily activities. Ineffective discipline was assessed as the degree of parental follow-up on disciplinary practices when the child misbehaved. Communication was assessed as parent-child openness of communication and

Continued on next page

creased learning efficiency[18,19] and increased motor activity.[11]

Evidence from studies of human neonates suggests that maternal smoking during pregnancy is associated with increased rates of neurobehavioral difficulties.[20-24] Several studies have linked maternal smoking during pregnancy with childhood inattention, impulsivity, and motor hyperactivity in offspring, using laboratory tasks and parent and teacher ratings,[24-28] and, recently, with attention deficit hyperactivity disorder (ADHD) in offspring, using diagnostic measures.[29] Similarly, maternal smoking during pregnancy has been associated with parent-teacher ratings of conduct problems in children[26,28,30,31] and a criminal record in young adults.[32]

We herein report analyses of data from the Developmental Trends Study[33,34] to determine if maternal smoking during pregnancy is associated with increased risk for 1 or more of the *DSM-III-R* disruptive behavior disorders. There is only 1 other study in which diagnostic measures were used; this study examined only ADHD as an outcome and not oppositional defiant disorder (ODD) or CD.[29] The existing evidence suggests the possibility that maternal smoking is linked to ADHD and CD. Alternatively, smoking may be specifically related to CD, with an apparent association between smoking and ADHD due to the high rates of comorbidity between ADHD and CD.[35]

In addition to using diagnostic measures, we add to previous investigations by extending the number of controlled variables. As noted by others,[26,28,30-32] the apparent relationship between maternal smoking and behavior problems in offspring could be a false correlate of a causal relationship between characteristics of women who smoke during pregnancy (eg, psychopathologic characteristics) and behavior problems in their offspring. The following 4 categories of risk factors for CD and other disruptive behavior disorders must be controlled to provide strong evidence of a direct association between maternal smoking during pregnancy and conduct problems in the offspring: demographic factors (eg, problem-solving skills. Items for each dimension were summed, and then the correlation of each item with the summed score was examined. Only those items that were correlated 0.50 or more with the summed score were retained. The scales demonstrated good internal consistency (Cronbach α for supervision, .87; for ineffective discipline, .68; for communication, .87). These measures were then dichotomized as to whether parenting was maladaptive along a particular dimension. Due to skewed distributions, parenting was coded as maladaptive for scores that fell within the upper 25% of each scale.[34] In addition, response to a question assessing the frequency with which parents used physical discipline (almost never, sometimes, and often) was used as a measure of harsh discipline.

Parental Psychopathologic Characteristic

Psychopathologic characteristics of the biological parents were assessed using structured diagnostic interviews of the biological mother about herself and about the biological father. The interview consisted of sections covering *DSM-III-R* diagnoses of antisocial personality disorder and alcohol and other drug abuse from the Schedule for Affective Disorders and Schizophrenia[41] and sections covering other Axis I disorders from the Structured Clinical Interview for *DSM-III-R*–Non-patient Version.[42] The Minnesota Multiphasic Personality Inventory (MMPI) also was administered to the biological mother because few women meet *DSM-III-R* criteria for antisocial personality disorder, and because using only the diagnosis of antisocial personality disorder has been found to underestimate maternal personality disturbances related to CD.[43,44] Based on previous findings, the sum of the *K*-corrected *T* scores on the MMPI F (Validity), Pd (Psychopathic Deviate), and Ma (Mania) scales was used as the index of maternal antisocial personality.[45,46] Parental abuse of alcohol and other drugs were collapsed into a composite variable (0 indicates no; 1, abuse). All measures except the biannual structured diagnostic interviews were obtained in year 1.

Child Diagnosis

Each child, his parent, and his teacher were interviewed separately each year using the National Institute of Mental Health Diagnostic Interview Schedule for Children.[47] Subjects were asked to report symptoms that had occurred during the previous 6 months. Information derived from these interviews led to determination of a child's diagnostic status based on criteria from *DSM-III-R*,[48] using a best estimate method of combining reports from parent, teacher, and child. All diagnoses for which the child met full criteria were assigned. A diagnosis of CD did not preclude a comorbid diagnosis of ODD in our study to assess association of maternal smoking with each disorder separately.

STATISTICAL ANALYSIS

The relation of maternal smoking during pregnancy to each of the disruptive behavior disorders was examined using Mantel-Haenzel χ^2 procedures. To select control variables for the multivariate analyses, the 3 smoking groups and children with and without CD were compared on the 4 groups of risk factors. The χ^2 and Mantel-Haenzel χ^2 procedures were used to examine the relation of CD and the level of maternal smoking to dichotomous risk factors. *t* tests were used to examine mean differences in smoking groups with and without CD on continuous risk factor variables, and analysis of variance was used to assess differences among the 3 smoking groups on these risk factors. Logistic regression analysis was then used to examine the relation of maternal smoking during pregnancy and CD when confounding and potential mediating variables were controlled. In addition, a logistic regression analysis was conducted to determine if adverse perinatal outcomes mediated the relationship between maternal smoking during pregnancy and CD. The α was set at the .05 level. All analyses were conducted using statistical software (Statistical Package for the Social Sciences, version 6.1.3, SPSS, Inc, Chicago, Ill).

socioeconomic status [SES]), parental psychopathologic conditions (eg, paternal antisocial personality disorder), pregnancy risk factors (eg, maternal age and low birth weight), and family and parenting risk factors (eg, number of children in the household and harsh discipline). These have not been comprehensively controlled in previous research; assessments of parental psychopathologic characteristics have been notably absent from most studies linking maternal smoking and children's behavior problems. Our study is the first to control for these 4 categories of potential confounds of the correlation between maternal smoking during pregnancy and behavior problems of offspring in a single sample.

RESULTS

Sixty-three percent of the mothers reported that they were nonsmokers or occasional smokers; 13% of the mothers reported that they smoked half a pack or less daily; and 24% of the mothers reported that they smoked more than half a pack daily.

One hundred five boys (59.3%) met *DSM-III-R* criteria for CD during at least 1 assessment during the 6 years of the study.[33] Within this group, 64.8% of the boys first received a diagnosis in year 1, 14.2% in year 2, 6.6% in year 3, 9.5% in year 4, and 4.8% in year 6. The diagnosis of CD was moderately persistent, with 63 (92.6%) of the 68 boys who met criteria for CD in year 1 receiving a second diagnosis in at least 1 subsequent year and continuing to exhibit antisocial symptoms even in years when full diagnostic criteria for CD were not met.[33]

BIVARIATE ANALYSES

Mothers who smoked more cigarettes during pregnancy were significantly more likely to have a child who met *DSM-III-R* criteria for CD at least once during the 6 years of the study (Mantel-Haenzel χ^2=13.74; df=1, 177; P=.001). Forty-nine percent of the mothers who did not smoke during pregnancy had offspring with CD as compared with 70% of the offspring of mothers who smoked half a pack or less daily and 81% of the offspring of mothers who smoked more than half a pack daily. Mothers who smoked more than half a pack daily during pregnancy were more than 4 times as likely to have a child with CD than mothers who did not smoke (odds ratio, 4.4; 95% confidence interval, 1.87-10.27; P=.001). Attention-deficit hyperactivity disorder was not significantly associated with maternal smoking (Mantel-Haenzel χ^2=0.09; df=1, 177; P=.76). There was a nonsignificant positive trend for ODD to be associated with maternal smoking during pregnancy (χ^2=2.79; df=1, 177; P=.09). The rate of maternal smoking during pregnancy for children with ODD who also had a diagnosis of CD was 49%. In contrast, the rate of maternal smoking among youth with ODD without CD (24%) was virtually the same as that for children without a diagnosis of ODD or CD (23%), suggesting that this nonsignificant trend for ODD was due to the frequent co-occurrence of ODD and CD.

The 4 groups of risk factors were then examined for their association with maternal smoking during pregnancy or CD. These variables included demographic factors (eg, SES and ethnicity), parental psychopathologic conditions (eg, paternal antisocial personality disorder, maternal MMPI antisocial index, and maternal and paternal depression and substance abuse), other pregnancy risk factors (eg, maternal age at birth of the child, use of illicit drugs and alcohol during pregnancy, pregnancy and birth complications, low birth weight, and prematurity), and family and parenting risk factors (eg, number of children in the household, marital status, poor communication, little supervision, and ineffective and harsh discipline). Variables associated with CD and/or smoking at the trend level or better (P=.10) are shown in **Table 1** and **Table 2**. These variables included a number of variables associated with smoking and/or CD in previous research (eg, SES, parental antisociality, and maladaptive parenting) and were included as control variables in the subsequent multivariate analyses.

Table 1. Risk Factors Significantly Associated With Childhood CD*

Risk Factors	Boys With No CD (n=72)	Boys With CD (n=105)	Tests of Significance
Demographics			
Mean SES index	3.5	2.6	t=4.76; P<.001
African American, %	18.1	38.1	χ^2=8.17; P=.004
Parental psychopathologic characteristic, %			
Paternal APD	12.5	29.5	χ^2=7.07; P=.008
Paternal substance abuse	22.2	45.7	χ^2=10.21; P=.001
Mean maternal MMPI	166.3	177.6	t=−3.14; P=.002
Perinatal variables			
Mean maternal age at birth of child, y	26.8	23.3	t=4.74; P<.001
Family and parenting variables			
Not married, %	44.4	72.4	χ^2=14.01; P<.001
Poor communication, %	11.1	35.2	χ^2=13.0; P<.001
Ineffective discipline, %	25.0	46.7	χ^2=8.5; P=.004
Harsh discipline, %	1.6	1.8	t=2.94; P=.004
Poor supervision, %	15.3	40.0	χ^2=12.4; P<.001

**CD indicates conduct disorder; SES, socioeconomic status; APD, antisocial personality diagnosis; MMPI, Minnesota Multiphasic Personality Inventory antisocial index; and marital status, biological parents' marital status in year 1.*

LOGISTIC REGRESSION ANALYSES

A logistic regression was conducted in which the relation of smoking to CD was examined when SES and parental antisocial personality were controlled. Maternal smoking during pregnancy was coded to allow contrasts of smoking no more than half a pack daily and smoking more than half a pack daily vs no smoking. This model

Table 2. Risk Factors Significantly Associated With Maternal Smoking During Pregnancy*

Risk Factors	Level of Maternal Smoking: None (n=112)	≤Half Pack Daily (n=23)	>Half Pack Daily (n=42)	Tests of Significance†
Demographics				
Mean SES index	3.24	2.65	2.38	F=8.48; P<.001
Parental psychopathologic characteristic %				
Paternal APD	16.1	30.4	35.7	χ^2=7.4; P=.007
Paternal substance abuse	26.8	43.5	57.1	χ^2=12.7; P<.001
Perinatal variables, %				
Maternal illicit drug use	1.8	0	11.9	χ^2=6.9; P=.008
Maternal alcohol use	8.9	26.1	28.6	χ^2=10.1; P=.001
Low birth weight	4.5	17.4	9.5	χ^2=5.1; P=.08
Family and parenting variables				
Mean No. of children	1.08	1.0	1.6	F=5.1; P=.007
Marital status, %	54.5	73.9	71.4	χ^2=4.5; P=.03
Poor communication, %	17.0	47.8	35.7	χ^2=7.9; P=.005
Ineffective discipline, %	30.4	52.0	50.0	χ^2=6.1; P=.01
Poor supervision, %	25.9	26.1	42.9	χ^2=3.7; P=.05

**Abbreviations are given in the footnote to Table 1.*
†χ^2 procedures are Mantel-Haenzel tests for linear association.

Table 3. Basic Model of Regressing Maternal Smoking During Pregnancy and Well-established Risk Factors for CD on Childhood CD*

Variables	B	Wald Statistic	P	Odds Ratio (95% Confidence Intervals)
Smokes ≤ half pack per day	0.40	0.57	.45	1.5 (0.53-4.25)
Smokes >half pack per day	1.2	6.1	.01	3.3 (1.27-8.58)
Paternal APD	0.68	2.2	.14	2.0 (0.81-4.79)
Maternal MMPI	0.01	3.3	.07	1.0 (1.00-1.03)
SES	0.40	0.57	.003	.65 (0.48-0.86

**Abbreviations are given in the footnote to Table 1. For the overall model, χ^2=36.2; df=5; P<.001.*

Table 4. Final Model of Regressing Maternal Smoking During Pregnancy and Identified Risk Factors for CD on Childhood CD*

Variables	B	Wald Statistic	P	Odds Ratio (95% Confidence Intervals)
Smokes ≤ half pack per day	0.50	0.74	.39	1.6 (0.53-5.11)
Smokes > half pack per day	1.2	5.3	.02	3.3 (1.2-9.07)
Paternal APD	0.55	1.3	.26	1.7 (0.67-4.5)
Maternal MMPI	0.01	1.4	.24	1.0 (0.99-1.03)
SES	−0.28	3.1	.08	0.76 (0.56-1.03)
Maternal age	−0.10	7.1	.01	0.90 (0.84-0.97)
Poor supervision	0.96	4.6	.03	2.6 (1.09-6.2)
Harsh discipline	0.74	4.3	.04	2.1 (0.56-2.2)

**Abbreviations are given in the footnote to Table 1. For the overall model, χ^2=56.1; df=8; P<.001.*

is shown in **Table 3**. In this model, smoking more than half a pack daily (*P*=.01), SES (*P*=.003), and maternal antisocial personality at the trend level (*P*=.07) were independent predictors of CD when other variables were controlled.

A subsequent series of logistic regression analyses were conducted by adding subsets of variables to this basic model. These included ethnicity and parental substance abuse, other pregnancy risk factors (ie, maternal age at birth of the proband, and use of alcohol and illicit drugs during pregnancy), perinatal adversity (ie, low birth weight and complications), and family and parenting factors (ie, marital status of the biological parents, number of children in the household, little supervision, harsh discipline, ineffective discipline, and poor communication). The contrast of smoking more than half a pack daily remained a significant predictor of CD in all of these models (*P* range, .02-.05). The new independent predictors of CD that emerged in these analyses were maternal age (*P*=.003), harsh discipline (*P*=.04), and little supervision at the trend level (*P*=.07).

A final regression analysis adding all of these significant independent predictors to the basic model was then conducted (**Table 4**). Smoking more than half a pack daily during pregnancy (*P*=.02), maternal age (*P*=.008), little parental supervision (*P*=.03), and harsh discipline (*P*=.04) were significant independent predictors of CD in this model.

COMMENT

Mothers who smoked more than half a pack daily during pregnancy were significantly more likely to have offspring who met *DSM-III-R* diagnostic criteria for CD during the preadolescent or adolescent years than women who did not smoke or smoked only occasionally during pregnancy. The *DSM-III-R* criteria for CD are based on a disturbance of conduct lasting at least 6 months, during which at least 3 conduct symptoms are present such as lying, setting fires, vandalism, physical cruelty, forcible sexual activity, and/or stealing. The *DSM-III-R* criteria for CD are quite comparable to those of *DSM-IV*, with more than 90% of youth who meet criteria under 1 definition meeting criteria under the other.[49]

These findings support previous work showing that maternal smoking during pregnancy is associated with increased rates of preschool and school-age behavior problems[21,28-31] and delinquency in the offspring.[32] Our findings extend previous work by providing evidence that maternal smoking during pregnancy is uniquely associated with CD rather than with disruptive behavior problems more generally and that the relation of maternal smoking during pregnancy and CD cannot be explained by a broad range of known risk factors for CD. Smoking during pregnancy was found to be associated with a number of other risk factors for CD, including having less affluent and less well-educated parents, larger family size, maternal use of alcohol and other drugs during pregnancy, having a biological father who met diagnostic criteria for antisocial personality and/or substance abuse disorders, and maladaptive parenting. Nonetheless, maternal smoking during pregnancy was associated with an increased risk for CD in the offspring, even when these other risk factors for CD were controlled. Thus, our findings suggest that the relation of maternal smoking during pregnancy and CD cannot be better explained by other variables that characterize "the type of mother who smokes during pregnancy."[50,51] Although these findings suggest that maternal smoking during pregnancy may be causally related to the development of CD in her offspring, the possibility that smoking is a marker for a causative maternal characteristic not measured herein cannot be ruled out.

Several other limitations of this study should be acknowledged. Our findings are based on a relatively small, clinical sample of boys. The regression analyses suggest that maternal smoking during pregnancy is an independent risk factor for CD, but replication in population-based samples is important to establish that maternal smoking is a risk factor for CD in samples that do not have high numbers of other risk factors for CD. On the other hand, the use of clinic control subjects (boys who never met criteria for CD in years 1-6) ensures that the association between CD and maternal smoking during pregnancy is specific to CD and not a nonspecific association with childhood psychopathologic characteristics in general. Thus, there are advantages to clinic comparison groups as well. Further research is also needed to explore the generalizability of these findings to girls. There is some evidence that effects of maternal smoking during pregnancy are stronger for boys than girls[52]; this may be particularly so in terms of the relation of smoking to CD, due to the already increased risk for disruptive behavior problems in boys.[53]

Data on the perinatal period in our study were based on maternal retrospective reports of pregnancies and births that had occurred 7 to 12 years previously. These data may be flawed by difficulties in recall and by underreporting, although retrospective recall of smoking has been demonstrated to be fairly reliable compared with recall of other substance use.[54,55] The absence of data on prenatal and postnatal environmental smoke exposure is another limitation of our findings, since emerging evidence suggests there may be a continuum of smoking effects depending on the level and type of exposure (eg, active and passive smoke exposure).[30] The strongest future studies will be prospective, longitudinal studies that use more sophisticated assessments of prenatal and postnatal smoke exposure, including biochemical assays of carbon monoxide in expired air and measurement of thiocyanate, nicotine, and cotinine levels in blood, urine, or saliva.

Unfortunately, our data did not allow us to examine the association of diagnostic status during the 6 years with the covariates at each time since, with the exception of diagnostic status, data are based on year 1 assessments only. Analytic strategies such as random-effects modeling may be useful in future studies to capture the relation of factors over time to the emergence and stability of the diagnosis.

Given the more than ample evidence from animal studies that suggests a role for nicotine exposure in altering the development of central and peripheral neurotransmitter systems, the possibility of a similar mechanism of action in human fetuses must be considered. Although our data are not sufficient to be fully conclusive, they strongly support an independent association between in utero nicotine exposure and the development of clinically significant behavioral abnormalities. Whereas there are clear indications for further investigation in this area, our findings are robust. If indeed maternal smoking during pregnancy has a direct biologic effect on neural systems that regulate behavior, prospective studies could identify manifestations of these effects as early as infancy.[56,57]

The scientific and social significance of identifying a relatively modifiable prenatal risk factor for CD clearly warrants testing in future correlational and preclinical studies. During their lifetime, youth with CD create extraordinary costs for society by being markedly more likely to use criminal justice, mental health, substance abuse, medical, and special education services. If smoking and CD are causally related, interventions designed to reduce maternal smoking during pregnancy could be quite powerful in reducing the prevalence of CD. If even a small attributable risk for CD is identified for maternal cigarette smoking, the savings to society in terms of economics and human misery from effective prenatal smoking reduction programs could be quite significant.

Accepted for publication August 28, 1996.

Supported by grant MH-42529 from the National Institute of Mental Health, Rockville, Md (Drs Loeber and Lahey), and by grants from the Walden and Jean Young Shaw Foundation (Department of Psychiatry, University of Chicago) and the Irving B. Harris Center for Developmental Studies (Department of Psychiatry, University of Chicago).

Presented in part at the 42nd Annual Meeting of the American Academy of Child and Adolescent Psychiatry, New Orleans, La, October 20, 1995.

Reprints: Lauren S. Wakschlag, PhD, Department of Psychiatry, MC 3077, University of Chicago, 5841 S Maryland Ave, Chicago, IL 60637 (e-mail: laurie@yoda.bsd.uchicago.edu).

REFERENCES

1. Kazdin A. Treatment of conduct disorder: progress and directions in psychotherapy research. *Dev Psychopathol.* 1993;5:277-310.
2. Cotton P. Smoking cigarettes may do developing fetus more harm than ingesting cocaine, some experts say. *JAMA.* 1994;271:576-577.
3. DiFranza J, Lew R. Effect of maternal cigarette smoking on pregnancy complications and sudden infant death syndrome. *J Fam Pract.* 1995;40:385-394.
4. Hagino N, Lee J. Effects of maternal nicotine on the development of sites for [3H]nicotine binding in the fetal brain. *Int J Dev Neurosci.* 1985;3:567-571.
5. Marks M, Burch J, Collins A. Effects of chronic nicotine infusion on tolerance development and nicotinic receptors. *J Pharmacol Exp Ther.* 1983;226:817-825.
6. Marks M, Grady S, Collins A. Down regulation of nicotinic receptor function after chronic nicotine infusion. *J Pharmacol Exp Ther.* 1993;266:1268-1276.
7. Seidler FJ, Albright ES, Lappi SE, Slotkin TA. In search of a mechanism for receptor-mediated neurobehavioral teratogenesis by nicotine: catecholamine release by nicotine in immature rat brain regions. *Dev Brain Res.* 1994;82:1-8.
8. Slotkin T. Prenatal exposure to nicotine: what can we learn from animal models. In: Zagon I, Slotkin T, eds. *Maternal Substance Abuse and the Developing Nervous System.* Orlando, Fla: Academic Press Inc; 1992:97-124.
9. Van de Kamp J, Collins A. Prenatal nicotine alters nicotinic receptor development in the mouse brain. *Pharmacol Biochem Behav.* 1994;47:889-900.
10. King J, Davila-Garcia M, Azmitia E, Strand F. Differential effects of prenatal and postnatal ACTH or nicotine exposure on 5-HT high affinity uptake in the neonatal rat brain. *Int J Dev Neurosci.* 1991;9:281-286.
11. Richardson S, Tizabi Y. Hyperactivity in the offspring of nicotine-treated rats: role of the mesolimbic and nigostriatal dopaminergic pathways. *Pharmacol Biochem Behav.* 1994;47:331-337.
12. Fung Y, Lau Y. Effects of prenatal nicotine exposure on rat striatal dopaminergic and nicotinic systems. *Pharmacol Biochem Behav.* 1989;33:1-6.
13. Navarro HA, Seidler FJ, Whitmore WL, Slotkin TA. Prenatal exposure to nicotine via maternal infusions: effects on development of catecholamine systems. *J Pharmacol Exp Ther.* 1988;244:940-944.

14. Navarro HA, Seidler FJ, Schwartz RD, Baker FE, Dobbins SS, Slotkin TA. Prenatal exposure to nicotine impairs nervous system development at a dose which does not affect viability or growth. *Brain Res Bull.* 1989;23:187-192.
15. Navarro HA, Mills E, Seidler FJ, Baker FE, Lappi SE, Tayyeb MI, Spencer JR, Slotken TA. Prenatal nicotine exposure impairs beta-adrenergic function: persistent chronotropic subsensitivity despite recovery from deficits in receptor binding. *Brain Res Bull.* 1990;25:233-237.
16. Zahalka EA, Seidler FJ, Yanai J, Slotkin TA. Fetal nicotine exposure alters ontogeny of M1-receptors and their link to G-proteins. *Neurotoxicol Teratol.* 1993;15: 107-115.
17. Slotkin TA, Greer N, Faust J, Cho H, Seidler FJ. Effects of maternal nicotine injections on brain development in the rat: ornithine decarboxylase activity, nucleic acids and proteins in discrete brain regions. *Brain Res Bull.* 1986;17:41-50.
18. Bertolini A, Bernardi M, Genedani S. Effects of prenatal exposure to cigarette smoke and nicotine on pregnancy, offspring development and avoidance behavior in rats. *Neurobehav Toxicol Teratol.* 1982;4:545-548.
19. Johns J, Louis T, Becker R, Means L. Behavioral effects of prenatal exposure to nicotine on guinea pigs. *Neurobehav Toxicol Teratol.* 1982;4:365-369.
20. Fried P, Watkinson B. 12- and 24-month neurobehavioral follow-up of children prenatally exposed to marijuana, cigarettes and alcohol. *Neurotoxicol Teratol.* 1988;10:305-313.
21. Fried P, O'Connell C, Watkinson B. 60- and 72-month follow-up of children prenatally exposed to marijuana, cigarettes, and alcohol: cognitive and language assessment. *J Dev Behav Pediatr.* 1992;13:383-391.
22. McCartney J, Fried P, Watkinson B. Central auditory processing in school-age children prenatally exposed to cigarette smoke. *Neurotoxicol Teratol.* 1994;16: 269-276.
23. Sexton M, Fox N, Hebel JR. Prenatal exposure to tobacco, II: effects on cognitive functioning at age three. *Int J Epidemiol.* 1990;19:72-77.
24. Naeye RL, Peters EC. Mental development of children whose mothers smoked during pregnancy. *Obstet Gynecol.* 1984;64:601-607.
25. Kristjansson E, Fried P, Watkinson B. Maternal smoking during pregnancy affects children's vigilance performance. *Drug Alcohol Depend.* 1989;24:11-19.
26. Fried P, Watkinson B, Gray R. A follow-up study of attentional behavior in 6-year-old children exposed prenatally to marijuana, cigarettes and alcohol. *Neurotoxicol Teratol.* 1992;14:299-311.
27. Streissguth AP, Martin DC, Barr HM, Sandman B, Kirchner GL, Darby B. Intrauterine alcohol and nicotine exposure: attention and reaction time in 4-year-old children. *Dev Psychol.* 1984;20:533-541.
28. Fergusson D, Horwood J, Lynskey M. Maternal smoking before and after pregnancy: effects of behavioral outcomes in middle childhood. *Pediatrics.* 1993;92: 815-822.
29. Milberger S, Biederman J, Faraone SV, Chen L, Jones J. Is maternal smoking during pregnancy a risk factor for attention deficit hyperactivity disorder in children? *Am J Psychiatry.* 1996;153:1138-1142.
30. Makin J, Fried P, Watkinson B. A comparison of active and passive smoking during pregnancy: long-term effects. *Neurotoxicol Teratol.* 1991;13:5-12.
31. Weitzman M, Gortmaker S, Sobol A. Maternal smoking and behavior problems of children. *Pediatrics.* 1992;90:342-349.
32. Rantakallio P, Laara E, Isohanni M, Moilanen I. Maternal smoking during pregnancy and delinquency of the offspring: an association without causation? *Int J Epidemiol.* 1992;21:1106-1113.
33. Lahey BB, Loeber R, Hart EL, Frick PJ, Applegate B, Zhang Q, Green SM, Russo MF. Four-year longitudinal study of conduct disorder in boys: patterns and predictors of persistence. *J Abnorm Child Psychol.* 1995;104:83-93.
34. Loeber R, Green S, Keenan K, Lahey BB. Which boys will fare worse? early predictors of the onset of conduct disorder in a six-year longitudinal study. *J Am Acad Child Adolesc Psychiatry.* 1995;34:499-509.
35. Hinshaw SP, Lahey BB, Hart EL. Issues of taxonomy and comorbidity in the development of conduct disorder. *Dev Psychopathol.* 1993;5:31-50.
36. Hollingshead A. *Four-Factor Index of Social Status.* New Haven, Conn: Yale University, Dept of Sociology; 1975.
37. Shiono P, Behrman R. Low birth weight: analysis and recommendations. In: Behrman R, ed. *Low Birth Weight.* Los Altos, Calif: Center for the Future of Children; 1995:4-18.
38. Barnes H, Olson D. Parent-adolescent Communication Scale. In: Olson D, McCubbin H, Barnes H, Larsen A, Muxen M, Wilson W, eds. *Family Inventories: Inventories Used in a National Survey of Families Across the Family Life Cycle.* St Paul, Minn: Family Social Science; 1982:33-48.
39. Capaldi D, Patterson G. *Psychometric Properties of Fourteen Latent Constructs From the Oregon Youth Study.* New York, NY: Springer-Verlag NY Inc; 1989.
40. Loeber R, Stouthamer-Loeber M. Family factors as correlates and predictors of juvenile conduct problems and delinquency. In: Tonry M, Morris N, eds. *Crime and Justice: An Annual Review of Research.* Chicago, Ill: University of Chicago Press; 1986:29-149.
41. Spitzer R, Endicott J. *Schedule for Affective Disorders and Schizophrenia.* New York: New York State Psychiatric Institute; 1978.
42. Spitzer R, Williams J, Gibbon M. *Structured Clinical Interview for DSM-III-R–Non-patient Version.* New York: New York State Psychiatric Institute; 1987.
43. Lahey B, Russo M, Walker J. Personality characteristics of the mothers of children with disruptive behavior disorders. *J Consult Clin Psychol.* 1989;57:512-515.
44. Rutter M, Harrington R, Quinton D, Pickles A. Adult outcome of conduct disorder in childhood: implications for concepts and definitions of patterns of psychopathology. In: Ketterlinus R, Lamb M, eds. *Adolescent Problem Behaviors: Issues and Research.* Hillsdale, NJ: Lawrence Erlbaum Associates; 1994:57-80.
45. Huesmann LR, Lefkowitz MM, Eron LD. Sum of MMPI F, 4, and 9 as a measure of aggression. *J Consult Clin Psychol.* 1978;46:1071-1078.
46. Hare RD. Comparison of procedures for the assessment of psychopathy. *J Consult Clin Psychol.* 1985;53:7-16.
47. Costello A, Edelbrock C, Kalas R, Dulcan M. *The NIMH Diagnostic Interview Schedule for Children (DISC): Development, Reliability and Comparison Between Clinical and Lay Interviewers.* Worcester: University of Massachusetts Medical School; 1984.
48. American Psychiatric Association. *Diagnostic and Statistical Manual of Mental Disorders, Third Edition, Revised.* Washington, DC: American Psychiatric Association; 1987.
49. Lahey BB, Applegate B, Barkley RA, Garfinkel B, McBurnett K, KerdyK L, Greenhill L, Hynd GW, Frick PJ, Newcorn J, Biederman J, Ollendick T, Hart EL, Perez D, Waldman I, Shaffer D. *DSM-IV* field trials for oppositional defiant disorder and conduct disorder in children and adolescents. *Am J Psychiatry.* 1994;151: 1163-1171.
50. Rantakallio P. A follow-up to the age of 14 of children whose mothers smoked during pregnancy. *Acta Paediatr Scand.* 1983;72:747-753.
51. Fogelman K. Smoking in pregnancy and subsequent development of the child. *Child Care Health Dev.* 1980;6:233-249.
52. Streissguth AP. Smoking and drinking during pregnancy and offspring learning disabilities: a review of literature and development of a research strategy. In: Lewis M, ed. *Learning Disabilities and Prenatal Risk.* Chicago: University of Illinois Press; 1986:28-67.
53. Loeber R, Keenan K. Interaction between conduct disorder and its comorbid conditions: effects of age and gender. *Clin Psychol Rev.* 1994;14:497-523.
54. Jacobson JL, Jacobson SW. Methodological issues in human behavioral teratology. In: Rovee-Collier C, Lipsitt LP, eds. *Advances in Infancy Research.* Norwood, NJ: Ablex; 1990:111-148.
55. Petitti DB, Friedman GD, Kahn W. Accuracy of information on smoking habits provided on self-administered research questionnaires. *Am J Public Health.* 1981; 71:308-311.
56. Bates J, Bayles K, Bennett D, Ridge B, Brown M. Origins of externalizing behavior at eight years of age. In: Pepler D, Rubin K, eds. *The Development and Treatment of Childhood Aggression.* Hillsdale, NJ: Lawrence Erlbaum Associates; 1991: 93-120.
57. Keenan K, Shaw D. The development of coercive family processes: the interaction between aversive toddler behavior and parenting factors. In: McCord J, ed. *Coercion and Punishment in Long-term Perspective.* New York, NY: Cambridge University Press; 1992:165-182.

The Ondine Curse, False Suffocation Alarms, Trait-State Suffocation Fear, and Dyspnea-Suffocation Fear in Panic Attacks

In a reply to my criticisms of the false suffocation–alarm theory of panic attacks,[1] Klein[2] stated that "Ley inexplicably ignores my discussion of Ondine's Curse." The explanation for this omission lies in my attempt to keep my letter within the 750-word limit recommended by the editor in his "Instructions for Authors," a limit that would have been grossly exceeded if I had used the same 600 words used in an earlier explanation[3] of why the Ondine curse does not prove the existence of a suffocation alarm and why the curse is not the "pharmacological converse of panic disorder."[4]

My criticism might best be presented in the format of 2 questions. If the Ondine curse (the arrestation of breathing during sleep) proves that sleep free of suffocation depends on the existence of a suffocation alarm (presumably true alarms activated by the buildup of carbon dioxide) and if a panic attack is triggered by this same suffocation alarm (false though it may be, activated by a relatively low level of carbon dioxide), then why are panic attacks not experienced during every respiratory cycle during sleep? And what accounts for death that arises from sleep apnea in people who do not suffer the Ondine curse (people presumably equipped with intact suffocation alarms), ie, asymptomatic adults who intermittently stop breathing for long intervals during sleep? Add sleep apnea to carbon monoxide poisoning, heroin overdoses, and inhalation of 100% nitrogen as another agent on the list of occasions when breathing stops, but the putative suffocation alarm fails.

Let me also address the remarks by Klein[2] that my theory "has nothing to do with chronic suffocation fear, which Taylor and Rachman[5] address." Contrary to Klein's impression, Rachman and Taylor[6] made no reference to chronic suffocation fear; their study attempted to analyze claustrophobia in 2 components, fear of restriction and fear of suffocation. Because occasions that signal restriction, suffocation, or both evoke anxiety in all, the issue is not one of chronic vs acute but rather one of degree of intensity of suffocation fear as a trait. When occasions arise that evoke a sense of impending suffocation, the strong presumption is that those on the high end of the trait scale of suffocation fear will respond faster and with greater intensity of state fear than those on the low end of the scale. Because dyspnea (the sense of difficulty breathing) is a harbinger of suffocation (the process by which breathing is restricted), occasions in which dyspnea is experienced would be expected to be accompanied by a more intense state of suffocation fear in individuals on the high end of the suffocation-fear trait scale than those on the low end. Thus, the data of Taylor and Rachman support my dyspneic fear theory of panic[7,8]: dyspneic fear and conditioned dyspneic fear (anticipation of suffocation) are states of suffocation fear.

Ronald Ley, PhD
State University of New York at Albany
1400 Washington Ave
Albany, NY 12222

1. Ley R. Panic attacks: Klein's false suffocation alarm, Taylor and Rachman's data, and Ley's dyspneic-fear theory. *Arch Gen Psychiatry.* 1996;53:83.
2. Klein DF. In reply. *Arch Gen Psychiatry.* 1996;53:83-85.
3. Ley R. The 'suffocation alarm' theory of panic attacks: a critical commentary. *J Behav Ther Exp Psychiatry.* 1994;24:269-273.
4. Klein DF. False suffocation alarms, spontaneous panics, and related conditions: an integrative hypothesis. *Arch Gen Psychiatry.* 1993;50:306-317.
5. Taylor S, Rachman S. Klein's suffocation theory of panic. *Arch Gen Psychiatry.* 1994;51:505-506.
6. Rachman S, Taylor S. Analyses of claustrophobia. *J Anxiety Disord.* 1993;7:281-291.
7. Ley R. Dyspneic-fear and catastrophic cognitions in hyperventilatory panic attacks. *Behav Res Ther.* 1989;27:549-554.
8. Ley R. The many faces of Pan: psychological and physiological differences among three types of panic attacks. *Behav Res Ther.* 1992;30:347-357.

In reply

The recent exchanges between Drs Ley and Klein[1-3] have been useful in clarifying aspects of Klein's[4] false suffocation alarm theory of panic; they also have stimulated testable extensions of the theory.[2] The commentaries by Ley[1,3] also raise the important question of whether alternative theories provide equally good or better accounts of panic attacks. Ley[1,3] claimed that our findings[5] not only support Klein's theory but also support Ley's[6,7] dyspneic fear theory. The latter states that

> *fear experienced during a hyperventilatory panic attack is a direct response to the sensation of severe dyspnea (ie, respiratory distress) in the context of a situation in which the sufferer believes that she has little or no control over the conditions that give rise to the dyspnea.[6]*

Our study was not designed to contrast the theories of Ley and Klein. We made no assumption about whether our suffocation fear scale is a trait or state measure; it was intended simply as a measure of sensitivity to claustrophobic provocation. We found that people with an intense fear of suffocation, compared with people with milder fears, were more likely to have a history of panic and more likely to panic in response to a dyspnea-inducing exercise (eg, breathing through a narrow straw). These results are consistent with Klein's theory and with Ley's emphasis on the role of dyspneic fear in panic attacks. The fact that our results were obtained from an experiment[8] performed for reasons unrelated to the theories of Klein and Ley, but which on later reanalysis[5] provided potentially important support for the idea of a suffocation monitor, is worth noting. If pressed to do so, Klein may well have deduced our findings from his theory—but Ley may have had similar success.

We believe that Ley is making an overstatement by asserting that our findings "point clearly to the significance of a sense of uncontrollable dyspnea/suffocation in panic attacks."[1] Ley's theory states that classic panic attacks occur "in the context of a situation in which the sufferer believes that she has little or no control over the conditions that give rise to the dyspnea."[6] Thus, Ley's theory suggests that classic panic attacks will occur when dyspnea is perceived as uncontrollable and will not occur when dyspnea is seen as controllable. Our dyspnea induction exercise provided subjects with a great deal of control. Our subjects were simply asked to breathe through a narrow straw for 2 minutes. They were told that they could discontinue the exercise at any time. The subjects simply held the straw in their mouths while occluding the nostrils; they could easily discontinue the dyspnea-inducing exercise at any time. Although we did not measure our subjects' perceived control, it seems unlikely that they would have seen themselves as having little or no control to discontinue the dyspnea-inducing exercise. Yet, panic attacks were reported by 18.4% of subjects with high suffocation fear compared with only 1.5% of subjects with low suffocation fear. This suggests that perceived uncontrollability is not a necessary requirement for dyspnea-induced panic. This is inconsistent with Ley's theory but is consistent with Klein's theory, which has a physiocentric emphasis.[9]

While we think there is considerable merit in the idea of a suffocation monitor and its relation to panic disorder, we should note that not all panic disorders may be suffocation related. In a preliminary analysis of an ongoing study (Steven Taylor, PhD, S. Rachman, PhD, and Adam Radomsky, unpublished data, 1997), we assessed the responses of 78 people with panic disorder to 4 suffocation challenges: (1) breathing through a narrow straw for 2 minutes, (2) rebreathing one's air into a bag for 1 minute, (3) breath holding for 20 seconds after exhaling (without previous hyperventilation), and (4) maximum duration breath holding after exhaling (without previous hyperventilation). Many subjects (36 [46.2%]) reported a full or limited symptom panic attack in response to one or more of the challenges. The moderately high incidence of panic is consistent with the importance of suffocation in panic disorder. However, theories of panic need to consider the possibility that some types of panic disorder may be unrelated to suffocation false alarms or dyspneic fear.

Further studies are needed to test predictions that differentiate between the theories of Klein and Ley. The relative merits of the theories also can be evaluated on other criteria. Ley's dyspneic fear theory, compared with Klein's theory, may be regarded as more parsimonious in that it does not assume a suffocation alarm system. However, Ley's theory, at least in its present form,[6,7] is not described in much detail and may not be more parsimonious once its assumptions are fully specified. Continued debate about the relative merits of these and other theories should prove fruitful in furthering our understanding of panic disorder and related phenomena.

Steven Taylor, PhD
S. Rachman, PhD
University of British Columbia
2255 Wesbrook Mall
Vancover, British Columbia
Canada V6T 2A1

1. Ley R. Panic attacks: Klein's false suffocation alarm, Taylor and Rachman's data, and Ley's dyspneic-fear theory. *Arch Gen Psychiatry*. 1996;53:83.
2. Klein DF. In reply. *Arch Gen Psychiatry*. 1996;53:83-85.
3. Ley R. The Ondine curse, false suffocation alarms, trait-state suffocation fear, and dyspnea-suffocation fear in panic attacks. *Arch Gen Psychiatry*. 1997;54:677.
4. Klein DF. False suffocation alarms, spontaneous panics, and related conditions: an integrative hypothesis. *Arch Gen Psychiatry*. 1993;50:306-317.
5. Taylor S, Rachman S. Klein's suffocation theory of panic. *Arch Gen Psychiatry*. 1994;51:505-506.
6. Ley R. Dyspneic-fear and catastrophic cognitions in hyperventilatory panic attacks. *Behav Res Ther*. 1989;27:549-554.
7. Ley R. The many faces of Pan: psychological and physiological differences among three types of panic attacks. *Behav Res Ther*. 1992;30:347-357.
8. Rachman S, Taylor S. Analyses of claustrophobia. *J Anxiety Disord*. 1993;7:281-291.
9. Klein DF. In reply. *Arch Gen Psychiatry*. 1994;51:506.

In reply

Ley[1] still inexplicably and evasively ignores my point that patients with the Ondine curse do not feel distressed while actually suffocating. He simply confuses the matter by gratuitously suggesting that an alarm system has to be either off or maximally on. Clearly many physiological alarm systems produce mounting discomfort and activation but do not lead to a full-fledged maximum reaction unless adaptive action has failed to be effective. Ley obscures the issue by a physiologically unwarranted dictum about how alarm systems work.

Central sleep apnea is a pathological feature of the breathing control mechanism; patients with central sleep apnea breathe insufficiently except during full wakefulness. Such patients are quite similar to patients with the Ondine curse, so this does not contradict my views. In obstructive sleep apnea, obesity or upper airway narrowing may result in hypoxia and hypercapnia, which may induce central apnea. During sleep apnea, the usual response is numerous awakenings in a gasping, often panicking, state that can be relieved by continuous positive airway pressure. The rare death seems due to progressive down-regulation of the suffocation alarm mechanism by persistent hypercapnia and hypoxia, quite analogous to "blue bloating."

Ley's lack of physiological understanding is shown by his use of a pathological condition (sleep apnea) to argue against the existence of a normal control mechanism. This is as logical as saying that diarrhea shows that there is no mechanism for peristaltic control. Central sleep apnea, like the Ondine curse, actually implies the existence of an impaired central respiratory regulator driven by suffocation signals, such as carbon dioxide level.

Taylor and Rachman[2] state, "Klein and Ley need to consider the possibility that some types of panic disorder may be unrelated to suffocation false alarms or dyspnea fear." I agree and, in fact, made this specific point in my article. As for the last 2 paragraphs in Ley's letter, simply repeating unwarranted assertions does not substantively advance the discussion.

Donald F. Klein, MD
New York State Psychiatric Institute
722 W 168th St
New York, NY 10032

1. Ley R. The Ondine curse, false suffocation alarms, trait-state suffocation fear, and dyspnea-suffocation fear in panic attacks. *Arch Gen Psychiatry*. 1997;54:677.
2. Taylor S, Rachman S. In reply. *Arch Gen Psychiatry*. 1997;54:677-678.

Drug Abuse and Addiction Treatment Research

The Next Generation

A GROUP of articles in this issue of the ARCHIVES focuses on drug abuse and addiction. Most of these articles deal with treatment in one aspect or another. In aggregate, they are a bit like a cafeteria, providing a sampling of some of the most important and difficult issues facing the field. These issues include the pervasiveness of comorbidity between mental disorders and substance abuse and the realities of polydrug use as the norm in drug abuse and addiction. Another issue addressed that has not received enough attention concerns matching treatments to the individual needs of the patient. Questions of treatment and services matching are particularly timely in the current climate, in which managed care is dominating health services provision systems and evolving rapidly.

See also pages 696, 700, 706, 713, 721, 730, and 737

These articles are a part of what might be thought of as a new generation of drug abuse research projects. These new research undertakings are helping us move beyond simplistic notions of drug addiction and allowing us to approach the problem with greater recognition of its complexity. The treatment studies exemplify the move beyond the focus on simplistic outcome measures, such as whether the individual keeps using a single drug. Newer generation drug treatment studies recognize the need for and focus on a greater set of outcomes and functionality measures. These broader functionality outcomes should be the target of most future drug treatment studies; after all, these are the measures that matter.

THE NATURE OF ADDICTION

This focus on functionality is particularly important as we recognize the nature of addiction as a chronic, relapsing disorder, rather than simply as a series of discreet, short-term drug-using episodes. That addiction is a chronic, relapsing disorder means there likely will be subsequent episodes of drug use—relapses. It also means that although total abstinence after a single treatment course may be a desired outcome, it typically is unreasonable to expect. A major task of treatment for many individuals is to increase the intervals between relapses and to reduce the intensity and duration of relapses when they do occur. It also means helping the individual manage the disorder and continue to function despite occasional relapses.

That addiction is a chronic disorder also means what it implies: that one remains addicted for a long period. Sustaining one's addiction actually becomes a way of life, and it pervades all aspects of life, including family, job, and community. Therefore, functioning is impaired in all spheres; treatment must address all of these functionality outcomes as well.

Understanding and treating addiction appropriately requires a clear sense of what addiction actually is and what really matters within the disorder. For example, many people still focus primarily on the physical dependence aspects of addiction. But physical dependence is not the most important feature of this disorder. Even the florid physical withdrawal symptoms of heroin and alcohol addiction can be relatively easily managed with medications. Moreover, some of the most addicting substances, like cocaine and amphetamines, do not produce traditional physical dependence as defined by the presence of dramatic physical withdrawal symptoms. It is no longer accurate to define addiction by physical withdrawal symptoms.

A more appropriate focus is the essence of addiction as defined by the American Medical Association, the Institute of Medicine, and the American Psychiatric Association: compulsive, uncontrollable drug craving, seeking, and use for no medical purpose, despite negative health and social consequences. It is this aspect—uncontrollable drug craving, seeking, and use—that is at the heart of all the functionality impairments that characterize addiction and its consequences for individuals, their families, and society.

Another core aspect of addiction should be mentioned. Although addiction is clearly a behavioral disorder that has imbedded social context aspects, it is ultimately a brain disease. The behavioral state of compulsive, uncontrollable drug craving, seeking, and use comes about as a result of fundamental and long-lasting changes in brain structure and function produced by prolonged, repeated drug use.[1] Therefore, any strategies for dealing with addicted individuals,

This article is also available on our Web site: www.ama-assn.org/psych.

particularly treatment approaches, must recognize that the addicted individual is in a different brain state. And an ultimate task for treatment is to reverse, or at least to somehow compensate for, those brain changes.

One interesting potential set of markers of the brain changes of addiction are some of the less dramatic consequences or side effects of the altered dopamine functioning that characterizes the addicted state. In this issue of the ARCHIVES, the study by Desai et al[2] about impaired color vision in cocaine addicts provides one such example of a potential side effect of altered dopamine neurotransmission accompanying cocaine addiction. Time will determine whether this is a characteristic of all addictions, as they all are accompanied by altered brain dopamine function, or whether it is unique to cocaine addiction.

COMORBIDITY OF MENTAL AND ADDICTIVE DISORDERS

All family members and most professionals in the field—whether scientists or clinicians—readily acknowledge that comorbidity is the usual, rather than the unusual, state of affairs.

Comorbidity is reality! Estimates vary by disorder, but more than 50% of people with mental disorders have also been found to abuse drugs, including alcohol[3]; there is also a widespread belief that many mentally ill people who abuse drugs may be actually attempting to medicate themselves. We do not know if that is actually true, but the sequence of onset between the mental disorder and substance use favors that hypothesis for many patients.

However, many of our causative models ignore the almost inevitability of comorbidity or at best treat it superficially. Worse, many of our treatment approaches ignore comorbidity or insist that mental and addictive disorders be treated separately. In many states, for example, the public treatment service systems are totally separate for mental and addictive disorders. This is particularly discouraging, as most research shows that whatever the cause both comorbid conditions need to be treated simultaneously and in an integrated way.[4-8]

Two articles in this issue of the ARCHIVES relate to comorbid mental and addictive disorders. The article by Cornelius et al[9] clearly demonstrates that fluoxetine can be effective in reducing the depressive symptomatology and the alcohol use of severely depressed alcoholics. The mechanisms of action are unclear. It could be that fluoxetine is affecting alcohol consumption because the patients had been medicating themselves for their depressive symptoms and fluoxetine is working by relieving their depression. Alternatively, fluoxetine may be working on some common causative mechanism for both types of disorder. Other antidepressants have been shown to be effective in reducing depressive symptoms but have not been consistent in reducing excessive drinking in depressed alcoholics.[10,11] Because altered serotonergic function has been implicated in depression and alcoholism, fluoxetine may be working on a common mechanism, rather than just through reducing the depression and, therefore, the need to medicate oneself.

Another study in this issue of the ARCHIVES focuses on the prediction of outpatient treatment compliance in newly released schizophrenic patients with comorbid substance use disorders. Miner et al[12] found that female patients and patients with negative syndrome schizophrenia were more compliant with outpatient referral than patients with mixed syndromes. This finding serves as an important base for developing strategies that may help a comorbid patient group that has been historically difficult to treat. Obviously, the better able we are to predict who will comply with outpatient treatment after release from the hospital, the more likely we are able to keep them living within their own community.

MEDICATIONS FOR POLYDRUG USE

Schottenfeld et al[13] studied another reality, polydrug use. In the real world, most addicts use more than 1 drug, yet most of our studies focus on only 1 substance. The authors compare the efficacy of buprenorphine, a partial μ-agonist, with that of traditional methadone treatment in controlling heroin and cocaine use. Buprenorphine has many attributes that suggest it might be a good alternative to methadone, including longer-lasting actions and somewhat reduced abuse liability and withdrawal symptoms.

This study found no differences between methadone and buprenorphine treatment in reducing heroin use. When the medications were administered at reasonable doses, both were quite effective. However, both were rather limited in reducing cocaine use, emphasizing the complexity of treating polydrug use, which is far more common than the use of only a single substance.

One question is whether we will ultimately need more than 1 medication to handle multiple drug addictions or whether we will discover a single medication to address whatever emerges to be the common essence of addiction. As the neuroscience of drug addiction progresses, there is increasing evidence that although there are differences in the mechanisms by which different drugs affect the brain, there also are many common effects that may underlie some common properties of all addictions.[14-16] If so, seeking a medication to address those common properties or mechanisms is not an unreasonable strategy.

The study by Schottenfeld et al also underscores the need to maintain adequate dosages of antiaddiction medications, particularly methadone. This point may seem obvious; however, surveys of the dosages actually used in methadone treatment programs have shown that a large fraction are using suboptimal or even subthreshold dosages, partly because of the stigma of using a substitution medication.

THE NEXT GENERATION OF BEHAVIORAL TREATMENT STUDIES

Despite the tremendous progress in brain research, it remains clear that no medication will ever control addiction all by itself. Although at its essence addiction is a brain disease, the phenomenon is far more complex than being simply a brain disease. It has truly imbedded behavioral and social context aspects, including all of the stimuli associated with initial drug use that actually become a part of the addiction. Simple exposure to environmental cues, or conditioning factors, that are associated with drug use can trigger tremendous craving and relapse to drug use, even after long periods of abstinence.

A useful analogy is the treatment of schizophrenia; no matter how effective the medications for this disorder become, we still need psychosocial rehabilitation to help patients handle their residual symptoms and to function fully in society. The same will always be true for long-term drug addicts, whose addiction can interfere greatly with all aspects of life. Therefore, just handling the physical brain changes will not be enough. Addicts will have to be able to handle later exposure to craving-eliciting cues in the environment and will need rehabilitation to either learn or relearn social skills or job skills. Moreover, it is likely that we will find combining behavioral and pharmacological medications to be truly synergistic, not just complimentary, in nature.[17]

The article by Crits-Christoph et al[18] describes the rationale, design, and methods of a major multisite clinical trial of different behavioral treatments for cocaine addiction. This study compares 2 therapies, cognitive therapy or supportive-expressive psychodynamic therapy and individual drug counseling; these therapies are then compared with group counseling (a control). To our knowledge, this is the largest clinical trial conducted to date on psychotherapy and drug counseling for cocaine dependence. It compliments a growing portfolio of National Institute on Drug Abuse–supported behavioral treatment studies, many of which will ultimately be used in combination with medications. The article in this issue of the ARCHIVES is only an appetizer, as data collection for this trial is scheduled to be completed by the end of 1997. But it does emphasize the kinds of clinical trial testing of drug treatments that are available. It includes the use of explicit treatment manuals for each of the treatments being studied. Manualizing therapies is a growing trend in drug abuse treatment.

TREATMENT MATCHING

There is widespread belief among clinicians and administrators in the substance abuse field that particular treatment approaches will be more or less successful for particular types of patients, the notion that types of treatments or treatment programs should be matched to types of patients. In a general sense, this notion also underlies some of the strategies studied in the articles discussed, in which the treatment approach is being tailored to address such traits as patients' comorbid mental disorders or their particular polydrug use. But these are not really treatment matching studies, looking in detail at whether one can in fact match the right type of treatment to particular individual patients. Actually, despite the widespread belief in treatment matching, there has been relatively little research to support the concept of matching, and the studies to date have not been conclusive. One example is the recently published study of alcohol treatment matching, Project MATCH (Matching Alcoholism Treatments to Client Heterogeneity),[19] which basically found similar efficacy rates for various alcohol treatment modalities, independent of the patient characteristics examined in that study.

The article by McLellan et al[20] in this issue of the ARCHIVES reports the results of a study that looks at treatment matching somewhat differently. The authors first acknowledged the extreme difficulty in even trying to match substance abuse patients to an overall optimal setting or program, in part because of logistic problems. Therefore, they turned to a different approach, what might be viewed as treatment matching within a program rather than across programs. Within each of 4 different programs used by an Employee Assistance Program, patients received either standard services or services that were matched to the problems presented by the patient at treatment admission.

This study showed that matching treatment services within a program can be quite effective. Matched patients had better outcomes than standard care patients. The findings were also consistent with the predictions that guided the matching strategy (ie, the problems that dictated the services to be provided). Thus, although we do not yet have the ability to do fine-grained matching of patients to the most appropriate overall treatment programs for them, we do have clear data that demonstrate that when we address the patients' specific needs within a program we can improve their outcomes.

COMMENT

These articles reflect the new direction in which drug addiction research is moving. They recognize the fact that treatment approaches have to address the full complexity of addiction and its effects on every aspect of the patient's life. Addiction is and must be seen by all as the quintessential biobehavioral disorder, with clear biological, behavioral, and social aspects. Combined biological, behavioral, and social, or whole person, treatments are clearly the direction we must continue to go.

Alan I. Leshner, PhD
National Institute on Drug Abuse
5600 Fishers Lane, Room 10-05
Rockville, MD 20857

REFERENCES

1. Leshner AI. Understanding drug addiction: implications for treatment. *Hosp Pract.* 1996;31:47-54, 57-59.
2. Desai P, Roy M, Roy A, Brown S, Smelson D. Impaired color vision in cocaine-withdrawn patients. *Arch Gen Psychiatry.* 1997;54:696-699.

3. Regier DA, Farmer ME, Rae DS, Locke BZ, Keith SJ, Judd LL, Goodwin FK. Comorbidity of mental disorders with alcohol and other drug abuse: results from the Epidemiologic Catchment Area (ECA) study. *JAMA.* 1990;264:2511-2518.
4. Drake RE, Osher FC, Wallach MA. Homelessness and dual diagnosis. *Am Psychol.* 1991;46:1149-1158.
5. Robbins LN, Regier DA. *Psychiatric Disorders in America, the Epidemiologic Catchment Area Study.* New York, NY: Free Press; 1991:356-366.
6. Kessler RC, Crum RM, Warner LA, Nelson CB, Schulenberg J, Anthony JC. Lifetime occurrence of *DSM-III-R* alcohol abuse and dependence with other psychiatric disorders in the National Comorbidity Survey. *Arch Gen Psychiatry.* 1997;54:313-321.
7. Kessler RC, McGonagle KA, Zhao S, Nelson CB, Hughes M, Eshelman S, Wittchen HU, Kendler KS. Lifetime and 12-month prevalence of *DSM-III-R* psychiatric disorders in the United States: results from the National Comorbidity Survey. *Arch Gen Psychiatry.* 1994;51;8-19.
8. Drake RE, Mueser KT, Clark RE, Wallach MA. The course, treatment and outcome of substance disorder in persons with severe mental illness. *Am J Orthopsychiatry.* 1996:66:42-51.
9. Cornelius JR, Salloum IM, Ehler JG, Jarrett PJ, Cornelius MD, Perel JM, Thase ME, Black A. Fluoxetine in depressed alcoholics: a double-blind, placebo-controlled trial. *Arch Gen Psychiatry.* 1997; 54:700-705.
10. McGrath PJ, Nunes EV, Stewart JW, Goldman D, Agosti V, Ocepek-Welikson K, Quitkin FM. Imipramine treatment of alcoholics with major depression: a placebo-controlled clinical trial. *Arch Gen Psychiatry.* 1996;53:232-240.
11. Mason BJ, Kocsis JH, Ritvo CE, Cutler RB. A double-blind, placebo-controlled trial of desipramine for primary alcohol dependence stratified on the presence or absence of major depression. *JAMA.* 1996;275:761-767.
12. Miner CR, Rosenthal RN, Hellerstein DJ, Muenz LR. Prediction of compliance with outpatient referral in patients with schizophrenia and psychoactive substance use disorders. *Arch Gen Psychiatry.* 1997;54:706-712.
13. Schottenfeld RS, Pakes JR, Oliveto A, Ziedonis D, Kosten TR. Buprenorphine vs methadone maintenance treatment for concurrent opioid dependence and cocaine abuse. *Arch Gen Psychiatry.* 1997;54:713-720.
14. Koob GF. Drug addiction: the yin and yang of hedonic homeostasis. *Neuron.* 1996;16:893-896.
15. Self DW, Nestler EJ. Molecular mechanisms of drug reinforcement and addiction. *Annu Rev Neurosci.* 1995;18:463.
16. Pich EM, Pagliusi SR, Tessari M, Talabot-Ayer D, Huijsduijnen RH, Chiamulera C. Common neural substrates for the addictive properties of nicotine and cocaine. *Science.* 1997:275:83-86.
17. McLellan AT, Arndt IO, Metzger DS, Woody GE, O'Brein CP. The effects of psychosocial services in substance abuse treatment. *JAMA.* 1993;269: 1953-1959.
18. Crits-Christoph P, Siqueland L, Blaine J, Frank A, Luborsky L, Onken LS, Muenz L, Thase ME, Weiss RD, Gastfriend DR, Woody G, Barber JP, Butler SF, Daley D, Bishop S, Najavits LM, Lis J, Mercer D, Griffin ML, Moras K, Beck AT. The National Institute on Drug Abuse Collaborative Cocaine Treatment Study: rationale and methods. *Arch Gen Psychiatry.* 1997;54:721-726.
19. Project MATCH Research Group. Matching alcoholism treatments to client heterogeneity: project MATCH posttreatment drinking outcomes. *J Stud Alcohol.* 1997;58:7-29.
20. McLellan AT, Grissom GR, Zanis D, Randall M, Brill P, O'Brein CP. Problem-service 'matching' in addiction treatment: a prospective study in 4 programs. *Arch Gen Psychiatry.* 1997;54:730-735.

Impaired Color Vision in Cocaine-Withdrawn Patients

Parul Desai, MD; Monique Roy, MD; Alec Roy, MD; Stafford Brown; David Smelson, PsyD

Background: The main reinforcing effect of cocaine happens by altering dopaminergic neurotransmission in the brain reward systems. Dopamine is found in high concentrations in the retina in which it plays an important role in color vision. Therefore, we investigated whether cocaine-dependent patients might have impaired color vision.

Methods: We compared patients recently withdrawn from cocaine (n=31) with matched normal controls (n=31) on 2 color vision tests.

Results: Cocaine-withdrawn patients had significantly higher error scores than matched controls on the Farnsworth-Munsell 100-hue and Lanthony desaturated D-15 color vision tests. Also, 23 of the 31 cocaine-withdrawn patients had blue-yellow color vision losses on the Farnsworth-Munsell 100-hue test compared with 3 controls ($P<.001$, χ^2 test) and 15 had blue-yellow color vision loss on the Lanthony desaturated D-15 test compared with 2 controls ($P<.001$, χ^2 test).

Conclusions: These significantly higher test error scores and blue-yellow color vision losses suggest that color vision is impaired in cocaine-withdrawn patients. Color vision testing may be useful in future studies of cocaine-dependent patients.

Arch Gen Psychiatry. 1997;54:696-699

THE MAIN reinforcing effects of cocaine are owing to its ability to inhibit the uptake of dopamine in the nucleus accumbens and reward systems of the brain.[1] Dopamine is also found in high concentration in the retina.[2] Retinal dopamine is a neuromodulator and neurotransmitter and is involved in color vision.[3-8] The electroretinogram (ERG) is a method of recording retinal responses to flashes of colored light. We previously reported ERG abnormalities in patients recently withdrawn from cocaine[9] that lasted up to 8 weeks.[10] Therefore, we wondered whether color vision might be impaired in cocaine-dependent patients. The Farnsworth-Munsell (FM) 100-hue[11] and Lanthony desaturated D-15 (DD-15)[12-14] tests are 2 reliable clinical color vision tests. We decided to administer them to patients recently withdrawn from cocaine. We hypothesized that the cocaine-withdrawn patients would show significantly higher error scores on these 2 color vision tests compared with age- and sex-matched normal controls.

From the Department of Ophthalmology, University of Medicine and Dentistry of New Jersey, New Jersey Medical School, Newark (Drs Desai and M. Roy and Mr Brown), and the Departments of Psychiatry (Dr A. Roy) and Psychology (Dr Smelson), Veterans Affairs Medical Center, East Orange, NJ.

RESULTS

The 31 cocaine-withdrawn patients had a mean duration (±SD) of cocaine abuse of 15.4±7.1 years (range, 7-29 years). Their mean age (±SD) was 39.8±5.8 years (range, 29-45 years) and the controls' mean age was 39.0±9.7 years (range, 26-45 years) (t=0.29, df=60, P=<.1). At the time of color vision testing, patients were withdrawn from cocaine for a mean (±SD) of 26.0±30.3 days (range, 2-180 days).

Cocaine-withdrawn patients had significantly higher FM 100-hue error scores than controls (mean [±SD], 133.7±66.9 vs 45.1±27.1; t=7.12; df=60; $P<.001$) (**Figure 1**).

See also page 691

Cocaine-withdrawn patients also had significantly higher Lanthony DD-15 test[12-14] error scores than controls (mean [±SD], 83.3±71.3 vs 11.8±14.5; t=6.22; df=60; $P<.001$) (**Figure 2**).

Twenty-three of the 31 cocaine-withdrawn patients had blue-yellow color vision loss on the FM 100-hue test compared with 3 controls ($P<.001$) and 15 had a blue-yellow color vision loss on the Lanthony DD-15 test[12-14] compared with 2 controls ($P<.001$). There were no significant differences between the groups for

SUBJECTS AND METHODS

Thirty-one cocaine-withdrawn inpatients, 30 men and 1 woman, from the locked drug and alcohol rehabilitation unit of the Veterans Affairs Medical Center, East Orange, NJ, were studied. We included subjects who met *DSM-III-R* criteria for cocaine dependence; reported having used at least 12 g of cocaine during the 3 months preceding their admission; and were drug-, alcohol-, and medication-free at the time of testing. Excluded were subjects who (1) were physically dependent on opiates, barbiturates, or alcohol or abused marijuana; (2) met *DSM-III-R* criteria for another Axis I psychiatric disorder other than phobic or anxiety disorder; (3) were taking any centrally acting medications; (4) had a preexisting ocular pathologic condition such as cataract, high intraocular pressure, or fundus abnormality or a macular pathologic condition such as abnormal pigmentation, pigment atrophy, age-related macular degeneration changes, abnormalities of pupil size, or visual acuity less than 20/25 OU; (5) had clinical evidence of any cognitive impairment; (6) had congenital color vision deficiency; or (7) had a family history of color vision deficiency. Random weekly urinalyses were performed to ensure that patients were not abusing illicit drugs while on the locked ward.

The 31 cocaine-withdrawn patients were matched for sex and age (within 7 years) with 31 normal controls. The controls were recruited from among normal volunteers and hospital personnel. The controls were enrolled in the study if they were medication-free and did not have a history of substance abuse, depression, or treatment of any psychiatric disorder. All of the subjects gave written informed consent.

In all of the subjects, an eye examination, including direct ophthalmoscopy, slit-lamp examination, applanation tonometry, and near visual acuity, was performed. The right eye was selected for testing. All subjects were given 4 color vision tests by a trained ophthalmologist (P.D.). These included Ishihara, FM D-15, Lanthony DD-15, and FM 100-hue color vision tests.[11] The first test was used to determine any congenital color vision deficiency and to exclude such patients. The FM D-15 color vision test was used to train the patient with monocular vision and to understand the process of test taking.

We used the Lanthony DD-15[12-14] and FM 100-hue tests[11] for evaluating color vision. We used northern daylight for illumination during color vision testing, which was performed between 10 AM and 2 PM. The illumination intensity was checked with a Luxmeter (Neuberger, Germany) and was maintained around 30 foot-candles. No time limit was enforced for the completion of the tests.

For the Lanthony DD-15[12-14] and FM 100-hue[11] tests we calculated the test error score and determined the axis of color vision defect. For the FM 100-hue test we used the computerized FM D-85 hue program (Department of Ophthalmology, Loma Linda University, Loma Linda, Calif) to obtain the score and used Smith and Pokorny quadrant analysis to determine the axis.[15] For the Lanthony DD-15 color vision test we used the Lanthony scoring system (P. Lanthony, personal communication).

In the statistical analysis, unpaired t and χ^2 tests were used. Because the error scores of the color vision tests were not normally distributed, we used their square roots.

either red-green or mixed (blue-yellow and red-green) color vision deficiencies.

There were no significant correlations between the Lanthony DD-15[12-14] or the FM 100-hue test error scores and either the number of days of substance withdrawal (r=0.31, n=31, P=<.1 and r=0.2, n=31, P<.1, respectively) or the number of years of alcohol use (r=0.01, n=26, P<.1 and r=0.23, n=26, P<.1, respectively).

COMMENT

We found that patients recently withdrawn from cocaine have blue-yellow color vision losses. The cocaine-withdrawn patients had significantly higher error scores than normal controls on the FM 100-hue and Lanthony DD-15[12-14] color vision tests. Also, significantly more of the cocaine-withdrawn patients had blue-yellow color vision loss than controls on both tests.

Color vision test results are known to be influenced by age, sex, and medication.[11,16,17] However, the patients in our study were carefully matched for age and sex with normal controls. No subject was taking any centrally acting medication because this may affect color vision. Because the cocaine-withdrawn patients were on a locked ward and subject to random urine drug screenings, which were consistently negative, we believe that the results of our study are owing to the cocaine intake in the weeks and months prior to admission to the drug and alcohol rehabilitation unit.

We suggest that the impaired color vision found in these cocaine-withdrawn patients is owing to the effect of the cocaine on retinal neurotransmission, particularly on the retinal dopamine system. This stems from preclinical studies showing that cocaine withdrawal leads to a hypodopaminergic state[18-20] and from our previous clinical studies showing that cocaine-withdrawn patients have significantly reduced blue cone b-wave ERG amplitudes (ie, the retinal response to flashes of blue light is decreased).[9,10,21] The retinal dopamine system is implicated because similarly decreased ERG amplitudes have been found with the administration of neuroleptic drugs, and other dopamine antagonists, to normal subjects[22,23] and primates[24] and in disorders that decrease dopaminergic function. For example, patients with Parkinson disease have a 50% decrease in retinal dopamine and show blue-yellow color vision losses and decreased ERG responses, particularly reduced blue cone amplitudes,[25,26] which normalize temporarily following treatment with levodopa.

We do not believe that the results of our study are owing to drugs other than cocaine. Alcohol intoxication is known to be associated with abnormal color vision test results.[27-29] Twenty-five of the 31 cocaine-withdrawn patients in our study had used alcohol.

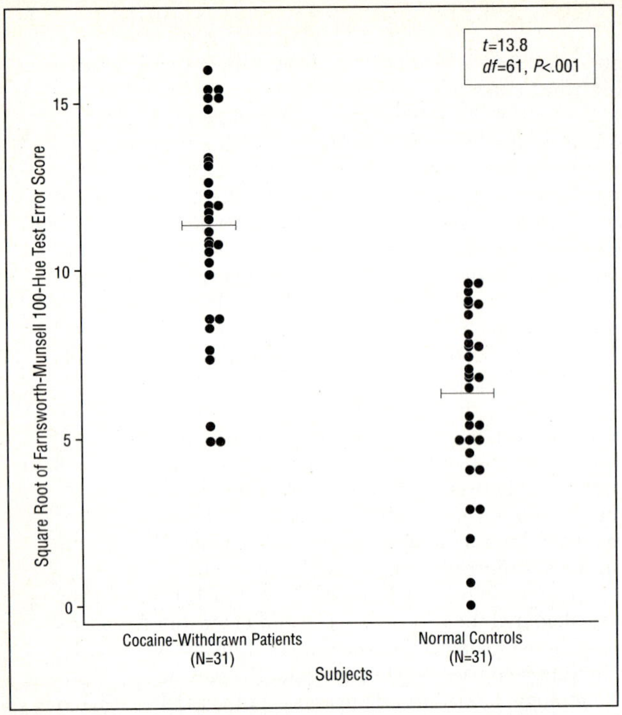

Figure 1. *Cocaine-withdrawn patients have a significantly higher mean square root of Farnsworth-Munsell 100-hue test error scores compared with matched normal controls (P<.001, t test).*

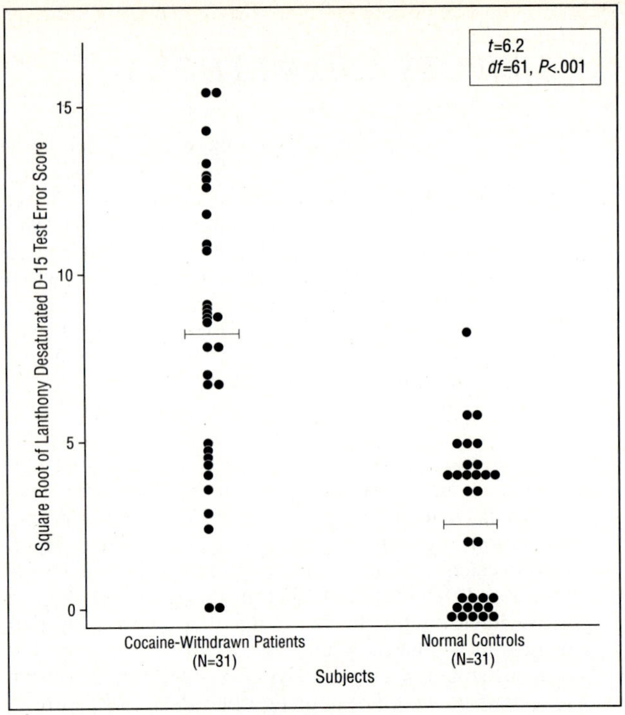

Figure 2. *Cocaine-withdrawn patients have a significantly higher mean square root of Lanthony desaturated D-15 test error scores compared with matched normal controls (P<.001, t test).*

However, the color vision deficits found in withdrawing alcoholics are transient, relate to alcohol intake, and attenuate and disappear during the first few days of withdrawal.[27,28] For example, Kapitany et al[30] found that 6 of 11 retested, color-deficient withdrawing alcoholics showed remission after 1 week, and significant improvement in color vision tests could be seen in all of the patients after 3 weeks. In contrast, our patients had been withdrawn from cocaine for a mean of more than 3 weeks and at that time still showed highly significant color vision deficits. Also, there were no significant correlations between color vision test error scores and either years of alcohol use or number of days of substance withdrawal. Furthermore, all 4 alcohol-using patients withdrawn from cocaine for 2 months or more had blue-yellow color vision losses; 1 had been abstinent for 6 months and 2 for 4 months. Additionally, 3 of the 4 cocaine-withdrawn patients who did not use alcohol had blue-yellow color vision losses.

We also do not believe that the results of our study are owing to an effect of cocaine on ocular blood vessels. Kosten[31] noted long-lasting decreases in cerebral cortical blood flow in cocaine-withdrawn patients examined with single photon emission computerized tomographic scan. This he attributed to the vasoconstrictive effects of cocaine leading to cerebral blood flow reduction. In fact, color vision losses have been reported in many retinal vascular diseases such as diabetes[32,33] and sickle cell disease.[34] However, detailed retinal examination by a trained ophthalmologist (P.D.) showed that none of our patients had any evidence of a retinal lesion, greatly diminishing the possibility that the color vision losses resulted from local abnormalities in retinal blood flow. In our previous ERG studies, the b-wave amplitude to blue flash was reduced but that to white flash was not significantly different between cocaine-withdrawn patients and controls.[9,10,21] This is relevant because inner retinal ischemia is usually associated with reduction in b-wave ERG responses to white flash.[35]

CONCLUSION

We found that cocaine-withdrawn patients showed evidence of color vision loss compared with matched normal controls. The lack of significant correlations between color vision test results and the number of days of cocaine withdrawal suggests the possibility that there may be a long-lasting residual effect of cocaine abuse on color vision. We previously reported that ERG changes in cocaine-withdrawn patients persist for at least 8 weeks[21] and Volkow et al[36] reported positron emission tomographic changes in D_2 dopamine receptor binding in patients withdrawn from cocaine for up to 4 months.

Accepted for publication November 6, 1996.

Corresponding author: Monique Roy, MD, University of Medicine and Dentistry of New Jersey, New Jersey Medical School, 90 Bergen St, Doctor's Office Center, Room 6164, Newark, NJ 07103.

REFERENCES

1. Ritz M, Lamb R, Goldberg S, Kuhar M. Cocaine receptors on dopamine transporters are related to self-administration of cocaine. *Science.* 1987;237:1219-1223.
2. Djamgoz M, Wagner H. Location and function of dopamine in the adult vertebrate retina. *Neurochem Int.* 1992;20:139-191.

3. Witkovsky P, Dearry A. Functional roles of dopamine in the vertebrate retina. *Prog Retina Res.* 1991;11:247-292.
4. Dowling J. Dopamine: a retinal neuromodulator? *Trends Neurosci.* 1986;9:236-240.
5. Bodis-Wollner I, Piccolino M. Dopaminergic mechanisms in vision. New York, NY: Alan R Liss Inc; 1998.
6. Bodis-Wollner I. Visual deficits related to dopamine deficiency in experimental animals and Parkinson's disease patients. *Trends Neurosci.* 1990;13:296-302.
7. Iuvone P, Galli C, Garrison-Gund C, Neff N. Light stimulates tyrosine hydroxylase activity and dopamine synthesis in retinal amacrine neurons. *Science.* 1978; 202:901-902.
8. Brainard G, Morgan W. Light-induced stimulation of retinal dopamine: a dose-response relationship. *Brain Res.* 1987;424:199-203.
9. Roy M, Roy A, Williams J, Weinberger L, Smelson D. Reduced blue cone electroretinogram in cocaine-withdrawn patients. *Arch Gen Psychiatry.* 1997;54: 153-156.
10. Roy M, Smelson D, Roy A. Abnormal electroretinogram in cocaine dependent patients: relationships to craving. *Br J Psychiatry.* 1996;168:507-511.
11. Verriest G, Van Laethem J, Uvijls A. A new assessment of the normal ranges of the Farnsworth-Munsell 100-hue test scores. *Am J Ophthalmol.* 1982;93:635-642.
12. Lanthony P. The desaturated panel D-15. *Doc Ophthalmol.* 1978;46:185-189.
13. Lanthony P. Evaluation du panel D-15 desature, I: methode de quantification et scores normaux. *J Fr Ophthalmol.* 1986;9:843-847.
14. Lanthony P. Evaluation du panel D-15 desature, II: comparison entre les tests panel D-15 desature et Farnsworth-Munsell 100-hue. *J Fr Ophthalmol.* 1987;10: 579-585.
15. Smith V, Pokorny J, Pass A. Color axis determination on the Farnsworth-Munsell 100-hue test. *Am J Ophthalmol.* 1985;100:176-182.
16. Weleber R. The effect of age on human cone and rod ganzfeld electroretinogram. *Invest Ophthalmol Vis Sci.* 1981;20:392-399.
17. Roy M, Podgor M, Collier B, Gunkel R. Color vision and age in a normal North American population. *Graefes Arch Clin Exp Ophthalmol.* 1991;229:139-144.
18. Ackerman J, White F. Decreased activity of rat A10 dopamine neurons following withdrawal from repeated cocaine. *Eur J Pharmacol.* 1992;218:171-173.
19. Cerruti C, Pilotte N, Uhl G, Kuhar M. Reduction in dopamine transporter mRNA after cessation of repeated cocaine administration. *Mol Brain Res.* 1991;22:132-138.
20. Karoum I, Egan M, Wyatt R. Selective reduction in dopamine turnover in the rat frontal cortex and hypothalamus during withdrawal from repeated cocaine exposure. *Eur J Pharmacol.* 1994;254:127-132.
21. Roy M, Smelson D, Roy A. Longitudinal study of blue cone retinal function in cocaine withdrawn patients. *Biol Psychiatry.* 1997;41:252-253.
22. Holopigian K, Clewer L, Seiple W, Kupersmith M. The effects of dopamine blockade on the human flash electroretinogram. *Doc Ophthalmol.* 1994;86: 1-9.
23. Muruiwa F, Kim SD, Nao-i N, Sawada A. Effect of metoclopramide, dopamine receptor blocker, on the EOG light peak. *Nippon Ganka Gakkai Zasshi.* 1992;96: 375-380.
24. Tagliati M, Bodis-Wollner I, Kovanecz I, Stanzione P. Spatial frequency tuning of the monkey pattern ERG depends on D_2 receptor—linked action of dopamine. *Vision Res.* 1994;34:2051-2057.
25. Gottlob I, Schneider E, Heider WI, Skrandies W. Alterations of visual evoked potentials and electroretinograms in Parkinson's disease. *Electroencephalogr Clin Neurophysiol.* 1987;66:349-357.
26. Ellis C, Allen T, Marden C, Ikeda H. Electroretinographic abnormalities in idiopathic Parkinson's disease and the effects of levodopa administration. *Clin Vis Sci.* 1987;1:347-355.
27. Verriest G, Franc P, Pierat P. Results of color vision tests in alcoholics and mentally disordered subjects. *Ophthalmologica.* 1980;180:247-256.
28. Mergler D, Blair L, LeMaire J, Lalande F. Color vision impairment and alcohol consumption. *Neurotoxicology.* 1988;10:255-260.
29. Russell R, Carney E, Feiock K, Garrett M, Karwoski P. Acute ethanol administration causes transient impairment of the blue-yellow color vision. *Alcohol Clin Exp Res.* 1980;4:396-399.
30. Kapitany T, Dietzel M, Gunberger J, Frey R, Koppensteiner L, Schleifer G, Marx B. Color vision deficiencies in the course of acute alcohol withdrawal. *Biol Psychiatry.* 1993;33:415-422.
31. Kosten T. Pharmacology of heroin and cocaine addiction. Paper presented at: Advances in Addiction Psychiatry Conference; 1994; Philadelphia, Pa.
32. Pokorny J, Smith V, Verriest G, Pinckers A, eds. *Congenital and Acquired Color Vision Defects.* New York, NY: Grune & Stratton Inc; 1979.
33. Roy M, Gunkel R, Podgor M. Color vision defects in early diabetic retinopathy. *Arch Ophthalmol.* 1986;104:225-228.
34. Roy M, Rodgers G, Gunkel R, Noguchi C, Schechter A. Color vision defects in sickle cell anemia. *Arch Ophthalmol.* 1987;105:1676-1678.
35. Karpe G, Uchermann A. The clinical electroretinogram, VII: the electroretinogram in circulatory disturbance of the retina. *Acta Ophthalmol.* 1955;33:496-516.
36. Volkow N, Fowler J, Wolf A. Effects of chronic cocaine abuse on postsynaptic dopamine receptors. *Am J Psychiatry.* 1990;147:719-724.

ORIGINAL ARTICLE

Fluoxetine in Depressed Alcoholics

A Double-blind, Placebo-Controlled Trial

Jack R. Cornelius, MD, MPH; Ihsan M. Salloum, MD, MPH; Joan G. Ehler, MD; Patricia J. Jarrett, MD, PhD; Marie D. Cornelius, PhD; James M. Perel, PhD; Michael E. Thase, MD; Ann Black, MS

Background: The selective serotonergic medication fluoxetine has demonstrated efficacy in the treatment of major depression and has suggested efficacy in the treatment of alcoholism. However, no completed trials with any selective serotonergic medication have been reported in patients who display both major depression and alcoholism, despite previous observations that both depression and alcoholism are associated with low serotonergic functioning.

Methods: Fifty-one patients diagnosed as having comorbid major depressive disorder and alcohol dependence were randomized to receive fluoxetine (n=25) or placebo (n=26) in a 12-week, double-blind, parallel-group trial. Weekly ratings of depression and alcohol consumption were obtained throughout the 12-week course of the study.

Results: The improvement in depressive symptoms during the medication trial was significantly greater in the fluoxetine group than in the placebo group. Total alcohol consumption during the trial was significantly lower in the fluoxetine group than in the placebo group.

Conclusions: Fluoxetine is effective in reducing the depressive symptoms and the alcohol consumption of patients with comorbid major depressive disorder and alcohol dependence. It is unknown whether these results generalize to the treatment of less depressed and less suicidal alcoholics.

Arch Gen Psychiatry. 1997;54:700-705

MAJOR DEPRESSION and alcohol dependence are the most common psychiatric disorders, and comorbidity between these disorders is common,[1] but surprisingly little is known about this dual-diagnosis population (hereafter referred to as depressed alcoholics). Information about more severely depressed alcoholics is especially scarce, because most studies of depressed alcoholics have been conducted in detoxification centers, where depressive symptoms would be expected to be less severe than in psychiatric hospitals. Moreover, patients with recent suicide attempts or prominent suicidal ideation are generally excluded from pharmacological trials involving alcoholics. Consequently, little is known about treatment response in alcoholics displaying depressive symptoms severe enough to necessitate inpatient treatment in a psychiatric hospital.

Depressed alcoholics are characterized by several symptoms associated with low serotonergic functioning. For example, studies evaluating cerebrospinal fluid levels of 5-hydroxyindoleacetic acid, the major metabolite of serotonin, implicate low serotonergic functioning in the cause of depression,[2,3] suicidality,[4,5] alcoholism,[6-8] and impulsivity,[9] all of which are observed in depressed alcoholics. Such findings led to speculation that abnormality of brain serotonin metabolism might be a factor causing the excessive alcohol intake and the depressive symptoms of depressed alcoholics.[3] Furthermore, cerebrospinal fluid levels of 5-hydroxyindoleacetic acid have been shown to be lower in depressed male alcoholics than in nondepressed male alcoholics, suggesting a more severe serotonergic dysfunction in depressed alcoholics.[10] Because of this more severe serotonergic dysfunction, a serotonergic medication such as fluoxetine might be more effective in depressed alcoholics than in nondepressed alcoholics.[11]

Various selective serotonin reuptake inhibitors have been shown to de-

See also page 691

From the Department of Psychiatry, Western Psychiatric Institute and Clinic, Pittsburgh, Pa.

SUBJECTS AND METHODS

SUBJECTS

This study was conducted at the Western Psychiatric Institute and Clinic of the University of Pittsburgh, Pittsburgh, Pa. This facility is a large, comprehensive, urban university psychiatric hospital. All patients were recruited from consecutive admissions on the inpatient services of this hospital. On admission to the hospital, all patients received a thorough medical and psychiatric evaluation by a psychiatrist unrelated to the study, and standard admission laboratory tests. A blood alcohol level and a urine drug screen were obtained at baseline, at the end of treatment, and at any week in which alcohol or drug use was suspected. Patients who had been diagnosed as having comorbid major depressive disorder and alcohol dependence were then reexamined by a research team–attending psychiatrist to establish the comorbid diagnoses, using *DSM-III-R*[20] criteria. Before entry into the protocol, the study was explained and written consent was obtained, in keeping with the requirements of the University of Pittsburgh Biomedical Institutional Review Board. Patients were recruited into the study without regard to sex, race, or ethnicity. Following a 2- to 3-day detoxification with minor tranquilizers and a subsequent 1-week washout period, the continued presence of the comorbid diagnoses was confirmed using the Structured Clinical Interview for *DSM-III-R*.[21] Only patients meeting the diagnostic criteria for current diagnoses of both major depressive disorder and alcohol dependence were included in the study. The depressive diagnosis was required to be primary diagnosis, defined by *DSM-III-R* as being "the condition that was chiefly responsible for occasioning the evaluation."

Exclusionary criteria included a diagnosis of bipolar disorder, schizoaffective disorder, schizophrenia, or nonalcohol substance dependence. Abuse of other substances was not an exclusionary criterion, provided that alcohol was clearly the main substance of abuse. Patients with hyperthyroidism or hypothyroidism, clinically significant liver disease (liver function tests ≥ 3× normal), notable cardiac or renal impairment, pregnancy, mental retardation, or clinically evident cognitive impairment were excluded. Patients who had received antipsychotic or antidepressant medication in the month before admission to the hospital were excluded, as were patients younger than 18 or older than 65 years of age.

TREATMENT AND ASSESSMENT

Patients were randomly assigned to receive fluoxetine (n=25) or placebo (n=26) administered in identical-looking opaque capsules. Patient randomization was stratified for sex and race, based on previous descriptive studies of depressed alcoholics at our facility.[22,23] All subjects were initially given 1 capsule (20 mg fluoxetine or placebo), which could be increased to 2 capsules after 2 weeks if substantial residual depressive symptoms persisted. The mean±SD maximal daily dose was 1.25±0.45 capsules per day, which did not differ between the treatment groups. Verification of compliance with medication was assessed by weekly pill counts and by plasma levels of fluoxetine and norfluoxetine at weeks 2, 4, and 12. Substantial blood levels of fluoxetine were observed in more than 99% of blood specimens of patients assigned to fluoxetine. All patients also received "usual care" for dual-diagnosis patients at our facility, consisting of weekly supportive psychotherapy sessions and weekly meetings with an attending psychiatrist (J.R.C., I.M.S., J.G.E., or P.J.J.) with expertise in evaluating and treating dual-disorder patients. Attendance at Alcoholics Anonymous also was encouraged for all patients. Weekly ratings of symptoms were performed by the same attending psychiatrist at baseline and at each of 12 weeks of the pharmacotherapy trial. The screening, the baseline ratings, and the first 2 weekly ratings were performed while the patient was still in the hospital, and the remaining 10 weekly ratings were conducted on an outpatient basis after discharge from the hospital.

Weekly ratings of depression and drinking were obtained throughout the course of the trial. Observer-rated depression was assessed with the 24-item Hamilton Rating Scale for Depression (HAM-D-24).[24] Self-rated depression was assessed using the Beck Depression Inventory (BDI).[25] Drinking behavior was evaluated using a timeline follow-back method[26] and the Addiction Severity Index.[27] Verification of level of drinking was obtained at baseline and at the end of the study from a relative or close friend specified by the patient. In the rare case of an unresolved discrepancy between self-report and significant-other report, the more adverse report was assumed accurate.

STATISTICAL ANALYSIS

All analyses were conducted using the Statistical Package for the Social Sciences.[28] Descriptive statistics were calculated for all variables. Continuous baseline measures were compared by analysis of variance. Categorical measures were compared by χ^2 analysis, corrected for continuity.

Outcome measures were compared by analysis of covariance, using baseline depression and drinking as the covariates. Outcome measures were calculated using intention-to-treat analyses including all randomized patients, and used the last-observation-carried-forward for dropouts. Within-group analyses were conducted using paired Student *t* tests. All tests of significance were 2-tailed. Variance estimates are given as SDs. An α level of ≤.05 was used in the study.

crease alcohol ingestion in laboratory animals. For example, studies with rats have reported decreases in alcohol ingestion that range from 18% to 84% for selective serotonergic agents including zimeldine hydrochloride, citalopram, fluvoxamine maleate, and viqualine.[12,13] Similarly, decreases in alcohol intake also have been shown after administration of serotonin precursors such as tryptophan, from administration of intracerebral serotonin, and from administration of postsynaptic serotonergic agonists such as MK-212 and quipazine maleate. No improvement was observed in laboratory animals after administration of tricyclic antidepressants.[13]

Several studies have been conducted to determine whether fluoxetine decreases the alcohol consumption of problem drinkers or alcoholics who do not have comorbid major depression. Naranjo et al[14-17] reported that several selective serotonergic medications (fluoxetine, zimeldine, viqualine, and citalopram) notably reduce drinking in nondepressed heavy social drinkers, although these decreases were modest. Subsequently, Gorelick and Paredes[18] showed a significant but modest decrease in drinking among 20 alcohol-dependent males during the first week of treatment with fluoxetine, although this improvement was not sustained in later weeks.

Our own research group recently reported a first open-label study of fluoxetine in 12 patients with comorbid major depression and alcohol dependence.[11] Treatment with 20 to 40 mg of fluoxetine resulted in a significant within-group decrease in depressive symptoms and in alcohol consumption. However, because no placebo control was used in that study, the investigators could not rule out the possibility that part or all of the therapeutic effect observed with fluoxetine was a placebo response or a response to inpatient detoxification, or that there was observer bias. Preliminary findings from the current double-blind study also were published previously, based on a sample size of only 21 patients.[19] The results of that preliminary analysis did not show a significant difference between treatment groups in depressive symptoms, probably because of the small sample size, although the magnitude of improvement in the 2 groups was similar to that currently being reported.

To our knowledge, no double-blind, placebo-controlled studies have been reported evaluating the efficacy of selective serotonergic medications in patients with comorbid major depression and alcohol dependence. In this article, we report data from a randomized double-blind, placebo-controlled study of a selective serotonergic medication (fluoxetine) for the treatment of depressed alcoholics. We hypothesized that fluoxetine would significantly reduce the depressive symptoms and the alcohol consumption of this dual-diagnosis population.

RESULTS

SAMPLE DESCRIPTION

Fifty-one patients participated in this study, including 25 who were randomly assigned to fluoxetine and 26 to placebo. Demographic, diagnostic, and baseline severity characteristics of randomized subjects are given in **Table 1**. These included 26 men and 25 women. Their mean age was 34.8±10.2 years. Twenty-seven of the patients were black and 24 were white. No significant differences were seen between treatment groups for sex, race, age, or marital or employment status. A total of 147 patients were screened to identify the 51 patients who participated in this study. Forty-six of these patients (90% of those randomized) completed the pharmacotherapy study; the other 5 patients (10%) dropped out before the end of the trial.

All 51 patients were actively drinking at the time they were admitted to the hospital, immediately before entry into the study. The patients met an average of 5.7±1.7 of the 9 *DSM-III-R* diagnostic criteria for alcohol dependence at baseline. Thus, the patients in this study generally met *DSM-III-R* criteria for severe alcohol dependence. The patients met an average of 6.8±1.1 of the 9 *DSM-III-R* diagnostic criteria for major depression. Thus, the patients in this study generally met *DSM-III-R* criteria for severe major depressive episode.

Twenty (39%) of the 51 patients made a suicide attempt in the current episode. Eighteen of those 20 patients (35% of the total sample) made a suicide attempt in the week before admission to the hospital. Thirty-one (61%) of the patients had made a suicide attempt in their lifetime. Forty-six (90%) of the patients reported suicidal ideations in the week before hospitalization. Thus, this sample showed a high level of current and past suicidal behavior and of current suicidal ideation on admission to the hospital, which is consistent with the findings of our previously published work describing the clinical characteristics of depressed alcoholics at our institution.[29,30]

Prominent depressive severity was observed on admission to the hospital. After detoxification and a subsequent 1-week medication-free washout period (baseline), a moderate level of depressive symptoms persisted. No significant differences were observed between the level of depressive symptoms in the 2 treatment groups on admission to the hospital or after detoxification and washout. However, the fluoxetine group was significantly more depressed than the placebo group following detoxification and washout on the BDI.

DEPRESSION OUTCOMES

Between-group measures of overall treatment outcome are given in **Table 2**. The change in the HAM-D-24 (improvement) during the medication trial was significantly greater in the fluoxetine group than in the placebo group. However, no significant between-group difference was observed on the BDI.

Within-group measures of treatment outcome also were calculated for each of the 2 treatment groups. The fluoxetine group showed a significant within-group decrease (improvement) in depression on the HAM-D-24 and the BDI during the 12-week course of the study. In contrast, the placebo group showed no significant improvement in depressive symptoms on either of these 2 measures.

The improvement in the Global Assessment Scale score during the medication trial was 3 times as great in the fluoxetine group as in the placebo group, which was a significant difference. Thus, at the end of the medication study, the mean Global Assessment Scale score for those in the placebo group was in the moderately impaired range, and the mean Global Assessment Scale score for those in the fluoxetine group was in the mildly impaired range.

None of the patients in either treatment group made a suicide attempt during the course of the pharmacotherapy trial, nor did they experience other adverse events. Also, no patients were discontinued from the study be-

Table 1. Demographic and Baseline Clinical Characteristics of Randomized Subjects

	Treatment Group		Difference Between Groups	
Variable	Fluoxetine (n=25)	Placebo (n=26)	Test Statistic	*P*
Female, %	48.0	50.0	χ^2=0.020	<.90
Mean age, y	35.7±10.4	34.0±10.0	F=0.378	.54
White, %	48.0	46.2	χ^2=0.017	<.90
Currently married, %	20.0	3.8	χ^2=3.204	.07
Employed, %	36.0	26.9	χ^2=0.488	<.50
No. of *DSM-III-R* criteria, AD	5.5±1.6	5.9±1.8	F=0.636	.43
No. of *DSM-III-R* criteria, MDD	6.7±1.1	6.8±1.1	F=0.223	.64
Suicide attempt in previous week, %	36.0	34.6	χ^2=0.011	<.92
Lifetime suicide attempt, %	70.8	60.9	χ^2=9.042	<.11
Current suicide ideation, %	92.0	88.5	χ^2=1.199	<.90
HAM-D-24 at presentation	33.2	33.0	F=0.005	.94
HAM-D-24 after detoxification and washout	19.2±8.2	17.9±8.1	F=0.485	.49
BDI at presentation	29.6±12.4	24.8±12.4	F=1.964	<.17
BDI after detoxification and washout	19.7±13.4	12.3±7.5	F=6.278	<.02
No. of days drinking in past 90 days	54.5±29.2	45.2±28.9	F=1.226	.27
No. of days drinking to drunkenness in past 90 days	40.1±27.7	32.0±26.4	F=1.061	<.31
GAS after detoxification and washout	53.3±8.7	49.6±6.6	F=2.919	.09

**Values are given as mean±SD, unless otherwise indicated. AD indicates alcohol dependence; MDD, major depressive disorder; HAM-D-24, 24-item Hamilton Rating Scale for Depression; BDI, Beck Depression Inventory; and GAS, Global Assessment Scale.*

Table 2. Between-Group Comparisons of Treatment Outcome*

Variable	Fluoxetine (n=25)	Placebo (n=26)	Test Statistic	*P*
Cumulative drinks during 12-week trial	70.2±100.7	215.5±248.5	F=5.12	<.03
Cumulative number of drinking days during trial	10.6±15.6	20.3±18.3	F=4.26	<.05
Drinks per drinking day during 12-week trial	2.4±2.9	5.4±5.5	F=4.13	<.05
Cumulative number of days of heavy drinking	4.8±7.0	16.0±18.0	F=4.51	.04
No. of weeks until first drink	5.5±4.5	3.9±4.0	F=3.14	.08
No. of weeks until first heavy drinking	8.0±4.8	4.7±4.2	F=6.03	<.02
No. of patients abstinent throughout entire trial	7 (28.0%)	4 (15.4%)	χ^2=1.20	.27
Change in HAM-D-24	−6.0±9.6	−2.0±13.3	F=4.17	<.05
Change in BDI	−6.5±12.8	−0.9±12.1	F=1.90	.17
Change in GAS	16.8±14.5	5.2±17.0	F=8.73	.005
Alcoholics Anonymous attendance, sessions	14.7±17.0	15.3±19.8	F=0.01	.92
Psychotherapy attendance, sessions	9.9±2.8	8.9±3.1	F=1.53	.22

**Abbreviations are given in the footnote to Table 1. Values are given as mean±SD unless otherwise indicated.*

cause of medication side effects. Fluoxetine was well tolerated by the patients in this study.

DRINKING OUTCOMES

Total alcohol consumption during the 12-week pharmacotherapy trial was 3 times higher in the placebo group than in the fluoxetine group, which was a significant difference. The cumulative number of drinking days during the trial was twice as high in the placebo group as in the fluoxetine group, which also was a significant difference. In addition, the number of drinks per drinking day was twice as high in the placebo group, which again was a significant difference. The number of days of heavy drinking, defined as drinking 5 or more drinks per day, was 3 times as high in the placebo group as in the fluoxetine group, which was a significant difference.

Outcome measures concerning the length of abstinence in the 2 treatment groups also were assessed. The number of weeks until first heavy drinking was significantly higher in the fluoxetine group than in the placebo group. Thus, those in the fluoxetine group avoided heavy drinking almost twice as long as those in the placebo group. However, the proportion of patients who were completely abstinent during the entire 12-week treatment study was low in both treatment groups. Specifically, 28% (n=7) of those in the fluoxetine group vs 15% (n=4) of those in the placebo group were totally abstinent during the entire 12-week study, which was not a significant difference.

The time course of treatment response was assessed by comparing levels of drinking in the 2 treatment groups during the first half (6 weeks) of the study, and then repeating these analyses for the second half of the study. The levels of drinking were significantly heavier in the placebo group in each of the 2 halves of the study, and the difference in level of drinking was 2- to 3-fold across both periods. Thus, the drinking patterns in each of the 2 halves of the study showed a significant treatment effect for fluoxetine that was similar in magnitude across both halves of the study.

Attendance at Alcoholics Anonymous meetings and at supportive psychotherapy sessions did not significantly differ between the treatment groups. Self-reported level of alcohol use significantly correlated with levels of liver function tests at baseline and at multiple timepoints throughout the study. Self-reported level of alcohol use also significantly correlated with level of alcohol use as reported by a relative or close friend at baseline and at the end of the study.

Sixteen patients (31%) had alcohol in their blood on admission to the hospital, of which about two thirds (n=11) had levels indicating legal intoxication (≥100 mg/100 mL). Only 2 patients had alcohol in their blood at any time during the course of the study. No patients had positive results of the urine drug screen on admission to the hospital or during the study. No significant difference between treatment groups was observed at any time for blood alcohol level or for liver function test levels.

CORRELATING DRINKING AND DEPRESSION

The association between drinking and depression was assessed by calculating Pearson correlation coefficients of change in depression vs change in drinking (number of drinks per week) during the 12-week study. In the placebo group, change in drinking was significantly correlated with change in depression on the HAM-D-24 (Pearson $r=0.618$; $P=.001$) and on the BDI (Pearson $r=0.594$; $P=.001$). In the placebo group, level of drinking was significantly correlated with level of BDI depression at midpoint (week 6) and at end point (week 12), but not at baseline. In the fluoxetine group, no significant correlation was observed for change in drinking vs change in depression on the HAM-D-24 or the BDI. In the fluoxetine group, no significant correlation was observed between level of drinking and level of depression at any time, such as at baseline, midpoint, or end point.

COMMENT

This study provides data from what we believe is the first double-blind, placebo-controlled study evaluating the efficacy of a selective serotonergic medication in the treatment of patients with comorbid major depression and alcohol dependence. The findings from this study show efficacy for fluoxetine in reducing the depressive symptoms and the alcohol consumption of these patients. These findings support the hypothesis that fluoxetine would significantly reduce both of these groups of symptoms in depressed alcoholics. Thus, the findings of this double-blind, placebo-controlled study are consistent with our previous pilot findings and preliminary findings in depressed alcoholics.[11,19]

The findings of the present study can be compared with those of a recent study by McGrath et al,[31] which evaluated the efficacy of the tricyclic antidepressant imipramine hydrochloride in alcoholics with primary major depression. That study showed efficacy for imipramine in treating the depressive symptoms of depressed alcoholics, but did not show efficacy for imipramine in treating the excessive drinking of these patients. Another recent study, by Mason et al,[32] evaluated the efficacy of the tricyclic antidepressant desipramine hydrochloride in alcoholics stratified on the presence or absence of major depression. That study showed efficacy for desipramine in treating both the depression and the alcohol relapse of depressed alcoholics. Thus, it seems that tricyclic antidepressants show efficacy in treating the depression of depressed alcoholics, but it is unclear whether they show efficacy in treating the excessive alcohol use of these patients. Further studies are warranted to clarify the efficacy of tricyclic antidepressants in depressed alcoholics and to assess whether factors such as primary vs secondary depression might account for differences in response to antidepressants.

The results of the present study also can be compared with those of a recent study by Kranzler et al,[33] which evaluated the efficacy of fluoxetine in a group of alcoholics, most of whom (86%) did not have comorbid depression. That study found that fluoxetine had no notable effects on alcohol consumption, but it reduced HAM-D-24 scores more than did placebo treatment among subjects with current major depression. The authors of that study concluded that fluoxetine is probably not useful for relapse prevention in alcoholics with mild to moderate alcohol dependence and no comorbid depression. They suggested that future studies with fluoxetine probably should focus on more severely alcohol-dependent subjects or those with comorbid depression. The important therapeutic effects observed for fluoxetine in our study were obtained in a sample with comorbid depression and severe alcohol dependence. Indeed, our current sample showed prominent baseline suicidality, which has been strongly linked to low serotonergic functioning.[4,5] Thus, our current findings, in conjunction with those of Kranzler et al,[33] suggest that fluoxetine shows efficacy for the drinking and the depression of alcoholics with comorbid major depression, but shows little if any efficacy for treating the drinking or the depression of alcoholics without comorbid depression.

The pharmacology of the antidrinking effects by fluoxetine for depressed alcoholics is unclear. This antidrinking effect may result from the more severe serotonergic dysfunction observed in depressed alcoholics compared with that seen in nondepressed alcoholics.[10] Alternatively, it is possible that the antidrinking effect of selective serotonergic medications such as fluoxetine in depressed alcoholics is due at least in part to their antidepressant effect. However, in this study, the change in drinking did not correlate significantly with the change in depression in the fluoxetine group. Also, the improvement in level of depressive symptoms was modest in the fluoxetine group. These findings suggest that the antidrinking effect of fluoxetine was not entirely due to its antidepressant effect. Further studies are warranted to clarify the nature of the antidrinking effect of fluoxetine in depressed alcoholics.

Finally, change in the level of depression was strongly correlated with change in the level of drinking in the placebo group in this study. In addition, the level of drinking was significantly correlated with the level of depression at multiple timepoints during the study in the placebo group. Also, large reductions in depressive symptoms occurred during detoxification and washout in both treatment groups. These findings suggest that there is a strong relation between depression and drinking in depressed alcoholics. These findings are consistent with our previous findings.[29,30] Further studies are warranted to clarify the nature of the relation between drinking and depression in depressed alcoholics.

The results of the present study should be interpreted in light of several limitations. First, the sample in this study was more depressed and more suicidal than most depressed alcoholics, who often are treated in alcohol detoxification centers rather than in psychiatric hospitals. Consequently, it is unclear to what extent the results of this study generalize to the treatment of less depressed and less suicidal alcoholics. Second, the period of observation in our trial was short in terms of the natural history of alcohol dependence. Continuation studies and long-term follow-up studies would be necessary to determine whether the benefits associated with fluoxetine treatment are sustained. Third, residual low levels of depressive symptoms and alcohol consumption persisted in both treatment groups. Thus, treatment with fluoxetine was associated with a significant reduction but not an elimination of alcohol consumption or depression. Fourth, the sample size in the present study was small. Large multisite trials of selective serotonergic medications appear to be warranted in depressed alcoholics.

Accepted for publication January 28, 1997.

This work was supported by grants AA09127 and AA10523 from the National Institute on Alcohol Abuse and Alcoholism and by grant MH30915 from the Mental Health Clinical Research Center, Rockville, Md.

Presented at the 149th Annual Meeting (New Research) of the American Psychiatric Association, New York, NY, May 7, 1996.

We thank David J. Kupfer, MD, and Roger F. Haskett, MD, for their helpful comments on the manuscript.

Reprints: Jack R. Cornelius, MD, Western Psychiatric Institute and Clinic, 3811 O'Hara St, Room 1092, Pittsburgh, PA 15213.

REFERENCES

1. Kessler RC, McGonagle KA, Zhao S, Nelson CB, Hughes M, Eshleman S, Wittchen H, Kendler KS. Lifetime and 12-month prevalence of *DSM-III-R* psychiatric disorders in the United States: results from the National Comorbidity Survey. *Arch Gen Psychiatry.* 1994;51:8-19.
2. Åsberg M, Traskman L, Thoren P. 5-HIAA in the cerebrospinal fluid. *Arch Gen Psychiatry.* 1976;33:1193-1197.
3. Takahashi S, Yamane H, Kondo H, Tani N, Kato N. CSF monoamine metabolites in alcoholism: a comparative study with depression. *Folia Psychiatr Neurol.* 1974;28:347-354.
4. Traskman L, Åsberg M, Bertilsson L, Sjostrand L. Monoamine metabolites in CSF and suicidal behavior. *Arch Gen Psychiatry.* 1981;38:631-636.
5. Mann JJ, Stanley M, McBride PA, McEwen BS. Increased serotonin$_2$ and β-adrenergic receptor binding in the frontal cortices of suicide victims. *Arch Gen Psychiatry.* 1986;43:954-959.
6. Ballenger JC, Goodwin FK, Major LF, Brown GL. Alcohol and central serotonin metabolism in man. *Arch Gen Psychiatry.* 1979;36:224-227.
7. Banki CM, Arato M, Papp Z, Kurcz M. Biochemical markers in suicidal patients. *J Affect Disord.* 1984;6:341-350.
8. Banki CM. Factors influencing monoamine metabolites and tryptophan in patients with alcohol dependence. *J Neural Transm Basic Neurosci Neurol Sect Psychiatry Sect.* 1981;50:89-101.
9. Soubrié P. Reconciling the role of central serotonin neurons in human and animal behavior. *Behav Brain Sci.* 1986;9:319-364.
10. Roy A, DeJong J, Lamparski D, Adinoff B, George T, Moore M, Garnett D, Kerich M, Linnoila M. Mental disorders among alcoholics. *Arch Gen Psychiatry.* 1991;48:423-427.
11. Cornelius JR, Salloum IM, Cornelius MD, Perel JM, Thase ME, Ehler JG, Mann JJ. Fluoxetine trial in suicidal depressed alcoholics. *Psychopharmacol Bull.* 1993;29:195-199.
12. Lawrin MO, Naranjo CA, Sellers EM. Identification and testing of new drugs for modulating alcohol consumption. *Psychopharmacol Bull.* 1986;22:1020-1025.
13. Naranjo CA, Sellers EM, Lawrin MO. Modulation of ethanol intake by serotonin uptake inhibitors. *J Clin Psychiatry.* 1986;47:16-22.
14. Naranjo CA, Kadlec KE, Sanhueza P, Woodley-Remus D, Sellers EM. Fluoxetine differentially alters alcohol intake and other consummatory behaviors in problem drinkers. *Clin Pharmacol Ther.* 1990;47:490-498.
15. Naranjo CA, Poulos CX, Bremner KE, Lanctot KL. Fluoxetine attenuates alcohol intake and desire to drink. *Int Clin Psychopharmacol.* 1994;9:163-172.
16. Naranjo CA, Sullivan JT, Kadlec KE, Woodley-Remus DV, Kennedy G, Sellers EM. Differential effects of viqualine on alcohol intake and other consummatory behaviors. *Clin Pharmacol Ther.* 1989;46:301-309.
17. Naranjo CA, Sellers EM, Sullivan JT, Woodley DV, Kadlec K, Sykora K. The serotonin uptake inhibitor citalopram attenuates ethanol intake. *Clin Pharmacol Ther.* 1987;41:266-274.
18. Gorelick DA, Paredes A. Effect of fluoxetine on alcohol consumption in male alcoholics. *Alcohol Clin Exp Res.* 1992;16:261-265.
19. Cornelius JR, Salloum IM, Cornelius MD, Perel JM, Ehler JG, Jarrett PJ, Levin RL, Black A, Mann JJ. Preliminary report: double-blind, placebo-controlled study of fluoxetine in depressed alcoholics. *Psychopharmacol Bull.* 1995;31:297-303.
20. American Psychiatric Association. *Diagnostic and Statistical Manual of Mental Disorders, Third Edition, Revised.* Washington, DC: American Psychiatric Association; 1987.
21. Spitzer RL, Williams JBW, Gibbon M, First MB. *Instructional Manual for the Structured Clinical Interview for DSM-III-R (SCID), Revised.* New York: Biomedical Research Division, New York State Psychiatric Institute; 1988.
22. Cornelius JR, Jarrett PJ, Thase ME, Fabrega H, Haas GL, Jones-Barlock A, Mezzich JE, Ulrich RF. Gender effects on the clinical presentation of alcoholics at a psychiatric hospital. *Compr Psychiatry.* 1995;36:435-440.
23. Cornelius JR, Fabrega H, Cornelius MD, Mezzich JE, Maher PJ, Salloum IM, Thase ME, Ulrich RF. Racial effects on the clinical presentation of alcoholics at a psychiatric hospital. *Compr Psychiatry.* 1996;37:102-108.
24. Hamilton M. A rating scale for depression. *J Neurol Neurosurg Psychiatry.* 1960;23:56-62.
25. Beck AT, Ward CH, Mendelson M, Mock J, Erbaugh J. An inventory for measuring depression. *Arch Gen Psychiatry.* 1961;4:561-571.
26. Sobell LC, Sobell MB, Leo GI, Cancilla A. Reliability of a timeline method: assessing normal drinkers' reports of recent drinking and a comparative evaluation across several populations. *Br J Addict.* 1988;83:393-402.
27. McLellan AT, Luborsky L, Woody GE, O'Brien CP. An improved diagnostic evaluation instrument for substance abuse patients: the addiction severity index. *J Nerv Ment Dis.* 1980;168:26-33.
28. Norusis MJ. *SPSS for Windows: Base System User's Guide, Release 5.0.* Chicago, Ill: SPSS; 1992.
29. Cornelius JR, Salloum IM, Mezzich J, Cornelius MD, Fabrega H, Ehler JG, Ulrich RF, Thase ME, Mann JJ. Disproportionate suicidality in patients with comorbid major depression and alcoholism. *Am J Psychiatry.* 1995;152:358-364.
30. Cornelius JR, Salloum IM, Day NL, Thase ME, Mann JJ. Patterns of suicidality and alcohol use in alcoholics with major depression. *Alcohol Clin Exp Res.* 1996;20:1451-1455.
31. McGrath PJ, Nunes EV, Stewart JW, Goldman D, Agosti V, Ocepek-Welikson K, Quitkin FM. Imipramine treatment of alcoholics with major depression: a placebo-controlled clinical trial. *Arch Gen Psychiatry.* 1996;53:232-240.
32. Mason BJ, Kocsis JH, Ritvo CE, Cutler RB. A double-blind, placebo-controlled trial of desipramine for primary alcohol dependence stratified on the presence or absence of major depression. *JAMA.* 1996;275:761-767.
33. Kranzler HR, Burleson JA, Korner P, Del Boca FK, Bohn MJ, Brown J, Liebowitz N. Placebo-controlled trial of fluoxetine as an adjunct to relapse prevention in alcoholics. *Am J Psychiatry.* 1995;152:391-397.

Prediction of Compliance With Outpatient Referral in Patients With Schizophrenia and Psychoactive Substance Use Disorders

Christian R. Miner, PhD; Richard N. Rosenthal, MD; David J. Hellerstein, MD; Larry R. Muenz, PhD

Background: Most patients with concurrent schizophrenia and psychoactive substance use disorders may be adequately treated as outpatients. However, many do not comply with outpatient referrals and are therefore at heightened risk for rehospitalization.

Method: Drawing on standardized interview data collected during an index hospitalization, we developed a logistic regression model to predict compliance with outpatient treatment. The model was tested on a confirmatory sample, and its sensitivity and specificity were further evaluated in a cross-validation study of 1000 random samples.

Results: In a reference sample, the logistic function distinguished compliant from noncompliant patients in 37 (76%) of 49 cases. In a confirmatory sample, compliance status was predicted for 11 (78%) of 14 patients with a sensitivity of 1.00 and a specificity of 0.67. Women and patients with negative syndrome schizophrenia were compliant with outpatient referral, whereas those with mixed syndromes were most likely to be noncompliant. Cross-validation supports the stability of the model.

Conclusion: While most persons with schizophrenia and concurrent substance abuse comply with integrated outpatient treatment, most who cannot may be predicted in advance.

Arch Gen Psychiatry. 1997;54:706-712

PERSONS WHO are mentally ill and have a psychoactive substance use disorder (PSUD) present several well-known, but daunting, public health problems. Many of these patients have frequent, "revolving door" inpatient stays on acute care services[1,2]; over the long term, this pattern of service utilization is costly and clinically unproductive.[3,4] Attempts to interrupt the cycle of relapse and repeated acute-care hospitalization by referral to a long-term care facility often fail because many patients no longer warrant institutionalization once they are appropriately medicated and constrained from substance abuse. While outpatient services may constitute the most humane and cost-effective alternative, they are often fragmented and inadequately geared to meet the needs of this class of patients.[5-7]

Previous studies suggest that patients with mental illness and a PSUD generally are less compliant with outpatient treatment than patients with similar psychiatric conditions but without PSUDs.[8,9] However, findings are qualified by the fact that in many parts of the country, mental health and substance abuse services are uncoordinated, presenting these patients with treatment options that are logistically complex and/or based on mutually contradictory premises.[10] Recently, however, we showed that a substantial proportion of patients with PSUDs and co-occurring schizophrenia (PSUD/S) may be adequately treated in a low-intensity, supportive group format that integrates features of both psychiatric and substance abuse services.[11]

We previously described the components of this treatment modality[12]

See also page 691

and outlined the characteristics of patients with PSUD/S for whom it seems effective. Concurrent with a schizophrenia-continuum diagnosis, most study patients simultaneously met PSUD criteria for "crack" cocaine, marijuana, and alcohol. In the present report, we describe the characteristics of early treatment dropouts. Although most patients complied with outpatient treatment,[11] some failed from the outset to engage with outpatient services, notwithstanding assisted transition from

From the Department of Psychiatry, Beth Israel Medical Center, New York, NY (Drs Miner, Rosenthal, and Hellerstein), and the Department of Psychiatry, University of Pennsylvania, Philadelphia (Dr Muenz).

PATIENTS AND METHODS

During an index acute-care hospitalization, patients with symptoms consistent with the *DSM-III-R* criteria[19] for schizophrenia-continuum disorder and at least 1 PSUD were referred as research candidates to an evaluation team for further assessment. Inclusion criteria were willingness to sign informed consent, chronological age between 18 and 50 years, a research diagnostic criteria (RDC)[20] diagnosis of schizophrenia-continuum disorder, at least 1 concurrent *DSM-III-R* PSUD, and an expressed desire for substance abuse treatment. Exclusion criteria were the presence of a life-threatening medical illness, *DSM-III-R* antisocial personality disorder, a Global Assessment Scale[19,21] score of 30 or less, and a Mini-Mental State Examination[22] score less than 24.

After at least 14 days of treatment on the inpatient unit, prospective subjects were assessed by 2 trained interviewers (unaware of study hypotheses) who administered the Schedule for Affective Disorders and Schizophrenia,[23] the Addiction Severity Index (ASI),[24,25] and the Brief Symptom Inventory.[26] The Schedule for Affective Disorders and Schizophrenia structured interview and a review of the medical record and index hospital course for each patient were the basis for judging RDC and also for completing the Schedule for the Assessment of Negative Symptoms (SANS)[27,28] and the Schedule for the Assessment of Positive Symptoms (SAPS).[29] Following the highly restrictive criteria of Andreasen and Olsen,[30,31] we classify subjects cross-sectionally at intake into those exemplifying positive, negative, or mixed schizophrenic syndromes. During the first year of the study, interviewers maintained acceptable interrater reliability across all instruments: for RDCs mean $\kappa=0.86$; for the ASI severity profiles, mean $\kappa=0.84$; for the SANS, the mean intraclass correlation coefficient[32] was 0.93; and for the SAPS, the mean intraclass correlation coefficient was 0.90.

On meeting study criteria, patients were randomized to 2 mode-of-service conditions, one providing experimental integrated psychiatric and substance abuse treatment and the other providing standard care as a control. Treatment conditions were balanced for intensity and levels of service were comparable across the 2 groups. Also, patients in both conditions were counseled about their aftercare and accompanied by staff to their first group therapy session before discharge from the inpatient service. Thus, before leaving the hospital, in addition to receiving scheduled follow-up appointments, all study patients became familiar with the treatment setting, met the treatment team, and became acquainted with other group patients. As expected under randomization, subjects in the 2 groups did not differ significantly on any measure at the time of index. Between-condition outcome effects have been described previously,[11] and, for the present report, data from the 2 conditions are pooled.

Ridgely[33] described the characteristics of the engagement phase of substance abuse treatment for mentally ill young adults. In our study, subjects who did not attend at least 2 initial postdischarge outpatient sessions were considered nonengaged. In practice, those in this category generally do not return for outpatient treatment once they leave the inpatient setting. Conversely, subjects who attended their first 2 outpatient sessions were considered to be engaged in treatment, and their subsequent dropout rate was low during the first 4 months.

After random assignment to treatment, discharge from the inpatient service, and intake at the outpatient site, 18 (37%) of the first 49 subjects were considered nonengaged because they did not attend at least 2 initial outpatient sessions. The nonengaged group included 7 patients receiving experimental treatment and 11 patients receiving the control treatment, a nonsignificant difference by Fisher's exact test.

Data analysis proceeded in 5 main steps. First, in an exploratory analysis, we used data from the first 49 randomized subjects to compute correlations between treatment engagement/nonengagement (a binary dependent variable) and 37 predictors drawn from the RDC, ASI, the Brief Symptom Inventory, SANS, SAPS, and demographic variables collected at index (**Table 1**). One subject was adopted early in life, knew nothing of her biological parents, and, therefore, had missing data on 2 ASI scales pertaining to substance use in the family of origin.

Because the magnitude of ϕ and point biserial correlation coefficients may be attenuated by highly skewed distribution forms, a conservative criterion (the absolute value of correlation coefficients of 0.15 or less) was used to remove only the most obviously irrelevant variables from further consideration. A variable retained by virtue of correlation at the low end of the range may account for less than 3% of outcome variance. After the exploratory step, 17 independent variables remained for inclusion into logistic regression procedures.[34] The 2 ASI scales indexing family substance abuse were screened out by this procedure, and, accordingly, there were no missing data on the independent variables included in the logistic model.

Second, candidate predictors were entered into a PROC LOGISTIC regression analysis[35] to derive a logistic discriminant function predicting treatment engagement. A backward stepwise elimination procedure removed unrelated predictors one at a time, and only those with significant Wald χ^2 values (criterion $\alpha<.05$) were retained. Because the sample was relatively small, the *P* values resulting from the usual large sample, "asymptotic" method were compared with an alternative algorithm for exact logistic regression.[36]

Third, after deriving a final logistic equation, its predictions were compared with true scores of the patients on engagement/nonengagement. The receiver-operating characteristics (ROC)[37-39] of the model were examined to determine the logistic regression criterion cutoff with optimal sensitivity and specificity (**Figure 1**). In this step, the logistic regression equation yields a probability, P_j, that subject j will engage with treatment, given the subject's scores on the independent variables in the model. The analyst then chooses the threshold P_0, such that if P_j is greater than P_0, the model classifies the subject as engaged. As the analyst varies the threshold, the sensitivity and specificity of the model also vary. Thus, in Figure 1, the 24 data points along the ROC curve indicate thresholds of *P*: the ROC curve plots 1–specificity against sensitivity and affords an appraisal of the optimal ("maximim") balance between the 2, ie,

Continued on next page

the point closest to the upper left corner of the graph. Optimal sensitivity and specificity define the criterion cutoff rule by an outcome probability value, which in turn may be used to predict compliance status in a new sample. Thus, in the fourth step, the model was applied to data from 14 new patients, predicted outcome scores were generated, and predicted engagement status was compared with true treatment engagement status.

Finally, a randomized cross-validation procedure[40] was performed. In this step, data from 42 (67%) subjects were randomly selected as a "training set," and a logistic regression was performed. Estimates of sensitivity and specificity derived from the training set were compared with estimates derived by applying the model to a "test set" that was comprised of data from the remaining 21 subjects (33%). This process was iterated 1000 times.

an inpatient unit and despite the efforts of study workers to follow up patients who missed appointments.

In a randomized controlled study with a sample of 49 patients with PSUD/S, we showed that outpatient treatment retention is significantly greater for integrated than for nonintegrated services.[11] Further, the linkage between inpatient and outpatient services is implicated as a key factor in successful treatment by either modality.[13] When subjects from the integrated and nonintegrated groups were pooled, patients who attended their first 2 outpatient sessions had an .86 probability of remaining in treatment at 4 months. At 8 months, the probability of retention is .55 (.79 for integrated treatment vs .46 for nonintegrated treatment). Treatment retention, in turn, takes on added importance because patients who remain engaged in either treatment condition demonstrated reduced severity of psychiatric symptoms, reduced substance use over time, and reduced hospitalization rates.

Conversely, across the integrated and nonintegrated treatment conditions, patients who do not attend their first appointments after discharge from an inpatient service demonstrated high rates of rehospitalization,[11] with readmission often occurring shortly after discharge. From the perspective of mental health services research, determining the subset of patients with mental illness and a PSUD who are unlikely to make the transition to community-based treatment is important. Clearly, this subset requires alternative innovative treatment planning. After assisted transition between inpatient and outpatient services, approximately one third of our sample did not follow up with outpatient appointments. Do these patients differ in clinical profile from more compliant patients with similar psychiatric and substance abuse disorders?

One might hypothesize that severity of psychiatric symptoms at index would predict poor outpatient treatment compliance in the PSUD/S population.[14] However, the current sample of patients with PSUD/S represents a highly restricted range of symptom severity; almost all demonstrate high levels of psychiatric symptoms, particularly at times when they require hospitalization.[7] Alternatively, one might suppose that patients with PSUD/S who have more severe substance abuse problems would more strenuously resist engagement with outpatient services.[15] In our current sample, such judgments were also problematic because most patients historically demonstrated extremely high levels of abuse with multiple substances,[7] and even low-intensity intake of psychoactive substances is associated with recurrence of symptoms.[16,17] A third possibility is that patients with PSUD/S vary by symptom pattern and that different patient subtypes respond differentially to treatment (and to treatment referral).

Table 1. Exploratory Correlations Relating Treatment Noncompliance to 37 Candidate Predictors (N=49)*

Variable	No. (%)	Mean	SD	r
Demographic and clinical history				
Age at index	...	32.08	6.62	0.10
Sex, M	37 (76)	...	...	0.36†
No. of treatments for PSUD	...	3.31	6.18	0.30†
Schizophrenia, y	...	10.71	5.83	0.23†
Drug abuse, y	...	12.83	8.35	0.18†
Alcohol abuse, y	...	15.57	7.93	0.08
Diagnostic category				
Negative syndrome	10 (20)	...	...	−0.30†
Mixed syndrome	28 (57)	...	...	0.27†
Positive syndrome	11 (22)	...	...	−0.03
Schizophrenia by RDC	14 (29)	...	...	−0.06
Schizoaffective disorder by RDC				
Manic type	9 (18)	...	...	0.27†
Depressed type	12 (24)	...	...	−0.16†
Mixed	14 (29)	...	...	−0.04
ASI				
Family drug history (N=48)	8 (17)	...	...	−0.13
Family alcohol history (N=48)	33 (69)	...	...	−0.01
Drug severity score	...	7.45	1.79	−0.08
Alcohol severity score	...	7.31	1.77	0.20†
Alcohol composite score	...	0.26	0.23	−0.03
Drug composite score	...	0.38	0.32	−0.18†
Family composite score	...	0.29	0.17	−0.15
Psychiatric composite score	...	0.52	0.22	−0.07
Brief Symptom Inventory				
Global severity index	...	1.21	0.89	−0.21†
Paranoia subscale	...	1.47	1.14	−0.16†
Depression subscale	...	1.42	1.21	−0.20†
Psychoticism subscale	...	1.28	1.11	−0.23†
SANS and SAPS global scores				
Affective flattening and blunting	...	2.06	1.39	−0.25†
Alogia	...	2.17	1.50	−0.15
Avolition	...	2.65	1.30	−0.08
Anhedonia	...	2.71	1.46	−0.08
Attention	...	2.51	1.29	−0.22†
Hallucinations	...	3.29	1.35	0.05
Delusions	...	3.22	1.09	−0.05
Bizarreness	...	1.90	1.19	0.07
Formal thought disorder	...	1.94	1.28	−0.06
SANS global summary	...	12.11	4.67	−0.23†
SAPS global summary	...	10.35	2.84	0.01

**Negative correlations indicate variables associated with compliance; ellipses, not applicable. PSUD indicates psychoactive substance use disorder; RDC, research diagnostic criteria; ASI, Addiction Severity Index; SANS, Schedule for the Assessment of Negative Symptoms; and SAPS, Schedule for the Assessment of Positive Symptoms.*

†Variable retained for further analysis.

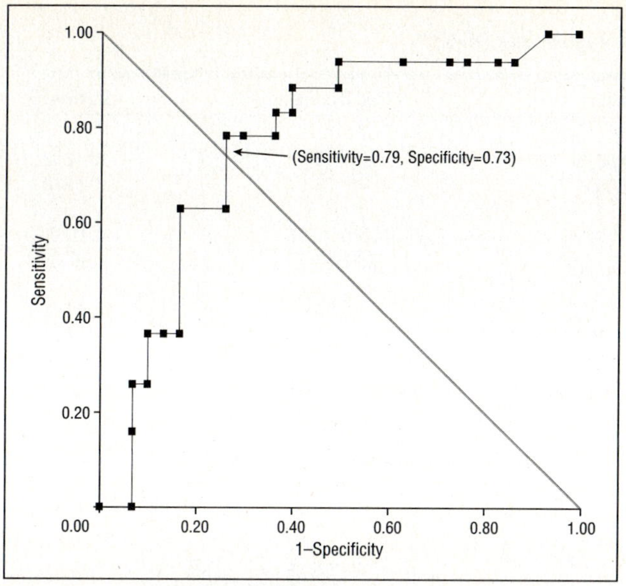

Figure 1. *Receiver-operating characteristics (ROC) curve for a logistic regression model predicting nonengagement in outpatient treatment among patients with schizophrenia and psychoactive substance use disorders (N=49).*

This report follows the suggestion that the population of patients with PSUD/S, like those with schizophrenia generally, may be analyzed into constituent subgroups according to schizophrenia syndrome type.[18] Could syndromal differences be used, before discharge from inpatient care, to predict which patients are least likely to follow up with outpatient services? We hypothesized that treatment compliance might be lowest among patients with negative (or deficit) syndrome. Those with the negative syndrome show several features that we expected to be especially troublesome, ie, marked social withdrawal, low levels of motivation, and a relative absence of severe positive symptoms that might impel compliance directly, through patients' subjective distress, or indirectly, through interventions by those in support networks. The ability to determine the patients likely to benefit from low-intensity outpatient services and those likely to require more intensive interventions is prerequisite for the rational design of psychiatric care that productively addresses the needs of patients with mental illness and PSUDs and those of the community at large.

RESULTS

The final logistic regression model includes 4 terms, including the intercept, and suggests that men, subjects who meet criteria for mixed-syndrome schizophrenia, and subjects who have low global scores on the SANS Affective Flattening and Blunting scale are those most likely to be noncompliant with outpatient treatment. None of the other candidate predictors yielded odds ratios differing significantly from the chance value of 1. Parameter estimates, odds ratios, and summary goodness of fit for the PROC LOGISTIC model are given in **Table 2**, and comparative results from the exact logistic regression are given in **Table 3**.

Table 2. Final Logistic Regression Model Predicting Nonengagement in Outpatient Treatment for Patients With PSUD/S From Index Inpatient Data (N=49)*

Predictor	B	SE	Wald χ^2	*P*	Odds Ratio
Male gender	2.67	1.18	5.15	.023	14.43
Mixed syndrome	1.78	0.78	5.17	.023	5.93
SANS affective flattening (global scores)	−0.52	0.26	3.88	.049	0.60†

**Intercept=−2.70±1.27 [−2 Log L criterion=49.54; χ^2 (df=3)=15.90; P<.001]. PSUD/S indicates psychoactive substance use disorder and co-occurring schizophrenia; SANS, Schedule for the Assessment of Negative Symptoms. See Table 3 for confidence intervals.*

†The odds ratio for this SANS variable is interpreted with reference to change of 1 point on the affective flattening global severity scale, in which 5 is severe; 4, marked; 3, moderate; 2, mild; 1, questionable; and 0, absent. A subject with a score of 3 on this scale has 0.6 the odds of being resistant to treatment as a subject who scores 2.

In the reference sample, we correctly identified treatment engagement status for 37 (76%) of 49 subjects, with a sensitivity of 0.79 and a specificity of 0.73. When the model described in Table 2 was applied to data from a confirmatory sample of 14 additional patients, the new set of predicted scores correctly classified 11 (78%) of 14 patients, with a sensitivity of 1.00 and a specificity of 0.67. The following tabulation shows gender by treatment engagement (number [percentage]). The reference and validation samples are combined (ϕ=.38; *P*<.01).

Gender	Compliant, No. (%)	Noncompliant, No. (%)	Total, No.(%)
F	14 (93)	1 (7)	**15 (100)**
M	24 (50)	24 (50)	**48 (100)**
Total	**38**	**25**	**6**

Schizophrenic syndrome type by treatment engagement status for the combined reference and validation samples are shown (number [percentage]) in the following tabulation (Pearson χ^2=7.32; *df*=(2,2), *P*<.05).

Syndrome Type	Compliant, No. (%)	Noncompliant, No. (%)	Total, No. (%)
Negative	11 (92)	1 (8)	**12 (100)**
Mixed	19 (49)	20 (51)	**39 (100)**
Positive	8 (67)	4 (33)	**12 (100)**
Total	**38**	**25**	**63**

Figure 2 shows results from the randomized cross-validation procedure. A horizontal line can readily be fit to each scatterplot, indicating stable sensitivity (Figure 2, left) and stable specificity (Figure 2, right). Thus, the cross-validation estimates suggest stable values of sensitivity and specificity across 1000 test sets of data. Over the 1000 iterations, 97.5% yielded a sensitivity of 0.67 or higher, 76.9% yielded a specificity of 0.67 or higher, and 74.4% yielded both values of 0.67 or higher.

Given the validity and stability of the logistic regression model for predicting treatment compliance, the following decision rules may be derived from our study:

1. Predict all women will be compliant with treatment;

2. Predict all negative syndrome patients will be compliant;

Table 3. Comparison of Large-Sample (Asymptotic) and Exact Logistic Regressions (N=63)*

	Intercept	Gender	Mixed Syndrome	SANS-AFB
Coefficient				
Exact	. . .	−2.6855	−1.7405	0.4302
Asymptotic	−2.9695	−2.8094	−1.8280	0.4532
95% confidence interval				
Exact	. . .	−6.57, −0.55	−3.48, −0.26	−0.01, 0.92
Asymptotic	0.5604,−5.378	−5.02, −0.60	−3.22, −0.26	0.00, 0.91
P				
Exact	. . .	.0051	.0166	0.0591
Asymptotic	.0157	.0129	.0110	0.0499

**SANS-AFB indicates Schedule for the Assessment of Negative Symptoms, Affective Flattening and Blunting scale.*

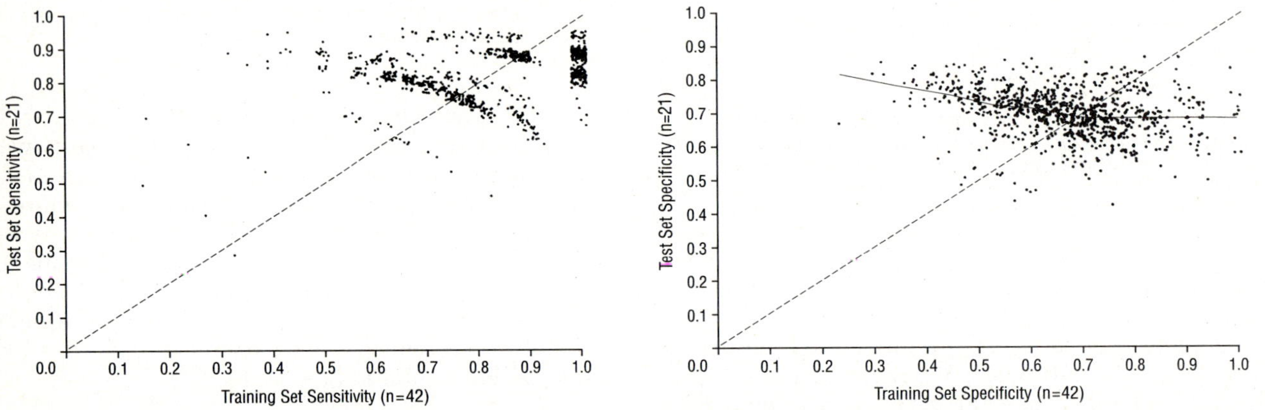

Figure 2. *Predicting treatment engagement. Left, Cross-validation of the sensitivity of a logistic regression with 63 subjects divided into 1000 training and test sets. Right, Cross-validation of the specificity of a logistic regression with 63 subjects divided into 1000 training and test sets.*

3. For all others, if the SANS Affective Flattening and Blunting scale scores indicate marked or severely flat affect, predict compliance, otherwise predict noncompliance.

In our sample, this heuristic device results in sensitivity and specificity approaching those of the underlying logistic regression model, yielding values of 0.84 and 0.65, respectively, in the context of a 75% accuracy rate (47/63).

COMMENT

Frequently, standard treatment for patients with severe mental illness and comorbid addictive disorders operates on the implicit assumption that patients with a dual diagnosis are a monolithic group with a single set of service requirements. The model for predicting treatment noncompliance described herein points toward a need for greater treatment differentiation, even among a relatively homogenous sample of patients with PSUD/S.

The results of our present study are as notable for identifying the patients who initially engage with outpatient treatment as they are for predicting those who never begin. Remarkably, although patients with negative syndrome schizophrenia may be more globally impaired than others,[41] 11 (92%) of 12 successfully engaged and remained in treatment. This is generally consistent with earlier findings that schizophrenia syndrome type apparently shapes the clinical trajectory of patients with PSUD/S.[18] Patients with PSUD/S who have negative syndrome schizophrenia demonstrate severely impaired social, affective, and motivational competencies, but, contrary to our expectations, most respond positively to appropriate structure and treatment, even in the context of a service that is neither comprehensive nor ideal.

The categorization of patients with schizophrenia into negative, positive, and mixed subtypes may fluctuate when based on serial cross-sectional assessments. This should be particularly true across episodes of exacerbation and during the early years of illness, but we found few empirical studies that addressed this issue, particularly with the PSUD/S population. Cross-sectional assessment is appropriate under the assumption that negative and positive syndrome clusters reflect 2 or more underlying disease processes that may combine heterogeneously in different patients.[41]

Carpenter[42] and Wagman et al[43] selected samples of patients with the deficit syndrome by rigorous longitudinal assessment, differentiating primary negative symptoms that remain stable during 6 to 12 months from secondary negative symptoms arising from depression, drugs, environmental deprivation, anxiety, or psychosis. However, empirically based procedures for making these distinctions are not well established, and little research in this area has been published. We plan to address this issue in future work with the PSUD/S population. In the present study, cross-sectional diagnostic assessments were made 14 days after inpatient admission in an effort to assure that short-term effects of substance abuse had abated and did not influence the RDC diagnosis or ratings of negative and positive symptoms.

In the model described herein, 3 variables (ie, gender, the presence of mixed syndrome, and lower scores on the SANS Affective Flattening and Blunting scale) together correctly predicted the treatment engagement status of three fourths (47/63; 75%) of our sample. Men are about 14 times more likely to be noncompliant for outpatient treatment referral than are women, almost all of whom are compliant. One might speculate that men are more likely than women to actively reject the help represented by treatment, fearing a loss of perceived independence in accordance with traditional gender-role stereotypes. Alternatively, because the incidence of PSUD is generally higher among men, they may be more likely to view their substance use as normative.

Patients meeting the criteria of Andreasen and Olsen[30] for mixed-syndrome schizophrenia are also more likely to be noncompliant than those with other syndrome types. In our sample, most patients in the mixed-syndrome schizophrenia category showed "marked" or "severe" levels of both positive and negative symptoms. Perhaps the combination of both sets of symptoms is synergistically more disorganizing than either set alone.

Even among men with mixed syndrome, the severity of core negative symptoms (eg, flat affect) predicted compliance. This result supports and illuminates the finding that patients meeting criteria for the negative syndrome are almost all compliant. Perhaps patients with severe negative symptoms are more willing than others to allow treatment services to supply auxiliary stimulation and structure when they cannot satisfactorily regulate their own emotional state.

Patients with comorbid schizophrenia and addictive disorders are generally believed to be difficult to engage and retain in outpatient treatment.[44] Nevertheless, previous results[11] suggest that once engaged, a substantial proportion remain in and make good use of integrated services. For those who have a poor outcome, a prime factor is resistance to outpatient treatment engagement at the very outset. That is, despite thorough preparation before discharge (including familiarization with the outpatient site and treatment staff, attendance of the first few sessions while still an inpatient,[12] and encouragement by family members and case managers), a significant proportion "disappear" and never return once they are discharged from the hospital. Current results suggest that many of these patients might be ascertained during the discharge planning phase of inpatient treatment.

The present report is based on a relatively small group of subjects and would be strengthened by replication with a larger sample. For example, the decision rules may offer greater clinical utility than statistical prediction by logistic regression, but the principal value of research with a limited sample size is to inform the design of larger, more definitive studies. Future outcome research should also focus on interventions that could have a useful clinical effect on the trajectory of illness in patients with PSUD/S. Enhanced intervention with men who have mixed-syndrome schizophrenia, regardless of their substance abuse history, could target characteristics that contribute to noncompliance and thereby improve treatment engagement, early retention, and, ultimately, longer-term outcome. For example, a form of assertive case management[45-47] incorporating aspects of the assertive community treatment model[48,49] might be designed specifically to locate these patients in the community and accompany them to their early treatment sessions. A second focus for assertive case management might be on early intervention in drug abuse relapse, ie, escorting patients to 12-step meetings, a detoxification facility, or other services when necessary, and otherwise intervening to support sobriety. We hope to use knowledge of patient characteristics at intake to design interventions for patients who are at especially high risk for early dropout.

Accepted for publication October 16, 1996.

This study was supported by Public Health Service grant R01MH46327 from the National Institute of Mental Health, Bethesda, Md.

We thank Miriam Moussatche, Maria Ferguson, and Lisa Nastase, the research assistants who assisted in clinical interviewing, and Jacob Cohen, PhD, and 3 anonymous reviewers who read earlier versions of the manuscript and offered valuable advice. While their suggestions improved the article, any remaining shortcomings are our responsibility.

Reprints: Christian R. Miner, PhD, 9 Fierman Hall, Beth Israel Medical Center, 1st Ave at 16th St, New York, NY 10003.

REFERENCES

1. Carpenter MD, Mulligan JC, Bader IA, Meinzer AE. Multiple admissions to an urban psychiatric center. *Hosp Community Psychiatry.* 1985;31:397-400.
2. Seibyl JP, Satel SL, Anthony D, Southwick SM, Krystal JH, Charney DS. Effects of cocaine on hospital course in schizophrenia. *J Nerv Ment Dis.* 1993;181:31-37.
3. Kivlahan DR, Heiman JR, Wright RC, Mundt JW, Shupe JA. Treatment cost and rehospitalization in schizophrenic outpatients with a history of substance abuse. *Hosp Community Psychiatry.* 1991;42:609-614.
4. Bartels SJ, Teague GB, Drake RE, Clark RE, Bush PW, Noordsy DL. Substance abuse in schizophrenia: service utilization and costs. *J Nerv Ment Dis.* 1993;181:227-232.
5. Mechanic D. Strategies for integrating public mental health services. *Hosp Community Psychiatry.* 1991;42:797-801.
6. Salloum IM, Moss HB, Daley DC. Substance abuse and schizophrenia: impediments to optimal care. *Am J Drug Alcohol Abuse.* 1991;17:321-336.
7. Rosenthal RN, Hellerstein DJ, Miner CR. Integrated services for treatment of schizophrenic substance abusers: demographics, symptoms and substance abuse patterns. *Psychiatr Q.* 1992;63:3-26.
8. Miller FT, Tannenbaum JH. Drug abuse in schizophrenia. *Hosp Community Psychiatry.* 1989;40:847-849.
9. Solomon P, Davis J, Gorson B. Discharged state hospital patient's characteristics and use of aftercare. *Am J Psychiatry.* 1984;141:1566-1570.
10. Ridgely MS, Goldman HH, Talbott JA. *Treatment of Chronic Mentally Ill Young Adults With Substance Abuse Problems: Emerging National Trends.* Baltimore, Md: University of Maryland School of Medicine, Department of Psychiatry; 1987. Mental Health Policy Studies.

11. Hellerstein DJ, Rosenthal RN, Miner CR. A prospective study of integrated outpatient treatment for substance-abusing schizophrenic patients. *Am J Addict.* 1995; 4:33-42.
12. Rosenthal RN, Hellerstein DJ, Miner CR: A model of integrated services for outpatient treatment of patients with comorbid schizophrenia and addictive disorders. *Am J Addict.* 1992;1:339-348.
13. Stickney SK, Hall RCW, Gardner ER. The effect of referral procedures on aftercare compliance. *Hosp Community Psychiatry.* 1980;31:567-569.
14. McLellan AT, Luborsky L, Woody GE, O'Brien CP, Druley KA. Predicting response to alcohol and drug abuse treatments: role of psychiatric severity. *Arch Gen Psychiatry.* 1983;40:620-625.
15. Wolpe PR, Gorton G, Serota R, Sanford B. Predicting compliance of dual diagnosis inpatients with aftercare treatment. *Hosp Community Psychiatry.* 1992; 44:45-49.
16. Lieberman JA, Kane JM, Alvir J. Provocative tests with psychostimulant drugs in schizophrenia. *Psychopharmacology (Berl).* 1987;91:415-433.
17. Drake RE, Osher FC, Noordsy DL, Hurlbut SC, Teague GB, Beaudett MS. Diagnosis of alcohol use disorders in schizophrenia. *Schizophr Bull.* 1990;16:57-67.
18. Rosenthal RN, Hellerstein DJ, Miner CR. Positive and negative syndrome typology in schizophrenic patients with psychoactive substance use disorders. *Compr Psychiatry.* 1994;35:91-97.
19. American Psychiatric Association. *Diagnostic and Statistical Manual of Mental Disorders, Third Edition, Revised.* Washington, DC: American Psychiatric Association, 1987.
20. Spitzer RL, Endicott J, Robins E. Research diagnostic criteria: rationale and reliability. *Arch Gen Psychiatry.* 1978;35:773-782.
21. Endicott J, Spitzer RL, Fleiss J, Cohen J. The Global Assessment Scale: a procedure for measuring overall severity of psychiatric disturbance. *Arch Gen Psychiatry.* 1976;33:766-771.
22. Folstein MF, Folstein SE, McHugh PR. 'Mini-Mental State': a practical method forgrading the cognitive state of patients for the clinician. *J Psychiatr Res.* 1975; 12:189-198.
23. Spitzer RL, Endicott J. *Schedule for Affective Disorders and Schizophrenia (SADS).* 3rd ed. New York, NY: New York State Psychiatric Institute, Biometrics Research; 1977.
24. McLellan AT, Luborsky L, Woody GE, O'Brien CP. An improved evaluation instrument for substance abuse patients: the Addiction Severity Index. *J Nerv Ment Dis.* 1980;168:26-33.
25. McLellan AT, Luborsky L, Cacciola J, Griffith J, Evans F, Barr HL, O'Brien CP. New data from the Addiction Severity Index: reliability and validity in three centers. *J Nerv Ment Dis.* 1985;173:412-423.
26. Derogatis LR, Spencer PM. *The Brief Symptom Inventory (BSI) Administration, Scoring & Procedures Manual.* Baltimore, Md: Johns Hopkins University School of Medicine; 1982.
27. Andreasen NC. Negative symptoms in schizophrenia: definition and reliability. *Arch Gen Psychiatry.* 1982;39:784-788.
28. Andreasen NC. *Scale for the Assessment of Negative Symptoms (SANS).* Iowa City: University of Iowa; 1983.
29. Andreasen NC. *Scale for the Assessment of Positive Symptoms (SAPS).* Iowa City: University of Iowa; 1984.
30. Andreasen NC, Olsen S. Negative v positive schizophrenia: definition and validation. *Arch Gen Psychiatry.* 1982;39:789-794.
31. Fenton WS, McGlashan TH. Testing systems for assessment of negative symptoms in schizophrenia. *Arch Gen Psychiatry.* 1992;49:179-184.
32. Kendall MG, Stuart A, Ord JK. *The Advanced Theory of Statistics.* 5th ed. New York, NY: Oxford University Press; 1991: vol 2.
33. Ridgely MS. Creating integrated programs for severely mentally ill persons with substance disorders. *New Dir Ment Health Serv.* 1991;50:29-41.
34. Fleiss JL, WIlliams JB, Dubro AF. The logistic regression analysis of psychiatric data. *J Psychiatr Res.* 1986;20:145-209.
35. PROC LOGISTIC. In: *SAS/Stat User Guide (Version 6) II.* 4th ed. Cary, NC: SAS Institute; 1992..
36. Mehta C, Patel N. *Users Manual for LogXact-Turbo.* Cambridge, Mass: Cytel Software; 1993.
37. Hanley JA, McNeil BJ. Maximal attainable discrimination and the utilization of radiologic examinations. *J Chronic Dis.* 1982;35:601-611.
38. Swets JA, Pickett RM. Evaluation of Diagnostic Systems: Methods From Signal Detection Theory. Orlando, Fla: Academic Press Inc; 1982.
39. Swets JA. Indices of discrimination or diagnostic accuracy: their ROCs and implied models. *Psychol Bull.* 1986;99:100-117.
40. Stone M. Cross-validatory choice and assessment of statistical prediction. *J R Stat Soc (Series B).* 1974;36:111-147.
41. Andreasen NC, Carpenter WT. Diagnosis and classification of schizophrenia. *Schizophr Bull.* 1993;19:199-214.
42. Carpenter WT Jr. The negative symptom challenge. *Arch Gen Psychiatry.* 1992; 49:236-237.
43. Wagman AMI, Heinrichs DW, Carpenter WT. Deficit and nondeficit forms of schizophrenia: neuropsychological evaluation. *Psychiatry Res.* 1987;22:319-330.
44. Roberts LJ, Shaner A, Eckman TA, Tucker DE, Vaccaro JV. Effectively treating stimulant-abusing schizophrenics: mission impossible? *New Dir Ment Health Serv.* 1992;53:55-65.
45. Clark RE, Fox TS. A framework for evaluating the economic impact of case management. *Hosp Community Psychiatry.* 1993;44:469-473.
46. Bachrach LL. Continuity of care and approaches to case management for long-term mentally ill patients. *Hosp Community Psychiatry.* 1993;44:465-468.
47. Robinson GK, Toff-Bergman G. *Choices in Case Management: Current Knowledge and Practice for Mental Health Programs.* Washington, DC: Mental Health Policy Resource Center; 1990.
48. Stein LI, Test MA. Alternative to mental hospital treatment, I: conceptual model, treatment program, and clinical evaluation. *Arch Gen Psychiatry.* 1980;37:392-397.
49. Stein LI, Test MA. The evolution of the training in community living model. *New Dir Ment Health Serv.* 1985;26:7-16.

Buprenorphine vs Methadone Maintenance Treatment for Concurrent Opioid Dependence and Cocaine Abuse

Richard S. Schottenfeld, MD; Juliana R. Pakes, MEd; Alison Oliveto, PhD; Douglas Ziedonis, MD; Thomas R. Kosten, MD

Background: Buprenorphine, a partial μ-agonist and κ-antagonist, has been proposed as an alternative to methadone for maintenance treatment of opioid dependence, especially for patients with concurrent cocaine dependence or abuse. This study evaluated whether higher maintenance doses of buprenorphine and methadone are superior to lower doses for reducing illicit opioid use and whether buprenorphine is superior to methadone for reducing cocaine use.

Methods: A total of 116 subjects were randomly assigned to 1 of 4 maintenance treatment groups involving higher or lower daily doses of sublingual buprenorphine (12 or 4 mg) or methadone (65 or 20 mg) in a double-blind, 24-week clinical trial. Outcome measures included retention in treatment and illicit opioid and cocaine use as determined by urine toxicology testing and self-report.

Results: There were significant effects of maintenance treatment on rates of illicit opioid use, but no significant differences in treatment retention or the rates of cocaine use. The rates of opioid-positive toxicology tests were lowest for treatment with 65 mg of methadone (45%), followed by 12 mg of buprenorphine (58%), 20 mg of methadone (72%), and 4 mg of buprenorphine (77%), with significant contrasts found between 65 mg of methadone and both lower-dose treatments and between 12 mg of buprenorphine and both lower-dose treatments.

Conclusions: The results support the superiority of higher daily buprenorphine and methadone maintenance doses vs lower doses for reducing illicit opioid use, but the results do not support the superiority of buprenorphine compared with methadone for reducing cocaine use.

Arch Gen Psychiatry. 1997;54:713-720

BUPRENORPHINE, a high-affinity partial μ-agonist and κ-antagonist,[1-9] represents a promising alternative to methadone for maintenance treatment of opioid dependence. Despite the overall success of methadone maintenance, it is associated with a number of problems, including the need for daily dosing, potential diversion of take-home doses and overdoses, difficulty in withdrawing from methadone, lack of availability, and limited patient and community acceptance in many areas of the country.[10-14] In addition, methadone is not a successful treatment for all patients: 1-year retention rates in methadone maintenance programs have declined to less than 50%, and illicit drug use, especially of cocaine, persists for 15% to 40% of patients.[15-24] Cocaine use during methadone maintenance treatment is of particular concern because of its prevalence and association with continued illicit opioid use, an increased risk for human immunodeficiency virus infection, increased family, medical, and vocational problems, and a continued focus on drug-related social interactions and criminal activity.[17,19,25-30]

See also page 691

The pharmacoogic profile of buprenorphine suggests that there may be a number of advantages to its use as a maintenance treatment. Buprenorphine attenuation of opioid self-administration is dose-dependent and long-lasting,[31-34] leading to the possibility of less than daily maintenance dosing.[35] Ceiling effects at higher doses result in a lower risk of overdose following short-term administration compared with methadone,[36,37] and buprenorphine may have a reduced abuse liability in heroin-dependent individuals because its use may precipitate withdrawal symptoms.[38,39] Withdrawal symptoms following the abrupt discontinuation of buprenorphine therapy are also usually

From the Department of Psychiatry, Yale University School of Medicine, and The APT Foundation, New Haven, Conn.

SUBJECTS AND METHODS

SUBJECTS

Subjects were recruited from individuals seeking methadone maintenance treatment at the Legion Avenue Program of The APT Foundation, New Haven, Conn, or from respondents to word-of-mouth advertisements about the availability of an experimental agonist maintenance program. Subjects were eligible for the study if they met Food and Drug Administration criteria for methadone maintenance, had a urine toxicology test that was positive for opioids, and met *DSM-III-R* criteria for both opioid dependence and cocaine dependence or abuse. A naloxone challenge test (intramuscular injection of 0.8 mg of naloxone) was used to verify current physiologic opioid dependence in subjects with no history of methadone maintenance (n=63). Exclusion criteria were as follows: (1) current alcohol or sedative dependence, (2) current psychosis or suicide risk, (3) inability to read or understand rating forms and symptom checklists, and (4) pregnancy. Women of childbearing age were included if they agreed to adequate contraception to prevent pregnancy during the course of the study and agreed to undergo monthly pregnancy tests during the study. The study protocol was approved by the Human Investigations Committee of Yale University School of Medicine.

After giving written informed consent, 132 subjects were randomly assigned to 1 of the 4 maintenance groups, using a computer-generated list of random numbers. At the conclusion of the study, 16 subjects were deemed ineligible because they did not satisfy the eligibility criteria regarding cocaine dependence or abuse (4 subjects from each of the 4 maintenance treatments), leaving 116 eligible subjects. Including these 16 subjects in the data analysis does not substantially alter the major findings of the study (analyses are available). There were no significant differences among the 4 groups in baseline demographic, social, drug abuse, or psychiatric features (**Table 1**).

MAINTENANCE TREATMENTS

Maintenance medications were dispensed daily, and ingestion was observed by the nursing staff. To maintain double-blind treatments, all subjects received 24 mL of oral medication (methadone or placebo) and 1 mL of SL medication (buprenorphine or placebo). A research pharmacist prepared all medications and was the only person with knowledge of drug assignment. Buprenorphine solutions were prepared in 30% ethanol (vol/vol) at concentrations ranging from 0 to 12 mg/mL. All subjects reached their full maintenance dose at the beginning of week 3. Induction during the first 2 weeks occurred as follows: for the 65-mg methadone group, subjects received 35 mg of methadone daily during the first week and 50 mg daily during the second week; for the 12-mg buprenorphine group, 4 mg daily during the first week and 8 mg daily during the second week; for the 4-mg buprenorphine group, 1 mg daily during the first week and 2 mg daily during the second week; and for the 20-mg methadone group, 20 mg daily, beginning the first week of the study. All subjects reached their full maintenance dose at the beginning of week 3. Subjects were either detoxified or transferred to methadone maintenance after completing the 24-week study.

All subjects were required to participate in a 1-hour weekly group counseling session to enhance motivation for abstinence from illicit drugs and to develop coping skills and behavioral techniques to prevent relapse. Subjects were not discharged from the study for continued illicit opioid or cocaine use. They were discharged from the study for medical reasons or if they missed 3 consecutive days of medication or 3 consecutive counseling sessions.

ASSESSMENTS

Baseline assessments included urine toxicology testing for opioids and cocaine metabolites, a structured drug use

relatively mild.[3,40-43] It is of particular interest that buprenorphine suppresses cocaine self-administration in rhesus monkeys,[44] and early studies have found lower rates of cocaine use among buprenorphine-maintained patients compared with methadone-maintained patients.[45,46] While subsequent studies have reported inconsistent results,[47-60] the initial findings of reduced cocaine use associated with buprenorphine led to the hypothesis that buprenorphine might be superior to methadone for maintenance treatment of patients with concurrent opioid dependence and cocaine dependence or abuse.

Results of random-assignment, double-blind clinical trials comparing buprenorphine with methadone for maintenance treatment of opioid dependence generally have supported the safety of buprenorphine and its efficacy when compared with lower-dose (20-30 mg orally) methadone maintenance.[54,58-62] These studies, however, have not clearly established that buprenorphine in the doses used (typical range, 2-8 mg sublingually [SL]) is as effective as methadone at higher maintenance doses (60-80 mg orally) for reducing illicit opioid use, nor have they fully evaluated the impact of maintenance treatment on cocaine use. Although no significant differences between buprenorphine and methadone in the rates of cocaine use were reported in any of those studies,[54,58-62] the power of the studies to detect significant differential effects of maintenance treatment on cocaine use is limited because of the heterogeneity of the patients with regard to the presence or absence of a diagnosis of cocaine dependence or abuse. Additionally, the doses of buprenorphine used may have been insufficient. A buprenorphine dose–ranging study in subjects who were dependent on opioids and cocaine documented robust dose-dependent effects on illicit opioid use and significant but less robust effects on cocaine use, with maximal reductions of illicit drug use at 12- to 16-mg SL daily doses of buprenorphine.[34]

To evaluate buprenorphine as an alternative to methadone maintenance for patients with concurrent opioid dependence and cocaine dependence or abuse, we conducted a random-assignment, double-blind clinical trial that compared daily maintenance with 12- or 4-mg SL buprenorphine or 65- or 20-mg oral methadone doses. The doses of buprenorphine were chosen to provide a significant contrast with regard to both illicit opioid and interview, the Addiction Severity Index,[65] and a psychiatric evaluation. Sections of the Structured Clinical Interview for *DSM-III-R*[66] that assessed substance use, mood, and antisocial personality disorders were administered by trained research interviewers; information with regard to lifetime depression and antisocial personality disorders was obtained on 111 and 108 of the 116 subjects, respectively. Supervised urine samples for toxicology testing were collected from subjects twice weekly during the first 9 months (January-September 1991) of the study, and then 3 times weekly from all subjects until the completion of the study in July 1993. Toxicology testing was performed using a fluorescent polarization immunoassay (Abbott Tdx, Abbott Diagnostics Diision of Abbott Laboratories, Abbott Park, Ill), with cutoff values for opiate-positive urine samples that were established at 200 ng/mL and for cocaine metabolites at 300 ng/mL.[67] Weekly self-report ratings of drug use and opiate withdrawal symptoms were collected by research staff with the use of the Weekly Drug Use Inventory and the Opiate Withdrawal Symptom Checklist. (Copies of all instruments are available on request.) In the Weekly Drug Use Inventory, subjects are asked to report the number of days during the past week that they used heroin, other illicit opioids, or cocaine; the routes of administration used for each drug; and the average amount used each day in grams or dollar value. The Opiate Withdrawal Symptom Checklist is a 20-item questionnaire that rates withdrawal symptoms experienced in the past 24 hours (eg, "My nose has been runny") on a scale from 1 ("not at all") to 4 ("very much"). Data were collected from subjects during the time in which they participated in the study.

STATISTICAL ANALYSIS

Analysis by χ^2 and analysis of variance were used to compare groups with regard to baseline characteristics. Differences in retention were analyzed using the Kaplan-Meier product-limit method and the generalized Wilcoxon test.[68,69] The χ^2 test was used to analyze maintenance treatment effects on the proportion of subjects who achieved 3 or more consecutive weeks of abstinence in each treatment. Random regression models were chosen for the principal analysis of medication effects on repeated urine toxicology results and self-report data with regard to drug use and opioid withdrawal symptoms.[70] This approach was specifically designed for unbalanced repeated measures with missing data, allowing for intrasubject serial correlation and unequal variance and covariance structures across time. Solution of these problems was accomplished by incorporating available trend data for each individual (individualized subject response pattern across time), with information on the behavior of the group from which the subject was drawn. The random regression models provided *P* values for the Wald statistics, which were expressed as χ^2 values. To evaluate pairwise differences among the 4 maintenance treatments, we used a modified Bonferroni method to adjust the significance level for the 5 planned comparisons.[71] To develop a continuous outcome measure with regard to the urine toxicology results, the results of urine toxicology testing were aggregated into 8 successive 3-week periods. The baseline value and the proportion of tests that were positive for illicit opioids or cocaine during each successive 3-week period were then calculated for each subject and used in the random regression model. During the time that subjects remained in the study, 6% (364/6067) of scheduled urine toxicology samples were not obtained and were coded as positive. Leaving missing values as "missing" or imputing them to the average value for the subject over the preceding weeks did not affect the significance of the major findings. Data were available for 678 three-week aggregates, or 73% of the total 928 expected 3-week aggregates if all 116 subjects remained in treatment for the 8 successive 3-week periods.

The primary data analyses were conducted on the 116 enrolled subjects who met eligibility criteria for opioid dependence and cocaine dependence or abuse. Additional data analyses were conducted on 58 of the original 116 subjects who completed the 24-week clinical trial (ie, subjects who completed the study).

Table 1. Baseline Characteristics of Sample*

	Treatment Group			
Variable	Methadone, 65 mg (n=28)	Buprenorphine, 12 mg (n=29)	Methadone, 20 mg (n=30)	Buprenorphine, 4 mg (n=29)
Age, y	32.6 (5.3)	32.6 (4.8)	31.6 (5.6)	33.7 (6.6)
Sex, M	16 (57)	20 (69)	21 (72)	23 (77)
Race, W	21 (75)	23 (79)	23 (79)	23 (77)
Employed	21 (75)	23 (82)	17 (57)	21 (72)
Education, y	12.0 (1.8)	11.82 (1.2)	11.67 (1.6)	12.1 (1.5)
Years of heroin use	7.1 (6.3)	9.5 (7.2)	6.8 (6.8)	6.1 (6.6)
Days of heroin use/last 30 d	29.32 (2.9)	28.18 (6.2)	29.9 (0.4)	28.41 (4.5)
Years of cocaine use	3.83 (5.3)	4.96 (4.9)	5.5 (5.6)	3.63 (5.0)
Days of cocaine use/last 30 d	9.29 (11.4)	9.82 (10.2)	6.67 (9.4)	8.72 (10.1)
Baseline cocaine-positive urine toxicology test†	20 (71)	17 (59)	17 (59)	20 (67)
Lifetime depression‡	4 (14.8)	4 (14.8)	2 (6.7)	4 (14.8)
Antisocial personality disorder‡	6 (22.2)	5 (20.0)	8 (26.7)	8 (30.7)

**Values expressed as mean (SD), except for sex, race, employment, baseline cocaine-positive urine toxicology test, lifetime depression, and antisocial personality disorder for which the number (percentage) of subjects is given. There were no statistically significant differences among the 4 treatment groups on any of the variables.*

†All subjects had baseline opioid-positive urine toxicology tests.

‡Data regarding lifetime depression and antisocial personality disorders were available for 111 and 109 subjects, respectively.

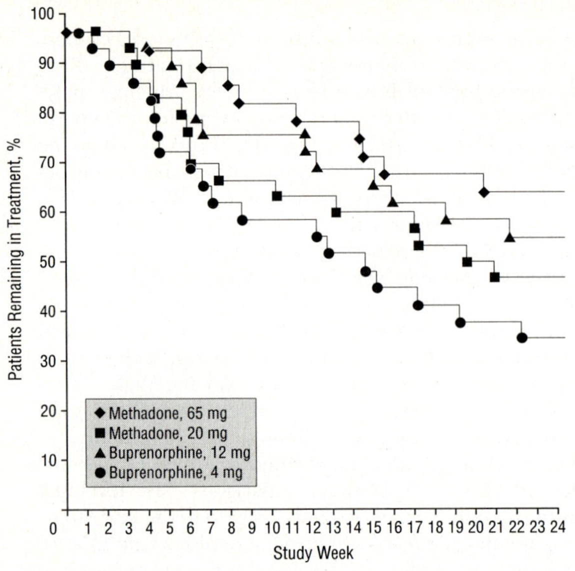

Figure 1. *Patients who remained in each maintenance group at the end of each study week.*

cocaine use. The 65-mg dose of methadone was chosen since it was approximately the average dose used in our methadone programs and allowed comparison with previous studies that compared methadone and buprenorphine.[54,61] The 20-mg dose of methadone, which is sufficient to suppress most symptoms of opioid withdrawal and prevent early attrition from treatment[63] and is the average dose used in many programs,[64] was chosen as an "active control," as in the study conducted by Johnson et al.[54] Since maintenance treatment often requires a prolonged period to achieve maximal effects,[16] subjects were treated for 24 weeks. We hypothesized that higher maintenance doses of buprenorphine and methadone are superior to lower doses for reducing illicit opioid use and buprenorphine is superior to methadone for reducing cocaine use.

RESULTS

RETENTION IN TREATMENT

Survival curves for the 116 subjects are shown in **Figure 1**. Differences in retention among the 4 maintenance treatments were not statistically significant (Wilcoxon χ^2=6.5, *df*=3; *P*=.09). (Differences in retention for the initially enrolled sample of 132 individuals were significant; Wilcoxon χ^2=7.84, *df*=3; *P*<.05.) Rates of completion of the 24-week clinical trial for the 65-mg methadone group, the 12-mg buprenorphine group, the 20-mg methadone group, and the 4-mg buprenorphine group were 64.3%, 55.2%, 46.7%, and 34.5%, respectively, and the mean (SD) number of weeks of completed treatment were 19.6 (8.1), 18.1 (8.5), 16.4 (9.3), and 14.3 (6.6), respectively. Reasons for premature termination from the clinical trial did not differ significantly among the 4 groups. Reasons included dropping out, as indicated by missing medications 3 days in a row (n=42), missing 3 consecutive counseling sessions (n=9), and detoxification for medical reasons that were unrelated to maintenance treatment (eg, pregnancy or persistent liver enzyme abnormalities [n=7]). No patients in any of the 4 maintenance treatments reported adverse effects that required dose reduction or termination from the study.

EFFECTS ON ILLICIT OPIOID USE

There were significant effects of maintenance treatment, time, and the interaction between maintenance treatment and time on the rates of opioid-positive urine samples (**Table 2**). The mean rates were lowest for the 65-mg methadone treatment group (45%) and the 12-mg buprenorphine group (58%), and they were highest for the 20-mg methadone group (72%) and the 4-mg buprenorphine group (77%). Significant contrasts were found between high-dose methadone treatments and both low-dose treatments and between high-dose buprenorphine and both low-dose treatments, but not between the 65-mg methadone treatment and the 12-mg buprenorphine treatment. The rates of opioid-positive samples decreased from baseline in all treatments during the first 6 weeks of the study; the rates continued to decline during the remaining 18 weeks in the high-dose methadone and buprenorphine treatments, while the rates increased slightly in the lower dose methadone and buprenorphine treatments (**Figure 2**).

The proportion of subjects who achieved 3 or more consecutive weeks of abstinence from illicit opioids, as determined by urine toxicology testing, was also higher in the high-dose treatments, and the average number of days per week of illicit opioid use was lowest in the high-dose treatments. There were significant contrasts for these outcomes between 65-mg methadone and both low-dose treatments and between the 12- and 4-mg buprenorphine treatments. Finally, there was a significant effect of time on opiate withdrawal symptoms (Wald χ^2=316.5, *df*=23; *P*<.001) but no significant effects of either maintenance treatment (Wald χ^2=2.11, *df*=3; *P*=.55) or of the interaction between maintenance treatment and time (Wald χ^2=75, *df*=69; *P*=.29). During the first 3 weeks, the mean weekly withdrawal scores for all subjects declined from 39.9 at baseline to 31.5 and then remained relatively stable throughout the remainder of the study.

For the subjects who completed the study, there were significant effects of maintenance treatment on the rates of illicit opioid use, with the lowest rates of opioid-positive urine samples for the 65-mg methadone treatment (44%) and the 12-mg buprenorphine treatment (51%), and higher rates for the 20-mg methadone treatment (73%) and the 4-mg buprenorphine treatment (66%). There were significant contrasts between both high-dose treatments and 20-mg methadone, while the differences between both high-dose treatments and buprenorphine (4 mg) and between methadone (65 mg) and buprenorphine (12 mg) were not significant.

EFFECTS ON COCAINE USE

There were no significant effects of maintenance treatment (Wald χ^2=2.5, *df*=3; *P*=.48) or time (Wald χ^2=10.9, *df*=8; *P*=.21) on the rates of cocaine-positive samples, while the interaction between maintenance treatment and

Table 2. Illicit Opioid Use During MT*

Variable	MT				Significance		
	Methadone, 65 mg	Buprenorphine, 12 mg	Methadone, 20 mg	Buprenorphine, 4 mg	MT, χ^2	Time, Wald χ^2	MT/Time Interaction, Wald χ^2
All subjects (N=116)							
No. of subjects in treatment group	28	29	30	29	. . .	. . .	. . .
Rates of opioid-positive tests, %	45†‡	58‡§	72	77	39.2‖; *df*=3	343.4‖; *df*=8	65.3‖; *df*=24
Proportion abstinent for ≥3 consecutive weeks	60.7†‡	41.4¶	23.3	13.8	16.3‖; *df*=3	. . .	. . .
Opioid use, d/wk	0.76‡§	1.44‡	1.73	2.98	31.7‖; *df*=3	842.6‖; *df*=23	136.4‖; *df*=69
Subjects who completed study (n=58)							
No. of subjects in treatment group	18	16	14	10	. . .	. . .	. . .
Rates of opioid-positive tests, %	44†	51§	73	66	14.0#; *df*=3	354.8‖; *df*=8	37.5**; *df*=24

*MT indicates maintenance treatment.
†Significant differences compared with methadone, 20 mg (P<.005).
‡Significant differences compared with buprenorphine, 4 mg (P<.005).
§Significant differences compared with methadone, 20 mg (P<.02).
‖P<.001.
¶Significant differences compared with buprenorphine, 4 mg (P<.02).
#P<.01.
**P<.05.

time was significant (Wald χ^2=39.7, *df*=24; *P*<.025). The rates remained relatively stable for the 12-mg buprenorphine treatment and both methadone treatments, while the rates increased over time in the 4-mg buprenorphine treatment (**Figure 3**). The proportion of subjects who achieved 3 or more documented consecutive weeks of abstinence from cocaine in the 65-mg methadone treatment, 12-mg buprenorphine treatment, 20-mg methadone treatment, and 4-mg buprenorphine treatment were 50.0%, 34.5%, 40.0%, and 20.7%, respectively, but these differences were not significant (χ^2=5.55, *df*=3; *P*=.14). Consistent with the urine toxicology test results, the reported days of cocaine use per week was not significantly affected by maintenance treatment (Wald χ^2=3.61, *df*=3; *P*=.31) or time (Wald χ^2=30.88, *df*=8; *P*=.13), while there was a significant interaction between maintenance treatment and time (Wald χ^2=107.75, *df*=69; *P*<.005). Similarly, for subjects who completed the study, there were no significant effects on the rates of cocaine-positive samples of maintenance treatment (Wald χ^2=1.09, *df*=3; *P*=.78), time (Wald χ^2=8.3, *df*=8; *P*=.40), or the interaction between maintenance treatment and time (Wald χ^2=33.11, *df*=24; *P*=.10).

COMMENT

The results of this study support the hypothesis that higher-dose maintenance treatments with oral methadone and SL buprenorphine are superior to lower-dose treatment with either agent for reducing illicit opioid use. Dose-related effects of maintenance treatment on illicit opioid use were independent of effects on retention, since higher doses of both buprenorphine and methadone were associated with greater reductions in illicit opioid use even among subjects who completed the study. The results of the study, however, do not support the hypothesis that buprenorphine is more effective than methadone for reducing cocaine use.

The study results are generally consistent with the other random-assignment, double-blind clinical trials comparing buprenorphine and methadone for maintenance treatment of opioid dependence.[54,58,59,61,62] Johnson et al[54] found no significant differences between 8-mg SL buprenorphine and 60-mg oral methadone, and both of these treatments were superior to 20-mg oral methadone with regard to retention and reducing illicit opioid use. Strain et al[58] also reported no significant differences in either retention or the rates of illicit opioid use in patients who were maintained with buprenorphine (mean SL dose, 8.9 mg/d) or methadone (mean oral dose, 54 mg/d), and Strain et al[59] reported similar findings in a second study that compared buprenorphine and methadone in opioid-dependent cocaine users. Kosten et al,[61] however, found that 6 mg of SL buprenorphine was superior to 2 mg of SL buprenorphine, but it was not as effective as the 65-mg oral dose of methadone for reducing illicit opioid use. Similarly, Ling et al[62] reported that buprenorphine (8 mg SL) was not significantly different from 30-mg oral methadone and that neither of these treatments was as effective as 80-mg oral methadone with regard to retention or reductions in illicit opioid use. Overall, these clinical trials document a clear dose response to maintenance with buprenorphine, with higher maintenance doses associated with greater reductions in illicit opioid use. In conjunction with the results of previous dose-ranging studies,[31-34] these studies suggest that the minimum effective daily maintenance dose of SL buprenorphine for reducing illicit opioid use ranges from 8 to 16 mg.

The finding in this study of a nonsignificant trend for higher rates of illicit opioid use with 12-mg SL buprenorphine compared with 65-mg oral methadone is consistent with the results reported by Kosten et al[61] and Ling et al,[62] and raises questions about whether a larger sample size would have detected a significant difference between these treatments and about the optimal daily dose of buprenorphine for maintenance treatment of opioid

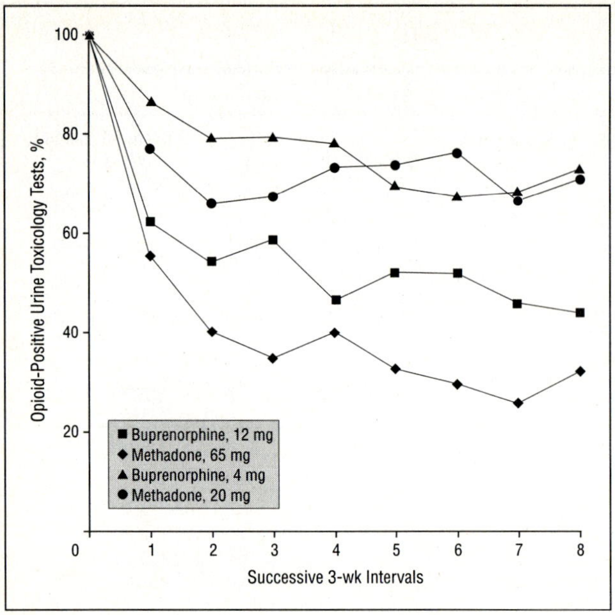

Figure 2. *Proportion of opioid-positive urine toxicology tests at baseline and during 8 successive 3-week intervals.*

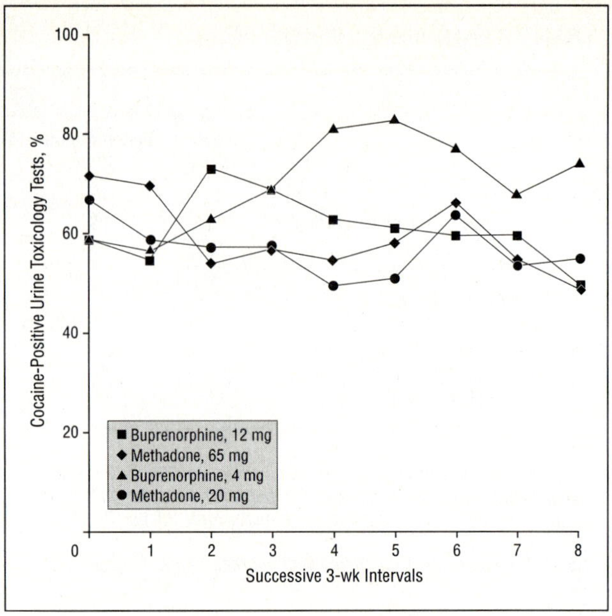

Figure 3. *Proportion of cocaine-positive urine toxicology tests at baseline and during 8 successive 3-week intervals.*

dependence. Consistent with its actions as a partial agonist at the μ-opiate receptor, the physiologic and subjective effects of buprenorphine reach a plateau at higher buprenorphine doses.[36,37] The ceiling dose above which no greater effect is observed differs, depending on the effect being measured, with respiratory depression maximally suppressed at 16 mg, while many subjective measures of euphoria peak at doses between 8 and 16 mg. However, whether there is a ceiling dose for reducing illicit opioid use has not been established. The results of the 1 dose-ranging study that directly compared daily SL doses of buprenorphine (4, 8, 12, and 16 mg) showed the superiority of the 16- and 12-mg doses and a nonsignificant trend for greater reductions of illicit opioid use at the 16-mg dose compared with the 12-mg dose.[35] The effects of even higher daily doses have not been systematically evaluated. Taken together, the available data suggest that daily maintenance doses of buprenorphine even higher than 12 mg, carefully titrated to patient response, may be required to achieve optimal results.

The study results also provide additional support for the dose-dependent efficacy of methadone when used for maintenance treatment of opioid dependence. In clinical practice, higher maintenance doses of methadone are generally associated with greater reductions in illicit opioid use.[16,72] The findings of the current study and other recent random-assignment, double-blind studies[54,62,63] provide compelling evidence that higher methadone doses lead to greater reductions in illicit opioid use and document the importance of using a sufficient methadone dose (of at least 50-60 mg) to achieve optimal response.

The findings in this and other clinical trials that buprenorphine is not more effective than methadone in reducing cocaine use are consistent with the results of recent cocaine challenge studies in buprenorphine- and methadone-maintained patients, demonstrating that neither agent leads to an attenuation of cocaine effects.[52,73-75] Foltin et al[75] reported that cocaine effects are augmented at higher maintenance doses of methadone; however, in the current study and prior clinical trials,[54,62] higher maintenance doses of methadone were not associated with increased rates of cocaine use. While there is often an association between continued illicit opioid and cocaine use during maintenance treatment,[15,25,26] in the current study, significant declines in the rates of illicit opioid use were not accompanied by similar declines in the rates of cocaine use. Maintenance with 4-mg SL buprenorphine, however, was generally associated with the worst outcome on all measures, including retention and the rates of illicit opioid and cocaine use.

Methadone and buprenorphine were well tolerated by patients, with no adverse effects that required dose reduction or termination from the study. Methadone maintenance has been available in New Haven since 1968; thus, it is notable that 48% of the 132 subjects who initially enrolled in the clinical trial had no prior treatment with methadone maintenance. While data regarding reasons for participating in the study were not collected systematically, many subjects reported a preference for buprenorphine and enrolled in the hope of being treated with buprenorphine rather than methadone. An interest in receiving a novel maintenance agent and long waiting lists that precluded rapid entry into methadone programs and recruitment outreach efforts may have contributed to the enrollment of these patients.

The limited efficacy of either methadone or buprenorphine maintenance for reducing cocaine abuse in opioid-dependent patients is relatively disappointing and points to the poor treatment prognosis of these patients when they are treated with fixed daily agonist maintenance doses and the current levels or type of counseling provided in most methadone maintenance programs. Comorbidity, especially the presence of antisocial personality disorder, may further contribute to a poor prognosis.[76] Some limitations should be considered in evaluating the results of this study. First, missing data, primarily due to attrition, create problems for data analysis that can only be partially resolved through the use of random regression models. Attrition appears to be associated with an adverse outcome, however, since subjects who terminated the study prematurely generally had higher rates of opioid- and cocaine-positive urine samples prior to termination. Second, fixed-dose maintenance treatment does not optimize the treatment response for individual patients, and better results may be obtained by titrating maintenance dose to clinical response. Finally, although weekly drug counseling may be sufficient to increase retention and reduce illicit opioid use compared with having entirely optional counseling, as in some studies,[54] it may still not be optimal. The level of services provided to patients in methadone maintenance programs has a substantial effect on treatment outcome, including retention in treatment and rates of illicit opioid, cocaine, and other drug use.[77] Additionally, Higgins et al[78] have documented a substantial impact for some behavioral interventions with primary cocaine abusers, and Silverman et al[79] reported that contingency management led to significant reduction in cocaine use among methadone-maintained patients. These considerations point to the need for additional studies to evaluate systematically the efficacy of using flexible and higher maintenance-dosing strategies and of combining buprenorphine or methadone maintenance treatment with structured behavioral, psychosocial, or additional pharmacologic interventions.

Accepted for publication August 20, 1996.

This research was supported by grants K02-DA0112, R18-DA06190, and R01-DA06266 from the National Institute on Drug Abuse.

The authors gratefully acknowledge the contributions of H. D. Kleber, MD, who was involved in the initiation of the study, and of the 4 anonymous reviewers, who provided thoughtful and helpful suggestions.

Reprints: Richard S. Schottenfeld, MD, 34 Park St, Room S103, New Haven, CT 06519.

REFERENCES

1. Blaine JD. Introduction. *NIDA Res Monogr.* 1992;121:1-4.
2. Jasinski DR, Pevnick JS, Griffith JD. Human pharmacology and abuse potential of the analgesic buprenorphine. *Arch Gen Psychiatry.* 1978;35:501-516.
3. Lewis JW, Walter D. Buprenorphine: background to its development as a treatment for opiate dependence. *NIDA Res Monogr.* 1992;121:120-141.
4. Kajiwara M, Aoki K, Ishii K, Numata H, Matsumiya T, Oka T. Agonist and antagonist actions of buprenorphine on three types of opioid receptor in isolated preparations. *Jpn J Pharmacol.* 1986;40:95-101.
5. Leander JD. Buprenorphine has potent kappa opioid receptor antagonist activity. *Neuropharmacology.* 1987;26:1445-1447.
6. Leander JD. Opioid agonist and antagonist behavioural effects of buprenorphine. *Br J Pharmacol.* 1983;78:607-615.
7. Lewis JW. Buprenorphine. *Drug Alcohol Depend.* 1985;14:363-372.
8. Cone EJ, Gorodetzky CW, Yousefnejad D, Buchwald WF, Johnson RE. The metabolism and excretion of buprenorphine in humans. *Drug Metab Dispos.* 1984;12:577-581.
9. Johnson RE, Fudala PJ. Development of buprenorphine for the treatment of opioid dependence. *NIDA Res Monogr.* 1992;121:120-141.
10. Newman RG. Methadone treatment. *N Engl J Med.* 1987;325:450.
11. Dole VP. Implications of methadone maintenance for theories of narcotic addiction. *JAMA.* 1988;260:3025-3029.
12. Dole VP. Methadone treatment and the acquired immunodeficiency syndrome epidemic. *JAMA.* 1989;262:161-162.
13. Schottenfeld RS, Kleber HD. Methadone maintenance. In: Kaplan HI, Sadock BJ, eds. *Comprehensive Textbook of Psychiatry VI.* Philadelphia, Pa: Williams & Wilkins; 1995:2031-2038.
14. Cooper JR. Ineffective use of psychoactive drugs: methadone treatment is no exception. *JAMA.* 1992;267:281-282.
15. Hartel Schoenbaum EE, Selwyn PA, et al. Heroin use during methadone maintenance treatment: the importance of methadone dose and cocaine use. *Am J Public Health.* 1995;85:83-88.
16. Ball JC, Ross A. *The Effectiveness of Methadone Maintenance Treatment.* New York, NY: Springer-Verlag NY Inc; 1991.
17. Kolar AF, Brown BS, Weddington WW, Ball JC. A treatment crisis: cocaine use by clients in methadone maintenance programs. *J Subst Abuse Treat.* 1990;7:101-107.
18. Cushman P. Cocaine use in a population of drug abusers on methadone. *Hosp Community Psychiatry.* 1990;39:1205-1207.
19. Hunt D, Spunt B, Lipton D, Goldsmith D, Strug D. The costly bonus: cocaine-related crime among methadone treatment clients. *Adv Alcohol Subst Abuse.* 1986;6:107-122.
20. Magura S, Siddiqi Q, Freeman RC, Lipton DS. Changes in cocaine use after entry to methadone treatment. In: Stimmel B, ed. *Cocaine, AIDS, and Intravenous Drug Use.* Binghamton, NY: Haworth Press Inc; 1991:31-45.
21. Pollack MH, Rosenbaum J. Fluoxetine treatment of cocaine abuse in heroin addicts. *J Clin Psychiatry.* 1991;52:31-33.
22. Chambers CD, Taylor WJR, Moffett AD. The incidence of cocaine abuse among methadone maintenance patients. *Int J Addict.* 1972;7:427-441.
23. Kaul B, Davidow B. Drug abuse patterns of patients on methadone maintenance treatment in New York City. *Am J Drug Alcohol Abuse.* 1981;8:17-25.
24. Hanbury R, Sturiano V, Cohen M, Stimmel B, Aguillaume C. Cocaine use in persons on methadone maintenance. *Adv Alcohol Subst Abuse.* 1986;6:97-106.
25. Condelli WS, Fairbank JA, Dennis ML, Rachal JV. Cocaine use by clients in methadone programs: significance, scope, and behavioral interventions. *J Subst Abuse Treat.* 1991;8:203-212.
26. Dunteman GH, Condelli WS, Fairbank JA. Predicting cocaine use among methadone patients: analysis of findings from a national study. *Hosp Community Psychiatry.* 1992;43:608-611.
27. Chaisson RE, Bacchetti P, Osmond D, Brodie B, Sande MA, Moss AR. Cocaine use and HIV infection in intravenous drug users in San Francisco. *JAMA.* 1989;261:561-565.
28. Meandzija B, O'Connor P, Fitzgerald B, Rounsaville BJ, Kosten TR. HIV infection and cocaine use in methadone maintained and untreated intravenous drug users. *Drug Alcohol Depend.* 1994;36:109-113.
29. Kosten TR, Rounsaville BJ, Kleber HD. A 2.5 year follow-up of cocaine use among treated opioid addicts. *Arch Gen Psychiatry.* 1987;44:281-284.
30. Kosten TR, Rounsaville BJ, Kleber HD. Antecedents and consequences of cocaine abuse among opioid addicts: a 2.5 year follow-up. *J Nerv Ment Dis.* 1988;176:176-181.
31. Bickel WK, Stitzer ML, Bigelow GE, Liebson IA, Jasinski DR, Johnson RE. Buprenorphine: dose related blockade of opioid challenge effects in opioid dependent humans. *J Pharmacol Exp Ther.* 1988;247:47-53.
32. Mello NK, Mendelson JH. Buprenorphine suppresses heroin use by heroin addicts. *Science.* 1980;207:657-659.
33. Mello NK, Mendelson JH, Kuehnle JC. Buprenorphine effects on human heroin self-administration: an operant analysis. *J Pharmacol Exp Ther.* 1981;223:30-39.
34. Schottenfeld RS, Pakes J, Ziedonis D, Kosten TR. Buprenorphine: dose-related effects on cocaine and opioid use in cocaine-abusing opioid-dependent humans. *Biol Psychiatry.* 1993;34:66-74.
35. Johnson RE, Eissenberg T, Stitzer ML, Strain EC, Liebson IA, Bigelow GE. Buprenorphine treatment of opioid dependence: clinical trial of daily versus alternate-day dosing. *Drug Alcohol Depend.* 1995;40:27-35.
36. Walsh SI, Preston KL, Stitzer ML, Cone EJ, Bigelow GE. Clinical pharmacology of buprenorphine: ceiling effects at high doses. *Clin Pharmacol Ther.* 1994;55:569-580.
37. Walsh SL, Preston KL, Bigelow GE, Stitzer ML. Acute administration of buprenorphine in humans: partial agonist and blockade effects. *J Pharmacol Exp Ther.* 1995;274:361-372.
38. Strain EC, Preston KL, Liebson IA, Bigelow GE. Buprenorphine effects in methadone-maintained volunteers: effects at two hours after methadone. *J Pharmacol Exp Ther.* 1995;272:628-638.
39. Walsh SL, June HL, Schuh KJ, Preston KL, Bigelow GE, Stitzer ML. Effects of

buprenorphine and methadone in methadone-maintained subjects. *Psychopharmacology (Berl).* 1995;119:268-276.
40. Amass L, Bickel WK, Higgins ST, Hughes JR. A preliminary investigation of outcome following gradual or rapid buprenorphine detoxification. *J Addict Dis.* 1994; 13:33-45.
41. Fudala PJ, Jaffe JH, Dax EM, Johnson RE. Use of buprenorphine in the treatment of opioid addiction, II: physiologic and behavioral effects of daily and alternate-day administration and abrupt withdrawal. *Clin Pharmacol Ther.* 1990;47:525-534.
42. San L, Cami J, Fernandez T, Olle JM, Peri JM, Torrens M. Assessment and management of opioid withdrawal symptoms in buprenorphine-dependent subjects. *Br J Addict.* 1992;87:55-62.
43. Negus SS, Woods JH. Reinforcing effects, discriminative stimulus effects, and physical dependence liability of buprenorphine. In: Cowan A, Lewis JW, eds. *Buprenorphine: Combatting Drug Abuse With a Unique Opioid.* New York, NY: John Wiley & Sons Inc; 1995:71-101.
44. Mello NK, Mendelson JH, Bree MP, Lukas SE. Buprenorphine suppresses cocaine self-administration by rhesus monkeys. *Science.* 1989;245:859-862.
45. Kosten TR, Kleber HD, Morgan C. Role of opioid antagonists in treating intravenous cocaine abuse. *Life Sci.* 1989;44:887-892.
46. Kosten TR, Kleber HD, Morgan C. Treatment of cocaine abuse with buprenorphine. *Biol Psychiatry.* 1989;26:637-639.
47. Carroll ME, Lac ST. Effects of buprenorphine on self-administration of cocaine and a nondrug reinforcer in rats. *Psychopharmacology (Berl).* 1992;106:439-446.
48. Carroll ME, Carmona GN, May SA, Buzalsky S, Larson C. Buprenorphine's effects on self-administration of smoked cocaine base and orally delivered phencyclidine, ethanol and saccharin in rhesus monkeys, *J Pharmacol Exp Ther.* 1992; 261:26-37.
49. Brown EE, Finlay JM, Wong JTF, Damsa G, Fibiger HC. Behavioral and neurochemical interactions between cocaine and buprenorphine: implications for the pharmacotherapy of cocaine abuse. *J Pharmacol Exp Ther.* 1991;256:119-162.
50. Kosten TA, Marby DW, Nestler EJ. Cocaine conditioned place reference is attenuated by chronic buprenorphine treatment. *Life Sci.* 1991;49:201-206.
51. Mendelson JH, Teoh SK, Mello NK, Ellingboe J. Buprenorphine attenuates the effects of cocaine on adrenocorticotropin (ACTH) secretion and mood states in man. *Neuropsychopharmacology.* 1992;7:157-162.
52. Rosen MI, Pearsall HR, McDougle CJ, Price LH, Woods SW, Kosten TR. Effects of acute buprenorphine on responses to intranasal cocaine: a pilot study. *Am J Drug Alcohol Abuse.* 1993;19:451-464.
53. Winger G, Skjoldager P, Woods JH. Effects of buprenorphine and other opioid agonists and antagonists on alfentanil- and cocaine-reinforced responding in rhesus monkeys. *J Pharmacol Exp Ther.* 1992;261:311-317.
54. Johnson RE, Jaffe JH, Fudala PJ, et al. A controlled trial of buprenorphine treatment for opioid dependence. *JAMA.* 1992;267:2750-2755.
55. Gastfriend DR, Mendelson JH, Mello NK, Teoh SK, Reif S. Buprenorphine pharmacotherapy for concurrent heroin and cocaine dependence. *Am J Addict.* 1993;4:1-11.
56. Gastfriend DR, Mendelson JH, Mello NK, Teoh SK, Reif S. Longitudinal dose comparison of buprenorphine for combined opiate and cocaine dependence. *NIDA Res Monogr.* 1996;162:179.
57. Comer SD, Lac ST, Curtis LK, Carroll ME. Effects of buprenorphine and naltrexone on reinstatement of cocaine-reinforced responding in rats. *J Pharmacol Exp Ther.* 1993;267:1470-1477.
58. Strain EC, Stitzer ML, Liebson IA, Bigelow GE. Comparison of buprenorphine to methadone in the treatment of opioid dependence. *Am J Psychiatry.* 1994;151: 1025-1030.
59. Strain EC, Stitzer ML, Liebson IA, Bigelow GE. Buprenorphine versus methadone in the treatment of opioid-dependent cocaine users. *Psychopharmacology (Berl).* 1994;116:401-406.
60. Olivetto A, Kosten TR, Schottenfeld RS, Ziedonis D, Falcioni J. Cocaine use in buprenorphine- vs methadone-maintained patients. *Am J Addict.* 1994;3:43-48.
61. Kosten TR, Schottenfeld R, Ziedonis D, Falcioni J. Buprenorphine versus methadone maintenance for opioid dependence. *J Nerv Ment Dis.* 1993;181:358-364.
62. Ling W, Wesson DR, Charavastra C, Klett CJ. A controlled trial comparing buprenorphine and methadone maintenance in opioid dependence. *Arch Gen Psychiatry.* 1996;53:401-407.
63. Strain EC, Stitzer ML, Liebson IA, Bigelow GE. Dose-response effects of methadone in the treatment of opioid dependence. *Ann Intern Med.* 1993;119:23-27.
64. D'Aunno T, Vaugn TE. Variation in methadone treatment practices: results from a national study. *JAMA.* 1992;267:253-258.
65. McLellan AT, Kushner H, Metzger D, et al. The fifth edition of the Addiction Severity Index. *J Subst Abuse Treat.* 1992;9:199-212.
66. Spitzer RL, Williams JBW, Gibbon M, First MB. *Structured Clinical Interview for* DSM-III-R. Washington, DC: American Psychiatric Press; 1990.
67. Poklis A. Evaluation of TDx cocaine metabolite assay. *J Anal Toxicol.* 1987;11: 228-230.
68. Dawson-Saunders B, Trapp RG. *Basic and Clinical Biostatistics.* East Norwalk, Conn: Appleton & Lange; 1990.
69. Selvin S. *Statistical Analysis of Epidemiologic Data.* New York, NY: Oxford University Press Inc; 1991.
70. Gibbons RD, Hedeker D, Elkin I, et al. Some conceptual and statistical issues in analysis of longitudinal psychiatric data. *Arch Gen Psychiatry.* 1993;50:739-750.
71. Keppel G. *Design and Analysis: a Researcher's Handbook.* 2nd ed. Englewood Cliffs, NJ: Prentice-Hall International Inc; 1982.
72. US General Accounting Office. *Methadone Maintenance: Some Treatment Programs Are Not Effective: Greater Federal Oversight Needed.* Washington, DC: Government Printing Office; 1990. publication GAO/HRD-90-104.
73. Strain EC, Stitzer ML, Liebson IA, Bigelow GE. The effects of cocaine in buprenorphine maintained outpatient volunteers: results from clinical experiences and laboratory challenges. *Am J Addict.* 1994;3:129-143.
74. Teoh SK, Mellow NK, Mendelson JH, et al. Buprenorphine effects on morphine- and cocaine-induced subjective responses by drug-dependent men. *J Clin Psychopharmacol.* 1994;14:15-27.
75. Foltin RW, Christiansen I, Levin FR, Fischman MW. Effects of single and multiple intravenous cocaine injections in humans maintained on methadone. *J Pharmacol Exp Ther.* 1995;275:38-47.
76. Cacciola JS, Rutherford MJ, Alterman AI, MaKay JR, Snider EC, et al. Personality disorders and treatment outcome in methadone maintenance patients. *J Nerv Ment Dis.* 1996;184:234-239.
77. McLellan AT, Arndt IO, Metzger DS, Woody GE, O'Brien CP. The effects of psychosocial services in substance abuse treatment. *JAMA.* 1993;269:1943-1959.
78. Higgins ST, Budney AJ, Bickel WK, Foeng FE, Donham R, Badger GJ. Incentives improve outcome in outpatient behavioral treatment of cocaine dependence. *Arch Gen Psychiatry.* 1994;51:568-576.
79. Silverman K, Higgins ST, Brooner RK, et al. Sustained cocaine abstinence in methadone maintenance patients through voucher-based reinforcement therapy. *Arch Gen Psychiatry.* 1996;53:409-415.

SPECIAL ARTICLE

The National Institute on Drug Abuse Collaborative Cocaine Treatment Study

Rationale and Methods

Paul Crits-Christoph, PhD; Lynne Siqueland, PhD; Jack Blaine, MD; Arlene Frank, PhD; Lester Luborsky, PhD; Lisa Simon Onken, PhD; Larry Muenz, PhD; Michael E. Thase, MD; Roger D. Weiss, MD; David R. Gastfriend, MD; George Woody, MD; Jacques P. Barber, PhD; Stephen F. Butler, PhD; Dennis Daley, MSW; Sarah Bishop, MA; Lisa M. Najavits, PhD; Judy Lis, MSN; Delinda Mercer, MA; Margaret L. Griffin, PhD; Karla Moras, PhD; Aaron T. Beck, MD

The National Institute on Drug Abuse Collaborative Cocaine Treatment Study is a large, multisite psychotherapy clinical trial for outpatients who meet the *DSM-IV* criteria for cocaine dependence. For 480 randomized patients, the outcomes of 4 treatments are compared for an 18-month period. All treatments include group drug counseling. One treatment also adds cognitive therapy, one adds supportive-expressive psychodynamic therapy, and one adds individual drug counseling; one consists of group drug counseling alone. In addition, 2 specific interaction hypotheses, one involving psychiatric severity and the other involving degree of antisocial personality characteristics, are being tested. This article describes the main aims of the project, the background and rationale for the study design, the rationale for the choice of treatments and patient population, and a brief description of the research plan.

Arch Gen Psychiatry. 1997;54:721-726

The National Institute on Drug Abuse (NIDA) Collaborative Cocaine Treatment Study is a multisite clinical trial investigating the efficacy of 4 treatments for outpatients with cocaine dependence. To our knowledge, it represents the largest clinical trial conducted to date on psychotherapy and counseling for cocaine dependence. This article describes the rationale for the study design, which was developed in response to 2 NIDA Requests for Application for a Cooperative Agreement research program.[1,2] The first phase of the project (conducted from October 1991 to July 1993) involved site selection, protocol development, and staff recruitment. The second phase (conducted from July 1993 to July 1994) involved training the staff to an acceptable level of competence, field testing the assessment procedures and protocol treatments, and obtaining preliminary pilot data relevant to the hypotheses of the study. The main clinical trial began in July 1994, and data collection is scheduled to end in January 1998. This article describes the main aims of the study, the background for the project, and a description of the main elements of the study design.

See also page 691

From the Department of Psychiatry, University of Pennsylvania (Drs Crits-Christoph, Siqueland, Luborsky, Woody, Barber, Moras, and Beck and Ms Mercer), and Philadelphia Veterans Hospital (Dr Woody), Philadelphia, Pa; the National Institute on Drug Abuse, Rockville, Md (Drs Blaine and Onken); Brookside Hospital, Nashua, NH (Drs Frank and Butler and Ms Bishop); Gaithersburg, Md (Dr Muenz); Western Psychiatric Institute and Clinic, University of Pittsburgh, Pittsburgh, Pa (Dr Thase, Mr Daley, and Ms Lis); and Harvard Medical School and McLean Hospital (Drs Weiss, Najavits, and Griffin) or Massachusetts General Hospital (Dr Gastfriend), Boston, Mass. A complete list of the members of the National Institute on Drug Abuse Collaborative Cocaine Treatment Study Group appears on page 722.

AIMS OF THE NIDA COLLABORATIVE COCAINE TREATMENT STUDY

This study investigates the relative efficacy of 4 manual-guided treatments for outpatients who meet the *DSM-IV* criteria for cocaine dependence: (1) group drug counseling (GDC) alone, (2) individual cognitive therapy (CT) plus GDC, (3) individual supportive-expressive (SE) psychodynamic therapy plus GDC, and (4) individual drug counseling (IDC) plus GDC. The following main effects and interaction hypotheses are being tested.

The National Institute on Drug Abuse Collaborative Cocaine Treatment Study Group

Coordinating Center, Principal Investigator, and Center Coordinators

University of Pennsylvania, Philadelphia: Paul Crits-Christoph, PhD (*principal investigator*); Lynne Siqueland, PhD (*project coordinator*); Karla Moras, PhD (*assessment unit director*); Jesse Chittams, MA (*director of data management/analysis*); Larry Muenz, PhD (*statistician*).

Collaborating Scientists

National Institute on Drug Abuse, Treatment Research Branch, Division of Clinical and Research Sevices, Rockville, Md: Jack Blaine, MD; Lisa Onken, PhD.

Clinical Centers, Principal Investigators, and Clinic Coordinators

University of Pennsylvania, Philadelphia: Lester Luborsky, PhD (*principal investigator*); Jacques Barber, PhD (*coprincipal investigator*); Delinda Mercer, MA (*project director*). *Brookside Hospital, Harvard Medical School, Boston, Mass:* Arlene Frank, PhD (*principal investigator*); Stephen F. Butler, PhD (*coprincipal investigator*); Sarah Bishop, MA (*project director*). *McLean Hospital/Massachusetts General Hospital, Harvard University Medical School:* Roger D. Weiss, MD (*principal investigator*); David R. Gastfriend, MD (*coprincipal investigator*); Lisa M. Najavits, PhD (*project director*). *University of Pittsburgh, Western Psychiatric Institute and Clinic, Pittsburgh, Pa:* Michael Thase, MD (*principal investigator*); Dennis Daley, MSW (*coprincipal investigator*); Ishan M. Salloum, MD (*coprincipal investigator*); Judy Lis, MSN (*project director*).

Training Unit Heads Cognitive Therapy

University of Pennsylvania, Philadelphia: Aaron T. Beck, MD. *University of Kansas Medical Center, Lawrence:* Bruce Liese, PhD.

Supportive-Expressive Psychodynamic Therapy

University of Pennsylvania, Philadelphia: Lester Luborsky, PhD; David Mark, PhD.

Individual Drug Counseling

Veterans Administration Medical Center, University of Pennsylvania School of Medicine, Philadelphia: George Woody, MD. *University of Pennsylvania, Philadelphia:* Delinda Mercer, MA.

Group Drug Counseling

University of Pennsylvania, Philadelphia: Delinda Mercer, MA; Gloria Carpenter, MEd. *University of Pittsburgh, Western Psychiatric Institute and Clinic, Pittsburgh, Pa:* Dennis Daley.

Monitoring Board

University of California, Santa Barbara: Larry Beutler, PhD. *Belair, Md:* Jim Klett, PhD. *Yale University, New Haven, Conn:* Bruce Rounsaville, MD. *Brown University, Providence, RI:* Tracie Shea, PhD.

Main Effects

One of the primary aims of this study is to compare the short- and long-term efficacy and patient acceptance of CT plus GDC, SE psychodynamic therapy plus GDC, IDC plus GDC, and GDC alone. The comparison of the combined individual and group treatments with GDC alone addresses the practical question of whether it is sufficient to treat cocaine-dependent patients with GDC alone. The IDC plus GDC treatment also addresses a practical question: if GDC needs to be supplemented with individual treatment, is a professional psychotherapist needed or are the services of a substance abuse counselor equally effective? The IDC plus GDC treatment is also included to control for the extra time with an individual counselor that those patients in CT and SE psychodynamic therapy will receive.

Interaction Hypotheses

There are 2 hypotheses: (1) Patients with higher levels of psychiatric severity (concurrent psychiatric symptoms) will show a better response to the psychotherapies (CT plus GDC and SE psychodynamic therapy plus GDC) compared with the drug counseling treatments (IDC plus GDC and GDC alone). (2) Patients with more antisocial personality characteristics will have a better response to CT plus GDC compared with SE psychodynamic therapy plus GDC, but patients without antisocial personality characteristics will have a better response to SE psychodynamic therapy plus GDC compared with CT plus GDC.

BACKGROUND

Developing and testing treatments for cocaine use disorders is a high national priority. The *National Institute on Drug Abuse Household Survey 1994*[3] indicates that the prevalence of frequent cocaine use has remained at 0.3% of the population since 1985. The effects of cocaine extend beyond the individual user and are wide ranging, especially in the areas of drug-related violence and risk behaviors associated with the human immunodeficiency virus. The development of successful treatments for cocaine use disorders, therefore, has the potential for a notable effect on the health of cocaine users; the larger social and medical problems associated with its use could also be affected. Given the magnitude of the problem, the NIDA determined that a controlled clinical trial of the most promising psychotherapy and counseling approaches for cocaine dependence was warranted. Selection of the treatments for study was based on practical considerations (eg, clinical relevance) and prior empirical work, particularly the studies by Woody et al[4,5] on psychotherapy and counseling approaches for opiate dependence. The treatments chosen for this study included IDC and GDC, SE psychodynamic therapy, and CT.

Some form of IDC or GDC by a nondoctoral-level provider is the standard treatment offered to substance abusers in most clinical settings.[6] Psychodynamically oriented psychotherapy continues to be the most widely used professional treatment.[7] In preparation for this project, NIDA staff conducted an informal survey of clinicians who work with substance abusers. This survey suggested that psychodynamic therapy was also frequently used in the community for the treatment of these patients. Cognitive-behavioral therapies are also used commonly in the community, with cognitive-behavioral relapse prevention strategies increasingly incorporated into the treatment of substance abusers in particular.[8] Cognitive-behavioral and psychodynamic therapies not only represent 2 approaches that are commonly used but also serve as contrasting theoretical perspectives because of their distinctiveness from each other.

It is not at all clear if these treatments are efficacious for cocaine dependence. In recent years, the results of several controlled trials testing these treatments, alone or in combination with psychopharmacological treatments for cocaine dependence, have been published; this literature has been reviewed elsewhere.[9,10] Several studies have supported the efficacy of cognitive-behavioral relapse prevention treatment for cocaine use disorders,[11,12] particularly for delayed effects emerging at follow-up.[13] Promising results using a behavioral therapy (contingency contracting and community reinforcement) have also been reported.[14] Less promising evidence concerning the use of interpersonal psychotherapy or psychodynamic therapy has been reported.[15,16]

The Role of Psychiatric Severity

Rather than focus solely on main effect comparisons between treatments in clinical trials, several researchers have suggested that it is more relevant to clinical practice to examine interaction effects, with an eye toward matching different treatment modalities to patient characteristics.[17-19] One known modifier of response to psychotherapy is level of psychiatric severity.[20] Substance-dependent patients with notable psychiatric symptoms may need a treatment that addresses these ongoing psychiatric problems that might be fueling the addictive process or making the substance use disorder more difficult to treat. In contrast, substance-abusing patients with low levels of psychiatric symptomatology might find more intensive psychotherapeutic treatments to be less relevant. For them, standard drug counseling may suffice.

The available literature tends to support these views. In an examination of outcomes in 6 rehabilitation programs, McLellan et al[21] found that patients with low levels of psychiatric severity improved in all treatment programs, whereas patients with high levels of psychiatric severity showed virtually no improvement. Rounsaville et al[22] found that higher psychiatric severity was associated with poorer outcome in current functioning and psychosocial adjustment but not substance use outcome in a 2.5-year follow-up of persons addicted to opiates. Most relevant to this study, Woody et al[23] found that opiate-dependent patients with a high psychiatric severity achieved better psychiatric and drug use outcomes when they received psychotherapy in addition to IDC than when they received only the latter. With the use of an alcohol-dependent sample, Kadden et al[24] and Cooney et al[25] found that patients with a higher psychiatric severity did better in coping skills training group therapy than in interactional group therapy, but both treatments were equally effective for patients with low psychiatric severity.

The previously described studies indicate consistently that patients with higher levels of psychiatric severity show greater improvement when their treatment includes professional psychotherapy. However, the benefits of this interactional model of treatment matching have not been studied prospectively in a cohort of cocaine-dependent patients.

The Role of Antisocial Personality Disorder

Beutler[18] reported that, in 8 of 9 studies, patients low on a trait measure of antisocial personality disorder did better in verbal psychotherapy compared with behavioral therapy. Several more recent studies found that patients with higher levels of traits associated with antisocial personality disorder fared better in more directive treatments.[24-27]

The likelihood that only a few cocaine abusers are likely to manifest few traits associated with antisocial personality disorder might explain the poor results from interpersonal and psychodynamic treatments in controlled studies. These findings serve as the basis for the hypothesis of the current project: patients who are more impulsive and who have more characteristics of antisocial personality disorder will have better outcomes in cognitive-behavioral therapy, whereas less impulsive patients will have better outcomes in psychodynamic therapy.

RESEARCH PLAN

Patient Selection

The selection criteria were designed to identify a representative group of primary cocaine-dependent patients who would be suitable for outpatient treatment and whose personal characteristics and life circumstances would not interfere with study participation. Patients aged 18 to 60 years are included if they have a principal current diagnosis of cocaine dependence or cocaine dependence in early partial remission (as determined by *DSM-IV* criteria). The principal diagnosis is established using a 0 to 8 severity rating scale adapted from the *Anxiety Disorders Interview Schedule-Revised*[28] that reflects the diagnostician's evaluation of the subjective distress and functional impairment associated with the diagnosis. In addition, patients must have used cocaine at least once in the 30 days before enrollment, have a current postal address and plan to live in the area for the next 2 years, be able to provide the name of at least 1 person who can generally locate their whereabouts, and be able to understand and complete the assessment measures. Explicit written, informed consent was obtained from all patients.

Patients are excluded if (1) they have a principal diagnosis of alcohol or polysubstance abuse or dependence; (2) they have a diagnosis of current opioid dependence or opioid dependence in early partial remission (sustained full remission is acceptable); (3) there is evidence of dementia or another irreversible organic brain syndrome; (4) they have a psychotic disorder; (5) they have any history of or current bipolar disorder; (6) they are at current imminent suicide or homicide risk, require hospitalization or residential treatment, or are in a halfway house; (7) they are unwilling to discontinue a current psychotherapeutic treatment; (8) they must continue to receive a psychotropic medication; (9) they have any life-threatening or unstable medical illness or a medical illness that can create marked change in mental state; (10) incarceration is impending; (11) they were hospitalized more than 10 days of the past 30 days for treatment of cocaine use; (12) they are currently legally mandated for treatment; or (13) they are more than 12 weeks pregnant.

Therapist and Drug Counselor Selection and Training

For the chosen treatments to have the best chance possible of demonstrating efficacy, they must be provided under optimal conditions (ie, by therapists and drug counselors with specialized expertise and training). Details of therapist and counselor selection and training will be reported in separate articles. Briefly, all therapists and counselors were first selected from a pool of applicants. Training then consisted of 4 weekend workshops plus supervised experience with 4 patients per therapist or counselor. Ratings of adherence and competence of treatment sessions by supervisors and independent raters were used to make final decisions about certifying each therapist or counselor as performing the treatment adequately enough to participate in the main trial.

Patient Screening and Randomization Procedures

Patients are initially screened for study participation via telephone or on a walk-in basis to determine if the basic inclusion criteria are met. If the criteria are met, patients return for an enrollment evaluation, which includes a urine drug screen. To be randomized, patients must complete the enrollment evaluation, still meet the inclusion criteria, and complete an orientation phase that includes attendance and assessment requirements. The patient is required to attend 3 visits at the clinic within 14 days, including 1 group session at which another urine drug screen is collected, and 2 case management visits. Group counselors suggest attendance at local self-help groups, such as Cocaine or Alcoholics Anonymous; promote human immunodeficiency virus risk reduction; and address housing, job, or financial needs. This orientation phase selects for treatment only those patients with enough motivation to attend at least a few sessions. Although it might ideally be of interest to test treatments on the full range of patients who contact a treatment program, it seems likely that psychotherapy treatments only have a chance of efficacy with patients sufficiently motivated to attend a minimal number of orientation sessions.

After satisfactory completion of the postorientation assessments, patients are randomized to treatment. Random assignment to treatment uses a special technique known as adaptive or "urn" randomization.[29] Urn randomization ensures equivalence of the groups on preselected variables that may relate to outcome across treatments or that may interact with type of treatment to affect outcome.

For this project, the following factors were included in the adaptive randomization algorithm: sex, marital status, employment status, mode of cocaine use, psychiatric severity, and degree of antisocial personality characteristics. Sex, marital status, employment status, and mode of cocaine use were chosen because these variables have been associated with outcome, retention, or both in prior studies[6,30] or within our pilot data. Psychiatric severity and degree of antisocial personality disorder were chosen because they were specifically hypothesized to interact with treatment modality in relation to outcome. The urn randomization was separate for each site to ensure that treatments were balanced on the relevant factors within each site.

Treatments

Format. All 3 individual treatments have a 6-month active phase and a 3-month booster phase. The same session schedule is followed in all 3 individual treatments. During the first 3 months, individual sessions are held twice per week; during the next 3 months, sessions are held weekly. During the booster phase, 1 session is held each month. For the GDC modality, group sessions are held once a week for the 6 months of the active phase. During the booster phase, patients in the GDC alone treatment group meet individually with the group counselor once per month for a half hour visit.

Cognitive Therapy. Cognitive therapy provided in this study follows a detailed manual.[31] This treatment is based on the assumption that substance use disorders are related to individuals' maladaptive beliefs and related thought processes. Cognitive therapy for substance abuse consists of 5 components: (1) collaboration, (2) case conceptualization, (3) structure, (4) socialization to the cognitive model, and (5) use of cognitive and behavioral techniques. Among the techniques used are Socratic questioning, advantages-disadvantages analysis, monitoring of drug-related beliefs, activity monitoring and scheduling, behavioral experiments, and role playing.

SE Psychodynamic Therapy. Brief SE psychodynamic therapy as conducted in this study follows the general SE psychodynamic therapy treatment manual[32] and a more specific variant of it developed for cocaine abusers.[33] According to this model, the problems associated with the use of cocaine and with its cessation are viewed in the context of an understanding of the person's interpersonal and intrapsychic functioning. The core conflictual relationship theme[34] concept provides the framework for this understanding. The patient's core conflictual relationship theme, defenses, and views of self influence complicate the steps needed to stop using cocaine and to address the problems involved with cocaine dependence. The therapist uses supportive and interpretive techniques, particularly interpretations related to aspects of patients' core conflictual relationship themes, that most interfere with the achievement of patients' goals.

Individual Drug Counseling. This modality[35] is based on a widely used approach to the treatment of drug addiction. It is time limited and focuses primarily on helping the patient achieve and maintain abstinence by encouraging behavioral changes, such as avoiding drug triggers, structuring one's life, and engaging in healthy behaviors (eg, exercise). Individual drug counseling is a staged approach with specific interventions keyed to the stages. In content and structure, it is consistent with the philosophy of the 12-step approach, specifically that addiction is a disease that damages the person physically, emotionally, and spiritually and that recovery is a gradual process. Participation in self-help groups is strongly encouraged.

Group Drug Counseling. This treatment[36] is designed to educate patients about the important concepts in addiction recovery, to strongly encourage participation in 12-step programs, and to provide a supportive group atmosphere in which members can express feelings, discuss problems, and learn to draw strength from one another. The group is progressive; the first 3-month phase is psychoeducational, and the second 3-month phase consists of open discussion with a focus on patients' helping each other solve problems in recovery.

Assessments

The assessment battery was designed to capture multiple domains: diagnoses, substance use patterns, psychopathological features or symptoms, quality of life, treatment services use, theory-specific measures of mediators of outcome, treatment process, attrition, and motivation for treatment. Most assessments are made at enrollment (or immediately following the orientation phase) and at monthly intervals during the active (months 1-6) and follow-up (months 9, 12, 15, and 18) phases. In addition, patients receive an assessment when they drop out of treatment or violate protocol.

The primary outcome measure is the Drug Use Composite Scale of the Addiction Severity Index, a measure commonly used in substance abuse treatment with available reliability and validity data.[37-40] This measure will be used to assess relative reduction in drug use during the active and follow-up phases of the protocol. Observed urine samples, collected once a week at group sessions, will be used as a secondary outcome measure. Urine samples will be used to assess time until remission (ie, 4 weeks of no drug use).

In addition to the main efficacy measures, a primary dependent variable of interest is retention in treatment. Days until a patient drops out of treatment or otherwise violates the protocol will be used as the measure of retention.

Psychiatric severity is assessed via the psychiatric severity composite score on the Addiction Severity Index. The degree of antisocial personality characteristics is assessed using the Socialization Scale of the California Psychological Inventory. These measures have been used successfully in previous research on psychiatric severity[21,23] and antisocial personality traits,[24,25] respectively.

Power Analysis and Sample Size Determination

There is no single power calculation for a large, complex study like this one. Power will vary as a function of distribution of outcome measure, main effects vs interactional effects, and expected effect size. For the Addiction Severity Index, as the outcome measure analyzed via an analysis of covariance, the power to detect main effects is high (0.90-0.96) assuming 120 patients (30 per site) randomized into each of 4 treatments, 33% attrition (ie, lack of data), a type I error of 0.05, and effect sizes of 0.30 to 0.50 for our contrasts of interest.

Analyzing each interaction separately (SE psychodynamic therapy vs CT at 2 levels of antisocial personality characteristics and SE psychodynamic therapy plus CT [pooled] vs IDC at 2 levels of psychiatric severity), we computed the size of the interaction effect that can be detected with a power of 0.80 and a Bonferroni-corrected type I error of 0.025. As previously described, the sample size is 120 per arm of the study and there is 33% attrition. We found a Cohen F=0.55 for degree of antisocial personality characteristics and F=0.48 for the psychiatric severity interaction. Thus, with our proposed sample size, and correcting for attrition, the Bonferroni-corrected interaction tests are sensitive to moderate-sized effects.

The statistical power for detecting differences in our other main outcome of interest, retention rates, was also examined. With the use of retention rates (in which dropout is defined as no contact with a patient for 4 consecutive weeks) from our training phase of 90% at 1 month, 70% at 3 months, and 50% at 6 months and a power of 80%, an exponential function predicting dropout at time *t* months was calculated and used for power analysis for survival data. With the use of the method of Zelen and Dannemiller,[41] the study's sample size was found to be adequate to detect a moderately small hazard ratio of 1.8 for each Bonferroni-corrected (2-tailed) pairwise comparison of the 4 treatments, with a power of 0.80.

Data Analysis

The initial analysis of the main treatment data will consist of analyses of the patterns of retention. This will be performed in a time-to-event analysis using the definition of retention previously given. Analyses of differences in efficacy using the Addiction Severity Index drug use composite score will be done via longitudinal regression approaches that allow for the use of all data collected. Additional cross-sectional analyses (analysis of covariance on 3- and 6-month outcomes) will be performed, as well as time-to-event analysis using the measure of days until abstinent determined from the urine data. Type of treatment, site, psychiatric severity, and degree of antisocial personality disorder will be the main independent variables for all of the previously described analyses. Statistically significant omnibus tests will be followed by post hoc comparisons of individual treatment modalities, as appropriate.

Several samples will be analyzed. An intent-to-treat pragmatic analysis that uses all data collected on patients, regardless of whether the patient was a dropout or a protocol violator, will be conducted.[42] Further analyses using only data available on patients up to dropout, protocol violation, or therapy completion will also be conducted. In this latter analysis, an attempt is made to discern the effects of the therapies themselves, free of the effects of other treatments that patients may have received after dropping out of the program or otherwise violating protocol.

Various secondary analyses examining other outcome measures, mediators of outcome, and predictors of outcome will also be performed. The details of these analyses will be discussed in subsequent reports.

SIGNIFICANCE

To our knowledge, this study is the largest, most well-controlled study of manual-guided psychotherapy and counseling for cocaine dependence yet conducted. The study is likely to yield practical information about the treatment of these patients, such as answers to these basic questions: Is professional psychotherapy a useful addition to the standard drug-focused group counseling? Are there patient characteristics (eg, psychiatric severity or degree of antisocial personality characteristics) that interact with type of treatment, thereby providing guidance to clinicians for making better matches between patients and treatments? The multisite nature of this project will allow for the examination of the extent to which answers to these questions are robust across different sites.

Accepted for publication November 6, 1996.

This study was supported in part by grants U18-DA07090, U18-DA07663, U18-DA07673, U18-DA07693, and U18-DA07085 from the National Institute on Drug Abuse, Rockville, Md; grant P50-MH-45178 and Career Development Awards K02-MH00756 and K05-DA00168 from the National Institute of Mental Health, Rockville.

We thank John Boren, PhD, National Institute on Drug Abuse, project officer for this cooperative agreement.

Reprints: Paul Crits-Christoph, PhD, Room 700, 3600 Market St, Philadelphia, PA 19104.

REFERENCES

1. *Maximizing the Efficacy of Psychotherapy and Drug Abuse Counseling Strategies in the Treatment of Cocaine Abusers.* Rockville, Md: National Institute on Drug Abuse; 1991. US Dept of Health and Human Services publication DA-91-04.
2. *Maximizing the Efficacy of Psychotherapy and Drug Abuse Counseling Strategies in the Treatment of Cocaine Abusers.* Rockville, Md: National Institute on Drug Abuse; 1990. US Dept of Health and Human Services publication DA-90-04.
3. *National Institute on Drug Abuse Household Survey 1994.* Rockville, Md: National Institute on Drug Abuse, US Dept of Health and Human Services; 1994.
4. Woody GE, Luborsky L, McLellan AT, O'Brien CP, Beck AT, Blaine J, Herman I, Hole A. Psychotherapy for opiate addicts: does it help? *Arch Gen Psychiatry.* 1983; 40:639-645.
5. Woody GE, McLellan AT, Luborsky L, O'Brien CP. Psychotherapy in community-based methadone programs: a validation study. *Am J Psychiatry.* 1995;152: 1302-1308.
6. Means LB, Small M, Capone DM, Capone TJ, Condren R, Peterson M, Hayward B. Client demographics and outcome in outpatient cocaine treatment. *Int J Addict.* 1989;24:765-783.
7. Jensen JP, Bergin AE, Greaves DW. The meaning of eclecticism: new survey and analysis of components. *Professional Psychol: Res Pract.* 1990;21:124-130.
8. Rawson RA, Obert JL, McCann MJ, Marinelli-Casey P. Relapse prevention strategies in outpatient substance abuse treatment. *Psychology Addict Behav.* 1993;7:85-95.
9. Crits-Christoph P, Siqueland L. Psychosocial treatment for drug abuse: selected review and recommendations for national health care. *Arch Gen Psychiatry.* 1996; 53:749-756.
10. Najavits LM, Weiss RD. The role of psychotherapy in the treatment of substance use disorders. *Harv Rev Psychiatry.* 1994;2:84-96.
11. Carroll KM, Rounsaville BJ, Gawin FH. A comparative trial of psychotherapies for ambulatory cocaine abusers: relapse prevention and interpersonal psychotherapy. *Am J Drug Alcohol Abuse.* 1991;17:229-247.
12. Carroll KM, Rounsaville BJ, Gordon LT, Nich C, Jatlow P, Bisighini RM, Gawin FH. Psychotherapy and pharmacotherapy for ambulatory cocaine abusers. *Arch Gen Psychiatry.* 1994;51:177-187.
13. Carroll KM, Rounsaville BJ, Nich C, Gordon LT, Wirtz PW, Gawin F. One-year follow-up of psychotherapy and pharmacotherapy for cocaine dependence. *Arch Gen Psychiatry.* 1994;51:989-997.
14. Higgins ST, Budney AJ, Bickel WK, Hughes JR, Foeg F, Badger G. Achieving cocaine abstinence with a behavioral approach. *Am J Psychiatry.* 1993;150:763-769.
15. Rounsaville BJ, Glazer W, Wilber CH, Weissman MM, Kleber HD. Short-term interpersonal psychotherapy in methadone-maintained opiate addicts. *Arch Gen Psychiatry.* 1983;40:629-636.
16. Kang SY, Kleinman PH, Woody G, Millman RB, Todd TC, Kemp J, Lipton DS. Outcomes for cocaine abusers after once-a-week psychosocial therapy. *Am J Psychiatry.* 1991;148:630-635.
17. Shoham-Salomon V. Introduction to special section on client-therapy interaction research. *J Consult Clin Psychol.* 1991;59:203-204.
18. Beutler LE. Toward specific psychological therapies for specific conditions. *J Consult Clin Psychol.* 1979;47:882-897.
19. Beutler LE. Have all won and must all have prizes? revisiting Luborsky et al's verdict. *J Consult Clin Psychol.* 1991;59:226-232.
20. Luborsky L, Diguer L, Luborsky E, McLellan AT, Woody G, Alexander L. Psychological health-sickness (PHS) as a predictor of outcomes in dynamic and other psychotherapies. *J Consult Clin Psychol.* 1993;61:542-548.
21. McLellan AT, Luborsky L, Woody GE, O'Brien CP, Druley KA. Predicting response to alcohol and drug abuse treatments: role of psychiatric severity. *Arch Gen Psychiatry.* 1983;40:620-625.
22. Rounsaville BJ, Kosten TR, Weissman MM, Kleber HD. Prognostic significance of psychopathology in treated opiate addicts: a 2.5-year follow-up study. *Arch Gen Psychiatry.* 1986;43:739-745.
23. Woody GE, McLellan AT, Luborsky L, O'Brien CP, Blaine J, Fox S, Herman I, Beck AT. Psychiatric severity as a predictor of benefits from psychotherapy: the Penn-VA study. *Am J Psychiatry.* 1984;141:1172-1177.
24. Kadden RM, Cooney NL, Getter H, Litt MD. Matching alcoholics to coping skills of interactional therapies: posttreatment results. *J Consult Clin Psychol.* 1989; 57:698-704.
25. Cooney NL, Kadden RM, Litt MD, Getter H. Matching alcoholics to coping skills or interactional therapies: two-year follow-up results. *J Consult Clin Psychol.* 1991; 59:598-601.
26. Beutler LE, Engle D, Mohr D, Daldrup RJ, Bergan J, Meredith K, Merry W. Predictors of differential response to cognitive, experiential, and self-directed psychotherapeutic procedures. *J Consult Clin Psychol.* 1991;59:333-340.
27. Beutler LE, Machado P, Engle D, Mohr D. Differential patient and treatment maintenance among cognitive, experiential and self-directed psychotherapies. *J Psychother Integr.* 1993;3:15-31.
28. DiNardo PA, Barlow DH. *Anxiety Disorders Interview Schedule-Revised (ADIS-R).* Albany, NY: Phobia and Anxiety Disorders Clinic; 1988.
29. Wei LJ. An application of an urn model to the design of sequential controlled trials. *J Am Stat Assoc.* 1978;73:559-563.
30. Gainey RR, Wells EA, Hawkins JD, Catalano RF. Predicting treatment retention among cocaine users. *Int J Addict.* 1993;28:487-505.
31. Beck AT, Wright FD, Newman CF, Liese BS. *Cognitive Therapy of Substance Abuse.* New York, NY: Guilford Press; 1993.
32. Luborsky L. *Principles of Psychoanalytic Psychotherapy: A Manual for Supportive-Expressive Treatment.* New York, NY: Basic Books Inc Publishers; 1984.
33. Mark D, Luborsky L. *A Manual for the Use of Supportive-Expressive Psychotherapy in the Treatment of Cocaine Abuse.* Philadelphia: Dept of Psychiatry, University of Pennsylvania; 1992.
34. Luborsky L. Core conflictual relationship themes (CCRT): a basic case formulation method. In: Eells T, ed. *Handbook of Psychotherapy Case Formulation.* New York, NY: Guilford Press. In press.
35. Mercer D, Woody G. *Addiction Counseling.* Philadelphia: Center for Studies of Addiction, University of Pennsylvania, Philadelphia Veterans Affairs Medical Center; 1992.
36. Mercer D, Carpenter G, Daley D, Patterson C, Volpicelli J. *Addiction Recovery Manual.* Philadelphia: Treatment Research Unit, University of Pennsylvania; 1994:2.
37. McLellan AT, Kushner H, Metzger D, Peters R, Smith I, Grissom G, Pettinati H, Argeriou M. The fifth edition of the Addiction Severity Index. *J Subst Abuse Treat.* 1992;9:199-213.
38. Kosten TR, Rounsaville BJ, Kleber HD. Concurrent validity of the Addiction Severity Index. *J Nerv Ment Dis.* 1983;17:606-610.
39. McLellan AT, Luborsky L, Cacciola J, Griffith JE. New data from the Addiction Severity Index: reliability and validity in three centers. *J Nerv Ment Dis.* 1985; 173:412-423.
40. Stoffelmayr BE, Mavis BE, Kasim RM. The longitudinal stability of the Addiction Severity Index. *J Subst Abuse Treat.* 1994;11:373-378.
41. Zelen M, Dannemiller MC. The robustness of life testing procedures derived from the exponential distribution. *Technometrics.* 1961;3:29-49.
42. Lavori PW. Clinical trials in psychiatry: should protocol deviation censor patient data? *Neuropsychopharmacology.* 1992;6:39-48.

Problem-Service 'Matching' in Addiction Treatment

A Prospective Study in 4 Programs

A. Thomas McLellan, PhD; Grant R. Grissom, PhD; David Zanis, PhD; Mary Randall, MA; Peter Brill, MD; Charles P. O'Brien, MD, PhD

Background: Our initial attempts to "match" substance-abuse patients from an employee assistance program to an optimal setting or program failed. Scientifically, we found no differential predictors of better outcomes by setting or program. From a practical perspective, it was impossible to place patients in the intended programs. This led to a second study, designed to identify specific patient problems and match professional services to those problems within each of the 4 programs.

Methods: Ninety-four new patients admitted to 4 substance-abuse treatment programs were randomly assigned to standard treatment and treated in the usual manner or were assigned to "matched" services, in which patients received at least 3 professional sessions directed at their important employment, family, or psychiatric problems.

Results: Matched patients stayed in treatment longer, were more likely to complete treatment, and had better posttreatment outcomes than did the standard patients treated in the same programs.

Conclusions: For logistical, financial, and clinical reasons, it is improbable that patients will be matched to specific types of programs. However, within any program, it is possible and practical to match appropriate services to patients' specific treatment problems. This strategy was clinically and administratively practical, attractive to patients, and responsible for a 20% to 30% increase in the effectiveness of this substance-abuse treatment system.

Arch Gen Psychiatry. 1997;54:730-735

Many evaluation studies show that substance-abuse treatments can be effective, not just in reducing use of alcohol, drugs, or both among those treated but also in relieving many of the medical, social, psychological, and family problems so often associated with addictive disorders.[1-5] Many or even most treatment programs may be effective with at least some of the patients they treat, but some programs may be particularly effective with specific types of patients. In fact, this idea of "matching" the right types of patients to the right kinds of programs has been as attractive to clinicians and administrators as it has been elusive to those who have tried to accomplish it. Although there have been several patient-treatment matching efforts, including a recent national treatment-matching study of alcohol-dependent patients,[6] only a few studies have shown evidence of improvement in matched patients compared with patients treated in standard treatment or with "mismatched" controls.[7-9] We report herein results from a 2-stage, prospective, matching study in a network of 4 private treatment programs used by a large employee assistance program (EAP). Our goal was to develop and test a clinically practical and scientifically sound matching procedure that would enable other treatment networks to assign patients to the most clinically appropriate options within their network.

See also page 691

In the initial phase of the study, we evaluated a large cohort of patients at admission, during treatment, and 6 months after treatment in the 4 previously described programs[10] in an attempt to find evidence of better outcomes for specific types of patients treated in a specific kind of treatment program. Unlike our earlier study of a decade ago that prompted the present work,[11,12] we were unable to find evidence of better outcomes for any type of patient in either setting in any specific program. From a practical perspective, we found it difficult to place patients into any treatment program, even when they wanted to go to that program.

From the Department of Psychiatry, Penn-VA Center for Studies of Addiction, the Department of Psychiatry, University of Pennsylvania, Philadelphia (Drs McLellan, Zanis, and O'Brien and Ms Randall) and Compass Information Services, King of Prussia, Pa (Drs Grissom and Brill).

SUBJECTS AND METHODS

Treatment programs in the network—4 private treatment programs from the Philadelphia, Pa, area—were used by the EAP. All 4 programs were accredited, licensed, and widely used as treatment providers by other referral agencies in the area. There were 2 inpatient and 2 outpatient programs, and 1 program in each setting espoused a traditional philosophy of substance-abuse care using education, 12 steps to sobriety, and group and individual counseling to stress a goal of abstinence. The other program in each setting espoused a psychiatric approach similar to that of mental health or general psychiatric clinics. These programs also included traditional components (eg, education, group therapy, 12-step teachings, and Alcoholics Anonymous referral), but also included professional psychiatric and family therapies. The planned length of stay for the inpatient programs was 21 days. The traditional outpatient program met 3 times during the week and once on weekends for a planned duration of 30 days. The psychiatric outpatient program met 3 times per week for a planned duration of 45 days.

SUBJECTS

Subjects were 130 adults who were dependent on alcohol, drugs, or both (*DSM-III-R* criteria),[14] referred by the EAP for treatment during 1994. All subjects were employed, insured persons drawn from businesses in the Philadelphia area. There were no exclusionary restrictions; all those accepted for treatment were eligible for the study; 93% of those approached agreed to enter the study.[10]

ADMISSION ASSESSMENT

At the EAP intake unit, all patients were interviewed with the Addiction Severity Index (ASI).[15,16] The ASI is a 1-hour, structured interview that measures the lifetime and recent (past 30 days) severity of problems in 7 areas: medical status, employment and self-support, alcohol use, drug use, legal status, family and social relationships, and psychiatric symptoms. The information collected at the initial evaluation was used clinically to determine referral and initial treatment plan and by the study investigators to collect quantitative estimates of pretreatment status.

MATCHING PROCEDURE

After placement in 1 of the 4 programs based on normal clinical and administrative procedures, each subject was randomly assigned to standard or matched treatment services.

Standard Services

For standard patients, the research staff provided the ASI information to the program clinical director, who was asked to treat the patient " . . . in the standard manner, as though there were no treatment study ongoing." No instructions were given to withhold any services from patients in the standard condition.

Matched Services

The ASI admission information also was provided to program clinical directors for the matched subjects. However, when the ASI data indicated significant problems in the areas of employment, family relations, or psychiatric status, staff were asked to provide a minimum of 3 individual sessions from a psychiatrist, psychologist, or social worker, as appropriate, to the target problem area. For example, patients who showed evidence of a significant psychiatric problem were targeted to receive at least 3 individual therapy sessions with a psychiatrist or psychologist.

A "significant" problem was defined operationally by an ASI baseline composite score of more than 1 SD above the mean for subjects in the earlier stage of the project.[10] These 3 problem areas were targeted for special services because a number of predictive studies[11-13,17-19] (including the first stage of this project[13]) had shown them to be among the most important patient characteristics in predicting poor outcome following treatment. Three sessions were considered a minimally appropriate "dose" of care, although it was acknowledged that 3 sessions probably would not be enough to address serious problems adequately. All programs were encouraged to provide more sessions if possible, and all programs had appropriate professional staff on site (at least part time) to provide these services.

DURING TREATMENT PROCEDURE

All subjects were telephoned by research staff each week during treatment to record the number of specialized

Continued on next page

The lack of scientific evidence for patient-*program* matching and the practical problems of placing patients into these programs caused us to drop our efforts at developing better patient-*program* placement decisions.

The positive findings from the first stage of the study were that the severity of patients' admission problems in the areas of employment, psychiatric health, and family relations were the best predictors of posttreatment outcome.[6,10,13] A second finding was that the 4 programs differed substantially in the nature and number of services provided to patients.[10] Finally, we found that the program that had provided the most services in a specific problem area generally showed the best outcomes in that problem area.[10]

These findings led to the prospective experiment reported herein, in which a new cohort of patients was evaluated at admission, placed into any 1 of the 4 programs in which the insurance, geography, availability, and patient preference would permit, and then randomly assigned to receive standard services or services that were matched to the problems the patient had at treatment admission.

RESULTS

PRETREATMENT

The demographic and background characteristics (**Table 1**) show that the average subject was about 38 years old, male (70%), white (71%), and with at least 12 years of education. Thirty-seven percent of patients were married and living with their families at the time of ad-services (eg, vocational therapy or family therapy medication) or general discussion sessions (group or individual counseling) that each patient received during the previous week. The Treatment Services Review (TSR),[20] a 10-minute, technician-administered patient interview, was used for that purpose. The TSR measured the services that were provided by the program and those that were received through referral in the same 7 problem areas covered by the ASI. The TSR sums the total amount of treatment activity received into a composite score in each problem area, providing a reliable and representative sample of the treatment received by a patient.[20]

FOLLOW-UP PROCEDURE

Six months after treatment discharge, subjects were recontacted by research staff and readministered the ASI interview by telephone, to measure outcome status. After the interview, subjects were asked to come in to our facility to receive a $25 reimbursement. When they did, they were asked to submit a urine and breathalyzer sample. One hundred eleven of the 130 patients were reinterviewed and complied with urine and breath sample requests (85%). Ninety-four subjects had urinalysis results that were consistent with their self-reported use (equally distributed across group and program) and these are the cases on which all analyses are based. The low number of total subjects eliminated the possibility of group-by-program, or group-by-setting analyses, so we have reported only between-group differences summed across programs.

STATISTICAL ANALYSIS

The 7 composite scores of the ASI served as the major measures of change and outcome. The 2 groups were compared at baseline and follow-up using repeated measures, multiple analysis of covariance (MANCOVA), with a 2-tailed α of .05 as indication of an overall significant difference. Where there was a significant main or interaction effect in the overall test, we followed with analyses of the individual ASI composite scores using ANCOVAs and Student *t* tests, again with α set to .05. We have performed this analytic strategy several times and find it more reasonable than simply adjusting individual ANOVAs or ANCOVAs for type I error rates using a Bonferroni correction.[1,10,12] Data are expressed as mean±SD.

mission to treatment, although 30% reported being separated or divorced. Despite the significant pattern of regular use of alcohol, drugs, or both, most of these patients never had been treated for alcohol abuse (56%) or drug abuse (65%). These patients also had serious and chronic medical problems (30%), psychiatric problems (37%), and legal problems (13%).

A between-groups MANOVA on the 7 ASI baseline composite scores disclosed no significant overall difference in problem severity (F<1). Legal status was the only problem area in which a statistically significant difference was found; the standard group showed a higher proportion of patients who were awaiting legal charges.

Table 1. Background Characteristics at Admission to Treatment Program*

Background Factors	Matched Services (n=45)	Standard Treatment (n=49)
Demographics		
Age, y	37 (5)	38 (6)
Male	77	65
White	79	64
Black	18	31
Hispanic	3	4
Education, y	13 (2)	12 (2)
Problem area		
Drug or alcohol abuse		
Alcohol use, y	13 (3)	14 (3)
Alcohol use to intoxication, y	11 (3)	12 (4)
Sedative abuse, y	1 (3)	0.97 (3)
Cocaine use, y	2 (3)	4 (4)
Amphetamine use, y	2 (3)	2 (2)
Marijuana use, y	6 (4)	8 (5)
Previous alcohol treatments, No.	1 (2)	1 (2)
Never treated for alcohol abuse	55	57
Prior drug treatments, No.	1 (2)	1 (2)
Never treated for drug abuse	80	57
Medical		
Chronic medical problems	28	33
Medical hospitalizations	2 (2)	4 (3)
Employment		
Longest continuous employment, y	9 (5)	9 (7)
Employed	80	81
Legal		
Awaiting charges†	5	21
Ever incarcerated	12	14
Family and social		
Married	37	38
Separated or divorced	27	33
Single, never married	34	27
Living with substance abuser	11	10
Sexual abuse, lifetime	2	11
Psychiatric		
Previous psychiatric treatments	32	39
Attempted suicide, lifetime	12	18
Depressed, lifetime	43	68
Problems controlling violence, lifetime	44	50

**Values are given as percentages or mean (±SD).*
†P=.01 by Student t test or χ^2.

DURING TREATMENT

The average length of inpatient stay was 11±3 days for the standard group and 12±3 days for the matched group, not significantly different (t<1; df=43; P>.10). The average length of stay in outpatient treatment was 20±5 days for the standard group and 26±3 days for the matched group, significantly different (t=2.11; df=46; P<.05). Also, significantly more matched patients completed treatment (93%) than standard patients (81%) (χ^2=3.91; df=1; P<.05).

Table 2 gives the average total TSR service scores for the matched and standard groups in 6 ASI problem areas during 4 weeks of treatment. As predicted, the matched patients received more of the 3 "targeted" matching services (family, employment, and psychiatric) than did the standard patients, significantly so in the family (t=2.35; df=93; P<.03) and employment areas (t=2.51; df=91; P<.02), but only a trend in the psychiatric area (P<.10). The 2 groups received approximately equal amounts of services in the other 4 areas.

POSTTREATMENT

Table 3 gives the baseline and follow-up composite scores from the ASI. A repeated measures MANCOVA across all of the follow-up ASI composite scores (baseline values were covariates) showed a significant main effect of time (F=6.67; df=1,89; P<.001) but a nonsignificant between-groups trend favoring the matched group (F=2.15; df=1,89; P<.09). The MANCOVA examining only the 3 target areas (employment, family, and psychiatric) showed a significant main effect favoring the matched group (F=6.15; df=1,91; P<.01).

The standard group showed significant improvements between admission to treatment and follow-up (paired Student t tests) in the alcohol, drug, family, and psychiatric areas, but failed to show improvement in medical status and showed significantly worsened status in employment (P<.05). The matched group showed statistically significant improvement in all of the ASI problem areas.

Table 2. Treatment Services Provided in Matched and Standard Groups*

Area	Mean (±SD) TSR Score: Standard Treatment	Matched Services
Problem		
Alcohol	50.5 (35.9)	47.4 (31.3)
Drug	33.0 (26.6)	30.8 (27.7)
Medical	3.2 (7.2)	5.7 (4.1)
Targeted		
Employment	1.8 (4.1)	4.2 (2.4)†
Family	2.2 (4.6)	4.2 (4.7)†
Psychiatric	3.9 (5.8)	6.8 (4.6)

*TSR indicates Treatment Services Review.
†P<.05 from within-group paired Student t test.

Analyses of covariance on the follow-up composite scores showed significant between-group differences in the employment and family areas (P<.01) and trends favoring the matched group in the medical and psychiatric areas (P<.10). **Table 4** gives comparisons of the 2 groups on positive status (eg, abstinent and working) and negative status (eg, retreated, hospitalized, and incarcerated) measures of outcome during the entire period from discharge to follow-up. The matched group had better outcomes on 9 of the 12 status measures (4 significant at P<.05), were tied on 1 measure, and were worse on 2 measures.

COMMENT

This 2-stage study of matching within a 4-program, network of substance-abuse treatment programs has shown that matched patients received more services in the targeted areas, stayed in treatment longer, were more likely to complete treatment, and had better 6-month outcomes than did the standard-care patients treated in the same programs. Because an intent-to-treat design was used with random assignment and analyses were not confined only to treatment completers, we believe that the experimental intervention was causally associated with the differential outcomes. The findings also were consistent with the a priori predictions guiding the matching strategy. Finally, with regard to the importance and robustness of the findings, 2 points are important. First, this was a health services evaluation of treatment effectiveness under *real-world* conditions rather than a clinical trial of treatment efficacy under more controlled but less realistic conditions. It is traditional for clinical trials of efficacy to show substantial reductions in effect size when transferred to field conditions. These data indicate a statistically significant matching effect under field conditions. Second, the control group here was not a "no-treatment" condition. In fact, the control patients were treated in programs that had shown evidence of effectiveness.[10] For these reasons, we believe the findings have potential practical value and impact for the contemporary treatment of addiction.

This study has limitations. Although the EAP-referred patients in this study are an important group,

Table 3. Change in Addiction Severity Index Scores*

Area	Standard Treatment (n=50): Baseline	Standard: 6 Months	Standard: P†	Matched Services (n=45): Baseline	Matched: 6 Months	Matched: P†	ANCOVA on ASI Scores at 6 Months
Problem							
Alcohol	0.45 (0.33)	0.12 (0.21)	<.001	0.49 (0.36)	0.10 (0.10)	<.001	...
Drug	0.14 (0.14)	0.04 (0.06)	<.001	0.13 (0.13)	0.02 (0.06)	<.001	...
Medical	0.24 (0.32)	0.21 (0.21)	...	0.25 (0.17)	0.14 (0.16)	<.01	.09
Targeted							
Employment	0.38 (0.29)	0.44 (0.27)	<.05	0.31 (0.27)	0.23 (0.21)	<.01	.00
Family	0.23 (0.26)	0.19 (0.20)	<.01	0.27 (0.15)	0.11 (0.17)	<.001	.01
Psychiatric	0.28 (0.24)	0.19 (0.22)	<.05	0.31 (0.21)	0.13 (0.11)	<.001	.11

Mean (±SD) Addiction Severity Score†

*ANCOVA indicates analysis of covariance; ASI, Addiction Severity Index. Scores vary from 0 (no problem) to 1 (extreme problem) in preceding 30 days.
†Within-group change in ASI scores by paired Student t tests.

Table 4. Six-Month Outcome Status Indicators

Status Indicators	Standard Treatment (n=49)	Matched Services (n=45)	P*
Positive			
Abstinence from alcohol	65	69	...
Abstinence from all drugs	77	76	...
Working ≥20 hours per week	69	83	<.05
No criminal activity	91	97	...
Not having family conflicts	51	64	<.05
Negative			
Re-treated for alcohol or drug abuse	35	24	<.05
Hospitalized for medical problem	4	2	...
Hospitalized for psychiatric problem	4	5	...
Receiving welfare	8	5	...
Arrested and charged for a crime	8	0	<.05
Incarcerated	2	0	...

*χ^2 analysis.

they probably differ in the amount of pressure to enter-treatment and in their background characteristics from other groups of insured patients, and they probably differ substantially from patients treated in the public sector. Thus, it is not possible to generalize these findings to other groups.

A major consideration in all studies using self-report data is the reliability and validity of the information collected. The data were based on confidential interviews at admission and follow-up using instruments and procedures that have been validated in many similar studies.[15,16,20-22] The self-reported data on drug and alcohol use were supported by the results of concurrent, independent urinalysis and breathalyzer readings. It is impossible to claim that there was no misrepresentation by any of the patients but it is unlikely that there were different rates of misrepresentation between the 2 groups.

Our choice of a 6-month follow-up was based on work during the past 15 years showing that 60% to 80% of patients who relapse following treatment do so within 3 to 4 months after discharge.[23] Because many of the patients who do relapse return to treatment, later follow-up evaluations of a single treatment episode may become contaminated by the effects of subsequent treatments.

Although the TSR has been shown to be a reliable and valid quantitative measure of services received during treatment,[20] it is not designed to measure the important domain of treatment quality. Aware of this limitation and sensitive to pressures to limit the amount and costs of services provided, we attempted to obtain quality treatment services in the target areas by specifically requesting professionally trained and experienced personnel to provide individual sessions in the employment, psychiatric, and family problem areas, although we are aware that not all professionals offer similar quality of care.[24,25] We do not know whether these services could be provided with equally positive effects by less experienced professionals or by paraprofessional counselors. Such a conclusion should not be extrapolated from these data.

Finally, a major limitation of the study was the low number of subjects, minimizing our statistical power to detect significant between-group differences within programs. Similarly, although there were trends indicating better results of matched services for the subgroup of patients with the most severe psychiatric, family, and employment problems (data not shown), there was insufficient power to test this important aspect of the study.

The results have led us to 3 conclusions. First, in the real world, there are many obstacles to placing patients into any treatment program, and attempts to match special types of patients to specific kinds of treatment programs are impractical.

Second, we continue to find that the nature and severity of the psychiatric, family, employment, medical, and legal problems of substance-abuse patients are major predictors of posttreatment outcome from substance-abuse treatment. This is not new; results of many studies during the past decade support this conclusion.[1-13,17,18] These problems can be identified easily and reliably at the time of treatment admission and can be targeted as part of the overall treatment.

Finally, we believe that strategies designed to direct professional services to these addiction-related problems are practical and transferable to other addiction-treatment settings and can be effective in improving the results of substance-abuse treatment. Again, this conclusion follows more than a decade of research showing that the addition of professional marital counseling,[26,27] psychotherapy,[28,29] employment counseling and skill training,[30,31] and medical care[32-34] produces clinically and significantly better outcomes from substance-abuse treatment than do drug and alcohol counseling alone.

Accepted for publication November 6, 1996.

This research was sponsored by Center grant V101 (91) from the Department of Veterans Affairs, Washington, DC, and center grants P506090R, P50 DA05186, and P50 DA07705 from the National Institute on Drug Abuse, Bethesda, Md.

Reprints: A. Thomas McLellan, MD, Center for Studies of Addiction, School of Medicine, University of Pennsylvania, Bldg 7 PVAMC, University Ave, Philadelphia, PA 19104.

REFERENCES

1. McLellan AT, Luborsky L, O'Brien CP, Woody GE, Druley KA. Is treatment for substance abuse effective? *JAMA.* 1982;247:1423-1427.
2. Ball JC, Ross A. *The Effectiveness of Methadone Maintenance Treatment.* New York, NY: Springer-Verlag NY Inc; 1991.
3. Anglin MD, Speckart GR, Booth MW. Consequences and costs of shutting off methadone. *Addict Behav.* 1989;14:307-326.
4. Hubbard RL, Marsden ME, Rachal JV, Harwood HJ, Cavanaugh ER, Ginzburg HM. *Drug Abuse Treatment: A National Study of Effectiveness.* Chapel Hill, NC: University of North Carolina Press; 1989.
5. Miller WR, Hester RK. Inpatient alcoholism treatment: who benefits? *Am Psychol.* 1986;41:794-805.
6. NIAAA Project MATCH Research Group. Matching alcoholism treatments to client heterogeneity: project MATCH posttreatment drinking outcomes. *J Stud Alcohol.* 1997;90:1179-1188.
7. Kadden RM, Cooney NL, Getter H, Litt MD. Matching alcoholics to coping skills or interactional therapies: post treatment results. *J Consult Clin Psychol.* 1989; 57:698-704.
8. Kadden RM, Cooney NL, Getter H, Litt MD. Matching alcoholics to coping skills

or interactional therapies: two-year follow-up results. *J Consult Clin Psychol.* 1991; 59:598-601.
9. McLachlan J. Therapy strategies, personality orientation, and recovery from alcoholism. *Can Psychiatr Assoc J.* 1974;19:25-30.
10. McLellan AT, Grissom G, Alterman AI, Brill P, O'Brien CP. Substance abuse treatment in the private setting: are some programs more effective than others? *J Subst Abuse Treat.* 1993;10:243-254.
11. McLellan AT, Luborsky L, Woody GE, Druley KA, O'Brien CP. Predicting response to alcohol and drug abuse treatments: role of psychiatric severity. *Arch Gen Psychiatry.* 1983;40:620-625.
12. McLellan AT, Luborsky L, Woody GE, O'Brien CP, Druley KA. Increased effectiveness of substance abuse treatment: a prospective study of patient-treatment 'matching.' *J Nerv Ment Dis.* 1983;171:597-605.
13. McLellan AT, Alterman AI, Metzger DS, Grissom G, Woody GE, Luborsky L, O'Brien CP. Similarity of outcome predictors across opiate, cocaine and alcohol treatments: role of treatment services. *J Clin Consult Psychol.* 1994;62: 1141-1158.
14. American Psychiatric Association. *Diagnostic and Statistical Manual of Mental Disorders, Third Edition, Revised.* Washington, DC: American Psychiatric Association; 1987.
15. McLellan AT, Luborsky L, Cacciola J, Griffith J. New data from the Addiction Severity Index: reliability and validity in three centers. *J Nerv Ment Dis.* 1985;173:412-423.
16. McLellan AT, Cacciola J, Kushner H, Peters F, Smith I, Pettinati H. The fifth edition of the Addiction Severity Index: cautions, additions and normative data. *J Subst Abuse Treat.* 1992;9:261-275.
17. Havassy BE, Hall SM, Wasserman D. Social support and relapse: commonalities among alcoholics, opiate users and cigarette smokers. *Addict Behav.* 1989;16: 233-246.
18. Rounsaville BJ, Dolinsky ZS, Babor TF, Meyer RE. Psychopathology as a predictor of treatment outcome in alcoholics. *Arch Gen Psychiatry.* 1987;44:505-513.
19. Institute of Medicine. *Broadening the Base of Treatment for Alcohol Problems.* Washington, DC: National Academy Press; 1990.
20. McLellan AT, Alterman AI, Woody GE, Metzger D. A quantitative measure of substance abuse treatments: the Treatment Services Review. *J Nerv Ment Dis.* 1992; 180:101-110.
21. Zanis D, McLellan AT, Randall M. Can you trust the self reports of drug users during treatment? *Drug Alcohol Depend.* 1995;38:121-125.
22. Ehrman RN, Robbins SJ. Reliability and validity of 6-month timeline reports of cocaine and heroin use in a methadone population. *J Consult Clin Psychol.* 1994;62: 843-850.
23. McLellan AT, Woody GE, Metzger D, McKay J, Alterman AI, O'Brien CP. Evaluating the effectiveness of treatments for substance use disorders: reasonable expectations, appropriate comparisons. *Milbank Q.* 1996;74:51-85.
24. McLellan AT, Woody GE, Luborsky L, O'Brien CP. Is the counselor an 'active ingredient' in substance abuse treatment? *J Nerv Ment Dis.* 1988;176:423-430.
25. Luborsky L, Crits-Cristoph P, McLellan AT, Woody GE. Do psychotherapists vary much in their effectiveness? the answer within four outcome studies. *Am J Orthopsychiatry.* 1986;56:211-223.
26. McCrady BS, Noel NE, Abrams DB, Stout RL, Nelson HF, Hay WM. Comparative effectiveness of three types of spouse involvement in outpatient behavioral alcoholism treatment. *J Stud Alcohol.* 1986;47:459-467.
27. Stanton MD, Todd T. *The Family Therapy of Drug Abuse and Addiction.* New York, NY: Guilford Press; 1982.
28. Carroll KM, Rounsaville BJ, Gordon LT, Nich C, Jatlow P, Bisighini RM, Gawin FH. Psychotherapy and pharmacotherapy for ambulatory cocaine abusers. *Arch Gen Psychiatry.* 1994;51:177-187.
29. Woody GE, Luborsky L, McLellan AT, O'Brien CP. Psychotherapy for opiate addicts: does it help? *Arch Gen Psychiatry.* 1983;40:639-645.
30. French MT, Rachal JV, Harwood HJ, Hubbard RL. Does drug abuse treatment affect employment and earnings of clients? *Benefits Q.* 1990;6:58-67.
31. French MT, Dennis ML, McDougal GL, Karountzos GT, Hubbard RL. Training and employment programs in methadone treatment: client needs and desires. *J Subst Abuse Treat.* 1992;9:293-303.
32. Schonberg SK, ed. *Substance Abuse: A Guide for Health Professionals.* Elk Grove Village, Ill; American Academy of Pediatrics Press; 1988.
33. Fleming MF, Barry KL, eds. *Addictive Disorders.* St Louis, Mo: Mosby–Year Book Inc; 1992.
34. McLellan AT, Arndt IO, Woody GE, Metzger D. Psychosocial services in substance abuse treatment? a dose-ranging study of psychosocial services. *JAMA.* 1993;269:1953-1959.

ORIGINAL ARTICLE

Naltrexone and Alcohol Dependence

Role of Subject Compliance

Joseph R. Volpicelli, MD, PhD; Karen C. Rhines; Jared S. Rhines; Laura A. Volpicelli; Arthur I. Alterman, PhD; Charles P. O'Brien, MD, PhD

Background: Two previous double-blind, placebo-controlled studies demonstrated that naltrexone (50 mg/d) reduces alcohol drinking in alcohol-dependent subjects. In both studies, treatment compliance was excellent. However, a robust treatment effect size for naltrexone relative to placebo has been shown for compliant subjects but not for subjects who missed research visits. The goal of this study was to determine the effectiveness of naltrexone in subjects who received psychosocial treatment in a more naturalistic setting with respect to the role of treatment attendance and medication compliance.

Methods: Ninety-seven alcohol-dependent subjects were randomly assigned to receive either naltrexone (n=48) or matching placebo (n=49) for 12 weeks. All subjects received individual counseling (twice per week for the first month followed by once per week).

Results: Overall, naltrexone showed only modest effects in reducing alcohol drinking for the 12 weeks of treatment. However, naltrexone treatment efficacy improved across a variety of outcome measures for subjects who completed treatment and were highly compliant with taking medication.

Conclusions: Naltrexone is clinically effective relative to placebo in individuals who comply with the treatment protocol and take medication. The modest treatment effects in the entire sample suggest that the clinical efficacy of naltrexone could be improved by enhancing treatment compliance.

Arch Gen Psychiatry. 1997;54:737-742

THE OPIOID antagonist naltrexone reduces alcohol drinking during the first 3 months of treatment after alcohol detoxification in double-blind, placebo-controlled studies.[1-4] These clinical results are consistent with preclinical animal studies that showed that opiate antagonists reduce alcohol preference in monkeys,[5-7] mice,[8] and rats,[9] particularly in strains bred for excessive alcohol drinking,[10] and after environmental stressors that increase alcohol drinking.[11] Furthermore, clinical studies have demonstrated that naltrexone may reduce the reinforcing or pleasurable effects of alcohol in social drinkers[12] and alcohol-dependent subjects who slip and sample alcohol.[13,14] Together, the preclinical and clinical data show that naltrexone reduces the reinforcing effects of alcohol and excessive alcohol drinking. Thus, naltrexone may be an effective medication to treat alcohol dependence.

One important limitation to any pharmacological treatment is patient compliance. While a treatment may be effective pharmacologically, it will not be effective clinically if patients are not compliant with taking the medication. The 2 published double-blind studies that used naltrexone for alcoholism treatment showed good medication compliance and adherence with the study protocol. For example, in the University of Pennsylvania/Veterans Affairs study,[2] nearly 60% of the naltrexone-treated subjects completed all 12 research visits, and in the Yale study,[1] more than 90% of subjects prescribed naltrexone had urine tests positive for the drug marker riboflavin.

See also page 691

It is not clear that the excellent compliance rates seen in the research trials can be extrapolated to clinical programs. Clinical programs that use naltrexone to treat opioid dependence typically observe poor compliance.[15-18] While formerly opioid-dependent patients consistently taking naltrexone show marked improvement, many patients are not compliant with taking prescribed naltrexone and simply drop out of treatment.[15-18] For example, 1 study reported that less than 10% of patients who

From the Department of Psychiatry, University of Pennsylvania, Philadelphia, and the Philadelphia Veterans Affairs Medical Center (Drs Volpicelli, Alterman, and O'Brien, Mr Rhines, and Ms Volpicelli), and the Department of Psychology, Rutgers University, Piscataway, NJ (Ms Rhines).

SUBJECTS AND METHODS

SUBJECTS

Subjects were newly admitted alcohol-dependent patients receiving outpatient treatment at the University of Pennsylvania/Veterans Affairs Treatment Research Center, Philadelphia. The study subjects were 21 to 65 years of age, met the *DSM-III-R*[20] criteria for alcohol dependence, and recently completed medical detoxification for alcohol withdrawal. Exclusionary criteria included a major psychiatric illness associated with psychosis or dementia at the time of the evaluation or being judged by a psychiatrist to be a danger to self or others; a history of unstable or serious medical condition; narcotic use in the past 30 days; laboratory evidence of significant hepatocellular injury as evidenced by elevated bilirubin level; current disulfiram treatment; female patients who were pregnant, nursing, or not using a reliable method of contraception; and abstinence from alcohol for longer than 21 days. This study was reviewed and approved by the University of Pennsylvania Human Subjects Committee, and all subjects provided written informed consent after a full explanation of the study.

TREATMENT

After they gave informed consent, subjects were randomized in computer number–generated blocks of 20 subjects into either naltrexone or placebo treatment groups. All subjects received an initial 1-week placebo lead-in to establish baseline measures. After this lead-in, subjects received naltrexone or placebo. Of the 127 subjects seen for an initial intake interview, 12 (9.4%) dropped out before eligibility could be ascertained, 1 dropped out because of work-related problems, 13 (10.2%) had either an inadequate or an excessive duration of abstinence, 1 was incarcerated, and 1 relocated. Of the remaining 99 eligible subjects, 1 declined participation. One subject was later dropped from analysis because of a medication error. This resulted in 97 subjects, 48 treated with naltrexone and 49 with placebo.

In addition to receiving naltrexone or placebo for 12 weeks, all subjects received counseling with a certified alcohol counselor or a postdoctoral fellow in substance abuse. Counseling consisted of individual psychotherapy modeled after Gorski and Miller's relapse prevention program.[21] During the first month of treatment, subjects met with their counselor twice per week. For the remainder of treatment, subjects had 1 individual session per week.

MEDICATION REGIMEN

Study medication was either naltrexone hydrochloride, 50 mg, or identical-appearing placebo tablets. All patients were instructed to take 1 pill orally per day for the duration of the study. A technician (K.C.R., J.S.R., or L.A.V.) counted the number of pills returned each week in the pill vial and also asked the subject if any pills were missed in the preceding week.

ASSESSMENT INSTRUMENTS

Subjects were seen for weekly visits to assess alcohol craving and consumption. Alcohol craving was assessed on a 10-point scale (0, not at all; 9, would have had a drink if one were available). Alcohol consumption reports were obtained by means of the alcohol use questionnaire, a technician-administered instrument that assessed the frequency and amount of alcohol consumed in the preceding week. If it was determined that a subject had consumed alcohol in the past week, an alcohol subjective response questionnaire was administered to assess the perceived feelings of "high" resulting from alcohol use. Subjects rated their subjective feelings of "high" on a 3-point scale; they felt an increased high (+1), no difference (0), or a decreased high (−1), compared with feelings while not taking medication. Finally, a side-effects checklist was administered by the technician to assess the duration and severity of treatment-emergent side effects. If a subject reported severe symptoms, the study psychiatrist was consulted.

Monthly research visits were also scheduled. During these visits, the 90-Item Symptom Checklist[22] was administered to assess psychiatric symptoms or disorders. A study physician ordered blood chemistry studies, including liver function tests, urine drug screens, and a complete blood cell count. Subjects were prematurely terminated from the study if they experienced severe and persistent side effects, experienced psychiatric or medical emergencies that required inpatient hospitalization, or required the use of narcotic medications for pain relief. To provide a safety net for subjects whose clinical condition deteriorated (at least 2 consecutive weeks with ≥3 days of excessive drinking, ie, ≥5 drinks in 1 day), subjects were given the opportunity to stop the study and receive standard ambulatory or inpatient treatment.

The major dependent measure used to determine naltrexone's effect was time to relapse to an episode of clinically significant drinking. Relapse was defined as at least 5 drinks during 1 drinking occasion or a documented breath alcohol level greater than 100 mg/dL. Other important outcome measures included alcohol craving, percentage of drinking days, liver enzyme levels, and psychological distress.

STATISTICAL ANALYSIS

In the results that follow, we used end-point analysis techniques, ie, the status of the dependent variable at either week 12 or the time of subject termination, to analyze alcohol craving, percentage of drinking days, liver enzyme results, and psychiatric symptoms. If data were not obtained beyond the baseline period, the subject was dropped from the analysis for that particular variable. Furthermore, results were analyzed for all 97 randomized subjects (intention-to-treat analysis) and separately for the 71 subjects who completed treatment (subjects who missed more than 2 research visits; modeled after the treatment completion criteria used in the Yale study[1]), or were dropped from the study because of clinical deterioration.

For continuous variables, such as the percentage of drinking days, alcohol craving, and liver enzyme levels, analyses of covariance were used with baseline values as the covariate. To normalize the data for statistical analysis for the liver enzyme data, a log transformation was used. Time to any alcohol drinking (alcohol slip) and time to alcohol relapse were measured by survival analysis with the use of the Mantel-Haenszel comparison of survival curves.[23] In addition, analysis of the subjective effects of alcohol was conducted by means of an ordered χ^2, the Mantel extension of the Mantel-Haenszel procedure.[24] Finally, interaction effects of medication compliance with alcohol drinking were analyzed by logistic regressions. All the analyses were 2-tailed, with significance levels at $P<.05$.

began naltrexone treatment for opioid dependence were still taking the medication after 2 months.[18] Thus, while naltrexone is effective pharmacologically to reduce the opiate high, its clinical utility is limited because of poor subject compliance.

The pooled results of a study of 99 subjects completed at the University of Pennsylvania/Veterans Affairs Center[19] demonstrate that patient compliance also limits the effectiveness of naltrexone for the treatment of alcohol dependence. While naltrexone was effective overall in reducing relapse to clinically significant drinking (risk reduction, 0.51), the relative effectiveness of naltrexone was higher for the subjects who completed all 12 research sessions (risk reduction, 0.74) than for the less compliant subjects (risk reduction, 0.27).

The present study attempts to extend the findings of our first University of Pennsylvania/Veterans Affairs study by examining the effectiveness of naltrexone in an outpatient treatment setting (similar to the clinical standard treatment in the community) with a more heterogeneous population of subjects, that is, with a nonveteran population, including women. Our primary hypothesis was that naltrexone treatment will reduce the rate of subjects who relapse to an episode of clinically significant drinking, particularly in those subjects who adhere to the treatment protocol and those subjects who are more compliant with taking their medications.

RESULTS

SOCIODEMOGRAPHICS

The baseline sociodemographics of the 2 study groups of the sample did not differ (**Table 1**).

Of the 49 subjects in the placebo group, 36 (73%) completed the treatment protocol, compared with 35 (73%) of 48 naltrexone-treated subjects. Of the 36 placebo-treated subjects who completed treatment, 12 subjects were dropped because of clinical complications. Clinical complications for the placebo group included clinical deterioration from excessive alcohol use in 10, side effects in 1, and cessation of treatment because of an injury that required narcotic medication in 1. Only 3 subjects of the 35 treatment completers failed to finish the study because of clinical complications; 1 subject was dropped because of clinical deterioration from excessive alcohol drinking and 2 subjects were dropped because of severe nausea.

OUTCOME FOR ALL SUBJECTS AND TREATMENT COMPLETERS

Naltrexone had a modest effect in reducing a return to excessive drinking for all subjects. Among placebo-treated subjects, 26 (53%) of the 49 relapsed during the 12 weeks of the study, compared with 17 (35%) of 48 naltrexone-treated subjects (χ^2=3.35, 1 *df*; *P*=.07) (survival analysis). For treatment completers, the effectiveness of naltrexone was more clearly established. Relapse occurred in 19 (53%) of the 36 placebo-treated subjects and in only 9 (26%) of the 35 naltrexone-treated subjects (χ^2=5.20, 1 *df*; *P*=.02). Naltrexone treatment did not significantly prevent subjects from sampling alcohol ("slipping") for all subjects or for the treatment completers (**Table 2**). Among placebo-treated subjects, 65% (32/49) of all subjects and 61% (22/36) of the completers reported a slip, compared with 56% (27/48) and 51% (18/35) of the subjects in the naltrexone group.

Table 1. Baseline Subject Sociodemographics and Clinical Characteristics in the Placebo and Naltrexone Treatment Groups*

	Placebo	Naltrexone†
Age, y	37.9±8.5	39.0±9.0
Race		
African American	2.0	6.1
White	40.0	34.7
Other	58.0	59.2
Male	82.0	73.5
Employed	64.0	71.4
Married	46.0	42.9
Years of regular drinking	15.8±9.7	15.0±8.6
Aspartate aminotransferase, U/L	34.6±38.1	28.8±13.9
γ-Glutamyltransferase, U/L	78.6±97.7	66.4±69.0
Baseline drinking days	14.8±8.9	13.3±8.9

*Data are given as mean±SD and percentage of subjects.

†None of these variables was significantly different for the naltrexone and placebo groups.

Similarly, in the intent-to-treat analysis for all subjects, placebo-treated subjects drank on an average of 10.8% of the study days, whereas naltrexone-treated subjects drank on 6.2% of the study days. This difference, while favorable for the naltrexone group, was not statistically significant by means of an analysis of covariance controlling for baseline drinking during the 30 days before the beginning of the study. However, placebo-treated subjects who completed treatment drank on 12.7% of the study days, whereas naltrexone-treated subjects who completed treatment drank on 5.40% of the study days ($F[1,68]=4.85$; *P*=.03). As Table 2 shows, liver enzyme (aspartate aminotransferase and γ-glutamyltransferase) levels for the naltrexone-treated group were significantly lower than for the placebo group in both the intent-to-treat sample and treatment completers. Since study dropouts often did not have follow-up liver enzyme levels determined, the intent-to-treat and treatment completer samples are virtually identical. Mean craving scores were generally lower in the naltrexone group, but these differences were not significantly different for either the intent-to-treat analysis or treatment completers.

The pharmacological effects of naltrexone on alcohol reward were assessed for subjects who consumed any alcohol during the study. Naltrexone significantly reduced the "high" associated with drinking. Eleven (50%) of the 22 naltrexone-treated subjects reported feeling a less-than-expected high from drinking, whereas only 7 (25%) of 28 placebo-treated subjects reported a decreased high. One (5%) of the 22 naltrexone-treated subjects reported an increased high from drinking, whereas 4 (14%) of the 28 placebo-treated subjects reported an increased high. Similar findings were observed for the treatment completers (χ^2=3.71 and 5.20, respectively).

Naltrexone treatment had no overall effect on psychopathology as assessed by the 90-Item Symptom

Table 2. Treatment Outcome for All Subjects and Subject Completers

	Placebo	Naltrexone	Effect Size	Significance
No. of subjects				
Total sample	49	48	...	...
Completers	36	35	...	...
% Relapse				
Total sample	53.1	35.4	0.375	χ^2=3.06, *P*=.08
Completers	52.8	27.7	0.557	χ^2=5.44, *P*=.02
% Slip				
Total sample	65.3	56.3	0.185	χ^2=0.83, *P*=.36
Completers	61.1	51.4	0.189	χ^2=0.68, *P*=.41
% Drinking days (mean±SE)				
Total sample	10.76±2.32	6.20±1.59	0.31	F(1,94)=2.31
Completers	12.66±2.99	5.40±1.78	0.57	F(1,68)=5.68, *P*=.02
Alcohol craving (mean±SE)				
Total sample	3.14±0.39	2.79±0.34	0.15	F(1,94)=0.38, *P*=.53
Completers	3.42±0.48	2.40±0.38	0.29	F(1,68)=1.52, *P*=.22
Aspartate aminotransferase, U/L (mean±SE)				
Total sample	34.4±4.45	27.1±2.3	0.58	F(1,58)=8.05, *P*=.006
Completers	34.6±4.68	25.7±2.1	0.70	F(1,53)=8.66, *P*=.005
γ-Glutamyltransferase, U/L (mean±SE)				
Total sample	66.2±15.0	45.1±7.4	0.52	F(1,57)=4.89, *P*=.03
Completers	69.6±16.3	43.7±8.2	0.61	F(1,52)=6.58, *P*=.01
Alcohol high (less, same, more), No.				
Total sample	7, 17, 4	11, 10, 1	0.56	χ^2=3.71, *P*=.05
Completers	5, 13, 3	9, 7, 0	0.96	χ^2=5.20, *P*=.02
Symptom Checklist 90 (mean±SE)				
Total sample	48.3±9.3	31.7±5.5	0.22	F(1,65)=1.16, *P*=.28
Completers	51.4±11.1	28.7±5.7	0.26	F(1,53)=2.24, *P*=.14

Checklist.[22] Controlling for baseline Symptom Checklist scores, there were no statistical differences between the placebo and naltrexone groups in total score overall (48.3 vs 31.7).

Side effects associated with naltrexone treatment were generally mild and did not differ with respect to naltrexone. Only 1 placebo-treated and 2 naltrexone-treated subjects reported side effects severe enough to terminate participation in the study. Among reported side effects, increased sexual desire was the only side effect reported more frequently by the naltrexone-treated subjects than by the placebo-treated subjects. Seventeen (35%) of the 48 naltrexone-treated subjects reported mild to moderate increased sexual desire, compared with 9 (18%) of the 49 placebo-treated subjects. This difference approached significance (χ^2=3.59, 1 *df*; *P*=.06).

OUTCOME BY MEDICATION COMPLIANCE

The effects of naltrexone on alcohol drinking were even more pronounced when subject medication compliance was taken into account. A significant interaction was found between compliance with medication for alcohol relapse (β=−0.071, *P*=.04). Similarly, the percentage of days on which a naltrexone pill was taken was negatively correlated with the percentage of days of drinking (*r*=−0.417, *P*=.003). There was no correlation, however, in the placebo group among percentage of days on which alcohol was consumed and compliance with taking placebo (*r*=−0.157, *P*=.28).

To better see the effects of medication compliance with treatment outcome, data for medication-compliant vs less compliant subjects were analyzed by means of a median split of medication compliance. Subjects who reported taking medication on 90% of the study days or better composed the high-compliance group, with 23 placebo-treated and 28 naltrexone-treated subjects. The remaining subjects, those who took less than 90%, composed the less compliant group, consisting of 26 placebo-treated and 20 naltrexone-treated subjects.

For medication-compliant subjects, naltrexone treatment significantly reduced alcohol relapse. More than half (12/23 [52%]) of the medication-compliant placebo-treated subjects relapsed, compared with only 4 (14%) of the 28 naltrexone-treated subjects. The Kaplan-Meier curves showing the distribution of the time to relapse are illustrated in the **Figure**. The survival analysis was significantly different (χ^2=9.25, 1 *df*; *P*=.002). Survival curves for the naltrexone-treated and placebo-treated medication-compliant subjects are shown in the Figure.

Fifteen (65%) of 23 highly compliant placebo-treated subjects admitted to sampling alcohol while they were actively taking medication, while only 10 (36%) of 28 highly compliant naltrexone-treated subjects admitted to sampling alcohol (**Table 3**). The Mantel-Haenszel comparison of survival curves showed χ^2=4.20, 1 *df* (*P*=.03). A comparison of the percentage of days on which drinking was reported during the study showed that highly medication-compliant placebo-treated subjects drank on an average of 11.02% of the study days, whereas highly compliant naltrexone-treated subjects drank only on 2.83% of the study days.

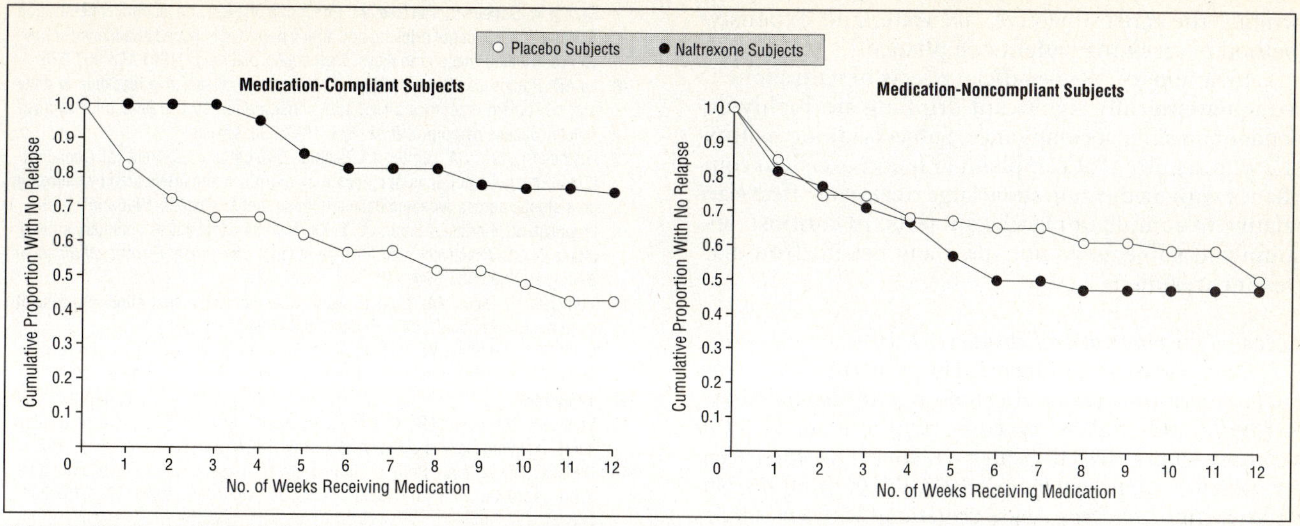

Return to clinically significant drinking in medication-compliant naltrexone- and placebo-treated subjects across the 12 weeks of the study.

Table 3. Treatment Outcome Variables for Medication-Compliant and Less-Compliant Subjects

	Compliant				Less Compliant			
Outcome Variable	Placebo (n=23)	Naltrexone (n=28)	Effect Size	*P*	Placebo (n=26)	Naltrexone (n=20)	Effect Size	*P*
% Relapse	52.2	14.3	0.73	.002	30.8	50.0	−0.63	.19
% Days drinking	11.0	2.83	0.69	.01	10.5	10.9	−0.02	.94

Controlling for baseline drinking during the 30 days before the study, the difference in percentage of days drinking was also statistically significant ($F[1,48]=6.49$, $P=.01$).

Of those subjects considered less compliant, there were no significant differences between the naltrexone and placebo groups in any of the dependent drinking measures. The number of less compliant placebo-treated subjects who returned to clinically significant drinking was 8 (31%) of 26, whereas 10 (50%) of the 20 less compliant naltrexone-treated subjects returned to clinically significant drinking while active in the study. The survival analysis was not statistically different. In addition, in the less compliant placebo group, 13 (50%) of 26 subjects sampled alcohol compared with 15 (75%) of 20 in the less compliant naltrexone group; survival analysis was not significant. The average percentage of drinking days during the study did not significantly differ between the 2 groups, with less compliant placebo-treated subjects drinking on 10.5% of the study days, compared with 10.9% of the study days for the less compliant naltrexone-treated subjects.

COMMENT

Overall, the results of this study are consistent with previous reports of the effectiveness of naltrexone in alcohol dependence treatment. Naltrexone treatment reduced the number of subjects who returned to clinically significant drinking (alcohol relapse), reduced the percentage of days of drinking, and improved liver enzyme results. Naltrexone did not prevent subjects from sampling alcohol, but once alcohol was consumed, subjects reported less "high" from drinking. Unlike our original study, we did not find that naltrexone reduced alcohol craving.

While compliance with taking the medication and completing the protocol was generally good in this heterogeneous population, the study found a significant negative correlation between medication compliance with naltrexone and the percentage of days of drinking during the study. Treatment outcome effect sizes for highly compliant subjects were clinically large and statistically significant. In contrast, for less compliant subjects, naltrexone did not improve treatment outcome. This finding raises 2 important implications. First, naltrexone is more likely to be clinically effective when used in conjunction with psychosocial programs that enhance medication compliance. Second, from a research perspective, the inclusion of less compliant subjects increases the noise in the data. As noncompliance increases, the intent-to-treat analysis increases the chance of a type II statistical error and may unfairly bias our attempts to find effective medications.

One limitation of the study is that the measure of medication compliance was pill count. While pill count is an inexpensive means of determining compliance, it can be inaccurate because pill count does not measure whether the pill was actually ingested and thus may overestimate actual compliance.[25,26] Thus, pill counts could be strengthened by additional measures, such as taking a riboflavin tablet at the same time the medication is taken so that urine assays of added riboflavin could provide a measure of compliance. Finally, blood or urine assays of the metabolite of naltrexone, β-naltrexol, would provide the most objective, accurate, and expensive method of assessing patient compliance.

In summary, the beneficial effects of naltrexone in reducing clinically significant drinking are highly dependent on subject compliance. Subjects taking naltrexone who are protocol-compliant or report excellent compliance with medication show large treatment effect sizes relative to compliant placebo subjects. In contrast, less compliant subjects do not show any benefit from naltrexone treatment.

Accepted for publication February 19, 1997.

This research was supported by grant AA-07517 from the National Institute on Alcoholism and Alcohol Abuse, Rockville, Md, and by the University of Pennsylvania/Veterans Affairs Medical Center, Treatment Research Center, which is supported by grant DA-06107 from the National Institute on Drug Abuse center and Veterans Affairs Merit Review research funds.

Both the naltrexone and placebo tablets were generously supplied by Dupont Pharma, Wilmington, Del.

Reprints: Joseph R. Volpicelli, MD, PhD, Treatment Research Center, 3900 Chestnut St, Philadelphia, PA 19104.

REFERENCES

1. O'Malley SS, Jaffe AJ, Chang G, Schottenfeld RS, Meyer RE, Rounsaville B. Naltrexone and coping skills therapy for alcohol dependence: a controlled study. *Arch Gen Psychiatry.* 1992;49:881-887.
2. Volpicelli JR, Alterman AI, Hayashida M, O'Brien CP. Naltrexone in the treatment of alcohol dependence. *Arch Gen Psychiatry.* 1992;49:876-880.
3. Volpicelli JR, Clay KL, Watson NT, O'Brien CP. Naltrexone in the treatment of alcoholism: predicting response to naltrexone. *J Clin Psychiatry.* 1995;56:39-44.
4. Volpicelli JR, O'Brien CP, Alterman AI, Hayashida M. Naltrexone and the treatment of alcohol dependence: initial observations. In: Reid L, ed. *Opioids, Bulimia, and Alcohol Abuse & Alcoholism.* New York, NY: Springer-Verlag; 1990: 195-214.
5. Altshuler HL, Phillips PE, Feinhandler DA. Alterations of ethanol self-administration by naltrexone. *Life Sci.* 1980;26:679-688.
6. Myers RD, Borg S, Mossberg R. Antagonism by naltrexone of voluntary alcohol selection in the chronically drinking macaque monkey. *Alcohol.* 1986;6:383-388.
7. Kornet M, Goosen C, Van Ree JM. Effect of naltrexone on alcohol consumption during chronic alcohol drinking and after a period of imposed abstinence in free-choice drinking rhesus monkeys. *Psychopharmacology.* 1991;104:367-376.
8. Le AD, Poulos CX, Quan B, Chow S. The effects of selective blockade of delta and mu opiate receptors on ethanol consumption by C57BL/6 mice in a restricted access paradigm. *Brain Res.* 1993;630:330-332.
9. Hubbell CL, Czirr SA, Hunter GA, Beaman CM, LeCann NC, Reid LD. Consumption of ethanol solution is potentiated by morphine and attenuated by naloxone persistently across repeated daily administrations. *Alcohol.* 1986;2(6):1-16.
10. Froehlich JC, Harts J, Lumeng L, Li TK. Naloxone attenuates voluntary ethanol intake in rats selectively bred for high ethanol preference. *Pharmacol Biochem Behav.* 1990;35:385-390.
11. Volpicelli JR, Davis MA, Olgin JE. Naltrexone blocks the post-shock increase of ethanol consumption. *Life Sci.* 1986;38:841-847.
12. Swift RM, Whelihan W, Kuznetsov O, Buongiorno G, Hsuing H. Naltrexone-induced alterations in human ethanol intoxication. *Am J Psychiatry.* 1994;151: 1463-1467.
13. Volpicelli JR, Watson NT, King AC, Sherman CE. Effect of naltrexone on alcohol 'high' in alcoholics. *Am J Psychiatry.* 1995;152:613-615.
14. O'Malley SS, Jaffe AJ, Rode S, Rounsaville BJ. Experience of a 'slip' among alcoholics treated with naltrexone or placebo. *Am J Psychiatry.* 1996;153:281-283.
15. Kleber HD, Kosten TR. Naltrexone induction: psychologic and pharmacologic strategies. *J Clin Psychiatry.* 1984;45(9):29-38.
16. Kosten TR, Kleber HD. Strategies to improve compliance with narcotic antagonists. *Am J Drug Alcohol Abuse.* 1984;10:249-266.
17. Greenstein RA, Arndt IC, McLellan AT, O'Brien CP, Evans B. Naltrexone: a clinical perspective. *J Clin Psychiatry.* 1984;45:25-28.
18. Greenstein RA, O'Brien CP, McLellan AT, Woody GE, Grabowski J, Long M, Coyle-Perkins G, Vittor A. Naltrexone: a short-term treatment for opiate dependence. *Am J Drug Alcohol Abuse.* 1981;8:291-300.
19. O'Brien CP, Volpicelli LA, Volpicelli JR. Naltrexone in the treatment of alcoholism: a clinical review. *Alcohol.* 1996;13:35-39.
20. American Psychiatric Association. *Diagnostic and Statistical Manual of Mental Disorders, Third Edition, Revised.* Washington, DC: American Psychiatric Association; 1987.
21. Gorski TT, Miller MM. *Staying Sober: Guide to Relapse Prevention.* Independence, Mo: Herald House; 1986.
22. Derogatis LR, Lipman RS, Rickels K. The Hopkins Symptom Checklist (HSCL): a self-report symptom inventory. *Behav Sci.* 1974;19:1-15.
23. Miller RG Jr. *Survival Analysis.* New York, NY: John Wiley & Sons Inc; 1981.
24. Mantel N. Chi-square tests with one degree of freedom: extensions of the Mantel-Haenszel procedure. *Am Stat Assoc J.* 1963;58:690-700.
25. Urquhart J. Ascertaining how much compliance is enough with outpatient antibiotic regimens. *Postgrad Med J.* 1992;68:S49-S59.
26. Cramer JA, Mattson RH, Prevey ML, Scheyer RD, Ouellette VL. How often is medication taken as prescribed? a novel assessment technique. *JAMA.* 1989;261: 3273-3277.

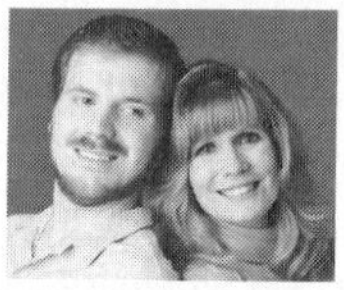

Double-blindness Procedures, Rater Blindness, and Ratings of Outcome

Observations From a Controlled Trial

Metin Başoğlu, MD, PhD; Isaac Marks, MD, FRCPsych; Maria Livanou; Richard Swinson, MD, FRCPsych

Background: We determined whether blindness in a double-blind randomized controlled trial of alprazolam and exposure therapies in patients with panic disorder and agoraphobia was maintained in assessors and patients, what were the factors related to "unblinding," and whether unblinding was associated with clinical outcome.

Method: In 129 patients with panic disorder and agoraphobia who were randomized to alprazolam-exposure, placebo-exposure, alprazolam-relaxation, or placebo-relaxation conditions, blindness was tested at the end of treatment by the independent assessors' and patients' classification of the treatment condition.

Results: Assessors' classifications were correct in 82% of the alprazolam group and 78% of the placebo group; corresponding figures for patients' classifications were 73% and 70%, respectively. Factors associated with unblinding included drug side effects but not assessors' ratings of treatment outcome.

Conclusion: Judgment of the validity of the outcome of a randomized controlled trial is easier if the report notes not only the use of a double-blindness procedure but also details how blind the raters remained and how any unblinding affected their ratings of clinical outcome.

Arch Gen Psychiatry. 1997;54:744-748

THE DOUBLE-BLIND procedure in clinical trials aims to reduce bias from the expectations of assessors and patients. Problems in maintaining assessor and/or patient blindness have been long known to researchers. Such problems have been experienced in drug trials involving medical conditions such as the common cold,[1] obesity,[2,3] myocardial infarction,[4-6] and smoking,[7] as well as psychiatric disorders such as schizophrenia,[8] aggressive behavior,[9] depression,[10] anxiety,[11-13] and panic disorder.[14,15] A comprehensive literature search[16] found that blindness was not maintained in 20 of the 23 double-blind studies of psychotropic drugs that tested blindness. Nevertheless, few studies report detailed tests of whether their double-blind procedures actually maintained blindness. Most researchers say their trial was double blind without reporting such testing.

Blindness may be invalidated in several ways. Patients and clinicians may be "unblinded" by the presence or absence of side effects.[2-4,7-9,13,15,17-23] Furthermore, patients may be alerted by the informed consent procedure telling them about potential side effects of the study drug.[2,7,14,15] Past experience with similar drugs may alert patients and clinicians to side effects of the trial drug.[3,10] Unblinding can also occur when the study tablets differ from each other in taste, color, or smell.[24] Finally, patients and clinicians may correctly identify the study tablets as active drug if improvement occurs and as placebo if there is no improvement.[1-3,5,10,12,13,15,25] Some argue for the testing of blindness from very early on in treatment on the assumption that ratings are then less influenced by clinical outcome.[7,10,15] However, improvement and unblinding may occur even early in treatment.[15]

In a trial based in London, England, and Toronto, Ontario,[26] our study examined how successfully a careful double-blind procedure maintained assessor blindness (at both sites) and patient blindness (at the London site only) and whether correct classification of the treatment related to side effects, drug dose, or clinical outcome. A 2×2 design was used involving combinations of drug and psychological treatments (alprazolam-exposure, alprazolam-relaxation, placebo-exposure, placebo-relaxation conditions). We aimed to draw attention yet again to the importance of testing blindness in clinical tri-

From the Section of Experimental Psychopathology, Department of Psychiatry, University of London, London, England (Drs Başoğlu and Marks and Ms Livanou); and the Department of Psychiatry, Clark Institute of Psychiatry, Toronto, Ontario (Dr Swinson).

PATIENTS, MATERIALS, AND METHODS

DESCRIPTION OF CLINICAL TRIAL

Details of study design, procedures, and assessment are reported by Marks et al.[26] In brief, 154 patients with panic disorder and agoraphobia were randomized to 1 of the 4 treatment conditions. Of the 154 patients, 82 were treated at the London site and 72 were treated at the Toronto site. Assessors and patients were unaware of alprazolam vs placebo conditions, whereas only assessors were unaware of psychological treatment.

Before trial entry, all prior psychotropic drug therapy was withdrawn, followed by screening and drug-free washout (mean time, 23 days; SD, 17 days) to week 0. Patients underwent individual outpatient treatment from weeks 0 to 8, tapering of medication therapy to discontinuation from weeks 8 to 16, and then follow-up to week 43. After baseline evaluation at week 0, a psychiatrist prescribed the medication, and a behavior therapist (psychiatrist, nurse, or other) gave the psychological treatment. Patients were alerted to potential drug side effects by the informed consent procedure.

Dose was as in phase 2 of the Cross-National Collaborative Panic Study.[29] Alprazolam tablet strengths were 1.0 mg from weeks 0 to 8 and 1.0, 0.5, 0.375, and 0.25 mg during tapering; placebo tablets were matched for taste, color, size, and smell. Tablet doses began at week 0 with 1 mg/d, rising to a mean of 6 mg/d or more (up to 10 mg/d) if needed to eliminate panic and markedly reduce phobic avoidance. Up to 3 attempts were made to raise medication doses to 10 tablets per day. Rise in dose ceased when patients became panic free, with much reduced avoidance. If patients had undue side effects, the dose was reduced stepwise until tolerance occurred, after which the dose was raised again. Side effects were monitored by the assessor throughout the treatment. The medication was prescribed and dose adjustments were made jointly by the assessor and the therapist.

From weeks 8 to 16, medication therapy was tapered no faster than 1 tablet per day for 3 days, to 4 mg; below that, taper was even slower, down to 0.25 mg (the patient was not told the dose). Dose at week 8 decided taper duration (mean time, 8.4 weeks; SD, 1.1), after which treatment ceased.

At each visit the number of remaining tablets was noted by the therapist. Venous blood (7 mL) samples were taken at weeks 0, 4, 8, 18 (2 weeks following slower taper), 23, and 43 to analyze plasma benzodiazepine and psychotropic drug levels (these were only made known at the end of the trial). By week 4, patients took a mean of 4.4 (SD, 1.7) mg of alprazolam; by week 8, 5.1 (SD, 2.2) mg/d of alprazolam; by week 4, 5.1 (SD, 2.2) tablets of placebo; and by week 8, 7.4 (SD, 2.2) tablets of placebo. Mean plasma alprazolam level was 45 ng/L at weeks 4 to 8 among the alprazolam group and 0 ng/L among the placebo group. The assessors had no knowledge of the patients' alprazolam plasma levels.

Ratings of clinical outcome were made at weeks 0, 2, 4, 6, and 8. To remain blind, the assessor was not told of and asked patients not to reveal their psychological treatment conditions. The classification of treatment condition by assessors and patients was performed at week 8. After the assessment was completed, assessors filled in a questionnaire consisting of 3 items (My guess is that this patient has been receiving [a] alprazolam or [b] placebo; My guess is that this patient has been receiving [a] exposure or [b] no exposure; and Did the patient reveal to you the type of psychological therapy s/he received during the treatment period? [a] yes or [b] no) and then asked patients whether they thought they were receiving alprazolam or placebo. Thus, certainty of classification was not rated, and a response of "don't know" was not allowed.

VARIABLES ANALYZED

Variables included classification of treatment condition by assessors and patients, the Clinician's Global Impression (CGI) scale, the Patient's Global Impression (PGI) scale (for both scales, 1 indicates very much improved; 2, much improved; 3, minimally improved; 4, no change; 5, minimally worse; 6, much worse; and 7, very much worse), and the assessor-rated Side Effects–Interference With Function scale (0 indicates none; 1, does not interfere significantly with patient function; 2, significantly interferes with patient function; and 3, nullifies therapeutic effect). A rating of 3 on the latter scale meant that the patient was unable to perform daily activities or homework exercises or avoided spontaneous or prescribed outings in phobic situations because of side effects such as sedation or drowsiness and impaired mental or motor coordination. The CGI and PGI were used in phases 1 and 2 of the Cross-National Collaborative Panic Study.[29,30] These variables correlate highly with other self- and assessor-rated clinical ratings, particularly of phobia.[31]

STATISTICAL ANALYSIS

Of the 154 patients who entered the trial, 134 underwent evaluation on clinical outcome ratings at week 6. Five patients dropped out between weeks 6 and 8, leaving 129 patients (67 patients in London and 62 patients in Toronto) for analysis at week 8. At week 8, data on the assessors' classification of treatment condition were available for the 129 patients; data on the patients' classification of drug treatment condition were available for 60 patients in London.

The frequencies of correct and incorrect classification regarding treatment group were computed. We determined whether the proportion of correct classifications in each group was above that expected by chance (50%) using χ^2 analyses with Yates correction. We examined whether correct vs incorrect classifications were related to side effects, treatment outcome, and drug dose at week 8 using 2-tailed t tests, separately for the alprazolam and placebo groups. There were so few instances of incorrect classification of psychological treatment condition that factors related to correct classification could not be examined. The .05 level of significance was used for all analyses.

Drug dose was analyzed because a higher alprazolam dose may have been more anxiolytic, thus unblinding the assessor, and dose increments were stopped or delayed if patients reported intolerable side effects during treatment. This led to the placebo group taking more tablets per day than did the alprazolam group at week 8 (mean number, 7.4 [SD, 2.2] vs 5.1 [SD, 2.2], respectively; t=6.1; P<.001). Assessors may have been unblinded by tablet counts being less than the maximum for the alprazolam group and near maximum for the placebo group (10 tablets per day).

als. In addition, concerns about maintaining blindness have been raised mainly in relation to drug treatment and have received inadequate attention in psychological treatment trials. Indeed, most studies of psychological treatment, with few exceptions,[27,28] did not report testing of blindness.

RESULTS

TREATMENT EFFECTS ON CGI-RATED IMPROVEMENT

Alprazolam and exposure therapies had a significant effect on CGI ratings of improvement at week 8 (F=9.2, *P*<.01 and F=24.0, *P*<.001, respectively). The interaction effect just failed to reach significance (F=3.3, *P*=.07), reflecting less improvement in the placebo-relaxation group than in the alprazolam-relaxation group.

Table 1. Percentage of Correct and Incorrect Classifications of Treatment

Classifications	Actual Treatment, No. (%) of Patients: Alprazolam Group	Placebo Group	Total	χ^2	*P*
Assessors					
Alprazolam	56 (82)*	12 (18)	**68 (100)**	44.8	<.001
Placebo	13 (22)	47 (78)*	**60 (100)**		
Patients†					
Alprazolam	24 (73)*	9 (27)	**33 (100)**	9.4	.002
Placebo	8 (30)	19 (70)*	**27 (100)**		
	Psychological Treatment: Exposure	**Relaxation**			
Assessors					
Exposure	60 (90)*	7 (10)	**67 (100)**	84.7	<.001
Relaxation	4 (7)	57 (93)*	**61 (100)**		

**The asterisk indicates correct classification.*
†Analyses based on London data only.

PERCENTAGES OF CORRECT CLASSIFICATIONS

Classifications by assessor and patient regarding treatment conditions appear in **Table 1**. Assessors' classifications were correct in 82% of the alprazolam group and 78% of the placebo group; corresponding figures for patients' classification were 73% and 70%, respectively. The proportion of assessors' correct classifications of psychological treatment condition was even higher (90% for exposure and 93% for relaxation). All χ^2 values were highly significant.

Table 2 compares patients who were correctly classified as receiving alprazolam or placebo with those incorrectly classified in terms of side effects, drug dose at week 8 (number of tablets per day), and improvement.

For the alprazolam group, assessors' correct classifications related to more side effects and to higher drug dose but not to treatment outcome. Patients' correct classifications also related to more side effects but not to drug dose or treatment outcome. For the placebo group, assessors' correct classifications related to fewer side effects and tended to relate to lower drug dose, but not to their own ratings of treatment outcome. Patients' correct classifications related to their own rating of less improvement (PGI), but not to side effects or drug dose.

EFFECT OF PAST DRUG USE

Of the 128 patients eligible for analysis, 75 (58.6%) had taken psychotropic medication before trial entry. Previous experience of drugs did not relate to patients' correct classifications in the alprazolam group (χ^2 after Yates correction, 0.20; *df*=1; *P*=.66) or in the placebo group (χ^2 after Yates correction, 0.87; *df*=1; *P*=.35).

SIDE EFFECTS VS RATINGS OF CLINICAL OUTCOME

Although the double-blind procedure did not fully maintain blindness because of side effects, correct classification did not relate to ratings of clinical outcome in the

Table 2. Relationship Between Classification of Treatment Condition and Side Effects, Drug Dose, and Clinical Improvement*

Ratings	Alprazolam Group: Classification: Correct	Incorrect	*t*	*P*	Placebo Group: Classification: Correct	Incorrect	*t*	*P*
Assessor								
No. of patients	56	12	...	...	47	13	...	...
Side effects†	0.9 (0.6)	0.3 (0.5)	−3.6	<.001	0.2 (0.4)	0.8 (0.9)	2.7	.02
Drug dose, mean (SD) No. of tablets per day	4.6 (2.0)	7.0 (2.0)	3.6	<.001	7.8 (1.8)	6.1 (3.0)	−1.9	.07
Mean (SD) CGI†	2.3 (0.9)	2.1 (0.9)	−0.8	.43	2.8 (1.2)	2.5 (1.2)	−0.9	.38
Patient								
No. of patients	24	8	...	...	19	9	...	...
Side effects†	1.0 (0.6)	0.3 (0.5)	−3.7	<.001	0.2 (0.5)	0.1 (0.3)	−0.3	.80
Drug dose, mean (SD) No. of tablets per day	5.4 (2.4)	6.3 (2.2)	0.98	.38	9.0 (1.4)	7.4 (2.6)	−1.7	.12
Mean (SD) PGI†	2.3 (1.2)	2.3 (1.2)	−0.1	.49	3.1 (1.0)	1.6 (0.9)	−3.9	<.001

**CGI indicates Clinician's Global Improvement scale; PGI, Patient's Global Improvement scale.*
†Scoring is described in the "Description of Clinical Trial" subsection of the "Materials and Methods" section of the text.

alprazolam group. Any bias by assessors and patients in favor of alprazolam may have been offset by antitherapeutic effects of side effects. Compared with the placebo group (*t* tests), the alprazolam group had higher scores for side effects at week 8 (mean scores, 0.8 [SD, 0.6] vs 0.3 [SD, 0.6]; $t=4.5$; $P<.001$). In the alprazolam group, more severe side effects correlated with less improvement at week 8 in the CGI ($r=0.23$; $P<.05$) and PGI ($r=0.26$; $P<.05$) scores.

COMMENT

In our study, double blindness was not fully maintained, as in most previous reports where this issue has been tested. The unblinding of assessors, however, did not necessarily invalidate their ratings of treatment outcome, because their outcome ratings were not associated with correct classification of the treatment condition. The latter finding should be interpreted with caution, however, because of the relatively few numbers of incorrect classifications (ranging from 8-13) on which the *t* tests were based.

Unblinding of the assessors may in part be due to the fact that they rated drug side effects repeatedly throughout treatment and adjusted drug dose in consultation with the therapist. Furthermore, they were not kept unaware of the number of tablets each patient was taking at any assessment week. Because a flexible drug dose regimen was used in the trial, the alprazolam group took fewer tablets per day at week 8 than did the placebo group (mean number of tablets, 5.1 vs 7.4, respectively). Assessors could deduce that someone taking nearly 10 tablets per day was more likely to be receiving placebo than alprazolam. These problems could have been avoided by having an independent psychiatrist, uninvolved in assessment of patients, monitor side effects and drug prescription. Furthermore, in future studies it might be useful to give both groups the same number of tablets (some of which would be placebo in the active drug group) and to increase the dose of active drug while always keeping the total number of pills constant. This procedure would blind everyone to drug status except the independent psychiatrist.

Unblinding, however, was not associated with the assessors' ratings of clinical response in the alprazolam group. This may be partly due to the drug side effects interfering with clinical improvement. In drug trials where the active drug has therapeutic and side effects independent of each other, assessor unblinding is more likely to affect ratings of clinical outcome. In our study, drug side effects such as impaired mental and behavioral coordination may have increased phobic avoidance by further undermining patients' sense of control over phobic situations. Indeed, lack of control over stressors can induce panic in patients with panic disorder.[32] This explanation is further supported by patient diaries; patients who had more side effects carried out less self-exposure and felt more anxious in phobic situations.[33] In addition, the fact that half of the placebo group had exposure therapy and that they improved as much as those in the alprazolam group who had exposure therapy[26] may have confounded any relationship between unblinding and ratings of clinical outcome. Furthermore, there was no drug effect on panic (due to a strong placebo effect on panic), which may have made it harder for assessors to identify the alprazolam group from clinical outcome alone.

Patients' correct classifications related to clinical outcome only in the placebo group. Of all 27 patients in the London placebo group, 19 who were unimproved correctly classified their placebo condition, whereas 8 patients who were markedly improved mistakenly classified an alprazolam condition. As we had no early ratings of blindness, we cannot tell if lack of improvement in the 19 patients led to their unblinding or vice versa. Similarly, it is unclear if the 8 patients' mistake was due to their improvement or vice versa.

We could not study factors related to correct classification of psychological treatment, as treatment condition was incorrectly classified in too few patients. Twenty of the 139 patients accidentally revealed their psychological treatment to the assessor during the trial. In other cases, it was fairly easy to be unblinded by the patients' accounts of progress on their target phobias, which best reflected the effects of exposure therapy on phobic avoidance. Thus, unblinding concerning psychological treatment may not necessarily have affected the ratings of clinical outcome, as these ratings may have reflected true treatment response.

Several conclusions arise from our study. Use of a double-blind procedure is no guarantee that rater blindness is maintained regarding medication or psychological treatment. The validity of trial results can therefore be better judged if blindness is tested in a repeated fashion, preferably starting early in treatment. A better way of testing blindness than that we used may be to ask the raters to classify the treatment condition and indicate their level of certainty. The raters would be allowed to respond "don't know" and asked to refrain from merely hazarding a guess. A high percentage of this response would indicate success of the blinding procedures. Information also needs to be obtained as to the reasons for raters' classifications, so that unblinding due to real treatment effects (eg, clinical response or side effects) can be distinguished from unblinding due to failures in blinding procedures. If unblinding has occurred but outcome ratings are not associated with correct classification, then the results can be accepted with some confidence. If there is an association between outcome ratings and correct classification, this may not necessarily indicate that the blindness procedures have failed, since this association may reflect true effect of treatment.

Accepted for publication October 8, 1996.

Supported by grants from the Upjohn Company, Kalamazoo, Mich, for the treatment phase.

Reprints: Metin Başoğlu, MD, PhD, Institute of Psychiatry, 99 Denmark Hill, London SE5 8AF, England.

REFERENCES

1. Karlowski TR, Chalmers TC, Frenkel LD, Kapikian AZ, Lewis TL, Lynch JM. Ascorbic acid for the common cold. *JAMA*. 1975;231:1038-1042.

2. Brownell KD, Stunkard AJ. The double-blind in danger: untoward consequences of informed consent. *Am J Psychiatry.* 1982;139:1487-1489.
3. Moscucci M, Byrne L, Weintraub M, Cox C. Blinding, unblinding and the placebo effect: an analysis of patients' guesses of treatment assignment in a double-blind clinical trial. *Clin Pharmacol Ther.* 1987;41:259-265.
4. Howard J, Whittemore AS, Hoover J, Panos M, and the Aspirin Myocardial Infarction Study Research Group. How blind was the patient blind in AMIS? *Clin Pharmacol Ther.* 1982;32:543-553.
5. Byington R, Curb DJ, Mattson ME. Assessment of blindness at the conclusion of the β-blocker heart attack trial. *JAMA.* 1985;253:1733-1736.
6. Jespersen CM, and the Danish Study Group on Verapamil in Myocardial Infarction. Assessment of blindness in the Danish Verapamil Infarction Trial II (DAVIT II): Danish Study Group on Verapamil in Myocardial Infarction. *Eur J Clin Pharmacol.* 1990;39:75-76.
7. Hughes JR, Krahn D. Blindness and validity of the double-blind procedure. *J Clin Psychopharmacol.* 1985;5:138-142.
8. Engelhardt DM, Margolis RA, Rudorfer L, Paley HM. Physician bias and the double-blind. *Arch Gen Psychiatry.* 1969;20:315-320.
9. Marini JL, Sheard MH, Bridges CI, Wagner E. An evaluation of the double-blind design in a study comparing lithium carbonate with placebo. *Acta Psychiatr Scand.* 1976;53:343-354.
10. Rabkin JG, Markowitz JS, Stewart J, McGrath P, Harrison W, Quitkin FM, Klein DF. How blind is blind? assessment of patient and doctor medication guesses in a placebo-controlled trial of imipramine and phenelzine. *Psychiatr Res.* 1986; 19:75-86.
11. Uhlenhuth EH, Canter A, Neustadt JO, Payson HE. The symptomatic relief of anxiety with meprobamate, phenobarbital and placebo. *Am J Psychiatry.* 1959;115: 905-910.
12. Rickels K, Cattell RB, Weise C, Gray B, Yee R, Mallin A, Aaronson HG. Controlled psychopharmacological research in private psychiatric practice. *Psychopharmacology (Berl).* 1966;9:288-306.
13. Rickels K, Lipman RS, Fisher S, Park LC, Uhlenhuth EH. Is a double-blind clinical trial really double-blind? a report of doctors' medication guesses. *Psychopharmacology (Berl).* 1970;16:329-336.
14. Munjack DJ, Brown RA, McDowell D, Palmer R. Actual medication versus therapist guesses: in a blind study, how blind is blind? *J Clin Psychopharmacol.* 1989; 9:148-149.
15. Margraf J, Ehlers A, Roth WT, Clark DB, Sheikh J, Agras WS, Taylor CB. How 'blind' are double-blind studies? *J Consult Clin Psychol.* 1991;59:184-187.
16. Fisher S, Greenberg RP. How blind is the double-blind design for evaluating psychotropic drugs? *J Nerv Ment Dis.* 1993;181:345-350.
17. White K, Kando J, Pharm D, Park T, Waternaux C, Brown WA. Side effects and the 'blindability' of clinical drug trials. *Am J Psychiatry.* 1992;149:1730-1731.
18. Oxtoby A, Jones A, Robinson M. Is your 'double-blind' design truly double-blind? *Br J Psychiatry.* 1989;155:700-701.
19. Naylor GJ, Martin B, Hopwood SE, Watson Y. A two-year double-blind cross-over trial of the prophylactic effect of methylene blue in manic-depressive psychosis. *Biol Psychiatry.* 1986;21:915-920.
20. Ney PG, Collins C, Spensor C. Double-blind: double-talk or are there ways to do better research? *Med Hypotheses.* 1986;21:119-126.
21. Adelman HS, Compas BE. Stimulant drugs and learning problems. *J Special Educ.* 1977;11:377-416.
22. Letemendia FJJ, Harris AD. The influence of side-effects on the reporting of symptoms. *Psychopharmacology (Berl).* 1959;1:39-47.
23. Wing L. The use of reserpine in chronic psychotic patients: a controlled study. *J Ment Sci.* 1956;102:530-541.
24. Hill LE, Nunn AJ, Fox W. Matching qualities of agents employed in double-blind controlled clinical trials. *Lancet.* 1976;1:352-356.
25. Krammer MS, Shapiro SH. Scientific challenges in the application of randomized trials. *JAMA.* 1986;252:2739-2745.
26. Marks IM, Swinson RP, Başoğlu M, Kuch K, Noshirvani H, O'Sullivan G, Lelliott P, Kirby M, McNamee G, Şengün S, Wickwire K. Alprazolam and exposure alone and combined in panic disorder with agoraphobia: a controlled study in London and Toronto. *Br J Psychiatry.* 1993;162:776-787.
27. Marks IM, Gray S, Cohen D, Hill R, Mawson D, Ramm E, Stern RS. Imipramine and brief therapist-aided exposure in agoraphobics having self-exposure homework. *Arch Gen Psychiatry.* 1983;40:153-162.
28. Marks IM, Stern RS, Mawson D, Cobb J, McDonald R. Clomipramine and exposure for obsessive-compulsive rituals, I. *Br J Psychiatry.* 1980;136:1-25.
29. Cross-National Collaborative Panic Study, Second Phase Investigators. Drug treatment of panic disorder: comparative efficacy of alprazolam, imipramine and placebo. *Br J Psychiatry.* 1992;160:191-202.
30. Ballenger JC, Burrows GD, DuPont RL Jr, Lesser IM, Noyes R, Pecknold JC, Rifkin A, Swinson RP. Alprazolam in panic disorder and agoraphobia: results from a multicenter trial, I: efficacy in short-term treatment. *Arch Gen Psychiatry.* 1988; 45:413-422.
31. Başoğlu M, Marks IM, Kiliç C, Noshirvani H, O'Sullivan G. The relationship between panic, anticipatory anxiety, agoraphobia, and global improvement in panic disorder with agoraphobia treated with alprazolam and exposure. *Br J Psychiatry.* 1994;164:647-652.
32. Sanderson W, Rapee R, Barlow D. The influence of an illusion of control on panic attacks induced via inhalation of 5.5% carbon dioxide-enriched air. *Arch Gen Psychiatry.* 1989;46:157-162.
33. Başoğlu M. *Patterns and Predictors of Treatment Outcome in Panic Disorder and Agoraphobia Treated With Alprazolam and Exposure.* London, England: University of London; 1993. Dissertation.

Noradrenergic and Serotonergic Function in Posttraumatic Stress Disorder

Steven M. Southwick, MD; John H. Krystal, MD; J. Douglas Bremner, MD; C. A. Morgan III, MD; Andreas L. Nicolaou, PhD; Linda M. Nagy, MD; David R. Johnson, PhD; George R. Heninger, MD; Dennis S. Charney, MD

Background: Yohimbine hydrochloride produces marked behavioral and cardiovascular effects in combat veterans with posttraumatic stress disorder (PTSD). In the present study, yohimbine was used as a probe of noradrenergic activity, and meta-chlorophenylpiperazine (m-CPP) as a probe of serotonergic activity. To our knowledge, this is the first study to describe the behavioral and cardiovascular effects of meta-CPP in patients with PTSD, and to compare these effects with those of yohimbine.

Method: Twenty-six patients with PTSD and 14 healthy subjects each received an intravenous infusion of yohimbine hydrochloride (0.4 mg/kg), m-CPP (1.0 mg/kg), or saline solution on 3 separate test days in a randomized balanced order and in double-blind fashion. Behavioral and cardiovascular measurements were determined at multiple times.

Results: Eleven (42%) of the patients with PTSD experienced yohimbine-induced panic attacks and had significantly greater increases compared with controls in anxiety, panic, and PTSD symptoms, but not in cardiovascular measurements. Eight patients (31%) with PTSD experienced m-CPP–induced panic attacks and had significantly greater increases compared with controls in anxiety, panic, and PTSD symptoms, and in standing diastolic blood pressure. Yohimbine-induced panic attacks tended to occur in different patients from m-CPP–induced panic attacks.

Conclusion: These data suggest the presence of 2 neurobiological subgroups of patients with PTSD, one with a sensitized noradrenergic system, and the other with a sensitized serotonergic system.

Arch Gen Psychiatry. 1997;54:749-758

THE NORADRENERGIC system has been the most intensively studied neural system in humans suffering from posttraumatic stress disorder (PTSD). This system was chosen as a focus of study because of extensive preclinical data linking it to fear and anxiety,[1-9] vigilance,[10-12] selective attention,[12-15] and consolidation of memory.[16-24] Persons with PTSD often suffer with analogous symptoms of hypervigilance, anxiety, fear, and recurrent intrusive memories. Norepinephrine also was selected because of its central role in the sympathetic nervous system and in what is commonly termed the "flight or fight response." Since 1918, many psychophysiological studies consistently have shown heightened sympathetic nervous system reactivity in combat veterans with trauma-related symptoms.[25-33]

Evidence of noradrenergic dysregulation in PTSD also has come from investigations of neuroendocrine and peripheral catecholamine receptor systems. Twenty-four–hour urine norepinephrine excretion[34,35] has been reported as significantly elevated and platelet α_2-adrenergic receptor number[36] and lymphocyte basal cyclic adenosine monophosphate and adenylate cyclase levels[37] as significantly decreased in combat veterans with PTSD compared with normal controls. In a study that simultaneously evaluated psychophysiological and peripheral noradrenergic activity in response to viewing a combat film, Blanchard et al[38] reported a parallel rise in blood pressure, heart rate, subjective distress, and plasma norepinephrine in combat veterans with PTSD.

We recently reported on the use of yohimbine hydrochloride as a probe of peripheral and central noradrenergic reactivity in 20 combat veterans with PTSD.[39] Yohimbine is an α_2-adrenergic receptor antagonist that activates noradrenergic neurons by blocking the presynaptic α_2-adrenergic autoreceptor.[40-42] Patients with PTSD had potentiated biochemical, behavioral, and cardiovascular responses to yohimbine. Indeed, 70% of patients expe-

From the Clinical Neurosciences Division, National Center for Post-Traumatic Stress Disorder, Veterans Affairs Medical Center, West Haven, Conn (Drs Southwick, Krystal, Bremner, Morgan, Nicolaou, Nagy, Johnson, Heninger, and Charney); and the Department of Psychiatry, Yale University School of Medicine, New Haven, Conn (Drs Southwick, Krystal, Bremner, Morgan, Nagy, Johnson, Heninger, and Charney).

PATIENTS AND METHODS

PATIENTS

Twenty-six male patients were recruited from a 4-month inpatient PTSD treatment program at the National Center for Post-Traumatic Stress Disorder located in the Connecticut Department of Veterans Affairs Medical Center, West Haven, Conn. Military records, including the DD214, were used to verify Vietnam combat experience. Exclusion criteria included organic mental disorders; neurologic disorders, such as seizures; cardiovascular disease, including hypertension, history of myocardial infarction, or significant electrocardiographic abnormalities; and serious medical illnesses, such as diabetes and chronic hepatitis.

Mean±SEM age was 41.8±0.5 years. Mean±SEM weight was 85.6±2.6 kg. A 4-week drug-free period, monitored by staff, was required of all patients before the first test session.

Each patient who gave voluntary written informed consent for participation in this study met criteria for PTSD using the structured clinical interview for *DSM-III-R*[92] and had a Mississippi Post-Traumatic Stress Disorder scale score greater than 107.[93] Mean±SEM severity of PTSD on the Mississippi scale was 132.9±3.8 of a possible 175. This is considered to be severe PTSD.[93]

A consensus diagnostic team finalized all diagnoses. Six patients and 15 patients met current *DSM-III-R* criteria for panic disorder and major depression, respectively, on admission to the study. Eighteen patients met lifetime *DSM-III-R* diagnostic criteria for major depression, 6 for lifetime panic disorder, and 20 for lifetime alcohol dependence.

HEALTHY SUBJECTS

Fourteen healthy male subjects, recruited from responses to advertisements, gave voluntary written informed consent for participation in the study and were determined to be free of mental disorder based on the results of a structured psychiatric interview. None reported a history of mental illness in first-degree relatives or use of psychoactive medication for at least 4 weeks. Mean±SEM age was 39.8±3.7 years. Mean±SEM weight was 81.0±2.7 kg.

None had a history of serious medical illness. All had normal results on physical examination, electrocardiogram, and laboratory tests of renal, hepatic, pancreatic, hematopoietic, and thyroid function. Healthy controls and patients were paid for participation in this study.

PROCEDURES

On 3 separate test days during 20-minute infusions in a randomized balanced order and in double-blind fashion, patients and healthy subjects received an intravenous infusion of yohimbine hydrochloride (0.4 mg/kg), m-CPP (0.1 mg/kg), or saline solution. On each test day, subjects received two 10-minute infusions. On the saline test day, both infusions consisted of 0.9% saline solution. On the m-CPP test day, both 10-minute infusions contained 0.05 mg/kg of m-CPP for a total of 0.1 mg/kg for 20 minutes. On the test day for yohimbine, one infusion contained yohimbine hydrochloride (0.4 mg/kg administered for 10 minutes), and the other infusion consisted of saline solution infused for 10 minutes. The m-CPP doses and rates of infusion were identical to those of previously reported studies in healthy subjects,[88] and in patients with panic disorder,[77] obsessive-compulsive disorder,[83] and schizophrenia.[90] Investigators and raters were not aware of the medication status except for the research pharmacist. The interval between infusions was generally 4 to 7 days.

Subjects arrived on the Neurobiological Studies Unit by 8:30 AM. They fasted overnight for 10 hours, were supine with their heads elevated during most of the 5-hour

rienced panic attacks and 40% experienced flashbacks after yohimbine administration. The 70% panic attack rate closely resembles the experience reported in patients with panic disorder,[43-45] raising the possibility that PTSD and panic disorder share a common neurobiological abnormality related to the noradrenergic system.[39]

Although yohimbine clearly has pronounced effects in combat veterans with PTSD, it is unclear whether other anxiogenic probes that alter the function of different neurotransmitter systems would produce similar reactions in this patient population. The present study was designed to test the specificity of the yohimbine response in combat veterans with PTSD and to evaluate potential serotonergic (5-HT) contributions to trauma-related symptoms. Altered 5-HT activity following severe stress or trauma has been reported in animal and human studies.[46-53] In humans, for example, platelet 5-HT uptake has been reported as significantly decreased in patients with PTSD compared with normal controls,[53] and specific 5-HT reuptake inhibitors have been found to be moderately efficacious in treating the full range of PTSD-specific symptoms in a subgroup of traumatized patients.[54-58] Furthermore, low 5-HT activity in humans has been associated with aggression,[59] impulsivity,[59] and suicide,[60] behaviors that often are reported in combat veterans with PTSD.

In the present study, yohimbine was used as a probe of noradrenergic activity, and meta-chlorophenylpiperazine (m-CPP) was used as a probe of 5-HT activity in combat veterans with PTSD compared with normal controls. The m-CPP interacts with the 5-HT transporter[61] and several 5-HT receptor subtypes, including, in descending affinity, the 5-HT$_3$, 5-HT$_{2C}$, 5-HT$_{2A/B}$, 5-HT$_7$, 5-HT$_{1A}$, and 5-HT$_{1D}$ receptors.[62-66] Meta-chlorophenylpiperazine is a partial agonist at 5-HT$_1$ receptors,[65-67] a partial agonist or antagonist of the 5-HT$_2$ receptor,[68-70] and an antagonist of 5-HT$_3$ receptors.[71,72] Relative to its potency at 5-HT$_{2C}$ receptors, m-CPP seems to possess markedly lower affinities for α_1, α_2, dopamine$_1$, and dopamine$_2$ receptors.[63,73] Meta-chlorophenylpiperazine has been used widely to investigate 5-HT function in neuropsychiatric disorders such as panic disorder,[74-77] obsessive-compulsive disorder,[78-83] schizophrenia,[84] depression,[85-87] and alcoholism.[88-91] These investigations disclose that, depending on the disorder under study,[74-91] m-CPP has a broad spectrum of behavioral test day, and stood only to use the bathroom and to permit recordings of their standing blood pressure and pulse rate. Sleep was not permitted. Blood pressure and pulse rate were measured in the usual clinical fashion at 15 and 0.5 minutes before and at 40, 60, 120, and 180 minutes following the dose.

Self-report behavioral ratings were administered 15 minutes before and at 20, 60, 120, and 180 minutes after infusion. Panic attack symptoms were assessed using a 27-item Panic Attack Symptom Scale (PASS) that includes the 13 *DSM-III-R* panic symptoms. Possible scores range from 27 to 108. Symptoms are rated on a 4-point scale (1=not present to 4=severe). The PTSD-specific symptoms were measured using a scale consisting of 8 *DSM-III-R* items (anger, difficulty concentrating, distant from others, emotionally numb, flashbacks, hypervigilance, intrusive thoughts, and startle). Symptoms are rated on a 5-point scale (1=not present to 5=worst ever), with possible scores ranging from 8 to 40.

To determine whether a panic attack or flashback had occurred during test sessions, all subjects were evaluated by a research psychiatrist (S.M.S. or J.H.K.) and a research nurse who were not aware of the medication status. This evaluation was based on direct clinical observation and patient self-report.

Panic attacks were determined using the following criteria: (1) increase in severity of 4 or more *DSM-III-R* panic attack symptoms on the PASS compared with baseline; (2) crescendo increase in severe subjective anxiety of at least 25 mm from baseline on a 100-mm visual analog scale for anxiety; (3) for patients with a history of panic attacks, the drug-induced anxiety state had to be similar to a naturally occurring panic attack in intensity and specific symptoms; (4) consensual agreement of the 2 research psychiatrists (S.M.S. and J.H.K.) that a panic attack had occurred based on the aforementioned 3 criteria and nursing notes.

Flashbacks were determined using the following criteria: (1) reexperiencing a past traumatic event during the course of drug or placebo infusion; (2) involvement of 1 or more sensory modalities (hearing, seeing, smelling, and/or feeling); (3) for patients with a history of flashbacks, the drug-induced reexperiencing state must have been similar to a naturally occurring flashback; and (4) consensual agreement of the 2 research psychiatrists that a flashback had occurred.

DATA ANALYSIS

Data were analyzed with standard Statistical Analysis System procedures. Effects of yohimbine and m-CPP on anxiety, PTSD symptom ratings, and cardiovascular variables were evaluated with repeated-measures analysis of variance (ANOVA). Initial analyses included all time points. Subsequent pairwise comparisons involved baseline and peak measurements between particular test days for individual items. Assessments of statistical significance included main effects of diagnosis, drug (placebo vs yohimbine or m-CPP), and time. The α levels were adjusted for multiple comparisons.

We used *t* tests to determine how and when patients differed from healthy subjects in response to both active agents compared with placebo and with each other. Baseline values were subtracted from values at each time point for the variable of interest, resulting in a change score for each time point. Subtracting this change score for placebo from that of yohimbine resulted in an estimate of the net yohimbine effect. Similar estimates were calculated comparing m-CPP with placebo and m-CPP with yohimbine.

Pearson correlation coefficients (for symptoms significantly increased in response to either or both active agents compared with placebo) evaluate the relations between peak changes from baseline in individual symptoms following m-CPP and yohimbine. The α levels were adjusted for multiple comparisons.

effects, including exacerbation of anxiety, psychosis, and obsessions.

In the present report, 26 combat veterans with *DSM-III-R* PTSD and 14 noncombat healthy controls were administered intravenous yohimbine, m-CPP, and placebo on 3 separate test days. Subjects were rated for panic attacks, flashbacks, anxiety symptoms and *DSM-III-R* PTSD-specific symptoms, and blood pressure and heart rate responses. To our knowledge, this is the first study to describe the subjective, behavioral, and cardiovascular effects of m-CPP in patients with PTSD and the first to compare these effects with those of yohimbine.

RESULTS

FREQUENCY OF PANIC ATTACKS AND FLASHBACKS

Yohimbine produced panic attacks in 11 (42%) of 26 patients and 1 (7%) of 14 controls. Eight patients (31%) and no controls had a panic attack in response to m-CPP. Three patients had panic attacks in response to both active compounds. No panic attacks occurred after placebo administration. Flashbacks occurred after yohimbine in 8 patients (31%) and no controls. In response to m-CPP, 7 patients (27%) and no controls had flashbacks. Four of these patients had flashbacks while receiving both drugs. Two patients had flashbacks during placebo administration, both of whom also had flashbacks while receiving yohimbine and 1 while taking m-CPP. The drug administered on the first day was neither more nor less likely to cause a panic attack or a flashback than the drug administered on the second day.

PANIC ATTACK SYMPTOM SCALE

Effects of Yohimbine

Change Over Time From Baseline (**Figure 1**). Total PASS score was significantly higher following yohimbine compared with placebo in patients with PTSD (F=14.84, *df*=4,100, *P*<.001; at 20 minutes—*t*=5.96, *df*=25, *P*<.001; at 60 minutes—*t*=3.04, *df*=25, *P*<.01) and in healthy controls (F=18.62, *df*=4,52, *P*<.001; at 20 minutes—*t*=5.54, *df*=13, *P*<.001; at 60 minutes—*t*=3.64, *df*=13,

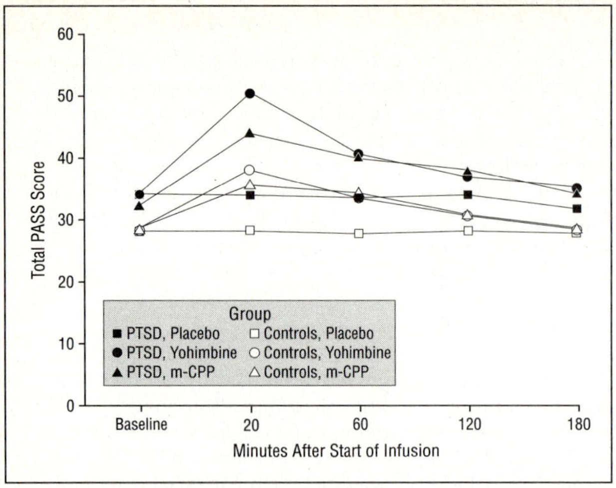

Figure 1. *Effects of yohimbine hydrochloride, meta-chlorophenylpiperazine (m-CPP), and placebo on total Panic Attack Symptom Scale (PASS) score in healthy controls and patients with posttraumatic stress disorder (PTSD).*

P<.005). The increased effects of yohimbine over placebo, however, were not significantly different in patients compared with controls (F=1.35, *df*=4,152, *P*=.56).

Peak Change From Baseline (**Table 1**). Patients and healthy controls were not significantly different on the total PASS score or on any of the individual items. However, patients who had yohimbine-induced panic attacks had significantly greater increases on the total PASS score compared with healthy controls and on 2 individual items: fear of going crazy and goose bumps. Compared with patients without yohimbine-induced panic attacks, patients with PTSD and panic attacks had significantly greater increases on the total PASS score, fear of losing control, fear of going crazy, and muscle twitching.

Effects of m-CPP

Change Over Time From Baseline (Figure 1). Total PASS score was significantly higher following m-CPP compared with placebo in patients (F=7.56, *df*=4,100, *P*<.001; at 20 minutes—*t*=4.13, *df*=25, *P*<.005; at 60 minutes—*t*=3.21, *df*=25, *P*<.005; at 120 minutes—*t*=2.96, *df*=25, *P*<.01; at 180 minutes—*t*=2.82, *df*=25, *P*<.01) and in healthy controls (F=9.10, *df*=4,52, *P*<.001; at 20 minutes—*t*=3.17, *df*=13, *P*<.01; at 60 minutes—*t*=2.98, *df*=13, *P*<.02), but not in patients compared with controls.

Peak Change From Baseline (Table 1). Change in total PASS score or in any of the individual items did not differ significantly between the total group of patients and controls. Patients with m-CPP–induced panic attacks had significantly greater increases on the total PASS score and on the items of choking or smothering sensation and feelings of unreality and irritability than did controls. Patients who experienced m-CPP–induced panic attacks, compared with patients who did not, had significantly greater increases on the total PASS score and on the following individual symptoms: choking or smothering sensation, feelings of unreality, muscle twitching, tremor or shakiness, uncoordination, and weakness.

Comparison of Yohimbine and m-CPP Behavioral Effects on PASS

In the group of 26 patients with PTSD, 11 individual PASS symptoms changed significantly over time in response to yohimbine or m-CPP. Responses to yohimbine were as follows (*df*=1,25 for all): sweating—F=27.12, *P*<.001; muscle aches—F=13.79, *P*<.001; nausea—F=9.35, *P*<.01; light-headedness—F=25.92, *P*<.001; dizziness—F=13.19, *P*<.002; restlessness—F=8.93, *P*<.01; hot or cold flashes—F=16.78, *P*<.001; uncoordination—F=4.89, *P*<.05; goose bumps—F=32.69, *P*<.001; tremor or shakiness—F=27.12, *P*<.001; and runny nose—F=18.65, *P*<.001. Responses to m-CPP were as follows (*df*=1,25 for all): sweating—F=4.38, *P*<.05; muscle aches—F=15.24, *P*<.001; nausea—F=14.25, *P*<.001; light-headedness—F=12.48, *P*<.01; dizziness—F=15.52, *P*<.001; restlessness—F=14.60, *P*<.001; hot or cold flashes—F=11.41, *P*<.01; uncoordination—F=15.72, *P*<.001; goose bumps—F=5.74, *P*<.05; tremor or shakiness—F=7.66, *P*<.01; and runny nose—F=4.38, *P*<.05. After adjusting for multiple comparisons (α=.004), Pearson correlations between peak changes over time were not significant for any of the symptoms.

PTSD SCALE

Effects of Yohimbine

Change Over Time From Baseline (**Figure 2**). Total PTSD score was significantly higher following yohimbine compared with placebo in patients (F=8.60, *df*=4,100, *P*<.001; at 20 minutes—*t*=4.09, *df*=25, *P*<.005; at 60 minutes—*t*=3.00, *df*=25, *P*<.01) and in healthy controls (F=6.83, *df*=4,52, *P*<.003; at 20 minutes— *t*=3.17, *df*=13, *P*<.01; at 60 minutes—*t*=2.31, *df*=13, *P*<.04). Patients with PTSD had a significantly greater yohimbine-placebo increase than did controls overall (F=2.68, *df*=4,152, *P*<.04) and at 20 minutes (*t*=−3.00, *df*=29.3, *P*<.01).

Peak Change From Baseline (**Table 2**). Peak change in total PTSD score and in individual items did not differ significantly between patients and controls. Patients with yohimbine-induced panic attacks had significantly greater increases in total PTSD score and intrusive thoughts than controls. On the other hand, there were no significant differences between patients with and without yohimbine-induced panic attacks.

Effects of m-CPP

Change Over Time From Baseline (Figure 2). Total PTSD score was significantly higher following m-CPP compared with placebo in patients with PTSD (F=4.61, *df*=4,100, *P*<.002; at 20 minutes— *t*=2.86, *df*=25, *P*<.01, at 60 minutes, *t*=3.27, *df*=25, *P*<.005; at 120 minutes—*t*=3.14, *df*=25, *P*<.005; at 180 minutes—*t*=2.47, *df*=25, *P*<.03) and in healthy controls (F=8.13, *df*=4,52, *P*<.001; at 20 minutes—*t*=3.28, *df*=13, *P*<.01; at 60 minutes—*t*=2.67, *df*=13, *P*<.02), but not in patients compared with healthy controls (F=1.31, *df*=4,152, *P*=.27).

Peak Change From Baseline (Table 2). There were no significant differences in any individual symptom or

Table 1. Effects of Intravenous Yohimbine or Meta-chlorophenylpiperazine Compared With Placebo on the Panic Attack Symptom Scale*

	Patients With Posttraumatic Stress Disorder†				Healthy Subjects (n=14)	
	With Panic Attacks		Without Panic Attacks			
Symptom	Baseline	Peak Change	Baseline	Peak Change	Baseline	Peak Change
Yohimbine hydrochloride vs placebo						
Fear of losing control						
Placebo	1.64 (0.30)	0.18 (0.14)	1.30 (0.14)	0.50 (0.23)‡	1.00 (0.00)	0.07 (0.07)
Yohimbine	1.68 (0.30)	1.41 (0.40)	1.50 (0.18)	−0.10 (0.11)	1.00 (0.00)	0.14 (0.10)
Fear of going crazy						
Placebo	1.50 (0.25)	−0.05 (0.08)	1.17 (0.09)	0.23 (0.17)‡	1.00 (0.00)	0.00 (0.00)§
Yohimbine	1.45 (0.24)	1.18 (0.35)	1.27 (0.15)	0.13 (0.10)	1.00 (0.00)	0.00 (0.00)
Goose bumps						
Placebo	1.09 (0.09)	0.00 (0.13)	1.17 (0.19)	0.03 (0.08)	1.00 (0.00)	0.00 (0.00)§
Yohimbine	1.09 (0.09)	1.55 (0.34)	1.03 (0.03)	1.03 (0.28)	1.00 (0.00)	0.21 (0.15)
Muscle twitching						
Placebo	1.18 (0.18)	0.18 (0.18)	1.20 (0.08)	0.47 (0.17)‡	1.07 (0.07)	0.00 (0.00)
Yohimbine	1.27 (0.19)	2.00 (0.36)	1.27 (0.17)	0.67 (0.24)	1.18 (0.14)	0.82 (0.29)
Total PASS score						
Placebo	33.45 (2.82)	3.00 (2.63)	34.20 (2.02)	2.73 (1.77)‡	27.79 (0.23)	0.71 (0.37)§
Yohimbine	34.05 (3.19)	28.05 (3.29)	33.97 (1.70)	11.10 (2.66)	28.54 (0.51)	9.89 (1.68)
m-CPP vs placebo						
Choking or smothering sensation						
Placebo	1.13 (0.13)	0.00 (0.00)	1.06 (0.06)	0.00 (0.00)‡	1.00 (0.00)	0.07 (0.07)§
m-CPP	1.06 (0.06)	1.44 (0.37)	1.06 (0.06)	0.22 (0.13)	1.00 (0.00)	0.14 (0.10)
Feelings of unreality						
Placebo	1.56 (0.26)	−0.19 (0.13)	1.17 (0.08)	0.33 (0.18)‡	1.00 (0.00)	0.07 (0.07)§
m-CPP	1.13 (0.13)	2.00 (0.38)	1.22 (0.10)	0.33 (0.16)	1.00 (0.00)	0.36 (0.17)
Irritability						
Placebo	1.69 (0.25)	−0.06 (0.24)	1.50 (0.17)	0.17 (0.19)	1.04 (0.04)	−0.04 (0.04)§
m-CPP	1.75 (0.30)	1.50 (0.28)	1.33 (0.13)	0.44 (0.16)	1.00 (0.00)	0.07 (0.07)
Muscle twitching						
Placebo	1.25 (0.13)	0.25 (0.13)	1.17 (0.11)	0.39 (0.17)‡	1.07 (0.07)	0.00 (0.00)
m-CPP	1.13 (0.13)	1.63 (0.38)	1.06 (0.06)	0.28 (0.14)	1.21 (0.21)	0.43 (0.25)
Tremor, shakiness						
Placebo	1.25 (0.16)	0.00 (0.00)	1.14 (0.07)	0.36 (0.16)‡	1.00 (0.00)	0.00 (0.00)
m-CPP	1.13 (0.08)	1.75 (0.35)	1.08 (0.06)	0.47 (0.16)	1.00 (0.00)	0.71 (0.27)
Uncoordination						
Placebo	1.31 (0.21)	0.06 (0.06)	1.14 (0.10)	0.08 (0.14)‡	1.00 (0.00)	0.00 (0.00)
m-CPP	1.06 (0.06)	1.44 (0.26)	1.14 (0.10)	0.36 (0.15)	1.00 (0.00)	0.36 (0.17)
Weakness						
Placebo	1.50 (0.21)	0.00 (0.16)	1.14 (0.08)	0.19 (0.16)‡	1.07 (0.05)	0.00 (0.09)
m-CPP	1.38 (0.25)	1.63 (0.36)	1.11 (0.09)	0.33 (0.11)	1.00 (0.00)	0.57 (0.17)
Total PASS score						
Placebo	35.81 (3.39)	2.44 (2.31)	33.03 (1.84)	3.03 (1.92)‡	27.79 (0.23)	0.71 (0.37)§
m-CPP	33.56 (2.62)	32.06 (4.13)	31.39 (1.41)	7.00 (1.73)	28.25 (0.39)	7.89 (2.11)

**Values are given as mean (±SEM). m-CPP indicates meta-chlorophenylpiperazine; PASS, Panic Attack Symptom Scale.*
†Patients with posttraumatic stress disorder and yohimbine-induced panic attacks, n=11; without yohimbine-induced panic attacks, n=15; with m-CPP–induced panic attacks, n=8; without m-CPP–induced panic attacks, n=18.
‡Statistically significant (P<.002) group×drug×time interaction (patients with panic attacks vs patients without panic attacks).
§Statistically significant (P<.002) group×drug×time interaction (patients with panic attacks vs healthy controls).

in total PTSD score between the patient group as a whole and controls. Compared with controls, patients who had m-CPP–induced panic attacks had a significantly greater increase in total PTSD score and in the following PTSD symptoms: anger, distant from others, flashbacks, hypervigilance, intrusive thoughts, and startle. Compared with patients without m-CPP–induced panic attacks, those with panic attacks had a significantly greater increase in total PTSD score and in the following specific symptoms: anger, difficulty concentrating, distant from others, and hypervigilance.

Comparison of Yohimbine and m-CPP Behavioral Effects on PTSD Scale

Relative to placebo, 4 symptoms (distant from others, intrusive thoughts, emotionally numb, and flashbacks) increased significantly in response to m-CPP or yohimbine in the group of 26 patients with PTSD. Responses to yohimbine were as follows (*df*=1,25 for all): distant from others, F=6.48, *P*<.05; intrusive thoughts, F=4.28, *P*<.05; emotionally numb, F=19.12, *P*<.001; and flashbacks, F=9.67, *P*<.01. Responses to m-CPP were as fol-

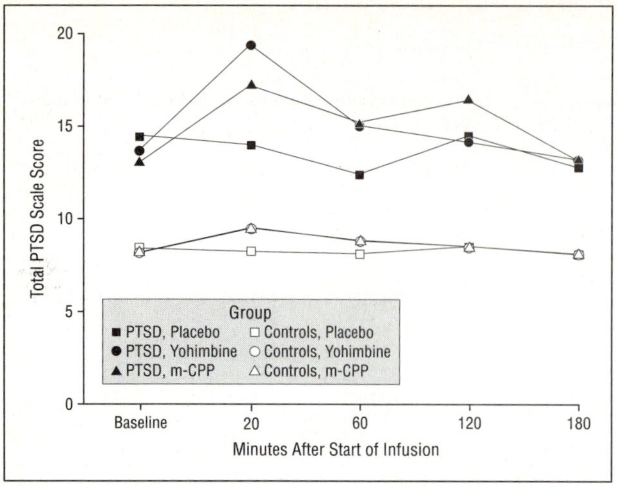

Figure 2. *Effects of yohimbine hydrochloride, meta-chlorophenylpiperazine (m-CPP), and placebo on total Post-Traumatic Stress Disorder (PTSD) scale score in healthy controls and patients with PTSD.*

lows (*df*=1,25 for all): distant from others, F=13.33, *P*<.01; intrusive thoughts, F=10.47, *P*<.01; emotionally numb, F=19.67, *P*<.001; and flashbacks, F=5.43, *P*<.05. Following adjustments for multiple comparisons (α=.013), the Pearson correlation between peak change over time for yohimbine and m-CPP was significant only for the symptom of distant from others (*r*=.49, *df*=24, *P*<.01).

BLOOD PRESSURE AND HEART RATE PEAK CHANGE FROM BASELINE

Effects of Yohimbine

Patients with PTSD did not differ significantly from healthy controls in changes in blood pressure and heart rate over time. Furthermore, no significant differences were observed in any blood pressure and heart rate measurements when comparing patients who had yohimbine-induced panic attacks with patients who did not have yohimbine-induced panic attacks and when comparing patients who had yohimbine-induced panic attacks with healthy controls.

Effects of m-CPP

When comparing the entire patient group with healthy controls, no significant differences were observed in measurement changes of blood pressure and heart rate over time. Similarly, there were no significant differences when comparing patients who had m-CPP–induced panic attacks with patients who did not have m-CPP–induced panic attacks, nor when comparing patients who had m-CPP–induced panic attacks with healthy controls.

COMMENT

Similar to previously published findings in combat veterans with PTSD, yohimbine infusion caused increases in anxiety, panic, and PTSD-specific symptoms. Although the incidence of yohimbine-induced panic attacks in patients with PTSD (42%) was lower than the 70% observed by Southwick et al[39] and the 60% by Bremner et al,[94] the rate was considerably higher than that found in the present control group (7%). Furthermore, the rate of yohimbine-induced flashbacks was similar among patients with PTSD in all 3 studies (31%, 40%, and 30%, respectively).

The subgroup of patients with yohimbine-induced panic attacks had significantly greater increases in total PASS and total PTSD scale scores than did healthy controls. These data suggest that a subgroup of patients with PTSD, and not the entire group, has a potentiated anxiogenic and PTSD symptom behavioral response to yohimbine. Because the primary action of yohimbine is on the noradrenergic system, these findings suggest that a subgroup of combat veterans with PTSD has increased reactivity of this system.[40-42,95,96]

Although the effect of yohimbine on blood pressure was greater in patients than controls, the difference was not significant. This contrasts with the observations in our earlier study.[39] This discrepancy potentially may be explained by differences in the 2 patient populations. In the first study, not all patients were elective admissions and therefore likely to be more acutely ill.

The present data indicate that m-CPP also causes increases in anxiety, panic, and PTSD-specific symptoms among combat veterans with PTSD. Metachlorophenylpiperazine induced panic attacks in 31% and flashbacks in 27% of patients. Because we believe this is the first report of m-CPP challenge in patients with PTSD, it is impossible to compare the present findings with earlier work. However, our findings concur with clinical data supporting a relation between 5-HT function and impulsivity,[59] aggression,[59] and suicide,[60] clinical features commonly associated with PTSD.

Like the subgroup of patients with yohimbine-induced panic attacks, the group with m-CPP–induced panic attacks also had significantly greater increases in total PASS and total PTSD scale scores compared with healthy controls. Thus, some but not all patients with PTSD have potentiated responses to m-CPP, with rapid increases in both panic and PTSD-specific symptoms. These data are consistent with preclinical studies showing that chronic stress results in increased behavioral responses to m-CPP[46-52] that seem to be mediated by 5-HT_{2C} receptors.[68-70] Thus, the current findings suggest that some patients with PTSD may have supersensitive 5-HT_{2C} receptors.

Yohimbine-induced panic attacks and m-CPP–induced panic attacks tended to occur in different patients. Only 3 (19%) of 16 patients with drug-induced panic attacks had the attacks on both active test days. The remaining 13 patients (81%) had their panic attacks following administration of yohimbine or m-CPP, but not both, suggesting the possibility of at least 2 biological subtypes of PTSD, one characterized by dysregulated noradrenergic and the other by dysregulated 5-HT function. These data indicate that panic attack and flashback induction in combat veterans with PTSD is not specific to yohimbine or m-CPP and suggest that these phenomena do not represent a specific response to α_2-adrenergic receptor blockade or 5-HT_{2C}–receptor stimu-

Table 2. Effects of Intravenous Yohimbine or Meta-chlorophenylpiperazine Compared With Placebo on the Posttraumatic Stress Disorder Scale*

	Patients With PTSD†					
	With Panic Attacks		Without Panic Attacks		Healthy Subjects (n=14)	
Symptom	**Baseline**	**Peak Change**	**Baseline**	**Peak Change**	**Baseline**	**Peak Change**
Yohimbine hydrochloride vs placebo						
Intrusive thoughts						
Placebo	1.64 (0.20)	0.27 (0.30)	1.87 (0.29)	0.33 (0.27)	1.07 (0.07)	−0.07 (0.07)§
Yohimbine	1.73 (0.22)	1.55 (0.33)	1.53 (0.20)	0.53 (0.26)	1.00 (0.00)	0.00 (0.00)
Total PTSD score						
Placebo	13.82 (1.57)	1.09 (1.53)	14.77 (1.55)	1.17 (0.87)	8.46 (0.22)	0.04 (0.22)§
Yohimbine	14.45 (1.60)	10.18 (1.82)	13.03 (1.21)	3.97 (1.49)	8.32 (0.19)	1.39 (0.41)
m-CPP vs placebo						
Anger						
Placebo	1.88 (0.39)	−0.13 (0.08)	1.83 (0.28)	0.50 (0.24)‡	1.00 (0.00)	0.00 (0.00)§
m-CPP	1.38 (0.21)	2.13 (0.57)	1.67 (0.22)	0.22 (0.13)	1.00 (0.00)	0.00 (0.00)
Difficulty concentrating						
Placebo	2.63 (0.42)	−0.13 (0.23)	2.00 (0.19)	0.39 (0.18)‡	1.18 (0.11)	−0.11 (0.06)
m-CPP	2.31 (0.33)	1.81 (0.41)	2.14 (0.15)	0.42 (0.23)	1.07 (0.05)	0.71 (0.21)
Distant from others						
Placebo	2.00 (0.41)	−0.13 (0.21)	1.94 (0.25)	0.33 (0.15)‡	1.07 (0.07)	−0.07 (0.07)§
m-CPP	1.88 (0.41)	1.88 (0.41)	1.78 (0.25)	0.72 (0.18)	1.00 (0.00)	0.14 (0.10)
Flashbacks						
Placebo	1.50 (0.37)	0.00 (0.16)	1.17 (0.12)	0.11 (0.21)	1.00 (0.00)	0.00 (0.00)§
m-CPP	1.31 (0.25)	1.19 (0.46)	1.03 (0.03)	0.42 (0.22)	1.00 (0.00)	0.00 (0.00)
Hypervigilance						
Placebo	1.69 (0.25)	0.31 (0.34)	1.83 (0.21)	0.39 (0.18)‡	1.14 (0.11)	−0.07 (0.05)§
m-CPP	1.56 (0.32)	1.81 (0.44)	1.75 (0.18)	0.42 (0.16)	1.07 (0.07)	0.00 (0.00)
Intrusive thoughts						
Placebo	1.88 (0.36)	0.13 (0.21)	1.72 (0.22)	0.39 (0.27)	1.07 (0.07)	−0.07 (0.07)§
m-CPP	1.69 (0.25)	1.69 (0.47)	1.44 (0.18)	0.83 (0.21)	1.04 (0.03)	−0.04 (0.03)
Startle						
Placebo	1.56 (0.31)	0.94 (0.29)	1.19 (0.12)	1.19 (0.29)	1.00 (0.00)	0.29 (0.16)§
m-CPP	1.50 (0.31)	1.88 (0.39)	1.06 (0.06)	1.00 (0.27)	1.00 (0.00)	0.07 (0.07)
Total PTSD score						
Placebo	15.31 (2.31)	0.19 (1.45)	13.94 (1.24)	1.56 (0.97)‡	8.46 (0.22)	0.04 (0.22)§
m-CPP	13.50 (1.99)	11.59 (2.55)	12.83 (1.02)	3.72 (1.11)	8.18 (0.10)	1.32 (0.48)

**Values are given as mean (±SEM). PTSD indicates posttraumatic stress disorder; m-CPP, meta-chlorophenylpiperazine.*
†No. of patients in each group given in footnote to Table 1.
‡Statistically significant (P<.006) group×drug×time interaction (patients with panic attacks vs patients without panic attacks).
§Statistically significant (P<.006) group×drug×time interaction (patients with panic attacks vs healthy controls).

lation. Instead, it seems that panic attacks and flashbacks can be induced in this population by multiple anxiogenic agents that have differing mechanisms of action. For example, Rainey et al[97] reported panic attacks and flashbacks in combat veterans after infusion of sodium lactate.

While yohimbine and m-CPP have marked effects on anxiety and PTSD-specific symptoms relative to placebo, there was little correlation between the behavioral responses to yohimbine and m-CPP in individual patients. Four PTSD-specific symptoms increased significantly relative to placebo in response to yohimbine and/or m-CPP in the entire patient group. After correction for multiple comparisons, in only 1 of the 4 symptoms was the peak change following yohimbine significantly correlated with the peak change following m-CPP. Similarly, none of the 11 PASS symptoms that changed significantly in response to yohimbine or m-CPP had peak changes following yohimbine that significantly correlated with peak changes following m-CPP. This suggests that m-CPP and yohimbine have distinct effects on anxiety and PTSD symptoms in individual patients with PTSD and further supports the concept of specific neurobiological subtypes in this disorder.

The possibility of neurobiological subtypes and differential behavioral responses to m-CPP and yohimbine has potential clinical relevance. To date, no one therapy consistently has been shown to be effective for the treatment of PTSD.[98-100]

From the results of the present study, it is possible to speculate that patients with increased behavioral sensitivity to yohimbine might benefit from drugs that reduce noradrenergic function, such as clonidine hydrochloride or propranolol hydrochloride, and might experience an initial exacerbation of symptoms if treated with noradrenergic reuptake inhibitors such as desipramine hydrochloride. Patients with increased behavioral sensitivity to m-CPP might respond preferentially to drugs with primary actions on 5-HT function. The behavioral effects of m-CPP have been shown to be reduced by chronic fluoxetine hydrochloride and clomipramine hydrochloride treatment in patients with obsessive-compulsive disorder.[80] The matching of biological subtypes with appropriate pharmacological agents may increase the efficacy of pharmacotherapy in the treatment of PTSD.

Intrusive memories and flashbacks were induced by yohimbine and m-CPP. These memories often were remarkably vivid and palpable. Identification of neurotransmitters and neuropeptides involved in memory encoding and retrieval has been the subject of considerable preclinical investigation. The tendency for yohimbine to elicit traumatic memory recall and flashbacks may relate to β-adrenergic–receptor stimulation in the amygdala and cortical structures.[16,17,24] Less is known about mechanisms by which m-CPP might effect traumatic memories and flashbacks, although other 5-HT agonists, such as lysergic acid diethylamide (LSD) are capable of inducing flashbacks[101-103] that seem to be mediated by the 5-HT_{2A} receptor. It may be that the induction of flashbacks by m-CPP and LSD share a common mechanism involving this 5-HT receptor.

There are a number of potential limitations in the present study. First, although yohimbine and m-CPP have been used as probes of noradrenergic and 5-HT function, respectively, both agents have effects on multiple neurotransmitter systems. For example, yohimbine binds to 5-HT receptors and m-CPP to adrenergic receptors.[73,95,96,104] However, m-CPP clearly has greater affinity than yohimbine for 5-HT receptors, and yohimbine has greater affinity than m-CPP for adrenergic receptors.[73,104]

Second, patients in this study were treatment-seeking veterans with chronic and pervasive trauma-related symptoms. They are not necessarily representative of the veteran population as a whole. It is unclear if the present results can be generalized to non–treatment-seeking combat veterans (with and without PTSD), civilians with noncombat PTSD, and persons who have been more recently traumatized.

Third, because our patients with PTSD had a high rate of comorbid panic disorder, major depression, and alcoholism, it could be argued that these comorbid disorders rather than PTSD accounted for the observed results. This is an especially important issue for panic disorder, because yohimbine and m-CPP are known to cause panic attacks in patients with panic disorder[43-45,74-77] but not in patients with major depressive disorder[105] or alcoholism.[88-91] In the present study, however, 8 of 11 patients with yohimbine-induced panic attacks and 6 of 8 with m-CPP–induced panic attacks did not meet comorbid criteria for panic disorder, making it unlikely that panic disorder alone can explain these findings. Similarly, because 4 of 11 and 7 of 11 patients with yohimbine-induced panic attacks, and 3 of 8 and 7 of 8 with m-CPP–induced panic attacks did not meet comorbid criteria for current major depression and current alcohol abuse, respectively, each of these 2 comorbid diagnoses alone cannot explain the above findings. Nevertheless, the influence of comorbid Axis I diagnoses on the behavioral effects of the 2 study agents cannot be definitively determined because of the small sample size.

Along with preclinical observations that stress profoundly alters the function of many neurotransmitter and neuropeptide systems, the aforementioned behavioral responses to yohimbine and m-CPP support the view of PTSD as a multisystem neurobiological disorder. There is now ample clinical evidence showing chronic alterations in the noradrenergic, 5-HT, and glucocorticoid systems in many traumatized persons even 25 years after exposure to traumatic stressors.[106] With the elucidation of biological subtypes, it is hoped that specific treatments can be developed and targeted toward underlying neurobiological disturbances, with the ultimate goal of reducing the level of suffering in persons who have been severely traumatized.

Accepted for publication October 8, 1996.

This work was supported by the National Center for Post-Traumatic Stress Disorder, Veterans Affairs Medical Center, West Haven, Conn, by Merit Review research grants funded by the Department of Veterans Affairs, Washington, DC (Drs Southwick and Krystal), and by grant R01-MH40140 from the National Institute of Mental Health, Bethesda, Md (Dr Charney).

Reprints: Steven M. Southwick, MD, National Center for Post-Traumatic Stress Disorder, Veterans Affairs Medical Center, Department of Psychiatry (116A), West Haven, CT 06516.

REFERENCES

1. Tsuda A, Tanaka M. Differential changes in noradrenaline turnover in specific regions of rat brain produced by controllable and uncontrollable shocks. *Behav Neurosci.* 1985;99:802-817.
2. Tsuda A, Tanaka M, Ida Y, Tsujimaru S, Ushijima I, Nagasaki N. Effects of preshock experience on enhancement of rat brain noradrenaline turnover induced by psychological stress. *Pharmacol Biochem Behav.* 1986;24:115-119.
3. Stone EA. Accumulation and metabolism of norepinephrine in rat hypothalamus after exhaustive stress. *J Neurochem.* 1973;21:589-601.
4. Tanaka M, Kohno Y, Nakagawa R, Ida Y, Takeda S, Nagasaki N, Noda Y. Regional characteristics of stress-induced increases in brain noradrenaline release in rats. *Pharmacol Biochem Behav.* 1983;19:543-547.
5. Tanaks M, Kohno Y, Nagagawa R, Ida Y, Takeda S, Nagasaki N. Time-related differences in noradrenergic turnover in rat brain regions by stress. *Pharmacol Biochem Behav.* 1982;16:315-319.
6. Redmond DE Jr. Studies of the nucleus locus-coeruleus in monkeys and hypotheses for neuropsychopharmacology. In: Meltzer HY, ed. *Psychopharmacology: The Third Generation of Progress.* New York, NY: Raven Press; 1987:967-975.
7. Abercrombie ED, Jacobs BL. Single-unit response of noradrenergic neurons in the locus coeruleus of freely moving cats, I: acutely presented stressful and nonstressful stimuli. *J Neurosci.* 1987;7:2837-2843.
8. Foote SL, Bloom FE, Aston-Jones G. Nucleus locus coeruleus: new evidence for anatomical and physiological specificity. *Physiol Rev.* 1983;63:844-914.
9. Levine ES, Litto WJ, Jacobs BL. Activity of cat locus coeruleus noradrenergic neurons during the defense reaction. *Brain Res.* 1990;531:189-195.
10. Aston-Jones G, Bloom FE. Activity of norepinephrine-containing locus coeruleus neurons in behaving rats anticipates fluctuations in the sleep-waking cycle. *J Neurosci.* 1981;1:876-886.
11. Grant SJ, Aston-Jones G, Redmond DJ. Responses of primate locus coeruleus neurons to simple and complex sensory stimuli. *Brain Res Bull.* 1988;21:402-410.
12. Aston-Jones G, Valentino R, Van Blockstaele EJ. Locus coeruleus, stress, and PTSD: neurobiological and clinical parallels. In: Murburg M, ed. *Catecholamine Function in PTSD: Emerging Concepts.* Washington, DC: American Psychiatric Press; 1994:17-62.
13. Foote SL, Bloom FE, Aston-Jones G. Nucleus locus coeruleus: new evidence of anatomical and physiological specificity. *Physiol Rev.* 1981;63:844-914.
14. Segal M, Bloom FE. The action of norepinephrine in the rat hippocampus, IV: the effects of locus coeruleus stimulation on evoked hippocampal unit activity. *Brain Res.* 1976;107:513-525.
15. Waterhouse BD, Moises HC, Woodward DJ. Noradrenergic modulation of so-

matosensory cortical neuronal responses to iontophoretically applied putative neurotransmitters. *Exp Neurol.* 1980;69:30-49.
16. McGaugh JI. Involvement of hormonal and neuromodulatory systems in the regulation of memory storage. *Annu Rev Neurosci.* 1989;2:255-287.
17. McGaugh JL. Significance and remembrance: the role of neuromodulatory systems. *Psychol Sci.* 1990;1:15-25.
18. Pitman RK. Posttraumatic stress disorder, hormones, and memory. *Biol Psychiatry.* 1989;26:221-223.
19. Squire LR. Mechanisms of memory. *Science.* 1986;232:1612-1619.
20. Devauges V, Sara SL. Memory retrieval enhancement by locus coeruleus stimulation: evidence for mediation by beta-receptors. *Behav Brain Res.* 1991;43: 93-97.
21. Sara SJ, Devauges V. Idazoxan, an alpha-2 antagonist, facilitates memory retrieval in the rat. *Behav Neurol Biol.* 1989;51:401-411.
22. LeDoux JE, Romanski L, Xagoraris A. Indelibility of subcortical emotional memories. *J Cogn Neurosci.* 1969;1:238-243.
23. Reiser M. *Memory in Mind and Brain: What Dream Imaging Reveals.* New York, NY: Basic Books Inc Publishers; 1991:2.
24. Cahil L, Prins B, Weber M, McGaugh S. B-Adrenergic activation and memory for emotional events. *Nature.* 1994;371:702-704.
25. Fraser F, Wilson EM. The sympathetic nervous system and the 'irritable heart of soldiers.' *BMJ.* 1918;2:27-29.
26. Dobbs D, Wilson WP. Observations on the persistence of neurosis. *Dis Nerv Syst.* 1960;21:40-46.
27. Blanchard EB, Kolb LC, Prins A, Gates S, McCoy GC. Changes in plasma norepinephrine to combat-related stimuli among Vietnam veterans with post traumatic stress disorder. *J Nerv Ment Dis.* 1991;179:371-373.
28. Malloy PF, Fairbank JA, Keane TM. Validation of a multimethod assessment of posttraumatic stress disorders in Vietnam veterans. *J Consult Clin Psychol.* 1983; 51:488-494.
29. Pallmeyer TP, Blanchard EB, Kolb LC. The psychophysiology of combat-induced posttraumatic stress disorder in Vietnam veterans. *Behav Res Ther.* 1986;24:645-652.
30. Pitman RK, Orr SP, Forgue DF, DeJong JB, Clairborn JM. Psychophysiologic assessment of posttraumatic stress disorder imagery in Vietnam combat veterans. *Arch Gen Psychiatry.* 1987;44;970-975.
31. Orr SP. Psychophysiologic studies of post traumatic stress disorder. In: Giller EL, ed. *Biological Assessment and Treatment of Post Traumatic Stress Disorder.* Washington, DC: American Psychiatric Press; 1990:135-157.
32. Shalev AY, Orr SP, Pitman RK. Psychophysiologic assessment of traumatic imagery in Israeli civilian patients with posttraumatic stress disorders. *Am J Psychiatry.* 1993;150:620-624.
33. Pitman RK, Orr SP, Forgue DF, Altman B, deJong JB, Herz LR. Psychophysiologic responses to combat imagery of Vietnam veterans with posttraumatic stress disorder versus other anxiety disorders. *J Abnorm Psychol.* 1990;99: 49-54.
34. Kosten TR, Mason JW, Giller EL, Ostroff RB, Harkness L. Sustained urinary norepinephrine and epinephrine elevation in post-traumatic stress disorder. *Psychoneuroendocrinology.* 1987;12:13-20.
35. Yehuda R, Southwick SM, Giller EL, Xiaowan MA, Mason JW. Urinary catecholamine excretion and severity of PTSD symptoms in Vietnam combat veterans. *J Nerv Ment Dis.* 1992;180:321-325.
36. Perry BD, Giller EL, Southwick SM. Altered platelet alpha2 adrenergic binding sites in post-traumatic stress disorder. *Am J Psychiatry.* 1987;144:1511-1512.
37. Lerer B, Ebstein RP, Shestatsky M, Shemesh Z, Greenberg D. Cyclic AMP signal transduction in post-traumatic stress disorder. *Am J Psychiatry.* 1987;144: 1324-1327.
38. Blanchard EB, Hickling EJ, Taylor AC. The psychophysiology of motor vehicle accident related posttraumatic stress disorder. *Biofeedback Self Regul.* 1991; 16:449-458.
39. Southwick SM, Krystal JH, Morgan AC, Johnson D, Nagy L, Nicolaou A, Heninger GR, Charney DS. Abnormal noradrenergic function in post traumatic stress disorder. *Arch Gen Psychiatry.* 1993;50:266-274.
40. Starke K, Borowski E, Endo T. Preferential blockade of presynaptic alpha-adrenoreceptors by yohimbine. *Eur J Pharmacol.* 1975;34:385-388.
41. Goldberg MR, Robinson D. Yohimbine: a pharmacological probe for study of the alpha$_2$-adrenoreceptor. *Pharmacol Rev.* 1983;35:143-180.
42. Ruffolo RR Jr, Waddell JE, Yaden EL. Postsynaptic alpha adrenergic receptor subtypes differentiated by yohimbine in tissues from the rat: existence of alpha-2 adrenergic receptors in rat aorta. *J Pharmacol Exp Ther.* 1981;217:235-240.
43. Charney DS, Heninger GR, Breier A. Noradrenergic functions in panic anxiety: effects of yohimbine in healthy subjects and patients with agoraphobia and panic disorder. *Arch Gen Psychiatry.* 1984;42:751-763.
44. Charney DS, Woods SW, Goodman WK, Heninger GR. Neurobiological mechanisms of panic anxiety: biochemical and behavioral correlates of yohimbine-induced panic attacks. *Am J Psychiatry.* 1987;144:1030-1036.
45. Gurguis GNM, Uhde IW. Plasma 3-methoxy-4-hydroxyphenylethylene glycol (MHPG) and growth hormone responses to yohimbine in panic disorder patients and normal controls. *Psychoneuroendocrinology.* 1990;15:217-224.
46. Dunn AJ. Changes in plasma and brain tryptophan and brain serotonin and 5-hydroxyindoleacetic acid after footshock stress. *Life Sci.* 1989;42:1847-1853.
47. Morgan WW, Rudden PK, Pfeil KA. Effect of immobilization stress on serotonin content and turnover in regions of the rat brain. *Life Sci.* 1975;17:143-150.
48. Shimizu N, Take S, Hori T, Oomura Y. In vivo measurement of hypothalamic serotonin release by intracerebral microdialysis: significant enhancement by immobilization stress in rats. *Brain Res Bull.* 1992;28:727-734.
49. Tanaka M, Kohno Y, Nakagawa R, Nishikawa T, Tsuda A, Nagasaki N. Immobilization stress increases serotonin turnover in the extended brain regions in the rat. *Kurume Med J.* 1983;30:35-43.
50. Moreau JL, Jenck F, Martin JR, Perrin S, Haefely WE. Effects of repeated mild stress and two antidepressant treatments on the behavioral response to $5HT_{1C}$ receptor activation in rats. *Psychopharmacology.* 1993;110:140-144.
51. Wright IK, Ismail H, Upton N, Marsden CA. Effect of isolation rearing on 5-HT agonist-induced responses in the rat. *Psychopharmacology.* 1991;105:259-263.
52. Kawahara H, Yoshida M, Yokoo H, Nishi M, Tanaka M. Psychological stress increases serotonin release in the rat amygdala and prefrontal cortex assessed by in vivo microdialysis. *Neurosci Lett.* 1993;162:81-84.
53. Arora RC, Fitchner CG, O'Connor F. Paroxetine binding in the blood platelets of posttraumatic stress disordered patients. *Life Sci.* 1993;53:919-928.
54. McDougle C, Southwick SM, Rorbaugh R, Charney DS, St James RJ. An open trial of fluoxetine in the treatment of post traumatic stress disorder. *J Clin Psychopharmacol.* 1991;1:325-327.
55. Nagy LM, Morgan CA, Southwick SM, Charney DS. Open prospective trial of fluoxetine for post traumatic stress disorder. *J Clin Psychopharmacol.* 1993; 13:107-113.
56. Davidson JRT, Ross S, Newman E. Fluoxetine in posttraumatic stress disorder. *J Trauma Stress.* 1991;4:419-423.
57. Shay J. Fluoxetine reduces explosiveness and elevates mood in Vietnam combat vets with PTSD. *J Trauma Stress.* 1992;5:97-102.
58. van der Kolk BA, Dreyfuss D, Michaels M, Shera D, Berkowitz R, Fisler R, Saxe G. Fluoxetine in posttraumatic stress disorder. *J Clin Psychiatry.* 1994;55:517-522.
59. Brown GL, Linnoila ML. CSF serotonin metabolite (5-HIAA) studies in depression, impulsivity, and violence. *J Clin Psychiatry.* 1990;51:31-41.
60. Stanley M, Stanley B. Postmortem evidence for serotonin's role in suicide. *J Clin Psychiatry.* 1990;51:22-28.
61. Wolf WA, Kuhn DM. The 5-HT transporter is an additional site of action for the 5-HT agonists RU 24969 and TFMPP. *Neurochem Int.* 1991;19:39-44.
62. Hoyer D. Functional correlates of serotonin $5\text{-}HT_1$ recognition sites. *J Recept Res.* 1988;8:59-81.
63. Hamik A, Peroutka SJ. 1-(*m*-chlorophenyl) piperazine interactions with neurotransmitter receptors in the human brain. *Biol Psychiatry.* 1989;25:569-575.
64. Glennon RA, Ismaiel AE-KM, McCarthy BG, Peroutka SJ. Binding of arylpiperazines to $5\text{-}HT_3$ serotonin receptors, results of a structure-affinity study. *Eur J Pharmacol.* 1989;168:387-392.
65. Schoeffter P, Hoyer D. Interaction of arylpiperazines with $5\text{-}HT_{1A}$, $5\text{-}HT_{1B}$, $5\text{-}HT_{1C}$ and $5\text{-}HT_{1D}$ receptors: do discriminatory $5\text{-}HT_{1B}$ receptor ligands exist? *Arch Pharmacol.* 1989;339:675-683.
66. Shen Y, Monsma FJ, Metcalf MA, Jose PA, Hamblin MW, Sibley DR. Molecular cloning and expression of a 5-hydroxytryptamine: receptor subtype. *J Biol Chem.* 1993;268:18200-18204.
67. Sheldon PW, Aghajanian GK. Excitatory responses to serotonin (5-HT) in neurons of the rat piriform cortex: evidence for mediation by $5\text{-}HT_{1C}$ receptors in pyramidal cells and $5\text{-}HT_2$ receptors in interneurons. *Synapse.* 1991;9:208-218.
68. Conn PJ, Sanders-Bush E. Relative efficacies of piperazines at the phosphoinositide hydrolysis-linked serotonergic ($5\text{-}HT_2$ and $5\text{-}HT_{1C}$) receptors. *J Pharmacol Exp Ther.* 1987;242:552-557.
69. Sheldon PW, Aghajanian GK. Serotonin (5-HT) induces IPSP's in pyramidal layer cells of rat piriform cortex: evidence for the involvement of a $5\text{-}HT_2$ activated interneuron. *Brain Res.* 1990;506:62-69.
70. Carver JG, Grahame-Smith DG, Johnson ES, Madgwick Z. The effects of 5-HT and *m*-chlorophenylpiperazine (m-CPP) on the efflux of [^{3}H]-5-HT from human perfused platelets. *Br J Clin Pharmacol.* 1993;35:473-478.
71. Ireland SJ, Tyers MB. Pharmacological characterization of 5-hydroxytryptamine–induced depolarization of the rabbit isolated vagus nerve. *Br J Pharmacol.* 1987; 90:229-238.
72. Robertson DW, Bloomquist W, Wong DT, Cohen ML. MCPP but not TFMPP is an antagonist at cardiac $5\text{-}HT_3$ receptors. *Life Sci.* 1991;50:599-605.

73. Hoyer D. Functional correlates of serotonin 5-HT_1 recognition sites. *J Recept Signal Transduct Res.* 1988;8:59-81.
74. Klein E, Zohar J, Geraci MF, Murphy DL, Uhde TW. Anxiogenic effects of m-CPP in patients with panic disorder: comparison to caffeine's anxiogenic effects. *Biol Psychiatry.* 1991;30:973-984.
75. Asnis GM, Wetzler S, Sanderson WC, Kahn RS, van Praag HM. Functional interrelationship of serotonin and norepinephrine: cortisol response to MCPP and DMI in patients with panic disorder, patients with depression, and normal control subjects. *Psychiatry Res.* 1992;43:65-76.
76. Kahn RS, Wetzler S, Asnis GM, Kling MA, Suckow RF, van Praag HM. Pituitary hormone responses to meta-chlorophenylpiperazine in panic disorder and healthy control subjects. *Psychiatry Res.* 1991;37:25-34.
77. Charney DS, Woods SW, Goodman WK, Heninger GR. Serotonin function in anxiety, II: effects of the serotonin agonist MCPP in panic disorder patients and healthy subjects. *Psychopharmacology.* 1987;92:14-24.
78. Barr LC, Goodman WK, Price LH, McDougle CJ, Charney DS. The serotonic hypothesis of obsessive compulsive disorder: implications of pharmacologic challenge studies. *J Clin Psychiatry.* 1992;53(suppl):17-28.
79. Hollander E, DeCaria CM, Nitescu A, Gully R, Suckow RF, Cooper TB, Gorman JM, Klein DF, Liebowitz MR. Serotonergic function in obsessive-compulsive disorder: behavioral and neuroendocrine responses to oral *m*-chlorophenylpiperazine and fenfluramine in patients and healthy volunteers. *Arch Gen Psychiatry.* 1992;49:21-28.
80. Hollander E, DeCaria C, Gully R, Nitescu A, Suckow RF, Gorman JM, Klein DF, Liebowitz MR. Effects of chronic fluoxetine treatment on behavioral and neuroendocrine responses to meta-chlorophenylpiperazine in obsessive-compulsive disorder. *Psychiatry Res.* 1991;36:1-17.
81. Barr LC, Goodman WK, Price LH. The serotonin hypothesis of obsessive compulsive disorder. *Int Clin Psychopharmacol.* 1993;2:79-82.
82. Hollander E, Cohen LJ, DeCaria C, Saoud JB, Stein DJ, Cooper TB, Islam NN, Liebowitz MR, Klein DF. Timing of neuroendocrine responses and effect of a m-CPP and fenfluramine plasma levels in OCD. *Biol Psychiatry.* 1993;34:407-413.
83. Charney DS, Goodman WK, Price LH, Woods SW, Rasmusson SA, Heninger GR. Serotonin function in obsessive-compulsive disorder: a comparison of the effects of tryptophan and *m*-chlorophenylpiperazine in patients and healthy patients. *Arch Gen Psychiatry.* 1988;45:177-185.
84. Krystal JH, Seibyl JP, Price LH, Woods SW, Heninger Gr, Aghajanian GK, Charney DS. *m*-Chlorophenylpiperazine effects in neuroleptic-free schizophrenic patients. *Arch Gen Psychiatry.* 1993;50:624-635.
85. Mellow AM, Lawlor BA, Sunderland T, Mueller EA, Molchan SE, Murphy DL. Effects of daily oral *m*-chlorophenylpiperazine in elderly depressed patients: initial experience with a serotonin agonist. *Biol Psychiatry.* 1990;28:588-594.
86. Anand A, Charney DS, Delgado PL, McDougle CJ, Heninger GR, Price LH. Neuroendocrine and behavioral responses to intravenous *m*-chlorophenylpiperazine (mCPP) in depressed patients and healthy comparison subjects. *Am J Psychiatry.* 1994;151:1626-1630.
87. Overstreet DH, Rezvani AH, Janowsky DS. Genetic animal models of depression and ethanol preference provide support for cholinergic and serotonergic involvement in depression and alcoholism. *Biol Psychiatry.* 1992;32:919-936.
88. Krystal JH, Webb E, Kranzler H, et al. Serotonergic and noradrenergic dysregulation in alcoholism: m-CPP and yohimbine effects in recently detoxified alcoholics and healthy subjects. *Am J Psychiatry.* 1996;153:83-92.
89. Krystal JH, Webb E, Cooney N, Kranzler HR, Charney DS. Specificity of ethanol-like effects elicited by serotonergic and noradrenergic mechanisms. *Arch Gen Psychiatry.* 1994;51:898-911.
90. Krystal JH, Webb E, Cooney NL, Kranzler HR, Southwick SM, Heninger GH, Charney DS. Serotonergic and noradrenergic dysregulation on alcoholism: m-chlorophenylpiperazine and yohimbine effects in recently detoxified alcoholics and healthy comparison subjects. *Am J Psychiatry.* 1996;153:83-92.
91. Benkelfat C, Murphy DL, Hill JL, George DT, Nutt D, Linnoila M. Ethanol-like properties of serotonergic partial agonist m-chlorophenylpiperazine in chronic alcoholic patients. *Arch Gen Psychiatry.* 1991;48:383.
92. Spitzer RL, Williams JBW. Structured clinical interview for *DSM-III-R.* New York, NY: Biometrics Research Department, NY State Psychiatric Institute; 1985.
93. Keane TM, Caddell JM, Taylor KL. Mississippi scale for combat-related post-traumatic stress disorder: three studies in reliability and validity. *J Consult Clin Psychol.* 1988;56:85-90.
94. Bremner JD, Ng CK, Staib L, Markey J, Duncan J, Zubal G, Krystal JH, Mazza S, Rich D, Southwick SM, Capelli S, Seibyl JP, Dey H, Soufer R, Charney DS, Innis RB. PET measurement of cerebral metabolism following a noradrenergic challenge in patients with posttraumatic stress disorder and in healthy subjects. *J Nucl Med.* 1993;3334:205-206.
95. Charney DS, Woods SW, Price LH, Goodman WK, Glazer WM, Heninger GR. Noradrenergic dysregulation in panic disorder. In: Ballenger JC, ed. *Neurobiology of Panic Disorder.* New York, NY: Wiley Liss; 1990:91-105.
96. Redmond DE Jr. New and old evidence for the involvement of a brain norepinephrine system in anxiety. In: Fann WE, ed. *The Phenomenology and Treatment of Anxiety.* New York, NY: Plenum Publishing Corp; 1979:153-203.
97. Rainey JM, Aleem A, Ortiz A, Yeragani V, Pohl R, Berchau R. A laboratory procedure for the induction of flashbacks. *Am J Psychiatry.* 1987;144:1317-1319.
98. Friedman MJ. Towards rational pharmacotherapy for post traumatic stress disorder. *Am J Psychiatry.* 1988;145:281-285.
99. Friedman MJ. Biological approaches to the diagnosis and treatment of post traumatic stress disorder. *J Traum Stress.* 1991;4:67-81.
100. Southwick SM, Yehuda R, Giller E, Charney DS. The effects of antidepressants in the treatment of post traumatic stress disorder: a quantitative review. In: Murburgh M, ed. *Catecholamine Function in Post-Traumatic Stress Disorder: Emerging Concepts.* Washington, DC; American Psychiatric Press; 1994:293-305.
101. Rasmussen K, Glennon RA, Aghajanian GK. Phenylethylamine hallucinogens in the locus coeruleus: potency of action correlates with rank order of 5-HT_2 binding affinity. *Eur J Pharmacol.* 1986;94:213-216.
102. Titeler M, Lyon RA, Glennon RA. Radioligand binding evidence implicates the brain 5-HT_1 receptor as a site of action for LSD and phenylisopropylamine hallucinogens. *Psychopharmacology.* 1988;94:213-216.
103. Buckholz MS, Zhou D, Freedman DX, Potter WZ. Lysergic acid diethylamide (LSD) administration selectively downregulates $serotonin_2$ receptors in rat brain. *Neuropsychopharmacology.* 1990;3:137-148.
104. Winter JC, Rabin RA. Yohimbine as a serotonergic agent: evidence for receptor binding and drug discrimination. *J Pharmacol Exp Ther.* 1992;263:682-689.
105. Heninger GR, Charney DS, Price LH. α_2 Adrenergic receptor sensitivity in depression: the plasma MHPG, behavioral, and cardiovascular responses to yohimbine. *Arch Gen Psychiatry.* 1988;45:718-726.
106. Southwick SM, Krystal JH, Johnson DR, Charney DS. Neurobiology of post traumatic stress disorder. In: Tasman A, Riba MG, eds. *Review of Psychiatry.* Washington, DC: American Psychiatric Press; 1992;11:347-370.

Clozapine Withdrawal: Serotonergic or Dopaminergic Mechanisms?

Baldessarini et al[1] note several case reports of rapid relapse after abrupt withdrawal of clozapine therapy and mention 5 cases of their own. They suggest that the mechanism could include 1 or more of the following: (1) rapid elimination of clozapine from the brain, (2) enhanced release of dopamine in the brain, and (3) stimulation by dopamine of D_4 dopamine receptors that may have become supersensitive and up-regulated because of prolonged blockade by clozapine therapy. They suggest, on this basis, that thioridazine therapy might be more effective than risperidone or haloperidol to treat clozapine withdrawal–induced relapse because thioridazine has some ability to block D_4 receptors and is administered in doses similar to those of clozapine.

We have carried out a randomized 2-year trial comparing clozapine and a typical neuroleptic drug (usually haloperidol) in recent onset schizophrenic patients who had minimal positive symptoms during prior treatment with neuroleptic drugs to assess the risk-benefit ratio for clozapine therapy in positive symptom responders to neuroleptic drugs. At the end of the 2 years of treatment during which the response to clozapine therapy was superior to prior treatment with neuroleptic drugs, in several important domains, eg, cognition,[2] according to the protocol, clozapine therapy was tapered in 10 patients during a 3-week period; in another 9 patients, clozapine therapy was tapered after the addition of perphenazine in doses of 24 mg/d for 7 days after a 6-day build-up of the dose of perphenazine. Four of the patients whose dose of clozapine was tapered without perphenazine relapsed while still taking clozapine. Relapse occurred within 3 to 14 days after the last dose of clozapine in 4 of the other 5 patients who were withdrawn from clozapine therapy without cross-tapering with perphenazine. Of the 90 patients treated with perphenazine prior to stopping clozapine, 6 patients relapsed, 5 patients within 1 week after the last dose of clozapine was received, and 1 patient, 6 weeks after the last dose was received. Thus, 15 (78.9%) of the 19 neuroleptic-responsive schizophrenic patients relapsed when clozapine therapy was tapered after a 2-year treatment period. We also noted relapse in 25 (39.1%) of the 64 neuroleptic-resistant patients who stopped treatment with clozapine abruptly because of noncompliance or side effects.

The reason for the higher rate of relapse in the neuroleptic-responsive patients compared with the neuroleptic-resistant patients is unclear. It strongly suggests that these 2 groups of patients have fundamental differences in neurochemistry, at least for those factors that are likely to be relevant to the antipsychotic effects of clozapine, eg, serotonin (5-hydroxytryptamine [5-HT]) and dopamine levels, turnover, and signal transduction mechanisms; the same may be true for acetylcholine, glutamate, and norepinephrine levels. This hypothesis is consistent with the differences in the responsivity of these 2 patient groups to the ability of neuroleptic drugs to diminish positive symptoms, an effect most likely due to their ability to block D_2 receptors.

It is, in my opinion, unlikely that D_4 receptor stimulation is a major factor in clozapine withdrawal psychosis. Loxapine has almost as much selectivity as clozapine for the D_4 receptor.[3] The ratio of the affinity constant (K_i) values for D_2 and D_4 receptors is approximately 4 nmol/L, whereas that of clozapine is approximately 8 nmol/L. Four of the 5 neuroleptic-responsive patients who had relapsed after stopping clozapine therapy responded only partially to loxapine in doses of 20 to 100 mg/d for periods of 6 weeks to 4 months. They did not return to their preclozapine or clozapine-treated state of remission while receiving loxapine therapy. However, 1 patient responded to loxapine therapy at a dose of 20 mg/d during a 3-month period to almost the same extent as he did while receiving clozapine therapy. He continued to do well for at least the next 6 months.

We have hypothesized that clozapine-induced relapse may be due, in part, to serotonergic-receptor alterations such that stimulation of various serotonin receptor subtypes, eg, $serotonin_{2A}$, $serotonin_{2C}$, $serotonin_6$, or $serotonin_2$, may be excessive during and after withdrawal of clozapine therapy.[4] Cyproheptadine, 4 mg 3 times a day, was added to perphenazine therapy in 4 of the patients who relapsed. Cyproheptadine therapy was begun within the first week of relapse. Improvement in the patient's condition was noted within 3 to 7 days and was persistent in 3 of the 4 patients. However, 1 of the 4 patients relapsed after 4 weeks. Increasing the dose of perphenazine was ineffective as was a prolonged trial of risperidone. This patient responded well after clozapine therapy was restarted. Five patients treated with risperidone after unsuccessful trials of typical neuroleptic drugs at usually effective doses had a satisfactory response to risperidone.

I agree with Baldessarini et al[1] that clozapine therapy should be slowly cross-tapered. However, I suggest that cyproheptadine or other serotonin-receptor antagonists, such as ritanserin (available in Europe), should be used along with typical neuroleptic drugs or risperidone to minimize the effects of withdrawal of clozapine therapy if psychosis emerges following tapering of the clozapine.

Herbert Y. Meltzer, MD
Department of Psychiatry
Psychiatric Hospital at Vanderbilt
1601 23rd Ave S
Suite 306
Nashville, TN 37212

1. Baldessarini RJ, Gardner DM, Garver DL. Conversions from clozapine to other antipsychotic drugs. *Arch Gen Psychiatry* 1995;52:1071-1072.
2. Lee MA, Thompson P, Meltzer HY. Effects of clozapine on cognitive function in schizophrenia. *J Clin Psychiatry*. 1994;55(suppl B):82-87.
3. Roth BL, Tandra S, Burgess LH, Sibley DR, Meltzer HY. D_4 dopamine receptor binding affinity does not distinguish between typical and atypical antipsychotic drugs. *Psychopharmacology*. 1995;120:365-368.
4. Meltzer HY, Lee MA, Ranjan R, Mason ED, Cola PA. Relapse following clozapine withdrawal: effect of cyproheptadine plus neuroleptic. *Psychopharmacology*. 1996;124:176-187.

In reply

Risk of exacerbation soon after discontinuing clozapine maintenance treatment of chronic psychotic illness evidently is high, though its quantification requires further study.[1] *Pharmacodynamic contributions to this response are probably complex, and any single mechanism, dopaminergic or serotonergic, is likely to be incomplete. Dr Meltzer's anecdotal observation of no early relapses in 4 of 4 patients switched from clozapine therapy to the typical neuroleptic perphenazine plus serotonin antagonist cyproheptadine is interesting and may support his thesis that antiserotonergic actions of clozapine are particularly important.*[2] *It also encourages systematic studies with selective antiserotonin agents.*

He also noted that risperidone protected against relapses after stopping clozapine therapy, although details were not provided, and suggested that its potent antiserotonin properties may account for this response, and lack of D_4 dopamine receptor selectivity, preclude involvement of dopaminergic mechanisms.[2] *This neuroleptic drug has very high serotonin$_2$ (5-hydroxytryptamine$_2$ [5-HT_2]) affinity (affinity constant, K_i=0.3 nmol/L),*[3] *and virtually identical high affinity at D_4 and D_2 receptors (K_i both 11 nmol/L) expressed in membranes of genetically transfected cells*[4] *(SF-1 and COS-7, Research Biochemicals International, Natick, Mass) tritium[^{3}H]-labeled spiperone (0.1-0.5 nmol/L) (DuPont-New England Nuclear, Boston, Mass) (N.S.K., R.J.B., and J. W. Kebabian, PhD, and J. L. Neumeyer, PhD, unpublished data, September 1995). We also found that patients can be successfully transferred from clozapine to risperidone therapy provided that clozapine was removed gradually while the dose of risperidone was slowly increased.*[1] *However, it is unclear whether the dosing technique or the actions of the drug replacing clozapine is more important.*

Dr Meltzer found that loxapine failed *to prevent psychotic relapses after withdrawal from clozapine therapy in 4 of 5 cases, and implied that it is clozapinelike, at least in having selectivity for D_4 receptors—again casting doubt on dopaminergic mechanisms in reactions to stopping clozapine therapy.*[2] *However, loxapine, though a dibenzepine like clozapine, is nonisosteric with clozapine due to 2- vs 8-chloro-substitution. In contrast to clozapine, it is an extrapyramidally active,* typical *neuroleptic drug with weak antimuscarinic activity and high D_2 affinity, with correspondingly greater potency.*[5] *It had selective affinity for serotonin$_2$-over-D_2 receptors (4.0-fold K_i ratio), like the more potent neuroleptic risperidone (5.8-fold), though both were less selective than clozapine (14-fold).*[3] *We found that loxapine lacked substantial D_4 selectivity in receptor-transfected membranes (D_2 and D_4, K_i=20-30 nmol/L), compared with clozapine's 6.5-fold D_4-over-D_2 selectivity (inverse K_i ratio=260/40 nmol/L). These findings do not indicate pharmacological similarity of loxapine and clozapine but, instead, suggest some similarities of loxapine and risperidone, with an expectation that neither may protect against effects of withdrawing clozapine.*

Unexpectedly, Dr Meltzer encountered early relapses in 15 (78.9%) of the 17 neuroleptic-responsive *patients stopping clozapine use* slowly *(some with perphenazine added), but in only 25 (39.1%) of the 64* neuroleptic-unresponsive *patients discontinuing clozapine treatment* abruptly *(P=.003, Fisher exact test).*[2] *This difference is difficult to interpret because it evidently involved clinically dissimilar patients as well as different rates of stopping clozapine therapy. Perhaps even slow discontinuation of clozapine therapy may not avoid relapses, or previously neuroleptic-responsive patients may be particularly vulnerable to removal of antipsychotics.*

Dopaminergic mechanisms remain plausible contributors to early clinical deterioration with removal of clozapine therapy. Potent blockade of inhibitory presynaptic D_2 autoreceptors by neuroleptic drugs given after clozapine administration may increase turnover of dopamine onto D_4 receptors made supersensitive by clozapine.[1] *Support for this hypothesis is provided by new evidence of apparently increased abundance (up-regulation) of putative D_4 sites in the brains of rats given clozapine (donated by Sandoz Research Institute, Bern, Switzerland) (20 mg/kg, twice daily for 3 weeks) or its vehicle intraperitoneally, and evaluated on the day after the last dose was received.*

Since highly D_4-selective radioligands are still in development,[6] *abundance of putative D_4 sites was estimated as the difference in binding of 2 radioligands—one nonselective for D_2/D_3/D_4 receptors and another, such as racloplide, selective for D_2/D_3 sites.*[7-10] *Alternatively, a nonselective radioligand can be combined with masking concentrations of unlabeled racloplide.*[11,12] *We used the D_2/D_3/D_4 ligand [^{3}H]-(±)-nemonapride (1 nmol/L) (DuPont-New England Nuclear) alone to assay mainly the abundant D_2 sites in frozen sections of rat forebrain, and with excess S(-)-raclopride (0.3 μmol/L) to selectively reveal D_4 receptors. Other sites where the radioligand may bind were also occluded, with 1,3-ditolylguanidine (0.5 μmol/L) for sigma sites (σ_1, σ_2) and pindolol (0.1 μmol/L) to mask serotonin$_{1A}$ sites, and 10-μmol/L S(-)-sulpiride was used to define nonspecific binding (drugs from Research Biochemicals International). Tissue sections were evaluated by computer-assisted densitometric autoradiography (MCID-M4 system; Imaging Research, St*

Catherines, Ontario); optical densities of silver grains produced by tritium in photographic film were converted to values of bound radioligand (expressed as femtomoles per milligram of tissue) for statistical analysis.[11,12]

Clozapine treatment induced a large increase of D_4-like binding in the limbic nucleus accumbens septi (mean[±SD], 171%±15% of controls; t=4.1, P<.005 [11 df]*), smaller increases in corpus striatum, and none in prefrontal cerebral cortex. In contrast, mainly D_2 binding without raclopride was increased in mesioprefrontal cortex (mean[±SD], 159%±12% of controls;* t=4.1, P<.005 [11 df]*), but in neither accumbens nor striatum. Similar results were obtained with alternative $D_2/D_3/D_4$ radioligand, [^{3}H]spiperone (DuPont-New England Nuclear) (with 40-nmol/L ketanserin to block serotonin$_2$ receptors), and after pretreatment (2 mg/kg thrice daily for 3 weeks) with another D_4-selective agent, S(+)-N-propylnorapomorphine ([+]-NPA) (Research Biochemicals International), whose pharmacological properties support its candidacy as an atypical antipsychotic agent.*[10,12-16] *These observations indicate that repeated treatment with clozapine and other D_4 antagonists can selectively increase the apparent abundance of D_4 receptors in specific regions of the mammalian limbic forebrain.*

In conclusion, special clinical caution is required when clozapine therapy is discontinued rapidly, pending quantification of the evident associated risks of early psychotic relapse, consideration of potential contributing pharmacological mechanisms, and testing of various treatment strategies. Options for safe management are needed as novel antipsychotic agents are introduced and more patients are switched from clozapine therapy to alternatives.

Ross J. Baldessarini, MD
Frank I. Tarazi, PhD
Nora S. Kula, MS
Harvard Medical School
Department of Psychiatry and Mailman Research Center
McLean Hospital
115 Mill St
Belmont, MA 02178

David M. Gardner, Pharm D
Faculty of Pharmaceutical Sciences and Medicine
Dalhousie University
Halifax, Nova Scotia

This work was supported, in part, by grants MH-31154, MH-34006, and MH-47370 from the National Institute of Mental Health, Washington, DC, by the Bruce J. Anderson Foundation, Boston, and the McLean Private Donors Neuropharmacology Research Fund, Belmont, Mass (Dr Baldessarini).

1. Baldessarini RJ, Gardner DM, Garver DL. Conversions from clozapine to other antipsychotic drugs. *Arch Gen Psychiatry.* 1995;52:1071-1072.
2. Meltzer HY. Clozapine withdrawal: serotonergic or dopaminergic mechanisms? *Arch Gen Psychiatry.* 1997;54:760-761.
3. Roth BL, Tandra S, Burgess LH, Sibley DR, Meltzer HY. D_4 dopamine receptor binding affinity does not distinguish between typical and atypical antipsychotic drugs. *Psychopharmacology.* 1995;120:365-368.
4. Kula NS, Baldessarini RJ, Kebabian JW, Neumeyer JL. S(+)-aporphines are not selective for human D_3 dopamine receptors. *Cell Mol Neurobiol.* 1994; 14:185-191.
5. Baldessarini RJ, Frankenburg FR. Clozapine, an atypical antipsychotic. *N Engl J Med.* 1991;324:746-754.
6. Kebabian JW, Tarazi FI, Kula NS, Baldessarini RJ. Compounds selective for dopamine receptor subtypes. *Drug Discovery Today.* In press.
7. Seeman P, Guan H-C, Van Tol HHM. Dopamine D_4 receptors elevated in schizophrenia. *Nature.* 1993;365:441-145.
8. Murray AM, Hyde TM, Knable MB, Herman MM, Bigelow LB, Carter JM, Weinberger DR, Kleinman JR. Distribution of putative D_4 dopamine receptors in postmortem striatum from patients with schizophrenia. *J Neurosci.* 1995;15:2186-2191.
9. Baldessarini RJ, Tarazi FI. Brain dopamine receptors: a primer on their current status, basic and clinical. *Harvard Rev Psychiatry.* 1996;3:301-325.
10. Baldessarini RJ. Dopamine receptors and clinical medicine. In: Neve RL, Neve KA, eds. *The Dopamine Receptors.* Totowa, NJ: Humana Press; 1997:457-498.
11. Tarazi FI, Florijn WJ, Creese I. Differential regulation of dopament receptors following chronic typical and atypical antipsychotic drug treatment. *Neuroscience.* In press.
12. Tarazi FI, Yeghiayan SK, Baldessarini RJ, Kula NS, Neumeyer JL. Long-term effects of S(+)N-*n*-propylnorapomorphine compared with typical and atypical antipsychotics: differential increases of cerebrocortical D_2-like and striatolombic D_4-like dopamine receptors. *Neuropsychopharmacology.* In press.
13. Campbell A, Yeghiayan SK, Baldessarini RJ, Neumeyer JL. Selective antidopaminergic effects of S(+)N-*n*-propylnoraporphines in limbic vs extrapyramidal sites in rat brain: comparisons with typical and atypical antipsychotic agents. *Psychopharmacology.* 1991;103:323-329.
14. Campbell A, Baldessarini RJ, Neumeyer JL. Altered spontaeous behavior and responses to apomorphine in rats following pretreatment with S(+)-aporphines or fluphenazine. *Psychopharmacology.* 1993; 111:351-358.
15. Seeman P, Van Tol HHM. Dopamine D_4 receptors bind inactive S(+)-aporphines, suggesting neuroleptic role: sulpiride not stereoselective. *Eur J Pharmacol.* 1993;233:173-174.
16. Lahti RA, Evans DL, Stratman NC, Figur LM. Dopamime D_4 vs D_2 receptor selectivity of dopamine receptor antagonists: possible therapeutic implications. *Eur J Pharmacol.* 1993;236:483-486.

In reply

The thoughtful comments of Dr Meltzer and Dr Baldessarini and colleagues are very important in advancing both the clinical practice and the therapeutic basis of antipsychotic medication. This letter provides some additional views and information that may be helpful in this discussion.

What is the basis of rapid relapse on clozapine withdrawal?

To explain those instances of rapid relapse of schizophrenic patients when clozapine therapy is withdrawn, Baldessarini et al[1] *give 3 reasonable hypotheses, as mentioned in Meltzer's letter.*

To consider these different possible mechanisms, it is first important to note that the inhibition constant (k_i) of a neuroleptic drug depends on the radioligand used to label the receptor.[2,3] *Clozapine, for example, at the D_2 dopamine receptor has a k_i of 390±70 nmol/L (mean[±SD]) using [^{3}H]nemonapride, 186±40 nmol/L using [^{3}H]spiperone, and 83±15 nmol/L using [^{3}H]raclopride. Haloperidol at the D_2 receptor has a k_i of 9.6±1.5 nmol/L using [^{3}H]nemonapride, 2.9±0.4 nmol/L using [^{3}H]spiperone, and 0.67±0.06 nmol/L using [^{3}H]raclopride.*[2,3] *These neuroleptic agent inhibition constants (K_is) are related to the tissue-buffer partition coefficients of the radioligands.*[2,3] *Thus, by extrapolating the relation between the neuroleptic agent k_i and the tissue-buffer partition, one obtains the true k_i of the neuroleptic drug in the absence of any competing radioligand. This extrapolated radioligand-independent k_i exactly agrees with the K_d of the neuroleptic drug obtained by direct measurement using either [^{3}H]clozapine or [^{3}H]haloperidol.*[2,3]

Hence, the neuroleptic drugs discussed by Meltzer and by Baldessarini et al have ligand-independent k_is at human cloned D_2 and D_4 receptors and serotonin$_{2A}$ (rat cerebral cortex) receptors that are as follows[2,3]*:*

Drug	Mean (±SD) Neuroleptic Receptor k_i, nmol/L*		
	D_2	D_4	$Serotonin_{2A}$
Clozapine	44±8	1.6±0.4	11±3.5
Loxapine	5.2±0.03	7.8±1.5	10.2±1.2
Haloperidol	0.35±0.05	0.84±0.5	25±8
Risperidone	0.3±0.1	0.25±0.1	0.14±0.1
Ritanserin	10±4	30±5	1±0.5
Thioridazine	0.4±0.12	1.5±0.5	60±15
Trifluperazine	0.96±0.2	44±6	135±50

A second preliminary point relevant to this discussion is that therapeutic doses of clozapine occupy high levels of brain D_2 receptors in patients.[4] This conclusion is a direct result of k_i of the neuroleptic drug being dependent on the tissue-membrane partition of the radioligand. This stems from the fact that clozapine occupies 50% of the D_2 receptors, as measured using radiolabeled carbon 11 [^{11}C]raclopride,[5] but a much lower percentage (0% to 22%) when using radioactive congeners of spiperone.[6-8] Thus, under clinical conditions in which the patient has no radioligand, clozapine occupies high levels of D_2 receptors. In addition, clozapine occupies high levels of D_4 and $serotonin_{2A}$ receptors. The blockade of each of these receptors by clozapine may contribute different components of antipsychotic action.

In the light of these 2 preliminary points, it may be seen that, of the neuroleptic drugs listed above, clozapine has the weakest association with D_2. Thus, clozapine is readily displaceable by endogenous dopamine at the D_2 receptor. This may be the reason for rapid relapse. That is, after the patient has stopped taking clozapine, any sudden surge of impulse-triggered release of dopamine will almost immediately displace any residual clozapine occupying the D_2 receptors, with an ensuing psychosis.

Which neuroleptic is best for replacing clozapine?

Only the extensive clinical experience of Drs Meltzer and Baldessarini et al can appropriately answer this question. However, if D_4 blockade has an antipsychotic role, then the above list indicates that only clozapine is D_4 selective. Loxapine is D_2 selective, as are most other neuroleptic drugs. Risperidone is equally potent at D_2 and D_4.

The suggestion by Meltzer to use ritanserin to minimize withdrawal psychosis is interesting. As indicated in the above tabulation, however, ritanserin has a 10-nmol/L K_d for the D_2 receptor. Thus, depending on the clinical dose used, one would expect ritanserin to occupy D_2 receptors and to allay psychotic symptoms. At low doses, however, ritanserin would be selective for $serotonin_{2A}$ receptors, occupying only about 1 D_2 receptor for every 10 $serotonin_{2A}$ receptors occupied.

Finally, the pharmacological nature of the D_4-like sites, elevated by clozapine or by haloperidol,[9] is unknown. Using tissues that have significant amounts of the D_4-like sites, preliminary findings in this laboratory with D_4-selective [^3H]ligands indicate that the actual amount of D_4 receptors in the human striatum is different and much lower than the amount of D_4-like sites. As explained elsewhere,[1,9,10] the D_4-like sites are defined by subtracting the densities of 2 radioligands, [^3H]nemonapride and [^3H]raclopride. It may be, however, that these radioligands detect different proportions of monomers and dimers of the D_2 receptors, yielding an apparent population of D_4-like sites. Further research is needed to determine the nature of the D_4-like binding sites as well as why they are elevated in schizophrenia.[10]

Philip Seeman, MD, PhD,
Departments of Pharmacology and Psychiatry
Medical Science Bldg
Room 4344
University of Toronto
8 Taddle Creek Rd,
Toronto, Ontario, Canada M5S 1A8

1. Baldessarini RJ, Gardner DM, Garver DL. Conversions from clozapine to other antipsychotic drugs. *Arch Gen Psychiatry.* 1995;52:1071-1072.
2. Seeman P, Van Tol HHM. Deriving the therapeutic concentrations for clozapine and haloperidol: the apparent dissociation constant of a neuroleptic at the dopamine D_2 or D_4 receptor varies with the affinity of the competing radioligand. *Eur J Pharmacol.* 1995;291:59-66.
3. Seeman P. Therapeutic receptor-blocking concentrations of neuroleptics. *Int Clin Psychopharmacol.* 1995;10(suppl 3):5-13.
4. Seeman P, Kapur S. Clozapine occupies high levels of dopamine D_2 receptors. *Life Sci.* 1997;60:PL207-PL216.
5. Nordström A-L, Farde L, Nyberg S, Karlsson P, Halldin C, Sedvall G. D_1, D_2, and 5-HT_2 receptor occupancy in relation to clozapine serum concentration: a PET study of schizophrenic patients. *Am J Psychiatry.* 1996;152:1444-1449.
6. Louwerens JW, Buddingh JA, Zijlstra S, Pruim J, Korf J, Paans AMJ, Vaalburg W, Slooff CJ. Dopamine (D_2)-receptor occupancy in clozapine-treated patients as measured by positron emission tomography using ^{18}FESP. In: Brunello N, Mendlewicz J, Racagni G, eds. *New Generation of Antipsychotic Drugs: Novel Mechanisms of Action.* Basel, Switzerland: S Karger AG; 1993; 4:130-135.
7. Conley R, Zhao M, Wong D, Tamminga C. ^{11}C NMSP receptor occupancy by clozapine and haloperidol in schizophrenic subjects. *Biol Psychiatry.* 1996; 39:513. Abstract.
8. Karbe H, Wienhard K, Hamacher K, Huber M, Herholz K, Coenen HH, Stöcklin G, Lövenich A, Heiss WD. Positron emission tomography with (^{18}F) methylspiperone demonstrates D_2 dopamine receptor binding differences of clozapine and haloperidol. *J Neural Transm.* 1991;86:163-173.
9. Schoots O, Seeman P, Guan H-C, Paterson A, Van Tol HHM. Long-term haloperidol elevates dopamine D_4 receptors by two-fold in rats. *Eur J Pharmacol.* 1995;289:67-72.
10. Seeman P, Guan H-C, Van Tol HHM. Schizophrenia: elevation of dopamine D_4-like sites, using [^{3}H]nemonapride and [^{125}I]epidepride. *Eur J Pharmacol.* 1995;286:R3-R5.

Anterior Paralimbic Mediation of Procaine-Induced Emotional and Psychosensory Experiences

Ketter et al[1] report on an increase in anterior paralimbic cerebral blood flow (CBF) associated with procaine-induced affective and perceptual symptoms. Changes in CBF and increased activation of left anterior paralimbic structures were associated with procaine-induced fear. Superior temporal activation occurred in the entire group of subjects, most of whom experience "hallucinations." Intense unformed visual hallucinations were associated with greater global CBF.

The clinical psychiatric symptoms of the toxic effects of lidocaine hydrochloride and procaine are similar, both showing dysphoric mood changes with fear of death or doom-related content and hallucinations.[2] Based on the work of Post et al,[3] it had been previously hypothesized that activation of the amygdala, hippocampus, and related structures might be involved in producing the symptoms of lidocaine toxicity.[4-6] The interesting finding by Ketter et al[1] that procaine-induced fear is related to activation of the left amygdala in experimental subjects suggests that the fears about death and doom anxiety seen in the clinical syndrome of the toxic effects of procaine, and perhaps lidocaine, may be similarly caused.

The authors' inferences regarding the procaine-induced auditory and visual sensory experiences which they term hallucinations may be more problematic. While it is true that formed hallucinations are part of the clinical syndromes of the toxic effects of lidocaine and procaine,[2] it is unclear that the unformed visual and auditory sensory perceptions reported by Ketter et al are hallucinations and could be a different class of perceptions altogether. Auditory experiences similar to those described in the article have also been described in alcohol withdrawal states.[7] These phenomena originally believed to be "elementary" hallucinations are actually entotic phenomena, ie, real sounds (objective tinnitus) caused by contractions of the muscles governing the function of the middle ear. Reports, popping, clicking, and fluttering noises were referable to contractions of the tensor tympani, stapedius, and tensor veli palitini muscles. The alcohol withdrawal states in some as yet undefined way increase or intensify these contractions, magnify their perception, or both and may distort their perceived point of origin making them appear to have arisen in the external environment.

In pursuing their aim of trying to relate the activation of cerebral structures to the generation of hallucinations, it would be important for the authors to determine whether the perceptions they report are internally derived or are of peripheral origin, such as objective tinnitus arising in the middle ear, or subjective tinnitus of cochlear or neural origin in the auditory sphere, or retinal phenomena in the visual sphere. It would be helpful to know whether the authors have considered these issues and whether they have been able to infer the origin of the auditory and visual sensations they describe on the basis of more detailed clinical data than they report in their article.

Stephen M. Saravay, MD
Consultation-Liasion Psychiatry
Long Island Jewish Medical Center
New Hyde Park, NY 11040

1. Ketter TA, Andreason PJ, George MS, Lee C, Gill DS, Parekh PI, Willis MW, Herscovitch P, Post RM. Anterior paralimbic mediation of procaine-induced emotional and psychosensory experiences. *Arch Gen Psychiatry.* 1986;53:59-69.
2. Saravay SM, Marke J, Steinberg MD, Rabiner CJ. 'Doom anxiety' and delirium in lidocaine toxicity. *Am J Psychiatry.* 1987;144:159-163.
3. Post RM, Kennedy C, Shinohara M, Squillace K, Miyaoka M, Suda S, Ingvar DH, Sokoloff L. Local cerebral glucose utilization of lidocaine-kindled seizures. *Soc Neurosci Abstr.* 1979;5:196. Abstract.
4. Lloyd B, Greenblatt D. Neuropsychiatric sequelae of pharmacotherapy of cardiac arrhythmias and hypertension. *J Clin Psychopharmacol.* 1981;1:394-398.
5. Mesulam MM. Lidocaine toxicity and the limbic system. *Am J Psychiatry.* 1987;144:1623.
6. Saravay SM, Marke J, Steinberg MD, Rabiner CJ. Lidocaine toxicity and the limbic system. *Am J Psychiatry.* 1987;144:1623-1624.
7. Saravay SM, Pardes H. Auditory elementary hallucinations in alcohol withdrawal psychosis. *Arch Gen Psychiatry.* 1967;16:652-658.

In reply

We appreciate Dr Saravay's comments regarding similarities between the acute clinical responses of some of our healthy volunteers to intravenous procaine[1] and the psychopathological features observed in some medical patients receiving more sustained intravenous lidocaine therapy.[2]

Dr Saravay raises the important issue of whether the perceptual changes induced by short-term procaine challenge in our subjects are of peripheral vs central origin. He describes the visual and auditory experiences of our subjects as unformed sensory perceptions and, hence, suggests that they may be of peripheral origin. However, these experiences were, in fact, more heterogeneous, and in some cases more complex, than Dr Saravay suggests. Some subjects did have unformed auditory (buzzing and ringing) and visual (flashing lights) experiences while others noted partially formed auditory (electronic music) and visual (swirls of color, thumbprintlike patterns) symptoms. Fully formed auditory (spoken words) or visual (faces, landscapes) hallucinations did not occur in our sample. As Dr Saravay acknowledges, formed hallucinations may be seen as the toxic effects of procaine and lidocaine. Indeed, patients in Dr Saravay's report on doom anxiety with lidocaine therapy had variable perceptual experiences, ranging from unformed to formed.[2]

Thus, although some of our subjects had unformed sensory perceptions consistent with (but not necessarily indicating) peripheral origin, others had partially formed perceptions more consistent with central origin. Patients with focal epilepsies describe unformed, partially formed, and fully formed auditory and visual experiences during partial seizures originating in the temporal and occipital lobes, respectively. The complexity of these events seems to depend on whether primary sensory, primary association, or secondary association cortices are involved. Thus, even unformed perceptual experiences can be of central origin. A parsimonious mechanistic hypothesis would be that procaine-induced sensory phenomena are of central origin and vary in complexity depending on the extent of brain regions activated. With this model, variability in clinical responses could be related to different degrees of overall procaine (global CBF) response, with more limited responses activating primary sensory cortices and yielding unformed perceptions, and more robust responses resulting in widespread activations that involve association cortices and, thus, more complex perceptual phenomena.

On the other hand, limited evidence suggests that local anesthetics can either attenuate or exacerbate tinnitus,[3] possibly by peripheral rather than central effects.[4] Hence another, albeit less parsimonious, possible explanation is that short-term procaine challenge could cause unformed perceptual experiences by peripheral effects and more complex sensory changes by central (or central plus peripheral) mechanisms. With this model, peripheral activation could occur at a lower threshold and yield unformed sensory experiences, while central activation could occur at a higher threshold and result in more complex sensory events in those subjects with more robust responses to procaine. Additional study is needed to clarify the roles of central vs peripheral mechanisms underlying procaine-induced perceptual phenomena.

Terence A. Ketter, MD
Department of Psychiatry and Behavioral Sciences
Stanford University School of Medicine
Stanford, CA 94305-5543

Paul J. Andreason, MD
Chulhee Lee, PhD
Debra S. Gill, MA
Priti I. Parekh
Mark W. Willis, MEng
Peter Herscovitch, MD
Robert M. Post, MD
National Institutes of Health
Bethesda, MD 20892-1272

Mark S. George, MD
Departments of Psychiatry
Radiology and Neurology
Medical University of South Carolina
Charleston, SC 29425-0720

1. Ketter TA, Andreason PJ, George MS, Lee C, Gill DS, Parekh PI, Willis MW, Herscovitch P, Post RM. Anterior paralimbic mediation of procaine-induced emotional and psychosensory experiences. *Arch Gen Psychiatry.* 1996;53:59-69.
2. Saravay SM, Marke J, Steinberg MD, Rabiner CJ. 'Doom anxiety' and delirium in lidocaine toxicity. *Am J Psychiatry.* 1987;144:159-163.
3. Duckert LG, Rees IS. Treatment of tinnitus with intravenous lidocaine: a double-blind randomized trial. *Otolaryngol Head Neck Surg.* 1983;91:550-555.
4. Lyttkens L, Larsson B, Wasterstrom SA. Local anesthetics and tinnitus: proposed peripheral mechanism of action of lidocaine. *J Otorhinolaryngol Relat Spec.* 1984;46:17-23.

Correction and Clarification

Our recently published Commentary "Current Therapeutic Profile of Lithium" (*Arch Gen Psychiatry.* 1997;54:16-20) was published with 2 errors. On page 16, third column, lines 12 and 13, the sentence that reads "Thus, patients with more severe cases and with lower proportions of cases of . . ." should have read "Thus, *patient samples* with more severe cases and with lower proportions of cases of. . . ." On page 17, third column, second paragraph, line 3, the sentence that reads "The measurement of in vivo brain lithium levels in patients was made with nuclear lithium-7 magnetic . . ." should have read "The measurement of in vivo brain lithium levels in patients was made *possible* with nuclear lithium-7 magnetic. . . ."

Samuel Gershon, MD
Jair C. Soares, MD
Western Psychiatric Institute and Clinic
University of Pittsburgh Medical Center
3811 O'Hara St
Pittsburgh, P 15213

Announcement

Free Patient Record Forms Available

Patient record forms are available free of charge to ARCHIVES readers by calling or writing FORMEDIC, 12D Worlds Fair Dr, Somerset, NJ 08873-9863, telephone (908) 469-7031.

THIS MONTH IN ARCHIVES OF GENERAL PSYCHIATRY

Lay-administered structured interviews and self-administered problem checklists are 2 types of instruments frequently used to measure psychopathology among children. These instruments are presumed to differ in cost (checklists—less expensive) and performance (interviews—more useful). **Boyle et al** (page 793) examined the reliability and validity of an interview and a checklist, using assessments collected from parents of children aged 6 to 16 years in the general population, and detected no differences in reliability and validity. These findings suggest that checklists might be able to substitute for interviews in some diagnosis-based epidemiological studies.

Simonoff et al (page 801) report rates of *DSM-III-R* disorder from clinical interviews of more than 1400 general population twin pairs from the Virginia Twin Study of Adolescent Behavioral Development. Imposing a standard additional impairment criterion decreases the rates of all disorders, especially anxiety and phobic disorders. High levels of comorbidity between anxiety and phobic disorders raise questions about the validity of diagnostic distinctions.

Do shyness, anxiety, and social withdrawal help prevent at-risk youths from becoming delinquent? Previous studies provide contradictory answers. **Kerr et al** (page 809) argue that behavioral inhibition is the protective factor, but it has sometimes been confounded with these other constructs. In a sample of boys from low socioeconomic areas, inhibited boys were less at risk for delinquency even if they were disruptive. Withdrawn boys, on the other hand, were more at risk for delinquency or delinquency with depression. These results, particularly if they are replicated, may guide the selection of youths for targeted preventive interventions.

Rey et al (page 817) describe a global scale to measure the quality of the environment in which a child was reared and they report that it has good interrater and test-retest reliability. They also present information about the scale's construct and predictive validity and suggest that this instrument may be valuable in clinical and outcomes research.

In the first magnetic resonance imaging study of frontostriatal anatomy in treatment-naive pediatric obsessive-compulsive disorder (OCD), **Rosenberg et al** (page 824) report that patients with OCD had significantly smaller striatal (caudate and putamen) volumes than controls. Lower striatal volumes were associated with greater OCD symptom severity but were unrelated to illness duration. These results suggest that abnormalities in striatal anatomy may be associated with the clinical presentation of OCD and that this pathological involvement may be a central neurobiological deficit in this illness.

In the first ever study of treatment-naive pediatric patients with obsessive-compulsive disorder (OCD) near onset of illness, **Rosenberg et al** (page 831) assessed 3 well-delineated aspects of prefrontal cortical function: the ability to suppress responses, the volitional execution of delayed responses, and the anticipation of predictable events. A selective disturbance in cognitive response suppression was observed in OCD that may underlie the repetitive symptomatic behavior that characterizes the illness.

Serotonin and adverse childhood rearing experiences relate to childhood-onset chronic aggression, but it is unclear if there are relationships among serotonin, rearing experiences, and aggression in children. **Pine et al** (page 839) report that aggression and adverse rearing in prepubertal boys positively correlate with prolactin response to fenfluramine hydrochloride challenge, a serotonergic measure. While the direction of the association between aggression and serotonin is opposite to findings in adults, it is consistent with prior studies in boys.

The introduction of noninvasive brain imaging techniques in the early 1980s permitted direct study of the relationship of perinatal brain injury to childhood psychopathology. **Whitaker et al** (page 847) examined this relationship in a large regional cohort of low-birth-weight infants screened as newborns using a cranial ultrasonogram. They found that one group of neonatal ultrasonogram abnormalities was related to psychiatric disorder at age 6 years, particularly attention deficit hyperactivity disorder, even in children of normal intelligence and with all competing predictors statistically controlled. These findings suggest that injury to subcortical structures may be involved in behavioral inhibition.

Stimulants are effective in the short-term treatment of attention deficit hyperactivity disorder (ADHD), but little is known about their ability to ameliorate symptoms of the disorder over a longer period. **Gillberg et al** (page 857) studied 62 children aged 6 to 11 years with severe ADHD symptoms who participated in a randomized double-blind placebo-controlled study of amphetamine. The drug was well tolerated and clearly superior to placebo in reducing inattention, hyperactivity, and other behavioral problems. Wechsler Intelligence Scale for Children–Revised scores tended to improve. Positive effects of the stimulant drug persisted 15 months after starting treatment.

The Collaborative Multimodal Treatment Study of Children With Attention Deficit Hyperactivity Disorder is the largest National Institute of Mental Health–originated clinical trial to date and the first with children. **Arnold et al** (page 865) present the overall design and the rationale for some critical design decisions made by investigators.

Progress in pediatric psychopharmacology research has suffered significant delay, especially when compared with the achievements in the adult field. The National Institute of Mental Health (NIMH) has coordinated systematic efforts to identify the major obstacles to research in this area of pharmacology and to propose feasible solutions. Aspects relevant to pediatric research, including methodological, ethical, legal, regulatory, financial, and family or community aspects, are discussed. **Vitiello** and **Jensen** (page 871) present possible solutions, together with initiatives recently undertaken by NIMH, to spur research in child psychopharmacology.

Little is known about the differential efficacy of commonly used psychotherapies for the treatment of adolescents with major depression. **Brent et al** (page 877) found that cognitive behavioral therapy (CBT) was more efficacious than either systemic-behavioral family therapy or nondirective supportive therapy for rapidity and completeness of depressive symptom relief. Parents also viewed CBT as more credible over time than either of the other 2 treatments. Cognitive behavioral therapy seems to be a viable treatment option for adolescents with major depression in clinical settings.

A Commentary by Michael Rutter, titled Child Psychiatric Disorder: Measures, Causal Mechanisms, and Interventions, is also included in this issue.

COMMENTARY

Child Psychiatric Disorder

Measures, Causal Mechanisms, and Interventions

DURING RECENT decades there has been a spectacular burgeoning of research into child psychiatric disorders. The results have changed clinical practice in child psychiatry[1] and have done much to aid understanding of the childhood roots of some adult psychiatric disorders.[2] The set of 12 articles in this issue of the ARCHIVES illustrate well the accomplishments and the serious challenges that remain. They cover a wide territory, but their key messages may be summarized under the headings of measurement, causal mechanisms, and therapeutic interventions.

MEASUREMENT

Psychiatric research continues to be troubled by difficulties in measurement.[3] At one time, many investigators thought that the use of standardized interviews and operationalized criteria for diagnosis would solve the problems, but it is evident that they have not. The study by Boyle et al[4] is helpful in focusing on the relative merits and demerits of structured respondent-based interviews and checklists. They conclude that there is not much to choose between the 2 methods for reliability and validity, note that checklists take much less time to complete, and point out that the approach of the 2 methods is basically similar. Nevertheless, there was substantial disagreement between the 2 about whether individuals met the criteria for caseness for particular diagnoses (κ values from 0.05 to 0.52); it was rightly inferred that both instruments are likely to involve considerable error.

Because previous research has shown similar levels of disagreement for a range of instruments, a consensus has developed that multiple measures are required, preferably involving different informants and repeated measures over time.[5] This approach reduces error, minimizes rater bias, and minimizes the effect of situation specificity. This has led to more robust findings[6,7]; however, major unresolved difficulties remain.

Most crucially, not only is there generally weak agreement between the ratings of different informants, such as parent and child,[8] but also the patterns of correlates vary by informant. This is most strikingly evident in the genetic findings.[9] It makes little sense to postulate a genetic difference between the same disorder as reported by parents and children, unless the 2 are reflecting some difference in the meaning of the disorder. Of course, there is no shortage of possible explanations. Parents may, for example, be unaware of their children's behavior outside the home or their inner feelings (and hence mood state). Also, they may provide a more balanced perspective on the extent to which their children's behavior or emotions are abnormal. But it is by no means obvious why any of these hypothesized differences should lead to such radically different genetic findings. Moreover, there is an extreme lack of research to test whether the proposed explanations are truly valid. Such research is urgently needed.

See also pages 793, 801, 809, 817, 824, 831, 839, 847, 857, 865, 871, and 877

In the meanwhile, there is the dilemma of how best to combine multiple measures given that they differ in their correlates. Two main solutions have been proposed. Either the "or" rule (ie, a symptom is counted as present if it is present on either the parent or the child report) is followed,[10] or structural equation modeling is used to derive a latent variable.[6] Both work reasonably well in many ways, but the first involves the likelihood that chalk and cheese are being mixed and the second means that the findings apply to a latent variable that accounts for a relatively small proportion of the population variance. Neither approach seems satisfactory, and the real need is to determine why ratings vary by informant.

Boyle et al[4] comment on the reduced reliability when symptom assessments need to include either duration or timing of onset. Similarly, Angold et al[10] found both to be highly unreliable and cautioned on the problems created by such criteria for many diagnoses in the prevailing classification systems. Boyle et al also note that although disruptive behavior disorders (whether assessed by interview or questionnaires) were strongly associated with impaired social functioning, the association was much weaker for anxiety disorders. Simonoff et al,[8] using data from the Virginia Twin Study of Adolescent Behavioral Development, similarly found that it was common to find children with multiple anxiety symptoms but without social impair-

This article is also available on our Web site: www.ama-assn.org/psych.

ment. It is generally accepted that the diagnosis of disorder needs to require the presence of such impairment if unrealistically high rates of disorder are to be avoided.[11]

A recurrent feature in studies using repeated ratings is that the levels of psychopathological features on the second occasion tend to be systematically lower than those on the first assessment; Boyle et al found that the effect was more marked with the checklist but it was present also with the structured interview. The reasons for the decline are ill understood, but presumably they reflect the fact that most symptoms concern behaviors that require relative judgments (such as on degree of depression or hyperactivity) and hence are open to rater sets and to the comparison groups used by raters. The latter seems to be important for reports of hyperactivity where the evidence indicates the likelihood of biases reflecting twin-contrast (and presumably also sibling-contrast) effects.[9,12,13] There is a need, when that is the case, to supplement ratings with psychometric assessments (such as the continuous performance test for inattention) and mechanical measures (such as actometers for activity level).

The article by Kerr et al[14] is noteworthy for its substantive and methodological implications. The key substantive result is that whereas behavioral inhibition protected boys against delinquency social withdrawal did not. This may serve to explain the puzzling reports in the literature suggesting that shyness protects against delinquency but the combination of shyness and aggression predisposes to it.[15,16] The implication is that, despite their surface similarities, behavioral inhibition (social anxiety) and social withdrawal (a nonanxious preference for solitary activity) constitute rather different constructs with different functions. Care needs to be taken to ensure that measures differentiate between the 2 and assess behavioral constellations as well as separate traits. Kerr et al properly caution on the limitations of their study (small sample size and quite limited questionnaire measures of their constructs), but the methodological messages echo those put forward previously by Stattin and Magnusson[17] based on other data sets.

Three measurement issues arise. First, it is an inherent feature of structured respondent-based interviews and questionnaires that they can tap only those constructs included. That is no problem when the features to be investigated are well established, but it does constitute a serious constraint for the discovery of clinically relevant phenomena that were not already recognized. That this matters is obvious from the frequency with which unexpected phenomena turn out to be clinically pertinent. The social abnormalities associated with an institutional rearing,[18,19] the different social features associated with severe developmental disorders of receptive language,[20] and the social anxiety associated with fragile X[21] illustrate this point. The investigator-based interviews, such as the Child and Adolescent Psychiatric Assessment,[22] that elicit descriptions of behavior rather than yes or no answers to structured questions on specific symptoms should avoid this constraint, but their advantages and disadvantages in relation to respondent-based interviews have yet to be assessed.

Second, the findings draw attention to the need to pay attention to the mechanisms involved in comorbidity.[23,24] Numerous studies have drawn attention to its high frequency. It is evident that much of the apparent comorbidity is artifactual (resulting from measurement problems and errors in the prevailing psychiatric diagnostic concepts). Nevertheless, the phenomenon is important with respect to the possibility that comorbid patterns may represent meaningfully different disorders and may also be used to investigate the mechanisms involved in the process by which one condition creates a risk for another.

Third, behind all of these issues lies the dilemma of when dimensional measures are to be preferred to categorical ones.[25,26] Unfortunately, all too often protagonists on both sides tend to assume that one is right and the other is wrong. That is misleading for a host of different reasons.[27,28] Nevertheless, the issue of whether extreme categories do or do not differ qualitatively from variations within the normal range remains an important question that is open to empirical testing.[29]

The report by Rey et al[30] deals with the separate issues involved in measuring children's rearing environment. They opted for a global scale of family qualities on the grounds that composite measures often provide the best prediction of psychopathological features and are cost-effective. Their findings indicate that they have developed a reliable and robust measure that is simple to apply. Nevertheless, the price paid is substantial. A growing amount of evidence suggests that environmental effects are best considered by the effect on individual children rather than as a familywide influence.[31,32] Also, the family variables that affect one sort of outcome are not necessarily the same as those that affect others.[33,34] Achieving family measures that are valid and discriminating, as well as reliable, probably requires systematic standardized questioning that covers the range of possible family risk features. Moreover, as with measures of psychopathological features, reports from parents and children are desirable, and observational measures are needed to assess certain sorts of family features.[35] As Rey et al note, these are time-consuming and expensive and for some purposes their much simpler composite index will suffice. It is primarily in the testing of specific hypotheses about environmental risk mediation that more intensive measures are needed. Their use will need to be in the context of designs that can take account of the fact that some supposedly environmental effects are, in actuality, partially mediated genetically[36,37] and that gene-environment correlations and interactions are likely to be operating.[38-40]

TESTING CAUSAL HYPOTHESES

The 5 articles testing causal hypotheses all raise interesting issues. Kovacs et al[41] used the family history method (plus direct interviewing of mothers) to compare the rates of psychopathological features in relatives of young people with an early-onset depressive or bipolar disorder vs those with some other psychiatric condition. As expected, affective disorders were more common in the first- and second-degree relatives of probands with affective disorder. The authors argue that pedigrees ascertained through affectively ill children are good candidates for genetic studies. That may well be so, although their data provide no indication that that is more the case with childhood- than adult-onset affective disorders. Other studies have shown that an onset before early adult life tends to be associated with a greater familial loading than that found when the onset is later,[42,43] but the increased loading is more evident with an adolescent than with a prepubertal onset.[44] The few twin data available for this age group suggest a greater genetic component to affective symptoms in adolescence than in childhood,[45,46] but whether that is also the case with major depressive disorders remains uncertain.

As WITH OTHER studies, comorbidity was frequent among the probands in the Kovacs et al study. Their findings on familial loading are provocative because of some curiosities in patterns. Thus, there was an increase for alcoholism and antisocial personality but not any type of affective disorder in male relatives. In female relatives, the odds ratio for substance abuse (3.45) was greater than that for either major depression (1.47) or recurrent unipolar depression (2.31), and that for alcoholism (2.15) was comparable. This increased familial loading for nonaffective disorders was not entirely a function of comorbidity in probands, but the presence of comorbidity in relatives was not reported. Harrington et al[44] found that comorbid depression was more frequent in the relatives of probands with a prepubertal onset of depression. As Kovacs et al note, the familial aggregation may reflect environmental, as well as genetic, mediation. The possible role of gene-environment correlations and interactions[46-48] also needs to be considered. Twin and adoptive studies of affective disorder in children and adolescents are greatly needed; the findings of Kovacs et al highlight the importance, when using them, of examining the effects of age of onset and comorbidity.

The 2 articles by Rosenberg et al[49,50] add to the growing evidence that neural abnormalities may play a role in the genesis of obsessive-compulsive disorder (OCD). One study compared young patients with OCD with matched healthy control subjects on 3 oculomotor tests thought to reflect prefrontal function. Group differences were found only for response suppression, and it is argued that a selective deficit in frontal-striatal function is implied. The overlap between groups was substantial, but the association found with the severity of OCD symptoms suggests that the between-group difference was meaningful. The other article used magnetic resonance imaging; patients with OCD had significantly smaller striatal volumes than controls, implying possible underlying striatal pathological features. Rosenberg et al[49,50] properly caution about the need for replication and determination of whether the findings are specific to OCD. Both are essential, particularly in view of the surprising inconsistency of biological findings in child psychiatry, as evident, for example, in the field of autism.[51] It may well be that the conjunction of molecular genetic findings with other biological investigations will help bring greater order to the field and facilitate the identification of neural causal mechanisms.[52] In making inferences about neural functioning from patterns of cognitive function, it will be necessary to appreciate that developmental considerations mean that findings in adult life cannot be extrapolated to childhood.[53]

The study by Pine et al[54] is innovative in its use of the brothers of convicted delinquents as subjects and in its focus on biosocial interplay. Their findings, using the fenfluramine challenge procedure to assess central serotonergic activity, showed that an increased prolactin response was associated with aggression and adverse rearing. The authors note several important methodological limitations to their study, but the findings are provocative in the suggestion that the patterns of serotonin activity associated with aggression vary by age, with an increase early in life but a decrease in childhood. The apparent developmental switch, if confirmed, might explain some of the contradictions in the literature. There are other puzzles, such as the possible sex difference in serotonin correlates, as evident in the Dunedin, New Zealand, study.[55] The association with adverse rearing is an important reminder that evidence of a biological correlate does not necessarily mean biological determination of the behavior.[56,57] Animal and human studies have repeatedly shown that psychosocial manipulations have biological consequences.[58]

It has long been assumed that social adversity increases the susceptibility of low-birth-weight infants to obstetric or perinatal risks.[59,60] This assumption is based on old studies with 2 major problems. First, in the absence of imaging data, it was not known when obstetric risk actually led to brain dysfunction; second, the apparent interaction between social adversity and obstetric risk could be an artifact of the correlation between the 2. The findings of Whittaker et al[61] are important in suggesting that there is no biosocial interaction in relation to psychiatric disorder at age 6 years. A parenchymatous lesion, ventricular enlargement, or both, as identified on neonatal ultrasonographic scans (but, strikingly, not germinal matrix hemorrhage or intraventricular bleeding), were accompanied by a 4-fold increase in risk of psychopathological features, mainly attention deficit hyperactivity disorder. Social disadvantage, contrary to most views, actually reduced this risk. Family dysfunction did independently predict attention deficit hyperactivity disorder, but, again, it did not increase the risk associated with parenchymatous damage. The article does not deal with the psychosocial effects in any detail, but the difference found between broad social variables and more proximal within-the-family features emphasizes the need to go beyond composite psychosocial adversity measures if we are to understand how environmental risks are mediated.

There is still much to learn about the mechanisms involved in the psychiatric risks associated with brain injury. In this study, the odds ratio decreased from 4.4 to 3.0 when children with low IQs were excluded, emphasizing the role of cognitive impairment in the psychopathological risk. The finding that the risk still remained high also underlines that the risk is by no means wholly mediated in this way. The role of motor dysfunction was not assessed; this needs to be investigated in view of other evidence of its prevalence as a consequence of early brain injury.[62]

THERAPEUTIC INTERVENTIONS

The last 4 articles round off the collection nicely in what they provide on the evaluation of treatment. The Swedish study[63] is informative in its demonstration that in 6- to 11-year-old children without major psychosocial adversity who were shown to be responders to amphetamine the benefits of continuing drug treatment were still evident at 15 months. The clinical implications of this finding are severely constrained by the heterogeneity of the sample, by the exclusion of children with major psychosocial problems, and, most of all, by 1 curious feature. The withdrawal of active drug at 15 months did not lead to any significant deterioration in behavior during the subsequent 3 months (unfortunately no details of this crucial finding are provided). Also, because the children received no nonpharmacological treatment, it is not known how the benefits of drugs compare with those of psychological intervention.

The impressive National Institute of Mental Health multisite study[64] promises much more. The challenge of maintaining treatment fidelity, cooperation, and scientific rigor during a 2-year period across 6 sites will be considerable, but it is clear that the appropriate steps have been taken to optimize the chances of success. It is odd that after half a century's experience with the use of stimulants and hundreds of randomized controlled trials showing substantial short-term benefits, we still lack good evidence of long-term benefits (a crucial issue with a chronic disorder like attention deficit hyperactivity disorder), especially in comparison with psychosocial interventions. Nevertheless, that is the state of affairs. The testing of treatments in combination, as well as individually, along with the 10-month follow-up after completion of treatment are particularly important features. Such large-scale collaborative enterprises are inevitably expensive, and the National Institute of Mental Health is to be congratulated on its recognition that this was the only way in which a really convincing answer to a vitally important question (regarding theory and practice) could be answered. The importance of pediatric psychopharmacological research, with the scientific issues, is emphasized by Vitiello and Jensen.[65]

In the face of evidence that antidepressants may be less effective in childhood or adolescence than in adult life, attention has turned to the use of psychological treatments. Brent et al,[66] in a well-planned study, show that cognitive-behavioral therapy is more effective than either family therapy or nondirective supportive therapy in the treatment of major depression in adolescence. The findings attest to the efficacy of cognitive-behavioral therapy and provide strong support for its greater use. The authors note the surprising finding that the major improvement in depressive symptoms did not seem to be accompanied by parallel gains in social functioning. What this means remains uncertain at present. One of the few limitations of this study is the lack of analysis of mediating variables. Treatment studies provide an invaluable means of testing causal mechanisms if there is within-group analysis to determine whether the outcome gains are a function of changes in the postulated mediating mechanism. This constitutes 1 of the key challenges for the future and provides the essential link between causal research and studies of treatment efficacy. As noted by the articles in this special issue, there needs to be an integration between the 2 if gains in knowledge on basic causal processes are to lead to the hoped for gains in clinical practice.

Michael Rutter, MD, FRS
Medical Research Council Child Psychiatry Unit
Institute of Psychiatry
De Crespigny Park
London SE5 8AF
England

REFERENCES

1. Rutter M. Research to clinical practice in child psychiatry: retrospect and prospect. *J Child Psychol Psychiatry.* In press.
2. Rutter M. Relationship between mental disorders in childhood and adulthood. *Acta Psychiatr Scand.* 1995;91:73-85.
3. Magnusson D, Bergman LR. *Data Quality in Longitudinal Research.* Cambridge, England: Cambridge University Press; 1990.
4. Boyle MH, Offord DR, Racine YA, Szatmari P, Sanford M, Fleming JE. Adequacy of interviews vs checklists for classifying childhood psychiatric disorder based on parent reports. *Arch Gen Psychiatry.* 1997;54:793-799.
5. Verhulst FC, Koot HM. *Child Psychiatric Epidemiology: Concepts, Methods, and Findings.* Newbury Park, Calif: Sage Publications Inc; 1992.
6. Fergusson DM, Horwood LJ, Lynskey MT. The stability of disruptive childhood behaviors. *J Abnorm Child Psychol.* 1995;23:379-396.
7. Moffitt TE, Caspi A, Dickson N, Silva P, Stanton W. Childhood-onset versus adolescent-onset antisocial problems in males: natural history from ages 3 to 18 years. *Dev Psychopathol.* 1996;9:399-424.
8. Simonoff E, Pickles A, Meyer J, Silberg JL, Maes HH, Loeber R, Rutter M, Hewitt JK, Eaves LJ. The Virginia Twin Study of Adolescent Behavioral Development: influences of age, sex, and impairment on rates of disorder. *Arch Gen Psychiatry.* 1997;54:801-808.
9. Eaves L, Silberg J, Meyer J, Maes H, Simonoff E, Pickles A, Rutter M, Neale MC, Reynolds C, Erikson M, Health A, Loeber R, Truett K, Hewitt J. Genetics and developmental psychopathology, 2: the main effects of genes and environment on behavioral problems in the Virginia Twin Study of Adolescent Behavioral Development. *J Child Psychol Psychiatry.* In press.
10. Angold A, Erklanis A, Costello EJ, Rutter M. Precision, reliability and accuracy in the dating of symptom onsets in child and adolescent psychopathology. *J Child Psychol Psychiatry.* 1996;37:657-664.
11. Shaffer D, Fisher P, Dulcan M, Davies M, Piacentini J, Schwab-Stone M, Lahey B, Lichtman J, Canino G, Rubio-Stipec M, Rae D. The NIMH Diagnostic Interview Schedule for Children Version 2.3 (DISC-2.3): description, acceptability, prevalence rates, and performance in the MECA study. *J Am Acad Child Adolesc Psychiatry.* 1996;35:865-877.
12. Thapar A, Hervas A, McGuffin P. Childhood hyperactivity scores are highly heritable and show sibling competition effects: twin study evidence. *Behav Genet.* 1995;25:537-544.
13. Simonoff E, Pickles A, Hervas A, Silberg J, Meyer J, Rutter M, Eaves L. Genetic influences on childhood hyperactivity: contrast effects imply parental rating bias, not sibling interaction. *Psychol Med.* In press.
14. Kerr M, Tremblay RE, Pagani L, Vitaro F. Boys' behavioral inhibition and the risk of later delinquency. *Arch Gen Psychiatry.* 1997;54:809-816.
15. Kellam SG, Simon MB, Ensminger ME. Antecedents in first grade of teenage substance use and psychological well-being: a ten-year community-wide prospective study. In: Ricks DF, Dohrenwend BS, eds. *Origins of Psychopathology.* Cambridge, England: Cambridge University Press; 1983:17-42.
16. Moskowitz DS, Schwartzmann AE. Painting group portraits: studying life outcomes for aggressive and withdrawn children. *J Pers.* 1989;57:723-746.
17. Stattin H, Magnusson D. Antisocial development: a holistic approach. *Dev Psychopathol.* 1996;8:617-645.
18. Chisholm K, Carter MC, Ames EW, Morison SJ. Attachment security and indiscriminately friendly

behavior in children adopted from Romanian orphanages. *Dev Psychopathol.* 1995;7:283-294.
19. Keaveney L, O'Connor T. The network of social relations of adoptees exposed to severe early deprivation. Presented at the Society for Research in Child Development Conference; April 5, 1997; Washington, DC.
20. Rutter M, Mawhood L, Howlin P. Language delay and social development. In: Fletcher P, Hall D, eds. *Specific Speech and Language Disorders in Children.* London, England: Whurr; 1992:63-78.
21. Cohen LL, Vietze PM, Sudhalter V, Jenkins EC, Brown WT. Parent-child dyadic gaze patterns in fragile X males and non-fragile X males with autistic disorder. *J Child Psychol Psychiatry.* 1989; 30:845-856.
22. Angold A, Prendergast M, Cox A, Harrington R, Simonoff E, Rutter M. The Child and Adolescent Psychiatric Assessment (CAPA). *Psychol Med.* 1995;25:739-753.
23. Caron C, Rutter M. Comorbidity in child psychopathology: concepts, issues and research strategies. *J Child Psychol Psychiatry.* 1991;32:1063-1080.
24. Rutter M. Comorbidity: concepts, claims and choices. In: Farrington D, Maughan B, eds. *Overlapping Disorder, Overlapping Risks.* New York, NY: Plenum Publishing Corp. In press.
25. Fergusson DM, Horwood LJ. Predictive validity of categorically and dimesionally scored measures of disruptive childhood behaviors. *J Am Acad Child Adolesc Psychiatry.* 1995;34:477-485.
26. Jensen FS. Predictive validity of categorically and dimensionally scored measures of disruptive childhood behaviors: comment. *J Am Acad Child Adolesc Psychiatry.* 1995;34:485-487.
27. Klein DN, Riso LP. Psychiatric disorders: problems of boundaries and comorbidity. In: Costello CG, ed. *Basic Issues in Psychopathology.* New York, NY: Guilford Press; 1993:19-66.
28. Cantwell DP, Rutter M. Classification: conceptual issues and substantive findings. In: Rutter M, Taylor E, Herzov L, eds. *Child and Adolescent Psychiatry: Modern Approaches.* Oxford, England: Blackwell Scientific Publications; 1994:3-21.
29. Rende R, Plomin R. Nature, nurture, and the development of psychopathology. In: Cicchetti D, Cohen D, eds. *Handbook of Developmental Psychopathology.* New York, NY: John Wiley & Sons Inc; 1995:291-314.
30. Rey JM, Singh M, Hung S, Dossetor DR, Newman L, Plapp JM, Bird KD. A global scale to measure the quality of the family environment. *Arch Gen Psychiatry.* 1997;54:817-822.
31. Plomin R, Daniels D. Why are children in the same family so different? *Behav Brain Sci.* 1987;10:1-15.
32. Reiss D, Hetherington M, Plomin R, Howe GW, Simmens SJ, Henderson SH, O'Connor TJ, Bussell DA, Anderson ER, Law T. Genetic questions for environmental studies: differential parenting and psychopathology in adolescence. *Arch Gen Psychiatry.* 1995;52:925-936.
33. Rutter M. Family and school influences on cognitive development. *J Child Psychol Psychiatry.* 1985;26:683-704.
34. Rutter M. *Maternal Deprivation Reassessed.* 2nd ed. Harmondsworth, England: Penguin Books; 1981.
35. Rutter M, Tuma AH, Lann IS, eds. *Assessment and Diagnosis in Child Psychopathology.* New York, NY: Guilford Press; 1988.
36. Plomin R, Bergeman CS. The nature of nurture: genetic influences on 'environmental' measures. *Behav Brain Sci.* 1991;14:373-386.
37. Plomin R. *Genetics and Experience: The Interplay Between Nature and Nurture.* Thousand Oaks, Calif: Sage Publications Inc; 1994.
38. Kendler KS. Genetic epidemiology in psychiatry: taking both genes and environment seriously. *Arch Gen Psychiatry.* 1995;52:895-899.
39. Rutter M. Nature-nurture integration: the example of antisocial behavior. *Am Psychol.* 1997; 52:390-398.
40. Rutter M, Dunn J, Plomin R, Simonoff E, Pickles A, Maughan B, Ormel J, Eaves L. Integrating nature and nurture: implications of person-environment correlations and interactions for developmental psychopathology. *Dev Psychopathol.* In press.
41. Kovacs M, Devlin B, Pollock M, Richards C, Mukerji P. A controlled family history study of childhood-onset depressive disorder. *Arch Gen Psychiatry.* 1997;54:613-623.
42. Rende R, Weissman M, Rutter M, Wickramaratne P, Harrington R, Pickles A. Psychiatric disorders in the relatives of depressed probands, II: familial loading for comorbid non-depressive disorders based upon proband age of onset. *J Affect Disord.* In press.
43. Weissman MM, Wickramaratne P, Merikangas KR, Leckman JF, Prusoff BA, Caruso KA, Kidd KK, Gammon GD. Onset of major depression in early childhood: increased familial loading and specificity. *Arch Gen Psychiatry.* 1984;34:98-111.
44. Harrington R, Rutter M, Weissman M, Fudge H, Groothues C, Bredenkamp D, Pickles A, Rende R, Wickramatne P. Psychiatric disorders in the relatives of depressed probands, I: comparison of prepubertal, adolescent and early adult onset cases. *J Affect Disord.* In press.
45. Thapar A, McGuffin P. A twin study of depressive symptoms in childhood. *Br J Psychiatry.* 1994; 165:259-265.
46. Silberg J, Rutter M, Eaves L. Pubertal status, life stress and depression in juvenile twins: a genetic investigation. Presented at the Society for Research in Child Development Conference; April 3, 1997; Washington, DC.
47. Kendler KS, Karkowski-Shuman L. Stressful life events and genetic liability to major depression: genetic control of exposure to the environment? *Psychol Med.* 1997;27:549-564.
48. McGuffin P, Katz R, Bebbington P. The Camberwell Collaborative Depression Study, III: depression and adversity in the relatives of depressed probands. *Br J Psychiatry.* 1988;152:775-782.
49. Rosenberg DR, Keshavan MS, O'Hearn KM, Dick EL, Bagwell WW, Seymour AB, Montrose DM, Pierri JN, Birmaher B. Frontostriatal measurement in treatment-naive children with obsessive-compulsive disorder. *Arch Gen Psychiatry.* 1997; 54:824-830.
50. Rosenberg DR, Averbach DH, O'Hearn KM, Seymour AB, Birmaher B, Sweeney JA. Oculomotor response inhibition abnormalities in pediatric obsessive-compulsive disorder. *Arch Gen Psychiatry.* 1997;54:831-838.
51. Bailey A, Phillips W, Rutter M. Autism: towards an integration of clinical, genetic, neuropsychological, and neurobiological perspectives. *J Child Psychol Psychiatry.* 1996;37:89-126.
52. Rutter M, Plomin R. Opportunities for psychiatry from genetic findings. *Br J Psychiatry.* In press.
53. Vargha-Khadem F, Isaacs E, van der Werf S, Robb S, Wilson J. Development of intelligence and memory in children with hemiplegic cerebral palsy: the deleterious consequences of early seizures. *Brain.* 1992;115:315-329.
54. Pine DS, Coplan JD, Wasserman GA, Miller LS, Fried JE, Davies M, Cooper TB, Greenhill L, Shaffer D, Parsons B. Neuroendocrine response to fenfluramine challenge in boys: associations with aggressive behavior and adverse rearing. *Arch Gen Psychiatry.* 1997;54:839-846.
55. Moffitt T, Caspi A, Fawcett P, Brammer GL, Raleigh M, Yuwiler A, Silva P. Whole blood serotonin and family background relate to male violence. In: Raine A, Farrington D, Brennan P, Mednick SA, eds. *Unlocking Crime: The Biosocial Key.* New York, NY: Plenum Publishing Corp. In press.
56. Kreuzi MJP, Jacobsen T. Serotonin and human violence: do environmental mediators exist? In: Raine A, Farrington D, Brennan P, Mednick SA, eds. *Unlocking Crime: The Biosocial Key.* New York, NY: Plenum Publishing Corp. In press.
57. Rutter M. Antisocial behavior: developmental psychopathology perspectives. In: Stoff D, Breiling J, Maser JD, eds. *Handbook of Antisocial Behavior.* In press.
58. Shively CA, Laber-Laird K, Anton RF. Behavior and physiology of social stress and depression in female cynomolgus monkeys. *Biol Psychiatry.* 1997; 41:871-882.
59. Sameroff AJ, Chandler MJ. Perinatal risk and the continuum of caretaking casualty. In: Horowitz F, Hetherington M, Scarr-Salapatek S, Siegel G, eds. *Review of Child Development Research.* Chicago, Ill: University of Chicago Press; 1975;4: 187-244.
60. Meisels SJ, Plunkett JW. Developmental consequences of preterm birth: are there long-term effects? In: Baltes PB, Featherman DL, Lerner RM, eds. *Life Span Development and Behavior.* Hillsdale, NJ: Lawrence A Erlbaum Associates; 1988;9:87-129.
61. Whitaker AH, Van Rossem R, Feldman JF, Schonfeld IS, Pinto-Martin JA, Torre C, Shaffer D, Paneth N. Psychiatric outcomes in low-birth-weight children at age 6 years: relation to neonatal cranial ultrasound abnormalities. *Arch Gen Psychiatry.* 1997;54:847-856.
62. Powls A, Botting N, Cooke RWI, Marlow N. Motor impairment in children 12 to 13 years old with a birthweight of less than 1250 g. *Arch Dis Child.* 1995;72:62-66.
63. Gillberg C, Melander H, von Knorring A-L, Janols L-O, Thernlund G, Hägglöf B, Eidevall-Wallin L, Gustafsson P, Kopp S. Long-term stimulant treatment of children with attention-deficit hyperactivity disorder symptoms: a randomized, double-blind, placebo-controlled trial. *Arch Gen Psychiatry.* 1997;54:857-864.
64. Arnold LE Abikoff HB, Cantwell DP, Conners CK, Elliott G, Greenhill LL, Hechtman L, Hinshaw SP, Hoza B, Jensen PS, Kraemer HC, March JS, Newcorn JH, Pelham, WE. National Institute of Mental Health Collaborative Multimodal Treatment Study of Children With ADHD (MTA): design challenges and choices. *Arch Gen Psychiatry.* 1997; 54:865-870.
65. Vitiello B, Jensen PS. Medication development and testing in children and adolescents: current problems, future directions. *Arch Gen Psychiatry.* 1997; 54:871-876.
66. Brent DA, Holder D, Kolko D, Birmaher B, Baugher M, Roth C, Iyengar S, Johnson BA. A clinical psychotherapy trial for adolescent depression comparing cognitive, family, and supportive therapy. *Arch Gen Psychiatry.* 1997;54;877-885.

Break the debilitating cycle of

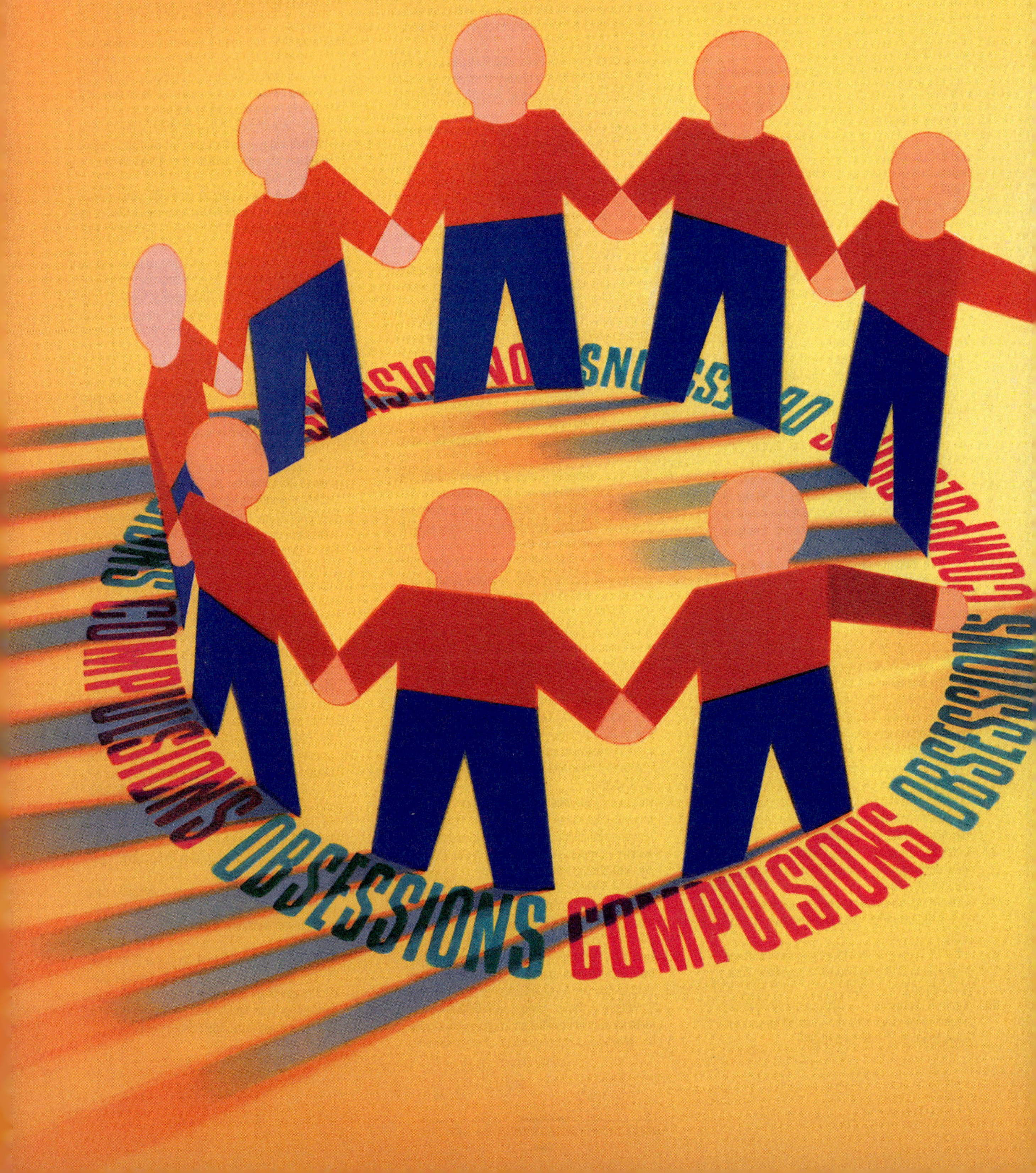

Adequacy of Interviews vs Checklists for Classifying Childhood Psychiatric Disorder Based on Parent Reports

Michael H. Boyle, PhD; David R. Offord, MD; Yvonne A. Racine, MA; Peter Szatmari, MD; Mark Sanford, MB, ChB; Jan E. Fleming, MD

Background: The advantages and disadvantages of lay-administered structured interviews and self-administered problem checklists for estimating prevalence and associated features of childhood psychiatric disorder have attracted little comment. This article compares the scientific adequacy of these 2 instruments for classifying *DSM-III-R* categories of childhood psychiatric disorder in general population samples.

Methods: Study data are from parental assessments of 251 children aged 6 to 16 years participating in a 2-stage measurement evaluation study. Reliability and validity were compared between the Diagnostic Interview for Children and Adolescents (the structured interview used in the study) and the revised Ontario Child Health Study scales (the self-administered problem checklist used in the study).

Results: Reliability estimates based on the κ statistic were comparable for the 2 instruments and ranged from 0.21 (conduct disorder) to 0.70 (depression) on the lay interview and from 0.27 (depression) to 0.61 (oppositional defiant disorder) on the self-administered checklist. Validity coefficients tended to favor the checklist categories, but only marginally.

Conclusions: On balance, differences in reliability and validity were small between the 2 instruments. These differences would appear to have no discernible impact on the knowledge about prevalence and associated features of disorder generated by use of such instruments in general population surveys.

Arch Gen Psychiatry. 1997;54:793-799

From the Centre for Studies of Children at Risk, Department of Psychiatry, McMaster University, and the Hamilton Health Sciences Corporation, Hamilton, Ontario.

SELF-ADMINISTERED problem checklists and lay-administered structured interviews have been used to study childhood psychiatric disorder in the general population.[1] The advantages and disadvantages of these 2 approaches for estimating prevalence and associated features of disorder have attracted little comment. Checklists are less expensive to use: for example, administration times for the parent version of the Child Behavior Checklist are about 10 to 15 minutes[2] vs 60 minutes[3] for the most recent version of the Diagnostic Interview Schedule for Children (DISC-2.3). Checklists have few, if any, training requirements for administration, unlike the weeks of training required by the newer interviewer-based assessments such as the Child and Adolescent Psychiatric Assessment.[4] Checklists also offer considerable flexibility of data collection—in person, by telephone, or by mail. In contrast, structured interviews provide an opportunity to motivate respondents and to overcome literacy problems, thus broadening the range of respondents from whom information can be obtained. In addition, an interview can be used to capture very detailed information because of its ability to navigate complex question sequences.

The usefulness of information obtained by checklists and interviews is difficult to compare and depends on the objectives for measurement.[5] In cross-sectional studies, the objective of measurement is to discriminate among individuals. Reliability in this context focuses on consistency or reproducibility of response—the extent to which measures can be replicated. Validity focuses on the meaningfulness of response—the extent to which measures generate useful and sensible discriminations. Meaningfulness is evaluated by testing hypotheses, based on theory, about how the measure should perform when applied to individuals. The few studies that have correlated "external validators" with disorders assessed by self-administered problem checklists and lay-administered structured interviews could find few differences between the 2 types of instruments.[6-8]

The objective of this article was to compare the reliability and validity of a self-administered problem checklist and a lay-administered structured interview for use in cross-sectional prevalence studies of childhood psychiatric disorder.

SUBJECTS AND METHODS

SUBJECTS

The design of the study has been described in other publications.[9,10] Briefly, a simple random sample of 2317 children aged 6 to 16 years was selected in 1989 from those attending all public schools in an industrialized, urban setting (Hamilton, Ontario) (94 schools and 27 629 students). Among the eligible sample of 2219 children, 1751 (78.9%) were from families who provided written, informed consent to participate in the study. All stage 1 participants (parents, teachers, and adolescents aged 12-16 years) completed self-administered problem checklists and questionnaires.

A stratified random sample of stage 1 families was selected for stage 2; an intensive follow-up was done, on average, 48 days later. The strata were age (6-11 years, 12-16 years), sex, and high vs low symptom scores in the index child, based on the original Ontario Child Health Study scales.[11,12] Among the 329 children selected for stage 2, 251 (76.3%) were from families who agreed to participate in stage 2. All participants completed the self-administered problem checklists and questionnaires a second time. Furthermore, each parent and child/adolescent dyad was administered, on average 17 days apart, the revised version of the Diagnostic Interview for Children and Adolescents (DICA-R).[13] The second administration of the checklist and the first administration of the interview were done independently, several days apart, with their order of completion randomized. Interviewers had no knowledge of the checklist responses.

MEASURES OF DISORDER

The following disorders were studied: conduct disorder (CD), oppositional defiant disorder (ODD), attention-deficit hyperactivity disorder (ADHD), overanxious disorder (OAD), separation anxiety disorder (SAD), and major depressive disorder (MDD). We revised the original Ontario Child Health Study scales to measure each disorder (OCHS-R scales).[9] Problem behavior items were matched to symptom criteria specified in *DSM-III-R*.[14] When no adequate match was found for a symptom, an abbreviated description of the symptom was generated by consensus. Each item is scored 0, 1, or 2, indicating responses of "never or not true," "sometimes or somewhat true," and "often or very true," respectively. The raw scores are added to form a scale score to measure each disorder. The time for assessment is the past 6 months. This study used only the parent version of the OCHS-R scales.

The lay-administered structured interview used in this study was the DICA-R,[13] which uses computer algorithms based on subject responses to determine if *DSM-III-R* criteria for individual disorders are met. The interviewer-training procedures, modifications to the interview itself, and psychometric properties of the DICA-R in our study are reported elsewhere.[10] This study used only the parent version of the DICA-R.

DIMENSIONAL AND CATEGORICAL REPRESENTATIONS OF DISORDER

The checklist represents disorder dimensionally. To construct categories, the checklist scale scores obtained during its second administration (subsequent to screening) were divided into binary classifications at each score and cross-tabulated with the interview classifications of disorder obtained during its first administration, and thresholds or cut points were identified to yield prevalences that were as similar as possible. This method removed the confounding effects of threshold differences on the comparison of the 2 instruments.[15] To construct dimensional measures of disorder from the interview, yes responses were coded 1 and summed to form symptom scores. There was 1 symptom for each *DSM-III-R* criterion irrespective of the number of interview questions addressed to each.

RELIABILITY

Test-retest reliability estimates were based on the Cohen κ for categories of disorder and on the intraclass correlation

RESULTS

The number of cases identified is similar for both instruments, which is a direct result of the method used to select thresholds on the checklist (**Table 2**). Percent prevalences were low for CD, SAD, and MDD. Agreement on cases between the 2 instruments was very low.

ATTENUATION AND RELIABILITY

Table 3 shows that attenuation (reduction in percent prevalence from the first to the second assessment) is present for both instruments and all disorders. Except for CD, attenuation is larger when the checklist instrument is used to classify disorder. Test-retest reliability estimates based on κ are higher for interview classifications of ADHD, OAD, and MDD and for checklist classifications of CD, ODD, and SAD. When the intraclass correlation coefficient and Pearson *r* are used to estimate the test-retest reliability of interview symptom counts and checklist scale scores, the checklist yields marginally higher estimates for all disorders except SAD, for which the difference is substantial.

VALIDITY

Table 4 shows that the positive predictive value of case identification for seeking help exceeds 50% for both instruments and all classes of disorder. Differences between the instruments for each type of disorder are small. The receiver operating characteristic analyses indicate that areas under the curve are consistently higher for the checklist and significantly different for CD and ODD.

As shown in **Table 5**, patterns of association between the disorders and measures of impairment are similar for the 2 instruments. The disruptive behavior disorders (CD, ODD, and ADHD) exhibit strong and statistically significant associations with parent assessments of impaired social functioning and poor school performance, and with teacher assessments of impaired social functioning. These strengths of association are considerably weaker for the emocoefficient and the Pearson *r* correlation for checklist scale scores and interview symptom counts. Checklist scale scores were derived from the raw scores (0, 1, 2) of individual items. Unlike the Pearson *r*, the intraclass correlation coefficient allocates systematic shifts, such as attenuation effects, to the error term.

VALIDITY

The validation exercise consisted of 3 steps. Step 1 examined discrimination between families who did and did not access help in the previous 6 months for emotional or behavioral problems in their children. Accuracy was estimated in 2 ways. The first centered on positive predictive value, which was defined as the number and percentage of children classified with a disorder (test positives) who also accessed help. This approach evaluates accuracy at a single point defined by the threshold for caseness. The second method arose from a receiver operating characteristic analysis,[16] which is based on the distribution of interview symptom counts and checklist scale scores among children accessing and not accessing help in our sample. This approach evaluates accuracy throughout the whole range of scores. The area under the curve served as the index of accuracy. The receiver operating characteristic curve was generated by plotting sensitivity (ie, the percentage of children accessing help who were classified test positive) against 1–specificity (ie, the percentage of children not accessing help who were classified as test positive) for all cut points throughout the range of symptom counts (DICA-R) vs scale scores (OCHS-R). The area under the curve was calculated according to the trapezoidal nonparametric method.[17] Because comparisons involved the same sample, the appropriate correction was made for estimating the SE of the difference between 2 areas.[18]

Step 2 examined the strength of association between disorders and measures of impairment. It was hypothesized that impaired social functioning and poor school performance assessed separately by parents and teachers should be associated with all categories of disorder, irrespective of type. Relative odds computed from 2×2 tables were used to estimate the strength of association between each disorder and binary measures of impairment. To examine effects attributable to the scale of measurement (categorical vs dimensional), the η (eta) coefficient was used to estimate strength of association between binary measures of impairment and interview symptom counts and checklist scale scores. We assumed that the larger association, the stronger the evidence of validity. Measures of impairment were respondent specific (not combined) so that cross-informant comparisons could be made. The sign test was used to determine overall whether the strengths of association with impairment favored one instrument or the other.

Step 3 examined the convergent and discriminant validity of the 2 instruments against associated features believed to differentiate among categories of disorder. The following linkages have some support in the literature and were hypothesized to exist in this study: discipline problems with disorders of conduct (CD and ODD),[19] slow development with attentional problems (ADHD),[20] and parental depressed mood with emotional disorders (OAD, SAD, and MDD).[21] These hypotheses were tested using relative odds derived from forward, stepwise logistic regressions to identify disorders (independent variables) having significant associations ($P<.05$) with each correlate (dependent variable). One logistic regression model was specified for each correlate, and disorders with nonsignificant relative odds were excluded. Large and statistically significant relative odds were hypothesized for disorders linked with specific correlates (convergent validity), and smaller, nonsignificant relative odds were hypothesized for disorders not linked with specific correlates (discriminant validity). These analyses were repeated using the interview symptom counts and checklist scale scores to examine differences that might be attributable to the level of measurement (ie, categorical vs dimensional). **Table 1** gives an abbreviated description of external variables used in the analyses with estimates of their prevalence at time 1 and test-retest reliabilities over an average interval of 48 days. All variables listed in Table 1 were measured on the basis of single informant assessments—parent or teacher, but not both.

tional disorders and most are nonsignificant. The 95% confidence intervals around the point estimates are too large for comparisons at the individual disorder level. Taken as a group, the relative odds between disorder and impairment are larger for the checklist in 9 of 12 comparisons (parent-assessed impairment) and 8 of 12 comparisons (teacher-assessed impairment). However, the magnitudes of these differences are nonsignificant when evaluated using the sign test. Evaluation of the interview symptom counts and checklist scale scores using the η coefficient yielded similar results and are not presented here.

The logistic regression models in **Table 6** display the dependent variables (correlates) at the top of each column and the independent variables (disorders) in the left column. The patterns of association are comparable for both instruments. Evidence of convergent validity (areas marked by a dagger) exists for each instrument on 5 of 6 occasions. There is one discriminant validity failure: developmental problems are associated more strongly with MDD than ADHD in the interview. When symptom counts and scale scores replace the classifications of disorder in the logistic regression analyses, the results are similar in that the evidence for convergent and discriminant validity are comparable for both instruments (data not shown).

COMMENT

There appear to be few differences in the usefulness of assessment data obtained by the interview and checklist used in this study. With the exception of ADHD, OAD, and MDD (higher for the interview), test-retest reliability estimates based on κ were marginally higher for the checklist. Test-retest reliability estimates of checklist scale scores vs the interview symptom counts were uniformly higher for the checklist. This result may seem surprising given the longer test-retest interval for the checklist (48 days) than for the interview (17 days). It is important to note, however, that symptoms assessed by the interview had to meet criteria for duration, severity, and, in some instances, age at onset. If they did not meet appropriate criteria, they were treated as absent for the construction of symptom counts. Despite the clinical importance of these criteria, they also serve to truncate the amount of variance available for measurement. When these criteria are set aside, the reliability of symptom scores generated by the DICA-R increase on average from 0.62 (the mean of Pearson r estimates for the interview in Table 3) to 0.74.

Although the validity evidence was nominally better for the checklist, the magnitudes of differences were small. The factors with the most influential impact on validity estimates were type of disorder (OAD and SAD performed least well) and respondent (validity estimates were highest when the parent also provided the data for the validity variable). In another report,[6] we used the same 2 instruments to compare assessment data collected from adolescents aged 12 to 16 years and found no appreciable differences in reliability and validity. The type of instrument that might be suitable for children younger than 12 years remains intractable because of problems associated with the reliability of their responses.[23]

Table 1. Description of Variables, Prevalence, and Test-Retest Reliability Based on κ*

Variable Name and Abbreviated Description†	Parent		Teacher	
	%	κ	%	κ
Use of help Use of consultation or help for any emotional or behavioral problems	32.0	0.60	NA	NA
Impaired social functioning Problems getting along with 1 or more of other children, teachers at school, and the family‡	14.9	0.65	20.2	0.58
Poor school performance Below average or poor student	17.9	0.63	30.0	0.72
Discipline problem Perceived need for outside help in disciplining child	21.3	0.66	NA	NA
Developmental delay Late age for first walking or talking or problems with coordination or clumsiness	16.2	0.64	NA	NA
Parental depressed mood Score of ≥20 on Centre for Epidemiologic Studies Depression Scale[22]	16.5	0.61	NA	NA

*NA indicates not applicable. The percentage is the percent prevalence. κ is the estimate of test-retest reliability; the average interval was 48 days.
†Full description and measurement are available from authors.
‡Family item not included in the teacher assessment.

METHODOLOGICAL ISSUES

The empirical findings of this report must be viewed in light of some important issues. The first issue concerns the small numbers of children for studying CD, SAD, and MDD. Low prevalences of these disorders in the general population make them difficult to study reliably. Consequently, statistical power for testing hypotheses using these classifications is low.

Second, the study experienced a relatively large sample loss that reaches 40% when nonresponse is compounded at stage 1 (78.9% response rate) and stage 2 (76.3% response rate). We examined a number of variables (eg, child sex and age, family status, maternal education, family dysfunction, and receipt of social assistance), but none of them discriminated between responders and nonresponders. Even if the groups were less alike and selection bias a greater concern, we would expect the impact to be similar for both instruments.

Third, the reliability comparisons between the interview and checklist were compromised by 2 factors: a longer average retest interval for the checklist (48 days) than for the interview (17 days) and larger attenuation effects for the checklist than for the interview. The direction of bias introduced by these factors is to reduce the size of the reliability coefficients of the checklist. Nevertheless, the checklist produced reliability coefficients comparable in size to the interview, indicating unequivocally that checklist classifications of childhood psychiatric disorder are at least as reliable as interview-generated classifications. This may be possible because checklist classifications are free of 2 sources of variation that can influence reliability: (1) interviewer error and (2) the absence of criteria for establishing the presence of symptoms, eg, duration, severity, and age at onset where applicable.

Fourth, the criteria for validation used in this study are limited in context to prevalence surveys. Different objectives, eg, to replicate clinical judgments or to evaluate sensitivity to change in treatment trials, would lead

Table 2. Children Classified With Disorder and Agreement on Cases Between the DICA-R and OCHS-R (N=223)*

	% of Cases		Agreement on Cases†			
Disorder	DICA-R	OCHS-R	++	+−,−+	−−	κ ($SE_κ$)
CD	5.4	5.8	6	13	204	0.45 (0.13)
ODD	24.7	28.3	38	42	143	0.52 (0.06)
ADHD	14.8	14.8	15	36	172	0.36 (0.09)
OAD	14.3	10.8	11	34	178	0.31 (0.09)
SAD	4.0	4.9	4	12	207	0.37 (0.14)
MDD	4.0	5.4	1	19	203	0.05 (0.09)

*DICA-R indicates revised version of Diagnostic Interview for Children and Adolescents; OCHS-R, revised Ontario Child Health Study scales; CD, conduct disorder; ODD, oppositional defiant disorder; ADHD, attention-deficit hyperactivity disorder; OAD, overanxious disorder; SAD, separation anxiety disorder; and MDD, major depressive disorder.
†Double plus signs indicate positive on both interview and checklist; plus/minus and minus/plus, positive on one instrument and negative on the other; and double minus signs, negative on both interview and checklist.

Table 3. Attenuation and Test-Retest Reliability Estimates (N=210)*

	Attenuation % (t_2–t_1)		Test-Retest Reliability					
			κ ($SE_κ$)		ICC		Pearson *r*	
Disorder	DICA-R	OCHS-R	DICA-R	OCHS-R	DICA-R	OCHS-R	DICA-R	OCHS-R
CD	−3.3	−1.4	0.21 (0.14)	0.44 (0.12)	0.67	0.69	0.67	0.72
ODD	−3.8	−11.0	0.51 (0.07)	0.61 (0.06)	0.70	0.76	0.71	0.81
ADHD	−2.4	−9.0	0.59 (0.08)	0.50 (0.07)	0.72	0.77	0.73	0.81
OAD	−1.0	−10.5	0.57 (0.08)	0.30 (0.08)	0.61	0.64	0.61	0.68
SAD	−1.5	−2.4	0.32 (0.18)	0.40 (0.13)	0.34	0.64	0.36	0.68
MDD	−0.9	−4.3	0.70 (0.14)	0.27 (0.11)	NA	0.61	NA	0.65

**κ is the estimate of test-retest reliability; ICC, intraclass correlation coefficient; DICA-R, revised version of Diagnostic Interview for Children and Adolescents; OCHS-R, revised Ontario Child Health Study scales; CD, conduct disorder; ODD, oppositional defiant disorder; ADHD, attention-deficit hyperactivity disorder; OAD, overanxious disorder;*
SAD, separation anxiety disorder; MDD, major depressive disorder; and NA, not available. Skip pattern for classifying DICA-R MDD precludes estimating meaningful symptom scores.

Table 4. Discrimination Between Cases Using and Not Using Consultation or Help for Emotional-Behavioral Problems During the Past 6 Months (N=218)*

	Positive Predictive Value, %		ROC Analysis, % of Area Under the Curve (SE)		
Disorder	DICA-R	OCHS-R	DICA-R	OCHS-R	*z*
CD	100 (12/12)	92 (12/13)	66.3 (3.9)	78.4 (3.2)	−3.27
ODD	68 (36/53)	70 (44/63)	74.2 (3.5)	79.0 (3.1)	−1.66
ADHD	81 (25/31)	73 (22/30)	69.9 (3.8)	73.7 (3.4)	−1.04
OAD	57 (17/30)	62 (15/24)	61.6 (4.0)	63.7 (3.9)	−0.50
SAD	71 (5/7)	73 (8/11)	56.9 (4.1)	62.4 (3.9)	−0.57
MDD	75 (6/8)	92 (11/12)	NA	73.5 (3.3)	NA

**ROC indicates receiver operating characteristic; DICA-R, revised version of Diagnostic Interview for Children and Adolescents; OCHS-R, revised Ontario Child Health Study scales; CD, conduct disorder; ODD, oppositional defiant disorder; ADHD, attention-deficit hyperactivity disorder; OAD, overanxious disorder; SAD, separation anxiety disorder; MDD, major depressive disorder; and NA, not available. Skip pattern for classifying MDD precludes estimating meaningful symptom scores.*

to different criteria. In the absence of a criterion standard for classifying disorder, it is important to have clear objectives for classification so that appropriate criteria can be identified for evaluation.[24]

CHECKLISTS VS INTERVIEWS

Despite the lack of empirical evidence, the belief is growing in child psychiatry that the structured interview is the method of choice for diagnosis-based epidemiological research in general populations.[25,26] This belief is grounded in the notion that the personal interview is a better conduit for obtaining subtle information of high clinical relevance and for meeting nosological requirements to date the onset and duration of psychiatric symptoms. It is possible, of course, that these theoretical advantages contribute little to useful classification in cross-sectional surveys. First, the evolution of the *DSM* has been accompanied by a concerted effort to make symptoms of disorder more contextually specific, concrete, and observable. Increasingly, symptoms are defined by events and observable behavior that are fairly explicit and understandable to most respondents. As attempts continue to simplify the data needed for classification, the descriptive content of interviews and checklists will become increasingly similar. Second, lay-administered structured interviews such as the DICA and the Diagnostic Interview Schedule for Children that require verbatim questioning and strict recording of answers (respondent-based approaches)[27] are not too dissimilar from problem checklists in the lack of opportunities to clarify the wording or intent of questions for respondents. Thus, person-to-person variation in the interpretation of questions and thresholds for giving a positive response will afflict these interviews and self-administered questionnaires in a similar way. Furthermore, the impact of error at the individual symptom or item level is diminished when multiple symptoms or items are used interchangeably for measurement. In measuring childhood disorder, the focus is on consistency of responses across many questions and not on individual questions per se. As a result, errors at the individual level tend to average out.[28] Finally, the nosological requirements for dating the onset and duration of symptoms may actually detract from useful classification. As noted earlier, applying the duration criterion to the construction of interview symptom counts had an adverse effect on test-retest reliability estimates. Furthermore, in this report and others,[6-8] incorporating interview data on symptom onset and duration into classifications of disorder offered no more discrimination against "external validators" than checklist classifications of disorder that are void of such data. The inaccuracy of long-term psychiatric recall data in cross-sectional studies of adults[29] suggests that retrospective data be used cautiously.

Table 5. Relative Odds (95% Confidence Intervals) Between Classifications of Disorder and Impaired Social Functioning and Poor School Performance Assessed by Parents and Teachers*

Respondent for Impairment	Impaired Social Functioning: DICA-R	Impaired Social Functioning: OCHS-R	Poor School Performance: DICA-R	Poor School Performance: OCHS-R
Parent† (N=213)				
CD	10.8‡ (3.2-37.0)	8.9‡ (2.5-31.4)	6.2§ (1.9-20.5)	7.5§ (2.1-26.1)
ODD	5.7‡ (2.5-12.9)	8.6‡ (3.7-20.3)	2.7‖ (1.2-5.8)	2.7§ (1.3-5.8)
ADHD	5.8‡ (2.4-13.8)	4.3‡ (1.8-10.6)	6.7‡ (2.9-15.6)	6.3‡ (2.7-14.9)
OAD	1.3 (0.4-3.6)	1.8 (0.6-5.4)	1.1 (0.4-3.0)	3.4‖ (1.3-8.7)
SAD	1.0 (0.1-8.8)	2.4 (0.6-9.7)	0.9 (0.1-7.5)	2.1 (0.5-8.2)
MDD	0.9 (0.1-7.3)	7.1§ (1.9-26.3)	1.8 (0.4-9.3)	9.4‡ (2.5-35.3)
Teacher¶ (N=184)				
CD	6.5§ (1.9-22.8)	13.3‡ (3.2-54.7)	1.4 (0.4-5.0)	3.9 (1.1-14.6)
ODD	2.4‖ (1.1-5.4)	3.5§ (1.6-7.7)	1.7 (0.8-3.4)	1.6 (0.8-3.2)
ADHD	4.0§ (1.7-9.4)	3.2‖ (1.3-7.8)	2.7‖ (1.2-6.1)	2.4 (1.1-5.5)
OAD	0.9 (0.3-2.7)	1.8 (0.6-4.9)	1.4 (0.6-3.5)	3.1‖ (1.3-7.5)
SAD	4.9 (1.0-25.6)	2.4 (0.6-10.2)	2.5 (0.5-12.8)	3.2 (0.8-12.5)
MDD	1.9 (0.4-10.2)	2.4 (0.6-10.2)	1.0 (0.2-5.1)	5.3‖ (1.3-22.0)

*DICA-R indicates revised version of Diagnostic Interview for Children and Adolescents; OCHS-R, revised Ontario Child Health Study scales; CD, conduct disorder; ODD, oppositional defiant disorder; ADHD, attention-deficit hyperactivity disorder; OAD, overanxious disorder; SAD, separation anxiety disorder; and MDD, major depressive disorder.

†Number of significant relative odds, 15 of 24. Number of times OCHS-R relative odds were greater than DICA-R relative odds, 9 of 12.

‡$P<.001$.

§$P<.01$.

‖$P<.05$.

¶Number of significant relative odds, 9 of 24. Number of times OCHS-R relative odds were greater than DICA-R relative odds, 8 of 12.

Table 6. Relative Odds (95% Confidence Intervals) Derived From Forward Stepwise Logistic Regressions Between Classifications of Disorder and Selected Correlates (N=214)*

Disorder	DICA-R: Discipline Problems	DICA-R: Developmental Delay	DICA-R: Depressed Mood	OCHS-R: Discipline Problems	OCHS-R: Developmental Delay	OCHS-R: Depressed Mood
CD	15.1†‡ (2.9-80.0)	§	§	4.4†‖ (1.1-18.1)	§	§
ODD	6.1†¶ (2.8-13.4)	2.8§‖ (1.2-6.6)	3.2‡§ (1.5-7.0)	7.4†¶ (3.3-16.6)	2.3§‖ (1.0-5.2)	§
ADHD	§	4.1†‡ (1.6-10.5)	§	§	4.9†¶ (2.0-12.1)	§
OAD	§	§	3.5†‡ (1.4-8.6)	§	§	†
SAD	§	§	4.6†‖ (1.0-22.0)	§	§	4.8†‖ (1.2-18.7)
MDD	§	7.3§‖ (1.6-34.8)	†	§	§	9.7†¶ (2.6-35.9)

*DICA-R indicates revised version of Diagnostic Interview for Children and Adolescents; OCHS-R, revised Ontario Child Health Study scales; CD, conduct disorder; ODD, oppositional defiant disorder; ADHD, attention-deficit hyperactivity disorder; OAD, overanxious disorder; SAD, separation anxiety disorder; and MDD, major depressive disorder.

†Variables hypothesized to yield large and statistically significant relative odds (convergent validity).

‡$P<.01$.

§Variables hypothesized to yield nonsignificant relative odds (discriminant validity).

‖$P<.05$.

¶$P<.001$.

WHAT IS A CASE?

This question is prompted by the substantial disagreement on caseness between the 2 instruments in this study. Is one instrument more likely to identify true cases than another? We think not. If this were so, we would expect the validity evidence to be stronger for one instrument than the other. We believe that both instruments contain a substantial amount of error in identifying cases and that this error makes it possible for both instruments to yield classifications that appear to be equally valid. The disagreement on caseness reflects both the limits of reliability associated with each instrument and procedural differences in collecting information. A recent study of psychiatric disorders in adults[30] has shown that simply altering diagnostic procedures, while holding constant operational criteria for classification, led to substantial disagreement on case status. Four procedures were studied, and, when each pair of procedures was compared, κ estimates of agreement fell between 0.53 and 0.67.

We believe that the "substantial error" found in our interview and checklist is not idiosyncratic but applicable to similar instruments in current use. The problem of total error (ie, the combination of random and systematic error) or, conversely, the issue of useful variance, has not been studied adequately in the classification of childhood psychiatric disorder. Our preoccupation with symptom description and nosological requirements has eclipsed debate on the objectives of classification and the development of external criteria for validation.[24]

FUTURE WORK

This study found no scientific basis for choosing one particular checklist over one particular interview in the context of an epidemiological survey of childhood psychiatric disorder. There were, however, fairly large differences in completion times between the 2 instruments used in this study—on average, 15 minutes for the checklist and 40 minutes for the interview—differences large enough to constitute an economic savings to investigators and a reduction in burden (time) for respondents. There are, of course, other practical considerations when selecting instruments for epidemiological studies: the cost of gaining access to households, the number of respondents within a household who are expected to contribute data, literacy and motivation among the sample, the total time available for data collection, and interviewer training requirements, to name just a few.

There are many interesting questions waiting to be addressed in child psychiatric epidemiology.[31] We believe that defining the limits of usefulness for different types of instruments (including a mix of diagnostic instruments) applicable to epidemiological research is an area that needs urgent attention. Many of these questions will require specialized approaches such as observational techniques, standardized tests, and best-estimate diagnoses. It is conceivable that checklists may be able to play a bigger role in the classification and measurement of childhood psychiatric disorder, given the current state of nosological practice. The generalizability of our work to instruments currently favored in psychiatric epidemiology, to the classification of rare disorders, and to the use of interviews vs checklists for classification in clinic populations and among adults are important issues to be addressed in future work.

Accepted for publication October 8, 1996.

This work was supported by funds from the National Health Research and Development Program, Ottawa, Ontario (grant 6606-3760-42), and the Ontario Ministry of Community and Social Services, Toronto.

When this work was done, support was provided by a William T. Grant Foundation Faculty Scholar Award, New York, NY (Dr Boyle), a National Health Scientist Award, Health and Welfare Canada, Ottawa (Dr Offord), a Research Fellowship, Ontario Mental Health Foundation, Toronto (Dr Szatmari), and a National Alliance for Research on Schizophrenia and Depression Young Investigator Award, Chicago, Ill (Dr Fleming).

The authors are grateful to anonymous reviewers for their helpful comments and wish to thank the Hamilton Board of Education, particularly Keith Reilly and Owen Jackson; principals and teachers of the Board; and parents and students for their help in this project.

Corresponding author: Michael H. Boyle, PhD, Centre for Studies of Children at Risk, Patterson Bldg, 1200 Main St W, Hamilton, Ontario, Canada L8N 3Z5.

REFERENCES

1. Costello EJ. Developments in child psychiatric epidemiology. *J Am Acad Child Adolesc Psychiatry.* 1989;28:836-841.
2. Barkley R. Child behavior rating scales and checklists. In: Rutter M, Tuma AH, Lann IS, eds. *Assessment and Diagnosis in Child Psychopathology.* London, England: Guilford Press; 1988:113-155.
3. Shaffer D, Fisher P, Dulcan MK, Davies M, Piacentini J, Schwab-Stone ME, Lahey BB, Bourdon K, Jensen PS, Bird HR, Canino E, Regier DA. The NIMH Diagnostic Interview Schedule for Children version 2.3 (DISC-2.3): description, acceptability, prevalence rates, and performance in the MECA Study. *J Am Acad Child Adolesc Psychiatry.* 1996;35:865-877.
4. Angold A, Prendergast M, Cox A, Harrington R, Simonoff E, Rutter M. The Child and Adolescent Psychiatric Assessment (CAPA). *Psychol Med.* 1995;25:739-753.
5. Guyatt GH, Feeny DH, Patrick DL. Measuring health-related quality of life. *Ann Intern Med.* 1993;118:622-629.
6. Boyle MH, Offord DR, Racine YA, Szatmari P, Sanford M, Fleming JE. Interviews versus checklists: adequacy for classifying childhood psychiatric disorder based on adolescent reports. *Int J Method Psychiatr Res.* 1996;6:309-319.
7. Jensen PS, Watanabe HK, Richters JE, Roper M, Hibbs ED, Salzberg AD, Liu S. Scales, diagnosis and child psychopathology, II: comparing the CBCL and the DISC against external validators. *J Abnorm Child Psychol.* 1996;24:151-168.
8. Gould MS, Bird H, Jaramillo BS. Correspondence between statistically derived behavior problem syndromes and child psychiatric diagnoses in a community sample. *J Abnorm Child Psychol.* 1993;21:287-313.
9. Boyle MH, Offord DR, Racine Y, Fleming JE, Szatmari P, Sanford M. Evaluation of the revised Ontario Child Health Study scales. *J Child Psychol Psychiatry.* 1993;34:189-213.
10. Boyle MH, Offord DR, Racine Y, Sanford M, Szatmari P, Fleming JE, Price-Munn N. Evaluation of the Diagnostic Interview for Children and Adolescents for use in general population samples. *J Abnorm Child Psychol.* 1993;21:663-681.
11. Boyle MH, Offord DR, Hofman HG, Catlin GP, Byles JA, Cadman DT, Crawford JW, Links PS, Rae-Grant NI, Szatmari, P. Ontario Child Health Study, I: methodology. *Arch Gen Psychiatry.* 1987;44:826-831.
12. Boyle MH, Offord DR, Racine Y, Sanford M, Szatmari P, Fleming JE. Evaluation of the original Ontario Child Health Study scales. *Can J Psychiatry.* 1993;38:397-405.
13. Reich W, Welner Z. *Revised Version of the Diagnostic Interview for Children and Adolescents (DICA-R).* St Louis, Mo: Dept of Psychiatry, Washington University School of Medicine; 1988.
14. American Psychiatric Association. *Diagnostic and Statistical Manual of Mental Disorders, Third Edition, Revised.* Washington, DC: American Psychiatric Association; 1987.
15. Boyle MH, Offord DR, Racine Y, Szatmari P, Fleming JE, Sanford M. Identifying thresholds for classifying childhood psychiatric disorder: issues and prospects. *J Am Acad Child Adolesc Psychiatry.* 1996;35:1440-1448.
16. Fombonne E. The use of questionnaires in child psychiatry research: measuring their performance and choosing an optimal cut-off. *J Child Psychol Psychiatry.* 1991;32:677-693.
17. Hanley JA, McNeil BJ. The meaning and use of the area under a receiver operating characteristic (ROC) curve. *Radiology.* 1982;143:29-36.
18. Hanley JA, McNeil BJ. A method of comparing the areas under receiver operating characteristic curves derived from the same cases. *Radiology.* 1983;148:839-843.
19. Earls F. Oppositional-defiant and conduct disorders. In: Rutter M, Taylor E, Hersov L, eds. *Child and Adolescent Psychiatry: Modern Approaches.* Oxford, England: Blackwell Scientific Publications; 1994:308-329.
20. Taylor E. Syndromes of attention deficit and overactivity. In: Rutter M, Taylor E, Hersov L, eds. *Child and Adolescent Psychiatry: Modern Approaches.* Oxford, England: Blackwell Scientific Publications; 1994:285-307.
21. Harrington R. Affective disorders. In: Rutter M, Taylor E, Hersov L, eds. *Child and Adolescent Psychiatry: Modern Approaches.* Oxford, England: Blackwell Scientific Publications; 1994:330-350.
22. Radloff LS. The CES-D Scale: a new self-report depression scale for research in the general population. *Appl Psychol Measure.* 1977;1:385-401.
23. Schwab-Stone M, Fallon T, Briggs M, Crowther B. Reliability of diagnostic reporting for children aged 6-11 years: a test-retest study of the Diagnostic Interview Schedule for Children–Revised. *Am J Psychiatry.* 1994;151:1048-1054.
24. Zarin DA, Earls F. Diagnostic decision making in psychiatry. *Am J Psychiatry.* 1993;150:197-206.
25. Hodges K. Structured interviews for assessing children. *J Child Psychol Psychiatry.* 1993;34:49-68.
26. Shaffer D, Schwab-Stone M, Fisher P, Cohen P, Piacentini J, Davies M, Conners CK, Regier D. The Diagnostic Interview Schedule for Children–Revised version (DISC-R), I: preparation, field testing, interrater reliability and acceptability. *J Am Acad Child Adolesc Psychiatry.* 1993;32:643-650.
27. Harrington R, Hill J, Rutter M, John K, Fudge H, Zoccolillo M, Weissman MM. The assessment of lifetime psychopathology: a comparison of two interviewing styles. *Psychol Med.* 1988;18:487-493.
28. Streiner DL, Norman GR. *Health Measurement Scales: A Practical Guide to Their Development and Use.* 2nd ed. Oxford, England: Oxford University Press; 1995:31.
29. Simon GE, VonKorff M. Recall of psychiatric history in cross-sectional surveys: implications for epidemiologic research. *Epidemiol Rev.* 1995;17:221-227.
30. McGorry PD, Mihalopoulos C, Henry L, Dakis J, Jackson HJ, Flaum M, Harrigan S, McKenzie D, Kulkarni J, Karoly R. Spurious precision: procedural validity of diagnostic assessment in psychotic disorders. *Am J Psychiatry.* 1995;152:220-223.
31. Canino G, Bird HR, Rubio-Stipec M, Bravo M. Child psychiatric epidemiology: what we have learned and what we need to learn. *Int J Method Psychiatr Res.* 1995;5:79-92.

ORIGINAL ARTICLE

The Virginia Twin Study of Adolescent Behavioral Development

Influences of Age, Sex, and Impairment on Rates of Disorder

Emily Simonoff, MD; Andrew Pickles, PhD; Joanne M. Meyer, PhD; Judy L. Silberg, PhD; Hermine H. Maes, PhD; Rolf Loeber, PhD; Michael Rutter, MD, FRS; John K. Hewitt, PhD; Lindon J. Eaves, Dsc

Background: The Virginia Twin Study of Adolescent Behavioral Development is a cohort-longitudinal epidemiological study that uses the genetic twin design to study the development and maintenance of child psychiatric disorders. We determined the rates of *DSM-III-R* disorders, disorders with impairment, and age, sex, and comorbidity effects.

Methods: Families of 2762 white twins aged 8 to 16 years participated. Twins and their parents were asked systematically about risk factors and current psychiatric symptoms by means of investigator-based psychiatric interviews and questionnaires. The *DSM-III-R* diagnoses were made for major depressive disorder, separation anxiety, overanxious disorder, simple phobia, social phobia, agoraphobia, oppositional defiant disorder, conduct disorder, and attention deficit hyperactivity disorder.

Results: The 3-month point prevalence for any *DSM-III-R* disorders was 413 per 1000, and that for disorders with associated impairment was 142 per 1000. Emotional disorders with impairment occurred in 89 per 1000, with girls being more commonly affected; behavioral disorders had a prevalence of 71 per 1000, with boys being more frequently affected. The proportion with disorder who also had functional impairment varied across disorders; anxiety and phobic disorders were particularly likely not to be accompanied by impairment. Rates of emotional and behavioral disorders increased over the age range. There was extensive comorbidity among disorders.

Conclusions: The prevalence rates and patterns of findings from this study of twins are consistent with those of other epidemiological studies, supporting previous findings of few differences in rates of psychiatric disorder between twins and singletons. The importance of including measures of functional impairment is evident by its effect on rates of disorder and patterns of comorbidity.

Arch Gen Psychiatry. 1997;54:801-808

From the Medical Research Council Child Psychiatry Unit and the Social, Genetic and Developmental Psychiatry Research Centre, Institute of Psychiatry, London, England (Drs Simonoff, Pickles, and Rutter); Virginia Institute of Psychiatric and Behavioral Genetics, Virginia Commonwealth University, Richmond (Drs Meyer, Silberg, Maes, and Eaves); Western Psychiatric Institute, Pittsburgh, Pa (Dr Loeber); and Institute of Behavioral Genetics, University of Colorado, Boulder (Dr Hewitt).

THE VIRGINIA Twin Study of Adolescent Behavioral Development (VTSABD) is the first large-scale epidemiological twin study of child psychiatric symptoms and disorders. This longitudinal study of twins aged 8 to 16 years combines developmental, epidemiological, and genetic strategies. The VTSABD was designed to explore the role of genetic and environmental variation in the development and persistence of child psychiatic disorders and to use the genetic twin design to test hypotheses about the ways in which risk factors operate. Child psychiatric epidemiologists[1,2] have highlighted the role of longitudinal general population samples in understanding these effects. These questions include reasons for sex differences and age trends in rates of disorder, the differences between early- and late-onset disorders, the role of shared genetic and/or environmental risk factors in comorbidity among disorders, and the relationship between symptoms as dimensions and psychiatric disorders as categories. Multiple waves of data collection will allow examination of the role of risk factors, changes in rates and patterns of disorder with age, and the stability of disorder.

Whereas twins have higher rates of prematurity, language delay, and reading retardation,[3] which could predispose them to higher rates of psychopathology, there is no evidence of such increased rates. A comparison of twins rated on the Child Behavior Checklist[4] with published norms showed small elevations in mean scores of twins.[5] However, 2 comparisons of twins with population- and informant-matched singletons have shown few or no differences on multiple comparisons and inconsistency in the direction of the effect.[6,7] A comparison of clinic attend-ers indicated that twins were more likely than singletons to receive a diagnosis of conduct disorder, although there were few twin-singleton differences in the rate of individual smptoms.[8]

The VTSABD uses the Child and Adolescent Psychiatric Assessment (CAPA)[9] administered to mothers, fathers, and children. Many other large studies have made diagnoses from questionnaires along with measures of impairment[10,11] or used respondent-based interviews.[12-15] Interviewer-based assessments have the advantage of applying clear and consistent definitions and thresholds for the presence of symptoms, which are determined by the interviewer through standardized but flexible questioning to elucidate behavioral examples from the informant.[16] For informants of all ages, this allows standardization of the description of behavior and emotions.[17] Interviewer-based methods are particularly important for younger children, where comprehension may be an issue.[18]

We present our 3-month prevalence rates of *DSM-III-R* diagnoses from the first wave of data collection and examine the effects of age and sex and the pattern of comorbidity among disorders. The effect of including functional impairment on rates of disorder is explored.

SUBJECTS AND METHODS

POPULATION

The VTSABD is an ongoing cohort-longitudinal study of twins born between 1974 and 1983; 1412 families were included in the first wave of data collection, with 2 subsequent waves of data collection occurring at approximately 1½-year intervals. The study was limited to white families because there were too few data from other ethnic groups to provide adequate power to detect differential effects.

Ascertainment and participation of the sample has been described in detail elsewhere.[19] A sample of 6837 putative twin pairs born between 1970 and 1985 was ascertained through the state school system and participating private schools in Virginia, and through families who contacted the VTSABD. Parents of these twins were sent a brief letter describing the study and asked to complete a questionnaire regarding zygosity. Nonresponders were followed up with 2 further mailings and attempted telephone contact. After the contact, 1424 putative pairs were removed for a variety of reasons, including having moved out of state, having moved and left no forwarding address, the children not being twins, and duplicate ascertainment. Of the 5413 twin families, 1894 were selected for interview in the main study. Others were excluded because they were not white, were outside the age range, had moved out of state by the time of interviewing, or had moved without leaving a forwarding address. A total of 1412 families (2824 children) participated, 75% of the targeted sample. At the time of the interview, 62 twins were older than 16 years and were excluded from the current analyses, leaving a total of 2762 individuals.

INFORMANTS

Because of the lack of consensus on which informants to use in rating child psychopathology,[20-23] the VTSABD maximized available sources by including child, mother, and father informants for interviews and questionnaires and teacher informants for questionnaires. Twins completed the assessment on themselves only, while parents completed a similar assessment on both twins. Teachers who knew the children well were selected by school principals to complete questionnaires on 1 or both twins. In addition to biological parents living with the twins, other parenting figures were used as informants when they knew the child well. Parenting figures were required to have lived with the child for at least 6 months. Biological parents not living with the twins were used as informants only when contact with the children was frequent and long-standing.

MEASURES

The VTSABD examines the common areas of psychopathology: anxiety disorders, phobias, major depressive disorder; conduct disorder; oppositional defiant disorder; and attention deficit hyperactivity disorder. Questionnaire measures include scales designed to elicit normal variation in the areas of psychopathology examined in the study and have been described elsewhere.[24,25] The CAPA is used to elicit symptoms of clinical severity and to make psychiatric diagnoses.

The CAPA was administered by lay interviewers, trained by 2 of us (J.L.S. and E.S.). Training consisted of a 3-week in-house course that included didactic sessions, audio and video examples of interviews, role play, and practice interviews supervised by trained staff members. Throughout the study, all interviews were audiotaped and a team of monitors reviewed all interviews. Particular attention was paid to ensure that there was no slippage in symptom thresholds, that interviewers obtained adequately detailed behavioral examples to justify their ratings, and that skipping out of screening sections was justified. Regular local and statewide update and revision meetings were held throughout the study.

Interviewers were assigned in pairs to families, with randomized allocation to interviewing of the twins and parents. Each interviewer obtained information from 1 twin and then from 1 parent. Assessments were carried out in a standardized order. In addition to assessments of the children's psychopathology, parents were asked about the pregnancy with the twins, the twins' early medical and developmental history, twin zygosity, and the similarity of the twins' early environment. Lifetime parental psychopathology was determined by the measures developed by Kendler et al[26] for parental anxiety and depressive disorders as well as alcohol and substance abuse. A further measure was designed by 2 of us (E.S. and M.R.) specifically for the study to elicit antisocial personality.

THE CAPA

The CAPA makes *DSM-III-R*[27] and, now, *International Classification of Diseases, 10th Revision* (*ICD-10*)[28] and *DSM-IV*[29] diagnoses by means of symptoms present in the last 3 months. At the time of the first wave of data collection, *ICD-10* and *DSM-IV* criteria were not available, and we limited ourselves to *DSM-III-R* in this wave. The CAPA and its development have been described in detail elsewhere.[9,16] The version used in the VTSABD focuses on common child psychiatric disorders. Computer algorithms for determining the presence of individual symptoms are in line with those used in the Great Smoky Mountain Study,[30] which also uses the CAPA. These algorithms use intensity, frequency, and duration of symptoms to determine whether they are of clinical severity. Other requirements for *DSM-III-R* diagnoses, such as age at onset, are also implemented.

In combining informants, we applied the "or" rule (parent *or* child response positive) used in many recent epidemiological studies that have multiple informants.[13,14,30] Under this rule, a symptom is endorsed when either parent or child information meets algorithm criteria. The *or* rule is particularly appropriate for the CAPA, where informants are required to give behavioral descriptions of potential symptoms, reducing the likelihood of false-positive responses. Two sources were used for each symptom: the child and 1 parent. The latter was preferentially selected from mothers, but father information was used when mother information was unavailable. This procedure takes account of families where only 1 parent was an informant and ensures that all subjects had the same number of informants contributing to the symptom rating. The *or* rule was applied to all areas of disorder except attention deficit hyperactivity disorder, where children were not used as informants.

In addition to making *DSM-III-R* diagnoses, we added an impairment requirement to each diagnosis. The coding of symptoms in the CAPA, particularly the emotional ones, requires the presence of impairment at the time symptoms occur. The CAPA also assesses psychosocial impairment more broadly. Psychosocial impairment is tied specifically to symptom areas, although the presence of comorbidity allows multiple symptom areas to be related to impairment. The CAPA covers psychosocial impairment in a range of 15 areas, including relationships with parents, siblings, peers, and teacher, ability to carry out homework and extracurricular activities, disciplinary action taken by school, and treatment and medication received. Each area of impairment is coded 0 (no impairment), 1 (partial impairment), or 2 (severe impairment). Symptom area–specific impairment scores were generated for child and parent informants and then summed across informants to form a combined score. A cutoff of 2 on the combined score was used as the criterion for the presence of impairment. This threshold could be reached in 3 ways: (1) an individual informant could report severe impairment in 1 area; (2) an individual informant could report partial impairment in 2 areas; and (3) the child and parent informants could each report partial impairment in 1 area. These impairment criteria were combined with the diagnoses to generate new diagnoses, with associated (symptom area–specific) impairment. We chose our threshold to reflect a moderate level of functional impairment; using a different instrument, Bird et al[13] selected a similar impairment threshold, on the grounds that it correlated best with other measures of severity and adaptive functioning.

DATA ANALYSIS

We are concerned here with the epidemiology of twins as individuals, and thus each twin pair contributes 2 observations. However, although each twin pair can be considered as independently sampled, individual twins within a pair cannot. The sampling design is equivalent to a simple 2-stage cluster design with twin pairs as the primary sampling unit. In light of the lack of independence of observations made on twins, we used a generalized estimating equation approach to provide consistent estimates of both prevalence and confidence intervals. Generalized estimating equation estimation was undertaken by the methods described by Liang and Zeger[31] as implemented in version 5 of the program Stata.[32] All significance levels and 95% confidence intervals were calculated by means of the robust parameter covariance matrix[33] from logistic regression models estimated with an "exchangeable" working correlation matrix, the form most appropriate to clustered data of this kind. Differences by age and sex were examined by first fitting models that allowed for their interactive effect. If no significant interaction was found, this term was dropped from the model, and main effects for age and sex were then estimated. We report results in which age is treated as a 3-level (8-10, 11-13, and 14-16 years) categorical factor (allowing nonlinear effects) and where age is treated as a simple 3-valued variable (providing more powerful tests of trend).

Corrections for lack of independence actually made little difference for these data, the twin correlations for current psychiatric diagnosis being relatively low. For the analysis of the comorbidity data, it seemed likely that low frequencies represented a more serious difficulty for standard methods than lack of independence. Therefore, we analyzed the comorbidity data by means of exact logistic regression as implemented in LogXact,[33,34] uncorrected for nonindependence. These analyses were stratified by the potentially confounding effects of age and sex (eg, hyperactivity and conduct disorder might have been associated purely because they are both more common in boys).

RESULTS

Of the 2762 twins included in the study, 1275 (46.3%) were male and 1478 (53.7%) were female. There were 2674 mother informants and 2148 father informants, whose relationship to the child is described in **Table 1**. There was no mother informant in 3.2% and no father informant in 22.2% of cases. In 99% of cases, at least 1 parent participated to some extent, and there would have been sufficient parent information to make diagnoses based on parent information alone in 95% to 97% of cases, depending on the disorder.

RATES OF DISORDER

The 3-month prevalence rates of disorder per 1000 in the VTSABD sample are given in **Table 2**, along with their 95% confidence intervals. Overall, 413 per 1000 in the VTSABD sample qualified for at least 1 of the *DSM-III-R* diagnoses assessed; 358 per 1000 had at least 1 emotional disorder and 106 per 1000 had at least 1 behavioral disorder. The rates of disorder associated with functional impairment were considerably lower: 142 per 1000 for any disorder, 89 per 1000 for emotional disorders, and 71 per 1000 for behavioral disorders. The decrease in rates when functional impairment was added were greater for the any emotional disorder category, where those with impairment were only 25% (89/356) of those who met *DSM-III-R* criteria, than for the any behavioral disorder category, where 67% of those who met *DSM-III-R* criteria also had functional impairment.

Within the emotional disorders, the proportion of *DSM-III-R* cases that also had functional impairment showed wide variation. For depression, 87% of those with a *DSM-III-R* diagnosis had functional impairment, compared with only 21% for simple phobia, 21% for separation anxiety, 30% for social phobia, 40% for agoraphobia, and 41% for overanxious disorder. In general, the most prevalent emotional disorders were least likely to be associated with functional impairment. This variation contrasted with the pattern for behavioral disorders, where the comparable proportions of those who met *DSM-III-R* criteria who had impairment were 88%, 65%, and 58% for oppositional defiant, conduct, and attention deficit hyperactivity disorders, respectively. Because of the increasing emphasis on disorder associated with functional impairment, such as severe emotional disturbance,[35] further analyses focused primarily on disorders with impairment.

In the participating sample, 1966 twins (71%) took part after initial contact, while 796 (29%) initially deferred but subsequently agreed to participate. The relationship between deferred participation and rates of disorder was examined by means of the χ^2 statistic. Of the 18 comparisons, 4 were significant, and none of these was for a *DSM-III-R* disorder with impairment. Of the 4, 3 showed a higher rate in the immediate participation group (separation anxiety, agoraphobia, and oppositional defiant disorder—all $P<.05$) and 1 (social phobia; $P<.001$) was higher in the deferred group.

Table 1. Type and Proportion of Parent Informants

Type	No. (%) Mother	Father
Biological	2606 (94.4)	1900 (68.8)
Stepparent	34 (1.2)	154 (5.6)
Grandparent	10 (0.4)	6 (0.2)
Adoptive parent	16 (0.6)	46 (1.6)
Parental partner	0 (0)	10 (0.4)
Foster parent	2 (0.1)	2 (0.1)
Legal guardian	4 (0.1)	30 (1.1)
No informant	88 (3.2)	614 (22.2)
Total	**2762 (100)**	**2762 (100)**

INFLUENCES OF SEX AND AGE

Rates of disorder with impairment by sex and age groups are shown in Table 2. For any disorder, there was a significant increase with age ($P<.001$ for both categorial and continuous age regressions, given in this order throughout) but no sex effect or sex×age interaction (hereafter, unless specified otherwise, the sex × age interactions are nonsignificant). The rate of any emotional disorder increased with age ($P<.005$ and $P<.001$) and was higher in girls ($P<.005$ for both regressions). The rates of any behavioral disorder also increased with age ($P=.03$) but were higher in boys ($P<.001$).

The results for depression were striking in finding only a significant age trend ($P=.001$ and $P<.005$). The decreasing rate of separation anxiety with age was significant only for continuous age regressions ($P<.05$). Overanxious disorder increased with age ($P<.001$) and had higher rates in girls ($P<.002$). Of the phobias, both simple and social phobias were more prevalent in girls ($P<.005$ and $P<.05$, respectively) but no significant sex difference was seen for agoraphobia. Only social phobia showed a main effect of age, with increasing disorder with age ($P<.05$).

Table 2. Prevalence Rates of Disorder per 1000

			Overall*			
			Impairment Not Required		Impairment Required	
Diagnosis	Main Effect or Interaction	No.	Rate	95% CI	Rate	95% CI
Depression	A, a†	2741	13	10-19	12	8-17
Separation anxiety	a	2723	72	62-83	15	11-21
Overanxious	A, a, S‡	2742	108	96-122	44	36-53
Simple phobia	S	2725	212	196-229	44	37-53
Agoraphobia	...	2738	27	22-34	11	8-16
Social phobia	A, a, S	2734	84	73-96	25	20-32
Any emotional	A, a, S	2674	358	338-378	89	78-101
Oppositional defiant	A, a	2742	39	32-47	34	27-42
Conduct	A, a, S	2742	66	56-78	43	35-53
Attention deficit hyperactivity	S	2636	24	18-30	14	10-19
Any behavioral	A, a, S	2674	106	94-120	71	61-82
Any disorder	A, a	2674	413	392-433	142	128-158

**Rates without and with functional impairment requirement. CI indicates confidence interval.*
†Main effect of age: A for categorical; a for continuous age regressions for disorders with impairment.
‡Main effect of sex (S) for disorders with impairment.

Regarding the behavioral disorders, there was a significant age effect ($P<.005$ and $P<.01$) for oppositional defiant disorder, but no effect of sex. Conduct disorder affected boys more frequently ($P<.005$) and increased with age ($P<.005$). Significantly more boys had attention deficit hyperactivity disorder ($P<.005$), but there was no age main effect or sex × age interaction.

COMORBIDITY AMONG DISORDERS

Of the 413 per 1000 with *DSM-III-R* disorders, 251 (61%) had 1 disorder only, 105 (25%) had 2 disorders, and 57 (14%) had 3 or more disorders. For *DSM-III-R* disorders with impairment, 76 from the total of 142 (53%) per 1000 had 1 disorder only, 41 (29%) had 2 disorders, and 25 (18%) had 3 or more disorders.

In general, the odds ratios for the associations between disorders, as shown in **Table 3**, were strikingly large and significant, although tending to be lower for the more prevalent disorders defined without the additional impairment criterion. For disorders with impairment, the odds ratios within the emotional disorder area were generally larger than those among behavioral disorders, which in turn tended to be larger than those between emotional and behavioral disorders. All were greater than 1, indicating that no disorder was protective for any other. Interestingly, the odds ratio of 3.2 between conduct disorder and attention deficit hyperactivity disorder was not significant and was quite low by the standards of the Table as a whole.

The **Figure** shows the patterns of comorbidity among disorders with impairment. Of the 89 per 1000 with an impairing emotional disorder, 17 (19%) also had a behavioral disorder. In contrast, of the 71 individuals per 1000 with a behavioral disorder, 17 (24%) also had an emotional disorder. This degree of overlap was highly significant ($P<.001$).

Depression was significantly comorbid with all other disorders except attention deficit hyperactivity disorder (Table 3). For depression, 77% of cases with impairment were comorbid with at least 1 other emotional disorder and 27% with 2 or more disorders; 55% were comorbid with overanxious disorder, 45% with phobias (simple, social, and agoraphobia combined), and only 9% with separation anxiety (Figure, B). Furthermore, cases of comorbidity between depression and separation anxiety also included comorbidity with overanxious disorder. Separation anxiety disorder showed significant comorbidity with all the emotional but none of the behavioral disorders. Of the cases of separation anxiety with impairment, 67% were comorbid with at least 1 other emotional disorder and 27% with 2 or more. However, only 7% were comorbid with depression, compared with 40% with overanxious disorder and 57% with phobias. Overanxious disorder showed a pattern generally similar to that of depression. Sixty-eight percent of impairing overanxious disorder was comorbid with another emo-

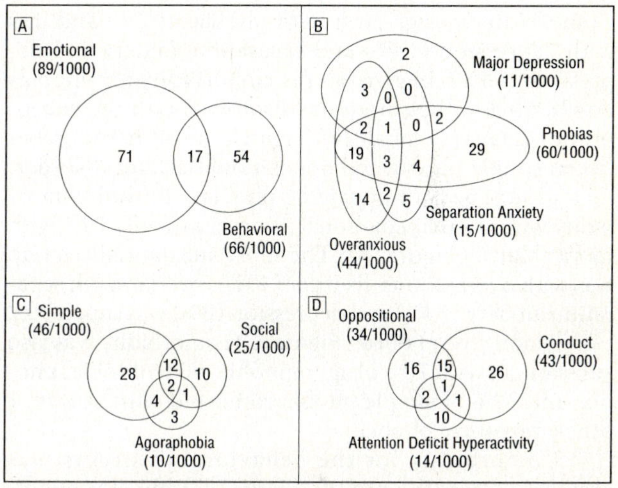

Comorbidity among disorders with impairment. Cell sizes indicate number of cases per 1000. All representations are based on the sample with complete data on all disorders with impairment; hence, there is slight variation in numbers from those given in Table 2.

Rates With Impairment by Sex and Age

Boys				Girls			
Overall	8-10 y	11-13 y	14-16 y	Overall	8-10 y	11-13 y	14-16 y
12	5	11	21	12	4	10	24
11	14	11	8	18	28	17	7
31	19	28	48	56	26	44	107
31	26	34	32	56	49	56	65
9	7	11	11	12	15	8	14
18	9	11	37	31	32	21	43
70	55	63	96	105	83	94	146
39	19	41	58	30	23	35	33
59	45	47	90	29	21	23	48
20	24	13	25	8	14	4	5
90	75	78	124	54	44	53	67
141	120	116	195	143	120	136	183

Table 3. Odds Ratios for Comorbidity Between Disorders*

Diagnosis	Depression OR	Depression 95% CI	Separation Anxiety OR	Separation Anxiety 95% CI	Overanxious OR	Overanxious 95% CI	Simple Phobia OR	Simple Phobia 95% CI
Depression	...	...	**7.0**	**2.9-15.9**	**7.3**	**3.5-15.2**	**1.8**	**0.8-3.9**
Separation anxiety	14.7	3.4-48.6	...	...	**5.2**	**3.6-7.5**	**3.2**	**2.3-4.3**
Overanxious	24.5	10.8-55.9	20.2	9.2-43.2	...	...	**2.6**	**2.0-3.4**
Simple phobia	10.4	4.2-24.0	20.9	10.1-42.6	27.3	16.9-44.3	...	...
Agoraphobia	14.7	3.4-48.2	39.6	14.4-103.2	12.3	4.8-29.6	32.3	14.2-75.0
Social phobia	4.9	1.2-15.0	11.2	4.1-26.9	19.0	10.6-34.1	26.2	14.9-46.1
Oppositional defiant	15.0	6.2-34.3	2.6	0.5-8.5	5.0	2.6-9.2	4.7	2.4-8.7
Conduct	11.2	4.6-25.6	1.4	0.2-5.8	3.7	1.9-6.8	2.9	1.4-5.6
Attention deficit hyperactivity	1.7	0.0-10.4	2.1	0.1-13.3	2.6	0.5-8.6	2.4	0.5-7.9

**Odds ratios (ORs) for comorbidity between disorders, stratified by age and sex (see text). CI indicates confidence interval. Upper triangular area (boldface) refers to disorders without the impairment requirement; lower triangular area,* DSM-III-R *disorders with associated impairment.*

tional disorder but only 14% with more than 1. Comorbidity was greatest with phobias (57%) and less with depression (13%) and separation anxiety and depression (14%). In general, the comorbidity for phobias was limited to the emotional disorders, with the exception of relatively small but significant odds ratios between simple phobia and oppositional defiant disorder. As a group, 52% of impairing phobias showed comorbidity with another emotional disorder but only 10% with more than 1 (Figure, B). The most substantial overlap was with overanxious disorder (40%); overlap with separation anxiety (13%) and depression (8%) was much less.

Among the phobias (Figure, C) comorbidity was also substantial, with 70% of agoraphobia, 60% of social phobia, and 39% of simple phobia comorbid with at least 1 other impairing phobia.

Comorbidity for the behavioral disorders was greatest within the group (Figure, D) but not exclusive to it. As well as significant comorbidity with conduct and attention deficit hyperactivity disorders, oppositional defiant disorder showed comorbidity with depression and overanxious disorder. Conduct disorder was significantly comorbid with oppositional defiant disorder, depression, and overanxious disorder, the association with attention deficit hyperactivity disorder being just short of significance ($P=.08$). The rate of overlap with at least 1 other behavioral disorder was 71%, 40%, and 29% for oppositional defiant, conduct, and attention deficit disorders. The greatest overlap was between oppositional defiant and conduct disorders.

COMMENT

Our findings indicate that, overall, disorder increases with age and, while boys have higher rates of behavioral disorders and girls of emotional disorders, there is no significant sex effect in the aggregated disorder. Requiring a further impairment criterion reduces the rate of disorder, particularly for the anxiety and phobic disorders. Comorbidity is substantial, even after age and sex effects are taken into account. Previous epidemiological studies have reported widely varying rates of disorder; rates will vary according to sample characteristics, instruments and informants used to identify disorder, the diagnostic criteria used, and the requirement or not of functional impairment. Despite the caution that must be placed on comparing rates across samples, the overall rates of disorder and patterns of age and sex effects seen in the VTSABD are in line with many previous studies.[12-14,30,36-40]

Other epidemiological studies have reported that 25% to 55% of those who have at least 1 psychiatric disorder have more than 1 such disorder[12,30,36,37,39,41]; our rates of 38% and 46% (for disorders without and with the additional impairment requirements, respectively) are consistent with those findings. Previous studies have suggested that comorbidity runs across domains of disorder and is not limited to comorbidity among emotional or among behavioral disorders. However, only a few of the previous studies have indicated the statistical significance of their findings,[30,37,41] which is crucial because the observed numbers may be small. Our findings show that the comorbidity between emotional and behavioral disorders is largely through depression and overanxious disorder on the one hand and oppositional defiant and conduct disorder on the other. The high rates of comorbidity, particularly among emotional disorders, must inevitably raise concerns as to the appropriateness of the classification scheme. Because our data are stratified by age and sex, the comorbid relationships observed are independent of these potentially shared risk factors.

Once all anxiety disorders were combined, we found significant comorbidity with oppositional defiant and with conduct disorders ($P<.001$ for both) but not attention deficit hyperactivity disorder. This places our findings in line with those of other studies.[13,30,37] Our failure to find significant comorbidity between depression and attention deficit is supported by Bird et al,[41] who found an inconsistent relationship, depending on the scoring method, but is different from the findings of Fergusson et al,[37] who reported a significant relationship. The mere marginal significance of the comorbidity between conduct and attention deficit hyperactivity disorder is surprising but may relate to the informants contributing to different diagnoses; attention deficit is reported on only by parents, while both informants are used for conduct

Agoraphobia		Social Phobia		Oppositional Defiant		Conduct		Attention Deficit Hyperactivity	
OR	95% CI	OR	95% CI	OR	95% CI	OR	95% CI	OR	95% CI
6.4	**1.8-17.7**	**1.1**	**0.3-3.2**	**11.0**	**4.7-24.4**	**5.9**	**2.5-13.2**	**0.9**	**0.0-5.5**
6.8	**3.9-11.7**	**2.7**	**1.8-4.1**	**2.4**	**1.2-4.4**	**1.5**	**0.8-2.7**	**1.2**	**0.4-3.1**
2.2	**1.1-4.0**	**2.4**	**1.6-3.4**	**3.0**	**1.8-4.9**	**1.9**	**1.2-3.0**	**2.0**	**0.9-4.0**
3.3	**2.0-5.4**	**2.7**	**2.0-3.7**	**2.5**	**1.6-3.8**	**1.1**	**0.8-1.7**	**2.0**	**1.1-3.6**
...	...	**3.9**	**2.1-6.8**	**2.4**	**0.8-5.7**	**1.7**	**0.6-3.8**	**3.3**	**1.0-8.8**
18.0	6.8-44.0	...	...	**1.8**	**1.0-3.3**	**1.1**	**0.6-1.9**	**0.9**	**0.2-2.4**
3.3	0.6-11.0	3.9	1.5-8.5	...	...	**13.7**	**8.6-21.9**	**3.8**	**1.5-8.5**
1.6	0.2-6.7	2.5	0.9-5.8	29.1	17.4-48.6	...	...	**1.7**	**0.7-3.7**
5.9	0.6-25.5	2.6	0.3-10.9	7.5	2.6-18.6	3.2	0.9-8.7	...	...

disorder, and the contribution from child reports is substantial.

The strengths of the VTSABD include its large sample size and wide age range, consisting of the resident 8- to 16-year-old white twin population of Virginia. An acceptable proportion of the target population participated in the study. The sample was investigated by means of the CAPA interviewer-based assessment with multiple informants. An advantage of the CAPA is its inclusion of ratings of functional impairment that are tied to specific symptom areas. Limitations of the study include the exclusion of minority groups (because the number of eligible twins was considered too small for useful comparisons, particularly in genetic analyses). The use of a single-phase general population sample, rather than a high-risk sample obtained after a preliminary screening assessment, meant that the numbers of individual cases of rare disorders would have been too small for analysis, and therefore only the more common disorders were assessed. Having pairs of subjects (twins) as the sample design unit makes 2-phase designs more complex and would have made longitudinal genetic analysis particularly difficult.

We find that the addition of further psychosocial impairment has a substantial effect on rates of disorder. Bird et al[13] previously reported a similar effect on the overall rate of aggregated disorders; our findings are the first to explore the effect on individual disorders. We used a conservative estimate of impairment, and more work is necessary to examine the impact of different thresholds. In relation to comorbidity, we found substantially higher odds ratios for diagnoses that require impairment. The effect is particularly strong for comorbidity involving anxiety and phobic disorders. It is unclear whether this reflects an important characteristic of the comorbid relationships among disorders or is merely a statistical phenomenon. Simulations indicate that, for disorders defined by the extremes of dimensions, and where the comorbidity is the result of the correlation between the 2 dimensions, raising the threshold for classification (thereby lowering the prevalence) would in itself increase the odds ratios. Impairment has the greatest impact on base rates for anxiety and phobic disorders, and it is here that the effect on odds ratios is greatest. Further work, involving reports from different informants and longitudinal data, is required to determine whether impairment conveys unique information or serves only as a way to increase diagnostic thresholds.

Accepted for publication April 24, 1997.

The VTSABD is supported by grant MH-45268 (principal investigator, Dr Eaves) from the National Institute of Mental Health, Bethesda, Md. Drs Silberg and Meyer are supported in part by Junior Faculty Awards from the John D. and Catherine T. MacArthur Foundation, Chicago, Ill.

Thanks to Cathy Coshall, MSc, for assistance with statistical analysis.

Reprints: Emily Simonoff, MD, Medical Research Council Child Psychiatry Unit, Institute of Psychiatry, De Crespigny Park, London SE5 8AF, England.

REFERENCES

1. Costello EJ, Angold A. Toward a developmental epidemiology of the disruptive behavior disorders. *Dev Psychopathol.* 1993;5:91-101.
2. Rutter M. Epidemiological approaches to developmental psychopathology. *Arch Gen Psychiatry.* 1988;45:486-495.
3. Rutter M, Redshaw J. Growing up as a twin: twin-singleton differences in psychological development. *J Child Psychol Psychiatry.* 1991;32:885-895.
4. Achenbach TM, Edelbrick C. *Manual for the Child Behavior Checklist.* Burlington: University of Vermont; 1985.
5. Gau JS, Silberg JL, Erickson MT, Hewitt JK. Childhood behavior problems: a comparison of twin and non-twin samples. *Acta Genet Med Gemellol.* 1992;41:53-63.
6. Gjone H, Novik TS. Parental ratings of behaviour problems: a twin and general population comparison. *J Child Psychol Psychiatry.* 1995;36:1213-1224.
7. Van Den Oord EJ, Koot HM, Boomsma DI, Verhulst FC, Orlebeke JF. A twin-singleton comparison of problem behaviour in 2-3-year-olds. *J Child Psychol Psychiatry.* 1995;36:449-458.
8. Simonoff E. A comparison of twins and singletons with child psychiatric disorders: an item sheet analysis. *J Child Psychol Psychiatry.* 1992;33:1319-1332.
9. Angold A, Costello E. A test-retest reliability study of child-reported psychiatric symptoms and diagnoses using the Child and Adolescent Psychiatric Assessment (CAPA-C). *Psychol Med.* 1995;25:755-762.
10. Offord DR, Alder RJ, Boyle MH. Prevalence and sociodemographic correlates of conduct disorder. *Am J Soc Psychiatry.* 1986;6:272-278.
11. Verhulst FC, Van Der Ende J. Six year developmental course of internalizing and externalizing problem behaviors. *J Am Acad Child Adolesc Psychiatry.* 1992;31:924-931.
12. Anderson JC, Williams S, McGee R, Silva PA. *DSM-III* disorders in preadolescent children. *Arch Gen Psychiatry.* 1987;44:69-76.
13. Bird HR, Canino G, Rubio-Stipec M, Gould MS, Ribera J, Sesman M, Woodbury

M, Huertas-Goldman S, Pagan A, Sanchez-Lacay A, Moscoso M. Estimates of the prevalence of childhood maladjustment in a community survey in Puerto Rico. *Arch Gen Psychiatry.* 1988;45:1120-1126.
14. Cohen P, Cohen J, Kasen S, Velez CN, Hartmark C, Johnson J, Rojas M, Brook J, Streuning EL. An epidemiological study of disorders in late childhood and adolescence, I: age- and gender-specific prevalence. *J Child Psychol Psychiatry.* 1993; 34:851-867.
15. Reinherz HZ, Giaconia RM, Lefkowitz ES, Pakiz B, Frost AK. Prevalence of psychiatric disorders in a community population of older adolescents. *J Am Acad Child Adolesc Psychiatry.* 1993;32:369-377.
16. Angold A, Prendergast M, Cox A, Harrington R, Simonoff E, Rutter M. The Child and Adolescent Psychiatric Assessment. *Psychol Med.* 1995;25:729-753.
17. Harrington R. The assessment of lifetime psychopathology: a comparison of two interviewing styles. *Psychol Med.* 1988;18:487-493.
18. Breton JJ, Bergeron L, Valla JP, Lepine S, Houde L, Gaudet N. Do children aged 9 through 11 years understand the DISC Version 2.25 questions? *J Am Acad Child Adolesc Psychiatry.* 1995;34:946-954.
19. Meyer JM, Silberg JL, Simonoff E, Kendler KS, Hewitt JK HJ. The Virginia Twin-Family Study of Adolescent Behavioral Development: assessing sample biases in demographic correlates of psychopathology. *Psychol Med.* 1996;26:1113-1133.
20. Achenbach TM, McConaughy SH, Howell CT. Child/adolescent behavioral and emotional problems: implications of cross-informant correlations for situational specificity. *Psychol Bull.* 1987;101:213-232.
21. Bird HR, Gould MS, Staghezza B. Aggregating data from multiple informants in child psychiatry epidemiology research. *J Am Acad Child Adolesc Psychiatry.* 1992;31:78-85.
22. Loeber R, Green SM, Lahey BB, Stouthamer-Loeber M. Optimal informants on childhood disruptive behaviors. *Dev Psychopathol.* 1989;1:317-337.
23. Reich W, Earls F. Rules for making psychiatric diagnoses in children on the basis of multiple sources of information: preliminary strategies. *J Abnorm Child Psychol.* 1987;15:601-616.
24. Hewitt JK, Silberg JL, Rutter M, Simonoff E, Meyer JM, Maes H, Pickles A, Neale MC, Loeber R, Erickson MT, Kendler KS, Heath AC, Truett KR, Reynolds CA, Eaves LJ. Genetics and developmental psychopathology, 1: phenotypic assessment in the Virginia Twin Study of Adolescent Behavioral Development. *J Child Psychol Psychiatry.* In press.
25. Eaves LJ, Silberg JL, Meyer JM, Maes HH, Simonoff E, Pickles A, Rutter M, Neale MC, Reynolds CA, Erickson MT, Heath AC, Loeber R, Truett KR, Hewitt JK. Genetics and developmental psychopathology, 2: the main effects of genes and environment on behavioural problems in the Virginia Twin Study of Adolescent Behavioral Development. *J Child Psychol Psychiatry.* In press.
26. Kendler KS, Neale MC, Kessler RC, Heath AC, Eaves LJ. A population-based twin study of major depression in women. *Arch Gen Psychiatry.* 1992;49:257-266.
27. American Psychiatric Association, Committee on Nomenclature and Statistics. *Diagnostic and Statistical Manual of Mental Disorders, Third Edition, Revised.* Washington, DC: American Psychiatric Association; 1987.
28. World Health Organization. *The ICD-10 Classification of Mental and Behavioural Disorders.* Geneva, Switzerland: World Health Organization; 1992.
29. American Psychiatric Association, Committee on Nomenclature and Statistics. *Diagnostic and Statistical Manual of Mental Disorders, Fourth Edition.* Washington, DC: American Psychiatric Association; 1994.
30. Costello EJ, Angold A, Burns B, Stangl D, Tweed D, Erkanli A. The Great Smoky Mountains Study of youth, I: prevalence and correlates of *DSM-III-R* disorders. *Arch Gen Psychiatry.* 1996;53:1137-1143.
31. Liang KY, Zeger SL. Longitudinal data analysis using generalized linear models. *Biometrika.* 1986;73:13-22.
32. *Stata Statistical Software Release 5.0.* College Station, Tex: Stata Corp; 1997.
33. Huber PJ. The behavior of maximum likelihood estimates under non-standard conditions. In: *Proceedings of the Fifth Berkeley Symposium in Mathematical Statistics and Probability.* Berkeley, Calif: University of California; 1967:221-233.
34. *LogXact.* Cambridge, Mass: Cytel Software Corp; 1995.
35. 58 *Federal Register.* 29425 (1993).
36. Feehan M, McGee R, Raja SN, Williams SM. *DSM-III-R* disorders in New Zealand 18-year-olds. *Aust N Z J Psychiatry.* 1994;28:87-99.
37. Fergusson DM, Horwood LJ, Lynskey MT. Prevalence and comorbidity of *DSM-III-R* diagnosis in a birth cohort of 15 year olds. *J Am Acad Child Adolesc Psychiatry.* 1993;32:1127-1134.
38. Fombonne E. The Chartres study, I: prevalence of psychiatric disorders among French school-aged children. *Br J Psychiatry.* 1994;164:69-79.
39. McGee R, Feehan M, Williams S, Partridge F, Silva PA, Kelly J. *DSM-III* disorders in a large sample of adolescents. *J Am Acad Child Adolesc Psychiatry.* 1990; 29:611-619.
40. Rutter M, Cox A, Tupling C, Berger M, Yule W. Attainment and adjustment in two geographical areas, I: the prevalence of psychiatric disorder. *Br J Psychiatry.* 1975;126:493-509.
41. Bird HR, Gould MS, Staghezza BM. Patterns of diagnostic comorbidity in a community sample of children aged 9 through 16 years. *J Am Acad Child Adolesc Psychiatry.* 1993;32:361-368.

ORIGINAL ARTICLE

Boys' Behavioral Inhibition and the Risk of Later Delinquency

Margaret Kerr, PhD; Richard E. Tremblay, PhD; Linda Pagani, PhD; Frank Vitaro, PhD

Of all passions, that which inclineth men least to break the laws is fear.
Thomas Hobbes
Leviathan

Background: In some studies, shyness and anxiety have protected at-risk boys from developing delinquency. In others, shyness and withdrawal have increased risk. We argue that this is because behavioral inhibition, which is the protective factor, has been confounded with social withdrawal and other constructs. Our study addresses 3 major questions: (1) is behavioral inhibition, as distinguished from social withdrawal, a protective factor in the development of delinquency; (2) does the protective effect depend on whether disruptiveness is also present; and (3) does inhibition increase the risk of later depressive symptoms even if it protects against delinquency?

Methods: The subjects were boys from low socioeconomic status areas of Montreal, Quebec. Age 10- to 12-year predictors were peer-rated inhibition, withdrawal, and disruptiveness; age 13- to 15-year outcomes were self-rated depressive symptoms and delinquency. Eight age 10- to 12-year behavioral profiles were compared with 4 age 13- to 15-year outcome profiles.

Results: Inhibition seemed to protect disruptive and nondisruptive boys against delinquency. Disruptive boys who were noninhibited were more likely than chance to become delinquent; disruptive boys who were inhibited were not. Inhibition did not increase the risk for depression among disruptive boys. Among nondisruptive boys, only nondisruptive-inhibited boys were significantly less likely than chance to become delinquent. However, withdrawal was not protective. Disruptive-withdrawn boys were at the greatest risk for delinquency or delinquency with depressive symptoms.

Conclusion: Inhibition and social withdrawal, although behaviorally similar, present different risks for later outcomes and, therefore, should be differentiated conceptually and empirically.

Arch Gen Psychiatry. 1997;54:809-816

From the Research Unit on Children's Psycho-Social Maladjustment, University of Montreal, Montreal, Quebec. Dr Kerr is now at Gannon University, Erie, Pa.

THE ROOTS of adolescent delinquency can be found in childhood personality and cognitive abilities.[1] Aggressive children, especially if they are also hyperactive, are most likely to become juvenile delinquents[2,3] and adult criminals.[4,5] Other childhood personality factors seem to reduce the risk of delinquency. In one study, anxiety and, to a lesser degree, prosociality protected kindergarten boys from becoming delinquent adolescents.[1] In other studies, shyness protected elementary school-aged and adolescent boys from becoming delinquent (J. McCord, unpublished data, 1987).[6-8] However, shyness paired with aggression has sometimes predicted higher, not lower, levels of later delinquency or other problems (J. McCord, unpublished data, 1987),[9] and similar results have been found for social withdrawal, a related construct.[10-12] In this article, we argue that the operational definitions of the variables that proved to be protective, whatever they were called, all included some measure of behavioral inhibition. We argue further that behavioral inhibition is the protective factor and that it should be distinguished from constructs such as social withdrawal, which, despite its behavioral similarity, might increase risk.

Behavioral inhibition is a tendency to react fearfully to strange people, objects, or situations[13] or to the threat of punishment or nonreward[14] and it has certain physiological correlates.[13,15-17] In studies in which anxiety and shyness protected against delinquency, their operational definitions included behavioral inhibition. One of 3 items used to measure anxiety[1] captured the essence of inhibition: "tends to be fearful or afraid of new things or new situations." Likewise, 1 of 3 items used to measure shyness,[6] "not speaking up much," is one behavioral indicator used to identify inhibited children.[13,15,16]

SUBJECTS AND METHODS

SUBJECTS

The subjects were from the Montreal Longitudinal-Experimental Study of boys at high risk for delinquent behavior.[1] In 1984, kindergarten teachers from French-speaking schools in areas of Montreal with the lowest socioeconomic indexes were asked to rate the boys in their classes. The teachers typically had about 8 boys in their morning classes and 8 in their afternoon classes. Of the teachers who were asked, 87% returned ratings on a total of 1116 boys from 53 schools. To control for cultural effects, only sons of white, French-speaking, native-born Canadians (1037 boys) were retained in the sample. Parents of these subjects had attained an average of 10.5 years of schooling. Average maternal age (±SD) at subject's birth was 25.3 years (±4.7 years) and average paternal age was 29.3 years (±5.7 years). Most parents were unskilled workers. On the Blishen and McRoberts occupational prestige scale,[28] mothers and fathers had mean scores of about 42 (on this scale the minimum possible score is 17.81 for a newspaper deliverer; the maximum score, 101.78 for a dentist). For our study, 778 subjects were retained. They were those for whom no missing data existed on any of the measures of interest, which covered ages 10 to 15 years.

Those 259 subjects for whom data were missing, and who were excluded from the analyses, differed in several ways from the 778 who were retained. Subjects not included were, according to kindergarten teachers' judgments, more aggressive ($F[1,1035]=24.4$, $P<.001$), less prosocial ($F[1,1035]=13.8$, $P<.001$), more anxious ($F[1,1035]=5.5$, $P=.02$), more inattentive ($F[1,1035]=20.8$, $P<.001$), more oppositional ($F[1,1035]=16.7$, $P<.001$), and more hyperactive ($F[1,1035]=28.2$ $P<.001$). Additionally, their mothers and fathers had attained about a year less schooling than those included in the study ($Fs[1,1035]>16.4$, $Ps<.001$); however, neither the mothers nor the fathers were lower in occupational prestige ($Fs[1,1035]<1.6$, $P>.05$). Thus, the sample with complete data was somewhat biased toward better adjusted kindergarten boys from low socioeconomic environments.

MEASURES

Disruptiveness, Inhibition, and Withdrawal

Peer ratings from the Pupil Evaluation Inventory (PEI)[29] were used to classify boys on disruptiveness, inhibition, and withdrawal for ages 10, 11, and 12 years. Researchers administered the PEI to all of the subjects' classmates. Each classmate (boy or girl) nominated 4 boys whom they thought best exemplified each of the 35 descriptive phrases. For these analyses, we transformed the scores into proportions. A boy's score on any given PEI item represented the proportion of classmates who thought he was 1 of 4 boys whom the item best described. A PEI score on a single item then represented views of multiple informants. Furthermore, because we averaged PEI scores over 3 ages, the disruptiveness, inhibition, and withdrawal measures used in this study represent views of multiple informants on multiple occasions during the 3-year period. For disruptiveness we selected items that captured aggression and hyperactivity, the combination most predictive of later delinquency.[2,3] The 3 items that composed our disruptiveness measure were (1) "those who are mean and cruel to other children," (2) "those who start fights over nothing," and (3) "those who cannot sit still." Internal consistency α for these 3 items ranged from 0.85 to 0.88 during the 3 years. Additionally, the 3 different groups of peers agreed substantially about which of their classmates were disruptive. The internal consistency α for the 3 years' composite measures was 0.91. The 2 items that composed our inhibition measure were (1) "those who are too shy to make friends easily" and (2) "those who are upset when called on to answer questions in class." Internal consistency α for these 2 items ranged from 0.74 to 0.82 during the 3 years. The 3 different groups of peers also agreed substantially about which boys were inhibited. The internal consistency α for the 3 years' composite measures was 0.86. One item ("those who often want to play alone") was taken to represent withdrawal, a nonanxious preference for solitary activity. The internal consistency α for the 3 withdrawal measures (ages 10, 11, and 12 years) was 0.74. We dichotomized mean (10-, 11-, and 12-year) disruptiveness, inhibition, and withdrawal using 70th percentile cutoffs. Those whose scores fell above the 70th percentile cutoffs were considered disruptive, inhibited, or withdrawn, and those whose scores fell below the 70th percentile cutoffs were considered nondisruptive, noninhibited, or nonwithdrawn.

Social withdrawal, in contrast, can be seen as a nonanxious preference for solitary activity[18] or a failure to be rewarded by social interaction or others' approval. This is conceptually equivalent to a lack of "reward dependence" in Cloninger's[19,20] terminology or "psychotocism" (toughmindedness) in Eysenck's[21] terminology. Cloninger's[20] "antisocial" personality profile describes people who are low on reward dependence (withdrawn), low on anxiety (not inhibited), and high on novelty seeking (aggressive-hyperactive). In other words, antisocial people are aggressive-withdrawn. We suggest then that inhibition and withdrawal should be distinguished because we should expect different outcomes when they are combined with aggression. Inhibited-aggressive children should be at lower risk for delinquency; withdrawn-aggressive children should be at higher risk. However, anxiety and shyness are often associated with depressed mood.[22-27] Either behavioral inhibition or social withdrawal might, therefore, pose a risk for later depression.

We used longitudinal data to test 3 hypotheses: (1) that behavioral inhibition will act as a protective factor in the development of delinquency, whereas social withdrawal will not; (2) that comorbidity of withdrawal and aggression will be associated with negative outcomes, whereas comorbidity of inhibition and aggression will not; and (3) that even if it protects against delinquency, behavioral inhibition might put children at greater risk for later depressive symptoms.

Depressive Symptoms

As the measure of depressive symptoms, we used age 15-years self-reported depressive symptoms from the Children's Depression Inventory[30] (M. Kovacs, PhD, unpublished data, 1983), which is a self-rated 27-item scale that assesses affective, cognitive, motivational, and somatic symptoms of depression in school-aged children. Subjects rated each item on a 0- to 2-point scale, with higher scores indicating more severe depressive symptoms. Total scores ranged from 0 to 43. Those scoring above the 70th percentile, which corresponded to a score of 12, were considered to have depressive symptoms. Those scoring below the 70th percentile were considered not to have depressive symptoms. Self-reports of depression have been shown to be reliable and valid in assessing depressive symptoms of adolescents.[31,32]

Delinquency

As the measure of delinquency, we used self-reports of behavior during 1-year periods prior to the 13-, 14-, and 15-year assessments. Subjects indicated that during the previous 12 months they had committed each of 7 crimes never (0), once or twice (1), often (2), or very often (3). The crimes included using a weapon in a fight, breaking and entering, arson, making coercive threats of violence, stealing something worth more than $100, vandalizing an automobile, and physically assaulting someone without provocation. Approximately 50% of the subjects scored 0 on the combined 13- to 15-year measure. We considered those whose scores fell above the 70th percentile as delinquent. Self-reported delinquency has proved to be a valid assessment of the frequency of delinquent acts in previous studies.[33,34]

PROCEDURE

Four disruptive predictor groups and 4 nondisruptive groups were formed: (1) disruptive-inhibited-withdrawn, (2) disruptive-inhibited, (3) disruptive-withdrawn, (4) disruptive, (5) inhibited-withdrawn, (6) inhibited, (7) withdrawn, and (8) no problems. Numbers observed and expected to fall in the 8 predictor groups are summarized under predictors in **Table 1**.

This distribution is significantly different from chance (likelihood ratio χ^2=121.5, P<.001). The disruptive-inhibited profile, which characterizes only 3% of the subjects, is the least likely combination. Only half as many boys as expected were found to be disruptive-inhibited (25 observed, 48.9 expected) or withdrawn-only (57 observed, 114.3 expected) and fewer than expected were inhibited-only (75 observed, 114.3 expected). In contrast, almost twice as many as expected were found to be disruptive-inhibited-withdrawn (40 observed, 20.9 expected) or inhibited-withdrawn (93 observed, 48.9 expected). Inhibition and withdrawal tend to co-occur; however, there are still many boys who are characterized by one and not the other.

Four outcome groups were formed: (1) depressed-delinquent, (2) depressed, (3) delinquent, and (4) no problems. The numbers observed and expected in these groups are summarized under outcomes in Table 1. This distribution is also unlike chance (likelihood ratio χ^2=47, P<.001). Fewer boys than expected were delinquent-only (107 observed, 145.1 expected) and depressed-only (117 observed, 155.1 expected). More boys than expected were delinquent-depressed (91 observed, 52.9 expected) and without problems (463 observed, 424.9 expected). Having both problems then occurred more often than expected and having either problem alone occurred less often than expected.

STATISTICAL ANALYSIS

A statistical software program (EXACON, Lars R. Bergman and Bassam M. El-Khouri, Department of Psychology, Stockholm University, Stockholm, Sweden)[35] was used to calculate exact probabilities for cell frequencies in the contingency table formed by the 8 predictor profiles and the 4 outcome profiles. Cells of this table contain numbers of subjects with all possible combinations of predictor and outcome profiles. The software program calculates the χ^2 component for each cell and an exact probability that the number of subjects is greater or fewer than would be expected if the predictors were independent of the outcomes. We used a .05 significance level after performing Bonferroni corrections within disruptive and nondisruptive groups. Thus, we identified significant types (predictor-outcome combinations for which there were more subjects than would be expected by chance) and significant antitypes (predictor-outcome combinations for which there were fewer subjects than would be expected by chance). For significant types and antitypes, we calculated odds ratios relative to chance.

RESULTS

Table 2 and the **Figure** summarize the results. Table 2 lists the numbers of subjects observed and expected for each predictor-outcome combination. The significant types and antitypes from the table are shown in the Figure. Predictor profiles appear in the center column of the Figure. Predictor-outcome combinations that are likely (types) appear to the right; predictor-outcome combinations that are unlikely (antitypes) appear to the left. Odds ratios relative to chance are also included in the Figure. They indicate how much greater the odds of a given outcome are for a given predictor group than for the other predictor groups.

PROTECTIVE EFFECT OF INHIBITION FOR DELINQUENCY

We now return to the first of our hypotheses: inhibition will protect against future delinquency, whereas withdrawal will not. Our results suggest that inhibition does act as a protective factor. In the top half of the Figure we see the protective effect of inhibition, but not withdrawal, for disruptive boys. In the Figure, the 2 disruptive profiles that do not include inhibition are significantly linked to outcome profiles that include delinquency; whereas, the 2 disruptive profiles that include inhibition are not linked to outcomes that include delinquency. Disruptive-withdrawn boys are likely to become delinquent-depressed (χ^2=9.7, P<.05). The odds

Table 1. Observed and Expected Numbers of Boys Characterized by Different Predictor and Outcome Profiles

Profile Groups	Observed, No. (%)	Expected, No. (%)
Predictors*		
Disruptive-inhibited-withdrawn	40 (5.1)	20.9 (2.7)
Disruptive-inhibited	25 (3.2)	48.9 (6.3)
Disruptive-withdrawn	43 (5.5)	48.9 (6.3)
Disruptive	125 (16.0)	114.3 (14.7)
Inhibited-withdrawn	93 (12.0)	48.9 (6.3)
Inhibited	75 (9.6)	114.3 (14.7)
Withdrawn	57 (7.3)	114.3 (14.7)
No problems	320 (41.1)	267.4 (34.4)
Outcomes†		
Delinquent	107 (13.8)	145.1 (18.7)
Depressed	117 (15.0)	155.1 (19.9)
Delinquent-depressed	91 (11.7)	52.9 (6.8)
No problems	463 (59.5)	424.9 (54.6)

*Likelihood ratio χ^2=121.5, P<.001.
†Likelihood ratio χ^2=47.0, P<.001.

ratio indicates that they are, in fact, 3.21 (1.59; 6.51) times more at risk than the rest of the sample; thus, withdrawal is not a protective factor. Also, disruptive boys are likely to become delinquent (χ^2=12.8, $P<.05$). Their risk is 2.65 (1.66; 4.24) times that of the rest of the sample. Furthermore, disruptive boys with profiles that do not include inhibition are unlikely to end up in the no problems outcome group. Antitypes to the no problems outcome appear for disruptive (χ^2=2.8, $P<.05$) and disruptive-withdrawn (χ^2=7.2, $P<.05$) boys. The odds of having a no problems outcome are only 0.24 (0.12; 0.48) as great for disruptive-withdrawn boys and 0.57 (0.39; 0.84) as great for disruptive-only boys as for the rest of the sample. In contrast, no antitypes appear for disruptive-inhibited-withdrawn or disruptive-inhibited boys.

One explanation for these findings, however, would be that disruptive-noninhibited boys were actually more disruptive than disruptive-inhibited boys, even though all 4 groups were above the 70th percentile on peer-rated disruptiveness. To address this issue, we compared the 4 disruptive groups on teacher- and mother-rated fighting and hyperactivity taken from mothers' responses to the Social Behavior Questionnaire.[36] Three items pertain to fighting: "fights with other children"; "bullies or intimidates other children"; and "bites, kicks, or hits friends, brothers, or sisters." Two items pertain to hyperactivity: "very restless, always running and jumping" and "squirmy and fidgety." One-way analysis of variance revealed no differences among groups on mother-rated fighting (F=0.84, $P>.05$) or hyperactivity (F=1.6, $P>.05$) or teacher-rated hyperactivity (F=0.63, $P>.05$). The groups did differ on teacher-rated fighting (F=2.6, $P=.05$), but not in a direction that would explain the results. Disruptive-withdrawn boys were highest on teacher-rated fighting but disruptive-only boys were lowest, lower than disruptive-inhibited or disruptive-inhibited-withdrawn boys. Furthermore, Scheffé tests revealed that no 2 groups differed significantly. A protective effect of inhibition then is suggested by the fact that disruptive-inhibited boys, whether they are withdrawn or not, are not likely to become delinquent; whereas, disruptive-noninhibited boys, whether they are withdrawn or not, are likely to become delinquent.

Another way in which a protective effect could be revealed is through antitypes to outcomes involving delinquency. There are 2 possible outcomes that involve delinquency: delinquency alone and delinquency with depressive symptoms. When we examine the antitypes on the left side of the Figure, we find that one predictor profile, the inhibited-only profile, has an antitype to an outcome involving delinquency (χ^2=6.7, $P=.01$). Their risk of becoming delinquent is only 0.16 (0.04; 0.65) that for the overall sample. Even though nondisruptive boys are generally not at high risk for delinquency, inhibition is a protective factor for them just as it is for disruptive boys.

COMORBIDITY OF INHIBITION AND DISRUPTIVENESS

In the studies cited earlier, inhibition combined with disruptiveness sometimes seemed to increase, rather than decrease, the likelihood of later delinquency. However, in those studies inhibition and withdrawal were confounded. What do we find when we distinguish disruptive-inhibited from disruptive-withdrawn boys and compare their outcomes? As reported previously, we find that disruptive-inhibited boys are not at increased risk for any negative outcome; whereas, disruptive-withdrawn boys are at increased risk for comorbid delinquency and depression. Comorbidity of inhibition and aggression or inhibition, withdrawal, and aggression then does not increase the risk of negative outcomes; comorbidity of withdrawal and aggression does increase the risk.

INHIBITION AS A RISK FACTOR FOR DEPRESSIVE SYMPTOMS

Even if inhibition decreases the risk of later delinquency, does it increase the risk of later depressive symptoms? To answer this question, we examine types to the 2 outcomes involving depressive symptoms: depressive symptoms alone and depressive symptoms with delinquency. Only disruptive-withdrawn boys are likely to develop depressive symptoms and their depressive symptoms are combined with delinquency (χ^2=9.7, $P<.05$). As noted previously, their risk of developing this combination is 3.21 (1.59; 6.51) times greater than the other boys' risk. Withdrawal, not inhibition, with comorbid disruptiveness poses a risk for later depressive symptoms with delinquency.

COMMENT

In previous studies, anxiety and shyness have been identified as protective factors in the development of delinquency,[1,6-9] but shyness and social withdrawal have also been identified as risk factors.[6,10-13] Because behavioral inhibition seemed to be part of the operational definitions of the variables that were protective, we hypothesized, and the present results suggest, that behavioral inhibition is the protective factor, whereas social withdrawal is a risk factor.

Table 2. Observed and Expected Numbers of Boys With All Combinations of Predictor and Outcome Profiles

Predictor Profiles	Outcome Profiles* Delinquent	Depressed	Delinquent-Depressed	No Problems	Total† (%)
Disruptive-inhibited-withdrawn					
Observed	7	8	8	17	40 (5.1)
Expected	6	6	5	24	
Disruptive-inhibited					
Observed	3	2	6	14	25 (3.2)
Expected	3	4	3	15	
Disruptive-withdrawn					
Observed	11	8	12	12	43 (5.5)
Expected	6	7	5 (T)‡	26 (A)§	
Disruptive					
Observed	32	19	14	60	125 (16.0)
Expected	17 (T)§	19	15	74 (A)‡	
Inhibited-withdrawn					
Observed	5	18	10	60	93 (11.9)
Expected	13	14	11	55	
Inhibited					
Observed	2	17	5	51	75 (9.6)
Expected	10 (A)§	11	9	45	
Withdrawn					
Observed	2	8	9	38	57 (7.3)
Expected	8	9	7	34	
No problems					
Observed	45	37	27	211	320 (41.1)
Expected	44	48	37	190 (T)†	
Total† (%)	107 (13.8)	117 (15.0)	91 (11.7)	463 (59.5)	778

*T indicates Bonferroni-corrected significant types; A, Bonferroni-corrected antitypes.
†Due to rounding error, some of the rows and columns do not equal the totals.
‡$P<.05$.
§$P<.01$ after Bonferroni corrections.

The developmental literature suggests at least 2 ways in which behavioral inhibition might decrease the risk of delinquency. First, in strange situations, behaviorally inhibited children might be less likely to perform socially deviant acts. In an experimental setting, inhibited 6-year-olds were less likely to cheat when given the opportunity and inhibited 7-year-olds were less likely to use unfair, nonverbal strategies to compete for a scarce resource.[37] The authors of that study proposed that inhibition to the unfamiliar experimenter and setting was responsible for the suppression of deviant behavior. Shy, anxious, inhibited boys then might become behaviorally inhibited in the types of unfamiliar situations in which delinquent behavior usually occurs. Consistent with this hypothesis is evidence that 15-year-olds who became 24-year-old criminals had lower resting heart rates and skin conductance activity than noncriminals.[38] These biological characteristics are opposite of those included in the behaviorally inhibited profile of Kagan et al[13,15] and Garcia-Coll et al.[16]

Another way in which behavioral inhibition might decrease the risk of delinquency is by interfering with exposure to deviant peers. Delinquency is a social phenomenon in that most delinquent acts take place in the company of deviant friends,[39] and associating with deviant peers is one step on the path to delinquency.[40-42] In some studies, associating with deviant peers has seemed to increase the risk of delinquency in and of itself.[41,43] This leads some to believe that mere association causes delinquency,[44] though causality has not been proved. However, if associating with deviant peers is a risk factor, then anything that interferes with a child's ability to form such alliances should be a protective factor. Behavioral inhibition might protect by impeding friendship formation with deviant peers.[40,45,46] By definition, however, socially withdrawn children should associate less with peers also. If lessened exposure to deviant peers was the mechanism, then withdrawn-aggressive and inhibited-

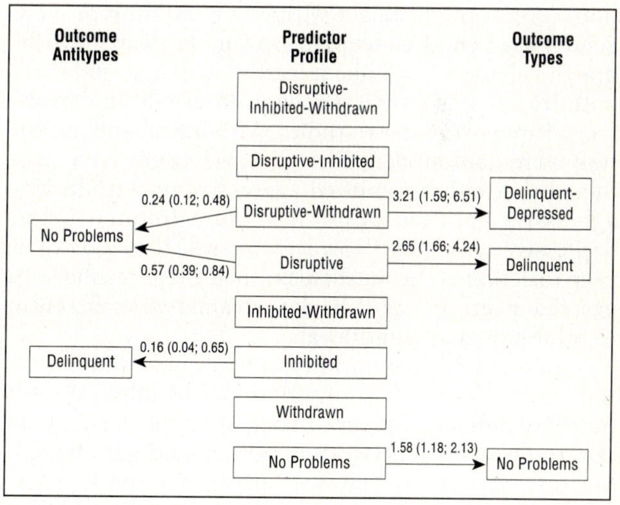

Predictor-outcome combinations that are likely (types) and unlikely (antitypes) along with odds ratios.

aggressive children should have been equally protected from delinquency and they were not. Consequently, these results suggest that behavioral inhibition rather than a lack of social connections with deviant peers is the protective factor. There is one alternative explanation for this effect that might still involve deviant peers, however. The friends that disruptive-inhibited and disruptive-withdrawn boys select might differ in some way that is important to the development of delinquency such as being less aggressive and less likely to model and reward deviant behavior. If so, then the influence of deviant peers might still be an important factor. In a follow-up study (unpublished data, 1996), however, we found that friends of disruptive-inhibited boys are not less aggressive, but they are more anxious and withdrawn. Perhaps disruptive-inhibited boys select friends who are also inhibited and thus similarly protected against delinquency.

In this sample we found no trade-off between protection against delinquency and risk for depression. Inhibited boys were protected against delinquency, but they were not at an increased risk for later depression, which was a reasonable prediction given that anxiety and shyness are often associated with depression or depressed mood.[22-27] Instead, disruptive-withdrawn boys were most at risk for later depression combined with delinquency, 2 outcomes that have been linked before.[47,48] The developmental literature suggests that social withdrawal and disruptiveness might produce later depressive symptoms through the same mechanism: peer rejection. Aggressive children are often rejected by their peers,[49-52] and this might lead to depressive symptoms. Increases in aggression have paralleled increases in depression and the relation was partly mediated by increased peer rejection.[53] Peers might reject withdrawn children as well. School-aged children seem to grow more aware of withdrawn behavior[54] and like it less[18,55] with age, and early withdrawal has predicted later internalizing problems.[56] In most of these studies, withdrawal and inhibition were confounded; therefore, we might have predicted that either inhibited-aggressive or withdrawn-aggressive children would develop delinquency and depressive symptoms. However, because they did not, if peer rejection is the mechanism then these results suggest that peers distinguish between and react differently to inhibition and withdrawal.

In our study, comorbid disruptiveness and inhibition and comorbid disruptiveness and withdrawal were linked to different outcomes, suggesting that it is important to distinguish between inhibition and withdrawal. Serious childhood behavior problems tend to co-occur,[57] as do psychiatric problems in general,[58] and they predict worse outcomes when they co-occur.[3,59] This is more pronounced in clinical samples[60]; however, in a general population sample, children's internalizing and externalizing problems have been shown to correlate positively and increasingly with age (H. Stattin and M.K., unpublished data, 1994). Additionally, youths with both types of problems differ biologically from those with externalizing problems alone.[61] Some have suggested that inhibition loses its protective power when combined with aggression and that inhibited-aggressive children are actually more at risk than noninhibited-aggressive children.[6] We find no support for that suggestion in our data. On the contrary, it was precisely the disruptive-inhibited boys who were protected against delinquency relative to other disruptive boys. In contrast, disruptive-withdrawn boys were at increased risk for future delinquency with depressive symptoms. If we had not distinguished inhibition from withdrawal we would not have discovered these differences.

We argued that withdrawal is comparable with lack of social reward dependence in Cloninger's[19,20] tridimentional theory, whereas behavioral inhibition is comparable with harm avoidance anxiety. Cloninger[20] postulates that specific brain systems, with their associated neuromodulators, underlie these dimensions. Furthermore, these systems interact differently with the system that underlies the third dimension: novelty seeking. Harm avoidance (behavioral inhibition) modulates novelty seeking (hyperactive-aggressive) tendencies, whereas low reward dependence (withdrawal) potentiates hyperactive-aggressive tendencies. This can explain why disruptive-inhibited boys would be protected against delinquency, whereas disruptive-withdrawn boys would not, and why disruptive-withdrawn boys would be more at risk than disruptive-only boys. Furthermore, according to Cloninger,[20] the harm avoidance system also modulates the reward dependence system. This can explain why disruptive-inhibited-withdrawn boys would be protected against delinquency instead of being at increased risk.

One must keep in mind that these results apply to a low socioeconomic status, male, French-speaking, Canadian sample. What is more, 33% of the subjects in the original sample were not included in these analyses because of missing data, and attrition was related to several personality and demographic characteristics. Some of the most at-risk boys in the original sample, that is the most aggressive and least prosocial, were excluded from these analyses. Although this probably had the effect of decreasing variability and weakening the observed effects, we need to see whether these effects can be found in different samples. The developmental literature suggests, however, that the same effects will be found in other samples. Previous studies have found that similar factors underlie adolescent adjustment in different aged samples from different countries.[3] Another possible limitation concerns the self-report delinquency measure. Although such measures have proved valid, in general,[33,34] inhibited boys might conceivably have been more anxious than uninhibited boys to conceal their delinquent acts from the researchers. Although this risk is minimized by the procedure—the measures were collected by questionnaire and the delinquency questions were embedded in a questionnaire about school, hobbies, and relationships with peers and parents—we would welcome a conceptual replication using different measures of delinquency.

To the extent that these results indicate that stronger effects would be observed in the population of males of low socioeconomic status, they should guide the selection of cases for targeted preventive interventions. Disruptive-only and disruptive-withdrawn preadolescent boys should be primary targets for intervention because they are clearly more at risk of seriously deviant behavior in early adolescence. However, these interventions should consider the differences in behavior profiles and the differences in outcomes. Disruptive-only and disruptive-withdrawn boys may need different forms of intervention.

Our study demonstrates the value of using a categorical approach. The outcomes are different for inhibited and withdrawn boys depending on whether they are disruptive. Moreover, among disruptive boys, the outcomes are different for inhibited vs withdrawn boys. If we had considered inhibition, withdrawal, and disruptiveness as linear variables that are equally relevant to everyone, we might not have seen that different combinations of characteristics carry different implications for future experience. However, large samples must be used to make this approach work, and profiles that include variables such as peer, family, and cognitive characteristics are needed to improve prediction. In a person-oriented approach, we still need to be able to explain why some people's outcomes deviate from the general trend.

Accepted for publication October 8, 1996.

This study was supported by grants from the government of Quebec's Conseil Québcois de la Recherche Sociale and Fonds pour la Formation de Chercheurs et l'Aide à la Recherche, Quebec City; the Social Sciences and Humanities Research Council of Canada, Ottawa, Ontario; and the University of Montreal.

We thank Pierre Charlebois, PhD, Claude Gagnon, PhD, Serge Larivée, PhD, and Marc LeBlanc, PhD, for participating in the planning and execution of the longitudinal study; Hélène Beauchesne, MSc, and Lucille David, MSc, for coordinating the data collection; Hélène Boileau, Lyse Desmarais-Gervais, MSc, Diane Héroux, and Maria Rosa for creating the data banks; Pierre McDuff, MSc, for performing the statistical analyses; Mihn T. Trinh, MSc, for providing the documentation; Bernard Boulerice, PhD, for statistical expertise; and Louise LeBlanc for secretarial assistance.

Reprints: Margaret Kerr, PhD, Department of Psychology, Gannon University, 109 University Sq, Erie, PA 16541.

REFERENCES

1. Tremblay RE, Pihl RO, Vitaro F, Dobkin PL. Predicting early onset of male antisocial behavior from preschool behavior. *Arch Gen Psychiatry.* 1994;51:732-738.
2. Farrington DP, Loeber R, Van Kammen WB. The long-term criminal outcomes of conduct problem boys with or without impulsive-inattentive behavior. In: Robins LN, Rutter M, eds. *Straight and Devious Pathways from Childhood to Adulthood.* New York, NY: Cambridge University Press; 1990:62-81.
3. Pulkkinen L, Tremblay RE. Patterns of boys' social adjustment in two cultures and at different ages: a longitudinal perspective. *Int J Behav Dev.* 1992;15:527-553.
4. Farrington DP. Childhood, adolescent, and adult features of violent males. In: Huesmann LR, ed. *Aggressive Behavior: Current Perspectives.* New York, NY: Plenum Publishing Corp; 1994:215-240.
5. Stattin H, Magnusson D. The role of early aggressive behavior in the frequency, seriousness and types of later crime. *J Consult Clin Psychol.* 1989; 57:710-718.
6. Ensminger ME, Kellam SG, Rubin BR. School and family origins of delinquency: comparisons by sex. In: Van Dusen KT, Mednick SA, eds. *Prospective Studies of Crime and Delinquency.* Norwell, Mass: Kluwer Academic Publishers; 1983: 73-97.
7. West DJ, Farrington DP. *Who Becomes Delinquent?* London, England: Heinemann Medical Books Ltd; 1973.
8. Blumstein A, Farrington DP, Moitra S. Delinquency careers: innocents, amateurs, and persisters. *Crime Justice Rev Res.* 1984;6:187-219.
9. Kellam SG, Simon MB, Ensminger ME. Antecedents in first grade of teenage substance use and psychological well-being: a ten-year community-wide prospective study. In: Ricks DF, Dohrenwend BS, eds. *Origins of Psychopathology.* New York, NY: Cambridge University Press; 1983:17-42.
10. Moskowitz DS, Schwartzman AE. Life paths of aggressive and withdrawn children. In: Cantor N, Buss D, eds. *Personality Psychology: Recent Trends and Emerging Directions.* New York, NY: Springer-Verlag NY Inc; 1989:99-114.
11. Serbin LA, Peters PL, McAffer VJ, Schwartzman AE. Childhood aggression and withdrawal as predictors of adolescent pregnancy, early parenthood, and environmental risk for the next generation. *Can J Behav Sci.* 1991;23:318-331.
12. Moskowitz DS, Schwartzman AE. Painting group portraits: studying life outcomes for aggressive and withdrawn children. *J Pers.* 1989;57:723-746.
13. Kagan J, Reznick JS, Snidman N. Biological bases of childhood shyness. *Science.* 1988;240:167-171.
14. Gray JA. Brain systems that mediate both emotion and cognition. *Cogn Emotion.* 1990;4:269-288.
15. Kagan J, Reznick JS, Snidman N. The physiology and psychology of behavioral inhibition in children. *Child Dev.* 1987;58:1459-1473.
16. Garcia-Coll C, Kagan J, Reznick JS. Behavioral inhibition in young children. *Child Dev.* 1984;55:1005-1019.
17. Rosenberg A, Kagan J. Iris pigmentation and behavioral inhibition. *Dev Psychobiol.* 1987;43:377-392.
18. Rubin KH, Mills RSL. The many faces of social isolation in childhood. *J Consult Clin Psychol.* 1988;6:916-924.
19. Cloninger CR. A unified biosocial theory of personality and its role in the development of anxiety states. *Psychiatr Dev.* 1986;3:167-226.
20. Cloninger CR. A systematic method for clinical description and classification of personality variants: a proposal. *Arch Gen Psychiatry.* 1987;44:573-588.
21. Eysenck HJ. The definition and measurement of psychotocism. *Pers Individual Differences.* 1992;13:757-785.
22. Traub GS. Correlations of shyness with depression, anxiety, and academic performance. *Psychol Rep.* 1983;52:849-850.
23. Alfano MS, Joiner TE, Perry M. Attributional style: a mediator of the shyness-depression relationship? *J Res Pers.* 1994;28:287-300.
24. Anderson CA, Arnoult LH. Attributional styles and everyday problems in living: depression, loneliness, and shyness. *Soc Cogn.* 1985;3:16-35.
25. Ishiyama FI. Shyness: anxious social sensitivity and self-isolating tendency. *Adolescence.* 1984;19:903-911.
26. Jones WH, Briggs SR, Smith TG. Shyness: conceptualization and measurement. *J Pers Soc Psychol.* 1986;51:629-639.
27. Stephan E, Fath M, Lamm H. Loneliness as related to various personality and environmental measures: research with the German adaptation of the UCLA Loneliness Scale. *Soc Behav Pers.* 1988;16:169-174.
28. Blishen BR, McRoberts HA. Revised socioeconomic index for occupations in Canada. *Can Rev Soc Anthropol.* 1976;13:71-79.
29. Pekarik EG, Prinz RJ, Liebert DE, Weintraub S, Neale JN. The Pupil Evaluation Inventory: a sociometric technique for assessing children's social behavior. *J Abnorm Child Psychol.* 1976;4:83-97.
30. Kovacs M. The Children's Depression Inventory (CDI). *Psychopharmacol Bull.* 1985;21:995-998.
31. Reynolds WM. Self-report methodology. In: Ollendick TH, Hersen M, eds. *Handbook of Child and Adolescent Assessment.* Boston, Mass: Allyn & Bacon Inc; 1993:98-123.
32. Costello AJ, Angold A. Scales to assess child and adolescent depression: checklists, screens, and nets. *J Am Acad Child Adolesc Psychiatry.* 1988;27:726-737.
33. Klein MW. *Cross-National Research in Self-Reported Crime and Delinquency.* Dordrecht, The Netherlands: Kluwer; 1989.
34. Hindelang MJ, Hirschi T, Weis JG. *Measuring Delinquency.* Beverly Hills, Calif: Sage Publishers Inc; 1981.
35. Bergman L, El-Khouri B. EXACON: a FORTRAN 77 program for the exact analysis of single cells in a contingency table. *Educ Psychol Meas.* 1987;47:155-161.
36. Tremblay RE, Loeber R, Gagnon C, Charlebois P, Larivée S, LeBlanc M. Disruptive boys with stable and unstable high fighting behavior patterns during junior elementary school. *J Abnorm Child Psychol.* 1991;19:285-300.
37. Asendorpf JB, Nunner-Winkler G. Children's moral motive strength and temperamental inhibition reduce their immoral behavior in real moral conflicts. *Child Dev.* 1992;63:1223-1235.
38. Raine A, Venables PH, Williams M. Relationships between central and autonomic measures of arousal at age 15 years and criminality at age 24 years. *Arch Gen Psychiatry.* 1990;47:1003-1007.
39. Gold M. *Delinquent Behavior in an American City.* Pacific Grove, Calif: Brooks/Cole Publishing Co; 1970.

40. Dishion TJ, Patterson GR, Stoolmiller M, Skinner ML. Family, school, and behavioral antecedents to early adolescent involvement with antisocial peers. *Dev Psychol.* 1991;27:172-180.
41. Elliott DS, Huizinga D, Ageton SS. *Explaining Delinquency and Drug Use.* Beverly Hills, Calif: Sage Publishers Inc; 1985.
42. Patterson GR, DeBaryshe BD, Ramsey E. A developmental perspective on antisocial behavior. *Am Psychol.* 1989;44:329-335.
43. Conger RD, Simons RL. Life-course contingencies in the development of adolescent antisocial behavior: a matching law approach. In: Thornberry TP, ed. *Developmental Theories of Crime and Delinquency.* New Brunswick, NJ: Transaction Publishers; 1997:55-99.
44. Hoge RD, Andrews DA, Leschied AW. Tests of three hypotheses regarding the predictors of delinquency. *J Abnorm Child Psychol.* 1994;22:547-559.
45. Boivin M, Vitaro F. The impact of peer relationships on aggression in childhood: inhibition through coercion or promotion through peer support. In: McCord J, ed. *Coercion and Punishment in Long-Term Perspectives.* New York, NY: Cambridge University Press; 1995:183-197.
46. Cairns RB, Cairns BD, Neckerman HJ, Gect SD, Gariépy J-L. Social networks and aggressive behavior: peer support or peer rejection? *Dev Psychol.* 1988;24:815-823.
47. Devine D, Kempton R, Forehand R. Adolescent depressed mood and young adult functioning: a longitudinal study. *J Abnorm Child Psychol.* 1994;22:629-640.
48. Chiles JA, Miller ML. Depression in an adolescent delinquent population. *Arch Gen Psychiatry.* 1980;37:1179-1184.
49. Roff JD. Childhood aggression, peer status, and social class as predictors of delinquency. *Psychol Rep.* 1992;70:31-34.
50. Cantrell VL, Prinz RJ. Multiple predictors of rejected, neglected, and accepted children: relation between sociometric status and behavioral characteristics. *J Consult Clin Psychol.* 1985;53:884-889.
51. Dodge KA, Coie JD, Brakke NP. Behavior patterns of socially rejected and neglected preadolescents: the roles of social approach and aggression. *J Abnorm Child Psychol.* 1982;10:389-410.
52. Roff JD, Wirt RD. Childhood social adjustment, adolescent status, and young adult mental health. *Am J Orthopsychiatry.* 1984;54:595-602.
53. Panak WR, Garber J. Role of aggression, rejection, and attributions in the prediction of depression in children. *Dev Psychopathol.* 1992;4:145-165.
54. Younger A, Boyko KA. Aggression and withdrawal as social schemas underlying children's peer perceptions. *Child Dev.* 1987;58:1094-1100.
55. Younger A, Piccinin AM. Children's recall of aggressive and withdrawn behaviors: recognition memory and likeability judgments. *Child Dev.* 1989;60:580-590.
56. Rubin KH, Hymel S, Mills RSL. Sociability and social withdrawal in childhood: stability and outcomes. *J Pers.* 1989;57:237-255.
57. Zoccolillo M. Co-occurrence of conduct disorder and its adult outcomes with depressive and anxiety disorder: a review. *J Am Acad Child Adolesc Psychiatry.* 1992;31:547-556.
58. Kessler RC, McGonagle KA, Zhao S, Nelson CB, Hughes M, Eshleman S, Wittchen HU, Kendler KS. Lifetime and 12-month prevalence of *DSM-III-R* psychiatric disorders in the United States: results from the National Comorbidity Survey. *Arch Gen Psychiatry.* 1994;51:8-19.
59. Harrington R, Fudge H, Rutter M, Pickles A, Hill J. Adult outcomes of childhood and adolescent depression, II: links with antisocial disorders. *J Am Acad Child Adolesc Psychiatry.* 1991;30:434-439.
60. McConaughy SH, Achenbach TM. Comorbidity of empirically based syndromes in matched general population and clinical samples. *J Child Psychol Psychiatry.* 1994;35:1141-1157.
61. Lahey BB, McBurnett K, Loeber R, Hart EL. Psychobiology of conduct disorder. In: Sholevar GP, ed. *Conduct Disorders in Children and Adolescents.* Washington, DC: American Psychiatric Press; 1995:27-44.

A Global Scale to Measure the Quality of the Family Environment

Joseph M. Rey, MD, FRANZCP; Michelle Singh, MPsychol(Clin); Se-fong Hung, FHKAM(Psychiatry), MRCPsych; David R. Dossetor, MD, MRCPsych; Louise Newman, MD, FRANZCP; Jon M. Plapp, PhD; Kevin D. Bird, PhD

Background: Simple, reliable measures of the quality of the environment in which a child was reared that can be used in clinical research and practice are lacking.

Method: The reliability and validity of a global scale to retrospectively appraise the quality of that environment were examined. Fifty-three clinicians from 4 centers in Australia and 1 in Hong Kong, People's Republic of China, used the scale to rate 7 case vignettes; 4 clinicians rated 20 medical records, and 49 rated 211 subjects after clinical interviews.

Results: Interrater reliability (intraclass correlation coefficient) was 0.82 (time 1) and 0.84 (time 2) for case vignettes, 0.90 for medical records, and 0.89 for clinical interviews. Consistency in time was high (r=0.91). Lower ratings, indicative of a less adequate environment, were associated with a clinical diagnosis of oppositional defiant or conduct disorder.

Conclusions: Our simple-to-use scale appears to measure reliably a relevant clinical construct and fills a gap among the instruments available. Ratings may be useful as a cost-effective index to consider in outcome studies, when examining response to treatment, or in other clinical research.

Arch Gen Psychiatry. 1997;54:817-822

HUMAN DEVELOPMENT and behavior are influenced by the quality of the family environment and interactions to which people are exposed, particularly during infancy and childhood. However, there are no yardsticks available in clinical practice to quantify this construct simply and reliably. A variety of proxies are used to estimate the quality of that environment. The most common is socioeconomic status (SES). More sophisticated studies use measures of psychosocial adversity.[1] In most cases, however, these scales do not capture the range of factors that constitute an adequate family environment. Other measures used include self-reported or interview-based instruments that estimate aspects of family functioning or patterns of relating believed to be clinically relevant.[2-4] Most are complex and time-consuming and produce scores on a variety of dimensions that are frequently collapsed into a summary score and used in analyses.[4]

Global instruments also have disadvantages. Multidimensional scales can measure different aspects of the child's environment that may influence specific facets of development or behavior. However, family processes and life events interact with each other in complex ways that are difficult to disentangle.[5] As Shaffer et al[6] pointed out, global measures can provide a summary statement and allow raters to assimilate and synthesize many aspects of the family's environment and condense it into a single, clinically meaningful index.

We herein report aspects of the reliability and validity of a global measure of the quality of a subject's familial psychosocial environment, the Global Family Environment Scale (GFES). The GFES seeks retrospectively to quantify the adequacy of the environment in which a child is reared. This encompasses the family's ability to provide physical and emotional care, secure attachment relationships, consistency, and appropriate, nonpunitive limits. It is widely accepted that these elements foster adaptive psychological development.

This instrument, like other global measures such as the Global Assessment Scale[7] and Axis V of *DSM-IV*,[8] was designed to be rated by clinicians following a standard assessment interview of a child, adolescent, or young adult or from charts in which adequate developmental and family information is available. It can be completed by

From the Department of Psychological Medicine, University of Sydney (Drs Rey, Dossetor, and Plapp), Rivendell Child, Adolescent and Family Services (Drs Rey and Plapp), Wentworth Area Health Service, Child and Adolescent Mental Health Team (Ms Singh), the Department of Psychological Medicine, Royal Alexandra Hospital for Children (Dr Dossetor); Liverpool Pediatric Mental Health (Dr Newman), and the School of Psychology, University of New South Wales (Dr Bird), Sydney, New South Wales; and the Yaumatei Child Psychiatric Center, Hong Kong, People's Republic of China (Dr Hung).

MATERIALS AND METHODS

THE SCALE

The GFES is a single-score measure with a structure similar to that of Axis V of *DSM-III-R*.[9] The following instructions were given to raters: "Consider family environment on a hypothetical continuum from 1 to 90 depending on the quality of the family environment in which the child was brought up. Give an overall rating of the lowest quality of family environment to which the index child was exposed during a substantial period (at least 1 year) before the age of 12. Use all the range of ratings (eg, 23, 57). Rating should focus on the overall quality of the family environment and not be influenced by the degree of pathology of the child."

Scores of 81 to 90 indicate an adequate family environment that is stable, secure, and nurturing for the child, with consistent care, affection, and discipline and reasonable expectations. Scores of 71 to 80 indicate a slightly unsatisfactory family environment that is mainly stable and secure but contains some conflicts and inconsistencies about discipline or expectations (ie, a parent may be often absent or unavailable because of illness or work; a child may be singled out for special treatment) or changes of residence and school. Scores of 51 to 70 reflect a moderately unsatisfactory environment. Moderate parental discord (which may have resulted in separation or divorce), inadequate or moderate conflict about discipline and expectations, moderately unsatisfactory parental supervision or care, and frequent changes of residence and school may be present. Scores of 31 to 50 reflect poor family environment. Persistent parental discord, hostile separation with problems about custody, exposure to more than 1 step-parent, substantial parental inconsistency or inadequate care, some abuse (by parental figures or siblings) or neglect, poor supervision, and very frequent changes of residence or school may be present. Scores of 11 to 30 indicate a very poor environment, including several usually short-term parental figures (ie, de facto fathers), severe parental conflict, inconsistent or inappropriate care, evidence of substantial abuse (ie, cruel discipline) or neglect, or grave lack of parental supervision may be present. Finally, scores of 1 to 10 reflect a very disturbed family environment, often resulting in the child being made a ward of the state, institutionalized, or placed in foster care more than once. Evidence of severe abuse or neglect or extreme deprivation are present.

Raters were asked to integrate information from all available sources and base ratings as much as possible on positive, objective evidence. Factors to consider were stability of the family background (residence, suburb, school), changes in parental figures, consistency of discipline and expectations, and appropriate care and affection (neither neglect nor overprotection). However, clinicians were free to consider other factors they believed to be important. Having a single-parent or a nontraditional family was not to be rated negatively in the absence of other factors.[5] A substantial period of exposure to the lowest quality environment was operationalized as 1 year. In this study, ratings were arbitrarily based on the first 12 years of life.

CENTERS AND RATERS

To avoid distortions that may result from testing an instrument in a single setting, 4 services from Sydney, New South Wales, and 1 service from Hong Kong, People's Republic of China, were recruited. The main center was a university-affiliated mental health service (Rivendell Child, Adolescent and Family Services, Sydney). The other Sydney centers were the Department of Psychological Medicine of the Royal Alexandra Hospital for Children, university-affiliated Liverpool Pediatric Mental Health service, and Wentworth Area Health Service. The last only provided ratings of case vignettes. These represent the type and range of mental health services for children and adolescents in Australia. To examine whether ratings were influenced by cultural factors, Yaumatei Child Psychiatric Mental Health, Hong Kong, was also involved.

With few exceptions (eg, clinicians who were unable to attend the training sessions), all clinicians working in these agencies participated in the study.

TRAINING

Minimal and standard levels of training were established. Minimal training lasted about 1 hour and consisted of a

practitioners from a variety of backgrounds (eg, psychiatrists, psychologists, social workers).

RESULTS

RELIABILITY

Case Vignettes

Median scores for the 7 case vignettes were 75, 68, 40, 82, 5, 70, and 75. Interrater agreement when clinicians rated the same 7 vignettes was consistently high across centers and times (**Table 1**). Center 2 showed the lowest reliability at time 1 (ICC=0.74). This was due to 1 of the 12 clinicians giving very atypical ratings. When that clinician was excluded from analysis, reliability was higher for times 1 (ICC=0.86) and 2 (ICC=0.88). Clinicians were very consistent in their ratings between times 1 and 2 (r=0.91).

Clinical Interviews

Descriptive information about the type of patients undergoing assessment in the various centers, ratings made by the different professionals, and reliability are presented in **Table 2**. The distribution of ratings was negatively skewed, with a mean of 61.2 (SD=22.6) and a median of 70. Half of the distribution fell outside the range of 50 to 80, indicating that the anchor points produced more variability of ratings than is typically obtained from global scales in clinic settings.[15] Clinicians preferred to give ratings ending with 0 or 5 (ie, 50 or 85), but more than a quarter of the ratings had other endings. There was a clear tail at the top of the distribution, so there was no suggestion of a ceiling effect. Agreement among clinicians was consistently high across centers. By comparison, agreement on PSAI scores was significantly lower.

description of the scale to the group of clinicians and explanation of the rules for making the ratings and the meaning of anchor points, with examples and answers to questions to clarify issues. Considering all aspects of the family environment—lack of affection, neglect, excessive criticism, unreasonable expectations, enmeshment, and overprotection—and not just disruptions of parenting were highlighted. Standard training consisted of this plus the ratings of 3 case vignettes and group discussion of the reasons for the ratings, until these and the meaning of the anchor points were clear to everyone. This group session lasted 2 to 3 hours. The GFES and a training kit are available on request.

RELIABILITY STUDIES

To estimate if raters were consistent in time, 7 case vignettes were prepared. These were based on real patients with potentially identifying data removed or changed. They included a wide range of family environments. Time 1 ratings were performed immediately after the training session, and time 2 ratings were performed 4 to 6 weeks later.

The following 3 aspects of interrater agreement were examined: case vignettes, actual clinical assessments, and medical records. Clinical assessment consisted of the standard diagnostic interview routinely administered at each service to newly referred patients aged 4 to 18 years. At least 2 clinicians needed to be present during the interview (this occurred regularly in the participating services, for training or clinical reasons). Raters were aware of all the information about a patient (eg, from referring agents, school, or previous treatment) but were instructed not to discuss the family environment between themselves before making the ratings. The ratings were completed on a form that described the anchor points and provided instructions for rating.

OTHER MEASURES

Raters involved in the clinical interview were requested to rate independently a Psychosocial Adversity Index (PSAI).[1,10,11] This index was obtained by giving 1 point for the presence of each of the following items: broken home or chronic family disharmony, breadwinner receiving welfare benefits, 4 or more siblings, and parent(s) with a psychiatric disorder or chronic physical illness. Other information collected included SES and clinical diagnosis. Up to 3 *DSM-IV* diagnoses were allowed per case, and these were obtained by consensus between the clinicians performing the assessment. The SES was computed on the basis of the breadwinner's occupation.[12]

STATISTICAL ANALYSIS

Reliability was examined using intraclass correlation coefficients (ICCs). Computation of agreement based on case vignettes and charts assumed that a random sample of clinicians had been selected from a larger population and that each clinician had rated each vignette or file (ICC[2,1]).[13] Agreement on clinical interview cases assumed that a set of raters—typically 2—randomly selected from a larger population judged each case (ICC[1,1]).[13] Because more than 2 clinicians rated a case in some centers, Haggard's[14(p14)] procedure was used to compute the mean number of judges. The consistency of clinicians' ratings at different times was examined by correlating the GFES ratings from the same clinicians at times 1 and 2. This correlation, as well as the correlation between PSAI and GFES scores, was based on the double-entry method[14(p3)] in which each pair of scores is entered twice, the second time in reverse order. The double-entry method ensures that these correlations are commensurate with the ICC indexes of generalizability across raters within occasions and within measures.

When subjects with oppositional defiant or conduct disorder were compared with those with other diagnoses, all the subjects with either of these diagnoses were included in the oppositional conduct group, irrespective of comorbidity. Because each subject was rated by at least 2 clinicians, 2 parallel analyses were performed, 1 for each set of raters (allocation to first or second set was random). Alpha was set at .05 for all analyses.

Ratings Based on Case Files

In a preliminary study (performed before the formal reliability study of the GFES, using an earlier version of the scale), 3 of us (J.M.R., M.S., and S.-f.H.) made ratings based on information in 21 case files. Agreement was good (ICC=0.77). This was repeated using the current version of the GFES, as in the other reliability studies. Four clinicians from center 1 (J.M.R., J.M.P., a research psychologist, and a trainee) rated 20 charts. Agreement between raters was high (ICC=0.90; 95% confidence interval [CI], 0.81-0.95). By comparison, reliability of *DSM-IV* Axis V ratings made at the same time was lower (ICC=0.57; 95% CI, 0.36-0.77).

Training

Interrater agreement on clinical interviews achieved in the center that had received minimal training was lower (ICC=0.84; 95% CI, 0.78-0.89) than among centers that had received standard training (ICC=0.93; 95% CI, 0.90-0.95). The extra training made a small but significant contribution to agreement among raters (CIs did not overlap). This difference was not found when case vignettes were rated.

Cultural Setting

Reliability for the Hong Kong center on ratings based on clinical interviews (ICC=0.95; 95% CI, 0.91-0.97) was not different from that of the Sydney centers (ICC=0.88; 95% CI, 0.84-0.91). The same occurred when rating of case vignettes were made.

CONCURRENT VALIDITY

Correlation between SES[12] and GFES ratings was moderate (r=0.40). Correlations were higher between

Table 1. Interrater Agreement on GFES Scores Based on 7 Case Vignettes*

	Center No.					
	1†‡	2§	3‖	4¶	5#‡	All Centers
No. (%) of raters	**16** (100)	**12** (100)	**9** (100)	**12** (100)	**4** (100)	**53** (100)
Psychiatrists	5 (31)	2 (17)	4 (44)	4 (33)	0	15 (28)
Psychologists	4 (25)	5 (42)	2 (22)	2 (17)	2 (50)	15 (28)
Social workers	2 (12)	3 (25)	2 (22)	2 (17)	1 (25)	10 (19)
Trainees	5 (31)	2 (17)	1 (11)	4 (33)	1 (25)	13 (24)
Time 1						
ICC, *r*	0.87	0.74	0.90	0.80	0.91	0.82
95% CI	...	...	...	...	...	0.65-0.96
Time 2						
ICC, *r*	0.85	0.84	0.93	0.75	0.96	0.84
95% CI	...	...	...	...	...	0.67-0.96
Time 1–time 2, *r***	0.92	0.86	0.96	0.88	0.94	0.91

*GFES indicates Global Family Environment Scale; ICC, intraclass correlation (2, 1)[13]; and CI, confidence interval.
†Rivendell Child, Adolescent and Family Services, Sydney, New South Wales.
‡Indicates minimal training, described in the "Training" subsection of the "Materials and Methods" section of the text.
§Royal Alexandra Hospital for Children, Sydney.
‖Yaumatei Child Psychiatric Center, Hong Kong, People's Republic of China.
¶Liverpool Pediatric Mental Health, Sydney.
#Wentworth Area Health Service, Sydney.
**Double entry method.[14(p3)]

GFES and PSAI scores (Table 2). The overall attenuation-corrected correlation[16] of 0.76 suggests that, if measurement error in both scales was removed, PSAI scores would account for 58% of the variance in GFES scores.

CONSTRUCT VALIDITY

It is widely accepted that oppositional defiant and conduct disorders are common among dysfunctional families and in environments with high levels of chronic adversity.[17] If that were the case and if the GFES actually measured a similar construct, it could be expected that patients in the oppositional conduct group would have lower GFES ratings than those outside. For the first set of raters, GFES scores were lower for subjects with a clinical diagnosis of oppositional conduct disorder (n=63; mean=51.62; SD=23.00) than for those with other diagnoses (n=148; mean=65.70; SD=21.54; t=4.26; df=209; P<.001). Comparable results were obtained for the second set of raters.

Since PSAI scores explained more than half of the variance on GFES ratings, it would appear that the GFES measures a construct similar to chronic adversity. On the other hand, at face value, it seems that the GFES captures a construct that is more accurate or goes beyond what is measured with the PSAI. If so, it could be expected that GFES ratings would be associated with oppositional conduct disorder even after taking into account the association between these disorders and the PSAI. This was tested by performing 2 parallel hierarchical logistic regression analyses (1 for each set of raters). Diagnosis (oppositional conduct vs other) was the dependent variable. The predictor variables were SES (entered at step 1), PSAI (step 2), and GFES scores (step 3). The SES scores did not show an association with diagnosis. The PSAI scores made a significant contribution to the predictability of diagnosis (χ^2=7.65; df=1; P=.006). Adding GFES scores to the model resulted in a further increase in the predictability of diagnosis (χ^2=8.85; df=1; P=.003). Results using the second set of raters were similar.

COMMENT

The GFES ratings made by a variety of mental health professionals working with children and adolescents were reliable across clinic settings and cultures, whether based on a routine assessment interview, case vignettes, or medical records. As expected, lower GFES ratings were associated with a diagnosis of oppositional conduct disorder.

Reliability of GFES ratings is as high as or higher than that reported for other global measures that have been valuable for clinical and research use.[6,7] Reliability of Axis V ratings across several studies in the same center for 10 years have been remarkably consistent (ICC=0.57 at present, and 0.58,[11] 0.54,[15] and 0.66[15] in previous studies).

The reasons for the lower reliability of adversity ratings are uncertain. However, reliability of PSAI scores was consistent with that reported when rating the PSAI from medical records (ICC=0.68).[11] Reliability of the PSAI may have been influenced negatively by lack of experience in its use,[11] the narrow range of scores (0-5), and the fact that adversity scores were positively skewed (almost half of the subjects had a score of 0).

Most clinic subjects, when rated on other global scales, receive scores that typically fall at about the moderate range. For example, in a study using the Global Assessment of Functioning,[15] we found that 59% of the ratings fell within 20 scale points (46-65) and 91% fell within 40 points. This may result in a restriction of range. The GFES was designed so that a larger section was given to the poor and moderately unsatisfactory environments (1-70) and a smaller section to the slightly unsatisfactory and ad-

Table 2. Descriptive Information and Results of Reliability Study Based on Clinical Patient Interviews*

	Center, No.†				
	1‡	2	3	4	All Centers
No. of subjects	117	31	39	24	211
Female, %	44	36	26	8	35
Age, y					
Mean	13	10	9	9	12
SD	2	3	3	3	3
Range	4-18	4-16	4-15	4-15	4-18
SES§					
Mean	4.83	5.03	5.39	6.19	5.15
SD	1.82	1.61	1.52	1.15	1.71
No. (%) of diagnoses‖	**159** (100)	**41** (100)	**40** (100)	**37** (100)	**277** (100)
Disruptive¶	66 (42)	9 (22)	11 (28)	12 (32)	98 (35)
Emotional#	45 (28)	7 (17)	2 (5)	16 (43)	70 (25)
Other	48 (30)	25 (61)	27 (68)	9 (24)	109 (39)
No. of raters	16	10	10	13	49
No. (%) of ratings	**234 (100)**	**65 (100)**	**83 (100)**	**62 (100)**	**444 (100)**
Social workers	75 (32)	1 (2)	12 (14)	6 (10)	94 (21)
Psychologists	66 (28)	19 (29)	24 (29)	15 (24)	124 (28)
Trainees	37 (16)	19 (29)	9 (11)	21 (34)	86 (19)
Psychiatrists	56 (24)	26 (40)	38 (46)	20 (32)	140 (32)
GFES					
Mean	63.12	58.60	69.14	46.21	61.22
SD	20.85	22.60	19.52	25.93	22.62
Range	5-90	8-88	6-90	3-80	3-90
ICC, *r*	0.84	0.92	0.95	0.91	0.89
95% CI	...	...	...	...	0.86-0.92
PSAI					
ICC, *r*	0.69	0.56	0.98	0.87	0.78
95% CI	...	...	...	...	0.71-0.82
Correlation between GFES and PSAI, *r***	0.48	0.64	0.64	0.76	0.62

**SES indicates socioeconomic status; GFES, Global Family Environment Scale; ICC, intraclass correlation (1, 1)[13]; CI, confidence interval; and PSAI, Psychosocial Adversity Index.*
†Described in Table 1. Center 5 was excluded.
‡Indicates minimal training, described in the "Training" subsection of the "Materials and Methods" section of the text.
§Ranges from 1 (highest) to 7 (lowest).[12]
‖There was more than 1 diagnosis per case.
¶Indicates attention-deficit, oppositional, and conduct disorders.
#Indicates anxiety disorders, depression, and dysthymia.
***Double entry method.[14(p3)]*

equate environments (71-90). It was hoped this change would produce a wider spread of ratings and avoid restrictions of range. Results suggest that this was achieved.

Once published, many instruments are used off-the-shelf or with minimal training. Therefore, estimating the influence of training on the reliability of GFES was necessary.[15] Differences in training did not make a large impact on agreement—although it was significant for ratings based on clinical interviews—once raters understood the basis for the ratings and the meaning of the anchor points.

The construct measured by the GFES is related to psychosocial adversity as measured by the PSAI. In fact, PSAI scores explain about half the variance in GFES ratings. However, PSAI ratings are cross-sectional (although some of the situations may be enduring), whereas the GFES takes into account the family environment during the first 12 years of life and rates the worst 12 months. The GFES appears to be a better, more reliable measure than the PSAI.

A full evaluation of the construct measured by the GFES will require more studies. These should include examining the emphasis given by clinicians to the various dimensions, overt and covert, of the family environment. There are preliminary data suggesting that GFES scores are associated with outcome and response to treatment. One hundred forty-five adolescents referred for treatment at a mean age of 14 years were interviewed at a mean age of 20 years to ascertain their functioning and whether they suffered from a personality disorder.[18] There was an association between GFES scores and personality disorder diagnoses after controlling for the effects of gender, family history of psychiatric disorders, drug and alcohol problems, and delinquency (M.S., unpublished data, 1994). Functioning (eg, employment situation, problems with the law, and problems in interpersonal relationships) was examined at follow-up in the same subjects.[19] Those with poor functioning had lower GFES ratings than subjects with good functioning, even after taking into account the effect of family type, discipline problems at school, number of externalizing symptoms between 4 and 12 years of age, and whether they had a personality disorder. Fifty-seven patients with obsessive-compulsive disorder aged 7 to 19 years underwent a combined treatment program (medication and cognitive behavior therapy) and were subsequently followed up for an average of 2 years.[20] Twenty-two subjects maintained treatment gains when medication therapy was ceased. They differed from those who had not been able to tolerate withdrawal from medication without a recurrence of symptoms in that they had a better family environment (higher GFES scores).

These results suggest that the GFES is a measure with some promise. It fills a gap among the instruments currently available to clinicians and researchers, its use is simple, and, more importantly in the current climate, it does not require much training, time, or resources. The GFES appears to be robust across cultures and has predictive value above other family and developmental variables, although this will require further research. The GFES scores may be useful as a cost-effective index to consider in outcome studies, when examining response to treatment or in other clinical research.

Accepted for publication December 11, 1996.

Presented in part as poster exhibit at the 10th World Congress of Psychiatry, Madrid, Spain, August 23-28, 1996.

Our colleagues in the various centers contributed to this work and made it possible but are too many to name individually. We are grateful for their generous help.

Corresponding author: Joseph M. Rey, MD, FRANZCP; Rivendell, Hospital Road, Concord West, New South Wales 2138, Australia.

REFERENCES

1. Biederman J, Milberger S, Faraone SV, Kiely K, Guite J, Ablon S, Warburton R, Reed F. Family-environment risk factors for attention-deficit hyperactivity disorder. *Arch Gen Psychiatry.* 1995,52:464-470.
2. Vaughn CE, Leff JP. The measurement of expressed emotion in the families of psychiatric patients. *Br J Soc Clin Psychol.* 1976;15:157-165.
3. Epstein NB, Baldwin LM, Bishop DS. The McMaster family assessment device. *J Marital Fam Ther.* 1983;9:171-180.
4. Mrazek DA, Mrazek P, Klinnert M. Clinical assessment of parenting. *J Am Acad Child Adolesc Psychiatry.* 1995;34:272-282.
5. Emery RE, Kitzmann KM. The child in the family: disruptions in family functions. In: Cicchetti D, Cohen DJ, eds. *Developmental Psychopathology.* New York, NY: John Wiley & Sons Inc; 1995;2:3-31.
6. Shaffer D, Gould MS, Brasic J, Ambrosini P, Fisher P, Bird H, Aluwahlia S. A Children's Global Assessment Scale (CGAS). *Arch Gen Psychiatry.* 1983;40:1228-1231.
7. Endicott J, Spitzer RL, Fleiss JL, et al. The Global Assessment Scale: a procedure for measuring overall severity of psychiatric disturbance. *Arch Gen Psychiatry.* 1976;33:766-771.
8. American Psychiatric Association. *Diagnostic and Statistical Manual of Mental Disorders, Fourth Edition.* Washington, DC: American Psychiatric Press; 1994.
9. American Psychiatric Association. *Diagnostic and Statistical Manual of Mental Disorders, Third Edition, Revised.* Washington, DC: American Psychiatric Press; 1987.
10. Shaffer D, Chadwick O, Rutter M. Psychiatric outcome of localized head injury in children. In: Porter R, Fitzsimons DW, eds. *Outcome of Severe Damage to the Central Nervous System.* Belle Mead, NJ: Excerpta Medica–Princeton; 1975:191-213. Ciba Foundation Symposium 34.
11. Rey JM, Plapp JM, Stewart G, Richards I, Bashir M. Reliability of the psychosocial axes of *DSM-III* in an adolescent population. *Br J Psychiatry.* 1987;150:228-234.
12. Daniel A. *Power, Privilege and Prestige: Occupations in Australia.* Melbourne, Victoria: Longman Cheshire; 1983.
13. Shrout PE, Fleiss JL. Intraclass correlations: uses in assessing rater reliability. *Psychol Bull.* 1979;86:420-428.
14. Haggard EA. *Intraclass Correlation and the Analysis of Variance.* New York, NY: Dryden Press; 1958.
15. Rey JM, Starling J, Wever BC, Dossetor D, Plapp JM. Reliability of global assessment of functioning in a clinical setting. *J Child Psychol Psychiatry.* 1995; 36:787-792.
16. Nunnally JC. *Psychometric Theory.* New York, NY: McGraw-Hill Book Co; 1978:237.
17. Vitiello B, Jensen PJ. Disruptive behavior disorders. In: Kaplan HI, Sadock BI, eds. *Comprehensive Textbook of Psychiatry.* Baltimore, Md: Williams & Wilkins; 1995;6:2311-2319.
18. Rey JM, Morris-Yates A, Singh M, Andrews G, Stewart GW. Continuities between adolescent disorder and personality disorder in young adults. *Am J Psychiatry.* 1995;152:895-900.
19. Rey JM, Singh M, Morris-Yates A, Andrews G. Referred adolescents as young adults: relationship between psychosocial functioning and personality disorder. *Aust N Z J Psychiatry.* 1997;31:219-226.
20. Wever C, Rey JM. Juvenile obsessive compulsive disorder. *Aust N Z J Psychiatry.* 1997;31:105-113.

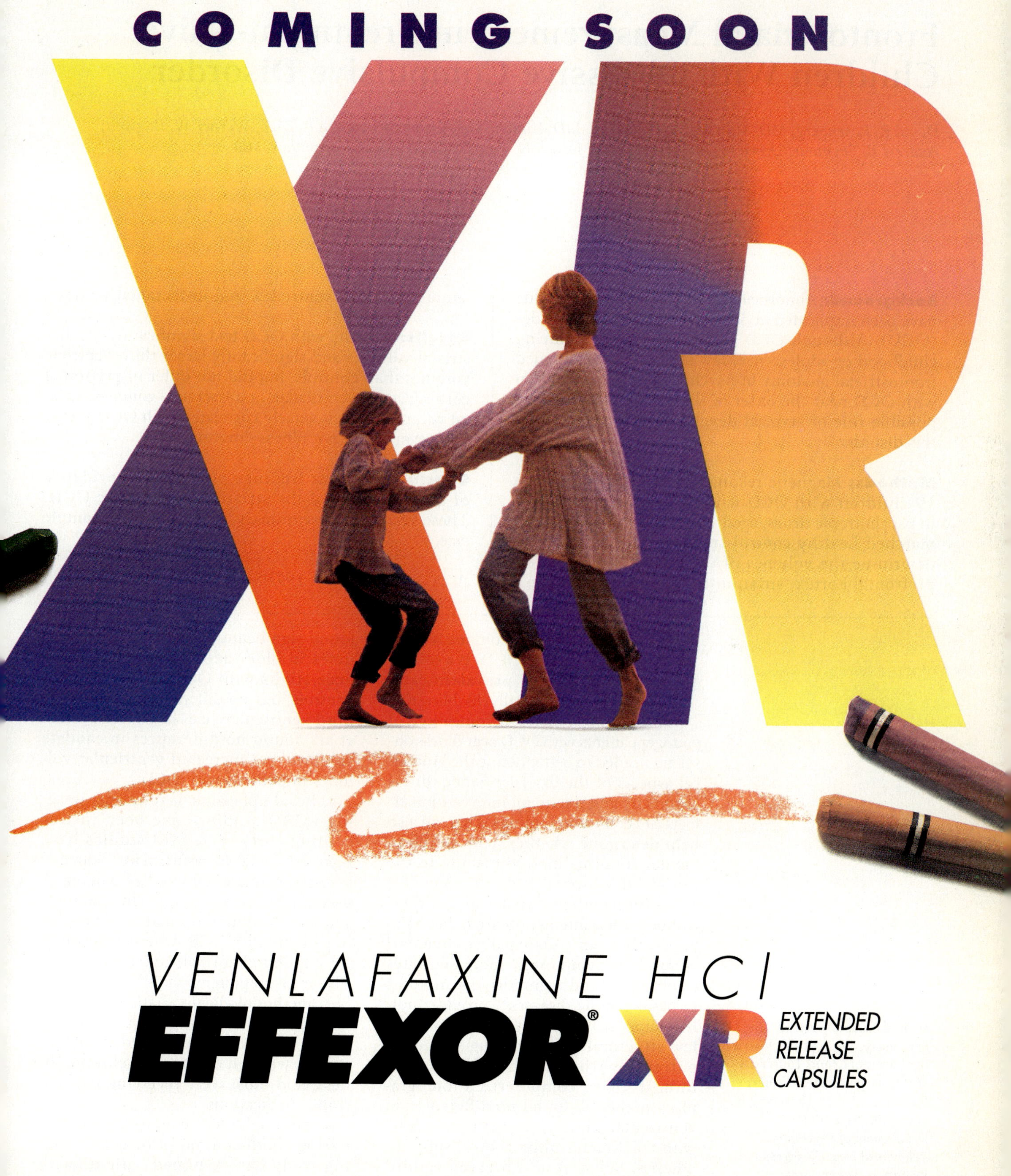
COMING SOON
XR
VENLAFAXINE HCl
EFFEXOR® XR
EXTENDED
RELEASE
CAPSULES
WYETH-AYERST
LABORATORIES
Philadelphia, PA 19101

Frontostriatal Measurement in Treatment-Naive Children With Obsessive-Compulsive Disorder

David R. Rosenberg, MD; Matcheri S. Keshavan, MD; Kirsten M. O'Hearn; Elizabeth L. Dick; Werner W. Bagwell; Andrew B. Seymour; Debra M. Montrose, MSW; Joseph N. Pierri, MS, MD; Boris Birmaher, MD

Background: Abnormalities in frontostriatal circuits have been implicated in obsessive-compulsive disorder (OCD). Although OCD commonly emerges during childhood or adolescence, few studies have examined frontostriatal anatomy in psychotropic-naive children with OCD near the onset of illness to determine the possible role of atypical developmental processes in this disorder.

Methods: Magnetic resonance imaging scans from 19 children with OCD who had not been exposed to psychotropic drugs, aged 7 to 18 years, and 19 case-matched healthy control subjects were analyzed to determine the volumes of the following structures: prefrontal cortex, striatum (caudate and putamen), lateral and third ventricles, and intracranial volume.

Results: Patients with OCD had significantly smaller striatal volumes and significantly larger third ventricle volumes than controls, but did not differ in prefrontal cortical, lateral ventricular, or intracranial volumes. Striatal volumes were inversely correlated with OCD symptom severity but not illness duration.

Conclusions: Our findings provide new evidence of abnormalities of the striatum in pediatric OCD. These results are preliminary, given the small sample size.

Arch Gen Psychiatry. 1997;54:824-830

OBSESSIVE-compulsive disorder (OCD) is a severe, highly prevalent, and chronically disabling disorder.[1-3] Investigations of younger patients with OCD near illness onset are needed to better define the biological aspects of the disorder, since illness chronicity and treatment intervention effects can confound findings. This can also help determine whether neurodevelopmental abnormalities contribute to the cause of the disorder.

Abnormalities in basal ganglia-frontal cortex interaction are believed to be involved in causing obsessive and compulsive symptoms.[4] Increased rates of obsessive and compulsive symptoms in basal ganglia diseases[5,6] provide indirect support for this hypothesis. Only a few structural brain imaging studies in patients with OCD have been performed. Using computerized tomography, Insel et al[7] found no differences in ventricular brain ratio between adults with OCD and healthy control subjects, whereas Behar et al[8] observed significantly greater ventricular brain ratios in adolescents with OCD. Luxenberg et al[9] found significantly smaller caudate volumes in older adolescents and young male adults with OCD compared with controls, but no differences in lateral or third ventricular size. In contrast, Stein et al[10] found no differences in caudate volumes, but increased ventricular volumes in patients with OCD.

Results of magnetic resonance imaging (MRI) studies have been just as contradictory. Five MRI studies have reported caudate measurements; 4 directly assessed caudate volume,[11-14] whereas 1 used the bicaudate ratio.[15] Three of the 5 studies[12,14,15] found normal caudate sizes in patients with OCD, whereas the other 2[11,13] found abnormal caudate volumes. These discrepancies may be related to MRI methodological variations between studies and the heterogeneous nature of OCD.[14] The patients examined in the MRI studies were all adults with chronic illness, and most were receiving psychotropic medications.

Although OCD commonly emerges during childhood, no prior neuroimaging study has examined patients with OCD near illness onset, before exposure to psychotropic medication. Studying

From the Department of Psychiatry, Western Psychiatric Institute and Clinic, University of Pittsburgh Medical Center, Pittsburgh, Pa. Dr Rosenberg is now affiliated with the Department of Psychiatry, Behavioral Neurosciences, and Pediatrics, Wayne State University School of Medicine, Detroit, Mich.

SUBJECTS AND METHODS

SUBJECTS

Twenty-one outpatients with OCD who had not been exposed to psychotropic medication, ranging in age from 7 to 18 years, and 21 healthy control subjects matched pairwise for age, sex, weight, height, and parental socioeconomic status were recruited (**Table 1**). Using parent(s) and the child as informants, the pediatric Schedule for Affective Disorders and Schizophrenia–Present Episode Version and the Schedule for Affective Disorders and Schizophrenia–Epidemiologic Version[23,24] were administered to all patients and controls to determine diagnoses. A board-certified child psychiatrist (D.R.R.) also confirmed the presence of *DSM-III-R*[25] criteria for OCD with the child and family and reviewed all other diagnostic information for each case. Exclusion criteria for patients and controls included lifetime history of psychosis, bipolar disorder, anorexia or bulimia, substance abuse, Sydenham chorea, Tourette syndrome or other tic-related conditions, epilepsy, head injury with sustained loss of consciousness, Huntington disease, dyskinesia, chronic debilitating medical illness, autism, mental retardation, and learning disabilities. No subject had had a major depressive episode within 4 months of MRI scanning. Eight of the 19 patients with OCD had comorbid anxiety disorders, 1 had attention-deficit hyperactivity disorder, 2 had dysthymia, 3 had oppositional or conduct disorders, and 5 had OCD as the sole diagnosis. Controls were free of all psychiatric illness and had no family history of mood disorder in any first-degree relative or mania or schizophrenia in any first- or second-degree relative. No more than 20% of their second-degree relatives had had a major depressive episode. Legal guardians gave written informed consent, and all children gave written assent.

Unless otherwise indicated, data are given as mean±SD.

CLINICAL MEASURES

The children's version of the Yale-Brown Obsessive-Compulsive Scale (CY-BOCS)[26,27] measured OCD symptom severity (for obsessive symptoms, mean score, 11 [SD, 4]; for compulsive symptoms, mean score, 11 [SD, 3]; total mean score, 23 [SD, 6]). All patients with OCD had a total CY-BOCS score of at least 12 and a 17-item Hamilton Depression Rating Scale[28] score of 12 or less (mean score, 6 [SD, 4]). The CY-BOCS score was derived from the first 10 items on the scale. Severity of anxiety was measured by the Hamilton Anxiety Rating Scale[29] (mean score, 9 [SD, 8]).

NEUROPSYCHOLOGICAL SCREENING

A screening neuropsychological examination measured general intelligence,[30] cerebral dominance,[31] manual dexterity,[32] and attention.[33] Patients with OCD had significantly higher left-handedness index scores than controls ($t[18]=2.65$; $P=.02$; 6.9±5.5 vs 10.4±1.2, respectively). Four patients with OCD identified themselves as being left-hand dominant, whereas all controls were right-hand dominant. No significant differences were observed between case-control pairs on the other neuropsychological measures.

MRI ACQUISITION

Magnetic resonance imaging was performed using a 1.5-T unit (Signa System, General Electric Medical Systems, Milwaukee, Wis) running version 5.4 software at the University of Pittsburgh's Magnetic Resonance Center, Pittsburgh, Pa. A sagittal scout series verified patient position, cooperation, and image quality and clarity. A 3-dimensional, spoiled-gradient recalled acquisition in the steady state pulse sequence was used to obtain 120 1.5-mm thick contiguous coronal images through the entire brain. Parameters were repetition time of 25 milliseconds; echo time, 5 milliseconds; acquisition matrix, 256×256; number of excitations, 1; field of view, 24 cm; and flip angle, 10°. Coronal sections were obtained perpendicular to the anterior-commissure–posterior-commissure line to provide a more reproducible guide for image orientation. Axial proton density and T_2-weighted images were obtained to enable exclusion of structural abnormalities on MRI. A neuroradiologist reviewed all scans to rule out clinically significant abnormalities. Subjects whose MRI scans on visual inspection showed artifacts due to movement and magnetic field inhomogeneities (n=2) were excluded. Thus, 19 case-control pairs underwent analysis.

IMAGE ANALYSIS

The imaging data were transferred from the MRI unit to a computer workstation (Macintosh, Apple Computer, Cupertino, Calif), and the data were analyzed using the IMAGE software (version 1.45) developed at the National Institute of Health,[34] which provides valid and reliable volume measurements of specific structures using a semiautomated segmentation approach.[35,36] All measurements were made by several of us who were trained and reliable raters (A.B.S., W.W.B., and K.M.O.) and unaware of identifying subject information.

NEUROANATOMIC MEASUREMENTS

The boundaries of the structures of interest were determined by reference to standard neuroanatomical atlases,[37,38] and definitions (available on request) were adapted from previously published psychiatric neuroimaging studies.[39-42]

Intracranial Volume

This was calculated by summing up areas of successive coronal slices, including gray and white matter and cerebrospinal fluid (CSF) volumes, and multiplying by slice thickness. All of the frontal, parietal, temporal, and occipital cortex were included. Separate measurements were obtained for gray and white matter volumes and total volume measurement. The cerebellum and brainstem were not included. These areas were traced manually to exclude their volume.

Continued on next page

Prefrontal Cortex

Separate measurements were obtained for gray matter, white matter, and total volume. The anterior boundary of the prefrontal cortex was defined as the most anterior coronal section containing gray matter (frontal pole). The most posterior coronal slice showing the genu of the corpus callosum was used to mark the posterior limit of the prefrontal cortex. Measurements were made on coronal slices, and the gray, white, and total prefrontal cortical volumes were computed by measuring areas of successive slices anterior to the genu up to the frontal poles.

Striatum (Caudate and Putamen)

Separate measurements were obtained for the left and right caudate nuclei using a manual tracing technique. The head and body of the caudate were measured, whereas the tail was excluded. The caudate nucleus was delineated medially by the lateral ventricle and was separated from the globus pallidus and putamen by white matter tracts. Superiorly, the caudate was delineated by white matter; inferiorly, it merged with the nucleus accumbens and putamen. All regions were measured in the coronal plane (**Figure 1**).

Separate measurements were obtained for the left and right putamen. The lenticular complex consists of the putamen and the globus pallidus. The putamen was delineated medially by the globus pallidus and laterally by white matter tracts. Measurements of the putamen were performed in the coronal plane.

Lateral Ventricle Volume

The lateral ventricles were measured simultaneously for both hemispheres. Each image was segmented into the brain and CSF compartments. The areas containing pixels of defined signal intensity (corresponding to CSF) were measured in coronal slices. These were summed up and multiplied by the slice thickness. Separate measurements were obtained for left and right lateral ventricles.

Third Ventricle Volume

The third ventricle was delineated laterally by the thalami and posteriorly by the pinae. It was measured in all coronal slices anterior to the cerebral aqueduct, up to and including the suprachiasmatic recess. The appearance of the anterior commissure defined the anterior boundary of the third ventricle. The infundibular, suprapineal, and posterior commissural recesses of the third ventricle were included in the measurements.

All regions were measured with coronal scans in the 3-dimensional, spoiled-gradient recalled acquisition in the steady state using a semiautomated segmentation algorithm. This computerized technique uses mathematically derived cutoffs for gray matter–white matter–CSF partitions derived with histograms of signal intensities; this method has been validated with a point-counting stereological method using the theorem of systematic sampling developed by Cavalieri[43] that is used extensively in biomedical research.[44-46] High correlations were observed between both techniques (r=0.96), and phantom studies showed excellent validity and sensitivity for both techniques.[37] Intraclass correlations of interrater reliability for the independent designation of regions on segmented images obtained from 12 subjects were 0.99 for intracranial volume (by K.M.O. and W.W.B.); from 16 subjects, 0.90 and 0.93 for the right and left striata (caudate and putamen), respectively (by A.B.S. and W.W.B.); from 16 subjects, 0.95 and 0.97 for the right and left caudate, respectively; from 16 subjects, 0.85 and 0.88 for the left and right putamen, respectively; from 25 subjects, 0.99 for prefrontal cortical white and gray matter and total prefrontal cortical volume (by A.B.S. and W.W.B.); and from 20 subjects, 0.99 for the right and left lateral ventricles and 0.97 for the third ventricle (by A.B.S. and K.M.O.).

DATA ANALYSIS

Because of the wide age range and significant difference in handedness index scores[31] between patients with OCD and controls, regional morphometric volumes (caudate, putamen, prefrontal cortex, and lateral and third ventricles) were analyzed using analyses of covariance (ANCOVAs) test for differences between case-control pairs. An ANCOVA with handedness score as a covariate was used to compare case-control intracranial volumes. Correlations of intracranial volume and regional morphometric volumes with age and clinical and neuropsychological inventories were also performed using Pearson, partial, and Spearman correlations. Bonferroni corrections were used to control for multiple correlates. Two-way (sex by diagnostic group) analyses of variance (ANOVAs) were performed in view of some previous studies suggesting gender-specific abnormalities in OCD.[9,47,48] Two-tailed significance tests are reported throughout.

As some neuroimaging[13,49,50] and neuropsychological studies[10] have reported significant laterality effects in OCD, we examined for differences in left and right structural volumes using repeated measures ANOVAs in which the main effects of laterality (left vs right) and the interaction of laterality with group were tested. There were no significant differences in laterality interaction effects, so left and right volumes were pooled for comparison purposes (**Table 2**).

To evaluate the sample size required to test our hypotheses, we computed effect sizes for some key measures. Data from a previous investigation[9] indicated a high effect size (d=1.35) for abnormalities in striatal anatomy in adolescents and young adults with OCD. Given the rigorous inclusion-exclusion criteria that precluded recruitment of a larger sample and the high effect size, we chose to cautiously report our preliminary results on this relatively small sample.

this population avoids potential confounds of illness progression and active medications in the central nervous system.[16,17] The prefrontal cortex, a primary site of metabolic abnormality in OCD,[18] sends prominent efferent projections to its striatal target fields and undergoes substantial developmental changes during adolescence.[19,20] Therefore, we performed a morphometric MRI study in children with OCD, focusing on selected brain regions within or adjacent to prefrontal-striatal circuits.

Table 1. Demographic and Clinical Data From Nondepressed Children With OCD and Case-Matched Normal Control Subjects*

	Patients (n=19)	Normal Controls (n=19)	t†	P
Age, y	12±3 (7-18)	12±3 (7-19)	1.52	.15
Sex, No. of subjects				
Male	13	13	...	...
Female	6	6	...	...
Weight, kg	45.7±16.0 (21.6-76.5)	50.4±18.8 (24.3-85.5)	1.01	.33
Height, cm	148.5±21.0 (107.5-172.5)	148.8±19.8 (120.0-177.5)	0.09	.93
Parental SES‡	1.9±0.70 (1-4)	1.9±0.52 (1-3)	0.32	.75
Age at onset of first clinical presentation,§ y	10±3 (5-17)	...	...	...
Duration of illness, y	2.7±2.0 (0.25-6.6)	...	...	...

Patients had not been exposed to psychotropic drugs. Data are given as mean±SD (range), unless indicated otherwise. OCD indicates obsessive-compulsive disorder.

†*Paired t statistic.*

‡*Parental SES indicates parental socioeconomic status, measured by assessment of parental education level and highest level of occupational functioning of the parents on a scale of 1 to 5, with 1 indicating highest parental SES and 5 indicating lowest parental SES.[21]*

§*Onset of OCD symptoms is based on extensive developmental data obtained from all families. One child's parents reported that their child started hoarding items excessively at 6 months of age and would become uncontrollably upset when the hoarded items were taken away. We recognize the inherent problems in defining the age at onset of the illness at such an early stage of development, given the retrospective nature of the assessment. Nonetheless, the parents were fairly insistent that this was when they first noted the condition and from that point on, 1 obsessive-compulsive ritual led to another. Childhood onset of OCD has been documented in the literature as early as 2 years of age.[22]*

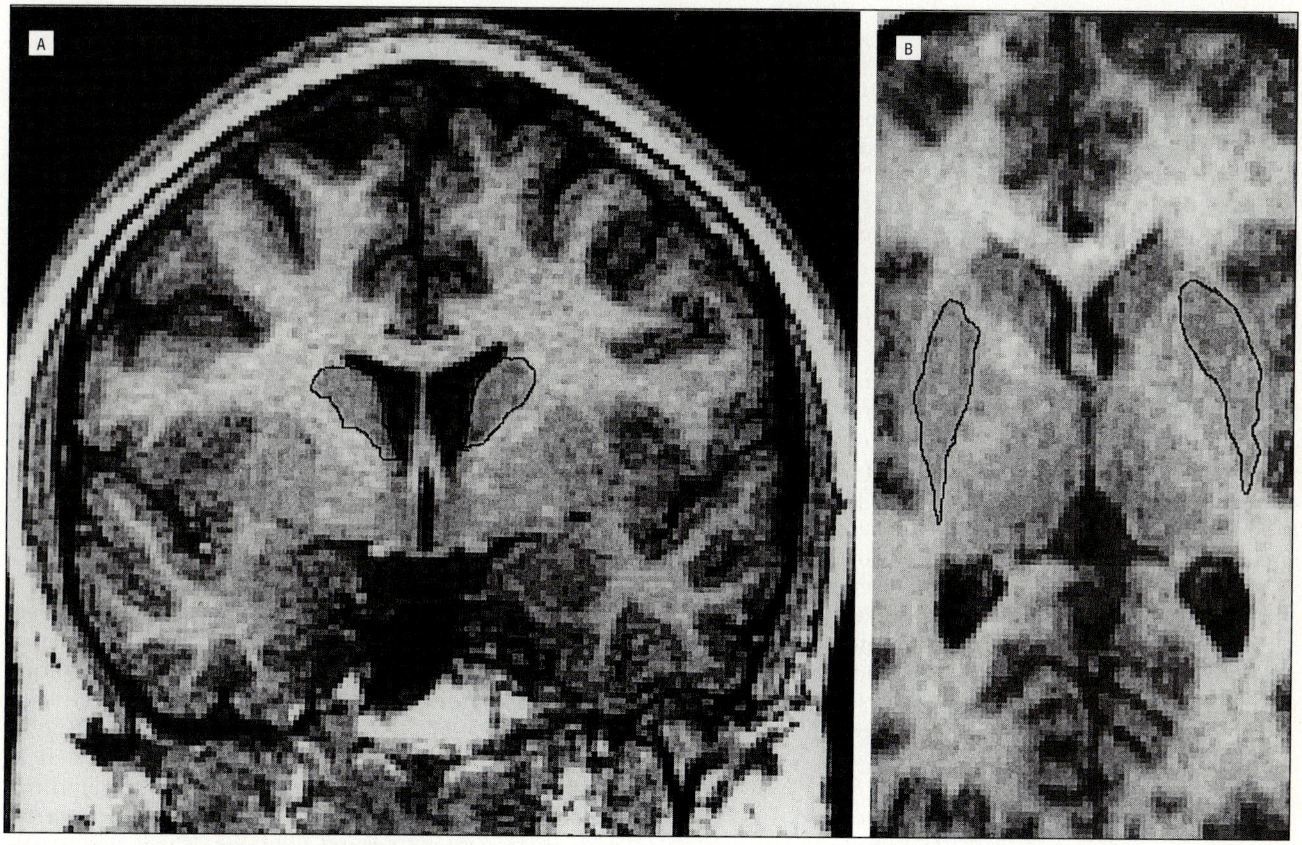

Figure 1. *Measurement of the striatum, caudate nucleus (A), and putamen (B) in the coronal plane using a manual tracing technique.*

RESULTS

VOLUMETRIC COMPARISONS BETWEEN PATIENTS WITH OCD AND CONTROLS

Patients with OCD had significantly smaller striatal volumes than controls (F[1,33]=9.33; *P*=.004) (Figure 1 and **Figure 2**). When we looked at the subcomponents of the striatum, significantly smaller putamen volumes were observed in patients with OCD than controls (F[1,33]=9.13; *P*=.005; 7.05±0.70 cm^3 vs 7.72±0.76 cm^3, respectively), whereas case-control pairs did not differ significantly in caudate volumes (F[1,33]=1.38; *P*=.25; 7.51±0.96 cm^3 vs 7.95±0.88 cm^3, respectively). Significantly larger third ventricle volumes were observed in patients with OCD than controls (F[1,33]=5.27; *P*=.03). Patients and controls did not differ significantly in prefrontal cortical gray matter (F[1,33]=0.30; *P*=.59), white

Table 2. Volumetric Results for Patients With OCD and Normal Control Subjects*

Region	Volume, cm³ Patients (n=19)	Volume, cm³ Controls (n=19)	95% Confidence Interval of Difference Between Groups
Intracranial volume	1199.20±113.94	1228.72±111.23	−107.70 to 48.66
Prefrontal cortical gray matter	18.28±2.29	19.37±2.34	−2.82 to 0.64
Prefrontal cortical white matter	8.00±1.67	8.37±1.64	−1.43 to 0.71
Total prefrontal cortex	26.28±3.24	27.73±3.40	−3.87 to 0.97
Striata	14.57±1.16	15.67±1.31	−2.01 to −0.21†
Left	7.20±0.61	7.82±0.69	−1.07 to −0.16‡
Right	7.37±0.63	7.86±0.67	−0.97 to −0.02§
Lateral ventricles	7.83±6.78	5.66±5.15	−6.69 to 2.36
Left	3.97±3.70	2.84±2.69	−3.56 to 1.32
Right	3.86±3.16	2.82±2.54	−1.09 to 3.17
Third ventricle	1.18±0.48	0.96±0.24	−0.05 to 0.48‖

**Data are given as mean±SD. OCD indicates obsessive-compulsive disorder.*
†*P=.004.*
‡*P=.007.*
§*P=.008.*
‖*P=.03.*

matter (F[1,33]=0.02; *P*=.90), total (F[1,33]=0.16; *P*=.69), lateral ventricular (F[1,33]=0.48; *P*=.49), or intracranial volume (F[1,34]=0.01; *P*=.91). Comparison of the 15 right-hand-dominant–case-control pairs also yielded significantly decreased total striatal (F[1,25]=6.92; *P*=.01) and putamen volumes (F[1,25]=7.66; *P*=.01) and increased third ventricular volumes (F[1,25]=4.49; *P*=.04). No significant differences were observed in other regional structural volumes.

CLINICAL CORRELATIONS

Significant inverse correlations were observed in patients with OCD between striatal volumes and severity of OCD symptoms as measured by the composite obsessive and compulsive scores on the CY-BOCS (partial *r*=−0.53; *P*=.02), and the obsessive (partial *r*=0.65; *P*=.004) but not compulsive CY-BOCS subscales. The inverse correlation between obsessive scores and striatal volumes persisted after Bonferroni correction, although the inverse correlation with the composite obsessive and compulsive score did not. Striatal volumes were not significantly correlated with illness duration, age at onset of illness, clinical ratings of depression or anxiety, parental socioeconomic status, or behavioral handedness scores.

GENDER

Comparable ages were observed in male (12.4±3.2) and female patients with OCD (12.4±3.5). Age at onset of illness did not differ between male and female patients (*t*[9.44]=0.70; *P*=.50; 7.4±5.0 years vs 9.3±5.2 years, respectively). There were no gender-related differences between patients in any of the structural volumes.

COMMENT

To our knowledge, this is the first neuroimaging study of children with OCD who had not been exposed to psychotropic medication to demonstrate reduced striatal volumes and increased third ventricular volumes. Our results support the hypothesis that abnormalities in striatal anatomy may be associated with the clinical presentation of OCD, and that this pathological involvement may be a central neurobiological deficit in this illness. Children with OCD had larger third ventricular volumes than controls. This is consistent with their reduced striatal volumes. There was a significant inverse correlation between striatal and third ventricle volumes in patients with OCD (partial *r*=−0.50; *P*=.03) but not controls. Depression, generalized anxiety, duration of illness, and age at onset of illness did not appear to have an impact on our findings, since there was no correlation between these measures and regional morphometric volumes.

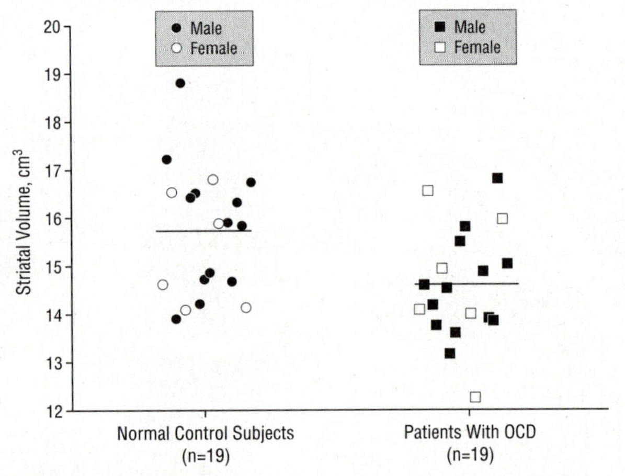

Figure 2. *Striatal volume by group. OCD indicates obsessive-compulsive disorder. Lines indicate means.*

Although the most widely accepted neurobiological model of OCD posits abnormalities in basal ganglia-frontal cortex interaction, not all structural neuroimaging studies have identified abnormalities in these brain regions. Different study methods and small sample sizes could in part account for these conflicting findings.[11]

Variability in the number of patients receiving medication in each study, the psychotropic medications used, how long patients had been treated, and comorbidity also may account for discrepant findings.[16,17,51] This underscores the importance of standardizing research protocols in patients with OCD and eliminating and/or controlling for potential confounds such as illness progression, comorbidity, and medication.

To our knowledge, our study is the first to report reduced putamen volumes in patients with OCD. The relation between abnormalities of the putamen and OCD is supported by several lines of observations. Putaminal lesions have been known to be associated with OCD symptoms.[52,53] Giedd et al[54] found that patients with Sydenham chorea and OCD symptoms had significantly greater putamen volumes than controls. Using fluorescent serum antibody determinations, Kiessling et al[55] found that children with OCD showed antibodies directed against the putamen at a rate significantly higher than that of controls.

We also observed significant inverse correlations in patients with OCD between putamen volumes and severity of obsessive but not compulsive symptoms. The caudate nucleus has typically been more implicated as being involved in complex cognitive functions, while the putamen has been thought to subserve primarily motor functions.[56,57] Thus, it is curious that putamen but not caudate volumes were reduced in patients with OCD and correlated significantly with obsessions but not compulsions. However, in a recent meta-analysis of the functional imaging literature in OCD, Aylward et al[14] found similar caudate function between patients with OCD and controls after normalizing for global metabolism. Specifically, caudate abnormalities disappeared when global metabolic values were taken into account. In our study, we covaried for total brain volume, which may eliminate differences observed when brain volume is not used as a covariate. Our methods, however, may not have been sensitive enough to detect subtle but potentially significant case-control differences in caudate volumes. The reduction in striatal volume in our patients with OCD was approximately 7%.

The reduced putamen volume in OCD may be a result of the putamen's receiving more projections from the amygdala than the caudate does. Lesions of the temporal lobe result in reduction of putamen volumes, whereas damage to the frontal lobes results in reduction of caudate volumes.[58] Therefore, we examined the relationship between putamen and amygdala volumes and observed a significant positive correlation in patients with OCD between putamen and amygdala volumes ($r=0.56$; $P=.03$) but not between amygdala and caudate volumes. Conversely, we observed significant positive correlations between caudate and prefrontal cortical volumes ($r=0.52$; $P=.05$[8]) but not between putamen and prefrontal cortical volumes. The full details of this temporal lobe structure and others will be presented elsewhere. Further study of larger samples and replication of our results are required before more definitive conclusions can be drawn.

Functional neuroimaging studies repeatedly have demonstrated increased metabolic rates in the prefrontal cortex of patients with OCD.[50] These abnormalities have been primarily localized to ventral prefrontal circuits, with no abnormalities observed in dorsal prefrontal regions. Our measurement of total prefrontal cortex may not have been sensitive enough to reliably detect more subtle localized volumetric differences. Alternatively, neurobehavioral probes that selectively activate the system during functional neuroimaging studies may be superior to resting state studies.[49,59,60]

Our results are consistent with evidence from other studies suggesting striatal abnormalities in OCD. Future volumetric MRI studies are needed to examine subdivisions of prefrontal cortex (ie, ventral and dorsal prefrontal cortex), other basal ganglia and temporal lobe structures, and the thalamus, which has also been implicated in the function of OCD.[61]

Accepted for publication October 8, 1996.

This study was supported by grants MH-01180 (Dr Keshavan) and MH-01372 (Dr Rosenberg) from the National Institute of Mental Health, Rockville, Md, and the National Obsessive Compulsive Foundation, Milford, Conn, and a grant from the Scottish Rite Foundation, Lexington, Mass (Dr Keshavan).

We thank Neal Ryan, MD, who referred us his carefully ascertained healthy young children, which allowed for pairwise case-control matching; Denise Davis, RN, and Patricia Erb, RN, for their assistance with MRI data acquisition; and David Kupfer, MD, David Lewis, MD, Ranga Krishnan, MD, Delbert Robinson, MD, Jay Giedd, MD, Jay Pettegrew, MD, Jeffrey Lowengrub, MD, Robert Moore, MD, PhD, and Jean Miewald for their consultation on these data.

Reprints: David R. Rosenberg, MD, Wayne State University School of Medicine, Psychiatry 9B, 4201 St Antoine Blvd, Detroit, MI 48201 (e-mail: Drosen@med.wayne.edu).

REFERENCES

1. Valleni-Basile LA, Garrison CZ, Jackson KL, Waller JL, McKeown RE, Addy CL, Cuffe SP. Frequency of obsessive-compulsive disorder in a community sample of young adolescents. *J Am Acad Child Adolesc Psychiatry.* 1994;33:782-791.
2. Hanna GL. Demographic and clinical features of obsessive-compulsive disorder in children and adolescents. *J Am Acad Child Adolesc Psychiatry.* 1995;34:19-27.
3. Flament MF, Whitaker A, Rapoport JL, Davis M, Berg CZ, Kalikow K, Sceery W, Schaffer D. Obsessive-compulsive disorder in adolescence: an epidemiological study. *J Am Acad Child Adolesc Psychiatry.* 1988;27:764-771.
4. Insel TR. Toward a neuroanatomy of obsessive-compulsive disorder. *Arch Gen Psychiatry.* 1992;49:739-744.
5. Pitman RE, Green RC, Jenike MA, Mesulam MM. Clinical comparison of Tourette's disorder and obsessive-compulsive disorder. *Am J Psychiatry.* 1987;144:1166-1171.
6. Swedo SE, Rapoport JL, Cheslow DL, Leonard H, Ayoub EM, Hosier DM, Wald ER. High prevalence of obsessive-compulsive symptoms in patients with Sydenham's chorea. *Am J Psychiatry.* 1989;146:246-249.
7. Insel TR, Donnelly EF, Lalakea ML, Alterman IS, Murphy DL. Neurological and neuropsychological studies of patients with obsessive-compulsive disorder. *Biol Psychiatry.* 1983;18:741-751.
8. Behar D, Rapoport JL, Berg CJ, Denckia MB, Mann L, Cox C, Fedio P, Zahn T, Wolfman MG. Computerized tomography and neuropsychological test measures in adolescents with obsessive-compulsive disorder. *Am J Psychiatry.* 1984;141:363-369.
9. Luxenberg JS, Swedo SE, Flament MF, Friedland RP, Rapoport J, Rapoport SI. Neuroanatomical abnormalities in obsessive-compulsive disorder determined with

quantitative x-ray computed tomography. *Am J Psychiatry.* 1988;145:1089-1093.

10. Stein DJ, Hollander E, Chan S, DeCaria CM, Hilal S, Liebowitz MR, Klien DF. Computed tomography and neurological soft signs in obsessive-compulsive disorder. *Psychiatry Res.* 1993;50:143-150.
11. Robinson D, Wu H, Munne RA, Ashtari M, Alvir JM, Lerner G, Koreen A, Cole K, Bogerts B. Reduced caudate nucleus volume in obsessive-compulsive disorder. *Arch Gen Psychiatry.* 1995;52:393-398.
12. Kellner CH, Jolley RR, Holgate RC, Austin L, Lydiard RB, Laraia M, Ballenger JC. Brain MRI in obsessive-compulsive disorder. *Psychiatry Res.* 1991;36:45-49.
13. Scarone S, Colombo C, Livian S, Abbruzzese M, Ronchi P, Locatelli M, Scotti G. Increased right caudate nucleus size in obsessive-compulsive disorder: detection with magnetic resonance imaging. *Psychiatry Res.* 1992;45:115-121.
14. Aylward EH, Harris GJ, Hoehn-Saric R, Barta PE, Machlin SR, Pearlson GD. Normal caudate nucleus in obsessive-compulsive disorder assessed by quantitative neuroimaging. *Arch Gen Psychiatry.* 1996;53:577-584.
15. Aylward EH, Schwartz J, Machlin S, Pearlson G. Bicaudate ratio as a measure of caudate volume on MR images. *Am J Neuroradiol.* 1991;12:1217-1222.
16. Keshavan MS, Bagwell WW, Haas GL, Sweeney JA, Schooler N, Pettegrew JW. Changes in caudate volume with neuroleptic treatment. *Lancet.* 1994;344:1434.
17. Chakos MH, Lieberman JA, Bilder RM. Increase in caudate nuclei volumes of first-episode schizophrenic patients taking antipsychotic drugs. *Am J Psychiatry.* 1994;151:1430-1436.
18. Swedo SE, Schapiro MB, Grady CL, Cheslow DL, Leonard HL, Kumar A, Friedland R, Rapoport S, Rapoport JL. Cerebral glucose metabolism in childhood-onset obsessive-compulsive disorder. *Arch Gen Psychiatry.* 1989;46:518-523.
19. Huttenlocher PR. Synaptic density in human frontal cortex: developmental changes and effects of aging. *Brain Res.* 1979;163:195-205.
20. Jernigan TL, Tallal P. Late childhood changes in brain morphology observable with MRI. *Dev Med Child Neurol.* 1990;32:379-385.
21. Hollingshead AB. *Four Factor Index of Social Status.* Available in: New Haven, Conn: Yale University Department of Sociology; 1978.
22. Rapoport JL, Swedo SE, Leonard HL. Childhood obsessive-compulsive disorder. *J Clin Psychiatry.* 1992;53:11-16.
23. Chambers WJ, Puig-Antich J, Hirsch M. The assessment of affective disorders in children and adolescents by semi-structured interview: test-retest reliability of the Schedule for Affective Disorders and Schizophrenia for School-age Children–Present Episode Version. *Arch Gen Psychiatry.* 1985;42:696-702.
24. Orvaschel H, Puig-Antich J, Chambers W, Tabrizi MA, Johnson R. Retrospective assessment of prepubertal major depression with the Kiddie-SADS-E. *J Am Acad Child Adolesc Psychiatry.* 1982;21:392-397.
25. American Psychiatric Association. *Diagnostic and Statistical Manual of Mental Disorders, Third Edition, Revised.* Washington, DC: American Psychiatric Association; 1987.
26. Goodman WK, Price LH, Rasmussen SA, Mazure C, Fleischmann RL, Hill CL, Heninger GR, Charney DS. Thc Yale-Brown Obsessive Compulsive Scale, I: development, use, and reliability. *Arch Gen Psychiatry.* 1989;46:1006-1011.
27. Wolff RP, Wolff LS. Assessment and treatment of obsessive-compulsive disorder in children. *Behav Modif.* 1991;15:372-393.
28. Hamilton M. Development of a rating scale for primary depressive illness. *Br J Soc Clin Psychol.* 1967;6:278-296.
29. Hamilton M. The assessment of anxiety states by rating. *Br J Med Psychol.* 1959;32:50-55.
30. Ammons RB, Ammons CH. *Ammons Quick IQ Test.* New York, NY: Psychological Test Specialists; 1962.
31. Annett M. The binomial distribution of right, mixed and left handedness. *Q J Exp Psychol.* 1967;19:327-333.
32. Knights RM, Norwood J. *Revised Smoothed Normative Data on the Neuropsychological Test Battery for Children.* Ottawa, Ontario: Carleton University; 1980.
33. Wechsler D. *Wechsler Intelligence Scale for Children.* New York, NY: Psychological Corporation; 1991.
34. Rasband W. *NIH IMAGE Manual.* Bethesda, Md: National Institutes of Health; 1996.
35. Keshavan MS, Beckwith C, Bagwell W, Pettegrew JW, Krishnan KRR. An objective method for edge detection in MRI morphometry. *Eur Psychiatry.* 1994;9:205-207.
36. Keshavan MS, Anderson S, Beckwith C, Nash K, Pettegrew JW, Krishnan KRR. A comparison of stereology and segmentation techniques for volumetric measurements of lateral ventricles in magnetic resonance imaging. *Psychiatry Res.* 1995;61:53-60.
37. Daniels DL, Haughton VM, Naidich TP. *Cranial and Spinal Magnetic Resonance Imaging: An Atlas and Guide.* New York, NY: Raven Press; 1987.
38. Talairach J, Tournoux P. *Co-planar Stereotaxic Atlas of the Human Brain.* New York, NY: Thieme-Stratton Inc; 1988.
39. Shenton ME, Kikinis R, Jolesz FA, Pollack SD, LeMay M, Wible CG, Hokama H, Martin J, Metcalf D, Coleman M. Abnormalities of the left temporal lobe and thought disorder in schizophrenia: a quantitative magnetic resonance imaging study. *N Engl J Med.* 1992;327:604-612.
40. Krishnan KRR, McDonald WM, Escalona PR, Doraiswamy PM, Na C, Husain MM, Figiel GS. Magnetic resonance imaging of the caudate nuclei in depression: preliminary observations. *Arch Gen Psychiatry.* 1992;49:553-557.
41. McCarley RW, Shenton ME, O'Donnell BF, Faux SF, Kikinis R, Nestor PG, Jolesz FA. Auditory P300 abnormalities and left posterior superior temporal gyrus volume reduction in schizophrenia. *Arch Gen Psychiatry.* 1993;50:190-197.
42. Zipursky RB, Marsh L, Lim KO, DeMent S, Shear PK, Sullivan EV, Murphy GM, Csernansky JG, Pfefferbaum A. Volumetric MRI assessment of temporal lobe structures in schizophrenia. *Biol Psychiatry.* 1994;35:501-516.
43. Cavalieri B. *Geometra degli indivisibili.* Torino, Italy: Unione Tipografico Editrice; 1966.
44. Chalkey J. Methods for quantitative morphological analysis of tissue. *J Natl Cancer Inst.* 1943;4:37-43.
45. Weibel ER. Practical methods for biological morphometry. *Stereological Methods.* 1979;1:14-15.
46. Gunderson HJG, Jenson EG. The efficacy of systematic sampling in stereology and its prediction. *J Microsc.* 1987;147:229-263.
47. Rasmussen SA, Tsuang MT. Clinical characteristics and family history in *DSM-III* obsessive-compulsive disorder. *Am J Psychiatry.* 1986;143:317-322.
48. Tien AY, Pearlson GD, Machlin SR, Bylsma FW, Hoehn-Saric R. Oculomotor performance in obsessive-compulsive disorder. *Am J Psychiatry.* 1992;149:641-646.
49. Rauch SL, Jenike MA, Alpert NM, Baer L, Breiter HCR, Savage CR, Fischman AJ. Regional cerebral blood flow measured during symptom provocation in obsessive-compulsive disorder using oxygen 15–labeled carbon dioxide and positron emission tomography. *Arch Gen Psychiatry.* 1994;51:62-70.
50. Baxter LR. Neuroimaging studies of obsessive-compulsive disorders. *Psychiatr Clin North Am.* 1992;15:871-884.
51. Fujimoto T, Nakano T, Fujii M, Okada A, Harada K, Yokoyama Y, Uchida T, Tsuji T, Igata A, Asakura T. Changes in proton T1 in dog brains due to the administration of haloperidol. *Magn Reson Imaging.* 1987;5:469-474.
52. Hebebrand J, Siemon P, Lutcke A, Mari BG, Remschmidt H. A putaminal lesion in an adolescent with obsessive-compulsive disorder and atypical anorexia nervosa. *J Nerv Ment Dis.* 1995;181:520-521.
53. Rothfield JM. Generalized dystonia and obsessive-compulsive disorder associated with bilateral circumscribed magnetic resonance signal changes in the putamen. *J Nerv Ment Dis.* 1995;183:113-114.
54. Giedd JN, Rapoport JL, Kruesi MJP, Parker C, Schapiro MB, Allen AJ, Leonard HL, Kaysen D, Dickstein DP, Marsh WL, Kozuch PL, Vaituzis AC, Hamburger SD, Swedo SE. Sydenham's chorea: magnetic resonance imaging of the basal ganglia. *Neurology.* 1995;45:2199-2202.
55. Kiessling LS, Marcotte AC, Culpepper L. Antineuronal antibodies: tics and obsessive-compulsive symptoms. *J Dev Behav Pediatr.* 1994;15:421-425.
56. Percheron F, Fenelon G, Leroux-Hugon V, Feve A. History of the basal ganglia system: slow development of a major cerebral system. *Rev Neurol.* 1994;150:543-554.
57. Kimura M, Aosaki T, Ishida A. Neurophysiological aspects of the differential roles of the putamen and caudate nucleus in voluntary movement. *Adv Neurol.* 1993;60:62-70.
58. Shedlack KJ, Lee E, Radtke RA, Friedman AH, Crain BJ, Boyko O, Krishnan KRR. Ipsilateral subcortical atrophy associated with temporal lobectomy. *Psychiatry Res.* 1994;54:295-304.
59. Leenders KL, Palmer AJ, Quinn N, Clark JC, Firnau G, Garnett ES, Nahmins C, Jones T, Marsden CD. Brain dopamine metabolism in patients with Parkinson's disease measured with positron emission tomography. *J Neurol.* 1986;49:853-860.
60. Weinberger DR, Berman KF, Zee RF. Physiologic dysfunction of dorsolateral prefrontal cortex in schizophrenia. *Arch Gen Psychiatry.* 1986;43:114-123.
61. Modell JG, Mountz JM, Curtis GC, Greden JF. Neurophysiologic dysfunction in basal ganglia/limbic striatal and thalamocortical circuits as a pathogenetic mechanism of obsessive-compulsive disorder. *J Neuropsychiatry.* 1989;1:27-36.

ORIGINAL ARTICLE

Oculomotor Response Inhibition Abnormalities in Pediatric Obsessive-Compulsive Disorder

David R. Rosenberg, MD; David H. Averbach, MD; Kirsten M. O'Hearn; Andrew B. Seymour; Boris Birmaher, MD; John A. Sweeney, PhD

Background: Disturbances in the orbital prefrontal cortex and its ventral striatal target fields have been identified in neuroimaging studies of obsessive-compulsive disorder (OCD). In animal models and studies of patients with lesions to this brain circuitry, a selective disturbance in the ability to suppress responses to irrelevant stimuli has been demonstrated. Such a deficit in response suppression might underlie the apparent inhibitory deficit suggested by the symptoms of OCD. To date, little direct evidence of such a deficit has been reported. Further, although OCD commonly emerges during childhood or adolescence, few studies have examined psychotropic-naive pediatric patients near the onset of illness to find the possible role of atypical developmental processes in this disorder.

Methods: Oculomotor tests were administered to 18 psychotropic medication–naive, nondepressed patients with OCD aged 8.8 to 16.9 years and 18 case-matched healthy comparison subjects to assess the following 3 well-delineated aspects of prefrontal cortical function: the ability to suppress responses, the volitional execution of delayed responses, and the anticipation of predictable events.

Results: A significantly higher percentage of response suppression failures was observed in patients with OCD ($P=.003$), particularly in younger patients compared with their case-matched controls. No significant differences between patients with OCD and controls were observed on other prefrontal cortical functions. Severity of OCD symptoms was related to response suppression deficits.

Conclusion: A basic disturbance of behavioral inhibition in OCD was detected that may underlie the repetitive symptomatic behavior that characterizes the illness.

Arch Gen Psychiatry. 1997;54:831-838

IN RECENT years, there has been increased recognition of obsessive-compulsive disorder (OCD) as a severe, highly prevalent, and chronically disabling disorder.[1-4] Because OCD emerges during childhood or adolescence in as many as 80% of the cases,[5] studies during childhood near the onset of illness are critical to delineate the psychobiology of the disorder before course of illness and treatment effects can confound findings and to determine whether neurodevelopmental abnormalities contribute to the cause of the disorder.

The most widely accepted neurobiological model of OCD posits abnormalities in basal ganglia–frontal cortex interaction.[6-8] Indirect support for this model comes from observations of increased rates of obsessive and compulsive symptoms in neuropsychiatric disorders that result primarily from basal ganglia disease (eg, Sydenham chorea and Tourette syndrome).[9,10] More direct evidence comes from functional neuroimaging studies that have demonstrated increased metabolic rates in the caudate nucleus and orbital prefrontal cortex associated with OCD symptom severity.[11-13]

Frontal cortical and basal ganglia circuits are critical for executing goal-directed behaviors. Monkey and human positron emission tomography studies have identified frontal lobe regions specifically related to reflexive and voluntary fast conjugate (saccadic) eye movements.[14-17] Performance of goal-directed saccadic eye movements is also especially vulnerable to frontostriatal lesions.[18,19]

The symptoms of OCD suggest a problem in the natural inhibition of repetitive thoughts and behaviors. The orbital prefrontal cortex, a site of metabolic abnormalities in OCD, has been shown in many monkey lesion and human neuropsychological studies[18-23] to play a crucial role in subserving the

From the Departments of Psychiatry (Drs Rosenberg, Averbach, Birmaher, and Sweeney; Ms O'Hearn; and Mr Seymour) and Neurology (Dr Sweeney), Western Psychiatric Institute and Clinic, University of Pittsburgh Medical Center, Pittsburgh, Pa. Dr Rosenberg is now affiliated with the Departments of Psychiatry and Behavioral Neurosciences and Pediatrics, Wayne State University School of Medicine, Detroit, Mich.

ability to suppress behavioral responses to irrelevant stimuli (also referred to as "neurobehavioral response inhibition"). Tien et al[24] observed an increased rate of response suppression errors using an antisaccadic eye movement paradigm in 11 adult, nondepressed, mostly medicated (10 of 11 subjects) patients with OCD. Thus, a disturbance in ventral frontostriatal circuitry may have a disinhibitory effect that could be influential in the cause of OCD. To date, however, few studies have evaluated disturbances in neurobehavioral functions subserved by frontostriatal circuits in OCD.

The prefrontal cortex subserves various key behavioral functions including response inhibition, initiating delayed responses, and the temporal integration of behavior.[25-27] To date, it has not been determined whether the response suppression function of the prefrontal cortex is selectively impaired relative to other prefrontal cortical functions in OCD. Therefore, we evaluated response inhibition as well as other cognitive functions subserved by the prefrontal cortex to determine whether there is a selective impairment in inhibitory controls of neurocognitive processes in OCD. Further, by studying pediatric patients with OCD, we were able to examine

SUBJECTS AND METHODS

SUBJECTS

Eighteen psychotropic medication–naive, pediatric, nondepressed outpatients with OCD (9 males, 9 females) aged 8.8 to 16.9 years and 18 age- and sex case-matched healthy comparison subjects were enrolled in our study (**Table**). Diagnoses were determined using the child version of the Schedule for Affective Disorders and Schizophrenia-Present Episode and the Schedule for Affective Disorders and Schizophrenia–Epidemiologic Version[12,28] with parent(s) and child as informants. In each case, a board certified child psychiatrist (D.R.R.) interviewed the child, confirmed the presence of each of the criteria symptoms for OCD with the child and family, and reviewed all other diagnostic information. Case-control pairs were matched within 1 year of age and had comparable parental socioeconomic status (A. B. Hollingshead, PhD, unpublished data, 1978). Eleven of the 18 patients with OCD also had comorbid *DSM-III-R* anxiety disorders (overanxious disorder), 2 had attention deficit hyperactivity disorder, 4 had dysthymia, and 4 had oppositional-conduct disorder. Only 1 subject had OCD as the sole diagnosis. None of the subjects had a major depressive episode within 4 months of testing. The controls had no family history of affective disorder in first-degree relatives. Legal guardians gave informed consent and all of the subjects gave written assent.

METHODS

Clinical Measurements

The severity of OCD symptoms was measured by the Leyton Obsessional Inventory[29] and the child version of the Yale-Brown Obsessive-Compulsive Scale–Revised Edition.[30] The severity of anxiety was measured by the Beck Anxiety Inventory[31] and the Hamilton Anxiety Rating Scale.[32] Depressive symptoms were measured with the Children's Depression Inventory[33] and the 17-item Hamilton Depression Rating Scale.[34] A neuropsychological screening examination assessed general intelligence,[35] cerebral dominance,[36] manual dexterity,[37] and attention.[38]

Neurocognitive Testing Procedures

Neurocognitive testing was performed using oculomotor tasks that are easy for children to understand. Three volitionally controlled saccadic eye movement tests were administered (ie, antisaccade, oculomotor delayed response [ODR], and predictive saccadic tasks). A test of reflexive visually guided saccades was administered to confirm that abnormalities in volitionally controlled eye movements could not be attributed to deficits in basic oculomotor function.

Testing Environment

Subjects were tested alone in a dark room to prevent distraction by extraneous information, to increase the compelling nature of the stimulus in the antisaccadic task, and to eliminate background spatial cues. Direct current electro-oculography recordings of each eye were obtained (Grass Neurodata 12 Acquisition System, Neurodata, Pasadena, Calif) to assess a wide extent of the horizontal visual field. Blinks were monitored using electrodes placed above and below the left eye. Stationary targets (LEDs) were presented to the left or right of center fixation at a distance of 1 m. Except for the brief presentation of the "to be remembered" target locations on the ODR task, the central fixation light was turned off concurrently with the presentation of peripheral targets in all of the tasks. Except for the predictive saccadic task, the spatial location and timing of the presentation of peripheral cues were unpredictable.

Visually Guided Saccadic Task

While fixating on a central cue, peripheral targets were presented at ±10°, ±20°, or ±30° from center fixation. Subjects were instructed to look as quickly as possible toward these targets. Peripheral targets were presented for 1.5 seconds. The latency, accuracy (ie, error in degrees of visual angle), and peak velocity of saccades were recorded. Fifty-four trials were administered.

Antisaccadic Response Suppression Task

This task, developed by Hallet[39] and Guitton et al[40] required subjects to fixate on a central target and then look the same distance but in the opposite direction from targets presented to the left or right of center fixation (±8°, ±16°, or ±24°). Thus, if a target appeared 8° to the left, subjects needed to move their eyes 8° to the right. This test requires the suppression of a powerful reflexive response to look toward novel peripheral targets and the ability to volitionally drive the eyes away from a target when no cue exists in the periphery to guide movement (**Figure 1**). The technician carefully explained the task and administered 8 practice trials, pointing manually to where the eyes should be focused when targets were presented. During the actual testing, subjects were realerted to task instructions after 2 consecutive errors (reflexive glances toward the target) to ensure that poor performance did not merely reflect uncertainty about the task or the subject's failure to pay attention. The percentage of trials in which the subject looked toward peripheral targets (response suppression errors) and the latency and accuracy of saccades toward the correct location were recorded. Antisaccadics following response suppression errors were excluded from the analyses of response latency and accuracy. One and a half seconds after the peripheral light was presented, it was turned off and a light at the correct location (where the subject should have been looking) was turned on. This provided subjects with feedback about their performance on an ongoing basis. Thirty-six trials were performed.

ODR TASK

The subjects began by fixating on a central cue. The targets were presented briefly (100 milliseconds) ±9°, ±18°, or ±27° from center. The subjects were told not to look at that target, but to remember its location while holding central fixation. After a varying delay (1, 2, 4, or 8 seconds), the central light was extinguished, which served as the subject's cue to look to where the peripheral target had been presented. As in the antisaccadic task, careful detailed discussion and slow practice trials preceded testing. The number of trials with saccadics toward the briefly presented peripheral targets (response suppression failures) and the latency and accuracy of saccadics toward the remembered target locations were recorded. Twenty-four trials were administered.

Predictive Saccadic Task

The subjects began by fixating on a central target, after which a light began to move back and forth from 7.5° to the left and right of center at a constant interval. This spaciotemporal predictability dramatically reduces response latency.[41,42] Two predictive saccadic tasks were used with the same features except that on 1 task, the target shifted position more rapidly (every 1.5 vs 0.75 seconds). Saccadic latency and accuracy were recorded. The saccadic from central fixation to the first peripheral cue was not used in the calculations. The 19 trials recorded in each task were clustered into 5 blocks of trials (trials 1-4, 5-8, 9-12, 13-16, and 17-19). The average saccadic latency in each block of trials was calculated. One subject with OCD did not perform these tasks as they were not operational at the time of testing, so they and their matched controls were excluded from these analyses.

Eye Movement Analysis

Eye movement recordings were analyzed off-line using custom programs developed in our laboratory. Eye position recordings were calibrated (converted from raw voltage data to eye position in degrees of visual angle) for each trial independently using data from the time subjects fixated on the central fixation cue and the peripheral location to which the subjects were to move their eyes. Quantitative assessment of oculomotor function was performed without the knowledge of subject age, sex, or diagnosis.

STATISTICAL ANALYSIS

The primary data analysis involved the use of repeated measurements of analysis of variance for comparisons of matched case-control pairs on each task, which effectively controlled for performance differences related to subject age. Correlations of oculomotor performance with age, sex, and clinical symptom inventories were also performed. Two-way (sex by diagnostic group) analysis of variance was performed in view of some previous studies suggesting sex-specific abnormalities in OCD.[24,43,44]

Eye movement measurements in the left and right visual fields were examined using repeated measurements of analysis of variance in which the main effects of laterality (left vs right) and the interaction of laterality with the groups were tested for each task. A significant interaction of laterality with the groups was observed for total antisaccadic response suppression failures ($F[1,16]=6.16$, $P=.02$) and were significant when targets were displaced ±8° from central fixation ($F[1,17]=10.51$, $P=.005$) but not at ±16° or ±24° from central fixation. Patients with OCD and controls had significantly more response suppression failures in the left visual field ($F[1,17]=8.91$, $P=.008$). Therefore, in the analysis of antisaccadic response suppression failures, laterality was treated as an additional independent variable. For the remaining variables, data from leftward and rightward saccadics were pooled.

the developmental acquisition of cognitive skills subserved by the prefrontal cortex in this illness.

RESULTS

VISUALLY GUIDED SACCADIC TASK

No significant differences were observed between patients with OCD and matched controls in peak velocity ($F[1,17]=0.27$, $P=.61$), latency ($F[1,17]=1.95$, $P=.18$), or accuracy ($F[1,17]=0.74$, $P=.40$) of visually guided saccadics.

ANTISACCADIC TASK

Patients with OCD made significantly more antisaccadic response suppression errors than did controls ($F[1,17]=11.85$, $P=.003$) (**Figure 2**). This effect held true regardless of how far targets were presented from central fixation, though response suppression errors increased for both groups as peripheral targets were presented closer to center fixation ($F[2,34]=23.11$, $P=.001$). Patients with OCD did not show any abnormalities in saccadic latency ($F[1,17]=0.05$, $P=.83$) or accuracy ($F[1,17]=0.89$, $P=.36$).

Demographic and Clinical Data From Nondepressed, Psychotropic Medication–Naive Pediatric Patients With OCD and Case-Matched Normal Controls*

Characteristic	Subjects† Patients With OCD, Mean±SD (Range)	Normal Controls, Mean±SD (Range)	t‡	P
Age, y	12.7±2.4 (8.8-16.7)	12.8±2.5 (8.7-16.8)	0.33	.74
Parental SES§	2.4±0.86 (1-4)	2.2±0.86 (1-3)	1.0	.33
Age of onset, y	10.0±4.0 (0.5-15)	...	...	...
Duration of illness, y	2.7±2.8 (0.4-11.3)	...	...	...
Leyton Obsessional Inventory	18.5±11.5 (1-35)	1.3±2.2 (0-7)	6.1	.001
CY-BOCS				
Obsessions	11.0±3.2 (5-16)	0	14.5	.001
Compulsions	10.1±3.6 (3-15)	0	11.8	.001
Total score	21.1±6.2 (9-29)	0	14.4	.001
CDI	7.6±8.6 (0-32)	2.3±4.0 (0-14)	2.6	.02
Hamilton Depression Rating Scale	5.5±3.9 (2-16)	1.9±0.5 (0-2)	3.9	.001
Beck Anxiety Inventory	11.0±10.0 (0-36)	2.6±3.0 (0-9)	3.8	.001
Hamilton Anxiety Rating Scale	11.7±8.2 (0-28)	1.3±1.6 (0-4)	5.8	.001

**OCD indicates obsessive-compulsive disorder; SES, socioeconomic status; CY-BOCS, child version of the Yale-Brown Obsessive-Compulsive Scale; CDI, Children's Depression Inventory; and ellipses, not relevant to controls (ie, age of onset and duration of illness).*

†There were 18 subjects enrolled in the group with OCD (9 males, 9 females) and 18 subjects enrolled in the control group (9 males, 9 females).

‡Paired t test, df=17.

§Measured by the assessment of parental educational level and highest level of occupational functioning on a scale of 1 to 5, with 1 indicating the highest and 5 indicating the lowest parental SES.[26]

ODR TASK

The trend for pediatric patients with OCD to display more response suppression failures on the ODR task than controls was not significant ($F[1,17]=3.61$, $P=.07$) (**Figure 3**). Only when targets were presented close to central fixation (±9°) did patients with OCD make significantly more ODR response suppression errors ($t[17]=2.12$, $P<.05$).

The overall accuracy of saccadics toward remembered target locations did not differ between patients with OCD and controls, though there was a trend toward a significant delay by group interaction effect ($F[3,51]=2.77$, $P=.051$). An exploratory analysis indicated that at the longest delay, performance of the controls deteriorated, but no drop-off in performance was seen in the patients with OCD ($t[17]=2.38$, $P=.03$) (**Figure 4**). There was no group difference in response latency ($F[1,17]=.64$, $P=.43$).

PREDICTIVE SACCADIC TASKS

Comparable significant reductions of saccadic latency across blocks of trials were observed in patients with OCD and controls on the 1.5-second ($F[4,64]=10.97$, $P=.001$) and 0.75-second ($F[4,64]=13.84$, $P=.001$) predictive saccadic tasks.

CLINICAL CORRELATIONS

There were no sex differences on any of the oculomotor measurements. Antisaccadic response suppression errors were related to the severity of OCD symptoms indexed by the total Yale-Brown Obsessive-Compulsive Scale–Revised Edition score ($r=0.49$, $P=.003$) and the obsessive ($r=0.48$, $P=.003$) and compulsive($r=0.49$, $P=.003$) Yale-Brown Obsessive-Compulsive Scale–Revised Edition subscales. On the ODR task, no significant correlations were observed between response suppression errors and OCD symptom severity even for trials when targets were presented close to central fixation. No significant correlations were observed between antisaccadic and ODR response suppression failures and clinical ratings of depression or anxiety, duration of illness, age of onset of illness, sex, parental socioeconomic status, manual dexterity (grooved pegboard test), or attention (digit span).

DEVELOPMENTAL TRENDS

Significant inverse correlations were observed between the age and rate of antisaccadic response suppression errors in patients with OCD ($r=-0.54$, $P=.02$) (Figure 2, right). A similar trend was observed in control subjects ($r=-0.44$, $P=.07$).

The slopes of the relationships between age and rates of antisaccadic response suppression failures were not significantly different between patients with OCD and controls ($F[1,32]=0.48$, $P=.49$). To provide some estimate of the degree of possible developmental delay in skill acquisition in the OCD sample, we calculated the approximate age at which a 40% overall error rate was achieved. Controls achieved this level of performance at approximately 11 years of age, while patients with OCD achieved this level at about 16 years of age.

COMMENT

To our knowledge, this is the first study designed specifically to contrast the functional integrity of different domains of prefrontal cortical functions in OCD and also the first cognitive study of young onset, nondepressed, psychotropic-naive patients with OCD. These findings replicate and extend the findings of Tien et al[24] in a study demonstrating increased antisaccadic response suppression errors in medicated adult patients with OCD. Our study provides important new data about disturbances in prefrontal neurocognitive functions in OCD without the confounds of central nervous system–active medications and with less potential influence of disease progression. Severity of depression and general anxiety did not seem to influence our findings.

Our results support the hypothesis that a selective deficit in response inhibition is associated with the clinical presentation of OCD and that a selective deficit in frontostriatal function may be a central and specific neurocognitive deficit in this illness. Our data also provide important new cross-sectional developmental information about a possible delay in the acquisition of this specific prefrontal cortical function in OCD because patients with OCD seemed to acquire this cognitive skill about 5 years later than their age-matched controls.

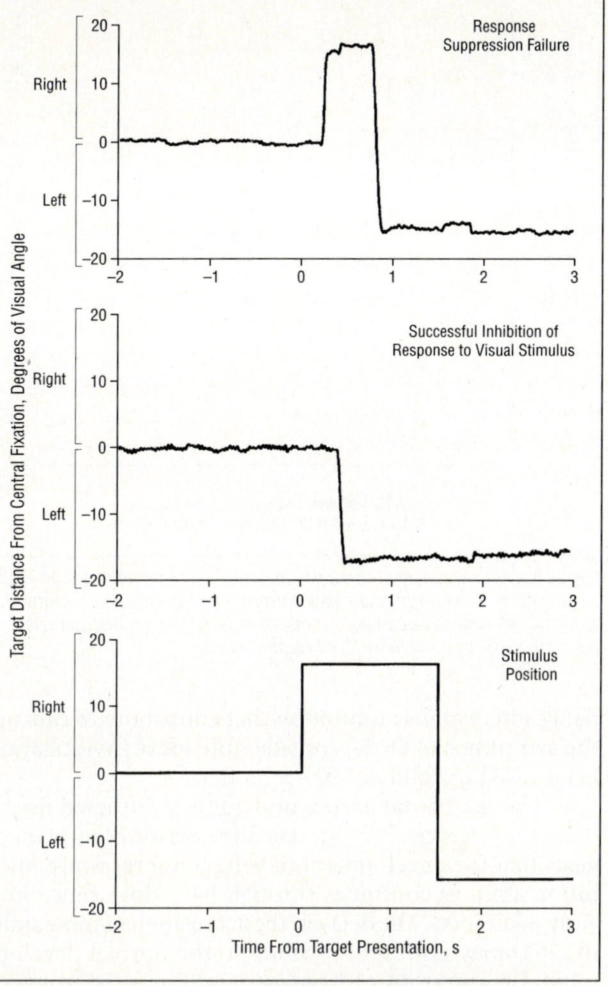

Figure 1. *Responses to an unpredictable visual target on the antisaccadic task. Note that the normal control (middle) correctly averts gaze from the target light to the opposite direction, while the patient with obsessive-compulsive disorder (top) makes a response suppression error by looking toward the light that they were instructed to look away from.*

POTENTIAL RELEVANCE FOR NEUROBIOLOGICAL MODELS OF OCD

Fuster[25] described response inhibition, maintaining preparatory set, and initiating delayed responses as core functions of the prefrontal cortex. Primate studies of the ventral and dorsal prefrontal cortex suggest a specific functional neuroanatomy for these functions. The orbital prefrontal cortex seems to facilitate the suppression of context-inappropriate responses[18-20,22,23,45] and mediates the ability to perform successive response inhibition and reversal tasks (eg, suppressing responses on the antisaccadic task).[18-21] Human clinical and monkey studies have observed a loss of inhibitory control over reflexive responses after lesions to the orbital prefrontal cortex.[26,27,46] The dorsolateral prefrontal cortex plays a more specific role in maintaining spatial information on-line for guiding future volitional action (eg, making saccadics based on remembered information on the ODR task).[14,47]

Neuroimaging[11,28,48] and neuropsychological studies[49,50] have most consistently localized dysfunctional areas in patients with OCD to the frontal cortex and the basal ganglia. Given the clinically apparent disinhibitory features of the ego-dystonic repetitive thoughts and

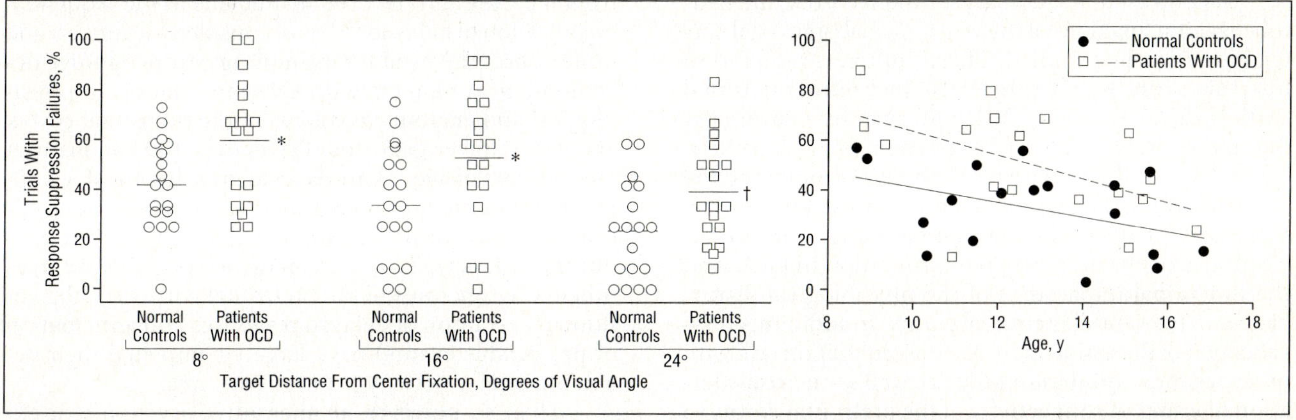

Figure 2. *Left, Mean response suppression failures for nondepressed, psychotropic medication–naive pediatric patients with obsessive-compulsive disorder (OCD) and normal controls performing the antisaccadic task. Lines through distributions represent the mean value. Asterisks indicate P=.01; dagger, P=.02. Right, Response suppression failures as a function of age for nondepressed, psychotropic medication–naive pediatric patients with OCD and normal controls performing the antisaccadic task. Note the marked inverse correlation between age and total number of response suppression errors in patients with OCD and a trend for such an effect in controls.*

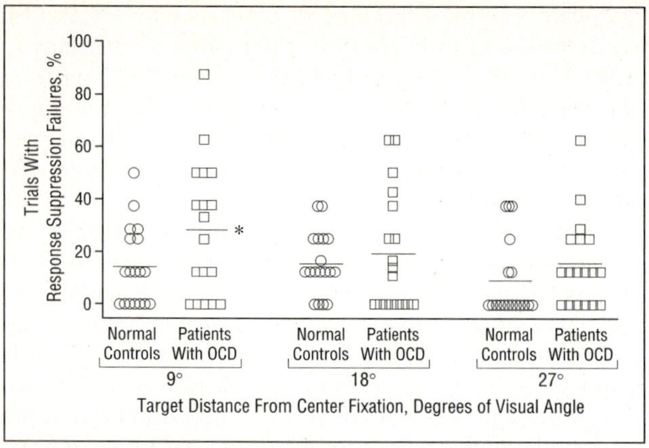

Figure 3. *Mean response suppression failures for nondepressed, psychotropic medication–naive pediatric patients with obsessive-compulsive disorder (OCD) and normal controls performing the oculomotor delayed response task. Lines through distributions represent the mean value. Asterisk indicates* $P = .05$.

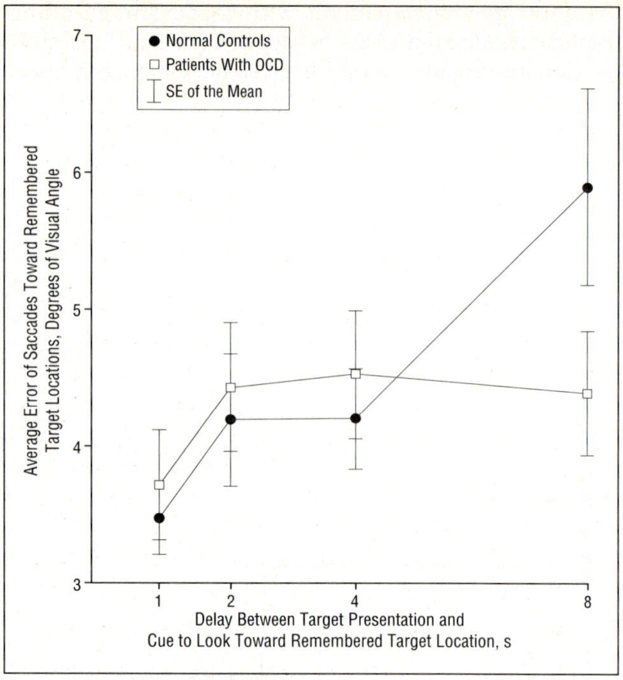

Figure 4. *Mean accuracy of saccadics to remembered target locations after varying delay for nondepressed, psychotropic medication–naive pediatric patients with obsessive-compulsive disorder (OCD) and normal controls performing the oculomotor delayed response task.*

behaviors that are the primary manifestations of OCD, a general disturbance in the ability to suppress context-inappropriate responses may be a critical neurobehavioral underpinning to the pathophysiology of OCD. The selective behavioral deficit in response inhibition suggests the possibility of a focal abnormality in ventral prefrontal cortex consistent with the suspected pathophysiology of OCD. Such a deficit could represent a neurocognitive mechanism explaining how physiological disturbances in the ventral prefrontal cortex could be related to symptom expression in OCD.

The fact that patients with OCD exhibited no impairment on the predictive and ODR tasks, functions believed to be subserved primarily by the dorsal prefrontal cortex, suggests that the dorsal prefrontal cortex may be intact in patients with OCD. The selective deficit in neurobehavioral response inhibition in pediatric patients with OCD is especially intriguing when one considers that some degree of selectivity has been established for the orbital prefrontal cortex in mediating this function.[17,26,27,47] Moreover, functional neuroimaging studies of patients with OCD[11-13,28] have revealed abnormalities in ventral but not dorsal prefrontal cortical regions.

In contrast to the dorsal prefrontal cortex, the neurobehavioral functions of the ventromedial prefrontal cortex have been less studied. Thus, caution is required in inferring a direct linkage between the ventral prefrontal cortical disturbances in OCD indicated by neuroimaging studies and problems of response suppression. Neuroimaging studies in patients with OCD employing the relevant tasks as activation paradigms are needed to further clarify the neurobiological importance of this deficit in neurobehavioral response inhibition in OCD and the functional importance of the physiological disturbances in the ventral prefrontal cortex. In addition, cross-validation of the antisaccadic response inhibition task with other response inhibition tasks, as well as the consideration of issues of connectivity of the prefrontal cortex to other brain regions, are necessary. Thus, while our findings support our neurocognitive hypothesis that physiological dysfunction in the ventral prefrontal cortex and its ventromedial striatal target fields leads to disturbances in response inhibition that contribute to causing the symptoms of OCD, considerably more investigation is required to validate such a model.

The prefrontal cortex undergoes protracted developmental changes.[51,52] Our data in pediatric controls suggests that the development of behavioral response inhibition abilities continues through late adolescence into early adulthood. The delay in the acquisition of these skills in OCD may represent a failure in the normal developmental maturation of frontostriatal circuitry, particularly orbital prefrontal–ventromedial striatal circuits. Replication of our observation with larger samples is needed, as is the assessment of subjects in younger and older age ranges than were enrolled in our study.

The growing evidence for the role of the orbital prefrontal cortex and the caudate nucleus in the sequential organization of behavior[53,54] is of considerable interest and underscores the need for examining neurocognitive development in patients with OCD in relation to physiological and anatomical studies of the prefrontal cortex and its striatal target fields. Typically, OCD has an onset after 7 years of age.[55] Our data suggest that the development of the core prefrontal function we believe most relevant to OCD (response inhibition) progresses throughout the risk period for the emergence of OCD, whereas other core functions of the prefrontal cortex (ie, the volitional execution of delayed responses and anticipation of predictable events) have largely completed their developmental trajectory prior to that time.

There is, however, an alternative psychometric explanation for the apparently selective antisaccadic response inhibition effect in pediatric patients with OCD. The antisaccadic task may have better sensitivity than the predictive saccadic and ODR tasks for detecting generalized prefrontal abnormalities. What seems to be a selective deficit for pediatric patients with OCD may, instead, reflect an increased sensitivity of the antisaccadic paradigm, rather than an impairment in a particular functional domain. Further studies using complementary strategies are necessary to confirm the specific linkage of response inhibition deficits to abnormalities in ventral prefrontal circuits in OCD.

Moreover, we cannot be certain that our findings are specific to OCD and not influenced by comorbid conditions, particularly other childhood anxiety disorders present in 11 of the 16 patients. Severity of anxiety and depression, however, did not seem to influence oculomotor function. Future studies controlling for comorbid conditions will be critical for determining whether the observed oculomotor deficits are specific to OCD or generalizable to anxiety or other comorbid conditions.

Our results suggest that established disturbances of the ventral prefrontal cortex in OCD may exert their clinical effect by disrupting a specific cognitive function, namely, the ability to suppress behavioral and ideational responses that would interfere with ongoing purposive behavior. Our data also provide important new cross-sectional developmental information suggesting a possible delay in the acquisition of this specific prefrontal cortical function in OCD as control subjects seemed to acquire this cognitive skill approximately 5 years earlier than their age-matched OCD counterparts.

Accepted for publication August 20, 1996.

This study was supported by grants R01-42969 (Dr Sweeeney), P50-45156 (Dr Sweeney), and MH-01372 (Dr Rosenberg) from the National Institute of Mental Health, Rockville, Md, and a grant from the National Obsessive Compulsive Foundation, Melford, Calif.

A previous version of this paper was a recipient of the Peter Henderson, MD, Memorial Award in 1995 for the best paper in the general area of child and adolescent psychiatry and was presented at the Society for Neuroscience Annual Meeting, San Diego, Calif, November 25, 1995, and the Society for Biological Psychiatry Annual Meeting, New York, NY, May 17-21, 1996.

We are grateful to Neal Ryan, MD, who referred his carefully ascertained healthy young pediatric patients to us, which allowed for pairwise case-control matching. We also thank Benjamin J. McCurtain and Elizabeth L. Dick for their assistance with data processing and analysis and David Kupfer, MD, and Joel Greenhouse, PhD, for their consultation on this data.

Reprints: David R. Rosenberg, MD, Wayne State University School of Medicine, Psychiatry 9B, 4201 St Antoine Blvd, Detroit, MI 48201 (e-mail: Drosen@med.wayne.edu).

REFERENCES

1. Valleni-Basile LA, Garrison CZ, Jackson KL, Waller JL, McKeown RE, Addy CL, Cuffe SP. Frequency of obsessive-compulsive disorder in a community sample of young adolescents. *J Am Acad Child Adolesc Psychiatry.* 1994;33:782-791.
2. Hanna GL. Demographic and clinical features of obsessive-compulsive disorder in children and adolescents. *J Am Acad Child Adolesc Psychiatry.* 1995;34:19-27.
3. Flament MF, Whitaker A, Rapoport JL. Obsessive-compulsive disorder in adolescence: an epidemiological study. *J Am Acad Child Adolesc Psychiatry.* 1988;27:764-771.
4. Robins LN, Helzer JI, Weissman MM, Orvgschel H, Gruenberg E, Burke JD, Regier MD. Lifetime prevalence of specific psychiatric disorders in three sites. *Arch Gen Psychiatry.* 1984;41:949-958.
5. Pauls DL, Alsobrook JP II, Phil M, Goodman W, Rasmussen S, Leckman JF. A family study of obsessive-compulsive disorder. *Am J Psychiatry.* 1995;152:76-84.
6. Khanna S. Obsessive-compulsive disorder: is there a frontal lobe dysfunction? *Biol Psychiatry.* 1988;24:602-613.
7. Modell JG, Mountz JM, Curtis GC, Greden JF. Neurophysiologic dysfunction in basal ganglia—limbic striatal and thalamocortical circuits as a pathogenetic mechanism of obsessive-compulsive disorder. *J Neuropsychiatry Clin Neurosci.* 1989;1:27-36.
8. Insel TR. Toward a neuroanatomy of obsessive-compulsive disorder. *Arch Gen Psychiatry.* 1992;49:739-744.
9. Pitman RE, Green RC, Jenike MA, Mesulam MM. Clinical comparison of Tourette's disorder and obsessive-compulsive disorder. *Am J Psychiatry.* 1987;144:1166-1171.
10. Swedo SE, Rapoport JL, Cheslow DL, Leonard HL, Ayoub EM, Hosier DM, Wald ER. High prevalence of obsessive-compulsive symptoms in patients with Sydenham's chorea. *Am J Psychiatry.* 1989;146:246-249.
11. Rauch SL, Jenike MA, Alpert NM, Breiter HCR, Savage CR, Fischman AJ. Regional cerebral blood flow measured during symptom provocation in obsessive-compulsive disorder using oxygen 15–labeled carbon dioxide and positron emission tomography. *Arch Gen Psychiatry.* 1994;51:62-70.
12. Baxter LR, Phelps ME, Mazziotta JC, Guze BH, Schwartz JM, Selin CE. Local cerebral glucose metabolic rates in obsessive-compulsive disorder: a comparison with rates in unipolar depression and normal controls. *Arch Gen Psychiatry.* 1987;44:211-218.
13. Swedo SE, Pietrini P, Leonard HL, Schapiro MB, Rettew DC, Goldberger EL, Rapoport SI, Rapoport JL, Grady CL. Cerebral glucose metabolism in childhood-onset obsessive-compulsive disorder: revisualization during pharmacotherapy. *Arch Gen Psychiatry.* 1992;49:690-694.
14. Funahashi S, Bruce CJ, Goldman-Rakic PS. Mnemonic coding of visual space in the monkey's dorsolateral prefrontal cortex. *J Neurophysiol.* 1989;61:331-349.
15. Funahashi S, Bruce CJ, Goldman-Rakic PS. Visuospatial coding in primate prefrontal neurons revealed by oculomotor paradigms. *J Neurophysiol.* 1990;63:814-831.
16. Goldman-Rakic PS. Circuitry of primate prefrontal cortex and regulation of behavior by representational knowledge. In: Plum F, Mountcastle V, eds. *Handbook of Physiology.* Bethesda, Md: American Physiological Society; 1987:373-417.
17. Sweeney JA, Mintun MA, Kwee S, Wiseman MB, Brown DL, Rosenberg DR, Carl JR. A positron emission tomography study of voluntary saccadic eye movements and spatial working memory. *J Neurophysiol.* 1996;75:454-468.
18. Rosvold HE, Mishkin M. Non-sensory effects of frontal lesions on discrimination learning and performance. In: Delafresnaye JF, ed. *Brain Mechanisms and Learning.* Oxford, England: Basil Blackwell Publishers; 1961:555-576.
19. Passingham RE. Visual discrimination learning after selective prefrontal ablations in monkeys. *Neuropsychologia.* 1972;10:27-39.
20. Diamond A. Developmental progression in human infants and infant monkeys, and the neural bases of, inhibitory control of reaching. In: Diamond A, ed. *The Development and Neural Bases of Higher Cognitive Functions.* New York, NY: Academy of Science Press; 1990:267-317.
21. Goodglass H, Kaplan E. *An Assessment of Aphasia and Related Disorders.* Philadelphia, Pa: Lea & Febiger; 1972:54.
22. Luria AR. *Higher Cortical Function in Man.* New York, NY: Basic Books Inc Publishers; 1966:246.
23. Stuss DT, Benson DF. Frontal lobe lesions and behavior. In: Kertesz A, ed. *Localization in Neuropsychology.* Orlando, Fla: Academic Press Inc; 1983:429-449.
24. Tien AY, Pearlson GD, Machlin SR, Bylsma FW, Hoehn-Saric R. Oculomotor performance in obsessive-compulsive disorder. *Am J Psychiatry.* 1992;149:641-646.
25. Fuster JM. *The Prefrontal Cortex: Anatomy, Physiology and Neuropsychology of the Frontal Lobe.* New York, NY: Raven Press; 1989:125-155.
26. Rosenkilde CE. Functional heterogeneity of the prefrontal cortex in the monkey: a review. *Behav Neural Biol.* 1979;25:301-345.
27. Cummings JL. Frontal-subcortical circuits and human behavior. *Arch Neurol.* 1993;50:873-880.
28. Baxter LR, Schwartz JM, Bergman KS, Szuba MP, Guze BH, Mazziotta JC, Alazraki A, Selin CE, Ferng H-K, Munford P, Phelps ME. Caudate glucose metabolic rate changes with both drug and behavior therapy for obsessive-compulsive disorder. *Arch Gen Psychiatry.* 1992;49:681-689.
29. Cooper J. The Leyton Obsessional Inventory. *Psychol Med.* 1970;1:48-64.

30. Riddle MA, Scahill L, King RA, Hardin MT, Anderson GM, Ort SI, Smith JC, Leckman JF, Cohen DJ. Double-blind, crossover trial of fluoxetine and placebo in children and adolescents with obsessive-compulsive disorder. *J Am Acad Child Adolesc Psychiatry.* 1992;31:1062-1069.
31. Beck AT, Epstein N, Brown G, Steer RA. An inventory for measuring clinical anxiety: psychometric properties. *J Consult Clin Psychol.* 1988;56:893-897.
32. Hamilton M. The assessment of anxiety states by rating. *Br J Med Psychol.* 1959; 32:50-55.
33. Kovacs M. Child's Depression Inventory. *Psychopharmacol Bull.* 1985;21:995-998.
34. Hamilton M. Development of a rating scale for primary depressive illness. *Br J Soc Clin Psychol.* 1967;6:278-296.
35. Ammons RB, Ammons CH. *Ammons Quick IQ Test.* New York, NY: Psychological Test Specialists; 1962.
36. Annett M. The binomial distribution of right, mixed and left handedness. *J Exp Psychol A.* 1967;19:327-333.
37. Knights RM, Norwood J. *Revised Smoothed Normative Data on the Neuropsychological Test Battery for Children.* Ottawa, Ontario: Carleton University; 1980.
38. Wechsler D. *Wechsler Intelligence Scale for Children.* New York, NY: Psychological Corp; 1991.
39. Hallet PE. Primary and secondary saccadics to goals defined by instructions. *Vision Res.* 1978;18:1279-1296.
40. Guitton D, Buchtel HA, Douglas RM. Frontal lobe lesions in man cause difficulties in suppressing reflexive glances and in generating goal-directed saccadics. *Exp Brain Res.* 1985;58:455-72.
41. Findlay JM. Spatial and temporal factors in the predictive generation of saccadic eye movements. *Vision Res.* 1981;21:347-354.
42. Ross SM, Ross LE. Children's and adults' predictive saccadics to square-wave targets. *Vision Res.* 1987;27:2177-2180.
43. Rasmussen SA, Tsuang M-T. Clinical characteristics and family history in *DSM-III* obsessive-compulsive disorder. *Am J Psychiatry.* 1986;143:317-322.
44. Luxenberg JS, Swedo SE, Flament MF, Friedland RP, Rapoport J, Rapoport SI. Neuroanatomical abnormalities in obsessive-compulsive disorder determined with quantitative x-ray computed tomography. *Am J Psychiatry.* 1988;145:1089-1093.
45. Iversen SD, Mishkin M. Perseverative interference in monkeys following selective lesions of the inferior prefrontal convexity. *Exp Brain Res.* 1970;11:376-386.
46. Malloy P, Birhrle A, Duffy J, Cimino C. The orbitomedial frontal syndrome. *Arch Clin Neuropsychol.* 1993;8:185-201.
47. Goldman PS, Rosvold HE. Localization of function within the dorsolateral prefrontal cortex of the rhesus monkey. *Exp Neurol.* 1970;27:291-304.
48. Swedo SE, Schapiro MB, Grady CL, Cheslow DL, Leonard HL, Kumar A, Friedland R, Rapoport S, Rapoport JL. Cerebral glucose metabolism in childhood-onset obsessive-compulsive disorder. *Arch Gen Psychiatry.* 1989;46:518-523.
49. Flor-Henry P, Yeudall LT, Koles ZJ, Howarth BG. Neuropsychological and power spectral EEG investigations of the obsessive-compulsive syndrome. *Biol Psychiatry.* 1979;14:119-130.
50. Gross-Isseroff R, Sasson Y, Voet H, Hendler T, Luca-Haimovici K, Kandal-Sussman H, Zohar J. Alternation learning in obsessive-compulsive disorder. *Biol Psychiatry.* 1996;39:733-738.
51. Huttenlocher PR. Synaptic density in human frontal cortex: developmental changes and effects of aging. *Brain Res.* 1979;163:195-205.
52. Jernigan TL, Tallal P. Late childhood changes in brain morphology observable with MRI. *Dev Med Child Neurol.* 1990;32:379-385.
53. Van Den Bercken JHL, Cools AR. Evidence for a role of the caudate nucleus in the sequential organization of behavior. *Behav Brain Res.* 1982;4:319-337.
54. Graybiel AM, Aosaki T, Flaherty AW, Kimura M. The basal ganglia and adaptive motor control. *Science.* 1994;265:1826-1831.
55. Rasmussen SA, Eisen JL. The epidemiology and clinical features of obsessive-compulsive disorder. *Psychiatr Clin North Am.* 1992;15:743-758.

ORIGINAL ARTICLE

Neuroendocrine Response to Fenfluramine Challenge in Boys

Associations With Aggressive Behavior and Adverse Rearing

Daniel S. Pine, MD; Jeremy D. Coplan, MD; Gail A. Wasserman, PhD; Laurie S. Miller, PhD; Jane E. Fried, MD; Mark Davies, MPH; Thomas B. Cooper, MS; Laurence Greenhill, MD; David Shaffer, MD; Bruce Parsons, PhD, MD

Background: There is evidence of relationships among serotonin, aggressive behavior, and a childhood history of socially adverse-rearing conditions. This study examines the prolactin response to fenfluramine hydrochloride challenge in young boys who show clinically significant aggressive behavior or who are raised in a social environment that is conducive to the development of chronic aggression.

Methods: A series of 34 younger brothers of convicted delinquents underwent standardized psychiatric and observation-based assessments of their social-rearing environments that were conducted during home visits. Approximately 2 years later, these boys underwent a reassessment of psychiatric status and an assessment of central serotonergic activity using the fenfluramine challenge procedure.

Results: Increasing degrees of aggressive behavior at either assessment were positively correlated with the prolactin response to fenfluramine challenge. Furthermore, adverse-rearing circumstances that were conducive to the development of aggressive behavior also exhibited positive correlations with the prolactin response. This association between adverse rearing and the prolactin response was statistically independent of that between aggression and the prolactin response.

Conclusion: In young boys, aggressive behavior and social circumstances that are conducive to the development of aggressive behavior are positively correlated with a marker of central serotonergic activity.

Arch Gen Psychiatry. 1997;54:839-846

HUMAN AGGRESSION is influenced by biological and environmental factors that are operating during childhood, but the manner in which these factors interact throughout development to ultimately shape aggressive behavior is poorly understood.[1-12] Biological factors may be especially important for aggression that arises during childhood and becomes chronic through adulthood.[4,5,10] There has been particular interest in the relationship between such early-onset chronic aggression and abnormalities in the serotonergic nervous system. In both animals[13,14] and adult humans,[15-20] deficits in central serotonergic activity facilitate impulsive aggression. For example, aggressive adults exhibit a reduced concentration of cerebrospinal 5-hydroxyindoleacetic acid (CSF 5-HIAA), which is the main metabolite of serotonin, and this deficit in CSF 5-HIAA may index reduced activity of the brainstem raphe neurons.[17-21] Similarly, Coccaro et al[16] noted inverse correlations between various indexes of aggression and the prolactin response to fenfluramine hydrochloride challenge in adults. Fenfluramine increases synaptic serotonin levels by releasing serotonin from nerve terminals and inhibiting serotonin reuptake. Increased synaptic serotonin stimulates a rise in the prolactin level, the magnitude of which indexes central serotonergic activity.[16,22]

Retrospective reports of chronic aggression that starts in childhood have predicted reduced CSF 5-HIAA concentrations and a blunted prolactin response to fenfluramine challenge among adults.[5,15,16,19] These results, coupled with the chronicity of early-onset aggression, suggest that the association between aggression and reduced serotonergic activity arises early in life.[3,4] Nevertheless, 2 recent studies in aggressive prepubertal children found positive, rather than inverse, associations between aggression and indexes of central serotonergic activity.[21,22] Castellanos et al[21] found a positive correlation between aggressivity and CSF 5-HIAA concentrations in 29 boys with attention deficit hyperactivity disor-

From the Departments of Child and Adolescent Psychiatry (Drs Pine, Wasserman, Miller, Fried, Greenhill, and Shaffer and Mr Davies), Analytic Neurochemistry (Mr Cooper), and Neuroscience (Dr Parsons), and the Biological Studies Unit (Dr Coplan), New York State Psychiatric Institute and the College of Physicians and Surgeons of Columbia University (Drs Pine, Coplan, Wasserman, Miller, Fried, Greenhill, and Shaffer and Mr Davies), New York, NY.

SUBJECTS AND METHODS

SUBJECTS

As described elsewhere,[26,35,36] subjects in this study were drawn from a sample of 126 boys who were all younger brothers of delinquents in New York, NY. Families were contacted after an older brother was identified through court records. At study intake in 1992 and 1993, we examined associations among rearing factors, children's behavior, and platelet 5-HT_{2A} receptor characteristics in 34 of these boys.[35] Fourteen to 24 months later, 109 boys (86.5%) underwent psychiatric reexaminations.

Exclusion criteria for the fenfluramine challenge study included any physical illness, abnormal blood chemistry values or complete blood cell counts, current use of any medication or illicit substance, and needle phobia. Fifty-six boys who were not excluded for any of these reasons were approached for the fenfluramine challenge study after psychiatric reexamination. To increase the base rates of psychiatric symptoms in the selected subsample, the first 10 boys were required to have at least 1 elevated subscale score on the Child Behavior Checklist (CBCL).[37] Thirty-six of the eligible 56 boys agreed to participate; 2 of these 36 were excluded when they failed to follow the prechallenge protocol. Therefore, this report is based on challenges in 34 boys, who were all from impoverished families; 44% were African American and 56% were Hispanic (**Table 1**). Eight of the 34 boys participated in our prior study of platelet 5-HT_{2A} receptor characteristics.[35]

PSYCHIATRIC ASSESSMENT

Subjects underwent 1 psychiatric assessment at intake and a second assessment in the weeks before the fenfluramine challenge. Both assessments were based on the CBCL[37] and the Diagnostic Interview Schedule for Children[38-40] that were administered to caretakers by a trained interviewer. The CBCL is composed of 2 broadband subscales, each of which subsumes a set of narrowband subscales. It possesses excellent psychometric properties and generates age- and sex-adjusted normative ratings.[37] Because we were interested in externalizing psychiatric symptoms, we selected the broadband CBCL Externalizing subscale and its 2 narrowband component subscales (Aggression and Delinquency). The Diagnostic Interview Schedule for Children generates diagnoses for 32 current *DSM-III-R* Axis I diagnoses with acceptable psychometry.[38-40] We selected diagnoses of oppositional defiant disorder (ODD), conduct disorder (CD), and ADHD. Oppositional defiant disorder and CD were combined into 1 category, since they may be part of a single underlying disorder in young children.[1-3,8-12]

REARING ENVIRONMENT ASSESSMENT

The rearing environment was assessed only at intake, when trained interviewers visited the home of each child for 4 hours. Interviewers completed the Home Observation and Measurement of the Environment Inventory (the HOME scale), which is a standardized 7-subscale measure based on 59 dichotomously coded observations and interview responses.[41] Each subscale exhibits excellent psychometric properties and is coded so that higher scores are given to healthier environments. Existing research, in this[26] and other samples,[27] has demonstrated associations between low HOME subscale scores and disruptive psychiatric symptoms.

For the present study, as in our prior work,[26,35] we selected 3 HOME subscales on an a priori basis: (1) the "Emotional Climate" subscale, which measures the degree to which parents control their temper when they are angry at their child; (2) the "Encouragement of Maturity" subscale, which measures the degree of proper parental limit setting on a child's behavior; and (3) the "Emotional Responsivity" subscale, which measures the degree of parental encouragement and praise exhibited to the child.

SEROTONERGIC ASSESSMENT

Serotonergic activity was assessed by use of the fenfluramine challenge.[16,22,42] All boys were free of medications for at least 1 month; none had prior exposure to psychopharmacological treatment. All boys followed low-monoamine diets for 4 days, fasted the night before the challenge, and received nothing by mouth during the challenge.

An intravenous catheter was inserted by 8:30 AM; baseline blood samples were collected at 9:45 and 10 AM. Oral fenfluramine hydrochloride (10 mg/kg) was given at 10 AM. Blood was sampled hourly until 2 PM. Fenfluramine and norfenfluramine levels were assayed at 4 points. Blood samples were centrifuged, placed on ice, and stored at −20°C to be assayed as a batch. All samples were run in duplicate with the use of previously described methods.[43,44] Prolactin was assayed with the use of a double-antibody radioimmunoassay with intra-assay and interassay coefficients of variation of 2.0% and 3.5%, respectively.[43] Fenfluramine and norfenfluramine levels were quantified by gas chromatography with the use of a nitrogen-selective detector,[44] with intra-assay and interassay relative standard deviation (RSD%) of 2.7% and 3.7%, respectively, for fenfluramine, and of 3.7% and 5.5%, respectively, for norfenfluramine.

DATA ANALYSIS

The prolactin response was quantified by use of the area under the curve (AUC) that was derived from the Simpson approximation,[45] minus the baseline prolactin value. The 2 baseline prolactin values were averaged in this calculation. Associations were also examined with the use of both the maximal prolactin ("prolactin-max") and the maximal minus baseline ("Δ-max") criteria.[16,22,42] Finally, associations were examined with baseline prolactin levels, and analyses of the prolactin response to fenfluramine were rerun while including the baseline prolactin value as a covariate, based on the complicated and incompletely understood relationships among serotonin, dopamine, baseline prolactin, and prolactin change measures.[13-16,46] To the extent that baseline prolactin and prolactin change measures are both influenced by serotonin,[13-16,46] it might be considered "overcontrol" to covary for the baseline prolactin value.[47]

We used Pearson correlations and unpaired Student *t* tests to examine univariate relationships and multiple linear regression or analysis of covariance to examine multivariate relationships. In all analyses, dependent measures were normally distributed, scattergrams were inspected to ensure that outliers were not present, and an a priori α of .05 was used.

der (ADHD), while Halperin et al[22] found larger prolactin responses to fenfluramine in 10 aggressive than in 14 nonagressive boys with ADHD.

At least 3 explanations have been offered for these different findings in children and adults. First, ADHD may play a role in the inconsistencies, since both studies that have found positive associations between prepubertal aggression and central serotonergic measures studied only children with ADHD, while other studies have used more heterogeneous samples. Second, since the serotonergic nervous system may exhibit considerable plasticity through adolescence (eg, down-regulating in response to high levels of endogenous serotonin),[23-25] enhanced serotonergic activity in early childhood could be a developmental precursor of a later serotonergic deficit.[22] Serotonin would then serve different functions in children and adults; this is an idea that is consistent with basic science research.[23-25] Third, differences could result because adverse-rearing conditions may affect the relationship between aggression and serotonin in children.[21] This would be consistent with the ample research that has noted associations between rearing and early-onset aggression.[26-30]

Research on the relationship between adverse rearing and serotonin may enhance understandings of the association between serotonin and aggression across development. Recent studies in nonhuman primates have suggested that rearing circumstances may impact on biology and behavior during development, producing both changes in serotonergic activity and a behavioral pattern analogous to human aggression.[31-34] Preliminary results from our group extended this line of research to humans, as we found that harsh parental discipline correlated with a reduced density of platelet 5-hydroxytryptamine$_{2A}$ (5-HT$_{2A}$) receptors and higher aggression in children.[35] Nevertheless, since most nonhuman primate studies used central rather than platelet serotonin measures, it is important to examine associations between rearing and serotonin in children with the use of central measures.

Based on this research, we entered the present study with the goal of replicating and extending 2 sets of findings. First, we attempted to replicate results that have suggested that aggression in prepubertal children is positively correlated with central serotonergic activity. Second, using a central measure, we attempted to extend findings of an association between adverse-rearing conditions and serotonin in children.[35]

Table 1. Characteristics of the Sample (N=34)*

Variable	Intake	Prechallenge
Age, y	8.4±1.5	10.0±1.5
Psychopathology		
CBCL subscale, *t* score		
Externalizing	55.3±15.1	57.4±12.0
Aggression	59.5±10.0	58.9±10.2
Delinquency	58.8±9.7	60.3±9.8
Internalizing	53.6±14.9	53.8±13.2
No. (%) with a diagnosis of current oppositional defiant or conduct disorder	10 (29)	7 (21)
No. (%) with a diagnosis of current attention deficit hyperactivity disorder	14 (41)	7 (21)
Rearing environment on home subscale, score		
Emotional Climate	4.7±1.5	...
Emotional Responsivity	6.9±2.4	...
Encouragement of Maturity	4.9±1.9	...
Response to fenfluramine challenge		
Prolactin level, ng/mL		
Baseline	...	5.7±1.4
Maximal	...	10.8±3.7
Prolactin response AUC, ng/mL×h	...	113.1±31.3
Maximal fenfluramine hydrochloride plus norfenfluramine level, ng/mL	...	88.0±18.0

**CBCL indicates Child Behavior Checklist; AUC, area under the curve. Data are given as the mean±SD unless otherwise indicated.*

RESULTS

UNIVARIATE ASSOCIATIONS

Stability of Behavior and Relationship With Rearing

The CBCL scores exhibited moderate stability; the HOME and CBCL subscale scores were correlated. As pre-

Table 2. Pearson Correlations Among Continuous Measures*

Measure	AUC_{PRL}	MAT_1	$EMOTV_1$	$EMOTC_1$	EXT_1	AGG_1	DEL_1	EXT_2	AGG_2
MAT_1	−0.59†								
$EMOTV_1$	−0.38‡	+0.62†							
$EMOTC_1$	−0.21	+0.38‡	+0.58†						
EXT_1	+0.49§	−0.16	−0.21	−0.25					
AGG_1	+0.54†	−0.17	−0.23	−0.28	+0.97†				
DEL_1	+0.25	−0.08	−0.10	−0.10	+0.82†	+0.66†			
EXT_2	+0.47§	−0.31	−0.43§	+0.03	+0.48§	+0.50§	+0.30		
AGG_2	+0.48§	−0.32	−0.40§	−0.02	+0.44§	+0.50§	+0.18	+0.96†	
DEL_2	+0.26	−0.22	−0.32	+0.14	+0.40§	+0.33‡	+0.48§	+0.71†	+0.49§

AUC_{PRL} indicates area under the curve, prolactin; MAT, Encouragement of Maturity Home Observation and Measurement of the Environment (HOME) subscale; subscript 1, measure collected at intake; EMOTV, Emotional Responsivity HOME subscale; EMOTC, Emotional Climate HOME subscale; EXT, Child Behavior Checklist (CBCL) Externalizing subscale; AGG, CBCL Aggression subscale; DEL, CBCL Delinquency subscale; and subscript 2, measure collected before challenge.
†$P<.001$.
‡$P<.05$.
§$P<.01$.

sented in **Table 2**, the associations between the HOME and CBCL subscale scores were significant only for the Emotional Responsivity subscale in the current sample. In the full sample, significant associations were documented between the CBCL scores and each HOME subscale score (G.A.W., unpublished data, August 1996).

AUC Prolactin Response and Behavior

The mean values for the prolactin indexes are given in Table 1; Table 2 presents the relationships between the AUC prolactin response and CBCL. The AUC was positively correlated with scores on both the broadband Externalizing and narrowband Aggression subscales, at intake and prechallenge, but with neither the intake nor prechallenge narrowband Delinquency subscale. The baseline prolactin level correlated with the Aggression subscale score, both at intake (r=0.47; P<.01) and prechallenge (r=0.34; P<.05). When the baseline prolactin value was included as a covariate, the partial correlation between the AUC and Aggression subscale score remained significant, both at intake (r=0.36; P<.05) and prechallenge (r=0.37; P<.05).

Given the possibility that ADHD may have accounted for the inconsistencies in prior studies, the AUC data were compared for boys who were classified with respect to ADHD and ODD or CD status. In this analysis, as given in **Table 3**, boys were considered to have ODD or CD or ADHD if they met criteria for these disorders at *either* of the 2 assessments. Boys with ODD or CD showed higher AUC prolactin responses than boys without ODD or CD. In contrast, boys with ADHD but no ODD or CD did not differ from boys with neither ADHD nor ODD nor CD. Boys with ADHD alone had a lower prolactin AUC response than boys with ODD or CD (t_{16}=2.6; P<.05; independent sample t test with the Fisher-Behrens adjustment). Because 12 of the 13 boys with ODD or CD also had ADHD, it was not possible to compare the prolactin response in boys with ODD or CD who had and did not have ADHD.

Beyond the data presented in Table 3, 6 boys had an anxiety disorder in the absence of ODD or CD, 2 had comorbid ADHD, and no boy had a mood disorder. There was a "no-diagnosis" group of 12 boys with no diagnosis at either assessment. The boys with ODD or CD at either assessment had a higher AUC than boys with no diagnosis (n=12; 104.0±23.9 μg/L [mean±SD] [104.0±23.9 ng/mL]×hour). Neither the AUC in the boys with anxiety disorders without ODD or CD (n=6; 104.3±25.6 μg/L [104.3±25.6 ng/mL]×hour) nor in the boys with ADHD without ODD or CD differed from the AUC in the boys with no diagnosis. No differences were found in the baseline prolactin level for all comparisons across diagnostic groups.

AUC Prolactin Response and Rearing Environment

As given in Table 2, the scores on the 2 HOME subscales were negatively correlated with the AUC. Because higher scores on the HOME subscales indicate healthier environments, negative correlations suggest that increasingly adverse-rearing circumstances correlate with larger prolactin responses. There were no significant correlations between the baseline prolactin value and HOME subscale scores.

Table 3. Prolactin Response Based on Diagnosis*

Diagnosis†	AUC_{PRL}, μg/L×h
ODD/CD, at intake assessment‡	
+ODD/CD (n=10)	136.5±35.0
−ODD/CD (n=23)	103.4±24.0, t_{32}=3.2§
ODD/CD, at prechallenge assessment‖	
+ODD/CD (n=7)	139.5±41.8
−ODD/CD (n=27)	106.3±24.6, t_{32}=2.7¶
ODD/CD vs ADHD vs neither, based on both intake and prechallenge assessments#	
+ODD/CD (n=13)	130.5±35.5[a]
−ODD/CD, +ADHD (n=5)	101.3±12.9[b]
−ODD/CD, −ADHD (n=16)	102.7±26.0[b], $F_{2,31}$=3.9¶

**AUC_{PRL}* indicates area under the curve prolactin response; ODD/CD, oppositional defiant or conduct disorder; ADHD, attention deficit hyperactivity disorder; and superscripts a and b, values with the same superscript do not significantly differ (P>.10) on post hoc independent sample t tests while those with different superscripts (a vs b) significantly differ (P<.05). Data are given as the mean±SD.*

†Four subjects met criteria for ODD or CD at both the intake and prechallenge assessments. Six subjects met criteria for ODD or CD only at the intake assessment, and 3 met criteria only at the prechallenge assessment. Data are shown for dichotomizing subjects using only the intake assessment, only the prechallenge assessment, and both the intake and prechallenge assessments.

‡Subjects are dichotomized based on a positive (+) or negative (−) diagnosis for ODD or CD on the Diagnostic Interview Schedule for Children using only the intake assessment.

§P<.05.

‖Subjects are dichotomized based on a positive (+) or negative (−) diagnosis for ODD or CD on the Diagnostic Interview Schedule for Children using only the prechallenge assessment.

¶P<.01.

#To compare groups cross-classified on ODD or CD and ADHD based on both assessments, subjects are categorized into 3 groups using the Diagnostic Interview Schedule for Children as (1) positive (+) on either ODD or CD at either *intake* or *prechallenge (+ODD/CD); (2) negative (-) on ODD* and *CD at* both *intake* and *prechallenge* but *positive (+) for a diagnosis of ADHD at* either *intake* or *prechallenge (−ODD/CD, +ADHD); and (3) negative (-) on ODD, CD,* and *ADHD at* both *the intake and prechallenge assessments (−ODD/CD, −ADHD).*

MULTIVARIATE ANALYSES

Rearing and AUC Response

To examine the specificity of the relationship between rearing measures and serotonergic activity, the AUC was regressed on the 3 HOME subscales in a single model. The step including the 3 subscales accounted for a significant proportion of the variance in the AUC (R^2=0.36; F[3,30]=5.3; P<.005), but only the Encouragement of Maturity subscale predicted the AUC (β=−.58; t=3.3, df=30; P<.005).

Rearing, Behavior, and AUC Response

Given that a child's AUC was predicted both by a pattern of parenting associated with a child's aggressive behavior and by the degree of aggression in the child, a model was fit to consider the statistical independence of these associations. To reduce multicollinearity,[47] we used the mean of the intake and prechallenge Aggression subscale scores. Hence, the AUC was regressed on the HOME subscales and the mean Aggression subscale score in 1 model. This model accounted for most of the variance in the AUC (R^2=0.60; F[4,29]=10.5; $P<.001$). The relationship between the Encouragement of Maturity subscale and AUC remained significant ($\beta=-.54$; t=3.5, df=29; P=.001), as did the relationship between the mean Aggression subscale score and AUC ($\alpha=+.52$; t=5.2, df=29; $P<.001$). Similar results were found when the baseline prolactin value was included as a covariate, namely, both the Encouragement of Maturity ($\beta=-.44$; t=3.6, df=28; P=.001) and Aggression ($\beta=+.32$; t=2.9, df=28; $P<.01$) subscale scores correlated with the AUC.

SUPPLEMENTARY ANALYSES

Prolactin-Max and Peak-Δ Criteria

We found comparable associations when we used prolactin-max or peak-Δ criteria[16,22,42] to define the prolactin response. However, relative to the AUC response, the prolactin-max response correlated somewhat more strongly with the HOME subscale scores ($r=-0.57$; $P<.001$ for the Encouragement of Maturity; $r=-0.52$; $P<.001$ for Emotional Responsivity; and $r=-0.38$; $P<.05$ for Emotional Climate), as did the peak-Δ response ($r=-0.59$; $P<.001$ for Encouragement of Maturity; $r=-0.55$; $P<.001$ for Emotional Responsivity; and $r=-0.39$; $P<.05$ for Emotional Climate). In contrast, the relationships with the CBCL Aggression subscale were slightly weaker than those that were found using the AUC criterion. This applied to correlations between the CBCL Aggression subscale and both the prolactin-max (r=0.52; $P<.001$ at intake; r=0.42; $P<.01$ at prechallenge) or peak-Δ criteria (r=0.43; $P<.01$ at intake; r=0.36; $P<.05$ at prechallenge).

Other Analyses

In a set of post hoc analyses, associations between serotonergic activity and behavior or rearing conditions could not be explained by a number of potentially confounding factors. These factors included fenfluramine or norfenfluramine levels, age, Tanner stage, body size, social class, ethnicity, season of fenfluramine challenge, the degree of psychiatric symptoms in parents (including substance abuse or antisocial behavior, measured with standardized interviews[48]), and the child's IQ (Wechsler Intelligence Scale for Children–III) or academic achievement (Wechsler Achievement Scale–III). No boy had a history of illicit drug or alcohol use. No changes had occurred in family composition due to trauma or violence between the intake HOME assessment and the fenfluramine challenge. Correlations between the prolactin response and CBCL Internalizing subscale score, which is a measure of anxiety and depressive symptoms, were markedly lower than those between the prolactin response and CBCL Externalizing subscale score (data available on request). Finally, there was no evidence of a relationship between psychiatric measures and the timing of the peak prolactin response. Associations between disruptive psychiatric disorder and the prolactin level were seen at both 3 and 4 hours, but not at 1 or 2 hours, after fenfluramine ingestion (data also available on request).

COMMENT

SEROTONIN AND AGGRESSION

This study found a positive correlation between aggression ratings and the prolactin response to fenfluramine challenge in prepubertal boys. This finding is consistent with that of 2 prior reports on the association between aggression and central serotonin measures in prepubertal boys: one report that relied on CSF 5-HIAA[21] and a second report that relied on the prolactin response to fenfluramine.[22] In a third study among 15 prepubertal boys, Stoff et al[49] found no significant correlation between the prolactin response to fenfluramine and scores on 2 aggression scales, although there was a nonsignificant positive correlation (r=0.38) between the prolactin response and score on one aggression scale. In contrast, Kruesi et al,[50] studying children and adolescents, found low CSF 5-HIAA levels in subjects with disruptive behavior disorders compared with those in subjects with obsessive-compulsive disorder. In the subjects with disruptive behavior disorders, the CSF 5-HIAA levels were negatively correlated with the severity of aggression at follow-up.[51] Viewed against evidence that extreme aggression before puberty predicts chronic aggression in adulthood[1-12] and evidence that chronically aggressive adults have a deficit in serotonin,[15-20] the present and prior[21,22,49-51] studies in children and adolescents raise the possibility of a developmental change in the relationship between serotonin and aggression.

SEROTONIN AND REARING FACTORS

The present study found a positive correlation between the prolactin response to fenfluramine and maladaptive parent-child interaction patterns that are implicated in aggression, as reflected by scores on the HOME subscales.[26,27] While this extends our prior cross-sectional results based on platelet 5-HT_{2A} receptor density at intake,[35] the 2 reports show both inconsistencies and consistencies. For example, the prolactin AUC response, but not the platelet 5-HT_{2A} receptor density, correlated with aggression ratings. Both the prolactin AUC response and platelet 5-HT_{2A} receptor density did correlate with the HOME subscale scores. However, unlike the prolactin AUC response, the intake platelet 5-HT_{2A} receptor density correlated most strongly with the Emotional Climate subscale at intake, although there was also a correlation with the Emotional Responsivity subscale scores (r=0.36; $P<.05$).

Differences in the relationship between the HOME subscale scores and the 2 serotonin measures might relate to the fact that each HOME subscale showed a unique relationship with aggression ratings in the full sample from which boys in the 2 reports were drawn. The Emotional Climate subscale predicted only intake aggression ratings, the Encouragement of Maturity subscale predicted only prechallenge ratings, and the Emotional Responsivity subscale predicted both intake and prechallenge ratings (G.A.W., unpublished data, August 1996). Differences also might relate to the sampling variability or to the unclear relationship between central and peripheral serotonin measures.[42]

These findings are consistent with those of nonhuman primate studies that have noted that a disruption of the parent-child relationship may produce behavior analogous to human aggression[34] and changes in central serotonergic activity.[31-33] The findings from the primate studies performed by Rosenblum et al[32,34,52,53] seem to be particularly relevant. Unlike studies that remove mothers from the social milieu,[33,54] Rosenblum and colleagues[32,34,52,53] housed mother and child bonnet macaques together while they examined the effect of stress on biology and behavior in these monkeys. In these studies, the stress of a "variable foraging demand" condition led a mother bonnet macaque to become preoccupied and uninvolved with the regulation of her child's behavior, but it did not increase overt hostility toward the child.[52,53] This pattern is similar to items on the Encouragement of Maturity and Emotional Responsivity HOME subscales. The change in maternal behavior associated with the stress of the variable foraging demand condition predicted an abnormal response to serotonergic challenge in the children of stressed mother bonnet macaques.[32] This is consistent with our findings that have linked the HOME subscales and the prolactin AUC response in human children. As a whole, the findings from these primate studies and our results suggest an association between serotonin and emotionally affiliative behavior; this is a conclusion supported by the results of other primate studies that have used social or pharmacological manipulations.[55,56]

While primate studies suggest associations between manipulated rearing conditions and serotonin, such experimental paradigms in humans are obviously ethically unfeasible. Therefore, a direct effect of rearing on serotonin remains only 1 of at least 2 other plausible explanations for the association that was found in this study between rearing factors and serotonin. First, childhood aggression might partially explain the association, since the boys' aggression ratings at intake in this study predicted HOME ratings at intake and the subsequent prolactin response to fenfluramine challenge. The results from the multivariate analyses, however, are not consistent with this possibility, where the association between rearing and serotonin would be expected to disappear after statistical control for child aggression.[47] Second, genetic or environmental factors that influence parent-child interactions, childhood aggression, and childhood serotonin in tandem could play a role. For example, a genetic monoamine oxidase deficit may produce familial serotonin abnormalities and impulsive aggression.[57] In animal studies, a congenital monoamine oxidase deficiency produces early-life elevations of serotonin activity, preceding an adulthood serotonin deficit.[23-25]

STUDY LIMITATIONS

Four features limit the conclusions from this study. First, it was not possible to study demographically matched comparison children without a family history of delinquency. Without such comparisons, we cannot designate 1 or another group of boys as abnormal on a serotonergic basis, and the correlational nature of our results should be kept in mind. A lack of comparison data does not preclude the delineation of biological correlates of aggression among children who are at familial risk for disruptive psychopathology.

Second, there are limitations to our assessment of serotonergic activity. We did not use placebo challenges, which are difficult to perform in prepubertal children.[22,58] Furthermore, the prolactin response to D,L-fenfluramine is probably influenced by dopaminergic and other neurobiological factors besides serotonergic activity. Nevertheless, the prolactin response to racemic and D-fenfluramine, which is the more specific serotonin probe, are highly correlated.[59]

Third, we focused on mother-son interactions and serotonin in boys. We did not examine the relationship between aggression and the pattern of interactions with fathers, who were rarely present during home visits. Future studies might consider if paternal behavior relates to both the behavior and biological characteristics of the child. Similarly, future studies might examine associations in girls, since gender differences have been found in serotonergic correlates of childhood depression.[58] It also may be important to examine maternal serotonin. Studies in humans[60] and nonhuman primates[61] suggest that both maternal behavior and maternal serotonin could play a role in associations among rearing factors, a boy's serotonin profile, and his behavioral profile.

Finally, we measured 2 dynamic constructs (ie, the rearing environment and serotonergic activity) at single time points. Although there were no changes in family composition due to trauma or violence, other aspects of parent-child interactions may change over time. Future studies attempting replications might conduct more extensive home observations at regular intervals. Nevertheless, the HOME subscales do predict psychiatric and cognitive constructs both cross-sectionally and over time,[26,27,41] and Plomin[62] has argued that the HOME ratings are influenced by genetic factors. This suggests that the HOME subscales may relate to some potentially enduring aspects of biology. We also conducted fenfluramine challenges at only 1 time point. Future studies might conduct challenges at multiple developmental stages to further understandings of longitudinal associations among serotonin, rearing factors, and childhood aggression.

Accepted for publication August 28, 1996.

This project was supported by a grant to the Lowenstein Center for the Study of Disruptive Disorders (Dr Wasserman, principal investigator) from the Lowenstein Foundation, New York, NY, and by Research Training Grant MH-16432, Center Grant MH-43878 to the Center to Study Youth Depression, Anxiety, and Suicide, and

Scientist Development Awards MH-01391 (Dr Pine) and MH-01039 (Dr Coplan) for Clinicians from the National Institute of Mental Health, Bethesda, Md.

Presented in part at "Understanding Aggressive Behavior in Children" conference by the New York Academy of Sciences, New York, NY, September 29 to October 2, 1995.

We acknowledge the helpful suggestions of Donald F. Klein, MD, and J. John Mann, MD, in preparing the manuscript and the help of Jack M. Gorman, MD, Laszlo A. Papp, MD, and the staff of the Biological Studies Unit, New York State Psychiatric Institute, New York, in conducting this study.

Corresponding author: Daniel S. Pine, MD, New York State Psychiatric Institute, 722 W 168th St, Unit 78, New York, NY 10032.

REFERENCES

1. Rutter M, Giller H. *Juvenile Delinquency: Trends and Perspective.* New York, NY: Guilford Press; 1980.
2. Moffit TE. Adolescence-limited and life-course–persistent antisocial behavior: a developmental taxonomy. *Psychol Rev.* 1993;100:674-701.
3. Lahey BB, Hart EL, Pliszka S, Applegate B, McBurnett K. Neurophysiological correlates of conduct disorder: a rationale and a review of research. *J Clin Child Psychol.* 1993;22:141-153.
4. Zubieta JK, Alessi NE. Is there a role of serotonin in the disruptive behavior disorders? a literature review. *J Child Adolesc Psychopharmacol.* 1993;3:11-35.
5. Brown GL, Goodwin FK, Ballenger JC, Goyer PF, Major LF. Aggression in humans correlates with cerebrospinal fluid amine metabolites. *Psychiatry Res.* 1979; 1:131-139.
6. Farrington D, Ohlin L, Wilson JQ. *Understanding and Controlling Crime.* New York, NY: Springer-Verlag NY Inc; 1986.
7. Caspi A, Elder GH, Bem DJ. Moving against the word: life-course patterns of explosive children. *Dev Psychol.* 1987;28:308-313.
8. Farrington DP. Early predictors of adolescent aggression and adult violence. *Violence Vict.* 1989;4:79-100.
9. Farrington DP. Age and crime. In: Tonry M, Morris N, eds. *Crime and Justice: An Annual Review of Research.* Chicago, Ill: University of Chicago Press; 1986;7: 189-250.
10. Moffit TE, Silva PA. Neuropsychological deficit and self-reported delinquency in an unselected birth cohort. *J Am Acad Child Adolesc Psychiatry.* 1988;27:233-240.
11. Robins LN. Sturdy childhood predictors of adult antisocial behavior: replications from longitudinal studies. *Psychol Med.* 1978;8:611-622.
12. Loeber R, Green SM, Keenan K, Lahey BB. Which boys will fare worse? early predictors of the onset of conduct disorder in a six-year longitudinal study. *J Am Acad Child Adolesc Psychiatry.* 1995;34:488-498.
13. Olivier B, Moss J, Tulp M, van der Poel A. Animal models of anxiety and aggression in the study of serotonergic agents. In: Langer SZ, Brunello N, Racagni G, Mendlewicz J, eds. *Serotonin Receptor Subtypes: Pharmacologic Significance and Clinical Implications.* Basel, Switzerland: S Karger AG; 1992; 1:67-79.
14. Soubire P. Reconciling the role of central serotonin neurons in human and animal behavior. *Behav Brain Sci.* 1986;9:319-364.
15. Brown GL, Ebert MH, Goyer PF, Jimerson DC, Klein WJ, Bunney WE, Goodwin FK. Aggression, suicide, and serotonin: relationships to CSF amine metabolites. *Am J Psychiatry.* 1982;139:741-746.
16. Coccaro EF, Siever LJ, Klar H, Maurer G, Cochrane K, Cooper TB, Mohs RC, Davis KL. Serotonergic studies in affective and personality disorder patients: correlates with suicidal and impulsive aggression. *Arch Gen Psychiatry.* 1989;43:587-599.
17. Virkkunen M, Rawlings R, Tokola R, Poland RE, Guidotti A, Nemeroff C, Bissette G, Kalogeras K, Daronen S, Linnoila M. CSF biochemistries, glucose metabolism, diurnal activity rhythms in alcoholic, violent offenders, fire setters, and healthy volunteers. *Arch Gen Psychiatry.* 1994;51:20-27.
18. Virkkunen M, Nuutila A, Goodwin FK, Linnoila M. Cerebrospinal fluid monoamine metabolite levels in male arsonists. *Arch Gen Psychiatry.* 1987;44:241-247.
19. Limson R, Goldman D, Roy A, Lamparski D, Ravitz B, Adinoff B, Linnoila M. Personality and cerebrospinal fluid monamine metabolites in alcoholics and controls. *Arch Gen Psychiatry.* 1991;48:437-441.
20. Linnoila M, Virkkunen M, Scheinin M, Nuutila A, Rimon R, Goodwin FK. Low cerebrospinal fluid 5-hydroxyindoleacetic acid differentiates impulsive from nonimpulsive violent behavior. *Life Sci.* 1983;33:2609-2614.
21. Castellanos J, Elia J, Kruesi M, Gulotta CS, Mefford IN, Potter WZ, Ritchie GF, Rapoport JL. Cerebrospinal fluid monamine metabolites in boys with attention-deficit hyperactivity disorder. *Psychiatry Res.* 1994;52:305-316.
22. Halperin JM, Sharma V, Siever LJ, Schwartz ST, Matier K, Wornell G, Newcorn JH. Serotonergic function in aggressive and nonaggressive boys with attention deficit hyperactivity disorder. *Am J Psychiatry.* 1994;151:243-248.
23. Whitaker-Azmitia PM, Zhang X, Clarke C. Effects of gestational exposure to monoamine oxidase inhibitors in rats: preliminary behavioral and neurochemical studies. *Neuropsychopharmacology.* 1994;11:125-132.
24. Shemer AV, Azmitia EC, Whitaker-Azmitia PM. Dose-related effects of prenatal 5-methoxytryptamine (5-MT) on development of serotonin terminal density and behavior. *Dev Brain Res.* 1991;59:59-63.
25. Whitaker-Azmitia PM, Azmitia E. Autoregulation of fetal serotonergic neuronal development: role of high affinity serotonin receptors. *Neurosci Lett.* 1986;67: 307-312.
26. Wasserman GA, Miller LS, Pinner E, Jaramillo B. Parenting predictors of early conduct problems in urban high risk boys. *J Am Acad Child Adolesc Psychiatry.* 1996;35:1227-1236.
27. Dubow EF, Ippolito MF. Effects of poverty and quality of the home environment on changes in the academic and behavioral adjustment of elementary school-aged children. *J Clin Child Psychol.* 1994;23:401-412.
28. Dodge KA, Coie JD, Brakke NP. Behavior patterns of socially rejected and neglected preadolescents: the role of social approach and aggression. *Dev Psychol.* 1982;10:389-410.
29. Cohen P, Brook J. Family factors related to the persistence of psychopathology in children and adolescents. *Psychiatry.* 1987;50:332-345.
30. Lewis DL. From abuse to violence: psychophysiological consequences of maltreatment. *J Am Acad Child Adolesc Psychiatry.* 1992;31:383-391.
31. Botchin B, Kaplan JR, Manuck SB, Mann JJ. Neuroendocrine responses to fenfluramine challenge are influenced by exposure to chronic social stress in adult male cynomolgus macaques. *Psychoneuroendocrinology.* 1994;19:1-11.
32. Rosenblum LA, Coplan JD, Bassoff T, Gorman JM, Andrews MW. Adverse early experiences affect noradrenergic and serotonergic functioning in adult primates. *Biol Psychiatry.* 1994;35:221-227.
33. Kraemer GW, Ebert MH, Schmidt DE, McKinney WT. A longitudinal study of the effect of different social rearing conditions on cerebrospinal fluid norepinephrine and biogenic amine metabolites in rhesus monkeys. *Neuropsychopharmacology.* 1989;2:175-189.
34. Rosenblum LA. Human aggression: a perspective drawn from nonhuman primates. In: Glick RA, Roose SP, eds. *Rage, Power, and Aggression.* New Haven, Conn: Yale University Press; 1993:194-211.
35. Pine DS, Wasserman G, Coplan JD, Fried JA, Huang Y, Kassir S, Greenhill L, Shaffer DS, Parsons B. Platelet 5-HT2A characteristics and rearing factors in boys at risk for delinquency—a preliminary report. *Am J Psychiatry.* 1996;153:538-544.
36. Pine DS, Wasserman G, Coplan JD, Staghezza-Jaramillo B, Davies M, Fried JA, Greenhill L, Shaffer DS. Cardiac factors and disruptive behavior in boys at risk for behavior disorders. *Psychosom Med.* 1997;58:342-353.
37. Achenbach TM. *Manual for the Child Behavior Checklist/4-18 and 1991 Profile.* Burlington, Vt: University of Vermont; 1991.
38. Shaffer D, Schwab-Stone M, Fisher P, Cohen P, Piacentini J, Davies M, Edelbrock C, Regier D. The Diagnostic Interview Schedule for Children Revised Version (DISC-R): preparation, field testing, inter-rater reliability, and acceptability. *J Am Acad Child Adolesc Psychiatry.* 1993;32:643-650.
39. Jensen P, Roper M, Fisher P, Piacentini J, Canino G, Richters J, Rubio-Stipec M, Dulcan M, Goodman S, Davies M, Rae D, Shaffer D, Bird H, Lahey B, Schwab-Stone M. Test-retest reliability of the Diagnostic Interview Schedule for Children (DISC 2.1): parent, child, and combined algorithms. *Arch Gen Psychiatry.* 1995; 52:61-71.
40. Schwab-Stone M, Fallon T, Briggs M, Crowther B. Reliability of diagnostic reporting for children aged 6-11 years: a test-retest study of the Diagnostic Interview Schedule for Children–Revised. *Am J Psychiatry.* 1994;151:1048-1054.
41. Bradley RH. The HOME Inventory: rationale and research. *J Child Psychol Psychiatry.* 1985;26(suppl 4):191-201.
42. Mann JJ, McBride PA, Brown RP, Linnoila M, Leon AC, DeMeo M, Mieczkowski T, Myers JE, Stanley M. Relationship between central and peripheral serotonin indexes in depressed and suicidal psychiatric inpatients. *Arch Gen Psychiatry.* 1992;49:442-446.
43. Sinha YN, Selba FW, Lewis OJ, Vanderlaan WP. A homologous RIA for human prolactin. *J Clin Endocrinol Metab.* 1973;36:509.
44. Krebs HA, Cheng LK, Wright GJ. Determination of fenfluramine and norfenflur-

amine in plasma using a nitrogen-sensitive detector. *J Chromatogr.* 1984;310: 412-417.

45. Press WH, Flannery BP, Teukolsky SA, Betterling WT. *Numeric Recipes for the Art of Scientific Computing.* New York, NY: Cambridge University Press; 1986.
46. Hanna GL, McCracken JT, Cantwell DP. Prolactin in childhood obsessive-compulsive disorder: clinical correlates and response to clomipramine. *J Am Acad Child Adolesc Psychiatry.* 1991;30;2:173-178.
47. Cohen J, Cohen P. *Multiple Regression/Correlation Analysis for the Behavioral Sciences.* 2nd ed. Hillsdale, NJ: Erlbaum; 1983.
48. Lisch JD, Weissman MM, Adams PB, Hoven CW, Bird H. Family history epidemiologic pilot testing and validation. *Psychiatr Res.* 1995;57:169-190.
49. Stoff DM, Pasatiempo AP, Yeung J, Cooper TB, Bridger WH, Raninovich H. Neuroendocrine response to D,L-fenfluramine and aggression in disruptive behavior disorders of children and adolescents. *Psychiatry Res.* 1992;43:263-276.
50. Kruesi MJP, Rapoport JL, Hamburger SD, Hibbs E, Potter WZ, Lenane M, Brown GL. Cerebrospinal fluid monoamine metabolites, aggression, and impulsivity in disruptive behavior disorders of children and adolescents. *Arch Gen Psychiatry.* 1990;47:419-426.
51. Kruesi MJP, Hibbs ED, Zahn TP, Keysor CS, Hamburger SD, Bartko JJ, Rapoport JL. A 2-year prospective follow-up study of children and adolescents with disruptive behavior disorders. *Arch Gen Psychiatry.* 1992;49:429-435.
52. Rosenblum LA, Paully GS. The effects of varying environmental demands on maternal and infant behavior. *Child Dev.* 1984;55:305-314.
53. Andrews MW, Rosenblum LA. Attachment in monkey infants raised in variable and low-demand environments. *Child Dev.* 1991;62:686-693.
54. Higley JD, Suomi SJ, Linnoila M. CSF monoamine metabolite concentrations vary according to age, rearing, and sex, and are influenced by the stressor of social separation in rhesus monkeys. *Psychopharmacology (Berl).* 1991;103:551-556.
55. Raleigh MJ, McGuire MT, Brammer GL, Yuwiler A. Social and environmental influences on blood serotonin concentration in monkeys. *Arch Gen Psychiatry.* 1984; 41:405-410.
56. Raleigh MJ, McGuire MT, Brammer GL, Pollack DB, Yuwiler A. Serotonergic mechanisms promote dominance acquisition in adult male vervet monkeys. *Brain Res.* 1991;559:181-190.
57. Brunner HG, Nelen M, Breakefield XO, Ropers HH, van Oost BA. Abnormal behavior associated with a point mutation in the structural gene for monoamine oxidase A. *Science.* 1993;262:578-580.
58. Ryan ND, Birmaher B, Perel JM, Dahl RE, Meyer V, Al-Shabbout M, Iyengar S, Puigh-Antich J. Neuroendocrine response to L-5-hydroxytryptophan challenge in prepubertal major depression: depressed vs normal children. *Arch Gen Psychiatry.* 1992;49:843-851.
59. Coccaro EF, Kovoussi RJ, Cooper TB, Hauger R. Hormonal response to D- and D,L-fenfluramine in human subjects. *Neuropsychopharmacology.* 1996;15:595-607.
60. Cook EH, Stein MA, Ellison T, Unis AS, Leventhal BL. Attention deficit hyperactivity disorder and whole-blood serotonin levels: effects of comorbidity. *Psychiatry Res.* 1995;57:13-20.
61. Higley JD, King ST, Hasert MF, Champoux M, Suomi SJ, Linnoila M. Stability of interindividual differences in serotonin function and its relationship to severe aggression and competent social behavior in rhesus macaque females. *Neuropsychopharmacology.* 1996;14:67-76.
62. Plomin R. *Genetics and Experience: the Interplay Between Nature and Nurture.* Thousand Oaks, Calif: SagePublications; 1994.

Correction

Error in Figure. In the article titled "Backward Masking Performance in Unaffected Siblings of Schizophrenic Patients: Evidence for a Vulnerability Indicator" published in the May issue (1997;54:465-472), the numbers given for the x-axis in Figure 5 (on page 469) were printed incorrectly. Figure 5 is reprinted correctly here. The journal regrets the error.

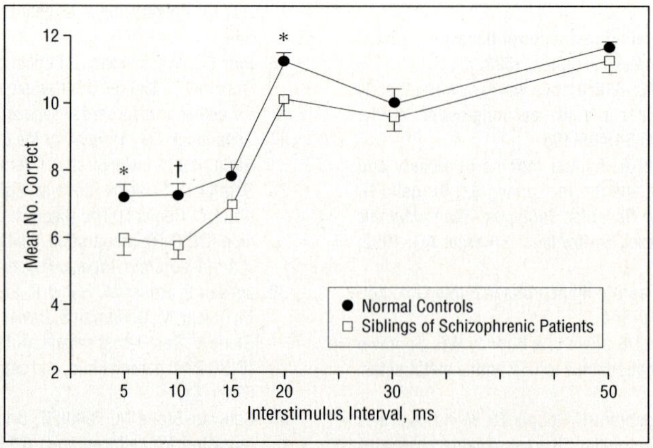

Figure 5. *Results for unaffected siblings of schizophrenic patients and control subjects on a location masking task with a focused target. The energy of the mask was equal to that of the target. Asterisk indicates* P<.05; *dagger,* P<.025.

ORIGINAL ARTICLE

Psychiatric Outcomes in Low-Birth-Weight Children at Age 6 Years: Relation to Neonatal Cranial Ultrasound Abnormalities

Agnes H. Whitaker, MD; Ronan Van Rossem, PhD; Judith F. Feldman, PhD; Irvin Sam Schonfeld, PhD, MPH; Jennifer A. Pinto-Martin, PhD; Carolyn Torre, RN, MA; David Shaffer, MD; Nigel Paneth, MD, MPH

Background: This study examined the relation of neonatal cranial ultrasound abnormalities to psychiatric disorder at age 6 years in a regional birth cohort of low-birth-weight children.

Methods: Neonatal cranial ultrasound abnormalities were classified as (1) isolated germinal matrix and/or intraventricular hemorrhage (suggestive of injury to glial precursors) or (2) parenchymal lesions and/or ventricular enlargement (suggestive of white matter injury) with or without germinal matrix–intraventricular hemorrhage. Psychiatric disorders by *DSM-III-R* at age 6 years were assessed by means of a structured parent interview. Children with severe mental retardation were excluded. Analyses were conducted first in the entire sample and then in children with normal intelligence.

Results: Twenty-two percent of the cohort had at least 1 psychiatric disorder, the most common being attention deficit hyperactivity disorder (15.6%). In the entire sample, parenchymal lesions and/or ventricular enlargement increased risk relative to no abnormality, independently of other biological and social predictors, for any disorder (odds ratio [OR], 4.4; 95% confidence interval [CI], 1.8-10.3; $P<.001$), attention deficit hyperactivity disorder (OR, 3.4; CI, 1.3-8.7; $P=.02$), and tic disorders (OR, 8.7; CI, 1.3-57.7; $P=.02$). In children of normal intelligence, parenchymal lesions/ventricular enlargement independently increased risk for any disorder (OR, 4.8; CI, 1.6-12.0; $P<.01$), attention deficit hyperactivity disorder (OR, 4.5; CI, 1.3-16.0; $P=.02$), and separation anxiety (OR, 5.3; CI, 1.1-24.8; $P=.03$). These effects were not ameliorated by female sex or social advantage. Isolated germinal matrix/intraventricular hemorrhage was not related to psychiatric disorder at age 6 years.

Conclusion: Neonatal cranial ultrasound abnormalities suggestive of white matter injury significantly increased risk for some psychiatric disorders at age 6 years in low-birth-weight children.

Arch Gen Psychiatry. 1997;54:847-856

From the Division of Child and Adolescent Psychiatry, Columbia University and New York State Psychiatric Institute (Drs Whitaker, Van Rossem, Feldman, and Shaffer and Ms Torre) and Gertrude H. Sergievsky Center, Columbia University (Dr Whitaker) New York, NY; Department of Sociology and Criminal Justice, University of Delaware, Newark (Dr Van Rossem); City College of the City University of New York (Dr Schonfeld); School of Nursing and Division of Biostatistics and Epidemiology, Department of Pediatrics, School of Medicine, University of Pennsylvania, Philadelphia (Dr Pinto-Martin); Program in Epidemiology and Department of Pediatrics and Human Development, College of Human Medicine, Michigan State University, East Lansing (Dr Paneth).

THE INTRODUCTION, in the early 1980s, of ultrasonography (US) as a noninvasive means of imaging the brain in low-birth-weight (LBW; <2.5 kg) newborns brought an unprecedented opportunity to study the sequelae of perinatal brain injury. While a substantial body of literature now exists on the motor and cognitive sequelae of neonatal cranial US abnormalities in LBW infants,[1-3] the relation of these abnormalities to childhood psychiatric disorders has been relatively neglected. Such research is timely because the balance of evidence suggests that behavior problems,[4-8] in particular those found in attention deficit hyperactivity disorder (ADHD),[9-17] are an important aspect of the morbidity found among schoolage LBW survivors, whose numbers continue to grow as a result of improved techniques of newborn intensive care.[18] Such research is important because an estimated 6.5% of children who will become of school age in the United States in 1997 were LBW infants (Nigel Paneth, MD, written communication, August 1996), and because term infants of normal birth weight may sustain similar types of brain injury during the late second and early third trimesters.[19,20]

In LBW neonates, perinatal brain injury is most commonly subcortical, reflecting site-specific vulnerabilities of the developing fetal brain in the late second and early third trimesters.[21,22] One site of vulnerability is the germinal matrix. The germinal matrix proliferates neuroblasts and glioblasts during early and middle gestation and provides the protomap for the columnar organization of the cortex; it then involutes by 34 weeks of gestation. In response to metabolic and hemodynamic stress, the fragile capillaries of the germinal matrix can easily bleed, sometimes into the adjacent ventricle. Such

SUBJECTS AND METHODS

BIRTH COHORT AND ATTRITION

Birth Cohort

Participants were members of the Neonatal Brain Hemorrhage Study birth cohort.[25,33] That study prospectively enrolled 1105 consecutive infants with birth weights of 501 to 2000 g who were cared for in the neonatal intensive care units of 3 New Jersey hospitals between September 1, 1984, and June 30, 1987. Enrollees accounted for 83% of all neonates weighing less than 2000 g and for about 90% of all those weighing less than 1500 g born in 3 New Jersey counties during that period. According to a protocol described elsewhere,[33] the cohort was screened with cranial US scans obtained at 4 hours, 24 hours, and 7 days of life; 98% of the cohort was scanned at least 1 of these times and 47% were also scanned between the third and fifth hospital weeks and/or before discharge. Scans were read independently by at least 2 radiologists who were unaware of all clinical information except birth weight and were submitted to a third reader in cases of disagreement. In 94% of cases, diagnostic agreement by 2 readers was obtained.[33] A maternal interview and systematic chart abstraction provided other important prenatal, perinatal, and neonatal information.[33] At about 2 years of age, 86% of survivors were assessed for major neurodevelopmental impairments[2] and for behavior problems, by means of a standardized parent questionnaire, the Child Behavior Checklist for 2- to 3-year-olds (CBCL/2-3).[34]

Age 6 Years

By age 6 years, 207 infants had died, leaving 898 children eligible for follow-up, of whom 685 (76%) participated in the study at age 6 years. Of the 213 nonparticipants, 45 families (5% of those eligible) refused, 143 (16%) could not be located, and 25 children (3%) had been adopted. While nonparticipants had higher scores on an index of maternal social disadvantage[3] (mean risk count, 1.8 vs 0.9; $P<.001$), they did not differ from participants in birth characteristics, including US status, or on behavior problems at age 2 years (CBCL/2-3 Total Problem Score).[34] Of the 685 participants, 597 (87%) were assessed at home visits, representing 66.5% of the eligible sample; the remainder were assessed by telephone (85 subjects) or mail (3 subjects). Birth characteristics, maternal social disadvantage, and total behavior problems at 2 and 6 years of age (as measured with the CBCL for 4- to 18-year-olds)[35] did not differ by mode of assessment.

The present report was limited to the 564 children seen at home for whom the psychiatric diagnostic interview was obtained and considered valid. The interview was not obtained on 12 children because of time constraints or other factors and was considered invalid for 21 children too severely disabled to be tested with the Stanford-Binet Intelligence Scale, Fourth Edition (SB).[36] These latter 21 children had a mean (±SD) composite score on the Vineland Adaptive Behavior Scale[37] of 39.4±8.5, indicating that they were truly disabled rather than uncooperative. There were no sociodemographic differences between the children having psychiatric interview data and the 33 children without it.

PROCEDURES

All procedures were approved by the New York State Psychiatric Institute institutional review board. A pediatric nurse practitioner (C.T.) and a psychologist, both unaware of US status, conducted the home visits after obtaining written informed consent. The nurse obtained parental reports on child psychiatric disorder, behavior problems and adaptive functioning, family functioning, and parental mental health. She examined the child for motor problems and rated the child's level of socioemotional impairment and the home environment. The psychologist administered the child cognitive assessments and rated the child's behavior during testing. Teacher report on behavior problems was also requested.

PREDICTORS

Neonatal Cranial US Status

Ultrasound abnormalities are defined as follows. A GMH was defined by focal echodensity in the thalamocaudate groove, just lateral to the frontal horns of the lateral ventricles. An IVH was defined by an echodense focus or foci within the lateral, third, or fourth ventricles separate from, and at least as echodense as, the choroid plexus. A parenchymal lesion (PL) was defined by focal or confluent echodense and/or echolucent areas in the parenchyma. A ventricular enlargement (VE) was defined by at least moderate enlargement, as judged by the radiologist, of at least 1 lateral ventricle on the final scan obtained.

On postmortem examination, both GMH and IVH are associated with destruction of the germinal matrix and its glial precursor cells,[38,39] while PLs and VEs are associated with evidence of ischemic injury to white matter.[26,27] Thus, 3 mutually exclusive groups, more consistent with pathological findings than the widely used Papile classification,[40] were formed: (1) no abnormality (NA); (2) isolated GMH and/or IVH (GMH/IVH); and (3) PL and/or VE, with or without GMH or IVH (PL/VE).

Non-US Predictors

Prenatal factors included maternal social disadvantage, defined by a composite index described elsewhere[3]; maternal tobacco use, measured by the average number of cigarettes smoked per day during this pregnancy (log transformed); and maternal alcohol consumption during pregnancy, scored as a 3-category variable (none; mild [1-6 drinks a week and <3 drinks on any occasion]; and severe [≥7 drinks a week or ≥3 drinks on any occasion]).[41] *Perinatal factors* included sex, 5-minute Apgar score, gestational age, and fetal growth ratio (birth weight relative to the median

hemorrhage occurs in up to 40% of very LBW (VLBW) neonates during the perinatal period.[23]

A second site of vulnerability is the developing subcortical white matter, which is especially sensitive to ischemic injury and metabolic insults before 32 weeks of gestation because of both vascular and cellular factors. From a vascular standpoint, the deep white matter has but a single arterial supply[24,25] and thus of the weight-for-gestational-age distributions compiled by Williams et al[42]). *Neonatal complications of prematurity* were indexed by fraction of inspired oxygen at the end of 24 hours,[43,44] and *neonatal chronic illness* by days receiving mechanical ventilation.[3] *Social disadvantage at age 6* was measured by means of 2 composite indexes. One index, "distal social disadvantage" (mean±SD, −0.02±0.68), was calculated as the sum of the standardized scores of the following variables: single-parent family, mother's education (reversed), household income (reversed), any income from welfare, and the Four Factor Index of Social Status (A. B. Hollingshead, PhD, unpublished data, 1975; scale reversed); if any of these variables were missing, the mean of the remaining variables was substituted. The second index, "proximal social disadvantage" (mean±SD, −0.03±0.69), was calculated similarly by means of the HOME[45] total score (reversed), the General Health Questionnaire,[46] and the Family Dysfunction Scale of the Family Health and Activity Questionnaire.[47]

CHILD OUTCOMES

Psychiatric Diagnoses at Age 6 Years

The Diagnostic Interview Schedule for Children–Parent version 2.1P (DISC 2.1P)[48] is a structured interview that assesses *DSM-III-R*[49] psychiatric disorders. The child version was not used because of the unreliability of self-report at this age.[50] The DISC 2.1P has been shown to have good sensitivity for rare disorders[48] and adequate test-retest reliability for common disorders in older children.[51]

In the present sample, DISC 2.1P diagnoses showed reasonable agreement with standardized assessments of behavior problems. For example, children with ADHD, when compared with children with other diagnoses, had higher ratings of attention problems from parents on the CBCL/4-18[35] (mean±SD T score, 65.4±8.8 vs 57.7±6.2; $t[121]=4.79$, $P<.001$) and from teachers on the Teacher's Report Form[52] (mean±SD T score, 61.8±8.8 vs 57.2±11.1; $t[83]=2.08$, $P=.04$). Moreover, children with ADHD were more likely to be rated as inattentive (31.0%) or hyperactive (42.9%) by the study psychologist on the Test Behavior Checklist[53] than were children with other diagnoses (5.9% [$P<.01$] and 17.6% [$P=.01$], respectively) (additional data available on request).

Table 1 shows the specific disorders assessed, grouped into diagnostic clusters consistent with *DSM-III-R*. Some *DSM-III-R* disorders were not assessed because of their rarity at this age. "Any disorder" was defined as any 1 of the 19 disorders listed. Diagnoses were derived by means of algorithms (available on request) that implemented diagnostic inclusion criteria in the *DSM-III-R*.[49] Psychiatric exclusion criteria were not used; developmental exclusion criteria were used for the elimination disorders. Consistent with other studies,[54,55] a diagnosis of disorder was not assigned on the basis of symptoms alone. It was also necessary to have at least mild psychosocial impairment (defined by a nurse's rating of <71 on the Children's Global Clinical Assessment Scale).[55] The diagnosis of ADHD, for example, was assigned only if the child had at least 8 of 14 possible symptoms of ADHD, each symptom had been present most of the time for at least 6 months, and the overall Children's Global Clinical Assessment Scale score was less than 71.

Other Child Characteristics

Intelligence at 6 years of age was defined as the composite score on the SB, and motor problems as the total score on the Riley Motor Problems Inventory.[56]

STATISTICAL ANALYSIS

The bivariate relations of US status to psychiatric outcomes were examined by means of logistic regression with 2 dummy variables as predictors, each encoding the comparison of 1 of the 2 US abnormality groups (GMH/IVH or PL/VE) with the NA group. The log odds of psychiatric disorder vs no disorder were the dependent variables. The bivariate relations of US status to other (non-US) predictors and the relations of diagnoses of disorders to non-US predictors and other child outcomes (eg, intelligence) were examined by means of χ^2 or Fisher exact tests for categorical variables and 1-way analyses of variance for continuous ones; the strength of these relations was assessed with correlations (ϕ, point-biserial, and product-moment, as appropriate).

Throughout this article, 2-tailed 5% significance levels were used. For the multivariate analysis, only diagnoses and diagnostic clusters having a bivariate relation to US status with a significance level of $P<.10$ were considered. When the number of cases of a given diagnosis was less than 10, the related diagnostic cluster was used instead, as long as it also showed a bivariate relation to US status. When the relation of a diagnostic cluster to US status was due primarily to 1 disorder in the cluster, that disorder was used. Explanatory variables were entered in 2 steps: first the US status variables and then the complete set of all non-US predictors. This strategy allowed evaluation of the robustness of the effect of US status when controlling for other potential risk factors. A subsequent logistic regression analysis included, in a third step, multiplicative terms representing the interaction of US status with sex and distal and proximal social disadvantage. Separate sets of logistic regressions were run for each interaction. The change in the −2 log likelihood (L^2) was used to evaluate the contribution of the interactions to the prediction of the outcome.[57] These analyses were repeated for a subsample of children with normal intelligence (SB composite scores ≥85) and for a subsample that excluded all children diagnosed at age 2 years with disabling cerebral palsy.[2]

To conserve cases and power, missing values were substituted with the sample mean or mode, while dummy-coded missing value indicators were added to equations.[58] None of the missing value indicators related significantly to any outcome.

may be especially susceptible to injury from hypoperfusion. From a cellular standpoint, the immature oligodendroglia that form myelin appear to be extremely sensitive to oxidative stress and injury from free radical formation.[26] Perinatal white matter injury, which occurs in 5% to 10% of VLBW infants,[26] is frequently found in association with, and often on the same side as, germinal matrix hemorrhage (GMH) and/or intra-

Table 1. Prevalence of DISC 2.1P Diagnoses Overall and by Ultrasound Status*

Diagnosis	Entire Sample (N=562-564)	Ultrasound Status: NA (n=453-454)	GMH/IVH (n=77-78)	PL/VE (n=31-32)
Any disorder	22.0	20.3	21.8	46.9†
Any disruptive disorder	17.2	15.9	19.2	31.3‡
Attention deficit hyperactivity disorder	15.6	14.3	16.7	31.3‡
Oppositional defiant disorder	6.0	5.7	7.7	6.3
Conduct disorder	1.4	1.3	1.3	3.1
Any anxiety disorder	10.3	9.9	10.3	15.6
Obsessive-compulsive disorder	6.6	6.8	3.8	9.4
Separation anxiety	4.1	3.7	3.8	9.4
Overanxious disorder	1.4	0.9	2.6	6.3‡
Simple phobia	0.7	0.7	1.3	0.0
Avoidant disorder	0.4	0.4	0.0	0.0
Panic disorder	0.0	0.0	0.0	0.0
Any elimination disorder	7.1	6.6	7.7	12.5
Nocturnal enuresis	6.0	5.7	7.7	6.3
Diurnal enuresis	1.2	1.1	1.3	3.1
Encopresis	1.2	1.3	0.0	3.1
Any tic disorder	2.0	1.8	0.0	9.4‡
Transient tics	0.4	0.4	0.0	0.0
Motor tics	0.9	0.7	0.0	6.3‡
Vocal tics	0.4	0.2	0.0	3.2
Tourette syndrome	0.4	0.4	0.0	0.0
Other disorders				
Major depressive disorder	0.2	0.2	0.0	0.0
Elective mutism	0.4	0.4	0.0	0.0
Pica	0.4	0.2	0.0	3.1
Any disorder other than attention deficit hyperactivity disorder and tic disorders	17.2	16.5	16.7	28.1

**Prevalence is given as the percentage of the group having the relevant diagnosis. The effective number for each group varies by diagnosis because occasionally the answer to a question required for the assignment of a particular diagnosis was missing for a child. Missing answers were most common for transient tics, for which the effective numbers for the entire sample, and for groups with no abnormalitity (NA), germinal matrix hemorrhage/intraventricular hemorrhage (GMH/IVH), and parenchymal lesions and/or ventricular enlargement (PL/VE) were, respectively, 554, 448, 78, and 28. DISC 2.1P indicates Diagnostic Interview Schedule for Children–Parent Version 2.1P.*

†P<.01 vs the NA group.

‡P<.05 vs the NA group.

ventricular hemorrhage (IVH) but probably represents a distinct pathophysiological process.[25] On postmortem examination, perinatal white matter lesions are correlated with ventricular enlargement[25,27] and with ischemic/infarctive lesions of the basal ganglia, brainstem, and cerebellum.[25,27] In premature neonates, unlike full-term neonates, cortical gray matter is limited in extent,[19] and distinct lesions of cortical gray matter are infrequently reported. However, cortical development might be adversely affected in preterms by both GMH/IVH and ischemic white matter injury because of their effects on late migration, organization, and myelination.[28]

Thus far, only 4 studies have examined the relation of neonatal cranial US abnormalities to behavioral outcomes at school age in LBW children; all used relatively small samples from individual hospitals. While 3 of these studies[29-31] found no relation of US abnormalities to behavior, a fourth found that attention problems and/or hyperactivity were related to those types of US abnormalities suggestive of white matter injury.[32] However, this last study did not control for other behavioral predictors, and none of these studies examined the possible moderating role of sex or social disadvantage on the relation of US status to behavioral outcome.

The present study examines the relation of neonatal cranial US abnormalities to psychiatric disorder at age 6 years in a large, regional LBW cohort. A range of child psychiatric diagnoses was assessed by means of a structured diagnostic interview of the parent, and detailed information was collected on other predictors and outcomes. The following questions are addressed: Which, if any, types of US abnormalities are related independently of other predictors to psychiatric disorder at age 6 years? Is the relation diagnostically specific? Does the relation differ by sex or social disadvantage? Does any relation remain when the sample is restricted to children of normal intelligence?

RESULTS

SAMPLE DESCRIPTION

Of the 564 children in the present sample, 454 (80.5%) had no US abnormalities, 78 (13.8%) had GMH/IVH, and 32 (5.7%) had PL/VE. Of those with PL/VE, 15 also had GMH/IVH. Fifty-one percent (287/564) of the sample were male, 21% (119/564) were black, 16% (89/559) lived in single-parent households, 7% (39/564) had a caretaker who received welfare benefits, and 9% (48/555) of the mothers had not finished high school. The mean (±SD) age at follow-up was 6.3±0.28 years (range, 5.2-8.7 years). Many of the children were in kindergarten (58% [325/564]) or first grade (32% [181/564]). Consistent with most LBW samples,[59] general intellectual functioning (mean±SD, 102.3±13.4 on the SB) was close to the national average, while nearly 21% (116/564) had excessive motor problems as defined by scores in the top second percentile of the Riley Motor Problems Inventory standardization sample. As noted earlier, children too severely disabled to be psychometrically tested were excluded, but 14 children in the present sample had some type of impairment: 9 had mental retardation (4 mild and 5 moderate) as defined in a previous report[3]; 9 required assistance with walking because of disabling cerebral palsy as diagnosed at age 2 years[2]; and 4 children had both conditions.

PREVALENCE OF PSYCHIATRIC DISORDER

As shown in Table 1, slightly more than one fifth of the sample (22%) had at least 1 psychiatric disorder, the most

Table 2. Nonultrasound Predictors by Ultrasound Status*

Predictors	Total (N=564)	NA (n=454)	GMH/IVH (n=78)	PL/VE (n=32)
		Ultrasound Status		
Prenatal factors				
Social disadvantage at birth	0.9±1.2	0.9±1.2	0.8±1.2	1.0±1.3
Cigarettes per day (ln)	0.7±1.2	0.8±1.2	0.4±0.9	0.9±1.2
No.	491	397	64	30
Alcohol consumption				
No.	476	384	62	30
Mild	45.8 (218)	45.6 (175)	50.0 (31)	40.0 (12)
Severe	2.7 (13)	2.3 (9)	3.2 (2)	6.7 (2)
Perinatal factors				
Sex (male)	50.9 (287)	50.2 (228)	50.0 (39)	62.5 (20)
Fetal growth ratio†	0.9±0.2	0.9±0.2	1.0±0.2	1.0±0.2
No.	563	454	77	32
Gestational age,† d	221.7±21.6	224.5±21.0	211.4±20.7	206.0±18.2
Apgar score (5 min)†	7.9±1.4	8.0±1.3	7.6±1.5	7.1±1.4
No.	547	440	76	31
Neonatal complications of prematurity				
Fraction of inspired O_2, %†‡	37.4±19.5	35.3±17.7	41.4±23.5	48.6±21.6
Neonatal chronic illness				
Days receiving ventilator assistance†	5.6±13.4	4.6±12.7	7.8±14.1	13.9±17.8
Social disadvantage (measured at age 6 y)				
Distal	0.0±0.7	0.0±0.7	0.0±0.6	0.2±0.7
Proximal	0.0±0.7	0.0±0.7	0.0±0.7	0.1±0.8
No.	563	453	78	32

**The data are presented as percentage (number) for categorical variables and as mean±SD for continuous variables. NA indicates no abnormality; GMH/IVH, germinal matrix hemorrhage and/or intraventricular hemorrhage; PL/VE, parenchymal lesions and/or ventricular enlargement; and ln, natural logarithm.*

†*F or* χ^2, $P<.001$ *for a comparison among the 3 groups.*

‡*Valid only for children receiving oxygen.*

common being ADHD (15.6%). More than two thirds of those with any disorder had more than 1. Boys were more likely than girls to have any disorder (28.9% vs 14.8%; *P*<.001), any disruptive disorder (23.8% vs 10.5%; *P*<.001), ADHD (22.0% vs 9.0%; *P*<.001), oppositional defiant disorder (8.0% vs 4.0%; *P*<.001), obsessive-compulsive disorder (8.7% vs 4.3%; *P*=.04), and nocturnal enuresis (9.4% vs 2.5%; *P*<.001).

RELATION OF US STATUS TO PSYCHIATRIC DISORDERS

The prevalences of several disorders and clusters of disorders were greater in the PL/VE than in the NA group, namely, any disorder (unadjusted odds ratio [OR], 3.5; 95% confidence interval [CI], 1.7-7.2; *P*<.001), any disruptive disorder (OR, 2.4; 95% CI, 1.1-5.3; *P*=.03), ADHD (OR, 2.7; 95% CI, 1.2-6.0; *P*=.01), overanxious disorder (OR, 7.5; 95% CI, 1.3-42.6; *P*=.02), any tic disorder (OR, 5.8; 95% CI, 1.4-22.9; *P*=.01), and motor tics (OR, 10.0; 95% CI, 1.6-62.15; *P*=.01); all *P*<.05. The GMH/IVH group did not differ significantly from the NA group for any psychiatric outcome. Of the disorders and clusters listed, 3 did not meet criteria for further consideration (see "Statistical Analysis" section): any disruptive disorder (because its relation to PL/VE was due primarily to ADHD) and overanxious disorder and motor tics (because of their low prevalence). For any disorder other than ADHD or tics, the comparison between the PL/VE and NA groups was nearly significant (OR, 2.0; 95% CI, 0.9-4.4; *P*=.10). Thus, the 4 outcomes considered further are any disorder, ADHD, tic disorders, and any disorder other than ADHD or tics.

RELATION OF NON-US PREDICTORS TO US STATUS

As shown in **Table 2**, the US groups did not differ by sex, by social disadvantage at birth or at age 6 years, or by maternal alcohol use during pregnancy. In general, the NA group tended to be at less perinatal and neonatal risk, having greater gestational age, higher 5-minute Apgar scores, lower fractions of inspired oxygen, and fewer ventilator days than either the GMH/IVH or PL/VE group. The lower fetal growth ratio in the gestationally more mature NA group, as compared with the other 2 groups, results from using birth weight to define the sample.[60]

PSYCHIATRIC OUTCOMES—MULTIVARIATE ANALYSIS

Effects of US Status on Psychiatric Disorder Controlling for Non-US Predictors

Table 3 presents the results of regression analysis with all non-US predictors included. The adjusted ORs comparing the PL/VE with the NA group were strikingly similar to the unadjusted ones given above. The

Table 3. Adjusted ORs and Confidence Intervals for Selected Disorders: Full Model*

Predictors	Any Disorder (N=564) OR	Any Disorder 95% Confidence Interval	ADHD (N=563) OR	ADHD 95% Confidence Interval	Tic Disorders (N=563) OR	Tic Disorders 95% Confidence Interval	Any Disorder Other Than ADHD or Tic Disorders (N=564) OR	Any Disorder Other Than ADHD or Tic Disorders 95% Confidence Interval
US status								
GMH/IVH	1.4	0.7-2.7	1.5	0.7-3.3	0.0	0.0-∞	1.1	0.5-2.2
PL/VE	4.4†	1.8-10.3	3.4‡	1.3-8.7	8.7‡	1.3-57.7	2.1	0.8-5.3
Prenatal factors								
Social disadvantage at birth	1.0	0.8-1.2	0.9	0.7-1.2	0.4	0.1-1.1	1.1	0.9-1.4
Cigarettes per day (ln)	1.5†	1.2-1.8	1.5†	1.2-1.9	2.0‡	1.0-3.8	1.3‡	1.0-1.6
Alcohol consumption (mild)	0.6	0.4-1.1	0.5‡	0.3-1.0	0.3	0.0-2.0	0.8	0.5-1.4
Alcohol consumption (severe)	1.4	0.4-4.9	0.2	0.0-1.7	3.4	0.2-54.4	1.7	0.4-6.3
MVI alcohol consumption	0.0	0.0-∞	0.0	0.0-∞	0.0	0.0-∞	0.0	0.0-∞
MVI smoking	664.9	0.0-∞	911.0	0.0-∞	5456.2	0.0-∞	436.1	0.0-∞
Perinatal factors								
Sex (male)	2.6†	1.7-4.2	3.4†	2.0-5.8	2.9	0.6-13.6	2.4†	1.5-4.0
Fetal growth ratio	0.8	0.2-3.4	0.6	0.1-3.0	0.1	0.0-5.1	0.8	0.2-3.7
Gestational age	1.0	1.0-1.0	1.0	1.0-1.0	0.9‡	0.9-1.0	1.0	1.0-1.0
Apgar (5 min)	1.0	0.8-1.2	1.0	0.8-1.3	1.5	0.8-2.7	1.1	0.9-1.3
MVI Apgar	2.6	0.5-13.9	2.7	0.3-22.5	109.4	0.3-35 205.9	3.7	0.5-26.8
Neonatal complications of prematurity								
Fraction of inspired O_2	1.0	1.0-1.0	0.6	1.0-1.0	1.0	0.9-1.0	1.0	1.0-1.0
MVI fraction of inspired O_2	0.7	0.4-1.2	1.0	0.6-1.8	1.7	0.3-9.2	0.7	0.4-1.2
Neonatal chronic illness								
Days receiving ventilatory assistance	1.0§	1.0-1.0	1.0	1.0-1.0	1.0	1.0-1.0	1.0	1.0-1.0
Social disadvantage (measured at age 6 y)								
Distal	0.8	0.5-1.3	0.9	0.5-1.5	1.7	0.4-8.0	0.7	0.5-1.2
Proximal	2.3†	1.6-3.3	2.1†	1.4-3.1	1.1	0.3-3.7	2.2†	1.5-3.1
MVI proximal	2128.6	0.0-∞	7808.8	0.0-∞	0.0	0.0-∞	4072.9	0.0-∞
Constant	0.0‡	0.0-0.4	0.0	0.0-1.5	86 933.6	0.0-∞	0.0	0.0-1.4

**ADHD indicates attention deficit hyperactivity disorder; OR, odds ratio; US, ultrasound; GMH/IVH, germinal matrix hemorrhage and/or intraventricular hemorrhage; PL/VE, parenchymal lesions and/or ventricular enlargement; and MVI, missing value indicator. The infinity sign (∞) stands for an extremely large number.*

†*P*<.001.

‡*P*<.05.

§*P*<.01.

presence of PL/VE still significantly increased the risk for any disorder, ADHD, and tic disorders, while GMH/IVH again did not affect risk for any psychiatric outcome.

Effects of Non-US Predictors on Psychiatric Disorder

Several of the non-US predictor variables were related independently to the 4 psychiatric outcomes of interest. Maternal smoking elevated risk for all 4 outcomes. Male sex and proximal (but not distal) social disadvantage predicted 2 of the outcomes: any disorder and ADHD. For both, the odds of disorder increased by a little more than 2 times for each unit increase in the scale for proximal social disadvantage. Days receiving mechanical ventilation, maternal alcohol use, and gestational age were each related to a single outcome.

Moderating Effect of Sex and Distal and Proximal Social Disadvantage on the Relation of US Abnormalities to Psychiatric Outcomes

Neither sex nor proximal social disadvantage modified the effect of US status on any psychiatric outcome. However, distal social disadvantage actually reduced the risk for ADHD associated with PL/VE (OR, 0.2; Wald χ^2=5.0; df=1; P=.05).

Relation of US Status to Psychiatric Disorder Among Children of Normal Intelligence

In the sample as a whole, intelligence was negatively related to psychiatric disorder (point-biserial r=−0.35, P<.001, for any disorder with the SB composite). Intelligence was also associated with US status; as reported elsewhere,[3] children in the PL/VE group had significantly lower SB composite scores than children in the NA group.

To address the possibility that the association between US status and psychiatric disorder might be influenced by the children with low intelligence in the sample, all analyses were repeated with the sample restricted to children of at least normal intelligence. In this subsample (n=521), as in the full sample, GMH/IVH (n=72) was not related to any psychiatric outcome. Also as in the full sample, PL/VE (n=20) was significantly related to any disorder (unadjusted OR, 3.0; 95% CI, 1.2-7.7; P=.02). Now, PL/VE was also significantly related to separation anxiety disorder (unadjusted OR, 4.9; 95% CI, 1.3-18.4; $P=.02$) but not to tic disorders. While the bivariate relation of PL/VE to ADHD was not significant, it did meet the .10 criterion for further examination (unadjusted OR, 2.5; 95% CI, 0.9-7.1; $P=.09$).

With all other predictors controlled, PL/VE was related to any disorder (adjusted OR, 4.8; 95% CI, 1.6-12.0; $P<.01$), ADHD (adjusted OR, 4.5; 95% CI, 1.3-16.0; $P=.02$), and separation anxiety disorder (adjusted OR, 5.3; 95% CI, 1.1-24.8; $P=.03$). Non-US predictors were related to any disorder and to ADHD among the children with normal IQ in essentially the same way as in the sample as a whole (data available on request). Also as in the intact sample, distal social advantage reduced the risk associated with PL/VE for ADHD (OR, 0.04; Wald $\chi^2=5.6$; $df=1$; $P=.04$). No other significant interactions between US status and sex or social disadvantage were found. When the sample was restricted to those who had not been diagnosed (at age 2 years) as having disabling cerebral palsy (n=530), the results were essentially identical to those obtained in this subsample of children with normal IQ.

COMMENT

This study examined the relation of perinatal brain injury, as detected on neonatal cranial US, to psychiatric disorder in LBW children at early school age. The study has several methodological strengths: children with neonatal US abnormalities were prospectively identified based on screening of a large regional birth cohort; a structured parent interview was used to diagnose a range of child psychiatric disorders at age 6 years; and detailed information was available on other social and biological predictors and other child outcomes.

Although the study has some limitations, these do not pose major threats to the validity of the findings. While our pathological studies[27] as well as those of others[61] have shown that US is not completely sensitive to milder forms of white matter injury, this limitation would lead to an underestimation of the effects of PL/VE on outcomes. Although the sample was limited to children seen on home visits, comprising only two thirds of those eligible to be seen at age 6 years, the effective sample remained reasonably representative, as discussed in the section on the birth cohort and attrition. Finally, although psychiatric diagnoses were based solely on parental interviews, parent, teacher, and psychologist ratings of behavior were in reasonable agreement.

The finding that isolated GMH/IVH did not increase risk for psychiatric disorder at age 6 years was surprising given that in most LBW infants, the germinal matrix is still proliferating (primarily glioblasts) at the time of birth.[62] It must be underscored that isolated GMH/IVH may have behavioral effects at age 6 years that are not captured by diagnosable psychiatric disorder or may be related to disorders that typically emerge later.

By constrast, PL/VE, which is indicative of ischemic injury to white matter,[27] increased by 4-fold the risk for having at least 1 psychiatric disorder, even after control for other predictors. However, the relation of PL/VE to any disorder was accounted for by its relation to specific disorders, most strongly and consistently ADHD. This study extends an earlier finding[32] to a rigorously diagnosed and population-based sample, while controlling for other predictors. As in other schoolage LBW cohorts[11,13,15] and among 6-year-olds in the general population,[63] ADHD was the most common disorder. The relation of PL/VE to ADHD was unlikely to have resulted from its greater frequency, however, because some other common disorders (eg, oppositional defiant disorder) were not related to PL/VE. Neither birth weight nor gestational age increased risk for ADHD independent of US status, suggesting that recent reports of elevated rates of ADHD in LBW cohorts[11,13,15] may reflect the higher rates of PL/VE likely to have been present in such groups.

Here, as in other other recent studies,[64-66] maternal smoking during pregnancy adversely affected childhood behavior; the present study shows this effect to be independent of PL/VE and social disadvantage. A recent review[66] of the effects of nicotine on the fetal brain points to functional alteration of receptors within the basal ganglia as a possible mechanism for this effect.[67] However, postnatal maternal smoking, a factor not assessed here, might also have played a role.

As in other population-based studies of childhood psychiatric disorder,[63] male sex independently predicted increased risk for ADHD, a finding that has been attributed to sex differences in the development of the dopaminergic system.[68-70] The advantage of female sex was constant across brain injury groups, however, and was not particularly pronounced in the presence of perinatal brain injury.

In the present study, proximal social disadvantage was an independent predictor of ADHD; previous studies on this point have been inconsistent.[71] Distal social disadvantage actually reduced the risk of ADHD among children with PL/VE; findings from a recent study[72] raise the possibility that this effect may result from selective mortality among LBW infants born to severely disadvantaged mothers.

From a theoretical standpoint, the findings of the present study are not consistent with the widely accepted interactional model of biological and social risk.[73-75] According to that model, among children who are not severely disabled, higher rates of psychiatric disorder would be expected with greater social disadvantage, and perinatal brain injury per se would have an effect only among socially disadvantaged children. Among advantaged children, inherent "self-righting tendencies" would counteract any adverse effects of perinatal risk factors,[73] including presumedly those of perinatal brain injury. Instead, in this study both PL/VE and social disadvantage raised the risk of psychiatric disorder independently of one another, and social advantage did not protect children with PL/VE from increased risk for psychiatric disorder. Of course, an interaction suggesting a protective effect of social advantage in the presence of some other aspects of perinatal risk might still exist. However, it does appear from the present results that the relation of PL/VE to psychiatric disorder at age 6 years is more consistent with a main effects model than an interactional model.

Consistent with modern neurodevelopmental models of psychiatric disorders, such as that proposed by Weinberger for schizophrenia,[76] the effects of PL/VE on ADHD, tic disorders, and separation anxiety disorder at age 6 years may reflect an effect of perinatal ischemic injury on brain maturational events that occurs at this age, in particular maturation of the striatum (caudate and putamen) of the basal ganglia. Maturation of the striatum is thought to play an important role in the improvement of behavioral inhibition that normally occurs in middle childhood[77] but is notably deficient in ADHD, tic disorders, and anxiety disorders.[78,79] In a postmortem study in this cohort,[25] ischemic/infarctive white matter lesions were statistically associated with ischemic/infarctive lesions of the basal ganglia, probably because they share with deep white matter the distinction of having only 1 arterial supply and thus are especially vulnerable to hypoperfusion.[24] Structural and functional brain imaging studies of children with ADHD[80-83] and tic disorders[84,85] have found abnormalities in the basal ganglia, specifically the corpus striatum (caudate and putamen), while subtle motor impairments in a subset of children with anxiety disorders[86] also suggest basal ganglia abnormalities. The striatum receives substantial dopaminergic input from the substantia nigra,[87] and dysregulation of the dopaminergic system has been implicated in both ADHD[78,88] and tic disorders.[78,89] Alterations of the dopaminergic system have been shown to accompany ischemic brain injury in human neonates[90] and in rats.[91] The striatal dopaminergic system appears to be more vulnerable to ischemic injury than other striatal neurotransmitter systems (eg, serotonin),[92] perhaps because, in the striatum, dopamine synapses are closely juxtaposed with glutamate synapses,[93] which are thought to play a key role in mediating the neurotoxic effects of ischemia.[94] As the cohort undergoes puberty, which is accompanied by cortical maturation[95] and synaptic pruning,[96-99] it is possible that PL/VE will increase risk for disorders that typically have a later onset and in which abnormalities of cortical–basal ganglionic circuits have been implicated, such as mood disorders,[100] obsessive-compulsive disorder,[101] and schizophrenia.[93,100,102,103] Certainly, further longitudinal follow-up of this cohort will be of great interest.

Accepted for publication January 28, 1997.

This work was supported by the John Merck Fund, the March of Dimes Birth Defects Foundation (grant 12-261), and the National Institute of Mental Health (grant 5-R01 MH4583-04).

We thank the children and families who made this study possible. We also thank Janet Baxendale and Dawn McCulloch, MS, for their contributions to data collection; Suzannah Blumenthal and Mary Rojas, PhD, for their contributions to data management and analysis; Prudence Fisher, MS, for assistance with the diagnostic interview; and Jim Johnson, PhD (deceased), Mark Davies, MPH, Michael Parides, PhD, Daniel Pine, MD, and Claudia Holzman, DVM, PhD, for their valuable suggestions.

Reprints: Agnes H. Whitaker, MD, Unit 78, New York State Psychiatric Institute, 722 W 168th St, New York, NY 10032.

REFERENCES

1. Levene MI. Cerebral ultrasound and neurological impairment: telling the future. *Arch Dis Child.* 1990;65:469-471.
2. Pinto-Martin JA, Riolo S, Cnaan A, Holzman C, Susser MW, Paneth N. Cranial ultrasound prediction of disabling and non-disabling cerebral palsy at age two in a low birthweight population. *Pediatrics.* 1995;95:249-254.
3. Whitaker AH, Feldman JF, Van Rossem R, Schonfeld IS, Pinto-Martin JA, Torre C, Blumenthal SR, Paneth NS. Neonatal cranial ultrasound abnormalities in LBW infants: relation to cognitive outcomes at age six. *Pediatrics.* 1996;98:719-729.
4. Breslau N, Klein N, Allen L. Very low birthweight: behavioral sequelae at nine years of age. *J Am Acad Child Adolesc Psychiatry.* 1988;27:605-612.
5. Klein NK. Children who were very low birthweight: cognitive abilities and classroom behavior at five years of age. *J Spec Educ.* 1988;22:41-54.
6. Rose SA, Feldman JF, Rose SL, Wallace IF, McCarton C. Behavior problems at 3 and 6 years: prevalence and continuity in full-terms and preterms. *Dev Psychopathol.* 1992;4:361-374.
7. Ross G, Lipper EG, Auld PAM. Social competence and behavior problems in premature children at school age. *Pediatrics.* 1990;86:391-397.
8. McCormick M, Workman-Daniels K, Brooks-Gunn J. The behavioral and emotional well-being of school-age children with different birthweights. *Pediatrics.* 1996;97:18-25.
9. Marlow N, Roberts BL, Cooke RWI. Motor skills in extremely low birthweight children at the age of 6 years. *Arch Dis Child.* 1989;64:839-847.
10. McCormick MC, Gortmaker SL, Sobol AM. Very low birth weight children: behavior problems and school difficulty in a national sample. *J Pediatr.* 1990;117:687-693.
11. Szatmari P, Saigal S, Rosenbaum P, Campbell D, King S. Psychiatric disorders at five years among children with birthweights <1000g: a regional perspective. *Dev Med Child Neurol.* 1990;32:954-962.
12. Scottish Low Birthweight Study Group. The Scottish Low Birthweight Study, II: language attainment, cognitive status, and behavioural problems. *Arch Dis Child.* 1992;67:682-686.
13. Szatmari P, Saigal S, Rosenbaum P, Campbell D. Psychopathology and adaptive functioning among extremely low birthweight children at eight years of age. *Dev Psychopathol.* 1993;5:345-357.
14. Pharoah POD, Stevenson CJ, Cooke RWI, Stevenson RC. Prevalence of behavior disorders in low birthweight infants. *Arch Dis Child.* 1994;70:271-274.
15. Breslau N, Brown GG, DelDotto JE, Kumar S, Ezthuthachan S, Andreski P, Hufnagle KG. Psychiatric sequelae of low birth weight at six years of age. *J Abnorm Child Psychol.* 1996;24:385-400.
16. Breslau N. Psychiatric sequelae of low birth weight. *Epidemiol Rev.* 1995;17:96-106.
17. Buka SL, Lipsitt LP, Tsuang MT. Emotional and behavioral development of low-birthweight infants. In: Friedman SL, Sigman MD, eds. *The Psychological Development of Low-Birthweight Children.* Norwood, NJ: Ablex Publishing Corp; 1992:187-214.
18. Hack M, Klein NK, Taylor HG. Long-term developmental outcomes of low birth weight infants. In: Behrman R, ed. *Low Birth Weight.* Los Altos, Calif: Center for the Future of Children, The David and Lucile Packard Foundation; 1995:176-196.
19. Truwit CL, Barkovich AJ, Koch TK, Ferriero DM. Cerebral palsy: MR findings in 40 patients. *Am J Neuroradiol.* 1992;13:67-78.
20. Niemann G, Wakat JP, Krageloh-Mann I, Grodd W, Michaelis R. Congenital hemiparesis and periventricular leukomalacia: pathogenic aspects on magnetic resonance imaging. *Dev Med Child Neurol.* 1994;36:943-950.
21. Volpe JJ. Intracranial hemorrhage: germinal matrix–intraventricular hemorrhage of the premature infant. In: Volpe JJ, ed. *Neurology of the Newborn.* Philadelphia, Pa: WB Saunders Co; 1994:403-446.
22. Johnston MV. Neurotransmitters and vulnerability of the developing brain. *Brain Dev.* 1995;17:301-306.
23. Paneth N, Pinto-Martin J. The epidemiology of germinal matrix–intraventricular hemorrhage. In: Kiely J, ed. *Reproductive and Perinatal Epidemiology.* Boca Raton, Fla: CRC Press; 1991:371-399.
24. Moody DM, Bell MA, Challa VR. Features of the cerebral vascular pattern that

predict vulnerability to perfusion or oxygenation deficiency: an anatomic study. *Am J Neuroradiol.* 1991;11:431-439.
25. Paneth N, Rudelli R, Kazam E, Monte W. *Brain Damage in the Preterm Infant.* London, England: MacKeith Press; 1994.
26. Leviton A, Paneth N. White matter damage in preterm newborns: an epidemiologic perspective. *Early Hum Dev.* 1990;24:1-22.
27. Paneth N, Rudelli R, Monte W, Rodriguez E, Pinto J, Kairam R, Kazam E. White matter necrosis in very low birth weight infants: neuropathologic and ultrasonographic findings in infants surviving six days or longer. *J Pediatr.* 1990;116: 975-984.
28. Evrard P, Gressens P, Volpe JJ. New concepts to understand the neurological consequences of subcortical lesions in the premature brain. *Biol Neonate.* 1992; 61:1-3.
29. Weisglas-Kuperus N, Baerts W, Fetter WPF, Sauer PJJ. Neonatal cerebral ultrasound, neonatal neurology and perinatal conditions as predictors of neurodevelopmental outcome in very low birthweight infants. *Early Hum Dev.* 1992; 31:131-148.
30. Roth SC, Baudin J, McCormick DC, Edwards AD, Townsend J, Stewart AL, Reynolds EOR. Relation between ultrasound appearance of the brain of very preterm infants and neurodevelopmental impairment at eight years. *Dev Med Child Neurol.* 1993;35:755-768.
31. Sostek AM. Prematurity as well as intraventricular hemorrhage influence developmental outcome at 5 years. In: Friedman SL, Sigman MD, eds. *The Psychological Development of Low-Birthweight Children.* Norwood, NJ: Ablex Publishing Corp; 1992:259-274.
32. Fawer CL, Calame A. Significance of ultrasound appearances in the neurological development and cognitive abilities of preterm infants at 5 years. *Eur J Pediatr.* 1991;150:515-520.
33. Pinto-Martin J, Paneth N, Witomski T, Stein I, Schonfeld S, Rosenfeld D, Rose W, Kazam E, Kairam R, Katsikiotis V. The Central New Jersey Neonatal Brain Haemorrhage Study: design of the study and reliability of ultrasound diagnosis. *Paediatr Perinat Epidemiol.* 1992;6:273-284.
34. Achenbach TM. *Manual for the Child Behavior Checklist/2-3 and 1992 Profile.* Burlington, Vt: University of Vermont Department of Psychiatry; 1992.
35. Achenbach TM. *Manual for the Child Behavior Checklist/4-18 and 1991 Profile.* Burlington, Vt: University of Vermont Department of Psychiatry; 1991.
36. Thorndike RL, Hagen EP, Sattler JM. *The Stanford-Binet Intelligence Scale: Fourth Edition—Guide for Administration and Scoring.* Chicago, Ill: Riverside Publishing Co; 1986.
37. Goodman S, Alegria M, Hoven C, Leaf P, Narrow W. *Core Service Utilization and Risk Factors (SURF) Modules: NIMH Multi-site Methodologic Survey of Child and Adolescent Populations Field Trials.* Rockville, Md: National Institute of Mental Health; 1992.
38. Larroche JC. Intraventricular hemorrhage in the premature neonate. In: Korobkin R, Guilleminault C, eds. *Advances in Perinatal Neurology.* New York, NY: SP Medical and Scientific Books; 1979:115-141.
39. Rorke LB. *Pathology of Perinatal Brain Injury.* New York, NY: Raven Press; 1982.
40. Papile LA, Burstein J, Burstein R. Incidence and evolution of subependymal and intraventricular hemorrhage. *J Pediatr.* 1978;92:529-534.
41. Holzman C, Paneth N, Little R, Pinto-Martin J. Perinatal brain injury in premature infants born to mothers using alcohol in pregnancy. *Pediatrics.* 1995;95: 66-73.
42. Williams RL, Creasy RK, Cunningham GC, Hawes WE, Norris FD, Tashiro M. Fetal growth and perinatal viability in California. *Obstet Gynecol.* 1982;59:624-632.
43. Tarnow-Mordi W, Ogston S, Wilkinson AR, Reid E, Gregory J, Saeed M, Wilke R. Predicting death from initial disease severity in very low birthweight infants: a method for comparing the performance of neonatal units. *BMJ.* 1990;300: 1611-1614.
44. Cimma R, Risemberg H, White JJ. A simple objective system for early recognition of overwhelming neonatal respiratory distress. *J Pediatr Surg.* 1980;15: 581-585.
45. Caldwell BM, Bradley RH. *Administration Manual—Home Observation for Measurement of the Environment.* Little Rock, Ark: University of Arkansas at Little Rock; 1984.
46. Goldberg DP. *The Detection of Psychiatric Illness by Questionnaire: A Technique for the Identification and Assessment of Non-psychotic Psychiatric Illness.* London, England: Oxford University Press; 1972.
47. Byles J, Byrne C, Boyle MH, Offord DR. Ontario Child Health Study: reliability and validity of the General Functioning Subscale of the McMaster Family Assessment Device. *Fam Process.* 1988;27:97-101.
48. Fisher PW, Shaffer D, Piacentini JC, Lapkin J, Kafantaris V, Leonard H, Herzog DB. Sensitivity of the Diagnostic Interview Schedule for Children, 2nd Edition (DISC-2.1) for specific diagnoses of children and adolescents. *J Am Acad Child Adolesc Psychiatry.* 1993;32:666-673.
49. American Psychiatric Association, Committee on Nomenclature and Statistics. *Diagnostic and Statistical Manual of Mental Disorders, Revised Third Edition.* Washington, DC: American Psychiatric Association; 1987.
50. Schwab-Stone M, Fallon T, Briggs T, Crowther B. Reliability of diagnostic reporting for children aged 6-11 years: a test-retest study of the Diagnostic Interview Schedule for Children–Revised. *Am J Psychiatry.* 1994;151:1048-1054.
51. Jensen P, Roper M, Fisher P, et al. Test-retest reliability of the Diagnostic Interview Schedule for Children (Version 2.1): parent, child and combined algorithms. *Arch Gen Psychiatry.* 1995;52:61-71.
52. Achenbach TM. *Manual for the Teacher's Report Form and 1991 Profile.* Burlington, Vt: University of Vermont Department of Psychiatry; 1991.
53. Aylward GP. *Test Behavior Checklist.* Brandon, Vt: Clinical Psychology Publishing Co Inc; 1986.
54. Bird H, Canino GJ, Rubio-Stipec M, Ribera JC. Further measures of the psychometric properties of the Children's Global Assessment Scale. *Arch Gen Psychiatry.* 1987;44:821-824.
55. Shaffer D, Gould MS, Brasic J, Ambrosini P, Fisher P, Bird H, Aluwahlia S. A Children's Global Assessment Scale (CGAS). *Arch Gen Psychiatry.* 1983;40: 1228-1231.
56. Riley GD. *Riley Motor Problems Inventory—Manual.* Los Angeles, Calif: Western Psychological Services; 1976.
57. Fleiss JL. *Statistical Methods for Rates and Proportions.* New York, NY: John Wiley & Sons Inc; 1981.
58. Cohen J, Cohen P. *Applied Multiple Regression/Correlation Analysis for the Behavioral Sciences.* Hillsdale, NJ: Lawrence Erlbaum Assoc; 1983.
59. Ornstein M, Ohlsson A, Edmonds J, Asztalos E. Neonatal follow-up of very low birthweight/extremely low birthweight infants to school age: a critical overview. *Acta Scand Paediatr.* 1991;80:741-748.
60. Arnold CC, Kramer MS, Hobbs CA, McLean FH, Usher RH. Very low birth weight: a problematic cohort for epidemiologic studies of very small or immature neonates. *Am J Epidemiol.* 1991;134:604-613.
61. Hope PL, Gould SJ, Howard S, Hamilton PA, Costello AM, Reynolds EOR. Precision of ultrasound diagnosis of pathologically verified lesions in the brains of very preterm infants. *Dev Med Child Neurol.* 1988;30:457-471.
62. Volpe JJ. Neuronal proliferation, migration, organization, and myelination. In: Volpe JJ, ed. *Neurology of the Newborn.* Philadelphia, Pa: WB Saunders Co; 1995:43-85.
63. Offord DR, Boyle MH, Szatmari P, Rae-Grant MI, Links PS, Cadman DT, Byles JA, Crawford JW, Blum HM, Byrne C, Thomas H, Woodward CA. Ontario Child Health Study, II: six-month prevalence of disorder and rates of service utilization. *Arch Gen Psychiatry.* 1987;44:832-836.
64. Nichols PL, Chen TC. *Minimal Brain Dysfunction: A Prospective Study.* Hillsdale, NJ: Lawrence Erlbaum Assoc; 1981.
65. Fergusson DM, Horwood LJ, Lynskey MT. Maternal smoking before and after pregnancy: effects on behavioral outcomes in middle childhood. *Pediatrics.* 1993; 92:815-822.
66. Weitzman M, Gortmaker S, Sobol A. Maternal smoking and behavior problems of children. *Pediatrics.* 1992;90:342-349.
67. Cairns NJ, Wonnacott S. 3H nicotine binding sites in fetal human brain. *Brain Res.* 1988;475:1-7.
68. Shaywitz BA, Cohen DJ, Leckman JF, Young JG, Bowers MB. Ontogeny of dopamine and serotonin metabolites in the cerebrospinal fluid of children with neurological disorders. *Dev Med Child Neurol.* 1980;22:748-754.
69. Wong DF, Wagner HN, Dannals RF, et al. Effects of age, dopamine and serotonin receptors measured by positron tomography in the living human brain. *Science.* 1984;226:1393-1396.
70. Seeman P, Bzowej NH, Guan HC, Bergeron C, Reynolds GP, Bird ED, Riederer P, Jellinger K, Watanabe S, Tourtellote W. Human dopamine receptors in children and aging adults. *Synapse.* 1987;1:399-405.
71. Szatmari P, Offord DR, Boyle MH. Correlates, associated impairments and patterns of service utilization of children with attention deficit disorder: findings from the Ontario Child Health Study. *J Child Psychol Psychiatry.* 1989; 30:205-217.
72. National Center for Health Statistics. *Perinatal Mortality in the United States, 1985-91.* Washington, DC: National Center for Health Statistics; 1995;922-927.
73. Sameroff AJ, Chandler MJ. Reproductive risk and the continuum of caretaking casualty. In: Horowitz FD, ed. *Review of Child Development Research.* Chicago, Ill: University of Chicago Press; 1975:187-244.
74. Rubin RA, Balow B. Perinatal influences on behavior and learning problems of children. In: Lahey BB, Kazdin AE, eds. *Advances in Clinical Child Psychology.* New York, NY: Plenum Press; 1977:119-160.
75. Horowitz FD. The concept of risk: a reevaluation. In: Friedman SL, Sigman MD, eds. *The Psychological Development of Low-Birthweight Children.* Norwood, NJ: Ablex Publishing Corp; 1992:61-88.
76. Weinberger D. Schizophrenia as a neurodevelopmental disorder. In: Hirsch S, Weinberger D, ed. *Schizophrenia.* Cambridge, Mass: Blackwell Science; 1995: 293-323.

77. Ornitz E. Developmental aspects of neurophysiology. In: Lewis M, ed. *Child and Adolescent Psychiatry: A Comprehensive Textbook*. Philadelphia, Pa: Williams & Wilkins; 1991:38-51.
78. Rogeness GA, Javors GA, Pliszka SR. Neurochemistry and child and adolescent psychiatry. *J Am Acad Child Adolesc Psychiatry*. 1996;31:765-781.
79. Gray JA, McNaughton N. The neuropsychology of anxiety: a reprise. In: Hope DA, ed. *Perspectives on Anxiety, Panic, & Fear*. Lincoln, Neb: University of Nebraska Press; 1996:61-134.
80. Lou HC, Henriksen L, Bruhn P, Borner H, Nielsen JB. Striatal dysfunction in attention deficit and hyperkinetic disorder. *Arch Neurol*. 1989;46:48-52.
81. Lou NC, Henriksen L, Bruhn P. Focal cerebral hypoperfusion in children with dysphasia and/or attention deficit disorder. *Arch Neurol*. 1984;41:825-829.
82. Castellanos FX, Giedd JN, Eckburg P, Marsh WL, Vaituzis C, Kaysen D, Hamburger SD, Rapoport JL. Quantitative morphology of the caudate nucleus in attention deficit hyperactivity disorder. *Am J Psychiatry*. 1994;151:1791-1796.
83. Hynd GW, Hern LK, Novey ES, Eliopulos D, Marshall R, Gonzalez JJ, Voeller KK. Attention deficit-hyperactivity disorder and asymmetry of the caudate nucleus. *J Child Neurol*. 1993;8:339-347.
84. Singer HS, Reiss AL, Brown JE, Aylward EH, Shih B, Chee E, Harris EL, Reader MJ, Chase GA, Bryan RN. Volumetric MRI changes in basal ganglia of children with Tourette's syndrome. *Neurology*. 1993;43:950-956.
85. Peterson B, Riddle MA, Cohen DJ. Reduced basal ganglia volumes in Tourette's syndrome using three-dimensional reconstruction techniques from magnetic resonance imaging. *Neurology*. 1993;43:941-949.
86. Pine D, Shaffer D, Schonfeld IS. Persistent emotional disorder in children with neurological soft signs. *J Am Acad Child Adolesc Psychiatry*. 1993;32:1229-1236.
87. Kitai ST, Kocsis JD, Preston RJ, Sugimori M. Monosynaptic inputs to caudate neurons identified by intracellular injection of horseradish peroxidase. *Brain Res*. 1976;109:601-606.
88. Castellanos FX, Rapoport JL. Etiology of attention-deficit hyperactivity disorder. *Child Adolesc Psychiatr Clin North Am*. 1992;1:373-384.
89. Singer HS. Neurobiological issues in Tourette syndrome. *Brain Dev*. 1994;16:353-364.
90. Blennow M, Zeman J, Dahlin I, Lagercrantz H. Monoamine neurotransmitters and metabolites in the cerebrospinal fluid following perinatal asphyxia. *Biol Neonate*. 1995;67:407-413.
91. Dell'Anna ME, Luthman J, Lindqvist E, Olson L. Development of monoamine systems after neonatal anoxia in rats. *Brain Res Bull*. 1993;32:159-170.
92. Gordon K, Statman D, Johnston MV, Robinson TE, Becker JB, Silverstein FS. Transient hypoxia alters striatal catecholamine metabolism in immature brain: an in vivo microdialysis study. *J Neurochem*. 1990;54:605-611.
93. Freed WJ. The therapeutic latency of neuroleptic drugs and nonspecific postjunctional supersensitivity. *Schizophr Bull*. 1988;14:269-277.
94. Johnston MV, Trescher WH, Taylor GA. Hypoxic and ischemic central nervous system disorders in infants and children. *Adv Pediatr*. 1995;42:1-45.
95. Fuster JM. *The Prefrontal Cortex*. New York, NY: Raven Press; 1989.
96. Huttenlocher PR. Synaptic density in human frontal cortex: developmental changes and effects in aging. *Brain Res*. 1979;163:195-205.
97. Feinberg I. Schizophrenia: caused by a fault in programmed synaptic elimination during adolescence? *J Psychiatr Res*. 1982;17:319-334.
98. Huttenlocher PR, deCourten C, Garey LJ, Van Der Loos H. Synaptogenesis in human visual cortex: evidence for synapse elimination during normal development. *Neurosci Lett*. 1982;33:247-252.
99. Purves D, Lichtman JW. Elimination of synapses in the developing nervous system. *Science*. 1980;210:153-157.
100. Swerdlow NR, Koob GF. Dopamine, schizophrenia, mania, and depression: toward a unified hypothesis of cortico-striato-pallido-thalamic function. *Behav Brain Sci*. 1987;10:197-245.
101. Brody AL, Saxena S. Brain imaging in obsessive-compulsive disorder: evidence for the involvement of frontal-subcortical circuitry in the mediation of symptomatology. *CNS Spectrums Int J Neuropsychiatr Med*. 1996;1:27-41.
102. Pettegrew JW, Keshavan MS, Minshew NJ. ^{31}P nuclear magnetic resonance spectroscopy: neurodevelopment and schizophrenia. *Schizophr Bull*. 1993;19:35-53.
103. Jernigan TL, Zisook S, Heaton RK, Moranville JT, Hesselink JR, Braff DL. Magnetic resonance imaging abnormalities in lenticular nuclei and cerebral cortex in schizophrenia. *Arch Gen Psychiatry*. 1991;49:238-243.

Long-term Stimulant Treatment of Children With Attention-Deficit Hyperactivity Disorder Symptoms

A Randomized, Double-blind, Placebo-Controlled Trial

Christopher Gillberg, MD, PhD; Hans Melander, MSc; Anne-Liis von Knorring, MD, PhD; Lars-Olof Janols, MD, PhD; Gunilla Thernlund, MD; Bruno Hägglöf, MD, PhD; Lena Eidevall-Wallin, MD; Peik Gustafsson, MD; Svenny Kopp, MD

Background: We wanted to study the effects of amphetamine on symptoms of attention-deficit hyperactivity disorder (ADHD) over a longer period than has been reported in previous studies of central stimulants in this condition.

Methods: Sixty-two children, aged 6 to 11 years, meeting *DSM-III-R* symptom criteria for ADHD participated in a parallel-group design, randomized, double-blind, placebo-controlled study of amphetamine treatment. Treatment was not restricted to children with "pure" ADHD, ie, some had comorbid diagnoses. In the amphetamine group, children received active treatment for 15 months.

Results: Amphetamine was clearly superior to placebo in reducing inattention, hyperactivity, and other disruptive behavior problems and tended to lead to improved results on the Wechsler Intelligence Scale for Children–Revised. Treatment failure rate was considerably lower and time to treatment failure was longer in the amphetamine group. Adverse effects were few and relatively mild.

Conclusion: The results of this long-term, placebo-controlled study of the central stimulant amphetamine in the treatment of ADHD indicate that there are remaining positive effects of the drug 15 months after starting treatment.

Arch Gen Psychiatry. 1997;54:857-864

From the Departments of Child and Adolescent Psychiatry, University of Göteborg, Göteborg (Drs Gillberg and Kopp), University of Uppsala, Uppsala (Drs von Knorring and Janols), University of Lund, Lund (Drs Thernlund, Eidevall-Wallin, and Gustafsson), University of Umeå, Umeå (Dr Hägglöf), and the Swedish Medical Products Agency, Uppsala (Mr Melander), Sweden.

STIMULANTS HAVE been used in the treatment of childhood attention deficits and hyperactivity for 60 years.[1] They are effective in the short term.[2,3] With the use of stimulant drugs, overactivity, aggressiveness, and impulsivity decrease and attention increases. Children's interactions with peers, teachers and parents, and mother-child emotional climate improve; parents and teachers exert less control over the child.[4,5] Stimulant medication added to behavior therapy increases efficacy.[6] Learning and achievements in arithmetic, reading, and fine motor skills improve.[7-9] The response rate to stimulant treatment varies from 70% to 96%.[10] Side effects are usually mild and dose dependent. Appetite and weight loss and insomnia are common. Seizures have been reported with methylphenidate, but the clinical significance of this remains unclear.[11] Increased tics are occasionally reported.[12,13] Stimulant treatment does not appear to increase the risk for later addiction or abuse.[14,15]

Methodologically acceptable studies have pertained to short-term effects. Two uncontrolled longer-term studies did not demonstrate clear benefits.[16,17] A long-term study of children with attention-deficit hyperactivity disorder (ADHD) receiving a multimodality treatment program (including medication with stimulants) indicated clear gains after 3 years.[18]

About 2% of all US school-aged children are treated with stimulants. In some states and in certain age groups the figure is higher.[19] In Europe, the practice of stimulant treatment varies. Stimulants are widely used by drug addicts. In Sweden, this has contributed to a negative attitude toward these drugs in treatment, especially in the treatment of children. Stimulant medication, at present, is only available on a named-patient basis with a special permission from the Medical Products Agency, the Swedish drug regulatory authority.[20]

A randomized, double-blind, placebo-controlled study was undertaken to study the long-term effects of stimulant treatment. The aims of this study were to (1) evaluate effects of amphetamine on behavior and cognition and (2) study adverse effects during 15 months of treatment.

SUBJECTS AND METHODS

SUBJECTS

Children considered for inclusion were consecutive cases referred for evaluation for treatment of ADHD symptoms. Sixty-two children (52 boys, 10 girls) aged 6 to 11 years participated in a 4-site study (the Child and Adolescent Psychiatric University departments in Malmö-Lund, Göteborg, Uppsala, and Umeå) in Sweden (**Table 1**). The study was performed in collaboration with the Swedish Medical Products Agency. Seventy-two children were assigned for the study. There was no refusal. Parents provided informed consent. Ten children were withdrawn before randomization (see the "Attrition" section).

Children were comprehensively examined in an outpatient clinic by a child psychiatrist and a psychologist before starting the study. The psychiatrists discussed the procedure in detail before the study was launched. The *DSM-III-R*[21] was used in the diagnostic procedure. Children aged between 6 and 11 years whose parents sought treatment for them because of severe hyperactivity or inattention problems and accepted randomized double-blind placebo-controlled conditions, who met at least 8 of the 14 *DSM-III-R* criteria for ADHD, and who had an IQ above 50 were assigned for study. Children were excluded if they had chronic medical conditions, such as diabetes, cardiovascular or neurological disorders; were receiving ongoing medication (except antiepileptic drug treatment); had height below −2 SDs of the norm; had major psychosocial problems; or had a history of alcohol or drug abuse themselves or of their principal caretaker(s).

PREVIOUS TREATMENTS

All 72 children assigned for study had been subjected to intervention prior to the study. Two children had received amphetamine therapy. Eight had been taking other drugs (neuroleptics, γ-linolenic-butyric acid, and folic acid). Three were taking carbamazepine and 1 was taking valproic acid at baseline and continued taking these drugs throughout the study. Thirty-two children (15 of whom had a personal assistant) were in classrooms for children with behavioral and academic problems or had special education help in their home classroom. Six families had received counseling as the only mode of treatment.

Fifty-two of the children met 10 or more of the 14 *DSM-III-R* criteria for ADHD. All had pervasive problems.

COMORBIDITY

In the 62 randomized children, a number of comorbid diagnoses were made, the most frequent being pervasive developmental disorders. One boy met 8 of the 16 symptom criteria for autistic disorder (and 13 of the 14 criteria for ADHD). Six additional boys with 6 to 7 symptoms of autistic disorder (and 9-12 symptoms of ADHD) met criteria for pervasive developmental disorders not otherwise specified/atypical autism.[22] Another 20 children had 1 to 5 such symptoms. This degree of comorbidity of attention deficits with autistic-type symptoms is similar to that in a general population sample.[23] Nine boys and 1 girl had mild mental retardation (ie, IQ 51-72). Eight children had oppositional defiant disorder. Three boys had conduct disorder. Three children had separation anxiety disorder. One of these also had oppositional defiant disorder. Two boys had Tourette syndrome and 1 boy had motor tic disorder before the study started. Tics were mild and not sufficient cause for exclusion. Thirty-six (58%) of the 62 children had no comorbid diagnoses.

ATTRITION

Ten children (7 boys, 3 girls)—of the same age as those who continued in the study—were withdrawn before randomization. Two of these had mild mental retardation, compared with 10 of the 62 who remained in the study ($P=.67$). One boy with Asperger syndrome (meeting 13 of the 14 ADHD criteria) was also withdrawn before randomization.

Reasons for leaving the study before randomization were the following: parents changed their mind about need for medication (n=1), no positive effects observed (n=4), difficulties falling asleep (n=1), loss of appetite (n=1), increased withdrawal (n=1), increased blood pressure with vertigo (n=1), and general rash (n=1).

STUDY DESIGN

The study comprised (1) a baseline evaluation (month 0), (2) a 3-month period—when dosage was titrated to optimal level—of single-blind amphetamine treatment (months 1-3), (3) randomization at the end of month 3, (4) a 12-month period of treatment with either amphetamine or placebo in double-blind fashion (months 4-15), and (5) a 3-month period of single-blind placebo. Clinical examinations and questionnaire screenings were performed at month 0 and at the end of months 3, 6, 9, 12, 15, and 18. The

RESULTS

BASELINE CHARACTERISTICS

There were no major differences between treatment groups (Table 1). There were no differences across sites in terms of degree of behavior impairment, need and use of services before the study started, amphetamine dosage, or overall outcome.

MISSING DATA

Data on time to treatment failure due to lack of efficacy were obtained for all children. In the intention-to-treat analyses, 1 child failed to provide at least 2 Conners parent ratings between months 3 and 15; the corresponding number for teacher ratings was 10. The WISC-R results from both 0 and 15 months were available for 43 subjects. Less than 10% of the data on adverse effects, other symptoms, and weight and height were missing.

SINGLE-BLIND AMPHETAMINE TREATMENT

All 62 children improved significantly during single-blind amphetamine treatment according to Conners parent and teacher ratings. Mean scores dropped by 27% to 47%.

parents and children were not aware of the time of randomization but were informed that some time during the study placebo might be given instead of amphetamine.

PROCEDURES

A 60- to 120-minute baseline structured interview covering all the symptoms listed in the childhood section of the *DSM-III-R* was used. Children underwent neurodevelopmental examination. Interrater reliability for ADHD symptoms and for the neurodevelopmental examination has been shown to be good to excellent.[23,24]

The physical examination included assessments of height, weight, pulse, and blood pressure, as well as side effects such as tics, stereotypies, and disturbances of appetite and sleep.

The neuropsychological testing included the Wechsler Intelligence Scale for Children–Revised (WISC-R).[25] Diagnoses were made by the child psychiatrist using the information obtained at interview and neurodevelopmental and physical examination.

The Conners Teacher Rating Scale and Conners Parent Rating Scale[26] have been used extensively in Sweden in school-aged children, and are valid measures of behavioral abnormality. At baseline, Conners teacher total scores were more than 2 SDs above the mean of normal Swedish 10-year-olds in all cases except 5 who had scores between 1 and 2 SDs above the mean. The same figures applied to Conners parent total scores, but the children with "intermediate high" scores on this scale were a different group than those who scored "intermediate high" on the teacher scale.

The Birleson Depression Self-report Scale[27] was used in children 10 years or older. For younger children, items were read aloud and responses were recorded by the interviewer. This scale is a valid measure of depressive symptoms in Swedish children and adolescents.

The McGrath Test[28] contains a series of 9 simple drawings of human faces depicting moods ranging from happiness to sadness. The child is asked, "How do you feel?" and is instructed to point to the appropriate face.

AMPHETAMINE DOSAGE

Amphetamine sulfate was used because this was the drug available in Sweden at the time of the present study. Amphetamine was chosen because it was believed to have less effect on seizure threshold than methylphenidate hydrochloride. With a possible treatment duration of more than 1 year and with some of the children at risk for seizure disorders, we wanted a drug with a relatively low risk of provoking epileptic seizures.

Dosage was titrated from 5 mg twice daily (breakfast and lunch). The allowable maximum daily dose was preset at 60 mg. The mean dose at the beginning of double-blind treatment was 17 mg/d (range, 5-35 mg/d), corresponding to 0.52 mg/kg of body weight (range, 0.20-1.10) per day. During double-blind treatment, the dosage was decreased for 8 children and increased for 11 children. The maximum dose administered was 45 mg/d.

Patients receiving high doses of amphetamine who were randomized to placebo had the active drug withdrawn gradually over a 2-week period.

STATISTICAL ANALYSIS

Randomization was balanced within each site and stratified for age (6- to 8-year-olds and 9- to 11-year-olds). The duration of randomized double-blind treatment and scores on the Conners rating scales for parents and teachers were prespecified as primary efficacy variables. Patients receiving randomized treatment whose symptoms deteriorated and returned to prestudy levels of behavior problems according to parent judgment (and corroborated by the research-clinician) were offered open treatment with amphetamine. Before such treatment was started, every effort was made to obtain new ratings on the Conners scales. Time from randomization to interruption of double-blind treatment was analyzed using the Kaplan-Meier method and the log rank test. Change on the Conners scales was evaluated using analysis of variance (ANOVA). In the primary intention-to-treat analysis, the last ratings before interruption of randomized treatment were carried forward and used as the score for the subsequent visits. For inclusion in this analysis, at least 2 ratings between times 3 and 15 months had to be available. If the 3-month score was missing, the average score for all patients at 3 months was used instead. As a complement to this procedure, an analysis of ratings obtained on randomized treatment was performed.

The preplanned analyses of the Conners scores were (1) treatment differences in change from months 3 through 15 and (2) change from months 15 through 18 in all patients receiving amphetamine at month 15.

In the analysis of other numerical and categorical variables, ANOVA and χ^2 methods were used. The Fisher exact test and *t* tests were used in the analysis of WISC-R results. Alpha levels of .01 or less were considered significant.

DURATION OF RANDOMIZED DOUBLE-BLIND TREATMENT

Patients in the placebo group were withdrawn from randomized treatment more often than those in the amphetamine group ($P<.001$). During the 12-month double-blind phase, 71% of the placebo group and 29% of the amphetamine group stopped treatment or went on to open treatment (**Figure 1**). A total of 32 children (8 in the placebo group and 24 in the amphetamine group) completed randomized treatment through month 15. Most withdrawals occurred during the first 3 months after randomization. A similar pattern was seen for both sexes and for younger (6-8 years) and older (9-11 years) children.

CONNERS PARENT AND TEACHER SCALES

The lower deviance level after the initial single-blind treatment was maintained in the amphetamine group but not in the placebo group ($P<.001$) through the follow-up visits 3 to 12 months after randomization (**Figure 2** and **Table 2**). This result pertained both to total and subscale scores.

Conners teacher total scores followed the same pattern as those of the parent scale (**Figure 3** and Table 2). The initial decrease during single-blind amphetamine treatment was followed by an increase in the placebo group, while the amphetamine group remained on a lower level ($P<.01$). With the exception of the anxious-

Table 1. Baseline Characteristics of Randomized Patients*

Characteristic	Amphetamine Group (n=32)	Placebo Group (n=30)	Total (N=62)
Male	26	25	51
Age, y	9 (1.6)	9 (1.5)	9 (1.6)
Height, cm	135 (10.5)	138 (12.7)	137 (11.6)
WISC-R IQ			
Verbal	90 (34.3)	92 (37.6)	91 (33.0)
Performance	86 (32.8)	91 (37.2)	88 (32.0)
Mild mental retardation (IQ, 51-72)	5	5	10
Autistic disorder	0	1	1
Pervasive developmental disorder NOS	3	3	6
Oppositional defiant disorder	7	1	8
Conduct disorder	3	0	3
Separation anxiety disorder	1	1	2
Tics or Tourette syndrome	1	2	3
No comorbid diagnosis	18	18	36

Data are given as number of patients or as mean (SD). WISC-R indicates Wechsler Intelligence Scale–Revised for Children; NOS, not otherwise specified.

fearful subscale, the results were similar for all the subscale scores.

Withdrawal at month 15 was not done for 3 patients in the amphetamine group (clinically contraindicated in 1 patient, 1 patient failed to show up at appointed time, administrative lapse in a third patient).

For all patients receiving amphetamine treatment at month 15, treatment withdrawal did not lead to change in average parent scores at month 18. Average teacher scores indicated (nonsignificant) deterioration of behavior.

All the significant results reported for boys and girls collapsed remained significant when analyzed separately for boys only. Change in Conners parent total scores was accounted for by older children (9-11 years) ($P<.001$). Conners teacher total scores declined in both age subgroups, but significant change ($P<.02$) occurred only in the older subgroup. The younger and older children in the study had the same mean number of attention-deficit problems at baseline.

DEPRESSED MOOD

There were no significant differences between the treatment groups on the Birleson and McGrath measures.

WISC-R RESULTS

Children who had been taking placebo for 6 months (n=8) or more were compared with those who had been taking amphetamine for 9 months or more (n=35) with respect to change in WISC-R scores. The prediction was that the latter group would show greater increases in IQ scores. The mean change in IQ from 0 to 15 months was +4.5 (SD, 4.7) in the group treated with amphetamine

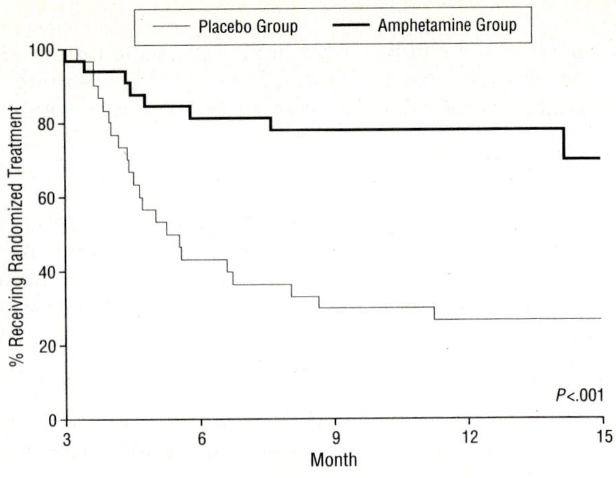

Figure 1. *Time to treatment failure after randomization to treatment with amphetamine or placebo.*

for 9 months or more and +0.7 (SD, 7.2) in the group receiving placebo for 6 months or more ($P<.05$, *t* test, 1 tailed). In the former group, 28 of 34 individuals changed in a positive direction, whereas in the latter group only 4 of 8 did ($P<.06$, Fisher exact test). Verbal scores did not increase more than performance scores in any of the groups.

ADVERSE EVENTS AND OTHER SYMPTOMS

Most side effects were recorded at a low rate and, with the exception of decreased appetite, did not differ between the amphetamine and placebo groups (Table 2).

Early awakenings and disturbed sleep tended to occur less frequently with single-blind amphetamine treatment than at baseline. Poor appetite was uncommon at baseline, but after 3 months of single-blind amphetamine treatment 56% (33/59) reported this side effect. The amphetamine group significantly more often had decreased appetite at 6 months.

Abdominal pains "occasionally" or "often" occurred in 32% (20/62) on at least 1 assessment (including at baseline). Of these, 3 children reported such problems only at baseline, 6 had at least the same degree of problems before any medication was used, and 1 had abdominal pain only at the 18-month follow-up (after taking placebo for 3 months). Of those who had an increase of abdominal pain symptoms during the double-blind phase, 5 received amphetamine and 5 received placebo at the time of reported problems ($P=.91$). Three children had tics or Tourette syndrome diagnosed before baseline. Their tics did not increase in frequency or severity while receiving double-blind amphetamine treatment. One boy with mild tics at baseline had an increase of severe tics on a 15-mg daily dose of amphetamine and had to discontinue use of the drug. He also experienced visual hallucinations while taking a higher dose of the drug (see below). Eighteen children developed tics during the study. Of these, 6 had tics that were observed at baseline. Four of the remaining 12 were receiving placebo, and 4 were receiving amphetamine on all occasions when tics were reported. None of these

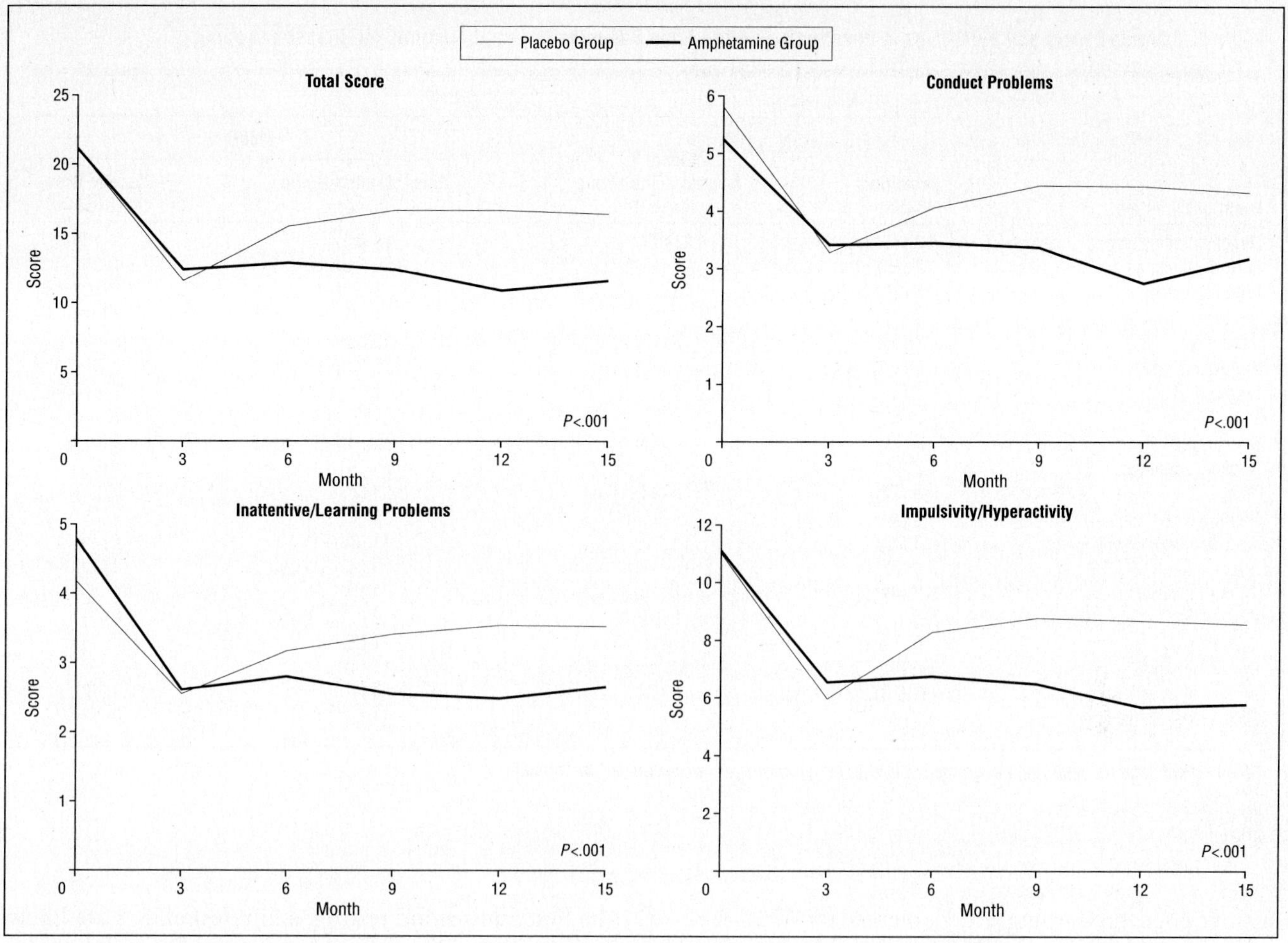

Figure 2. *Results of the Conners Parent Rating Scale for children in the amphetamine and placebo groups. Total scores decreased from month 0 to month 3 for all individuals, and increased up to month 6 in the placebo group.*

showed increase of tic frequency or severity. Four children had tics observed only toward the end of single-blind treatment with amphetamine. Two of these were then given (double-blind) active amphetamine treatment, and no more tics were observed. Two received (double-blind) placebo and had no further tics. Four children showed stereotypies clearly separable from tics, but not related to amphetamine treatment. Several children were described as "euphoric" or "hypomanic" at baseline. Most of these were considered not euphoric or hypomanic after 3 months of single-blind amphetamine treatment. Four boys experienced hallucinations, 3 during treatment with amphetamine and 1 with placebo. One (6 years old) had to stop amphetamine treatment. His behavior improved promptly, but his mother would not let him have another trial of medication. An 11-year-old boy who was receiving amphetamine developed acute, severe visual hallucinations that disappeared on dose reduction from 25 to 15 mg daily. A week later, severe tics developed and the drug had to be discontinued (see above). Another amphetamine-treated boy experienced visual hallucinations toward the end of the active treatment period. When the drug was discontinued, hallucinations subsided immediately. A boy receiving placebo (9 years old) with an abnormal electroencephalogram was among the most psychiatrically disturbed in the study, meeting all 14 of the diagnostic criteria for ADHD. Average weight gain from baseline through month 15 (1.7 kg) was less than expected (4.0 kg). There was a weak linear relation between weight gain and months on amphetamine treatment. One month of amphetamine treatment inhibited weight gain by an average of 0.2 kg ($P<.04$). Average height gain (6.5 cm) was close to that expected (7.0 cm). There was no significant relation between height development and duration of amphetamine treatment.

EFFECTS OF COMORBID DIAGNOSES

Subgroups with and without comorbid diagnoses were compared with regard to Conners parent and teacher total and subscale scores and adverse events and symptoms. No significant differences were found. The WISC-R scores at baseline did not contribute to outcome.

COMMENT

To our knowledge, this is the first prospective, randomized, double-blind, placebo-controlled, long-term study of stimulant treatment for childhood attention-deficit problems. Amphetamine was clearly superior to placebo in improving behavior. There was a trend toward a

Table 2. Adverse Events and Symptoms at Baseline and After 3 and 6 Months for Amphetamine and Placebo Groups

	No. (%) of Patients*			
			Month 6	
Event or Symptom	Baseline (n=54)	Month 3, Amphetamine Group (n=60)	Amphetamine Group (n=40)	Placebo Group (n=16)
Difficulty falling asleep	18 (33)	23 (39)	14 (35)	3 (19)
Early awakenings	13 (25)	8 (13)†	6 (15)	4 (25)
Disturbed sleep	15 (28)	10 (17)‡	9 (23)	2 (12)
Increased need to sleep	6 (11)	5 (8)	1 (2)	2 (12)
Headache	7 (13)	8 (13)	10 (25)	3 (19)
Abdominal pain	9 (17)	6 (10)	5 (12)	1 (6)
Diarrhea	3 (6)	0	1 (2)	1 (6)
Constipation	3 (6)	3 (5)	1 (2)	0
Dry mouth	4 (7)	6 (10)	5 (12)	1 (6)
Nausea, vomiting	3 (6)	3 (5)	5 (12)	1 (6)
Tics	9 (17)	14 (23)	8 (20)	5 (31)
Stereotypies	2 (4)	9 (15)‡	5 (12)	1 (6)
Anxiety, nervousness	18 (33)	14 (23)	11 (28)	7 (44)
Dysthymia	4 (7)	10 (17)‡	9 (23)	2 (13)
Euphoria, hypomania	22 (41)	8 (13)§	4 (10)	4 (25)
Palpitation	0	2 (3)	2 (5)	0
Dizziness	0	1 (2)	1 (2)	0
Decreased appetite	2 (4)	33 (55)§	17 (42)	2 (12)†
Increased appetite	7 (13)	8 (13)	4 (10)	2 (12)
Hallucinations, delusions	0	0	1 (2)	0

*Data reflect patients' reporting occurrence of events or symptoms as "occasionally" or "often."
†$P<.05$
‡$P<.10$.
§$P<.001$.

positive effect on learning as documented by WISC-R results. Ten of the original cohort of 72 children assigned for study dropped out while receiving single-blind treatment with amphetamine before randomization. Three of these had severe side effects and 4 did not respond to treatment. Unwanted reactions were clinically nonsignificant in the randomized cases, except in a minority who had severe—but reversible—side effects. Tics were not associated with stimulant treatment. As in previous long-term follow-up studies, height was not affected.[29]

We chose amphetamine because we did not want to restrict our study to children with normal electroencephalograms and no history of seizures. No child experienced seizures during the study.

Behavioral improvement was most marked in the homes (with Conners score declines ranging from 43%-47%) and slightly less obvious in the classroom (declines of 27%-40%). Short-term studies have usually demonstrated more improvement based on teacher ratings than on parent ratings. This could be associated with behavior in the classroom being particularly difficult to regulate for children with attention deficits or with teachers being more observant of the type of symptoms shown by such children. Our findings also could be associated with the teacher scale being longer, including many items not specifically pertaining to attention-activity-impulsivity problems. Nevertheless, short-term studies[19,30] have indicated that general behavior as well as attention deficits improves with stimulant treatment.

Improvements on the WISC-R on retesting were expected, but more than 12 months elapsed between the first and second testing, and retest effects are likely to be minor after such a long time. Only the group receiving amphetamine for more than 9 months tended to improve. This suggests that the findings are not an artifact of retesting. However, the improvement on the WISC-R should not be taken as proof of academic success.[19]

It is difficult to maintain double-blind conditions for an extended period for a cohort of children with attention deficits participating in a randomized comparative study of an effective drug and placebo. Only 27% of the original cohort assigned to placebo completed randomized treatment through month 15. Children receiving amphetamine usually remained on treatment for the whole double-blind active treatment period of 12 months. Children receiving placebo, on the other hand, required open treatment with amphetamine in a majority of the cases before the blinded period was over. This was anticipated, and time to treatment failure was prechosen as a primary efficacy variable. Indeed, this finding strongly suggests the superiority of amphetamine over placebo. However, the high withdrawal rate causes some problems for the analysis of the results obtained, particularly on the Conners scales. Therefore, caution is warranted in the interpretation. Nevertheless, the findings of the intention-to-treat analyses received some support by the results from the randomized treatment analysis. The small number of patients still receiving placebo after 6 months did allow for some random fluctuations, but the overall pattern was similar, even though the differences obtained tended to be less marked.

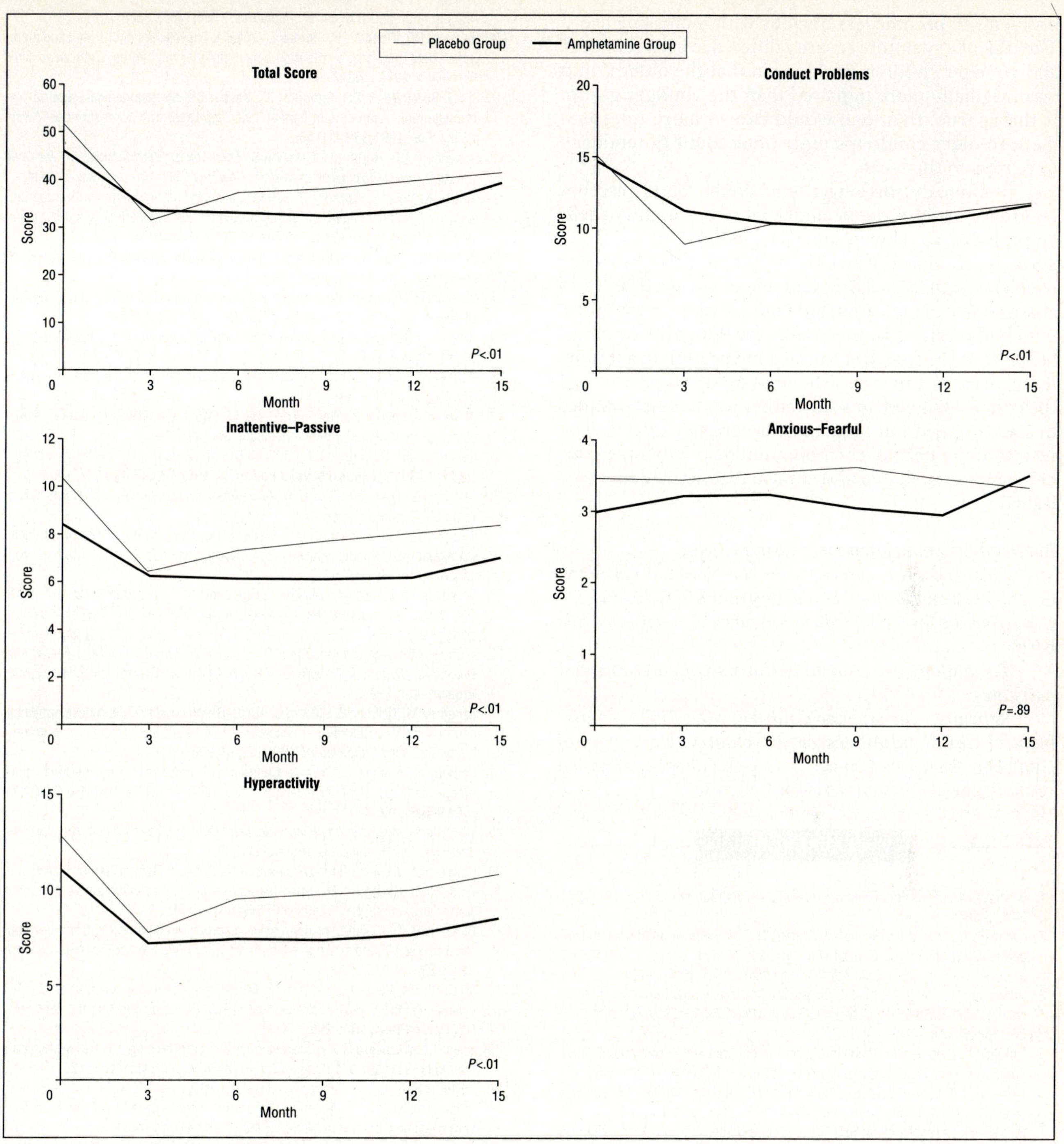

Figure 3. *Results of the Conners Teacher Rating Scale for children in the amphetamine and placebo groups. Total scores decreased from month 0 to month 3 and increased up to month 6 in the placebo group.*

The children suffered from severe attention deficits. A considerable subgroup (42%) had comorbid diagnoses, including mild mental retardation, autistic features, oppositional defiant disorder, and tic disorders. This is a reflection of clinical realities; "pure" ADHD cases are relatively rare. Clinical improvement was equally good in the "comorbid" group (and in the individual diagnostic subgroups) as in the "pure" ADHD group, agreeing with previous studies that have suggested that neurological disorders and pervasive developmental disorders do not influence response to treatment.[31-33] This suggests that stimulant treatment should not be "disorder geared" but rather seen as a possible adjunct in the treatment of attention deficits with or without comorbid symptoms/disorders. However, caution is warranted in the interpretation of these findings, since numbers were small, and type II errors cannot be excluded.

Behavior was more improved in older children than in the younger ones. This could be a reflection of greater parent and teacher tolerance for deviance in younger children or of true age effect differences. Younger and older children were equally impaired on clinical examination and had similar types and degrees of comorbidity at baseline. There is normally a tendency for attention-deficit problems to become less obvious with increasing age.[34] The lack of a symptom severity difference between older and younger children could mean that the older group was originally more impaired than the younger group. If this is true, then one would expect more improvement in older children simply on account of tendency to regress to the mean.

In summary, this longer-term, double-blind, placebo-controlled study of amphetamine for severe attention deficit problems has shown some promising results with regard to reduction of overactivity and other behavior problems both in the home and school setting. There was also a tendency for learning to improve more in the group who had received amphetamine for 9 months or more. Side effects precluded continued medication in a minority of all cases, but were otherwise mild. About 1 in 7 of the cohort assigned for study either was a nonresponder or had dropped out because of severe side effects. The results are in need of corroboration before definite conclusions can be drawn and clinical recommendations be issued.

Accepted for publication December 11, 1996.

This study was supported by the National Corporation of Swedish Pharmacies and by grant K97-21X-11251-03C from the Swedish Medical Research Council (Dr Gillberg).

The authors are grateful to Carina Löf for secretarial assistance.

Reprints: Christopher Gillberg, MD, PhD, Department of Child and Adolescent Psychiatry, University of Göteborg, Annedals Clinics, S 413 45 Göteborg, Sweden (e-mail: christopher.gillberg@pediat.gu.se).

REFERENCES

1. Bradley C. The behavior of children receiving benzedrine. *Am J Psychiatry.* 1937; 94:577-585.
2. Jacobvitz D, Sroufe LA, Stewart M, Leffert N. Treatment of additional and hyperactivity problems in children with sympathomimetic drugs: a comprehensive review. *J Am Acad Child Adolesc Psychiatry.* 1990;29:677-688.
3. Stevenson RD, Wolraich MD. Stimulant medication therapy in the treatment of children with attention deficit hyperactivity disorder. *Pediatr Clin North Am.* 1989; 36:1183-1197.
4. DuPaul GJ, Barkley RA. Social interaction of children with attention deficit hyperactivity disorder: effects of methylphenidate. In: McCord R, Tremblay RE, eds. *Preventing Antisocial Behavior: Interventions From Birth Through Adolescence.* New York, NY: Guilford Press; 1992:89-116.
5. Barkley RA. The social interactions of hyperactive children: developmental changes, drug effects and situational variation. In: McMahon R, Peters R, eds. *Childhood Disorders: Behavioral-Developmental Approaches.* New York, NY: Brunner/Mazel; 1985:218-243.
6. DuPaul GJ, Barkely RA. Behavioral contributions to pharmacotherapy: the utility of behavioral methodology in medication treatment of children with attention deficit hyperactivity disorder. *Behav Ther.* 1993;24:47-65.
7. Douglas VI, Barr RG, O'Neill ME, Britton BG. Short-term effects of methylphenidate on the cognitive learning academic performance of children with attention deficit disorder in the laboratory and the classroom. *J Child Psychol Psychiatry.* 1986;27:191-211.
8. Sebrechts MM, Shaywitz SD, Shaywitz BA, Jatlow P, Anderson GM, Cohen DJ. Components of attention, methylphenidate dosage and blood levels in children with attention deficit disorder. *Pediatrics.* 1986;77:222-228.
9. Garfinkel BD, Wender PH, Sloman L, O'Neill I. Tricyclic antidepressant and methylphenidate treatment of attention deficit disorder in children. *J Am Acad Child Psychiatry.* 1983;22:343-348.
10. Elia J, Borcherding BG, Rapoport JL, Keysor CS. Methylphenidate and dextroamphetamine treatments of hyperactivity: are there true nonresponders? *Psychiatry Res.* 1991;36:141-155.
11. Rosenberg DR, Holttum J, Gershon S. *Textbook of Pharmacotherapy for Child and Adolescent Psychiatric Disorders.* New York, NY: Brunner/Mazel; 1994.
12. Gadow K, Nolan E, Sprafkin J. School observations of children with attention-deficit hyperactivity disorder and comorbid tic disorder: effect of methylphenidate treatment. *J Dev Behav Pediatr.* 1995;16:167-176.
13. DuPaul GJ, Stoner G. *ADHD in the Schools: Assessment and Intervention Strategies.* New York, NY: Guilford Press; 1994.
14. Dulcan MK. Using psychostimulants to treat behavioral disorders of children and adolescents. *J Child Adolesc Psychopharmacol.* 1990;1:7-22.
15. Fulton A, Yates WR. Family abuse of methylphenidate. *Am Fam Physician.* 1988; 38:143-145.
16. Riddle KD, Rapoport JL. A 2-year follow-up of 72 hyperactive boys. *J Nerv Ment Dis.* 1976;162:126-134.
17. Weiss G, Kruger E, Danielson U, Elman M. Effect of long-term treatment of hyperactive children with methylphenidate. *Can Med Assoc J.* 1975;112:159-165.
18. Satterfield JH, Satterfield BT, Cantwell DP. Three-year multimodality treatment study of 100 hyperactive boys. *J Pediatrics.* 1981;98:143-144.
19. Barkley RA. *Hyperactive Children: A Handbook for Diagnosis and Treatment.* New York, NY: Guilford Press; 1990.
20. Swedish Medical Products Agency. Medikamentell behandling av uppmärksamhetsstörningar med hyperaktivitet hos barn. Uppsala, Sweden: Swedish Medical Products Agency; 1991;1:7-11.
21. American Psychiatric Association. *Diagnostic and Statistical Manual of Mental Disorders, Third Edition, Revised.* Washington, DC: American Psychiatric Association; 1987.
22. World Health Organization. *The ICD-10 Classification of Mental and Behavioural Disorders: Diagnostic Criteria for Research.* Geneva, Switzerland: World Health Organization; 1993.
23. Landgren M, Kjellman B, Gillberg C. ADHD, DAMP and other neurodevelopmental/neuropsychiatric disorders in six-year-old children: epidemiology and comorbidity. *Dev Med Child Neurol.* 1996;38:891-906.
24. Gillberg IC, Gillberg C, Groth J. Children with preschool minor neurodevelopmental disorders, V: neurodevelopmental profiles at age 13. *Dev Med Child Neurol.* 1989;31:14-24.
25. Wechsler D. *Wechsler Intelligence Scale for Children, Third Edition–Revised.* New York, NY: Psychological Corporation; 1992.
26. Conners CK. *Conners Rating Scales Manual, Conners Teacher Rating Scales, Conners Parent Rating Scales: Instruments for Use With Children and Adolescents.* North Tonawanda, NY: Multihealth Systems; 1990.
27. Birleson P. The validity of depressive disorder in childhood and the development of a self-rating scale: a research report. *J Child Psychol Psychiatry.* 1981; 22:73-88.
28. McGrath PA, Veber LL, Hearth MT. Multidimensional pain assessment in children. In: Fidds HL, et al, eds. *Advances in Pain Research and Therapy.* New York, NY: Raven Press; 1985;9:387-393.
29. Klein RG, Mannuzza S. Hyperactive boys almost grown up, III: methylphenidate effects on ultimate height. *Arch Gen Psychiatry.* 1988;45:1131-1134.
30. Taylor E, Schachar R, Thorley G, Wieselberg HM, Everitt B, Rutter M. Which boys respond to stimulant treatment? a controlled trial of methylphenidate in boys with disruptive behaviour. *Psychol Med.* 1987;17:121-143.
31. Handen BL, Janosky J, McAuliffe S, Breaux AM, Feldman H. Prediction of response to methylphenidate among children with ADHD and mental retardation. *J Am Acad Child Adolesc Psychiatry.* 1994;33:1185-1193.
32. Mayes SD, Crites DL, Bixler EO, Humphrey FJ II, Mattison RE. Methylphenidate and ADHD : influence of age, IQ and neurodevelopmental status. *Dev Med Child Neurol.* 1994;36:1099-1107.
33. Quintana H, Firmaher B, Stedge D, Lennon S, Freed J, Bridge J, Greenhill L. Use of methylphenidate in treatment of children with autistic disorder. *J Autism Dev Disord.* 1995;25:283-294.
34. Gillberg C, Hellgren L. Outcome of attention disorders. In: Sandberg S, ed. *Hyperactivity Disorders.* Cambridge, England: Cambridge University Press; 1996: 473-499.

National Institute of Mental Health Collaborative Multimodal Treatment Study of Children With ADHD (the MTA)

Design Challenges and Choices

L. Eugene Arnold, MEd, MD; Howard B. Abikoff, PhD; Dennis P. Cantwell, MD; C. Keith Conners, PhD; Glen Elliott, MD, PhD; Laurence L. Greenhill, MD; Lily Hechtman, MD; Stephen P. Hinshaw, PhD; Betsy Hoza, PhD; Peter S. Jensen, MD; Helena C. Kraemer, PhD; John S. March, MD, MPH; Jeffrey H. Newcorn, MD; William E. Pelham, PhD; John E. Richters, PhD; Ellen Schiller, PhD; Joanne B. Severe, MS; James M. Swanson, PhD; Donald Vereen, MD; Karen C. Wells, PhD; for the MTA

The Collaborative Multimodal Treatment Study of Children With Attention Deficit Hyperactivity Disorder (ADHD), the MTA, is the first child multisite cooperative agreement treatment study of children conducted by the National Institute of Mental Health, Rockville, Md. It examines the long-term effectiveness of medication vs behavioral treatment vs both for treatment of ADHD and compares state-of-the-art treatment with routine community care. In a parallel-groups design, 576 children (age, 7-9 years) with ADHD (96 at each site) are thoroughly assessed and randomized to 4 conditions: (1) medication alone, (2) psychosocial treatment alone, (3) the combination of both, (4) or community comparison. The first 3 groups are treated for 14 months and all are reassessed periodically for 24 months. Designers met the following challenges: framing clinically relevant primary questions; defining the target population; choice, intensity, and integration and combination of treatments for fair comparisons; combining scientific controls and standardization with clinical flexibility; and implementing a controlled clinical trial in a nonclinical setting (school) controlled by others. Innovative solutions included extensive decision algorithms and manualized adaptations of treatments to specific needs.

Arch Gen Psychiatry. 1997;54:865-870

The Multimodal Treatment Study of Children With Attention Deficit Hyperactivity Disorder (ADHD), the MTA study, is a multisite cooperative agreement sponsored by the National Institute of Mental Health (NIMH), Rockville, Md, cosponsored by the Office of Special Education Programs of the US Department of Education, Washington, DC. A landmark study, it is the first cooperative child treatment study ever undertaken by NIMH and the largest NIMH clinical trial to date.

We described the background and rationale in a previous report.[1] Briefly, ADHD is one of the most common (3% to 5%) childhood mental disorders.[2] Previous study has demonstrated short-term efficacy of pharmacological and behavioral (psychosocial [PS]) treatments for ADHD, but their relative merits and long-term effectiveness are unknown. The field's diagnostic and therapeutic expertise had progressed to the point of warranting a multisite study to answer critical questions that could not be answered by single-site studies. The Request for Applications (RFA MH-92-03) was released in February 1992, and grants were awarded to 6 sites (listed at the end of this article) in September 1992. The first subjects enrolled in 1994; the last will finish in 1998.

During the first project year, we developed a common protocol based on the original 6 competing proposals, augmented by new ideas from group discussion. Several methodological challenges re-

A complete list of the members of the MTA study with their affiliations appears at the end of this article.

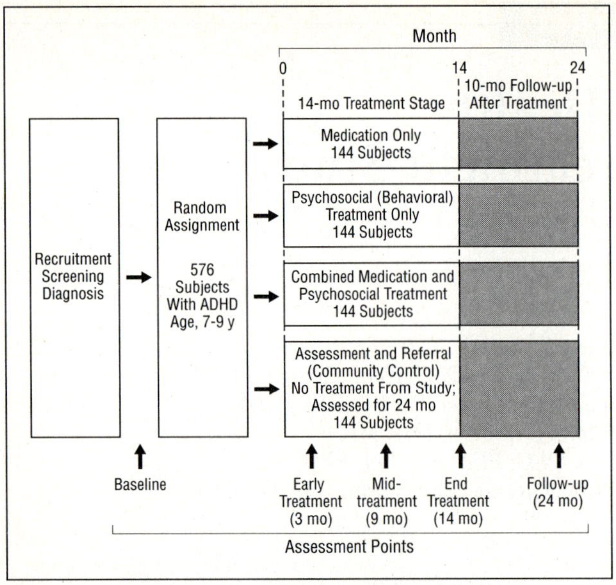

Figure 1. *Basic design and subject flow of Multimodal Treatment Study of Children With Attention Deficit Hyperactivity Disorder (ADHD), the MTA study. A 1-way 4-group design is necessary to allow long-term follow-up comparison of outcome. Three of the 4 groups are treated for 14 months. The medication strategy includes a 1-month blind titration with methylphenidate for best dose, open titration with other drugs if necessary, monthly maintenance visits with algorithmic dose adjustments, supplementary general advice and selected readings, case management by the pharmacotherapist, and emergency services as needed. The psychosocial (behavioral) treatment strategy is an intense and multicomponent one (see Figure 2), which includes parent training, structured teacher consultation, an 8-week full-time summer treatment program, 12 weeks of having a half-time behavioral specialist in the classroom, case management by the therapist/consultant, and emergency services as needed. The combined strategy includes both of the other strategies. At the end of 14 months of MTA treatment, recommendations and referrals are made for any indicated further treatment, which is not provided by the MTA. The assessment and referral group receives no MTA treatment but seeks their own in the community, and is assessed at the same times as the 3 treated groups.*

quired critical choices. This article reports the resolution of 5 of these in addition to describing the design: (1) choice of primary questions, (2) definition of target population, (3) the choice and intensity of treatment modalities (giving each a fair chance in comparisons and combining them in ways that respect their relative strengths), (4) promoting the relevance of research findings to clinical practice and policy while maintaining scientific standards, and (5) carrying out a controlled clinical trial in the nonclinical school setting.

MTA DESIGN

Five hundred seventy-six boys and girls (age, 7-9 years) with ADHD (96 at each of 6 sites) are randomly assigned to 1 of 4 treatment conditions in a parallel-groups design, as shown in **Figure 1** and are assessed periodically for 2 years. Three of the groups are treated for the first 14 months in specified protocols and the fourth group (assessment and referral, or community control) is referred for community treatment of the parents' choosing.

This design allows long-term (14 and 24 months) outcome comparisons among state-of-the-art pharmacotherapy, state-of-the-art behavioral treatment, and the combination (first primary question), as well as comparison of such systematic intensive treatments with treatment provided in the community (second primary question). A comprehensive multidomain assessment battery at baseline, 3 months, 9 months, treatment end point (14 months), and 24 months (10-month follow-up) will support subsidiary analyses of effects of severity, comorbidity, sex, socioeconomic status, ethnicity, parental psychopathology, and domain of dysfunction on outcome, palatability, and compliance; it also will allow examination of predictor, mediator, and moderator variables. This design resulted from the following considerations.

CHOICE OF PRIMARY QUESTIONS

Candidates for primary question included cost-effectiveness questions: How intense a treatment is needed and at what point do returns diminish, especially for the labor-intensive behavioral treatments? What is the relative effectiveness of various behavioral treatment components, eg, parent training (PT) vs teacher consultation vs classroom aide vs child treatment? Clinically, is it better to tailor specific PS treatment components to the apparent needs of each child or to give everyone the same manualized package of proved components? As attractive as such questions are, the current controversies about medication use, relative advantages of medication and behavioral treatment, and long-term utility of various treatments suggested that the first priority should be a long-term comparing of the 2 basic modalities (drug and PS treatment) and their combination. Later studies could explore intensity thresholds, dismantle components, and explore the potential benefits of tailoring specific components. A second priority for public policy is finding whether state-of-the-art intensive treatment is any better than the highly variable (often minimal) treatment available in the community. Therefore, the 2 primary issues are (1) the relative advantages of medication vs PS treatment vs combined treatment over time (long-term) and (2) the advantage of systematic state-of-the-art treatment relative to routine community treatments.

INCLUSION OF A PS-TREATMENT-ONLY CONDITION

Few clinical issues have been more hotly debated than the relative values of medication and PS treatment for ADHD. Our decision to include a PS-treatment-only condition in the main comparison was unusual for an ADHD treatment study of this length, because stimulant medication with or without PS treatment is the generally accepted standard. Inclusion of a PS-treatment arm is scientifically efficient, answering 2 additional questions besides what PS treatment adds to medication (the usual ADHD study question); we can also find what medication adds to PS treatment and compare the 2 modalities. The relevant literature[1,3-8] suggested that, with sufficiently intense behavioral intervention, it had become feasible to manage ADHD without medication. Whether it is advisable is an empirical question begging for an answer. Clinical assumptions that combined pharmacological and PS treatments are better for ADHD in the long run than either modality alone have not been definitively tested in well-controlled trials; they are based on 1 poorly controlled unreplicated trial[9] and extrapolations from short-term studies suggesting such an additive effect.[1,3,6,10-14] However, in addition to the possibility of additive effects, alternate possibilities include reciprocal effects, in which the combination's effects are the same as either modality alone,[14] and interference, in which one modality eventually interferes with the other.[15,16] For example, could successful medication reduce parents' motivation to implement a behavioral program that might have more lasting benefit? Only a design including a PS-treatment-only group can yield information to settle this important issue.

DEFINITION OF TARGET POPULATION

The desire for a broad, representative sample for clinical and public health relevance was balanced by the need for a well-defined sample whose subjects could participate in the treatments and assessments. This tension was partially resolved by deciding that the only exclusion criteria are conditions or situations that would interfere with treatment, assessment, or the design (the complete list will be published in an article on recruitment and assessment). For example, a child in the same classroom as an already enrolled MTA subject is ineligible because of the risk of cross-arm contamination by teacher consultation if one pupil is assigned PS treatment and the other is not. No exclusions are made for comorbidity, which commonly occurs in the clinical ADHD population, unless it requires treatment incompatible with MTA treatment.

Diagnosis

A more difficult choice was to take only the *DSM-IV* combined type 2[2] of ADHD (the full syndrome, with symptoms of both inattentiveness and impulsivity or hyperactivity). This sacrificed a higher proportion of girls (more likely to have inattentive type) as potential subjects. It seemed necessary, however, to ensure that subjects have ADHD of sufficient severity to allow the demonstration of potential treatment effects across outcome domains (behavioral, academic, or family).

Age Range

The age restriction (age, 7-9 years; school grade, 1-4) relinquished considerably the opportunity to study age effects on differential treatment response, but a narrow age range is needed to group children effectively for PS treatments.

CHOICE, INTENSITY, AND INTEGRATION OF TREATMENTS

Guiding principles in choice of treatments were that they must be (1) state-of-the-art, with research evidence of at least short-term efficacy; (2) manualized and transportable; (3) sufficiently intense, integrated, and flexible to credibly stand alone; and (4) capable of individualization and adjustment to make them suitable for long-term participation. Distinctions between modalities have to be drawn sharply enough to support the comparisons required by the primary questions. Several challenges arose in designing the treatment strategies for each arm, and they are outlined below.

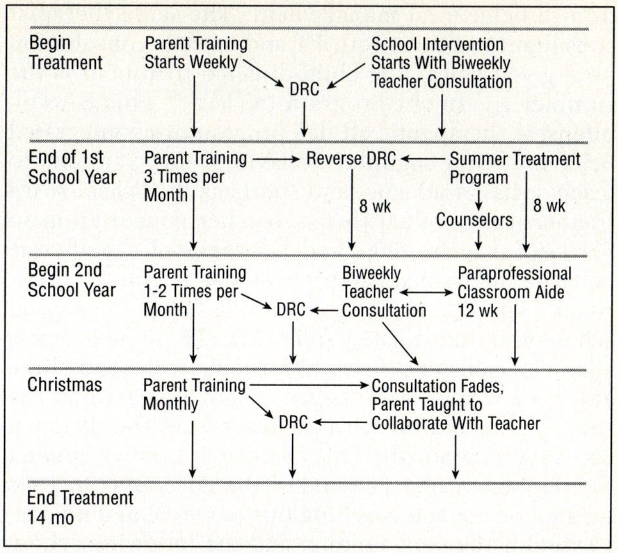

Figure 2. *Flow of intense behavioral treatment. Diagonal and horizontal arrows show some ways in which components are integrated. Parent training provides continuity throughout the 14 months. DRC indicates daily report card. See the "Integrating Components" subsection of the "Choice, Intensity, and Integration of Treatments" section for more details.*

Treatment Strategies for Ensuring Fair Comparisons

Pursuit of the first question requires that each treatment be given its "best shot." To meet this requirement (and ethical obligations to subjects who stop a successful pre-MTA medication regimen to be randomized to PS treatment), a multicomponent package of intense behavioral interventions is required. To give the medication condition its optimal chance, we chose a medication *strategy* rather than a single drug. This strategy, similar to that of a good clinician, systematically tries various drugs and doses until a satisfactory result is found.[17]

Integrating Components

The PS treatment needs to address several domains of function. This requires several components—direct treatment of the child, PT, and school-based intervention—that must be integrated. They are organized in a flow (**Figure 2**) designed to capitalize on the strengths of each at the appropriate time.

The PT regimen developed for the MTA (based on work by Barkley[18] and Forehand and McMahon[19]) involves 27 group and 8 individual sessions for each family during a 14-month period, first weekly and then less frequently. It begins after randomization the first spring, in concert with biweekly teacher consultation in behavioral management. The same therapist consultant conducts both PT and teacher consultation for a given child. The child-directed treatment is the summer treatment program (STP).[8,20] This 8-week intensive therapeutic all-day program uses integrated behavioral and cognitive-behavioral interventions to teach social, academic, and sports skills. *School-based treatment* has a dual thrust: teacher consultation in behavioral techniques and 12 weeks of a half-time behaviorally trained paraprofessional aide in the classroom.[5] The aide is scheduled in the fall of the second school year, immediately following STP, to help generalize STP gains to the new classroom. At the end of the aide's 12 weeks, parents are coached to assume the role of collaborating with the teacher, as the therapist consultants gradually fade their own teacher contact to telephone calls. The end of the PT course focuses on supporting and coaching this new role and on preparing for the next summer and the following school year.

To promote integration of components, the same behavioral specialists function as counselors in the STP and as paraprofessional aides in the fall classroom. They are supervised in both settings by the same therapist consultant who does the PT and teacher consultation. The school, STP, and home efforts are linked by a daily report card[10,21]: a list of target behaviors is checked yes or no and sent home daily with the child for reinforcement by parents, using a reward menu devised in PT. The STP and home efforts are also linked by a "reverse daily report card," in which success on parent-checked home behaviors is reinforced at STP.

Combining Modalities

Medication and PS Treatment. Combining medication and PS treatment to allow a fair comparison to each unimodal treatment presented a difficult integration challenge. At first, it seemed best to ensure that the 2 modalities in combined treatment were identical to the homologous treatments in the unimodal treatment arms. This would theoretically support valid comparisons of additive effects. However, we soon realized that this approach would be artificial, lacking in ecological validity. If combined treatment has advantages, these must include the complementarity of modalities, the increased flexibility each affords the other, and the superior data base available to guide treatment.

Therefore, the 2 modalities are integrated by algorithms that respect and capitalize on the characteristics of each. Once titrated, medication dose should not often need adjustment, while increases carry the risk of side effects. Conversely, PS treatment is more slowly "titrated," with more cumulative "dosage," by its nature is continually adjusted to the patient's changing status, and carries less risk from "dosage escalation." This contrast suggests that when a problem arises during treatment that is not clearly medication related (eg, side effects), PS treatment should be adjusted first, avoiding the risk of unnecessary dose or drug changes. Thus, a clinical problem that in the medication-only arm calls for prompt adjustment of dose can be delayed in combined treatment for a month, while the problem is addressed through PS-treatment adjustments. The comparability for analyses of additive effects was preserved by the rule that combined treatment may not involve any therapeutic procedure not available to 1 of the unimodal arms.

Synchronization. Another problem in combining modalities was the proper timing of the methylphenidate titration[17] relative to beginning PS treatment. Completing titration before beginning PS treatment or delaying titration 1 month until the PS treatment takes effect would have controlled for the historical effect of PS treatment. The decision to start both modalities together has the advantages of making both modalities the same length as the unimodal arms and giving the children and caretakers some immediate relief while the PS treatment starts. The multiple-repeat titration[17] that we use controls for the historical effect of the concomitant PS treatment.

SCIENTIFIC STANDARDIZATION VS CLINICAL FLEXIBILITY AND RELEVANCE

Treatment fidelity has 2 aspects: adherence—how well the standardized treatment protocol is followed—and competence—how well the treatment is done clinically.[22] These introduce a tension between competent clinical care and scientific rigor. Good clinical treatment is individualized, compatible with the clinician's style, intuitive as well as logical, and attentive to the affective relationship. Good science requires that the treatment be uniform, manualized, explicit, and logical, with the patient-clinician relationship a variable to be examined. A multisite study has an additional tension, between desire for site flexibility and the need for a common protocol. Site flexibility would make the best use of each site's strengths, might maximize efficiency, and might be argued to produce the best clinical outcome. However, a common protocol demonstrates portability of treatment, shows its effectiveness "in adoptive hands," and enables any site differences that nonetheless arise to be informative. To resolve such tensions for both treatment modalities, fidelity structures include not only the usual manuals, checklists, weekly supervision, cross-site training, and site visits, but also 4 weekly cross-site clinical teleconference panels for all therapists and supervisors, one panel for each of the treatment arms and one for adjunct (emergency) services. These panels support a common cross-site "clinical culture," with "case law" precedents in recorded minutes to prevent drift over time. The treatment strategies themselves were constructed with algorithmized flexibility.[23]

Medication involves systematic individualized titration to find the best dose,[17] manualized algorithms guiding further dosage adjustments in response to monthly clinical assessment, and algorithms for systematically trying other drugs in pursuit of a defined standard of response. The order established for drugs to be tried was methylphenidate, dextroamphetamine, pemoline, and imipramine. Even nonprotocol drugs, combinations of drugs, or deviations from the manual order can be approved at the discretion of the cross-site pharmacology panel, offering a compromise between clinical flexibility and the need for standardization across sites. To meet individual patient needs, the pharmacotherapist can provide informative readings and/or manual-defined supportive counseling to medication-only subjects within the allotted time of the monthly visit.

Psychosocial treatment is adjusted to the individual needs of the child in several ways: Child-specific daily report card target behaviors are individually selected. Individual PT sessions and telephone calls supplementing the group PT allow for fine-tuning each family's program and emphasizing techniques especially relevant for a given family. The therapist consultant has the option (through manualized algorithms) of skipping ahead to relevant PT or teacher consultation modules if needed for a child's emergent problem.

MAINTAINING SCIENTIFIC CONTROL IN THE SCHOOL SETTING

The school setting is key to the symptomatic impairment of ADHD and constitutes the main crucible for distilling treatment effectiveness. We devoted a substantial part of the PS treatment package to school intervention: 2 of the 4 components are school based (teacher consultation and paraprofessional aide), and a third (STP) includes rehearsal in a classroom setting of skills and behavior required for regular school. The fourth component (PT) includes modules that train parents to collaborate with teachers and to support good school behavior by home-based reinforcement. Therefore, we faced the challenge of planning a controlled clinical trial in a nonclinical setting that we could not control, a setting that was the "turf" of a nonclinical profession with its own values, concepts, and procedures.

Recognition of this challenge prompted us to solicit the consultation and cosponsorship of the US Department of Education's Office of Special Education Programs (OSEP). An OSEP representative attended steering committee meetings during protocol planning, and educational consultants sponsored by the OSEP helped develop the school interventions, ensuring their validity, practicality, and palatability in school settings.

Another important decision was to accept only subjects whose main teacher and principal made a firm commitment to participate. The agreement to cooperate follows the format of an informed consent and results in an informed agreement. The principal's commitment is key to the success of the school intervention in the second year, which includes teacher consultation and 12 weeks of a paraprofessional aide; the principal's commitment to assign the subject the second year to a teacher who will cooperate is essential.

Finally, the importance of teacher ratings and other in-school assessments persuaded us to let the school calendar constrain our decisions about treatment length, recruitment window, and length of titration. Such constraints are the price of capturing the ecological validity of the school setting.

CONCLUSIONS

There are considerable challenges in designing a long-term clinical trial to be both scientifically valid and responsive to clinicians' needs. Many clinicians, at least psychotherapists,[24] do not apply research findings to their practice, probably because they perceive much research as irrelevant, performed on purified samples unlike clinical populations, and using artificial treatments.[24-27] Actually, investigators and clinicians have much to offer each other. Recognizing this complementarity, the MTA attempted to fold clinical wisdom, flexibility, and relevance into a rigorous randomized design, using manualized clinical strategies and algorithmized responsiveness to emergent clinical needs. We believe that such solutions will advance the field of clinical trials and open a 2-way path of enrichment between research and clinical practice. Further, although some of the challenges presented by child and adolescent research differ from those in adult research,[28] we hope that this first NIMH child multisite clinical trial will also open a 2-way path of enrichment between adult and child and adolescent research methodology.

Accepted for publication January 28, 1997.

The MTA is a cooperative treatment study performed by 6 independent research teams in collaboration with the staff of the Division of Clinical and Treatment Research of the NIMH and the OSEP of the US Department of Education (DOE). The NIMH Principal Collaborators: *Peter S. Jensen, MD; L. Eugene Arnold, MEd, MD; John E. Richters, PhD; and Joanne B. Severe, MS.* Six Sites Principal Investigators and Coinvestigators: *Stephen P. Hinshaw, PhD, and Glen Elliott, MD, PhD, from the University of California at Berkeley and San Francisco (grant UO1 MH50461); C. Keith Conners, PhD, Karen C. Wells, PhD, and John S. March, MD, MPH, from Duke University, Durham, NC (grant UO1 MH50447); James M. Swanson, PhD, and Dennis P. Cantwell, MD, from the University of California at Irvine and Los Angeles (grant UO1 MH50440); Howard B. Abikoff, PhD, and Lily Hechtman, MD, from the Long Island Jewish Medical Center, New York, and Montreal Children's Hospital, Montreal, Quebec (grant UO1 MH50453); Laurence L. Greenhill, MD, and Jeffrey H. Newcorn, MD, from the New York State Psychiatric Institute, Columbia University, and Mount Sinai Medical Center, New York (grant UO1 MH50454); and William E. Pelham, PhD, and Betsy Hoza, PhD, from the University of Pittsburgh, Pittsburgh, Pa (grant UO1 MH50467).* Statistical and Design Consultant: *Helena C. Kraemer, PhD, Stanford University, Stanford, Calif.* The OSEP/DOE Principal Collaborator: *Ellen Schiller, PhD.*

Reprints: Peter S. Jensen, MD, Chief, Child and Adolescent Disorders Research Branch, National Institute of Mental Health, Parklawn 18C-17, 5600 Fishers Ln, Rockville, MD 20857.

REFERENCES

1. Richters JE, Arnold LE, Jensen PS, Abikoff H, Conners CK, Greenhill LL, Hechtman L, Hinshaw SP, Pelham WE, Swanson JM. The NIMH collaborative multimodal treatment study of children with attention-deficit/hyperactivity disorder (MTA): background and rationale. *J Am Acad Child Adolesc Psychiatry.* 1995; 34:987-1000.
2. American Psychiatric Association. *Diagnostic and Statistical Manual of Mental Disorders, Fourth Edition.* Washington, DC: American Psychiatric Association; 1994.
3. Pelham WE, Schnedler RW, Bender M, Nilsson D, Miller J, Budrow M, Ronnei M, Paluchowski C, Marks D. The combination of behavior therapy and methylphenidate in the treatment of attention deficit disorder: a therapy outcome study. In: Bloomingdale L, ed. *Attention Deficit Disorder III: New Research in Attention, Treatment, and Psychopharmacology.* Oxford, England: Pergamon Press; 1988:29-48.
4. Pelham WE, Hinshaw SP. Behavioral intervention for ADHD. In: Turner SM, Calhoun KS, Adams HE, eds. *Handbook of Clinical Behavior Therapy.* 2nd ed. New York, NY: John Wiley & Sons Inc; 1992:259-283.
5. Swanson JM. *School-Based Assessments and Interventions for ADD Students.* Irvine, Calif: KC Publications; 1992.
6. Pelham WE, Carlson CL, Sams SE, Vallano G, Dixon MJ, Hoza B. Separate and combined effects of methylphenidate and behavior modification on boys with attention-deficit hyperactivity disorder in the classroom. *J Consult Clin Psychol.* 1993;61:506-515.
7. Pfiffner LJ, O'Leary SG. Psychological treatments: school based. In: Matson JL, ed. *Hyperactivity in Children: A Handbook.* Boston, Mass: Allyn & Bacon; 234-255.
8. Pelham WE, Hoza B. Comprehensive treatment for ADHD: a proposal for intensive summer treatment programs and outpatient follow-up. In: Hibbs E, Jensen P, eds. *Psychosocial Treatment Research of Child and Adolescent Disorders.* New York, NY: APA Press; 1996:311-340.
9. Satterfield JH, Satterfield BT, Cantwell DP. Three-year multimodality treatment study of 100 hyperactive boys. *J Pediatr.* 1981;98:650-655.
10. Pelham WE, Schnedler R, Bologna N, Contreras A. Behavioral and stimulant treatment of hyperactive children: a therapy study with methylphenidate probes in a within-subject design. *J Appl Behav Anal.* 1980;13:221-236.
11. Pelham WE, Murphy DA. Behavioral and pharmacological treatment of hyperactivity and attention deficit disorders. In: Herson M, Bruening SE, eds. *Pharmacological and Behavioral Treatment: An Integrative Approach.* New York, NY: John Wiley & Sons Inc; 1986:108-147.
12. Horn WF, Ialongo NS, Pascoe JM, Greenberg G, Packard T, Lopez M, Wagner A, Puttler L. Additive effects of psychostimulants, parent training, and self-control therapy with ADHD children. *J Am Acad Child Adolesc Psychiatry.* 1991;30:233-240.
13. Abikoff H. Interaction of methylphenidate and multimodal therapy in the treatment of attention-deficit hyperactivity disorder. In: Greenhill L, Osman BO, eds. *Ritalin: Theory and Patient Management.* New York, NY: Mary Ann Liebert; 1991: 147-154.
14. Abikoff H, Hechtman L. Multimodal therapy and stimulants in the treatment of children with ADHD. In: Hibbs ED, Jensen PS. *Psychosocial Treatments for Child and Adolescent Disorders: Empirically Based Approaches.* Washington, DC: American Psychological Association; 1996:346-369.
15. Craighead LW, Stunkard AJ, O'Brien RM. Behavior therapy and pharmacotherapy for obesity. *Arch Gen Psychiatry.* 1981;38:763-768.
16. Craske MG. An Integrated treatment approach to panic disorder. *Bull Menninger Clin.* 1996;60(suppl A):A87-A104.
17. Greenhill LL, Abikoff HB, Arnold LE, Cantwell DP, Conners CK, Elliott G, Hechtman L, Hinshaw SP, Hoza B, Jensen PS, Kraemer HC, March JS, Newcorn JH, Pelham WE, Richters JE, Schiller EP, Severe JB, Swanson JM, Vereen D, Wells KC. Medication treatment strategies in the MTA: relevance to clinicians and researchers. *J Am Acad Child Adolesc Psychiatry.* 1996;35:1304-1313.
18. Barkley RA. *Defiant Children: A Clinician's Manual for Parent Training.* New York, NY: Guilford Press; 1987.
19. Forehand R, McMahon R. *Helping the Noncompliant Child: A Clinician's Guide to Parent Training.* New York, NY: Guilford Press; 1981.
20. Pelham WE, Gnagy B, Greiner A, Hoza B, Sams S, Martin L, Wilson T. A summer treatment program for children with ADHD. In: Roberts M, LaGreca A, eds. *Model Programs for Service Delivery for Child and Family Mental Health.* Hillsdale, NJ: Lawrence A. Erlbaum Associates; 1996:193-213.
21. O'Leary KD, Pelham WE, Rosenbaum A, Price G. Behavioral treatment of hyperkinetic children: an experimental evaluation of its usefulness. *Clin Pediatr.* 1976; 5:510-515.
22. Waltz J, Addis ME, Koerner K, Jacobson NS. Testing the integrity of a psychotherapy protocol: assessment of adherence and competence. *J Consult Clin Psychol.* 1993;61:620-630.
23. Arnold LE, Hoagwood K, Jensen PS, Vitiello B. Towards clinically relevant clinical trials. *Psychopharmacol Bull* 1997;33:135-142.
24. Morrow-Bradley C, Elliott R. Utilization of psychotherapy research by practicing psychotherapists. *Am Psychol.* 1986;41:188-197.
25. Howard GS. The scientist-practitioner in counseling psychology: toward a deeper integration of theory, research, and practice. *Couns Psychol.* 1986;14:61-105.
26. Barlow, DH. On the relation of clinical research to clinical practice: current issues, new directions. *J Consult Clin Psychol.* 1981;49:147-155.
27. Jacobson NS, Truax P. Clinical significance: a statistical approach to defining meaningful change in psychotherapy research. *J Consult Clin Psychol.* 1991;59: 12-19.
28. Arnold LE. Treatment research methodology comparisons: adult vs child and adolescent, and psychopharmacological vs psychosocial treatments. *Psychopharmacol Bull.* 1993;29:5-17.

Medication Development and Testing in Children and Adolescents

Current Problems, Future Directions

Benedetto Vitiello, MD; Peter S. Jensen, MD

Progress in pediatric psychopharmacological research has suffered notable delay, especially compared with the achievements in adult psychopharmacology. Although safety and efficacy of the use of many psychotropic agents in children remain largely unproved, their pediatric use has been increasing and their widespread off-label prescribing by practitioners has raised some important concerns. The National Institute of Mental Health, in cooperation with the Food and Drug Administration and leading researchers, has coordinated systematic efforts to identify the major obstacles to research in pediatric psychopharmacology and to propose feasible solutions. In 1995, a conference cosponsored by the National Institute of Mental Health and the Food and Drug Administration gathered more than 100 research experts, family and patient advocates, and representatives of mental health professional associations. Participants met in working groups focused on specific aspects of child research and reached consensus on various recommendations. Each of the various aspects relevant to conducting research in this area (methodological, ethical, legal, regulatory, financial, and family or community context) presents specific challenges, which are herein outlined. Recommendations for possible solutions are presented, some of which are being implemented. Because data about drug safety and efficacy in adults can rarely be extrapolated to children, there is no substitute for pediatric psychopharmacological research. Successful strategies for overcoming the many obstacles with which this research has to contend must enlist the concerted efforts of all the relevant parties (investigators, clinicians, industry, federal agencies, ethicists, families, and community representatives).

Arch Gen Psychiatry. 1997;54:871-876

Despite a substantial and increasing use of psychotropic medications in children and adolescents, only few of these drugs have been systematically studied for efficacy and safety in patients of pediatric age.[1,2] With the exception of the stimulants, whose effects have been extensively studied in children with attention deficit hyperactivity disorder, most of the remaining psychotropic drugs do not have any specific labeling for pediatric patients, other than a standard exclusionary statement that "safety and efficacy have not been established in children." This lack of data has forced physicians and families to make difficult choices, based on the extrapolation of information from studies of adults with similar conditions, resulting in considerable "off-label" use of these drugs.[3] In some instances (eg, tricyclic agents in attention deficit hyperactivity disorder), off-label use is supported by research[4]; however, the soundness of other treatments (eg, clonidine in attention deficit hyperactivity disorder) is poorly documented, thus raising the concern in lay and professional communities.[5] The pediatric use of psychotropic medications is of enormous pub-

This article is also available on our Web site: www.ama-assn.org/psych.

From the Child and Adolescent Disorders Research Branch, National Institute of Mental Health, Rockville, Md.

lic health relevance: given the estimates of approximately 8 million children who suffer from some form of severe emotional, behavioral, or mental disorder,[6] many of them may benefit from the judicious use of medications.

The National Institute of Mental Health (NIMH), with the National Plan for Research on Child and Adolescent Mental Disorders,[7] had already identified pediatric psychopharmacology as an important, but understudied, area. Recently, many initiatives have been undertaken by NIMH to define obstacles to pediatric psychopharmacological research and identify possible solutions.[8] In 1995, a large conference cosponsored by NIMH and the Food and Drug Administration (FDA) gathered more than 100 researchers from universities, National Institutes of Health, and industry; experts in ethical, legal, and regulatory aspects of pediatric research; family and patient advocates; and representatives of mental health professional associations. In 1996, pursuant to recommendations from this conference, NIMH commissioned a review of pediatric psychopharmacological data, awarded supplemental funds to existing grants to study psychotropic medications in children, and established a network of Research Units of Pediatric Psychopharmacology.

We review critical issues and obstacles faced by the field of pediatric psychopharmacological research and highlight the major recommendations emerging from the 1995 conference and currently appearing in the implementation phase.

SAFETY AND EFFICACY

Evidence for drug efficacy must come from adequate and well-controlled studies in the targeted patient population, unless this requirement is waived or modified by the FDA.[9] Recent regulations[10] allow evidence of drug efficacy in children to be derived from data about drug efficacy in adults, if convincing proof of similarity in psychopathological features and pharmacological response exists across the age groups. Such continuity in psychopathological features has been shown for some disorders, such as obsessive-compulsive disorder, major depression, and schizophrenia,[11,12] but not for others. However, similar treatment response cannot be inferred across the age groups based only on similar psychopathological or associated biological features. For instance, the phenomenology of major depressive disorder is similar across the age groups,[13] but an apparent discrepancy remains between the efficacy of tricyclic antidepressants in adults vs that in children.[2]

Safety of drugs must always be supported by appropriate research in the targeted age group. Some medications may be safe in adults but can produce toxic effects in children. In infants, chloramphenicol can result in the "gray syndrome." In young children, valproic acid can cause liver failure; tetracyclines, tooth discoloration; and phenobarbital, delay in intellectual development.[14] Because of the influence of development on psychopathologic features and pharmacological effects,[15] there is no substitute for clinical research in children. In particular, our knowledge of long-term drug effects is grossly incomplete. For most drugs, it is practically unknown if a long-term use results in sustained improvement and salutary effects on prognosis, or possible toxic side effects. In children, research on the long-term pharmacological effects is particularly important, owing to potentially longer exposure to drug and negative influence on development. Directly related to drug safety in children is the current lack of knowledge bridging between preclinical and clinical drug toxicology. As shown in animal models, permanent changes can result from exposure of animals' developing brain to some psychotropic agents,[16,17] but the relevance of these findings to humans remains unclear. The validation of drug toxicity in animal models remains an important priority.

Safety and Efficacy of Already Marketed Medications

Because many psychotropic agents are used off label, some data about their safety and efficacy in children already exist. These data, however, have never been systematically reviewed to update drug labeling. In 1994, the FDA requested that pharmaceutical companies review the extant data relevant to pediatric use of marketed medications and propose revisions to current labeling information.[10] These reviews are in progress. In parallel, NIMH has asked leading researchers to review the current evidence for safety and efficacy of psychotropic drugs in children and to determine whether continuity exists between children and adults in psychopathologic features and response to drug use. These reviews are likely to conclude that data to determine safety and efficacy in children are insufficient, especially data about long-term effects, and that more research is needed. For drugs still under patent, this research should be supported by the pharmaceutical industry. In return, financial incentives, such as extensions of patent life, may be considered and legislation about this issue is pending in Congress. For off-patent drugs, other funding sources need to be identified, including generic drug manufacturers, health maintenance organizations, private foundations, and public agencies. For medications under premarketing development, the FDA has started to recommend that basic safety and efficacy studies be conducted in children, if pediatric use is anticipated, even if not explicitly targeted by pharmaceutical companies. It is, therefore, likely that the labeling of future drugs will more often include specific information for pediatric use.

Combination Therapies

Polypharmacy has become common in child psychiatry, partially as a result of frequent comorbidity. Children with concurrent attentional, affective, and tic disorders may be prescribed various drugs, including stimulants, antidepressants, clonidine, and mood stabilizers. Almost no data, however, exist about the efficacy and safety of these combinations, and the rationale for their use is not always sound. Moreover, the combined use of pharmacological with psychosocial therapies is ubiquitous, but traditionally understudied. Research on combined treatment is clearly needed.

METHODOLOGICAL AND LOGISTIC ISSUES

Recruitment of children and adolescents into controlled clinical trials is difficult and has often resulted in small sample sizes. For instance, only 4 placebo-controlled studies of tricyclic agents in childhood depression have enrolled more than 15 patients into each treatment arm.[2] Several factors may contribute to this low enrollment rate, including (1) parents' reluctance to accepting the limitations associated with placebo-controlled trials, especially if marketed drugs can be prescribed off label; (2) excessively restrictive protocols, which exclude common comorbidity or limit concomitant treatment; (3) insufficient referrals from practitioners; and (4) minimal support from managed care organizations. To reach valid conclusions about drug effects, it is often impossible to avoid the inclusion of a placebo arm. It becomes, therefore, crucial to educate families about the power of placebo effects (which make placebo treatment quite different from no treatment!) and about the need to control for them. In parallel, the feasibility of alternative study designs (such as dose response, discontinuation strategies, and combined treatment approaches that may minimize parental resistance)should be continuously explored.[18] There is also an increased awareness that studies should be sensitive to clinical reality. Excessively restrictive protocols not only make enrollment difficult, but also may actually result in samples not representative of the patients they aim to study. Multisite studies can help obviate recruitment difficulties. The 7 Pediatric Pharmacology Research Units of the National Institute of Child and Human Development are a model,[19] after which the network of NIMH Research Units on Pediatric Psychopharmacology has been recently established. In addition to academic settings, practitioners' research networks (eg, Pediatric Research in the Office Setting) could be used for psychopharmacology, as they had been for cancer studies.[20]

It is unclear if the failure to replicate in children certain findings of adult psychopharmacological studies (eg, antidepressant efficacy of tricyclic agents) is related to the lack of sensitive and specific rating instruments that can detect drug effects in a developmentally appropriate manner. Besides the rating scales for attention deficit hyperactivity disorder, there are few universally accepted scales that are reliable and valid indicators of clinical change and pharmacological response in children. Continuous efforts are needed to develop and refine our research methodology.[21]

Pediatric age, ranging from birth to the 18th year of life, encompasses diverse phases of physiological and psychosocial development. To date, no consensus exists on how to subdivide pediatric age for research purposes. The FDA has traditionally distinguished among newborns (age, <1 month), infants (age, 1 month to 2 years), children (age, 2-12 years), and adolescents (age, 12-16 years). At the 1995 pediatric psychopharmacology conference, there was consensus to separate neonates (age, <1 years), toddlers (age, 1-3 years), preschoolers (age 3-6), schoolers (age, 6-12), early adolescents (age, 12-15), and late adolescents (age, 15-18). In pharmacokinetic studies, newborns and infants are considered quite different from children, who, in turn, differ from adolescents,[22] whereas minimal differences have been found between late adolescents and adults.[23] In drug efficacy studies, age groups should be selected based on developmentally determined physiological and psychopathological variables.[24] Practically, puberty is used to separate children from adolescents. Because Tanner staging[25] may be impractical and intrusive, a chronological cutoff around 12 years is often used to separate children from adolescents (even if girls have, on average, earlier sexual maturation than do boys).

Pediatric drug dosing has been often empirically determined by practitioners through trial and error. Dose-response and pharmacokinetic studies are needed urgently to rationally identify the appropriate dosing for drug efficacy trials.

The dearth of researchers in pediatric psychopharmacology is a major obstacle to the development of this discipline. Training programs in child psychiatry should emphasize psychopharmacology as a main area of both research and clinical activities.

ETHICAL AND LEGAL ISSUES

Children and adolescents are, as minors, unable to give full and independent *consent* to participate in research. Subjects with a mental age of at least 7 years can usually give *assent*. Consent and assent forms are the 2 documents that most institutional review boards require for pediatric research.[26] While research in minors has raised multiple concerns,[27,28] the current pediatric use of medications without adequate safety and efficacy data should, by itself, raise at least as much concern.

CLARITY AND APPLICABILITY OF ETHICAL GUIDELINES

Research guidelines allow children to be exposed to more than minimal risk only if direct benefit can accrue directly to them from their participation.[24] The interpretation of "minimal risk" and "direct benefit" varies across institutional review boards. Minimal risk is often defined as risk for harm "not greater than that normally encountered by the child in normal daily life or during routine medical examinations," even though procedures "reasonably commensurate" to the subjects' medical situation can be allowed under special conditions (a "minor" increase over minimal risk and potential for acquiring "vitally important" knowledge).[26] Practically, it helps to consider the risk-benefit ratio of research participation vs nonparticipation; such factors as illness severity, prognosis, and efficacy and safety of standard treatment are weighed against risks and benefits of the research.[29] Minimal risk can vary with patients' age, and institutional review boards may consider using different criteria for children and adolescents. Adolescents have the legal right to make health-related decisions (eg, about birth control or sexually transmitted diseases), and it may be inappropriate to impose on them the same limitations to research participation as to children.[30]

The use of placebo has some opponents, because no potential benefit can accrue to children randomized to it.[31] Practically, it is helpful to examine what the alternatives to placebo would be, if the child were not to enter the research protocol: if efficacious and safe treatments were available, the use of placebo might be unethical; but if no treatment, or treatments of dubious efficacy or potential toxic effects were the alternatives, then it would be legitimate to use a placebo. Realistically, not all situations are likely to be clear-cut, as the weight of evidence and standards of clinical practice are in flux. The NIMH has recently coordinated the publication of a casebook that illustrates the ethical aspects of situations commonly encountered in pediatric research.[32]

Consent forms are criticized by some parents for being often obscure, lengthy, and unnecessarily frightening. These documents should be realistically informative and developmentally appropriate, without being overburdensome or frightening. It is possible that the increasing length of these documents may be inversely proportional to their effectiveness in informing patients. Research aimed at validating structure and format of consent forms is needed.

Traditionally, children have been considered at high risk for product liability litigation. This perception may contribute to discouraging pharmaceutical companies from developing pediatric products. In fact, the statute of limitations, as it applies to minors, extends the time during which a suit can be filed until the age of majority *plus* the normal adult time frame, as defined by each state's statute of limitations. The extent to which product liability is indeed a problem is unknown, largely because few suits about the pediatric use of psychotropic agents have been brought to trial. To establish a legal precedent, a case must go to trial, be appealed, and finally have a judge's opinion issued. None of these steps occur for out-of-court settlements, and industry sources suggest that many such suits have been settled. Moreover, it is unclear if liability for off-label use of medications rests only with the prescribing physician, or also with the drug manufacturer. The labeling generic disclaimer that "safety and effectiveness have not been proved in children" seems unlikely to limit liability to the practitioner, especially since it has been common knowledge that the drug in question had been prescribed to children and has become, de facto, part of the current pharmacopeia. Protection from liability litigation may be best achieved by conducting the appropriate studies in pediatric age, rather than using a disclaimer.

MARKETING AND FINANCIAL ASPECTS

Pharmaceutical companies have traditionally considered the pediatric market of psychotropic drugs as too small and of scarce interest. Several indicators, however, suggest that psychotropic drugs are prescribed to children and adolescents with increasing frequency[1,33] and that the pediatric market might have been underestimated. Reliable data about the prevalence of medication use in children are needed. Databases of health maintenance organizations and insurance companies can be useful,[34] and epidemiological studies can help define patterns and intensity of use. In cases in which the small market size is a significant obstacle to drug development, the FDA orphan drug program can be considered. This program provides tax advantages, financial incentives (eg, up to a 5-year extension of patent life), and simplified and expedited review processes for potential treatments for "orphan" disorders (disorders that affect $<$200 000 people, or $<$1 per 1000 of the US population). Some psychiatric disorders, such as Tourette syndrome, qualify for this program. Still uncertain is the availability of health maintenance organizations to fund clinical trials, especially studies of the effectiveness of different treatment strategies.

In any case, the critical role of pediatric psychopharmacologic expertise within the industry cannot be overemphasized. It has been largely through the vision and efforts of a few key industry leaders that a medication like clomipramine was investigated and developed for use in children with obsessive-compulsive disorder.[35]

REGULATORY ASPECTS

The FDA mission is to assure that marketed drugs are safe, effective, and adequately labeled. Several steps have been taken by the FDA to stimulate pediatric drug research. The 1979 FDA guidelines,[36] although now somewhat outdated in diagnostic classification, contain useful information for investigators. Other initiatives have been directed at improving pediatric labeling. The first initiative, which established the pediatric use subsection in 1979,[9] did not have the desired effect of stimulating pediatric research, and a second initiative was launched in 1992[37] and then finalized in 1994.[10] This latter effort emphasized that, for diseases that are similar in children and adults and for which response to drug seems to be comparable, efficacy data from adult studies may be extrapolated to pediatric populations. In such instances, supplementary pharmacokinetic and safety data would still be needed from pediatric studies. The initiative includes 2 provisions that may have a dramatic influence on pediatric pharmacology. Sponsors of approved medications are given 2 years to examine available pediatric data to determine if the "Pediatric Use" subsection of labeling can be updated and, if so, to submit a supplemental application to support such modifications. The rule states that, in certain cases (eg, the drug is widely used, represents a potential hazard, or is therapeutically important in children), the FDA may actually require further pediatric studies and that, for certain drugs under development, the FDA may require sponsors to conduct studies in pediatric populations as a condition of approval. Unfortunately, the rule is somewhat ambiguous, suggesting that the conduct of specific pediatric studies is voluntary, yet implying that FDA has the authority to require research for certain drugs. It is still uncertain whether pediatric studies are or are not a regulatory requirement and to which extent the FDA can require such research.[38] Indeed, the FDA authority on these regulations of pediatric use labeling needs to be clarified. In the meantime, it is encouraging that several companies have already initiated pediatric drug studies.

PARENTAL AND COMMUNITY RELATIONS WITH PSYCHOPHARMACOLOGICAL RESEARCH

Families, teachers, community representatives, patient advocates, pediatricians, and other practitioners are central to all aspects of research, including hypothesis development, study design, implementation, and knowledge exchange. Without their input and support, pediatric psychopharmacological research will be difficult to conduct and of limited influence.

Lack of communication between community and researchers has been a serious obstacle and often translated into suspiciousness toward research and misconceptions about its purposes. Under such conditions, the stigma traditionally attached to mental illness renders psychopharmacological research even more difficult to conduct. Some investigators still do not evidence adequate understanding of the family context and appreciation of the importance of ethnic and cultural factors in determining attitudes, expectations, concerns, and biases. The training of clinical investigators has so far ignored these essential aspects of research communication. Confusion between the roles of researcher and medical provider can generate misunderstanding and disappointment, especially if research participation is seen as the only opportunity to receive care. Adequate feedback is not always given to parents and physicians during and after studies, thus inducing a feeling of being "used" for academic exercises of little personal relevance. Involvement of representatives of patients and families (eg, Tourette Syndrome Association, Obsessive Compulsive Disorders Foundation, Children and Adults With Attention Deficit Disorder) in designing and conducting research protocols can help address these deficiencies. Effectiveness studies, by adopting outcome points that are relevant to families (eg, level of functioning) can make research more salient and transportable to "real-world" situations. The NIMH multimodal treatment study[39,40] now in progress, has many of these characteristics. Similar efforts are needed for other disorders. Ultimately, participation in research should be viewed by children and families as an opportunity to gain personally relevant knowledge, in addition to a contribution to the advancement of science.[41] Currently, only few reports have addressed postresearch attitudes of children or families.[42-44]

CONCLUSIONS

Three major points emerge as central to pediatric psychopharmacological research. First, adult data about drug safety and efficacy can be seldom extrapolated to children. Hence, increased pediatric research must parallel the recent increases in pediatric prescribing. Second, the current use of many psychotropic agents in children without supporting data raises at least as many ethical concerns as conducting research in minors. Third, successful advancement of this research must recruit the concerted support of all the stakeholders, including families and patient representatives. Since the 1995 NIMH-FDA–sponsored conference, many activities relevant to pediatric psychopharmacology have been mounted. Besides the above-mentioned initiatives by NIMH (eg, research supplements, Research Units of Pediatric Psychopharmacology network), an increase in industry-sponsored research in pediatric psychopharmacology has occurred, with the completion of at least 2 pharmacokinetic studies and 2 efficacy trials of recently marketed antidepressants, and the initiation of several controlled studies on anxiety and mood disorders. Research in pediatric pharmacoepidemiology is developing. More attention is given to improving communications with families during and after studies at research institutions. The efforts of the Academy of Pediatrics in the general area of pediatric pharmacology[3,45] are noteworthy. The National Institutes of Health is actively considering the systematic inclusion of children in all research projects, including clinical trials. Under this approach, the exclusion of children from research protocols may have to be justified on scientific or ethical reasons.

Speaking on behalf of the other pharmaceutical companies present at the 1995 conference, one industry spokesperson said to the assembled participants, "We pledge to you to go back to our corporations and to be strong advocates for the development of safe and effective pediatric psychopharmacology agents." One parent spokesperson noted, "It's very evident to me, after listening to everybody else that . . . our issues are your issues, and your issues are our issues." The level of consensus reached among the diverse parties on the current needs for research in this area is promising, and the interim progress since the meeting is encouraging. These initiatives, if further pursued, should allow cautious optimism for the future of pediatric psychopharmacology.

Accepted for publication December 18, 1997.

The opinions and assertions contained in this article are the private views of the authors and are not to be construed as official or as reflecting the views of the Department of Health and Human Services, the NIMH.

We are indebted to Thomas Laughren, MD (FDA), for providing consultation on several regulatory aspects and to the participants of the conference "Pediatric Psychopharmacology: Current Aspects, Future Prospects," held January 24-25, 1995, in Washington, DC. We particularly acknowledge the contribution of the following participants who served as presenters, chairpersons, or reporters: Howard Abikoff, PhD; Virginia Anthony; L. Eugene Arnold, MD; Joseph Biederman, MD; Magda Campbell, MD; Dennis Cantwell, MD; Gabrielle Carlson, MD; Donald Cohen, MD; Keith Conners, PhD; Rex Cowdry, MD; Edwin Cook, MD; Harold Dent, PhD; Albert Derivan, MD; Joseph DeVeaugh-Geiss, MD; Nancy Domenici; Andrea Eberle, MD; Glen Elliott, MD, PhD; Julie Feliciano, JD; Bonnie Fell; Barbara Geller, MD; Samuel Gershon, MD; Leonard Glanz, JD; Laurence Greenhill, MD; John Heilingenstein, MD; Ralph Kauffman, MD; Kimberly Hoagwood, PhD; Martin Keller, MD; Paul Leber, MD; Thomas Laughren, MD; Henrietta Leonard, MD; Jeffrey Lieberman, MD; John March, MD; Cynthia Pfeffer, MD; Charles Popper, MD; Mark Riddle, MD; Neal Ryan, MD; Elizabeth Scanlon, MPH; Lana Skirboll, PhD; Jane Steinberg, PhD; James Swanson, PhD; Donald Vereen, MD; Elizabeth Wher, JD; Muriel Young, MD; and Deborah Zarin, MD.

Reprints: Peter S. Jensen, MD, Child and Adolescent Disorders Research Branch, Parklawn Bldg, Room 18-C-17, National Institute of Mental Health, 5600 Fishers Ln, Rockville, MD 20857.

REFERENCES

1. Jensen PS, Vitiello B, Leonard H, Laughren T. Child and adolescent psychopharmacology: expanding the research base. *Psychopharmacol Bull.* 1994;30:3-8.
2. Jensen PS, Ryan ND, Prien R. Psychopharmacology of child and adolescent major depression. *J Child Adolesc Psychopharmacol.* 1992;2:31-45.
3. American Academy of Pediatrics Committee on Drugs. Unapproved uses of approved drugs: the physician, the package insert, and the Food and Drug Administration: subject review. *Pediatrics.* 1996;98:143-145.
4. Biederman J, Baldessarini RJ, Wright V, Knee D, Hazmatz JS. A double-blind placebo controlled study of desipramine in the treatment of ADD, I: efficacy. *J Am Acad Child Adolesc Psychiatry.* 1989;28:777-784.
5. Swanson JM, Flockhart D, Udrea D, Cantwell D, Connor D, Williams L. Clonidine in the treatment of ADHD: questions about safety and efficacy. *J Child Adolesc Psychopharmacol.* 1996;5:301-304.
6. Institute of Medicine. *Research on Children and Adolescents With Mental, Behavioral, and Developmental Disorders.* Washington, DC: National Academy Press; 1989. Publication IOM-89-07.
7. Committee for the Study of Research on Child and Adolescents Mental Disorders. Report card on the National Plan for Research on Child and Adolescent Mental Disorders. *Arch Gen Psychiatry.* 1995; 52:715-723.
8. Cowdry RW, Jensen PJ. Grading the progress of child and adolescent mental health research: NIMH perspectives. *Arch Gen Psychiatry.* 1995;52:732-734.
9. Food and Drug Administration. Labeling and prescription drug advertising: content and format of labeling for human prescription drugs. *Federal Register.* June 26, 1979;44:37434-37467.
10. Food and Drug Administration. Specific requirements on content and format of labeling for human prescription drugs: revision of pediatric use subsection in the labeling. *Federal Register.* December 13, 1994;59:64240-64250.
11. Harrington R, Fudge H, Rutter M, Pickles A, Hill J. Adult outcomes of childhood and adolescent depression, I: psychiatric status. *Arch Gen Psychiatry.* 1990;47:465-473.
12. Maziade M, Gingras N, Rodrigue C, Bouchard S, Cardinal A, Gauthier B, Tremblay G, Cote S, Fournier C, Boutin P, Hamel M, Roy MA, Martinez M, Merette C. Long-term stability of diagnosis and symptom dimensions in a systematic sample of patients with onset of schizophrenia in childhood and early adolescence, I: nosology, sex and age of onset. *Br J Psychiatry.* 1996;169:361-370.
13. Ryan ND, Puig-Antich J, Ambrosini P, Rabinovich H, Robinson D, Nelson B, Iyengar S, Twomey J. The clinical picture of major depression in children and adolescents. *Arch Gen Psychiatry.* 1987; 44:854-861.
14. Farwell RF, Lee YJ, Hirtz DG, Sulzbacher SI, Ellenberg JH, Nelson JB. Phenobarbital for febrile seizures: effects on intelligence and on seizure recurrence. *N Engl J Med.* 1990;322:364-369.
15. Vitiello B, Jensen PS: Developmental perspectives in pediatric psychopharmacology. *Psychopharmacol Bull.* 1995;31:75-81.
16. Ricaurte GA, McCann UD. Neurotoxic amphetamine analogues: effects in monkeys and implications for humans. *Ann N Y Acad Sci.* 1992;648: 371-382.
17. Whitaker-Azmitia PM, Zhang X, Clarke C. Effects of gestational exposure to monoamine oxidase inhibitors in rats: preliminary behavioral and neurochemical studies. *Neuropsychopharmacology.* 1994;11:125-132.
18. Fava M. Traditional and alternative research designs and methods in clinical pediatric psychopharmacology. *J Am Acad Child Adolesc Psychiatry.* 1996;35:1292-1303.
19. Wilson JY. Pediatric pharmacology: the path clears for a noble mission. *J Clin Pharmacol.* 1993;33: 210-212.
20. Kung FH, Desai SJ, Dickerman JD, Goorin AM, Harris MB, Inoue S, Krisher, Murphy SB, Pratt CB, Toledano S, Wiley JM, Yu AL. Ifosfamide/carboplatin/etoposide (ICE) for recurrent malignant solid tumor of childhood: a pediatric oncology group phase I/II study. *J Pediatr Hematol Oncol.* 1995;17:265-269.
21. Conners CK. Methodology of antidepressant drug trials for treating depression in adolescents. *J Child Adolesc Psychiatry.* 1992;2:11-22.
22. Gibaldi M, Perrier D. *Pharmacokinetics.* 2nd ed. New York, NY: Marcel Dekker Inc; 1982.
23. Geller B, Cooper TB, Schluchter MD, Warham JE, Carr, LG. Child and adolescent nortriptyline single dose pharmacokinetics parameters: final report. *J Clin Psychopharmacol.* 1987;7:321-323.
24. Smith Rogers A. A research agenda for the study of therapeutic agents in adolescents. *J Adolesc Health.* 1994;15:672-678.
25. Tanner JM, Whitehouse RH. Clinical longitudinal standards for height, weight, height velocity, and stages of puberty. *Arch Dis Child.* 1976;51:170-182.
26. Office of the Federal Register. *Code of Federal Regulations 45 (Public Welfare), Part 46: Protection of Human Subjects.* Washington, DC: Office of the Federal Register, National Archives and Records Administration; October 1, 1994(45 CFR Subtitle A):116-135.
27. Arnold LE, Stoff DM, Cook E, Cohen DJ, Kruesi M, Wright C, Hattab J, Graham P, Zametkin A, Castellanos FX, McMahon W, Leckman JF. Ethical issues in biological psychiatric research with children and adolescents. *J Am Acad Child Adolesc Psychiatry.* 1995;34:929-939.
28. Coffey BJ. Ethical issues in child and adolescent psychopharmacology. *Child Adolesc Psychiatr Clin North Am.* 1995;4:793-807.
29. American Academy of Pediatrics Committee on Drugs. Guidelines for the ethical conduct of studies to evaluate drugs in pediatric populations. *Pediatrics.* 1995;95:286-294.
30. Leikin S. Minors' assent, consent, or dissent to medical research. *IRB Rev Hum Subj Res.* 1993; 15:1-7.
31. Glantz LH. Conducting research with children: legal and ethical issues. *J Am Acad Child Adolesc Psychiatry.* 1996;35:1283-1291
32. Hoagwood K, Jensen PS, Fisher CB, eds. *Ethical Issues in Mental Health Research with Children and Adolescents.* Mahwah NJ: Lawrence Erlbaum Inc Press; 1996.
33. Safer D, Krager JM. The increased rate of stimulant treatment for hyperactive/inattentive students in secondary schools. *Pediatrics.* 1994;94: 462-464
34. Zito JM, Riddle MA. Psychiatric pharmacoepidemiology for children and adolescents. *Child Adolesc Psychiatr Clin North Am.* 1995;4:77-95.
35. DeVeaugh-Geiss J, Moroz G, Biederman J, Cantwell D, Fontaine R, Greist JH, Reichler R, Katz R, Landau P. Clomipramine hydrochloride in childhood and adolescent obsessive-compulsive disorder: a multicenter trial. *J Am Acad Child Adolesc Psychiatry.* 1992;31:45-49.
36. Food and Drug Administration: FDA Bureau of Drugs Clinical Guidelines. *Guidelines for the Clinical Evaluation of Psychoactive Drugs in Infants and Children.* Washington, DC: Superintendent of Documents, US Government; 1979. FDA publication 79-3055.
37. Food and Drug Administration. Specific requirements on content and format of labeling for human prescription drugs: proposed revision of pediatric use subsection in the labeling. *Federal Register.* October 16, 1992;57:47423-47428.
38. Laughren TP. Regulatory issues in pediatric psychopharmacology. *J Am Acad Child Adolesc Psychiatry.* 1996;35:1276-1282.
39. Richters J, Arnold LEA, Jensen PS, Abikoff H, Conners CK, Greenhill L, Hechtman L, Hinshaw S, Pelham W, Swanson J. NIMH Collaborative Multisite, Multimodal Treatment Study of Children with ADHD, I: background and rationale. *J Am Acad Child Adolesc Psychiatry.* 1995;34: 987-1000.
40. Greenhill LL, Abikoff HB, Arnold LE, Cantwell DP, Conners CK, Elliott G, Hechtman L, Hinshaw SP, Hoza B, Jensen PS, March JS, Newcorn J, Pelham WE, Severe JB, Swanson JM, Vitiello B, Wells K. Medication treatment strategies in the MTA study: relevance to clinicians and researchers. *J Am Acad Child Adolesc Psychiatry.* 1996;35: 1304-1313.
41. Jensen PS, Hoagwood, Fisher CB. Bridging scientific and ethical perspectives: toward synthesis. In: Hoagwood K, Jensen PS, Fisher CB, eds. *Ethical Issues in Mental Health Research with Children and Adolescents.* Mahwah, NJ: Lawrence Erlbaum Inc Press; 1996:287-297.
42. Kruesi MJP, Swedo SE, Coffey ML, Hamburger SD, Leonard H, Rapoport JL. Objective and subjective side effects of research lumber punctures in children and adolescents. *Psychiatr Res.* 1988; 25:59-63.
43. Frader C, MacGrath PJ, Kay J, Adams S, Luke B, A prospective survey of reaction to blood tests by children and adolescents. *Pain.* 1990;40:53-60.
44. Smith M. Taking blood from chidden causes no more than minimal harm. *J Med Ethics.* 1985;11: 127-131.
45. Coté CJ, Kauffman RE, Troendle GJ, Lambert GH. Is the 'therapeutic orphan' about to be adopted? *Pediatrics.* 1996;98:118-123.

A Clinical Psychotherapy Trial for Adolescent Depression Comparing Cognitive, Family, and Supportive Therapy

David A. Brent, MD; Diane Holder, MSW; David Kolko, PhD; Boris Birmaher, MD; Marianne Baugher, MA; Claudia Roth, MSW; Satish Iyengar, PhD; Barbara A. Johnson, MD

Background: Previous studies in nonclinical samples have shown psychosocial treatments to be efficacious in the treatment of adolescent depression, but few psychotherapy treatment studies have been conducted in clinically referred, depressed adolescents.

Methods: One hundred seven adolescent patients with *DSM-III-R* major depressive disorder (MDD) were randomly assigned to 1 of 3 treatments: individual cognitive behavior therapy, systemic behavior family therapy (SBFT), or individual nondirective supportive therapy (NST). Treatments were 12 to 16 sessions provided in as many weeks. Intent-to-treat analyses were conducted using all follow-up data.

Results: Of the 107 patients enrolled in the study, 78 (72.9%) completed the study, 4 (3.7%) never initiated treatment, 10 (9.3%) had exclusionary criteria that were undetected at entry, 8 (7.5%) dropped out, and 7 (6.5%) were removed for clinical reasons. Cognitive behavior therapy showed a lower rate of MDD at the end of treatment compared with NST (17.1% vs 42.4%; $P=.02$), and resulted in a higher rate of remission (64.7%, defined as absence of MDD and at least 3 consecutive Beck Depression Inventory scores <9) than SBFT (37.9%; $P=.03$) or NST (39.4%; $P=.04$). Cognitive behavior therapy resulted in more rapid relief in interviewer-rated (vs both treatments, $P=.03$) and self-reported depression (vs SBFT, $P=.02$). All 3 treatments showed significant and similar reductions in suicidality and functional impairment. Parents' views of the credibility of cognitive behavior therapy improved compared with parents' views of both SBFT ($P=.01$) and NST ($P=.05$).

Conclusion: Cognitive behavior therapy is more efficacious than SBFT or NST for adolescent MDD in clinical settings, resulting in more rapid and complete treatment response.

Arch Gen Psychiatry. 1997;54:877-885

MAJOR DEPRESSION is a common and serious disorder in adolescence, with an estimated point prevalence ranging between 2.8% and 8.2%.[1] Moreover, due to a secular trend, this condition may be becoming more common, and beginning earlier in life.[2,3] Early-onset major depression is recurrent and is associated with significant long-term impairment, including early parenthood, divorce, work and legal difficulties, substance abuse, and suicidal behavior.[4-11] Therefore, the treatment of adolescent depression has major public health implications.

Almost all published treatment trials in clinically referred adolescents with major depression have focused on psychopharmacological treatments.[12-17] Only one, a large placebo-controlled clinical trial of fluoxetine in depressed children and adolescents, showed superior efficacy of this antidepressant,[12] with improvement and remittance rates on medication of 56% and 31%, respectively. The lack of definitively efficacious pharmacological interventions for depressed adolescents in most studies, coupled with the low response rate in the 1 positive study, makes the search for effective psychosocial treatments compelling.

In contrast to the psychopharmacological literature, most of the published psychosocial intervention studies for depressed adolescents have focused on samples obtained through screenings in schools or by advertisement. Cognitive behavior therapy (CBT) often has been used because of the role of cognitive distortion in the onset of depression.[18] In 3 studies in nonclinical samples, group CBT was superior to the wait-list control condition, but not to alternative active treatments.[19-21] In contrast, in a clinic-based sample, CBT was superior to relaxation training for the treatment of children and adolescents with depression.[22]

From the Western Psychiatric Institute and Clinic (Drs Brent, Kolko, Birmaher, and Johnson and Mss Holder, Baugher, and Roth) and the Department of Statistics, University of Pittsburgh (Dr Iyengar), Pittsburgh, Pa.

SUBJECTS AND METHODS

SAMPLE AND RECRUITMENT

Subjects eligible for this clinical trial were of normal intelligence, between the ages of 13 and 18 years, living with at least 1 parent or guardian, and met criteria for *DSM-III-R*[28] major depressive disorder (MDD), with an intake Beck Depression Inventory (BDI)[29] score of 13 or more. The following conditions resulted in exclusion from the study: psychosis, bipolar I or II disorder, obsessive-compulsive disorder, eating disorder, substance abuse within the past 6 months, ongoing physical or sexual abuse, pregnancy, and chronic medical illness.

Subjects were recruited from the Child and Adolescent Mood and Anxiety Disorder Clinic at Western Psychiatric Institute and Clinic, Pittsburgh, Pa, from October 1, 1991, through May 31, 1995. Of 122 adolescents who were eligible, 107 (87.7%) agreed to randomization. Nine of the 15 who refused to participate in the study did so because they did not want family therapy. About one third of subjects entering the protocol were recruited by an advertisement (35/107 or 32.7%); the remainder were self-referred or referred by parents or professionals. No demographic or clinical differences were observed between the subjects responding to advertisements and those recruited by clinical referral. Incentives for participation included free treatment and participant payment for the completion of evaluations.

RANDOMIZATION

Once the patient and family had given informed consent, they were randomized to 1 of the 3 treatments. To ensure comparability among the groups, the Begg and Iglewicz[30] modification of the Efron biased coin toss[31] was used, balancing on sex, number of parents in the household, and clinically significant suicidality (ie, ideation with a plan or an attempt).

TREATMENT

Overview of Treatment

Treatment consisted of 2 phases: active, in which patients received 12 to 16 sessions provided in 12 to 16 weeks, and a booster phase, in which patients received 2 to 4 sessions in as many months. In this article, we focus exclusively on the active phase. The 3 treatment cells were similar on almost all treatment variables related to treatment intensity and duration and the number, characteristics, and experience of therapists (**Table 1**). All therapists had master's degrees and a median of 10 years of clinical experience.

Family Psychoeducation for All 3 Cells

Patients in all 3 treatment cells received family psychoeducation about affective illness and its treatment.[32] In the first 3 treatment sessions, parents were given a psychoeducational manual and invited to discuss questions and concerns about the treatment of depression with up to 1 treatment hour devoted to psychoeducational issues.

Cognitive Behavior Therapy

Cognitive behavior therapy (CBT)[33] as used in this study adapts the approach of Beck et al[34] to the specific developmental needs of adolescents. Like the Beck CBT from which it is derived, this treatment emphasizes collaborative empiricism, the importance of socializing the patient to the cognitive therapy model, and the monitoring and modification of automatic thoughts, assumptions, and beliefs. To adapt CBT for adolescents, we provided more emphasis on the following: use of concrete examples to illustrate points, education about the nature of psychotherapy and socialization to the treatment model, active exploration of issues of autonomy and trust, focus on cognitive distortions and affective shifts that occur during sessions, and acquisition of problem solving, affect regulation,[35] and social skills.

Systemic Behavior Family Therapy

Systemic behavior family therapy (SBFT)[33] is a combination of 2 treatment approaches that have been used effectively for dysfunctional families of adolescents. The first phase of treatment is drawn from functional family therapy,[36] in which the therapist clarifies the concerns that brought the family into treatment and provides a series of reframing statements designed to optimize engagement in therapy and identification of dysfunctional behavior patterns. During the second phase, which was adapted from the problem-solving model developed by Robin and Foster,[37] the family members focus on communication and problem-solving skills and the alteration of family interactional patterns. Systemic behavior family therapy provides extensive socialization to the treatment model and education about depression, parenting and developmental issues and emphasizes skill building and positive practice in sessions and at home.

Nondirective Supportive Treatment

Nondirective supportive treatment[33] is designed to control for the nonspecific aspects of treatment, namely, the passage of time, amount of contact with a therapist, and the support of an empathic, concerned, and skilled professional.[26] The main goals of NST are to establish, maintain, and build rapport, provide support, and aid the patient in affect identification and expression of feelings through reflective listening, provision of accurate empathy, and discussion of patient-initiated options for addressing personal problems. In contrast to the other 2 treatments, NST therapists refrained from giving advice, setting limits, or teaching specific skills.

Treatment Distinctness and Flexibility

There were times when it was clinically indicated for a therapist in the CBT or NST cells to meet with the parents or other family members, or for a therapist in the SBFT cell to meet with individual family members. Up to 25% of the total treatment time (4 hours) could be allocated for these auxiliary sessions. In SBFT, consistent with the family focus of the treatment model, less time was devoted to auxiliary sessions than in either CBT or NST ($F[2,104]=17.31$; $P<.01$; pairwise comparisons using the Tukey procedure, $P<.01$).

Maintenance of Treatment Integrity

Each therapist had 6 months of intensive training using a cell-specific treatment manual and a library of training videotapes, and was required to treat 2 cases in adherence to the treatment model before becoming a therapist for the study. The supervisors, master's-level therapists expert in the treatment model, provided 1 hour of group and 1 hour of individual supervision per week for all protocol therapists. Videotapes were rated using a therapy-specific scale to ensure adherence to the model. Adherence to CBT was monitored by the 11-item Cognitive Therapy Rating Scale,[38] to SBFT by a modification of the 12-item Family Therapist Rating Scale,[39] and to NST by 8 items adapted from the Vanderbilt Psychotherapy Process Scale.[40] All 3 instruments had Likert responses from 0 (poor) to 6 (excellent), with increasing scores for more adherence and a 4 on each item as the lowest acceptable score.

Twenty-five percent of the videotapes, including those from auxiliary sessions, using the aforementioned scales, were reviewed by an external consultant, a doctoral-level professional with established expertise in the treatment. The internal and external consultants rated more than 90% of treatment sessions in each cell as "acceptable." The consultants also reviewed, at random, videotapes that were from a different modality, to establish discriminative validity.[26] The external consultants successfully discriminated psychoeducational sessions in CBT and NST cells from SBFT family sessions ($F[2,80]=146.80$; $P<.01$; the Tukey procedure, pairwise contrasts, $P<.01$) and CBT from NST and individual sessions conducted in SBFT ($F[2,165]=36.25$; $P<.001$; the Tukey procedure, pairwise contrasts, $P<.01$).

Referral for Open Treatment and Removal From Study

Patients who made a suicide attempt were removed from the protocol. In addition, patients who were still seriously symptomatic at midpoint (BDI $\geq$13 and persistent *DSM-III-R* MDD) were evaluated by 1 of the project psychiatrists (B.B. or B.A.J.). A clinical decision for removal was based on a failure to achieve notable improvement from intake to midpoint, resulting in a recommendation for open treatment, usually pharmacotherapy. This approach was used because it reflected our usual clinical practice.

Treatment of Parents

In the course of the intake assessment, the Lifetime Version of the Schedule for Affective Disorders and Schizophrenia, many parents were identified as currently depressed (38.8% of mothers and 6.6% of fathers).[41] Parents who had a Hamilton Depression Rating Scale score of 15 or more and serious functional impairment and who were not already in treatment were offered pharmacotherapy in our clinic at no cost, but only 10 of 31 mothers (3 of 12 in CBT, 2 of 6 in SBFT, 5 of 13 in NST) and 0 of 2 fathers who were identified as depressed elected to pursue our treatment recommendations.

Treatment Expectancy

Treatment expectancy (T×E) is a self-report measure that was used to assess the extent to which patients and parents endorsed the importance of elements of cognitive, family, and supportive treatment. For this construct, we used a measure similar to one used in the National Psychotherapy of Depression Collaborative Study,[42] in which the respondent rated preferences (on a 1-to-5 Likert scale) for elements of the 3 treatments offered (Paul Pilkonis, PhD, oral communication, February 5, 1990). This was administered to the patient and the parent before the beginning of treatment, at the sixth session, and at termination to determine whether expectancies were similarly distributed across treatment cells and whether there were significant treatment×time interactions.

Treatment Credibility

Treatment credibility (T×C) is a measure derived from Borkovec and Nau[43] to tap the extent to which patients or parents believe that the specific treatment to which they have been assigned sounds logical, seems likely to be helpful, and is an intervention that they would recommend to a friend. We administered the T×C to the parents and patients after session 1, at the sixth session, and at termination of treatment. Confirmatory factor analysis indicated the presence of only 1 factor with high internal consistency for patients and parents ($\alpha=.84$-$.92$) forms. For the goodness-of-fit tests, the *P* values ranged from .14 to .31, with 56% to 65% of the total variance explained, indicating that 1 factor is adequate.

ASSESSMENT AND OUTCOMES SCHEDULE

All of the following assessments were administered at intake, the sixth session, and the end of treatment (12th-16th session), with an attempt to interview the subjects who left the protocol at the time they would have finished treatment. In addition, the BDI[29] was obtained at every session.

Of the 107 subjects who entered the protocol, 94 (88%) received a 6-week interview and BDI, 99 (93%) received final interview, and 97 (91%) had a final BDI. There were no differences across cells with respect to proportions with missing data. Subjects for whom data were missing were dropouts or those who were removed from the study because of the discovery after entry into the protocol of preexisting exclusionary criteria.

PSYCHIATRIC SYMPTOMS

The School Age Schedule for Affective Disorders and Schizophrenia, Present and Lifetime Versions (K-SADS-P/E)[44,45] were used by interviewers unaware of treatment status to assess current and past diagnoses using *DSM-III-R* criteria.

Depression

From the K-SADS-P/E were derived the proportion meeting *DSM-III-R* MDD at the end of treatment, and the mean severity on 13 items related to depression. The patient's report of depressive symptoms was assessed by the BDI,[29] a widely used self-report questionnaire. One additional dichotomous measure of depressive outcome was defined by the sustained (at least 3 consecutive sessions) achievement of a BDI score less than 9 (BDI<9), a clinically meaningful cutpoint supported by previous studies,[46,47] and our own receiver operator curve analyses in this sample of the BDI against K-SADS-P/E diagnosis of MDD (optimal cutpoint of 10, area under the curve=0.91; $P<.001$).[48] Finally, we defined clinical remission as no longer fulfilling criteria for MDD and a BDI<9 for at least 3 consecutive sessions and sustained until the end of treatment.

Suicidality

The presence of clinically significant suicidality, corresponding to ideation with a plan or an attempt, was assessed by use of the K-SADS-P/E.

Continued on next page

Functional Impairment

The interviewer-generated Children's Global Assessment Scale (CGAS)[49] was used as a measure of functional impairment, both as a continuous measure, and as a marker of clinical impairment (CGAS<60).

DATA ANALYSIS

The data were analyzed using an intent-to-treat approach, defined as "the inclusion of all eligible patients regardless of compliance with the protocol."[50] Therefore, the 107 subjects randomized into the protocol were included, and follow-up continued even for those subjects who left the protocol to preserve, as much as possible, the effects of initial randomization.[51] Of these 107 subjects, 10 were found to have previously undetected exclusionary criteria, and 7 were removed on clinical grounds. Because these subjects were not removed from the protocol blind to treatment status, they were included in all analyses to guard against possible bias in the removal process. Moreover, data analyses using 103 subjects (excluding the 4 who never came for treatment) and 93 subjects (excluding the 4 who never came for treatment, and the 10 who, subsequent to enrollment, were found to have previously undetected exclusionary criteria) yielded the same results as our primary analyses.

The differential effect of the treatments on continuous outcomes was assessed by use of random effects regression,[32] with statistically significant treatment×time interactions indicating differences in the rates of change (ie, slope) in outcomes among the treatment groups. Only treatment×time interactions are reported in the text. Random effects regression allowed for the use of all observations, a flexibility not afforded by standard repeated measures analysis of variance.[52] The differential effects of the treatments on the time to recovery, using a defined dichotomous end point, was assessed by use of survival analysis and the Mantel-Cox log rank test.[53]

Changes over time in dichotomous outcomes were examined across groups by use of the McNemar χ^2. Dichotomous outcomes at the end of treatment (eg, presence of depression) were compared among the 3 groups by use of the Pearson χ^2, with follow-up pairwise tests.

For contrasts specified in our original hypotheses, namely, all pairwise contrasts among the 3 treatment groups, α was set at .05. To correct for multiple comparisons from post hoc analyses, the Tukey procedure was used in the case of analyses of variance and the Bonferroni procedure was used for every other type of test.

Family therapy seems to be a logical alternative treatment choice for adolescent depression, because it is a commonly used method of treatment for adolescents, and because parental depression, poor perceived support, and parent-child discord are associated with onset, prolonged course, and recurrence of depression and suicidality in youth.[23-25] In 1 study, the addition of a group for parents did not increase the efficacy of group CBT for adolescents.[20] However, despite compelling theoretical evidence, no study has used a family-focused intervention for the treatment of adolescent depression.

Table 1. Variables of Treatment Across Cells*

Variable	CBT (n=37)	SBFT (n=35)	NST (n=35)
Sessions, No.	12.1 (3.6)	10.7 (4.7)	11.2 (4.2)
Primary treatment, h	11.0 (3.4)	11.5 (5.0)	10.1 (4.0)
Auxiliary treatment, h†	1.5 (1.1)	0.3 (0.5)	1.5 (1.3)
Total time, h	12.5 (3.9)	11.7 (5.1)	11.6 (4.3)
Distribution hours, %			
0-2	2.7	11.4	2.9
3-5	2.7	2.9	8.6
6-8	8.1	2.9	8.6
9-11	5.4	11.4	5.7
>12	81.1	71.4	74.3
Treatment duration, wk	13.9 (3.9)	12.0 (5.4)	12.9 (4.9)
No. of therapists	4	4	4
Female therapists, %	75.0	50.0	75.0
Age of therapists, y	32.8 (5.0)	35.5 (7.9)	35.3 (4.1)
Experience of therapists, y	8.8 (4.7)	8.0 (3.9)	9.3 (6.5)

*CBT indicates cognitive behavior therapy; SBFT, systemic behavior family therapy; NST, nondirective supportive therapy. Values are given as mean (SD) unless otherwise indicated.

†CBT vs SBFT and SBFT vs NST significant at the .01 level using Tukey studentized range method.

Previous studies of the efficacy of psychotherapy have emphasized the importance of a supportive relationship with a therapist.[26,27] Furthermore, several pharmacological clinical trials of adolescent depression have been characterized by high placebo-response rates.[13,15,17] Therefore, we attempted to control for the salutary effect of having a therapeutic relationship by the use of supportive therapy. To examine the efficacy of different psychotherapeutic approaches, we compared individual CBT and family treatment approaches to adolescent depression with nondirective supportive therapy (NST) as a third cell to control for the nonspecific effects of psychotherapy. We hypothesized that at the end of treatment, patients treated with CBT or family therapy would show more rapid improvement and be more likely to achieve clinical remission than those treated with supportive therapy for depression, suicidality, and functional impairment, because CBT and family therapy specifically target factors associated with the onset, persistence, and recurrence of depression.

RESULTS

COMPARISON OF THE 3 TREATMENT GROUPS AT INTAKE

The 3 treatment groups were well balanced on demographic and almost all clinical variables (**Table 2**). Overall, there was a trend for the proportion of subjects that was seriously functionally impaired (CGAS<60) to differ among the groups (χ^2=5.60; df=2; P=.06), with a significant difference between CBT and the NST cell (40.5% vs 65.7%; χ^2=4.57; df=1; P=.03). Analyses were performed with the CGAS<60 included as a covariate, with no changes in the results; therefore, only the unadjusted analyses are given.

PROTOCOL DEVIATIONS

There were no significant differences across cells with respect to dropout, removal for ineligibility, or removal for clinical reasons (**Table 3**). Altogether, 7 of 37 subjects left CBT, 11 of 35 subjects left SBFT, and 11 of 35 subjects left NST. Of 107 subjects randomized, 4 never returned for treatment, 8 dropped out, 7 were removed for clinical reasons, and 10 were removed because they were discovered to have preexisting conditions that rendered them ineligible for the study (substance abuse [n=5], bipolar II disorder [n=1], did not live with parent or guardian [n=1], pregnancy [n=1], and obsessive-compulsive disorder [n=2]).

Of the 8 dropouts, 3 were noncompliant, 1 moved, 3 did not like the therapy or the therapist, and 1 believed the problem was "irritable bowel syndrome." Dropouts compared with nondropouts were found to be more likely to be hopeless on the Beck Hopelessness Scale[54] (15.9[1.4] vs 11.4[5.7]; separate variance t=5.96; df=36.6; P<.001; Bonferroni corrected α=.05/10=.005).

The 7 subjects who were removed on clinical grounds and referred for open treatment were referred because of persistent MDD; 1 subject also was suicidal. The 7 subjects referred for open treatment, compared with 29 who, although not referred, also had BDI>13 and MDD at week 6, were more likely to have comorbid dysthymic disorder (71.4% vs 20.7%; χ^2=6.84; df=1; P=.009; Bonferroni corrected α=.05/5=.01) and showed a much smaller mean decrease on the BDI from intake to 6 weeks (−0.8[5.1] vs −6.3[6.8]; separate variance t=2.23; df=9.2; P=.05).

Table 2. Demographic and Clinical Characteristics of Subjects*

Characteristic	CBT (n=37)	SBFT (n=35)	NST (n=35)
Mean (SD) age, y	15.7 (1.3)	15.4 (1.4)	15.7 (1.5)
Female, %	75.7	77.1	74.3
White, %	75.7	88.6	85.7
Mean (SD) socioeconomic distribution, %†	39.9 (13.0)	39.0 (12.5)	39.6 (15.1)
I	5.4	11.4	8.6
II	16.2	5.7	1.4
III	21.6	34.3	31.4
IV	43.2	45.7	34.3
V	13.5	2.9	14.3
Live with 2 parents, %	56.8	57.1	57.1
Comorbid diagnoses, %			
Dysthymic disorder	16.2	25.7	25.7
Anxiety disorder	37.8	28.6	28.6
Disruptive disorder	16.2	22.9	22.9
Current suicidality, %	35.1	34.3	40.0
History of suicide attempt, %	21.6	22.9	25.7
Mean duration of depression, mo (median quartile deviation)	7.0 (3.0)	5.9 (3.0)	5.0 (2.0)
Mean (SD) No. of previous depressive episodes	1.2 (0.5)	1.2 (0.6)	1.4 (0.8)

Explanations of the abbreviations are given in the first footnote to Table 1.
†*Hollingshead A.* Four-Factor Index of Social Status. *New Haven, Conn: Yale University Press; 1975.*

OUTCOME

Depression

For the presence of MDD at the end of treatment, there was a trend for a difference among the 3 groups (χ^2=5.22; df=2; P=.07), with a pairwise difference between CBT and NST (17.1% vs 42.4%; χ^2=5.23; df=1; P=.02) (**Table 4**). There was an overall treatment×time effect in interview-rated depressive symptoms (13 items related to depression, χ^2=6.15; df=2; P=.05), with CBT showing more rapid treatment response than both SBFT (treatment×time effect, χ^2=4.74; df=1; P=.03) and NST (treatment×time effect, χ^2=4.84; df=1, P=.03). There was a trend for a group difference in the rate of decline of self-rated symptoms (BDI, treatment×time effect, χ^2=5.70; df=2; P=.06), with a significant pairwise difference between CBT and SBFT (treatment×time effect, χ^2=5.10; df=1; P=.02) (**Figure 1**).

Table 3. Protocol Deviations After Randomization

	Session																	
Type of Therapy	0	1	2	3	4	5	6	7	8	9	10	11	12	13	14	15	16	Total
Cognitive behavior																		
Never came	1	...	...	...	...	...	...	...	...	...	...	...	...	...	...	...	...	1
Censored	...	...	...	...	...	...	...	1	...	1	...	...	...	...	...	...	...	2
Open	...	...	...	...	...	...	1	...	...	...	...	...	...	...	...	...	...	1
Dropped out	...	...	...	1	...	...	1	...	...	1	...	...	...	...	...	...	...	3
Systemic behavior family																		
Never came	3	...	...	...	...	...	...	...	...	...	...	...	...	...	...	...	...	3
Censored	...	1	1	...	...	...	...	1	...	...	...	...	...	...	...	...	...	3
Open	...	...	...	...	...	...	...	...	1	1	...	1	...	...	...	...	...	3
Dropped out	...	...	...	...	...	...	1	...	...	...	1	...	...	...	...	...	...	2
Nondirective supportive																		
Never came	...	...	...	...	...	...	...	...	...	...	...	...	...	...	...	...	...	0
Censored	...	...	...	2	...	1	...	...	...	1	...	...	...	1	...	...	...	5
Open	...	1	...	...	...	...	2	...	...	...	...	...	...	...	...	...	...	3
Dropped out	...	...	...	1	...	...	...	...	1	...	1	...	...	...	...	...	...	3
Total	**4**	**2**	**1**	**4**	**0**	**1**	**5**	**2**	**2**	**4**	**2**	**1**	**0**	**1**	**0**	**0**	**0**	**29**

Table 4. Treatment Outcome*

	Intake				6 Weeks				12-16 Weeks	
	CBT	SBFT	NST	*P*	CBT	SBFT	NST	*P*	CBT	SBFT
MDD episode, %	n=37	n=35	n=35	...	n=35	n=29	n=30	.90	n=35	n=31
	100	100	100		60.0	65.5	63.3	...	17.1	32.3
BDI	n=37	n=35	n=35	.28	n=35	n=30	n=29	.44	n=35	n=29
	24.3 (8.1)	22.6 (8.2)	25.7 (7.8)	...	10.7 (11.1)	13.7 (9.3)	13.4 (10.7)	...	5.7 (8.6)	9.1 (9.1)
DEP13	n=37	n=35	n=35	.35	n=35	n=29	n=30	.91	n=35	n=31
	2.9 (0.5)	2.7 (0.5)	2.8 (0.5)	...	2.1 (0.7)	2.1 (0.6)	2.1 (0.5)	...	1.5 (0.5)	1.7 (0.6)
Remission, %	n=37	n=35	n=35	...	n=36	n=32	n=30	.37	n=35	n=31
	0	0	0		16.7	6.2	16.7	...	60.0	29.0
Suicidality >4,	n=37	n=35	n=35	.91	n=35	n=29	n=30	.31	n=35	n=31
%	35.1	37.1	40.0	...	5.7	3.4	13.3	...	8.6	6.5
CGAS <60, %	n=37	n=35	n=35	.06	n=35	n=29	n=30	.76	n=35	n=31
	40.5	62.9	65.7	.03†	34.3	37.9	43.3	...	25.7	35.5
	58.8 (8.3)	54.5 (8.0)	56.3 (8.6)	... (0.9)	61.4 (8.9)	60.7 (5.9)	59.8 (8.0)	... (.70)	65.4 (10.1)	63.5 (8.2)
Child TxC	n=31	n=29	n=29	.50	n=34	n=26	n=28	...	n=34	n=28
	3.8 (1.0)	4.0 (0.8)	3.9 (1.0)	...	4.2 (0.7)	4.0 (0.9)	4.0 (0.8)	... (.47)	4.1 (0.8)	4.0 (1.0)
Parent TxC	n=36	n=31	n=29	.49	n=33	n=29	n=29	...	n=33	n=28
	4.3 (0.6)	4.5 (0.6)	4.5 (0.6)	...	4.3 (0.06)	4.2 (0.08)	4.1 (0.7)	... (.71)	4.4 (0.5)	4.3 (0.8)

Values are given as mean (SD) unless otherwise indicated. Abbreviations for therapies are given in the footnote to Table 1. MDD indicates Major Depressive Disorder; BDI, Beck Depression Inventory; DEP13, 13 depression items from the School Age Schedule for Affective Disorders and Schizophrenia, Present and Lifetime versions; CGAS, Children's Global Assessment Schedule; TxC, treatment credibility; and ANOVA, analysis of variance.

†*CBT vs NST.*

‡*CBT vs SBFT.*

There was a trend for overall differences in the rate of achievement of clinical response, defined as a BDI<9 sustained for at least 3 consecutive sessions and until the end of treatment, using survival analysis (Mantel-Cox χ^2=5.28; *df*=2; *P*=.07) (**Figure 2**) with a significant pairwise difference favoring CBT over SBFT (Mantel-Cox χ^2=4.84; *df*=1; *P*=.03). There was a difference among the 3 treatments in the achievement of remission defined by the absence of MDD and 3 consecutive scores on the BDI<9 sustained through remaining sessions (χ^2=5.96; *df*=2; *P*=.05). Pairwise comparisons showed a higher remission rate for CBT (60%) than for SBFT (37.9%; χ^2=4.50; *df*=1; *P*=.03) or NST (39.4%; χ^2=4.30; *df*=1; *P*=.04.

Suicidality

There was no significant difference among the 3 treatments for their effect on suicidality, although there were significant decreases in suicidality across all 3 groups (McNemar χ^2=21.78; *df*=1; *P*<.001).

Functional Impairment

There was no treatment×time interaction on the CGAS and no group differences in the proportion of subjects with a CGAS<60 at the end of treatment, although there was overall improvement in functional status across the 3 treatment groups (McNemar χ^2=11.26; *df*=1; *P*<.001).

Treatment Expectancy and Credibility

There were no differences among the groups in parent- or patient-rated treatment expectancies at intake, and no significant time or treatment×time effects. There was an overall group difference in the way parents' views of treatment credibility changed over time (treatment×time effect, χ^2=12.90; *df*=2; *P*=.002). Pairwise analyses showed that parents' views of treatment credibility improved over time in CBT relative to SBFT (χ^2=3.97; *df*=1; *P*=.05) and NST (χ^2=13.08; *df*=1; *P*<.001).

COMMENT

In this comparison of 3 psychosocial treatments for adolescent MDD, CBT emerged as more efficacious than SBFT or NST for the treatment of adolescent depression, with respect to effect on clinical recovery, rate of symptomatic improvement, and parent-rated treatment credibility. However, no group differences were seen for effect on suicidality or on functional status. These findings contrast with the more common occurrence in clinical psychotherapy trials that "everyone has won, and all must have prizes."[55] The implications of these findings will be discussed after placing them in the context of the limitations of this study.

The limitations of the study are those typical of most clinical trials based in university settings, in which there are numerous trade-offs between experimental control and generalizability.[56] For example, we had few suicide attempters in our study because suicide attempters tended to go to our emergency department, resulting in admission to an inpatient unit and almost certain treatment with an antidepressant, making these potential subjects ineligible. This limits our ability to generalize our findings to the treatment of more seriously suicidal patients. The exclusion of patients with comorbid substance abuse, or

NST	Posttreatment Differences P	Random Effects Regression: Treatment	Time	Treatment × Time
n=33	.07	...	...	...
42.4	.02†			
n=33	.19	NS	<.01	<.06
9.8 (11.4)	...			.02‡
n=33	.15	NS	<.01	.05
1.8 (0.8)	...			.03†
				.03‡
n=33	.05	...	...	...
36.4	.04†			
	.03‡			
n=33	.48	...	...	...
15.2				
n=33	.66	NS	<.01	NS
33.3	...			
63.3 (10.0)	... (.61)			
n=28	...	NS	NS	NS
4.2 (0.6)	.69			
n=27	.04	NS	.01	.002
4.0 (0.8)	.02†			<.01†
	ANOVA			.05‡

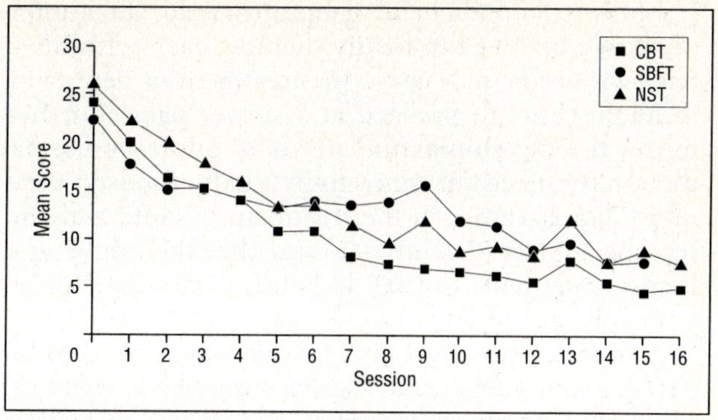

Figure 1. *Random effects regression for Beck Depression Inventory. CBT indicates cognitive behavior therapy; SBFT, systemic behavior family therapy; and NST, nondirective supportive therapy. Group×time,* P=*.06; CBT vs SBFT group×time,* P=*.02.*

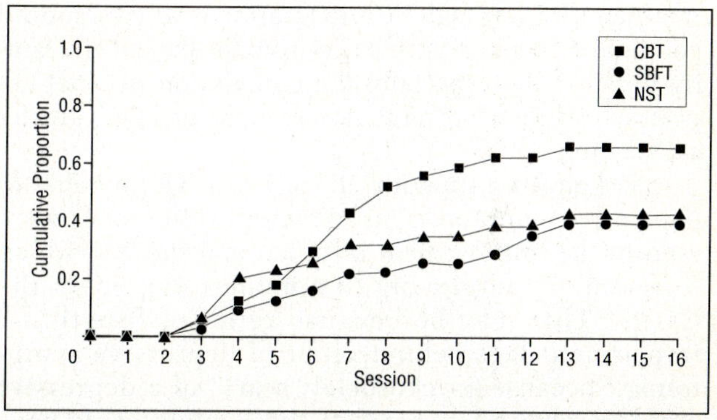

Figure 2. *Time to Beck Depression Inventory score less than 9 for at least 3 consecutive sessions and sustained for the remainder of treatment. Abbreviations are given in the legend for Figure 1. Mantel-Cox* χ^2*=5.28;* df=2; P=*.07. CBT vs SBFT, Mantel-Cox* χ^2*=4.84;* df=1; P=*.03.*

with ongoing physical or sexual abuse, while defensible on experimental grounds, makes our findings less generalizable to the full range of patients with depressive symptoms who may go to a typical service setting. The generous amount of weekly supervision (2 hours per therapist) and low caseload (4 ongoing cases for a 40% effort) were much more luxurious than any supervisory or staffing pattern found in area agencies, including our own. Although this supervisory time was built into the study to ensure high quality and fidelity, the question of the transferability of any of these interventions must be addressed. Finally, decisions to remove subjects for clinical reasons and for protocol violations were not made blind to treatment condition. Our intent-to-treat analyses were designed to protect our findings against possible bias in decisions to remove subjects from the protocol.

The rate of clinical remission was considerably better in the CBT cell than in the other 2 cells, providing support for the superior efficacy of CBT relative to NST or SBFT. This indicates that having a good therapeutic relationship, as in NST, may be necessary, but is not sufficient to result in optimal clinical improvement of adolescent depression. These results also indicate that insistence on the treatment of the family as a unit, as in SBFT, will cause a certain proportion of families to refuse treatment, and, in general, is not indicated, because individual CBT was more efficacious than SBFT for adolescent depression. These findings are consistent with those of Wood et al,[22] who found CBT superior to an alternative psychosocial intervention for child and adolescent patients with depression. Our remission rate was consistent with reported clinical response rates across a wide range of clinical and nonclinical studies in adolescent depression of 50% to 60%, regardless of dose, format, and type of intervention.[12,20,22] This indicates that further work is needed to find more efficacious psychosocial and psychopharmacological interventions, including combinations of both modalities. However, CBT or fluoxetine yielded responses that were superior to no treatment; in the study by Lewinsohn and Clarke,[20] 95% of subjects in the wait-list control condition were still depressed after 7 weeks.

Cognitive behavior therapy also showed greater rapidity of relief of depressive symptoms, compared with the other 2 treatments. This is of great clinical significance given that a significant proportion of depressed adolescents who commit suicide do so in the midst of their first episode.[9] The rapidity of response of CBT also represents an economic advantage at a time when patients, families, and clinicians are facing greater scrutiny and restriction of the number of mental health sessions available for treatment. The slower clinical response of patients' depressive symptoms in NST may be due to the strong dependency of the model on the therapeutic relationship, which takes time to build. In SBFT, slower response of depression may be attributable to the focus of the model on the identification and expression of family conflict, thereby causing patients to experience some recrudescence of symptoms at mid-treatment, before resolution of conflict and symptoms. Also, the number of people involved in family therapy, each with his or her own needs, may cause the treatment of depression in adolescents to proceed at a slower pace. Furthermore, the developmental needs of adolescents may dictate the need for more individually focused treatment. For example, in the treatment of child and adolescent anxiety, 1 study showed that the addition of family treatment to CBT is helpful only in children under the age of 10.[57]

In measures of parent-reported treatment credibility, CBT showed the greatest gains in credibility over time. In contrast to all other measures, focused on psychopathological symptoms, this measure comes closest to measuring satisfaction with treatment over time, because it taps the extent to which the subject felt helped and the likelihood that the subject would recommend this treatment for a friend. Future treatment studies should continue to focus on satisfaction from the patient and family perspective, especially the elucidation of what aspects of treatment are most closely associated with greater satisfaction.

Despite the superior efficacy of CBT for relief of depressive symptoms, no treatment differences were seen in the improvement of functional status, with all 3 treatments improving to a modest degree on the CGAS. This may be because relief of functional impairment lags behind relief of depressive symptoms,[58] because psychosocial "scars" of a depressive episode remain,[7] or because these adolescents have other problems, including nondepressive comorbidity, that require additional or different interventions. Further follow-up is indicated to elucidate whether providing symptomatic relief is sufficient for eventual improvement of functional status, or whether other psychosocial or pharmacological interventions are required. Similarly, all 3 treatments provided similar reductions in suicidality, suggesting that the processes for reduction of depression and suicidality in adolescents may be different.[25]

Two important outcomes and their predictors deserve mention. Dropouts were more hopeless than those who continued in treatment, highlighting the importance of targeting hopelessness about treatment early in the course of intervention to enhance compliance. Second, those who were removed from the protocol for clinical reasons were much more likely to have had "double depression." The malignant effect of dysthymia on subsequent course has now been well documented,[6,59] and its proper treatment may require a more intensive and multimodal approach.

Given the strong showing of CBT, studies comparing CBT and psychopharmacological interventions, separately and together, for the treatment of adolescent depression are indicated. Efforts also should be directed at the development of effectiveness studies of psychotherapy in real-world settings. In subsequent reports, we will describe, for each treatment, the patient characteristics that predict the best outcome, identify the specific effects and "active ingredients," and examine the effect of these 3 treatments on longer term course, service use, and outcome.

Accepted for publication January 28, 1997.

This work was supported by grant MH46500 from the National Institute of Mental Health, Bethesda, Md.

The expert assistance of Patricia Nuss in preparation of the manuscript is appreciated. In addition, we gratefully acknowledge the following colleagues who aided in the design or conduct of this study: Robert Berchick, PhD, Carl Bonner, PhD, Mary Beth Boylan, MA, Marlane Cully, MEd, Tom Devereaux, MSW, Terry Feinberg-Steinberg, MSW, Ellen Frank, PhD, Tom Gigliotti, MSW, Denise Harper, Susan Hogarty, MSN, Hope Jacobs, MEd, Ann Kolar, PhD, Marika Kovacs, PhD, Philip Lavori, PhD, Maureen Maher, MSW, James Matta, MA, Barbara McDonnell, Apryl Miller, LSW, Elizabeth Perkins, MSW, Paul Pilkonis, PhD, Randy Phelps, PhD, Kim Poling, MSW, Matt Scaife, MA, Joy Schweers, MEd, Bill Sherman, Jeannie Starzynski, MSW, Susan Wesner, MSN, and Karen Woodall, PhD. Above all, we thank the patients and families for their participation in this study.

Reprints: David A. Brent, MD, University of Pittsburgh School of Medicine, Western Psychiatric Institute and Clinic, 3811 O'Hara St, Pittsburgh, PA 15213.

REFERENCES

1. Lewinsohn PM, Hops H. Adolescent psychopathology, I: prevalence and incidence of depression and other *DSM-III-R* disorders in high school students. *J Abnorm Psychol.* 1993;102:133-144.
2. Kovacs M, Gatsonis C. Secular trends in age at onset of major depressive disorder in a clinical sample of children. *J Psychiatr Res.* 1994;28:319-329.
3. Ryan ND, Williamson DE, Iyengar S, Orvaschel H, Reich T, Dahl RE, Puig-Antich J. A secular increase in child and adolescent onset affective disorder. *J Am Acad Child Adolesc Psychiatry.* 1992;31:600-605.
4. Harrington R, Fudge H, Rutter M, Pickles A, Hill J. Adult outcomes of childhood and adolescent depression, I: psychiatric status. *Arch Gen Psychiatry.* 1990;47:465-473.
5. Kandel DB, Davies M. Adult sequelae of adolescent depressive symptoms. *Arch Gen Psychiatry.* 1986;43:255-262.
6. Kovacs M, Feinberg T, Crouse-Novak M, Paulauskas S, Pollock M, Finkelstein R. Depressive disorders in childhood, II: a longitudinal study of the risk for a subsequent major depression. *Arch Gen Psychiatry.* 1984;41:643-649.
7. Rohde P, Lewinsohn PM, Seeley JR. Are adolescents changed by an episode of major depression? *J Am Acad Child Adolesc Psychiatry.* 1994;33:1289-1298.
8. Andrews JA, Lewinsohn PM. Suicidal attempts among older adolescents: prevalence and co-occurrence with psychiatric disorders. *J Am Acad Child Adolesc Psychiatry.* 1992;31:655-662.
9. Brent DA, Perper JA, Moritz G, Allman C, Friend A, Roth C, Schweers J, Balach L, Baugher M. Psychiatric risk factors for adolescent suicide: a case-control study. *J Am Acad Child Adolesc Psychiatry.* 1993;32:521-529.
10. Fergusson DM, Lynskey MT. Suicide attempts and suicidal ideation in a birth cohort of 16-year-old New Zealanders. *J Am Acad Child Adolesc Psychiatry.* 1995;34:1308-1317.
11. Shaffer D, Gould MS, Fisher P, Trautman P, Moreau D, Kleinman M, Flory M. Psychiatric diagnosis in child and adolescent suicide. *Arch Gen Psychiatry.* 1996;53:339-348.
12. Emslie GJ, Rush AJ, Weinberg WA, Kowatch RA, Hughes CW, Carmody T, Rintelmann J. A double-blind, randomized, placebo-controlled trial of fluoxetine in children and adolescents with depression. *Arch Gen Psychiatry.* 1997;54:In press.
13. Kramer AD, Feiguine RJ. Clinical effects of amitriptyline in adolescent depression: a pilot study. *J Am Acad Child Adolesc Psychiatry.* 1981;20:636-644.
14. Kye C, Waterman MD, Ryan N, Birmaher B, Williamson D, Iyengar S, Dachille S. A randomized, controlled trial of amitriptyline in the acute treatment of adolescent major depression. *J Am Acad Child Adolesc Psychiatry.* 1996;35:1139-1144.
15. Kutcher S, Boulos C, Ward B, Marton P, Simeon J, Ferguson HB, Szalai J, Katic M, Roberts N, Dubois C, Reed K. Response to desipramine treatment in adolescent depression: a fixed-dose, placebo-controlled trial. *J Am Acad Child Adolesc Psychiatry.* 1994;33:686-694.
16. Geller B, Cooper MA, Graham DL, Marsteller FA, Bryant DM. Double-blind placebo-controlled study of nortriptyline in depressed adolescents using a 'fixed plasma level' design. *Psychopharmacol Bull.* 1990;26:85-90.

17. Simeon JG, Dinicola VF, Ferguson B, Copping W. Adolescent depression: a placebo-controlled fluoxetine treatment study and follow-up. *Prog Neuropsychopharmacol Biol Psychiatry.* 1990;14:791-795.
18. Garber J, Hilsman R. Cognitions, stress, and depression in children and adolescents. *Mood Disorders.* 1992;1:129-167.
19. Reynolds WM, Coates KI. A comparison of cognitive-behavioral therapy and relaxation training for the treatment of depression in adolescents. *J Consult Clin Psychol.* 1986;54:653-660.
20. Lewinsohn PM, Clarke GN. Cognitive-behavioral treatment for depressed adolescents. *Behav Ther.* 1990;21:385-401.
21. Kahn JS, Kehle TJ, Jenson WR, Clark E. Comparison of cognitive-behavioral relaxation, and self-modeling interventions for depression among middle-school students. *School Psychol Rev.* 1990;19:196-211.
22. Wood A, Harrington R, Moore A. Controlled trial of a brief cognitive-behavioral intervention in adolescent patients with depressive disorders. *J Child Psychol Psychiatry.* 1996;37:737-746.
23. Diamond GS, Serrano AC, Dickey M, Sonis WA. Current status of family-based outcome and process research. *J Am Acad Child Adolesc Psychiatry.* 1996;35:6-16.
24. Asarnow JR, Goldstein MJ, Tompson M, Guthrie D. One-year outcomes of depressive disorders in child psychiatric in-patients: evaluation of the prognostic power of a brief measure of expressed emotion. *J Child Psychol Psychiatry.* 1993;34:129-137.
25. Hollis C. Depression, family environment, and adolescent suicidal behavior. *J Am Acad Child Adolesc Psychiatry.* 1996;35:622-630.
26. Luborsky L, McLellan T, Woody GE, O'Brien CP, Auerbach A. Therapist success and its determinants. *Arch Gen Psychiatry.* 1985;42:602-611.
27. Burns DD, Nolen-Hoeksema S. Therapeutic empathy and recovery from depression in cognitive-behavioral therapy: a structural equation model. *J Consult Clin Psychol.* 1992;60:441-449.
28. American Psychiatric Association. *Diagnostic and Statistical Manual of Mental Disorders, Third Edition, Revised.* Washington, DC: American Psychiatric Association; 1987.
29. Beck AT, Steer RA, Garbin MG. Psychometric properties of the Beck Depression Inventory: twenty-five years of evaluation. *Clin Psychol Rev.* 1988;8:77-100.
30. Begg CB, Iglewicz B. A treatment allocation procedure for sequencial clinical trials. *Biometrics.* 1980;36:81-90.
31. Efron B. Forcing a sequential experiment to be balanced. *Biometrika.* 1971;58:403-417.
32. Brent DA, Poling K, McKain B, Baugher M. A psychoeducational program for families of affectively ill children and adolescents. *J Am Acad Child Adolesc Psychiatry.* 1993;32:770-774.
33. Brent DA, Roth C, Holder D, Kolko DJ, Birmaher B, Johnson BA, Schweers J. Psychosocial interventions for treating adolescent depression: a comparison of three psychosocial interventions. In: Hibbs ED, Jensen PS, eds. *Psychosocial Treatment for Child and Adolescent Disorders: Empirically Based Strategies for Clinical Practice.* Washington, DC: American Psychiatric Press Inc; 1996:187-206.
34. Beck AT, Rush AJ, Shaw BF, Emery G. *Cognitive Therapy of Depression.* New York, NY: Guilford Press; 1979.
35. Rotheram MJ. Evaluation of imminent danger for suicide among youth. *Am J Orthopsychiatry.* 1987;57:102-110.
36. Alexander J, Parsons BV. *Functional Family Therapy.* Pacific Grove, Calif: Brooks/Cole Publishing Co; 1982.
37. Robin AL, Foster SL. *Negotiating Parent-Adolescent Conflict: A Behavioral-Family Systems Approach.* New York, NY: Guilford Press; 1989.
38. Vallis TM, Shaw BF, Dobson KS. The Cognitive Therapy Scale: psychometric properties. *J Consult Clin Psychol.* 1986;54:381-385.
39. Piercy FP, Liard RA, Mohammed Z. A Family Therapist Rating Scale. *J Marital Fam Ther.* 1983;9:49-59.
40. Suh CS, Strupp HH, O'Malley SS. The Vanderbilt Process Measures: the Psychotherapy Process Scale (VPPS) and the Negative Indications Scale (NIS). In: Greenberg LS, Pinsof WM, eds. *The Psychotherapeutic Process: A Research Handbook.* New York, NY: Guilford Press; 1986:285-323.
41. Endicott J, Spitzer RL. A diagnostic interview: the Schedule for Affective Disorders and Schizophrenia. *Arch Gen Psychiatry.* 1978;35:837-844.
42. Elkin I, Shea T, Watkins JT, Imber SD, Sotsky SM, Collins JF, Glass DR, Pilkonis PA, Leber WR, Docherty JP, Fiester SJ, Parloff MB. National Institute of Mental Health Treatment of Depression Collaborative Research Program: general effectiveness of treatments. *Arch Gen Psychiatry.* 1989;46:971-982.
43. Borkovec TD, Nau SD. Credibility of analogue therapy rationales. *J Behav Ther Exp Psychiatry.* 1972;3:257-260.
44. Chambers WJ, Puig-Antich J, Hirsch M, Paez P, Ambrosini PJ, Tabrizi MA, Davies M. The assessment of affective disorders in children and adolescents by semistructured interview: test-retest reliability of the Schedule for Affective Disorders and Schizophrenia for School-age Children, Present Episode Version. *Arch Gen Psychiatry.* 1985;42:696-702.
45. Orvaschel H, Puig-Antich J, Chambers W, Tabrizi MA, Johnson R. Retrospective assessment of prepubertal major depression with the Kiddie-SADS-E. *J Am Acad Child Psychiatry.* 1982;21:392-397.
46. Ambrosini PJ, Metz C, Bianchi MD, Rabinovich H, Undie A. Concurrent validity and psychometric properties of the Beck Depression Inventory in outpatient adolescents. *J Am Acad Child Adolesc Psychiatry.* 1991;30:51-57.
47. Strober M, Green J, Carlson G. Utility of the Beck Depression Inventory with psychiatrically hospitalized adolescents. *J Consult Clin Psychol.* 1981;49:482-483.
48. Somoza E, Soutullo-Esperon L, Mossman D. Evaluation and optimization of diagnostic tests using receiver operating characteristic analysis and information theory. *Int J Biomed Comput.* 1989;24:153-189.
49. Shaffer D, Gould MS, Brasic J, Ambrosini P, Fisher P, Bird H, Aluwahlia SA. A Children's Global Assessment Scale (CGAS). *Arch Gen Psychiatry.* 1983;40:1228-1231.
50. Pocock SJ. *Clinical Trials: A Practical Approach.* New York, NY: John Wiley & Sons Inc; 1983:182.
51. Lavori PW. Clinical trials in psychiatry: should protocol deviation censor patient data? *Neuropsychopharmacology.* 1992;6:39-48.
52. Gibbons RD, Hedeker D, Elkin I, Waternaux C, Kraemer HC, Greenhouse JB, Shea T, Imber SD, Sotsky SM, Watkins JT. Some conceptual and statistical issues in analysis of longitudinal psychiatric data: application to the NIMH Treatment of Depression Collaborative Research Program dataset. *Arch Gen Psychiatry.* 1993;50:739-750.
53. Mantel N. Evaluation of survival data and two new rank order statistics arising in its consideration. *Cancer Chemother Rep.* 1966;50:163-170.
54. Beck AT, Weissman A, Lester D, Trexler L. The measurement of pessimism: the Hopelessness Scale. *J Consult Clin Psychol.* 1974;42:861-865.
55. Luborsky L, Singer B. Comparative studies of psychotherapies: is it true that 'everyone has won and all must have prizes?' *Arch Gen Psychiatry.* 1975;32:995-1008.
56. Weisz JR, Weiss B, Donenberg GR. The lab versus the clinic: effects of child and adolescent psychotherapy. *Am Psychol.* 1992;47:1578-1585.
57. Barrett PM, Dadds MR, Rapee RM. Family treatment of childhood anxiety: a controlled trial. *J Consult Clin Psychol.* 1996;64:333-342.
58. Puig-Antich J, Lukens E, Davies M, Goetz D, Brennan-Quattrock J, Todak G. Psychosocial functioning in prepubertal major depressive disorders, II: interpersonal relationship after sustained recovery from affective episode. *Arch Gen Psychiatry.* 1985;42:511-517.
59. Kovacs M, Akiskal HS, Gatsonis C, Parrone PL. Childhood-onset dysthymic disorder. *Arch Gen Psychiatry.* 1994;51:365-374.

Interference with Cognitive and Motor Performance: Because of initial sedation, CLOZARIL® (clozapine) may impair mental and/or physical abilities, especially during the first few days of therapy. The recommendations for gradual dose escalation should be carefully adhered to, and patients cautioned about activities requiring alertness.

Use in Patients with Concomitant Illness: Clinical experience with CLOZARIL® (clozapine) in patients with concomitant systemic diseases is limited. Nevertheless, caution is advisable in using CLOZARIL® (clozapine) in patients with renal or cardiac disease.

Use in Patients Undergoing General Anesthesia: Caution is advised in patients being administered general anesthesia because of the CNS effects of CLOZARIL® (clozapine). Check with the anesthesiologist regarding continuation of CLOZARIL® (clozapine) therapy in a patient scheduled for surgery.

Information for Patients: Physicians are advised to discuss the following issues with patients for whom they prescribe CLOZARIL® (clozapine):

– Patients who are to receive CLOZARIL® (clozapine) should be warned about the significant risk of developing agranulocytosis. They should be informed that weekly blood tests are required to monitor for the occurrence of agranulocytosis, and that CLOZARIL® (clozapine) tablets will be made available only through a special program designed to ensure the required blood monitoring. Patients should be advised to report immediately the appearance of lethargy, weakness, fever, sore throat, malaise, mucous membrane ulceration or other possible signs of infection. Particular attention should be paid to any flu-like complaints or other symptoms that might suggest infection.
– Patients should be informed of the significant risk of seizure during CLOZARIL® (clozapine) treatment, and they should be advised to avoid driving and any other potentially hazardous activity while taking CLOZARIL® (clozapine).
– Patients should be advised of the risk of orthostatic hypotension, especially during the period of initial dose titration.
– Patients should be informed that if they stop taking CLOZARIL® (clozapine) for more than 2 days, they should not restart their medication at the same dosage, but should contact their physician for dosing instructions.
– Patients should notify their physician if they are taking, or plan to take, any prescription or over-the-counter drugs or alcohol.
– Patients should notify their physician if they become pregnant or intend to become pregnant during therapy.
– Patients should not breast feed an infant if they are taking CLOZARIL® (clozapine).

Drug Interactions: The risks of using CLOZARIL® (clozapine) in combination with other drugs have not been systematically evaluated.

The mechanism of CLOZARIL® (clozapine) induced agranulocytosis is unknown; nonetheless, the possibility that causative factors may interact synergistically to increase the risk and/or severity of bone marrow suppression warrants consideration. Therefore, CLOZARIL® (clozapine) should not be used with other agents having a well-known potential to suppress bone marrow function.

Given the primary CNS effects of CLOZARIL® (clozapine), caution is advised in using it concomitantly with other CNS-active drugs or alcohol.

Orthostatic hypotension in patients taking clozapine can, in rare cases (approximately 1 case per 3,000 patients), be accompanied by profound collapse and respiratory and/or cardiac arrest. Some of the cases of collapse/respiratory arrest/cardiac arrest during initial treatment occurred in patients who were being administered benzodiazepines; similar events have been reported in patients taking other psychotropic drugs or even CLOZARIL® (clozapine) by itself. Although it has not been established that there is an interaction between CLOZARIL® (clozapine) and benzodiazepines or other psychotropics, caution is advised when clozapine is initiated in patients taking a benzodiazepine or any other psychotropic drug.

Because CLOZARIL® (clozapine) is highly bound to serum protein, the administration of CLOZARIL® (clozapine) to a patient taking another drug which is highly bound to protein (e.g., warfarin, digitoxin) may cause an increase in plasma concentrations of these drugs, potentially resulting in adverse effects. Conversely, adverse effects may result from displacement of protein-bound CLOZARIL® (clozapine) by other highly bound drugs.

Cimetidine and erythromycin may both increase plasma levels of CLOZARIL® (clozapine), potentially resulting in adverse effects. Although concomitant use of CLOZARIL® (clozapine) and carbamazepine is not recommended, it should be noted that discontinuation of concomitant carbamazepine administration may result in an increase in CLOZARIL® (clozapine) plasma levels. Phenytoin may decrease CLOZARIL® (clozapine) plasma levels, resulting in a decrease in effectiveness of a previously effective CLOZARIL® (clozapine) dose.

A subset (3%-10%) of the population has reduced activity of certain drug metabolizing enzymes such as the cytochrome P450 isozyme P450 2D6. Such individuals are referred to as "poor metabolizers" of drugs such as debrisoquin, dextromethorphan, the tricyclic antidepressants, and clozapine. These individuals may develop higher than expected plasma concentrations of clozapine when given usual doses. In addition, certain drugs that are metabolized by this isozyme, including many antidepressants (clozapine, selective serotonin reuptake inhibitors, and others), may inhibit the activity of this isozyme, and thus may make normal metabolizers resemble poor metabolizers with regard to concomitant therapy with other drugs metabolized by this enzyme system, leading to drug interaction.

Concomitant use of clozapine with other drugs metabolized by cytochrome P450 2D6 may require lower doses than usually prescribed for either clozapine or the other drug. Therefore, co-administration of clozapine with other drugs that are metabolized by this isozyme, including antidepressants, phenothiazines, carbamazepine, and Type 1C antiarrhythmics (e.g., propafenone, flecainide and encainide), or that inhibit this enzyme (e.g., quinidine), should be approached with caution.

CLOZARIL® (clozapine) may also potentiate the hypotensive effects of antihypertensive drugs and the anticholinergic effects of atropine-type drugs. The administration of epinephrine should be avoided in the treatment of drug induced hypotension because of a possible reverse epinephrine effect.

Carcinogenesis, Mutagenesis, Impairment of Fertility: No carcinogenic potential was demonstrated in long-term studies in mice and rats at doses approximately 7 times the typical human dose on a mg/kg basis. Fertility in male and female rats was not adversely affected by clozapine. Clozapine did not produce genotoxic or mutagenic effects when assayed in appropriate bacterial and mammalian tests.

Pregnancy Category B: Reproduction studies have been performed in rats and rabbits at doses of approximately 2-4 times the human dose and have revealed no evidence of impaired fertility or harm to the fetus due to clozapine. There are, however, no adequate and well-controlled studies in pregnant women. Because animal reproduction studies are not always predictive of human response, and in view of the desirability of keeping the administration of all drugs to a minimum during pregnancy, this drug should be used only if clearly needed.

Nursing Mothers: Animal studies suggest that clozapine may be excreted in breast milk and have an effect on the nursing infant. Therefore, women receiving CLOZARIL® (clozapine) should not breast feed.

Pediatric Use: Safety and effectiveness in pediatric patients have not been established.

ADVERSE REACTIONS: Associated with Discontinuation of Treatment: Sixteen percent of 1080 patients who received CLOZARIL® (clozapine) in premarketing clinical trials discontinued treatment due to an adverse event, including both those that could be reasonably attributed to CLOZARIL® (clozapine) treatment and those that might more appropriately be considered intercurrent illness. The more common events considered to be causes of discontinuation included: CNS, primarily drowsiness/sedation, seizures, dizziness/syncope; cardiovascular, primarily tachycardia, hypotension and ECG changes; gastrointestinal, primarily nausea/vomiting; hematologic, primarily leukopenia/granulocytopenia/agranulocytosis; and fever. None of the events enumerated accounts for more than 1.7% of all discontinuations attributed to adverse clinical events.

Commonly Observed: Adverse events observed in association with the use of CLOZARIL® (clozapine) in clinical trials at an incidence of greater than 5% were: central nervous system complaints, including drowsiness/sedation, dizziness/vertigo, headache and tremor; autonomic nervous system complaints, including salivation, sweating, dry mouth and visual disturbances; cardiovascular findings, including tachycardia, hypotension and syncope; and gastrointestinal complaints, including constipation and nausea; and fever. Complaints of drowsiness/sedation tend to subside with continued therapy or dose reduction. Salivation may be profuse, especially during sleep, but may be diminished with dose reduction.

Incidence in Clinical Trials: The following table enumerates adverse events that occurred at a frequency of 1% or greater among CLOZARIL® (clozapine) patients who participated in clinical trials. These rates are not adjusted for duration of exposure.

Treatment-Emergent Adverse Experience Incidence Among Patients Taking CLOZARIL® (clozapine) in Clinical Trials (N = 842) (Percentage of Patients Reporting)

Body System / Adverse Event[a]	Percent
Central Nervous System	
Drowsiness/Sedation	39
Dizziness/Vertigo	19
Headache	7
Tremor	6
Syncope	6
Disturbed sleep/Nightmares	4
Restlessness	4
Hypokinesia/Akinesia	4
Agitation	4
Seizures (convulsions)	3[b]
Rigidity	3
Akathisia	3
Confusion	3
Fatigue	2
Insomnia	2
Hyperkinesia	1
Weakness	1
Lethargy	1
Ataxia	1
Slurred speech	1
Depression	1
Epileptiform movements/Myoclonic jerks	1
Anxiety	1

(Continued)

Treatment-Emergent Adverse Experience Incidence Among Patients Taking CLOZARIL® (clozapine) in Clinical Trials (N = 842) (Percentage of Patients Reporting)

Body System / Adverse Event[a]	Percent
Cardiovascular	
Tachycardia	25[b]
Hypotension	9
Hypertension	4
Chest pain/Angina	1
ECG change/Cardiac abnormality	1
Gastrointestinal	
Constipation	14
Nausea	5
Abdominal discomfort/Heartburn	4
Nausea/Vomiting	3
Vomiting	3
Diarrhea	2
Liver test abnormality	1
Anorexia	1
Urogenital	
Urinary abnormalities	2
Incontinence	1
Abnormal ejaculation	1
Urinary urgency/frequency	1
Urinary retention	1
Autonomic Nervous System	
Salivation	31
Sweating	6
Dry mouth	6
Visual disturbances	5
Integumentary (Skin)	
Rash	2
Musculoskeletal	
Muscle weakness	1
Pain (back, neck, legs)	1
Muscle spasm	1
Muscle pain, ache	1
Respiratory	
Throat discomfort	1
Dyspnea, shortness of breath	1
Nasal congestion	1
Hemic/Lymphatic	
Leukopenia/Decreased WBC/Neutropenia	3
Agranulocytosis	1[b]
Eosinophilia	1
Miscellaneous	
Fever	5
Weight gain	4
Tongue numb/sore	1

[a]Events reported by at least 1% of CLOZARIL® (clozapine) patients are included.

[b]Rate based on population of approximately 1700 exposed during premarket clinical evaluation of CLOZARIL® (clozapine).

Other Events Observed During the Premarketing Evaluation of CLOZARIL® (clozapine): This section reports additional, less frequent adverse events which occurred among the patients taking CLOZARIL® (clozapine) in clinical trials. Various adverse events were reported as part of the total experience in these clinical studies; a causal relationship to CLOZARIL® (clozapine) treatment cannot be determined in the absence of appropriate controls in some of the studies. The table above enumerates adverse events that occurred at a frequency of at least 1% of patients treated with CLOZARIL® (clozapine). The list below includes all additional adverse experiences reported as being temporally associated with the use of the drug which occurred at a frequency less than 1%, enumerated by organ system.

Central Nervous System: loss of speech, amentia, tics, poor coordination, delusions/hallucinations, involuntary movement, stuttering, dysarthria, amnesia/memory loss, histrionic movements, libido increase or decrease, paranoia, shakiness, Parkinsonism, and irritability.

Cardiovascular System: edema, palpitations, phlebitis/thrombophlebitis, cyanosis, premature ventricular contraction, bradycardia, and nose bleed.

Gastrointestinal System: abdominal distention, gastroenteritis, rectal bleeding, nervous stomach, abnormal stools, hematemesis, gastric ulcer, bitter taste, and eructation.

Urogenital System: dysmenorrhea, impotence, breast pain/discomfort, and vaginal itch/infection.

Autonomic Nervous System: numbness, polydypsia, hot flashes, dry throat, and mydriasis.

Integumentary (Skin): pruritus, pallor, eczema, erythema, bruise, dermatitis, petechiae, and urticaria.

Musculoskeletal System: twitching and joint pain.

Respiratory System: coughing, pneumonia/pneumonia-like symptoms, rhinorrhea, hyperventilation, wheezing, bronchitis, laryngitis, and sneezing.

Hemic and Lymphatic System: anemia and leukocytosis.

Miscellaneous: chills/chills with fever, malaise, appetite increase, ear disorder, hypothermia, eyelid disorder, bloodshot eyes, and nystagmus.

Postmarketing Clinical Experience: Postmarketing experience has shown an adverse experience profile similar to that presented above. Voluntary reports of adverse events temporally associated with CLOZARIL® (clozapine) not mentioned above that have been received since market introduction and that may have no causal relationship with the drug include the following:

Central Nervous System: delirium; EEG abnormal; exacerbation of psychosis; myoclonus; overdose; paresthesia; possible mild cataplexy; and status epilepticus.

Cardiovascular System: atrial or ventricular fibrillation and periorbital edema.

Gastrointestinal System: acute pancreatitis; dysphagia; fecal impaction; intestinal obstruction/paralytic ileus; and salivary gland swelling.

Hepatobiliary System: cholestasis; hepatitis; jaundice.

Hepatic System: cholestasis.

Urogenital System: acute interstitial nephritis and priapism.

Integumentary (Skin): hypersensitivity reactions: photosensitivity, vasculitis, erythema multiforme, and Stevens-Johnson Syndrome.

Musculoskeletal System: myasthenic syndrome and rhabdomyolysis.

Respiratory System: aspiration and pleural effusion.

Hemic and Lymphatic System: deep vein thrombosis; elevated hemoglobin/hematocrit; ESR increased; pulmonary embolism; sepsis; thrombocytosis; and thrombocytopenia.

Miscellaneous: CPK elevation; hyperglycemia; hyperuricemia; hyponatremia; and weight loss.

DRUG ABUSE AND DEPENDENCE: Physical and psychological dependence have not been reported or observed in patients taking CLOZARIL® (clozapine).

Store and Dispense: Storage temperature should not exceed 86°F (30°C). Drug dispensing should not ordinarily exceed a weekly supply. Dispensing should be contingent upon the results of a WBC count.

Novartis Pharmaceuticals Corporation
East Hanover, New Jersey 07936

REV: JUNE 1997 P30118907

THIS MONTH IN

ARCHIVES OF GENERAL PSYCHIATRY

Childhood onset schizophrenia is a rare and severe form of the illness. In the first longitudinal brain imaging study of childhood onset schizophrenic patients, **Rapoport et al** (page 897) report a marked differential increase in ventricular volume across ages 14 to 16 years for a group of schizophrenic patients with mean onset at age 10 compared with healthy, yoked controls. In this sample, there was evidence suggesting a progressive brain abnormality. This suggests that early adolescence may be a critical period in which to observe abnormal brain development in schizophrenia, and that it is important to test in other samples whether these findings are generalizable.

Whether early-onset schizophrenia is basically the same illness as the later-onset variety has been questioned. **Zahn et al** (page 904) report high heart rates, elevated spontaneous fluctuations of skin conductance, greatly attenuated autonomic nervous system reactions to challenges and stimuli, and slow adaptation and habituation in 20 patients who developed schizophrenia before age 13 years compared with 54 age-matched controls. These findings are similar to those typically found in adult-onset schizophrenia and support the fundamental similarity of the 2 disorders. *A Commentary by Nasrallah and Tolbert, titled "Neurobiology and Neuroplasticity in Schizophrenia: Continuity Across the Life Cycle," also appears in this issue.*

Geriatric depression often occurs in the context of vascular disease or risk factors. **Alexopoulos et al** (page 915) hypothesized that cerebrovascular disease may predispose, precipitate, or perpetuate geriatric depressive syndromes. Disruption of prefrontal systems or their modulating pathways by single lesions or by the accumulation of lesions exceeding a threshold are hypothesized to be central mechanisms in "vascular depression." Prevention or treatment of cerebrovascular disease may reduce the risk of vascular depression or improve its outcomes. The choice of antidepressants may depend on their effect on recovery from ischemic lesions.

Medications are rarely implemented without psychotherapy or some form of psychosocial support. However, psychotherapy is rarely used optimally in studies evaluating medications for psychiatric disorders. **Carroll** (page 923) reviews the advantages of providing standardized psychotherapy in medication trials and points out problems that are associated with neglecting psychosocial aspects of treatment. *A Commentary about this article by Klein and Smith, titled "Psychotherapeutic Context for Clinical Trials is Promising, But Manualization Is Not," also appears in this issue.*

While many studies show that children of depressed parents are at increased risk for major depression, none of them have followed the offspring into adulthood to obtain more precise estimates of risk. In a 10-year follow-up, **Weissman et al** (page 932) show that the offspring of depressed parents are at high risk for the onset of anxiety disorders in childhood, major depression in adolescence, and alcohol dependence in adolescence and early adulthood. The findings support the potential value of early detection in the offspring of depressed parents.

It is not known for how long neuroleptics remain in the brain after the discontinuation of depot treatment. Four schizophrenic patients were withdrawn from haloperidol decanoate and examined repeatedly with positron emission tomography for up to 1 year. In 3 patients followed for 6 months, **Nyberg et al** (page 953) found that D_2 dopamine receptor occupancy decreased only slowly and was still 24%, 32%, and 34%. Remaining receptor occupancy may confound clinical evaluation of new antipsychotic treatments and the results of controlled clinical trials for several months after depot treatment is withdrawn.

Many studies have recently found glutamatergic abnormalities in schizophrenia. In an in vivo proton (^1H) magnetic resonance spectroscopy study, **Bartha et al** (page 959) report increased glutamine levels in the medial prefrontal cortex of never-treated schizophrenic subjects compared with controls. As glutamine is the primary precursor of the neurotransmitter glutamate, increased levels of glutamine in the medial prefrontal cortex provide the first in vivo evidence of aberrant glutamatergic metabolism in schizophrenic patients.

Childhood-Onset Schizophrenia

Progressive Ventricular Change During Adolescence

Judith L. Rapoport, MD; Jay Giedd, MD; Sanjiv Kumra, MD; Leslie Jacobsen, MD; Amy Smith; Paul Lee; Jean Nelson, MHS; Susan Hamburger, MS

Background: There is controversy about progression in brain abnormalities in later-onset schizophrenia. This study looked for more striking progression in brain abnormalities during adolescence in a chronically ill, treatment-refractory sample of patients with childhood-onset schizophrenia who had had more prepsychotic developmental disturbance, but clinical and neurobiological characteristics similar to those of patients with treatment-refractory adult-onset schizophrenia who have poor outcome.

Methods: Anatomic brain magnetic resonance images were obtained for 16 children and adolescents with onset of schizophrenia by 12 years of age and 24 temporally yoked, age- and sex-matched healthy controls. Subjects were scanned on initial admission and rescanned after 2 years with the identical equipment and measurement methods.

Results: Childhood schizophrenics showed a significantly greater increase in ventricular volume than did controls, for whom ventricles did not increase significantly (analysis of variance, diagnosis×time, $F=16.1$, $P<.001$). A significant decrease in midsagittal thalamic area was also seen for the schizophrenics ($P=.03$), which was unchanged at rescan for controls. These differential brain changes correlated significantly with each other and tended to be predicted by both prepsychotic developmental abnormality (Premorbid Assessment Scale, $P=.06$) and Brief Psychiatric Rating Scale at follow-up ($P=.07$).

Conclusions: More consistent progressive ventricular enlargement was seen during adolescence for this childhood-onset sample than has been reported for adult-onset populations. The brain imaging results support other clinical data showing both early and late deviations in brain development for at least this rare subgroup of treatment-refractory, very-early-onset schizophrenic patients.

Arch Gen Psychiatry. 1997;54:897-903

From the Child Psychiatry Branch, National Institute of Mental Health, Bethesda, Md.

CHILDHOOD-ONSET schizophrenia (COS), defined herein as schizophrenia with onset by 12 years of age, provides a unique research opportunity. Investigation into clinical and neurobiological features of this rare but severe form of the illness may reveal more salient risk factors and/or more striking neurodevelopmental abnormalities that can shed light on the parent disorder.

Clinical follow-up studies of patients with COS have shown continuing chronic schizophrenia as the patients progressed through adolescence into adulthood.[1,2] These data are consistent with the hypothesis that childhood- and later-onset schizophrenia represent the same illness or illnesses.

Since 1990, an ongoing study of COS has supported findings from previous clinical reports of schizophrenia with very early onset (at or before 12 years of age). The patients are severely ill and have more frequent prepsychotic developmental problems, such as motor and speech delay, than those seen for later-onset (ie, onset after 18 years of age) schizophrenia, and insidious onset of psychosis was most common.[3-5] Clinically, this treatment-refractory population resembled treatment-refractory adult patients with respect to severity of premorbid dysfunction and equal numbers of males and females in the group.[6]

See also page 913

Neurobiological studies also indicate patterns of abnormalities similar to those seen in adult patients for autonomic activity and

This article is also available on our Web site: www.ama-assn.org/psych.

SUBJECTS AND METHODS

SUBJECTS

Recruiting and diagnostic assessment have been presented in detail elsewhere.[3,9] Subjects were sought who met *DSM-III-R*[29] criteria for schizophrenia with documented onset of psychosis by 12 years of age (mean$\pm$SD, 10.23$\pm$1.75 years) who had not responded to treatment with typical neuroleptics. More than 800 records were reviewed and 150 in-person screenings were carried out to identify 30 patients who met unmodified diagnostic criteria. These subjects all participated in a double-blind comparison study of haloperidol and clozapine.[30] All patients agreed to return after 2 years for follow-up evaluation and repeated MR imaging. The 16 subjects who underwent rescanning in this study did not differ significantly from the 14 not yet due for rescanning on any clinical or demographic measure. A parallel study of brain development in a large sample of healthy pediatric controls is ongoing. The study used the Diagnostic Interview for Children and Adolescents (DICA) and DICA–Parent Version as screening instruments,[25,31,32] and thus, 2-year rescan data were available for 16 patients with COS and 24 yoked matched healthy controls.

Dates of initial and repeated MR imaging for the control group were within 6 months of those for the patient group for both the first and second scans. The range of rescan intervals was 1.5 to 4 years (mean$\pm$SD, 2.23$\pm$0.23 years). The groups did not differ significantly with respect to age, sex, or handedness. There was a significant difference, however, with regard to race: all of the controls were white, whereas 7 of the schizophrenics were black and 1 was Asian; socioeconomic status also differed, with that of the patients being significantly lower. Descriptive information for patients and controls is given in **Table 1**. At time of the first scan, all but 3 patients were being treated with typical neuroleptics.

At follow-up, all subjects were interviewed and rescanned while taking neuroleptic medication. As seen in Table 1, schizophrenic subjects had gained more weight in the interim and so were heavier than controls at the time of rescan (*P*=.008), but there was no significant difference in height. The protocol was approved by the National Institute of Mental Health institutional review board, and all subjects gave assent and their parents gave signed consent.

INTERIM MEDICAL HISTORY

At 2-year follow-up, 13 of the 16 patients were living at home, 2 were being maintained in residential treatment centers, and 1 was still hospitalized. Although most patients were considerably more stable clinically, most continued to experience moderate psychotic symptoms, as indicated by baseline and follow-up clinical rating scale scores on the Scale for Assessment of Positive Symptoms,[33] Scale for Assessment of Negative Symptoms,[34] and Brief Psychiatric Rating Scale[35] (Table 1). Eleven of the 16 subjects were rated as very much or much improved on the Clinical Global Impression Scale, 4 were rated minimally improved, and 1 was considered very much worse.

Diagnoses at follow-up were based on interviews of the children and parents that included portions of the Schedule for Affective Disorders and Schizophrenia for School-Age Children–Epidemiological Version of the DICA (*DSM-III-R* Version).[31] Thirteen of 16 patients met *DSM-III-R* criteria for chronic schizophrenia at follow-up, while 3 were diagnosed as having schizophrenia in partial or full remission. Comorbid diagnoses at follow-up included the following: Tourette disorder (2 patients), autistic disorder (1 patient), Asperger disorder (1 patient), and obsessive-compulsive disorder (1 patient). These disorders were mild, and in no case were they a focus of treatment. Prepsychotic developmental disturbance had been common for the group, with motor and language delays most common, as summarized by the Premorbid Adjustment Scale.[36]

Twelve patients were taking clozapine at follow-up, with an average ($\pm$SD) daily dose of 357$\pm$75 mg. The remaining 4 were taking an average of 8 mg of risperidone per day. However, only 6 patients were receiving monotherapy; additional medications included valproate, haloperidol, fluoxetine, lithium carbonate, and imipramine.

MR IMAGING PROTOCOL

All baseline and follow-up scans were obtained on the same 1.5-T scanner (Signa, General Electric Co, Milwaukee, Wis) with the use of a spoiled gradient recalled echo in the steady state imaging sequence with echo time of 5 milliseconds, time to repeat of 24 milliseconds, flip angle of 45°, acquisition matrix of 192$\times$256, 1 excitation, and field of view of 24 cm. T_1-weighted sagittal images with slice thickness of 1.5 mm in the axial and sagittal planes and 2.0 mm in

reactivity,[7] smooth-pursuit eye movements,[8] anatomic brain magnetic resonance (MR) images,[9] and spectral brain MR images.[10] Both smaller total cerebral volume and larger ventricular volume were seen for childhood schizophrenics, with greater effect size for cerebral volume reduction than that reported for adults.[11] These findings are compatible with a model of schizophrenia in which a very early onset of psychosis is associated with a more striking earlier abnormality of brain development. These questions of whether there are also more consistent progressive changes in brain anatomy, however, were not addressed.

The existence of ongoing change in brain morphologic characteristics has been the focus of several studies of later-onset schizophrenia: the results have generally not supported continued change.[12-17] When anatomic brain rescans have indicated change, they have been subtle,[18-20] although recent refined techniques have been more consistent in showing progression in some patients[21,22] and support older adult pneumoencephalographic studies suggesting that poor-outcome subgroups are likely to show progressive ventricular enlargement.[23,24] Virtually all studies, however, note individual schizophrenic patients showing ventricular volume increases that are outside the range for the controls.

To examine later brain development in COS, repeated MR images were obtained as part of a 2-year prospective follow-up study. Two lines of reasoning prompted this study. Childhood-onset schizophrenia typically has insidious rather than episodic onset,[3] with continuing severe illness in about half the cases.[5] In addition, independent of age at onset, the early adolescent years are a time of normal acceleration of ventricular enlargement,[25] and some models of schizophrenia[26-28] postulate the coronal plane were obtained. Vitamin E capsules, wrapped in gauze, were placed in the meatus of each ear, and a third capsule was taped to the lateral aspect of the left inferior orbital ridge to help standardize head placement. If no slice of a multiecho axial series contained all 3 capsules, the patient was realigned until this criterion was met. To control for possible head tilt within the coronal plane, each subject's nose was aligned at the 12-o'clock position. (External landmark–based alignment criteria do not guarantee standardization of internal structures.)

Subjects were scanned in the evening to promote their falling asleep in the scanner. Younger children were allowed to bring blankets or stuffed animals into the scanner and have their parents read to them. Patients who needed sedation were given chloral hydrate (2.0-3.0 g orally) or lorazepam (1.0-2.0 mg orally) and monitored with a pulse oximeter. No sedation was used for control subjects.

IMAGE ANALYSIS

The brain was separated from the intracranial cavity by means of a program that models the brain as an active surface template that then conforms to the individual brain through a series of energy minimization functions.[37] Subjective operator involvement includes choosing the midsagittal anterior commissure and posterior commissure points and placing boundaries for a box around the brain. The output of this program was then edited to remove artifacts related to eyeballs or patches of dura to yield our measures of left and right cerebral hemisphere volumes. This measure does not include ventricular volume, brain stem, or cerebellum. To avoid biases related to the rater's measurements changing over time, all scans were blinded with respect to diagnosis, any identifying characteristics, and time of scan and remeasured during the same 2-month period. Intrarater and interrater intraclass correlation coefficients (ICCs) were 0.94 and 0.89, respectively.

Lateral/ventricle volume was quantified on all coronal slices (2-mm slice thickness, contiguous) on which these structures were visible by an experienced rater using a supervised thresholding technique available in National Institutes of Health Image.[38] Intrarater and interrater ICCs for this highly automated procedure were 0.99 and 0.97, respectively.

The caudate, putamen, and globus pallidus were quantified in the coronal plane by experienced raters using a mouse-driven tracing tool available in National Institutes of Health Image to outline the perimeter of each of these structures. The caudate is bounded medially by the lateral ventricles and laterally by the internal capsule, the putamen is bounded medially by the globus pallidus and laterally by the external capsule, and the globus pallidus is bounded medially by the internal capsule and laterally by the putamen. Interrater reliabilities (ICCs) for the caudate, putamen, and globus pallidus, for 2 raters and 20 cases, were 0.87, 0.84, and 0.82, respectively.

Midsagittal area of the thalamus was measured by manually outlining this structure on a single midsagittal slice reconstructed from the axial series. Interrater reliability for this structure was 0.85.

Gray matter, white matter, and cerebrospinal fluid were separately quantified by means of a probabilistic segmentation program developed in our laboratory.[39] Cortical gray matter was distinguished from subcortical matter by a rater who examined the gray matter on each axial slice by means of ANALYZE (Mayo Clinic, Rochester, Minn). Interrater reliability (ICC) for this cortical vs subcortical procedure was 0.97 for 2 raters who measured 20 brains.

STATISTICAL ANALYSIS

Differences between the patients with COS and normal controls were analyzed with the Student t test (demographic variables) or repeated-measures analysis of variance (brain imaging variables) using a diagnosis×time of scan design. When significant, a diagnosis×time×side analysis of variance was also carried out. Within-group comparisons were done with paired t tests on the difference scores between scans 1 and 2. All variables were normally distributed within groups.

Because of the normal distribution of data, Pearson correlation coefficients were obtained to examine the associations within the scan 2–scan 1 difference scores, and between these changes in brain imaging measures and baseline and follow-up clinical and demographic data for the patients with COS. Within the schizophrenic group, stepwise linear regression was used to examine which baseline and/or follow-up brain and/or behavioral variables were best related to differential changes in brain anatomy.

The SAS statistical package (SAS Institute Inc, Cary, NC) was used for all statistical analyses. An α level of .05 was used for significance.

that group differences might be most apparent during adolescence when normal ventricular expansion begins. The availability of a childhood-onset cohort and our normative longitudinal study of brain development permitted such a study to be carried out. This is an initial report of 2-year rescanning for 16 patients with COS and 24 matched yoked controls, and represents the only brain rescan study during adolescence for any psychiatric disorder.

RESULTS

Values for total cerebral volume, lateral ventricular volume, ventricle-brain ratio, globus pallidus, caudate, and putamen, as well as midsagittal thalamic area, at initial and follow-up scans are given in **Table 2** and the **Figure** for the COS and control groups.

The patients with COS tended to differ at initial scan with respect to total cerebral volume (P=.02) and ventricular volume (P=.11). In addition, globus pallidus, caudate, and putamen volumes tended to be larger for schizophrenics (P=.03, .11, and .07, respectively).

Some significant changes with time were seen for the healthy controls with decrease in total cerebral volume (P=.03), caudate (P=.002), putamen (P=.02), and globus pallidus (P<.001). There was no significant change in ventricular volume or thalamic area for the controls.

For the schizophrenics, there were decreases in total cerebral volume and decreases in globus pallidus (P<.001) and caudate and midsagittal thalamic area (P=.004), as well as highly significant increases in ventricular volume (P=.002) and ventricle-brain ratio (P=.001). While ventricular size was greater on the left

Table 1. Demographic Data for Patients With Childhood-Onset Schizophrenia and Healthy Controls*

	Patients (n=16)	Controls (n=24)	*t* or χ^2	*P*
Socioeconomic status	67±34	30±16	*t*=3.48	.004
Sex, No.				
Male	10	18	χ^2=0.714	.40
Female	6	6		
Race, No.				
White	8	24	χ^2=15.000	.0005
Black	7	0		
Asian	1	0		
Handedness, No.				
Right	12	21	χ^2=1.932	.38
Left	3	3		
Mixed	1	0		
Age, y				
Scan 1				
Mean	14.8±2.4	14.3±1.9	*t*=−0.06872	.50
Range	9.2-19.1	10.8-17.8		
Scan 2				
Mean	16.8±2.4	16.7±2.1	*t*=−0.0844	.93
Range	10.7-21.3	13.3-21.2		
Weight, kg				
Scan 1				
Mean	62.1±19.6	55.1±14.0	*t*=−1.3124	.20
Range	26.2-114.2	33.3-93.6		
Scan 2				
Mean	79.2±17.7	64.7±14.6	*t*=−2.8253	.008
Range	47.7-104.9	41.9-112.5		
Height, cm				
Scan 1				
N	15	24		
Mean	167.4±11.9	164.8±12.7	*t*=−0.6009	.55
Range	150.1-198.9	139.7-184.2		
Scan 2				
N	11	22		
Mean	169.4±10.7	172.2±10.2	*t*=0.7555	.46
Range	152.4-190.5	147.3-188.0		
Tanner stage				
Scan 1				
N	16	23		
Mean	3.8±1.2	3.6±1.5	*t*=−0.4621	.65
Range	1.0-5.0	2.0-5.0		
Scan 2				
N	10	14		
Mean	4.9±0.3	4.7±0.8	*t*=−0.7667	.45
Range	4.0-5.0	2.0-5.0		
Ratings scales				
SAPS				
Scan 1				
Mean	55.4±20.4	...	...	...
Range	27-111	...		
Scan 2				
Mean	24.8±16.7	...	...	...
Range	5-78	...		
SANS				
Scan 1				
Mean	83.8±25.4	...	...	...
Range	38-117	...		
Scan 2				
Mean	58.1±25.8	...	...	...
Range	13-111	...		
BPRS				
Scan 1				
Mean	81.2±15.8	...	...	...
Range	48-110	...		
Scan 2				
Mean	55.0±9.6	...	...	...
Range	41-71	...		

**SAPS indicates Scale for Assessment of Positive Symptoms; SANS, Scale for Assessment of Negative Symptoms; and BPRS, Brief Psychiatric Rating Scale. Mean values are given ±SD.*

Table 2. Anatomic Brain MR Imaging Measures for Patients With Childhood-Onset Schizophrenia and Healthy Controls at Baseline and 2-Year Rescan*

	Controls (n=24)				Patients (n=16)				ANOVA			
									Diagnosis		Diagnosis ×Time	
	Time 1	Time 2	*t*	*P*	Time 1	Time 2	*t*	*P*	F†	*P*	F†	*P*
Total cerebral volume, mL	1137±137	1107±107	2.3	.03	1025±147	972±156	2.6	.02	8.5	.006	1.1	.31
Lateral ventricles, mL	12.5±6.4	12.5±5.8	0.02	.98	16.0±7.4	19.1±8.7	3.8	.002	5.3	.03	16.1	<.001
VBR	0.01±0.006	0.01±0.006	0.79	.44	0.015±0.006	0.019±0.009	3.4	.001	9.7	.003	19.6	<.001
Globus pallidus, mL	3.28±0.37	2.70±0.36	6.57	<.001	3.67±0.62	2.94±0.66	8.1	<.001	6.09	.02	3.22	.08
Caudate, mL	9.69±0.7	9.40±0.7	3.5	.002	10.26±1.2	9.42±1.2	2.8	.01	1.3	.26	6.5	.02
Putamen, mL	10.47±1.2	10.87±1.2	2.8	.01	11.29±1.6	11.23±1.3	0.3	.77	1.84	.18	0.7	.41
Thalamus area, mm^2	145±40	139±35	0.5	.65	120±15.9	103±22	3.5	.004	8.6	.006	5.2	.03

**MR indicates magnetic resonance; ANOVA, analysis of variance; and VBR, ventricle-brain ratio. Values are given as mean±SD. Values for* t *are by paired* t *test; all* P *values are 2 tailed.*
†df=*1,38.*

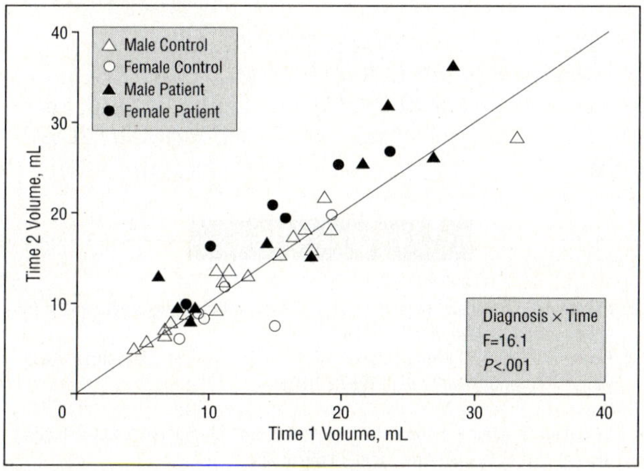

Brain ventricular volumes at baseline and 2-year follow-up for patients with childhood-onset schizophrenia (n=16) and age-matched, temporally yoked, healthy controls (n=24).

for both groups (F=7.28, *df*=1,38, *P*=.01), there was no significant relationship between side and diagnosis. There was, however, a trend for greater left-sided progressive enlargement in the patients with COS (time×side×diagnosis, F=2.48, *df*=1,38, *P*=.12).

Thus, there were several significant diagnostic differences with respect to brain changes on rescan as indicated by the diagnosis×time interaction (Table 2 and Figure) for ventricular volume (*P*<.001) and thalamic area (*P*=.03). There were greater decreases in globus pallidus (*P*=.05) and caudate (*P*=.02) volumes on rescan for the schizophrenic group, particularly for those in interim maintenance with atypical neuroleptics. Thus, rescan values did not differ significantly between the groups for these basal ganglia structures.

Progressive changes in ventricular volume and thalamic area correlated significantly with each other (*r*=−0.52, *P*=.05), but neither correlated significantly with change in total cerebral volume. (These relationships were not significant for controls.) Increase in ventricular volume showed a significant relationship to prepsychotic adjustment (higher scores on the Premorbid Adjustment Scale, *r*=0.46, *P*=.06)[36] and higher total Brief Psychiatric Rating Scale scores at follow-up (*r*=0.51, *P*=.04). There was no significant association with socioeconomic status, age at first scan, language delay, or prepsychotic autistic symptoms.

COMMENT

This report indicates a consistent pattern of progressive brain change for this rare, COS population. While in keeping with a few studies of patients with later-onset schizophrenia,[18-21] these results appear more consistent than those for any previous group.[20,21]

The findings are also in agreement with other clinical data for this sample, indicating a continuous process of disease progression for about half, although some have shown a good response to clozapine.[30]

There are a number of qualifications, however, to add to these conclusions. It will be most important to replicate these findings. The differential changes seen here may be unrelated to age at onset and certainly are not the "trigger" of psychoses, as this very-early-onset population had been seriously ill for a mean of 4 years at the time of their initial scan at the National Institutes of Health. It is possible that early case identification prompted the scanning and rescanning of a schizophrenic population during a developmental period uniquely sensitive to pathological effects.[25] As others have speculated,[27,28] the differential ventricular enlargement might possibly be seen only over a very limited period, as, in general, ventricular volume when measured later in life is not related to age at onset.[40] It is unlikely that the degree of change for the childhood schizophrenics shown in the Figure would be sustained, as that would produce improbably large ventricular volume in later life.

Other interpretations of these findings are also possible. While clinically and neurobiologically similar to adult populations,[3,5] these subjects represent a rare, and severely ill, treatment-refractory subgroup of COS who were participating in a clozapine trial. As a group, they were more ill than the predominantly outpatient subjects in the studies of adults with "negative" brain rescans reviewed above. Thus, the group might represent a truly different population and/or the effects of such severe illness might be more adverse on brain development. In fact, recent reports of brain rescanning find that adult patients with poor outcomes are more likely to show ventricular enlargement.[22] On follow-up, however, a number of our pediatric subjects were doing well and were no longer institutionalized, and their total medication had been reduced because of the beneficial effects of clozapine. While there is little indication from adult studies that institutionalization or medication could account for these findings, the possibility that clozapine treatment accelerates adolescent brain change cannot be ruled out.

The decrease in basal ganglia volume for these schizophrenic subjects on rescanning has been reported for this group previously.[41] This finding was a replication of previous work with adult patients, showing that initial enlargement of basal ganglia structures is related to lifetime exposure to typical neuroleptics and that these structures normalize with maintenance with atypical neuroleptics.[42,43]

We were concerned that the differential decrease in caudate volume with maintenance with clozapine might artifactually confound ventricular increase. However, this appears to be unlikely. The 4 patients who had also been maintained with typical neuroleptics showed similar ventricular increases; for the rest, reduction in basal ganglia volume did not correlate significantly with ventricular volume increase. Moreover, a previous rescan study of adult patients initially treated with typical neuroleptics and rescanned after 1 year of maintenance with atypical neuroleptics showed a 10% reduction in basal ganglia volume with no significant change in ventricular volume (M. Chakos, MD, oral communication, April 1997).

The correlation between ventricular increase and the decrease in our crude thalamic measure is intriguing, but until we have further refinement of our thalamic measure, this remains difficult to interpret.

Finally, the lack of socioeconomic and ethnic matching is regrettable. However, there was no significant difference in ventricular volume progression for the 7 black and 1 Asian patients compared with that of the white patients. The ethnic groups also did not differ from the other patients on any demographic or clinical variable, and socioeconomic status did not correlate significantly with ventricular change. The imbalances in our control population are being corrected.

This group of patients with COS, as with other COS populations,[44,45] had somewhat more striking albeit nonspecific early developmental delays and abnormalities than those seen for adult patients, as well as transient symptoms of pervasive developmental disorder. It is of particular interest, therefore, that those with higher Premorbid Adjustment Scale scores (including early transient autistic features) were among those with the greatest ventricular enlargement, suggesting that a more severe prepsychotic deviation in brain development is related to a greater degree of postpsychotic developmental deviance. However, autistic features per se did not predict enlargement, nor did any particular comorbidity contribute to these findings.

Models for early and late brain changes in schizophrenia are not mutually exclusive; they may reflect a continuous underlying process expressed differently during early and later neuronal development.[46,47] A growing body of studies have documented how the same neurotropic functions can have different effects at different periods in brain development,[48,49] and it seems most economical to assume a single continuous process from fetus through adult life.

In summary, COS presents a unique opportunity to examine abnormal neurodevelopment during a period of normally accelerated brain changes. In an extension of Murray's sense that neurodevelopmental schizophrenia will lead us to the "true" dementia precox,[50] the longitudinal study of childhood-onset cases may bring us closer to the core of the process eroding brain function. Continuing prospective clinical and brain imaging follow-up studies of these cases, and of adolescent patients with other childhood psychiatric disorders, are ongoing.

Accepted for publication May 27, 1997.

Reprints: Judith L. Rapoport, MD, Child Psychiatry Branch, National Institute of Mental Health, Bldg 10, Room 6N240, 10 Center Dr, MSC 1600, Bethesda, MD 20892-1600.

REFERENCES

1. Asarnow J, Thompson M, Goldstein M. Childhood onset schizophrenia: a follow-up study. *Schizophr Bull.* 1994;20:599-617.
2. Eggers C, Bunk D. The longterm course of childhood-onset schizophrenia: a 42-year followup. *Schizophr Bull.* 1997;23:105-117.
3. Gordon CT, Frazier J, McKenna K, Giedd J, Zametkin A, Zahn T, Hommer D, Hong W, Kaysen D, Albus K, Rapoport J. Childhood onset schizophrenia: an NIMH study in progress. *Schizophr Bull.* 1994;20:697-712.
4. Alaghband-Rad J, McKenna K, Gordon CT, Albus KE, Hamburger SD, Rumsey JM, Frazier JA, Lenane MC, Rapoport JL. Childhood-onset schizophrenia: the severity of premorbid course. *J Am Acad Child Adolesc Psychiatry.* 1995;34:1273-1283.
5. Jacobsen LK, Rapoport JL. Childhood onset schizophrenia: implications of clinical and neurobiological research. *J Child Psychol Psychiatr.* In press.
6. Meltzer H, Rabinowitz J, Lee MA, Cola P, Ranjon R, Findling R, Thompson P. Age at onset and gender of schizophrenic patients in relation to neuroleptic resistance. *Am J Psychiatry.* 1997;154:475-482.
7. Zahn TP, Jacobsen LK, Gordon CT, McKenna K, Frazier JA, Rapoport JL. Autonomic nervous systems markers of psychopathology in childhood-onset schizophrenia. *Arch Gen Psychiatry.* 1997;54:904-912.
8. Jacobsen L, Hong W, Hommer DW, Castellanos FX, Frazier JA, Giedd JN, Gordon CT, Karp BI, McKenna K, Rapoport JL. Smooth pursuit eye movements in childhood-onset schizophrenia: comparison with attention-deficit hyperactivity disorder and normal controls. *Biol Psychiatry.* 1996;40:1144-1154.
9. Frazier J, Giedd J, Hamburger S, Albus K, Kaysen D, Vaituzis C, Rajapakse J, Lenane M, McKenna K, Jacobsen L, Gordon C, Breier A, Rapoport JL. Brain anatomic magnetic resonance in childhood onset schizophrenia. *Arch Gen Psychiatry.* 1996;53:617-624.
10. Bertolino A, Kumra S, Callicot J, Maltoy V, Jacobsen L, Frank J, Rapoport JL, Weinberger DA. Proton magnetic resonance imaging in childhood onset schizophrenia. *Biol Psychiatry.* In press.
11. Alaghband-Rad J, Hamburger SD, Giedd JN, Frazier JA, Rapoport JL. Childhood-onset schizophrenia: biological markers in relation to clinical characteristics. *Am J Psychiatry.* 1997;154:64-68.
12. Nasrallah J, Olson S, McCalley-Whitters M, Chapman S, Jacoby C. Cerebral ventricular enlargement in schizophrenia. *Arch Gen Psychiatry.* 1986;43:157-159.
13. Ilowsky B, Juliano D, Bigelow L, Weinberger D. Stability of CT scan findings in schizophrenia: results of an 8 year followup study. *J Neurol Neurosurg Psychiatry.* 1988;51:209-213.
14. Vita A, Sacchetti E, Valvassori C, Cazzullo CL. Brain morphology in schizo-

phrenia: a 2-5 year CT scan followup study. *Acta Psychiatr Scand.* 1988;78: 618-621.
15. Degreef G, Ashtari M, Wu H, Borenstein M, Geisler S, Lieberman J. Follow-up MRI study in first episode schizophrenia. *Schizophr Res.* 1991;5:204-206.
16. DeLisi L, Stritzke R, Riordan H. The timing of brain morphological changes in schizophrenia and their relationship to clinical outcome. *Biol Psychiatry.* 1992; 31:241-254.
17. Jaskiw G, Juliano D, Goldberg T, Hertzman M, Urow-Hamell E, Weinberger D. Cerebral ventricular enlargement in schizophreniform disorder does not progress: a seven year followup study. *Schizophr Res.* 1994;14:23-28.
18. Kemali D, Maj M, Galderisi S, Milici N, Salvati A. Ventricle to brain ratio in schizophrenia: a controlled followup study. *Biol Psychiatry.* 1989;26:753-756.
19. Woods B, Yurgelun-Todd D, Benes FM, Frankenburg FR, Pope HG, McSparren J. Progressive ventricular enlargement in schizophrenia: comparison to bipolar affective disorder and correlation with clinical course. *Biol Psychiatry.* 1990;27: 341-352.
20. DeLisi L, Tew W, Shu-hong X, Hoff A, Sakuma M, Kusher M, Lee G, Shedlack K, Smith A, Grimson R. A prospective follow-up study of brain morphology and cognition in first-episode schizophrenic patients: preliminary findings. *Biol Psychiatry.* 1995;38:349-360.
21. DeLisi L, Sakuma M, Tew W, Kushrer M, Hoff A, Grimson R. Schizophrenia as a chronic active brain process: a study of progressive brain structural change subsequent to onset of schizophrenia. *Psychiatry Res Brain Imaging.* In press.
22. Lieberman JA, Alvir JMA, Koreen A, Geisler S, Chakos M, Sheitman B, Woerner M. Psychobiotic correlates of treatment response in schizophrenia. *Neuropsychopharmacology.* 1996;14:13S-21S.
23. Huber G. *Pneumoencephalographische und psychopathologische Bilder beii endogen Psychosen.* Berlin, Germany: Springer International; 1975.
24. Haug O. Pneumoencephalographic studies in mental disease. *Acta Psychiatr Scand.* 1962;165:1-114.
25. Giedd J, Snell J, Lange N, Rajapakse J, Kaysen D, Vaituzis C, Vauss Y, Hamburger S, Kozuch P, Rapoport J. Quantitative magnetic resonance imaging of human brain development: ages 4-18. *Cereb Cortex.* 1996;6:551-560.
26. Feinberg I. Schizophrenia: caused by a fault in programmed synaptic elimination during adolescence? *J Psychiatr Res.* 1982-83;17:319-339.
27. Keshavan M. Neurodevelopment and schizophrenia: quo vadis? In: Keshavan M, Murray R, eds. *Neurodevelopment and Adult Psychopathology.* New York, NY: Cambridge University Press. In press.
28. Keshavan M, Anderson S, Pettigrew J. Is schizophrenia due to excessive pruning of the prefrontal cortex? The Feinberg hypothesis revisited. *J Psychiatr Res.* 1994;28:239-265.
29. American Psychiatric Association. *Diagnostic and Statistical Manual of Mental Disorders, Third Edition, Revised.* Washington, DC: American Psychiatric Association; 1987.
30. Kumra S, Frazier JA, Jacobsen LK, McKenna K, Gordon CT, Lenane MC, Hamburger SD, Smith AK, Albus KE, Alaghband-Rad J, Rapoport JL. Childhood-onset schizophrenia: a double-blind clozapine-haloperidol comparison. *Arch Gen Psychiatry.* 1996;53:1090-1097.
31. Reich W, Welner Z. *Diagnostic Interview for Children and Adolescents–RC (*DSM-III-R *Version).* St Louis, Mo: Washington University; 1988.
32. Giedd JN, Kozuch P, Kaysen D, Vaituzis AC, Hamburger SD, Bartko J, Rapoport JL. Reliability of cerebral measures in repeated examinations with magnetic resonance imaging. *Psychiatr Res Neuroimaging.* 1995;61:113-119.
33. Andreasen NC. *The Scale for the Assessment of Positive Symptoms (SAPS).* Iowa City, Iowa: University of Iowa; 1984.
34. Andreasen NC. *The Scale for the Assessment of Negative Symptoms (SANS).* Iowa City, Iowa: University of Iowa; 1983.
35. Overall JE, Gorham DE. The Brief Psychiatric Rating Scale. *Psychol Rep.* 1961; 10:799-812.
36. Cannon-Spoor HE, Potkin SG, Wyatt RJ. Measurement of premorbid adjustment in chronic schizophrenia. *Schizophr Bull.* 1982;8:470-484.
37. Snell J, Merickel M, Ortega J, Goble J, Brookerman J, Kassell N. Boundary estimation of complex objects using hierarchical active surface templates. *Pattern Recognit.* 1995;28:1599-1609.
38. Rasband W. *Image, Version 1.6.* Bethesda, Md: National Institutes of Health; 1993.
39. Rajapakse JC, Giedd JN, DeCarli C, Snell JS, McLaughlin A, Vauss YC, Krain AL, Hamburger SD, Rapoport JL. A technique for single-channel MR brain tissue segmentation: application to a pediatric sample. *Magn Reson Imaging.* 1996;14: 1053-1065.
40. Lim K, Harris D, Beal M, Hoff A, Kyungtak M, Csernansky J, Faustman W, Marsh L, Sullivan E, Pfefferbaum A. Grey matter deficits in young onset schizophrenia are independent of age of onset. *Biol Psychiatry.* 1996;40:4-31.
41. Frazier J, Giedd J, Kaysen D, Albus K, Hamburger SD, Alaghband-Rad J, Lenane M, McKenna K, Breier A, Rapoport J. Childhood onset schizophrenia: brain MRI rescan after 2 years of clozapine maintenance treatment. *Am J Psychiatry.* 1996; 153:564-566.
42. Chakos MH, Lieberman JA, Bilder RM, Borenstein M, Lerner G, Bogerts B, Wu H, Kinon B, Ashtari M. Increase in caudate nuclei volumes of first-episode schizophrenic patients taking antipsychotic drugs. *Am J Psychiatry.* 1994;151:1430-1436.
43. Chakos MH, Lieberman JA, Alvir J, Bilder R, Ashtari M. Caudate nuclei volumes in schizophrenic patients with typical antipsychotics or clozapine. *Lancet.* 1995; 345:456-457.
44. Russell A, Bott L, Sammons C. The phenomenology of schizophrenia occurring in childhood. *J Am Acad Child Adolesc Psychiatry.* 1989;28:399-407.
45. Watkins J, Asarnow R, Tanguey P. Symptom development in childhood onset schizophrenia. *J Child Psychol Psychiatry.* 1988;29:865-878.
46. Waddington J, Scully P, Youssef H. Developmental trajectory and disease progression in schizophrenia: the conundrum, and insights from a 12 year prospective study in the Monaghan 101. *Schizophr Res.* 1997;23:107-118.
47. Pogue-Geile M. Developmental aspects of schizophrenia. In: Keshavan M, Murray R, eds. *Neurodevelopment and Adult Psychopathology.* New York, NY: Cambridge University Press. In press.
48. Vicario-Abejon C, Johe K, Hazel T, Collazo D, McKay RD. Functions of basic fibroblast growth factor and neurotrophins in the differentiation of hippocampal neurons. *Neuron.* 1995;15:105-114.
49. Mangiarini L, Sathasiuam K, Sellar M, Cozens B, Harper A, Hetherington G, Lawton M, Trottier Y, Lehrach H, Davies S, Bates G. Exon 1 of the HD gene with an expanded CAG repeat is sufficient to cause a progressive neurobiological phenotype in transgenic mice. *Cell.* 1996;87:493-506.
50. Murray R. Neurodevelopmental schizophrenia: the rediscovery of dementia praecox. *Br J Psychiatry.* 1994;165:6-12.

Autonomic Nervous System Markers of Psychopathology in Childhood-Onset Schizophrenia

Theodore P. Zahn, PhD; Leslie K. Jacobsen, MD; Charles T. Gordon, MD; Kathleen McKenna, MD; Jean A. Frazier, MD; Judith L. Rapoport, MD

Background: Consistent abnormalities in peripheral indicators of autonomic activity, ie, skin conductance (SC) and heart rate (HR), have been reported in adult-onset schizophrenia. Herein, we use these markers to test the hypothesis of continuity between childhood-onset schizophrenia and adult-onset schizophrenia.

Methods: Skin conductance and HR were recorded from 21 severely ill children and adolescents (mean age, 14.1 years) with childhood-onset (≤12 years) schizophrenia (patient group) and from 54 age-matched controls (control group) during a rest period, a series of innocuous tones, reaction time insructions, and a simple warned reaction time task.

Results: During rest, patients had higher rates of spontaneous SC responses (SCRs) and HRs than controls, but their SC level was marginally lower and declined more slowly over time. Half of the patients, compared with 4% of the controls, failed to give SC-orienting responses to the first 2 tones. Patients who responded had impaired SCR magnitudes, and their habituation was more erratic than that of controls. The increase in SC level and SCR frequency at the onset of the task period was greatly attenuated in the patients, so that both variables were higher in controls. Patients had smaller SCRs and anticipatory HR responses to the reaction time stimuli. Skin conductance nonresponding was associated with negative and total symptoms, and spontaneous SCR frequency was associated with positive symptoms.

Conclusions: The findings show similar abnormalities in autonomic nervous system activity in childhood-onset schizophrenia to those found in adult chronic schizophrenia, thus supporting the hypothesis of continuity of the childhood and adult forms of the illness. Comparisons with data from other childhood disorders suggest that the combination of low-elicited SC activity with high levels of spontaneous SC activity may be specific to schizophrenia.

Arch Gen Psychiatry. 1997;54:904-912

From the Laboratory of Brain and Cognition (Dr Zahn) and Child Psychiatry Branch (Drs Jacobsen, Gordon, McKenna, Frazier, and Rapoport), National Institute of Mental Health, Bethesda, Md. Dr Gordon is now with the Department of Psychiatry, University of Maryland School of Medicine, Baltimore; Dr McKenna, the Department of Psychiatry, Northwestern University School of Medicine, Chicago, Ill; and Dr Frazier, the Department of Psychiatry, Massachusetts Mental Health Center and Harvard Medical School, Boston.

Although *DSM-III-R*[1] requires no minimum age at onset for a diagnosis of schizophrenia, illness onset prior to late adolescence is rare.[2,3] On the basis of the clinical phenomenology and course of the disorder, there has been a growing consensus that childhood-onset schizophrenia (defined here as having an onset at age ≤12 years) is continuous with schizophrenia with a late-adolescent or later onset.[4-7] However, there are some quantitative differences including higher rates of poor prognosis indicators such as insidious onset and poor premorbid adjustment, less well-organized delusional systems, and more retarded developmental milestones in childhood-onset schizophrenia.[6,8] These suggest that childhood-onset schizophrenia may be a severe form of the disorder.

The continuity hypothesis may also be tested by studying objective cognitive and biological markers in childhood-onset schizophrenia that have been validated on adult patients. The small amount of previous research using this approach has supported continuity. Thus, similar deficiencies were reported in childhood-onset and adult-onset schizophrenia in attention and information processing using a span of apprehension task[9,10] and in event-related potentials recorded during that task.[11] The subjects in the present cohort have shown similar abnormalities in smooth pursuit eye movements[12] and in brain morphology[13] as found in adult patients.

SUBJECTS AND METHODS

PATIENTS

The group of patients with schizophrenia (patient group) consisted of 23 patients (13 male and 10 female). Two patients (1 male and 1 female) became too psychotic to participate in the protocol when they were medication free. The remaining 21 patients were tested after at least 10 days (mean [±SD], 21.2±4.8 days) without neuroleptic medication, although 20 (95%) were medication free for at least 2 weeks and 15 (71%) for 3 weeks or more. Their age at onset of psychotic symptoms was 12 years or younger (mean[±SD], 10.1±1.5 years); at testing, their mean age was 14.1±2.0 years. Consensus diagnoses using *DSM-III-R* criteria were made by 2 child psychiatrists on the basis of information obtained from medical records, referring physicians, and unstructured and structured interviews of the child and parent. We used the *Diagnostic Interview for Children and Adolescents*[27](*DICA-RC*) and the portions of the *Schedule for Affective Disorders and Schizophrenia for School-Age Children—Epidemiologic Version (Kiddie-SADS-E)*,[28] which assess symptoms of depression, mania, hallucinations, delusions, thought disorder, separation anxiety disorder, overanxious disorder, panic attacks, social phobia, specific phobias, obsessive-compulsive disorder, anorexia, and bulimia. All subjects had both positive and negative schizophrenic symptoms. They were selected for a lack of clinical response to, or intolerance of, conventional neuroleptics and were recruited nationally primarily for a clinical trial of clozapine. Owing to the rarity of the disorder,[2,3,29] it was possible to obtain a sufficient sample with unequivocal diagnoses only through the availability of an inpatient drug trial with an agent not generally available at the time. Further details about patient selection and characteristics are presented elsewhere.[7,22,29]

CONTROLS

The control group consisted of 54 subjects (35 male and 19 female; mean [±SD] age, 13.8±1.9 years) who were screened using the *DICA-RC*[30] and the Diagnostic Interview for the Parents of Children and Adolescents.[31] Controls who met criteria for any disorder (current or past) on either of those scales were excluded. In addition, any history of an Axis I disorder, learning disability, or mental retardation in a first-degree relative, as determined by structured interviews, was exclusionary for this group.

METHODS

Apparatus and Procedure

Physiological recording was made on a polygraph (Model 7B, Grass Instrument Co, Quincy, Mass), the output of which was digitized by a computer (PDP-11, Chrislin Industries Inc, Westlake Village, Calif) for off-line editing and analysis. Skin conductance was recorded by a constant voltage (0.5-V) method from the distal phalanges of the middle and ring fingers of the left hand, using silver–silver chloride electrodes (Beckman Instruments, Schiller Park, Ill), electrode collars 0.8 cm in diameter, and 0.5% potassium chloride electrode paste. Heart rate was recorded by a tachograph from the electrocardiogram (lead II).

The procedure began at least 10 minutes after the SC electrodes were applied to allow for hydration. There were 4 periods in the protocol:

1. A 3-minute rest period, at the outset of which subjects were told that they should try to relax, but stay awake, that after a few minutes there would be a series of tones or beeps, and that they did not have to do anything except to continue to relax.
2. A tones period, in which ten 1000-Hz, 80-dB

Continued on next page

Our study extends this strategy to measures of autonomic nervous system (ANS) activity and reactivity. Measures of ANS activity have not only discriminated adult patients with schizophrenia from normal controls and other groups but have been related also to clinical outcome.[14,15] Studies of the electrodermal-orienting response show that novel, moderate intensity stimuli frequently fail to elicit skin conductance (SC)–orienting reactions (OR) (SCORs) in about half of patients with

See also page 913

chronic schizophrenia in contrast to a smaller number of normal controls (10%-15%).[14,16] Patients who do respond give smaller amplitude SCORs than controls. This marker may be less extreme in acutely ill patients, especially those with a favorable outcome.[17,18] However, its specificity to schizophrenia has been questioned, especially vis-à-vis major depression.[19,20] Thus, adequate sensitivity and specificity may require a combination of several markers.

Adult patients with schizophrenia have also shown slower rates of habituation of the SCOR, elevated base levels of electrodermal activity (EDA) and heart rate (HR), slow declines in base levels across a rest period, and attenuated increments in ANS activity during task performance. Several studies have also shown less frequent and smaller ANS reactions to task-related stimuli in schizophrenia, sometimes even to a greater extent than the deficits in responding to nonsignal stimuli.[15,20] Many of these markers have been related to clinical outcome.[17,18,21]

The present protocol includes a resting baseline condition and the response to task performance addition to an OR paradigm. The subjects had failed previous trials of typical neuroleptic medications and were recruited for participation in a clozapine treatment trial.[22,23] They were tested in an unmedicated state. It was hypothesized that compared with age-matched controls this group would show abnormalities similar to those found in adult-onset chronic schizophrenia.

We also attempt to confirm findings, mostly in patients taking medication, that deficiencies in the OR, especially nonresponding, are related to the severity of negative symptoms of schizophrenia.[24-26] Further, it was speculated, on the basis of indirect evidence, that the frequency of spontaneous or nonspecific SC fluctuations during rest periods might reflect the severity of positive symptoms.[15]

($r=0.0002$ dynes/cm^2) pure tones of 1.5-second duration were presented every 20 to 30 seconds through a speaker.

3. Reaction-time (RT) instructions, by which subjects were instructed that: on each trial a ready light would come on; when he or she was ready, he or she should depress a telegraph key and keep it down until a tone (beep) sounded; at this time he or she should release the key as quickly as possible; and we were timing how fast he or she responded to the beep. The instructions were followed by a demonstration and at least 4 practice trials to ensure that the procedure was understood.

4. A simple warned RT task, in which 9 trials with 4-second foreperiods were followed by 9 trials with 8-second foreperiods. The intertrial interval was randomly distributed between 8 and 14 seconds by the computer (mean, 11 seconds).

Rating Scales

The extended Brief Psychiatric Rating Scale (BPRS),[32,33] Scale for the Assessment of Negative Symptoms (SANS),[34] and Scale for the Assessment of Positive Symptoms (SAPS)[35] were administered to the patients in all but 2 cases during the same week as the psychophysiological test, but always when the patient was in the unmedicated condition. The BPRS Positive Symptom Subscale (BPPOS) was the sum of Conceptual Disorganization–Disorganized Speech, Hallucinatory Behavior–Hallucinatory Statements, Unusual Thought Content, and Distractibility. The BPRS Negative Symptom Subscale (BPNEG) was the sum of Emotional Withdrawal, Motor Retardation, Blunted Affect, and Loss of Functioning. The latter is an overall measure of level of functioning.

Data Analysis

For the rest period, the intervals between tone presentations, and the task instruction period, we computed the rate of "spontaneous" SC responses (SCRs) per minute, for SCRs of at least 0.02 microsiemens (μS) in amplitude, and their mean amplitude. Levels of SC (SCLs) (in microsiemens), measured at 1-minute intervals during rest and instruction periods and before each tone and RT trial, were averaged for each period. Changes in SCL per minute (slope) were evaluated for rest and instruction periods. These periods were divided into 10-second "epochs." The mean, maximum, and minimum HR for each epoch were used to compute the mean HR and HR variability, defined as the mean difference between HR maxima and minima. Elicited SCRs had a minimum amplitude of 0.02 μS and an onset latency of 0.8 to 4 seconds as in previous studies.[36,37] The SCR magnitude is the total amplitude divided by the number of stimuli. The SCRs to the RT ready signal and stimulus were evaluated separately.

Heart rate decelerative and accelerative responses to the tones were measured as the difference between 10-second prestimulus minima or maxima and the corresponding poststimulus values. Heart rate deceleration during the RT foreperiod was defined as the level at the time of the warning stimulus minus that at the time of the RT stimulus. We also measured the mean and median of the RTs and their SD in milliseconds, and recorded 2 measures of extraneous key presses: the number of intertrial presses of the RT key and the number of trials that were aborted by premature release of the key.

An attempt to reduce type I error was made, when possible, by analyzing data for several dependent variables and for repeated measures initially by groups × sex multivariate analysis of covariance (MANCOVA), with age as a covariate by BMDP Program 4V.[38] These were followed up by univariate analyses of covariance (ANCOVA) using the Huynh-Feldt ϵ correction of the degrees of freedom for repeated measures when appropriate. Relationships between ANS and clinical variables were tested by Pearson correlations and *t* tests.

RESULTS

BASELINE ANS ACTIVITY

There were no significant differences in the 2 baseline electrodermal measures across the rest, tones, and instruction periods, but there was a multivariate effect for the groups × conditions interaction ($F[6, 272]=11.7$, $P<.001$) and univariate interaction effects for both SCRs per minute ($F[2, 138]=36.03$, $\epsilon=.82$, $P<.001$) and SCL ($F[2, 138]=9.48$, $\epsilon=.87$, $P<.001$). This was due to an attenuated effect of the task instructions on the patients (**Figure 1** and **Table 1**). The patients had more SCRs per minute than controls for the rest and tones periods ($F[1, 69]=6.92$, $P<.02$ and $F[1, 69]=11.76$, $P=.001$, respectively) but fewer SCRs per minute during the instructions ($F[1, 69]=11.17$, $P<.002$). Skin conductance levels during the rest and tones periods did not differ significantly, but the patients had lower SCL during the instructions ($F[1, 69]=10.03$, $P<.003$).

Heart rate (Table 1) was evaluated separately because EDA could not be recorded for one subject who wore mitts to prevent self-injury. Heart rate was higher in the patients (mean[±SD], 81.0±13.8) than in the controls (74.8±11.2, $F[1,69]=4.47$, $P<.04$), but it did not interact with conditions. For just the rest and tones periods, however, the group effect was larger during the tones period ($F[1, 70]=7.44$, $P<.009$) than during the first rest period ($F[1, 70]=4.74$, $P<.04$). The group × period interaction ($F[1, 70]=5.45$, $P<.03$) reflected a small decline in the controls and a small increase in the patients.

Skin conductance levels declined rapidly during the first rest period in the controls but not in the patients (Figure 1). There were group differences in both linear ($F[1, 72]=17.89$, $P<.001$) and quadratic trends ($F[1, 72]=4.69$, $P<.04$). The controls also showed a larger increase in SCL after the first tone than did the patients ($F[1, 69]=6.31$, $P<.02$). While the controls showed the largest increment in SCL during the first minute of instructions, many patients had their major increase in SCL at the beginning of the task. The difference between this point (RT1) and the last OR trial (T10), which minimizes the group difference and includes just subjects who were able to do the RT task, was still much smaller for the patients ($F[1, 63]=24.59$, $P<.001$).

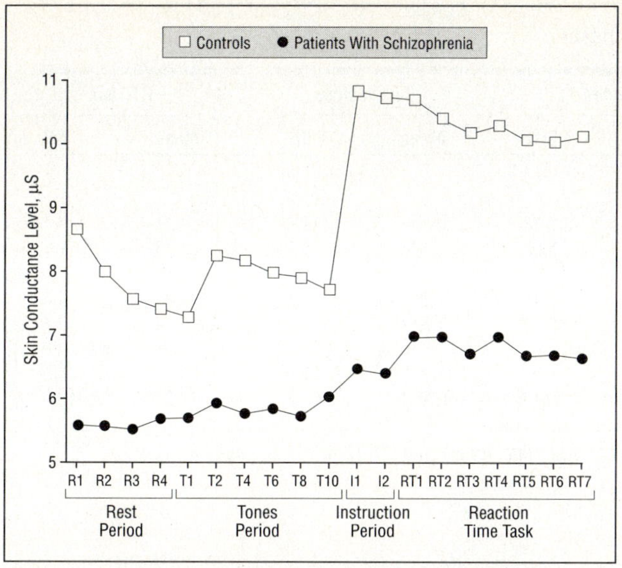

Figure 1. *Skin conductance levels (in microsiemens [µS]) across the study. The levels at R1 to R4 were obtained at the beginning of the rest (R) period and at subsequent 1-minute intervals; T1 to T10, just before the indicated tone (T) presentation; I1 and I2, at the end of the first and second minute of the instruction (I) period or at the end of the period if that occurred before 2 minutes; and RT1 to RT7, periodically during the reaction time (RT) task at approximately equal intervals.*

ORIENTING RESPONSES

The SCORs were evaluated by several criteria. First, nonresponding was defined as the absence of an OR on the first 2 trials. For SCORs defined by a minimum amplitude of 0.02 µS and an onset latency of 0.8 to 4 seconds, 7 of the 20 patients and none of the 54 controls were nonresponders ($P<.001$, Fisher exact test). If the criteria for an SCOR are made more stringent (minimum of 0.05 µS, 1-to 3-second latency) as sometimes recommended,[39] then 10 patients and 2 controls were nonresponders ($P<.001$). If a 3-trial criterion is used for nonresponding, $P<.005$ and $P<.002$ were obtained, respectively, for the 2 sets of criteria. Thus, more patients were SCOR nonresponders regardless of the criteria.

Lower responsivity in the patients (**Table 2**) was also shown by fewer total SCORs, fewer trials to habituation (2-trial criterion), smaller amplitude of the SCOR to the first tone, and smaller mean SCOR magnitudes and amplitudes. The ratio of the number of SCORs to spontaneous SCR rate (corrected for the time available for each response) is lower for the patients (Table 2), especially after the scores were transformed to reduce skewness.

The group difference in SCOR frequency is primarily on the first 3 to 4 trials (**Figure 2**). While the controls habituated to the first 5 tones as shown by a Cochran Q statistic (distributed like χ^2 with 4 *df*)[40] of 31.3 ($P<.001$), about half of the patients responded to each of the first 5 tones ($Q=0.74$, $P>.9$). Thus, the patients can be said to exhibit not only more nonresponding but also slower habituation rates.

Retarded habituation rates in schizophrenia have been shown to be due to an irregular stop-and-go pattern of responding.[36,37,41] Several such indexes were analyzed (Table 2): (1) for subjects who habituated in 3 or more trials (ie, the first instance of 2 consecutive nonresponse trials started at trial 4 or later), the proportion of tones that elicited an SCOR in the *prehabituation* period was lower in the patients than in the controls; (2) for subjects who habituated in less than 7 trials, the proportion of tones that elicited an SCOR in the *posthabituation* period was greater in patients; (3) a reversal in amplitude was scored when an SCOR (after the first tone) was larger than the SCOR to the preceding tone. The number of these did not differ, probably because of the many fewer total SCORs given by the patients, but the proportion of reversals to total responses was larger in the patients; and (4) a z statistic for the number of runs of responses and nonresponses over the series of trials did not differ, possibly also because of the patients' fewer SCORs. These analyses, in general, suggest that habituation was more erratic in the patient group than in the control group.

RESPONSIVITY TO RT STIMULI

Six patients could not master the RT procedure, usually because they did not keep the response key down for the entire foreperiod or because they needed prompting to release it at tone onset. One patient was not tested because he was in restraints. This rate of noncompliance is similar to that in adult patients with chronic schizophrenia (8 of 25).[42] Skin conductance responses to the task stimuli, especially to the RT stimulus (**Table 3**), were attenuated in the patients. An MANCOVA on the frequency and magnitude of SCRs to the RT ready signal and RT stimulus with foreperiod and sex as other dimensions showed a multivariate effect for the group difference ($F[2, 63]=8.09$, $P<.001$), and univariate effects for frequency ($F[1, 64]=14.62$, $P<.001$) and magnitude ($F[1, 64]=10.56$, $P<.002$). Group × stimulus interactions (overall: $F[1,64]=5.39$, $P<.007$; frequency: $F[1,64]=8.81$, $P<.005$; magnitude: $F[1,64]=6.60$, $P<.02$) indicated larger group differences for the RT stimulus. For the ready signal, there was a group effect only for magnitude; but for the RT stimulus, both frequency and magnitude were smaller for the patients (Table 3). There were no interactions with foreperiod or sex. Comparing SCORs to simple tones with SCRs to the RT stimulus yielded a groups × stimulus interaction for frequency ($F[1, 64]=5.10$, $P<.03$) but not for magnitude. Thus, the patients' deficit in SCR frequency is disproportionately greater for the RT stimulus than for simple tones. The patients also had smaller SCR amplitudes to both ready signal and stimulus, especially the latter (groups × stimulus interaction: $F[1,56]=4.50$, $P<.04$) and longer SCR latencies to the RT stimulus (Table 3). The patients also had fewer "anticipatory" SCRs and smaller HR deceleration during the RT foreperiod (Table 3).

The patients had more key presses during intertrial intervals than controls and nonsignificantly more premature key releases (Table 3). Reaction time was much longer (Table 3) and more variable (not shown) for the patients, and it showed a greater percent increment from the 4- to 8-second foreperiod in the patients (Table 3).

Table 1. Means of the Tonic Level Measures for the 4 Periods of the Protocol

Variable and Group	Rest Mean	Rest SD	Tones Mean	Tones SD	Instructions Mean	Instructions SD	RT Task* Mean	RT Task* SD
Skin conductance responses per minute								
Controls	2.43	2.84	2.88	2.48	11.44	4.21	4.11	3.44
Patients with schizophrenia	4.44†	4.27	5.25‡	3.82	7.53‡	4.39	3.75	2.18
Skin conductance level, μS								
Controls	7.82	4.87	7.95	4.88	10.80	5.16	10.28	4.80
Patients with schizophrenia	5.61	3.50	5.87	3.52	6.46‡	3.62	6.79	3.74
Heart rate, bpm								
Controls	74.6	11.5	73.9	11.0	76.1	11.1	73.9	10.6
Patients with schizophrenia	81.0†	14.4	82.1§	15.4	81.0	12.2	77.5	10.9

*For the reaction time (RT) task, n=13 for the patient group; otherwise n=20, except for heart rate, for which n=21. For controls, n=54 for all entries. μS indicates microsiemens.
†Different from controls at P<.05.
‡Different from controls at P<.005.
§Different from controls at P<.01.

Table 2. Indexes of Orienting Responses and Habituation

Variable	Patients With Schizophrenia Mean	Patients With Schizophrenia SD	Controls Mean	Controls SD	F	*P*
SCOR data						
Percent SCORs	43.5	27.0	61.9	27.0	6.36	.02
Trials to habituation	3.50	3.6	6.26	2.0	9.87	.003
Amplitude, trial 1, μS	0.576	0.94	1.412	1.02	13.07	.001
SCOR magnitude, μS	0.170	0.18	0.537	0.56	10.76	.002
SCOR amplitude, μS	0.378	0.34	0.797	0.64	9.61	.003
Specific/nonspecific SCR rate	3.02	5.79	7.40	7.32	6.42	.02
Ln specific/nonspecific SCR rate	1.02	0.72	1.89	0.64	26.43	.001
Habituation indexes						
Proportion of prehabituation SCORs	83.8	11.9	91.6	10.3	6.24	.02
Proportion of posthabituation SCORs	39.6	30.1	20.7	25.4	6.50	.02
No. of amplitude reversals	3.0	1.3	2.8	1.5	0.37	.55
Proportion of amplitude reversals	60.8	24.3	42.6	17.0	11.82	.002
z-Statistic for runs	0.607	1.13	0.110	1.34	1.92	.18

*SCOR indicates skin conductance–orienting response; SCR, skin conductance response; Ln, natural logarithm; and μS, microsiemens.

RELATIONSHIPS TO CLINICAL STATE

Using the restrictive criteria for SCORs, the mean (±SD) SANS scores for the 10 responders was 69.0±30.0 and for the 10 nonresponders it was 97.1±20.0 ($t[18]=2.46$, $P<.03$); for BPNEG the means were 15.4±3.8 and 19.3±4.0 ($t[18]=2.23$, $P<.04$). However, nonresponders also had nonsignificantly higher SAPS and BPPOS scores than responders. The totals of positive plus negative symptoms did separate the groups ($P<.03$ and $P<.02$, respectively). The BPRS Thinking Disturbance subscale (BPPOS minus Distractibility) differentiated the groups in the same direction ($P<.02$). Thus, while responder status was related to negative symptoms as hypothesized,[15] it may also, or better, reflect total schizophrenic pathology. In accord with this, SCOR magnitude across all trials was correlated with the SANS ($r=-0.63$, $P<.003$), BPNEG ($r=-0.51$, $P<.03$) and also with the SAPS ($r=-0.45$, $P<.05$). The hypothesis that spontaneous SCRs would be related to positive symptoms[15] was not confirmed for the SAPS, but it was confirmed for BPPOS ($r=0.57$, $P<.008$).

Exploratory analyses revealed that SCL distinguished between positive and negative symptoms. Mean SCL in rest and tones periods was related inversely to SANS ($r=-0.44$, $P=.05$) and to BPNEG ($r=-0.59$, $P<.006$) but positively to the comparable positive scales ($r=0.34$ and 0.36, $P=.14$ and .12). The differences between correlations with the positive and negative scales were at $P<.01$ in each case. Similar results were obtained for mean SCL during the RT instruction period. However, SCR frequency during the instructions was not related to any scale. The increment in SCR frequency from the rest and tones to instruction periods was inversely correlated with Thinking Disturbance ($r=-0.57$, $P<.02$), suggesting that baseline SCR frequency and its increment to task performance are related to symptoms in opposite directions. Heart rate was not related to any summary scale, even when corrected for age.

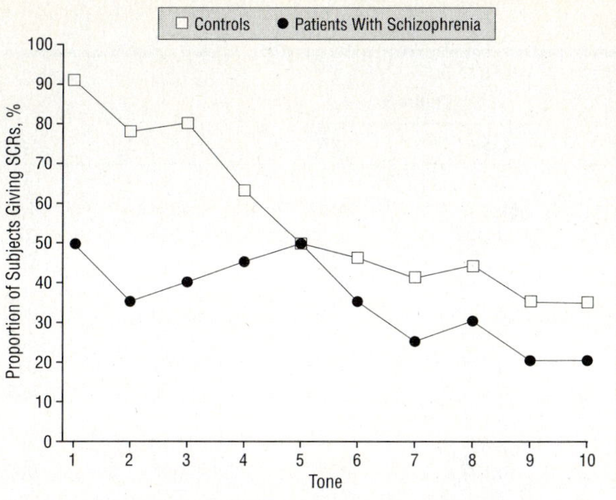

Figure 2. *Percentage of each group giving a skin conductance response (SCR) (minimum amplitude, 0.05 microsiemens; latency, 1-3 seconds) to each tone.*

COMMENT

BASELINE LEVELS

While spontaneous SCR frequency and HR were elevated in the patients, SCL showed a nonsignificant trend in the opposite direction. Thus, the data do not suggest high resting autonomic arousal or anxiety or stress about the test situation in the patients. Spontaneous SCRs are frequently elevated in schizophrenia, particularly in patients who are not taking medication and/or have positive symptoms.[15] They may be associated with auditory hallucinations,[43,44] other internally generated stimuli, or irrelevant external stimuli.[15] Elevated HR is a consistent finding in adult schizophrenia, but high SCL is not.[20] Similar dissociations between these 3 indexes of arousal have also been reported.[37,45]

The slow decline in resting SCL in the patients is consistent with many previous studies of patients with adult-onset schizophrenia.[18,24,25,36,37,41,46,47] In addition to their greater SCR frequency and HR in the tones period than in the first rest period compared with that in controls, this suggests a slower adaptation to the test situation and/or a smaller initial response to it.

The marked impairment in the tonic EDA response to the RT instructions in our patients cannot be attributed to differences in baseline levels because the curves for spontaneous SCRs cross over, and pretask SCL was lower for the patients. While similar to previous results from this laboratory with adult cases,[37,47,48] these findings do not find unequivocal support in the literature.[15,20] Tonic HR responses to stressors have been found to be impaired in schizophrenia,[37,49,50] but here the RT instructions did not produce a marked HR increase in either group.

ORIENTING RESPONSES

About half of the adult patients with chronic schizophrenia, but fewer controls, fail to give SCORs.[14,51] However, SCORs may have been attenuated in many studies by medication,[52-54] use of low-intensity tones,[14] or instructions to ignore the tones.[55] Also, SCORs may be more frequent in acute schizophrenia.[17,18,37,46] Given this, the 50% nonresponding in the present no–medication-taking patients, who had psychotic symptoms, compared with 4% nonresponding in controls is a large difference. Attenuated responsivity is also indicated by markedly lower SCOR magnitudes and amplitudes in the patients, especially to the maximally novel first tone.

Although patients had fewer trials to habituation, their rate of habituation was slower because of fewer prehabituation SCORs and more posthabituation SCORs than in controls. Of the 10 who were nonresponders by conventional criteria 7 gave posthabituation SCORs meeting the stricter criteria for an OR. Neither of the 2 control nonresponders did so. In addition, the patients' SCOR amplitudes were less likely to take a gradually diminishing course. These findings confirm previous research in adult cases.[36,37,41,46] Despite the large number of posthabituation SCORs for the patients, the ratio of elicited to spontaneous SCRs was a powerful discriminator of the groups, confirming previous studies.[36,37,56,57]

The OR to a novel stimulus may reflect a switch in attention to a potentially important event.[58] A deficiency in orienting suggests a basic defect in attention to the external environment. The patients showed deficiencies of 2 kinds: failure to respond to novel stimuli and failure to cease responding to familiar stimuli. Along with the patients' elevated rates of spontaneous SCRs, the SCOR data confirm the suggestion that patients with schizophrenia have difficulty distinguishing between internally generated events and external events.[15,59]

Deficient ORs could reflect a specific disorder in cerebral activity. Relationships of SCORs with prefrontal area in normal subjects[60] and with frontal and thalamic glucose metabolism in patients with schizophrenia[61] have been reported. In our patients, anterior frontal volume, total cerebral volume, and thalami were smaller than in controls[13] and the latter 2 measures correlated negatively with negative symptoms[13] as did SCOR frequency and magnitude. This suggests the possibility of frontal and/or thalamic mediation of SCOR abnormalities.

RT TASK

The greater attenuation of SCRs to the RT stimuli compared with SCRs to simple tones or the RT ready signal in the patients is consistent with previous studies from this laboratory,[37,47,48] particularly in patients with poor prognosis,[18] but hyporesponsivity in schizophrenia is not an unequivocal finding.[15] These studies suggest that the ANS in schizophrenia is impaired in distinguishing more important from less important stimuli. Along with the attenuated tonic ANS response to the instructions and studies of event-related potentials[11] and smooth pursuit eye tracking,[62] this may indicate an inability to allocate attentional resources in an appropriate manner. All 6 of the patient SCOR nonresponders who did the RT task gave some SCRs in that task, suggesting, as does the high incidence of posthabituation SCORs, that SCOR "nonresponding" reflects a central rather than a peripheral deficiency.

Table 3. Psychophysiology and Behavior in the RT Task*

Variable	Patients With Schizophrenia		Controls			
	Mean	SD	Mean	SD	F	*P*
SCRs to RT ready signal						
Percent SCRs	46.1	30.0	60.4	30.0	2.33	.14
SCR magnitude, μS	0.097	0.09	0.238	0.20	6.39	.02
SCR amplitude, μS	0.205	0.10	0.354	0.22	5.52	.03
SCRs to RT stimulus						
Percent SCRs	47.0	30.0	84.0	21.0	32.84	.001
SCR magnitude, μS	0.159	0.19	0.502	0.38	10.65	.002
SCR amplitude, μS	0.278	0.18	0.581	0.36	9.67	.003
SCR latency, s	1.89	0.55	1.48	0.41	9.06	.004
Anticipatory activity in long foreperiod						
No. of SCRs	2.92	2.8	5.36	4.6	3.40	.07
SCR magnitude, μS	0.031	0.04	0.102	0.13	4.95	.03
HR deceleration, bpm	0.6	4.3	3.1	3.5	5.03	.03
Behavior in the RT task						
Intertrial key presses	6.1	6.0	1.7	3.4	15.03	.001
Early key releases	1.9	2.4	1.3	1.6	2.64	.11
Median RT, ms	467	238	247	47	50.64	.001
Percent increase in RT	27.4	41	7.6	11	9.24	.004

**RT indicates reaction time; SCR, skin conductance response; μS, microsiemens; and HR, heart rate.*

Another indicator of attention in the RT task—slowing of HR during the RT foreperiod—was also attenuated in the patients, but not to the degree reported in a previous study of adult-onset schizophrenia.[18,37] This was largely due to a small deceleration in the controls, possibly resulting from greater effects of respiration, body movements, and other factors on HR fluctuations in children than in adults.[63]

CORRELATIONS WITH SYMPTOMS

The patients who were SCOR nonresponders were higher in negative symptoms than those who were SCOR responders as hypothesized, confirming studies of adult-onset schizophrenia.[24-26] Their trend to be higher in positive symptoms, also confirmed studies of adult-onset schizophrenia,[26,56] and they were significantly higher in the total of positive and negative symptoms. The magnitude of SCORs was similarly correlated with symptoms. Relationships between SCOR responding and various other BPRS scales[25,26,64] reported in adult-onset schizophrenia were not replicated here.

Our data confirmed a prediction, based mainly on indirect evidence, that spontaneous SCR frequency would be related to positive symptoms.[15] Correlations of spontaneous SCRs with BPRS Activation (r=0.31) and Thought Disturbance (r=0.35) were consistent with studies of adult-onset schizophrenia,[64-66] but that variable's correlations with BPRS Hallucinations (r=0.42, P<.06), and Blunted Affect (r=-0.48, P<.05) were not.[64-66] Only SCL showed significantly opposite correlations with positive and negative symptoms, similar to a previous finding.[65]

Although our major results were similar to and/or were predicted from the evidence from studies on adult-onset schizophrenia, there are many differences from those studies in these and other variables, possibly attributable to the generally greater severity of psychopathology, the presence of both positive and negative symptoms, and lack of medication in the present subjects.

CONCLUSIONS

The close similarities of our data to those from comparable studies of adult-onset schizophrenia are consistent with the hypothesis of continuity between childhood-onset schizophrenia and the more common adult-onset illness. This, of course, does not prove a common etiology for these 2 forms of schizophrenia because the pattern of results obtained could be produced by different underlying mechanisms, and these are not well understood at present, but the results are consistent with that hypothesis.

The fact that the present subjects were selected for poor response to conventional neuroleptic medications may limit the generality of the findings. However, the phenomenologic similarities between our sample and other samples of childhood-onset schizophrenia,[22,29,67-69] which describe pediatric schizophrenia as a severe unremitting disorder with a poor prognosis, suggests that our findings may be at least fairly typical of this group. In general, our findings resemble those in adult chronic and poor-outcome cases more than those in acute and good-outcome cases.[14,16-18,21,46] Unlike the data about adults, these markers here cannot be attributed to many years of hospitalization. Compared with similar studies of adults, the medication-free period was long, particularly given the severe illness of the patient group. In the experience of one of us (T.P.Z), the deviations from control values on many of the measures shown by the present patient group were remarkably consistent as schizophrenia studies go.[7] However, unselected samples of children with schizophrenia might not be as extremely deviant. The correlations of the ANS markers with severity of symptoms are consistent with this point.

Finally, are these markers specific to schizophrenia? Although low SCR amplitudes, small increments in EDA during task performance, and slow declines of resting SCL have been reported in attention deficit hyperactivity disorder,[20] disruptive behavior disorders,[70] and partially in autism,[71] ANS baseline values and SCOR habituation were within normal limits in those disorders. Children with obsessive-compulsive disorder did not differ from controls in ANS activity.[72,73] Elevated ANS baseline levels (including SCL) are found in many patients with anxiety disorders and in patients with agitated and neurotic depression, but such subjects also show enhanced SCORs and retarded habituation.[20] High rates of SCOR nonresponding have been reported in endogenous depression,[20,74-76] but this is accompanied by low spontaneous SCRs and SCLs. Thus, the discordance of lower elicited reactivity but elevated resting spontaneous EDA may be specific to schizophrenia.

Accepted for publication November 12, 1996.

We thank Thalene T. Mallus for expert technical assistance.

Reprints: Theodore P. Zahn, PhD, National Institute of Mental Health, Federal Bldg, Room B1A14, 7550 Wisconsin Ave, Bethesda, MD 20892.

REFERENCES

1. American Psychiatric Association. *Diagnostic and Statistical Manual of Mental Disorders, Third Edition, Revised.* Washington, DC: American Psychiatric Association; 1987.
2. Karno M, Norquist GS. Schizophrenia: epidemiology. In: Kaplan HI, Sacock BJ, eds. *Comprehensive Textbook of Psychiatry.* 5th ed. Baltimore, Md: Williams & Wilkins; 1989;1:699-705.
3. Kramer M. Population changes and schizophrenia, 1970-1985. In: Wynne LC, Cromwell RL, Matthysse S, eds. *The Nature of Schizophrenia: New Approaches to Research and Treatment.* New York, NY: John Wiley & Sons Inc; 1978:545-571.
4. Asarnow JR. Annotation: childhood-onset schizophrenia. *J Child Psychol Psychiatr.* 1994;35:1345-1371.
5. Rutter M. Childhood schizophrenia reconsidered. *J Aut Child Schizophr.* 1972; 2:315-337.
6. Werry JS. Child and adolescent (early onset) schizophrenia: a review in light of *DSM-III-R. J Aut Dev Dis.* 1992;22:601-624.
7. Gordon CT, Frazier JA, McKenna K, Giedd J, Zametkin A, Zahn T, Hommer D, Hong W, Kaysen D, Albus KE, Rapoport JL. Childhood-onset schizophrenia: an NIMH study in progress. *Schizophr Bull.* 1994;20:697-712.
8. Alaghband-Rad J, McKenna K, Gordon CT, Albus KE, Hamburger SD, Rumsey JM, Frazier JA, Lenane MC, Rapoport JL. Childhood onset schizophrenia: the severity of premorbid course. *J Am Acad Child Adolesc Psychiatry.* 1995;34:1273-1283.
9. Asarnow RF, Grandholm E, Sherman T. Span of apprehension in schizophrenia. In: Steinhauer SR, Gruzelier JH, Zubin J, eds. *Handbook of Schizophrenia.* Amsterdam, the Netherlands: Elsevier Science Publishers; 1991;5:335-370.
10. Asarnow RF, Sherman T. Studies of visual information processing in schizophrenic children. *Child Dev.* 1984;55:249-261.
11. Strandburg RJ, Marsh JT, Brown WS, Asarnow RF, Guthrie D. Information-processing deficits across childhood- and adult-onset schizophrenia. *Schizophr Bull.* 1994;20:685-695.
12. Jacobsen LK, Hong WL, Hommer DW, Hamburger SD, Castellanos FX, Frazier JA, Giedd JN, Gordon CT, Karp BI, McKenna K, Rapoport JL. Smooth pursuit eye movements in childhood onset schizophrenia: comparison with ADHD and normal controls. *Biol Psychiatry.* 1996;40:1144-1154.
13. Frazier JA, Giedd JN, Hamburger SD, Albus KE, Kaysen D, Vaituzis AC, Rajapakse JC, Lenane MC, McKenna K, Jacobsen LK, Gordon CT, Breier A, Rapoport JL. Brain anatomic magnetic resonance imaging in childhood-onset schizophrenia. *Arch Gen Psychiatry.*1996;53:617-624.
14. Bernstein AS, Frith CD, Gruzelier JH. An analysis of the skin conductance–orienting response in samples of American, British, and German schizophrenics. *Biol Psychol.* 1982;14:155-211.
15. Zahn TP, Frith CD, Steinhauer SR. Autonomic functioning in schizophrenia: electrodermal activity, heart rate, pupillography. In: Steinhauer SR, Gruzelier JH, Zubin J, eds. *Handbook of Schizophrenia.* Amsterdam, the Netherlands: Elsevier Science Publishers; 1991;5:185-224.
16. Ohman A. Electrodermal activity and vulnerability to schizophrenia: a review. *Biol Psychol.* 1981;12:87-145.
17. Frith CD, Stevens M, Johnstone EC, Crow TJ. Skin conductance responsivity during acute episodes of schizophrenia as a predictor of symptomatic improvement. *Psychol Med.* 1979;9:101-106.
18. Zahn TP, Carpenter WTJ, McGlashan TH. Autonomic nervous system activity in acute schizophrenia, II: relationships to short-term prognosis and clinical state. *Arch Gen Psychiatry.* 1981;38:260-266.
19. Iacono WG, Lykken DT, Peloquin LJ, Lumry AE, Valentine RH, Tuason VB. Electrodermal activity in euthymic unipolar and bipolar affective disorders. *Arch Gen Psychiatry.* 1983;40:557-565.
20. Zahn TP. Psychophysiological approaches to psychopathology. In: Coles MGH, Donchin E, Porges SW, eds. *Psychophysiology: Systems, Processes, and Applications.* New York, NY: Guilford Press; 1986:508-610.
21. Straube ER, Schied HW, Rein W, Breyer-Pfaff U. Autonomic nervous system differences as predictors of short-term outcome in schizophrenics. *Pharmacopsychiatry.* 1987;20:105-110.
22. Frazier JA, Gordon CT, McKenna K, Lenane MC, Jih D, Rapoport JL. An open trial of clozapine in 11 adolescents with childhood-onset schizophrenia. *J Am Acad Child Adolesc Psychiatry.* 1994;33:658-663.
23. Kumra S, Frazier JA, Jacobsen LK, McKenna K, Gordon CT, Lanane MC, Hamburger SD, Smith AK, Albus KE, Alaghband-Rad J, Rapoport JL. Childhood-onset schizophrenia: a double-blind clozapine-haloperidol comparison. *Arch Gen Psychiatry.* 1996;53:1090-1097.
24. Bernstein AS, Taylor KW, Starkey P, Juni S, Lubowsky J, Paley H. Bilateral skin conductance, finger pulse volume, and EEG orienting response to tones of differing intensities in chronic schizophrenics and controls. *J Nerv Ment Dis.* 1981; 169:513-528.
25. Straube E. On the meaning of electrodermal nonresponding in schizophrenia. *J Nerv Ment Dis.* 1979;167:601-611.
26. Kim DK, Shin YM, Kim CE, Cho HS, Kim YS. Electrodermal responsiveness, clinical variables, and brain imaging in male chronic schizophrenics. *Biol Psychiatry.* 1993;33:786-793.
27. Reich W, Welner Z. *DICA-RC (DSM-III-R Version), Revised Version V-R.* St Louis, Mo: Washington University; 1988.
28. Orvaschell H, Tabrizi MA, Chambers W. *Schedule for Affective Disorders and Schizophrenia for School-Age Children—Epidemiologic Version (Kiddie-SADS-E).* 3rd ed. New York, NY: New York State Psychiatric Institute and Yale University School of Medicine; 1980.
29. McKenna K, Gordon CT, Lenane MC, Kaysen D, Rapoport JL. Looking for childhood-onset schizophrenia: the first 71 cases screened. *J Am Acad Child Adolesc Psychiatry.* 1994;33:636-644.
30. Herjanic B, Campbell W. Differentiating psychiatrically disturbed children on the basis of a structured interview. *J Abnorm Child Psychol.* 1977;5:127-134.
31. Herjanic B, Reich W. Development of a structured psychiatric interview for children: agreement between child and parent on individual symptoms. *J Abnorm Child Psychol.* 1982;10:307-324.
32. Overall JE, Hollister LE, Pichot P. Major psychiatric disorders: a four-dimensional model. *Arch Gen Psychiatry.* 1967;24:146-151.
33. Pickar D, Labarca R, Doran AR, Wolkowitz OM, Roy A, Breier A, Linnoila M, Paul SM. Longitudinal measurement of plasma homovanillic acid in schizophrenic patients: correlation with psychosis and response to neuroleptic treatment. *Arch Gen Psychiatry.* 1986;43:669-676.
34. Andreasen NC. *The Scale for the Assessment of Negative Symptoms (SANS).* Iowa City: University of Iowa; 1983.
35. Andreasen NC. *The Scale for the Assessment of Positive Symptoms (SAPS).* Iowa City: University of Iowa; 1984.
36. Zahn TP, Rosenthal D, Lawlor WG. Electrodermal and heart rate orienting reactions in chronic schizophrenia. *J Psychiatr Res.* 1968;6:117-134.
37. Zahn TP, Carpenter WT, McGlashan TH. Autonomic nervous system activity in acute schizophrenia, I: method and comparison with normal controls. *Arch Gen Psychiatry.* 1981;38:251-258.
38. Dixon WJ. *BMDP Statistical Software Manual.* Berkeley, Calif: University of California Press; 1992.
39. Levinson DF, Edelberg R, Bridger WH. The orienting response in schizophrenia: proposed resolution of a controversy. *Biol Psychiatry.* 1984;19:489-507.
40. Siegel, S. *Nonparametric Statistics for the Behavioral Sciences.* New York, NY: McGraw-Hill Book Co; 1956.

41. Gruzelier J, Eves F, Connolly J, Hirsch S. Orienting, habituation, sensitisation, and dishabituation in the electrodermal system of consecutive, drug free, admissions for schizophrenia. *Biol Psychol.* 1981;12:187-209.
42. Zahn TP, Pickar D, Haier RJ. Effects of clozapine, fluphenazine, and placebo on reaction time measures of attention and sensory dominance in schizophrenia. *Schizophr Res.* 1994;13:133-144.
43. Toone BK, Cooke E, Lader MH. Electrodermal activity in the affective disorders and schizophrenia. *Psychol Med.* 1981;11:497-508.
44. Cooklin R, Sturgeon D, Leff J. The relationship between auditory hallucinations and spontaneous fluctuations of skin conductance in schizophrenia. *Br J Psychiatry.* 1983;142:47-52.
45. Ohman A, Nordby H, d'Elia G. Orienting in schizophrenia: habituation to auditory stimuli of constant and varying intensity in patients high and low in skin conductance responsivity. *Psychophysiology.* 1989;26:48-61.
46. Bartfai A, Levander S, Edman G, Schalling D, Sedvall G. Skin conductance responses in unmedicated recently admitted schizophrenic patients. *Psychophysiology.* 1983;20:180-187.
47. Zahn TP. *Autonomic Reactivity and Behavior in Schizophrenia: Psychiatric Research Report 19.* Washington, DC: American Psychiatric Association; 1964.
48. Zahn TP. Psychophysiological concomitants of task performance in schizophrenia. In: Kietzman ML, Sutton S, Zubin J, eds. *Experimental Approaches to Psychopathology.* New York, NY: Academic Press; 1975:109-131.
49. Albus M, Ackenheil M, Engel RR, Muller F. Situational reactivity of autonomic functions in schizophrenic patients. *Psychiatry Res.* 1982;6:361-370.
50. Kelly D. *Anxiety and Emotions.* Springfield, Ill: Charles C Thomas Publisher; 1980.
51. Gruzelier JH, Venables PH. Skin conductance orienting activity in a heterogeneous sample of schizophrenics: possible evidence of limbic dysfunction. *J Nerv Ment Dis.* 1972;155:277-287.
52. Spohn HE, Coyne L, Wilson JK, Hayes K. Skin-conductance orienting response in chronic schizophrenics: the role of neuroleptics. *J Abnorm Psychol.* 1989;98: 478-486.
53. Zahn TP, Pickar D. Autonomic effects of clozapine in schizophrenia: comparison with placebo and fluphenazine. *Biol Psychiatry.* 1993;34:3-12.
54. Zahn TP, Pickar D. Effects of a low-anticholinergic neuroleptic on autonomic activity in schizophrenia. Presented at the meeting of the Society for Psychophysiological Research;October 13, 1995; Toronto, Ontario.
55. Iacono WG, Lykken DT. The orienting response: importance of instructions. *Schizophr Bull.* 1979;5:11-14.
56. Alm T, Lindstrom LH, Ost LG, Ohman A. Electrodermal non-responding in schizophrenia: relationships to attentional, clinical, biochemical, computed tomographical and genetic factors. *Int J Psychophysiol.* 1984;1:195-208.
57. Ohman A, Ohlund LS, Alm T, Wieselgren IM, Ost LG, Lindström LH. Electrodermal nonresponding, premorbid adjustment, and symptomatology as predictors of long-term social functioning in schizophrenics. *J Abnorm Psychol.* 1989;98: 426-435.
58. Ohman A. The orienting response, attention and learning: an information-processing perspective. In: Kimmel HD, van Olst EH, Orlebeke JF, eds. *The Orienting Reflex in Humans.* Hillsdale, NJ: Erlbaum; 1979:443-472.
59. Frith CD. The positive and negative symptoms of schizophrenia reflect impairments in the perception and initiation of action. *Psychol Med.* 1987;17:631-648.
60. Raine A, Reynolds GP, Sheard C. Neuroanatomical correlates of skin conductance orienting in normal humans: a magnetic resonance imaging study. *Psychophysiology.* 1991;28:548-558.
61. Hazlett EA, Dawson ME, Buchsbaum MS, Nuechterlein KH. Reduced regional brain glucose metabolism assessed by positron emission tomography in electrodermal nonresponder schizophrenics: a pilot study. *J Abnorm Psychol.* 1993;102: 39-46.
62. Levy DL, Holzman PS, Matthysse S, Mendell NR. Eye tracking dysfunction in schizophrenia: a critical perspective. *Schizophr Bull.* 1993;19:461-536.
63. Porges SW, Fox NA. Developmental psychophysiology. In: Coles MGH, Donchin E, Porges SW, eds. *Psychophysiology: Systems, Processes, and Applications.* New York, NY: Guilford Press; 1986:611-625.
64. Dawson ME, Nuechterlein KH, Schell AM, Mintz J. Concurrent and predictive electrodermal corelates of symptomatology in recent-onset schizophrenic patients. *J Abnorm Psychol.* 1992;101:153-164.
65. Green MF, Nuechterlein KH, Satz P. The relationship of symptomatology and medication to electrodermal activity in schizophrenia. *Psychophysiology.* 1989;26: 148-157.
66. Olbrich R, Mussgay L. Spontaneous fluctuations of electrical skin conductance and the actual clinical state in schizophrenics. *Psychopathology.* 1987;20:18-22.
67. Green WH, Padron-Gayol M, Hardesty AS, Bassiri M. Schizophrenia with childhood onset: a phenomenological study of 38 cases. *J Am Acad Child Adolesc Psychiatry.* 1992;31:968-976.
68. Russel AT. The clinical presentation of childhood-onset schizophrenia. *Schizophr Bull.* 1994;20:631-646.
69. Spencer EK, Campbell M. Children with schizophrenia: diagnosis, phenomenology, and pharmacotherapy. *Schizophr Bull.* 1994;20:713-725.
70. Zahn TP, Kruesi MJP. Autonomic activity in boys with disruptive behavior disorders. *Psychophysiology.* 1993;30:605-614.
71. Zahn TP, Rumsey JM, Van Kammen DP. Autonomic nervous system activity in autistic, schizophrenic, and normal men: effects of stimulus significance. *J Abnorm Psychol.* 1987;96:135-144.
72. Zahn TP, Leonard HL, Swedo SE, Rapoport JL. Autonomic activity in children and adolescents with obsessive-compulsive disorder. *Psychiatry Res.* 1996;60: 67-76.
73. Berg CJ, Zahn TP, Behar D, Rapoport JL. Childhood obsessive-compulsive disorder: an anxiety disorder? In: Gittelman R, eds. *Anxiety Disorders of Childhood.* New York, NY: Guilford Press; 1986:126-135.
74. Bernstein AS, Riedel JA, Graae F, Seidman D, Steele H, Connolly J, Lubowsky J. Schizophrenia is associated with altered orienting activity: depression with electrodermal (cholinergic?) deficit, and normal orienting response. *J Abnorm Psychol.* 1988;97:3-12.
75. Bernstein AS, Schnur DB, Bernstein P, Yeager A, Wrable J, Smith S. Differing patterns of electrodermal and finger pulse responsivity in schizophrenia and depression. *Psychol Med.* 1995;25:51-62.
76. Thorell LH, Kjellman BF, d'Elia G. Electrodermal activity in antidepressant medicated and unmedicated depressive patients and in matched healthy subjects. *Acta Psychiatr Scand.* 1987;76:684-692.

Correction

Error in Reference Section. In the article titled "Increased Concentrations of Presynaptic Proteins in the Cingulate Cortex of Subjects With Schizophrenia," published in the June ARCHIVES (1997;54:559-566), there was an error in the publication information of reference 26. It should have read: Honer WG, Falkai P, Young C, Wang T, Xie J, Bonner J, Hu L, Boulianne GL, Lu Z, Trimble WS. Cingulate cortex synaptic terminal proteins and neural cell adhesion molecule in schizophrenia. *Neuroscience.* 1997;78:99-110.

COMMENTARY

Neurobiology and Neuroplasticity in Schizophrenia

Continuity Across the Life Cycle

Truth is revealed gradually lest it blinds!
Emily Dickinson

THE LONG-HELD notion that childhood-onset schizophrenia before the age of 12 years is a different disorder than adult-onset schizophrenia continues to crumble in the face of new data. The articles by Zahn et al[1] and Rapoport et al[2] not only provide important scientific data to that effect but also represent an incremental step in establishing that the psychotic clinical brain disorder that we call "schizophrenia" is one illness that may manifest throughout the life cycle. Accumulating evidence related to phenomenological, neurobiological, and pharmacological characteristics and course and outcome strongly indicate that the onset of schizophrenia may occur at age 10, 20, 30, or even 60 or 70 years.[3]

See also pages 897 and 904

As always, new knowledge enlightens but also provokes additional questions. The continuity of neurophysiological and neuroanatomical findings in childhood- and adult-onset schizophrenia underscores the structural and functional primary brain "lesion" in schizophrenia. For that reason, repeated measures over time, as in the study of Rapoport et al,[2] are particularly valuable in characterizing the evolution of the structural pathological changes. Thus, the neurophysiological measures used by Zahn et al must be repeated over time to detect maturational changes and ideally to be also correlated with the morphological changes. Such a paradigm for neurobiological research is essential to understand the neurodevelopmental and clinical trajectories of schizophrenia. Cognitive measures of regional brain function must also be included as a longitudinal study of the evolving neurobiological characteristics of schizophrenia.

An important fact emerges from both studies: only 50% of the schizophrenia samples fail to show skin conductance–orienting reactions just as 50% of patients with early-onset schizophrenia show neuroanatomical abnormalities such as large ventricles or reduced cerebral volume. But, rather than simply attribute that to the "heterogeneity of the syndrome" or "subtypes of the illness," consideration should be given to a possible continuum of neurodevelopmental lesions in time and space. As such, the most severe form of schizophrenia (clinically and biologically) is expressed in childhood and the less severe form in the sixth or seventh decade of life.

Since the publication of the first rescanning follow-up brain imaging study in schizophrenia,[4] there have been several reports that generally confirmed the lack of progressive ventricular enlargements. The study by Rapoport et al is the first rescanning report in childhood-onset schizophrenia. Their findings of several morphological changes during a 2-year period in midadolescence will fuel the debate as to whether the structural brain changes in schizophrenia are static (neurodevelopmental) or progressive (neurodegenerative). Given that the studies involving adult-onset schizophrenia do not support an ongoing progressive "atrophic" process, it is possible to speculate that what Rapoport et al[2] observed was an exaggerated neurodevelopmental and time-specific "subtractive" central nervous system process.[5] Synaptic pruning is well-known to peak in midadolescence, and there have been speculations about the possible role of this neuroplastic process in triggering schizophrenia in late adolescence or early adulthood.[6] Because the reduction in cerebral volume and enlargement in ventricular volume during midadolescence of subjects with childhood-onset schizophrenia occurred *after* the onset of their psychosis (at age <12 years), then there are 3 possible explanations: (1) synaptic pruning is excessive in the brains of subjects with childhood-onset schizophrenia as a result of a preexisting neurodevelopmental lesion, (2) the brain volume reduction in childhood-onset schizophrenia during midadolescence may somehow be related to antipsychotic drug treatment (in this case, clozapine), or (3) a combination of 1 and 2. However, reduced cerebral volume may not necessarily signify a deleterious neuroplastic event, just as with the reduction by clozapine of neuroleptic-induced caudate hypertrophy.[7] Clearly, the nature of what may or may not be an atrophic process in childhood-onset schizophrenia needs to be investigated using in vivo functional imaging such as magnetic resonance spectroscopy.[8] The regional distribution (such as frontal, tem-

This article is also available on our Web site: www.ama-assn.org/psych.

poral, or thalamic) of cerebral volume reduction in childhood-onset schizophrenia and whether gray and white matter are differentially affected are also important research questions generated by the findings of Rapoport et al.[2]

The abnormal changes in peripheral indicators of autonomic activity by Zahn et al[1] are consistent with putative frontal and thalamic distribution of pathologic changes in schizophrenia. The rescanning study by Rapoport et al,[2] which shows a striking decrease in thalamic volume in childhood-onset schizophrenia compared with that in healthy adolescents both at baseline and at follow-up, underscores the potential relevance of the thalamus in schizophrenia. The accelerated reduction in thalamic volume is also matched by a concomitant enlargement of ventricular volume in childhood-onset schizophrenia. The total cerebral volume is decreased in both groups over time, but twice as much (5.2% reduction) in the group with childhood-onset schizophrenia compared with the healthy adolescents (2.6%) who, in turn, had a 10% volume advantage at baseline. Replication of these findings should also be coupled with cognitive reassessments over time. Consideration should also be given to parental socioeconomic status or educational attainment as a potential covariant of proband cerebral size[9] and sex, which has been shown to be associated with differential neuroplastic change over time in normal populations.[10]

The data of the 2 articles discussed above will contribute to reframing the debate about the continuity of schizophrenia across the life cycle regardless of age at onset. They may also shift the neurodevelopemental vs neurodegenerative pathogenesis controversy into a novel model of an evolving neuroplasticity with ongoing (not merely prenatal) neurodevelopemental changes in brain morphology in childhood- and adult-onset schizophrenia. It is reasonable to postulate that structural brain development throughout the life cycle of individuals with schizophrenia may be anomalous because of deviant neuronal histoarchitecture during fetal life.[11]

Finally, bipolar disorder, which is another major psychosis with a childhood-onset form and neurodevelopmental features [12] should also be studied using the same paradigms as those used by Zahn et al and Rapoport et al. The specificity of the above findings to schizophrenia can then be assessed.

Henry A. Nasrallah, MD
Herman A. Tolbert, MD
Department of Psychiatry
The Ohio State University
College of Medicine
1670 Upham Dr
Columbus, OH 43210

REFERENCES

1. Zahn, TP, Jacobsen LK, Gordon CT, McKenna K, Frazier JA, Rapoport JL. Autonomic nervous system markers of psychopathology in childhood-onset schizophrenia. *Arch Gen Psychiatry.* 1997;54:904-912.
2. Rapoport JL, Giedd J, Kumra S, Jacobsen L, Smith A, Lee P, Nelson J, Hamburger S. Childhood-onset schizophrenia: progressive ventricular change during adolescence. *Arch Gen Psychiatry.* 1997;54:897-903.
3. Jeste DV, Harris MJ, Pearlson GD, Rabins P, Lesser I, Miller B, Coles C, Yassa R. Late-onset schizophrenia: studying clinical validity. *Psychiatr Clin North Am.* 1988;11:1-13.
4. Nasrallah HA, Olson SC, McCalley-Whitters M, Chapman S, Jacoby CG. Cerebral ventricular enlargement in schizophrenia: a preliminary follow-up study. *Arch Gen Psychiatry.* 1986,43:157-159.
5. Nowakowski RS. Basic concepts of CNS development. *Child Dev.* 1987;58:568-595.
6. Feinberg I. Schizophrenia: caused by a fault in programmed synaptic elimination during adolescence? *J Psychiatr Res.* 1982;17:319-339.
7. Chakos MH, Lieberman JA, Bilder RM, Bornstein M, Lerner G, Bogerts B, Wult, Kinon B, Ashtari M. Increase in caudate nuclei volumes of first-episode schizophrenic patients taking antipsychotic drugs. *Am J Psychiatry.* 1994;151:1430-1436.
8. Nasrallah HA, Skinner TE, Schmalbrock P, Robitaille PM. In vivo ^{1}H nuclear magnetic resonance spectroscopy of the hippocampal formation in schizophrenia. *Br J Psychiatry.* 1994;165:481-485.
9. Andreasen NC, Flaum M, Swayze V, O'Leary DS, Alliger R, Cohen G, Ehrhardt J, Yuh WTC. Intelligence and brain structure in normal individuals. *Am J Psychiatry.* 1993;150:130-134.
10. Cowell PE, Turetsky B I, Gur RC, Grossman RI, Shtasel DL, Gur RE. Sex differences in aging of the human frontal and temporal lobes. *J Neurosci.* 1994;14:4748-4755.
11. Nasrallah HA. Neurodevelopmental pathogenesis of schizophrenia. *Psychiatr Clin North Am.* 1993;16:269-280.
12. Nasrallah HA. Neurodevelopmental aspects of bipolar affective disorder. *Biol Psychiatry.* 1991;29:1-2.

'Vascular Depression' Hypothesis

George S. Alexopoulos, MD; Barnett S. Meyers, MD; Robert C. Young, MD; Scott Campbell, PhD; David Silbersweig, MD; Mary Charlson, MD

We propose that cerebrovascular disease may predispose, precipitate, or perpetuate some geriatric depressive syndromes. The "vascular depression" hypothesis is supported by the comorbidity of depression, vascular disease, and vascular risk factors and the association of ischemic lesions to distinctive behavioral symptoms. Disruption of prefrontal systems or their modulating pathways by single lesions or by an accumulation of lesions exceeding a threshold are hypothesized to be central mechanisms in vascular depression. The vascular depression concept can generate studies of clinical and heuristic value. Drugs used for the prevention and treatment of cerebrovascular disease may be shown to reduce the risk for vascular depression or improve its outcomes. The choice of antidepressants in vascular depression may depend on their effect on neurologic recovery from ischemic lesions. Research can clarify the pathways to vascular depression by focusing on the site of the lesion, the resultant brain dysfunction, the presentation of depression and time of onset, and the contribution of nonbiological factors.
Arch Gen Psychiatry. 1997;54:915-922

Earlier we suggested that late-onset depression encompasses a high percentage of patients with underlying neurologic brain disorders.[1] We now propose that cerebrovascular disease can predispose, precipitate, or perpetuate a depressive syndrome in many elderly patients. We have introduced the term "vascular depression"[2] because it is broad and encompasses entities with diverse pathogenetic mechanisms. Direct testing of the vascular depression hypothesis is impossible because the mechanisms of depression are unknown. However, the hypothesis can generate studies of the epidemiology, clinical presentation, outcomes, pathogenesis, and treatment of a large subgroup of geriatric patients with depression. What follows is a review of findings relevant to the vascular depression hypothesis and a discussion of their clinical and heuristic implications.

LATE-ONSET DEPRESSION

We have proposed that late-onset depression is heterogeneous and includes a subgroup of patients with neurologic disorders that may not be clinically evident when the depression first appears.[1] This position has been supported by studies showing that patients with late-onset depression have more neuropsychological[3,4] and neuroradiological abnormalities,[5-7] greater disability,[8] medical morbidity and mortality,[9,10] and lower familial prevalence of mood disorders than elderly patients with early-onset depression.[11] However, some studies failed to confirm the association between late-onset depression and high neurologic morbidity,[12-14] perhaps owing to the heterogeneity of late-onset depression.

Limitations of research on late-onset depression include difficulties in the identification of age at onset[15] and the assumption that depression is homogeneous over time, when in fact patients may experience episodes with different causes during different periods of their lives. Nevertheless, research on late-onset depression has provided a conceptual step for

This article is also available on our Web site: www.ama-assn.org/psych.

From the Cornell Institute of Geriatric Psychiatry, Cornell University Medical College, White Plains, NY.

identifying more homogeneous groups of geriatric depression. Depression occurring in the context of vascular disease may account for many geriatric depression cases with rather homogeneous causes.

COMORBIDITY OF DEPRESSION AND VASCULAR DISEASE

Cerebrovascular disease is frequent in elderly patients with depression. Early studies observed that cerebrovascular disease occurring 2 to 3 years prior to admission to a psychiatric hospital may have contributed to the development of depression.[16,17] In 15 186 primary care patients, those who received the diagnosis of depression had vascular diseases more frequently than nondepressed patients.[18] In a sample of 248 coronary bypass patients, 107 (43%) had significant depressive symptoms prior to surgery and 68% had depressive symptoms after surgery.[19]

Depression is highly prevalent in patients with hypertension,[20] coronary artery disease,[21] and vascular dementia.[22] Patients who have vascular dementia have more retardation, depression, and anxiety than patients with Alzheimer disease with similar cognitive impairment.[22] Therefore, there is evidence that patients with vascular disease often have depressive symptoms and that a large percentage of depressed elderly patients have vascular disease.

DEPRESSION AND ISCHEMIC BRAIN LESIONS

Depression is a frequent complication of stroke.[23-26] Stroke with neurologic symptoms and signs occurs in a small number of elderly patients with depression. However, "silent stroke" without neurologic signs is frequent in elderly depressed populations. In a Japanese sample, silent stroke greater than 5 mm in diameter was found in 86 (83%) of the 104 patients with major depression who were older than 65 years.[27] Silent stroke was observed in 59 (94%) of the 63 patients with depression onset after 65 years of age. A study of white populations (N=203) found that silent stroke occurs in 23% of persons older than 65 years; in 79% of them, the lesions exceeded 3 mm in diameter.[28]

The silent stroke data are in agreement with the pioneering findings of Krishnan et al[29] and Coffey et al,[30-33] who noted that elderly patients with depression have white matter hyperintensities (WMHs) more frequently than nondepressed patients. White matter hyperintensities correspond to areas of arteriolar ectasia, enlargement of perivascular spaces, and myelin pallor associated with arteriosclerotic changes of perforating arteries.[34] In asymptomatic patients, WMHs were found to be associated with extracranial carotid artery disease, reduced cerebral blood flow, and a history of hypertension, diabetes, and cardiac disease.[35] Not all WMHs are due to vascular disease. Demyelinating disorders frequently cause nonvascular WMHs and antidepressant treatment may conceivably contribute to WMHs. However, elderly depressed patients without cerebrovascular risk factors were found to have a similar degree of WMHs to nondepressed controls.[36] Therefore, WMHs are most frequent in elderly patients with depression with vascular disease. It is unclear whether WMHs can cause depression, but in one case depression developed following a large increase in WMHs.[37]

In addition to WMHs, 14 (40%) of 35 depressed elderly patients without neurologic history were found to have lesions of the thalamus and basal ganglia.[32] In contrast, only 1 of 22 normal elderly volunteers had such lesions, and their lesions are far less extensive than the lesions of elderly patients with depression.

CLINICAL CORRELATES OF VASCULAR LESIONS

Depression of patients with silent stroke, as a rule, has late onset and is accompanied by hypertension.[38] Patients with late-onset depression were found to have more vascular risk factors than elderly patients with early-onset depression,[39] although negative findings also exist.[40] In silent stroke, depression was associated with infrequent family history of mood disorders.[38] Similar findings have been reported in late-onset bipolar disorder. Late-onset bipolar disorders often are associated with vascular and degenerative brain disease, negative family history of mood disorders, and poor response to treatment.[41]

Patients with late-onset major depression and vascular risk factors seem to have more psychomotor retardation and lack of insight and less agitation and guilt than elderly patients with early-onset depression without vascular risk factors.[42] Moreover, the vascular depression group had greater impairment in frontal functions and more disability. Identification of relationships among specific symptoms, lesion location, and overall damaged tissue can provide information about the pathogenesis of vascular depression.

COGNITIVE IMPAIRMENT AND VASCULAR DEPRESSION

Vascular disease appears to be associated with depression and cognitive impairment. Stroke[23-26] and vascular dementia[22] often are accompanied by depression. The incidence of dementia 1 year after the first cerebral infarct was found to be 9 times greater than expected.[43] Lacunar infarcts in the basal ganglia, thalamus, and deep white matter, but not cortical infarcts, seem to be associated with a high prevalence of dementia in patients with Alzheimer disease.[44] Declining cognitive performance, perhaps due to unrecognized vascular disease, was found to be a stroke risk factor.[45]

In normal populations, WMHs correlated with impaired attention, mental speed, and executive functions,[46-49] although negative findings exist.[50,51] In cortical (28) or basal ganglia stroke, cognitive impairment was associated with high incidence and increased severity of depression.[23] In vascular dementia, a syndrome frequently associated with depression, the extent of WMHs correlated with cognitive impairment.[52] Patients with late-onset depression and vascular risk factors were described as having greater cognitive impairment than elderly patients with early-onset depression without vascular risk factors.[42,53] Executive functions were most affected. These findings suggest that cerebrovascular lesions lead to depression or cognitive impairment through related mechanisms.

COURSE OF VASCULAR DEPRESSION

The course of vascular depression has been insufficiently investigated. Late-onset depression, an entity that often occurs in the context of vascular disease, is a rather chronic disorder.[54] In elderly patients with depression, leukoencephalopathy was found to be associated with low quantitative electroencephalogram coherence[55,56]; low quantitative electroencephalogram coherence predicted failure to recover, residual symptoms and signs, increased mortality, and disability.[55,56]

Preliminary studies observed that abnormal initiation-perseveration scores and prolonged P300 latency predict poor antidepressant response in elderly patients with depression.[57] Similarly, abnormal initiation-perseveration scores predict early relapse in elderly patients with depression receiving controlled continuation treatment with nortriptyline.[57] Abnormal initiation-perseveration scores and long P300 latency are thought to reflect frontal systems impairment, an abnormality often caused by vascular disease.[58] While direct studies are needed, these findings suggest that vascular depression has a chronic and relapsing course.

Vascular lesions may lead to cognitive impairment and behavioral disability even in patients with mild mood disturbance.[46-49] Characterization of the clinical profile of vascular depression may have prognostic implications because vascular depression seems to have poor outcome.

LOCALIZATION OF LESIONS AND NEUROTRANSMITTER ABNORMALITIES

Subcortical lesions appear to be associated with depression.[59-65] Stroke of the caudate head may be the most likely to result in depression, while thalamic stroke has a rather low incidence of depression.[63] Most depressed patients with silent cerebral infarction have lesions either in the perforating arteries area or cortical and perforating artery areas.[38] Similarly, WMHs of elderly patients with depression are most prominent in subcortical and frontal areas.[30-32] Reduced size of the head of the caudate[66] and putamen[67] has been observed in neurologically unimpaired depressed patients. In elderly patients with depression, small caudate size was associated with impairment in construction, visual retention, and visual naming.[68] These findings may be explained by an impairment of the cortico-striato-pallido-thalamo-cortical (CSPTC) systems that disrupt visual attention, visual scanning, and motor planning, leading to memory and construction dysfunction.

Cortical lesions, especially lesions of the left hemisphere, often result in depression.[23] Young patients with depression seem to have reduced metabolism at the left anterolateral prefrontal cortex and cingulate.[69-76] Depression may occur after right hemisphere stroke,[77,78] despite difficulties in the recognition of depression owing to anosognosia. Depressed mood is infrequent in right hemisphere stroke, but vegetative signs and abnormal results of dexamethasone suppression tests are equally frequent in left and right hemisphere stroke.[77] In left hemisphere stroke, anterior lesions were associated with depression more often than posterior lesions.[23] A more complex lesion-location relationship was observed in right hemisphere stroke. Immediately after right hemisphere stroke, depression was more severe in patients with posterior lesions,[79] while the severity of depression occurring within 3 to 6 months after right hemisphere stroke was associated with anterior lesions.[79,80] These observations suggest that poststroke depression is mediated by different mechanisms, especially in patients with right hemisphere lesions.

Neurotransmitter changes following ischemic lesions may be related to depression. Animal studies suggest a biphasic serotonin response following ventrolateral lesions. Within 6 days from the development of the lesion, serotonin levels were found to be decreased and 5 hydroxyindolacetic acid levels were increased in the ipsilateral hemisphere.[81] In contrast, 12 weeks after the development of the lesion, serotonin levels were decreased and 5 hydroxyindolacetic acid levels were increased.[81] Lower cerebrospinal fluid 5 hydroxyindolacetic acid levels were observed in depressed patients within 5 days after stroke compared with nondepressed stroke patients and nonstroke controls.[82] A positron emission tomography study noted increased serotonin$_2$-receptor binding in the parietal and temporal cortex 16 months after left hemisphere stroke and speculated that increased serotonin$_2$-binding results from receptor up-regulation owing to low serotonin levels.[83] These observations parallel findings of increased serotonin$_2$-binding autopsy studies of non–stroke-related suicides.[84] Investigation of serotonin dysfunction after stroke may elucidate the mechanisms of vascular depression.

Changes in other neurotransmitters may be relevant to vascular depression. Animal studies observed that norepinephrine levels are decreased in the cortex and hippocampus and increased in the striatum and midbrain after ipsilateral ventrolateral lesions.[81] These changes were most pronounced 6 days after lesioning and persisted, although not as prominently, at 12 weeks. It has been suggested that lesions of the frontal pole and the caudate head lead to depression by damaging the ascending monoamine pathways through the ventral striatum and the pathways that run anteriorly to posteriorly.[23] Increases in dopamine[81,85] and acetylcholine[86] have been observed after ischemic lesions in animals, but their role in poststroke depression is unclear. Finally, animal research suggests a change in γ-aminobutyric acid (GABA) uptake after ischemic injury[87] and a neuroprotective effect of $GABA_A$ receptor agonists when administered soon after ischemic lesioning.[88] Further research may clarify the relevance of these findings in vascular depression.

Some aspects of the depressive syndrome are associated with rather specific functional brain abnormalities in younger patients with depression. Psychomotor slowing was found to be correlated with decreased flow in the left anterolateral cortex, while cognitive impairment correlated with decreased activity in the left medial prefrontal area.[72] Anxi-

Clinical Presentation of 'Vascular Depression'*

Cardinal Features

- Clinical and/or laboratory evidence of vascular disease or vascular risk factors. Clinical manifestations may include history of stroke or transient ischemic attacks, focal neurologic signs, atrial fibrillation, angina, history of myocardial infarction, carotid bruit, hypertension, and hyperlipidemia. Laboratory findings may include significant white matter hyperintensities at the territory of the perforating arteries, infarcts, or evidence of carotid occlusion or stenosis of the Willis circle arteries
- Depression onset after 65 years of age or change in the course of depression after the onset of vascular disease in patients with early-onset depression; development of more frequent and persistent depressive episodes

Secondary Features

- Cognitive impairment consisting of but not limited to disturbance of executive functions, ie, planning, organizing, sequencing, and abstracting
- Psychomotor retardation
- Limited depressive ideation, eg, guilt
- Poor insight
- Disability
- Absence of family history of mood disorders

**The cardinal features are expected in all patients. The secondary features may be present in most but not all patients with "vascular depression."*

ety occurring in the context of depression was associated with increased activity in the right posterior cingulate and bilateral inferior parietal areas.[71] These observations suggest that distinctive depressive syndromes may result from vascular lesions that disrupt specific prefrontal-subcortical circuits.

PREFRONTAL SYSTEM ABNORMALITIES IN DEPRESSION

The prefrontal cortex integrates sensory, emotional, and neuroendocrine functions that often are impaired during depression.[75] The frontal lobe is connected to the basal ganglia through 5 contiguous, nonoverlapping, parallel zones (CSPTC).[89] In each of these circuits, glutaminergic excitatory neurons from specific cortical sites project to the striatum. Inhibitory neurons from the striatum project to the globus pallidus and the substantia nigra. Efferent inhibitory neurons from these structures project to the thalamus and from the thalamus to the cortex. Stimulation at the cortical level has the net effect of disinhibiting the thalamus and exciting the cortex. In addition to the direct CSPTC pathways, indirect pathways exist with an inhibitory net effect on the cortex. Imbalance favoring the indirect inhibitory pathway of specific CSPTC circuits has been postulated in depression.[90,91]

Three CSPTC pathways may be relevant to depression.[75,76,89] Damage of the orbitofrontal circuit may lead to disinhibition, irritability, and diminished sensitivity to social cues.[75] Damage of the anterior cingulate may result in apathy and reduced initiative.[75] Damage of the dorsolateral circuit may result in difficulties in set shifting, learning, and word list generation.[75] These behavioral abnormalities resemble in part the depressive syndrome.

Krishnan[64] proposed that vascular lesions may confer vulnerability to depression through mechanisms that act alone or in synergy. Vascular white matter lesions may damage glutaminergic projections from cortical areas to the striatum or the GABAergic neurons of the limbic-basal ganglia interface and alter the input to the cortex.[64] Because these systems are "redundant," depressive symptoms may appear if the overall damage exceeds a critical level and leads in increased inhibitory CSPTC input.

Another mechanism may involve the damage of catecholamine neurons by white matter lesions at the pons, resulting in the reduction of stress responses.[72] A third mechanism postulates the disruption of control exerted by the orbitofrontal cortex on the serotoninergic raphe nuclei.[62] A recent study has shown that patients with depression who have vascular risk factors have greater dysfunction in auditory transmission at the pons than elderly patients with depression without vascular risk factors or elderly normal controls.[92] These hypotheses suggest that lesions at various sites may result in depression through mechanisms disrupting CSPTC circuits or their modulating systems.

Prefrontal and limbic dysfunction in depression has been suggested by positron emmission tomography activation studies of younger adults. Intravenous administration of procaine can induce emotional experiences associated with increased blood flow in the anterior temporal lobes, inferior frontal lobes, and anterior cingulate gyri in normal subjects.[93] However, minimal activation of these regions was noted in patients with depression who have the same experiences as the normal subjects.[93] Depressed patients had a more robust activation of the anterolateral prefrontal cortex than the normal subjects.[94-96]

Left prefrontal areas may participate in the development of sad moods. Transient sadness increases the activity of the left anterolateral prefrontal cortex,[97] left anterior cingulate, left medial frontal cortex, and left anterior limbic system.[98] The relationship of these findings to depression is unclear. However, they suggest that the left prefrontal system and its connections to limbic areas mediate some aspects of depressive symptoms.

DEFINITION OF VASCULAR DEPRESSION

Clinical studies suggest that patients with vascular depression have common characteristics (**Table**). Vascular disease or risk factors, late onset or change in the course of early-onset depression after the onset of vascular disease, are viewed as cardinal features. Neurologic signs and clinical and neuropsychological abnormalities having manifestations resembling frontal lobe syndrome may be found in most patients with vascular depression, but their presence and severity depend on the location and extent of the lesions. Late-onset and a negative family history for depression are expected in most cases but personal or family history of mood disorders should not preclude vascular depression. Family history of mood disorders seems to predispose patients to poststroke depression.[23] Moreover, a personal history of depression may not protect patients from and may even predispose them to vascular depression.

The proposed cardinal characteristics of vascular depression include cerebrovascular disease and vascular risk factors. A narrow definition, limiting vascular depression to patients with vascular lesions in specific brain areas, eg, basal ganglia, would have identified syndromes with a rather clear lesion-syndrome relationship. However, such a definition would have excluded depression resulting from metabolic or microanatomic changes associated with vascular risk factors. We believe that future research can be served best by the proposed broad definition because it allows focused studies to select criteria suitable to their objectives.

HYPOTHESES ON THE MECHANISMS OF VASCULAR DEPRESSION

The proposed vascular depression hypothesis unifies the poststroke and WMH findings and views vascular depression as a heterogeneous entity mediated by several mechanisms. Specific hypotheses on the mechanisms of vascular depression should consider the location of lesions, the clinical presentation, the time of depression onset, the presence of cognitive impairment, and the contribution of nonbiological factors.

Two broad hypotheses can be advanced and tested regarding the localization of lesions in vascular depression. The first hypothesis is that small lesions disrupting critical pathways may precipitate vascular depression. This hypothesis is supported by stroke studies showing that lacunar infarcts of the left caudate head or the left frontal pole often lead to depression.[23] The direct lesion-depression pathway may account for a minority of vascular depression cases, mainly those developing after stroke.[99]

The second hypothesis is that the accumulation of lesions exceeding a threshold predispose to depression. This hypothesis is most applicable to patients with neurologically silent lesions or an old stroke. The threshold concept is supported by the observation that a total area of WMHs exceeding 10 cm^2 may result in impaired attention and executive skills.[58] Similar impairments have been noted in late-onset depression with vascular risk factors.[100-103] The "threshold hypothesis" postulates vulnerability that may be conferred by the lesions themselves or by a broader cerebrovascular disturbance that compromises pathways relevant to depression. Nonbiological factors may be required to trigger depression in patients so predisposed. Depression developing 3 months after stroke was found to be predicted by impairment in activities of daily living, while depression occurring 12 months after stroke was predicted by social isolation.[99] Other studies have shown that reverse occipital asymmetry (the right side larger than the left side), absence of ventriculomegaly, and absence of family history of mood disorders are associated with low frequency of poststroke depression.[23] Studies of outcomes of patients with vascular disease or risk factors can identify biological and nonbiological mechanisms that mediate or protect from depression.

PHARMACOLOGY OF CEREBROVASCULAR DISEASE

The concept of vascular depression provides a potential opportunity for the primary prevention of geriatric depression by modifying risk factors for cerebrovascular disease. The Framingham Study[104] and the Copenhagen City Heart Study[105] have shown that hypertension is a significant risk factor for stroke. Effective treatment of hypertension[106,107] and hypercholesterolemia[108] reduces cerebrovascular morbidity and mortality. Warfarin and aspirin seem to reduce the risk of stroke in patients with atrial fibrillation.[109] Ticlopidine,[110] aspirin,[110,111] and dipyridamole[111] may prevent future stroke in patients with transient ischemic attacks or ischemic stroke. Studies are needed to ascertain whether antihypertensive, antihypercholesterolemia, and antiplatelet agents improve the outcome of vascular depression. Antiplatelet agents may prove to be effective in preventing further vascular damage occurring during depressive episodes, when the serotonin-mediated thrombogenic platelet response is enhanced.[112,113] In addition, longitudinal assessment of depressive symptoms during antiplatelet secondary prevention trials can evaluate the efficacy of these agents in improving the course of vascular depression.

Agents that reduce damage after stroke may be relevant to vascular depression. Animal studies suggest that several agents have cytoprotective action during ischemia and reperfusion. These include thrombolytic agents, calcium- and sodium-channel antagonists, N-methyl-D-aspartate (NMDA) receptor antagonists, glutamate synthesis inhibitors, glutamate-release inhibitors, GABA antagonists, gangliocides, aminosteroids, antioxidants, growth factors, and antiapoptotic agents.[114] The efficacy of these agents in stroke patients is under investigation. Recombinant tissue plasminogen activator administered within 6 hours from the onset of stroke may improve outcome in selected patients.[115] Nimodipine, a calcium channel blocker, may improve the outcome of ischemic stroke when administered within the first 12 hours.[116] Similarly, the monosialoganglioside-1 (GM-1) seems to be effective in reducing neurologic sequelae of ischemic stroke when given early.[117,118] Prophylactic use of free radical scavengers may be beneficial in patients at risk for cerebrovascular disease,[119] but definitive human studies are lacking. The role of the above-mentioned agents in the prevention and treatment of vascular depression can be examined in patients with ischemic events participating in acute interventional and secondary prevention trials.

PSYCHOTROPIC DRUGS IN VASCULAR DEPRESSION

Drugs that alter monoamine neurotransmitter function may influence postischemic recovery. Animal studies suggest that the dopamine receptor blocker haloperidol, the α_1 adrenergic receptor antagonist prazosin, the α_2-adrenergic receptor clonidine, and

GABA agonists such as diazepam and phenytoin interfere with motor recovery after ischemic lesions.[119-121] In contrast, amphetamine, the dopamine agonist bromocriptine, and the α_2 adrenergic receptor antagonists yohimbine and idazoxan may be beneficial to recovery from ischemic injury.[119-121] Early clinical observations suggest that the use of drugs shown to interfere with ischemic recovery in animals may hinder the recovery of motor function in patients with ischemic stroke. Studies of stroke victims may examine whether these agents influence the incidence of poststroke depression or alter the course of vascular depression.

Several drugs have been found effective in poststroke depression,[122] including trazodone,[123] nortriptyline,[124,125] amphetamine,[126] and methylphenidate.[127,128] Animal experiments suggest that antidepressants have different effects on recovery following the occurrence of ischemic lesions. In animals, desipramine[129] was noted to promote motor recovery after ischemic damage while fluoxetine had no significant effect.[130] In contrast, trazodone and amitriptyline seemed to slow recovery or reinstate postischemia motor function deficits.[129,130] These effects were thought to be mediated by antagonism of the α_1 noradrenergic receptor.[130] A clinical study has observed that fluoxetine may facilitate and maprotiline may hinder recovery in poststroke hemiplegic patients undergoing rehabilitation.[131] Further studies are needed to examine whether specific antidepressants influence the recovery of neurologic deficits in patients with poststroke depression. Such studies can identify antidepressants suitable for prophylaxis of vascular depression.

COMMENT

Converging evidence suggests that cerebrovascular disease or risk factors may lead to late-life depression syndromes. The vascular depression hypothesis is supported by the high frequency of depression in patients with hypertension, diabetes, and coronary artery disease and stroke[18-26]; the frequent occurrence of silent stroke and WMHs in geriatric depression[27,29-33]; and the association of depression with lesions impairing the integrity or regulation of CSPTC systems.[62,72,90-92]

The clinical value of the vascular depression concept can be tested by studies of the clinical presentation, course, and outcomes of a subgroup of elderly patients with depression who may have this syndrome. Elderly patients with depression treated in primary care settings may be particularly suitable for such studies because they frequently have vascular disease or risk factors. It is impossible to identify a homogeneous group of patients whose depression mainly is contributed by vascular disease because the cause of depression remains unknown. However, if it is demonstrated that vascular disease is associated with a more or less consistent presentation and outcomes, specific interventions may become available.

The vascular depression hypothesis can provide the impetus for focused pharmacological research. Drugs used in the prevention and treatment of cerebrovascular disease may be shown to reduce the risk of depression in patients with vascular risk factors or reduce chronicity, recurrence, cognitive impairment, and disability in vascular depression. Moreover, the long-term efficacy of specific antidepressants can be investigated in depressed patients at risk for new vascular lesions because basic research suggests that some antidepressants and not others promote recovery after ischemic brain lesions.

Vascular depression may be an entity particularly suitable for studies of mechanisms of depression. Lesions at specific locations may promote, have no effect on, or even protect patients from depression. The total "lesion burden" hypothesis may be relevant for some cases of vascular depression. Developments in structural and functional imaging, electrophysiology, and chronobiology permit the quantitative assessment of lesions and the sophisticated study of brain function changes associated with specific lesions. Course of illness studies can identify models of interaction between compromise in brain function, disability, and psychosocial factors leading to vascular depression.

Accepted for publication June 18, 1997.

This work was supported by grants RO1 MH42819, RO1 MH51842, P20 MH49762, and T32 MH19132 from the National Institute of Mental Health, Bethesda, Md (Dr Alexopoulos).

Reprints: George S. Alexopoulos, MD, Cornell Institute of Geriatric Psychiatry, Cornell University Medical College, 21 Bloomingdale Rd, White Plains, NY 10605.

REFERENCES

1. Alexopoulos GS. Clinical and biological findings in late-onset depression. In: Tasman A, Goldfinger SM, Kaufman CA, eds. *Review of Psychiatry.* Washington, DC: American Psychiatric Press; 1990;9:249-262.
2. Alexopoulos GS, Meyers BS, Young RC, Charlson M, Silversweig D. The clinical presentation of 'vascular depression.' In: New research program and abstracts, annual meeting of the American Psychiatric Association; May 4-9, 1996; New York, NY.
3. Alexopoulos GS, Young RC, Meyers BS. Geriatric depression: age of onset and dementia. *Biol Psychiatry.* 1993;34:141-145.
4. Alexopoulos GS, Meyers BS, Young RC, Mattis S, Kakuma T. The course of geriatric depression with 'reversible dementia.' *Am J Psychiatry.* 1993;150:1693-1699.
5. Alexopoulos GS, Young RC, Shindledecker R. Brain computed tomography in geriatric depression and primary degenerative dementia. *Biol Psychiatry.* 1992;31:591-599.
6. Jacoby RJ, Levy R. Computed tomography in the elderly, 3: affective disorder. *Br J Psychiatry.* 1980;136:270-275.
7. Coffee CE, Figiel GS, Djang WT, Cress M, Saunders WB, Weiner RD. Leukoencephalopathy in elderly depressed patients referred for ECT. *Biol Psychiatry.* 1988;24:143-161.
8. Alexopoulos GS, Vrontou C, Kakuma T, Meyers BS, Young RC, Klausner E, Clarkin J. Disability in geriatric depression. *Am J Psychiatry.* 1996; 153:877-885.
9. Roth M, Kay DWK. Affective disorders arising in the senium, II: physical disability as an etiological factor. *J Ment Sci.* 1956;102:141-150.
10. Jacoby RJ, Levy R, Bird JM. Computed tomography and the outcome of affective disorder: a follow-up study of elderly subjects. *Br J Psychiatry.* 1981;139:288-292.
11. Baron M, Mendlewicz J, Klotz J. Age of onset and genetic transmission in affective disorders. *Acta Psychiatr Scand.* 1981;64:373-380.
12. Conwell Y, Nelson JC, Kim KM, Majure CM. Depression in late life: age of onset as marker of a subtype. *J Affect Dis.* 1989;17:189-195.
13. Greenwald BS, Kramer-Ginsberg E. Age of onset in geriatric depression: relationship to clinical variables. *J Affect Dis.* 1988;15:61-68.
14. Herrmann N, Lieff S, Silberfeld M. The effect of age of onset on depression in the elderly. *J Geriatr Psychiatry Neurol.* 1989;2:182-187.
15. Wiener P, Alexopoulos GS, Kakuma T, Meyers BS, Rosendhal E, Chester J. The limits of history taking in geriatric depression. *Am J Geriatr Psychiatry.* 1997;5:116-125.
16. Post F. *The Significance of Affective Disorders in Old Age.* London, England: Institute of Psychiatry; 1962. Maudsley Monograph 10.
17. Post F, Schulman K. New views on old age affective disorder. In: Aire T, ed. *Recent Advances in Psychogeriatrics.* New York, NY: Churchill Livingstone Inc; 1985:119-140.
18. Luber MP, Alexopoulos GS, Hollenberg J, Charlson ME, Callahan M. Recognition, treatment, co-

morbidity and resource utilization of depressed patients in a general medical practice. In: Program and abstracts of the annual meeting of the Society of General Internal Medicine; May 2-4, 1996; Washington, DC.
19. Peterson JC, Williams-Russo PG, Charlson ME, Meyers BS. Longitudinal course of new onset depression after cardiac bypass surgery. In: Programs and abstracts of the 10th Annual International Conference on Mental Health Problems in the General Health Care Sector, National Institute of Mental Health; July 15-16, 1996; Bethesda, Md.
20. Rabkin JG, Charles E, Kass F. Hypertension and *DSM-III* depression in psychiatric outpatients. *Am J Psychiatry.* 1983;140:1072-1074.
21. Carney RM, Rich WM, Tevelde A, Saini J, Clark K, Jaffe AS. Major depressive disorder in coronary artery disease. *Am J Cardiol.* 1987;60:1273-1275.
22. Sulzer DL, Levin HS, Mahler ME, High WM, Cummings JL. A comparison of psychiatric symptoms in vascular dementia and Alzheimer's disease. *Am J Psychiatry.* 1993;150:1806-1812.
23. Starkstein SE, Robinson RG. Depression in cerebrovascular disease. In: *Depression in Neurological Disease.* Baltimore, Md: The Johns Hopkins University Press; 1993:28-49.
24. Folstein MF, Maiberger R, McHugh PR. Mood disorders as a specific complication of stroke. *J Neurol Neurosurg Psychiatry.* 1971;40:1018-1020.
25. Ebrahim S, Barer K, Nouri F. Affective illness after stroke. *Br J Psychiatry.* 1987;154:170-182.
26. Mendez MF, Adams NL, Lewandoski KS. Neurobehavioral changes associated with caudate lesions. *Neurology.* 1989;39:349-354.
27. Fujikawa T, Yamawaki S, Touhouda Y. Incidence of silent cerebral infarction in patients with major depression. *Stroke.* 1993;24:1631-1634.
28. Ryan RN, Manolio TA, Schertz LD, Jungteis C, Poirier VC, Elster AD, Kronmal RA. A method of using MR to evaluate the effects of cardiovascular disease on the brain: the cardiovascular health study. *Am J Neuroradiol.* 1994;15:1625-1633.
29. Krishnan KRR, Goli V, Ellinwood EH, France RD, Blazer DZ, Nemeroff CB. Leukoencephalopathy in patients diagnosed as major depressive. *Biol Psychiatry.* 1988;23:519-522.
30. Coffey CE, Figiel GS, Djang WT, Cross M, Saunders WB, Weiner RD. Leukoencephalopathy in elderly depressed patients referred for ECT. *Biol Psychiatry.* 1988;23:519-522.
31. Coffey CE, Figiel GS, Djang WT, Saunders WB, Weiner RD. White matter hyperintensity on MRI clinical and neuroanatomic correlates in the depressed elderly. *J Neuropsychiatry Clin Neurosci.* 1989;1:135-144.
32. Coffey CE, Figiel FS, Djang WT, Weiner RD. Subcortical hyperintensity on MRI: a comparison of normal and depressed elderly subjects. *Am J Psychiatry.* 1990;147:187-189.
33. Coffey CE, Wilkinson WE, Weiner RD, Paraschos IA, Djang WT, Webb MC, Figiel GS, Spritzer CE. Quantitative cerebral anatomy in depression: a controlled magnetic resonance imaging study. *Arch Gen Psychiatry.* 1993;50:7-16.
34. Braffman BH, Zimmerman RA, Trojanowski JQ, Gonatas NK, Hickey WF, Schlaepler WW. Brain MRI: pathologic correlation with gross and histopathology, 2: hyperintense white-matter foci in the elderly. *AJNR Am J Neuroradiol.* 1988; 151:559-566.
35. Fazekas F, Niederkorn K, Schmidt R, Offenbacher H, Honner S, Bertha G, Lechner H. White matter signal abnormalities in normal individuals: correlation with carotid ultrasonography, cerebral blood flow, measurements, and cerebrovascular risk factors. *Stroke.* 1988;19:1285-1288.
36. Miller DS, Kumar A, Yousem DM, Gottlieb GL. MRI high-intensity signals in late-life depression and Alzheimer's disease: a comparison of subjects without major vascular risk factors. *Am J Geriatr Psychiatry.* 1994;2:332-337.
37. Lesser IM, Hill-Gutierrez E, Miller BL, Boone KB. Late-onset depression with white matter lesions. *Psychosomatics.* 1993;34:364-367.
38. Fujikawa T, Yamawaki S, Touhouda Y. Background factors and clinical symptoms of major depression with silent cerebral infarction. *Stroke.* 1994;25:798-801.
39. Baldwin RC, Tomenson B. Depression in later life: a comparison of symptoms and risk factors in early and late onset cases. *Br J Psychiatry.* 1995; 167:649-652.
40. Krishnan KRR, Hays JC, Tupler LA, George LK, Blazer DG. Clinical and phenomenological comparisons of late-onset and early-onset depression. *Am J Psychiatry.* 1995;152:785-788.
41. Young RC, Klerman GL. Mania in late life: focus on age at onset. *Am J Psychiatry.* 1992;4:73-78.
42. Alexopoulos GS, Meyers BS, Young RC, Kakuma T, Sibersweig D, Charlson M. Clinically defined vascular depression. *Am J Psychiatry.* 1997; 154:562-565.
43. Kokmen E, Whisnant JP, O'Fallon WM, Chu C-P, Beard CM. Dementia after ischemic stroke: a population study in Rochester, Minnesota (1960-1984). *Neurology.* 1996;19:154-159.
44. Snowdon DA, Greiner LH, Mortimer JA, Riley KP, Greiner PA, Markesbery WR. Brain infarction and the clinical expression of Alzheimer's disease. *JAMA.* 1997;277:813-817.
45. Ferruzzi L, Guralnik JM, Salive ME, Pahor M, Corti MC, Baroni A, Havlik RJ. Cognitive impairment and risk of stroke in the older population. *J Am Geriatr Soc.* 1996;44:237-241.
46. Åstrom MG, Thompson RF, Hendrie HC, Norton J, Farlow MR, Edwards MK, Dean R. Foci of increased T_2 signal intensity in MR images of healthy elderly subjects: a follow-up study. *J Am Geriatr Soc.* 1990;38:1131-1138.
47. Harell LE, Duvall E, Folks DG, Duke L, Bartolucci A, Conboy T, Callaway R, Kerns D. The relationships of high-intensity signals on magnetic resonance images to cognitive and psychiatric state in Alzheimer's disease. *Arch Neurol.* 1991;48:1136-1140.
48. Van Swieten JC, Geyskes GG, Derix MMA, Peeck BM, Ramos LMP, van Latum JC, van Gijn J. Hypertension in the elderly is associated with white matter lesions and cognitive decline. *Ann Neurol.* 1991;30:825-830.
49. Ylikoski R, Ylikoski A, Erkinjuntti T, Sulkava R, Raininko R, Tilvis R. White matter changes in healthy elderly persons correlate with attention and speed of mental processing. *Arch Neurol.* 1993;50:818-824.
50. Fein G, van Dyke C, Davenport L, Turetsky B, Brant-Zawadzki M, Zatz L, Dillon W. Preservation of normal cognitive functioning in elderly subjects with extensive white matter lesions of long duration. *Arch Gen Psychiatry.* 1990;47:220-223.
51. Tupler LA, Coffey CE, Logue PE, Djang WT, Fagan M. Neuropsychological importance of subcortical white matter hyperintensity. *Arch Neurol.* 1992;49:1248-1252.
52. Meyers JS, Kawamura J, Terayama Y. White matter lesions in the elderly. *J Neurol Sci.* 1992;110: 1-7.
53. Lesser IM, Hill-Gutierrez E, Miller RL, Boone KB. Late-onset depression with white matter lesions. *Psychosomatics.* 1993;34:364-367.
54. Alexopoulos GS, Meyers BS, Young RC, Kakuma T, Feder M, Einhorn A, Rosendahl E. Recovery in geriatric depression. *Arch Gen Psychiatry.* 1996;53:305-312.
55. Leuchter AF, Dunkin JJ, Lufkin RB, Anzai Y, Cook IA, Newton TF. Effect of white matter disease on functional connections in the aging brain. *J Neurol Neurosurg Psychiatry.* 1994;57:1347-1354.
56. Leuchter A, Simon SL, Daly KA, Abrams M, Rosenberg-Thompson S, Dunkin JJ, Cook IA, Newton TF, Spar JE. Quantitative EEG correlates of outcome in older psychiatric patients, II: two-year follow-up of patients with depression. *Am J Geriatr Psychiatry.* 1994;2:290-299.
57. Alexopoulos GS. The subtypes of geriatric depression. In: Programs and abstracts of the annual meeting of the American Geriatric Association; March 5, 1997; Orlando, Fla.
58. Boone KB, Miller BL, Lesser IM, Merhinger CM, Hill-Gutierrez E, Goldberg M, Berman NG. Neuropsychological correlates of white matter lesions in healthy elderly subjects. *Arch Neurol.* 1992;49:549-554.
59. Damasio AR, Van Hoesen GW. Emotional disturbances associated with focal lesions of the limbic frontal lobe. In: Heilman KM, Satz P, eds. *Neuropsychology of Human Emotion.* New York, NY: Guilford Press; 1983:85-110.
60. Grafman J, Vance SC, Weingartner H, Salazar AM, Amin D. The effects of lateralized frontal lesions on mood regulation. *Brain.* 1986;109: 1127-1148.
61. Eslinger PJ, Damasio AR. Severe bilateral disturbance of higher cognition after bilateral frontal lobe ablation: patient EVR. *Neurology.* 1985; 35:1731-1741.
62. Mayberg HS, Solomon DH. Depression in Parkinson's disease: a biochemical and organic viewpoint. In: Weiner WJ, Lang AE, eds. *Behavioral Neurology of Movement Disorders: Advances in Neurology.* New York, NY: Raven Press; 1995; 65:49-60.
63. Starkstein SE, Robinson RG, Berthier ML, Parikh RM, Price TR. Differential mood changes following basal ganglia vs thalamic lesions. *Arch Neurol.* 1988;45:725-730.
64. Krishnan KRR. Neuroanatomic substrates of depression in the elderly. *J Geriatr Psychiatry Neurol.* 1993;6:39-58.
65. Krishnan KRR, McDonald WM. Arteriosclerotic depression. *Med Hypotheses.* 1995;44:111-115.
66. Krishnan KRR, McDonald WM, Escalona PR, Doraiswamy PM, Na C, Husain MM, Figiel GS, Boyko OB, Ellinwood EH, Nemeroff CB. Magnetic resonance imaging of the caudate nuclei in depression. *Arch Gen Psychiatry.* 1992;49:553-557.
67. Husain MM, McDonald WM, Doraiswamy PM, Figiel GS, Escalona PR, Boyko OB, Nemeroff CB, Krishnan KRR. A magnetic resonance imaging study of putamen nuclei in major depression. *Psychiatry Res Neuroimaging.* 1991;40:95-99.
68. Alexopoulos GS, Meyers BS, Bajulaiye R, Elkin C, Khouri P, Kakuma T. Caudate size in geriatric depression. In: New research program and abstracts, annual meeting of the American Psychiatric Association; May 20-25, 1995; Miami, Fla.
69. Baxter LR Jr, Phelps ME, Mazziotta JC, Schwartz JM, Gerner RH, Selin CE, Smida RM. Cerebral metabolic rates for glucose in mood disorders: studies with positron emission tomography and fluorodeoxyglucose. *Arch Gen Psychiatry.* 1985; 42:441-447.
70. Martinot JL, Hardy P, Feline A, Huret JD, Mazoyer B, Attar-Levy D, Pappata S, Syrota A. Left prefrontal glucose hypometabolism in the depressed state: a confirmation. *Am J Psychiatry.* 1990;147:1313-1317.
71. Bench CJ, Friston KJ, Brown RG, Scott LC, Frackowiak RSJ, Dolan RJ. The anatomy of melancholia: focal abnormalities of cerebral blood flow in major depression. *Psychol Med.* 1992;22: 607-615.
72. Dolan RJ, Bench CJ, Brown RG, Scott LC, Friston KJ, Frackowiak RSJ. Regional cerebral blood flow abnormalities in depressed patients with cognitive impairment. *J Neurol Neurosurg Psychiatry.* 1992;55:768-773.
73. Drevets WC, Videen TO, Preskorn SH, Price JL, Carmichael ST, Raichle ME. A functional anatomical study of unipolar depression. *J Neurosci.* 1992;12:3628-3641.
74. Ketter TA. Andreason PJ, George MS, Pazzaglia PJ, Marangell LM, Post RM. Blunted CBF response to procaine in mood disorders. In: New research program and abstracts, annual meeting of the American Psychiatric Association; May 22-27, 1993; San Francisco, Calif. Abstract NR297.
75. George MS, Ketter TA, Post RM. Prefrontal cortex dysfunction in clinical depression. *Depression.* 1994;2:59-72.
76. Baxter LR Jr, Schwartz JM, Phelps ME, Mazzi-

otta JC, Guze BH, Selin CE, Gerner RH, Sumida RM. Reduction of prefrontal cortex glucose metabolism common to three types of depression. *Arch Gen Psychiatry.* 1989;46:243-250.
77. Finkelstein SP, Benowitz LI, Baldessarini RJ, Arana GW, Levine D, Woo E, Bear D, Moya K, Stoll AL. Mood, vegetative disturbance, and dexamethasone suppression after stroke. *Ann Neurol.* 1982;12:463-468.
78. Starkstein SE, Robinson RG, Honig MA, Parikh RM, Joselyn J, Price TR. Mood changes after right hemisphere lesions. *Br J Psychiatry.* 1989;155:79-85.
79. Robinson RG, Starr LB, Lipsey JR, Rao K, Price TR. A two-year longitudinal study of poststroke mood disorders: dynamic changes in associated variables over the first six months of follow-up. *Stroke.* 1984;15:510-516.
80. House A, Dennis M, Warlow C, Hawton K, Molyneux A. Mood disorders after stroke and their relation to lesion location: a CT scan study. *Brain.* 1990;113:1113-1130.
81. Finkelstein S, Campbell A, Baldessarini R, Moya KL, Haber SN. Late changes in cerebral metabolism following focal ventrolateral cerebrocortical lesions in rats. *Brain Res.* 1985;344:205-210.
82. Bryer JB, Starkstein SE, Votypka V, Parikh RM, Price TR, Robinson RG. Reduction of CSF monoamine metabolites in poststroke depression: a preliminary report. *J Neuropsychiatry Clin Neurosci.* 1992;4:440-442.
83. Mayberg HS, Robinson RG, Wong DF, Parikh R, Bolduc P, Starkstein SE, Price T, Dannals RF, Links JM, Wilson AA, et al. PET imaging of cortical S2 serotonin receptors following stroke: lateralized changes and relationship to depression. *Am J Psychiatry.* 1988;145:937-943.
84. Mann JJ, Stanley M, McBride P, McEwen BS. Increased serotonin$_2$ and β-adrenergic receptor binding in the frontal cortices of suicide victims. *Arch Gen Psychiatry.* 1986;43:954-959.
85. Ishii H, Stanmirovic DB, Chang CJ, Mrsulja BB, Spatz M. Dopamine metabolism and free-radical related mitochondrial injury during transient brain ischemia. *Neurochem Res.* 1993;18:1193-1201.
86. Bertrand N, Ishii H, Beley A, Spatz M. Biphasic striatal acetylcholine release during and after transient cerebral ischemia in gerbils. *J Cereb Blood Flow Metab.* 1993;13:789-795.
87. Kuroda H, Baskin DS, Matsui T, Loh HH, Hosobuchi Y, Lee NM. Effects of dynorphin 1-13 on opiate binding and dopamine and GABA uptake in stroked cat brain. *Brain Res.* 1986;376:68-74.
88. Lyden P, Lonzo L, Nunez S. Combination chemotherapy extends the therapeutic window to 60 minutes after stroke. *J Neurotrauma.* 1995;12:223-230.
89. Alexander GE, DeLong MR, Strick PL. Parallel organization of functionally segregation circuits linking basal ganglia and cortex. *Ann Rev Neurosci.* 1986;9:357-381.
90. Baxter LR Jr, Schwartz LM, Guze BH, Bergman K, Szuba MP. PET imaging in obsessive-compulsive disorder with and without depression. *J Clin Psychiatry.* 1990;51(suppl):61-69.
91. Baxter LR Jr. Brain imaging as a tool in establishing a theory of brain pathology in obsessive-compulsive disorder. *J Clin Psychiatry.* 1990;51(suppl):22-25.
92. Kalayam B, Alexopoulos GS, Musiek FE, Kakuma T, Toro A, Silbergsweig D, Young RC. Brainstem evoked response abnormalities in late-life depression with vascular disease. *Am J Psychiatry.* 1997;154:970-975.
93. Ketter TA, Andreason PJ, George MS, Marangell LM, Pazzaglia PJ, Post RM. Reduced resting frontal lobe cerebral blood flow in mood disorders. In: New research program and abstracts, annual meeting of the American Psychiatric Association; May 22-27, 1993; San Francisco, Calif. Abstract NR298.
94. George MS, Ketter TA, Gill D, Haxby JV, Ungerleider L, Herscovitch P, Post RM. Brain regions involved in recognizing facial emotion or identity: an 015 PET study. *J Neuropsychiatry Clin Neurosci.* 1993;54:1-10.
95. George MS, Ketter TA, Gill DS, Marangell LB, Pazzaglia PJ, Post RM. Blunted cerebral blood flow with emotion recognition in depression. In: New research program and abstracts, annual meeting of the American Psychiatric Association; May 22-27, 1993; San Francisco, Calif. Abstract NR114.
96. Berman KF, Doran AR, Pickar D, Weinberger DR. Is the mechanism of prefrontal hypofunction in depression the same as in schizophrenia: regional cerebral blood flow during cognitive activation. *Br J Psychiatry.* 1993;162:183-192.
97. Pardo JV, Pardo PJ, Ratchle ME. Neural correlates of self-induced dysphoria. *Am J Psychiatry.* 1993;150:13-19.
98. George MS, Ketter TA, Parekh PI, Horwitz B, Herscovitch P, Post RM. Regional brain activity during transient sadness or happiness in healthy women. *Am J Psychiatry.* 1995;152:341-351.
99. Åstrom M, Adolfson R, Asplund K. Major depression in stroke patients: a three-year longitudinal study. *Stroke.* 1993;24:976-982.
100. Zubenko GS, Sullivan P, Nelson JP. Brain imaging abnormalities in mental disorders of late life. *Arch Neurol.* 1990;47:1107-1113.
101. Figiel GS, Krishnan KRR, Doraiswamy PM, Rao VP, Nemeroff CB, Boyko OB. Subcortical hyperintensities on brain magnetic resonance imaging: a comparison between late age onset and early onset elderly depressed subjects. *Neurobiol Aging.* 1991;12:245-247.
102. Churchill CM, Priolo CV, Nemeroff CB, Krishnan KRR, Breitner JCS. Occult subcortical magnetic resonance imaging in elderly depressives. *Int J Geriatr Psychiatry.* 1991;6:213-214.
103. Krishnan KRR, McDonald WM, Doraiswamy PM, Tupler LA, Husain M, Boyko OB, Figiel GS, Ellinswood EH. Neuroanatomical substrates of depression in the elderly. *Eur Arch Psychiatry Clin Neurosci.* 1993;243:41-46.
104. Kannel WB, Wolf PA, Verter J, McNamara PM. Epidemiologic assessment of the role of blood pressure in stroke: the Framingham Study. *JAMA.* 1996;276:1269-1278.
105. Lindenstrom E, Boysen G, Nyboe J. Influence of systolic and diastolic blood pressure on stroke risk: a prospective observational study. *Am J Epidemiol.* 1995;142:1279-1290.
106. Kannel WB. Cardioprotection and antihypertensive therapy: the key importance of addressing the associated coronary risk factors (the Framingham experience). *Am J Cardiol.* 1996;77:6B-11B.
107. Whisnant JP. Effectiveness versus efficacy of treatment of hypertension for stroke prevention. *Neurology.* 1996;46:301-307.
108. Sirtori CR. The treatment of hypercholesterolemia in primary and secondary prevention. *Ann Ital Med Int.* 1995;10(suppl):48S-52S.
109. Stroke Prevention in Atrial Fibrillation Investigators. Warfarin versus aspirin for prevention of thromboembolism in atrial fibrillation: Stroke Prevention in Atrial Fibrillation Study II. *Lancet.* 1994;343:687-691.
110. Bellavance A. Efficacy of ticlopidine and aspirin for prevention of reversible cerebrovascular ischemic events: the ticlopidine aspirin stroke study. *Stroke.* 1993;24:1452-1457.
111. Sivenius J, Riekkinen PJ, Laasko M, Smets P, Lowenthal A. European Stroke Prevention Study: antithrombotic therapy is also effective in the elderly. *Acta Neurol Scand.* 1993;87:111-114.
112. Kusumi I, Koyama A, Yamashita I. Serotonin-stimulated Ca_2^+ response is increased in the blood platelets of depressed patients. *Biol Psychiatry.* 1991;30:310-312.
113. Mikuni K, Kagaya A, Takahashi K, Meltzer HY. Serotonin but not norepinephrine-induced calcium mobilization of platelets is enhanced in affective disorders. *Psychopharmacology.* 1992;106:311-314.
114. Silver B, Weber J, Fisher M. Medical therapy for ischemic stroke. *Clin Neuropharmacol.* 1996;19:101-128.
115. Hacke W, Kaste M, Fiechi C, Toni D, Lesaffre E, von Kummer R, Boysen G, Bluhmki E, Hoxter G, Mahagne MH, Hennerici M, for the ECASS Study Group. Intravenous thrombolysis with recombinant tissue plasminogen activator for acute hemispheric stroke: the European Cooperative Acute Stroke Study (ECASS). *JAMA.* 1995;274:1017-1025.
116. Gelmers HJ, Hennerici M. Effect of nimodipine in acute ischemic stroke: pooled results from five randomized trials. *Stroke.* 1990;21(suppl 22):81-84.
117. Lenzi GL, Grigoletto F, Gent M, Roberts RS, Walker MD, Easton JD, Carolei A, Dorsey FC, Rocca WA, Bruno R, et al. Early treatment with monosialoganglioside GM-1: efficacy and safety results of the Early Stroke Trial. *Stroke.* 1994;25:1552-1558.
118. Svennerholm L. Gangliosides: a new therapeutic agent against stroke and Alzheimer's disease. *Life Sci.* 1994;55:2125-2134.
119. Goldstein LB. Pharmacologic modulation of recovery after stroke: clinical data. *J Neurol Rehab.* 1991;5:129-140.
120. Goldstein LB. Basic and clinical studies of pharmacologic effects on recovery from brain injury. *J Neural Transplant Plast.* 1993;3:175-192.
121. The Sygen in Acute Stroke Study Investigators, Goldstein LB. Common drugs may influence motor recovery after stroke. *Neurology.* 1995;45:865-871.
122. Finkelstein SP, Weintraub RJ, Karmouz N, Askinazi C, Davar G, Baldessarini RJ. Antidepressant drug treatment for poststroke depression: retrospective study. *Arch Phys Med Rehabil.* 1987;68:772-776.
123. Reding MJ, Orto LA, Winter SW, Fortuna IM, Di Ponte P, McDowell FH. Antidepressant therapy after stroke: a double-blind trial. *Arch Neurol.* 1986;43:763-765.
124. Lipsey JR, Spencer WC, Rabins PV, Robinson RG. Phenomenological comparison of poststroke depression and functional depression. *Am J Psychiatry.* 1986;143:527-529.
125. Lazarus LW, Moberg PJ, Langsley PR, Lingam V. Methylphenidate and nortriptyline in the treatment of poststroke depression: a retrospective comparison. *Arch Med Rehab.* 1994;75:403-406.
126. Masand P, Murray GB, Pickett P. Psychostimulants in poststroke depression. *J Neurol Psychiatry Clin Neurosci.* 1991;3:23-27.
127. Lingham VR, Lazarus LW, Groves L, Oh SH. Methylphenidate in treating poststroke depression. *J Clin Psychiatry.* 1988;49:151-153.
128. Lazarus LW, Winemiller DR, Lingam VR, Robinson RG. Efficacy and side effects of methylphenidate for poststroke depression. *J Clin Psychiatry.* 1992;53:447-449.
129. Boyerson MG, Harmon RL. Effects of trazodone and desipramine on motor recovery in brain-injured rats. *Am J Phys Med Rehab.* 1993;72:286-293.
130. Boyerson MG, Harmon RL, Jones JL. Differential effects of fluoxetine, amitriptyline and serotonin S2 antagonist markedly reduces infarct size following middle cerebral artery occlusion in the rat. *Neurology.* 1988;38:1667-1673.
131. Dam M, Tonon P, De Boni A, Pizzolato G, Casson S, Ermani M, Freo U, Piron L, Battistin L. Effects of fluoxetine and maprotilene on functional recovery in poststroke hemiplegic patients undergoing rehabilitation therapy. *Stroke.* 1996;27:1211-1214.

Manual-Guided Psychosocial Treatment

A New Virtual Requirement for Pharmacotherapy Trials?

Kathleen M. Carroll, PhD

The conduct of randomized clinical trials to evaluate the efficacy of pharmacotherapies for mental disorders is guided by research standards (at a high level of rigor) that govern most design elements, including randomization of subjects, use of placebo controls, formulation and dosage of the therapeutic agent, and monitoring of serum levels. In contrast, no such widely accepted guidelines are recognized for standardization of an essential, if unacknowledged, element of all such studies: the concomitant provision of at least a minimal form of psychosocial treatment. Standardized provision of psychosocial treatments in pharmacotherapy trials will foster replicability of findings and address several common problems (eg, attrition, medication noncompliance, reduction of error variance, and ethical issues associated with placebo controls). Careful selection and standardization of the psychosocial context in which medications are delivered will improve the validity, precision, and power of pharmacotherapy efficacy research, and should be considered a virtual requirement in research design.

Arch Gen Psychiatry. 1997;54:923-928

Why should psychosocial treatments be specified in pharmacological trials? Substantial levels of protocol deviation in clinical pharmacotherapy efficacy trials are the rule rather than the exception in most areas of psychiatry. Rates of attrition in recent short-term ambulatory trials range from 15% to 40% among patients with anxiety, depressive, and eating disorders[1-6] to as high as 60% to 80% for patients with personality or substance use disorders.[7-10] Similarly, detected rates of medication nonadherence are usually estimated to be approximately 50%[11,12]; however, these rates have been shown to be higher in some rigorous studies of treatments of depressive,[13,14] panic,[15] schizophrenic,[16] and bipolar[17] disorders, and as high as 80% in some studies of alcohol treatments.[18] Compliance is likely to be poorer in cases in which it may take several weeks to achieve therapeutic blood levels, the trial extends throughout months, or the medication has substantial adverse effects.[19]

Protocol deviation, in the form of differential attrition or compliance across treatments, undermines internal validity,[20] particularly if retention or compliance varies across conditions. Protocol deviation is also extremely costly in terms of statistical power and the actual expense of a trial. **Figure 1** illustrates the effect of sample size decreases (through either attrition or noncompliance) on a hypothetical placebo-controlled pharmacotherapy trial with a sample size of 100. Protocol deviation reduces power and leads to the need for severalfold increases in sample size,[21-25] particularly for smaller effect sizes.

See also page 929

However, the most popular and persistent methods for coping with the effects of protocol deviation are not methodologically defensible. One of the most commonly used strategies (ie, conducting analyses only based on the subsample of patients who complete treatment or comply fully with medications) is unacceptable because it leads to sample bias and undermines the validity of statistical tests.[20,26] Furthermore, findings from analyses based on compliant subsamples are frequently inconsistent with those based on intention-to-treat samples.[27-29] The preferred strategy for unbiased analyses of study treatments is an intention-to-treat analysis,[26,30,31] which requires assessment of all subjects who are randomized, regardless of protocol deviation. However, in trials with high dropout and nonadherence rates, intention-to-treat analyses will be based, to a large de-

From the Division of Substance Abuse, Yale University School of Medicine, New Haven, Conn.

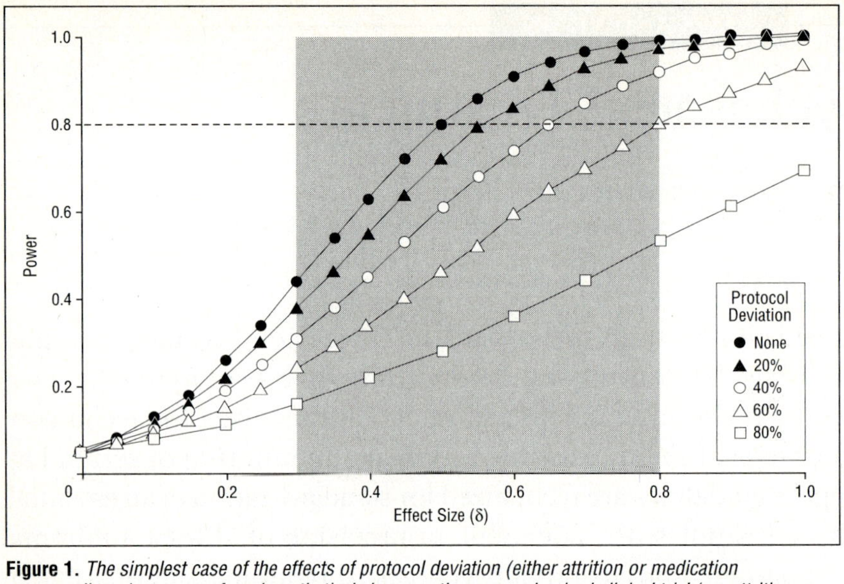

Figure 1. *The simplest case of the effects of protocol deviation (either attrition or medication noncompliance) on power for a hypothetical pharmacotherapy randomized clinical trial (eg, attrition or noncompliance considered as all-or-nothing events) (N=100 [medication, 50; placebo, 50]; α level set at .05 [1-tailed]).*

gree, on subjects who have had minimal, or even no, exposure to study treatments.

PSYCHOSOCIAL TREATMENT AS A STRATEGY TO PREVENT PROTOCOL DEVIATION

Prevention of protocol deviation is far preferable to coping with its effects. Two principal methods for the prevention of nonadherence are (1) the use of a "run-in" and (2) the use of procedures to foster better adherence. Run-ins reduce noncompliance by selecting patients who demonstrate their ability to adhere to the protocol.[32] However, because compliant subjects are often different from low compliers,[33] the ultimate result of a run-in is usually to reduce the generalizability of a study by evaluating treatment effects only on a select sample of compliant subjects.

The second strategy is to include procedures that foster protocol compliance. This recognizes that (1) the strategies that enhance protocol adherence in pharmacotherapy trials are principally psychosocial,[34] and (2) pharmacotherapies are necessarily delivered and evaluated within a psychosocial context. That the nature of that context can modify treatment adherence and outcome has long been recognized,[35-39] and numerous studies have established the strong influence of a psychosocial context on medication compliance and effects. For example, differences in outcome for methadone maintenance have been shown to be associated largely with program and staff characteristics.[40,41] Similarly, the addition of a primary care–based intervention that consisted of 4 brief visits to a physician and psychiatrist plus compliance monitoring resulted in antidepressant compliance rates of 88% compared with 57% for treatment as usual.[42]

There are few pharmacotherapy trials that include no psychosocial "context" whatsoever. An example would be a study in which the patients underwent a screening and were randomized to treatment, provided a study medication and instructions, and reassessed at termination, with little or no contact with staff in between. Here, unless the medication itself was highly reinforcing, the likelihood of achieving acceptable levels of compliance or retention would be low. At the other extreme would be a study that included a broad spectrum of procedures intended to enhance retention and compliance. These might include the following: regular monitoring of medication compliance through pill counts and medication serum levels; encouragement of patient self-monitoring of compliance (eg, medication diaries); extensive communication between the patient and staff about study medications, expected effects, side effects, and benefits; repeated stressing of the importance of adherence; contracting for adherence; direct reinforcement of adherence through incentives or rewards; provision of telephone or written reminders about appointments or taking medication; preparing and educating patients about the disorder and its treatment; and frequent contact and provision of extensive support and encouragement.[43-45] Such a study might approach full retention and compliance for patients who are assigned both to active medication and placebo treatment conditions. However, because compliance has been shown to have a positive effect on outcome, *even for placebo conditions*,[18,46,47] the inclusion of too intensive or broad a range of compliance-enhancing psychosocial interventions could produce ceiling effects and obscure the detection of medication effects (much as the lack of a psychosocial intervention could also obscure medication effects).

VARIABILITY IN PROVISION OF PSYCHOSOCIAL TREATMENTS

In practice, most pharmacotherapy trials fall somewhere between those extremes, in that some form of at least minimal psychosocial treatment is offered and intended to foster compliance and treatment retention. Inasmuch as the effectiveness of nonpharmacological aspects of treatment is of secondary interest in most pharmacotherapy trials, psychosocial components of treatment are rarely implemented according to current standards of psychotherapy research.[48] It is too often reported that a psychosocial treatment was offered, with only meager description of the type of therapy that was offered, its intensity, the therapy providers, or how much therapy the patients actually received.

A lack of specification of the psychosocial context in which medications are delivered is likely to increase the overall level of "noise" or variability in a pharmacotherapy trial for several reasons. First, when it is not specified or monitored, the provision of psychosocial treatment is likely to vary widely, with some patients receiving meager support, while others may receive fairly intensive treatment. Because the provision of psychotherapy has repeatedly been shown to affect adherence and outcome,[1,44-46,49] variability in the provision of nonpharmacological dimensions of treatment across patients is likely to lead to variability in protocol adherence and outcome. Moreover, the provision of psychotherapy may not be random, as patients in placebo conditions or who respond poorly to active medication may receive more ancillary care.

Second, the delivery of adequate dosing of study medications within the context of a clinical trial with psychiatric populations is often complex. Some patients may not be able to tolerate desired dosages, some report adverse effects that are difficult to attribute to the study medication, some require high levels of support, others have comorbid disorders that complicate treatment, and so on. Without clear guidelines about how to manage these issues, interventions are likely to vary across subjects and introduce noise into the conduct of the study.

Third, the failure to specify or monitor these dimensions may have a profound influence on the interpretation of outcome and, hence, on the detection of medication effects. Interventions that are usually included to foster greater retention and compliance with pharmacotherapy (eg, support and encouragement) are often seen as the "ground" against which medication effects are evaluated—in other words, necessary but essentially inert. However, the term *nonspecific* is not the same as *inert*.[50] Factors such as the patient-therapist relationship have been shown to have consistent and robust effect sizes that are often larger than the discernible effect of "active ingredients" of different psychotherapies.[51,52]

The effect of variability in the psychosocial context on power is illustrated in **Figure 2**, which presents power curves for the same hypothetical pharmacotherapy trial as for Figure 1. Particularly for what Cohen[53] would describe as medium pharmacotherapy effect sizes (d=0.3-.6), comparatively small increases in within-group variability would reduce power to a level such that medication effects, even if they existed,

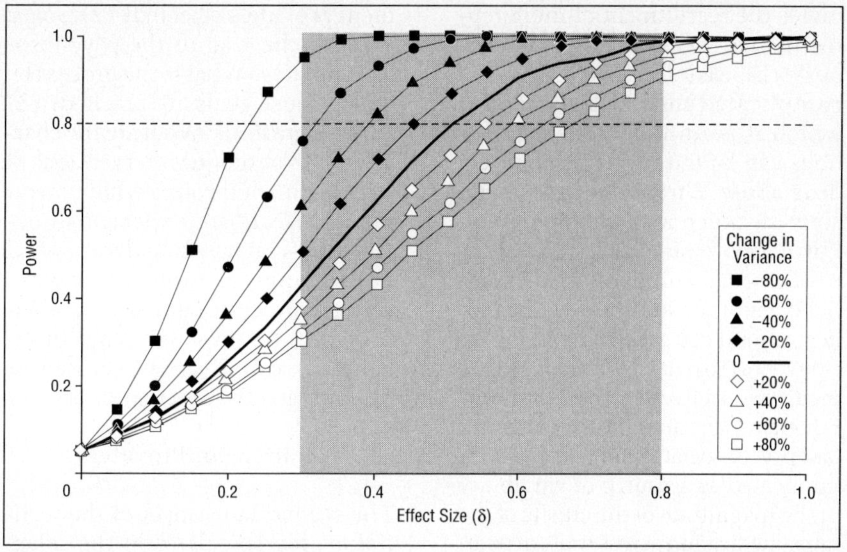

Figure 2. *Effect on power of reducing or increasing variance (N=100 [medication, 50; placebo, 50]; α level set at .05 [1-tailed]).*

would not be detectable. Conversely, modest reductions in noise variance (through a reduction of variability associated with the provision of psychosocial treatment) would increase power substantially. This effect is most pronounced for small-to-medium effects, in which many medication effects for psychiatric disorders lie. These estimates are hypothetical because direct systematic evaluation of the effect of controlled vs uncontrolled psychosocial treatment on variability in medication outcome has not yet been done (although the significance of this issue suggests it is a line that is worth pursuing). Moreover, these are likely to be conservative estimates, as data from a recent meta-analysis suggested that the effects of different therapists could account for as much as 73% of outcome variance and, on average, accounted for a medium effect size; furthermore, the use of manual-guided training was associated with reductions in this source of outcome variance.[54]

ETHICAL DILEMMAS ASSOCIATED WITH PLACEBO TREATMENTS

There is increasing criticism of placebo controls for those disorders in which a standard treatment exists.[55,56] It has been argued that it is unethical to withhold a known effective treatment; to evaluate new pharmacotherapies, a comparison of the novel medication with a standard or reference therapy is preferable.[57,58] However, without placebo controls, interpretation of findings is difficult in cases in which main effects between experimental and reference therapy are not found, and placebo controls continue to confer many advantages.

Moreover, for many types of mental disorders, a principally psychosocial treatment remains standard care, and withholding of a preferred psychosocial treatment—even in the context of powerful pharmacotherapies—requires full disclosure and consent, in addition to raising critical ethical concerns. A strictly medication-only study would be neither feasible nor ethical,[38,50] as it would withhold several dimensions of standard care for mental disorders. Not merely the provision, but also the standardization, of psychotherapy would promote consistent delivery of ethical care to treatment-seeking, symptomatic patients in placebo-controlled trials.

GENERALIZABILITY AND REPRODUCIBILITY

Generalizability of findings from pharmacotherapy trials may be limited when little attention is paid to the control of the psychosocial context. Klein[39] has noted that the embedding of pharmacotherapy trials within a psychotherapy framework promotes the recruitment of more representative samples. This is particularly the case for those chronic, complicated mental disorders in which it is unlikely that medications can be the sole treatment (eg, drug abuse, chronic posttraumatic stress disorder, and schizophrenia). Furthermore, standardization of the psychosocial context is also essential if results of studies are to be replicated, and can greatly aid in the interpretation of differences in medication effects across studies.[59] For example, variability in concomitant psychosocial treatments has been implicated as a source of variability in the magnitude of the effects of the same medication across trials of treatment of cocaine dependence.[60,61]

WHAT FEATURES SHOULD BE REQUIRED FOR PHARMACOTHERAPY TRIALS?

The technology model of psychotherapy research (ie, a strategy to reduce extraneous sources of variability in psychotherapy efficacy studies) specifies psychotherapies in a manner analogous to specification of a drug's formulation in pharmacological trials. This specification has greatly enhanced the ability of researchers to address differentiated questions concerning the conditions under which specified types of subjects will respond to particular types of treatments,[62] and has revolutionized the evaluation of the effectiveness of different forms of psychotherapy.[63] The following 3 key components of the technology model, each intended to reduce variability in the provision of treatment, are relevant to nearly all pharmacotherapy trials.

Standardization

Specification of treatment in manuals is a requirement of psychotherapy research[64] and has been used to provide both pharmacotherapies and psychotherapies uniformly in large-scale clinical trials.[65-67] Manuals define psychotherapies along several dimensions[68]: (1) *Structural*: What are the ideal and the minimum adequate number, duration, and frequency of sessions? Who provides the contact? How are treatment providers selected? (2) *Goals*: What is the goal of the psychosocial contacts? What is the process by which those goals are reached? (3) *Active ingredients*: What are the characteristics or unique interventions of this treatment through which therapeutic effects are expected to occur? (4) *Treatment boundaries*: What is the range of topics, interventions, or processes that would be expected to be present? What interventions would be proscribed or discouraged in this treatment?

Training of Providers

The second key aspect of the technology model relates to the selection and training of treatment providers. Training usually involves both didactic seminars and closely supervised "practice" cases, provided to help therapists modify their usual technique to adapt to manual guidelines. Training is supplemented with ongoing supervision to prevent therapist "drift" in the provision of treatment and to help therapists manage difficult cases in a manner that is consistent with the study protocol. Such training has been shown to foster consistent provision of treatment after even a single training case for experienced therapists.[69-71] Moreover, the perception that experienced pharmacotherapists do not need training to deliver pharmacotherapy uniformly and skillfully was contradicted by experience in the National Institute of Mental Health Treatment of Depression Collaborative Research Program, where, contrary to expectations, pharmacotherapists actually required more training and supervision than did psychotherapists to deliver pharmacotherapy competently and consistently.[72]

Monitoring of the Provision of Treatment

Akin to the monitoring of serum levels of medications to assess patients' compliance with pharmacotherapy, the monitoring of the provision of psychotherapy entails assessment of (1) patient participation in treatment sessions and (2) adequacy of treatment implementation, including both adherence (eg, Did the therapist follow the treatment manual?) and competence (eg, Did she or he do so skillfully?).[66,72-74] This typically requires the monitoring of taped treatment sessions, but less costly methods (eg, a therapist's self-monitoring of adherence) may be possible.[75] Even minimal compliance checks, if done randomly, are likely to produce greater compliance by providers and thus reduce variability in the provision of treatment.

WHAT TYPES OF PSYCHOSOCIAL TREATMENT ARE APPROPRIATE FOR PHARMACOTHERAPY TRIALS?

While application of the methodological features associated with the technology model may confer a number of advantages to the rigor and precision of pharmacotherapy trials, the appropriate selection of the psychosocial intervention itself is also of great importance. The advent of the technology model has enhanced the identification of specific psychosocial therapies that are relevant to pharmacological researchers in several ways. First, detailed treatment manuals that describe clearly defined principles and techniques that can address specific target problems for a variety of disorders are widely available. Second, there is a much greater variety of empirically validated treatments available that are compatible with pharmacotherapy and thus appropriate for use in pharmacotherapy trials.[76-78]

In general, cost and power considerations would encourage the selection of the lowest intensity treatment appropriate for the study population, medication type, and research questions that are being addressed. Minimal standards of acceptable psychosocial care will vary, of course, with different clinical populations and settings. For some clinical populations, standard psychosocial care can be fairly minimal (eg, nonrefractory, nonmelancholic depression), while in other populations, standard care may be comparatively intensive (eg, chronic schizophrenia with comorbid substance abuse).

An exemplary model of a low-intensity approach was developed by Fawcett and colleagues[79] to provide a standardized procedure for administration of imipramine or placebo in the National Institute of Mental Health Treatment of Depression Collaborative Research Program.[72] Clinical management[79] includes the specification of treatment goals (ie, medication management and enhancement of compliance and retention), concrete guidelines for the conduct of sessions, prescription of study medication, management of side effects, and, most important, the interpersonal context. The manual also specifies interventions that are prescribed to produce the desired relationship and outcomes (ie, support, advice, and encouragement), as well as proscribed behaviors of therapists. Thus, this type of approach can be conceived as forming the minimal "base" to which more targeted or intensive interventions could be added, as indicated.

Finally, the anticipation of a small medication effect is often invoked as a reason for not including a psychotherapy component (as it might reduce the differences between the active and placebo conditions). However, while a robust or intensive psychosocial treatment could overwhelm pharmacotherapy effects, minimal psychosocial interventions would not do so. If standardized and provided consistently, they would only add a "constant" to the medication conditions. Moreover, a psychotherapy's effect on reducing the differences between the active and placebo conditions would be offset by its advantages, particularly in protecting internal validity and power. It should also be noted that negative effects of psychotherapy and pharmacotherapy combinations have rarely been seen.[80,81]

IS THE COST JUSTIFIED?

Beyond adding complexity, a potential drawback for the addition of standardized psychotherapy in a pharmacotherapy trial is cost. However, expenses associated with standardizing psychosocial treatment should be evaluated in the context of other costs of any pharmacological trial. Recruitment, screening, and assessment of single subjects can cost thousands of dollars in staff and laboratory expenses, irrespective of the cost of the treatment itself. Because of the need to provide adequate clinical care to patients, costs for clinical personnel are built into most studies. The argument here is that the provision of that contact should be systematized and monitored. Therefore, additional expenses associated with the model would be limited chiefly to clinician training and treatment monitoring.

Estimating clinical and research-related costs in an outpatient randomized clinical trial at $5000 per patient, returning to the hypothetical randomized clinical trial with 100 patients, the total direct costs would be approximately $500 000. If the rates of attrition and noncompliance are assumed to be 30% and 40%, respectively, the total level of protocol deviation, might be approximately 50% (assuming there is some overlap between subjects who drop out and those who are noncompliant) for an effective loss of about 50 patients, or $250 000.

Next, estimating that the provision of standardized psychosocial treatment reduces the level of total protocol deviation by 25%, savings would be approximately $125 000. These savings would be offset by the cost of training and monitoring of the treatments, estimated at our center at $30 000, or $300 per patient.[67,68] Thus, the expenses associated with manual-guided psychosocial treatment, training, and monitoring of implementation are likely to be small compared with the costs of lost subjects, lost data, noise variance, reduced power, reduced replicability, and undermining of internal validity for which these methods are not used. Manual-guided psychosocial treatment should be a virtual requirement of pharmcotherapy trials, on par with essential design elements (eg, randomization and placebo controls).

Accepted for publication October 8, 1996.

This study was supported by grants P50-DA09241 and K02-DA00248 from the National Institute on Drug Abuse, Rockville, Md.

The comments of Bruce Rounsaville, MD, Alan Feingold, PhD, and Charla Nich, MS, are gratefully appreciated.

Reprints: Kathleen M. Carroll, PhD, Division of Substance Abuse, 34 Park St, Substance Abuse Center 208, New Haven, CT 06519.

REFERENCES

1. Clum GA, Clum GA, Surls R. A meta-analysis of treatments for panic disorder. *J Consult Clin Psychol.* 1993;61:317-326.
2. Conte HR, Plutchik R, Wild KV, Karasu TB. Combined psychotherapy and pharmacotherapy for depression: a systematic analysis of the evidence. *Arch Gen Psychiatry.* 1986;43:471-479.
3. Greist J, Chouinard G, DuBoff E, Halaris A, Kim SW, Koran L, Liebowitz M, Lydierd B, Rasmussen S, White K, Sikes C. Double-blind parallel comparison of three dosages of sertraline and placebo in outpatient with obsessive-compulsive disorder. *Arch Gen Psychiatry.* 1995;52:289-295.
4. Mitchell JE, Raymond N, Specker S. A review of the controlled trials of pharmacotherapy and psychotherapy in the treatment of bulimia nervosa. *Int J Eat Disord.* 1993;14:229-247.
5. Reynolds CF, Frank E, Perel JM, Imber SD, Cernes C, Morycz RK, Mazumdar S, Miller MD, Pollock BG, Rifai AN. Combined pharmacotherapy and psychotherapy in the acute and continuation treatment of elderly patients with recurrent major depression: a preliminary report. *Am J Psychiatry.* 1992;149:1687-1692.
6. Stack JA, Paradis CF, Reynolds CF, Houck PR, Frank E, Anderson B, Mayo AL, Miller MD, Rifai AH, Perel JM. Does recruitment method make a difference? effects on protocol retention and treatment outcome in elderly depressed patients. *Psychiatry Res.* 1995;56:17-24.
7. Callahan EJ. The treatment of heroin addiction: naltrexone alone with behavior therapy. *Am J Drug Alcohol Abuse.* 1980;7:795-807.
8. Cornelius JR, Soloff PH, Perel JM, Ulrich RF. Continuation pharmacotherapy of borderline personality disorder with haloperidol and phenelzine. *Am J Psychiatry.* 1993;150:1843-1848.
9. Cowdry RW, Gardner DL. Pharmacotherapy of borderline personality disorder: alprazolam, carbamazepine, trifluoperazine, and tranylcypromine. *Arch Gen Psychiatry.* 1988;45:111-119.
10. Mason BJ, Ritvo EC, Morgan RO, Salvato FR, Goldberg G, Welch B, Mantero-Atienza E. A double-blind, placebo-controlled pilot study to evaluate the efficacy and safety of oral nalmefene HCl for alcohol dependence. *Alcohol Clin Exp Res.* 1994; 18:1162-1167.
11. Sackett DL, Snow JC. The magnitude of compliance and noncompliance. In: Haynes RB, Taylor DW, Sackett DL, eds. *Compliance in Health Care.* Baltimore, Md: Johns Hopkins University Press; 1979:chap 1.
12. Kelly GR, Scott JE. Medication compliance and health education among outpatients with chronic mental disorders. *Med Care.* 1990;28:1181-1197.
13. Kupfer DJ, Perel JM, Frank E. Adequate treatment with imipramine in continuation treatment. *J Clin Psychiatry.* 1989;50:250-255.
14. Meterissian GB, Bradwejn J. Comparative studies on the efficacy of psychotherapy, pharmacotherapy, and their combination in depression: was adequate pharmacotherapy provided? *J Clin Psychopharmacol.* 1989;9:334-339.
15. Ballenger J, Burrows G, Dupont R, Lesser IM, Noyes R, Pecknold JC, Rifkin A, Swinson RP. Alprazolam in agoraphobia with panic attacks and panic disorder: results from a multicenter trial. *Arch Gen Psychiatry.* 1988;45:413-422.
16. Kane JM, Borenstein M. Compliance in the long-term treatment of schizophrenia. *Psychopharmacol Bull.* 1985;21:23-27.
17. Gelenberg A, Kane J, Keller M, Lavori P, Rosenbaum JF, Cole K, Lavelle J. Comparison of standard and low serum levels of lithium for mainte-

nance treatment of bipolar disorder. *N Engl J Med.* 1989;321:1489-1493.
18. Fuller RK, Branchey L, Brightwell DR, Derman RM, Emrick CD, Iber FL, James KE, Lacoursiere RB, Lee KK, Lowenstam I. Disulfiram treatment for alcoholism: a Veterans Administration cooperative study. *JAMA.* 1986;256:1449-1455.
19. Frank E, Kupfer DJ, Siegel LR. Alliance not compliance: a philosophy of outpatient care. *J Clin Psychiatry.* 1995;56(suppl 1):11-16.
20. Feinstein AR. 'Compliance bias' and the interpretation of therapeutic trials. In: Haynes RB, Taylor DW, Sackett DL, eds. *Compliance in Health Care.* Baltimore, Md: Johns Hopkins University Press; 1979:309-322.
21. Lackin JM, Foulkes MA. Evaluation of sample size and power for analyses of survival with allowance for nonuniform patient entry, losses to follow-up, noncompliance, and stratification. *Biometrics.* 1986;42:507-519.
22. Lakatos E. Sample size determination in clinical trials with time-dependent rates of losses and noncompliance. *Control Clin Trials.* 1986;7:189-199.
23. Freedman LS. The effect of partial noncompliance on the power of a clinical trial. *Control Clin Trials.* 1990;11:157-168.
24. Pledger GW. Compliance in clinical trials: impact on design, analysis, and interpretation. In: Schmidt D, Leppick IE, eds. *Compliance in Epilepsy.* Amsterdam, the Netherlands: Elsevier Science Publishers; 1988.
25. Goldsmith CH. The effect of compliance distributions on therapeutic trials. In: Haynes RB, Taylor DW, Sackett DL, eds. *Compliance in Health Care.* Baltimore, Md: Johns Hopkins University Press; 1979:297-308.
26. Lavori PW. Clinical trials in psychiatry: should protocol deviation censor patient data? *Neuropsychopharmacology.* 1992;6:39-48.
27. Lee YJ, Ellenberg JH, Hirtz DG, Nelson KB. Analysis of clinical trials by treatment actually received: is it really an option? *Stat Med.* 1991:10:1595-1605.
28. Newell DJ. Intention-to-treat analysis: implications for quantitative and qualitative research. *Int J Epidemiol.* 1992;21:837-841.
29. Nich C, Carroll KM. Now you see it, now you don't: a comparison of traditional versus random regression models in the analysis of longitudinal follow-up data from a clinical trial. *J Consult Clin Psychol.* 1997;65:252-261.
30. Kraemer HC, Pruyn JP, Gibbons RD, Greenhouse JB, Grochinski VJ, Waternaux C, Kupfer DJ. Methodology in psychiatric research: report on the 1986 MacArthur Foundation Network I Methodology Instititute. *Arch Gen Psychiatry.* 1987;44:1100-1106.
31. Rabeneck L, Viscoli CM, Horwitz RI. Problems in the conduct and analysis of randomized clinical trials: are we getting the right answers to the wrong questions? *Arch Intern Med.* 1992;152:507-512.
32. Lang JM. The use of a run-in to enhance compliance. *Stat Med.* 1990;9:87-95.
33. Hennekens CH, Buring JE. Methodologic considerations in the design and conduct of randomized trials: the U.S. Physicians' Health Study. *Control Clin Trials.* 1989;10:142S-150S.
34. Epstein LH, Cluss PA. A behavioral medicine perspective on adherence to long-term medical regimens. *J Consult Clin Psychol.* 1982;50:950-971.
35. Howard K, Rickels K, Mock JE, Lipman RS, Covi L, Baumm NC. Therapeutic syle and attrition rate from psychiatric drug treatment. *J Nerv Ment Dis.* 1970;150:102-110.
36. Klerman GL. Assessing the influence of the hosptial milieu upon the effectiveness of psychiatric drug therapy: problems of conceptualization and of research methodology. *J Nerv Ment Dis.* 1963; 137:143-154.
37. Uhlenhuth EH, Lipman RS, Covi L. Combined pharmacotherapy and psychotherapy: controlled studies. *J Nerv Ment Dis.* 1969;148:52-64.
38. Elkin I, Pilkonis PA, Docherty JP, Sotsky SM. Conceptual and methodological issues in comparative studies of psychotherapy and pharmacotherapy, I: active ingredients and mechanisms of change. *Am J Psychiatry.* 1988;145:909-917.
39. Klein DF. Improvement of phase III psychotropic drug trials by intensive phase II work. *Neuropsychopharmacology.* 1991;5:251-258.
40. Ball JC, Ross A. *The Effectiveness of Methadone Maintenance Treatment.* New York, NY: Springer-Verlag NY Inc; 1991.
41. McLellan AT, Arndt IO, Metzger DS, Woody GE, O'Brien CP. The effects of psychosocial services in substance abuse treatment. *JAMA.* 1993;269: 1953-1959.
42. Katon W, Von Korff MV, Lin E, Walker E, Simon GE, Bush T, Robinson P, Russo J. Collaborative managment to achieve treatment guidelines: impact on depression in primary care. *JAMA.* 1995; 273:1026-1031.
43. DiMatteo RM, DiNicola DD. *Achieving Patient Compliance.* Elmsford, NY: Pergamon Press Inc; 1982.
44. Haynes RB, Taylor DW, Sackett DL, eds. *Compliance in Health Care.* Baltimore, Md: Johns Hopkins University Press; 1979.
45. Meichenbaum D, Turk DC, eds. *Facilitating Treatment Adherence.* New York, NY: Plenum Publishing Corp; 1987.
46. Horwitz RI, Horwitz SM. Adherence to treatment and health outcomes. *Arch Intern Med.* 1993;153: 1863-1868.
47. Fawcett J, Clark DC, Aagesen CA, Pisani VD, Tilkin JM, Sellers D, McGuire M, Gibbens RD. A double-blind, placebo-controlled trial of lithium carbonate therapy for alcoholism. *Arch Gen Psychiatry.* 1987;44:248-256.
48. Waskow IE. Specification of the technique variable in the NIMH Treatment of Depression Collaborative Research Program. In: Williams JBW, Spitzer RL, eds. *Psychotherapy Research: Where Are We and Where Should We Go?* New York, NY: Guilford Press; 1984.
49. Meyer RE, Mirin SM, Altman JL, McNamee HB. A behavioral paradigm for the evaluation of narcotic antagonists. *Arch Gen Psychiatry.* 1976;33: 371-377.
50. Lambert MJ, Bergin AE. The effectiveness of psychotherapy. In: Bergin AE, Garfield SL, eds. *Handbook of Psychotherapy and Behavior Change.* 4th ed. New York, NY: John Wiley & Sons Inc; 1994: chap 7.
51. Horvath AO, Luborsky L. The role of the therapeutic alliance in psychotherapy. *J Consult Clin Psychol.* 1993;61:561-573.
52. Luborsky L, McLellan AT, Woody GE, O'Brien CP, Auerbach A. Therapist success and its determinants. *Arch Gen Psychiatry.* 1985;42:602-611.
53. Cohen J. *Statistical Power Analysis for the Behavioral Sciences.* 2nd ed. Hillsdale, NJ: Lawrence Erlbaum Associates Inc; 1988.
54. Crits-Christoph P, Baranackie K, Kurcias J, Beck AT, Carroll K, Perry K, Luborsky L, McLellan AT, Woody GE, Thompson L, Gallagher D, Zitrin C. Meta-analysis of therapist effects in psychotherapy outcome studies. *Psychother Res.* 1991;1:81-91.
55. Freedman B. Equipoise and the ethics of clinical research. *N Engl J Med.* 1987;317:141-145.
56. Schafer A. The ethics of the randomized clinical trial. *N Engl J Med.* 1982;307:719-724.
57. Levine RJ. The use of placebos in randomized clinical trials. *IRB Rev Hum Subst Res.* 1985;7:1-4.
58. Rothman KJ, Michels KB. The continued unethical use of placebo controls. *N Engl J Med.* 1994; 331:394-398.
59. Kraemer HC, Pruyn JP. The evaluation of different approaches to randomized clinical trials: report on the 1987 MacArthur Foundation Network I Methodology Workshop. *Arch Gen Psychiatry.* 1990;47:1163-1169.
60. Levin FR, Lehman AF. Meta-analysis of desipramine as an adjunct in the treatment of cocaine addiction. *J Clin Psychopharmacol.* 1991;11:374-378.
61. Meyer RE. New pharmacotherapies for cocaine dependence . . . revisited. *Arch Gen Psychiatry.* 1992; 49:900-904.
62. Williams JBW, Spitzer RL, eds. *Psychotherapy Research: Where Are We and Where Should We Go?* New York, NY: Guilford Press; 1984.
63. Luborsky L, DeRubeis RJ. The use of psychotherapy treatment manuals: a small revolution in psychotherapy research style. *Clin Psychol Rev.* 1984;4:5-15.
64. Kazdin AE. Methods of psychotherapy research. In: Bongar B, Beutler LE, eds. *Comprehensive Textbook of Psychotherapy: Theory and Practice.* New York, NY: Oxford University Press Inc; 1995: chap 11.
65. Elkin I, Shea MT, Watkins JT, Imber SD, Sotsky SM, Collins JF, Glass DR, Pilkonis PD, Leber WR, Docherty JP, Fiester SJ, Parloff MD. National Institute of Mental Health Treatment of Depression Collaborative Research Program: general effectiveness of treatments. *Arch Gen Psychiatry.* 1989; 46:971-982.
66. Hill CE, O'Grady KE, Elkin I. Applying the Collaborative Study Psychotherapy Rating Scale to rate therapist adherence in cognitive-behavior therapy, interpersonal therapy, and clinical management. *J Consult Clin Psychol.* 1992;60:73-79.
67. Carroll KM, Kadden R, Donovan D, Zweben D, Rounsaville BJ. Implementing treatment and protecting the validity of the independent variable in treatment matching studies. *J Stud Alcohol.* 1994; suppl 12:149-155.
68. Carroll KM, Nuro K. Treatment manuals and treatment compliance. In: Carroll KM, ed. *Facilitating Compliance in Alcohol Treatment.* Rockville, Md: National Institute on Alcoholism and Alcohol Abuse. In press. National Institute on Alcoholism and Alcohol Abuse Project MATCH Monograph Series.
69. Chevron E, Rounsaville BJ. Evaluating the clinical skills of psychotherapists: a comparison of techniques. *Arch Gen Psychiatry.* 1983;40:1129-1132.
70. Rounsaville BJ, Chevron E, Weissman MM, Prusoff BA, Frank E. Training therapists to perform interpersonal psychotherapy in clinical trials. *Compr Psychiatry.* 1986;27:364-371.
71. Weissman MM, Rounsaville BJ, Chevron E. Training psychotherapists to participate in psychotherapy outcome studies. *Am J Psychiatry.* 1982; 139:1442-1446.
72. Elkin I, Parloff MB, Hadley SW, Autry JH. NIMH Treatment of Depression Collaborative Research Program: background and research plan. *Arch Gen Psychiatry.* 1985;42:305-316.
73. Waltz J, Addis ME, Koerner K, Jacobson NS. Testing the integrity of a psychotherapy protocol: assessment of adherence and competence. *J Consult Clin Psychol.* 1993;61:620-630.
74. DiClemente C, Carroll KM, Connors G, Kadden R. Process assessment in treatment matching research. *J Stud Alcohol.* 1994;12(suppl):156-162.
75. Carroll KM, Rounsaville BJ, Nich C. Use of observer and therapist ratings to monitor delivery of coping skills treatment for cocaine abusers: utility of therapist session checklists. *Psychother Res.* In press.
76. Beck AT, Rush AJ, Shaw BF, Emery G. *Cognitive Therapy of Depression.* New York, NY: Guilford Press; 1979.
77. Klerman GL, Weissman MM, Rounsaville BJ, Chevron ES. *Interpersonal Psychotherapy of Depression.* New York, NY: Basic Books Inc Publishers; 1984.
78. Luborsky L. *Principles of Psychoanalytic Psychotherapy: A Manual for Supportive-Expressive (SE) Treatment.* New York, NY: Basic Books Inc Publishers; 1984.
79. Fawcett J, Epstein P, Fiester SJ, Elkin I, Autry JH. Clinical management—imipramine/placebo administration manual: NIMH Treatment of Depression Collaborative Research Program. *Psychopharmacol Bull.* 1987;23:309-324.
80. Klerman GL, Weissman MM, Markowitz J, Glick I, Wilner PJ, Mason B, Shear MK. Medication and psychotherapy 1&2. In: Bergin AE, Garfield SL, eds. *Handbook of Psychotherapy and Behavior Change.* 4th ed. New York, NY: John Wiley & Sons Inc; 1994.
81. Rounsaville BJ, Klerman GL, Weissman MM. Do psychotherapy and pharmacotherapy for depression conflict? empirical evidence from a clinical trial. *Arch Gen Psychiatry.* 1981;38:24-29.

A Psychotherapeutic Context for Clinical Trials Is Promising, But Manualization Is Not

IN THIS issue of the ARCHIVES, Carroll[1] argues for a psychotherapeutic context, standardized by manualization, for pharmacotherapy trials. This may well succeed in lowering the attrition rate and improving compliance,[2] but the superiority of detailed manuals over goal-oriented, supportive therapy has not been demonstrated. Therefore, standardization by manuals is premature.

THE ADOPTION OF MANUALS

Manual-based psychotherapy has become standard in psychotherapy research, to provide a distinct, operationalized, replicable structure. In comparative psychotherapy trials, manuals ensure adequate differentiation between therapies, thus allowing strong statements as to what was actually done.[3,4] However, since it has not been shown that manuals increase the treatment efficacy or diminish outcome variance, their required use compared with manual-free, supportive psychotherapy has not been shown to be necessary. Such a manual requirement may expensively address a nonexistent problem.

See also page 923

RESEARCH ON THE EFFICACY OF MANUALS

Schulte et al[5] compared the treatment of phobia using manualized exposure therapy vs nonmanualized psychotherapy. The subjects given manualized treatment fared the best; however, the subjects who received nonmanualized psychotherapy and happened to receive exposure therapy did as well as the subjects who received manualized treatment. It was the group of patients who received nonmanualized psychotherapy and lacked exposure therapy that accounted for group differences. Furthermore, a study of obsessive-compulsive disorder by Emmelkamp and colleagues[6] found no differences between structured exposure with response prevention therapy and individualized treatment. This suggests that strategic planning for exposure-responsive disorders (eg, simple phobia and obsessive-compulsive disorder) could suffice without manualization. A study by Jacobson and colleagues[7] compared highly structured vs individualized, flexible forms of social learning–based marital therapy. There were no significant differences at the end of the trial, but at 6-month follow-up, the subjects who were treated with individualized therapy were less likely to have experienced a relapse. In a meta-analysis of child and adolescent psychotherapy, Weisz and colleagues[8] found no significant difference in the mean effect size between structured and unstructured therapy studies.

Much of the literature consists of theoretical rather than empirical justifications of manuals.[9,10] Wilson[9] supports their use by citing research on the fallibility of clinical judgment; yet, these arguments may not apply to goal-oriented treatment plans. Luborsky and DeRubeis,[10(p10)] although proponents of manuals, noted that "qualities not explicitly described in a manual may turn out to be those qualities that are most crucial to the success of the therapy."

Roth and Fonagy[11(p42)] noted that, "the capacity of the therapist to achieve [manual] adherence depended, at least to some extent, on the patient's orientation to and willingness to accept the technique. The same therapist sometimes carried out the therapy 'well,' sometimes less so." This suggests that manual adherence is not a characteristic of superior therapists; rather, a lack of adherence is due to poor therapeutic progress or a bad match of therapy with patient.

MANUALS AND THERAPIST EFFECTS

Carroll[1] cites Crits-Christoph et al[12] as demonstrating that manuals diminish therapist effects. However, of the 27 studies in that meta-analysis,[12] two thirds were psychodynamic. There was a substantial negative correlation between the length of treatment and manualization. This correlation renders any causal interpretation suspect since longer treatments (less manualization) seem likely to incur larger therapist effects. In addition, 8 of the 9 cognitive treatments vs 5 of the 18 psychodynamic treatments were manualized. Thus, the manualization effect may actually reflect a type of treatment effect. The authors[12] attempt to handle this by partialing, but this is problematic with heavily skewed 2×2 tables.

DISADVANTAGES OF MANUALS

Many therapists argue that manualization impedes clinical flexibility and increases training costs.[13] There may be other disadvantages. Henry and colleagues[14] studied therapist behaviors associated with training in manualized, time-limited dynamic psychotherapy. They found an increase in the therapeutic elements emphasized in time-limited dynamic psychotherapy training;

however, there was also a statistically significant decrease in the expression of optimism and support, less time was spent assessing feelings, and the therapy had a more authoritarian tone. A follow-up study found that the therapists who adhered most strictly to the guidelines of the manual were the most likely to express hostility during therapy sessions.[15]

Svartberg and Stiles[16] studied short-term anxiety-provoking psychotherapy, which is a focused, psychoanalytically oriented treatment that was developed by Sifneos[17] for the resolution of oedipal, separation, and grief problems. The principal therapist strategies were anxiety-provoking clarifications and confrontations during a 20-week period. Symptomatic improvement was negatively correlated with ratings of manual adherence. The authors suggest that rigidity may be the deleterious element.

Research has not established the outcome superiority of manualized over nonmanualized forms. This should be investigated before any required adoption for pharmacotherapy trials. This also raises questions regarding the design of comparative psychotherapy trials, which have rarely systematically compared degrees of therapeutic structure.

Jacobson and colleagues[18] recently did a large dismantling study of the complex cognitive treatment of depression. The manualized cognitive therapy was not superior to its behavioral activation component. Drastic simplification of this treatment did not lessen its efficacy. Thus, it is unlikely that deviation from a manualized framework, in nonessential detail, has a significant impact, and it is not clear what the essential details are.

It is debatable whether there are "active ingredients" that are specific to various psychotherapies. Evidence for outcome superiority has been found primarily for behavioral, exposure-focused treatments of avoidant conditions. If significant outcome differences are rarely found in comparisons of psychotherapies, there is no a priori reason for concern that within-treatment psychotherapeutic variations may increase variability or skew effect sizes in pharmacotherapy trials. Supportive psychotherapy, including clarification, education, and raising of positive expectancies, without the use of manuals, would be a conservative, promising, preliminary initiative.

CONCLUSIONS

We agree that the development of such psychotherapeutic contexts for pharmacotherapy research is likely to lower dropout rates, promote compliance, and facilitate long-term follow-up. Furthermore, it seems ethically and empirically preferable to provide active treatment of subjects given placebo.[2] However, mandating the adoption of specific manualized guidelines is premature and may be counterproductive for establishing such psychotherapeutic contexts. Less expensive innovations are more likely to be accepted than more expensive ones.

However, this advance need not await the series of manualized vs nonmanualized therapy trials that are needed to empirically determine the best strategy. Less expensive, antidemoralizing psychotherapeutic contexts should be introduced while awaiting definitive findings. Each research center could make an initial appraisal by estimating, in comparable trials, whether their attrition rate, compliance, and effect sizes have improved.

Donald F. Klein, MD
Department of Psychiatry
Columbia University College of Physicians and Surgeons and New York State Psychiatric Institute
722 W 68th St, Room L-224
New York, NY 10032
Lauren B. Smith
New York

This work was supported in part by grant MH-30906 from the Public Health Service, Washington, DC.

REFERENCES

1. Carroll KM. Manual-guided psychosocial treatment: a new virtual requirement for pharmacotherapy trials? *Arch Gen Psychiatry.* 1997;54:923-928.
2. Klein DF. Improvement of phase III psychotropic drug trials with intensive phase II work. *Neuropsychopharmacology.* 1991;4:251-258.
3. Luborsky L, Woody G, McLellan AT, O'Brien CP, Rosenzweig J. Can independent judges recognize different psychotherapies? *J Consult Clin Psychol.* 1982;50:49-62.
4. Elkin I, Parloff MB, Hadley SW, Autry JH. NIMH Treatment of Depression Collaborative Research Program: background and research program. *Arch Gen Psychiatry.* 1985;42:305-316.
5. Schulte D, Kunzel R, Pepping G, Schulte-Bahrenberg T. Tailor-made versus standardized therapy of phobic patients. *Adv Behav Res Ther.* 1992;14:67-92.
6. Emmelkamp PM, Bouman TK, Blaauw E. Individualized versus standardized therapy: a comparative evaluation with obsessive-compulsive patients. *Clin Psychol Psychother.* 1994;1:95-100.
7. Jacobson NS, Schmaling KB, Holtzworth-Munroe A, Katt JL, Wood LF, Follette VM. Research-structured vs clinically flexible versions of social learning–based marital therapy. *Behav Res Ther.* 1989;27:173-180.
8. Weisz JR, Donenberg GR, Weiss B, Han SS. Bridging the gap between laboratory and clinic in child and adolescent psychotherapy. *J Clin Consult Psychol.* 1995;63:688-701.
9. Wilson GT. Manual-based treatments: the clinical application of research findings. *Behav Res Ther.* 1996;34:295-314.
10. Luborsky L, DeRubeis, RJ. The use of psychotherapy treatment manuals: a small revolution in psychotherapy research style. *Clin Psychol Rev.* 1984;4:5-14.
11. Roth A, Fonagy P. *What Works for Whom? A Critical Review of Psychotherapy Research.* New York, NY: Guilford Press; 1996.
12. Crits-Cristoph P, Baranackie K, Kurcias JS, Beck AT, Carroll K, Perry K, Luborsky L, McLellan AT, Woody GE, Thompson L, Gallagher D, Zitrin C. Meta-analysis of therapist effects in psychotherapy outcome studies. *Psychother Res.* 1991;1:81-91.
13. Dobson KS, Shaw BF. The use of treatment manuals in cognitive therapy: experience and issues. *J Consult Clin Psychol.* 1988;56:673-680.
14. Henry WP, Strupp HH, Butler SF, Schact TE, Binder JL. Effects of training in time-limited dynamic psychotherapy: changes in therapist behavior. *J Consult Clin Psychol.* 1993;61:434-440.
15. Henry WP, Schact TE, Strupp HH, Butler SF, Binder JL. Effects of training in time-limited dynamic psychotherapy: mediators of therapists' responses to training. *J Consult Clin Psychol.* 1993;61:441-447.
16. Svartberg M, Stiles TC. Therapeutic alliance, therapist competence, and client change in short-term anxiety-provoking psychotherapy. *Psychother Res.* 1994;4:20-33.
17. Sifneos PE. *Short-term Dynamic Psychotherapy: Evaluation and Technique.* New York, NY: Plenum Publishing Corp; 1979.
18. Jacobson NS, Dobson KS, Truax PA, Addis ME, Koerner K, Gollan JK, Gortner E, Prince SE. A component analysis of cognitive-behavioral treatment for depression. *J Consult Clin Psychol.* 1996; 64:294-304.

ORIGINAL ARTICLE

Offspring of Depressed Parents

10 Years Later

Myrna M. Weissman, PhD; Virginia Warner, MPH; Priya Wickramaratne, PhD; Donna Moreau, MD; Mark Olfson, MD

Background: There have been numerous studies that have shown that offspring of depressed parents are at a high risk for major depressive disorder (MDD) and impairment. None have followed up the offspring into adulthood to obtain more precise estimates of risk.

Method: One hundred eighty-two offspring from 91 families, in which 1 or more parents had MDD (high risk) or in which neither parent was depressed (low risk), were blindly reassessed in the third follow-up, using a structured diagnostic instrument 10 years after their initial identification.

Results: Compared with the offspring for whom neither parent was depressed, the offspring of depressed parents had increased rates of MDD, particularly before puberty, and phobias (both at approximately a 3-fold risk), panic disorder, alcohol dependence (at a 5-fold risk), and greater social impairment. The peak age at onset for MDD in both high- and low-risk offspring ranged from 15 to 20 years. The peak age at onset for anxiety disorder was considerably earlier, especially in female offspring in the high-risk group. The onset of alcohol dependence in the offspring in the high-risk group peaked in adolescence and then after the age of 25 years. The depressed offspring of depressed parents, compared with nondepressed parents, had more serious and impairing depressions during the follow-up period but were *less* likely to go for treatment.

Conclusions: The offspring of depressed parents are a high-risk group for onset of anxiety disorder and MDD in childhood, MDD in adolescence, and alcohol dependence in adolescence and early adulthood. The findings support the potential value of early detection in the offspring of depressed parents.

Arch Gen Psychiatry. 1997;54:932-940

From the Department of Psychiatry, College of Physicians and Surgeons of Columbia University (Drs Weissman, Wickramaratne, Moreau, and Olfson), and Division of Clinical and Genetic Epidemiology, New York State Psychiatric Institute (Drs Weissman, Wickramaratne, and Olfson and Ms Warner), New York, NY.

MAJOR DEPRESSIVE disorder (MDD) is highly prevalent, impairing, and familial.[1,2] Recent studies have shown that the onset of MDD initially occurs in persons at an early age, often in the age range from their teens to 20s, although it can occur prepubertally, and the most familial form is that of an early onset before the age of 20 years.[3-7] Major depressive disorder most frequently affects women in their childbearing years.[5,8] Thus, study of their offspring has treatment and public health implications.[9] The increased risk of MDD in the offspring of depressed parents has been well documented. Although some of these studies have been criticized on methodological grounds (eg, small samples, cross-sectional design, absence of control groups, or assessment of both biological parents), they all have shown an increased rate of MDD in the offspring of depressed parents. Two short-term (ie, 18 months and 3 years) longitudinal offspring studies have shown an increased and continuing risk of MDD for offspring of depressed parents.[10-12]

There have also been longitudinal studies of depressed children or adolescents. These studies have not included assessment of parental psychiatric status and control groups, and with few exceptions, the studies have not followed up the children into adulthood.[13-20] Longitudinal studies of depressed children, even those that include assessment of family psychiatric history,[21] unlike high-risk studies, cannot provide age-specific rates of illness onset. To calculate rates of onset, the follow-up of cohorts of patients who are not ill at the time of subject ascertainment is required.

We have been following up a cohort of offspring, for whom either 1 or both parents have MDD or for whom neither parent has MDD. At the initial interview, we found that the offspring (age range, 6-23 years) of depressed, compared with nondepressed, parents had a significantly increased risk for MDD, anxiety disorders, and markedly poorer overall functioning.[22-26]

METHODS

SAMPLE

The offspring were initially selected for the presence or absence of a lifetime history of MDD based on Research Diagnostic Criteria in their parents.[22,23] The depressed probands had received treatment at the Yale University Depression Research Unit, New Haven, Conn. The normal control subjects came from a 1975 community survey that was conducted in New Haven, and they had no history of psychiatric illness, based on at least 4 direct interviews (the last 2 used the Schedule for Affective Disorders and Schizophrenia–Lifetime version[31] during a 10-year period). All probands were white and group-matched for age and sex.

At the initial interview (time 1), the sample consisted of 220 offspring between the ages of 6 and 23 years from 91 families, including 153 offspring from 65 families with 1 or more depressed parent and 67 offspring from 26 families with neither parent depressed.[22]

Two years after the initial interview (time 2), all 91 families were contacted for a second interview. Eighty-five (93%) of the 91 families consented to participate. Of the 220 offspring interviewed at time 1, 174 (79%) of them were reinterviewed at time 2.[26] An additional sample of 43 offspring who were not age-eligible at time 1 were interviewed also, but they are not described in the present study.

Ten years after the initiation of the study (time 10), families were recontacted for a reassessment. Among the 220 offspring interviewed at time 1, there were 2 deaths, and 1 offspring was found to have Down syndrome. Eighty-four percent (182/217) of those offspring who were interviewed at time 1 were reinterviewed at time 10. There were 4 deaths among the 91 probands who were eligible to be interviewed. Of the remaining 87 living probands, 73 (84%) were interviewed. Sixty-six spouses of probands were eligible to be interviewed. There were 5 deaths, and of the remaining 61 living spouses, 52 (85%) were interviewed. There were no deaths by suicide. There were no significant differences in the attrition rate of probands, spouses, or offspring by parental status.

Attrition for the probands and spouses did not vary significantly by sex or age. Attrition of offspring did not differ by sex. However, at time 10, older offspring were more likely to be interviewed than younger offspring (mean age, 28.5 vs 26.4 years; $t=-2.09$; $df=54.9$; $P=.04$). There were 2 first onsets of MDD (determined by use of the independent best estimate [BE] diagnosis that was made, blind to initial proband and offspring data) in the spouses in the nondepressed group between times 2 and 10. These 2 families had 4 offspring and were reassigned to the groups of depressed parents.

ASSESSMENT

Probands, spouses of probands, and offspring were independently interviewed with the Schedule for Affective Disorders and Schizophrenia–Lifetime version that was modified to include Research Diagnostic Criteria and *DSM-III* and *DSM-III-R* criteria.[32] All interviews of offspring were conducted blind to the parents' status and the offsprings' previous assessments. The interview covered a period of assessment from the last interview until the present and included the following additional data. Overall functioning was assessed by the interviewer on the Global Assessment Scale.[33] The Global Assessment Scale is scored on a scale from 0 to 100, with lower scores indicating impairment in overall functioning. Life charts were used to record all episodes of illness that occurred during the period of assessment. Adults completed the Social Adjustment Scale–Self-Report, which contained questions in major areas of functioning on a 4-point scale, with a higher score indicating more impairment.[34]

INTERVIEWERS

Interviewers (ie, PhD- and master's-level experienced mental health professionals) were located in Connecticut, where most of the subjects lived. The training of the interviewers took place during 4 group sessions (each session was 8 hours) and included supervised field interviews. Periodic interviews were monitored by the supervisor to limit interviewer drift. Interviewers participated in joint interviews in which 1 interviewer conducted the interview and the other corated the interview. A total of 80 cases were corated (in all possible pairs) by 4 interviewers at time 10. Using probable or definite *DSM-III-R* criteria, κ coefficients (SEs) were as follows: MDD, 0.78 (0.09); panic disorder, 0.79 (0.20); any anxiety, 0.65 (0.12); suicide attempts, 0.80 (0.11); alcohol abuse or dependence, 0.81 (0.09); drug abuse or dependence, 0.96 (0.03); and any psychiatric disorder, 0.80 (0.07).[35]

THE BE DIAGNOSIS

Diagnoses of offspring were based on the BE procedure.[36] To derive the BE diagnoses, an experienced clinician who was not involved in the interviewing, and who was blind to the diagnostic status of the parent and the previous assessments, independently reviewed all available information, including direct and informant interviews and medical records that were obtained at time 10, and assigned a *DSM-III-R* diagnosis for each offspring. A similar procedure was completed for parents who were independent and blind to offspring data. Six clinicians (3 psychiatrists, 2 psychologists, and 1 psychiatric nurse) with extensive diagnostic experience completed the BE diagnosis procedure. If there was disagreement, a consensus diagnosis was made. One hundred seventy-three cases across 3 samples using the same procedures and best estimators were reviewed independently by a second best estimator who was also blind. The number of cases for the second review was determined by calculating the number of cases necessary to have an 80% chance to detect a 0.2 difference between κ coefficients. Using probable or definite *DSM-III-R* criteria, κ coefficients (SEs) were as follows: MDD, 0.86 (0.03); panic disorder, 0.88 (0.11); any anxiety, 0.68 (0.06); suicidal behavior or attempts, 0.80 (0.07); alcohol abuse or dependence, 0.92 (0.03); drug abuse or dependence, 0.89 (0.03); any psychiatric disorder, 0.85 (0.04); and no history of mental illness, 0.80 (0.06).

The diagnoses used for this study were cumulative across times 1, 2, and 10. At times 1 and 2, *DSM-III* criteria were used. At time 10, *DSM-III-R* criteria was used. Impairment was considered to be a necessary criterion. Offspring were considered to be impaired if they sought treatment, took medication, were hospitalized, or had impaired functioning at work, school, or home.

DATA ANALYSIS

Sample differences in the means of continuous outcomes, by parental MDD, were tested by use of the *t* test and, for

Continued on next page

categorical outcomes, by use of the the χ^2 test. To test for the potential confounding effects of age and sex for continuous outcomes (ie, Social Adjustment Scale–Self-Report, number of days that person was depressed), a procedure for unbalanced analysis of covariance (Statistical Analysis System General Linear Model, SAS Institute Inc, Cary, NC)[37] was used to assess the means by parental MDD with the age and sex of the offspring in the model. The age and sex of the offspring were retained in the model if they were significant at the .05 level. Cross-sectional categorical data (eg, treatment, parental MDD) were examined by use of maximum likelihood logistic regressions (using the SAS LOGISTIC procedure), controlling for the age and sex of the offspring.[37] The antilogarithm of the regression coefficient for parental MDD yields an odds ratio (OR) for evaluating the magnitude of the association with parental MDD. Cumulative lifetime rates of disorder were computed in each of the 2 groups (at high and low risk) using standard methods of survival analysis.[38] These methods were adjusted for the fact that (1) the risk of disorder varied with the age of the offspring, (2) there was a wide variation in the ages of the offspring at the end of the follow-up period (age range, 16-34 years), and (3) the age distribution of the offspring in the 2 groups may have varied. A limitation of this method is that at the older ages, there may be relatively few offspring at risk; as a result, onsets of disorder at these ages may artificially inflate the estimates of cumulative survival rates. The equality of survival distributions for the offspring of depressed parents compared with that of the offspring of nondepressed parents was tested by means of the log rank test for homogeneity, which weighs greater survival times more heavily, and by means of the Wilcoxon test, which places more weight on early survival times. The age-specific incidence rates of psychiatric disorder were estimated in 5-year intervals using the life-table method.[39] Where there were a sufficient number of cases of psychiatric disorder, the Cox multivariate proportional hazards model was used to assess the rates of psychiatric disorder by parental MDD with the age and sex of the offspring in the model.[40] The proportional hazards model applies the multiple regression method to a survival distribution and yields a ratio of the hazards of the outcome variables (ie, offspring diagnoses) for groups of interest (ie, parental MDD).

Two years later, the differences between the groups of offspring were more pronounced, with the offspring of depressed parents continuing to have an increased incidence of depression, high recurrence rates, and slower recovery.[27-29] Although there were few differences in symptom profiles among the depressed offspring by the clinical status of the parents, there were striking age-at-onset differences. All the prepubertal onsets occurred in the offspring of depressed parents who themselves had early onsets (age, <20 years).[24] There were no sex differences in the rates of prepubertal-onset MDD. After puberty, the female offspring showed a marked increase in onset of MDD that peaked between the ages of 15 and 20 years. For the male offspring, there was a gradual rise in onset after puberty.[29,30] The results also suggested that the depressed offspring of nondepressed parents have a different course of illness and that longer follow-up is required to capture clinically significant differences between the 2 groups.

The goal of the original study was to determine whether the lifetime rates of psychopathology (specifically MDD) in the offspring of depressed probands were greater than in the offspring of nondepressed parents. Comparisons were made in the overall lifetime rates of disorder (from birth to the time of interview) in the 2 groups. Because subjects were between the ages of 6 and 23 years, there was a wide variation in their stage of development at the first interview (time 1). As a consequence, many of the offspring at time 1 had not yet passed through the critical period of risk for the onset of depression, and the estimates of age-specific risks were unstable. With the availability of the 10-year follow-up, more precise estimates can be made of age-specific and cumulative lifetime rates.

Table 1. Demographic Characteristics of Probands (Parents) at Time 10 by Parental Diagnosis*

	Parental Diagnosis				
Characteristic	≥1 With MDD (n=52)	Neither Had MDD (n=21)	Statistic†	df	P
Female, No. (%)	30 (58)	14 (67)	0.503	1	.47
Mean (SD) age, y	54.8 (8.3)	56.9 (6)	1.23	51.6	.22
Current marital status, No. (%)					
Single, never married	0	0	3.12	2	.21
Married, remarried	41 (79)	15 (75)			
Separated, divorced	9 (17)	2 (10)			
Widowed	2 (4)	3 (15)			
Current religion, No. (%)					
Protestant	11 (21)	5 (24)	2.95	3	.39
Catholic	34 (65)	14 (67)			
Jewish	2 (4)	2 (10)			
Other	5 (10)	0			
Employment status, No. (%)					
Full-time (≥35 h)	24 (46)	8 (38)	0.397	2	.82
Part-time (<35 h)	11 (21)	5 (24)			
Irregular, not employed	17 (33)	8 (38)			
Mean (SD) household income, $	49 801 (26 095)	59 393 (23 492)	1.45	36.5	.15

*Numbers may vary due to missing data. MDD indicates major depressive disorder.

†t Statistic when the variable is continuous; χ^2 statistic when the variable is dichotomous.

RESULTS

CHARACTERISTICS OF PROBANDS AND OFFSPRING

At the 10-year follow-up, the depressed and nondepressed probands and their offspring did not differ by the major demographic variables, with 1 exception: the offspring of depressed compared with nondepressed par-

Table 2. Demographic Characteristics of Offspring at Time 10 by Parental Diagnosis*

Characteristic	Parental Diagnosis: ≥1 With MDD (n=129)	Parental Diagnosis: Neither Had MDD (n=53)	Statistic†	*df*	*P*
Female, No. (%)	71 (55.0)	29 (55)	0.002	1	.96
Age, No. (%)					
17-20 y	13 (10.1)	3 (6)	0.956	2	.62
21-28 y	56 (43.4)	25 (47)			
29-36 y	60 (46.5)	25 (47)			
Current marital status, No. (%)					
Single, never married	59 (46.8)	19 (36)	2.43	2	.29
Married, remarried	53 (42.1)	29 (55)			
Separated, divorced	14 (11.1)	5 (9)			
Ever divorced	14 (10.8)	7 (13)	0.204	1	.65
Current religion, No. (%)					
Protestant	27 (21.8)	7 (14)	4.90	3	.17
Catholic	72 (58.1)	38 (75)			
Jewish	4 (3.2)	2 (4)			
Other	21 (16.9)	4 (8)			
Educational level completed, No. (%)					
<High school	18 (13.9)	3 (6)	3.94	3	.26
High school only	48 (37.2)	21 (40)			
Some college or trade	23 (17.8)	14 (27)			
≥4 y college	40 (31.0)	14 (27)			
Employment status, No. (%)					
Full-time (≥35 h)	79 (61.7)	34 (64)	0.182	2	.91
Part-time (<35 h)	20 (15.6)	7 (13)	...	...	...
Irregular, not employed	29 (22.7)	12 (23)	...	...	...
Mean (SD) annual income, $					
Individual	22 759 (18 529)	26 179 (19 572)	1.06	86.1	.29
Household	49 214 (24 304)	54 158 (23 016)	1.18	96.4	.24
No. of children, mean (SD)	1.6 (0.79)	2.3 (1)	2.54	27.7	.02

*Numbers may vary due to missing data in some categories. MDD indicates major depressive disorder.
†*t* Statistic when the variable is continuous; χ^2 statistic when the variable is dichotomous.

ents had significantly *fewer children* (**Table 1** and **Table 2**).

CUMULATIVE RATES

During the 10-year follow-up, the offspring of depressed compared with nondepressed parents had higher rates of MDD and phobias (both at about 3-fold differences), panic disorder, and alcohol dependence (nearly a 5-fold difference) (**Table 3**). There was no significant interaction between parental depression status and parental and offspring gender for the risk of depression, anxiety, or alcohol dependence in offspring (data not given in Table 3).

AGE-SPECIFIC RATES

Figure 1 clearly shows that the peak time for the incidence period for both sexes for MDD was between the ages of 15 and 20 years. At all ages, the incidence by sex was higher in the offspring of depressed parents. There was a decline in the incidence after the age of 20 years. Prepubertal onset was uncommon and occurs in the high-risk offspring. The incidence rates were higher in female than male adolescents. After the age of 20 years, the incidence rates were similar in both sexes.

Figure 2 shows a different pattern for any anxiety disorder (including panic disorder, generalized anxiety disorder, agoraphobia, social phobia, simple phobia, separation anxiety, obsessive-compulsive disorder, and overanxious disorder). The peak incidence of anxiety in the offspring for both sexes was much earlier than that for MDD (age range, 5-10 years), especially in the offspring of depressed parents. Anxiety disorders that have an early onset are mostly phobias and separation anxiety disorder (mean ages at onset, 5.2 and 6.6 years, respectively). The incidence rates decline after the age of 12 years and converge by the sex of the offspring and parental diagnosis.

The incidence rate for alcohol dependence in both sexes of depressed probands increased at the ages of 15 to 20 years and after the age of 25 years (**Figure 3**).

SYMPTOMS OF DEPRESSION

Symptom patterns of depression (not shown) by the age at first onset (age, <14 and ≥14 years) in the offspring at time 10 showed only 1 significant difference (from a list of 27 symptoms) (χ^2=7.78; *df*=1; *P*=.005). These analyses were rerun by comparing symptom patterns in persons with onsets that occurred at younger than 18 years with symptom patterns that occurred in persons with onsets at age 18 years and older, and the results were similar. There were few differences in depressive symptoms in the offspring by

Table 3. Cumulative Rates of Disorder (Using *DSM-III-R*) (Applying Impairment Criteria) in Offspring by Parental Diagnosis*

Diagnoses in Offspring	Parental Diagnosis, No. (%) of Offspring: ≥1 With MDD (n=129)	Parental Diagnosis, No. (%) of Offspring: Neither Had MDD (n=53)	Relative Risk† (95% Confidence Interval)
Any mood disorder	87 (85.3)	20 (38)	2.39 (1.46-3.89)
MDD	64 (56.4)	13 (25)	2.50 (1.38-4.54)
Bipolar	3 (2.3)	0	. . .‡
Dysthymia	7 (6.1)	3 (6)	0.922 (0.238-3.58)
Any anxiety	51 (41.7)	8 (15)	2.96 (1.41-6.24)
Phobias	27 (21.0)	4 (8)	2.94 (1.03-8.41)
Panic disorder	14 (13.4)	0	. . .§
OCD	1 (1.9)	1 (2)	. . .‖
GAD	0	0	
ADHD	5 (3.9)	2 (4)	0.882 (0.166-4.67)
Any substance abuse	40 (32.0)	14 (28)	1.32 (0.715-2.42)
Alcohol abuse	18 (14.5)	8 (16)	0.934 (0.406-2.15)
Alcohol dependence	21 (21.6)	2 (7)	4.93 (1.16-21.06)
Drug abuse	7 (5.5)	7 (14)	0.414 (0.145-1.18)
Drug dependence	16 (14.5)	1 (2)	6.98 (0.925-52.74)
Schizophrenia	2 (1.8)	0	. . .¶
Childhood disorders			
Separation anxiety	16 (12.4)	6 (11)	1.08 (0.424-2.78)
Conduct disorder	44 (34.1)	11 (21)	1.88 (0.969-3.64)#
Overanxious disorder	17 (13.6)	1 (2)	7.22 (0.959-54.28)
Any of the previously cited diagnoses	99 (78.4)	25 (47)	2.18 (1.40-3.38)

**If the offspring reported (in the Schedule for Affective Disorders and Schizophrenia), during an episode of disorder, that they sought help, took medication, were hospitalized, or had impaired functioning at work, school, or home, they were considered to be impaired. MDD indicates major depressive disorder; OCD, obsessive-compulsive disorder; GAD, generalized anxiety disorder; and ADHD, attention deficit hyperactivity disorder.*
†*Relative risk adjusted for age and sex of offspring.*
‡*Two-tailed Fisher exact test=1.25,* df=*1,* P=*.56.*
§*Two-tailed Fisher exact test=6.23,* df=*1,* P=*.004.*
‖*Two-tailed Fisher exact test=0.427,* df=*1,* P>*.99.*
¶*Two-tailed Fisher exact test=0.831,* df=*1,* P>*.99.*
#*Data on impairment were not collected for conduct disorder.*

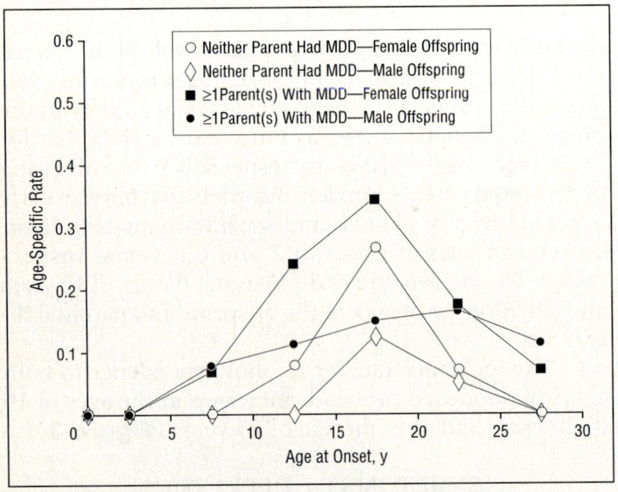

Figure 1. *Age-specific rates of major depressive disorder (MDD) by parental MDD and sex of offspring (N=182 [lifetime]).*

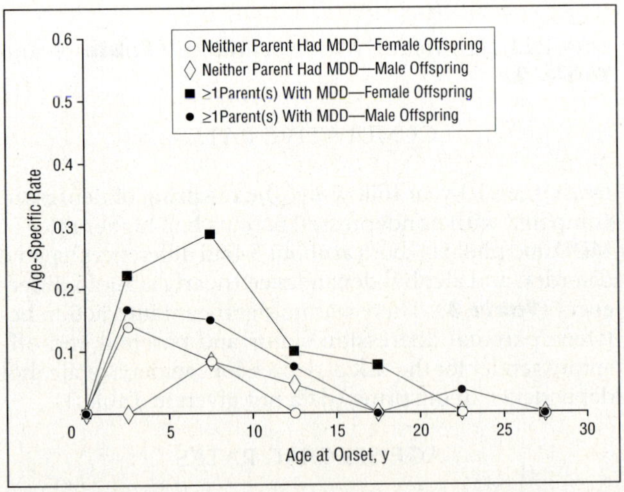

Figure 2. *Age-specific rates of any anxiety disorder by parental major depressive disorder (MDD) and sex of offspring (N=182 [lifetime]).*

proband group. Of 27 symptoms, the offspring of depressed parents more frequently reported feelings of worthlessness (χ^2=3.86; *df*=1; *P*=.05), and the offspring of nondepressed parents more frequently reported a loss of interest in sex (χ^2=7.63; *df*=1; *P*=.006). The significant differences that were found could have been due to chance because of the large number of comparisons made.

COMORBIDITY

Comorbidity of other disorders with MDD was high in the offspring from both groups (**Table 4**). While the stratified ORs suggest that there are higher rates of comorbidity in the offspring of *nondepressed* parents, our small sample size does not give adequate power to test whether the ORs differ significantly. Using the Breslow-

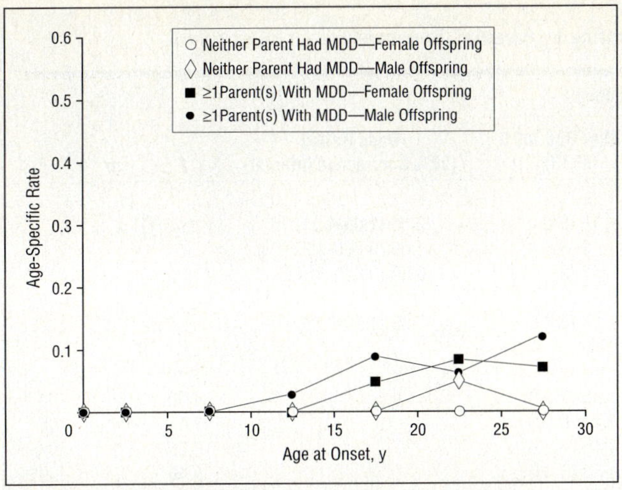

Figure 3. *Age-specific rates of alcohol dependence by parental major depressive disorder (MDD) and sex of offspring (N=182 [lifetime]).*

Day test for homogeneity of the ORs, there was only a suggestion that the ORs for comorbidity of dysthymia (χ^2=2.61; df=1; P=.11), any drug abuse or dependence (χ^2=1.88; df=1; P=.17), any phobias (χ^2=2.43; df=1; P=.12), and any of the previously described diagnoses with MDD (χ^2=2.40; df=1; P=.12) were higher in the offspring of nondepressed parents.

TREATMENT AND IMPAIRMENT

Throughout the 10 years, the offspring of depressed compared with nondepressed parents received slightly more outpatient treatment, and they had poorer overall functioning, as well as poorer functioning in work, family, and marriage (**Table 5**).

SEVERITY OF OUTCOME IN DEPRESSED OFFSPRING

Table 6 takes into account the depression status of the offspring and shows that the illness severity at time 10, in the offspring who were depressed at time 1 or 2, was greater in the offspring of depressed compared with nondepressed parents. The depressed offspring of depressed parents were *less* likely to go for treatment when they felt that they needed it, and *less* likely to receive treatment when they were depressed. More than 30% of the depressed offspring of depressed parents never received any treatment. They also had more impairment overall, in work and marriage, and more days on which they felt depressed.

Table 4. Comorbidity of Offspring MDD With Other *DSM-III-R* Diagnoses by Parental Diagnosis (Cumulative Rates for Times 1, 2, and 10)*

Parental Diagnosis	MDD in Offspring, No. (%) No	MDD in Offspring, No. (%) Yes	Odds Ratio (95% Confidence Interval)
≥1 Parent(s) depressed	60 (100)	69 (100)	
Any anxiety	17 (28)	43 (62)	4.18 (2.02-8.67)
Dysthymia	12 (20)	26 (38)	2.42 (1.09-5.33)
Any phobia	5 (8)	22 (32)	5.14 (1.92-13.76)
Any alcohol abuse	9 (15)	23 (33)	2.83 (1.21-6.64)
Panic disorder	2 (3)	13 (19)	6.73 (1.71-26.46)
OCD	0	3 (4)	. . .†
Any drug abuse	9 (15)	14 (20)	1.44 (0.57-3.62)
Any substance abuse	12 (20)	28 (41)	2.73 (1.24-5.98)
Any of the previously cited diagnoses	30 (50)	57 (83)	4.75 (2.18-10.33)
Neither parent depressed	39 (100)	14 (100)	
Any anxiety	3 (8)	6 (43)	9.00 (2.11-38.22)
Dysthymia	5 (13)	8 (57)	9.07 (2.42-33.91)
Any phobia	0	4 (29)	. . .‡
Any alcohol abuse	6 (15)	6 (43)	4.12 (1.09-15.61)
Panic disorder	0	0	
OCD	0	1 (7)	. . .§
Any drug abuse	4 (10)	5 (36)	4.86 (1.15-20.47)
Any substance abuse	9 (23)	8 (57)	4.44 (1.26-15.66)
Any of the previously cited diagnoses	13 (33)	13 (93)	26.00 (4.81-140.47)

**MDD indicates major depressive disorder; OCD, obsessive-compulsive disorder.*
†Two-tailed Fisher exact test=2.67, df=1, P=.25.
‡Two-tailed Fisher exact test=12.05, df=1, P=.03.
§Two-tailed Fisher exact test=2.84, df=1, P=.26.

COMMENT

Like previous investigators, we found that parental depression increases the risk of offspring depression, that the course of depression in children (as in adults) is protracted, that the morbidity rate is high, and that the overall symptom picture in offspring does not vary by the age at onset of the symptoms and does not differ by proband group.[11,12,15,16,41,42]

The overall rates and burden of illness are greater in the offspring of depressed parents, and their offspring continue to have higher rates of MDD (ie, a 3-fold increase) and anxiety disorders. As they mature, they also have high rates of alcohol dependence (ie, 5-fold increases) and poorer functioning in work, family, and marriage. The cumulative rate of MDD in the offspring of nondepressed parents (25.1/100) for the ages of 6 to 36 years is higher than that in the community sample for the ages of 15 to 34 years (17.1/100),[5,6] and it may be explained by our closer surveillance of the sample (ie, 3 interviews), as well as by their younger ages when the interviewing began.

The recurrent nature of depression that was found is consistent with findings from longitudinal studies of depressed adults and children.[16,17,43,44] The increased risk of MDD in the offspring of depressed parents is consistent with that found in numerous studies in which the offspring were minors.[9,11,44,45] The familial nature of depression was consistent with that of studies in which the probands were depressed children or adults.[21,46,47] While the absolute rates vary with the design and criteria used, the magnitude of the effect of familial depression (ie, a 2- to 3-fold increased risk) is consistent across high-risk and family studies.

There were more shifts to bipolar disorders in the offspring of depressed than nondepressed parents, but the overall rate of bipolar disorder (2.3% in the off-

Table 5. Treatment, Work Impairment, and Overall Functioning in Offspring by Parental Diagnosis*

Parameter	Parental Diagnosis: ≥1 With MDD (n=129)	Parental Diagnosis: Neither Had MDD (n=53)	Odds Ratio† (95% Confidence Interval)	F	df	P
Lifetime treatment for emotional problems, No. (%)						
Outpatient treatment	67 (52)	18 (34)	2.11 (1.08-4.11)	...	...	...
Hospitalization	8 (6)	3 (6)	1.09 (0.280-4.32)	...	...	...
Ever out of work in last 5 y due to psychopathologic disorder, No. (%)	13 (10)	1 (2)	6.50 (0.820-51.62)	...	...	...
Overall functioning (Global Assessment Scale score, ≤71), No. (%)	42 (33)	6 (11)	3.78 (1.50-9.56)	...	...	...
Social Adjustment Scale, mean (SD) score‡						
Work	1.80 (1.1)	1.45 (0.63)	...	4.50	1	.04
Social and leisure	1.97 (0.52)	1.81 (0.41)	...	3.47	1	.06
Extended family	1.66 (0.48)	1.45 (0.35)	...	8.05	1	.005
Marital	1.89 (0.58)	1.53 (0.35)	...	8.16	1	.005
Parental	1.44 (0.39)	1.26 (0.42)	...	1.94	1	.17
Family	1.75 (0.58)	1.73 (0.63)	...	0.03	1	.85
Overall	1.79 (0.42)	1.59 (0.33)	...	8.88	1	.003

Numbers may vary due to missing data. MDD indicates major depressive disorder.
†*Odds ratio adjusted for age and sex of offspring.*
‡*Means adjusted for age of offspring.*

Table 6. Severity of Outcome at Time 10 in Offspring With Any Depression at Time 1 or 2 by Parental Diagnosis*

Parameter	Parental Diagnosis: ≥1 With MDD (n=80)	Parental Diagnosis: Neither Had MDD (n=26)	Odds Ratio (95% Confidence Interval)†	Statistic‡	df	P
Did not go for treatment when felt it was needed, No. (%)	23 (33)	1 (4)	12.85 (1.61-102.54)	...	...	...
Global Assessment Scale score, ≤71, No. (%)	32 (40)	4 (15)	4.34 (1.33-14.14)	...	...	...
Social Adjustment Scale, mean (SD) score						
Work	1.84 (1.07)	1.30 (0.324)	...	−3.66	88.5	<.001
Social and leisure	1.97 (0.567)	1.89 (0.450)	...	−0.689	49	.49
Extended family	1.68 (0.509)	1.46 (0.314)	...	−2.54	64.6	.01
Marital	1.88 (0.630)	1.47 (0.358)	...	−3.05	46.1	.003
Parental	1.44 (0.402)	1.22 (0.405)	...	−1.44	23.2	.16
Family	1.78 (0.601)	1.61 (0.502)	...	−1.37	44.3	.18
Overall	1.80 (0.455)	1.59 (0.332)	...	−2.56	55.2	.01
No. of days depressed during follow-up, mean (SD)	118 (401)	11 (49)	...	−2.33	86	.02
Ever out of work in last 5 y due to psychopathologic disorder, No. (%)	11 (14)	1 (4)	...	1.92	1	.29§
No. of MDD episodes during follow-up, No. (%)						
0	53 (66)	23 (88)	...	...	...	...
1	23 (29)	2 (8)	...	...	...	...
2+	4 (5)	1 (4)	...	5.10	2	.08
Suicidal gestures or attempts, No. (%)	13 (16)	3 (12)	...	0.340	1	.75§
Treatment during 10 y, No. (%)∥						
Outpatient treatment	33 (67)	6 (100)	...	2.76	1	.16§
Hospitalization	4 (8)	3 (50)	...	8.42	1	.02§
Any treatment	33 (67)	6 (100)	...	2.76	1	.16§

Numbers may vary due to missing data. Odds ratios that were adjusted for age and sex of offspring (95% confidence interval) were as follows: offspring who did not go for treatment, 12.85 (1.61-102.54); Global Assessment Scale score, 4.34 (1.33-14.14). MDD indicates major depressive disorder.
†*Adjusted for age and sex of offspring.*
‡*t Statistic is used for continuous variables; χ^2 statistic is used for dichotomous.*
§*Two-tailed Fisher exact test.*
∥*Treatment of MDD for offspring with any depression at time 10: 1 or more parent(s) with MDD (n=49) and neither parent had MDD (n=6).*

spring of depressed parents) was lower than that reported by other investigators.[15,16] Of note, some of the offspring have not fully passed through the age at risk for the onset of bipolar disorder.

A prepubertal onset of MDD is uncommon, and it did not occur in the offspring of the nondepressed parents. The peak first onset of MDD in middle and late adolescence is consistent with the findings from epidemiologic studies of adolescents and adults.[3,6,45,48,49] This peak is consistent in female offspring regardless of proband diagnosis, suggesting a consistent vulnerability period for focus on detection and intervention. Why the rates should increase so abruptly in young females in middle and late adolescence and early adulthood is still unclear and is an area for further research. Parental affective disorders further increase the risk of first onset in adolescents. However, as noted by Beardslee et al,[45] affective disorders in parents may serve as an identifier of a constellation of risk factors. Symptoms by themselves do not discriminate risks.[45] Studies of the phenomenology of depressive disorders across childhood and adulthood have generally found similar symptoms across the ages.[20,42,50,51] The finding that anxiety disorder precedes the onset of MDD and is markedly increased in the offspring of depressed parents may be due to high rates of comorbid anxiety disorders in the parents. Alternately, early expression of anxiety disorders could constitute an underlying vulnerability to psychopathology by shared genetic or environmental factors.[52] Our analysis of sibling resemblance for MDD, anxiety, and conduct disorder at time 1 found that sibling resemblance in the high-risk cohort was substantially greater than in the low-risk cohort for anxiety disorders but not MDD, suggesting that anxiety disorders may reflect the most pronounced familial influences common to siblings at high risk for MDD.[53]

While, to our knowledge, this is the largest published offspring study of depressed parents and has the longest follow-up period, our sample of offspring with a broad age range is still small, and there were few offspring with a prepubertal onset of depression. The selection of parents from treatment settings may have resulted in more serious cases.[54] On the other hand, the similarity of findings from several studies that used different methods suggests the validity of the findings.

The current findings support initiatives aimed at early detection and possible treatment intervention in the parents of depressed offspring and the offspring of depressed parents. Physicians who specialize in pediatrics and adolescent medicine, as well as internists, family physicians, and child psychiatrists, are particularly well positioned to inquire about the mental health history of their patient's parents.[55]

Alternately, psychiatrists who treat adult patients should inquire about the clinical status of the offspring. Successful treatment of parental depression may provide primary prevention by reducing the symptoms of depression that may impair parenting.[56] A recent study suggested that depressed mothers who give negative self-reports may be more negative than their directly observed parenting behavior.[57] However, women who were chronically or severely depressed had both negative self-reports and observed negative parent-child relationships, suggesting that this is a particularly high-risk group for intervention. Secondary prevention may be achieved through the early detection and treatment of high-risk offspring who exhibit early or minor forms of anxiety, depressive, or substance abuse disorders. Finally, the aggressive treatment of established MDD (ie, tertiary prevention) may reduce the high level of social impairment that characterizes the depressed offspring of depressed parents.

Only a small proportion of young people with mental disorders receive adequate mental health treatment.[58-60] In the current study, a large number of the offspring who perceived a need for mental health care utilized no treatment whatsoever. One possible explanation is that the offspring of depressed parents develop negative attitudes toward mental health treatment because they associate it with their parents' chronic course of illness. Alternately, the depressed parent may deny that their offspring have the same disorder. A better understanding of how parental factors influence the seeking of health care for their offspring may help public health planners extend treatment to this vulnerable and underserved population.[61]

There are now strong financial incentives to limit treatment, and the assessment of clinical outcomes focuses on short-term treatment costs.[62] Our data suggest that outcomes should assess the impact of parental depression on the offspring over time.

Accepted for publication January 28, 1997.

This work was supported in part by grants MH-36197 (Dr Weissman) and 5P30MH43878 (Dr Weissman), and by Research Scientist Development Award K20-MH01042 (Dr Olfson) from the National Institute of Mental Health, Rockville, Md.

Corresponding author: Myrna M. Weissman, PhD, College of Physicians and Surgeons of Columbia University, New York State Psychiatric Institute, 722 W 168th St, New York, NY 10032 (e-mail: weissman@child.cpmc.columbia.edu).

REFERENCES

1. Klerman GL, Weissman MM. Increasing rates of depression. *JAMA.* 1989;261:2229-2235.
2. Weissman MM, Klerman GL. Depression: current understanding and changing trends. *Annu Rev Public Health.* 1992;13:319-339.
3. Christie KA, Burke JD, Regier DA, Rae DS, Boyd JH, Locke BZ. Epidemiologic evidence for early onset of mental disorders and higher risk of drug abuse in young adults. *Am J Psychiatry.* 1988;145:971-975.
4. Lahey BB, Flagg EW, Bird HR, Schwab-Stone M, Canino G, Dulcan MK, Leaf PJ, Davies M, Bourdon K, Horwitz S, Rubio-Stipec M, Freeman DH, Shaffer D, Goodman SH, Narrow WE, Weissman MM, Kandel D, Jensen PS, Richters JE, Regier DA. The NIMH Methods for the Epidemiology of Children and Adolescents (MECA) Study: background and methodology. *J Am Acad Child Adolesc Psychiatry.* 1996;35:855-864.
5. Kessler RC, McGonagle KA, Nelson CB, Hughes M, Swartz M, Blazer DG. Sex and depression in the National Comorbidity Survey, II: cohort effects. *J Affect Disord.* 1994;30:15-26.
6. Kessler RC, McGonagle KA, Shanyang Z, Nelson CB, Hughes M, Eshleman S, Wittchen HU, Kendler KS. Lifetime and 12-month prevalence of *DSM-III-R* psychiatric disorders in the United States. *Arch Gen Psychiatry.* 1994;51:8-19.
7. Weissman MM, Gershon ES, Kidd KK, Prusoff BA, Leckrnan JF, Dibble E, Harnovit J, Thompson WD, Pauls DL, Guroff JJ. Psychiatric disorders in the relatives of probands with affective disorders: the Yale University–National Institute of Mental Health Collaborative Study. *Arch Gen Psychiatry.* 1984;41:13-21.
8. Weissman MM, Olfson M. Depression in women: implications for health care research. *Science.* 1995;269:799-801.
9. Beardslee WR, Keller MB, Klerman GL. Children of parents with affective disorder. *Int J Fam Psychiatry.* 1985;6:283-299.
10. Orvaschel H, Walsh-Allis G, Ye W. Psychopathology in children of parents with recurrent depression. *J Abnorm Child Psychol.* 1988;16:17-28.
11. Hammen C, Burge D, Bumey E, Adrian C. Longitudinal study of diagnoses in children of women with unipolar and bipolar affective disorder. *Arch Gen Psychiatry.* 1990;47:1112-1117.
12. Hammen C, Burge D, Adrian C. Timing of mother and child depression in a longitudinal study of children at risk. *J Consult Clin Psychol.* 1991;59:341-345.
13. Lewinsohn PM, Gotlib IH, Seeley JR. Adolescent psychopathology, IV: specificity of psychosocial risk factors for depression and substance abuse in older adolescents. *J Am Acad Child Adolesc Psychiatry.* 1995;34:1221-1229.

14. Rao U, Weissman MM, Martin JA, Hammond RW. Childhood depression and risk of suicide: a preliminary report of a longitudinal study. *J Am Acad Child Adolesc Psychiatry.* 1993;32:21-27.
15. Rao U, Ryan ND, Birmaher B, Dahl RE, Williamson DE, Kaufman J, Rao R, Nelson B. Unipolar depression in adolescents: clinical outcome in adulthood. *J Am Acad Child Adolesc Psychiatry.* 1995;34:566-577.
16. Kovacs M, Feinberg TL, Crouse-Novak MA, Paulauskas SL, Finkelstein R. Depressive disorders in childhood, I: a longitudinal prospective study of characteristics and recovery. *Arch Gen Psychiatry.* 1984;41:229-237.
17. Kovacs M, Goldston D, Gatsonis C. Suicidal behaviors and childhood-onset depressive disorders: a longitudinal investigation. *J Am Acad Child Adolesc Psychiatry.* 1993;32:8-20.
18. Ferdinand RF, Verhulst FC. Psychopathology from adolescence into young adulthood: an 8-year follow-up study. *Am J Psychiatry.* 1995;152:1586-1594.
19. Orvaschel H, Lewinsohn PM, Seeley JR. Continuity of psychopathology in a community sample of adolescents. *J Am Acad Child Adolesc Psychiatry.* 1995;34:1525-1535.
20. Harrington R, Fudge H, Rutter M, Pickles A, Hill J. Adult outcomes of childhood and adolescent depression, I: psychiatric status. *Arch Gen Psychiatry.* 1990;47:465-473.
21. Harrington RC, Fudge H, Rutter ML, Bredenkamp CG, Pridham J. Child and adult depression: a test of continuities with data from a family study. *Br J Psychiatry.* 1993;162:627-633.
22. Weissman MM, John K, Merikangas KR, Prusoff BA, Wickramaratne P, Gammon GD, Angold A, Warner V. Depressed parents and their children: general health, social and psychiatric problems. *AJDC.* 1986;140:801-805.
23. Weissman MM, Gammon GD, John K, Merikangas KR, Warner V, Prusoff BA, Sholomskas D. Children of depressed parents: increased psychopathology and early onset of major depression. *Arch Gen Psychiatry.* 1987;44:847-853.
24. Weissman MM, Warner V, Wickramaratne P, Prusoff BA. Early onset major depression in parents and their children. *J Affect Disord.* 1988;15:269-278.
25. Chang G, Weissman MM, Warner V. Physicians' recognition of psychiatric disorders in children and adolescents. *AJDC.* 1988;142:736-739.
26. Fendrich M, Warner V, Weissman MM. Family risk factors, parental depression and childhood psychopathology. *Dev Psychol.* 1990;26:40-50.
27. Warner V, Weissman MM, Fendrich M, Wickramaratne PJ, Moreau D. The course of major depression in the offspring of depressed parents: incidence, recurrence, recovery. *Arch Gen Psychiatry.* 1992;49:797-801.
28. Weissman MM, Fendrich M, Warner V, Wickramaratne PJ. Incidence of psychiatric disorder in offspring at high and low risk for depression. *J Am Acad Child Adolesc Psychiatry.* 1992;31:640-648.
29. Fendrich M, Weissman MM, Warner V. Longitudinal assessment of major depression and anxiety disorders in children. *J Am Acad Child Adolesc Psychiatry.* 1991;30:67-74.
30. Fendrich M, Weissman MM, Warner V, Mufson L. Two-year recall of lifetime diagnoses in offspring at high and low risk for major depression: the stability of offspring reports. *Arch Gen Psychiatry.* 1990;47:1121-1127.
31. Endicott J, Spitzer RL. A diagnostic interview: the Schedule for Affective Disorders and Schizophrenia. *Arch Gen Psychiatry.* 1978;35:837-844.
32. Mannuzza S, Fyer AJ, Klein DF, Endicott J. Schedule for Affective Disorders and Schizophrenia–Lifetime version modified for the study of anxiety disorders (SADS-LA): rationale and conceptual development. *J Psychiatr Res.* 1986;20:317-325.
33. Endicott J, Spitzer RL, Fleiss JL, Cohen J. The Global Assessment Scale: a procedure for measuring overall severity of psychiatric disturbance. *Arch Gen Psychiatry.* 1976;33:766-771.
34. Weissman MM, Bothwell S. The assessment of social adjustment by patient self-report. *Arch Gen Psychiatry.* 1976;33:1111-1115.
35. Cohen JA. A coefficient of agreement for nominal scales. *Educ Psychol.* 1960;20:37-46.
36. Leckman JF, Sholomskas D, Thompson D, Belanger A, Weissman MM. Best estimate of lifetime psychiatric diagnosis: a methodological study. *Arch Gen Psychiatry.* 1982;39:879-883.
37. SAS Institute Inc. *SAS/STAT User's Guide: Version 6.* 4th ed. Cary, NC: SAS Institute Inc; 1990:2.
38. Cox DR, Oakes D. *Analysis of Survival Data.* New York, NY: Chapman & Hall; 1984.
39. Kalbfeisch JD, Prentice RL. *The Statistical Analysis of Failure Time Data.* New York, NY: John Wiley & Sons Inc; 1980.
40. Cox DR. Regression models and life tables. *J R Stat Soc Ser B.* 1972;34:187-220.
41. Lewinsohn PM, Hoberman HM, Rosenbaum M. A prospective study of risk factors for unipolar depression. *J Abnorm Psychol.* 1988;97:251-264.
42. Ryan ND, Puig-Antich J, Ambrosini P, Rabinovich H, Robinson D, Nelson B, Lyengar S, Twomey J. The clinical picture of major depression in children and adolescents. *Arch Gen Psychiatry.* 1987;44:854-861.
43. Lavori PW, Keller MB, Mueller TI, Scheftner W, Fawcett J, Corvell W. Recurrence after recovery in unipolar MDD: an observational follow-up study of clinical predictors and somatic treatment as a mediating factor. *Int J Methods Psychiatr Res.* 1994;4:211-229.
44. Keller MB, Beardslee WR, Dorer DJ, Lavori PW, Samuelson H, Klerman GL. Impact of severity and chronicity of parental affective illness on adaptive functioning and psychopathology in children. *Arch Gen Psychiatry.* 1986;43:930-937.
45. Beardslee WR, Keller MB, Seifer R, Lavori PW, Staley J, Podoresfsky D, Shera D. Prediction of adolescent affective disorder: effects of prior parental affective disorders and child psychopathology. *J Am Acad Child Adolesc Psychiatry.* 1996;35:279-288.
46. Weissman MM, Wickramaratne P, Merikangas KR, Leckman JF, Prusoff BA, Caruso KA, Kidd KK, Gammon GD. Onset of major depression in early adulthood: increased familial loading and specificity. *Arch Gen Psychiatry.* 1984;41:1136-1143.
47. Williamson DE, Ryan ND, Birmaher B, Dahl RE, Kaufman J, Rao U, Puig-Antich J. A case-control family history study of depression in adolescents. *J Am Acad Child Adolesc Psychiatry.* 1995;34:1596-1607.
48. Angold A. Childhood and adolescent depression, I: epidemiological and aetiological aspects. *Br J Psychiatry.* 1988;152:601-617.
49. Fleming J, Offord DR, Boyle MH. Prevalence of childhood and adolescent depression in the community: Ontario Child Health Study. *Br J Psychiatry.* 1989;155:647-654.
50. Carlson GA, Kashani JH. Phenomenology of major depression from childhood through adulthood: analysis of three studies. *Am J Psychiatry.* 1988;145:1222-1225.
51. Roberts RE, Lewinsohn PM, Seeley JR. Symptoms of *DSM-III-R* major depression in adolescence: evidence from an epidemiological survey. *J Am Acad Child Adolesc Psychiatry.* 1995;34:1608-1617.
52. Merikangas KR. Genetic epidemiologic studies of affective disorders in childhood and adolescence. *Eur Arch Psychiatry Clin Neurosci.* 1993;243:121-130.
53. Rende R, Wickramaratne P, Warner V, Weissman MM. Sibling resemblance for psychiatric disorders in offspring at high and low risk for depression. *J Child Psychol Psychiatry.* 1995;36:1353-1363.
54. Kendler K. Is seeking treatment for depression predicted by a history of depression in relatives? implications for family studies of affective disorder. *Psychol Med.* 1995;25:807-814.
55. Takeuchi DT, Bui KV, Kin L. The referral of minority adolescents to community mental health centers. *J Health Soc Behav.* 1993;34:153-164.
56. Weissman MM, Paykel ES, Klerman GL. The depressed woman as a mother. *Soc Psychiatry Psychiatr Epidemiol.* 1982;7:98-108.
57. Frankel KA, Harmon RJ. Depressed mothers: they don't always look as bad as they feel. *J Am Acad Child Adolesc Psychiatry.* 1996;35:289-298.
58. Keller MB, Lavori PW, Beardslee WR, Wunder J, Ryan N. Depression in children and adolescents: new data on 'undertreatment' and a literature review on the efficacy of available treatments. *J Affect Disord.* 1991;21:163-171.
59. Burns BJ. Mental health services use by adolescents in the 1970s and 1980s. *J Am Acad Child Adolesc Psychiatry.* 1991;30:144-150.
60. Bird HR, Canino G, Rubio-Stipec M, Gould MS, Ribera J, Sesman M, Woodbury M, Hertas-Goldman S, Pagan A, Sanchez-Lacay A, Moscoso M. Estimates of the prevalence of childhood maladjustment in a community survey in the relevance of childhood maladjustment in a community survey in Puerto Rico: the use of combined measures. *Arch Gen Psychiatry.* 1988;45:1120-1126.
61. Leaf PJ, Bruce ML, Tischler GL. The differential effect of attitudes on the use of mental health services. *Soc Psychiatry Psychiatr Epidemiol.* 1986;21:187-192.
62. Schowalter JE. Managed care: income to outcome. *J Am Acad Child Adolesc Psychiatry.* 1995;34:1123.

ORIGINAL ARTICLE

Reduction of Synaptophysin Immunoreactivity in the Prefrontal Cortex of Subjects With Schizophrenia

Regional and Diagnostic Specificity

Leisa A. Glantz, MS; David A. Lewis, MD

Background: Multiple lines of evidence indicate that the prefrontal cortex is a site of dysfunction in schizophrenia. However, the apparent absence of gross structural abnormalities in this area suggests that the pathophysiological characteristics of schizophrenia may involve more subtle disturbances in prefrontal cortical circuitry, such as alterations in synaptic connectivity and transmission. In this study, immunoreactivity for synaptophysin, an integral membrane protein of small synaptic vesicles, was used to assess the integrity of cortical synaptic circuitry in schizophrenia.

Methods: Using immunocytochemical techniques and adjusted optical density measurements, we examined synaptophysin immunoreactivity in prefrontal cortical areas 9 and 46 and in area 17 (the primary visual cortex) from 10 pairs of case subjects with schizophrenia and control subjects matched on a pairwise basis for age, sex, race, and postmortem interval, and in 5 matched pairs of nonschizophrenic psychiatric case subjects and normal control subjects.

Results: Compared with levels found in matched control subjects, synaptophysin immunoreactivity in areas 46 and 9 was significantly decreased ($P<.001$ and $P<.008$, respectively) across all cortical layers in the case subjects with schizophrenia. In contrast, no differences were observed in area 17. In addition, levels of synaptophysin immunoreactivity in areas 46, 9, and 17 did not differ between 5 nonschizophrenic psychiatric case subjects and their matched controls, suggesting that decreased synaptophysin levels in the prefrontal cortex of patients with schizophrenia may be specific to that disorder.

Conclusions: Additional studies are required to determine if the decrease in levels of synaptophysin immunoreactivity is caused by a decrease in the number or size of presynaptic terminals, a decrease in the number of synaptic vesicles per terminal, or a decrease in the expression of synaptophysin. However, all of these potential explanations are consistent with a disturbance in synaptic transmission in the prefrontal cortex of patients with schizophrenia.

Arch Gen Psychiatry. 1997;54:943-952

Correction

This article appeared in the July issue of the ARCHIVES (1997;54:660-669) and contained numerous errors created during the editorial and production process. We are now rerunning this article as it should have appeared. The ARCHIVES regrets the errors.

From the Departments of Neuroscience (Ms Glantz and Dr Lewis) and Psychiatry (Dr Lewis), University of Pittsburgh, Pittsburgh, Pa.

MULTIPLE lines of evidence have implicated the prefrontal cortex (PFC) as a site of dysfunction in schizophrenia. For example, many of the negative or deficit symptoms of schizophrenia are similar to those exhibited by patients with frontal lobe lesions.[1] In addition, a variety of functional neuroimaging and neuropsychological studies have identified abnormalities in the prefrontal cortex of subjects with schizophrenia.[2-8]

Attempts to identify the neuroanatomical basis for this dysfunction of the PFC have included both structural imaging and postmortem investigations. Many,[9-13] but not all,[14] structural imaging studies have revealed a decrease in PFC gray matter volume in subjects with schizophrenia. Similar differences in the thickness or volume of the PFC[15-18] between subjects with schizophrenia and control subjects have also been observed in postmortem measurements, although these differences did not reach statistical significance in every study. In addition, postmortem investigations have revealed that the density,[18] but not the number,[15,17] of PFC neurons is increased in subjects with schizophrenia compared with control subjects, although some investigators have observed decreased numbers of certain populations of PFC neurons.[19,20] The combination of decreased

PFC volume and increased cell packing density suggests that the amount of neuropil in this cortical region may be diminished in at least a subpopulation of subjects with schizophrenia. The cortical neuropil is composed of small dendrites, dendritic spines, and axon terminals,[21] critical elements in the structure of most cortical synapses. Consequently, a decrease in PFC neuropil volume in subjects with schizophrenia is likely to involve alterations in the synaptic connectivity of this region.

One way to test the hypothesis that the synaptic connectivity of the PFC is disturbed in schizophrenia is to assess the integrity of specific proteins that are known to be essential for synaptic function. For example, synaptophysin, a 38-kd integral membrane protein of small synaptic vesicles,[22-24] seems to be critical for calcium-dependent synaptic transmission.[25,26] Synaptophysin is present in more than 95% of cortical synaptic terminals,[22,23] and levels of synaptophysin immunoreactivity have been shown to be reliable measures of synaptic density.[27-29] Consequently, we used immunocytochemical techniques and optical density measurements to address the following 3 questions: Is synaptophysin immunoreactivity decreased in the PFC of subjects with schizophrenia compared with matched control subjects? If so, is the decrease selective to this region? Is the decreased synaptophysin immunoreactivity specific to the disease process of schizophrenia?

SUBJECTS AND METHODS

SUBJECTS

Specimens from 32 human brains were obtained during autopsies conducted at the Allegheny County Coroner's Office, Pittsburgh, Pa, or the University of Pittsburgh Medical Center. No neuropathological abnormalities were detected in any subjects except for 2 brains (Nos. 207 and 313) in which thioflavin S staining revealed a few senile plaques. The density of the plaques was insufficient to meet diagnostic criteria for Alzheimer disease,[30] and there was no clinical history of dementia in either subject. An independent committee of experienced clinicians made consensus *DSM-III-R* diagnoses for each subject using information obtained from clinical records, and, whenever possible (for 20 subjects), a structured interview with a surviving relative of the subject. All procedures were approved by the University of Pittsburgh's Institutional Review Board for Biomedical Research.

The first set of experiments (**Table 1**) used tissue specimens from 10 subjects with schizophrenia, 5 of whom also met diagnostic criteria for an alcohol-related disorder at some point during their life. This frequency of alcoholism is comparable with that observed in clinical studies of schizophrenia.[31] Eight subjects were receiving treatment with antipsychotic medications at the time of death. Case subject 207 had not taken antipsychotic medications for 10 years prior to death. Case subject 185 was known to be noncompliant with prescribed medications, and toxicology studies at autopsy failed to detect evidence of antipsychotic medications.

Each subject with schizophrenia was matched to 1 control subject on a pairwise basis for age, sex, race, and postmortem interval (PMI). Interviews with relatives confirmed that 8 control subjects had no history of any neurologic or psychiatric disorder. One subject (No. 230) had a history of alcohol dependence, and the other subject (No. 249) met diagnostic criteria for recurrent major depressive disorder with psychotic features. This individual had been treated intermittently for 25 years with antipsychotic medications.

The second study involved 5 case subjects in whom organic delusional disorder, major depressive disorder, or alcohol dependence or abuse had been diagnosed (**Table 2**). Case 217 was receiving antipsychotic treatment at the time of death, but the other 4 case subjects had no history of exposure to antipsychotic medications. These case subjects were matched with 5 control subjects who had no history of neurologic or psychiatric disease.

Finally, 1 additional pair of cases was studied. A 68-year-old white man (PMI, 16.8 hours) in whom major depression had been diagnosed and who had been receiving antipsychotic medications at the time of death, was matched with a 70-year-old white man (PMI, 16.5 hours) in whom major depression had been diagnosed, but who had never received antipsychotic medications.

PREPARATION OF TISSUE

The left hemisphere of each brain was cut into coronal blocks and immersed in a solution of 4% paraformaldehyde for 48 hours at 4°C.[32] Tissue blocks were then washed in a series of sucrose solutions in phosphate-buffered saline and stored in an antifreeze solution at −30°C. Mean (±SD) storage time did not differ between the case subjects with schizophrenia and their controls (29.3±14.0 and 29.5±12.3 months, respectively), or between the nonschizophrenic psychiatric case subjects and their controls (42.0±15.5 and 36.2±22.4 months, respectively). Previous studies have also shown that storage under these conditions does not affect immunoreactivity.[33] Sections (40 µm) were cut on a motor-driven cryostat to ensure maximal consistency in section thickness, and every 10th section was stained using the Nissl method.

AREAS EXAMINED

To assess the regional specificity of any changes in synaptophysin immunoreactivity, 3 areas with substantial differences in cytoarchitecture and afferent input were examined: PFC areas 9 and 46 and area 17, the primary visual cortex. These areas were identified using published cytoarchitectonic criteria.[32,34,35] Camera lucida drawings were made of Nissl-stained sections from each case subject, and the boundaries of each region were plotted to establish the appropriate zones for analysis on the sections labeled for synaptophysin immunoreactivity.

IMMUNOCYTOCHEMICAL PROCEDURES

Tissue sections from each pair of case and control subjects were pretreated in aqueous 1% hydrogen peroxide for 7½ minutes to remove endogenous peroxidase activity, washed, and then incubated at room temperature for 30 minutes in phosphate-buffered saline containing 0.3% Triton X-100 and 4.5% normal horse serum. Sections were incubated for 40 to 48 hours at 4°C in phosphate-buffered saline containing 0.3% Triton X-100, 0.05% bovine serum albumin, 3% normal horse serum, and 1 of 2 mouse monoclonal antibodies (Sigma, St Louis, Mo, diluted 1:1000 or Boehringer Mannheim, Indianapolis, Ind, diluted 1:100) that specifically recognize[24,36] synaptophysin. Sections were then processed using a standard Vectastain ABC kit (Vector Laboratories, Burlingame, Calif) and diaminobenzidine.

Control experiments involved replacing each primary antibody with normal mouse serum and processing the tissue as usual. No immunoreactivity was observed in these experiments. Specificity of the labeling was further indicated by the identical regional and laminar patterns of immunoreactivity produced by both antibodies.

Using the synaptophysin antibody from Sigma, 5 separate immunocytochemical experiments were performed for each cortical area of the case subjects with schizophrenia and their matched control subjects. A total of 4 experiments were performed for each area for the nonschizophrenic psychiatric case subjects and their matched controls. For each experiment, sections from a matched pair of subjects were processed together throughout the entire immunocytochemical procedure. Thus, for each of the 3 regions of interest, a total of 100 sections were prepared for the schizophrenia case-control study, and a total of 40 sections were prepared for the nonschizophrenia psychiatric case-control study. All of these sections were used in the quantitative analyses described herein.

ANALYSIS

Slide-mounted sections from each pair were randomly coded and scanned together, and the images were imported into an image analysis software program (Bioscan Inc, Edmonds, Wash) to obtain light transmittance measurements of synaptophysin immunoreactivity. Within each cytoarchitectonic region, rectangles that extended for 5 to 10 mm across the cortical surface and from the pial surface into the subjacent white matter were drawn. Rectangles varied in size because measurements were restricted to those portions of the areas of interest that were cut perpendicular to the pial surface and that were free of any discontinuities in the tissue. The average light transmittance (ranging 0-255) was determined in 3 different rectangles for each area on each section. The values from each rectangle were then averaged to produce a mean cortical and a mean white matter light transmittance value from each section of each cortical area of each subject. Because synaptophysin immunoreactivity was virtually absent in the white matter of all subjects, light transmittance measurements in the white matter were used to control for possible differences between subjects in nonspecific labeling. Adjusted optical density values were calculated from the mean light transmittance values according to the equation: adjusted optical density=log (light transmittance in white matter/light transmittance in cortex).[37] The adjusted optical density values were then used for comparisons between the matched pairs of subjects. Light transmittance values within the cortex were also divided into superficial and deep halves to determine adjusted optical density values for the supragranular and infragranular cortical layers.

Rescanning and remeasurement of the same coded sections produced mean adjusted optical density values that differed from the previous measurements by less than 1%. As an additional check on the reliability of these measurements, 5 neuroanatomists were asked to examine coded sections from 1 immunocytochemical experiment involving each of the subjects shown in Table 1, and to determine which section of a pair was more intensely immunoreactive, or if there was no discernible difference. In 49 of the resulting 50 comparisons, these ratings agreed with the findings of the quantitative comparisons (98% concordance).

STATISTICAL ANALYSES

For each of the 3 cortical regions, analysis of variance (ANOVA) was used to assess the significance (α=.05) of differences in adjusted optical density measurements between matched pairs of case subjects with schizophrenia and their control subjects, and between matched pairs of nonschizophrenic psychiatric case subjects and their control subjects. The ANOVA model factors were diagnostic group, matched pair, immunocytochemical experiment, and their second-order interactions. Diagnostic group effect, adjusting for pairing and immunocytochemical experiment, used F-statistics obtained from corresponding SAS Type III (SAS, Cary, NC) sums of squares. Linear regression analyses were used to evaluate the effects of age and PMI on adjusted optical density values.

RESULTS

QUALITATIVE COMPARISONS OF SYNAPTOPHYSIN IMMUNOREACTIVITY IN THE BRAINS OF SUBJECTS WITH SCHIZOPHRENIA AND MATCHED CONTROL SUBJECTS

Examination of the brains of subjects with schizophrenia and control subjects revealed a punctate pattern of synaptophysin immunoreactivity throughout the cortical neuropil (**Figure 1**). In contrast, cell bodies and the proximal portions of dendrites were not labeled. This pattern of immunoreactivity is consistent with the location of synaptophysin in small synaptic vesicles that aggregate in presynaptic axon terminals.

For each case subject, the laminar distribution of synaptophysin immunoreactivity differed consistently between the prefrontal and visual cortices. In areas 9 and 46, synaptophysin immunoreactivity was intense in layer 1, progressively decreased from the pial surface to the layer 6/white matter border (**Figure 2**, B), and then sharply declined to undetectable levels in the white matter. In contrast, a more complex laminar pattern of immunoreactivity was present in area 17, the primary visual cortex (Figure 2, D). These laminar changes were clearly reflected in adjusted optical density measurements of synaptophysin immunoreactivity in this region (**Figure 3**).

Table 1. Characteristics of Matched Pairs of Subjects With Schizophrenia and Control Subjects*

	Subjects With Schizophrenia					Control Subjects			
Pair	Subject No.	*DSM-III-R* Diagnosis	Sex/Race/ Age, y	Postmortem Interval, h	Cause of Death	Subject No.	Sex/Race/ Age, y	Postmortem Interval, h	Cause of Death
1	131	Chronic undifferentiated schizophrenia†	M/B/62	3.9	Pneumonia	249	M/B/57	4.3	ASCVD‡
2	153	Chronic paranoid schizophrenia§	M/B/24	18.3	Suicide by drowning	230	M/W/33	18.2	ASCVD‡
3	185	Schizophrenia§	M/W/64	8.6	ASCVD‡	313	M/W/60	11.0	ASCVD‡
4	236	Residual schizophrenia	M/W/69	17.0	Thermal burns	321	M/W/71	14.0	Aortic aneurysm
5	317	Chronic undifferentiated schizophrenia	M/W/48	8.3	Bronchopneumonia	278	M/W/50	4.5	ASCVD‡
6	398	Schizoaffective disorder	F/W/41	10.3	Pulmonary embolus	247	F/W/38	6.8	Pulmonary embolus
7	207	Schizophrenia	M/W/72	3.8	Subdural hematoma	168	M/W/77	6.2	ASCVD‡
8	377	Chronic undifferentiated schizophrenia‖	M/W/52	10.0	Gastrointestinal tract bleeding	178	M/W/48	7.4	ASCVD‡
9	341	Chronic undifferentiated schizophrenia¶	F/W/47	14.5	Suicide by drug overdose	208	F/W/56	18.0	ASCVD‡
10	333	Chronic undifferentiated schizophrenia	F/W/66	17.9	ASCVD‡	420	F/B/67	19.5	Carbon monoxide intoxication#
		Mean (±SD)	**54.5 (±15.0)**	**11.3 (±5.4)**		**Mean (±SD)**	**55.7 (±14.0)**	**10.9 (±6.0)**	

**Results of toxicology screening were available for all subjects, excluding subjects 131 and 207, and were negative except for prescription drugs or alcohol in some subjects.*

†Also met criteria for alcohol abuse, in remission at time of death.

‡ASCVD indicates atherosclerotic coronary vascular disease.

§Also met criteria for alcohol dependence, in remission at time of death.

‖Also met criteria for alcohol dependence, current at time of death.

¶Also met criteria for alcohol abuse, current at time of death.

#Accidental due to defective stove.

Within each region, similar laminar patterns of synaptophysin immunoreactivity were found in subjects with schizophrenia and control subjects. However, in areas 9 and 46, the intensity of immunoreactivity seemed to be decreased, especially in the superficial layers, in many of the case subjects with schizophrenia (Figure 2, A) compared with the matched controls (Figure 2, B). In contrast, no differences in the intensity of label were apparent between subjects with schizophrenia (Figure 2, C) and control subjects in area 17 (Figure 2, D).

QUANTITATIVE COMPARISONS OF SYNAPTOPHYSIN IMMUNOREACTIVITY IN THE BRAINS OF SUBJECTS WITH SCHIZOPHRENIA AND MATCHED CONTROL SUBJECTS

The mean (±SE) adjusted optical density value of synaptophysin immunoreactivity in area 46 (**Figure 4**, A) of the brains of subjects with schizophrenia (0.169±0.018) was significantly decreased ($F_{1,19}$=23.0; $P<.001$) compared with those of control subjects (0.198±0.027). Levels of synaptophysin immunoreactivity were decreased by 15% to 30% in the brains of subjects with schizophrenia relative to those of the matched control subjects in 6 of the 10 pairs (Figure 4, B). Similarly, in area 9 (Figure 4, C), the mean adjusted optical density value was significantly decreased ($F_{1,19}$=8.78; $P<.008$) in the brains of subjects with schizophrenia (0.164±0.017) compared with those of control subjects (0.192±0.030). In 8 pairs, the brains of subjects with schizophrenia exhibited a reduction in the amount of synaptophysin immunoreactivity relative to those of the matched control, with the reduction ranging from 10% to 35% in 5 pairs (Figure 4, D).

The intense synaptophysin immunoreactivity present in layer 1, which might represent surface artifact staining, could confound comparisons across subjects. Exclusion of values from layer 1 resulted in lower mean adjusted optical density measurements for the brains of subjects with schizophrenia (area 9, 0.152±0.015; area 46, 0.159±0.017) and those of the control subjects (area 9, 0.180±0.029; area 46, 0.185±0.025). These differences in adjusted optical density measurements between the brains of subjects with schizophrenia and those of control subjects remained statistically significant ($P<.005$)and were identical in magnitude to those found with measurements of the entire cortical thickness.

In contrast with these differences in the PFC, no group differences in levels of synaptophysin immunore-

Table 2. Characteristics of Matched Pairs of Nonschizophrenic Psychiatric Subjects and Normal Control Subjects*

	Nonschizophrenic Psychiatric Subjects					Control Subjects			
Pair	Subject No.	*DSM-III-R* Diagnosis	Sex/ Age, y	Postmortem Interval, h	Cause of Death	Subject No.	Sex/ Age, y	Postmortem Interval, h	Cause of Death
1	217	Organic delusional disorder†	M/29	9.0	Acute ethanol intoxication	187	M/32	7.6	Myocarditis
2	223	Major depression†	M/29	27.5	Suicide by drug overdose	457	M/25	17.0	Carbon monoxide intoxication‡
3	228	Major depression	F/66	5.4	Asphyxiation	365	M/68	10.0	ASCVD§
4	248	Major depression and somatization disorder	F/48	6.3	Suicide by hanging	250	F/47	5.3	ASCVD§
5	282	Alcohol abuse	M/58	11.5	Suicide by hanging	166	M/63	8.2	ASCVD§
		Mean (±SD)	**46.0 (±16.8)**	**11.9 (±9.0)**		**Mean (±SD)**	**47.0 (±18.7)**	**9.6 (±4.5)**	

**Results from toxicology screening were available for all subjects and were negative except for prescription drugs or alcohol in some subjects. All nonschizophrenic psychiatric and control subjects were white.*

†Also met criteria for alcohol dependence, current at time of death.

‡Accidental due to explosion.

§ASCVD indicates atherosclerotic coronary artery disease.

activity were observed in area 17 (Figure 4, E). Only 1 pair showed a decrease of more than 10% in the brain of the subject with schizophrenia (Figure 4, F).

In both prefrontal regions, neither age (area 46, $r=-0.07$; area 9, $r=-0.38$) nor PMI (area 46, $r=-0.36$; area 9, $r=-0.06$) was significantly correlated with the magnitude of the difference in synaptophysin immunoreactivity between subjects with schizophrenia and control subjects. In addition, there was no effect of sex on the group differences in synaptophysin immunoreactivity, although only 3 pairs of female subjects were available for this study.

LAMINAR COMPARISONS OF SYNAPTOPHYSIN IMMUNOREACTIVITY IN THE BRAINS OF SUBJECTS WITH SCHIZOPHRENIA AND OF MATCHED CONTROL SUBJECTS

To determine if the decrease in synaptophysin immunoreactivity in the subjects with schizophrenia was greater in the superficial cortical layers (Figure 2), adjusted optical density values for the superficial half (approximately layers 1-3) and deep half (layers 4-6) of the prefrontal areas were analyzed. The 2 pairs of subjects (pairs 5 and 10) that showed an increase in synaptophysin immunoreactivity in the brain of the subject with schizophrenia were excluded from this analysis. The magnitude of the absolute differences in mean adjusted optical density values was greater in the superficial cortical layers than in the deep layers for both areas 46 and 9 (**Figure 5**, A). However, when expressed as a percentage of the matched control value, the superficial and deep layers of the brains of subjects with schizophrenia exhibited a 20% decrease in adjusted optical density values in both prefrontal regions (Figure 5, B). These findings suggest that synaptophysin immunoreactivity was decreased across all cortical layers in the brains of subjects with schizophrenia, and that the greater absolute difference in adjusted optical density levels in the superficial layers may reflect the relatively higher synaptic density in these cortical layers.[21]

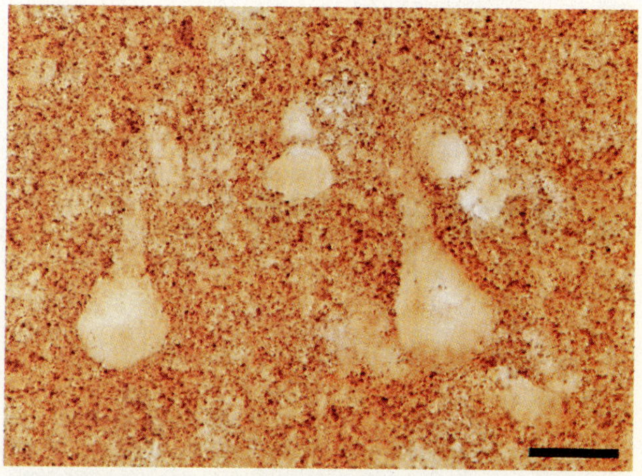

Figure 1. *Brightfield photomicrograph illustrating the typical appearance of synaptophysin immunoreactivity in area 46 of the prefrontal cortex of control subject 247. Synaptophysin immunoreactivity typically labels the neuropil in a punctate manner. Cell bodies and proximal dendrites are outlined by the terminal labeling. Calibration bar is equivalent to 20 μm.*

SYNAPTOPHYSIN IMMUNOREACTIVITY IN THE BRAINS OF NONSCHIZOPHRENIC PSYCHIATRIC CASE SUBJECTS AND OF MATCHED NORMAL CONTROL SUBJECTS

Similar studies were conducted on the brains of nonschizophrenic psychiatric case subjects and of matched normal control subjects to determine the diagnostic specificity of the observations on the brains of subjects with schizophrenia. In contrast with the findings in the schizophrenia case-control studies, levels of synaptophysin immunoreactivity were not decreased in any region of the brains of nonschizophrenic psychiatric case subjects (**Figure 6**). In areas 9 and 46, the brains of all nonschizophrenic psychiatric case subjects exhibited either no difference or an increase in the levels of synaptophy-

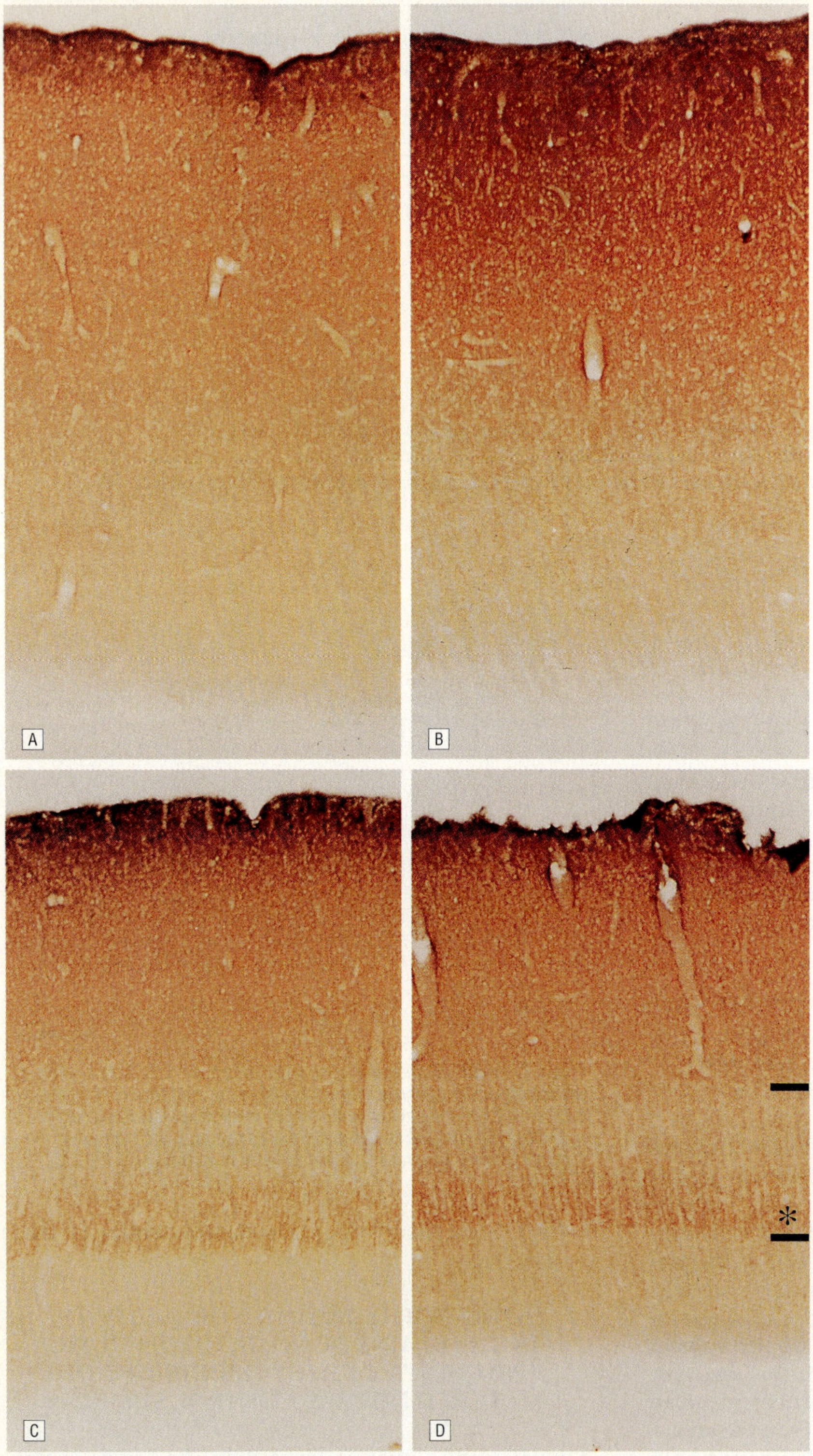

Figure 2. *Brightfield photomicrographs of synaptophysin immunoreactivity in areas 46 (A,B) and 17 (C,D) of a subject with schizophrenia (A and C) and the matched normal control subject (B and D; pair 1 in Table 1). Compared with the matched control subject, the intensity of synaptophysin immunoreactivity seems to be decreased in area 46, but not in area 17, of the subject with schizophrenia. Also apparent is the different laminar distribution of synaptophysin immunoreactivity in areas 46 and 17 in both subjects. D, Hash marks indicate the locations of the borders between layers 3 and 4 and layers 4 and 5, and the asterisk indicates the band of increased synaptophysin immunoreactivity located in layer 4cβ. Calibration bar is equivalent to 500 μm.*

sin immunoreactivity compared with their control subjects. The only exception was area 9 of pair 4, where synaptophysin levels were 7% lower in the brain of the nonschizophrenic psychiatric subject. These findings suggest that the reduction in synaptophysin immunoreactivity is not a common characteristic of individuals with psychiatric disorders, raising the possibility that it may be specific to schizophrenia.

COMMENT

These findings demonstrate that synaptophysin immunoreactivity is decreased in at least 2 regions of the PFC in most subjects with schizophrenia compared with matched control subjects, but is unchanged in the primary visual cortex. These results suggest that the reduc-

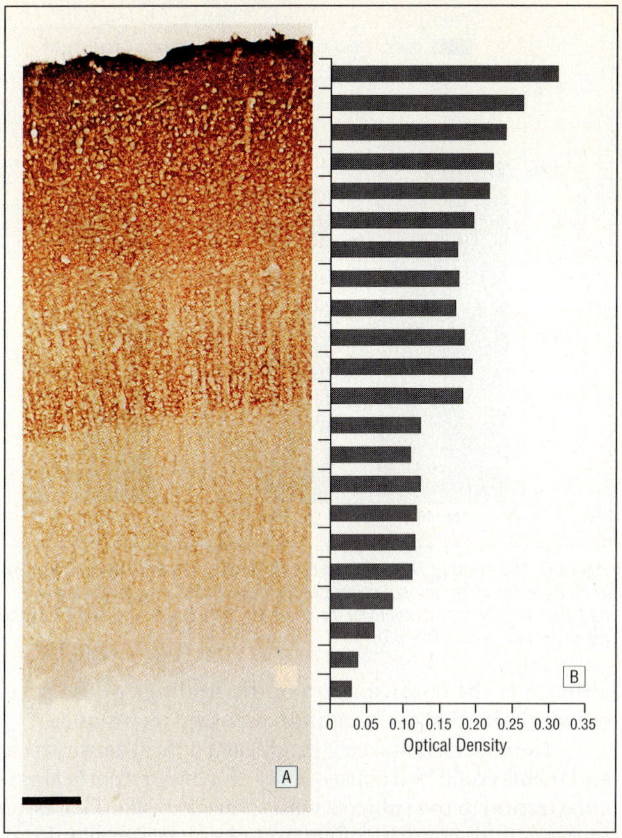

Figure 3. *A, Brightfield photomicrograph of synaptophysin immunoreactivity in area 17, the human primary visual cortex. Synaptophysin immunoreactivity progressively decreased from the pial surface through layer 3. At the border between layers 3 and 4, the intensity of immunoreactivity seemed to decrease stepwise, to remain relatively low in layers 4a and 4b, and then to increase again in layer 4c, with a particularly striking band in sublayer 4cβ. The border between sublayer 4cβ and layer 5 was defined by a sharp decline in immunoreactivity that continued throughout layer 5. The synaptophysin immunoreactivity then increased slightly in layer 6 before declining abruptly at the border between layer 6 and the white matter. Calibration bar in A is equivalent to 200 µm. The distinctive laminar pattern of synaptophysin immunoreactivity in this region is reflected in the optical density values shown in the 100-µm-deep bins, in panel B.*

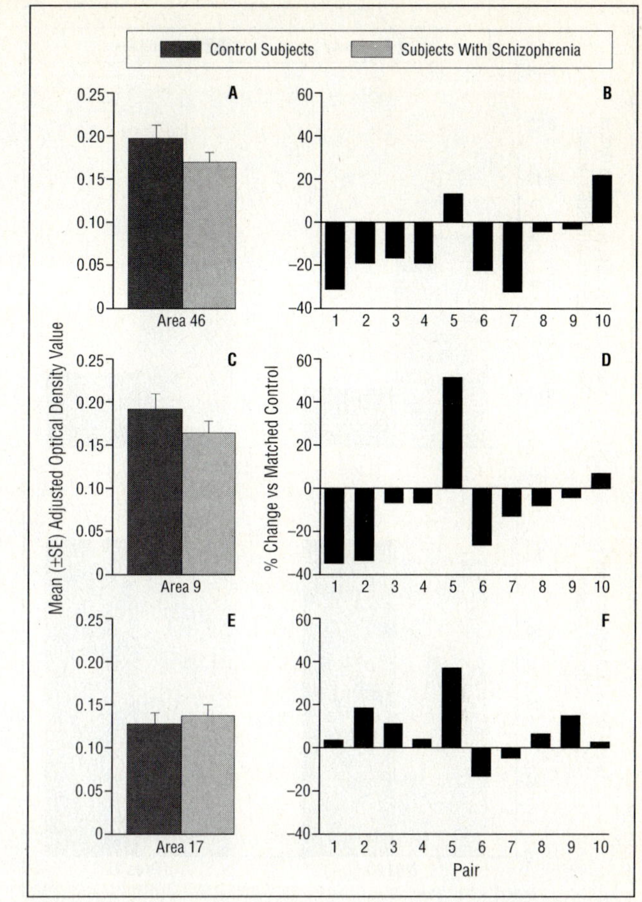

Figure 4. *The mean (±SE) adjusted optical density values of synaptophysin immunoreactivity for the 10 subjects with schizophrenia and matched control subjects in areas 46 (A; $F_{1,19}$=23.0; P<.001), 9 (C; $F_{1,19}$=8.78; P<.008), and 17 (E; $F_{1,23}$; P>.05). The percentage change in adjusted optical density of each subject with schizophrenia relative to the matched control subject for areas 46, 9, and 17 is shown in B, D, and F, respectively.*

tion of synaptophysin immunoreactivity in schizophrenia is not a global cortical effect, but exhibits regional selectivity. Consistent with these observations, synaptophysin protein levels have been reported to be significantly decreased in the PFC and inferior temporal cortex, but not in the primary visual cortex, of subjects with schizophrenia.[38] Other investigators have also observed a decrease in synaptophysin immunoreactivity in the hippocampal formation of subjects with schizophrenia.[39,40] In contrast with these findings of regional specificity, both the PFC and the primary visual cortex of subjects with schizophrenia have been reported to exhibit similar alterations in neuronal density.[18]

Although synaptophysin immunoreactivity was decreased in the PFC of most of the subjects with schizophrenia, levels were clearly increased in 1 subject with schizophrenia (No. 317) compared with the matched control subject (No. 278) in all 3 areas. To determine whether this finding reflected heterogeneity across subjects with schizophrenia or abnormally low levels of synaptophysin immunoreactivity in the matched control, we measured synaptophysin immunoreactivity in control subject 278 and 4 other closely matched normal white men (age range, 45-50 years; PMI range, 5.1-7.8 hours). This comparison suggested that adjusted optical density levels of synaptophysin immunoreactivity in control subject 278 were unusually low. For example, in area 9, mean adjusted optical density levels in control subject 278 were only 61% of the value for the matched case subject with schizophrenia, whereas in the other 4 matched controls, these values ranged from 88% to 95% of the levels for case subject 317. Thus, the apparent marked elevation (Figure 4) of adjusted optical density values in all 3 cortical areas of case subject 317 seems to have been an artifact of the matched control subject used in the initial study.

The decreased synaptophysin immunoreactivity in the PFC may be specific to schizophrenia, since no differences were observed between the brains of nonschizophrenic psychiatric case subjects and of matched normal control subjects. In addition, 2 of the control subjects (Nos. 230 and 249) used in the first study had a history of a psychiatric disorder, but levels of synaptophysin immunoreactivity were substantially reduced in both prefrontal regions of the case subjects with schizophrenia matched to these control subjects (pairs 1 and 2 of Figure 4, B and D). Several lines of evidence also indicate that the coexistence of a diagnosis of alcohol dependence or abuse in 5 schizophrenic subjects is unlikely to account for our findings. First, synaptophysin levels in the PFC of 2 of the subjects with schizophre-

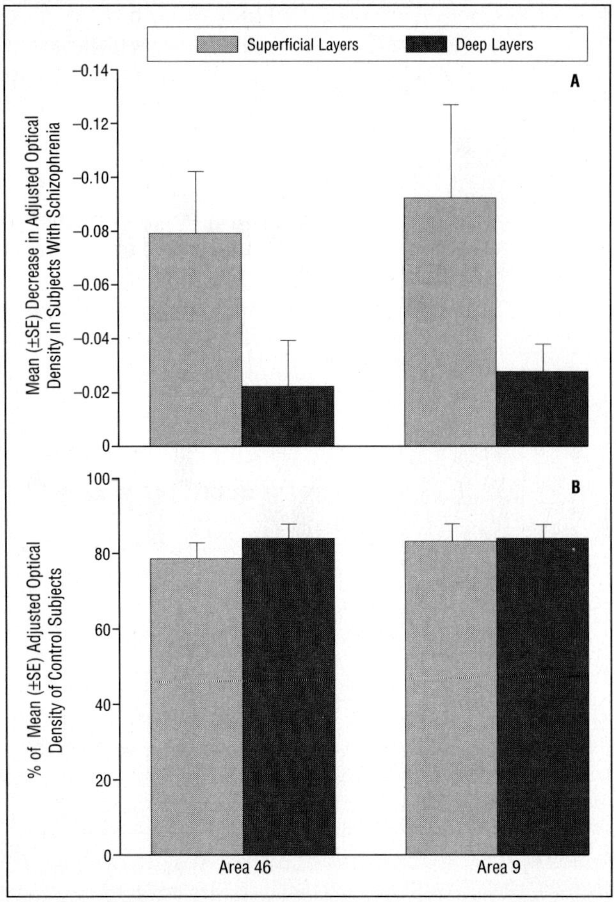

Figure 5. *Comparison of adjusted optical density values in the superficial and deep layers of areas 46 and 9 for 8 pairs of subjects with schizophrenia and their matched control subjects (see text). A, Mean (±SE) decrease in the adjusted optical density of the 8 subjects with schizophrenia relative to their matched control subjects. B, Mean (±SE) adjusted optical density of 8 subjects with schizophrenia as a percentage of the mean adjusted optical density of the 8 matched control subjects.*

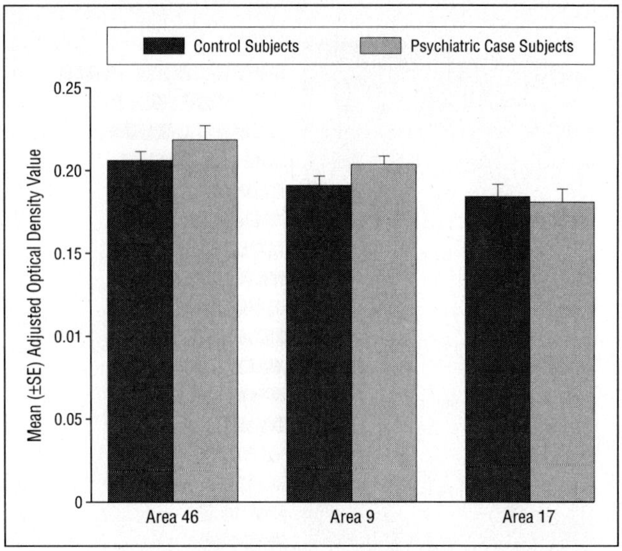

Figure 6. *The mean (±SE) adjusted optical density values of synaptophysin immunoreactivity for the nonschizophrenic psychiatric case subjects and matched normal control subjects for areas 46 (left), 9 (center), and 17 (right) (in each comparison,* P>*.05).*

nia who met criteria for alcohol abuse did not differ from the matched controls (pairs 8 and 9 of Figure 4). Second, in 1 subject with schizophrenia (No. 153) who had a history of alcoholism, PFC synaptophysin immunoreactivity was decreased compared with the matched control subject (No. 230) who also had a history of alcohol dependence. Third, none of the 5 subjects with schizophrenia who had a history of alcoholism showed decreased synaptophysin immunoreactivity in the primary visual cortex. Finally, the 3 nonschizophrenic psychiatric case subjects who met diagnostic criteria for alcohol dependence or abuse did not show decreased levels of synaptophysin immunoreactivity. Together, these findings strongly suggest that the decrease in synaptophysin immunoreactivity in schizophrenia may be specific to that disorder and not a general correlate of psychiatric illness or a consequence of alcoholism.

POSSIBLE CONFOUNDING VARIABLES

As indicated previously, multiple technical controls were used to minimize the potential pitfalls of quantitative immunocytochemical techniques.[41] Although we cannot completely exclude the influence of such potential confounding variables, perhaps the best evidence for their absence is the confirmation of the findings of the present study by the use of complementary techniques.[38]

The observed decrease in adjusted optical density measurements could be a consequence of increased cortical vascularization in the subjects with schizophrenia. That is, an increase in the density of cortical blood vessels would result in fewer axon terminals per unit area of cortex and, consequently, decreased adjusted optical density measurements of synaptophysin immunoreactivity. However, 2 observations argue against this explanation for our findings. First, the primary visual cortex is more highly vascularized than the PFC in the human brain[42] and might be expected to exhibit an even larger difference between subjects with schizophrenia and control subjects than would the PFC. However, no differences in levels of synaptophysin immunoreactivity in the visual cortex were detected. Second, quantitative measurements were made of blood vessel cross-sectional area for the 5 pairs of case subjects in whom the greatest decrease in synaptophysin levels was found in area 46 (Figure 4, B). In these pairs, the mean (±SE) area (per 1.0 mm^2 of cortex) of blood vessels in the subjects with schizophrenia (0.017±0.002 mm^2) was actually smaller than that of the controls (0.022±0.004 mm^2). Thus, the observed decrease in adjusted optical density measurements of synaptophysin immunoreactivity does not seem to be attributable to increased vasculature in the PFC of subjects with schizophrenia.

Finally, several lines of evidence suggest that the findings of this study are not due to medication effects. First, in 2 case subjects with schizophrenia not receiving antipsychotic medications at the time of death (Nos. 207 and 185), levels of synaptophysin immunoreactivity were decreased in the PFC. Second, case subject 341 who committed suicide by taking an overdose of chlorpromazine did not show a decrease in synaptophysin levels. Third, adjusted optical density measurements of synaptophysin immunoreactivity were more than 30% lower in the PFC of case subject 131 than in the matched control (No. 249), a subject who did not have schizophrenia but who had received treatment with antipsychotic medications. Fourth, synaptophysin levels were not decreased in control subject 217, who did not have schizophrenia and who had also been treated with antipsychotic medications. Fifth, in an additional pair of subjects (see "Subjects and Methods" section), in whom major depressive disorder had been diagnosed, synaptophysin levels in the PFC were not lower in the subject who had received treatment with antipsychotic medications. Sixth, administration of haloperidol for 2 weeks had no effect on synaptophysin protein levels in rodent cerebral cortex specimens.[40] Finally, although the decrease in synaptophysin immunoreactivity in schizophrenia could be due to a decrease in the number or size of axon terminals or in the density of synaptic vesicles per terminal, these types of changes are unlikely to be a consequence of antipsychotic medications. For example, although chronic treatment of rats with haloperidol or clozapine may cause a shift in the relative percentages of the types of postsynaptic membrane specializations, they do not change the total number or average size of cortical axon terminals or the density of synaptic vesicles per terminal.[43]

POSSIBLE MECHANISMS UNDERLYING DECREASED LEVELS OF SYNAPTOPHYSIN IMMUNOREACTIVITY

The findings of this study suggest several possible mechanisms that could impair synaptic transmission in the PFC of subjects with schizophrenia. First, decreased synaptophysin immunoreactivity could be due to a decrease in the number of presynaptic terminals, and consequently in the number of synapses, in the PFC of subjects with schizophrenia. Presynaptic terminals are major components of the cortical neuropil, and a variety of recent studies, though not all,[14,15,19,20] have produced findings consistent with a decreased amount of neuropil in the PFC of subjects with schizophrenia. First, both imaging and postmortem studies have revealed a decrease in PFC volume in subjects with schizophrenia.[9-13,16-18] Second, increased phospholipid turnover in the PFC of patients with schizophrenia observed with magnetic resonance spectroscopy[44-47] may also reflect a loss of neuropil.[45,46] Third, an increase in neuronal density[18] without a change in total cell number[15,17] has also been observed in the PFC of subjects with schizophrenia. Finally, the density of dendritic spines, the major sites of excitatory synapses on pyramidal neurons, is decreased in the PFC of subjects with schizophrenia.[48,49] These findings and those of the present study converge on the common hypothesis that the number of presynaptic terminals and synaptic contacts is decreased in the PFC of subjects with schizophrenia. This interpretation is consistent with previous suggestions that PFC dysfunction in schizophrenia is related to the elimination of cortical synapses during adolescence.[50-52]

Alternatively, a reduction in the number of synaptic vesicles per terminal could produce the observed decrease in synaptophysin immunoreactivity. Because the size of an axon terminal is directly correlated with the number of vesicles it contains,[53] a decrease in the number of synaptic vesicles per terminal in subjects with schizophrenia would be associated with a decrease in terminal size and a decrease in synaptophysin immunoreactivity. Such a decrease in axon terminal size might also contribute to a decrease in PFC neuropil and volume in schizophrenia.

Finally, the results of this study could be caused by a decrease in the expression of synaptophysin messenger RNA, as has been observed in the hippocampal formation of subjects with schizophrenia.[40] Although such changes might not produce structural alterations in the PFC, they would likely disrupt neurotransmission in this region, given the critical role of synaptophysin in exocytosis.[25]

What elements of PFC circuitry might contribute to the altered synaptophysin immunoreactivity in subjects with schizophrenia? The decreased synaptophysin immunoreactivity across all cortical layers suggests that the involved system or systems must have axon terminals distributed throughout the cortical gray matter. Thus, it seems unlikely that abnormalities in projections from the mediodorsal thalamic nucleus, which terminate in the middle layers of the PFC,[54] could, at least in isolation, account for these findings. However, abnormalities in these afferents could have secondary effects on synaptophysin levels across all cortical layers. Projections to the PFC from many other cortical regions terminate across all cortical layers.[55] Thus, decreased synaptophysin immunoreactivity could reflect alterations in corticocortical input, which would certainly impair the function of the PFC.

In addition, although they comprise a variety of different subtypes, as a group, PFC γ-aminobutyric acid (GABA) neurons provide axon terminals in all cortical layers.[56] Thus, alterations in GABA terminals might also account for the findings of the present study, an interpretation supported by studies demonstrating alterations in GABA systems in the PFC of subjects with schizophrenia.[15,57-59]

Clearly, it is impossible to determine from the results of this study exactly which neural system(s) are altered in the PFC of subjects with schizophrenia. In addition, although a decline in synaptophysin immunoreactivity could lead to altered function of the PFC in schizophrenia,[2-4,6-8] it is also possible that impaired activation of this region may induce a reduction in markers of synaptic transmission. However, whatever pathological mechanism(s) lead to these alterations, disturbances in the levels of synaptophysin, a critical component of synaptic transmission, are likely to have profound effects on PFC synaptic function in schizophrenia.

Accepted for publication June 21, 1996.

This work was supported in part by the Independent Scientist Award MH00519 (Dr Lewis) and the Center for the Neuroscience of Mental Disorders grant MH45156, from the National Institute of Mental Health (Dr Lewis), and by a grant from the Scottish Rite Schizophrenia Research Program, Northern Masonic Jurisdiction, Lexington, Mass (Ms Glantz).

Presented as a poster exhibit at the Society for Neuroscience Meeting, Miami, Fla, November 15, 1994.

We thank Mayada Akil, MD, and Larry Glanz, PhD, for their help in obtaining the clinical information on the subjects used in this study, and Gretchen Haas, PhD, Matcheri Keshavan, MD, and Nina Schooler, PhD, for their participation in the diagnostic conferences. We also thank Allan Sampson, PhD, and Kris Schmidt, MA, for statistical consultation, Mary Brady for photographic assistance, and Dr Akil and Michele Pucak, PhD, for helpful comments on the manuscript.

Corresponding author: David A. Lewis, MD, Western Psychiatric Institute and Clinic, W1651 BST, 3811 O'Hara St, Pittsburgh, PA 15213.

REFERENCES

1. Levin S. Frontal lobe dysfunctions in schizophrenia, II: impairments of psychological and brain functions. *J Psychiat Res.* 1984;18:57-72.
2. Berman KF, Torrey EF, Daniel DG, Weinberger DR. Regional cerebral blood flow in monozygotic twins discordant and concordant for schizophrenia. *Arch Gen Psychiatry.* 1992;49:927-934.
3. Buchsbaum MS, Haier RJ, Potkin SG, Neuchterlein K, Bracha HS, Katz M, Lohr J, Wu J, Lottenberg S, Jerabek PA, Trenary M, Tafalla R, Reynolds C, Bunney WE Jr. Frontrostriatal disorder of cerebral metabolism in never-medicated schizophrenics. *Arch Gen Psychiatry.* 1992;49:935-942.
4. Ingvar DH, Franzen G. Abnormalities of cerebral blood flow distribution in patients with chronic schizophrenia. *Acta Psychiat Scand.* 1974;50:425-462.
5. Park S, Holzman PS. Schizophrenics show spatial working memory deficits. *Arch Gen Psychiatry.* 1992;49:975-982.
6. Rubin P, Holm S, Friberg L, Videbech P, Anderson HS, Bendsen BB, Stromso N, Larsen JK, Lassen NA, Hemmingsen R. Altered modulation of prefrontal and subcortical brain activity in newly diagnosed schizophrenia and schizophreniform disorder: a regional cerebral blood flow study. *Arch Gen Psychiatry.* 1991;48:987-995.
7. Wolkin A, Sanfilipo M, Wolf AP, Angrist B, Brodie JD, Rotrosen J. Negative symptoms and hypofrontality in chronic schizophrenia. *Arch Gen Psychiatry.* 1992; 49:959-965.
8. Weinberger DR, Berman KF, Zec RF. Physiologic dysfunction of dorsolateral prefrontal cortex in schizophrenia, I: regional cerebral blood flow evidence. *Arch Gen Psychiatry.* 1986;43:114-124.
9. Andreasen NC, Flashman L, Flaum M, Arndt S, Swayze V II, O'Leary DS, Ehrhardt JC, Yuh WT. Regional brain abnormalities in schizophrenia measured with magnetic resonance imaging. *JAMA.* 1994;272:1763-1769.
10. Breier A, Buchanan RW, Elkashef A, Munson RC, Kirkpatrick B, Gellad F. Brain morphology and schizophrenia: a magnetic resonance imaging study of limbic, prefrontal cortex, and caudate structures. *Arch Gen Psychiatry.* 1992;49:921-926.
11. Schlaepfer TE, Harris GJ, Tien AY, Peng LW, Lee S, Federman EB, Chase GA, Barta PE, Pearlson GD. Decreased regional cortical gray matter volume in schizophrenia. *Am J Psychiatry.* 1994;151:842-848.
12. Shelton RC, Karson CN, Doran AR, Pickar D, Bigelow LB, Weinberger DR. Cerebral structural pathology in schizophrenia: evidence for a selective prefrontal cortical defect. *Am J Psychiatry.* 1988;145:154-163.
13. Zipursky RB, Lim KO, Sullivan EV, Brown BW, Pfefferbaum A. Widespread cerebral gray matter volume deficits in schizophrenia. *Arch Gen Psychiatry.* 1992; 49:195-205.
14. Wible CG, Shenton ME, Hokama H, Kikinis R, Jolesz FA, Metcalf D, McCarley RW. Prefrontal cortex and schizophrenia: a quantitative magnetic resonance imaging study. *Arch Gen Psychiatry.* 1995;52:279-288.
15. Akbarian S, Kim JJ, Potkin SG, Hagman JO, Tafazzoli A, Bunney WE Jr, Jones EG. Gene expression for glutamic acid decarboxylase is reduced without loss of neurons in prefrontal cortex of schizophrenics. *Arch Gen Psychiatry.* 1995;52:258-266.
16. Pakkenberg B. Post-mortem study of chronic schizophrenic brains. *Br J Psychiatry.* 1987;151:744-752.
17. Pakkenberg B. Total nerve cell number in neocortex in chronic schizophrenics and controls estimated using optical disectors. *Biol Psychiatry.* 1993;34:768-772.
18. Selemon LD, Rajkowska G, Goldman-Rakic PS. Abnormally high neuronal density in the schizophrenic cortex: a morphometric analysis of prefrontal area 9 and occipital area 17. *Arch Gen Psychiatry.* 1995;52:805-818.
19. Benes FM, Davidson J, Bird ED. Quantitative cytoarchitectural studies of the cerebral cortex of schizophrenics. *Arch Gen Psychiatry.* 1986;43:31-35.
20. Benes FM, McSparren J, Bird ED, SanGiovanni JP, Vincent SL. Deficits in small interneurons in prefrontal and cingulate cortices of schizophrenic and schizoaffective patients. *Arch Gen Psychiatry.* 1991;48:996-1001.
21. Bourgeois J-P, Goldman-Rakic PS, Rakic P. Synaptogenesis in the prefrontal cortex of rhesus monkeys. *Cereb Cortex.* 1994;4:78-96.
22. Jahn R, Schiebler W, Ouimet C, Greengard P. A 38,000-dalton membrane protein (p38) present in synaptic vesicles. *Proc Natl Acad Sci U S A.* 1985;82:4137-4141.
23. Navone F, Jahn R, DiGioia G, Stukenbrok H, Greengard P, DeCamilli P. Protein p38: an integral membrane protein specific for small vesicles of neurons and neuroendocrine cells. *J Cell Biol.* 1986;103:2511-2527.
24. Wiedenmann B, Franke WW. Identification and localization of synaptophysin, an integral membrane glycoprotein of M_r 38,000 characteristic of presynaptic vesicles. *Cell.* 1985;41:1017-1028.
25. Alder J, Lu B, Valtorta F, Greengard P, Poo M. Calcium-dependent transmitter secretion reconstituted in *Xenopus* oocytes: requirement for synaptophysin. *Science.* 1992;257:657-661.
26. Alder J, Kanki H, Valtorta F, Greengard P, Poo M. Overexpression of synaptophysin enhances neurotransmitter secretion at xenopus neuromuscular synapses. *J Neurosci.* 1995;15:511-519.
27. Hamos JE, DeGennaro LJ, Drachman DA. Synaptic loss in Alzheimer's disease and other dementias. *Neurology.* 1989;39:355-361.
28. Masliah E, Terry RD, Alford M, DeTeresa R. Quantitative immunohistochemistry of synaptophysin in human neocortex: an alternative method to estimate density of presynaptic terminals in paraffin sections. *J Histochem Cytochem.* 1990;38:837-844.
29. Masliah E, Terry RD, Alford M, DeTeresa R, Hansen LA. Cortical and subcortical patterns of synaptophysinlike immunoreactivity in Alzheimer's disease. *Am J Pathol.* 1991;138:235-246.
30. Khachaturian ZS. Diagnosis of Alzheimer's disease. *Arch Neurol.* 1985;42:1097-1105.
31. Dixon L, Haas G, Weiden PJ, Sweeney J, Frances AJ. Drug abuse in schizophrenic patients: clinical correlates and reasons for use. *Am J Psychiatry.* 1991;148:224-230.
32. Daviss SR, Lewis DA. Local circuit neurons of the prefrontal cortex in schizophrenia: selective increase in the density of calbindin-immunoreactive neurons. *Psychiatry Res.* 1995;59:81-96.
33. Rosenberg DR, Lewis DA. Postnatal maturation of the dopaminergic innervation of monkey prefrontal and motor cortices: a tyrosine hydroxylase immunohistochemical analysis. *J Comp Neurol.* 1995;358:383-400.
34. Lewis DA, Campbell MJ, Terry RD, Morrison JH. The laminar and regional distribution of neurofibrillary tangles and neuritic plaques in Alzheimer's disease: a quantitative study of visual and auditory cortices. *J Neurosci.* 1987;7:1799-1808.
35. Rajkowska G, Goldman-Rakic PS. Cytoarchitectonic definition of prefrontal areas in the normal human cortex, I: remapping of areas 9 and 46 using quantitative criteria. *Cereb Cortex.* 1995;5:307-322.
36. Devoto SH, Barnstable CJ. SVP38: a synaptic vesicle protein whose appearance correlates closely with synaptogenesis in the rat nervous system. *Ann N Y Acad Sci.* 1987;493:493-496.
37. Smolen AJ. Image analytic techniques for quantification of immunohistochemical staining in the nervous system. In: Conn PM, ed. *Quantitative and Qualitative Microscopy.* Orlando, Fla: Academic Press Inc; 1990:208-229.
38. Perrone-Bizzozero NI, Sower AC, Bird ED, Benowitz LI, Ivins KJ, Neve RL. Levels of the growth-associated protein GAP-43 are selectively increased in association cortices in schizophrenia. *Proc Natl Acad Sci U S A.* 1996;93:14182-14187.
39. Browning MD, Dudek EM, Rapier JL, Leonard S, Freedman R. Significant reductions in synapsin but not synaptophysin specific activity in the brains of some schizophrenics. *Biol Psychiatry.* 1993;34:529-535.
40. Eastwood SL, Harrison PJ. Decreased synaptophysin in the medial temporal lobe in schizophrenia demonstrated using immunoautoradiography. *Neuroscience.* 1995;69:339-343.
41. Peretti-Renucci R, Feuerstein C, Manier M, Lorimier P, Savasta M, Thibault J, Mons N, Geffard M. Quantitative image analysis with densitometry for immunohistochemistry and autoradiography of receptor binding sites—methodological considerations. *J Neurosci Res.* 1991;28:583-600.
42. Duvernoy H, Delon S, Vannson JL. Cortical blood vessels of the human brain. *Brain Res Bull.* 1981;7:519-579.
43. Vincent SL, McSparren J, Wang RY, Benes FM. Evidence for ultrastructural changes in cortical axodendritic synapses following long-term treatment with haloperidol or clozapine. *Neuropsychopharmacology.* 1991;5:147-155.
44. Deicken RF, Calabrese G, Merrin EL, Meyerhoff DJ, Dillon WP, Weiner MW, Fein G. ^{31}Phosphorus magnetic resonance spectroscopy of the frontal and parietal lobes in chronic schizophrenia. *Biol Psychiatry.* 1994;36:503-510.
45. Pettegrew JW, Keshavan MS, Panchalingam K, Strychor S, Kaplan DB, Tretta MG, Allen M. Alterations in brain high-energy phosphate and membrane phospholipid metabolism in first-episode, drug-naive schizophrenics: a pilot study of the dorsal prefrontal cortex by in vivo phosphorus 31 nuclear magnetic resonance imaging. *Arch Gen Psychiatry.* 1991;48:563-568.
46. Stanley JA, Williamson PC, Drost DJ, Carr TJ, Rylett RJ, Malla A, Thompson RT. An *in vivo* study of the prefrontal cortex of schizophrenic patients at different stages of illness via phosphorus magnetic resonance spectroscopy. *Arch Gen Psychiatry.* 1995;52:399-406.
47. Williamson P, Drost D, Stanley J, Carr T, Morrison S, Merskey H. Localized phosphorous 31 magnetic resonance spectroscopy in chronic schizophrenic patients and normal controls. *Arch Gen Psychiatry.* 1991;48:578.
48. Glantz LA, Lewis DA. Assessment of spine density on layer III pyramidal cells in the prefrontal cortex of schizophrenic subjects. *Soc Neurosci Abstr.* 1995;21:239.
49. Garey LJ, Ong WY, Patel TS, Kanani M, Davis A, Hornstein C, Bauer M. Reduction in dendritic spine number on cortical pyramidal neurons in schizophrenia. *Soc Neurosci Abstr.* 1995;21:237.
50. Feinberg I. Schizophrenia: caused by a fault in programmed synaptic elimination during adolescence? *J Psychiat Res.* 1982;17:319-334.
51. Hoffman RE, Dobscha SK. Cortical pruning and the development of schizophrenia: a computer model. *Schizophr Bull.* 1989;15:477-490.
52. Hoffman RE, McGlashan TH. Parallel distributed processing and the emergence of schizophrenic symptoms. *Schizophr Bull.* 1993;19:119-140.
53. Pierce JP, Lewin GR. An ultrastructural size principle. *Neuroscience.* 1994;58: 441-446.
54. Giguere M, Goldman-Rakic PS. Mediodorsal nucleus: areal, laminar, and tangential distribution of afferents and efferents in the frontal lobe of rhesus monkeys. *J Comp Neurol.* 1988;277:195-213.
55. Goldman-Rakic PS, Schwartz ML. Interdigitation of contralateral and ipsilateral columnar projections to frontal association cortex in primates. *Science.* 1982; 216:755-757.
56. Lund JS, Lewis DA. Local circuit neurons of developing and mature macaque prefrontal cortex: golgi and immunocytochemical characteristics. *J Comp Neurol.* 1993;328:282-312.
57. Sherman AD, Davidson AT, Baruah S, Hegwood TS, Waziri R. Evidence of glutamatergic deficiency in schizophrenia. *Neurosci Lett.* 1991;121:77-80.
58. Benes FM, Vincent SL, Alsterberg G, Bird ED, SanGiovanni JP. Increased $GABA_A$ receptor binding in superficial layers of cingulate cortex in schizophrenics. *J Neurosci.* 1992;12:924-929.
59. Benes FM, Vincent SL, Marie A, Khan Y. Up-regulation of $GABA_A$ receptor binding on neurons of the prefrontal cortex in schizophrenic subjects. *Neuroscience.* 1996;75:1021-1031.

Delayed Normalization of Central D_2 Dopamine Receptor Availability After Discontinuation of Haloperidol Decanoate

Preliminary Findings

Svante Nyberg, MD, PhD; Lars Farde, MD, PhD; Christer Halldin, PhD

Background: Antipsychotic drugs in depot formulations may prevent psychotic relapses, even after complete withdrawal. To examine the duration of drug remaining in the brain, central D_2 dopamine receptor occupancy was measured with positron emission tomography for a year after discontinuation of depot neuroleptic treatment.

Methods: Four schizophrenic patients were withdrawn from low-dose treatment with haloperidol decanoate (30-50 mg every 4 weeks). They were examined repeatedly with positron emission tomography and the radioligand carbon 11-labeled raclopride during the following year. At end point, a Scatchard analysis was performed to determine the density and affinity of D_2 dopamine receptors.

Results: Occupancy of D_2 dopamine receptors was highest 1 week after depot injection (66%, 77%, 82%, and 78% in 4 patients) and then decreased slowly. Six months after discontinuation of treatment, D_2 dopamine receptor occupancy was 24%, 32%, and 34% in 3 patients. After 1 year, D_2 dopamine receptor density and affinity in 2 patients were within the ranges of control subjects, suggesting no remaining haloperidol.

Conclusions: Our preliminary finding of persistence of D_2 dopamine receptor occupancy indicates that commonly used doses of haloperidol decanoate (200 mg every 4 weeks) maintain antipsychotic levels of receptor occupancy even 16 weeks after discontinuation of treatment. This may explain the lower relapse rates in patients withdrawn from depot neuroleptic treatment compared with those withdrawn from oral treatment. In addition, the remaining occupancy may confound the clinical evaluation of subsequent treatments. For controlled clinical trials of new antipsychotic drugs, we suggest a minimum washout of 6 months after the last depot injection.

Arch Gen Psychiatry. 1997;54:953-958

MAINTENANCE treatment with antipsychotic drugs clearly reduces the risk for psychotic relapses in schizophrenia.[1] However, the benefit of treatment does not apply to all patients, since some patients relapse despite continued treatment, and some do not relapse for extended periods even when medication is withdrawn. These observations and highly prevalent side effects have prompted the development of strategies for dose reduction or discontinuation of antipsychotic treatment.

The risk for recurrence of psychotic symptoms after withdrawal of treatment and the time before an eventual relapse may be influenced by the nature of previous treatment. In particular, previous treatment with depot formulations appears to reduce the risk for psychotic relapse for many dosage intervals after discontinuation.[1,2] Furthermore, remaining amounts of drugs from previous depot treatment may influence both therapeutic effects and adverse events of any subsequent treatment and thus confound the clinical evaluation of optimal dose and adverse events of the new treatment. These issues should also be of importance in the design of controlled clinical trials of new antipsychotic drugs. However, studies of long-term effects after discontinuation of treatment are scarce and may have been hampered by the lack of sufficiently sensitive methods.

In previous studies using positron emission tomography (PET), we have demonstrated quantitative relations between the degree of striatal D_2 dopamine receptor occupancy and clinical effects of classical antipsychotic drugs and proposed that 70% to 80% may be the optimal therapeutic interval for the treatment of acute schizophrenic psychoses.[3,4] Recently, we found D_2 dopamine receptor occupancy above 70% in schizophrenic patients the week after administration of low doses (30-50 mg every 4 weeks) of haloperidol decanoate.[5]

The persistence of D_2 dopamine receptor occupancy after discontinuation of

From the Psychiatry Section, Department of Clinical Neuroscience, Karolinska Institutet, Karolinska Hospital, Stockholm, Sweden.

SUBJECTS AND METHODS

This open study was approved by the Ethics and the Radiation Safety committees of the Karolinska Hospital, Stockholm, Sweden, and was a continuation of a previously reported PET study in 8 schizophrenic patients.[5] The PET examinations were performed at the Psychiatry Section, Department of Clinical Neuroscience, Karolinska Hospital.

DESIGN AND STUDY SCHEDULE

Patients were included at the time of a scheduled depot injection 8 weeks before the start of the study. From week 0 to week 52, the patients were observed without medication for up to 1 year as their clinical status permitted. The PET examinations were performed at 1, 4, 8, 16, and about 26 and 52 weeks after the last depot injection. At end point, the density of D_2 dopamine receptors (B_{max}) and the apparent dissociation constant $K^{app}{}_d$ was determined with a Scatchard analysis[8,9] in the remaining patients.

PATIENTS

Four patients were recruited from a specialized outpatient unit treating more than 400 schizophrenic patients at the Karolinska Hospital. In the whole outpatient population, 122 patients were treated with depot neuroleptics, 39 of whom were treated with haloperidol decanoate in the dose range of 20 to 100 mg (median, 50 mg) every 4 weeks. The patients had requested that medication be withdrawn, and were included after giving their informed consent. Particular care was taken to ensure that patients were cautioned of the risk for psychotic relapse. The patients had previously participated in a psychoeducational program on schizophrenia and were judged to fully understand the potential hazards of drug discontinuation. Monthly visits were scheduled to facilitate early recognition of recurrent psychotic symptoms and reinstatement of treatment if necessary.

The patients fulfilled *DSM-III-R*[10] diagnostic criteria for schizophrenia and had been ill for 3 to 11 years, but had not been hospitalized for at least 1 year before the study (**Table**). They did not have any other mental or physical illness or any substance abuse disorder. Urine samples for screening of metabolites of opiates, amphetamine, cocaine, and cannabis were collected at the time of each PET experiment, and screening yielded negative results in all cases. Psychotic symptoms were assessed using the Brief Psychiatric Rating Scale for Schizophrenia (BPRS)[11] (Kolakowska version, 18 items, with scores ranging from 1-7 [1 indicates not present; 7, maximal]) and the Clinical Global Impression (CGI) scale (with scores ranging from 1-7).[12] The patients had to be judged as responders to neuroleptic treatment and in stable clinical remission, which was indicated by low total BPRS and CGI scores (Table).

DRUG TREATMENT

At inclusion, the patients had received monotherapy consisting of haloperidol decanoate (Haldol Depot, 50 mg/mL, Janssen Pharmaceutica, Beerse, Belgium), 30 to 50 mg every 4 weeks, for at least 10 months with no change in dosage within the last 7 months (Table). The treatment was stopped after the last depot injection at week 0. The dose had previously been titrated so that extrapyramidal side effects should be minimal or absent.[5] Monotherapy had been ensured by requesting the patients to deposit previously prescribed drugs at the outpatient ward during the study. No anticholinergics were administered. Patient 4 was continuously treated with diazepam, 2 mg twice a day, for about 6 months after the last depot injection.

BLOOD ANALYSES

Blood samples for the determination of haloperidol concentrations were collected at 8 and 4 weeks before the start of the study, at week 0, and subsequently in connection with the PET experiments. Haloperidol plasma concentrations were analyzed using high-performance liquid chromatography with UV detection.[13] The limit of determination was 1 nmol/L.

Each patient's disposition of haloperidol by the polymorphic debrisoquin hydroxylase (CYP2D6) was determined by analysis of the *CYP2D6* genotype.[14,15] Patient 4 was homozygous for the mutated *CYP2D6B* allele and was thus a "poor metabolizer" genotype. The other patients were homozygous for the nonmutated wild-type allele and thus "extensive metabolizer" genotypes.

PET EXPERIMENTAL PROCEDURE

The PET experiments with the radioligand carbon 11-labeled raclopride were performed as previously described.[16,17] The specific radioactivity at the time of injection was higher than 500 Ci/mmol when tracer doses were used. The injected radioactivity was 230 to 340 MBq. In 2 experiments with higher doses of raclopride (patients 3 and 4 at 57 weeks), the specific radioactivity was 5.24 and 5.28 Ci/mmol, respectively. Radioactivity in brain tissue was measured for 51 minutes in each experiment with the PET camera system (model

depot treatment has only been studied in single cases, and not for more than a few weeks longer than a treatment interval.[6,7] Our exploratory study followed the time course of D_2 dopamine receptor occupancy after discontinuation of haloperidol decanoate treatment in 4 patients for 1 year, provided that they did not relapse and require reinstatement of treatment.

RESULTS

Four patients entered the study and had their last injection of haloperidol decanoate (30-50 mg) at week 0. All patients had a low degree of overt psychotic symptoms at inclusion and had been stable for more than a year (Table). Patient 2 had a moderate increase of psychotic symptoms 8 weeks after his last depot injection (CGI increase from mildly to moderately ill). Treatment was resumed, and he recovered without hospitalization. Patients 1 and 3 remained in remission for 45 and 57 weeks, respectively, when they had severe psychotic relapses (CGI increase from mildly to severely ill). They were both hospitalized, and after resuming treatment they recovered within 3 weeks. Patient 4 has been monitored clinically for more than 3 years and has not relapsed.

PC2048-15B, Scanditronix, Uppsala, Sweden), which has a resolution of 4.5 mm in the reconstructed images.[18]

REGIONS OF INTEREST

A head fixation system with individually made plastic helmets was used throughout all examinations, so that the same regions of interest could be used for all experiments in each subject.[19] Regions of interest were drawn on the reconstructed PET images, bilaterally for the putamen in 2 adjacent sections. Data from the 4 putamen regions were pooled before calculation of regional radioactivity. The cerebellum was drawn in 1 section. To obtain uptake curves, regional radioactivity was calculated for each scan, corrected for decay, and plotted vs time.

CALCULATIONS

Receptor Occupancy

The theory for equilibrium analysis of D_2 dopamine receptor occupancy using ^{11}C-labeled raclopride has been presented earlier.[16,20] The total radioactivity in the cerebellum, Cf(t), was used as an estimate of the free radioligand concentration in the brain. Radioactivity representing ligand bound specifically to D_2 dopamine receptors, $C_b(t)$, was defined as follows:

$$C_b(t)=C_{put}(t)-C_f(t)$$

where $C_{put}(t)$ is the regional radioactivity in the putamen.

The curves for $C_b(t)$ and $C_f(t)$ were integrated from 9 to 45 minutes (scans 12-18) after radioligand injection and the putamen-cerebellum (P/C) ratio (R) was obtained according to the following:

$$R = \int_9^{45} C_b(t) / \int_9^{45} C_f(t)$$

Occupancy of D_2 dopamine receptors was defined as the percent reduction in R during drug treatment compared with the mean±SD R of 3.77±0.57 previously obtained in 34 healthy subjects (age, 18-50 years).[8,21] In addition, for patients 3 and 4, the experiments at 57 weeks were used as their individual baseline measurements, and D_2 dopamine receptor occupancy was recalculated as the percent reduction in R during the previous experiments.

B_{max} and Apparent K_d

To separately calculate the total number of available D_2 dopamine receptors and B_{max}, additional information was required from experiments with low specific radioactivity, ie, a high total mass of injected radioligand. In such conditions, radioligand binding approaches saturation of the receptor population.[3,9] In summary, the relation between receptor binding and the concentration of ligand at equilibrium is described by the following hyperbolic function:

$$B=(B_{max}{}^*F)/(K_d^{app}+F)$$

where B_{max} is the number of available receptors, B is the concentration of ligand bound to receptors, K_d^{app} is the apparent equilibrium dissociation constant, and F is the concentration of unbound ligand. Rearrangement of this equation gives the following linear equation (Scatchard plot):

$$B/F=(B_{max}-B)/K_d^{app}$$

A series with at least 2 PET experiments with different specific radioactivity results in a series of B/F ratios and B values. The B_{max} is defined by the intercept with the x-axis; K_d^{app}, by the slope of the line. In our study, 2 consecutive PET experiments were performed during the same day using first high and then low specific radioactivity of ^{11}C-labeled raclopride.

The B/F ratios were measured at the time of equilibrium of specific ^{11}C-labeled raclopride binding in each experiment.[16] The ratio was thus obtained by calculating the ratio of C_b to C_f at maximum C_b ($C_b[t_{max}]$), as follows:

$$B/F=(C_b \times t_{max})/(C_f \times t_{max})$$

The 2 pairs of B/F values were plotted in a Scatchard diagram against the corresponding B value to obtain the B_{max} and K_d^{app}.

Remaining Haloperidol

The purpose of the Scatchard analysis was to examine whether there was remaining haloperidol bound to D_2 dopamine receptors at 57 weeks after discontinuation of therapy. In the presence of 2 ligands competing for binding sites, K_d^{app} should be expressed as the following:

$$K^*_d(1+[F/K_d])$$

and equation 4 should be expanded to the following:

$$\frac{B^*}{F^*}=\frac{B_{max}}{K_d^*\left(1+\frac{F}{K_d}\right)+F^*}$$

where the asterisk marks values for raclopride binding and F and K_d represent values for haloperidol. Thus, remaining haloperidol would be reflected in a higher K_d^{app}, ie, a lower apparent affinity of D_2 dopamine receptors.

The plasma levels of haloperidol are presented in **Figure 1**. Haloperidol could not be detected at week 16 or any later time in patients 1 and 4. In patient 3, the concentration was 2.6 nmol/L at weeks 16 and 29, but was not detectable at week 57.

Images representing a transverse section of the brain at the level of the basal ganglia were reconstructed for visualization of ^{11}C-labeled raclopride distribution (**Figure 2**).

The D_2 dopamine receptor binding ratios were plotted vs time after the last depot injection (**Figure 3**). The lowest ratios, indicating the highest receptor occupancies, were found at week 1. Thereafter, the binding ratios increased. At 6 and 12 months after the last depot injection, the ratios were still lower than −1 SD of the control group. The estimated D_2 dopamine receptor occupancy based on the baseline ratio of 3.77 is shown in Figure 3.

In patients 3 and 4, D_2 dopamine receptor occupancy was recalculated using the ratio found at 57 weeks as the individual baseline. In these patients, the D_2 dopamine receptor occupancies were 79% and 72%, respectively, at week 1; 35% and 33%, respectively, at week 16; and 23% and 12%, respectively, at week 26.

A Scatchard analysis was performed at 57 weeks in patients 3 and 4. In these patients, the calculated B_{max} was

Patient and Treatment Characteristics*

Patient No.	Schizophrenia Subtype	Age, y/Sex	Duration of Illness, y	Months Since Last Hospital Discharge	Haloperidol Decanoate Dose, mg Every 4 wk	Duration of Dose, mo	Total Score at Inclusion in Study: BPRS	Total Score at Inclusion in Study: CGI	Time to End Point, mo†	Total Score at End Point, CGI
1	Undifferentiated	42/F	3	28	30	9	24	2	11	6
2	Paranoid	46/M	11	131	30	7	22	3	2	4
3	Paranoid	36/M	8	13	50	13	26	3	13	6
4	Disorganized	45/M	9	107	50	15	34	4	13	3

*BPRS indicates Brief Psychiatric Rating Scale; CGI, Clinical Global Impressions scale.

†Defined in patients 1, 2, and 3 when the patient had a recurrence of psychotic symptoms, and neuroleptic treatment was restarted. The end point in patient 4 was defined by the last positron emission tomography examination at 13 months. Patient 4 did not relapse for 3 years following discontinuation of treatment.

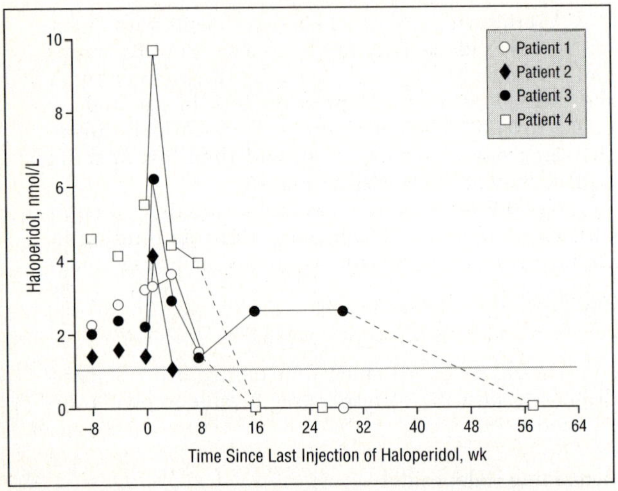

Figure 1. *Plasma concentrations of haloperidol in 4 schizophrenic patients 8 and 4 weeks before (-8 and -4 weeks) and after final administration of treatment with haloperidol decanoate (30-50 mg every 4 weeks) at week 0. The limit of determination, 1 nmol/L, is indicated as a dotted line.*

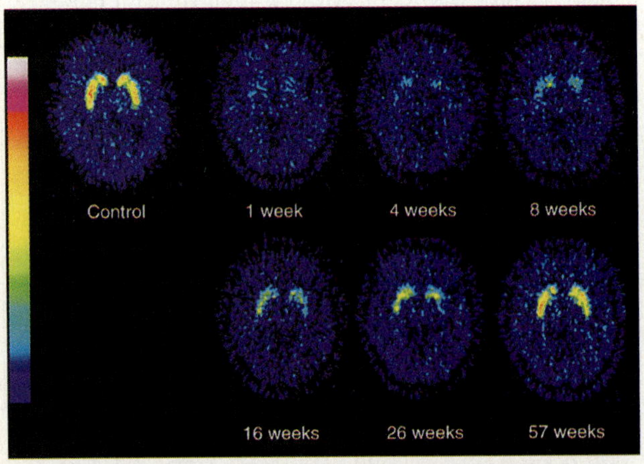

Figure 2. *Reconstructed positron emission tomography images representing a transverse section of the brain at the level of the basal ganglia in a healthy control subject (top left) and patient C, 1 to 57 weeks after discontinuation of treatment with haloperidol decanoate (50 mg every 4 weeks).*

24 and 23 pmol/mL, respectively, and the K_d^{app} was 6.5 and 7.1 pmol/mL, respectively.

COMMENT

Central D_2 dopamine receptor occupancy was measured with PET for up to 1 year in 4 patients after the discontinuation of haloperidol treatment. To the best of our knowledge, this is the first in vivo study spanning such a long time. A considerable D_2 dopamine receptor occupancy was found even 6 months after the last drug administration. Although the number of patients in the study is small, a methodological strength is that all were examined repeatedly and thus serve as their own controls. The differences between examinations were considerably larger than the methodological error. In addition, results were similar among patients, so some tentative conclusions may be drawn. Our findings suggest an explanation for the difference in relapse rates in patients discontinuing oral or depot neuroleptic treatment and have implications for the design of clinical drug trials.

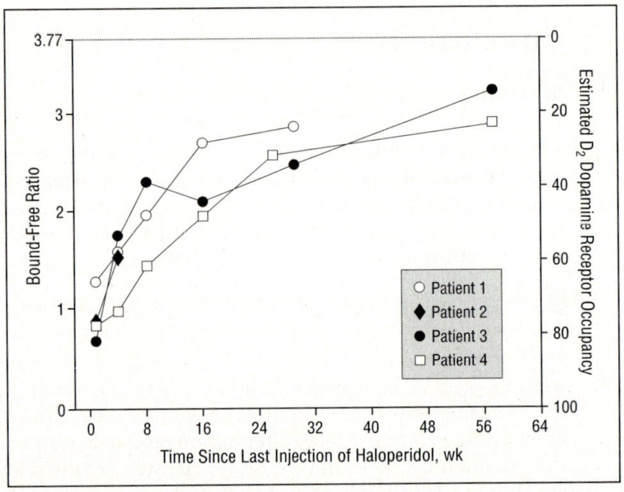

Figure 3. *Positron emission tomography determination of binding potentials (bound-free ratio) in 4 patients as a function of time after the last injection of haloperidol decanoate. The baseline in the mean ratio of 3.77 found in 34 healthy subjects is indicated. The estimated D_2 dopamine receptor occupancy using the baseline 3.77 is indicated on the right y-axis.*

HALOPERIDOL IN PLASMA AND D_2 DOPAMINE RECEPTOR OCCUPANCY

All patients would have concentrations well below the limit of determination (1 nmol/L) at 16 weeks, as predicted from the concentrations measured at week 1 and the previously reported half-life of 3 weeks for haloperidol when administered as decanoate.[22] This was the case in patients 1 and 4. In patient 3, however, detectable amounts of haloperidol were found at 16 and 29 weeks.

Such slow elimination of drug plasma levels has been reported after discontinuation of fluphenazine decanoate treatment.[23,24]

The relation between drug plasma concentration and central receptor occupancy can be described by the law of mass action (equation 3), given that there is a linear relationship between drug in brain and plasma, that the free plasma fraction of the drug is constant, and that the pharmacokinetics are linear. At 1 nmol/L of haloperidol in plasma, D_2 dopamine receptor occupancy should be 37%, based on a previous series of 16 determinations of D_2 dopamine receptor occupancy and haloperidol plasma concentration.[5] Thus, even after the apparent disappearance of haloperidol from plasma, there may be sufficient amounts present to induce receptor occupancy in the brain. This illustrates the high sensitivity of PET for the measurement of drug effects on central neuroreceptors, even at very low drug blood concentrations.

Patient 4 had a poor metabolizer *CYP2D6* genotype. This predicts a slow disposition of haloperidol.[13] Interestingly, this patient had the highest plasma concentrations of haloperidol, from 8 weeks before the study to week 8 (Figure 1).

EXTRAPOLATION TO COMMONLY USED DOSES OF HALOPERIDOL

In our study, the patients had been treated with low doses of haloperidol decanoate (30-50 mg every 4 weeks). However, considerably higher doses are commonly used. Extrapolating our data (equation 3) to the recommended doses of 200 mg every 4 weeks, D_2 dopamine receptor occupancy would be about 70% 16 weeks after discontinuation. Such high levels of D_2 dopamine receptor occupancy should still suffice to prevent psychotic relapses and explain the low risk of relapse the first months after discontinuation of depot treatment.[1,2]

The remaining high levels of receptor occupancy may also be expected to confound the clinical evaluation of optimal dosing and adverse events of any subsequent treatment. In particular, new drugs with low propensity to induce extrapyramidal side effects by themselves may be judged unfairly due to remaining receptor occupancy. To avoid carryover effects in clinical trials of new antipsychotic drugs, we suggest a washout from previous depot treatment for at least 6 months, or even longer if particularly high doses have been used. In addition, previous depot treatment should be included as a potential source of variance in the analysis of randomized patient samples.

CALCULATION OF D_2 DOPAMINE RECEPTOR OCCUPANCY

We have previously examined the test-retest reproducibility of PET-measured P/C ratio both in subjects not receiving medication[21] and haloperidol-treated patients.[25] Even at high D_2 dopamine receptor occupancy, the test-retest reproducibility was high. A difference between 2 P/C ratios greater than 0.121 in the same subject is required to reach significance at the 5% level.[25] This corresponds to a difference in D_2 dopamine receptor occupancy of 3.2%.

Experimental studies in animals show that the administration of high doses of antipsychotic drugs may increase D_2 dopamine receptor density.[26-28] A binding ratio 50% higher than the control group average was demonstrated with PET in a patient 2 weeks after withdrawal from high doses of sulpiride (1600 mg/d).[8] Seven weeks later, the ratio was only 2% above the control average. These findings suggest an increase of the D_2 dopamine receptor density during clinical treatment with neuroleptic drugs.

The error introduced by using the standard baseline P/C ratio is dependent on receptor occupancy and decreases linearly to 0% when the true occupancy is 100%.[3] Thus, if 70% D_2 dopamine receptor occupancy was calculated based on the healthy controls' average ratio of 3.77, then ±1 SD of the average ratios (3.20 and 4.34) gives a difference in occupancy of −5.3% and +3.9%. A higher-than-average receptor density in the examined subjects would introduce a systematic underestimation of D_2 dopamine receptor occupancy. If a 70% occupancy was calculated using the 3.77 average ratio, but the true baseline is increased by 50% to 5.66, the occupancy would be underestimated by about 10%. A higher density of receptors may have been present at the beginning of the study, thus leading to a slight underestimation of D_2 dopamine receptor occupancy at that time.

BINDING RATIOS AND RECEPTOR NUMBERS

To further examine if there were elevated receptor densities or remaining haloperidol in the brain of the patients after 1 year, experiments were performed to determine B_{max} and K^{app}_d. The densities of D_2 dopamine receptors in patients 3 and 4, 24 and 23 pmol/mL, respectively, were within the range of the 28.0±6.9 pmol/mL (mean±SD) found in 20 healthy subjects.[9] The apparent affinity constants of 6.5 and 7.1 pmol/mL were slightly lower than the 9.1±1.9 pmol/mL of healthy controls. Remaining haloperidol would rather have been reflected in a higher K^{app}_d. One year after treatment discontinuation, there was thus no evidence of haloperidol in the brains of these 2 patients.

In patients 3 and 4, D_2 dopamine receptor occupancy was also calculated with the binding ratio found after 1 year as their individual baselines. These individual baselines were slightly lower than the mean values of normal controls and schizophrenic patients, and thus yielded lower values for D_2 dopamine receptor occupancy. Clearly, irrespective of the baseline chosen, our findings indicate remaining occupancy of D_2 dopamine receptors even 6 months after treatment discontinuation, despite the low clinical doses of haloperidol.

Accepted for publication October 8, 1996.

Supported by grant MH 41205-05 from the National Institute of Mental Health, Rockville, Md, and grant 9114 from the Swedish Medical Research Council.

We gratefully acknowledge the members of the PET group at Karolinska Institutet. We also thank Leif Bertilsson, PhD, and Marja-Liisa Dahl, MD, PhD, from the Division of Clinical Pharmacology at Huddinge Hospital for analyses of plasma haloperidol levels and CYP2D6 genotypes.

Reprints: Svante Nyberg, MD, PhD, Karolinska Institutet, Department of Clinical Neuroscience, Psychiatry Section, Karolinska Hospital, S-171 76 Stockholm, Sweden (e-mail: svanten@psyk.ks.se).

REFERENCES

1. Gilbert PL, Harris J, McAdams LA, Jeste DV. Neuroleptic withdrawal in schizophrenic patients: a review of the literature. *Arch Gen Psychiatry.* 1995;52:173-188.
2. Baldessarini RJ, Viguera AC. Neuroleptic withdrawal in schizophrenic patients: commentary. *Arch Gen Psychiatry.* 1995;52:189-191.
3. Farde L, Nordström A-L, Wiesel F-A, Pauli S, Halldin C, Sedvall G. Positron emission tomographic analysis of central D_1 and D_2 dopamine receptor occupancy in patients treated with classical neuroleptics and clozapine: relation to extrapyramidal side effects. *Arch Gen Psychiatry.* 1992;49:538-544.
4. Nordström A-L, Farde L, Wiesel F-A, Forslund K, Pauli S, Halldin C, Uppfeldt G. Central D_2-dopamine receptor occupancy in relation to antipsychotic drug effects: a double-blind PET study of schizophrenic patients. *Biol Psychiatry.* 1993;33:227-235.
5. Nyberg S, Farde L, Halldin C, Dahl M-L, Bertilsson L. D_2 dopamine receptor occupancy during low-dose treatment with haloperidol decanoate. *Am J Psychiatry.* 1995;152:173-178.
6. Baron JC, Martinot JL, Cambon H, Boulenger JP, Poirier MF, Caillard V, Blin J, Huret JD, Loc'h C, Maziere B. Striatal dopamine receptor occupancy during and following withdrawal from neuroleptic treatment: correlative evaluation by positron emission tomography and plasma prolactin levels. *Psychopharmacology.* 1989;99:463-472.
7. Harasko-van der Meer C, Brücke T, Wenger S, Fischer P, Deecke L, Podreka I. Two cases of long-term dopamine D_2 receptor blockade after depot neuroleptics. *J Neural Transm Gen Sect.* 1993;94:217-221.
8. Farde L, Wiesel F-A, Stone-Elander S, Halldin C, Nordström A-L, Hall H, Sedvall G. D_2 dopamine receptors in neuroleptic-naive schizophrenic patients. *Arch Gen Psychiatry.* 1990;47:213-219.
9. Farde L, Hall H, Pauli S, Halldin C. Variability in D_2-dopamine receptor density and affinity: a PET study with [^{11}C]raclopride in man. *Synapse.* 1995;20:200-208.
10. American Psychiatric Association. *Diagnostic and Statistical Manual of Mental Disorders, Third Edition, Revised.* Washington, DC: American Psychiatric Press; 1987.
11. Overall JE, Gorham DR. The Brief Psychiatric Rating Scale. *Psychol Rep.* 1962;10:799-812.
12. Guy W. *Clinical Global Impressions: ECDEU Assessment Manual for Psychopharmacology.* Bethesda, Md: Early Clinical Drug Evaluation Unit, National Institute of Health; 1976:218-222.
13. Llerena A, Alm C, Dahl M-L, Ekqvist B, Bertilsson L. Haloperidol disposition is dependent on debrisoquin hydroxylation phenotype. *Ther Drug Monit.* 1992;14:92-97.
14. Dahl M-L, Johansson I, Porsmyr Palmertz M, Ingelman-Sundberg M, Sjöqvist F. Analysis of the *CYP2D6* gene in relation to debrisoquin hydroxylation in a Swedish population. *Clin Pharmacol Ther.* 1992;51:12-17.
15. Heim M, Meyer U. Genotyping of poor metabolizers of debrisoquin by allele-specific PCR amplification. *Lancet.* 1990;336:529-532.
16. Farde L, Eriksson L, Blomquist G, Halldin C. Kinetic analysis of central [^{11}C]raclopride binding to D_2-dopamine receptors studied by PET: a comparison to the equilibrium analysis. *J Cereb Blood Flow Metab.* 1989;9:696-708.
17. Halldin C, Farde L, Högberg T, Hall H, Ström P, Ohlberger A, Solin O. A comparative PET study of five carbon-11– or fluorine-18–labelled salicylamides: preparation and in vitro dopamine D-2 binding. *Int J Radiat Appl Instrum B.* 1991;18:871-881.
18. Litton JE, Holte S, Eriksson L. Evaluation of the Karolinska new positron camera system: the Scanditronix PC2048-15B. *IEEE Trans Nucl Sci.* 1990;37:743-748.
19. Bergstöm M, Boëthius J, Eriksson L, Greitz T, Ribbe T, Widén L. Head fixation device for reproducible position alignment in transmission CT and positron emission tomography. *J Comput Assist Tomogr.* 1981;5:136-141.
20. Farde L, Wiesel F-A, Halldin C, Sedvall G. Central D_2-dopamine receptor occupancy in schizophrenic patients treated with antipsychotic drugs. *Arch Gen Psychiatry.* 1988;45:71-76.
21. Nordström A-L, Farde L, Pauli S, Litton J-E, Halldin C. PET analysis of central [^{11}C]raclopride binding in healthy young adults and schizophrenic patients: reliability and age effects. *Hum Psychopharmacol.* 1992;7:157-165.
22. Reyntjens AJM, Heykants JJP, Woestenborghs RJH, Gelders YG, Aerts TJL. Pharmacokinetics of haloperidol decanoate: a 2-year follow-up. *Int Pharmacopsychiatry.* 1982;17:238-246.
23. Wistedt B, Jorgensen A, Wiles D. A depot neuroleptic withdrawal study: plasma concentration of fluphenazine and flupenthixol and relapse frequency. *Psychopharmacology.* 1982;78:301-304.
24. Gitlin MJ, Midha K, Fogelson D, Nuechterlein KH. Persistence of fluphenazine in plasma after decanoate withdrawal. *J Clin Psychopharmacol.* 1988;8:53-56.
25. Nyberg S, Farde L, Halldin C. Test-retest reliability of central [^{11}C]raclopride binding at high D_2 receptor occupancy: a PET study in haloperidol-treated patients. *Psychiatry Res.* 1996;67:163-171.
26. Burt D, Creese I, Snyder S. Antischizophrenic drugs: chronic treatment elevates dopamine receptor binding in brain. *Science.* 1977;196:326-328.
27. Clow A, Theodorou A, Jenner P, Marsden CD. Changes in rat striatal dopamine turnover and receptor activity during one years neuroleptic administration. *Eur J Pharmacol.* 1980;63:135-144.
28. Owen F, Cross AJ, Waddington JL. Dopamine-mediated behaviour and 3H-spiperone binding to striatal membranes in rats after nine months' haloperidol administration. *Life Sci.* 1980;26:55-59.

ORIGINAL ARTICLE

Measurement of Glutamate and Glutamine in the Medial Prefrontal Cortex of Never-Treated Schizophrenic Patients and Healthy Controls by Proton Magnetic Resonance Spectroscopy

Robert Bartha, BSc; Peter C. Williamson, MD; Dick J. Drost, PhD; Ashok Malla, MB; Tom J. Carr, MD; Len Cortese, MD; Gita Canaran, MA; R. Jane Rylett, PhD; Richard W. J. Neufeld, PhD

Background: Positron emission tomographic and postmortem studies comparing schizophrenic patients with healthy control subjects have found medial prefrontal cortical and anterior cingulate abnormalities that suggest dysfunction in glutamatergic neurons. The glutamate used for nerve signal transduction is predominantly derived from glutamine. After signal transduction, glutamate released into the synapse is converted to glutamine in glial cells, transported back to the presynaptic neuron, and reconverted to glutamate for reuse. In this study, levels of glutamate and glutamine were examined by means of in vivo proton (^{1}H) magnetic resonance spectroscopy.

Methods: Localized in vivo ^{1}H spectra were acquired from a 4.5-cm^3 volume in the left medial prefrontal cortex encompassing portions of Brodmann areas 24, 32, and 9 in 10 never-treated schizophrenic subjects and 10 healthy controls of comparable age, sex, handedness, education, and parental education. From each spectrum, metabolite levels were estimated for glutamate and glutamine, as well as 10 other metabolites and 3 macromolecules, by means of a noninteractive computer program that combined modeled in vitro spectra of every metabolite to reconstruct each in vivo spectrum.

Results: A significant increase in glutamine level was found in the medial prefrontal cortex of the schizophrenic patients compared with controls. *N*-acetylaspartate and other measured metabolites and macromolecules were not significantly changed in schizophrenics.

Conclusion: Increased glutamine levels in the medial prefrontal region most likely reflect decreased glutamatergic activity in this region in never-treated schizophrenic patients compared with healthy controls.

Arch Gen Psychiatry. 1997;54:959-965

THE MEDIAL prefrontal and anterior cingulate cortical regions have been implicated in the pathogenesis of schizophrenia by a number of in vivo and postmortem investigations. Recent in vivo studies using positron emission tomography and single photon emission computed tomography have shown decreased cerebral blood flow or glucose uptake in these regions in both medicated and unmedicated schizophrenic patients compared with healthy control subjects.[1-6] Other investigators have reported deficits only for patients with negative symptoms[7,8] or have failed to confirm these findings.[9,10] Increased cerebral blood flow in the right anterior cingulate cortex has also been observed in schizophrenic patients[11] with positron emission tomography in association with verbal reports of auditory hallucinations.

Postmortem studies of schizophrenic brains have found abnormalities in cell populations that include increased glutamate-immunoreactive vertical axons and decreased small interneurons and neurons.[12,13] Other postmortem studies have found conflicting evidence implicating glutamatergic function in schizophrenia. For example, studies have shown increased kainate receptor binding[14] (Brodmann areas 9 and 10), decreased prefrontal glutamate (Glu) levels and *N*-acetyl-α–linked–acidic dipeptidase activity, and increased prefrontal *N*-acetylaspartyl-glutamate (NAAG),[15] suggesting reduced glutamatergic activity in schizophrenics, while other findings of increased binding of D-[^{3}H] aspartate to glutamate uptake sites and [^{3}H] kainate to postsynaptic glutamate receptors[16] suggest an overabundant glutamatergic innervation in the same region.

The medial prefrontal cortex and anterior cingulate regions receive glutamatergic afferents from the thalamus as well as other cortical regions that have also been implicated in schizophrenia.[17] Therefore, it would be of interest to examine levels of glutamate and its metabolites in the me-

From the Department of Nuclear Medicine and Magnetic Resonance, St Joseph's Health Centre (Mr Bartha and Drs Williamson, Drost, and Carr), and Departments of Psychiatry (Drs Williamson, Malla, and Cortese and Ms Canaran), Physiology (Dr Rylett), and Psychology (Dr Neufeld), University of Western Ontario.

SUBJECTS AND METHODS

SUBJECTS

Fourteen never-treated, first-episode schizophrenic patients and 10 control subjects participated in the study, which was approved by the Review Board for Health Sciences Research Involving Human Subjects of the University of Western Ontario, London. Patients were referred for evaluation by their treating psychiatrist in the community, who was aware of the study. All participants gave their informed written consent. However, 2 subjects withdrew consent during the study and were not included. One patient was excluded because the data acquired were of insufficient quality for accurate quantification. Another was excluded because a large temporal lobe cyst was discovered on clinical magnetic resonance (MR) imaging. Eight of the remaining 10 were inpatients and 2 were outpatients. None of these patients had participated in a previous study.[23]

Clinical information for subjects is provided in **Table 1**. Subjects were classified as schizophrenic patients (*DSM-III-R* criteria) or control by a psychiatrist (P.C.W.) and a psychometrist (G.C.) with the use of the Structured Clinical Interview for *DSM-III-R* (SCID).[24] Both interviewers had to agree with the diagnosis for the subject to be included. Six patients were classified as paranoid and 4 as having an undifferentiated subtype. A follow-up SCID interview 6 months after the study by a psychiatrist (P.C.W.) confirmed the diagnosis of schizophrenia in 8 patients (1 had committed suicide and 1 could not be located). Along with the SCID, schizophrenic patients were also examined immediately before the imaging procedure by a psychiatrist (P.C.W.) by means of the Scale for the Assessment of Negative Symptoms (SANS)[25] and the Scale for the Assessment of Positive Symptoms (SAPS),[26] based on symptoms experienced during the previous week.

Schizophrenic patients ranged in age from 17 to 33 years (mean±SD age, 24±5 years). Eight of 10 schizophrenic patients experienced their first positive symptoms 1 year or less before imaging. One schizophrenic patient had positive symptoms for 17 months before imaging. One had heard voices occasionally for 7 years but did not develop other symptoms of schizophrenia until 3 months before imaging. Six schizophrenic patients received between 1 and 4 mg of lorazepam in the 24 hours before scanning. None of these subjects had been exposed to any antipsychotic medication before the MRS examination. The education level of each subject was rated on a 4-point scale (1, grade 10 or less; 2, grades 11-13; 3, 1-3 years of college or university; 4, 4 or more years of college or university). Parental education ratings were also evaluated as above for the most educated parent. The handedness of each subject was defined by a handedness questionnaire.[27]

Ten control subjects were chosen from a pool of subjects recruited by advertisement. Subjects were chosen to minimize demographic differences between the patient and control groups (Table 1). The criteria used included sex, age, education, parental education, and handedness assessed in the same manner as for patients. An SCID interview was also conducted on each control by the same 2 interviewers who conducted patient interviews; the absence of psychiatric symptoms in these subjects was confirmed by consensus. Five control subjects had participated in previous studies that included MR imaging and MRS examination.

No patients or controls had a history of head injury, drug or alcohol abuse, or serious medical illness based on the information provided during the SCID interview. As part of the MR study, routine clinical images were collected and viewed by a radiologist (T.J.C.), who detected no gross abnormalities on any scans of the 20 subjects who were included in the data analysis.

PROTON MRS EXAMINATION

Each subject was positioned within a whole-body MR imager (Siemens SP4000 Helicon, Siemans AG, Erlangen, Germany, 1.5 T) and taped under the chin and across the forehead to reduce motion. The same circularly polarized head coil was used to obtain all images and spectra. Every study began with an iterative computer algorithm[28] that directly set the currents in 12 resistive shim coils to improve magnetic field homogeneity over the entire head and thereby improve spectral quality. A series of sagittal and coronal images were then acquired for placing a $15 \times 15 \times 20$-mm^3 volume of interest (VOI) in the medial prefrontal region of the brain (**Figure 1**). In Tailairach coordinates,[29] the VOI was placed to lie within the region between $x=0$ to -15, $y=30$ to 50, and

dial prefrontal region (including anterior cingulate) of living patients. Levels of Glu and metabolites such as glutamine (Gln), NAAG, and aspartate (Asp) can be measured simultaneously in vivo by means of short-echo proton magnetic resonance spectroscopy (MRS),[18-20] which is not possible with positron emission tomography or single photon emission computed tomography. Abnormalities in Gln have been observed with in vivo short-echo ^{1}H MRS in other diseases.[21,22] An earlier ^{1}H MRS study of the dorsolateral prefrontal region by our group found increased Gln levels in patients with chronic but not never-treated schizophrenia compared with controls.[23] However, a decrease in Gln was observed in these never-treated patients after neuroleptic therapy. As Gln is a precursor of the neurotransmitter Glu, this decrease in Gln suggests increased levels of glutamate available for neurotransmission after treatment with neuroleptics.

We hypothesized that in the medial prefrontal and anterior cingulate region (including portions of Brodmann areas 24, 32, and 9), schizophrenic patients would show altered metabolite levels, suggesting decreased glutamatergic activity compared with controls. In this study, we report preliminary short-echo ^{1}H MRS medial prefrontal (including anterior cingulate) findings in 10 never-treated schizophrenic patients compared with 10 healthy controls of comparable age, sex, handedness, education, and parental education levels.

RESULTS

A typical spectrum (after water removal) from 1 subject is shown in **Figure 2**. It is displayed in the frequency domain after Fourier transform, although all quantification was done in the time domain. The average signal-

$z=0$ to 20. This volume encompassed parts of Brodmann areas 24, 32, and 9. After placement of the VOI, a stimulated echo acquisition mode (STEAM)[30] localized manual shim was done to further increase magnetic field homogeneity within the VOI. Both water-suppressed[31] and water-unsuppressed spectroscopy data were acquired with a STEAM sequence (repetition time, 1500 milliseconds; echo time, 20 milliseconds; mixing time, 30 milliseconds; 4096 points; 250-microsecond dwell time; 550 and 30 suppressed and unsuppressed averages, respectively).

SPECTRAL PROCESSING

All spectra were processed identically without operator interaction by means of our own software.[32] Each spectrum was eddy current corrected,[33] with the water unsuppressed spectrum used as a reference. Residual water was then subtracted by means of the results of an initial fit of the data in the time domain[34] (0-0.512 seconds) with a Hankel Lanczos singular value decomposition algorithm.[35] The resulting spectrum was then fit in the time domain (0-0.512 seconds) by means of a nonlinear Marquardt algorithm[36] to a complete spectrum model composed of 12 metabolites[18-20] and 3 macromolecules[37] with resonances between 1.9 and 3.5 ppm. The metabolites *N*-acetylaspartate (NAA), Glu, Gln, γ-aminobutyric acid (GABA), taurine (Tau), *myo*-inositol (Myo), glucose (Glc), Asp, NAAG, phosphocreatine plus creatine (PCr+Cr), choline-containing compounds including mostly phosphorylcholine, glycerophosphorylcholine, and free choline[20,38] (Cho), and scyllo-inositol (Syl) were all modeled with exponentially damped sinusoids. Macromolecule (M) resonances at 3.00 ppm (M 3.00), 2.29 ppm (M 2.29), and 2.05 ppm (M 2.05)[37] were modeled with gaussian damped sinusoids. The full-width half-maximum of these macromolecule peaks was fixed at 24 Hz. Six resonances with shifts of less than 1.9 ppm and 4 resonances with shifts of greater than 3.5 ppm were included in the spectrum model to account for minor baseline distortions and resonances adjacent to our spectral region of interest (1.9-3.5 ppm with NAA_{CH3} referenced to 2.01 ppm). These 10 resonances were unrestricted in amplitude, shift, width, and phase, and independent of the modeled metabolites except in delay time, which was linked.

By adjusting the amplitude parameters of each metabolite as well as the overall width, shift, zero-order phase, and delay time, the computer fitting algorithm minimized the difference between the complete spectrum model and the original data. Metabolite amplitudes were then scaled by the total MR-visible water[39] obtained from the unsuppressed water spectrum (corrected for 3% cerebrospinal fluid[18]), and the approximate concentration of water in the VOI (H_2O=55.12 mmol/mL, corrected for 41% gray matter and 56% white matter),[18] to yield relative metabolite levels in arbitrary units. This measure represents the average metabolite level in the volume studied uncorrected for the MR relaxation parameters T_1 and T_2 (since these parameters are unavailable for each metabolite in each individual).

STATISTICAL ANALYSIS

All statistical tests were performed with SPSS, release 6.0.[40] The subject characteristics age, education level, and parental education were comparable between subject groups according to a 2-tailed *t* test ($P>.10$). These variables were covariates for all statistical comparisons to reduce the extraneous variance in error terms, without removing genuine group effects.[41,42]

Although 12 metabolites and 3 macromolecules were modeled for each data set, some metabolites and macromolecules had large SDs. Therefore, we decided that only metabolites and macromolecules with coefficients of variation of less than 75% should be included in between-group comparisons. As Glu and Gln composed the focus of hypothesized differences, values of these metabolites were compared by analysis of covariance; the remaining metabolites were compared by multivariate analysis of covariance. *P* values of .05 or less were considered statistically significant.

To establish whether estimated metabolite levels were correlated (because of physiological changes or quantification artifact), bivariate correlations were made between all metabolites included in the analysis as well as between each metabolite and the SANS and SAPS scores for the schizophrenic patients. These correlations were carried out on each subject group independently. *P* values for significance were determined with a Bonferroni-based correction,[42,43] as no prior hypotheses were made.

to-noise ratio[32] for all data before preprocessing was 20±5:1. The mean (±SD) full-width half-maximum of the unsuppressed water spectra was 5.74±1.02 Hz. Five of the 12 quantified metabolites (NAA, Glu, Gln, PCr+Cr, and Cho) had coefficients of variation of less than 75% and were included in the statistical analysis. **Figure 3** shows the average estimated metabolite levels ±SD for each group. These metabolite levels represent average resting levels from the entire volume under investigation and are uncorrected for the MR relaxation parameters T_1 and T_2, or changes in cerebrospinal fluid, gray matter, and white matter ratios.

A significant increase was observed in the level of Gln among never-treated schizophrenic patients as compared with controls (7.2±3.7 vs 3.7±2.0 arbitrary units; N=10; *df*=15; F=6.1; *P*=.03), while no differences were observed in Glu. The multivariate analysis of covariance

Table 1. Subject Characteristics*

	Controls (n=10)	Never-Treated Schizophrenics (n=10)
Age, y (mean±SD)	26.3±6.4	24.4±5.1
Sex, No. M/F	8/2	8/2
Hand, No. R/L	9/1	10/0
Education level† (mean±SD)	2.7±0.7	2.7±0.9
Parental education level† (mean±SD)	3.0±0.8	2.5±0.9
SANS (mean±SD)	. . .	32.2±16.0
SAPS (mean±SD)	. . .	24.4±9.5

*SANS indicates Scale for the Assessment of Negative Symptoms; SAPS, Scale for the Assessment of Positive Symptoms.

†Level 1 indicates grade 10 or less; 2, grades 11 to 13; 3, 1 to 3 years of college; and 4, 4 or more years of college.

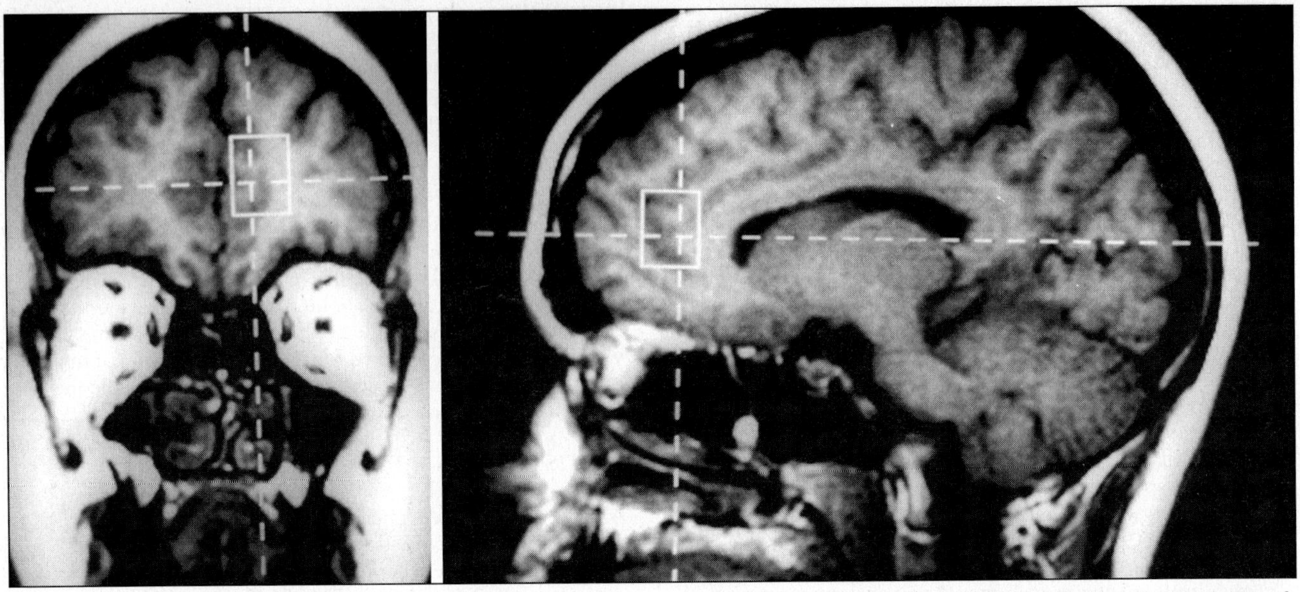

Figure 1. *Coronal (left) and sagittal (right) proton (^1H) magnetic resonance images showing the placement of the volume of interest in 1 subject. The 15×15×20-mm³ volume of interest is outlined by a white box positioned in the left medial prefrontal cortex and anterior cingulate regions (Brodmann areas and Tailairach coordinates are specified in the text). The vertical dotted line in the coronal image gives the position of the sagittal slice. The vertical dotted line in the sagittal image gives the position of the coronal slice. The horizontal lines in both images give the position of a transverse slice also used for positioning but not shown here.*

on the 3 remaining metabolites did not show a statistically significant difference between never-treated schizophrenic patients and controls ($P=.42$). The analyses of covariance on individual metabolite groups gave the *P* values shown in Figure 3. Never-treated schizophrenics showed a trend toward higher PCr+Cr levels (11.3±1.7 vs 9.9±1.1 arbitrary units; n=10; $df=15$; $F=3.4$; $P=.09$) compared with controls. Patients treated with lorazepam (n=6) and those not so treated (n=4) had Gln levels of 6.0±4.1 and 9.1±2.5 arbitrary units, respectively, and PCr+Cr levels of 10.9±1.7 and 11.9±1.7 arbitrary units, respectively. These metabolite levels were not significantly different between patients treated and not treated with lorazepam by means of a 2-tailed *t* test ($P=.21$ and $P=.40$ for Gln and PCr+Cr, respectively; the power of this test was necessarily low, but the *direction* of differences was contrary to lorazepam being the agent of elevated patient values).

Bivariate correlations between measured metabolites and clinical symptoms (SANS[25] and SAPS[26]) were done separately for healthy controls and never-treated schizophrenic patients. *P* values less than .02 and less than .01 were considered statistically significant for the healthy control and never-treated schizophrenic groups, respectively. One significant positive correlation was found between the metabolites Gln and Cho in the control group ($r=0.753$, $P=.01$). Pearson correlation coefficients for the correlation of clinical symptoms with metabolite levels are summarized in **Table 2**. No significant correlations were found between estimated metabolite levels and SANS scores. The SAPS scores correlated negatively with NAA levels ($P=.02$); however, this correlation was not significant after Bonferroni correction.

COMMENT

Although these results must be considered preliminary, this study showed a significant Gln increase in the medial prefrontal cortex (encompassing portions of Brodmann areas 24, 32, and 9) of never-treated schizophrenic patients compared with healthy controls. It has been estimated that 80% of stimulus-released glutamate is derived from Gln.[44] In this cycle, stimulus-released glutamate is taken up by astrocytes and converted to Gln, which is transported back to the presynaptic neuron and reconverted to glutamate.[45,46] This small neurotransmitter pool of glutamate does not equilibrate quickly with a larger pool of cellular glutamate.[44,47]

Our observation of increased Gln in schizophrenic patients may indicate an abnormality in the cycle of conversion of Gln to glutamate. This would decrease the glutamate available for signal transduction while the overall level of glutamate would appear unchanged, since the larger pool of cellular glutamate is unaltered. Thus, higher Gln levels could suggest decreased glutamatergic activity in the medial prefrontal region of schizophrenic patients. Conversely, increased Gln could indicate increased glutamatergic activity in keeping with increased D-[^{3}H] aspartate binding[16] (although caution must be taken when the results of this study are compared with those of previous postmortem studies, since the volume studied here includes several distinct regions of cortex). This possibility seems unlikely, as most functional imaging studies have shown decreased metabolic activity in this region[1-6] and the increase in receptor sites found on postmortem analysis could be interpreted as a compensatory effect of decreased glutamatergic activity. Increased glial cell volumes could also account for increased Gln levels in schizophrenic subjects, since ^{1}H MRS measures Gln for both neurons and glial cells,[48] but recent postmortem studies have not found increased glial cell volumes in the prefrontal cortex.[49]

As some patients received lorazepam in the 24 hours before assessment, there is a possibility that this medication could have affected Gln levels in patients, accounting for the difference from controls. However, this does not appear to be the case, as Gln levels tended to be lower

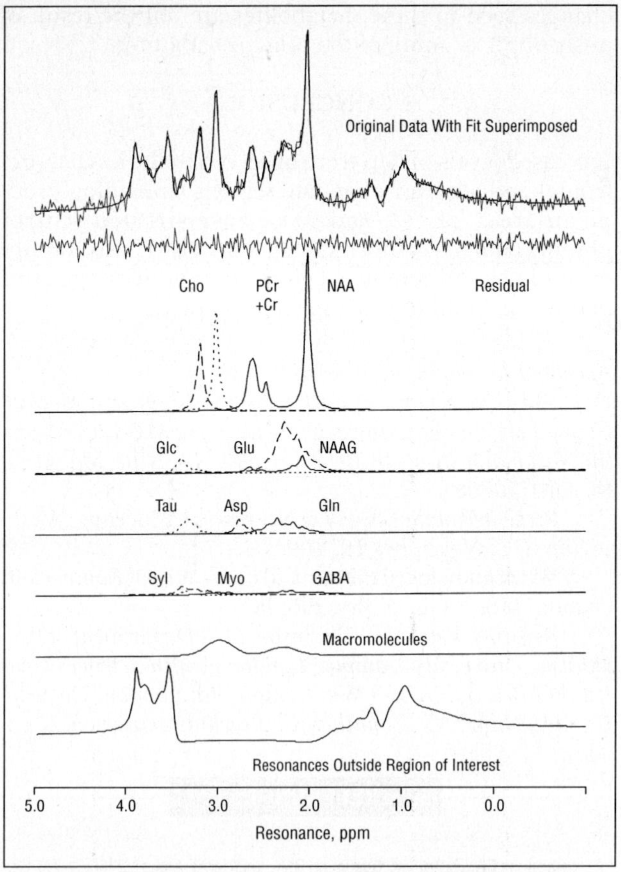

Figure 2. *Typical in vivo ¹H data after water subtraction in top trace (light line) with corresponding fit result superimposed (dark line). Data were fit in the time domain but are shown here in the frequency domain for interpretation. The difference between the two is shown beneath (residual). The individual metabolite components are displayed beneath the residual. The first line shows* N*-acetylaspartate (NAA; solid), phosphocreatine plus creatine (PCr+Cr; dotted), and choline-containing compounds (Cho; dashed). The second line shows* N*-acetylaspartyl glutamate (NAAG; solid), glutamate (Glu; dashed), and glucose (Glc; dotted). The third line shows glutamine (Gln; solid), aspartate (Asp; dashed), and taurine (Tau; dotted). The fourth line shows γ-aminobutyric acid (GABA; solid), myoinositol (Myo; dashed), and scyllo-inositol (Syl; dotted). The fifth line shows the macromolecules, while the sixth line shows the resonances fit outside the spectral region of interest (<1.9 ppm and >3.5 ppm).*

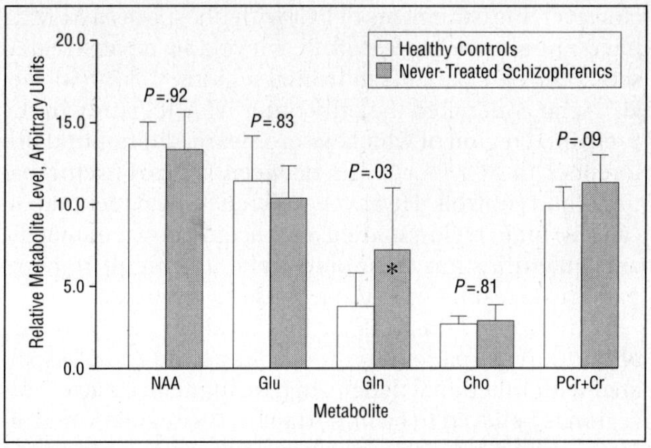

Figure 3. *Mean metabolite levels in arbitrary units after normalization to total magnetic resonance–visible water for the medial prefrontal cortex (encompassing portions of Brodmann areas 24, 32, and 9) of healthy control subjects (n=10) and never-treated schizophrenic patients (n=10). Errors represent ±1 SD. NAA represents* N*-acetylaspartate; Glu, glutamate; Gln, glutamine; Cho, choline-containing compounds (phosphorylcholine, glycerophosphorylcholine, and free choline[20,38]); and PCr plus Cr, phosphocreatine+creatine. Asterisk marks statistically significant analysis of covariance (*P *values shown on plot), with covariates consisting of age, education, and parental education.*

Table 2. Metabolite Correlations With Clinical Symptom Scores*

	Pearson Correlation	
Metabolite	**SANS**	**SAPS**
NAA	0.304	−0.730†
Glu	0.358	0.104
Gln	−0.261	−0.507
Cho	−0.334	−0.037
PCr+Cr	−0.345	0.181

**SANS indicates Scale for the Assessment of Negative Symptoms; SAPs, Scale for the Assessment of Positive Symptoms; NAA,* N*-acetyl aspartate; Glu, glutamate; Gln, glutamine; Cho, choline-containing compounds; PCr, phosphocreatine; and Cr, creatine.*
*†*P*=.02, not significant after Bonferroni-based correction.*

in the patients who had received lorazepam than in the patients who had not received lorazepam.

If the finding of increased Gln levels reflects decreased glutamatergic activity, this would be consistent with N-methyl-D-aspartate receptor hypofunction, which has been hypothesized in schizophrenia.[50,51] Olney and Farber[50] suggested that any mechanism that impairs the functional status of NMDA receptors of GABAergic neurons could result in widespread damage to the limbic system. This damage would be expected to be associated with decreased NAA levels in the medial prefrontal region, in keeping with reports of decreased NAA levels in the temporal regions of schizophrenic patients.[52,53] No differences were observed, but neuronal loss by this process could be subtle and not detectable by this technique. Differences in levels of GABA cannot be ruled out, as this metabolite is poorly resolved at this field strength.

The anterior cingulate cortex receives inputs from many parts of the brain, so it is impossible to determine the origin of glutamatergic projections that could account for the increase in Gln in patients. However, the anterior cingulate cortex receives glutamatergic afferents from the thalamus via basal ganglia–thalamocortical pathways.[54,55] It is possible that excitatory glutamatergic thalamic afferents to the anterior cingulate and medio-orbital cortex could be damaged early in brain development. Early neurodevelopmental lesions to the mediodorsal thalamus[56] or ventral hippocampus[57] in rats results in behaviors associated with dopaminergic supersensitivity in the nucleus accumbens at maturity, by a mechanism likely involving glutamatergic afferents to the medial prefrontal region. Our findings of increased Gln in never-treated patients could result from either type of neurodevelopmental lesion.

Proton MRS measures total PCr+Cr,[58] although the proportion of PCr is higher in most tissues.[20] The trend toward an increase in PCr levels in never-treated schizophrenics could be the result of an increase in PCr or Cr. The trend to increased PCr+Cr levels could indicate reduced metabolic activity, which has been demonstrated with functional imaging studies,[1-6] since PCr is an energy reserve used to produce adenosine triphosphate.

However, measurements of PCr with phosphorus 31 MRS have not shown increased PCr levels in never-treated schizophrenic patients in frontal regions.[59-61] Buckley et al,[62] who conducted the only other ^{1}H MRS study in the prefrontal region of which we are aware, did not find differences in PCr+Cr levels between schizophrenic patients and controls. However, differences in patient medications, brain region studied, data acquisition parameters, and quantification technique make it difficult to compare these results with those presented here.

Increased Gln and PCr+Cr levels in never-treated schizophrenic patients would be expected to be associated with functional deficits in the cingulate cortex. This region is believed to be important in the regulation of affect, motivation, selective attention, social interactiveness, and rational thought processes, functions that are impaired in schizophrenic patients.[63] Although none of the metabolite levels were significantly correlated with symptom scores, SAPS scores were inversely correlated with NAA levels before Bonferroni correction. While NAA levels did not differ between groups in this study, patients with positive symptoms may have a change in neuronal integrity in this region reflected in NAA levels. However, a larger study is necessary to confirm this correlation.

LIMITATIONS

Although the volume used was small (4.5 cm^3) and positioning was done with the aid of images to place the volume in gray matter, there was still a significant amount of white matter present in each volume, which could decrease the sensitivity of measurements. To exclude partial volume effects as the cause of metabolite level changes, the partial volume must be equal in controls and schizophrenics. Studies comparing metabolite levels in gray and white matter have generally shown increased PCr+Cr and Glu levels and decreased Cho levels in gray matter compared with white matter.[18,20,38] Although a trend toward increased PCr+Cr levels was observed, this increase was not accompanied by a corresponding increase in Glu and decrease in Cho levels. Therefore, it is unlikely that the changes reported here are the result of increased gray matter in the schizophrenic volume.

The inclusion of prior knowledge reduced the uncertainty of metabolite level estimates, but the overlapping resonances in the region of the spectrum containing Glu, Gln, and GABA were difficult to resolve. This lack of resolution led to metabolite estimates with high SDs for some metabolites (ie, approximately 53% for Gln), although the SDs of other metabolites (NAA, approximately 14%; Glu, approximately 21%) were comparable to those obtained from postmortem analysis (NAA, approximately 20%; Glu, approximately 40%)[15] and larger-volume spectroscopy studies (NAA+NAAG, approximately 9%; Glu, approximately 14%).[19] Future studies may show more pronounced results because of improvements in equipment and quantification, which will lead to decreased metabolite SDs. Although 1 positive correlation between Gln and Cho was observed in the control group, the lack of negative correlations between Gln and any other metabolite, as well as PCr+Cr and any other metabolite, in either subject group suggests that the changes seen in these metabolites are not the result of misfitting 1 or more of the other metabolites.

CONCLUSION

Increased levels of Gln were observed in the medial prefrontal and anterior cingulate regions (including Brodmann areas 24, 32, and 9) of never-treated schizophrenic patients compared with controls. These findings most likely reflect reduced glutamatergic activity in this part of the brain in schizophrenic patients.

Accepted for publication April 8, 1997.

This work was supported by the Medical Research Council of Canada, Ottawa, Ontario (grant MT-12078), and the National Institute of Mental Health, Rockville, Md (grant R01-MH50768).

Presented at the Society of Neuroscience Meeting, Washington, DC, November 19, 1996.

We acknowledge the clinical assistance of Rahul Manchanda, MB, BS, MRCPsy, FRCPC.

Reprints: Peter C. Williamson, MD, Department of Psychiatry, University Campus, London Health Sciences Centre, PO Box 5339, 339 Windermere Rd, London, Ontario, Canada N6A 5A5 (e-mail: williams@julian.uwo.ca).

REFERENCES

1. Tamminga CA, Thaker GK, Buchanan R, Kirkpatrick B, Alphs LD, Chase TN, Carpenter WT. Limbic system abnormalities identified in schizophrenia using positron emission tomography with fluorodeoxyglucose and neocortical alternations with deficit syndrome. *Arch Gen Psychiatry.* 1992;49:522-529.
2. Ebmeier KP, Blackwood DHR, Murray C, Souza V, Walker M, Dougall N, Moffoot APR, O'Carroll RE, Goodwin GM. Single-photon emission computed tomography with ^{99m}Tc exametazime in unmedicated schizophrenic patients. *Biol Psychiatry.* 1993;33:487-495.
3. Kawasaki Y, Maeda Y, Suzuki M, Urata K, Higaskima M, Kiba K, Yamaguchi N, Matsuda H, Hisada K. SPECT analysis of regional cerebral blood flow changes in patients with schizophrenia during the Wisconsin Card Sorting Test. *Schizophr Res.* 1993;10:109-116.
4. Siegel BV, Buchsbaum MS, Bunney WE, Gottschalk LA, Haier RJ, Lohr JB, Lottenberg S, Najafi A, Nuechterlein KH, Potkin SG, Wu JC. Cortical-striatal-thalamic circuits and brain glucose metabolic activity in 70 unmedicated male schizophrenic patients. *Am J Psychiatry.* 1993;150:1325-1336.
5. Ebmeier KP, Lawrie SM, Blackwood DHR, Johnstone EC, Goodwin GM. Hypofrontality revisited: a high resolution single photon emission computed tomography study in schizophrenia. *J Neurol Neurosurg Psychiatry.* 1995;58:452-456.
6. Dolan RJ, Fletcher P, Frith CD, Friston KJ, Frackowiak RSJ, Grasby PM. Dopaminergic modulation of impaired cognitive activation in the anterior cingulate cortex in schizophrenia. *Nature.* 1995;378:180-194.
7. Liddle PF, Friston KJ, Frith CD, Hirsch SR, Jones T, Frackowiak SJ. Patterns of cerebral blood flow in schizophrenia. *Br J Psychiatry.* 1992;160:179-186.
8. Andreasen NC, Rezai K, Alliger R, Swayze VW, Flaum M, Kirchner P, Cohen G, O'Leary DS. Hypofrontality in neuroleptic-naive patients and in patients with chronic schizophrenia. *Arch Gen Psychiatry.* 1992;49:943-958.
9. Gur RE, Mozley D, Resnick SM, Harper Mozley L, Shtasl DL, Gallacher F, Arnold SE, Karp JS, Alavi A, Reivich M, Gur RC. Resting cerebral glucose metabolism in first-episode and previously treated patients with schizophrenia relates to clinical features. *Arch Gen Psychiatry.* 1995;52:657-667.
10. Frith CD, Friston KJ, Herold S, Silbersweig D, Fletcher P, Cahill C, Dolan RJ, Frackowiak RSJ, Liddle PF. Regional brain activity in chronic schizophrenic patients during the performance of a verbal fluency task. *Br J Psychiatry.* 1995;167:343-349.
11. Silbersweig DA, Stern E, Frith C, Cahill C, Holmes A, Grootoonk S, Seaward J, McKenna P, Chua SE, Schnorr L, Jones T, Frackowiak RSJ. A functional neuroanatomy of hallucinations in schizophrenia. *Nature.* 1995;378:176-179.
12. Benes FM, Sorensen I, Vincent SL, Bird ED. Increased density of glutamate-

immunoreactive vertical process in superficial laminae in cingulate cortex of schizophrenic brain. *Cerebral Cortex.* 1992;2:503-512.
13. Benes FM, McSparren J, Bird ED, SanGiovanni JP, Vincent SL. Deficits in small interneurons in prefrontal and cingulate cortices of schizophrenic and schizoaffective patients. *Arch Gen Psychiatry.* 1991;48:996-1001.
14. Nishikawa T, Takashima M, Toru M. Increased [^{3}H] kainic acid binding in the prefrontal cortex in schizophrenia. *Neurosci Lett.* 1983;40:245-250.
15. Tsai G, Passani LA, Slusher BS, Carter R, Baer L, Kleinman JE, Coyle JT. Abnormal excitatory neurotransmitter metabolism in schizophrenic brains. *Arch Gen Psychiatry.* 1995;52:829-836.
16. Deakin JFW, Slater P, Simpson MDC, Gilchrist AC, Skan WJ, Royston MC, Reynolds GP, Cross AJ. Frontal cortical and left temporal glutamatergic dysfunction in schizophrenia. *J Neurochem.* 1989;52:1781-1786.
17. Vogt BA. Structural organization of cingulate cortex: areas, neurons, and somatodendritic transmitter receptors. In: Vogt BA, Gabriel M, eds. *Neurobiology of Cingulate Cortex and Limbic Thalamus.* Boston, Mass: Birkhauser; 1993:19-70.
18. Stanley JA, Drost DJ, Williamson PC, Thompson RT. The use of a priori knowledge to quantify short echo in vivo ^{1}H MR spectra. *Magn Reson Med.* 1995;34: 17-24.
19. Provencher SW. Estimation of metabolite concentrations from localized in-vivo proton NMR spectra. *Magn Reson Med.* 1994;30:672-679.
20. Michaelis T, Merboldt K, Bruhn H, Hanicke W, Frahm J. Absolute concentrations of metabolites in the adult human brain in vivo: quantification of localized proton MR spectra. *Radiology.* 1993;187:219-227.
21. Ernst T, Ross BD, Flores R. Cerebral MRS in infants with suspected Reye's syndrome. *Lancet.* 1992;340:486.
22. Kreis R, Ross BD, Farrow NA, Ackerman Z. Metabolic disorders of the brain in chronic hepatic encephalopathy detected with H-1 MR spectroscopy. *Neuroradiology.* 1992;182:19-27.
23. Stanley JA, Williamson PC, Drost DJ, Rylett J, Carr T, Malla A, Thompson RT. An in vivo proton magnetic resonance spectroscopy study of schizophrenic patients. *Schizophr Bull.* 1996;22:597-609.
24. Spitzer R, Williams J. *Structured Clinical Interview for* DSM-III-R. New York, NY: New York Psychiatric Institute; 1985.
25. Andreasen N. *Scale for the Assessment of Negative Symptoms (SANS).* Iowa City, Iowa: University of Iowa; 1994.
26. Andreasen N. *Scale for the Assessment of Positive Symptoms (SAPS).* Iowa City, Iowa: University of Iowa; 1994.
27. Bryden P. Measuring handedness with questionnaires. *Neuropsychologia.* 1977; 15:617-624.
28. Liu Z, Javaid T, Hu J, Brown TR. CSI—autoshim procedures for body and surface coil. In: Proceedings of the Society of Magnetic Resonance 2nd Annual Meeting; August 6-12, 1994; San Francisco, Calif; Page 1174. Abstract.
29. Tailairach J, Tournoux P. *Co-Planar Stereotaxic Atlas of the Human Brain.* New York, NY: Thieme Medical Publishers Inc; 1988.
30. Frahm J, Merboldt KD, Hanicke W. Localized proton spectroscopy using stimulated echoes. *J Magn Reson.* 1987;72:502-508.
31. Frahm J, Michaelis T, Merboldt KD, Bruhn H, Gyngell ML, Hanicke W. Improvements in localized proton NMR spectroscopy of human brain: water suppression, short echo times, and 1 ml resolution. *J Magn Reson.* 1990;90:464-473.
32. Bartha R, Drost DJ, Stanley J, Williamson PC. A comparison between time and frequency domain quantification of short echo ^{1}H MR spectra. In: Proceedings of the 3rd Society of Magnetic Resonance Meeting; August 19-25,1995; Nice, France. Page 1946. Abstract.
33. Klose U. In vivo proton spectroscopy in presence of eddy currents. *Magn Reson Med.* 1990;14:26-30.
34. De Beer R, van Ormondt D. Analysis of data using time domain fitting procedures. *NMR Basic Principles Prog.* 1992;26:201-248.
35. Van den Boogaart A, Ala-Korpela M, Jokisaari J, Griffiths JR. Time and frequency domain analysis of NMR data compared: an application to 1D ^{1}H spectra of lipoproteins. *Magn Reson Med.* 1994;31:347-358.
36. Marquardt DW. An algorithm for least-squares estimations of non-linear parameters. *J Soc Indust Appl Math.* 1963;11:431-441.
37. Behar KL, Rothman DL, Spencer DD, Petroff OAC. Analysis of macromolecule resonances in ^{1}H NMR spectra of human brain. *Magn Reson Med.* 1994;32:294-302.
38. Ross B, Michaelis T. Clinical applications of magnetic resonance spectroscopy. *Magn Reson Q.* 1994;10:191-247.
39. Christiansen P, Henriksen O, Stubgaard M, Gideon P, Larsson HBW. In vivo quantification of brain metabolites by 1H-MRS using water as an internal standard. *Magn Reson Imag.* 1993;11:107-118.
40. *SPSS for Windows: Release 6.0.* Chicago, Ill: SPSS Inc; 1993.
41. Cochran WG. Analysis of covariance: its nature and uses. *Biometrics.* 1957;13: 261-281.
42. Lees MC, Neufeld RWJ. Matching the limits of clinical inference to the limits of quantitative methods: a formal appeal to practice what we persistently preach. *Can Psychol.* 1994;35:268-282.
43. Larzelere RE, Mulaik SA. Single sample tests for many comparisons. *Psychol Bull.* 1977;4:557-569.
44. Bradford HF, Ward HK, Thomas AJ. Glutamine: a major substrate for nerve endings. *J Neurochem.* 1978;30:1453-1459.
45. Erecinska M, Silver IA. Metabolism and role of glutamate in mammalian brain. *Prog Neurobiol.* 1990;35:245-296.
46. Ross B. Biochemical considerations in ^{1}H spectroscopy: glutamate and glutamine; myo-inositol and related metabolites. *NMR Biomed.* 1991;4:59-63.
47. Hamberger AC, Chiang GH, Nylen ES, Scheff SW, Cotman CW. Glutamate as a CNS transmitter, I: evaluation of glucose and glutamine as precursors for the synthesis of preferentially released glutamate. *Brain Res.* 1979;168:513-530.
48. Urenjak J, Williams SR, Gadian DG, Noble M. Proton nuclear magnetic resonance spectroscopy unambiguously identifies different neural cell types. *J Neurosci.* 1993;13:981-989.
49. Selemon LD, Rajkowska G, Goldman-Rakic PS. Abnormally high neuronal density in the schizophrenic cortex. *Arch Gen Psychiatry.* 1995;53:805-818.
50. Olney JW, Farber NB. Glutamate receptor dysfunction in schizophrenia. *Arch Gen Psychiatry.* 1995;52:998-1007.
51. Javitt DC, Zukin SR. Recent advances in the phencyclidine model of schizophrenia. *Am J Psychiatry.* 1991;148:1301-1308.
52. Nasrallah PM. In vivo proton magnetic resonance spectroscopy of the hippocampal amygdala region in schizophrenics. *Schizophr Res.* 1992;6:150.
53. Renshaw PF, Yurgelum-Todd DA, Tohen M, Gruber S, Cohen BM. Temporal lobe proton magnetic resonance spectroscopy of patients with first-episode psychosis. *Am J Psychiatry.* 1995;152:444-446.
54. Alexander GE, De Long MR, Strick PL. Parallel organization of functionally segregated circuits linking basal ganglia and cortex. *Annu Rev Neurosci.* 1986;9: 357-381.
55. Alexander EA, Crutcher MD, De Long MR. Basal ganglia-thalamocortical circuits: parallel substrates for motor, oculomotor, 'prefrontal' and 'limbic' functions. *Prog Brain Res.* 1990;85:119-146.
56. Rajakumar N, Williamson P, Stoessl J, Flumerfelt B. Neurodevelopmental pathogenesis of schizophrenia. In: Proceedings of the Society of Neuroscience Meeting; 1996; Washington, DC. Vol 2, p 1187.
57. Lipska BK, Jaskiw GE, Chrapasta S, Karoum F, Weinberger DR. Ibotenic acid lesion of the ventral hippocampus differentially affects dopamine and its metabolites in the nucleus accumbens in prefrontal cortex. *Brain Res.* 1992;585(1-2): 1-6.
58. Miller BL. A review of chemical issues in ^{1}H NMR spectroscopy: N-acetyl-L-aspartate, creatine, and choline. *NMR Biomed.* 1991;4:47-52.
59. Pettegrew JW, Keshavan MS, Panchalingam K, Strychor S, Kaplan DB, Tretta MG, Allen M. Alternations in brain high-energy phosphate and membrane phospholipid metabolism in first-episode, drug-naive schizophrenics: a pilot study of the dorsal prefrontal cortex by in vivo phosphorus 31 nuclear magnetic resonance spectroscopy. *Arch Gen Psychiatry.* 1991;48:563-568.
60. Potwarka J, Drost DJ, Williamson PC. A study of schizophrenia using 2D ^{31}P chemical shift imaging with ^{1}H decoupling. In: Proceedings of the Society of Magnetic Resonance Meeting; April 27-May 3, 1996; New York, NY. Page 998. Abstract.
61. Stanley JA, Williamson PC, Drost DJ, Carr TJ, Rylett RJ, Malla A, Thompson RT. An in vivo study of the prefrontal cortex of schizophrenic patients at different stages of illness via phosphorus magnetic resonance spectroscopy. *Arch Gen Psychiatry.* 1995;52:399-406.
62. Buckley PF, Moore C, Long H, Larkin C, Thompson P, Mulvany F, Redmond O, Stack JP, Ennis JT, Waddington JL. ^{1}H-magnetic resonance spectroscopy of the left temporal and frontal lobes in schizophrenia: clinical, neurodevelopmental, and cognitive correlates. *Biol Psychiatry.* 1994;36:792-800.
63. Benes FM. Relationship of cingulate cortex to schizophrenia and other psychiatric disorders. In: Vogt BA, Gabriel M, eds. *Neurobiology of Cingulate Cortex and Limbic Thalamus.* Boston, Mass: Birkhauser; 1993:581-605.

Major Theories of Personality Disorder

edited by John F. Clarkin and Mark F. Lenzenweger, 390 pp, ISBN 1-57230-082-5, New York, NY, Guilford Press, 1996.

The editors have compiled a useful and timely volume. It is useful because it brings together some of the more important theories of personality disorder in a single volume, thereby facilitating comparison and analysis. The editors express the hope that this will fill the conceptual and theoretical void in the study of personality disorder. It is timely because the study of personality disorder is at an interesting juncture; after a period of steady growth, the field seems to lack direction. The editors suggest that the field is progressing to a second stage of its development in which greater emphasis is placed on etiology and development. The problem that the field faces is that the impetus and conceptual support for recent empirical work was largely provided by the *DSM-III*. The decision to classify personality disorders on a separate axis drew attention to the importance of personality disorder and promoted interest in the topic. The *DSM-III* also offered specific diagnostic criteria and distinguished personality pathology from other forms of psychopathologic conditions. These developments established the research agenda. But the *DSM* classification does not provide the theoretical framework required to organize the resulting findings; indeed, the *DSM* approach rejects the idea that theory has a role in classification. Nor does it provide the conceptual clarity required to sustain empirical research and promote theory development. Moreover, the many empirical studies stimulated by the *DSM* classification have produced little by way of substantive findings; data are many, but facts are few. Nevertheless, these studies are raising troublesome questions about the validity of the *DSM-IV* approach. Little evidence has accumulated to justify the continued use of categorical diagnoses based on phenotypic features or to support the validity of organizing the features of personality disorder into the 10 diagnoses proposed for Axis II disorders. This threatens the conceptual foundations on which many contemporary approaches rest.

Under these circumstances, Clarkin and Lenzenweger's contribution is especially important—it draws attention to theory at a time when the study of personality disorder needs a new theoretical and conceptual framework. Therefore, the question is whether the theories presented provide the conceptual integration needed to establish a coherent research agenda to replace that based on the *DSM-IV*. The volume does not offer an exhaustive account of all relevant theories. Given the diversity of personality pathology, the editors had to exercise selectivity, and one cannot fault their choice. Included are chapters about the cognitive approach by Pretzer and Beck, Benjamin's structural model of interpersonal behavior, Kernberg's psychoanalytic model, the social learning cum evolutionary theory by Millon and Davis, and a biological perspective by Depue. Together they provide a reasonable sampling of contemporary ideas. Nevertheless, they primarily reflect the contemporary American clinical scene. Important omissions are European perspectives, especially the contributions of the classic phenomenologists, and normal personality theory, especially trait theory.

Although the work of classic phenomenologists is barely referenced, Jaspers, Kretschmer, Schneider, and others made important contributions that are as relevant today as they were when first published. The conceptual issues that they grappled with, such as the definition and conceptualization of personality disorder, the relationship between personality disorder and other forms of psychopathology, and the relationship between normal and abnormal personality, are still key issues that are unresolved. Similarly, little attention is paid to the relevance of theories of normal personality to theorizing about disordered personality. Yet, the study of normal personality has made important progress in recent years and pertinent questions include whether theories of normal personality structure provide a viable alternative to the *DSM-IV* and what the relationship is between normal and disordered personality. A gap exists between the study of personality and clinical studies of personality disorder that must be closed if we are to develop a coherent theory of personality disorder.

With these omissions in mind, it is important to consider the extent to which the theories described provide the integration needed. Unfortunately, the answers that we seek do not lie between the covers of this volume. This is not a reflection on the work of the editors, but on the state of the field. Although the answers are not here, on finishing this text, one has a clear sense of what is needed—greater conceptual and theoretical rigor. It is instructive to consider the reasons why the theories described do not provide the foundation for integration or establish the research agenda. First, they offer different approaches to understanding personality disorder and focus on different aspects of psychopathology. Thus, it is often difficult to identify any common ground that is more than superficial. Most theories focus on a limited facet of personality pathology such as cognitions, interpersonal behaviors, dynamic processes, or biological processes. Only Millon and Davis' approach begins to offer the breadth and scope required. It is not that these theories are unimportant or uninteresting, rather that they are so circumscribed. To be fair, theorists who focus on cognitions or interpersonal difficulties would probably argue that these are the primary deficits and that other important aspects of psychopathology are a consequence of these difficulties. Even so, most theories offer a limited explanation of personality disorder.

Part of the difficulty is that several theories were originally developed to account for other phenomena and extended to personality disorder without much modification. In principle this need not be a problem, but in this case it means that important features of personality pathology are either neglected or inadequately explained. Benjamin's theory, for example, was developed to account for the structure of interpersonal behavior. Because interpersonal dysfunction is an inherent feature of personality disorder, the theory has obvious relevance. But interpersonal pathology is not the whole story—other features are also important and these are inadequately discussed. Similarly, Beck's approach was developed to account for the psychopathology of some Axis I disorders. Cognitive dysfunctions of various kinds are involved in personality disorder, but Beck's account does not provide comprehensive coverage. Thus, Benjamin and Beck address important issues and many of the concepts that they propose are likely to prove useful in a more comprehensive model because they involve relatively low-level generalizations. But neither model addresses important issues of the type that the editors raise in their introductory chapter.

A second reason why this volume does not provide the basis for integration is that the general state of theory construction is disappointing. Ideally, the different theories should be articulated with sufficient precision and clarity that a comparative analysis would identify important similarities and differences. Areas of similarity would then provide the basis for integration, and points of difference would provide opportunities to perform critical tests that would permit theoretical and empirical advance. In their introductory chapter, Clarkin and Lenzenweger identify issues that a satisfactory theory should address, for example, substantive foundations, formal structure, associated taxonomy, and development. Most models, however, fail to explicate their underlying assumptions and to address the fundamental issues confronting personality disorder research and theory. In addition to these shortcomings, some theories still rely excessively on broad generalizations and fuzzy concepts that offer little by way of detailed explanation.

Although the state of theorizing is generally disappointing, the real value of this volume is that it makes the problems confronting the field obvious. By putting theories together in a single volume, the editors have provided a valuable service. Reading these theories side by side highlights the issues and draws attention to the strengths and limitations of each approach in ways that are not readily apparent when they are read independently. This, itself, is a valuable contribution. Those in the field often behave as if the problems of classifying and theorizing about personality disorder have been solved to a greater degree than is actually the case. New perspectives and ideas about theory and therapy are often adopted enthusiastically and uncritically so that they rapidly attain near cultlike status. But clearly we have yet to come to grips with fundamental conceptual problems. In some ways, this volume clears the decks for new developments by making the limitations of contemporary theorizing so apparent. Thus, Clarkin and Lenzenweger force us to realize that the central problems facing the field are conceptual. The contemporary zeitgeist assumes that empirical analyses will inevitably yield progress. But as Millon and Davis argue in their chapter, empirical research that is not guided by theory is unlikely to yield substantive findings and the editors begin their introduction with the following quotation:

> In the dialogue between theory and experience, theory always has the first word. It determines the form of the question and thus the limits to the answer. (Jacop F. *The Logic of Life: A History of Heredity*. New York, NY: Pantheon Books; 1982.)

This is apparent with personality disorder; the problem is not lack of data but lack of conceptual and theoretical clarity; hence, a failure to ask the right questions. Although increased conceptual research is needed, it is difficult to fund and support. Nevertheless, progress is likely to be limited until it occurs.

This forces us to consider the question: what constitutes a good theory of personality disorder? In addition to the usual criteria of parsimony, explicitness, and precision, a good theory of personality disorder should also be comprehensive. Considered together, the theories described indicate the range of phenomena to be explained. They also indicate the forms of explanation required to provide a comprehensive account. In this sense, this volume charts the course for future theorizing. Theories and therapies that fail to recognize the multidimensional nature of personality disorder and its complex biological and psychosocial etiology lack credibility. It should be acknowledged, however, that it may be premature to consider developing a comprehensive and integrated theory of personality. Perhaps all that is possible is an overall framework for understanding personality disorder that organizes current knowledge using low-level concepts, establishes a conceptual understanding of the nature of personality disorder and its relationship to normality and other forms of pathology, and provides a guide for therapeutic activity and future research. Within this framework, specific or microtheories could be developed to account for focal aspects of psychopathology as exemplified by some of the theories in this volume. Under these circumstances, it would be important to acknowledge that these are microtheories and not overstate their range of application, as often occurs.

This is a volume that should be read by all involved in the research and clinical practice of personality disorder. After reading it, the issues are apparent and the limitations of current theories are all too obvious. Positions advanced with such confidence are seen to be limited. This realization can only be healthy for research and practice. It should pave the way for the conceptual and theoretical work that is required for the field to advance.

W. J. Livesley, MD, PhD
Department of Psychiatry
University of British Colombia
2255 Wesbrook Mall
Vancouver, British Columbia
Canada V6T 2A1

Treatment of Bulimia Nervosa With Ondansetron

Bulimia nervosa, a chronic psychiatric disorder, is characterized by frequent episodes of binge eating followed by purging (usually in the form of self-induced vomiting) with a loss of volitional control over these behaviors. This disorder occurs in 3% to 5% of young women.[1] Our research group has previously suggested that the pathophysiological characteristics driving the abnormal behaviors involve an increase in the basal tone of the vagus nerve as a result of repeated and aggressive stimulation of the gastric branch of the vagus nerve by binge eating and vomiting.[2] This hypothesis led us to treat a total of 5 women who met the *DSM-III-R* criteria for bulimia nervosa (binge-purge subtype) with ondansetron hydrochloride (a 5-hydroxytryptamine type 3 receptor antagonist that pharmacologically decreases vagal transmission[3]). All of these patients were considered to have severe bulimia nervosa due to the chronicity of the disease, a history of previous drug and psychotherapeutic treatment failures, or both.

All 5 patients were seeking treatment for bulimia nervosa as private patients and were not receiving any concurrent psychotherapeutic or drug treatment. Their clinical characteristics are provided in the **Table**. Treatment with ondansetron hydrochloride was initiated with 4 mg given 3 times daily as a base dose. The patients were instructed to take additional 4-mg doses as needed (up to a total of 24 mg/d) when experiencing intense urges to binge eat. The only notable side effect was constipation, which was treated with psyllium mucilloid (Metamucil). These patients displayed a marked reduction of symptoms during the first month of treatment with ondansetron (Table). After the first month, patient 1 had a total of 6 sporadic binge-vomit cycles during months 2 to 9 and has been free from binge-purge episodes; she has not required treatment with ondansetron for the last 7 months. Patient 2 elected to discontinue treatment with the drug prematurely after 6 weeks and relapsed immediately. She admittedly enjoyed binge eating and purging and was ambivalent about becoming totally abstinent. Instead, she tried to use ondansetron only when necessary, when it was inconvenient or embarrassing for her to engage in bulimic behaviors. Patient 3 did not have any binge-vomit episodes during months 2 to 3.5, and ondansetron treatment had been discontinued for 1.5 months when we lost contact with her when she received a scholarship to study abroad. Of the 2 remaining patients, patient 4 has been abstinent for 6 weeks and is not receiving ondansetron. Patient 5 did not return after week 6. Our attempt to reach her was unsuccessful.

These patients attributed the effectiveness of ondansetron to a decrease in the urge to engage in the binge-vomit behavior. This decrease in the uncontrollable urge to binge-vomit was accompanied by a resumption of normal hunger and normal satiation.

Responses of 5 Patients With Bulimia Nervosa to Treatment With Ondansetron*

Variable	Patient 1	Patient 2	Patient 3	Patient 4	Patient 5
Age, y	20	24	23	23	26
Illness duration, y	8	4	10	3	4
Past hospitalizations	Electrolyte imbalance, suicide attempt	None	None	None	None
Past psychotherapy	Multiple settings	Individual	Group	Group	None
Past drug treatment	Twice (SSRIs)	SSRIs	SSRIs	None	None
Date OND treatment was initiated	7/94	2/95	3/95	8/95	8/95
Bulimic episodes per week†					
Baseline	42	42	49	10	16
After treatment with OND, wk					
1	4	10	7	4	13
2	3	8	3	2	8
3	1	3	1	5	5
4	0	1	0	1	3
Current status	OND discontinued, symptom free	Elected to terminate treatment after 6 weeks and relapsed	OND discontinued, symptom free at last contact	Received OND for 8 weeks, currently not receiving OND, abstinent for the last 6 weeks	Lost contact after week 6, symptoms fluctuated between weeks 4 and 6

*SSRIs indicates selective serotonin reuptake inhibitors; OND, ondansetron hydrochloride.
†A bulimic episode is a behavioral cycle consisting of binge eating followed by self-induced vomiting.

Unlike traditional psychiatric drug treatment strategies that typically require 2 to 3 weeks for efficacy to emerge and often only result in partial improvement in the condition, the response to ondansetron in all 5 patients was more pronounced and evident during the first week. While double-blind, placebo-controlled experiments are necessary, the results from these 5 patients provide preliminary evidence supporting our hypothesis that an increase in vagal tone drives the binge-vomit cycles in bulimia nervosa.

Boyd K. Hartman, MD
Patricia L. Faris, PhD
Suck Won Kim, MD
Nancy C. Raymond, MD
Robert L. Goodale, MD
William H. Meller, MD
Elke D. Eckert, MD
University of Minnesota Medical School–Minneapolis
420 Delaware St SE
Minneapolis, MN 55455

This study was supported by grant R01 DK52291 from The National Institute of Diabetes and Digestive Kidney Diseases, National Institutes of Health, Washington, DC; and the Mark A. Nugent Research Foundation, St Paul, Minn.

1. Fairburn CG, Beglin SJ. Studies of the epidemiology of bulimia nervosa. *Am J Psychiatry*. 1990;147:401-408.
2. Faris PL, Raymond NC, De Zwaan M, Howard LA, Eckert ED, Mitchell JE. Nociceptive, but not tactile, thresholds are elevated in bulimia nervosa. *Biol Psychiatry*. 1992;32:462-466.
3. Figg WD, Graham CL, Hak LJ, Dukes GE. Ondansetron: a novel antiemetic agent. *South Med J*. 1993;86:497-502.

Patent Laws: Could Changes Enhance Drug Development?

Having spent the past 8 years conducting clinical trials for pharmaceutical companies, I have the impression that current patent laws often inhibit optimal research. One of the most common reasons for discontinuing development of a drug, or not evaluating a drug for a new indication, is "limited patent life."

The patent laws were intended to encourage the development of new drugs by providing financial incentives (ie, patent protection). These laws, however (understandably), did not consider current issues related to drug development, eg, the average time from patent application to Food and Drug Administration approval for marketing is 10 years. Much of the delay in having drugs approved for marketing is due to increased Food and Drug Administration requirements, eg, the need for extensive safety and efficacy data, studies of the minimum effective dose, and others. I think that most clinicians and researchers would agree that it is good for the Food and Drug Administration to require such data, because it greatly expands the scientific basis for the practice of medicine. On the other hand, related changes in patent life may be appropriate.

One result of the short effective patent life is that pharmaceutical companies are skipping or skimping on phase 2 studies, which are intended to provide initial evidence of efficacy and help to determine the optimal dosage regimen. Because phase 2 studies take time, many pharmaceutical companies have opted to gamble, spending more on larger phase 3 studies, with the expectation of having a longer effective patent life if they are successful. This has been most evident, I think, in Alzheimer disease studies, an area of potentially large profits. From the pharmaceutical company's perspective, this may be a reasonable gamble, but this is an extremely inefficient way to find a treatment for Alzheimer disease.

Further, given the large number of potential new compounds, it is impossible for pharamceutical companies to test all new compounds for all possible indications expeditiously. Issues may arise in animal safety studies or in early human trials that slow development; pharmaceutical companies should not have to rush to decide whether to develop a drug, if more data would help with the decision. Patent law changes could allow pharmaceutical companies to proceed with drug evaluation in a more measured, rational, and cost-effective manner; one option is to guarantee a minimum patent life after the drug has been approved, regardless of how many years were spent in drug development.

Changes in patent laws need not increase pharmaceutical company profits, which may be adequate. Pharmaceutical companies might agree to keep prices lower if they could be assured of longer patent life, although the issues involved in adjusting price based on patent life are complex.

Changing the patent laws would be difficult because it would require congressional action; however, changes could enhance the original intent of the laws, ie, to foster the optimal development of promising medications. Research-oriented physicians could initiate this effort.

Jeffrey A. Mattes, MD
Psychopharmacology Research Association of Princeton, PC
601 Ewing St
Suite A-12
Princeton, NJ 08540

The Identification and Validation of Distinct Depressive Syndromes in a Population-Based Sample of Female Twins

Since Aubrey Lewis' classic study there has been debate about whether the distinction between depressive subtypes is categorical or dimensional.[1-6] A recent article by Kendler et al[7] supports a categorical classification of depressive subtypes. Using a different means of validating nosological distinctions, our group reached similar conclusions and we think it relevant to review the similarities and differences between our findings and those of Kendler et al.

In a prospective epidemiological study of adult female twins, Kendler et al used latent class analysis and identified 3 depressive subtypes—mild typical, atypical, and severe typical depression. Subjects with atypical depression were characterized by reversed vegetative depressive symptoms (overeating and oversleeping). These groups differed on many validating criteria, supporting a categorical distinction.

We reached a similar conclusion using psychopharmacologic dissection, a distinctly different method.[8] In a series of 6 studies, patients with nonautonomous mood were randomized to receive imipramine, phenelzine, or placebo.[9-13] Nonresponders to their first treatment were crossed over double-blind to an active drug. There were approximately 475 patient trials. Our work suggested 3 depressive subtypes, strikingly similar to the subtypes of Kendler et al. Specifically, we identified a subgroup with atypical depression (overeating and oversleeping) characterized by poor tricyclic antidepressant (TCA) (44% [65/147]) and a good monoamine oxidase inhibitor (MAOI) response (72% [118/165]) and a second group, simple mood reactive depression (similar to the mild typical classification of Kendler et al) characterized by a good response to both TCAs (80% [24/30]) and MAOIs (75% [18/24]). In both groups, placebo response was approximately 25%. Using items from the Hamilton Depression Rating Scale (HAM-D), a measure of endogeneity was constructed. The response of patients with simple mood reactive depression to tricyclic drugs was similar if they had many or virtually no positive vegetative symptoms. This suggested that melancholic symptoms did not seem to be a precondition for imipramine benefit in this group, suggesting mild typical depression may differ from severe typical depression (melancholia). Clearly this distinction is not as well supported as that of atypical vs other groups.

Adherents to a dimensional view attribute observed differences in depressive subtypes to severity. If atypical depression were mild melancholia, a robust TCA response would be expected. Our work supported a categorical distinction between severe typical (melancholic) and atypical depression since their poor TCA response is inconsistent with a dimensional view. Could other factors interfere with these patients' ability to benefit from drug treatment? Chronicity or maladaptive character traits (superimposed on mild melancholia) did not seem to preclude TCA responsivity and explain the low TCA improvement rate, because the high MAOI improvement rate is consistent with a drug responsive group. Because the 44% TCA response rate was observed in 147 subjects with atypical depression, the confidence limits (95% confidence interval, 34-54) are narrow and a good approximation of what exists in the population. A preliminary family study also supports the distinction between atypical depression and melancholia.[14] Most prior discussion of the binary vs the unitary view of depression focused on patients with psychotic and melancholic symptoms, ie, are mood congruent delusions sufficient for inclusion in a particular categorical type?[15] Of particular interest is that these current studies offer a nosological distinction of patients formerly considered in the neurotic pole of the distribution, where categorical difference seemed unlikely.[7,13]

The 2 approaches resulted in other similarities and some minor differences. Contrary to previous anecdotal observation, we concluded, as did Kendler et al, that the atypical syndrome occurred independent of the presence of anxiety.[16] A robust MAOI effect occurred independent of anxiety.[11]

Kendler et al[7] found an association between bulimia nervosa and atypical depression. We reported that in atypical patients with bulimia, phenelzine therapy was superior to imipramine therapy and amelioration of depressive symptoms was associated with improvement of the eating disorder.[17] This suggested a possible link between depression and bulimia nervosa in subjects with atypical depression.

One difference is that the overwhelming majority of patients we identified as having atypical depression had a chronic course. Kendler et al indicate the course of atypical depression is characterized by short, frequent episodes. An epidemiologic approach is more likely to accurately assess the entire population than a clinic sample. However, it is possible assessment techniques that describe short, frequent episodes, may have missed between episode dysthymia.[7]

In summary, the salient aspects of the subtypes defined by Kendler et al using latent class analysis (in a female population sample of twins) are strikingly similar to the subtypes that we have identified using psychopharmacologic dissection (in male and female treatment seekers). The similar outcome in men and women in our studies suggests the findings by Kendler et al in women may also be applicable to men. The work of Kendler et al adds further support to including atypical as a parenthetical modifier of major depression in *DSM-IV*. Both sets of data support the possibility of categorically distinct depressive subtypes.

Frederic M. Quitkin, MD
Jonathan W. Stewart, MD
Patrick J. McGrath, MD
Edward V. Nunes, MD
Donald F. Klein, MD
New York State Psychiatric Institute
777 W 168th St
New York, NY 10032

1. Lewis AJ. *A Clinical and Historical Survey of Depressive States: Based on the Study of 61 Cases.* Adelaide, Australia: University of Adelaide; 1931. Thesis.
2. Lewis AJ. Melancholia: prognostic studies and case material. *J Ment Sci.* 1936; 82:488-558.
3. Kiloh LG, Andrews G, Neilson M, Bianchi GN. The relationship of the syndromes called endogenous and neurotic depression. *Br J Psychiatry.* 1972; 121:183-196.
4. Kiloh LG, Garside RF. Depression: a multivariate study of Sir Aubrey Lewis's data on melancholia. *Aust N Z J Psychiatry.* 1977;11:149-156.
5. Kendell RE. Clinical validity. In: Robins LN, Barrett JE, eds. *The Validity of Psychiatric Diagnosis.* New York, NY: Raven Press; 1989:305-323.
6. Parker G, Hadzi-Pavlovic D. Old data, new interpretation: a re-analysis of Sir Aubrey Lewis' MD thesis. *Psychological Med.* 1993;23:859-870.
7. Kendler KS, Eaves LJ, Walters EE, Neale MC, Heath AC, Kessler RC. The identification and validation of distinct depressive syndromes in a population-based sample of female twins. *Arch Gen Psychiatry.* 1996;53:391-399.
8. Klein DF. The pharmacological validation of diagnoses. In: Robins LN, Barrett JE, eds. *The Validity of Psychiatric Diagnoses.* New York, NY: Raven Press; 1989:203-217.
9. Quitkin FM, Stewart JS, McGrath PJ, Liebowitz MR, Harrison WM, Tricamo E, Klein DF, Markowitz JS, Rabkin JG, Wager SG. Phenelzine versus imipramine in the treatment of probable atypical depression: defining syndrome boundaries of selective MAOI responders. *Am J Psychiatry.* 1988;145:306-311.
10. Quitkin FM, McGrath PJ, Stewart JW, Harrison W, Wager SG, Nunes E, Rabkin JG, Tricamo E, Markowitz J, Klein DF. Phenelzine and imipramine in mood reactive depressives: further delineation of the syndrome of atypical depression. *Arch Gen Psychiatry.* 1989;46:787-793.
11. Quitkin FM, McGrath PJ, Stewart JW, Harrison W, Tricamo E, Wager SG, Ocepek-Welikson K, Nunes E, Rabkin JG, Klein DF. Atypical depression, panic attacks, and response to imipramine and phenelzine: a replication. *Arch Gen Psychiatry.* 1990;47:935-941.
12. Quitkin FM, Harrison W, Stewart JW, McGrath PJ, Tricamo E, Ocepek-Welikson K, Rabkin JG, Wager SG, Nunes E, Klein DF. Response to phenelzine and imipramine in placebo nonresponders with atypical depression: a new application of the crossover design. *Arch Gen Psychiatry.* 1991;48:319-323.
13. Quitkin FM, Stewart JW, McGrath PJ, Tricamo E, Rabkin JG, Ocepek-

Welikson K, Nunes EV, Harrison W, Klein DF. Columbia atypical depression: a subgroup of depressives with better response to MAOI than to tricyclic antidepressants or placebo. *Br J Psychiatry*. 1993;163(suppl 21):30-34.
14. Stewart JW, McGrath PJ, Rabkin JG, Quitkin FM. Atypical depression: a valid clinical entity? *Psychiatr Clin North Am*. 1993;16:479-495.
15. Glassman A, Kantor S, Shostak M. Depressions, delusions and drug response. *Am J Psychiatry*. 1975;132:716-719.
16. Joyce PR, Paykel ES. Predictors of drug response in depression. *Arch Gen Psychiatry*. 1989;46:89-99.
17. Rothschild R, Quitkin HM, Quitkin FM, Stewart JW, Ocepek-Welikson K, McGrath PJ, Tricamo E. A double-blind placebo-controlled comparison of phenelzine and imipramine in the treatment of bulimia in atypical depressives. *Int J Eating Disord*. 1994;15:1-9.

D_2 Dopamine Receptor Occupancy: A Crossover Comparison of Risperidone With Clozapine Therapy in Schizophrenic Patients

The atypical antipsychotic agents, clozapine and risperidone, have a similar pharmacological profile of D_2 dopamine receptor affinity, α_2, and serotonin$_2$ antagonism.[1] Despite this similarity, the clinical profile of these 2 drugs are quite different. For instance, risperidone produces dose-dependent extrapyramidal side effects,whereas clozapine does not.[2] Moreover, there may be differences in the antipsychotic efficacy of these 2 drugs n treatment-resistant patients. One possibility for this difference in clinical profile is that these drugs produce different levels of D_2 receptor occupancy. Previous estimates of D_2 receptor occupancy of these atypical agents have examined different individuals and do not account for interindividual variation.[3,4] We are, therefore, conducting a double-blind, randomized, crossover sodium iodide I 123-benzamide–single photon emission computed tomographic study with schizophrenic patients treated with fixed doses of clozapine and risperidone to investigate the degree of D_2 receptor occupancy by these drugs.

To date, we have examined 4 chronic schizophrenic male patients diagnosed using *DSM-III-R* criteria. Patients were scanned using single photon emission computed tomography after 4 weeks of receiving treatment with risperidone (6 mg/d) and clozapine (400 mg/d) in a double-blind, crossover study. Brief Psychiatric Rating Scale (BPRS) ratings were conducted by physicians blind to antipsychotic drug status prior to scanning. Estimates of D_2 receptor occupancy are based on the comparison of specific-binding potential during drug treatment to an independent reference normal control group.[5]

Significantly greater striatal D_2 receptor occupancies were observed during risperidone treatment (74% ± 3% [mean ± SD]) compared with clozapine treatment (51% ± 8%) (Student $t = 4.4$, $df = 3$, $P<.03$) in these 4 patients (**Table**). We also observed that each patient had a similar or higher BPRS total score when treated with risperidone compared with clozapine despite uniformly higher levels of D_2 receptor occupancy on risperidone.

To our knowledge, this is the first study that uses a fixed-dose, crossover design to minimize individual variation in D_2 receptor occupancy and is consistent with previous data indicating that risperidone is a more potent D_2 receptor antagonist than its atypical counterpart, clozapine. Moreover, we do not observe a relationship between higher D_2 receptor occupancy and lower BPRS scores. Although these data suggest that factors other than D_2 receptor occupancy are predictive of relative antipsychotic efficacy, no drug has yet been identified with antipsychotic action without a significant affinity for the D_2 receptor.[1]

This apparent paradox remains an intriguing question for the understanding of the mechanism of action of antipsychotic drugs and, particularly, for psychopharmacologists involved in the design of the next generation of these agents.

Tung-Ping Su, MD
Anil K. Malhotra, MD
Kayleen Hadd, RN, MSN
Alan Breier, MD
David Pickar, MD
Experimental Therapeutics Branch
National Institute of Mental Health
Bldg 10, Room 4N212
10 Center Dr
MSC 1380
Bethesda, MD 20892-1380

Presented in part at the 50th Annual Meeting of the Society of Biological Psychiatry, San Francisco, Calif, May 2, 1996.

Corresponding author: David Pickar, MD, National Institute of Mental Health, Bldg 10, Room 4N212, 10 Center Dr, MSC 1380, Bethesda, MD 20892-1380.

1. Pickar D. Prospects for the pharmacotherapy of schizophrenia. *Lancet*. 1995;345:557-562.
2. Marder SR, Meibach RC. Risperidone in the treatment of schizophrenia. *Am J Psychiatry*. 1994;151:825-835.
3. Farde L, Nordstrom A-L, Wiesel F-A, Pauli S, Halldin C, Sedvall G. PET-

Comparison of ^{123}I-BZM–Specific Binding, Estimated Percentage of D_2 Dopamine Receptor Occupancy, and BPRS During Risperidone and Clozapine Therapy in a Crossover Design*

	Risperidone			Clozapine		
Patient No./Age, y	^{123}I-BZM–Specific Binding	Estimated % of D_2 Dopamine Receptor Occupancy†	BPRS Total	^{123}I-BZM–Specific Binding	Estimated % of D_2 Dopamine Receptor Occupancy†	BPRS Total
1/31	0.41	75	33	0.95	43	36
2/48	0.43	74	44	0.68	59	45
3/26	0.49	70	59	0.70	58	41
4/41	0.38	77	40	0.90	44	38
Mean±SD 36.5±9	0.43±0.04	74±3.0	44±11	0.82±0.15	51±8	40±4

**All of the schizophrenic patients were men who received 6 mg/d of risperidone and 400 mg/d of clozapine in this crossover study. ^{123}I-BZM indicates sodium iodide I123-benzamide;. BPRS, Brief Psychiatric Rating Scale.*

†Estimated percentage of D_2 dopamine receptor occupancy equals [1−(patient specific binding/averaged normal control specific binding)] × 100.

analysis of central D_1- and D_2-dopamine receptor occupancy in patients treated with classical neuroleptics and clozapine-relation to extrapyramidal side effects. *Arch Gen Psychiatry.* 1992;49:538-844.
4. Farde L, Nyberg S, Oxenstierna G, Nakashima Y, Halldin C, Ericsson B. Positron emission tomography studies on D_2 and 5-HT_2 receptor binding in risperidone-treated schizophrenic patients. *J Clin Psychopharmacol.* 1995;15:19S-23S.
5. Pickar D, Su T-P, Weinberger DR, Coppola R, Malhotra AK, Knable MB, Lee KS, Gorey J, Breier A, Hsiao J. Individual variation in D_2 dopamine receptor occupancy in clozapine treated patients. *Am J Psychiatry.* 1996;153:1571-1578.

Sertraline and Imipramine for the Treatment of Dysthymia

In their article titled "A Placebo-Controlled, Randomized Clinical Trial Comparing Sertraline and Imipramine for the Treatment of Dysthymia," Thase et al[1] come to the conclusion that pharmacotherapy provides considerable relief from the symptoms of dysthymia, with both sertraline and imipramine being more effective than placebo.

However, they do not mention—and, therefore, I calculated for the readers of your journal—that the mean 17-item Hamilton Depression Rating Scale (HAM-D) end point score is (12.7-5.6=) 7.1 in the sertraline-treated group, (13.4-5.9=) 7.5 in the imipramine-treated group, and (12.7-3.9=) 8.8 in the placebo group. These active drug-placebo differences (1.7 and 1.3, respectively) may be statistically significant, but in my opinion they are clinically not relevant. The same may be said for the differences found in the mean Montgomery-Asberg Depression Rating Scale end scores: 18.5–9.6=–8.9 in the sertraline-treated group, 18.6–9.5=9.1 in the imipramine-treated group, and 19.0–6.7=12.3 in the placebo group. In short, Thase et al may overestimate the benefits of short-term treatment by antidepressants in primary, early-onset, pure dysthymia. In addition, they may underestimate its "costs" in side effects. They certainly do not stress the excess percentage over placebo of side effects. To give some examples, this excess percentage in the sertraline-treated group is 33%–13%=20% for male sexual dysfunction, 23%–12%=11% for somnolence, 21%–10%=11% for diarrhea, 10%–0.7%=9.3% for tremor, 26%–17%=9% for dry mouth, 12%–3%=9% for anorexia, and 10%–2%=8% for agitation. I hope this letter may contribute to a more balanced view on the possibilities and limitations of pharmacotherapy in this disorder.

Frans de Jonghe, MD, PhD
Psychiatric Hospital Amsterdam
S.P.D.C. C/OW
2^e Constatijn
Huygensstraat, 37
1054 AG Amsterdam
the Netherlands

1. Thase ME, Fava M, Halbreich U, Kocsis JH, Koran L, Davidson J, Rosenbaum J, Harrison W. A placebo-controlled, randomized clinical trial comparing sertraline and imipramine for the treatment of dysthymia. *Arch Gen Psychiatry.* 1996;53:777-784.

In reply

Dr de Jonghe is absolutely correct to point out that the drug-placebo differences on the HAM-D scale were small, albeit, statistically significant. I would also agree that a mean drug-placebo difference of about 2 points on the HAM-D scale has questionable clinical significance as an isolated finding. However, the pattern of differences across clinician-administered scales and patients' self-report measures in favor of the active medications was broad and consistent. Such a pattern of results adds to our confidence in the clinical significance of the study. Perhaps more importantly, the groups differed by 15% (sertraline-treated vs placebo) and 20% (imipramine-treated vs placebo) on global response rates. Differences of this magnitude are meaningful to clinicians and patients. The "cost" in terms of significant side effects was relatively high for imipramine therapy, but generally not much different for sertraline therapy and placebo.

Part of the problem in interpreting these data may be that we are not yet very good at assessing the core elements of dysthymia. For example, the HAM-D original scale was derived and validated in studies of older and preponderantly melancholic inpatients. Another part of the problem is probably contextual. Our patients who received placebo had up to 12 visits with board-certified psychiatrists, as well as weekly clinical contact with independent evaluators. This was a very labor-intensive and expensive nonspecific treatment. In clinical practice, psychiatrists' options would include doing nothing, offering psychotherapy, or beginning an active medication. For fair balance, I would agree that controlled studies of various psychotherapies are overdue in dysthymia. Until adequate comparative data are available, however, our patients with dysthymia are much better served by a trial of a modern antidepressant with proved efficacy, such as sertraline, than by doing nothing.

Michael E. Thase, MD
Western Psychiatric Institute and Clinic
University of Pittsburgh Medical Center
3811 O'Hara St
Pittsburgh, PA 15213-2593

The Idiosyncratic Definition of Nicotine Dependence

In an issue of the ARCHIVES, Fergusson et al[1] reported on the association between depressive disorders and nicotine dependence in a cohort of 16-year-olds in Christchurch, New Zealand. The authors state that subjects were classified as meeting *DSM-III-R* criteria if they smoked at least 5 cigarettes per day and reported 2 or more symptoms of nicotine dependence. They add that these criteria "broadly correspond to the criterion of mild nicotine dependence used by Breslau et al."[2] The symptoms of nicotine dependence used in this definition are described in the text as "concerned with failure to quit or reduce smoking, irritability when cigarettes were unavailable, difficulties in going a day without a cigarette, morning cough, needing a cigarette first thing in the morning, continued smoking despite medical advice, and stealing money or using savings to obtain cigarettes."[1] Although these 7 symptoms seem to be related to level of involvement with smoking and probably nicotine dependence, they bear a vague resemblance to the 9 criterion symptoms of psychoactive substance dependence in *DSM-III-R*, of which 3 are required to make the diagnosis. The relationship of the authors' definition of nicotine dependence to the definition in *DSM-III-R* nicotine dependence is unknown. Furthermore, the authors' statement that their criteria "broadly correspond to the criterion of mild nicotine dependence used by Breslau et al" is in error, as we used *DSM-III-R* criteria, measured by the *Diagnostic Interview Schedule, 3rd Edition, Revised*.[3] The criterion for mild nicotine dependence in *DSM-III-R* is identical to that for nicotine dependence, ie, 3 of the 9 symptoms, whereas more severe levels of dependence require more symptoms. In other words, mild nicotine dependence in our study was defined as *DSM-III-R* nicotine dependence.

Naomi Breslau, PhD
Department of Psychiatry
Henry Ford Hospital
3A-1 Ford Pl
Detroit, MI 48202

1. Fergusson DM, Lynskey MT, Horwood LJ. Comorbidity between depressive disorders and nicotine dependence in a cohort of 16-year-olds. *Arch Gen Psychiatry*. 1996;53:1043-1047.
2. Breslau N, Kilbey MM, Andresky P. Nicotine dependence, major depression, and anxiety in young adults. *Arch Gen Psychiatry*. 1991;48:1069-1074.
3. Robins LN, Helzer JE, Cottler L, Golding E. *NIMH Diagnostic Interview Schedule, 3rd Edition, Revised*. St Louis, Mo: Washington University; 1989.

In reply

We agree that the criteria for nicotine dependence used in our article were more liberal than those applied by Breslau et al and may not strictly meet applied DSM-III-R *criteria. The reason for our use of this more liberal criteria was that our sample (aged 16 years) was younger than the sample of 21 to 30 year olds studied by Breslau et al and showed less strongly established patterns of cigarette smoking. To address this issue, we employed the somewhat less stringent definition of nicotine dependence described in our article.*

Dr Breslau's comments raise the issue of the extent to which associations between nicotine dependence and depression are sensitive to minor variations in the criteria used to define nicotine dependence. To examine this, we have varied the criteria for nicotine dependence from the 2 symptoms used in our article to up to 4 symptoms. This analysis shows that the odds ratio (OR) between nicotine dependence and depression progressively declines with increasing stringency of the criteria used to define nicotine dependence. For a criteria using 2 symptoms the OR is 4.6, whereas a criteria using 4 or more symptoms decreases the OR to 1.9. The reasons for this become evident when the relationship between the number of symptoms of nicotine dependence and risk for depression is examined. The **Table** *demonstrates the relationship between the number of symptoms of nicotine dependence and rates of depression. There is evidence of a clear discontinuity in the dose-response distribution, with subjects having 1 or more symptoms of nicotine dependence being at far higher risk of depression than subjects without symptoms. There is relatively little variation in the risk for depression amongst those with symptoms. This Table clearly suggests that, for our data at least,* DSM-III-R *criteria for nicotine dependence were not the best way of describing the data. The optimum dichotomous classification is to contrast those subjects with any symptom of nicotine dependence with those subjects without symptoms. This property explains why the ORs decline with increasing stringency of criteria. The probable reason for this is that the association being investigated is in fact not between nicotine dependence and depression, but rather between regular smoking and depression. While all of the subjects meeting criteria for nicotine dependence will be regular smokers, not all regular smokers will meet criteria for nicotine dependence but are likely to have some symptoms of dependence. This is particularly likely to be the case amongst adolescents who are just beginning regular smoking.*

Relationship Between Number of Symptoms of Nicotine Dependence and Risk for Depression*

	No. of Symptoms				
	0	1	2	3	4
% Depressed	6.9	24.1	19.4	33.3	25.0

*χ^2 (4 df)=48.7; $P<.001$.

In summary, we agree with Dr Breslau that our criteria for nicotine dependence were less stringent than those used in her study. However, this lack of stringency does not threaten the validity of our results. To the contrary, our findings suggest that the use of more stringent criteria would have attenuated the association between smoking and depression. Our results suggest that, in the analysis of smoking and depression, it may be desirable to abandon the use of measures of nicotine dependence and instead analyze relationships between the frequency and regularity of smoking and risk for depression. In samples of older subjets this distinction may be unimportant, but in samples of adolescents who are just beginning regular smoking it would appear to be the regularity of smoking rather than the extent of nicotine dependence that defines the relationship between smoking behaviors and risk for depression.

David M. Fergusson, PhD
Michael T. Lynskey, MSc
John L. Horwood, MSc
Christchurch Health and Development Study
PO Box 4345
Christchurch, New Zealand

Interference with Cognitive and Motor Performance: Because of initial sedation, CLOZARIL® (clozapine) may impair mental and/or physical abilities, especially during the first few days of therapy. The recommendations for gradual dose escalation should be carefully adhered to, and patients cautioned about activities requiring alertness.

Use in Patients with Concomitant Illness: Clinical experience with CLOZARIL® (clozapine) in patients with concomitant systemic diseases is limited. Nevertheless, caution is advisable in using CLOZARIL® (clozapine) in patients with renal or cardiac disease.

Use in Patients Undergoing General Anesthesia: Caution is advised in patients being administered general anesthesia because of the CNS effects of CLOZARIL® (clozapine). Check with the anesthesiologist regarding continuation of CLOZARIL® (clozapine) therapy in a patient scheduled for surgery.

Information for Patients: Physicians are advised to discuss the following issues with patients for whom they prescribe CLOZARIL® (clozapine):

- Patients who are to receive CLOZARIL® (clozapine) should be warned about the significant risk of developing agranulocytosis. They should be informed that weekly blood tests are required to monitor for the occurrence of agranulocytosis, and that CLOZARIL® (clozapine) tablets will be made available only through a special program designed to ensure the required blood monitoring. Patients should be advised to report immediately the appearance of lethargy, weakness, fever, sore throat, malaise, mucous membrane ulceration or other possible signs of infection. Particular attention should be paid to any flu-like complaints or other symptoms that might suggest infection.
- Patients should be informed of the significant risk of seizure during CLOZARIL® (clozapine) treatment, and they should be advised to avoid driving and any other potentially hazardous activity while taking CLOZARIL® (clozapine).
- Patients should be advised of the risk of orthostatic hypotension, especially during the period of initial dose titration.
- Patients should be informed that if they stop taking CLOZARIL® (clozapine) for more than 2 days, they should not restart their medication at the same dosage, but should contact their physician for dosing instructions.
- Patients should notify their physician if they are taking, or plan to take, any prescription or over-the-counter drugs or alcohol.
- Patients should notify their physician if they become pregnant or intend to become pregnant during therapy.
- Patients should not breast feed an infant if they are taking CLOZARIL® (clozapine).

Drug Interactions: The risks of using CLOZARIL® (clozapine) in combination with other drugs have not been systematically evaluated.

The mechanism of CLOZARIL® (clozapine) induced agranulocytosis is unknown; nonetheless, the possibility that causative factors may interact synergistically to increase the risk and/or severity of bone marrow suppression warrants consideration. Therefore, CLOZARIL® (clozapine) should not be used with other agents having a well-known potential to suppress bone marrow function.

Given the primary CNS effects of CLOZARIL® (clozapine), caution is advised in using it concomitantly with other CNS-active drugs or alcohol.

Orthostatic hypotension in patients taking clozapine can, in rare cases (approximately 1 case per 3,000 patients), be accompanied by profound collapse and respiratory and/or cardiac arrest. Some of the cases of collapse/respiratory arrest/cardiac arrest during initial treatment occurred in patients who were being administered benzodiazepines; similar events have been reported in patients taking other psychotropic drugs or even CLOZARIL® (clozapine) by itself. Although it has not been established that there is an interaction between CLOZARIL® (clozapine) and benzodiazepines or other psychotropics, caution is advised when clozapine is initiated in patients taking a benzodiazepine or any other psychotropic drug.

Because CLOZARIL® (clozapine) is highly bound to serum protein, the administration of CLOZARIL® (clozapine) to a patient taking another drug which is highly bound to protein (e.g., warfarin, digitoxin) may cause an increase in plasma concentrations of these drugs, potentially resulting in adverse effects. Conversely, adverse effects may result from displacement of protein-bound CLOZARIL® (clozapine) by other highly bound drugs.

Cimetidine and erythromycin may both increase plasma levels of CLOZARIL® (clozapine), potentially resulting in adverse effects. Although concomitant use of CLOZARIL® (clozapine) and carbamazepine is not recommended, it should be noted that discontinuation of concomitant carbamazepine administration may result in an increase in CLOZARIL® (clozapine) plasma levels. Phenytoin may decrease CLOZARIL® (clozapine) plasma levels, resulting in a decrease in effectiveness of a previously effective CLOZARIL® (clozapine) dose.

A subset (3%-10%) of the population has reduced activity of certain drug metabolizing enzymes such as the cytochrome P450 isozyme P450 2D6. Such individuals are referred to as "poor metabolizers" of drugs such as debrisoquin, dextromethorphan, the tricyclic antidepressants, and clozapine. These individuals may develop higher than expected plasma concentrations of clozapine when given usual doses. In addition, certain drugs that are metabolized by this isozyme, including many antidepressants (clozapine, selective serotonin reuptake inhibitors, and others), may inhibit the activity of this isozyme, and thus may make normal metabolizers resemble poor metabolizers with regard to concomitant therapy with other drugs metabolized by this enzyme system, leading to drug interaction.

Concomitant use of clozapine with other drugs metabolized by cytochrome P450 2D6 may require lower doses than usually prescribed for either clozapine or the other drug. Therefore, co-administration of clozapine with other drugs that are metabolized by this isozyme, including antidepressants, phenothiazines, carbamazepine, and Type 1C antiarrhythmics (e.g., propafenone, flecainide and encainide), or that inhibit this enzyme (e.g., quinidine), should be approached with caution.

CLOZARIL® (clozapine) may also potentiate the hypotensive effects of antihypertensive drugs and the anticholinergic effects of atropine-type drugs. The administration of epinephrine should be avoided in the treatment of drug induced hypotension because of a possible reverse epinephrine effect.

Carcinogenesis, Mutagenesis, Impairment of Fertility: No carcinogenic potential was demonstrated in long-term studies in mice and rats at doses approximately 7 times the typical human dose on a mg/kg basis. Fertility in male and female rats was not adversely affected by clozapine. Clozapine did not produce genotoxic or mutagenic effects when assayed in appropriate bacterial and mammalian tests.

Pregnancy Category B: Reproduction studies have been performed in rats and rabbits at doses of approximately 2-4 times the human dose and have revealed no evidence of impaired fertility or harm to the fetus due to clozapine. There are, however, no adequate and well-controlled studies in pregnant women. Because animal reproduction studies are not always predictive of human response, and in view of the desirability of keeping the administration of all drugs to a minimum during pregnancy, this drug should be used only if clearly needed.

Nursing Mothers: Animal studies suggest that clozapine may be excreted in breast milk and have an effect on the nursing infant. Therefore, women receiving CLOZARIL® (clozapine) should not breast feed.

Pediatric Use: Safety and effectiveness in pediatric patients have not been established.

ADVERSE REACTIONS: Associated with Discontinuation of Treatment: Sixteen percent of 1080 patients who received CLOZARIL® (clozapine) in premarketing clinical trials discontinued treatment due to an adverse event, including both those that could be reasonably attributed to CLOZARIL® (clozapine) treatment and those that might more appropriately be considered intercurrent illness. The more common events considered to be causes of discontinuation included: CNS, primarily drowsiness/sedation, seizures, dizziness/syncope; cardiovascular, primarily tachycardia, hypotension and ECG changes; gastrointestinal, primarily nausea/vomiting; hematologic, primarily leukopenia/granulocytopenia/agranulocytosis; and fever. None of the events enumerated accounts for more than 1.7% of all discontinuations attributed to adverse clinical events.

Commonly Observed: Adverse events observed in association with the use of CLOZARIL® (clozapine) in clinical trials at an incidence of greater than 5% were: central nervous system complaints, including drowsiness/sedation, dizziness/vertigo, headache and tremor; autonomic nervous system complaints, including salivation, sweating, dry mouth and visual disturbances; cardiovascular findings, including tachycardia, hypotension and syncope; and gastrointestinal complaints, including constipation and nausea; and fever. Complaints of drowsiness/sedation tend to subside with continued therapy or dose reduction. Salivation may be profuse, especially during sleep, but may be diminished with dose reduction.

Incidence in Clinical Trials: The following table enumerates adverse events that occurred at a frequency of 1% or greater among CLOZARIL® (clozapine) patients who participated in clinical trials. These rates are not adjusted for duration of exposure.

Treatment-Emergent Adverse Experience Incidence
Among Patients Taking CLOZARIL® (clozapine) in Clinical Trials
(N = 842)
(Percentage of Patients Reporting)

Body System / Adverse Event[a]	Percent
Central Nervous System	
Drowsiness/Sedation	39
Dizziness/Vertigo	19
Headache	7
Tremor	6
Syncope	6
Disturbed sleep/Nightmares	4
Restlessness	4
Hypokinesia/Akinesia	4
Agitation	4
Seizures (convulsions)	3[b]
Rigidity	3
Akathisia	3
Confusion	3
Fatigue	2
Insomnia	2
Hyperkinesia	1
Weakness	1
Lethargy	1
Ataxia	1
Slurred speech	1
Depression	1
Epileptiform movements/Myoclonic jerks	1
Anxiety	1
Cardiovascular	
Tachycardia	25[b]
Hypotension	9
Hypertension	4
Chest pain/Angina	1
ECG change/Cardiac abnormality	1
Gastrointestinal	
Constipation	14
Nausea	5
Abdominal discomfort/Heartburn	4
Nausea/Vomiting	3
Vomiting	3
Diarrhea	2
Liver test abnormality	1
Anorexia	1
Urogenital	
Urinary abnormalities	2
Incontinence	1
Abnormal ejaculation	1
Urinary urgency/frequency	1
Urinary retention	1
Autonomic Nervous System	
Salivation	31
Sweating	6
Dry mouth	6
Visual disturbances	5
Integumentary (Skin)	
Rash	2
Musculoskeletal	
Muscle weakness	1
Pain (back, neck, legs)	1
Muscle spasm	1
Muscle pain, ache	1
Respiratory	
Throat discomfort	1
Dyspnea, shortness of breath	1
Nasal congestion	1
Hemic/Lymphatic	
Leukopenia/Decreased WBC/Neutropenia	3
Agranulocytosis	1[b]
Eosinophilia	1
Miscellaneous	
Fever	5
Weight gain	4
Tongue numb/sore	1

(Continued)

Treatment-Emergent Adverse Experience Incidence
Among Patients Taking CLOZARIL® (clozapine) in Clinical Trials
(N = 842)
(Percentage of Patients Reporting)

[a]Events reported by at least 1% of CLOZARIL® (clozapine) patients are included.

[b]Rate based on population of approximately 1700 exposed during premarket clinical evaluation of CLOZARIL® (clozapine).

Other Events Observed During the Premarketing Evaluation of CLOZARIL® (clozapine): This section reports additional, less frequent adverse events which occurred among the patients taking CLOZARIL® (clozapine) in clinical trials. Various adverse events were reported as part of the total experience in these clinical studies; a causal relationship to CLOZARIL® (clozapine) treatment cannot be determined in the absence of appropriate controls in some of the studies. The table above enumerates adverse events that occurred at a frequency of at least 1% of patients treated with CLOZARIL® (clozapine). The list below includes all additional adverse experiences reported as being temporally associated with the use of the drug which occurred at a frequency less than 1%, enumerated by organ system.

Central Nervous System: loss of speech, amentia, tics, poor coordination, delusions/hallucinations, involuntary movement, stuttering, dysarthria, amnesia/memory loss, histrionic movements, libido increase or decrease, paranoia, shakiness, Parkinsonism, and irritability.

Cardiovascular System: edema, palpitations, phlebitis/thrombophlebitis, cyanosis, premature ventricular contraction, bradycardia, and nose bleed.

Gastrointestinal System: abdominal distention, gastroenteritis, rectal bleeding, nervous stomach, abnormal stools, hematemesis, gastric ulcer, bitter taste, and eructation.

Urogenital System: dysmenorrhea, impotence, breast pain/discomfort, and vaginal itch/infection.

Autonomic Nervous System: numbness, polydypsia, hot flashes, dry throat, and mydriasis.

Integumentary (Skin): pruritus, pallor, eczema, erythema, bruise, dermatitis, petechiae, and urticaria.

Musculoskeletal System: twitching and joint pain.

Respiratory System: coughing, pneumonia/pneumonia-like symptoms, rhinorrhea, hyperventilation, wheezing, bronchitis, laryngitis, and sneezing.

Hemic and Lymphatic System: anemia and leukocytosis.

Miscellaneous: chills/chills with fever, malaise, appetite increase, ear disorder, hypothermia, eyelid disorder, bloodshot eyes, and nystagmus.

Postmarketing Clinical Experience: Postmarketing experience has shown an adverse experience profile similar to that presented above. Voluntary reports of adverse events temporally associated with CLOZARIL® (clozapine) not mentioned above that have been received since market introduction and that may have no causal relationship with the drug include the following:

Central Nervous System: delirium; EEG abnormal; exacerbation of psychosis; myoclonus; overdose; paresthesia; possible mild cataplexy; and status epilepticus.

Cardiovascular System: atrial or ventricular fibrillation and periorbital edema.

Gastrointestinal System: acute pancreatitis; dysphagia; fecal impaction; intestinal obstruction/paralytic ileus; and salivary gland swelling.

Hepatobiliary System: cholestasis; hepatitis; jaundice.

Hepatic System: cholestasis.

Urogenital System: acute interstitial nephritis and priapism.

Integumentary (Skin): hypersensitivity reactions: photosensitivity, vasculitis, erythema multiforme, and Stevens-Johnson Syndrome.

Musculoskeletal System: myasthenic syndrome and rhabdomyolysis.

Respiratory System: aspiration and pleural effusion.

Hemic and Lymphatic System: deep vein thrombosis; elevated hemoglobin/hematocrit; ESR increased; pulmonary embolism; sepsis; thrombocytosis; and thrombocytopenia.

Miscellaneous: CPK elevation; hyperglycemia; hyperuricemia; hyponatremia; and weight loss.

DRUG ABUSE AND DEPENDENCE: Physical and psychological dependence have not been reported or observed in patients taking CLOZARIL® (clozapine).

Store and Dispense: Storage temperature should not exceed 86°F (30°C). Drug dispensing should not ordinarily exceed a weekly supply. Dispensing should be contingent upon the results of a WBC count.

Novartis Pharmaceuticals Corporation
East Hanover, New Jersey 07936

REV: JUNE 1997 P30118907

THIS MONTH IN ARCHIVES OF GENERAL PSYCHIATRY

Eaton et al (page 993) provide community-based information about the onset and course of major depression, from a follow-up of the Baltimore Epidemiologic Catchment Area sample. In 1 year, 3 adults in 1000 have an episode of depression for the first time in their lives. Many new episodes begin slowly, over many years; and new episodes are longer than recurrent episodes. Women have higher incidence, but the pattern after initial onset is similar for male and female subjects.

Using data from the Collaborative Depression Study, **Solomon et al** (page 1001) prospectively studied the process of recovery from major depression across multiple episodes that occurred in a large cohort followed for up to 10 years. Up to 5 recurrent mood episodes were observed. The average duration of illness was highly consistent, with a median of approximately 20 weeks for each episode.

Major depressive episodes are often treated with the combination of psychotherapy and pharmacotherapy, although the cost-effectiveness of routinely combining these strategies is controversial. **Thase et al** (page 1009) conducted a meta-analysis of original data of the outcomes of 595 depressed outpatients treated with standardized 16-week trials of psychotherapy alone or in combination with tricyclic antidepressants. Results indicate a significant advantage for combined treatment only in more severe depressions. These findings suggest that relatively simple assessments of symptom severity and history may identify patients who warrant combined treatment.

Anecdotal observation suggest that, even among elderly subjects receiving the same form and intensity of treatment for major depressive illness, trajectories toward recovery can differ dramatically. **Dew et al** (page 1016) report empirical evidence suggesting 4 dominant profiles of recovery from depression in the elderly followed during 18 weeks of standardized treatment with combined nortriptyline and interpersonal psychotherapy. Moreover, patient characteristics prior to treatment—including psychosocial, clinical, and electroencephalographic sleep variables—predicted which persons would show relatively more rocky vs smoother courses toward recovery.

This issue also includes a Commentary by L. Judd, titled "The Clinical Course of Unipolar Major Depressive Disorders."

A previous controlled trial on patients with anorexia nervosa of early onset and short duration established that the outcome at 1 year was better after family therapy than the control individual therapy, but it remained uncertain whether the benefits would be sustained. **Eisler et al** (page 1025) followed up the same patients for 5 years and found that the improved response to family therapy was still evident.

No study has shown any antidepressant to be clearly superior to placebo in children and adolescents with severe depression. **Emslie et al** (page 1031) report on a placebo-controlled trial of fluoxetine in severely depressed child and adolescent outpatients. During this 8-week trial, fluoxetine was superior to placebo in overall response rate and in improving depressive symptoms. This is the first study to show an antidepressant to be safe and effective in treating depressed children and adolescents. The response rate of fluoxetine treatment was similar to that seen in adults with depression.

The homeless with severe mental illnesses are common in many large American cities and are often viewed as evidence of failed efforts at deinstitutionalization. **Lehman et al** (page 1038) studied the effectiveness of assertive community treatment (ACT) for these patients. Compared with patients who continued with the usual array of services, the ACT patients substantially reduced their use of inpatient and emergency department services and experienced better clinical, quality-of-life, and housing outcomes.

In the general population, posttraumatic stress disorder (PTSD) occurs more frequently in women than in men, although women do not experience more traumatic events. **Breslau et al** (page 1044) report that within a sample of young adults the sex difference in PTSD was, in part, due to women's higher rates of anxiety disorders or major depression preceding the trauma. The sex difference in PTSD was found to be markedly greater if the trauma occurred in childhood than after age 15 years.

Seldom has an entire generation of patients with an incurable fatal disease suddenly been offered the prospect of extended survival. The advent of protease inhibitors (in combination with other antiviral drugs) may signal such a turning point for patients with HIV/AIDS. Although good news, this treatment breakthrough raises multiple issues. **Rabkin** and **Ferrando** (page 1049) delineate such challenges as promoting treatment adherence, restructuring of lives and expectations, effects of restored health on appraisal of HIV risk behaviors, consequences for neurocognitive functioning, and possibilities of psychotropic–protease inhibitor drug interactions.

The Clinical Course of Unipolar Major Depressive Disorders

A FUNDAMENTAL paradigmatic shift is occurring in the understanding of unipolar major depressive disorders (MDD) among the general public, by many public health experts, and by the practicing psychiatric community. Most people in our society no longer view depression as a mysterious sickness of spirit or emotional weakness, but rather as a disease of the brain and an important health problem.[1] International public health experts acknowledge the high prevalence of unipolar MDD[2] combined with the pervasive human misery and impairment associated with it, and have identified this disease in 1990 as the fourth-ranked cause of disability and premature death worldwide.[3] In parallel, the treatment of unipolar MDD has evolved from incarceration, exorcism, and prayer to classic psychoanalysis, and now in the modern era to treatment with empirically proven, effective antidepressant medications and depression-specific brief psychotherapies. Meta-analyses of 6 standardized treatment studies by Thase et al[4] have helped move the treatment of depression forward by demonstrating significant therapeutic advantages when specific antidepressant medications and psychotherapies are combined in an integrated treatment algorithm.

Among practicing psychiatrists, the most recent and important paradigm shift is the acceptance of unipolar MDD as primarily a chronic rather than an acute illness. However, the field has been relatively slow to recognize the treatment implications of the natural tendency in patients with unipolar MDD for chronicity and episode recurrence. In part, this is because of the lack of cumulative and convincing scientific evidence from prospective longitudinal studies designed to follow up patients systematically from the first lifetime major depressive episode (MDE) into late life. Apart from the study by Angst and colleagues,[5,6] now completed, the National Institutes of Mental Health (NIMH) Collaborative Depression Study (CDS)[7,8] is the only ongoing *prospective* longitudinal study of unipolar mood disorders currently available. This is surprising, because study of the course of unipolar MDD is essential to understanding the fundamental nature of the disease and is the foundation for more effective

See also pages 993, 1001, 1009, and 1016

treatment strategies. For example, it was observations of clinical course that stimulated development of a newer treatment approach for unipolar MDD that includes acute, continuation, and maintenance treatments.[9,10] However, valuable information on the course of unipolar MDD has been contributed, both directly and indirectly, by retrospective, cross-sectional, and epidemiological studies. Although careful retrospective analyses of course have been reported,[11,12] the best example of this research strategy is the Iowa 500 study of Winokur and Tsuang and colleagues, the findings of which have been summarized recently in a seminal monograph[13] and article.[14] The pioneering treatment studies of Kupfer, Frank, and their colleagues[15-18] are notable examples of how cross-sectional studies can contribute information on course and outcome. By extending treatment studies to include continuation and maintenance phases, they demonstrated that recurrent unipolar MDD requires maintenance at the acute antidepressant dosage level for up to 5 years to prevent MDE recurrence, an observation simultaneously documenting course chronicity. Secondary analyses of national epidemiological databases have also gleaned information on course from the large numbers of community-based subjects diagnosed as having unipolar MDD in these studies. The NIMH Epidemiological Catchment Area (ECA)[19] has been uniquely useful in studying the short-term outcome of unipolar MDD because ECA respondents were followed up 1 year later with repeated diagnostic interviews.[20-25] Although these 3 research strategies have made contributions to our understanding of the course of unipolar MDD, all have notable methodological limitations restricting generalization. Much of what has been empirically established during the last 15 years on the natural history of unipolar MDD has been derived from the study by Angst[5,6] and the NIMH CDS.[7,8] As established by the Framingham Cardiovascular Disease Survey,[26] there is no substitute for prospective longitudinal investigations of diseases that are chronic in nature and have lifelong patterns of illness.

There is general agreement that first onset of unipolar MDD initially peaks late in the third decade of life[27-29] and specifically at a median of 25 years of age for community-dwelling subjects[30] and a mean of 29 years of age

This article is also available on our Web site: www.ama-assn.org/psych.

in clinically treated patients.[31] Approximately 8 of 10 people experiencing an MDE will have at least 1 more during their lifetime and, if episodes of minor or subsyndromal depression are included, the prevalence of recurrence would likely reach 100%.[5,6,11,12,25,27-29,32,33] Single isolated MDEs during a patient's life course are rare (14%)[27-29]; however, Mueller et al[34] have shown that 38% of CDS patients with unipolar MDD, experiencing MDEs of at least 5 years' duration, recover within the subsequent 5 years. The median number of MDEs during the lifetime of a patient with unipolar MDD is 4, with 25% of Angst's sample experiencing 6 or more episodes during 26 years' follow-up.[27-29] Solomon et al,[35] in a recent analysis of CDS patients with unipolar MDD, found a remarkable uniformity in the duration of multiple recurrent MDEs of a median of 20 weeks, consistent with earlier reports by Angst.[6,27-29] Recovery patterns from MDEs vary substantially from patient to patient,[5,6,18,28,32,33] but Keller et al[33] report that MDEs are resolved by gradual stepwise reductions of depressive symptoms over time, with 54% of patients recovering at 6 months, 70% within 1 year, and 88% by 5 years. Approximately 12% of patients will have chronic unremitting courses from the first MDE to the end of follow-up.[6,27-29,32] Angst and Preizig[27,28] have observed that patients with unipolar MDD spend about 23% of their follow-up time experiencing MDEs; however, Keller et al,[32] analyzing MDEs in detail, found that patients with unipolar MDD met full MDE criteria for only a median of 32% of the episode's total duration.

Winokur[14] has proposed that unipolar MDD is an etiologically heterogeneous but clinically homogeneous disease. Consistent with this proposition, various unipolar depressive subtypes, in addition to MDEs, can be observed during the course of illness, such as dysthymic disorder,[36] minor depressive disorder,[37] double depression,[38,39] recurrent brief depression,[40] and subsyndromal depressive symptoms.[21-25] This has fueled debate about whether unipolar MDD is a single disease whose clinical picture is characterized by different course patterns and clinical subtypes, or a heterogeneous cluster of distinct depressive disorders, each with different biological substrates and clinical characteristics. Recently, support for the single-illness hypothesis has been provided by a confluence of empirical evidence indicating that unipolar depressive subtypes occur in the same patients over time. One example is double depression,[38,39] in which patients with preexisting chronic dysthymic disorder have an increase of symptoms to meet criteria for MDE. Dysthymic disorder is a risk factor for MDE, and patients with double depression appear to oscillate between these 2 depressive subtypes, resulting in another course pattern or subtype labeled double depression.[38,39] In a follow-up study of Baltimore, Md, ECA subjects, Eaton et al[41] identified cases of MDE preceded by prodromal depressive symptoms, consistent with the depressive subtype of double depression.

Additional support for the single-disease hypothesis has been reported by Kessler et al,[42] who observed that minor depressive disorders and MDD among National Comorbidity Survey subjects were remarkably similar in clinical characteristics, suggesting that MDD and minor depression are on a symptomatic continuum and are depressive subtype expressions of the same illness. Sherbourne et al[43] found that Medical Outcomes Study patients with subsyndromal depressive symptoms and those with MDD shared many clinical characteristics and patterns of comorbidity and proposed subsyndromal depression as a subthreshold variant of unipolar MDD. Angst and Merikangas,[44] conducting new analyses of the Zurich Study, found little diagnostic stability in patients with unipolar MDD over time, since many patients met diagnostic criteria for multiple different depressive subtypes during 26 years of follow-up. Akiskal et al[45] described significant similarity between depressive subtypes in neurophysiological sleep parameters, high rates of family history of mood disorders, responses to antidepressants and sleep deprivation, and prospective courses leading to MDEs, indicating continuity between subthreshold depressive subtypes and the full syndrome of MDD. Comparison of depressive disorder diagnoses at ECA wave 1 with the diagnoses at wave 2 by myself and colleagues[25] revealed a striking number of changes in depressive subtype diagnoses. In our analysis, subjects diagnosed with one depressive subtype at wave 1 very frequently changed diagnoses, meeting criteria for another depressive subtype 1 year later. Depressive subtypes presenting during the course of unipolar illness seem to represent common alternate clinical manifestations of the same disease process of unipolar MDD.[46]

Although the recent monograph by Akiskal and Cassano[47] summarizes the current status and consensus on course and chronicity, there is still much to learn about unipolar MDD. Additional information on course and outcome are necessary to establish increasingly effective treatment strategies for keeping patients with unipolar MDD episode- and symptom-free during their lifetimes. *Prospective*, detailed, systematic studies of clinical course variations must be conducted to facilitate early identification of patients who will have more malignant courses of illness from those who will not. Empirically proved risk factors of outcome and course need to be identified to allow clinicians to anticipate and prevent early episode relapse, increased episode severity, frequent episode recurrence, and episode and symptomatic chronicity that may lead to dysthymia and double depression. However, it has been established that unipolar MDD is a chronic, lifelong illness, the risk for repeated episodes exceeds 80%, patients will experience an average of 4 lifetime MDEs of 20 weeks' duration each, and that this disease is dynamic, variable, and pleomorphic in its clinical presentation, with patients commonly experiencing a variety of depressive subtypes during their courses of illness.

Lewis L. Judd, MD
Department of Psychiatry
University of California, San Diego
9500 Gilman Dr
La Jolla, CA 92093-0603

Funds to conduct this study were provided in part by NIMH Mental Health Clinical Research Grant PHSMH30914 and by the Roehr Fund of the University of California, San Diego.

REFERENCES

1. National Mental Health Association. *National Opinion Poll on Depression.* Washington DC: NMHA; 1992 1992.
2. Kessler RC, McGonagle KA, Zhao S, Nelson CD, Hughes M, Eshelman S, Wittchen HU, Kendler KS. Lifetime and 12-month prevalence of *DSM-III-R* psychiatric disorders in the United States. *Arch Gen Psychiatry.* 1994;151:8-19.
3. Murray CJL, Lopez AD, eds. *The Global Burden of Disease.* Geneva, Switzerland: The Harvard School of Public Health on behalf of The World Health Organization and The World Bank; 1996.
4. Thase ME, Greenhouse JB, Frank E, Reynolds CF, Pilkonis PA, Hurley K, Grochocinski V, Kupfer DJ. Treatment of major depression with psychotherapy or psychotherapy-pharmacotherapy combinations. *Arch Gen Psychiatry.* 1997;54:1009-1015.
5. Angst J, Baastrup P, Grof H, Hippius W, Poldinger W, Weiss P. The course of monopolar depression and bipolar psychoses. *Psychiatr Neurol Neurschir (Amst).* 1973;76:489-500.
6. Angst J. The course of affective disorders. *Psychopathology.* 1986;19(suppl 2):47-52.
7. Katz M, Klerman GL. Introduction: overview of clinical studies programs. *Am J Psychiatry.* 1979; 136:49-51.
8. Katz M, Secunda SK, Hirschfeld RMA, Koslow SH. NIMH clinical research branch collaborative program on psychology of depression. *Arch Gen Psychiatry.* 1979;36:765-771.
9. NIMH/NIH Consensus Development Panel. Mood disorders: pharmacologic prevention of recurrences. *Am J Psychiatry.* 1985;142:469-476.
10. Frank E, Prien RF, Jarrett RB, Keller MB, Kupfer DJ, Lavori PW, Rush AJ, Weissman MM. Conceptualization and rationale for consensus definitions of terms in major depressive disorder: remission, recovery, relapse, and recurrence. *Arch Gen Psychiatry.* 1991;48:851-855.
11. Lehmann HE, Fenton FR, Deutsch M, Feldman S, Englesmann F. A 22-year follow-up study of 110 depressed patients. *Acta Psychiatr Scand.* 1988; 78:57-65.
12. Kiloh LG, Andrews G, Neilson M. The long-term outcome of depressive illness. *Br J Psychiatry.* 1988;153:752-757.
13. Winokur G, Tsuang MT. The natural history of mania, depression, and schizophrenia. Washington, DC: American Psychiatric Press Inc; 1996.
14. Winokur G. All roads lead to depression: clinically homogenous, etiologically heterogeneous. *J Affect Disord.* 1997;45:97-108.
15. Frank E, Kupfer DJ, Perel JM, Cornes C, Jarret JB, Mallinger AG, Thase ME, McEachran AB, Grochocinski VJ. Three-year outcomes for maintenance therapies in recurrent depression. *Arch Gen Psychiatry.* 1990;47:1093-1099.
16. Frank E, Kupfer DJ, Wagner EF, McEachran AB, Cornes C. Efficacy of interpersonal psychotherapy as a maintenance treatment of recurrent depression. *Arch Gen Psychiatry.* 1991;48:1053-1059.
17. Kupfer DM, Frank E, Perel JM, Cornes C, Mallinger AG, Thase ME, McEachran AB, Grochocinski VJ. Five-year outcome for maintenance therapies in recurrent depression. *Arch Gen Psychiatry.* 1992; 49:769-773.
18. Dew MA, Reynolds CF, Houck PR, Hall M, Buysse DJ, Frank E, Kupfer DJ. Temporal profiles of the course of depression during treatment: predictors of pathways toward recovery in the elderly. *Arch Gen Psychiatry.* 1997;54:1016-1024.
19. Eaton W, Holzer C III, VonKorff M, Anthony JC, Helzer JE, George L, Burr A, Boyd JH, Kessler LG, Locke BZ. The design of the ECA surveys: the control and measurement of error. *Arch Gen Psychiatry.* 1984;41:942-948.
20. Broadhead WE, Blazer DG, George LK, Tse CK. Depression, disability days, and days lost from work in a prospective epidemiologic survey. *JAMA.* 1990;264:2524-2528.
21. Howarth E, Johnson J, Klerman GL, et al. Depressive symptoms as relative and attributable risk factors for first-onset major depression. *Arch Gen Psychiatry.* 1992;49:817-823.
22. Johnson J, Weissman MM, Klerman GL. Service utilization and social morbidity associated with depressive symptoms in the community. *JAMA.* 1992;267:1478-1483.
23. Judd LL, Rapaport MH, Paulus MP, Brown JL. Subsyndromal symptomatic depression: a new mood disorder? *J Clin Psychiatry.* 1994;55:18-28.
24. Judd LL, Paulus MP, Wells KB, Rapaport MH. Socio-economic burden of subsyndromal depressive symptoms and major depression in a sample of the general population. *Am J Psychiatry.* 1996; 153:1411-1417.
25. Judd LL, Akiskal HS, Paulus MP. The role and clinical significance of subsyndromal depressive symptoms (SSD) in unipolar major depressive disorder. *J Affect Disord.* 1997;45:5-18.
26. Margolis JR, Gillum RF, Feinleib M, Brasch RC, Fabsitz RR. Community surveillance for coronary heart disease: the Framingham Cardiovascular Disease Survey. *Am J Epidemiol.* 1974;100: 425-436.
27. Angst J, Preizig M. Course of a clinical cohort of unipolar, bipolar and schizoaffective patients: results of a prospective study from 1959 to 1985. *Schweiz Archiv Neurol Psychiatr.* 1995;146:1-16.
28. Angst J, Preizig M. Outcome of a clinical cohort of unipolar bipolar and schizoaffective patients: results of a prospective study from 1959 to 1985. *Schweiz Archiv Neurol Psychiatr.* 1995;146:17-23.
29. Angst J. Clinical course of affective disorders. In: Helgason T, Daly RJ, eds. *Depressive Illness: Prediction of Course and Outcome.* Berlin, Germany: Springer-Verlag; 1988:1-44.
30. Burke KC, Burke JD Jr, Regier DA, Rae DS. Age at onset of selected mental disorders in five community populations. *Arch Gen Psychiatry.* 1990; 47:511-518.
31. Judd LL, Akiskal HS, Maser JD, Zeller PJ, Endicott J, Coryell W, Paulus MP, Kunovac JL, Leon AC, Mueller T, Rie JA, Keller MB. A prospective 12-year study of subsyndromal and syndromal depressive symptomatology in 431 patients with unipolar major depressive disorder. *Arch Gen Psychiatry.* In press.
32. Keller MB, Shapiro RW, Lavori PW, et al. Relapse in major depressive disorder: analysis with the life table. *Arch Gen Psychiatry.* 1982;39:911-915.
33. Keller MB, Lavori PW, Mueller TI, Endicott J, Coryell W, Hirshfeld RMA, Shay T. Time to recovery, chronicity, and levels of psychopathology in major depression. *Arch Gen Psychiatry.* 1992;49: 809-816.
34. Mueller T, Keller MB, Leon AC, Solomon DA, Shea MT, Coryell W, Endicott J. Recovery after 5 years of unremitting major depressive disorder. *Arch Gen Psychiatry.* 1996;53:794-799.
35. Solomon DA, Keller MB, Leon AC, Mueller TI, Shea MT, Warshaw M, Maser JD, Coryell W, Endicott J. Recovery from major depression: a 10-year prospective follow-up across multiple episodes. *Arch Gen Psychiatry.* 1997;54:1001-1006.
36. Akiskal HS. Dysthymic disorder: psychopathology of proposed chronic subtypes. *Am J Psychiatry.* 1983;140:11-20.
37. Skodol AE, Schwartz S, Dorenwend BP, Levav I, Shrout PE. Minor depressions in a cohort of young adults in Israel. *Arch Gen Psychiatry.* 1994;51: 542-551.
38. Keller MB, Lavori PW, Endicott J, et al. Double depression: two-year follow-up. *Am J Psychiatry.* 1983;140:689-694.
39. Keller MB, Hirschfeld RMA, Hanks DL. Double depression: a distinctive subtype of unipolar depression. *J Affect Disord.* 1997;45:65-73.
40. Angst J, Merikangas K, Scheidegger P, Wicki W. Recurrent brief depression: a new subtype of affective disorder. *J Affect Disord.* 1990;19:87-98.
41. Eaton WW, Anthony JC, Gallo J, Cai G, Tien A, Romanoski A, Lyketsos C, Chen L-S. Natural history of Diagnostic Interview Schedule/*DSM-IV* major depression: the Baltimore Epidemiologic Catchment Area follow-up. *Arch Gen Psychiatry.* 1997; 54:993-999.
42. Kessler RC, Zhao SY, Blazer DG, Swartz M. Prevalence, correlates and courses of minor depression and major depression in the National Comorbidity Survey. *J Affect Disord.* 1997;45:19-30.
43. Sherbourne CD, Wells KB, Hays RD, Rogers W, Burnam MA, Judd LL. Subthreshold depression and depressive disorder: clinical characteristics of general medical and mental health specialty outpatients. *Am J Psychiatry.* 1994;151:1777-1784.
44. Angst J, Merikangas K. The depressive spectrum: diagnostic classification and course. *J Affect Disord.* 1997;45:31-40.
45. Akiskal HS, Judd LL, Lemmi H, Gillin JC. Subthreshold depressions: clinical and sleep EEG, validation of dysthymic, residual and masked forms. *J Affect Disord.* 1997;45:53-63.
46. Judd LL. Pleomorphic expressions of unipolar depressive disease: summary of the 1996 CINP President's Workshop. *J Affect Disord.* 1997;45:109-116.
47. Akiskal HS, Cassano GB, eds. *Dysthymia and the Spectrum of Chronic Depressions.* New York, NY; Guilford Press: 1997.

Natural History of Diagnostic Interview Schedule/*DSM-IV* Major Depression

The Baltimore Epidemiologic Catchment Area Follow-up

William W. Eaton, PhD; James C. Anthony, PhD; Joseph Gallo, MD; Guojun Cai, MD; Allen Tien, MD; Alan Romanoski, MD; Constantine Lyketsos, MD; Li-Shiun Chen, MD

Background: Natural history can be characterized by incidence, recurrence, and duration of episodes. Research on the incidence of major depression is rare; studies of recurrence and duration are limited to clinical samples.

Methods: The Baltimore, Md, site of the Epidemiologic Catchment Area Program followed up its 1981 baseline cohort of 3481 respondents with an additional assessment in 1993 to 1996. Interviews were obtained from 1920 respondents (73% of the survivors). The Diagnostic Interview Schedule and the same survey procedures as in 1981 were used, augmented with a Life Chart Interview for dating the onset and duration of syndromes.

Results: There were 71 new cases of Diagnostic Interview Schedule/*DSM-IV* major depression and 23 698 person-years of exposure, generating an estimated incidence of 3.0 per 1000 per year. Incidence peaked while subjects were in their 30s, with a smaller peak when they were in their 50s. Prodromal symptoms often occurred many years before the full criteria for diagnosis were met. Women were at higher risk for becoming new cases but had neither higher risk for recurrence nor longer episodes than men. Episodes of depression lasted for 12 weeks. The duration of an episode, and time to an episode-free year, was longer in the first episode than in recurrent episodes.

Conclusions: The incidence estimated in this study is consistent with that found in the few other similar studies performed. The bimodality of onset suggests the value of further exploring the heterogeneity of depression via its natural history. Reported differences in prevalence between men and women seem to be due to differences in incidence, not chronicity.

Arch Gen Psychiatry. 1997;54:993-999

From the Departments of Mental Hygiene, School of Hygiene and Public Health (Drs Eaton, Anthony, Gallo, Cai, Tien, and Chen); and Psychiatry and Behavioral Sciences, School of Medicine (Drs Romanoski and Lyketsos), The Johns Hopkins University, Baltimore, Md.

THE NATURAL history of an illness consists of onset and chronicity, studied without intervention by the observer.[1] Onset includes the rate at which new cases form—incidence—and the prodrome. Chronicity consists of episode durations and recurrence after recovery. Incidence and chronicity combine to determine prevalence.[2] Estimates of natural history parameters help to explain prevalence differences between populations; where intervention might be cost-effective; and how episodes are generated and endure. Estimates for natural history are best obtained in a community survey in which cases are identified irrespective of treatment, as only approximately half of the individuals with major depression obtain treatment.[3,4]

Reviews about the incidence of depressive disorder draw on psychiatric case registers[5,6] and population-based studies.[7-9] Evidence on duration of episodes and recurrence is limited to clinical samples.[10] In the Epidemiologic Catchment Area (ECA) Program,[11-13] a baseline assessment of 13 538 respondents with the Diagnostic Interview

See also page 989

Schedule (DIS),[14] and a follow-up 1 year later, produced incidence estimates.[15] In 1993 to 1996, the Baltimore, Md, ECA site followed up its sample. The findings on the natural history of major depression from the Baltimore ECA follow-up are provided in this article.

RESULTS

INCIDENCE

Diagnostic Interview Schedule/*DSM-IV* major depression developed in 71 adults during the follow-up, yielding a cumulative

PARTICIPANTS AND METHODS

SAMPLING AND RESPONSE

The target population at baseline was 175 211 adult household residents of east Baltimore. In 1981, 4238 residents were probabilistically designated; 3481 (82%) completed interviews. These 3481 residents were the target for follow-up in 1993.

During the follow-up, 848 respondents died. Depression predicts mortality[16,17] but in this sample, only weakly (W. W. E., M. Kramer, ScD, and M. Badawi, ScD, unpublished data, 1997). Respondents who died between baseline and follow-up were excluded, as there is no evidence about onset of depression in the years after baseline but before death. The address of 415 individuals from the baseline sample of 3481 could not be established (W. W. E., J. G., J. Myllyluoma, and L. G. Weimer, unpublished data, 1997). Of the 2218 individuals located, 1920 (87%) participated in interviews (W. W. E., J. G., J. Myllyluoma, and L. G. Weimer, unpublished data, 1997). Thus, approximately 73% (1920/2633) of those alive were interviewed (W. W. E., J. G., J. Myllyluoma, and L. G. Weimer, unpublished data, 1997). The median time between baseline and follow-up interviews was 12.6 years.

The target population for follow-up was the survivors of the 1981 population of east Baltimore, represented by 2633 sample survivors. Poststratification weights were computed by comparing the 1981 age-race-sex distribution of the 1993 interviewees with the 1981 age-race-sex distribution of the 1993 survivors and multiplying the result by the 1981 sample weights, using procedures identical to those used in 1981.[18] An effective sample size was estimated by down-weighting by the ratio of the sum of the squared weights to the sum of the weights squared.[19]

There were 153 respondents who could not complete full interviews, for whom data on depressive disorder were missing. Forty-four completed short interviews; 83 interviews were conducted with informants because the respondent was ill; 15 were conducted with the short interview followed by informant interview; 6 were terminated early; and, in 5 more, the data required for diagnosis were missing in an idiosyncratic manner. These 153 respondents were older (61% were >65 years in 1981 vs 14% who were >65 years in 1981 for the group with complete responses). The informant and short-form group had less education (37% with lower than an elementary school level vs 9% for those with complete responses), presumably because older cohorts in this country have lower levels of educational attainment. There were no differences for race, sex, or marital status at the level of $P \leq .05$.

INTERVIEW METHOD

The same survey diagnostic instrument (DIS) was used, with the same survey contractor (SRA/Battelle, Baltimore, Md) and the same leader of the interviewer training, as in 1981. All subjects gave informed consent to be interviewed. Diagnostic algorithms for *DSM*, created by the originators of the DIS, were used.

ESTIMATING ONSET, DURATION, AND RECOVERY

The Baltimore ECA Follow-up addressed the problem of deterioration of recall with time, via a new instrument called the Life Chart Interview (LCI).[20] The LCI generates age- and calendar-linked personal memory cues for the respondent at the beginning of the interview, using an interactive visually oriented life calendar to focus on each of the 13, 14, or 15 years between 1981 and 1993-1996. Memory cues include occupation, residence, spouse, and *landmarks*, defined as "significant events that help you mark the passage of time."[20] Subsequently, if evidence of psychiatric disturbance is uncovered via the DIS, the LCI memory cues are used to date its onset, course, and offset. The LCI establishes the presence of a depressive episode in any given year via the subject's report of "a time when you felt sad or blue and had some of these other problems (eg, weight loss or sleeplessness)," as reported earlier by the respondent. A positive response to this question requires as a minimum that sadness or anhedonia and 2 other symptoms are present. This response is referred to as the "depression syndrome"[21] and is used to date the onset of new and recurrent episodes and the beginning of recoveries.

incidence proportion of 4.3% (Table 1). The highest risk period for men is the young adult and middle years (Table 1); for women, the highest risk is localized in the younger age category. Estimates for cumulative incidence with attrition weights (Table 1, right column) do not differ appreciably from unweighted data.

A total of 23 698 years of exposure to the risk of onset was experienced by the sample throughout all ages, with 71 onsets, yielding an annual incidence of 3.00 per 1000 person-years. Women have almost twice the incidence as men (3.62 vs 1.98 per 1000 per year). Curves for age at onset (**Figure 1**) reveal a peak at approximately 30 years for women and 40 years for men and a bimodality that is obscured by the broad categories of age in Table 1. The trough between the peaks is approximately at age 50 years for men and women, and the second peak occurs at approximately age 55 years. Confidence bands for these estimates are not provided because they are too broad to be informative.

The greater incidence for women and younger persons is confirmed in the proportional hazards regression (**Table 2**, left column). The proportional hazards procedures included examination of the effects of marital status, years of educational attainment, and interactions, but none of these were significant at the level of $P \leq .05$.

PRODROMAL PERIODS

The prodromal period is the period during which symptoms are present but the full criteria for major depression are not yet met.[24] The prodrome concept has been applied to the 71 new cases, whose recall period is more limited in time and, therefore, presumably more accurate than would be true for lifetime cases identified in a cross-sectional study. The beginning of the prodrome is the minimum age of onset reported for any DIS symptom in the *DSM-IV* symptom group.

The duration of the prodrome varies by symptom group (**Figure 2**). For 6 of the 9 groups, the median du-

New cases in the 1981 to 1993-1996 period are operationally defined by comparing lifetime diagnoses in 1981 with those in 1993-1996. The group at risk for incidence is those who have never in their lifetime met the full criteria for major depression. Once the full criteria of disorder have been met, the onset can be dated in 2 ways: (1) when the full criteria for diagnosis are first met or (2) at the time of the earliest syndromal spell. Complications arise in multiwave surveys of psychopathological features because manifestations of distress that seem to be precursors of depressive disorder are widespread in the population[22] and because there are discrepancies in reporting from wave to wave. One type of discrepancy occurs when respondents recall an episode at a later wave, which is reported to have occurred before the earlier wave but which contradicts the response in the earlier wave that no episode ever occurred. Twenty-one of the 71 new cases described had this pattern of apparently slow transition from syndrome to full-blown disorder. They are defined as at risk, from the baseline negative response; and as having had a new episode, due to the follow-up response. This resolution is consistent with the 2 different notions of onset: syndrome vs full criterion. For the 21 slow-onset cases, using the year of syndrome onset to estimate the year when full criteria were met would be inconsistent with the 1981 report and biased in the direction of early onset. Therefore, the year when the full criteria for depression were met was estimated from the average for the 46 who reported onset during the follow-up (ie, 1988), for these 21, and for 4 others who did not complete the LCI. Another discrepancy was the 17 subjects for whom onset was reported in the 1982 wave but who did not report any lifetime onset in the 1993-1996 follow-up. These subjects are not included in the numerator of incidence rates.

The operational definition of recovery is a period of 1 year in which there has been no depressive episode. Recurrence is the first episode following a recovery defined in this manner.[23] Once it has been determined that 1 or more episodes have occurred during a given year, the duration of the first episode during that year is estimated by asking the respondent "How long did that spell last?" and recording the answer in weeks.

STATISTICAL TECHNIQUES

Cumulative incidence analyses show proportions of the sample at risk who have first lifetime onsets during the follow-up, using unweighted and weighted methods and SEs estimated with an effective sample size. The actuarial approach, used in earlier studies,[7-9] estimates annual incidence by calculating the years at risk for individuals as they pass through each year of their life, for age-years that occurred during the period 1981 until their interview in 1993-1996. Precision in dating episodes is limited to year intervals because pilot work showed that respondents were unable to date onsets more precisely than in years. It was assumed that the 71 onsets of disorder occurred halfway through the age-year reported by the respondent and that the interviews in 1981, and in the follow-up, occurred halfway through the respondent's age at the interview. These assumptions are common to the life-table method used.[24] Curves for age of onset were estimated using a kernel smoothing procedure with a band width of 5.0 years.[25,26]

The relationships of sex, age, marital status, and educational level with risk of becoming a new or recurrent case were analyzed with proportional hazards regression.[24] The relationship of sex, age, marital status, educational level, and recurrence with duration of episodes was analyzed with linear regression.[27] The distribution of durations suggested that log transformation might enhance power, but it had little effect, so the duration in weeks was used.

FOLLOW-UP SAMPLE

The follow-up sample had approximately the same percentage of women as the baseline sample but fewer persons older than 65 years (**Table 1**). The race distribution was similar in 1981 and in the follow-up—approximately two thirds white. There were fewer widowed persons in the follow-up (10.9% vs 16.4% in 1981). In the follow-up, the levels of education achieved in 1981 were distributed away from the lower end of years of schooling (27.4% elementary school graduates in the baseline sample vs 18.7% in those followed up). The differences in age, marital status, and educational level are consistent with a higher rate of mortality among the elderly respondents.

ration of the prodrome is 1 year; it is only 2 years for appetite and suicidal thoughts or behavior. For dysphoria, the median is 5 years. For anhedonia, psychomotor retardation or agitation, and feelings of guilt and worthlessness, 75% or more have median durations shorter than 5 years. For dysphoria, appetite disturbance, and suicidal thoughts or behavior, the prodrome durations are more varied; the 75th percentile is 14 years for dysphoria, 13 years for suicidal thoughts or behaviors, and 12 years for appetite.

DURATION, RECOVERY, AND RECURRENCE

The duration of episodes varied for the first vs later episodes. The 25th, 50th, and 75th percentiles for the 71 incident episode durations were 4, 12, and 30 weeks, respectively; they were 4, 8, and 16 weeks for the 28 recurrent episodes. The linear regression, which adjusts for possible effects of age and sex (Table 2), shows that later episodes were shorter by approximately 11 weeks than incident episodes (coefficient of −11.25, significant at the $P=.05$ level). The model for duration was estimated with parameters for marital status, educational level, and all 2-way interactions; however, they had no important effect.

Among 54 subjects who were active cases in 1981, and the 71 new cases, the time to recovery was recorded on the life chart for 114 subjects. Ninety-seven of these subjects recovered during the follow-up, with a median time to an episode-free year of 1 year (**Figure 3**). Four fifths had recovered by 5 years. Incident cases have longer median times to recovery than prevalent cases (2 vs 1 year; significantly different via the log-rank test, $P<.001$). The time by which 80% recover (Figure 3, lower reference line) is substantially longer for new cases than prevalent cases—1 vs 8 years.

There were 89 subjects with a history of major depression at baseline (54 active cases and 35 recovered cases). Data from the life chart were recorded for 81 of these subjects. Eighty subjects recovered and were, there-

Table 1. Cumulative Incidence During the Entire Follow-up Period of Diagnostic Interview Schedule/*DSM-IV* Major Depressive Disorder: Frequencies, Percentages, and SEs for the Sample*

Age in 1981, y	Baseline Sample	Total Followed up	Total at Risk	At Risk, New Cases	Cumulative Incidence		SE
					Unweighted	Weighted	
			Men				
18-29	359	248	237	9	3.8	3.3	1.2
30-44	309	203	186	7	3.8	3.5	1.4
45-64	303	146	145	2	1.4	1.4	1.0
≥65	351	62	62	0	0.0	0.0	...
Missing diagnosis	...	48	...	...	...	...	...
Total	**1322**	**707**	**630**	**18**	2.9	2.7	0.7
			Women				
18-29	566	356	332	31	9.3	8.9	1.7
30-44	482	338	305	16	5.2	6.2	1.7
45-64	539	294	281	4	1.4	1.9	1.0
≥65	572	120	117	2	1.7	1.9	1.9
Missing diagnosis	...	105	...	...	...	...	...
Total	**2159**	**1213**	**1035**	**53**	4.6	5.7	0.9
			Men and Women				
Total (for all ages)	**3481**	**1920**	**1665**	**71**	3.9	4.3	0.6

Ellipses indicate no entries possible.

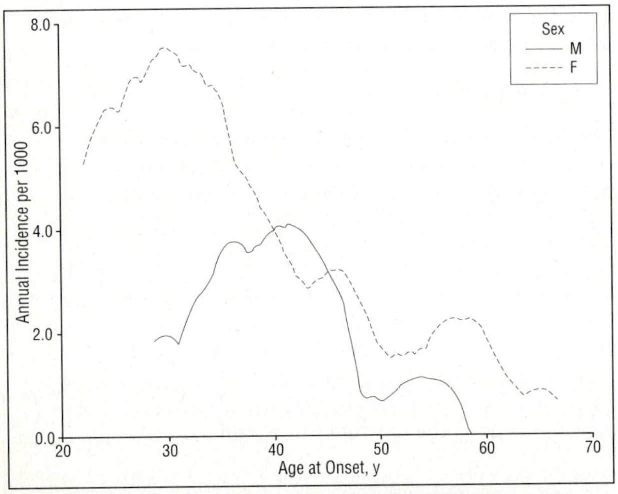

Figure 1. *Baltimore, Md, Epidemiologic Catchment Area Follow-up data, 1981 to 1996. The incidence of Diagnostic Interview Schedule/*DSM-IV *major depression per 1000 per year. The figure shows curves smoothed with a 5-year band width.*

fore, at risk of recurrence. Among the 46 respondents with active symptoms at baseline, there were 14 who had recurrent episodes. In the 34 who reported an episode during their lifetime, who had recovered 1 year or more before baseline, there were 14 who reported a recurrence. The time to recurrence between the 2 groups did not differ significantly ($P \leq .05$)when assessed by the log-rank test, suggesting that time-to-event models could be used with the 2 samples combined (**Figure 4**). Fewer than half the lifetime cases (28/80) actually had a recurrence. The median survival time is not quite reached after 20 years (Figure 4).

The 18- to 29-year-old group had the highest risk for recurrence; those older than 45 years had a lower risk for recurrence, as with incidence (Table 2). The risk for recurrence was almost identical for men and women (relative risk=0.95, $P \geq .05$). The effects of marital status, educational attainment, and interactions were examined in the recurrence model; none had an effect that was significant at P=.05.

COMMENT

This is the first estimate of the incidence of *DSM-IV* major depression based on a community survey with a prospective design. The 4-site ECA study used *DSM-III* criteria, estimating an incidence of 15.9 per 1000 person-years of follow-up.[15] There were 148 new cases of major depression in an earlier ECA analysis, of which 24 came from Baltimore.[15] The incidence for Baltimore was lower than the rate for all 4 sites combined: 24 of 2550 person-years of exposure (9.4 per 1000 per year). Thus, the current estimate of 3.0 per 1000 per year is approximately one third that estimated earlier from the same Baltimore cohort.

The higher ECA incidence rate is consistent with a curiously high lifetime prevalence. If 15.9 individuals in each 1000 persons in the population has a new episode of major depression for each year, a lifetime prevalence of more than 50% is projected during 40 years of exposure, say, from age 18 through 58 years. The 50% lifetime prevalence is substantially higher than lifetime prevalence estimates from the same ECA study or from later population-based field studies.[28] The discrepancy between incidence projection and lifetime prevalence might be explained by failure to recall episodes that occurred before the baseline interviews.[15,29] If such recall failure occurred, lifetime prevalence estimates would be biased low.[29,30]

The difference between 1-year ECA and Baltimore ECA follow-ups is not due to aging, as age-specific incidence rates in the 1981 to 1982 period, from the same Baltimore sample,[15] are higher than the age-equivalent rates from this follow-up, by approximately the same degree. The difference is unlikely to be an effect of birth

Table 2. Incidence, Recurrence, and Duration of Depressive Episodes by Age and Sex*

Variable	Proportional Hazards Regression				Linear Regression Duration, wk	
	Incidence Rate		Recurrence Rate			
	Relative Risk	95% Confidence Interval	Relative Risk	95% Confidence Interval	Regression Coefficient	SE
Sex						
M	1.00	. . .	1.00	. . .	0.00	. . .
F	1.98	1.16-3.38	0.95	0.42-2.12	4.23	4.38
Age, y						
18-29	1.00	. . .	1.00	. . .	0.00	. . .
30-44	0.64	0.39-1.07	0.75	0.35-1.63	7.98	4.13
≥45	0.18	0.08-0.38	0.11	0.01-0.88	−0.23	7.38
Recurrence	. . .	. . .	. . .	. . .	−11.25	4.26
Intercept	. . .	. . .	. . .	. . .	10.89	8.37

*Ellipses indicate no entries possible.

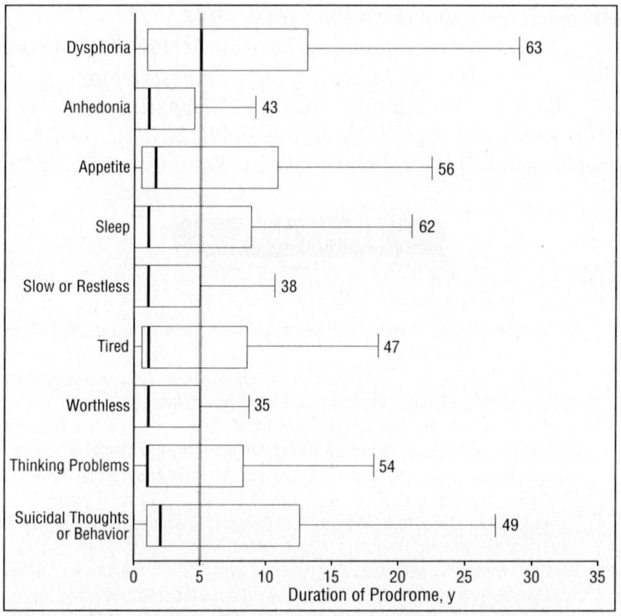

Figure 2. *Baltimore, Md, Epidemiologic Catchment Area Follow-up data, 1981 to 1996. Duration of prodrome for Diagnostic Interview Schedule/* DSM-IV *major depression, by symptom group, in 71 new cases. Boxes contain 50% of the cases. Vertical bars indicate median durations; right end of box, 75th percentile; and T at right, duration of outliers. A reference line at 5 years is indicated. The number of cases in which a symptom in the group occurred is at the right of T.*

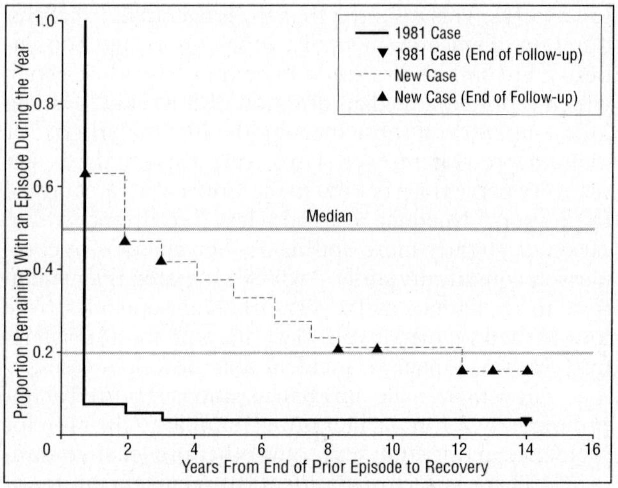

Figure 3. *Baltimore, Md, Epidemiologic Catchment Area Follow-up data, 1981 to 1996. The time to recovery from an episode of Diagnostic Interview Schedule/*DSM-IV *major depression for 71 cases with onset during the follow-up and 54 cases active in 1981. Reference lines at the median and the 20th percentile are indicated.*

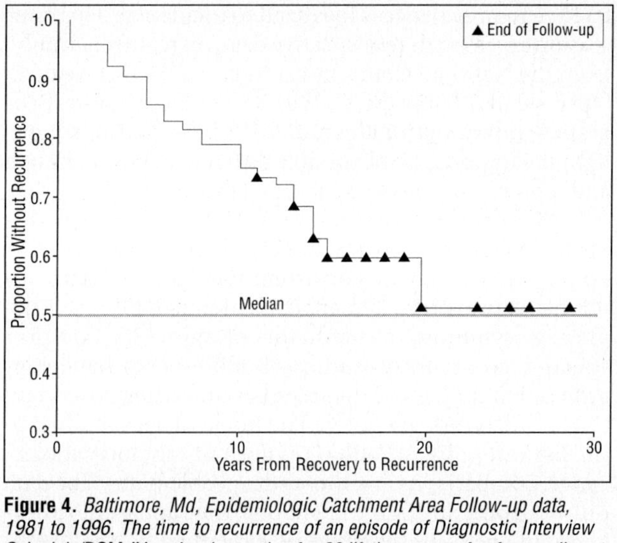

Figure 4. *Baltimore, Md, Epidemiologic Catchment Area Follow-up data, 1981 to 1996. The time to recurrence of an episode of Diagnostic Interview Schedule/*DSM-IV *major depression for 80 lifetime cases. A reference line at the median is indicated.*

cohort,[31,32] as the calendar period differs by little more than a decade (1982 vs 1994). The difference is not due to diagnostic criteria, because algorithms for *DSM-III* and *DSM-IV* produce only trivial differences in numbers of cases in this data set. Differential attrition is an unlikely explanation because depression is not strongly associated with attrition among survivors.[19,33]

The most important difference is the 1-year vs 13- to 15-year period of follow-up. Seventeen of 22 episodes of depression reported by at-risk respondents in 1982 were not reported in the follow-up. The not confirmed or "forgotten" episodes are presumed to be less severe than other episodes recalled in the follow-up. Excluding them from the numerator yielded comparability of design with other prospective studies that have longer than 1 year of follow-up. The rate reported in this article would be approximately 20% higher if the 17 not confirmed new cases were added into the numerator and 3 times as high (approximately matching the 1-year ECA incidence rate from Baltimore previously reported) if this number were added to the numerator for each year of follow-up.

There is consistency of incidence estimates for the 4 available studies with longer than a decade of follow-up. In the Lundby, Sweden, study,[8,9] the cases closest to the *DSM-IV* criteria are those with severe or medium impairment, with an incidence of 2.0 per 1000 per year for 1947 to 1957 and 4.4 per 1000 per year for 1957 to 1972. In Stirling County, Nova Scotia, the rate was 2.3 per 1000 per year.[7] Our estimate of 3.0 is approximately midway in the reported range between 2.0 and 4.4 per 1000. The length of the recall period is a critical aspect of design, which affects the threshold of reporting episodes, and should be considered in reporting results from incidence studies.

The median length of episodes was approximately 8 to 12 weeks. This is shorter than the longer than 6 months' duration of episodes in studies based on treated populations[10] but similar to a study in community adolescents, which reported a median duration of 8 weeks.[34] During follow-up, 80% of those meeting the lifetime criteria for major depression recovered in 5 years, close to the 5-year recovery percentage of 88% in the Collaborative Study of Depression.[10] Not quite 50% had at least 1 recurrence within 20 years, slightly more optimistic than the closest comparison community study,[35] which estimated the median time to recurrence as 15 years. Incident episodes were longer than recurrent episodes; the time to an episode-free year was longer for incident than prevalent cases.

The female-male prevalence ratio is reported at approximately 2:1 in the literature,[36] similar to the ratio for incidence in this study and some other prospective studies.[9,15] There is a virtually identical recurrence rate for men and women and almost identical episode durations and rates of recovery. The recall of depressive episodes may be different for men and women,[37] but a general sex-linked recall difference would not explain this pattern, which is differential according to whether the episodes are first or recurrent. The conclusion is that the sex difference in prevalence is localized to incidence. This conclusion agrees with retrospective data, on recurrence only, from the National Comorbidity Survey,[38] with 1-year relapse results from the Collaborative Depression Program,[39] but not with all studies.[34] These findings highlight the importance of possible differences between men and women in causes of the first episode.[40]

Many cases have slow onset, enduring years of prodromal symptoms before an episode meeting full diagnostic criteria occurs, consistent with the literature on double depression[41] and analyses of personality[42] or depressive symptoms as predictors of onset.[43,44] Two prospective community studies of adolescents have suggested that depressive disorder has an earlier onset than the middle years of life.[45,46] The range of ages studied in the Baltimore ECA Follow-up does not include adolescence; comparisons are, therefore, problematic. The data on prodrome in Figure 2 suggest that apparent differences in age of onset could be explained by the operational definition of onset.

The age distribution of incidence is bimodal, with peaks when subjects are in their 30s and 50s. The bimodality of age of onset for women was revealed in earlier analyses of 1 year of follow-up of the 4-site ECA data.[47] The current data overlap only slightly with that earlier analysis (~1600 of >23 000 person-years of risk), and the current finding should be considered a partial replication. The National Comorbidity Survey also revealed an upward shift in the rate of onset in women aged 50 to 54 years (the oldest age group in that study), based on retrospective recall, with "very small" sample size.[38] Several studies indicate that depressive disorders with early onset have higher genetic loading for depression and panic.[48,49] In this study, the analysis of age of onset was opportunistic and the sample was small. In view of the consistency with other epidemiological data, and results from genetic studies, further efforts to characterize depressive disorders in terms of natural history may be useful.[50]

Accepted for publication March 19, 1997.

This study was supported by grant MH47447 from the National Institute of Mental Health, Bethesda, Md.

Reprints: William W. Eaton, PhD, Department of Mental Hygiene, School of Hygiene and Public Health, The Johns Hopkins University, 624 N Broadway, Baltimore, MD 21205.

REFERENCES

1. Eaton WW. Studying the natural history of psychopathology. In: Tsuang M, Tohen M, Zahner G, eds. *Textbook in Psychiatric Epidemiology.* New York, NY: Wiley-Liss Inc; 1995:157-177.
2. Kleinbaum DG, Kupper LL, Morgenstern H. *Epidemiologic Research: Principles and Quantitative Methods.* Belmont, Calif: Wadsworth Inc; 1982.
3. Shapiro S, Skinner EA, Kessler LG, Von Korff M, German PS, Tischler GL, Leaf PJ, Benham L, Cottler L, Regier DA. Utilization of health and mental health services, three epidemiologic catchment area sites. *Arch Gen Psychiatry.* 1984;41:971-978.
4. Marino S, Gallo JJ, Ford DE, Anthony JC. Filters on the pathway to mental health care, I: incident mental disorders. *Psychol Med.* 1995;25:1135-1148.
5. Boyd JH, Weissman MM. Epidemiology. In: Paykel ES, ed. *Handbook of Affective Disorders.* New York, NY: Churchill Livingstone Inc; 1982:109-125.
6. Der G, Bebbington P. Depression in inner London: a register study. *Soc Psychiatry.* 1987;22:73-84.
7. Murphy JM, Olivier DC, Monson RR, Sobol AM, Leighton AH. Incidence of depression and anxiety: the Stirling County Study. *Am J Public Health.* 1988;78:534-540.
8. Hagnell O. *A Prospective Study of the Incidence of Mental Disorder.* Stockholm, Sweden: Svenska Bokforlaget; 1966.
9. Hagnell O, Essen-Moller E, Lanke J, Ojesjo L, Rorsman B. *The Incidence of Mental Illness Over a Quarter of a Century.* Stockholm, Sweden: Almqvist & Wiksell International; 1990.
10. Keller MB, Lavori PW, Mueller TI, Endicott J, Coryell W, Hirschfeld RM, Shea T. Time to recovery, chronicity, and levels of psychopathology in major depression: a 5-year prospective follow-up of 431 subjects. *Arch Gen Psychiatry.* 1992;49:809-816.
11. Eaton WW, Regier DA, Locke BZ, Taube CA. The Epidemiologic Catchment Area Program of the National Institute of Mental Health. *Public Health Rep.* 1981;96:319-325.
12. Regier DA, Myers JK, Kramer M, Robins LN, Blazer DG, Hough RL, Eaton WW, Lock BZ. The NIMH Epidemiologic Catchment Area program: historical context, major objectives, and study population characteristics. *Arch Gen Psychiatry.* 1984;41:934-941.
13. Eaton WW, Kessler LG, eds. *Epidemiologic Field Methods in Psychiatry: The NIMH Epidemiologic Catchment Area Program.* Orlando, Fla: Academic Press Inc; 1985.
14. Robins LN, Helzer JE, Croughan J, Ratcliff KS. National Institute of Mental Health Diagnostic Interview Schedule: its history, characteristics, and validity. *Arch Gen Psychiatry.* 1981;38:381-389.
15. Eaton WW, Kramer M, Anthony JC, Dryman A, Shapiro S, Locke BZ. The inci-

dence of specific DIS/*DSM-III* mental disorders: data from the NIMH Epidemiologic Catchment Area Program. *Acta Psychiatr Scand.* 1989;79:163-178.
16. Bruce ML, Leaf PJ, Rozal GP, Florio L, Hoff RA. Psychiatric status and 9 year mortality data in the New Haven Epidemiologic Catchment Area Study. *Am J Psychiatry.* 1994;151:716-721.
17. Kouzis A, Eaton WW. Psychopathology and mortality in the general population. *Soc Psychiatry Psychiatr Epidemiol.* 1995;30:165-170.
18. Kessler LG, Folsom R, Royall R, Forsythe A, McEvoy L, Holzer CE, Rae DS, Woodbury M. Parameter and variance estimation. In: Eaton WW, Kessler LG, eds. *Epidemiologic Field Methods in Psychiatry: The NIMH Epidemiologic Catchment Area Program.* Orlando, Fla: Academic Press Inc; 1985:327-349.
19. Leaf PJ, Myers JK, McEvoy LT. Procedures used in the Epidemiologic Catchment Area Study. In: Robins LN, Regier DA, eds. *Psychiatric Disorders in America.* New York, NY: Free Press; 1991:11-32.
20. Lyketsos CG, Nestadt G, Cwi J, Heithoff K, Eaton WW. The Life Chart Interview: a standardized method to describe the course of psychopathology. *Int J Methods Psychiatr Res.* 1994;4:143-155.
21. Anthony JC, Petronis KR. Suspected risk factors for depression among adults 18-44 years old. *Epidemiology.* 1991;2:123-132.
22. Eaton WW, Badawi M, Melton B. Prodromes and precursors: epidemiologic data for primary prevention of disorders with slow onset. *Am J Psychiatry.* 1995;152:967-972.
23. Frank E, Prien RF, Jarrett RB, Keller MB, Kupfer DJ, Lavori PW, Rush AJ, Weissman MM. Conceptualization and rationale for consensus definition of terms in major depressive disorder. *Arch Gen Psychiatry.* 1991;48:851-855.
24. Lawless JF. *Statistical Models and Methods for Lifetime Data.* New York, NY: John Wiley & Sons Inc; 1982.
25. Breslow NE, Day NE. *Statistical Methods in Cancer Research: Design and Analysis of Cohort Studies.* Lyons, France: International Agency for Research on Cancer; 1987:2.
26. Statistics and Epidemiology Research Corporation. *EGRET.* Seattle, Wash: Statistics and Epidemiology Research Corporation; 1990.
27. Draper N, Smith H. *Applied Regression Analysis.* 2nd ed. New York, NY: John Wiley & Sons Inc; 1981.
28. Kessler RC, McGonagle KA, Zhao S, Nelson CB, Hughes M, Eshleman S, Wittchen HU, Kendler KS. Lifetime and 12-month prevalence of *DSM-III-R*: psychiatric disorders in the United States. *Arch Gen Psychiatry.* 1994;51:8-19.
29. Parker G. Are the lifetime prevalence estimates in the ECA Study accurate? *Psychol Med.* 1987;17:275-282.
30. Simon GE, VonKorff M. Recall of psychiatric history in cross-sectional surveys: implications for epidemiologic research. *Epidemiol Rev.* 1995;17:221-227.
31. Wickramaratne PJ, Weissman MM, Leaf PJ, Holford TR. Age, period and cohort effects on the risk of major depression: results from five United States communities. *J Clin Epidemiol.* 1989;42:333-343.
32. Cross-National Collaborative Group. The changing rate of major depression: cross-national comparisons. *JAMA.* 1992;268:3098-3105.
33. Eaton WW, Anthony JC, Tepper S, Dryman A. Psychopathology and attrition in the Epidemiologic Catchment Area surveys. *Am J Epidemiol.* 1992;135:1051-1059.
34. Lewinsohn PM, Clarke G, Seeley JR, Rohde P. Major depression in community adolescents: age at onset, episode duration, and time to recurrence. *J Am Acad Child Adolesc Psychiatry.* 1994;33:809-818.
35. Lewinsohn PM, Zeiss AM, Duncan EM. Probability of relapse after recovery from an episode of depression. *J Abnorm Psychol.* 1989;98:107-116.
36. Burville PW. Recent progress in the epidemiology of major depression. *Epidemiol Rev.* 1995;17:21-31.
37. Wilhelm K, Parker G. Sex differences in lifetime depression rates: fact or artefact? *Psychol Med.* 1994;24:97-111.
38. Kessler RC, McGonagle KA, Swartz M, Blazer DG, Nelson CB. Sex and depression in the National Comorbidity Survey, I: lifetime prevalence, chronicity and recurrence. *J Affect Disord.* 1993;29:85-96.
39. Keller MB, Shapiro RW. Major depressive disorder: initial results from a one-year prospective naturalistic follow-up study. *J Nerv Ment Dis.* 1981;169:761-768.
40. Post RM. Transduction of psychosocial stress into the neurobiology of recurrent affective disorder. *Am J Psychiatry.* 1992;149:999-1010.
41. Keller MB, Shapiro RW. 'Double depression': superimposition of acute depressive episodes on chronic depressive disorders. *Am J Psychiatry.* 1982;139:438-442.
42. Hirshfeld RM, Klerman GL, Lavori P, Keller MB, Griffith P, Coryell W. Premorbid personality assessments of first onset of major depression. *Arch Gen Psychiatry.* 1989;46:345-350.
43. Dryman A, Eaton WW. Affective symptoms associated with the onset of major depression in the community: findings from the US NIMH Epidemiologic Catchment Area Program. *Acta Psychiatr Scand.* 1991;84:1-5.
44. Horwath E, Johnson J, Klerman G, Weissman M. Depressive symptoms as relative and attributable risk factors for first-onset major depression. *Arch Gen Psychiatry.* 1992;49:817-823.
45. Lewinsohn PM, Hops H, Roberts RE, Seeley JR, Andrews JA. Adolescent psychopathology, I: prevalence and incidence of depression and other *DSM-III-R* disorders in high school students. *J Abnorm Psychol.* 1993;102:133-144.
46. Giaconia RM, Reinherz HZ, Silverman AB, Pakiz B, Frost AK, Cohen E. Ages of onset of psychiatric disorders in a community population of older adolescents. *J Am Acad Child Adolesc Psychiatry.* 1994;33:706-717.
47. Anthony JC, Aboraya A. The epidemiology of selected mental disorders in later life. In: Birren JE, Sloane RB, Cohen GD, eds. *Handbook of Mental Health and Aging.* 2nd ed. Orlando, Fla: Academic Press Inc; 1992:27-73.
48. Weissman MM, Wickramaratne P, Merikangas KR, Leckman JF, Prusoff BA, Caruso KA, Kidd KK, Gammon GD. Onset of major depression in early adulthood: increased familial loading and specificity. *Arch Gen Psychiatry.* 1984;41:1136-1143.
49. Goldstein RB, Weissman MM, Adams PB, Horwath E, Lish JD, Charney D, Woods SW, Sobin C, Wickramaratne PJ. Psychiatric disorders in relatives of probands with panic disorder and/or major depression. *Arch Gen Psychiatry.* 1994;51:383-394.
50. Merikangas KR, Wicki W, Angst J. Heterogeneity of depression: classification of depressive subtypes by longitudinal course. *Br J Psychiatry.* 1994;164:342-348.

Announcement

Free Patient Record Forms Available

Patient record forms are available free of charge to ARCHIVES readers by calling or writing FORMEDIC, 12D Worlds Fair Dr, Somerset, NJ 08873-9863, telephone (908) 469-7031.

Recovery From Major Depression

A 10-Year Prospective Follow-up Across Multiple Episodes

David A. Solomon, MD; Martin B. Keller, MD; Andrew C. Leon, PhD; Timothy I. Mueller, MD; M. Tracie Shea, PhD; Meredith Warshaw, MSS, MA; Jack D. Maser, PhD; William Coryell, MD; Jean Endicott, PhD

Background: Major depressive disorder is often marked by repeated episodes of depression. We describe recovery from major depession across multiple mood episodes in patients with unipolar major depression at intake and examine the association of sociodemographic and clinical variables with duration of illness.

Methods: A cohort of 258 subjects treated for unipolar major depressive disorder was followed up prospectively for 10 years as part of the Collaborative Depression Study, a multicenter naturalistic study of the mood disorders. Diagnoses were made according to the Research Diagnostic Criteria, and the course of illness was assessed with the Longitudinal Interval Follow-up Evaluation. Survival analyses were used to calculate the duration of illness for the first 5 recurrent mood episodes after recovery from the index episode.

Results: Diagnosis remained unipolar major depressive disorder for 235 subjects (91%). The median duration of illness was 22 weeks for the first recurrent mood episode, 20 weeks for the second, 21 weeks for the third, and 19 weeks for the fourth and fifth recurrent mood episodes; the 95% confidence intervals were highly consistent. From one episode to the next, the proportion of subjects who recovered by any one time point was similar. For subjects with 2 or more recoveries, the consistency of duration of illness from one recovery to the next was low to moderate. None of the sociodemographic or clinical variables consistently predicted duration of illness.

Conclusion: In this sample of patients treated at tertiary care centers for major depressive disorder, the duration of recurrent mood episodes was relatively uniform and averaged approximately 20 weeks.

Arch Gen Psychiatry. 1997;54:1001-1006

THE COURSE of illness in unipolar major depression is usually characterized by recovery from the initial episode, with subsequent recurrences and recoveries. Kraepelin[1] described this " . . . tendency to multiple repetition . . ." as one of the most consistent features of depressive illness.

Only a few studies have prospectively collected data on large samples at periodic intervals over a span of many years to describe recovery from multiple episodes of major depression. One such study[2] reported the median length of each episode was approximately 23 weeks. Another study[3] examined the duration of the index episode and the first, second, and third prospectively observed recurrent mood episodes and found no consistency in the length of these episodes.

The episodic course of illness in major depression has been carefully investigated by the ongoing National Institute of Mental Health–Collaborative Program on the Psychobiology of Depression (Collaborative Depression Study [CDS]), a naturalistic, prospective, longitudinal study of the mood disorders.[4] Follow-up of CDS subjects with unipolar major depression at intake showed that the cumulative probability of recovering from the index episode within 26 weeks of enrollment in the study was 54%; within 1 year, 70%; and within 5 years, 88%.[5]

See also page 989

Many of the CDS subjects who recovered from the index episode subsequently suffered 1 or 2 prospectively observed recurrences of major depression. Recovery from the first recurrent mood episode (the first episode of depression after recovery from the index episode) was slower for subjects with a longer index episode, less family income, and older age at the time of recurrence.[6] The duration of the first prospective recurrence (averaged across subjects) was almost identical to the duration of the second prospective recurrence, and, for both of these episodes, 60% of the subjects recovered within 6 months and 80% recovered within 1 year.[7]

From the Department of Psychiatry and Human Behavior, Brown University, Providence, RI (Drs Solomon, Keller, Mueller, and Shea and Ms Warshaw); Department of Psychiatry, Cornell University, New York, NY (Dr Leon); National Institute of Mental Health, Washington, DC (Dr Maser); Department of Psychiatry, University of Iowa College of Medicine, Iowa City (Dr Coryell); and Department of Research and Training, New York State Psychiatric Institute, New York, NY (Dr Endicott). The names of the investigators participating in the National Institute of Mental Health–Collaborative Program on the Psychobiology of Depression (Collaborative Depression Study) are listed at the end of this article.

This article is also available on our Web site: www.ama-assn.org/psych.

SUBJECTS AND METHODS

SUBJECTS

From 1978 to 1981, the CDS recruited individuals receiving inpatient or outpatient treatment for a mood disorder at academic medical centers in Boston, Mass; Chicago, Ill; Iowa City, Iowa; New York, NY; and St Louis, Mo. Patients must have sought psychiatric treatment through the customary referral mechanisms, and there was no special solicitation of research subjects. In addition, subjects were at least 17 years of age, with an intelligence quotient higher than 70, English speaking, white, and without signs of a mood or psychotic disorder secondary to a general medical condition. Written informed consent was obtained after complete description of the study to the subjects. Of the 955 patients who were enrolled in the CDS, 431 were in an episode of major depression, with no underlying minor depression of at least 2 years' duration, no chronic intermittent depressive disorder, and no history of mania, hypomania, or schizoaffective disorder. Of these 431 subjects, 258 recovered and subsequently suffered at least 1 additional episode of major depression. The sociodemographic and clinical characteristics of the sample at intake are listed in **Table 1**.

METHODS

Assessments

Trained professional clinical interviewers assessed subjects with the Schedule for Affective Disorders and Schizophrenia–Lifetime Version.[9] Diagnoses were made according to the Research Diagnostic Criteria (RDC).[10]

Follow-up evaluations were performed every 6 months for the first 5 years of the study and annually thereafter, using the Longitudinal Interval Follow-up Evaluation (LIFE).[11] The LIFE measures the severity of psychopathology on a weekly basis and the type and dose of all prescribed medication. Severity of psychopathology is quantified on 6-point scales called the "psychiatric status ratings" (PSRs), which are assigned to each psychiatric disorder. A PSR of 1 corresponds to no symptoms. A PSR of 2 corresponds to 1 or 2 symptoms of a mild degree, with no impairment of functioning. A PSR of 3 corresponds to moderate psychopathology considerably less than that meeting the full criteria for the RDC disorder, with no more than moderate impairment in functioning. A PSR of 4 denotes marked symptoms not meeting the full criteria for the RDC disorder, with major impairment of functioning. A PSR of 5 corresponds to symptoms meeting the full criteria for the RDC disorder, and a PSR of 6 indicates full criteria for the RDC disorder along with psychosis or extreme impairment in functioning. The rater assigned a PSR for each week of the study, starting with the time of the last interview. To accomplish this, the rater first identified chronological anchor points such as holidays to assist the subject in remembering those times when significant improvement or deterioration occurred. Whenever possible, corroborative data were obtained from medical records.

The analyses reported in this article are based on the PSR scores for the 258 subjects with unipolar major depression at intake who experienced at least 1 recurrent mood episode; the analyses span up to 520 weeks of follow-up. *Recovery* was defined as at least 8 consecutive weeks with either no symptoms of any major mood disorder (major depressive disorder, mania, schizoaffective depression, and schizoaffective mania) or only 1 or 2 symptoms at a mild level of severity (PSR of 1 or 2). Thus, during a mood episode, the weekly level of psychopathology may have varied from a PSR of 1 to 6. However, a minimum of 8 consecutive weeks at a PSR of 1 or 2 was required for the outcome of recovery. Recurrence was the reappearance of a major RDC mood disorder (major depressive disorder, mania, schizoaffective depression, or schizoaffective mania) at full criteria (PSR of 5 or 6) for at least 2 consecutive weeks, beginning with the first of these 2 weeks. Recurrence occurred only after the individual had first recovered from the preceding mood episode.

Continued assessment of CDS subjects with unipolar major depression has yielded complete data for the first 10 years of follow-up. Since intake, many of the subjects have suffered multiple recurrences of mood episodes. Herein, we describe recovery from these recurrent episodes, each of which was observed prospectively.

The study focuses on duration of illness (time to recovery) of recurrent mood episodes in a sample identified as unipolar major depression at intake and examines the association of concurrent comorbidity, severity of illness, and treatment with duration of illness. Based on previous work,[2,7] it was expected that the duration of illness would average approximately 6 months. Duration of illness was hypothesized to be longer for older subjects[6] and for subjects with more severe mood episodes,[6] comorbid conditions,[8] less intense treatment, and lower socioeconomic status.[6]

RESULTS

The sample comprised 258 subjects with unipolar major depression at intake and at least 1 recurrent mood episode during 10 years of follow-up. The mean (SD) length of follow-up was 458 (126) weeks. Of the original sample, 91% of the subjects were followed up for at least 5 years, and 76% for the entire 10-year period. During the follow-up period, 27 subjects (10%) died. Diagnosis for major RDC mood disorder changed for 23 subjects (9%): mania developed in 15 subjects (6%) and schizoaffective disorder developed in 8 subjects (3%). These 23 subjects remained in follow-up for the present study.

The 258 subjects suffered 658 recurrent mood episodes during the 10-year follow-up period. The 235 subjects whose diagnosis remained unipolar major depressive disorder accounted for 587 (89%) of the 658 recurrent mood episodes, with a mean (SD) of 2.50 (2.04). The 23 subjects whose diagnosis changed had a mean (SD) of 3.09 (2.33) recurrent mood episodes, which was not significantly different (Mann-Whitney test $Z=1.23$, $P=.22$).

The mean (SD) PSR for the first recurrent episode was 4.3 (0.6), and 57% of the PSRs were 5 or 6, meaning that subjects met full criteria for the mood episode for 57% of the weeks they were in episode. The mean (SD) PSR for each of the second through fifth episodes was 4.4 (0.6), and 59% to 65% of the PSRs were 5 or 6.

The survival analyses of recovery from the first 5 recurrent mood episodes are given in **Table 2**. Based on

Treatment

This was a naturalistic study in that treatment was not assigned by design and not controlled by anyone connected with the study. However, all psychotropic treatment was assessed with the LIFE and described for each week of the study. To rate the intensity of somatic treatment, equivalent dose ranges were established for different classes of antidepressant somatic therapies (including lithium carbonate and electroconvulsive therapy). These dose ranges were then summarized on a 5-point scale to generate a composite antidepressant (CAD) score[12] for each week of the study. A CAD score of 0 indicated that no antidepressant somatic treatment was provided, and CAD scores 1 through 4 indicated the following daily doses of imipramine or its equivalents: score 1, 1 to 99 mg; score 2, 100 to 199 mg; score 3, 200 to 299 mg; and score 4, 300 mg or more.

Statistical Analysis

Duration of illness was calculated using survival analysis.[13] Separate analyses were conducted for each of the first 5 recurrent mood episodes from baseline through year 10, owing to the limited number of subjects (16 [6%] of 258) who experienced more than 5 recurrent mood episodes during the follow-up period. The index episode, described elsewhere,[5] has not been included, as it was not entirely prospective; subjects were enrolled in the study after the onset of the intake episode. Furthermore, the duration of the index episode may have reflected length-biased sampling, given that subjects were recruited on the basis of seeking treatment. That is, the intake episode may have been longer because patients with mood episodes of longer duration may be more likely to seek treatment.[14]

The survival time (duration of illness) began with the first week of recurrence for each mood episode. The event that ended each episode was either recovery or, for censored cases, end of follow-up period (10 years) or dropout. The cumulative probability of recovery was estimated with the Kaplan-Meier product limit.[15] The interval-specific probabilities of recovery for each mood episode, which are similar to hazards, were also calculated. These analytic techniques account for varying lengths of follow-up and the changing probability of recovery at different times.[16]

Subjects were stratified into 3 groups according to the number of major depressive episodes prior to intake: 0 episodes, 1 to 2 episodes, and 3 or more episodes. Survival curves (duration of illness) for these groups were compared using the generalized Wilcoxon test.[17]

In addition to analyzing the duration of illness for each recurrence across groups of subjects, length of illness for multiple mood episodes was examined within each individual subject. Consistency in the duration of illness between episodes, for each individual subject, was assessed through estimates of the intraclass correlation coefficient.[18] These were calculated for all subjects with 2 or more recurrent mood episodes.

A stepwise Cox proportional hazards model[19] was used to test the association between hypothesized explanatory variables and the duration of each episode. The explanatory variables were intake site, outpatient vs inpatient status at intake, age, sex, marital status, socioeconomic status, primary depression at intake, psychotic depression at intake, comorbid anxiety disorder (generalized anxiety disorder, panic disorder, phobic disorder, or obsessive-compulsive disorder) during the episode, comorbid substance use disorder (alcohol or other substance dependence) during the episode, mean psychiatric status rating during the episode, and total number of weeks subjects were ill with a major RDC mood disorder since intake into the study. Each episode was analyzed with a Cox proportional hazards model, and a Bonferroni correction was used to adjust the level of α for the 12 independent variables within-episode, resulting in a 2-tailed α level of $.05/12=.004$.

Kaplan-Meier estimates, 92% of the subjects recovered from the first recurrent mood episode during the 10-year follow-up period. Of those with a second recurrent episode, 88% recovered from that episode. Of those with a third, fourth, or fifth recurrent episode, approximately 90% recovered. From one recovery to the next, the proportion of subjects remaining ill at any time point after onset of illness was similar; in every instance, the 95% confidence intervals (CIs) overlap. The corresponding survival curves for the duration of the first 5 recurrent mood episodes are shown in the **Figure**, based on cumulative recovery probabilities (Kaplan-Meier estimates) for up to 10 years. The curves are virtually identical.

For the entire sample, the median duration of illness for each of the 5 recurrent mood episodes was very similar: for the first mood episode, 22 weeks; for the second, 20 weeks; for the third, 21 weeks; and for the fourth and fifth mood episodes, 19 weeks. Each of the 95% CIs for the median duration of illness overlapped.

The median duration of illness was also analyzed using data from only those subjects whose diagnosis remained unipolar major depressive disorder (n=235). There was little change; the median duration of illness for the first episode of major depression was 21 weeks; for the second, 20 weeks; for the third, 19 weeks; for the fourth, 21 weeks; and for the fifth, 20 weeks.

For each of the 5 recurrent mood episodes, the annual interval-specific probability of recovery (the probability that a person still ill at the start of a year will recover during that year) was highest in the first year after onset of the mood episode. During the first year after onset, the rate of recovery for the first recurrent episode was 73%; for the second, 70%; for the third, 76%; for the fourth, 78%; and for the fifth, 88%. The weighted mean (SD) for the probability of recovery across the 5 recurrent mood episodes was 74% (4%). This suggests that, on average, of the subjects at risk for recovery, 74% recovered in the first year after onset of the mood episode. In subsequent years, the rates of recovery declined steadily. Across all 5 recoveries, the weighted means (SDs) for the probability of recovery after onset of the mood episode were as follows: in the second year, 38% (8%); in the third year, 27% (8%); and in the fourth year, 16% (9%).

The median duration of illness was examined with regard to history of major depressive disorder prior to the index episode (**Table 3**). Subjects were classified into 3 groups:

those with no history of major depressive disorder prior to intake, those with a history of 1 or 2 episodes prior to intake, and those with 3 or more episodes prior to intake. For each recovery, the 3 groups were compared, and no statistically significant difference in the median duration of illness was observed.

Table 1. Sociodemographic and Clinical Characteristics of 258 Probands With MDD at Intake*

Characteristics	No. (%) of Patients
Sex	
Male	91 (35)
Female	167 (65)
Status at intake	
Inpatient	198 (77)
Outpatient	60 (23)
No. of previous episodes of MDD	
0	84 (33)
1	61 (24)
2	36 (14)
3+	77 (30)
RDC subtypes of MDD	
Endogenous	
Probable or definite	227 (88)
Definite	152 (59)
Psychotic, current	
Probable or definite	27 (10)
Definite	25 (10)
Primary, current	152 (59)
Current marital status	
Never married	83 (32)
Married or live in	120 (47)
Divorced, separated, or widowed	55 (21)
Socioeconomic status, Hollingshead-Redlich scale	
I	12 (5)
II	42 (16)
III	75 (29)
IV	82 (32)
V	47 (18)
Intake medical center location	
New York, NY	37 (14)
St Louis, Mo	71 (28)
Boston, Mass	75 (29)
Iowa City, Iowa	30 (12)
Chicago, Ill	45 (17)
Global Assessment Scale score†	38/38/10/5/65
Severity of depressive syndrome, Hamilton score†	26/26/6/9/42
Age at entry, y†	38/34/15/17/76

**MDD indicates major depressive disorder; RDC, Research Diagnostic Criteria.*

†Data are given as mean/median/SD/minimum/maximum.

Within-subject variability in duration of illness was examined, using data from the 224 subjects who recovered from 2 or more mood episodes. The intraclass correlation coefficient was 0.38.

Table 4 lists the highest level of treatment received for at least 4 consecutive weeks during each recurrent mood episode. Across the 5 recoveries, 54% to 78% of the subjects received at least 100 mg of imipramine or its equivalent. Approximately 33% of the subjects received at least 200 mg of imipramine or its equivalent, for the first 3 recurrences. This increased to 51% for the fifth recurrent mood episode. Mean (SD) CAD scores for the 8 weeks immediately preceding recovery ranged from 1.9 (1.3) to 2.2 (1.2) across the 5 recoveries, and all of the 95% CIs overlapped.

The association of sociodemographic and clinical variables with the probability of recovery from each of the 5 recurrent mood episodes was also examined. None of the independent variables consistently predicted a shorter duration of illness. The mean PSR during the episode was associated with a significantly shorter duration of illness for only the first recurrent mood episode (exp[B]=1.65; 95% CI, 1.14-2.37), and outpatient status at intake predicted a significantly shorter duration of illness for only the fourth recurrent mood episode (exp[B]=4.59; 95% CI, 1.17-18.00).

COMMENT

Few studies comparable to the CDS have been mounted to describe recovery from multiple episodes of major depressive disorder. When patient observations were considered collectively, the duration of illness across multiple recurrent mood episodes was highly consistent, with a median of approximately 20 weeks. However, consistency in the duration of illness across multiple episodes for the same individual was low to moderate, as shown by the intraclass correlation coefficient.

Diagnosis for some subjects changed during follow-up, and time to recovery was reanalyzed without this group, using data from only those subjects whose diagnosis remained unipolar major depressive disorder. From one episode to the next, the median duration of illness was still about 20 weeks.

Previous research from the CDS by Coryell et al[7] found striking consistency in the duration of illness for 2 prospectively observed mood episodes. The present article extends their work by describing a larger sample followed up during a longer period, analyzing the duration of illness within subjects and with regard to number of major depressive episodes prior to intake, and examining the association of hypothesized explanatory variables with duration of illness.

Table 2. Proportion of Subjects Remaining Ill

Recovery No.	No. of Subjects at Start of Mood Episode	Time From Onset of Episode, Proportions of Subjects (95% CI)* 1 mo	3 mo	6 mo	1 y	2 y	5 y
1	258	0.94 (0.89-0.97)	0.62 (0.56-0.68)	0.46 (0.40-0.52)	0.27 (0.22-0.33)	0.15 (0.11-0.20)	0.08 (0.05-0.12)
2	153	0.92 (0.84-0.96)	0.63 (0.54-0.71)	0.42 (0.34-0.50)	0.30 (0.23-0.38)	0.18 (0.13-0.25)	0.12 (0.08-0.18)
3	89	0.92 (0.80-0.97)	0.62 (0.50-0.72)	0.41 (0.31-0.52)	0.23 (0.16-0.33)	0.15 (0.09-0.24)	0.08 (0.04-0.16)
4	62	0.92 (0.75-0.97)	0.57 (0.43-0.70)	0.41 (0.29-0.54)	0.22 (0.14-0.34)	0.18 (0.11-0.33)	0.12 (0.07-0.23)
5	40	0.95 (0.60-0.99)	0.64 (0.46-0.79)	0.29 (0.17-0.45)	0.09 (0.04-0.22)	. . .†	. . .†

**Proportions represent Kaplan-Meier product limit estimates; CI indicates confidence interval.*

†Empty cells were not calculated because of limited number of subjects at risk for recovery.

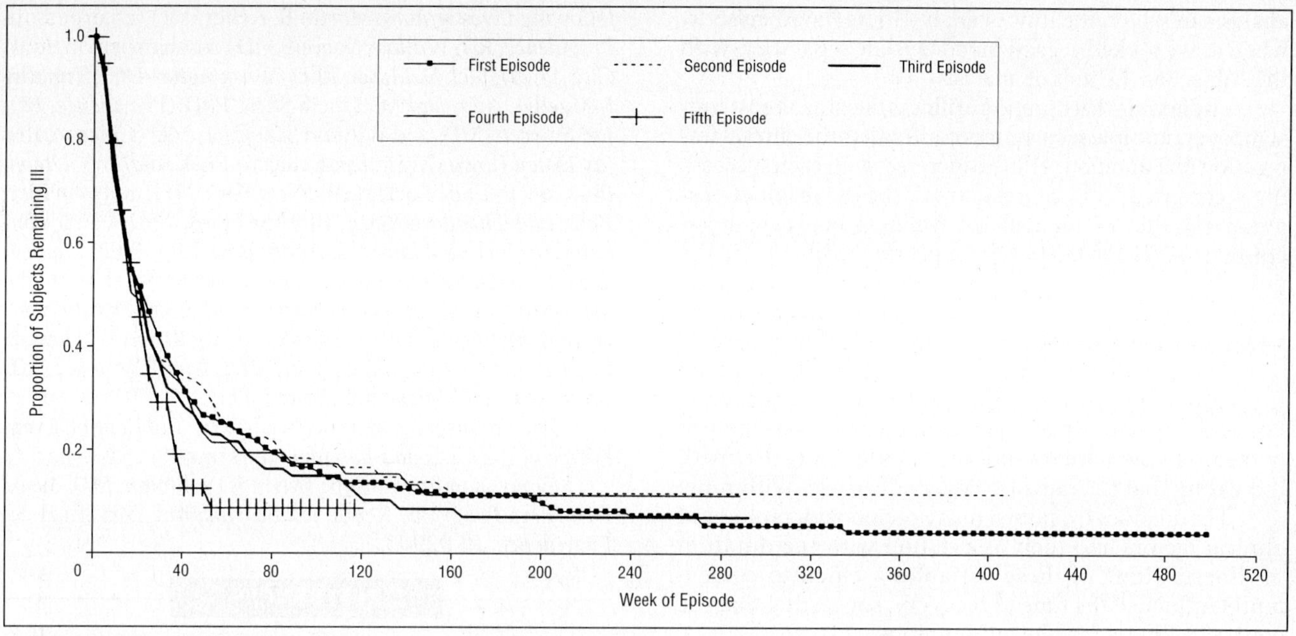

Survival curves for subjects who had 1 to 5 recurrent mood episodes.

Table 3. Median Time to Recovery and History of MDD Prior to Intake*

Recovery No.	No History of MDD: No. of Subjects	No History of MDD: Median Time to Recovery, wk	History of 1-2 Episodes of MDD Prior to Index Episode: No. of Subjects	History of 1-2 Episodes of MDD Prior to Index Episode: Median Time to Recovery, wk	History of ≥3 Episodes of MDD Prior to Index Episode: No. of Subjects	History of ≥3 Episodes of MDD Prior to Index Episode: Median Time to Recovery, wk	Wilcoxon Test†	*P*
1	84	21	97	25	77	16	3.12	.21
2	44	19	59	23	50	16	1.18	.55
3	21	29	34	23	34	20	0.73	.70
4	13	10	22	36	27	16	2.66	.27
5	10	19	13	18	17	18	0.07	.96

**MDD indicates major depressive disorder.*
†In all instances, df=2.

Table 4. Highest Level of Treatment for at Least 4 Consecutive Weeks During Each Mood Episode: Composite Antidepressant (CAD) Scores*

		No. (%) of Subjects†					
Recovery No.	Total No. of Subjects	No Treatment: CAD Score=0	Minimal Treatment‡	CAD Score=1	CAD Score=2	CAD Score=3	CAD Score=4
1	**224**	70 (31)	8 (4)	25 (11)	52 (23)	41 (18)	28 (13)
2	**125**	34 (27)	5 (4)	17 (14)	25 (20)	29 (23)	15 (12)
3	**77**	22 (29)	2 (3)	6 (8)	22 (29)	16 (21)	9 (12)
4	**53**	14 (26)	0 (0)	8 (15)	9 (17)	12 (23)	10 (19)
5	**33**	4 (12)	0 (0)	3 (9)	9 (27)	9 (27)	8 (24)

**Dosages for treatment with imipramine or its equivalents for CAD scores 1 through 4 were as follows: score 1, 1 to 99 mg/d; score 2, 100 to 199 mg/d; score 3, 200 to 299 mg/d; and score 4, 300 mg/d or more.*
†Numbers differ from those in other tables because of missing data. Percentages do not always add to 100 because of rounding.
‡Treatment at 1 or more levels for a total of less than 4 weeks during the episode.

Remarkably, the findings are roughly consistent with those of Kraepelin, who stated: "The duration of individual attacks is extremely varied. . . . For the most part, however, a simple attack usually lasts six to eight months."[1] The results are quite similar to those of Angst,[2] who found that the median length of each episode of major depression was about 23 weeks.

In contrast, Maj et al[3] noticed no consistent pattern in the duration of recurrences observed during their follow-up study. The inconsistency may be the result of differences in analytic techniques. We used survival analysis to account for observations of all subjects; it is unclear how the linear regression model used by Maj et al[3] could account for censored cases. Also, they performed a global analysis in which the unit of analysis was mood episode, whereas we looked at each mood episode separately, with the subject as the unit of analysis.

The finding that duration of illness remains almost constant over multiple recurrences contradicts the clinical impression that duration of illness increases with each succeeding recurrence. This impression may be the result of progressively shorter intervals of wellness between mood episodes, with one recurrence appearing to blend into the next. Such an idea is supported by the finding from previous work that the probability of recurrence in major depressive disorder increased with the number of prior episodes.[20]

Another finding from the present study involved the annual interval–specific probability of recovery. For each mood episode, the rate of recovery was highest in the first year of follow-up, and subsequently declined, indicating that the rate of recovery decreases with time.

The analyses examined many sociodemographic and clinical factors and their association with the duration of illness. None of these variables seemed to consistently influence the time to recovery, suggesting that the course of illness may be autonomous.

Most of the sample was treated, and the highest level of treatment received for at least 4 consecutive weeks seemed to increase as the number of episodes increased. This may have artificially controlled time to recovery and obscured differences that might otherwise have emerged.

This was a naturalistic study, and pharmacotherapy was not controlled. As such, the results reflect "effectiveness" of ordinary clinical practice, rather than the "efficacy" of treatment administered under controlled conditions. Although some may consider this a limitation, there is growing importance attached to this type of work.[21,22]

Most subjects enrolled in the study had a history of 1 or more mood episodes prior to intake, and the index episode was not analyzed. Therefore, the first 5 prospectively observed recurrent mood episodes did not represent the first 5 lifetime episodes, and the first recurrence in the present analyses represents a mixture of second, third, fourth, and more lifetime episodes. As a result, the analyses may have missed an initial increase in duration of illness that eventually plateaued (if, for example, the median duration of illness for the first lifetime episode was 5 weeks; for the second, 10 weeks; and for all subsequent episodes was 20 weeks). Another limitation is that the analyses were restricted to episodes of major depression, mania, schizoaffective depression, and schizoaffective mania (major RDC mood disorders) and therefore excluded episodes of minor depression, intermittent depression, or hypomania.

In summary, a sample of 258 patients treated for unipolar major depression at baseline was followed up prospectively for 10 years. Across multiple recurrent mood episodes, the duration of illness was consistent, with a median of approximately 20 weeks to recovery. In the context of this naturalistic study, none of the hypothesized sociodemographic or clinical factors seemed to influence the duration of illness. Fortunately, most patients recovered.

Accepted for publication December 18, 1996.

The National Institute of Mental Health–Collaborative Program on the Psychobiology of Depression (Collaborative Depression Study) was conducted with the participation of the following investigators: Martin B. Keller, MD (chairperson, *Providence, RI); William Coryell, MD* (co-chairperson, *Iowa City, Iowa); Jack D. Maser, PhD (Washington, DC); Timothy I. Mueller, MD, and M. Tracie Shea, PhD (Providence, RI); Jan Fawcett, MD, and William Scheftner, MD (Chicago, Ill); Jay Haley (Iowa City); Jean Endicott, PhD, Andrew C. Leon, PhD, and Jo-Ellen Loth, MSW (New York, NY); and John Rice, PhD, and Theodore Reich, MD (St Louis, Mo). Other contributors include Nancy C. Andreasen, MD, PhD; Paula J. Clayton, MD; Jack Croughan, MD; Robert M. A. Hirschfeld, MD; Martin M. Katz, PhD; Gerald L. Klerman, MD (deceased); Eugene Robins, MD (deceased); Robert W. Shapiro, MD (deceased); Robert L. Spitzer, MD; George Winokur, MD (deceased); and Michael A. Young, PhD.*

The manuscript was reviewed by the Publication Committee of the CDS and has its endorsement.

Corresponding author: David A. Solomon, MD, Mood Disorders Program, Rhode Island Hospital, 593 Eddy St, Providence, RI 02903.

REFERENCES

1. Kraepelin E. *Manic-Depressive Insanity and Paranoia.* Robertson GM, ed; Barclay RM, trans. Edinburgh, Scotland: E & S Livingstone; 1921.
2. Angst J. The course of affective disorders. *Psychopathology.* 1986;19(suppl 2):47-52.
3. Maj M, Veltro F, Pirozzi R, Lobrace S, Magliano L. Pattern of recurrence of illness after recovery from an episode of major depression: a prospective study. *Am J Psychiatry.* 1992;149:795-800.
4. Katz MM, Secunda SK, Hirschfeld RMA, Koslow SH. NIMH Clinical Research Branch Collaborative Program on the Psychobiology of Depression. *Arch Gen Psychiatry.* 1979;36:765-771.
5. Keller MB, Lavori PW, Mueller TI, Endicott J, Coryell W, Hirschfeld RMA, Shea MT. Time to recovery, chronicity, and levels of psychopathology in major depression: a 5-year prospective follow-up of 431 subjects. *Arch Gen Psychiatry.* 1992;49:809-816.
6. Keller MB, Lavori PW, Rice J, Coryell W, Hirschfeld RMA. The persistent risk of chronicity in recurrent episodes of nonbipolar major depressive disorder: a prospective follow-up. *Am J Psychiatry.* 1986;143:24-28.
7. Coryell W, Akiskal HS, Leon AC, Winokur G, Maser JD, Mueller TI, Keller MB. The time course of nonchronic major depressive disorder: uniformity across episodes and samples. *Arch Gen Psychiatry.* 1994;51:405-410.
8. Mueller TI, Lavori PW, Keller MB, Swartz A, Warshaw M, Hasin D, Coryell W, Endicott J, Rice J, Akiskal H. Prognostic effect of the variable course of alcoholism on the 10-year course of depression. *Am J Psychiatry.* 1994;151:701-706.
9. Endicott J, Spitzer RL. A diagnostic interview: the Schedule for Affective Disorders and Schizophrenia. *Arch Gen Psychiatry.* 1978;35:837-844.
10. Spitzer RL, Endicott J, Robins E. Research Diagnostic Criteria: rationale and reliability. *Arch Gen Psychiatry.* 1978;35:773-782.
11. Keller MB, Lavori PW, Friedman B, Nielsen E, Endicott J, McDonald-Scott P, Andreasen NC. The Longitudinal Interval Follow-up Evaluation: a comprehensive method for assessing outcome in prospective longitudinal studies. *Arch Gen Psychiatry.* 1987;44:540-548.
12. Keller MB. Undertreatment of major depression. *Psychopharmacol Bull.* 1988;24:75-80.
13. Kalbfleisch JD, Prentice RL. *The Statistical Analysis of Failure Time Data.* New York, NY: John Wiley & Sons Inc; 1980.
14. Coryell W, Endicott J, Winokur G, Akiskal H, Solomon D, Leon A, Mueller TI, Shea T. Characteristics and significance of untreated major depressive disorder. *Am J Psychiatry* 1995;152;1124-1129.
15. Kaplan EL, Meier P. Nonparametric estimation from incomplete observations. *J Am Stat Assoc.* 1958;53;457-481.
16. Leon AC, Friedman RA, Sweeney JA, Brown RP, Mann JJ. Statistical issues in the identification of risk factors for suicidal behavior: the application of survival analysis. *Arch Gen Psychiatry.* 1990;31:99-108.
17. Gehan EA. A generalized Wilcoxon test for comparing arbitrarily singly-censored samples. *Biometrika.* 1965;52:203-223.
18. Shrout PE, Fleiss JL. Intraclass correlations: uses in assessing rater reliability. *Psychol Bull.* 1979;86:420-428.
19. Cox DR. Regression models and life tables. *J R Stat Soc B.* 1972;34:187-220.
20. Keller MB, Lavori PW, Lewis CE, Klerman GL. Predictors of relapse in major depressive disorder. *JAMA.* 1983;250:3299-3304.
21. Hoagwood K, Hibbs E, Brent D, Jensen P. Introduction to the special section: efficacy and effectiveness in studies of child and adolescent psychotherapy. *J Consult Clin Psychol.* 1995;63:683-687.
22. Guscott R, Taylor L. Lithium prophylaxis in recurrent affective illness: efficacy, effectiveness and efficiency. *Br J Psychiatry.* 1984;164:741-746.

Treatment of Major Depression With Psychotherapy or Psychotherapy-Pharmacotherapy Combinations

Michael E. Thase, MD; Joel B. Greenhouse, PhD; Ellen Frank, PhD; Charles F. Reynolds III, MD; Paul A. Pilkonis, PhD; Katharine Hurley, MS; Victoria Grochocinski, PhD; David J. Kupfer, MD

Background: Few reliable correlates of treatment response in depression have emerged despite nearly 40 years of research. We examined the correlates of recovery in a "mega-analysis," or meta-analysis of original data, of 595 patients with major depressive disorder enrolled in 6 standardized treatment protocols.

Methods: All patients (mean age, 44 years; 31% male and 69% female) met criteria for nonbipolar, nonpsychotic primary major depressive disorder and were treated for 16 weeks with either cognitive behavior therapy or interpersonal psychotherapy alone (psychotherapy alone; n=243) or interpersonal psychotherapy plus antidepressant pharmacotherapy (combined therapy; n=352). The impact of treatment type, severity, study, and other covariates on recovery rates or time to recovery were examined by means of χ^2, log-rank tests, the Cox proportional hazards model, and sensitivity analyses.

Results: Whereas combined therapy was not significantly more effective than psychotherapy alone in milder depressions, a highly significant advantage was observed in more severe recurrent depressions. Poorer outcomes were also observed in women and older patients, although these effects were dependent on inclusion of particular studies.

Conclusions: Mega-analysis is a powerful method for comparing the efficacy of treatments and examining correlates of response. Using this method, we found new evidence in support of the widespread clinical impression that combined therapy is superior to psychotherapy alone for treatment of more severe, recurrent depressions.

Arch Gen Psychiatry. 1997;54:1009-1015

ALTHOUGH randomized clinical trials (RCTs) are the mainstay for testing the relative efficacy of various treatments for depression, the external validity and generalizability of findings from RCTs is limited by many of the same methodologic controls that ensure their internal validity.[1] Factors such as study-specific age limitations, restrictive inclusion and exclusion criteria, and a limited range and flexibility of treatments constrain the relevance of research findings to the patients seen outside of research settings. Studies of the correlates of treatment response derived from RCTs also have been hampered by the types of assessments collected. For example, the large RCTs funded by the pharmaceutical industry, which serve as the major source of data about new antidepressants, have relatively narrow assessment domains. Conversely, investigator-initiated projects typically have sample size limitations that preclude powerful tests of more than a few key hypotheses. Thus, 40 years after the discovery of the first effective antidepressant compounds, surprisingly few variables have been established as either general or specific correlates of treatment response.[2,3]

Traditional means to identify predictors of treatment response include expert opinion, qualitative reviews of empirical studies, and correlational studies of larger, "open-label" (uncontrolled) series of patients. More recently, the statistical technique of meta-analysis has been widely used.[4-6] In meta-analysis, average effect sizes of particular treatments are estimated by abstracting means and SDs or categorical response rates from relevant research studies. Meta-analyses are clearly more quantitative than these other methods, yet the conclusions drawn from them may be biased by systematic differences in methods or study design.[7] Although the impact of such differences also may be studied with meta-analysis,[5,6] the unit of observation is the study (ie, N=the number of studies reviewed), which necessitates that a large body of research must exist before meaningful conclusions can be drawn.

See also page 989

From the Western Psychiatric Institute and Clinic and Department of Psychiatry, University of Pittsburgh School of Medicine, Pittsburgh, Pa.

METHODS

Our Mental Health Clinical Research Center coordinated 5 outpatient research protocols conducted between 1982 and 1992: Maintenance Therapies of Recurrent Depression (MTRD),[19] Maintenance Therapies of Late-Life Depression (MTLD),[20] Psychobiology of Recovery From Depression (PRD),[21] Nocturnal Penile Tumescence in Depression Study (NPT),[22] and Social Zeitgebers in Depression (SZD).[23] A sixth protocol, the Pittsburgh, Pa, site of the TDCRP,[10] was performed jointly under the auspices of the Mental Health Clinical Research Center and the National Institute of Mental Health. Reports concerning the main hypotheses of each of these studies have been published previously.[10,19-23] All of the federally funded outpatient studies of major depressive disorder conducted at our facility during this period are included in this report.

The 6 studies shared the following common methods: (1) an intake diagnosis of major depressive disorder (nonpsychotic, nonbipolar subtypes) was made according to either *DSM-III* (TDCRP and MTRD) or *DSM-III-R* (MTLD, PRD, NPT, and SZD) criteria on the basis of a semistructured clinical interview conducted by a clinician and faculty psychiatrist team; (2) this diagnosis was confirmed according to Research Diagnostic Criteria[24] after an independent interview that used the Schedule for Affective Disorders and Schizophrenia[25]; (3) medical stability was determined by a physical examination, laboratory studies, and electrocardiogram; and (4) all patients provided explicit written informed consent. Five studies[19-23] required that patients score at least 14 on the first 17 items of the Hamilton Rating Scale for Depression (HRSD)[26] during a 14-day, psychotropic-free assessment interval. The TDCRP required a persistent score of 15 or higher on a modified 20-item HRSD during a 7-day interval. This version of the HRSD also assessed hypersomnia, hyperphagia, and weight gain.[10] Another difference concerned enrollment of patients suffering from antecedent dysthymia or chronic major depressive episodes (≥2 years' duration). Patients with chronic depression were enrolled in 3 studies (TDCRP, SZD, and NPT) and excluded from the remaining studies. The specific aims of the individual protocols virtually guaranteed that large differences would be apparent across studies on demographic variables (ie, age, sex, and marital status), clinical characteristics (ie, history of past episodes of depression, history of antecedent dysthymia, and age at onset of first depression), and recovery rates (**Table 1**). When pooled, our study group was larger and more heterogeneous than is typically possible for any single study.

TREATMENT

All 6 studies provided 16-week treatment protocols. In the TDCRP (n=79), patients were randomly assigned to treatment with interpersonal psychotherapy (IPT[27]), cognitive behavior therapy (CBT[28]), imipramine plus clinical management,[29] or placebo plus clinical management.[29] All 91 patients in the SZD study were treated with IPT. The 56 patients in the PRD protocol and the first 53 patients in the NPT protocol were treated with CBT. Patients in the MTRD (n=230) and MTLD (n=122) protocols received IPT in combination with either imipramine (MTRD; mean acute-phase dose, 218 mg/d) or nortriptyline (MTLD; mean acute-phase dose, 77 mg/d). Across the 6 studies, 243 patients were treated with psychotherapy alone and 352 patients received the combination of IPT and antidepressant medication. The relatively small number of TDCRP patients treated with placebo (n=20) or pharmacotherapy alone (n=20) led us to exclude these groups from the final analyses. Patient characteristics for the final sample of 595 patients are described in Table 1.

The grouping of patients in this manner was justified by the larger conceptual issue, ie, the relative efficacy of psychotherapy alone vs combined therapy. Overall comparability of IPT and CBT was found in the TDCRP.[10] Preliminary comparisons between the CBT and IPT with the use of the current data set revealed similar recovery rates and symptomatic outcomes (M.E.T., E.F., J.B.G., C.F.R., P.A.P., and D.J.K., unpublished data, May 23, 1996). Finally, there was no reason to believe that imipramine and

An alternate approach involves pooling the data of individual subjects participating in studies that use similar treatments, assessment methods, and time frames. Examples of such "mega-analyses," or meta-analyses of original data, include articles on antidepressant efficacy in atypical depression[8] and the incidence of treatment-emergent suicidal behavior.[9] In contrast to conventional meta-analysis, the data of each individual are retained, which permits testing for interactions between types of treatment and patient characteristics.

To date, mega-analyses of treatments for depression have focused on studies of pharmacotherapy, emphasizing short-term efficacy (ie, response over 4 to 6 weeks) and relatively narrow assessment domains (eg, diagnostic subtypes, symptoms, and side effects). Unfortunately, mega-analyses of large databases from industry-sponsored RCTs may be compromised by methods that pay insufficient attention to the reliability of assessments or standardization of treatment contacts. Standardization of treatments is a particularly important requirement before mega-analysis can be applied to psychotherapy studies, for which procedural specification and assurance of treatment fidelity are critical issues.[10,11]

We recently conducted a mega-analysis of the outcome of nearly 600 depressed outpatients, who ranged in age from 18 to 80 years and were pooled from 6 studies conducted during a 10-year period (1982-1992). In the first report based on this series, the relationships between clinical outcome and treatment type, symptom severity, demographic variables, and other pretreatment characteristics are examined. Our principal focus is on the differential efficacy of psychotherapy, alone, in comparison with the combination of psychotherapy and pharmacotherapy. Qualitative reviews have tended to emphasize the additive value of combined treatment strategies,[12-16] yet a majority of RCTs directly comparing monotherapy and combined regimens have failed to find significant differences (see, for example, the review by Persons et al[17]).

We suspected that the disparity between expert opinion and the results of empirical studies is the result of nortriptyline would have differential efficacy in the combined treatment cells.[4]

All psychotherapists had completed at least 1 year of supervised training in their respective modalities, leading to external certification of competence according to the guidelines originally developed by the TDCRP.[30,31] Combined treatment was provided by an IPT therapist and faculty psychiatrist, with the latter typically joining for the final 15 minutes of 60-minute sessions.

ASSESSMENT OF OUTCOME

Patients were assessed at least every 4 weeks with the 17-item HRSD, Global Assessment Scale,[32] and Beck Depression Inventory.[33] The HRSD and Global Assessment Scale ratings were performed by independent clinical evaluators, who had achieved and maintained intraclass correlation coefficients of 0.80 or greater on these measures (mean intraclass correlation coefficients on the HRSD and Global Assessment Scale exceeded 0.9).[34] Recovery, the primary dependent variable used in this report, was defined as a 4-week period with HRSD scores less than 7, maintained until week 16.[35] This relatively conservative definition of outcome was chosen to ensure that responses were complete and clinically meaningful.

STATISTICAL ANALYSES

The primary explanatory variables were treatment condition and pretreatment HRSD severity. With the use of the same method as the TDCRP,[10] patients were stratified into less severe (ie, pretreatment HRSD scores ≤19) and more severe (ie, pretreatment HRSD scores ≥20) subgroups. Missing severity data led to post hoc exclusion of 2 cases from the psychotherapy-alone condition. The number of patients in the 4 treatment×severity cells were as follows: more severe–psychotherapy alone, n=119; more severe–combined therapy, n=250; less severe–psychotherapy alone, n=122; and less severe–combined therapy, n=102.

The data were analyzed by 4 progressively more sophisticated methods. A critical α level of $P \leq .05$ was used for all statistical tests. We first compared simple recovery rates by means of contingency tables and χ^2 tests. While not an efficient analysis, this method provides an idea of what is going on in the data.[36] We next performed a univariate survival analysis of time to recovery by means of modified Kaplan-Meier survival curves and the log-rank χ^2 test.[36,37] The third step applied the Cox proportional hazards model[37] to determine the effect of treatment and severity while simultaneously controlling for other effects. Pretreatment HRSD score was entered as a continuous independent variable, and age, sex, age at onset, number of previous depressive episodes, and length of current episode were entered as covariates.

Finally, sensitivity analyses[38] were used to address the impact of each of the 6 studies on the overall findings. The Cox model regression coefficients were reestimated after each study was removed, one at a time. If any single study distorted or unduly influenced the overall pattern of results, the regression coefficients would be altered substantially. Conversely, regression coefficients that remained stable despite such perturbations of the data set would represent uniform effects.[38] This analysis was particularly important because patients were not randomly assigned to particular studies and 2 potential correlates of outcome, sex and age, were confounded with specific studies: only men entered the NPT study and only older patients with recurrent depression entered the MTLD study.

The validity of using the Cox model to control for interstudy differences depends in part on the overlap in the distributions of the covariates of interest. As summarized in Table 1, there was considerable overlap across studies on all variables except age and sex, for which there was 1 "outlier" study for each covariate. These particular confounds would be addressed in the sensitivity analyses by the removal of the outlier studies. However, because the combined-therapy condition included only patients with recurrent depression, it was essential to ensure that an adequate number of patients with recurrent depression were represented in the psychotherapy-alone condition. There were 158 patients with recurrent depression in this condition (less severe, n=73; more severe, n=85), ensuring valid comparisons between treatment conditions.

lack of adequate statistical power to detect the additive effect of combining 2 effective treatments. We also hypothesized that there is an interaction between pretreatment symptom severity and response to psychotherapy alone or combined treatment. Drawing on the findings of the National Institute of Mental Health Treatment of Depression Collaborative Research Program (TDCRP),[10,18] we predicted that psychotherapy alone and combined treatment would be equally effective in milder depressions, whereas combined treatment would be superior in more severe cases.

RESULTS

UNADJUSTED RECOVERY RATES

A comparison of simple recovery rates as a function of treatment and severity conditions demonstrated the predicted effect: the treatments were not significantly different in the less severe cells (psychotherapy alone [37%, or 46/122] vs combined therapy [48%, or 49/102]; χ^2=2.8, *df*=1, *P*=.10), whereas there was a significant difference between the more severe cells (psychotherapy alone [25%, or 29/119] vs combined therapy [43%, or 108/250]; χ^2=10.2, *df*=1, *P*=.001). A comparison of recovery rates within the psychotherapy-alone condition approached significance (more severe [25%] vs less severe [37%]; χ^2=3.5, *df*=1, *P*=.06), while combined therapy was equally effective in more severe (43%) and less severe (48%) cases (χ^2=0.7, *df*=1, *P*=.41).

UNIVARIATE SURVIVAL ANALYSIS

Figure 1 displays the cumulative recovery curves for the 4 treatment×severity conditions. The overall comparison across these cells did not reach statistical significance (log-rank χ^2=7.1, *df*=3, *P*=.07). However, pairwise comparisons demonstrated that patients in the more severe group had significantly faster recoveries when treated with combined therapy than when treated with

Table 1. Sociodemographic and Pretreatment Clinical Characteristics in the Treatment Studies Included in the Pittsburgh 600 Series Comparative Treatment Trials*

Study	No.	Sex, No. F/M	Age, y, Mean±SD	Age at Onset, y, Mean±SD	No. of Previous Episodes, Mean±SD	Duration of Index Episode, wk, Mean±SD	HRSD Score, Mean±SD	Antecedent Dysthymia, %	Chronic Depression, %	Remission Rate, %
MTRD	230	180:50	39.5±10.6	26.9±10.3	6.6±5.3	23.9±18.1	22.1±4.6	0	0	51
SZD	91	66:25	35.3±8.7	24.5±7.5	5.3±5.8	23.7±19.2	19.6±4.2	0	1.1	23
MTLD	122	88:34	67.6±6.0	48.2±17.5	5.5±5.6	22.7±20.8	22.3±3.7	0	0	32
PRD	56	42:14	37.9±8.7	30.8±11.1	1.5±2.0	41.4±19.3	21.3±3.9	0	0	43
NPT	53	0:53	38.4±10.5	33.9±11.3	1.2±2.7	41.7±47.2	19.2±3.9	11.5	34.1	38
TDCRP	43	32:11	34.1±7.5	28.5±8.4	1.1±1.9	51.6±56.7	19.5±3.7	7.0	23.3	30
Total	**595**	**408:187**	44.0±15.2	32.2±14.7	4.6±5.3	29.0±28.7	21.2±4.3	1.5	4.9	39

**MTRD indicates Maintenance Therapies of Recurrent Depression[19]; SZD, Social Zeitgebers in Depression[23]; MTLD, Maintenance Therapies of Late-Life Depression[20]; PRD, Psychobiology of Recovery From Depression[21]; NPT, Nocturnal Penile Tumescence in Depression Study[22]; TDCRP, Treatment of Depression Collaborative Research Program[10]; and HRSD, pretreatment 17-item Hamilton Rating Scale for Depression.*

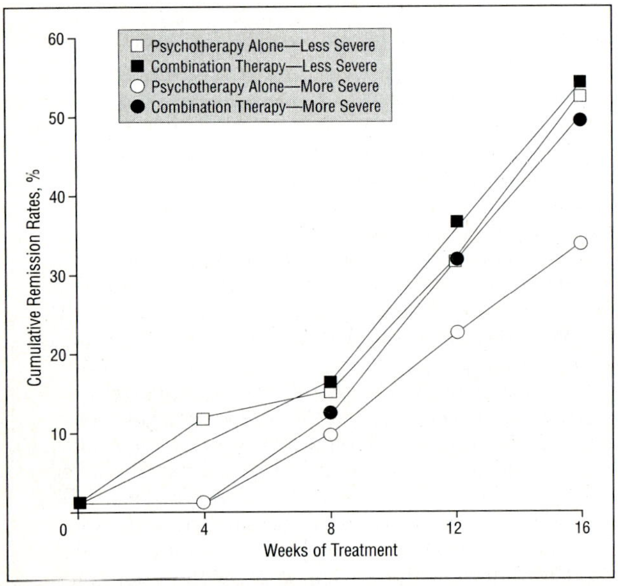

Figure 1. *Cumulative time to recovery curves as a function of pretreatment severity and treatment type. Outcome in the psychotherapy alone—more severe condition was significantly worse than those in the other 3 groups.*

psychotherapy alone (log-rank χ^2=4.8, df=1, P=.03). The clinical significance of this difference is illustrated by the following: the 75th percentile of the time to recovery was reached by 9 weeks (±0.25 weeks) in the more severe–combined therapy group, compared with 13 weeks (±1.6 weeks) for patients in the more severe–psychotherapy-alone group. There were no statistically significant differences between the more severe–combined therapy, less severe–combined therapy, and less severe–psychotherapy-alone groups.

COX MULTIPLE REGRESSION ANALYSES

Table 2 summarizes the Cox proportional hazards model analyses. Model 1 included only treatment and severity. Models 2 through 6 examined the other variables, added one at a time to model 1. Model 7 included all of the significant covariates.

Combined therapy was associated with significantly shorter times to recovery in 6 of the 7 models. Higher severity predicted slower recovery in all 7 models. Only age and sex were significantly related to time to recovery after the effects of treatment and severity were taken into account. Specifically, older patients and women had slower recoveries. When treatment, severity, age, and sex were fit simultaneously (model 7), all were significantly related to time to recovery (see Table 2).

SENSITIVITY ANALYSES

The significance of the regression coefficients for treatment and severity did not change after the sequential exclusion of each of the 6 studies (**Table 3**). This indicated that no particular study was overly influential in accounting for the superiority of combined therapy for treatment of more severe depressions. The effects of sex and age were less robust. The significance of the effect for sex was negated by removal of any 1 of 4 studies (SZD, MTLD, PRD, or TDCRP). The age effect was negated by removal of either the MTRD or MTLD study. The latter finding suggests that the negative prognostic effect of age was limited to the comparison of combined therapy outcomes in midlife vs late-life patients with recurrent depression.

COMMENT

Recent practice guidelines for treatment of major depressive disorder emphasize the importance of symptom severity in determining the need for antidepressant medication.[4,16] These guidelines recommend pharmacotherapy, alone or in combination with psychotherapy, for patients with more severe depressions. Although these recommendations are compatible with the findings of the TDCRP,[10,18] a number of other outpatient RCTs have not found the newer psychotherapies to be less effective treatments of more severe depressions.[39-44] Empirical evidence of the additive benefits of combined therapy is similarly limited.[17,39-41,43,45,46] As a result, the practice guidelines have been criticized as being biased in favor of pharmacotherapy.[17,47,48] As one of us (M.E.T.) coauthored one of these critiques,[17] it is important to note that the current study provides the strongest empirical evidence ever marshaled to indicate that combined therapy is superior

Table 2. Summary Table for the Cox Proportional Hazards Model Analyses: Regression Coefficients for Time to Remission

	Model*						
Variable/Covariate	1	2	3	4	5	6	7
Treatment	0.27†	0.42‡	0.31†	0.26†	0.32†	0.18	0.46‡
Severity	−0.04‡	−0.04‡	−0.04‡	−0.04‡	−0.04†	−0.04‡	−0.04†
Age (models 2 and 7)	...	−0.01‡	...	...	...	...	−0.01‡
Sex (models 3 and 7)	...	...	0.27†	...	...	...	0.28†
Age at onset (model 4)	...	...	...	−0.004	...	...	...
No. of episodes (model 5)	...	...	...	...	−0.002	...	...
Duration of index episodes (model 6)	...	...	...	...	...	−0.005	...

*Model 1: treatment + severity (no covariates); models 2 through 6: treatment + severity + 1 designated covariate; model 7: treatment + severity + age + sex.
†P≤.05.
‡P≤.01.

Table 3. Sensitivity Analysis: Impact of Study on Regression Coefficients for Time to Remission

	Study Removed*						
Variable/ Covariate	None†	MTRD	SZD	MTLD	PRD	NPT	TDCRP
Treatment	0.46‡	0.53§	0.40§	0.50‖	0.51‡	0.41§	0.47‡
Severity	−0.04§	−0.03§	−0.04§	−0.05‡	−0.04§	−0.04§	−0.04§
Age	−0.01‡	−0.02	−0.01‡	0.002	−0.01‡	−0.01‡	−0.01‡
Sex	0.28§	0.55‡	0.28	0.20	0.24	0.33§	0.23

*See Table 1 for explanation of studies.
†This is model 7 from Table 2.
‡P≤.01.
§P≤.05.
‖P≤.001.

to psychotherapy alone for treatment of more severely depressed outpatients, in terms of both overall recovery rates and shorter time to recovery.

Interpretation of these findings is limited by 3 "holes" in the data set. Specifically, no patient older than 60 years received psychotherapy alone, no patients with single-episode (nonrecurrent) depression were treated with combined therapy, and no patient received the combination of CBT and antidepressants. It seems unlikely that the lack of patients treated with both CBT and antidepressants biased results. For example, in 2 studies of more severely depressed inpatients, the combination of CBT and antidepressants yielded significantly better short-term[49] and longer-term[50] outcomes than did pharmacotherapy alone. To assess the impact of the imbalances between groups in terms of the numbers of younger, single-episode patients and older patients with recurrent depression, an additional post hoc analysis was performed. This analysis included only patients with recurrent depression who were younger than 60 years. **Figure 2** illustrates that the advantage favoring combined therapy over psychotherapy alone was particularly large among patients with more severe, recurrent depression (ie, 66/110 [60%] vs 16/85 [19%]; χ^2=33.4, *df*=1, *P*<.001). This 41% difference in recovery rates is larger than the typical drug vs placebo effect observed in outpatient RCTs.[4]

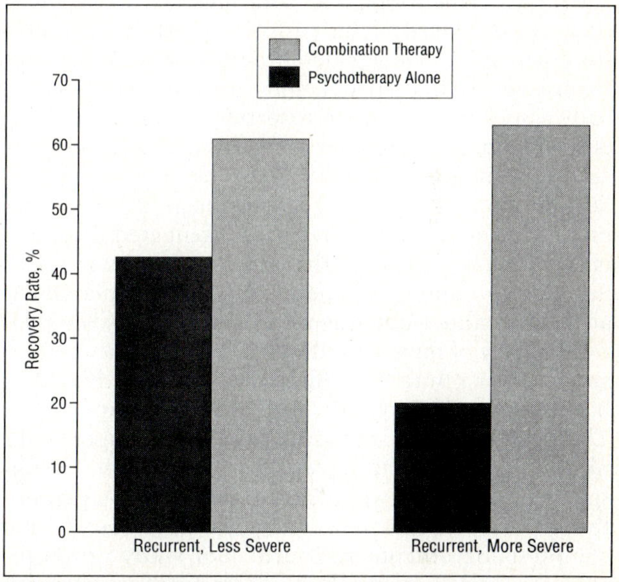

Figure 2. *Recovery rates in patients in midlife (younger than 60 years) with recurrent major depression as a function of severity and treatment type.*

Our results, however, do not fully support the American Psychiatric Association Practice Guideline's assertion that "most patients" do best when treated with either pharmacotherapy plus clinical management or combined regimens.[16] Less severely depressed patients treated with IPT or CBT alone achieved results comparable with those who received combined therapy. In ambulatory settings where HRSD scores are often less than 20, a practice policy that emphasizes combined therapy or pharmacotherapy first may not be justified for "most" patients, particularly if IPT or CBT is available as an alternative.

Our study also provides new data regarding 2 other potential correlates of recovery: women and older patients had less favorable outcomes. Both older age[51,52] and female sex[53,54] have been associated with poorer outcomes in previous reports, although neither correlate has been widely replicated. In the current study, the predictive value of sex was rather weak, as it was significant in only 2 of the models used in the sensitivity analysis. The negative impact of age specifically resulted from the contrast between the midlife and late-life patients with recurrent depression treated with combined therapy. A more detailed comparison of these groups has been published elsewhere.[55]

Consistent with previous studies,[2-4] no associations were found between outcome and either age at onset or number of previous depressive episodes. Such characteristics may be more relevant to long-term vulnerability than to response to acute-phase therapies. We did not observe the expected poorer outcomes among patients with chronic depression.[2-4] However, as only 6.4% of our study group was chronically depressed, the statistical power to detect such a difference was relatively low. Chronicity was associated with a significantly lower recovery rate in an earlier report from our group that focused on CBT treatment of depressed men.[56]

Several limitations of this study warrant further consideration. First, patients with the most serious forms of comorbidity were excluded from research participation, which limits the generalizability of these findings to unselected clinical populations. As comorbidity is typically associated with poorer treatment outcomes,[2-4,57] it is likely that lower recovery rates would have been observed in a study of an unselected population. Nevertheless, it is most unlikely that the advantage favoring combined treatment would have been attenuated if we had enrolled more patients with more complicated illness.[57] Second, the number of patients who received placebo or antidepressants alone was too small to assess the relative efficacy of these conditions. Thus, our data neither support nor refute the widely held opinion that combined therapy is superior to pharmacotherapy alone. Third, our findings are based on a fairly stringent definition of recovery during acute-phase therapy. In subsequent reports, we will compare the impact of psychotherapy alone and combined therapy on psychosocial and symptomatic outcomes. Fourth, our study group included a disproportionately large number of patients with recurrent depression, which may have skewed the overall results in favor of the combined strategy. If the advantage of combined therapy is pronounced only in more severe, recurrent depressions, this may help to further explain the disparity between the results of single-site RCTs and practice guideline recommendations. And fifth, the relatively low recovery rates observed across studies (ranging from 23% to 51%) point to the continued need for development of better treatments for depression.

A final issue concerns the validity of mega-analysis itself. In combining information from different studies, it is tacitly assumed that the information being combined is similar or "sufficiently" similar. When this is only approximately true, for example, when treatment groups differ on baseline characteristics, statistical methods such as the Cox proportional hazards model are necessary to make valid comparisons among treatment groups. In the current report, the ability to covary individual patient characteristics enabled adjustments to control statistically for differences across studies. Such statistical control was complemented by the sensitivity analyses, which demonstrated that the key findings were not dependent on inclusion of any particular study. Several other aspects of our mega-analysis decrease the chances that the results are not attributable to some unrecognized confound or artifact. For example, patients came from the same stable community population, they were diagnosed and assessed with standard, reliable measures, and they were treated at the same institution by means of standardized treatment protocols. These features are clearly strengths when compared with a conventional meta-analysis of unrelated studies.

Is there a future for mega-analysis? Olkin[58] recently proposed that meta-analysis of original data sets is the strongest empirical method available to determine the relative efficacy of treatments. By pooling the samples of studies conducted by affiliated investigators, we were able to address questions otherwise unanswerable by a single study, a large multicenter RCT, or, for that matter, conventional meta-analysis.[59] We found a clinically meaningful advantage for combined therapy (when compared with psychotherapy alone) for treatment of more severely depressed patients, particularly those with recurrent depressions.

Cornfield[60] noted more than 40 years ago that

> medical knowledge (and, one suspects, many other kinds of knowledge as well) has always advanced by a combination of many different kinds of observations, some controlled, and some uncontrolled, some directly and some only tangentially relevant to the problem at hand. Although some methods of observation and analysis are clearly to be preferred to others when a choice is possible, there are no magical methods that invariably lead to the right answer.

Mega-analysis replaces neither the RCT for testing specific hypotheses nor the use of meta-analysis for comparing treatment outcomes across unrelated studies. Rather, it provides a powerful alternative for researchers who are willing to adopt common assessments and standardized treatment protocols. We hope that more investigators will establish such linkages so that the scientific yield of scarce research funding and time-consuming RCTs can be increased.

Accepted for publication December 4, 1996.

This research was supported in part by grants MH-41884 (Dr Thase), MH-40023 (Drs Reynolds, Thase, and Frank), MH-15758 (Dr Greenhouse and Ms Hurley), MH-43832 (Drs Reynolds and Frank), MH-29618 (Drs Frank, Kupfer, and Thase), MH-33753 (Dr Pilkonis), and MH-30915 (the Mental Health Clinical Research Center; principal investigator, Dr Kupfer) from the National Institute of Mental Health, Bethesda, Md, as well as the support of a grant from the John D. and Catherine T. MacArthur Foundation, Chicago, Ill.

We thank all of the patients, faculty, and staff who participated in the studies reported herein. We also acknowledge Janice J. Jozefov and Lisa Stupar for their assistance in preparation of the manuscript. We thank Helena Kraemer, PhD, and several anonymous reviewers for their helpful critiques of earlier drafts.

Reprints: Michael E. Thase, MD, Western Psychiatric Institute and Clinic, Department of Psychiatry, University of Pittsburgh School of Medicine, 3811 O'Hara St, Pittsburgh, PA 15213.

REFERENCES

1. Persons JB. Psychotherapy outcome studies do not accurately represent current models of psychotherapy: a proposed remedy. *Am Psychol.* 1991;2:99-106.
2. Joyce PR, Paykel ES. Predictors of drug response in depression. *Arch Gen Psychiatry.* 1989;46:89-99.
3. Thase ME, Kupfer DJ. Characteristics of treatment-resistant depression. In: Zohar J, Belmaker RH, eds. *Treating Resistant Depression.* New York, NY: PMA Publishing; 1987:23-45.
4. Depression Guideline Panel. *Depression in Primary Care, Vol 2: Treatment of Major Depression, Clinical Practice Guideline Number 5.* Rockville, Md: Agency for Health Care Policy and Research; 1993. Publication 93-0551.
5. Chalmers TC, Levin H, Sacks HS, Reitman D, Berrier J, Nagalingam R. Meta-analysis of clinical trials as a scientific discipline, I: control of bias and comparison with large cooperative trials. *Stat Med.* 1987;6:315-325.
6. Smith ML, Glass GV. Meta-analysis of psychotherapy outcome studies. *Am Psychol.* 1977;32:752-760.
7. Greenhouse J. Meta-analysis review from a psychiatric statistical perspective. In: Schneider LS, Reynolds CF III, Lebowitz BD, Friedhoff AJ, eds. *Diagnosis and Treatment of Depression in Late Life.* Washington, DC: American Psychiatric Press; 1994:353-359.
8. Quitkin FM, Stewart JW, McGrath PJ, et al. Columbia atypical depression: a subgroup of depressives with better response to MAOI than to tricyclic antidepressants or placebo. *Br J Psychiatry.* 1993;163:30-34.
9. Beasley CM, Dornseif BE, Bosomworth JT, et al. Fluoxetine and suicide: a meta-analysis of controlled trials of treatment for depression. *BMJ.* 1991;303:685-692.
10. Elkin I, Shea MT, Watkins JT, et al. National Institute of Mental Health Treatment of Depression Collaborative Research Program: general effectiveness treatments. *Arch Gen Psychiatry.* 1989;46:971-982.
11. Jacobson NS, Hollon SD. Prospects for future comparisons between drugs and psychotherapy: lessons from the CBT versus pharmacotherapy exchange. *J Consult Clin Psychol.* 1996;64:104-108.
12. Hollon SD, Beck AT. Psychotherapy and drug therapy: comparison and combinations. In: Garfield SL, Bergin AE, eds. *Handbook of Psychotherapy and Behavior Change: An Empirical Analysis.* 2nd ed. New York, NY: John Wiley & Sons Inc; 1978:437-490.
13. Weissman MM. The psychological treatment of depression. *Arch Gen Psychiatry.* 1979;36:1261-1269.
14. Klerman GL. Psychotherapies and somatic therapies in affective disorders. *Psychiatr Clin North Am.* 1983;3:85-103.
15. Shea MT, Elkin I, Hirschfeld RMA. Psychotherapeutic treatment of depression. In: Frances AJ, Hales RE, eds. *American Psychiatric Press Review of Psychiatry, Volume 7.* Washington, DC: American Psychiatric Press; 1988:235-255.
16. American Psychiatric Association. Practice guideline for major depressive disorder in adults. *Am J Psychiatry.* 1993;150:207-228.
17. Persons JB, Thase ME, Crits-Christoph P. The role of psychotherapy in the treatment of depression. *Arch Gen Psychiatry.* 1996;53:283-290.
18. Klein DF, Ross DC. Reanalysis of the National Institute of Mental Health Treatment of Depression Collaborative Research Program General Effectiveness Report. *Neuropsychopharmacology.* 1993;8:241-251.
19. Frank E, Kupfer DJ, Perel JM, et al. Three year outcomes for maintenance therapies in recurrent depression. *Arch Gen Psychiatry.* 1990;47:1093-1099.
20. Reynolds CF III, Frank E, Perel JM, et al. Combined pharmacotherapy and psychotherapy in the acute and continuation treatment of elderly patients with recurrent major depression: a preliminary report. *Am J Psychiatry.* 1992;149:1687-1692.
21. Simons AD, Thase ME. Biological markers, treatment outcome, and 1-year follow-up in endogenous depression: electroencephalographic sleep studies and response to cognitive therapy. *J Consult Clin Psychology.* 1992;60:392-401.
22. Nofzinger EA, Thase ME, Reynolds CF III, et al. Sexual function in depressed men: assessment using self-report, behavioral and nocturnal penile tumescence measures before and after treatment with cognitive behavior therapy. *Arch Gen Psychiatry.* 1993;50:24-30.
23. Buysse DJ, Kupfer DJ, Frank E, Monk TH, Ritenour A. Electroencephalographic sleep studies in depressed outpatients treated with interpersonal psychotherapy, II: longitudinal studies at baseline and recovery. *Psychiatry Res.* 1992;40:27-40.
24. Spitzer RL, Endicott J, Robins E. Research Diagnostic Criteria: rationale and reliability. *Arch Gen Psychiatry.* 1978;35:773-782.
25. Endicott J, Spitzer RL. A diagnostic interview: the schedule for affective disorders and schizophrenia. *Arch Gen Psychiatry.* 1978;35:837-848.
26. Hamilton M. A rating scale for depression. *J Neurol Neurosurg Psychiatry.* 1960;23:56-62.
27. Klerman GL, Weissman MM, Rounsaville BJ, Chevron ES, eds. *Interpersonal Psychotherapy of Depression.* New York, NY: Basic Books; 1984.
28. Beck AT, Rush AJ, Shaw BG, Emery G. *Cognitive Therapy of Depression.* New York, NY: Guilford Press; 1979.
29. Fawcett J, Epstein P, Fiester SJ, Elkin I, Autry JH. Clinical management–imipramine/placebo administration manual: NIMH Treatment of Depression Collaborative Research Program. *Psychopharmacol Bull.* 1987;23:309-324.
30. Rounsaville BJ, Chevron ES, Weissman MM, Prusoff BA, Frank E. Training therapists to perform interpersonal psychotherapy in clinical trials. *Compr Psychiatry.* 1986;27:364-371.
31. Shaw BF. Specification of the training and evaluation of cognitive therapists for outcome studies. In: Williams JBW, Spitzer RL, eds. *Psychotherapy Research: Where We Are and Where We Should Go.* New York, NY: Guilford Publications; 1984:173-189.
32. Endicott J, Spitzer RL, Fleiss JL, Cohen J. The Global Assessment Scale: a procedure for measuring the overall severity of psychiatric disturbance. *Arch Gen Psychiatry.* 1976;33:66-71.
33. Beck AT, Ward CH, Mendelson M, Mock J, Erbaugh J. An inventory for measuring depression. *Arch Gen Psychiatry.* 1961;4:561-571.
34. Thase ME, Simons AD, Cahalane J, McGeary J. Cognitive behavior therapy of endogenous depression, part 1: an outpatient clinical replication series. *Behav Ther.* 1991;22:457-467.
35. Frank E, Prien RF, Jarrett DB, et al. Conceptualization and rationale to consensus definitions of terms in major depressive disorder: response, remission, recovery, relapse, and recurrence. *Arch Gen Psychiatry.* 1991;48:851-855.
36. Greenhouse J, Stangl D, Bromberg J. An introduction to survival analysis: statistical methods for the analysis of clinical trial data. *J Consult Clin Psychol.* 1989;57:536-544.
37. Cox DR, Oakes D. *Analysis of Survival Data.* London, England: Chapman & Hall; 1984.
38. Greenhouse J, Iyenar S. Sensitivity analysis and diagnostics. In: Cooper H, Hedges L, eds. *The Handbook of Research Synthesis.* New York, NY: Russell Sage Foundation; 1994:383-398.
39. Blackburn IM, Bishop S, Glen AIM, Whalley LJ, Christie JE. The efficacy of cognitive therapy in depression: a treatment trial using cognitive therapy and pharmacotherapy, each alone and in combination. *Br J Psychiatry.* 1981;139:181-189.
40. Murphy GE, Simons AD, Wetzel RD, Lustman PJ. Cognitive therapy and pharmacotherapy, singly and together in the treatment of depression. *Arch Gen Psychiatry.* 1984;41:33-41.
41. Hersen M, Bellack AS, Himmelhoch JM, Thase ME. Effects of social skill training, amitriptyline, and psychotherapy in unipolar depressed women. *Behav Ther.* 1984;15:21-40.
42. McKnight DL, Nelson-Gray RO, Barnhill J. Dexamethasone suppression test and response to cognitive therapy and antidepressant medication. *Behav Ther.* 1992;1:99-111.
43. Hollon SD, DeRubeis RJ, Evans MD, Wiemer MJ, Piasecki JM, Garvey MJ, Grove WM, Tuason VB. Cognitive therapy and pharmacotherapy for depression: singly and in combination. *Arch Gen Psychiatry.* 1992;49:774-781.
44. McLean P, Taylor S. Severity of unipolar depression and choice of treatment. *Behav Res Ther.* 1992;30:443-451.
45. Manning DW, Frances AJ. Combined therapy for depression: critical review of the literature. In: Manning DW, Frances AJ, eds. *Combined Pharmacotherapy and Psychotherapy for Depression.* Washington, DC: American Psychiatric Press; 1990:3-33.
46. Conte HR, Plutchik R, Wild KV, Karasu TB. Combined psychotherapy and pharmacotherapy for depression. *Arch Gen Psychiatry.* 1986;43:471-479.
47. Muñoz RF, Hollon SD, McGrath E, Rehm LP, VendenBos GR. On the AHCPR *Depression in Primary Care Guidelines:* further considerations for practitioners. *Am Psychol.* 1994;49:42-61.
48. Antonuccio D, Danton WG, DeNelsky GY. Psychotherapy for depression: no stronger medicine. *Sci Pract.* 1994;4:2-18.
49. Bowers WA. Treatment of depressed inpatients: cognitive therapy plus medication, relaxation plus medication, and medication alone. *Br J Psychiatry.* 1990;156:73-78.
50. Miller IW, Norman WH, Keitner GI. Cognitive-behavioral treatment of depressed inpatients: six- and twelve-month follow-up. *Am J Psychiatry.* 1989;146:1274-1279.
51. Brown RP, Sweeney J, Frances A, Kocsis JH, Loutsche E. Age as a predictor of treatment response in endogenous depression. *J Clin Psychopharmacol.* 1983;3:176-178.
52. Abou-Saleh MT, Coppen A. Classification of depression and response to antidepressant therapies. *Br J Psychiatry.* 1983;143:601-603.
53. Old Age Depression Interest Group. How long should the elderly take antidepressants? A double-blind placebo-controlled study of continuation/prophylaxis therapy with dothiepin. *Br J Psychiatry.* 1993;162:175-182.
54. Sargeant JK, Bruce ML, Florio LP, Weissman MM. Factors associated with 1-year outcome of major depression in the community. *Arch Gen Psychiatry.* 1990;47:519-526.
55. Reynolds CF III, Frank E, Kupfer DJ, et al. Treatment outcome in recurrent major depression: a post-hoc comparison of elderly ('young old') and mid-life patients. *Am J Psychiatry.* 1996;153:1288-1292.
56. Thase ME, Reynolds CF III, Frank E, et al. Response to cognitive behavior therapy in chronic depression. *J Psychother Pract Res.* 1994;3:204-214.
57. Thase ME, Howland RH. Refractory depression: relevance of psychosocial factors and therapies. *Psychiatr Ann.* 1994;24:232-239.
58. Olkin I. Meta-analysis: reconciling the results of independent studies. *Stat Med.* 1995;14:457-472.
59. Gaver DP, Draper D, Goel P, et al. *Combining Information: Statistical Issues and Opportunities for Research.* Washington, DC: National Academy Press; 1992.
60. Cornfield J. Statistical relationships and proof in medicine. *Am Stat.* 1954;8:19-21.

Temporal Profiles of the Course of Depression During Treatment

Predictors of Pathways Toward Recovery in the Elderly

Mary Amanda Dew, PhD; Charles F. Reynolds III, MD; Patricia R. Houck, MS; Martica Hall, PhD; Daniel J. Buysse, MD; Ellen Frank, PhD; David J. Kupfer, MD

Background: Predictors of treatment response and recovery from depression in late life remain poorly understood. Previous studies have focused on a narrow range of response and recovery variables; namely, whether patients achieve or do not achieve a defined outcome or time to achieve the outcome. Whether patients vary in their pathways toward those outcomes—and the extent to which such variation can be anticipated by patient characteristics prior to treatment—has not been empirically examined.

Methods: Depression symptom levels were monitored for 18 weeks in 95 persons aged 60 years or older who were experiencing a recurrence of major depression. Subjects received standardized combined nortriptyline treatment and interpersonal psychotherapy throughout the period. Cluster analysis was used to identify depression recovery patterns. Multivariate analyses considered whether recovery patterns were predicted by pretreatment psychosocial, clinical, and electroencephalographic sleep characteristics.

Results: Four subgroups of elders were identified who differed in rate, stability, and direction of recovery, ie, those showing (1) rapid sustained improvement, (2) delayed but sustained improvement, (3) partial or mixed response, or (4) no response. Pretreatment characteristics reliably predicted subjects' group membership. Higher levels of acute and chronic stressors, poorer social supports, younger age at first depressive episode, endogenous depression, higher current anxiety, older current age, and poorer subjective and objective (electroencephalographic) sleep predicted poorer response profiles.

Conclusions: There are multiple pathways by which individuals begin to emerge from depression; these pathways can be identified empirically. Variables from diverse psychobiologic domains can be used to predict which persons are likely to advance along which trajectories toward recovery.

Arch Gen Psychiatry. 1997;54:1016-1024

DEPRESSION is associated with neurobiologic factors, such as electroencephalographic (EEG) sleep alterations and cognitive impairment,[1-4] and with psychosocial characteristics pertaining to life stressors and supports.[5-7] Moreover, many of these associations grow more pronounced across the life span.[8-10] Given the influence of such factors on the occurrence and severity of depression in adults aged 60 years and older,[11-18] it is surprising that the correlates and predictors of *response to treatment of* or *recovery from* major depressive episodes in late life remain poorly understood. One might expect that key predictors of depression onset would also impede recovery.[16] However, except for the influence of medical burden,[11,13,19] controlled studies have been largely unable to identify baseline or pretreatment variables that robustly predict treatment response or recovery in depressed elders.[19-23] Instead, factors related to either diagnostic heterogeneity or treatment modulation have been most often assigned responsibility for course and timing of recovery.[24]

See also page 989

Yet clinical observation suggests that, even among depressed elders who are in homogeneous diagnostic categories and who receive nominally the same form and intensity of treatment, trajectories toward recovery can differ dramatically. Empirical studies may have failed to correspond with clinical acumen because such studies have focused on a narrow range of treatment response and depression recov-

From the Departments of Psychiatry (Drs Dew, Reynolds, Hall, Buysse, Frank, and Kupfer and Ms Houck), Epidemiology (Dr Dew), and Psychology (Dr Dew), University of Pittsburgh School of Medicine, Western Psychiatric Institute and Clinic, Pittsburgh, Pa.

SUBJECTS AND METHODS

SUBJECTS

Ninety-five persons aged 60 years or older were studied. **Table 1** lists clinical criteria for study enrollment.[28-32] At intake, subjects' mean (±SD) age was 67.1±5.5 years (range, 60-82 years), 22 (23%) were men, most subjects (56 [59%]) had completed high school (averaging 12.6 years of education), and 89 (94%) were white.

The subjects had been recruited for an investigation of maintenance therapies in late-life depression[22,28]; data described herein were gathered during the period prior to maintenance therapy assignment. During this preassignment period, subjects were treated openly with combined nortriptyline (steady-state target level, 80-120 ng/mL) and standardized interpersonal psychotherapy,[33,34] the latter having been provided weekly through week 12 and biweekly thereafter. There were no large or significant differences between any study groups (defined below) in time to reach target nortriptyline levels ($F[3,90]=0.67$, $P=.57$; mean [±SD] period, 5.6±4.2 weeks).

The design of the maintenance trial required that patients continue in open therapy until they achieved 16 continuous weeks of the Hamilton Depression Rating Scale (HAM-D) ratings of 10 or lower before assignment to maintenance therapy.[28] No patients met the 16-week criterion until they had been in open therapy for at least 18 weeks. Thus, our study focuses on the 18-week interval before any subjects advanced to randomization. Nine additional elders who had been lost to follow-up before 18 weeks (dropouts [n=5] and those with intercurrent medical conditions contraindicating further treatment with nortriptyline [n=4]) were excluded from analyses. These persons did not differ from other subjects on baseline variables examined in this study.

METHODS

Procedure

Baseline data were collected prior to inception of open therapy. Subjects kept a daily sleep-wake log[28] for a 14-day psychotropic drug-free and alcohol-free period before the baseline assessment. They then had 3 consecutive nights of polysomnography performed using standard procedures[35] at Western Psychiatric Institute and Clinic, Pittsburgh, Pa. Bedtime and wake time were at subjects' habitual times as determined by their sleep-wake logs. Polysomnographic technologists used standard scoring criteria[36] with periodic checks of interrater reliability.[37] Automated delta-wave and rapid eye movement (REM) activity analyses were conducted using standard methods of period and amplitude analysis.[37] Psychosocial data were collected while subjects were at Western Psychiatric Institute and Clinic. Written informed consent for the assessments and for participation in open therapy was obtained after study procedures were fully explained.

Measures: Dependent Measure

Depressive symptoms were evaluated at each clinic visit with the 17-item HAM-D.[31] Clinical raters were monitored to maintain interrater reliability (intraclass $r=0.89$). Because the HAM-D was administered weekly initially but biweekly after week 12, we averaged each subject's HAM-D scores for each 2-week interval through week 12 and used the biweekly HAM-D score thereafter. This yielded a total of 9 successive HAM-D scores per subject across the study period.

Baseline Predictors

Psychosocial Characteristics. In addition to demographic characteristics, social supports and stressors were assessed.

Continued on next page

ery variables. These variables include: (1) whether patients were defined at a given time point as treatment *responders* and (2) absolute time either to some initial response (eg, symptom improvement) or to recovery from an episode. Exclusive focus on such outcomes obscures any possibility of observing that individual elders vary widely in their temporal pathways to reach those outcomes. For example, among persons with the same total time to "recovery" (however defined), some may show steady, relatively rapid response, others more gradual improvement punctuated by symptom exacerbations, and still others may remain depressed for an extended period and quite suddenly improve. Individuals who fail to recover may also differ in whether they show no change over time, or a noisier pattern of frequent ups and downs, with no overall sustained change in course.

It has not been previously possible to empirically identify such temporal profiles in elderly patients. In controlled clinical studies, while statistical power may be sufficient to compare probability and timing of recovery across treatment groups, within-treatment samples have generally been too small to reliably examine the "natural history" of the depressive illness under uniform conditions of a single treatment (or no treatment) group. In nonexperimental observational studies, large samples of depressed persons followed up during long periods theoretically should provide good data for identifying distinct recovery profiles. However, the logistical reality that cohort follow-up assessments can be performed only relatively infrequently means that these latter studies essentially rely on retrospective data collected at each follow-up regarding the (sometimes lengthy) period since last assessment.[13,25-27] Thus, such studies lack the sensitivity to examine a fine-grained profile of symptom change over time.

In this study, we had the unusual opportunity to explore temporal profiles of depressive illness course and treatment response in a diagnostically homogeneous cohort of elders, all of whom received a controlled treatment package and were followed up closely during an extended, naturalistic observation period. This opportunity arose because the elders had enrolled in a trial of maintenance therapies for recurrent depression[28] and all received standardized (open) treatment for a prolonged period prior to assignment to maintenance conditions.

Perceived support from others was determined using the Interpersonal Support Evaluation List,[38] adapted for older adults[39] (score 0=low support; score 12=high support).

Concerning stressors, severity of chronic medical (nonpsychiatric) burden was determined from trained nurses' evaluations using the Cumulative Illness Rating Scale for older adults (score 0= low severity of medical burden across organ systems; score 52= high burden).[17] Whether subjects had experienced a recent acute life event or stressor that directly contributed to the onset of current depression was ascertained using the Schedule for Affective Disorders and Schizophrenia–Lifetime Version (episode met Research Diagnostic Criteria for situational depression). The Perceived Stress Scale[40] assessed subjects' appraisals of their daily lives as chronically stressful during the past month (score 0=low; score 56=high). The Perceived Stress Scale is conceptually distinct from depression[40,41] and was not correlated strongly with the HAM-D in the present sample (r=0.18).

Depression History Characteristics. The Schedule for Affective Disorders and Schizophrenia–Lifetime Version ascertained current episode characteristics and psychiatric history. Additional measures of baseline psychiatric status included the HAM-D to assess pretreatment symptoms, the Brief Symptom Inventory anxiety subscale,[42] and the Pittsburgh Sleep Quality Index.[43] The latter assesses subjective quality of sleep during the past month (score 0=excellent; score 21=poor quality).

Polysomnography. Measures represent averages over nights 2 and 3, with night 1 considered an adaptation night. Three categories of measures were included: sleep continuity, architecture, and REM. These are discussed further below.

Analyses

Identification of Depression Recovery Patterns. Hierarchical agglomerative cluster analysis[44,45] was applied to subjects' HAM-D scores across the 18-week period to identify any distinct recovery profiles. The analysis used the unweighted pair-group method, with arithmetic averages and squared Euclidean distance coefficients.[45]

Two data procedures were performed in preparation for this analysis. First, because cluster analysis requires complete data, we evaluated subjects' 9 waves of HAM-D scores for missing values. There averaged only 2 missing scores across the 95 subjects per assessment interval. We applied unbalanced repeated-measures modeling,[46,47] assuming a first-order autoregressive, within-subject covariance matrix, to the 9 waves of HAM-D data to impute missing scores. (Data were examined prior to this analysis; analytic assumptions, eg, homoscedasticity, were met.)

Second, because our conceptual interest concerned whether subjects had depression levels above or below a clinically significant threshold, we dichotomized each subject's HAM-D score at each assessment according to whether it was below 11. This allowed us to identify and tag persons with low vs clinically significant depression levels at each assessment and use this tagging in the cluster analysis.[45] (Cluster analysis was also undertaken with subjects' original HAM-D scores and yielded comparable results to those noted below; they are available from one of us [M.A.D.]. See Opdyke et al[48] for an examination of individual depressive symptom items in this cohort.)

Evaluation of Baseline Predictors of Depression Recovery Patterns. The 4 groups identified through cluster analysis were examined for differences in potential predictors assessed at baseline. Univariate tests were initially performed to evaluate group differences on each predictor. Then, direct discriminant function analysis with Varimax rotation[49] was performed to determine whether the set of predictors could reliably discriminate between groups.

We sought to determine whether unique patterns or profiles of recovery from depression could be identified during open treatment. Moreover, a major goal was to identify pretreatment psychosocial, clinical, and EEG sleep variables that predicted whether elders would have one temporal profile of recovery vs another. These 3 classes of pretreatment factors—and the specific variables within them—were chosen because each has been observed to influence incidence and recurrence of depression across the life span.[1-18]

RESULTS

IDENTIFICATION AND CROSS-VALIDATION OF DEPRESSION PATTERN-OF-RECOVERY GROUPS

Cluster analysis revealed distinct groups of elders. Based on the degree of change in the amalgamation coefficient as cluster agglomeration proceeded,[44] a 10-cluster solution was optimal. However, most individuals (n=75) were included in 1 of 3 dominant clusters. The largest cluster included persons whose HAM-D scores dropped below threshold rapidly after treatment inception and who then sustained low scores throughout the observation period (n=29; 30.5% of the sample). This group's recovery profile is depicted in the **Figure**, which plots proportions of the group with HAM-D scores below threshold across the 9 assessment intervals. The Figure shows that 62% of the group already had below-threshold HAM-D scores by the end of week 6; by weeks 8 through 10, all of these subjects had low scores.

The second cluster included persons responding more gradually (n=21; 22.1% of the sample); the proportion of this group with below-threshold HAM-D scores was small (0%-19%) until week 10. Thereafter, all persons in the group maintained low scores. A third cluster included the 23 persons (24.2%) who showed little or no evidence of response; generally, small proportions of this group had HAM-D scores below threshold at any assessment. The remaining 22 subjects (23.2%) were dispersed across 7 small clusters that showed varying patterns of fluctuation in HAM-D scores over time, without evidence of consistent change in any direction. These clusters were too small to study individually (each n≤5), and they were combined into a single—albeit heterogeneous—group of 22 elders, all of whom showed a variable pattern of partial or mixed response. The proportion of this group with HAM-D scores below threshold at any given assessment varied from 9% to 64% (Figure).

To further characterize temporal differences in HAM-D scores across the 4 defined groups, the proportions of each group with below-threshold scores were compared at each of the 9 assessments. As shown at the bottom of the Figure, while the groups could not yet be differentiated at week 2 ($\chi^2[3]=0.37$), they reliably differed at all subsequent assessments. Furthermore, a simple count of the number of subjects in each group whose HAM-D score never went below threshold, and the numbers with low HAM-D scores at a total of 1 to 3, 4 to 6, or 7 to 9 assessments also revealed marked differences (**Table 2**, upper section). In the rapid, sustained response group, almost all subjects scored below threshold on 7 to 9 assessments, while the delayed, sustained response and partial or mixed response groups had fewer such periods. Nonresponders had the fewest periods with low HAM-D scores. Finally, numbers of subjects with low HAM-D scores across *consecutive* observation periods were tallied (Table 2). Almost all rapid sustained responders had 6 to 9 consecutive periods of low HAM-D scores, while none of the nonresponders had any consecutive low periods.

In sum, the 4 identified groups differed on their distribution of HAM-D scores during the observation period; the proportions with HAM-D scores below threshold varied at specific assessments, and the profile of change in these proportions suggested distinct patterns of recovery (or lack thereof) in different subjects. The stability of the cluster solution was evaluated using a cross-validation procedure, in which a random 25% of subjects were withheld from the cluster solution. For the remaining 75%, a new cluster analysis replicated the pattern noted for the complete sample; the degree of change in the amalgamation coefficient as cluster agglomeration proceeded was virtually identical to that for the full sample, and 88% of subjects in the subsample (all but 8 respondents) were optimally classified into the same clusters merging from the full sample. For the 25% cross-validation subsample, the solution again replicated; 92% of the subsample (all but 2 subjects) were classified into the cluster in which they had been included in the full-sample analysis. These results suggest good stability, hence generalizability, of the cluster solution.[48]

BASELINE DIFFERENCES IN DEPRESSION PATTERN-OF-RECOVERY GROUPS

Could subjects' likelihood of showing one recovery pattern vs another be predicted by baseline psychosocial, depressive history, and EEG sleep characteristics? **Table 3** displays baseline data for subjects in each depression pattern-of-recovery group. As shown in the last column of Table 3, univariate analyses indicate that the groups differed on a variety of measures. These univariate tests, however, do not evaluate whether the groups can be reliably distinguished from each other across the *complete array* of interrelated predictors. Multivariate, discriminant function analysis was used to accomplish this goal.

Table 1. Eligibility Criteria for Enrollment in the Open Treatment Phase of a Clinical Trial of Maintenance Therapies for Recurrent Depression in Elderly Patients*

At intake
- Meet Research Diagnostic Criteria[29] for nondelusional unipolar major depression, determined by the Schedule for Affective Disorders and Schizophrenia[30]
- Current episode is at least the second lifetime episode of major depression
- One or more previous episodes occurred within 3 years of current episode
- Score above 16 on the Hamilton Depression Rating Scale[31]
- No evidence of dementia (Mini-Mental State Examination[32] score ≥27)
- No evidence of current substance abuse or dependence
- No evidence of serious or uncontrolled physical problems, based on results of physical examinations, electrocardiogram, and laboratory studies
- Chronic medical conditions (eg, heart disease), if present, are stable either without medication or with medications not known to have significant mood or sleep effects†

*Adapted from Reynolds et al.[28]

†Sixty-three percent (n=60) of the sample of 95 elders took at least 1 medication, including analgesics, diuretics, gastrointestinal medications, digoxin, calcium channel-blocking agents, estrogen, β-blockers, thyroid hormone, β-agonists, and oral hypoglycemics.

The small sample size (especially within each group) precluded use of the full set of risk factors in the discriminant analysis. Adopting a conservative approach, we evaluated the relative importance of only those variables that had been revealed in the preceding univariate analyses to have at least moderately sized effects (the effect size associated with each statistical test in Table 3 was at least moderately large, eg, $F>0.30$ for F values from analysis of variances).[49] Therefore, the analysis compared the 4 depression pattern-of-recovery groups on a subset of 14 risk factors in Table 3, including 4 psychosocial, 6 depressive history, and 4 EEG sleep characteristics. This subset of risk factors is listed in **Table 4**.

The discriminant analysis extracted 2 underlying dimensions. The first discriminated among elders according to speed and stability of response during the study period. Along this dimension, persons with a rapid, sustained response (group centroid of 0.96) were maximally separated from persons showing no response (centroid of −0.93), with the delayed response group and the partial or mixed response group lying between these extremes (centroids of −0.32 and −0.11, respectively). The second dimension distinguished persons with a partial or mixed response profile (group centroid of 1.36) from all remaining groups (centroids of −0.55, −0.58, and −0.01 for the rapid response, delayed response, and nonresponse groups, respectively).

Each dimension accounted for a significant portion the discriminating power of the risk factors (prior to removal of either function: $\chi^2[42]=83.69$, $P<.001$; after removal of first function: $\chi^2[26]=39.39$, $P<.05$). The

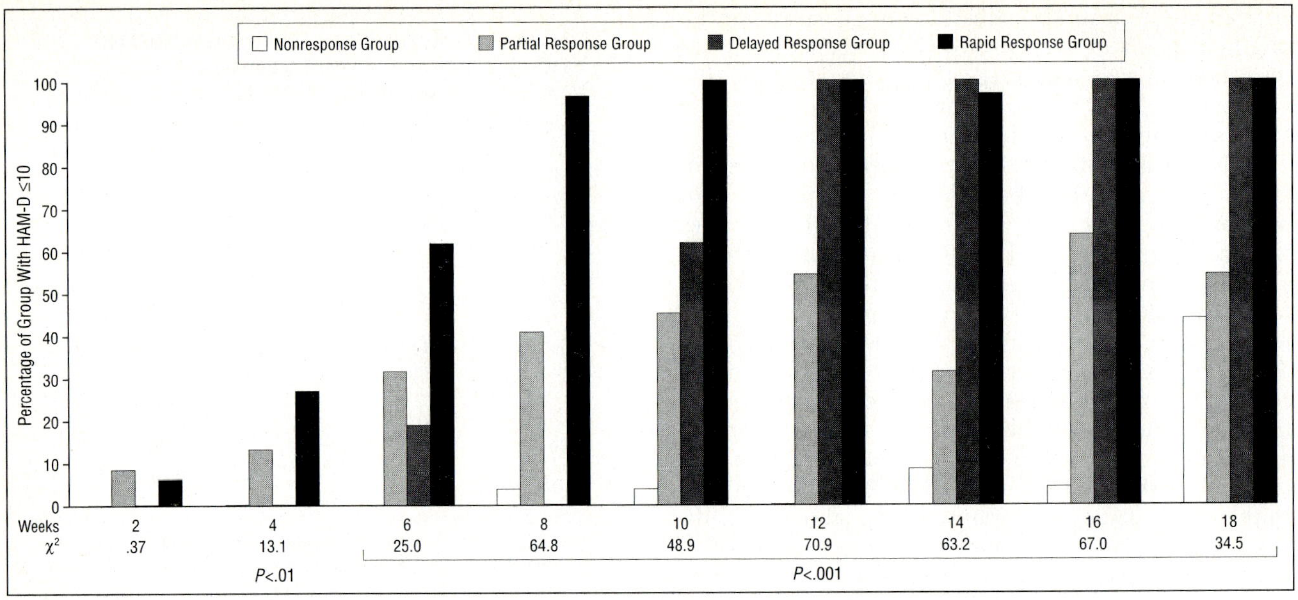

Hamilton Depression Rating Scale (HAM-D) scores over time in 4 groups reflecting patterns of recovery from major depression.

Table 2. Distribution of Subjects in Each Study Group According to Occasions on Which HAM-D* Scores Were Below Threshold (Score ≤10)

Distribution of Subjects	Groups Defined by Pattern of Recovery: Nonresponse (n=23)	Partial or Mixed Response (n=22)	Delayed Sustained Response (n=21)	Rapid Sustained Response (n=29)	χ^2
Subjects with HAM-D scores below threshold across total of nine 2-week periods, No. (%)					
0 periods	11 (47.8)	0 (0.0)	0 (0.0)	0 (0.0)	174.13†
1-3 periods	12 (52.2)	10 (45.4)	0 (0.0)	0 (0.0)	
4-6 periods	0 (0.0)	11 (50.0)	21 (100.0)	10 (34.5)	
7-9 periods	0 (0.0)	1 (4.5)	0 (0.0)	19 (65.5)	
Subjects with HAM-D scores below threshold across consecutive 2-week periods					
0 consecutive periods	23 (100.0)	4 (18.2)	0 (0.0)	0 (0.0)	193.68†
2 consecutive periods	0 (0.0)	10 (45.4)	0 (0.0)	0 (0.0)	
3-5 consecutive periods	0 (0.0)	8 (36.4)	21 (100.0)	2 (6.9)	
6-9 consecutive periods	0 (0.0)	0 (0.0)	0 (0.0)	27 (93.1)	

*HAM-D indicates Hamilton Depression Rating Scale.
†*P*<.001.

existence of 2 significant dimensions characterizing the pattern-of-recovery groups resulted in statistically significant pairwise differences between the 4 groups (tests available from M.A.D.).

The predictors' loadings on the 2 discriminant functions are listed in Table 4. These are interpretable in the same manner as factor loadings in factor analysis. They indicate that the most important predictors (with loadings exceeding an absolute value of 0.20) of having a relatively more rapid, sustained response were lower chronic stress levels at baseline (eg, loading=−0.37), a low likelihood that the current depression was precipitated by a life stressor, older age at first lifetime episode of depression, less severe depressive symptoms at baseline, lower anxiety levels, less subjective sleep impairment, a higher percentage of time in stage 2 sleep, a lower percentage of REM sleep, and less REM activity. Along the second dimension, subjects with a partial or mixed response profile (vs not) were older (eg, loading=0.32), had poorer social support, had a major life stressor precipitate the depressive episode, had depression characterized as endogenous, and had a longer sleep latency.

In summary, predictors related primarily to depressive symptoms and associated sleep factors were most strongly linked to subsequent rapidity of sustained improvement from depression; variables related primarily to psychosocial status predicted greater likelihood of a partial or mixed response rather than any other response profile.

The set of predictors in the discriminant analysis classified 63% of subjects correctly. Group-specific classification accuracy was 72% for the rapid response group,

Table 3. Baseline Psychosocial, Depression History, and EEG Sleep Characteristics in 4 Groups Defined by Pattern of Recovery From Current Depression (N=95)*

	Groups Defined by Pattern of Recovery				
Baseline Predictor	**Nonresponse (n=23)**	**Partial or Mixed Response (n=22)**	**Delayed Sustained Response (n=21)**	**Rapid Sustained Response (n=29)**	**Test Statistic#**
Psychosocial characteristics					
Current age, y	66.6 (5.4)	68.9 (6.8)	65.5 (4.7)	67.3 (4.8)	1.42
Social support	7.64 (1.5)	6.63 (1.8)	7.38 (1.6)	8.31 (1.7)	4.42**
Chronic medical burden	6.65 (2.2)	7.18 (2.9)	6.86 (3.9)	6.28 (2.9)	0.41
Perceived chronic stress	32.9 (7.4)	32.8 (7.4)	36.9 (9.6)	28.9 (7.5)	3.99**
Occurrence of major life stressor prior to episode onset, %	47.8	63.6	30.0	13.8	14.93††
Depression history					
Age at first episode, y	41.1 (16.7)	44.5 (17.9)	47.0 (15.4)	53.8 (15.9)	2.72**
No. of past episodes†	4.7 (2.3)	4.5 (2.2)	5.5 (3.5)	4.6 (5.0)	0.96
Lifetime comorbidity with any other RDC disorder, %	17.4	18.2	28.6	10.3	2.76
Remission prior to current episode, wk	51.9 (46.4)	49.6 (30.4)	69.3 (42.2)	59.0 (48.1)	1.15
Duration of current episode, % >16 wk	69.6	77.3	57.1	51.7	4.25
Severity of current depressive symptoms	23.1 (3.9)	22.9 (3.9)	21.5 (5.1)	20.3 (4.0)	2.45
Current episode RDC endogenous, ‡ %	56.5	81.8	42.9	55.2	7.23
Severity of current anxiety symptoms	1.94 (0.9)	1.67 (0.7)	1.87 (1.1)	1.04 (0.9)	5.42††
Severity of current perceived sleep impairment	12.8 (4.1)	11.1 (4.6)	10.3 (4.0)	9.8 (3.5)	2.45
EEG sleep					
Sleep latency, min†	29.5 (26.5)	38.3 (39.8)	18.6 (11.7)	24.5 (15.3)	1.61
Sleep efficiency,† % of recording period asleep	80.0 (8.7)	75.4 (13.1)	80.3 (11.6)	79.9 (10.1)	0.62
Percent stage 1†	6.8 (5.9)	9.1 (11.1)	6.4 (3.4)	5.6 (3.1)	0.63
Percent stage 2	55.3 (8.9)	58.8 (11.2)	60.8 (7.4)	63.0 (8.6)	3.27**
Percent REM	28.4 (7.1)	23.9 (6.2)	23.9 (4.3)	23.9 (6.2)	2.95**
Percent delta	9.6 (8.8)	8.2 (7.8)	8.8 (8.4)	7.4 (7.1)	0.33
Delta Ratio§	1.36 (0.5)	1.21 (0.3)	1.31 (0.3)	1.24 (0.5)	0.65
Total delta wave count $\times 10^{-2}$	49.4 (32.4)	51.3 (34.2)	52.1 (32.0)	47.4 (29.5)	0.11
REM latency, min‖	49.9 (23.2)	48.8 (21.9)	50.6 (24.7)	51.4 (25.1)	0.02
REM activity,‖ REM frequency/min of REM	170.8 (85.0)	134.3 (80.3)	138.6 (66.9)	126.3 (92.0)	1.63
REM density, REM activity/REM time	1.62 (0.5)	1.55 (0.6)	1.67 (0.7)	1.44 (0.5)	0.81
REM count/min, period 1	7.59 (6.2)	7.44 (7.0)	7.70 (5.8)	6.12 (5.0)	0.41
REM ratio†¶	1.29 (1.0)	2.94 (4.1)	1.72 (1.8)	1.81 (2.4)	0.65

**EEG indicates electroencephalographic; RDC, Research Diagnostic Criteria; and REM, rapid eye movement. Values are mean (±SD) unless otherwise noted.*
†*Transformation used prior to F tests; ln(x+1).*
‡*RDC for endogenous depression requires the presence of a constellation of vegetative symptoms and is judged without regard to the presence or absence of precipitating events.*[29]
§*Delta Ratio indicates ratio of delta wave counts per minute in non-REM period 1 to delta wave counts per minute in non-REM period 2.*[50]
‖*Transformation used prior to F tests; square root of x.*
¶*REM ratio indicates ratio of REM counts per minute in REM period 1 to REM counts per minute in REM period 2.*
#*F tests for continuous measures, χ^2 tests for dichotomous measures.*
**$P<.05$.
††$P<.01$.

53% for the delayed response group, 75% for the partial or mixed response group, and 48% for the nonresponse group. Most misclassifications in the latter group resulted in subjects' assignment to the partial or mixed response group. Although the discriminant functions do not classify 100% of subjects accurately, the large canonical correlation associated with each function (Table 4) indicates that the risk factors, as a set, are important predictors of depression pattern-of-recovery group membership.

To determine whether any one predictor category (psychosocial, depression history, or EEG sleep) contributed relatively more to the classification rate, the discriminant model was reestimated with each of the 3 categories of predictors omitted separately. All 3 categories contributed statistically significantly and to similar degrees to the final model (Table 4).

COMMENT

This study provides the first application of latent structure techniques in general—and cluster analysis in particular—to establish distinct temporal profiles of the course of depression and progress toward recovery in late life. The variation in temporal response profiles among elders was complex and striking. Across an 18-week period, 4 subgroups emerged who showed either (1) rapid, sustained response, with a level of depressive symptoms that quickly declined and remained low, (2) more delayed but ultimately sustained response, (3) partial or mixed response with HAM-D scores fluctuating above and below threshold, or (4) nonresponse, with little evidence of change in HAM-D scores during the observation period. By 4 weeks into treatment, there was already evidence that the 4 groups'

Table 4. Relationship of Baseline Predictors to Subsequent Pattern of Recovery From Depression*

Baseline Predictor	Discriminant Function Loading: Dimension 1: Rapidity of Recovery†	Discriminant Function Loading: Dimension 2: Partial or Mixed Response vs Other 3 Groups
Set I: psychosocial characteristics		
Older current age	−0.17	0.32‡
Higher social support	0.18	−0.38‡
Higher perceived chronic stress	−0.37‡	−0.06
Occurrence of major life stressor prior to episode onset	−0.33‡	0.41‡
Contribution of set I to final model: F(30,224)=1.19§		
Set II: depression history		
Older age at first episode	0.31‡	−0.16
Duration of current episode >16 wk	−0.11	0.19
Greater severity of current depressive symptoms	−0.30‡	0.19
Current episode RDC endogenous	0.14	0.40‡
Greater severity of current anxiety symptoms	−0.57‡	0.00
Greater severity of current perceived sleep impairment	−0.33‡	0.06
Contribution of set II to final model: F(24,227)=2.33§		
Set III: EEG sleep		
Longer sleep latency	0.03	0.24‡
Greater percent stage 2	0.36‡	−0.09
Greater percent REM	−0.31‡	−0.09
More REM activity	−0.32‡	−0.09
Contribution of set III to final model: F(30,224)=2.48§		
Canonical correlation	0.66‖	0.54¶

Six persons with incomplete data on 1 or more predictors were excluded from the discriminant analysis. They did not differ from remaining subjects on other study characteristics. Before the discriminant analysis, predictors were examined and found to meet analytic assumptions adequately.[49] RDC indicates Research Diagnostic Criteria; REM, rapid eye movement; and EEG, electroencephalographic.

†*Groups were arrayed along this dimension in the following order: rapid response group; delayed response group; partial/mixed response group; nonresponse group.*

‡*Loadings meeting criterion for interpretation.*

§$P<.001$.

‖$P<.01$.

¶$P<.05$.

temporal trajectories were diverging. Subsequently, while 3 of the groups showed relatively consistent, unidirectional change (or complete lack thereof), the group identified as partial or mixed responders was heterogeneous, composed of elders whose depressive symptom levels did not clearly move toward either sustained improvement or deterioration.

The profiles that we identified demand replication in other cohorts of elders, and younger persons, to determine their generalizability. For younger cohorts, while our own and others' work has considered time to response and remission in detail,[49,51,52] specific temporal pathways toward response have not yet been examined.

We studied elders with recurrent unipolar, nondelusional disease as opposed to other forms of depressive illness, and we focused on persons with relatively low medical burden, all of whom received 1 highly standardized treatment package. While control over treatment provided the homogeneity necessary to examine temporal changes in depression independent of treatment differences, future work is needed to determine the extent to which various treatments—or the receipt of any treatment—influence the nature of temporal profiles. Finally, due to the design of the larger trial,[27] we had only 18 weeks of observational data. A longer temporal focus is required to fully chart all relevant change points in the course of a single depressive episode or across multiple episodes.[53,54] In particular, some of the individuals whom we identified as nonresponders may have had variations of our delayed responder profile, but with an even more prolonged period (>18 weeks) prior to stable improvement.

These limitations notwithstanding, multivariate modeling suggested that the temporal profiles that we identified were highly predictable from pretreatment psychosocial, clinical, and biological variables. A core group of such characteristics predicted elders' likelihood of showing a more rapid, more sustained response vs brief, unstable, or no response. Thus, the more rapid and sustained the response, the less likely were elders to have had high baseline chronic stress or to have experienced a major life stressor that precipitated their depression. Both acute and chronic stressors increase risk for and timing of depression onset,[4,6] and such stressors may also increase time to initial treatment response.[21] Our finding that they affect rapidity and stability of response underscores the importance of considering such factors in efforts to avert or shorten new depressive episodes.

Pretreatment clinical characteristics also predicted the rapidity and sustained nature of response. Persons who were older at their first lifetime episode of depression, were less severely ill during their current episode, and had less biological perturbation at baseline (as indexed by EEG sleep architecture and REM-related parameters) showed a more rapid sustained response profile. These findings are important because, as noted earlier, controlled clinical studies have been unable to show that such factors were prognostic after treatment effects were considered. The findings are, however, consistent with data from naturalistic longitudinal cohort studies.[24,25] Nevertheless, the role that clinical history and status factors played in the present sample and in these naturalistic studies may differ from what would be observed in medically or neurologically impaired elders. For example, when onset of first lifetime depressive episode is linked to such impairments,[11,18] the effect of late age at onset on subsequent recovery pattern may be quite different from what we and others have observed in essentially healthy elders.

Our analyses further suggested that the partial or mixed response group was distinct from all other groups that we identified—including the nonresponder group. Thus, elders in the former group were older and most likely to meet the Research Diagnostic Criteria for endogenous depression. They also had the most negative social circumstances at baseline, as evidenced by low levels of social supports and a high rate of major life stressors prior to depression onset. These predictors, combined with their longer sleep latencies compared with those in other elders, suggest that this group entered treatment under the highest degree of psychosocial stress. Just as such stress is pathogenic for depression,[4,7] so it may lead to a particularly rocky, unstable course during treatment.

Together, our results begin to clarify both the range of temporal profiles of the course of depressive illness in elders and the predictors of which elders are likely to advance along which trajectories of response during treatment. In short, just as there are many pathways *to* depression, there seem to be many pathways *from* depression. Moreover, multiple variables, from different domains, impinge on rate and stability of response. It will be critical in future work to expand the measurement of these domains. In particular, neurobiological assessments well beyond polysomnography are likely to be needed to fully predict response patterns in the elderly.

More sensitive identification and prediction of the temporal course of depression provides a strong therapeutic challenge: how to compress response time and better maintain stable response to alleviate suffering. Few patients in our sample had low depression symptom levels at 2 weeks or even 4 weeks into state-of-the-art combined pharmacotherapy and psychotherapy. This implies that additional interventions may be needed to provide early symptomatic relief or to accelerate antidepressant treatment response.[55,56] With respect to maintaining the response, recognition that certain constellations of baseline psychosocial and stress-related characteristics bode for a more rocky course toward recovery may enable clinicians to better tailor psychotherapeutic interventions to address these factors directly.

Accepted for publication March 19, 1997.

This research was supported in part by grants MH37869, MH00295, MH43832, MH52247, MH16804, and MH30915 from the National Institute of Mental Health, Bethesda, Md; and by a grant from the John D. and Catherine T. MacArthur Foundation Mental Health Research Network on the Psychobiology of Depression and Other Affective Disorders, Chicago, Ill.

Reprints: Mary Amanda Dew, PhD, Department of Psychiatry, University of Pittsburgh School of Medicine, 3811 O'Hara St, Pittsburgh, PA 15213 (e-mail: DEW1@vms.cis.pitt.edu).

REFERENCES

1. Gillin JC, Borbely AA. Sleep: a neurobiological window in affective disorders. *Trends Neurosci.* 1985;8:537-542.
2. Kupfer DJ, Ehlers CL. Two roads to rapid eye movement latency. *Arch Gen Psychiatry.* 1989;46:945-948.
3. Reynolds CF, Kupfer DJ. Sleep research in affective illness: state of the art circa 1987. *Sleep.* 1987;10:199-215.
4. Dew MA. Psychiatric disorder in the context of physical illness. In: Dohrenwend BP, ed. *Adversity, Stress and Psychopathology.* New York, NY; Oxford University Press. In press.
5. Brown GW, Harris TO, eds. *Life Events and Illness.* New York: Guilford Press; 1989.
6. Frank E, Anderson B, Reynolds CF, Ritenour A, Kupfer DJ. Life events and the Research Diagnostic Criteria endogenous subtype: a confirmation of the distinction using the Bedford College Methods. *Arch Gen Psychiatry.* 1994;51:519-524.
7. Kessler RC, Price RH, Wortman CB. Social factors in psychopathology. *Ann Rev Psychol.* 1985;36:531-572.
8. Knowles JB, MacLean AW. Age-related changes in sleep in depressed and healthy subjects: a meta-analysis. *Neuropsychopharmacology.* 1990;3:251-259.
9. National Institutes of Health. *Consensus Development Conference on the Diagnosis and Treatment of Sleep Disorders in Late Life.* Washington, DC: US Government Printing Office; 1990.
10. Bazargan M, Hamm-Baugh VP. The relationship between chronic illness and depression in a community sample of urban black persons. *J Gerontol.* 1995;50B: S119-S127.
11. Caine ED, Lyness JM, King DA. Reconsidering depression in the elderly. *Am J Geriatr Psychiatry.* 1993;1:2-18.
12. Carpiniello B, Carta MG, Rudas N. Depression among elderly people: a psychosocial study of urban and rural populations. *Acta Psychiatr Scand.* 1989;80:445-450.
13. Cole MG. The prognosis of depression in the elderly. *Can Med Assoc J.* 1990; 143:633-639.
14. Reynolds CF, Hoch CC, Buysse DJ, Houck PR, Schlernitzauer M, Frank E, Mazumdar S, Kupfer DJ. Electroencephalographic sleep in spousal bereavement and bereavement-related depression of late life. *Biol Psychiatry.* 1992;31:69-82.
15. Dew MA, Reynolds CF, Buysse DJ, Houck PR, Hoch CC, Monk TH, Kupfer DJ. Electroencephalographic sleep profiles during depression: effects of episode duration and other clinical and psychosocial factors in older adults. *Arch Gen Psychiatry.* 1996;53:148-156.
16. George LK. Social and economic factors. In: Busse EW, Blazer DB, eds. *Geriatric Psychiatry.* Washington, DC: American Psychiatric Press Inc; 1989:202-234.
17. Miller MD, Paradis CF, Houck PR, Mazumdar S, Stack JA, Rifai AH, Mulsant B, Reynolds CF. Rating chronic medical illness burden in geropsychiatric practice and research: application of the Cumulative Illness Rating Scale. *Psychiatry Res.* 1992;41:237-248.
18. National Institutes of Health. Diagnosis and treatment of depression in late life: the NIH consensus development conference. *Psychopharmacol Bull.* 1993;29: 87-100.
19. Zubenko GS, Mulsant BH, Rifai AH, Sweet RA, Pasternak RE, Marino LJ, Tu X-M. Impact of acute psychiatric inpatient treatment on major depression in late life and prediction of response. *Am J Psychiatry.* 1994;151:987-994.
20. Georgotas A, McCue RE, Cooper T, Chang I, Mir P, Welkowitz J. Clinical predictors of response to antidepressants in elderly patients. *Biol Psychiatry.* 1987; 22:733-740.
21. Hinrichsen GA, Hernandez NA. Factors associated with recovery from and relapse into major depressive disorder in the elderly. *Am J Psychiatry.* 1993;150: 1820-1825.
22. Karp JF, Frank E, Anderson A, George CJ, Reynolds CF, Mazumdar S, Kupfer DJ. Time to remission in late-life depression: analysis of effects of demographic, treatment, and life-events measures. *Depression.* 1993;1:250-256.
23. Kennedy GJ, Kelman HR, Thomas C. Persistence and remission of depressive symptoms in late life. *Am J Psychiatry.* 1991;148:174-178.
24. Guscott R, Grof P. The clinical meaning of refractory depression: a review for the clinician. *Am J Psychiatry.* 1991;148:695-704.
25. Brodaty H, Harris L, Peters K, Wilhelm K, Hickie I, Boyce P, Mitchell P, Parker G, Eyers K. Prognosis of depression in the elderly: a comparison with younger patients. *Br J Psychiatry.* 1993;163:589-596.
26. Brugha TS, Bebbington PE, MacCarthy B, Sturt E, Wykes T, Potter J. Gender, social support and recovery from depressive disorders: a prospective clinical study. *Psychol Med.* 1990;10:147-156.
27. McLeod JD, Kessler RD, Landis KR. Speed of recovery from major depressive episodes in a community sample of married men and women. *J Abnorm Psychol.* 1992;101:277-286.
28. Reynolds CF, Frank E, Perel JM, Imber SD, Cornes C, Morycz RK, Mazumdar S, Miller MD, Pollock BG, Rifai AH, Stack JA, George CJ, Houck PR, Kupfer DJ. Combined pharmacotherapy and psychotherapy in the acute and continuation treatment of elderly patients with recurrent major depression: a preliminary report. *Am J Psychiatry.* 1992;149:1687-1692.
29. Spitzer RL, Endicott J, Robins E. Research Diagnostic Criteria: rationale and reliability. *Arch Gen Psychiatry.* 1978;35:773-782.
30. Endicott J, Spitzer RL. A diagnostic interview: the Schedule for Affective Disorders and Schizophrenia. *Arch Gen Psychiatry.* 1978;35:837-844.
31. Hamilton M. Development of a rating scale for primary depressive illness. *Br J Soc Clin Psychol.* 1967;6:278-296.
32. Folstein MF, Folstein SE, McHugh PR. Mini-mental state: a practical method for grading the cognitive state of patients for the clinician. *J Psychiatr Res.* 1975; 35:189-198.

33. Frank E, Frank N, Cornes C, Imber SD, Miller MD, Morris SM, Reynolds CF. Interpersonal psychotherapy in the treatment of late-life depression. In: Klerman GL, Weissman MM, eds. *New Applications of Interpersonal Psychotherapy.* Washington, DC: American Psychiatric Press Inc; 1993:167-168.
34. Klerman GL, DiMascio A, Weissman M, Prusoff B, Paykel E. Treatment of depression by drugs and psychotherapy. *Am J Psychiatry.* 1974;131:186-191.
35. Reynolds CF, Monk TH, Hoch CC, Jennings JR, Buysse DJ, Houck PR, Jarrett DB, Kupfer DJ. Electroencephalographic sleep in the healthy 'old-old': a comparison with the 'young-old' in visually scored and automated measures. *J Gerontol.* 1991;46:M39-M46.
36. Rechtschaffen A, Kales A. *A Manual of Standardized Terminology, Techniques, and Scoring System for Sleep Stages of Human Subjects.* Washington, DC: Department of Health, Education, and Welfare; 1965. National Institutes of Health publication 204.
37. Campbell PI, Reynolds CF, Berman SR, Hoch CC, Stack JA, Houck PR. Assessment of sleep fragmentation in the elderly: a reliability study. *Sleep Res.* 1987;16:547.
38. Cohen S, Mermelstein R, Kamarck T, Hoberman HM. Measuring the functional components of social support. In: Sarason IG, Sarason B, eds. *Social Support: Theory, Research and Applications.* The Hague, the Netherlands: Martinus Nijhoff; 1985:73-94.
39. Williamson GM, Schulz R. Relationship orientation, quality of prior relationship, and distress among caregivers of Alzheimer's patients. *Psychol Aging.* 1990;5:502-510.
40. Cohen S, Kamarck T, Mermelstein R. A global measure of perceived stress. *J Health Soc Behav.* 1983;24:385-396.
41. Cohen S, Williamson GM. Perceived stress in a probability sample of the United States. In: Spacapan S, Oskamp S, eds. *The Social Psychology of Health.* Newbury Park, Calif: Sage Publications; 1988:31-67.
42. Derogatis LR. *Brief Symptom Inventory: Administration, Scoring and Procedures Manual.* Towson, Md: Clinical Psychometrics Research; 1977.
43. Buysse DJ, Reynolds CF, Monk TH, Berman SR, Kupfer DJ. The Pittsburgh Sleep Quality Index (PSQI): a new instrument for psychiatric research and practice. *Psychiatry Res.* 1989;28:193-213.
44. Aldenderfer MS, Blashfield RK. *Cluster Analysis.* Beverly Hills, Calif: Sage Publications; 1984.
45. Romesburg HC. *Cluster Analysis for Researchers.* Belmont, Calif: Sage Publications; 1984.
46. Dixon WJ, Merdian KL. *ANOVA and Regression with BMDP 5V.* Los Angeles, Calif: Dixon Statistical Associates; 1992.
47. Gibbons RD, Hedeker D, Elkin I, Waternaux C, Kraemer HC, Greenhouse J, Shea MT, Imber SD, Sotsky SM, Watkins JT. Some conceptual and statistical issues in the analysis of longitudinal psychiatric data: application to the NIMH Treatment of Depression Collaborative Research Program dataset. *Arch Gen Psychiatry.* 1993;50:739-750.
48. Opdyke KS, Reynolds CF, Frank E, Begley AE, Buysse DJ, Dew MA, Mulsant BH, Shear MK, Mazumdar S, Kupfer DJ. The effect of continuation of treatment on residual symptoms in late-life depression: how well is 'well'? *Depression and Anxiety.* 1997;4:312-319.
49. Tabachnick BG, Fidell LS. *Using Multivariate Statistics.* 3rd ed. New York, NY: Harper Collins; 1996.
50. Kupfer DJ, Frank E, McEachran AB, Grochocinski VJ. Delta sleep ratio: a biological correlate of early recurrence in unipolar affective disorder. *Arch Gen Psychiatry.* 1990;47:1100-1105.
51. Cohen J. *Statistical Power Analysis for the Behavioral Sciences.* 2nd ed. Hillsdale, NJ: Lawrence Erlbaum; 1988.
52. Greenhouse JB, Kupfer DJ, Frank E, Jarrett DB, Rejman KA. Analysis of time to stabilization in the treatment of depression: biological and clinical correlates. *J Affect Disord.* 1987;13:259-266.
53. Frank E, Prien RF, Jarrett RB, Keller MB, Kupfer DJ, Lavori PW, Rush AJ, Weissman MM. Conceptualization and rationale for consensus definitions of terms in major depressive disorder: remission, recovery, relapse, and recurrence. *Arch Gen Psychiatry.* 1991;48:851-855.
54. Reynolds CF, Frank E, Kupfer DJ, Thase ME, Perel JM, Mazumdar S, Houck PR. Treatment outcome in recurrent major depression: a post hoc comparison of elderly ('young old') and midlife patients. *Am J Psychiatry.* 1996;153:1288-1292.
55. Kupfer DJ. Long-term treatment of depression. *J Clin Psychiatry.* 1991;52:28-34.
56. Baxter LR, Liston EH, Schwartz JM, Altshuler LL, Wilkins JN, Richeimer S, Guze BH. Prolongation of the antidepressant response to partial sleep deprivation by lithium. *Psychiatry Res.* 1986;19:1-23.

Family and Individual Therapy in Anorexia Nervosa

A 5-Year Follow-up

Ivan Eisler, PhD; Christopher Dare, FRCPsych; Gerald F. M. Russell, MD; George Szmukler, MD; Daniel le Grange, PhD; Elizabeth Dodge, MSc

Background: There is evidence that specific psychological treatments are effective in patients with eating disorders. Our goal was to determine by means of a controlled trial whether psychological treatments, previously found to be effective in anorexia nervosa, gave rise to enduring benefits.

Methods: A 5-year follow-up was conducted on patients who had participated in a previous trial of family therapy for anorexia and bulimia nervosa. Family therapy or individual supportive therapy had been administered to 80 outpatients for 1 year beginning on discharge from hospital after weight restoration. The 80 patients had been subdivided into 4 prognostically homogeneous groups of which 2 turned out to be the most important: patients with early onset and short history of anorexia nervosa, and patients with late-onset anorexia nervosa. At the 5-year follow-up, the efficacy of the outpatient therapies was again assessed by the maintenance of weight, and the categories of general outcome and dimensions of clinical functioning defined by the Morgan-Russell scales.

Results: Significant improvements were found in the group of 80 patients as a whole, mainly attributable to the natural outcome of anorexia nervosa, and most evident in the early onset and short history group, as expected. Within 2 of the prognostic groups, significant benefits attributable to the previous psychological treatments were still evident, favoring family therapy for patients with early onset and short history of anorexia nervosa and favoring individual supportive therapy for patients with late-onset anorexia nervosa.

Conclusions: Much of the improvements found at a 5-year follow-up can be attributed to the natural outcome of the illness. Nevertheless, it was still possible to detect long-term benefits of psychological therapies completed 5 years previously.

Arch Gen Psychiatry. 1997;54:1025-1030

From the Insitute of Psychiatry and the Maudsley Hospital, London, England.

It is widely believed[1,2] that psychotherapy (broadly conceived) is the major modality of treatment that is likely to achieve long-term improvement for patients with eating disorders. There is growing evidence that psychological treatments are effective in the short term and that different treatments offer specific benefits for specific subgroups of patients.[3-6] The task for research is the pursuit of long-term investigations of such treatments. We determined whether the benefits of family therapy found in a subgroup of patients with anorexia nervosa at the end of 1 year of treatment are still discernible at a 5-year follow-up.

In previous publications,[4,7,8] we have described the results of a controlled trial comparing family therapy and supportive individual therapy in the management of patients with eating disorders at the end of 1 year of treatment. The main conclusions were as follows[4]:

Patients with anorexia nervosa with an early onset (≤18 years old) and a short history of illness (<3 years) had a significantly better outcome if they had received family therapy than if they were treated individually. The differences were for weight gain and the more general outcome categories and clinical dimensions of the Morgan-Russell scales.[9,10]

Patients with anorexia nervosa with a late onset of illness (>18 years old) benefited more from individual therapy than family therapy. Those treated individually gained notably more weight.

Patients with anorexia nervosa whose illness had started early, but in whom it had continued for more than 3 years, and patients with severe bulimia nervosa had a poor outcome regardless of the treatment modality.

PATIENTS AND METHODS

In the original end-of-treatment study,[4] details were given of the design of the trial and the treatments provided.

DESIGN OF THE ORIGINAL TRIAL

The purpose of the trial was to compare the efficacy of family therapy and a control individual supportive therapy. These outpatient treatments were begun at the point of discharge of the patients from the hospital. A previous admission to the hospital was considered essential from the ethical point of view in a randomized trial on severely ill patients. At the time of discharge from the hospital, all patients had improved substantially, especially with marked increases in body weight. The subsequent outpatient therapies, lasting 1 year, were compared for their efficacy in preventing weight loss. The inpatient and outpatient therapies were provided in the Eating Disorders Unit at the Maudsley Hospital, London, England.

PATIENTS

The patients enrolled in the trial were from 80 consecutive hospital admissions: 57 patients with anorexia nervosa and 23 patients with bulimia nervosa. They satisfied the diagnostic criteria of *DSM-III-R*.[16] Most of the patients were severely ill, many with a history of multiple previous hospital admissions, and (especially the bulimia nervosa group) complicated by episodes of self-harm, severe depression, or personality disorder. The patients ranged in age from 14 to 55 years, and the duration of illness ranged from 1 to 14 years.

From the outset of the trial, it was appreciated that the patient population was not homogeneous. It was decided to subdivide the patients with anorexia into subgroups according to 2 factors known to influence outcome: a late age of onset and a longer duration of illness have been shown to be associated with an unfavorable prognosis.[9,17-19] The aim was to allocate the patients randomly within each subgroup to the family therapy or the control therapy, expecting that the 4 groups would differ in their outcome, but facilitating the comparison of the 2 therapies within each group rendered prognostically more homogeneous.

The 4 subgroups were as follows:

1. Anorexia nervosa of early onset (≤18 years old) and short history (duration <3 years) (EOSH).
2. Anorexia nervosa of early onset (≤18 years old) and long history (≥3 years) (EOLH).
3. Anorexia nervosa of late onset (>18 years old) (LO).
4. Bulimia nervosa of low weight (BN) as defined by Russell.[20]

The mean body weight on first assessment, expressed as percentage of average body weight (ABW) was EOSH, 65.9%; EOLH, 66.0 %; LO, 63.1%; and BN, 80.3%.

PATIENT ASSESSMENT AT 1- AND 5-YEAR FOLLOW-UPS

At the end of 1 year of outpatient therapy, an assessment was conducted and was reported in our previous articles.[4,7] This 1-year follow-up included all patients who had terminated their outpatient treatment early or had refused follow-up treatment (7 patients) and those who had continued their treatment for the full year. The reasons for including the treatment dropouts in the analysis were discussed in the earlier article.[4] The findings were similar whether dropouts were included or excluded.

About 5 years after the end of the outpatient treatment (mean=5.2; SD=2.1) the patients were followed up once more. This follow-up included dropouts from treatment, but only to assess the 5-year outcome for the entire cohort. Seven patients refused the follow-up at 5 years. In each case, an earlier, 3-year follow-up was available and the derived data were used. Patient status was assessed by 1 of 2 independent research psychologists (I.E. or D.LeG.). To facilitate objective assessments, the assessors were not involved in the provision of treatment. They had trained together in the same eating disorder unit, assessing videotaped patient interviews, which ensured a high reliability in their ratings.

Of the 80 patients originally enrolled in the study, 3 had died by the time of the 5-year follow-up. Information was obtained on all 77 remaining patients. Sixty-three patients had a clinical interview, 1 patient had a telephone interview and returned a questionnaire, and 3 patients returned a detailed questionnaire. Indirect information on 10 patients was obtained from a parent (6 patients) and a general practitioner or psychiatrist (4 patients).

At the 5-year follow-up, the patients were weighed, and structured interviews were conducted according to the Morgan-Russell method. The value of this method has been shown in several studies of anorexia nervosa.[4,9,10,18,19] Detailed clinical information is obtained, gauging the patient's adjustment along 5 dimensions: nutritional status, menstrual functioning, mental state, psychosexual adjustment, and socioeconomic status. The assessments are based on the 6-month period preceding the interview. Two sets of data were obtained.

Categories of General Outcome

The following categories were used to assess general outcome: Good, body weight is maintained within 15% of the ABW and menstrual cycles are regular; intermediate, body weight has risen to within 15% of the ABW but amenorrhea persists; poor, the patient weighs less than 15% below the ABW or bulimic symptoms have developed. Henceforth, the terms "good," "intermediate," and "poor" will qualify the outcome according to these definitions.

Separate and Aggregated Clinical Dimensions

The 5 Morgan-Russell dimensions already listed were used to evaluate clinical progress, scores being allocated on a 12-point scale, with a high score indicating improved functioning. To assess overall progress, an average outcome score was calculated as the mean of scores on the 5 scales.

DATA ANALYSIS

The data were analyzed using the STATISTICA for Windows computer program (Statsoft, Letchworth, England). The stratified randomization design of the study and the presence of a significant interaction between type of treatment and prognostic group required the analysis to be done separately for each subgroup (using the χ^2 or the Fisher exact probability test for categorical data and Student *t* tests for continuous data). A significance level of .05 was used in all analyses.

Table 1. Comparison of Outcome at End of Treatment and at 5-Year Follow-up

End of Treatment	5-Year Follow-up: Good (n=28)	Intermediate (n=18)	Poor (n=34)
Good (n=15)	13	2	0
Intermediate (n=12)	5	6	1
Poor (n=53)	10	10	33

Table 2. Outcome at 5-Year Follow-up by Prognostic Group and Therapy

Subgroup	Type of Therapy	Outcome: Good	Intermediate	Poor
1, Onset ≤18 y, duration <3 y (EOSH)	Individual*	4	2	5
	Family*	9	0	1
	Total	**13**	**2**	**6**
2, Onset ≤18 y, duration >3 y (EOLH)	Individual	1	4	4
	Family	3	1	6
	Total	**4**	**5**	**10**
3, Onset >18 y (LO)	Individual	4	2	1
	Family	2	2	3
	Total	**6**	**4**	**4**
4, Bulimia nervosa (BN)	Individual	3	2	5
	Family	0	4	5
	Total	**3**	**6**	**10**

Good vs intermediate + poor outcome, $P<.02$; Fisher probability test.

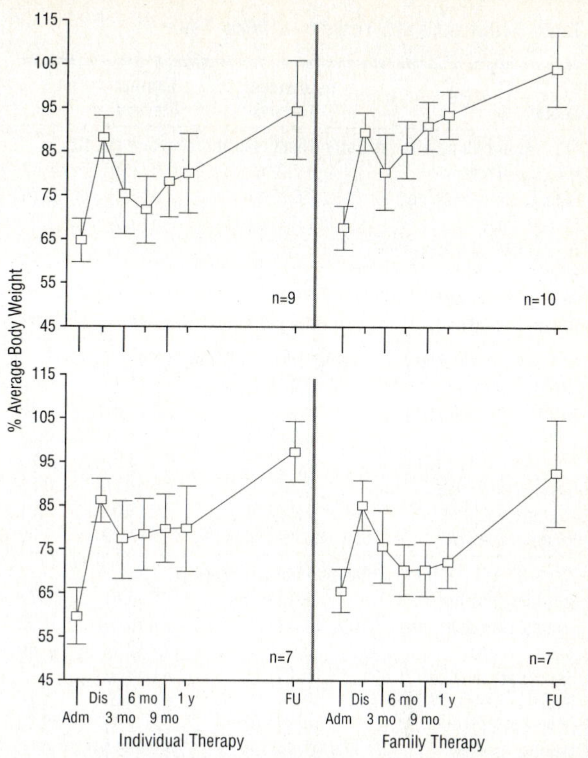

Weight gain during treatment and follow-up (FU) in patients with anorexia nervosa of early onset and short history (top) and late onset (bottom). Bars indicate 95% confidence interval. Data points (left to right) are from the original study: inpatient treatment from hospital admission (Adm) to discharge (Dis) from the hospital, and outpatient therapy at 3, 6, and 9 months and 1 year. The follow-up data points of the present study extend from 1 year to the follow-up (far right) 5 years later.

We did not examine in detail wider issues such as the characteristics of the families of the patients under treatment. In previous publications, we have reported on the assessments of parents measuring their level of "expressed emotion" (EE).[11,12] In our work with patients suffering from anorexia nervosa, we found that a high EE level in mothers was associated with dropping out of family therapy but not from individual therapy.[7,11] We have reported a possible connection between EE and response to treatment at 1 year in this cohort[8] and in separate studies in adolescent anorexia nervosa.[13,14] The findings suggested that in families with high EE scores, family therapy led to a less favorable outcome than individual therapy.[15]

We extended the evaluation of the 2 therapies used in the original controlled trial to a 5-year follow-up, when it can be expected that the effects of natural outcome may obscure the benefits of the early treatment.

RESULTS

THE 5-YEAR FOLLOW-UP

Table 1 gives the general outcome at the end of treatment and at the 5-year follow-up for all 80 patients. The overall improvement of the patients comparing the 2 follow-ups is highly significant ($\chi^2=34.98$; $P<.001$). When patients who refused the outpatient treatment are excluded from the analysis, the pattern of results remains substantially unchanged. In all subsequent analyses, the 7 patients who refused outpatient treatment are excluded.

COMPARISON OF THE 2 THERAPIES IN THE 4 PROGNOSTIC GROUPS

Table 2 gives the results in the 2 treatment groups at the 5-year follow-up separately for the 4 prognostic subgroups. The most important results are for patients in the EOSH and LO groups. The patients in the EOLH and BN groups fared badly with both treatments, with about 50% of patients in each group being classified as having a "poor" outcome.

EOSH GROUP

The EOSH patients generally did well, and the patients who received family therapy fared better than those given individual therapy, with respect to the preponderance of good and "intermediate" outcomes ($P\leq.02$) (Table 2).

Figure, top, shows the patients' changes in weight in response to each treatment during the course of the treatment and after it had come to an end. The average weight of the patients after each treatment was in the near-normal range at 5 years. **Table 3** shows that the patients who had family therapy achieved a mean weight of 103.4% ABW, but

Table 3. Outcome at 5 Years on Clinical Scales*

Scale	Individual Therapy	Family Therapy	t
Anorexia Nervosa of Early Onset and Short History (9, 10)			
Nutritional status	8.7 (2.8)	9.4 (1.8)	0.62
Menstrual functioning†	7.0 (5.1)	12.0 (0.0)	2.76
Mental state	11.5 (1.4)	12.0 (0.0)	1.07
Psychosexual adjustment	9.2 (2.2)	10.5 (2.1)	1.28
Social adjustment	10.2 (1.6)	11.1 (1.2)	1.30
Average outcome†	9.3 (2.1)	11.0 (0.4)	2.43
Weight, % ABW	94.4 (16.8)	103.4 (13.2)	1.32
Anorexia Nervosa of Early Onset and Long History (9, 9)			
Nutritional status	7.2 (3.3)	7.4 (4.4)	0.07
Menstrual functioning	4.5 (5.0)	3.4 (5.9)	0.38
Mental state	9.5 (2.1)	9.1 (3.8)	0.23
Psychosexual adjustment	8.1 (3.0)	8.5 (3.0)	0.24
Social adjustment	8.7 (2.9)	9.6 (2.1)	0.69
Average outcome	7.6 (2.5)	7.6 (3.0)	0.01
Weight, % ABW	95.7 (11.5)	86.9 (11.9)	1.60
Anorexia Nervosa of Late Onset (7, 7)			
Nutritional status	9.2 (2.0)	7.6 (4.8)	0.73
Menstrual functioning	11.3 (1.6)	7.4 (5.4)	1.70
Mental state†	12.0 (0.0)	9.7 (2.1)	2.60
Psychosexual adjustment†	10.1 (1.4)	6.0 (4.3)	2.21
Social adjustment	10.5 (1.6)	8.8 (3.0)	1.24
Average outcome†	10.6 (1.0)	7.8 (2.8)	2.35
Weight, % ABW	97.5 (9.0)	93.7 (18.0)	0.50
Bulimia Nervosa of Low Weight (9, 9)			
Nutritional status	7.4 (4.2)	6.2 (2.5)	0.74
Menstrual functioning	7.5 (5.4)	8.5 (5.4)	0.37
Mental state	10.2 (2.1)	8.0 (3.0)	1.78
Psychosexual adjustment	9.0 (3.3)	8.5 (4.1)	0.27
Social adjustment	9.5 (3.0)	7.0 (2.5)	1.86
Average outcome	8.5 (2.8)	7.6 (2.7)	0.66
Weight, % ABW	98.9 (8.8)	93.4 (8.9)	1.31

**Values are given as mean (SD) unless otherwise indicated. ABW indicates average body weight. More normal functioning is shown by a higher score (range, 0-12). The n values of each group for individual and family therapy, respectively, are given in parentheses.*

†$P \leq .05$.

the patients who had individual therapy reached a mean weight of 94.4% ABW. The difference between the 2 treatments favoring family therapy diminished with time so that at 5 years it was no longer statistically significant (t=1.32; P=.21).

Table 3 shows that if a broader assessment of the clinical progress of patients is made, there is a similar pattern, with patients in family therapy scoring consistently higher, the difference reaching statistical significance in the case of menstrual functioning and the average outcome score.

EOLH GROUP

Tables 2 and 3 show that there was no difference in the benefits of family therapy and individual therapy at the end of 5 years.

LO GROUP

There were only 14 patients in this prognostic group. Overall, this group of patients fared reasonably well with almost three fourths having a "good" or "intermediate" outcome at 5 years (Table 2). The differences in distribution between general outcome categories showed a somewhat better outcome after individual than family therapy but not reaching statistical significance.

The weight charts in the Figure, bottom, show that patients who had both family and individual therapy continued to improve after the treatment ended, with a somewhat higher weight being achieved at 5 years in the patients who had individual therapy. The comparison of the weights achieved then is given in Table 3, but the difference did not reach statistical significance.

Table 3 gives the clinical progress using the Morgan-Russell scales and completes the picture. The clinical ratings on all scales favored patients who were in individual therapy, reaching statistical significance in 2 of the subscales (mental state and psychosexual adjustment) and in the average outcome score.

BN GROUP

On the whole, these patients showed a disappointing outcome. Tables 2 and 3 give no significant difference between the effects of family therapy and individual therapy at the end of 5 years.

UNPLANNED TREATMENT IN THE INTERVENING 4 YEARS

On completion of the 1-year treatment at the Maudsley Hospital, most of the patients returned to their local medical services. For this reason, it was impossible to obtain detailed information on further unplanned treatments, such as possible courses of antidepressant medication. Nevertheless, general information was obtained from interviewing the patients at the 5-year follow-up and is summarized in **Table 4**.

The data should be interpreted with caution, because there was no information for 16 of the 80 patients and it was impossible to assess these treatments in depth because they ranged from brief individual therapy to hospital admissions. The patients who had received additional treatment tended to have a less favorable outcome (χ^2=11.27; P=.004) (**Table 5**).

FAMILY FACTORS AS POSSIBLE INDICATORS OF RESPONSE TO TREATMENT

In view of the lack of control for levels of EE between treatments in this study, it was not surprising to find an uneven distribution of high EE and low EE families between the 2 treatments. No correlation was found between EE score and outcome at 5 years for the 80 patients. Moreover a family with high EE was not predictive of a less favorable response to family therapy or a more favorable response to individual therapy.

COMMENT

This study shows enduring benefits during a period of 5 years after psychological treatments that previously[4] had been shown to be specifically effective in the treatment

Table 4. Additional Treatments During Follow-up Period*

Prognostic Group	Treatment Group	No Additional Treatment	Additional Treatment	Total
EOSH	Individual	5	3	**8**
	Family	9	1	**10**
EOLH	Individual	3	5	**8**
	Family	3	4	**7**
LO	Individual	6	0	**6**
	Family	2	5	**7**
BN	Individual	5	5	**10**
	Family	2	6	**8**

**EOSH indicates anorexia nervosa of early onset and short history; EOLH, anorexia nervosa of early onset and long history; LO, anorexia nervosa of late onset; and BN, bulimia nervosa of low weight.*

of anorexia nervosa: family therapy in EOSH anorexia nervosa, and individual supportive therapy in LO anorexia nervosa.

The previous end-of-treatment study had given rise to taxing methodological problems. This long-term follow-up of the original patients produced 3 further major difficulties: the completeness of the follow-up, the unplanned administration of intervening treatments, and the natural outcome of the illness, partly obscuring the late benefits of the therapies.

COMPLETENESS OF FOLLOW-UP

Although we were able to obtain follow-up data on all 80 patients, in some patients this information was incomplete. Most of the information was from face-to-face contact with the patients by investigators who had not been involved in the treatment program. The quality of information from the general practitioners and parents was sufficient to allow us at least to make a reliable categorization of general outcome on the Morgan-Russell scales for every patient. The more detailed information about clinical progress is less complete and has to be viewed more cautiously.

UNPLANNED INTERVENING TREATMENTS

The treatments obtained during the 5 years after the end of treatment at the Maudsley Hospital ranged widely in their intensity. One useful observation indicated that the patients who had obtained further treatment tended to be those whose progress was worse. This is not surprising, because residual disability is likely to lead to treatment-seeking behavior by the patients. We conclude that intervening treatments are more a sign of poor progress than of an effective therapeutic input.

NATURAL OUTCOME AND LONG-TERM EFFECTS OF THERAPIES

Overall, the patients showed the natural trend toward improvement, but with clear differences between the 4 prognostic groups. It was to allow for variations in natural outcome that these 4 groups were delineated to maximize the chances of detecting differences in the efficacy of the 2 therapies within each group.

Table 5. Additional Treatments During Follow-up by Outcome

Outcome Category	No Additional Treatments	Additional Treatments
Good	20	5
Intermediate	7	8
Poor	8	16

The patients in the EOSH group showed a good outcome at the end of 5 years, as had been predicted. This does not detract from the more important finding that the benefits of family therapy compared with individual therapy have endured until the 5-year follow-up of the patients within that group. The enduring nature of this benefit provides a powerful argument for family therapy being the treatment of choice in adolescent patients with anorexia nervosa.

The most surprising results were those for patients in the LO anorexic group. Late onset of illness has been shown to be a consistent predictor of poor outcome,[9,17-19] yet this group of patients progressed reasonably well. The 5-year follow-up confirms that the individual supportive therapy, found to be beneficial at 1 year, conferred benefits still detectable at 5 years. This result must be viewed with caution because of the small number of patients studied. Some of the negative findings in the LO group regarding the effects of the 2 therapies, as measured on the Morgan-Russell clinical scales, might be due to insufficient statistical power. For example, the ratings of menstrual functioning showed a difference that was not statistically significant but was large enough to be clinically meaningful.

The poor results of the EOLH group and the BN group were not unexpected. Patients with a long history of anorexia nervosa have not responded to previous treatments. Similarly, the BN group was an especially difficult group of patients, often of low weight and complicated by factors known from other studies[21,22] to contribute to a poor prognosis.

This report describes what we believe is the first clinical trial of psychological treatments in anorexia nervosa with positive findings sustained during the course of 5 years. So far, there have been few controlled trials of psychological treatments in anorexia nervosa, presumably because they raise ethical and practical difficulties. The restrictions and advantages of working as a research therapist in our setting have been ably discussed by Colahan.[23] It is easier to point to several comparable trials of psychological treatments in bulimia nervosa,[3,24-27] especially the long-term evaluation of cognitive behavior therapy and interpersonal therapy by Fairburn et al.[28]

Accepted for publication March 20, 1997.

The original study and the follow-up work was supported by the Medical Research Council of Great Britain.

Reprints: Gerald F. M. Russell, MD, Hayes Grove Priory Hospital, Prestons Road, Hayes, Kent, England BR2 7AS.

REFERENCES

1. Garner DM, Garfinkel PE. *Handbook of Psychotherapy for Anorexia Nervosa and Bulimia.* New York, NY: Guilford Press; 1985.
2. Mitchell JE, Raymond NC. Cognitive-behavioural therapy in the treatment of bulimia nervosa. In: Halmi KA, ed. *Psychobiology and Treatment of Anorexia Nervosa and Bulimia Nervosa.* Washington, DC: American Psychiatric Press; 1992.
3. Fairburn CG, Jones R, Peveler RC, Carr SJ, Solomon RA, O'Connor JB, Hope RA. Three psychological treatments for bulimia nervosa. *Arch Gen Psychiatry.* 1991;48:463-469.
4. Russell GFM, Szmukler GI, Dare C, Eisler I. An evaluation of family therapy in anorexia nervosa and bulimia nervosa. *Arch Gen Psychiatry.* 1987;44:1047-1056.
5. Freeman C, Sinclair F, Turnbul J, Annandale A. Psychotherapy for bulimia: a controlled study. *J Psychiatr Res.* 1985;19:423-433.
6. Crisp AH, Norton K, Gowers S, Halek C, Bowyer C, Yeldham D, Levett G, Bhat A. A controlled study of the effect of therapies aimed at adolescent and family pathology in anorexia nervosa. *Br J Psychiatry.* 1991;159:325-333.
7. Dare C, Eisler I, Russell GFM, Szmukler GI. Family therapy for anorexia nervosa: implications from the results of a controlled trial of family and individual therapy. *J Marital Fam Ther.* 1990;16:39-57.
8. Szmukler GI, Dare C. The Maudsley study of family therapy in anorexia and bulimia nervosa. In: Woodside DB, Shekter-Wolfson, eds. *Family Approaches in Treatment of Eating Disorders.* Washington, DC: American Psychiatric Press; 1991.
9. Morgan HG, Russell GFM. Value of family background and clinical features as predictors of long-term outcome in anorexia nervosa: four-year follow-up study of 41 patients. *Psychol Med.* 1975;5:355-371.
10. Morgan HG, Hayward AE. Clinical assessment of anorexia nervosa: the Morgan-Russell Outcome Assessment Schedule. *Br J Psychiatry.* 1988;152:367-371.
11. Szmukler GI, Eisler I, Russell GFM, Dare C. Anorexia nervosa: parental-expressed emotion and dropping out of treatment. *Br J Psychiatry.* 1985;147:265-271.
12. Vaughn CE, Leff JP. The influence of family and social factors on the course of psychiatric illness: a comparison of schizophrenic and depressed neurotic patients. *Br J Psychiatry.* 1976;129:125-137.
13. Le Grange D, Eisler I, Dare C, Russell GFM. Evaluation of family treatments in adolescent anorexia nervosa: a pilot study. *Int J Eat Disord.* 1992;12:347-357.
14. Dare C, Eisler I, Colahan M, Crowther C, Senior R, Asen K. The listening heart and the chi square: clinical and empirical perceptions in the family therapy of anorexia nervosa. *J Fam Ther.* 1995;17:31-57.
15. Dare C, Szmukler GI. The family therapy of early onset, short history anorexia nervosa. In: Woodside DB, Shekter-Wolfson, eds. *Family Approaches in Treatment of Eating Disorders.* Washington, DC: American Psychiatric Press; 1991.
16. American Psychiatric Association. *Diagnostic and Statistical Manual of Mental Disorders, Third Edition, Revised.* Washington, DC: American Psychiatric Association; 1987.
17. Theander S. Anorexia nervosa: a psychiatric investigation of 94 female patients. *Acta Psychiatr Scand.* 1970;214(suppl):7-194.
18. Hsu LKG, Crisp AH, Harding B. Outcome of anorexia nervosa. *Lancet.* 1979;1:61-65.
19. Ratnasuriya RH, Eisler I, Szmukler GI, Russell GFM. Anorexia nervosa: outcome and prognostic factors after 20 years. *Br J Psychiatry.* 1991;158:495-502.
20. Russell GFM. Bulimia nervosa: an ominous variant of anorexia nervosa. *Psychol Med.* 1979;9:429-448.
21. Lacey JH, Evans DH. The impulsivist: a multi-impulsive personality disorder. *Br J Addict.* 1986;81:641-649.
22. Fahy TA, Eisler I, Russell GFM. Personality disorder and treatment response in bulimia nervosa. *Br J Psychiatry.* 1993;162:765-770.
23. Colahan M. Being a therapist in eating disorder treatment trials: constraints and creativity. *J Fam Ther.* 1995;17:79-96.
24. Russell GFM. Evolution et evaluation des traitements de l'anorexie mentale. *Neuropsychiatrie Enfance Adolesc.* 1993;41:341-350.
25. Freeman CPL, Barry F, Dunkeld-Turnbull J, Henderson A. Controlled trial of psychotherapy for bulimia nervosa. *BMJ.* 1988;296:511-525.
26. Mitchell JE, Pyle RL, Eckert ED, Hatsukami D, Pomeroy C, Zimmerman R. A comparison study of antidepressants and structured intensive group psychotherapy in the treatment of bulimia nervosa. *Arch Gen Psychiatry.* 1990;47:149-157.
27. Agras WS, Rossiter EM, Arnow B, Schneider JA, Telch CF, Raeburn SD, Bruce B, Perl M, Koran LM. Pharmacologic and cognitive-behavioural treatment for bulimia nervosa: a controlled comparison. *Am J Psychiatry.* 1992;149:82-87.
28. Fairburn CG, Norman PA, Welch SL, O'Connor ME, Doll HA, Peveler RC. A prospective study of outcome in bulimia nervosa and the long-term effects of three psychological treatments. *Arch Gen Psychiatry.* 1995;52:304-312.

A Double-blind, Randomized, Placebo-Controlled Trial of Fluoxetine in Children and Adolescents With Depression

Graham J. Emslie, MD; A. John Rush, MD; Warren A. Weinberg, MD; Robert A. Kowatch, MD; Carroll W. Hughes, PhD; Tom Carmody, PhD; Jeanne Rintelmann

Background: Depression is a major cause of morbidity and mortality in children and adolescents. To date, randomized, controlled, double-blind trials of antidepressants (largely tricyclic agents) have yet to reveal that any antidepressant is more effective than placebo. This article is of a randomized, double-blind, placebo-controlled trial of fluoxetine in children and adolescents with depression.

Method: Ninety-six child and adolescent outpatients (aged 7-17 years) with nonpsychotic major depressive disorder were randomized (stratified for age and sex) to 20 mg of fluoxetine or placebo and seen weekly for 8 consecutive weeks. Randomization was preceded by 3 evaluation visits that included structured diagnostic interviews during 2 weeks, followed 1 week later by a 1-week, single-blind placebo run-in. Primary outcome measurements were the global improvement of the Clinical Global Impressions scale and the Children's Depression Rating Scale—Revised, a measure of the severity depressive symptoms.

Results: Of the 96 patients, 48 were randomized to fluoxetine treatment and 48 to placebo. Using the intent to treat sample, 27 (56%) of those receiving fluoxetine and 16 (33%) receiving placebo were rated "much" or "very much" improved on the Clinical Global Impressions scale at study exit (χ^2=5.1, df=1, P=.02). Significant differences were also noted in weekly ratings of the Children's Depression Rating Scale—Revised after 5 weeks of treatment (using last observation carried forward). Equivalent response rates were found for patients aged 12 years and younger (n=48) and those aged 13 years and older (n=48). However, complete symptom remission (Children's Depression Rating Scale—Revised ≤28) occurred in only 31% of the fluoxetine-treated patients and 23% of the placebo patients.

Conclusion: Fluoxetine was superior to placebo in the acute phase treatment of major depressive disorder in child and adolescent outpatients with severe, persistent depression. Complete remission of symptoms was rare.

Arch Gen Psychiatry. 1997;54:1031-1037

DEPRESSION IS a major cause of morbidity and mortality in children and adolescents.[1] School failure and school dropout are common outcomes for children and adolescents with depression,[2,3] and suicide remains one of the leading causes of death in adolescents.[4-6] The age of onset of depression is decreasing in those more recently born,[7] with the result that many individuals will experience their first episodes of depression during their adolescent years. Puberty marks a substantial rise in the overall prevalence of depression and is associated with a shift in the sex ratio, with a preponderance of females.

A meta-analysis of all available placebo-controlled trials (n=12) of tricyclic antidepressants (TCAs) in patients between the ages 6 and 18 years concluded that the difference between active treatment and placebo is too small to be clinically significant.[8] This lack of efficacy, as well as the prevalence of side effects of more noradrenergic antidepressants, has led to an increased interest in selective serotonin reuptake inhibitors.[8] Published articles about selective serotonin reuptake inhibitors in adolescent depression include 2 studies of "treatment-resistant" depression with fluoxetine[9,10]; 2 retrospective medical record reviews with fluoxetine[11] and sertraline treatment[12]; and 1 negative, double-blind, placebo-controlled study of fluoxetine.[13] Despite the lack of evidence of effectiveness in randomized control trials, antidepressant medications continue to be prescribed widely in this age group primarily based on adult data. For adults, the efficacy of antidepressant medications for major depressive disorder (MDD) is well established.[14,15] No one antidepressant is clearly more effective than another, except that monoamine oxidase inhibitors are more effective than TCAs for depression with atypical features.[16,17]

From the Departments of Psychiatry (Drs Emslie, Rush, and Kowatch and Ms Rintelmann), Neurology (Dr Weinberg), and Academic Computing (Dr Carmody), University of Texas Southwestern Medical Center at Dallas, and Terrell State Hospital (Dr Hughes), Terrell, Tex.

PATIENTS AND METHODS

PATIENTS

Child and adolescent outpatients (aged 7-17 years) who were self-referred or referred by other practitioners to our mood disorders program and who met *DSM-III-R* criteria for nonpsychotic MDD, single and recurrent. They were in good general medical health and of normal intelligence. Patients with bipolar I and II disorder, psychotic depression (lifetime), independent sleep-wake disorder, alcohol and other substance abuse (within the last year), anorexia nervosa or bulimia (lifetime), or previous adequate treatment with fluoxetine (20 mg/d for at least 3 weeks) were excluded. Any patient with at least 1 first-degree relative with bipolar I disorder (based on family history by a parent) was also excluded.

Possible patients for study were scheduled for a full evaluation after telephone screening for inclusion and exclusion criteria. Prior to the initial interview, the study was explained and written informed consent was obtained from the parent(s) and assent from the patient. The study was approved by the institutional review board at the University of Texas Southwestern Medical Center at Dallas. In addition to a structured psychiatric interview, the initial evaluation included a medical review of systems, a physical and neurological examination, and laboratory tests (blood chemistry study using an automated multiple analysis system, complete blood cell and differential cell counts, urinalysis, thyroid panel, and electrocardiogram). The evaluation was completed during a 3-week period.

METHODS

At the initial visit, each patient and parent(s) were interviewed separately using the Diagnostic Interview for Children and Adolescents,[25,26] a semistructured *DSM-III-R*–based diagnostic interview to establish that the patient met *DSM-III-R* criteria for MDD and to identify other concurrent and lifetime psychiatric disorders. The final diagnoses were based on information from interviews of the parent(s) and child. Additionally, criterion depressive symptoms and depressive symptom severity were assessed using the depressive items of the Kiddie Schedule for Affective Disorders and Schizophrenia[27] and the Children's Depression Rating Scale–Revised (CDRS-R),[28] respectively. Patients completed 2 self-report scales for depression, either the Children's Depression Inventory[29] (all patients ≤12 years) or the 21-item Beck Depression Inventory[30] (all patients ≥13 years) and the Weinberg Screening Affective Scale.[31] Overall functioning was assessed using the Children's Global Assessment Scale (CGAS).[32]

Following the initial diagnostic interview, the patients were seen for 2 additional follow-up interviews, 1 at visit 2 and 1 at visit 3. During the follow-up interviews, the patient and parent(s) were interviewed separately by 1 of 3 of us experienced in evaluating children and adolescents (G.J.E., W.A.W., and R.A.K.). The Diagnostic Interview for Children and Adolescents was reviewed. The Kiddie Schedule for Affective Disorders and Schizophrenia depressive items were scored for the past week and for the nadir of the present episode and were used primarily as a criteria measure at baseline. The CDRS-R and Brief Psychiatric Rating Scale–Children (BPRS-C),[33] a clinician-rated measure of general psychopathologic characteristics, were also completed. The course of illness, including the number, length, and timing of prior and current episodes, was established and the family history was reviewed.

Final consensus diagnoses were determined following visit 3 in a research conference that has been meeting weekly for the past 10 years. To enroll in the 1-week, single-blind, placebo run-in at visit 4 (3 weeks from initial interview), all patients had to continue to meet criteria for MDD, have a CDRS-R score greater than 40, and meet the previous inclusion-exclusion criteria. At the end of the placebo run-in week, the patients were randomized to either fluoxetine treatment or placebo if they still met all of the enrollment criteria, including a CDRS-R score greater than 40 the preceding week. Randomization was by a table of random numbers stratified for age and sex. Randomization was conducted by the pharmacy and clinicians, who remained blind to assignment until the end of the study. Those patients whose conditions improved (n=7) during the 1-week placebo run-in period continued to receive placebo for an additional week to determine if the symptoms returned. If the patients' conditions still improved, they were withdrawn from the study (n=7).

The possible reasons for the differences between adults and adolescents have been reviewed.[18,19] Ryan[19] noted that medications studied to date have been primarily noradrenergic or were metabolized quickly to noradrenergic metabolites. Based on limited animal studies, it is suggested that the noradrenergic system does not develop fully until early adulthood,[20,21] suggesting that serotonergic agents may be more effective in this age group.[19] Alternatively, high levels of hormones during puberty may decrease the effectiveness of TCAs.[18] Several articles have also commented on design issues,[22-24] small sample sizes, definitions of response, comorbidity, length of treatment, and large placebo response in children and adolescents. A primary concern is whether the populations studied are sufficiently homogeneous to allow a study of the efficacy of medication. The major concerns are that (1) the populations studied are abnormally treatment resistant (incipient bipolar, subjects with atypical depression, and substantial comorbidity), (2) the populations are overly treatment responsive, (3) the samples are too heterogeneous to detect medication effects, or (4) the wrong medications have been evaluated.

Our study was undertaken to evaluate the comparative efficacy, safety, and tolerability of fluoxetine treatment compared with placebo in child and adolescent outpatients with nonpsychotic MDD.

RESULTS

Five hundred eighty-three patients were screened by telephone during the course of the study (April 1, 1991 to January 31, 1995), 256 of whom were interviewed at least once. Of these, 106 patients completed the initial evaluation visits and enrolled in the placebo run-in period. Of the 150 ineligible patients, 34 (23%) refused to participate in the treatment study, 55 (37%) did not meet in-

OUTCOME MEASURES

Outcome was measured weekly. The Clinical Global Impressions (CGI) scale improvement rating and the CDRS-R were selected, a priori, as the major outcome measures. Additionally, the clinician completed the CGAS and the BPRS-C weekly. The patient completed the Beck Depression Inventory or Children's Depression Inventory and the Weinberg Screening Affective Scale at the beginning and the end of treatment. All subjects continued in the study for 8 weeks unless continued nonresponsiveness or adverse events dictated a change in treatment.

Following randomization, each patient was given 1 capsule of placebo or 20 mg of fluoxetine every morning. All patients were seen weekly for 8 consecutive weeks. Serum levels were collected on all patients at weeks 1, 2, 4, 6, and 8, approximately 8 hours after the last dose; however, results of blood chemistry levels were not provided to clinicians. Compliance was monitored by counting returned pills. New bottles were provided weekly, with 2 extra pills in the event of scheduling difficulties for the next visit. The pharmacy provided blinded medication based on the random assignment. Electrocardiograms and routine laboratory work (repeat of baseline studies) were repeated at weeks 4 and 8 (or at last visit) of the study.

STATISTICAL ANALYSIS

The data were computerized and managed using screen- and menu-guided Statistical Analysis System software (SAS, Cary, NC). Throughout our study, quality control procedures were in place to ensure accurate and complete data (eg, dual entry and multiple manual comparisons).

To assess interrater reliability specific for our study, the CGI scale and CDRS-R scores were assessed in the same interviews by 2 experienced clinicians during various stages of the evaluation and treatment phases of the study. Patients receiving dual assessments were selected solely on the availability of clinicians at the time of appointment, though patients were seen by 2 clinicians on completion of the study if at all possible. As the CGI scale improvement score is not completed during evaluation, paired scores are available for 48 patients for the CDRS-R and 41 patients for the CGI scale, 35 of which were performed at visit 8. The intraclass correlation[34] for the CDRS-R was 0.95 and the CGI improvement rating was 0.93. If the CGI scale improvement rating is used as a categorical variable[35] (ie, responder vs nonresponder), then $\kappa=0.951$.

The primary outcome measures for the study were categorical. The proportion of patients who were randomized (intent to treat) who responded in each group (drug and placebo) as defined by a CGI scale improvement rating of 1 or 2 ("very much" or "much" improved, respectively) and dimensional (the group mean weekly) CDRS-R scores. Secondary analyses to explore in more depth the pattern of response to fluoxetine treatment and placebo included a survival analysis of time to remission (defined as the first of 2 consecutive weekly CGI scale ratings of 1 or 2) and repeated-measures of analyses of variance using weekly CDRS-R scores with the last observation carried forward (LOCF).

However, the results of the LOCF method are not always reliable owing to the creation of "carried forward" data for weeks after discontinuation. This could bias the between-group comparison depending on how the pattern of dropouts varies between groups. Therefore, an additional method of analysis was used to obtain results based on all of the data but without the bias inherent in the LOCF method. For this analysis, the rate of change in the CDRS-R score was estimated for each patient (fluoxetine-treated or placebo) individually using all data available for that patient. The rates of change for all patients in each group (fluoxetine-treated or placebo) were averaged together. The averages for these 2 groups were then compared using a *t* test. The rate of change (or slope) was first estimated using linear regression (which also produces an estimated baseline CDRS-R score). Kraemer and Thieman[36] recommend analysis of linear regression slopes as an efficient method for use with "soft" data. As a check on the validity of this method, the average slope in each group and the variability of the average was estimated using the more sophisticated empirical Bayesian analysis described by Mori et al.[37] The empirical Bayesian analysis was selected because it adjusts for the correlation between the probability of dropout and the true unobservable rate of change (ie, informative right censoring). Such correlation can be tested[37] and was significant in our data ($P=.02$). Secondary outcome measures were compared based on the last available measurement using analysis of covariance with the baseline measurement as the covariate. All tests were 2-sided with $P<.05$ used for significance. Means are presented as ±SD.

clusionary criteria; 24 (16%) met exclusionary criteria; the condition of 22 (15%) improved during the evaluation, thereby, becoming ineligible; and 15 (10%) needed immediate treatment. Of the 106 patients enrolled in the placebo run-in period, 96 were randomized. Of the 10 not randomized, the condition of 7 improved, 2 refused further study, and 1 had significant side effects while receiving placebo. Of the 96 patients randomized, 48 received fluoxetine treatment and 48 received placebo.

As mentioned previously, the sample was stratified by age (≤12 years and and ≥13 years) and by sex. Of the 48 patients randomized to fluoxetine treatment, 24 were aged 12 years and younger and 24 were aged 13 years and older. Of those randomized to placebo, 24 were aged 12 years and younger and 24 were aged 13 years and older. The 2 groups, fluoxetine-treated and placebo, were not different in any demographic or clinical features, except that those assigned to fluoxetine treatment had a greater lifetime incidence of comorbid anxiety disorders ($\chi^2=4.2$, $df=1$, $P=.04$). **Table 1** lists the demographic and clinical characteristics of these 2 groups (fluoxetine treatment and placebo).

Table 2 lists the timing and basis for patients not completing the 8-week trial. The most common reason for discontinuation was continued nonresponse (19 patients who were receiving placebo and 7 who were receiving fluoxetine). Side effects, as a reason for discontinuation, were minimal, affecting only 4 patients who were receiving fluoxetine and 1 who was receiving placebo. The side effects leading to discontinuation of fluoxetine treatment were in 3 patients in whom manic symptoms developed and 1 patient who developed a severe rash.

Based on a CGI scale improvement rating of 1 or 2 (very much or much improved) to define response, 27 (56%) of 48 patients receiving fluoxetine treatment and 16 (33%) of 48 patients on placebo responded to treatment at exit from the study ($\chi^2=5.097$, $df=1$, $P=.02$). On the other hand, of

Table 1. Clinical and Demographic Characteristics

Features	Patient Group*	
	Fluoxetine-Treated	Placebo
Demographics		
Age, y	12.2±2.7	12.5±2.6
(Range)	(7-17)	(8-17)
Female, No. (%)	22 (46)	22 (46)
White, No. (%)	35 (72.9)	41 (85.4)
Socioeconomic status, No. (%)†		
1-2	14 (29.2)	16 (33.3)
3	16 (33.3)	18 (37.5)
4-5	18 (37.5)	14 (29.2)
Clinical characteristics		
CDRS-R score‡	58.5±10.5	57.6±10.4
(Range)	(42-90)	(42-82)
Melancholic, *DSM-III-R* (%)	7 (14.6)	12 (25)
First episode, No. (%)	23 (47.9)	23 (47.9)
No. of episodes	1.7±0.7	1.8±0.8
(Range)	(1-3)	(1-4)
Duration, current episode, wk	14.6±9.7	13.7±7.5
(Range)	(4-56)	(4-32)
Length of illness, mo	18.8±20.9	18.0±19.7
(Range)	(1-84)	(1-72)
Age at onset, y	10.6±2.7	11.0±2.6
(Range)	(6-16)	(5-17)
Positive family history, No. (%)§	25 (52.1)	29 (60.4)
CGAS score‖	47.9±8.3	48.4±7.8
(Range)	(25-65)	(35-80)
Comorbid diagnoses, lifetime, No. (%)		
None	7 (14.6)	11 (22.9)
Dysthymia	20 (41.7)	14 (29.2)
Anxiety disorders	32 (66.7)	22 (45.8)
ADHD	16 (33.3)	13 (27.1)
Oppositional/conduct	13 (27.1)	16 (33.3)

*There were 48 patients enrolled in each group (mean±SD).
†Two-factor index (A. B. Hollingshead, unpublished data, 1975).
‡CDRS-R indicates Children's Depression Rating Scale–Revised; CGAS, Children's Global Assessment Scale; and ADHD, attention deficit hyperactivity disorder.
§A first-degree relative with affective disorder treated with either hospitalization or medication.
‖Based on average of scores during evaluation.

Table 2. Reasons for Discontinuation Following Randomization

Patient Group	Week 1	2	3	4	5	6	7	8	Total
Fluoxetine-treated									
Lack of efficacy	...	...	...	...	1	3	2	1	**7**
Side effects	...	...	...	1	2	...	1	...	**4**
Protocol violation*	...	...	1	...	1	1	...	...	**3**
Placebo									
Lack of efficacy	...	1	1	1	5	5	5	1	**19**
Side effects	...	...	...	1	...	...	...	...	**1**
Protocol violation	1	...	...	1	...	...	...	...	**2**
Total	**1**	**1**	**2**	**4**	**9**	**9**	**8**	**2**	**36**

*Protocol violations included taking nonstudy medications and missing appointments. Ellipses indicate no patients discontinued.

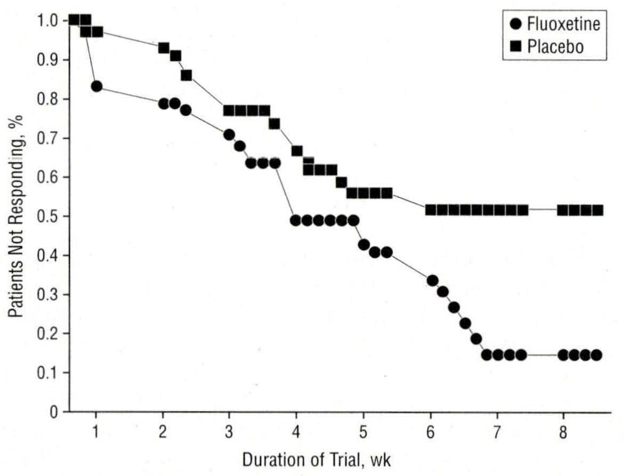

Figure 1. *Survival curve for time to response comparing fluoxetine and placebo. Response is Clinical Global Impressions scale (improvement) rating of 2 or less for 2 consecutive weeks.*

those who completed the entire 8 weeks of treatment 25 (74%) of 34 patients responded to fluoxetine treatment and 15 (58%) of 26 patients responded to placebo (χ^2=1.663, *df*=1, *P*=.20). This result is influenced by the differential dropout of nonresponders in the placebo group. While the condition of many patients improved during the study, only 15 (31%) of 48 patients of the fluoxetine-treated group and 11 (23%) of 48 patients of the placebo group had minimal symptoms (ie, a CDRS-R score ≤28) by end of the study.

To examine the pattern of change in the 2 groups, time to response was defined categorically as the first of 2 consecutive weeks when the CGI scale rating was a 1 or a 2 (much or very much improved). Kaplan-Meier survival curves[38] were compared using the log-rank test and were found significantly different (χ^2=5.66, *df*=1, *P*=.017) (**Figure 1**).

The other primary outcome measure, the weekly CDRS-R score, was examined as a continuous variable. **Figure 2** shows the traditional method of dealing with patient attrition during the course of the treatment (ie, weekly CDRS-R scores for each group are presented with the LOCF). The last available observation is filled in for the values for patients who discontinued study participation before 8 weeks. A repeated measure (analysis of variance) using all 96 patients showed a significant drug by time interaction (F=3.66; *df*=8, 752; *P*=.01). Age group by treatment interaction was also examined but was not significant (*P*=.76). Comparing the weekly CDRS-R scores for each treatment group using *t* tests, the first week that the groups were significantly different was week 5. At week 5, the mean CDRS-R score for the fluoxetine-treated group (39.8±13.2) was lower than the placebo group (46.8±16.6) (*t*=−2.28, *df*=94, *P*=.03).

To make the most efficient use of the available data[36] without resorting to a completion analysis or LOCF analysis, the rate of change (slope) and baseline CDRS-R score (intercept) were estimated from linear regressions on each patient and for each group. The estimated baselines were similar (54.2 for the fluoxetine-treated group vs 53.8 for the placebo group). However, the fluoxetine-treated group slope of −2.75±−2.52 was significantly different from the placebo group slope of −1.27±−2.86 (*t*=2.68, *df*=94, *P*<.001).

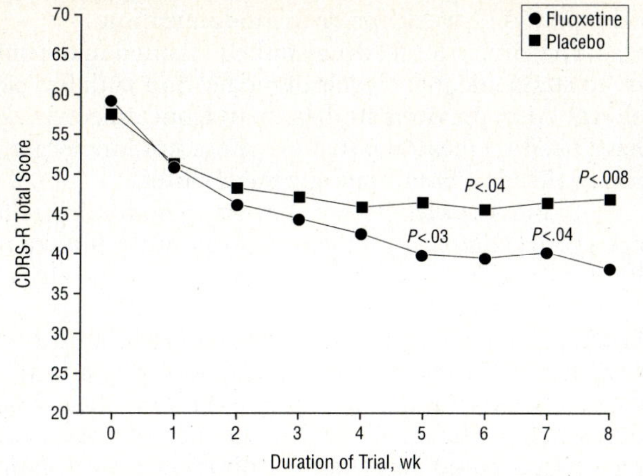

Figure 2. *Weekly Children's Depressive Rating Scale—Revised (CDRS-R) scores (last observation carried forward) for fluoxetine and placebo.*

These results may be interpreted as follows. The fluoxetine-treated group began with an average CDRS-R score of 54.2 and their scores improved by 2.75 U per week to end with an estimated week 8 score of 32.2. While placebo patients began with a similar average CDRS-R score (53.8), their score improved only 1.27 U per week to the end of the study with an estimated exit score of 43.6. Using the empirical Bayesian analysis of estimating slopes (intercept estimates were unavailable) gives an estimated slope of -2.60 ± 2.36 for the fluoxetine-treated group and a significantly smaller slope of -1.32 ± 3.56 for the placebo group ($t=2.08$, $df=94$, $P=.04$).

To further evaluate the effect of age and sex on response, regression lines were calculated for patients aged 12 years and younger and 13 years and older in each group. There were no significant drug by age interactions ($F=0.12$, $df=1, 92$, $P=.73$), though the younger patients independent of the treatment group started with lower CDRS-R scores ($F=8.77$, $df=1, 92$, $P=.004$). Similarly, if the sample is divided by sex, using the same analyses, there was no drug by sex interaction ($F=.001$; $df=1, 92$; $P=.96$).

Finally, for descriptive purposes, **Table 3** lists the initial and last available scores for all 96 patients on the clinician measures and self-report depression scales by groups. Fluoxetine treatment and placebo were associated with significant decreases between baseline and exit scores on these measures. As noted previously, improvement in the CDRS-R scores were greater in the fluoxetine-treated group (final CDRS-R score, 38.4 ± 14.8) than in the placebo group (final CDRS-R score, 47.1 ± 17.0) and the analysis of covariance ($F=10.58$; $df=1, 93$; $P=.002$). However, on measurements of general psychiatric symptoms (BPRS-C) and global functioning (CGAS), there were significant improvements in the condition of the patients in both groups during the course of the study, but the improvement in the fluoxetine-treated group was not significantly superior to the placebo group. Furthermore, self-reported depressive symptom measurements also showed improvement in both groups, but the between-group differences were not significant. However, given the wide variability of initial child self-reports, these findings are difficult to interpret.

Table 3. Baseline to Exit Outcomes

	Patient Group Scores*			
	Fluoxetine-Treated		Placebo	
Scale†	Baseline	Final	Baseline	Final
CDRS-R	58.5±10.5	38.4±14.8	57.6±10.4	47.1±17.0
(Range)	(42-90)	(19-71)	(42-82)	(17-78)
CDI/BDI	15.8±10.6	9.9±12.0	15.3±11.9	11.2±10.8
(Range)	(0-41)	(0-56)	(0-54)	(0-42)
WSAS	20.6±11.8	13.1±12.0	20.6±12.8	16.7±13.5
(Range)	(1-45)	(0-42)	(0-47)	(0-46)
BPRS-C	47.3±7.7	38.9±10.0	46.2±8.9	41.0±10.4
(Range)	(34-65)	(21-58)	(24-69)	(21-67)
CGAS	47.9±8.3	63.9±12.9	48.4±7.8	60.1±14.8
(Range)	(25-65)	(40-89)	(35-80)	(40-95)

**There were 48 patients enrolled in each group (mean±SD).*
†CDRS-R indicates Children's Depression Rating Scale–Revised; CDI, Children's Depression Inventory; BDI, Beck Depression Inventory; WSAS, Weinberg Screening Affective Scale; BPRS-C, Brief Psychiatric Rating Scale–Children; and CGAS, Children's Global Assessment Scale.

COMMENT

Fluoxetine treatment was superior to placebo in relieving depressive symptoms. The difference between fluoxetine treatment and placebo was evident in clinician assessment of clinical global improvement (the CGI scale) and in weekly clinician depressive symptom severity ratings (the CDRS-R). Differences between fluoxetine treatment and placebo became statistically significant after 5 weeks.

There was no clear difference in patient responsiveness to either fluoxetine treatment or placebo based on age or sex. The overall rates of response were similar to those reported in adults for fluoxetine treatment and placebo using comparable analyses. For example, the Depression Guideline Panel[11] reports that a meta-analysis of all available double-blind studies of fluoxetine treatment, with intent-to-treat samples, reveals a 46% response rate to fluoxetine treatment and a 22% difference between fluoxetine treatment and placebo.

Despite improvements in depressive symptoms, relatively complete remission of depressive symptoms (a CDRS-R score ≤28) was uncommon, which is not dissimilar to adult data in 6- to 8-week efficacy trials. Differences between the fluoxetine-treated group and the placebo group were less evident in self-report scales (Children's Depression Inventory, Beck Depression Inventory, and Weinberg Screening Affective Scale) and in clinician ratings of general psychiatric symptoms (the BPRS-C) and global functioning (the CGAS).

COMPARISON WITH FINDINGS FROM PREVIOUS STUDIES OF CHILDREN AND ADOLESCENTS

Several factors may explain a positive result in our study compared with previous studies of children and adolescents. While depressed at baseline evaluation, as evidenced by CDRS-R scores, the sample as a whole was neither overly responsive (ie, the placebo response rate of 33%) nor treatment resistant (ie, the fluoxetine-treated group response rate of 56%).

In the study of 38 children by Puig-Antich et al,[39] 56% (9/16) of the children responded to imipramine therapy and 68% (15/22) responded to placebo. Four patients in the imipramine-treated group, but none in the placebo group, failed to complete the 5-week protocol. An open extension of this study suggested that in addition to the high placebo response rate, failure to achieve therapeutic levels of imipramine limited effectiveness.[40]

In part, as a result of this study, Geller et al[41] designed their study of nortriptyline in children to be longer (8 weeks) and controlled for blood chemistry levels. The randomization was preceded by a 2-week placebo washout phase. The patients had severe depression, had a chronic course, and had a high rate of comorbidity including family histories of bipolar disorder. Of the 50 children randomized, 30.8% responded to active treatment and 16.7% responded to placebo based on an earlier version of the CDRS. The mean unrevised CDRS scores at the end of the study for active and placebo were 32.9 ± 11.4 and 32.0 ± 9.8, respectively.

In adolescents, using the same design as for children, Geller et al[42] enrolled 52 patients, 35 of whom were randomized. Response was defined as a CDRS score of less than 25 and a Kiddie Schedule for Affective Disorders and Schizophrenia depressive items score of 2 or less, except concentration. One active treatment patient and 4 placebo patients responded despite mean nortriptyline levels for the active treatment group of 350 ± 70 nmol/L. Kutcher et al[18] reported on a randomized, double-blind, placebo-controlled study of 750 nmol/L of desipramine per day in adolescent outpatients, which was an extension of an earlier report. Of 60 adolescents randomized, 18 dropped out before 6 weeks, 13 of whom were receiving desipramine. With response defined as a 50% or greater decrease in the Hamilton Depression Rating Scale, 48% responded to desipramine treatment compared with 35% to placebo, a difference that failed to reach significance.

Simeon et al[13] described 40 adolescent outpatients with MDD in a double-blind, placebo-controlled study of fluoxetine. All of the patients completed a 1-week, single-blind placebo run-in prior to randomization, though the length of time prior to enrolling in the single-blind placebo run-in was not described. Patients' dosages were titrated to 60 mg of fluoxetine by week 2 and studied for 6 weeks. Fifteen patients in each group completed the study. Simeon et al reported that 2 of every 3 patients showed mild to moderate improvement with either fluoxetine treatment or placebo. All clinical measures showed a greater improvement with fluoxetine treatment than placebo except sleep although none were statistically significant, perhaps owing to the relatively few patients tested. Similar to the study by Puig-Antich et al,[39] the placebo response rate was high.

The design of our study benefited from the experience of previous studies. Factors possibly contributing to a positive result included sample characteristics such as a relatively large sample, the exclusion of patients with psychotic depression, bipolar symptoms or a family history of bipolar disorder, and the recruitment of patients from a range of socioeconomic backgrounds, including those who were able to pay for treatment. All patients were self-identified patients. None were recruited by media methods. Methodologic issues included an extensive evaluation period (3 weeks) and a single-blind placebo period (1 week) prior to randomization.

The choice of the drug studied resulted in the ability to attain adequate levels of medication with few side effects. Also, previous studies, apart from Simeon et al,[13] have used medications that are more noradrenergic or metabolized to noradrenergic metabolites.

To our knowledge, there have been no studies in this age group comparing selective serotonin reuptake inhibitors and TCAs directly. However, in an open trial of 15 adolescents and young adults (aged 16-24 years) who had failed to respond to a TCA, Boulos et al[9] found a 64% response rate to fluoxetine treatment during a 6- to 7-week trial. Also, it has been proposed theoretically that differences in the rate of development of neurotransmitter systems could contribute to differences in response to antidepressants. Data from studies of nonprimates[20] and rhesus monkeys[21] suggest that the development of monoaminergic storage capacity and synthesis continues through childhood and is generally more rapid for serotonin than for catecholamines.

STUDY LIMITATIONS

The patients recruited evidenced relatively severe and persistent symptoms of depression and would not be representative of all children and adolescents with MDD. Of 150 patients who did not enroll in the treatment phase of the study following the initial interview, only 55 (37%) had not met MDD criteria initially. The rest improved, met exclusionary criteria, or refused enrollment in the study. Twenty-nine patients responded to the evaluation or single-blind placebo.

Following randomization, attrition during the study resulted in greater attrition from the placebo group because of failure to respond. Most patients had been seen weekly for at least 8 visits and discontinuation from the study came at the patient's or parent's request and it would have been unethical to continue studying these patients. Every effort was made to have the patients continue with the study as long as possible. It is impossible to know whether nonresponders at week 4 or later would have become responders if they had continued longer in the study in either group, which would effect the result of the χ^2 test of the CGI scale at exit. However, data in adults suggest that placebo responders are more likely to occur early in treatment and the placebo response rate in this study parallels adult findings and is not excessively low. Additionally, the analysis of the CDRS-R using slopes from individual regressions should not be effected much by attrition. Several simulation studies have shown that an unweighted average of individual slopes is subject to little bias owing to dropouts.[37,38] Also, an additional slopes analysis was performed using the procedure of Mori et al[37] that was designed specifically to adjust for nonrandom dropouts. Both of these analyses showed significant treatment effect.

Finally, the study may have been too short to demonstrate significant differences between the groups in global functioning (the CGAS) and, as comorbid disorders were frequent, measurements assessing other symptoms, not only depression (the BPRS-C), might change differentially as a function of treatment, although both groups improved on both measurements. Self-report measurements for children and adolescents, as mentioned previously, did not significantly differentiate the 2 groups, presumably in part because of relatively poor reliability. For example, some patients rated themselves on self-report as having minimal or no symptoms, whereas on clinical interview, they met criteria for MDD.

CONCLUSION

These data indicate that fluoxetine at 20 mg/d is safe and effective in children and adolescents with MDD. Replication is needed to evaluate the certainty of this finding. In addition, whether long-term treatment would result in the amelioration of school, general functioning, or concurrent comorbidities is unknown. How long to continue fluoxetine treatment, assuming it is effective, deserves study. Subsequent analyses to evaluate predictors of response are planned.

Accepted for publication August 20, 1996.

This study was supported by grants MH-39188 (Dr Emslie) and MH-41115 (Department of Psychiatry, University of Texas Southwestern Medical Center at Dallas) from the National Institute of Mental Health, National Institutes of Health, Bethesda, Md.

Presented in part at the annual New Clinical Drug Evaluation Unit Meeting, Orlando, Fla, June 2, 1995, and the Annual Meeting of the American Academy of Child & Adolescent Psychiatry, New Orleans, La, October 19, 1995.

We thank Kenneth Z. Altshuler, MD, Stanton Sharp Distinguished Chair and Chairman, Department of Psychiatry, for his administrative support; the staff of the Child and Adolescent Psychiatry Service at Children's Medical Center for their clinical assistance; Melody Brummett, for her secretarial support; and Christina Gullion, PhD, for design, management of the randomization procedures, and data management advice.

Reprints: Graham J. Emslie, MD, Department of Psychiatry, University of Texas Southwestern Medical Center at Dallas, 5323 Harry Hines Blvd, Dallas, TX 75235-9070.

REFERENCES

1. Fleming JE, Offord DR. Epidemiology of childhood depressive disorders: a critical review. *J Am Acad Child Adolesc Psychiatry.* 1990;29:571-580.
2. Weinberg W, Rehmet A. Childhood affective disorder and school problems. In: Cantwell DP, Carlson GA, eds. *Affective Disorders in Childhood and Adolescence: An Update.* Jamaica, NY: Spectrum Publishing Inc; 1983:109-128.
3. Weinberg W, Emslie G. Adolescents and school problems: depression, suicide, and learning disorders. *Adv Adolesc Ment Health.* 1988;3:181-205.
4. Brent DA. Correlates of the medical lethality of suicide attempts in children and adolescents. *J Am Acad Child Adolesc Psychiatry.* 1987;26:87-91.
5. Pfeffer CR, Klerman GL, Hurt SW, Lesser M, Peskin JR, Siefker CA. Suicidal children grow up: demographic and clinical risk factors for adolescent suicide attempts. *J Am Acad Child Adolesc Psychiatry.* 1991;30:609-616.
6. Rao U, Weissman MM, Martin JA, Hammond RW. Childhood depression and risk of suicide: a preliminary report of a longitudinal study. *J Am Acad Child Adolesc Psychiatry.* 1993;32:21-27.
7. Kovacs M, Gatsonis C. Secular trends in age at onset of major depressive disorder in a clinical sample of children. *J Psychiatr Res.* 1994;28:319-329.
8. Hazell P, O'Connell D, Heathcote D, Robertson J, Henry D. Efficacy of tricyclic drugs in treating child and adolescent depression: a meta-analysis. *BMJ.* 1995; 310:897-901.
9. Boulos C, Kutcher S, Gardner D, Young E. An open naturalistic trial of fluoxetine in adolescents and young adults with treatment-resistant major depression. *J Child Adolesc Psychopharmacol.* 1992;2:103-111.
10. Ghaziuddin N, Naylor MW, King CA. Fluoxetine in tricyclic refractory depression in adolescents. *Depression.* 1995;2:287-291.
11. Jain U, Birmaher B, Garcia M, Al-Shabbout M, Ryan N. Flouxetine in children and adolescents with mood disorders: a chart review of efficacy and adverse effects. *J Child Adolesc Psychopharmacol.* 1992;2:259-265.
12. Tierney E, Paramjit JT, Leinas JF, Rosenberg LA, Riddle MA. Sertraline for major depression in children and adolescents: preliminary clinical experience. *J Child Adolesc Psychopharmacol.* 1995;5:13-27.
13. Simeon J, Dinicola V, Ferguson HB, Copping W. Adolescent depression: a placebo-controlled fluoxetine treatment study and follow-up. *Prog Neuropsychopharmacol Biol Psychiatry.* 1990;14:791-795.
14. Baldessarini RJ. Current status of antidepressants: clinical pharmacology and therapy. *J Clin Psychiatry.* 1989;50:117-126.
15. Trivedi MH, Rush AJ. Efficacy of antidepressant medications, part 1: a meta-analysis. *Neuropsychopharmacology.* In press.
16. Thase ME, Trivedi MH, Rush AJ. MAOIs in the contemporary treatment of depression. *Neuropsychopharmacology.* 1995;12:185-219.
17. *Clinical Practice Guideline Number 5: Depression in Primary Care, 2: Treatment of Major Depression.* Rockville, Md: US Dept of Health and Human Services, Agency for Health Care Policy and Research; 1993. Health Care Policy and Research publication 93-0551.
18. Kutcher S, Boulos C, Ward B, Marton P, Simeon J, Ferguson HB, Szalai J, Katic M, Roberts N, Dubois C, Reed K. Response to desipramine treatment in adolescent depression: a fixed-dose, placebo-controlled trial. *J Am Acad Child Adolesc Psychiatry.* 1994;33:686-694.
19. Ryan ND. Pharmacotherapy of adolescent major depression: beyond TCAs. *Psychopharmacol Bull.* 1990;26:75-79.
20. Black IB, Hendry IA, Iversen LL. Trans-synaptic regulation of growth and development of adrenergic neurons in a mouse sympathetic ganglion. *Brain Res.* 1971; 24:229-240.
21. Goldman-Rakic CP, Brown RM. Postnatal development of monoamine content and synthesis in the cerebral cortex of rhesus monkeys. *Dev Brain Res.* 1982;4:339-349.
22. Conners CK. Methodology of antidepressant drug trials for treating depression in adolescents. *J Child Adolesc Psychopharmacol.* 1992;2:11-22.
23. Jensen PS, Ryan ND, Prien R. Psychopharmacology of child and adolescent major depression: present status and future directions. *J Child Adolesc Psychopharmacol.* 1992;2:31-45.
24. Strober M. The pharmacotherapy of depressive illness in adolescents, III: diagnostic and conceptual issues in studies of tricyclic antidepressants. *J Child Adolesc Psychopharmacol.* 1992;2:23-29.
25. Herjanic B, Reich W. Development of a structured psychiatric interview for children: agreement between child and parent on individual symptoms. *J Abnorm Child Psychol.* 1982;10:307-324.
26. Welner Z, Reich W, Herjanic B, Jung KG, Amado H. Reliability, validity, and parent-child agreement studies of the Diagnostic Interview for Children and Adolescents (DICA). *J Am Acad Child Adolesc Psychiatry.* 1987;26:649-653.
27. Chambers WJ, Puig-Antich J, Hirsch M, Paez P, Ambrosini PJ, Tabrizi MA, Davies M. The assessment of affective disorders in children and adolescents by semistructured interview: test-retest reliability of the K-SADS-P. *Arch Gen Psychiatry.* 1985;42:696-702.
28. Poznanski EO, Freman LN, Mokros HB. Children's Depression Rating Scale–Revised (September 1984). *Psychopharmacol Bull.* 1985;21:979-989.
29. Kovacs M. The Children's Depression Inventory (CDI). *Psychopharmacol Bull.* 1985;21:995-998.
30. Beck AT, Ward CH, Mendelson M, Mock J, Erbaugh J. An inventory for measuring depression. *Arch Gen Psychiatry.* 1961;4:561-571.
31. Weinberg WA, Emslie GJ. Weinberg Screening Affective Scale (WSAS and WSAS-SF). *J Child Neurol.* 1988;3:294-296.
32. Shaffer D, Gould MS, Brasic J, Ambrosini P, Fisher P, Bird H, Aluwahlia S. A Children's Global Assessment Scale (CGAS) (for children 4 to 16 years of age). *Psychopharmacol Bull.* 1985;21:747-748.
33. Overall JE, Pfefferbaum B. The Brief Psychiatry Rating Scale for Children. *Psychopharmacol Bull.* 1982;18:10-16.
34. Fleiss JL. *The Design and Analysis of Clinical Experiments.* New York, NY: John Wiley & Sons Inc; 1986.
35. Fleiss JL. *Statistical Methods for Rates and Proportions.* 2nd ed. New York, NY: John Wiley & Sons Inc; 1981.
36. Kraemer HC, Thieman S. A strategy to use soft data effectively in randomized controlled clinical trials. *J Consult Clin Psychol.* 1989;57:148-154.
37. Mori M, Woodworth GG, Woolson RF. Application of empirical Bayes inference to estimation of rate of change in the presence of informative right censoring. *Stat Med.* 1992;11:621-631.
38. Kaplin EL, Meier P. Nonparametric estimation from incomplete observations. *J Am Stat Assoc.* 1958;53:457-481.
39. Puig-Antich J, Perel JM, Lupatkin W, Chambers WJ, Tabrizi MA, King J, Goetz R, Davies M, Stiller RL. Imipramine in prepubertal major depressive disorders. *Arch Gen Psychiatry.* 1987;44:81-89.
40. Puig-Antich J, Perel JM, Lupatikin W, Chambers WJ, Shea C, Tabrizi MA, Stiller RL. Plasma levels of imipramine (IMI) and desmethylimipramine (DMI) and clinical response in prepubertal major depressive disorder: a preliminary report. *J Am Acad Child Psychiatry.* 1979;18:616-627.
41. Geller B, Cooper TB, McCombs HG, Graham DL, Wells J. Double-blind, placebo-controlled study of nortriptyline in depressed children using a 'fixed plasma level' design. *Psychopharmacol Bull.* 1989;25:101-108.
42. Geller B, Cooper TB, Graham DL, Marsteller FA, Bryant DM. Double-blind, placebo-controlled study of nortriptyline in depressed adolescents using a 'fixed plasma level' design. *Psychopharmacol Bull.* 1990;26:85-90.

A Randomized Trial of Assertive Community Treatment for Homeless Persons With Severe Mental Illness

Anthony F. Lehman, MD, MSPH; Lisa B. Dixon, MD; Eimer Kernan, MSW; Bruce R. DeForge, PhD; Leticia T. Postrado, PhD

Background: This experiment evaluated the effectiveness of an innovative program of assertive community treatment (ACT) for homeless persons with severe and persistent mental illnesses.

Methods: One hundred fifty-two homeless persons with severe and persistent mental illness were randomized to either the experimental ACT program or to usual community services. Baseline assessments included the Structured Clinical Interview for *DSM-III-R*, Quality-of-Life Interview, Colorado Symptom Index, and the Medical Outcomes Study 36-Item Short Form Health Survey. All assessments (except the Structured Clinical Interview) were repeated at the 2-, 6-, and 12-month follow-up evaluations.

Results: Subjects in the ACT program used significantly fewer psychiatric inpatient days, fewer emergency department visits, and more psychiatric outpatient visits than the comparison subjects. The ACT subjects also spent significantly more days in stable community housing, and they experienced significantly greater improvements in symptoms, life satisfaction, and perceived health status.

Conclusions: Relative to usual community care, the ACT program for homeless persons with severe and persistent mental illness shifts the locus of care from crisis-oriented services to ongoing outpatient care and produces better housing, clinical, and life satisfaction outcomes.

Arch Gen Psychiatry. 1997;54:1038-1043

From the Center for Mental Health Services Research (Drs Lehman, Dixon, and Postrado and Ms Kernan) and the Department of Family Medicine (Dr DeForge), University of Maryland, Baltimore.

NO ISSUE has done more to focus public concerns about the care of persons with severe and persistent mental illness (SPMI) in the community than the substantial numbers of these persons who are visibly homeless in our cities. Although estimates vary, data suggest that 20% to 35% of homeless persons suffer from SPMI.[1,2] The need for more effective community-based services to engage these persons in treatment and to help them achieve stable housing is compelling.

This article reports an experiment to evaluate the effect of an assertive community treatment (ACT) program on the service patterns and outcomes of homeless persons with SPMI. Two avenues of research led to this project. First, a series of studies have documented the prevalence of serious mental disorders among homeless persons and the failure of conventional community-based service systems to engage these patients and address their needs.[1-3] Second, prior studies have demonstrated the effectiveness of ACT programs for persons with SPMI who are frequent users of crisis-oriented services (emergency departments and hospitals) and who are at high risk of relapse.[4,5] Only 1 of these ACT program studies specifically addressed its application to homeless persons.[6] That study showed promising results, but it suffered from a variety of methodologic problems, especially subject attrition. Therefore, it seemed timely to test the proposition that an ACT program can benefit homeless persons with SPMI.

This study tests the hypotheses that an ACT program, compared with the usual array of community-based services for homeless persons with SPMI, (1) reduces use of crisis-oriented health care services; (2) enhances use of continuous, comprehensive community-based services; (3) reduces homelessness and enhances stable community-based housing; (4) reduces adverse social events (incarceration); (5) improves clinical outcomes; and (6) improves functional status and quality of life.

SUBJECTS AND METHODS

SAMPLE

Study participants met enrollment criteria for SPMI and homelessness. The SPMI criteria were based on diagnosis, duration of illness, and level of disability, as defined in prior studies.[7-9] The criteria were hierarchical.

Persons were automatically eligible if they were receiving Supplemental Security Income, Social Security Disability Income, or 100% Veterans Administration disability benefits because of a mental disorder (other than substance use disorder only) or if they had a diagnosis of schizophrenia (*DSM-III-R*[10] codes 295.1, 295.2, 295.3, 295.6, or 295.9) or schizoaffective disorder (code 295.7).

Persons who did not meet the first criterion were considered eligible if they had another Axis I mental disorder (other psychotic disorder, major affective disorder, anxiety disorder) and had an extensive prior hospitalization history (at least 2 prior psychiatric hospitalizations of >21 days within the prior 3 years, a total of at least 42 days prior to a current hospitalization, or ≥90 total days in a psychiatric hospital or nursing home during the past 3 years).

Persons not meeting either of the first 2 criteria were eligible if they had a history of mental disorder lasting for at least the past year, during which they had been unable to spend at least 75% of their time in some gainful activity (competitive employment, student in a regular educational program, or primary homemaker) owing to the mental disorder.

To qualify as homeless, participants had to have been literally homeless (ie, on the streets or in a shelter or mission) for at least 5 of the past 45 days or 14 of the past 180 days, or in temporary accommodations with at least 2 residential moves during the past 6 months. These criteria were based on the National Institutes of Mental Health definition of homelessness and prior studies of the homeless,[11] and excluded persons who were simply at risk of homelessness.

Subjects were recruited during a 19-month period from March 1, 1991, to September 30, 1992. Project staff screened all persons acutely admitted to inner-city psychiatric hospitals and screened all referrals from agencies serving homeless persons in metropolitan Baltimore, Md (primary health care agencies, shelters, missions, and soup kitchens). After providing a complete description of the study to participants, written informed consent was obtained. Of the persons screened, 183 were eligible and 152 (83%) agreed to participate. These included 44 (90%) of 49 eligible inpatients and 108 (80.6%) of 134 eligible persons from community-based agencies for the homeless. Those refusing to participate were more likely to be women (58% of refusers vs 35% of consenters; $\chi^2=5.50$, $df=1$, $P=.02$). Those refusing and those consenting to participation did not differ significantly on age, race, or referral diagnosis. Through stratified random assignment, 77 participants (22 inpatients and 55 community-based subjects) were randomly assigned to the ACT program, and 75 (22 inpatients and 53 community-based subjects) were assigned to usual comparison services.

INTERVENTIONS

The experimental condition was the ACT program, modeled after the ACT program first developed by Stein and Test.[12] Consistent with the their philosophy, the ACT program defined its mission broadly to integrate assertive, community-based clinical treatment with intensive case management and advocacy. The ACT team's long-term commitment was to promote continuity of care, and the team was available 24 hours every day. The ACT team consisted of 12 full-time equivalent staff, including a program director with a masters' degree in social work, a full-time psychiatrist and medical director, 6 clinical case managers (social workers, psychiatric nurses, and rehabilitation counselors), 2 consumer advocates, a secretary-receptionist, a part-time family outreach worker from the Alliance for the Mentally Ill of metropolitan Baltimore, and a part-time nurse practitioner to treat chronic medical problems. Each patient was assigned to a "mini-team" consisting of a clinical case manager (case load, 10-12 patients), an attending psychiatrist, and a consumer advocate. The entire ACT team, including the consumer advocates, worked together in decision making and each staff member was knowledgeable about most of the patients. Teamwork was fostered through daily sign-out rounds and twice-weekly treatment planning meetings.

The ACT program was implemented according to guidelines provided by ACT program consultants in Madison, Wis. The ACT team adhered closely to this model; however, the consumer advocates and the family outreach worker are not standard components of ACT programs. After the first year of operation, a site visit by an ACT program expert from Wisconsin confirmed our adherence to the ACT program model. As a result of the site visit, certain aspects of the program were further refined; specifically, implementation of daily sign-out rounds. The ACT program has been described in more detail elsewhere.[13]

The comparison condition consisted of services as usual in Baltimore. The public mental health system in Baltimore encompasses 7 community mental health centers operating under a nonprofit, private, local mental health authority, which was developed as part of the Robert Wood Johnson Foundation Program on Chronic Mental Illness.[14] Several community-based psychiatric inpatient and emergency facilities, including those affiliated with 2 major teaching institutions, provide acute inpatient and crisis-oriented care. A variety of community agencies in Baltimore focus specifically on serving the homeless. Health Care for the Homeless offers outreach, advocacy, case management, primary health care, and walk-in mental health counseling and some long-term outpatient mental health care. The goal of Health Care for the Homeless is to encourage homeless persons to seek health care and to facilitate their transition to mainstream health care services. The provider network for homeless persons also includes several privately run shelters, missions, and soup kitchens.

To document that the 2 intervention conditions differed on critical process variables, staff from the ACT team (n=11) and from the various community programs (n=83) serving the comparison patients completed the Community Program Philosophy Scale (CPPS),[15] a standardized measure of staff practices. The ACT program scored significantly higher than the comparison services on the 3 subscales known to differentiate ACT programs from clinic-based psychotherapy and medication services and from case management services. These subscales include emergency access (ACT program mean=16.0, SD=2.53; comparison mean=13.2, SD=3.01; $t=3.35$,

Continued on next page

$df=1,91$, $P=.005$); longitudinality of care (ACT program mean=15.5, SD=1.64; comparison mean=14.8, SD=2.90; $t=4.60$, $df=1,92$, $P<.001$); and team model (ACT program mean=16.5, SD=3.41; comparison mean=14.7, SD=2.62; $t=2.13$, $df=1,92$, $P=.04$). The ACT program also scored significantly higher than the comparison programs on some CPPS subscales that distinguish case management from routine clinic services, including housing assistance, linking to entitlements, and referral advocacy. The ACT team and the usual services did not differ on 2 other CPPS case management subscales, outreach orientation and vocational emphasis. These CPPS data indicate that we compared a well-developed ACT program with usual services that included generic case management services but did not adhere to the ACT model. At the time this study was designed and implemented, the most recently developed standardized fidelity measures for ACT programs were unavailable.[16,17]

CITYWIDE ENHANCEMENT OF HOUSING

The project grant enhanced housing opportunities for all subjects in the study. Specifically, 40 additional Housing and Urban Development Section 8 housing vouchers were allocated by the citywide mental health authority for the project and were available to either experimental or comparison subjects on a first-come, first-served basis. Also, the grant expanded a transitional homeless shelter by 10 beds to provide more access to immediate temporary shelter for ACT and comparison subjects. This shelter program provided case management for the comparison patients. Hence, the experiment occurred in a somewhat enriched housing environment than that which existed for other homeless persons in Baltimore.

ASSESSMENTS

Major assessments were conducted at baseline (after randomization) and at 2-, 6-, and 12-month follow-up points. Subjects were also contacted briefly once per month to collect interim housing and service usage data and to maintain tracking information. These monthly contacts were focused around a structured service report form to reduce the reactivity of these contacts as service episodes, a risk with persons who lack adequate contacts with the formal service system. When service needs or requests were made by subjects at these contacts, the research assistants provided the subject with a list of service agencies but did not intervene on the subject's behalf.

At baseline, subjects completed the Structured Clinical Interview for *DSM-III-R* (SCID),[18] the Lehman Quality-of-Life Interview (QOLI),[19] the Colorado Symptom Index (CSI),[20] and the Medical Outcomes Study 36-Item Short Form Health Survey (SF-36).[21] All are standardized instruments with good psychometric properties among persons with SPMI. The QOLI subjective measures provided the assessments of life satisfaction, and the QOLI objective measures provided the assessments of functional status and access to resources and opportunities. The QOLI, CSI, and SF-36 were repeated at each of the follow-up points. Subjects were paid $40 for the baseline assessment and $20 for each of the major follow-up assessments. Food vouchers were offered at the monthly tracking contacts.

FOLLOW-UP RATES AND ATTRITION

Two-, 6-, and 12-month follow-up rates were 94%, 88%, and 83%, respectively. Attrition by 12 months was higher among comparison subjects (23%) than among ACT program subjects (13%). However, there were no significant differences between study completers and noncompleters on any of the demographic, diagnostic, or homeless variables, as given in **Table 1**.

DATA ANALYSES

Data analyses were designed to examine differences between the 2 intervention groups on demographics, diagnoses, and histories of homelessness at baseline, and on service usage, housing, clinical measurements, and quality-of-life outcomes during the 1-year follow-up period. Baseline group comparisons were accomplished using χ^2 analysis for categorical variables and *t* tests for continuous variables. Because the 2 groups differed by chance on race (Table 1), all of the following analyses included race as a covariate. All analyses were conducted with and without imputation of missing data (methods described below); no significant differences between these analyses were found, although the imputation improved statistical power.

The follow-up data were of 2 general types. First, data on housing status and service usage were collected on a monthly basis (client monthly checklist) and, hence, produced cumulative outcomes during the 1-year follow-up period (eg, cumulative days of inpatient treatment, cumulative outpatient visits, and cumulative days living on the streets). For these variables, missing data were imputed using the mean for each person for the months in which data were obtained. The amount of data imputed for individuals ranged from none to 20%. The groups were compared on these cumulative housing and service usage outcomes by analysis of covariance (ANCOVA) with race (white or African American) as a covariate.

Second, the assessments of symptoms, health status, and quality of life were "point-in-time" outcomes repeated at baseline and at the 2-, 6-, and 12-month follow-up. Missing values were imputed at the 2- and 6-month follow-up points, using individual respondent means of the outcome at the time points bracketing the missing point. For example, a missing 6-month value would be imputed from the mean of the 2- and 12-month values for that person. If this could not be done owing to lack of 2 bracketing values, no imputation was performed. Therefore, missing values were not replaced for the 1-year follow-up. The proportion of missing values at any given time point ranged from 6% to 17%.

Repeated-measures 1-way ANCOVAs were used initially to test group, time, and group × time interaction effects on the CSI total symptom score. We conducted repeated-measures multiple ANCOVAs (MANCOVAs), assessing group, time, and group × time effects with race as a covariate for the multidimensional outcomes generated by the QOLI and SF-36. Even with imputation of missing values, the power of these repeated-measures analyses was limited, raising concern about type II errors.[22] Therefore, we also conducted ANCOVAs for all sets of measures at each time point to explore possible point-in-time group differences. All analyses were performed using SAS-PC[23] and SPSS/PC.[24]

Table 1. Subject Characteristics*

Characteristic	ACT Subjects (n=77)	Comparison Subjects (n=75)
Men	65	70
African American	61†	84
White	35	12
Mean (SD) age, y	39 (9.5)	36 (8.3)
Mean (SD) education, y	11 (2.9)	11 (2.5)
Never married	58	66
Veterans	20	19
Diagnoses		
Schizophrenia‡	46	43
Schizoaffective	14	14
Bipolar	17	24
Depressive disorder	6	11
Other Axis I disorder	17	8
Comorbid substance use disorder	71	71
Total time homeless, y		
<1	25	26
1-9	63	63
>10	12	11
Homeless >1 year	76	74

*ACT indicates assertive community treatment. Data are given as percentage of the total unless otherwise indicated.
†$\chi^2(3)=11.8$, $P<.01$.
‡Diagnoses are from the baseline Structured Clinical Interview for DSM-III-R.[18]

Table 2. Housing Locations During the Follow-up Year

Housing Location	Adjusted* Mean (SEM) Days in Location: ACT Subjects	Comparison Subjects
Psychiatric hospital	35.4 (8.7)†	66.9 (8.9)
Substance abuse hospital	5.3 (1.6)	3.8 (1.6)
General medical hospital	4.1 (2.0)	3.7 (2.0)
Homeless on streets	10.1 (5.2)	24.3 (5.3)
Homeless shelter	83.3 (10.3)	89.5 (10.5)
Jail	9.0 (6.1)	19.3 (6.2)
Community housing	210.2 (12.3)‡	160.1 (12.5)

*Adjusted for race as covariate. ACT indicates assertive community treatment.
†ANCOVA (analysis of covariance) $F=6.22$, $df=1,144$, $P=.01$.
‡ANCOVA $F=7.86$, $df=1,144$, $P=.006$.

RESULTS

SAMPLE CHARACTERISTICS

The demographics, SCID diagnoses, and homelessness patterns of the sample are given in Table 1. The 2 groups are comparable except for a higher percentage of African Americans randomized to the comparison condition.

SERVICE OUTCOMES

The ACT program subjects accumulated significantly fewer inpatient days than the comparison subjects (**Table 2**) and fewer emergency department visits (ACT program subjects adjusted mean=0.8 visits, SEM=0.3; comparison subjects adjusted mean=2.0, SEM=0.3; ANCOVA $F=6.96$, $df=1,144$, $P=.009$). The ACT program subjects used significantly more outpatient mental health visits (ACT program subjects adjusted mean=102.7, SEM=6.4; comparison subjects adjusted mean=39.5, SEM=6.6; ANCOVA $F=45.6$, $df=1,144$, $P<.001$).

With regard to use of general medical services, the groups did not differ significantly on cumulative general medical inpatient days (Table 2), emergency department visits, or outpatient visits for general medical care. Moreover, the 2 groups were similar in the amounts of inpatient care and emergency department visits for substance use disorders (data not shown). The ACT program subjects did accumulate more outpatient visits for substance abuse treatment (ACT program subjects adjusted mean=19.0 visits, SEM=3.0; comparison subjects adjusted mean=4.9, SEM=3.1; ANCOVA $F=10.8$, $df=1,144$, $P=.001$).

HOUSING OUTCOMES

During the follow-up period, the ACT program subjects spent significantly more days in stable community housing (Table 2) than the comparison subjects. The ACT subjects spent on average 58% fewer days on the streets without shelter and 53% fewer days in jail, but these differences were not statistically significant ($P>.05$) (Table 2).

The ACT program subjects were significantly more satisfied with their housing at the 6-month follow-up point, but not at either the 2- or 12-month follow-up points. Housing satisfaction mean adjusted ratings (1=terrible to 7=delighted) at 2 months were: ACT program subjects=4.60, SEM=0.15 vs comparison subjects=4.39, SEM=0.16; at 6 months: ACT program subjects=4.99, SEM=0.16 vs comparison subjects=4.46, SEM=0.17 (ANCOVA $F=5.18$, $df=1,139$, $P=.02$); and at 12 months: ACT program subjects=5.19, SEM=0.16 vs comparison subjects=5.07, SEM=0.18.

CLINICAL OUTCOMES

Repeated-measures ANCOVA for the CSI total score revealed significant group ($F=5.14$, $df=1,122$, $P<.001$) and time ($F=9.16$, $df=3,363$, $P<.001$) effects but no significant group × time effect. Similarly, repeated-measures ANCOVA for the SF-36 yielded significant group ($F=6.61$, $df=1,119$, $P=.01$) and time ($F=7.87$, $df=3,357$, $P<.001$) effects but no group × time interaction effect.

Point-in-time comparisons of the ACT and comparison subjects revealed no differences at baseline. At the 2-, 6-, and 12-month follow-up points, the ACT program subjects had better clinical outcomes as measured by the CSI. Adjusted mean CSI ratings (a lower CSI score means more symptoms) for the ACT and comparison groups, respectively, at 2 months were: 4.10 (SEM=0.10) vs 3.61 (SEM=0.10) (ANCOVA $F=11.88$, $df=1,147$, $P=.001$); at 6 months, 4.24 (SEM=0.10) vs 3.68 (SEM=0.10) (ANCOVA $F=15.34$, $df=1,147$, $P<.001$); and at 12 months, 4.12 (SEM=0.11) vs 3.77 (SEM=0.11) (ANCOVA $F=5.04$, $df=1,121$, $P=.03$). On the SF-36, ACT program subjects had better self-rated health status outcomes at 2 and 6 months, but this difference was not present at 1 year (**Table 3**).

Table 3. Medical Outcomes Study 36-Item Short Form Health Survey (MOS SF-36) Adjusted* Mean Scores

MOS Subscale	Follow-up Period, mo		
	2	6	12
General health			
Comparison subjects	42.4 (1.6)	42.4 (1.7)	39.1 (1.8)†
ACT program subjects	44.4 (1.5)	45.3 (1.6)	45.9 (1.7)
Physical functioning			
Comparison subjects	79.0 (2.8)	83.0 (2.7)	83.6 (3.7)
ACT program subjects	86.2 (2.8)	88.4 (2.6)	84.5 (3.5)
Mental health			
Comparison subjects	47.2 (1.9)‡	45.7 (1.9)§	46.8 (2.2)
ACT program subjects	53.2 (1.9)	53.6 (1.9)	51.7 (2.0)
Bodily pain			
Comparison subjects	60.6 (4.4)	59.6 (4.4)	64.7 (4.8)
ACT program subjects	69.3 (4.3)	66.1 (4.3)	68.7 (4.6)
Social functioning			
Comparison subjects	41.1 (2.1)	41.7 (1.9)	42.4 (2.3)
ACT program subjects	46.0 (2.0)	46.0 (1.9)	42.7 (2.1)
Vitality			
Comparison subjects	41.8 (1.9)∥	40.4 (1.9)¶	43.0 (2.1)
ACT program subjects	48.2 (1.8)	46.0 (1.9)	46.6 (1.9)

*Adjusted for race as covariate. All scales range from 0 (poorest) to 100 (best). Numbers inside parentheses are SE of adjusted means. ACT indicates assertive community treatment.

†ANCOVA (analysis of covariance) F=7.45, df=1,147, P=.01.

‡ANCOVA F=4.75, df=1,147, P=.03.

§ANCOVA F=8.39, df=1,147, P=.004.

∥ANCOVA F=5.84, df=1,147, P=.02.

¶ANCOVA F=4.14, df=1,147, P=.04.

QUALITY OF LIFE

Quality of life was assessed using the QOLI. Repeated-measures MANCOVAs revealed no between-group differences on the objective quality-of-life variables, including the number of daily activities, frequency of family and social contacts, and employment rates. Subjects in both groups did increase the frequency of their contacts with their families over the year, but this did not differ between the 2 groups.

For the life satisfaction variables, repeated-measures MANCOVAs showed that both groups of patients improved significantly on all areas of life satisfaction between the baseline and 12-month follow-up. The MANCOVAs for the life satisfaction subscales revealed no between-group differences at baseline (MANCOVA F=0.33, *df*=8,124, *P*=.97), 2 months (MANCOVA F=1.55, *df*=8,139, *P*=.14), and 12 months (MANCOVA F=1.19, *df*=8,103, *P*=.32). However, at the 6-month follow-up, ACT patients expressed greater life satisfaction than the comparison patients (MANCOVA F=2.93, *df*=8,139, *P*=.005). Results of ANCOVAs revealed that the ACT patients were more satisfied than the comparison patients with their general well-being (ACT program subjects adjusted mean=4.70, SEM=0.16; vs comparison subjects adjusted mean=4.17, SEM=0.16; ANCOVA F=5.51, *df*=1,147, *P*=.02), their neighborhoods (ACT program subjects adjusted mean=4.89, SEM=0.16 vs comparison subjects adjusted mean=4.13, SEM=0.16; ANCOVA F=10.67, *df*=1,147, *P*=.001), and their health (ACT program subjects adjusted mean=4.98, SEM=0.12 vs comparison subjects adjusted mean=4.50, SEM=0.12; ANCOVA F=7.66, *df*=1,147, *P*=.006). No between-group differences were found on satisfaction with safety, family relations, social relations, or finances.

COMMENT

The ACT program was associated with significant shifts in the patterns of housing, mental health services, and patient outcomes. The sample was a very high-risk group. About 75% had accumulated more than 1 year of homelessness. More than half had a diagnosis of schizophrenia or schizoaffective disorder and another one quarter had a diagnosis of major affective disorder. More than 70% had a comorbid substance use disorder. The ACT program subjects spent significantly more days stably housed, and they used fewer crisis-oriented services (inpatient days and emergency department visits) and more outpatient visits than did the comparison patients. These effects on patterns of care are consistent with prior ACT studies.[4,5] The ACT program subjects also experienced greater symptom reduction and greater improvements in life satisfaction and perceived health status.

The observed patterns of care confirm that the 2 service conditions differed in the ways hypothesized for ACT programs vs usual community care. Conceptually, ACT programs are designed to provide continuous, comprehensive care that can intervene rapidly to avert emerging crises and that can reduce the risk for future ones. This is achieved through the complete integration of case management and clinical care (including substance abuse treatment) on the ACT team. In the comparison condition, subjects received clinical care and case management from various community agencies. These services, with their inherent barriers to coordination and continuity, are less able than an ACT program to deal with crises.

No differences were found in the areas of work and interpersonal relations, and in related areas of life satisfaction. These findings are also consistent with prior studies of ACT programs.[4,5] In this study, lack of influence on such outcomes as employment is not surprising because the ACT team focused instead on clinical stabilization and housing. However, longer-term improvements in functional status are important, and the ACT team has recently been enhanced to include employment specialists with the goal of assisting subjects to find jobs if they so desire and are able. This is the focus of a new federally funded employment demonstration project.

The improvements among the comparison group raise an additional issue. To what degree did the services for the comparison group represent services as usual? The fact that the conditions of many of the subjects improved over time may indicate that the existing service system, while not optimal, afforded a reasonable safety net for this population. However, there are some reasons to believe that the comparison condition was not typical. As mentioned in the "Subjects and Methods" section, funding for the project enhanced housing options for both intervention groups. The project funded an additional 10 shelter beds with attached case management and 40 Housing and Urban Development Section 8 housing certificates that were available to the comparison group as well as the ACT program subjects. These housing opportunities provided better short- and long-term housing markets for the comparison group than would have been available to homeless persons not in the study.

In addition, a confound was introduced partway through the study when the city itself funded an additional ACT-style program for homeless persons with mental illness at another community mental health center. This made an intervention similar to the experimental program available to some of the comparison subjects.

Both the enhanced housing and the "contamination" of the comparison condition with an ACT-style program could attenuate any differences between the ACT program and the "services as usual" comparison. Unfortunately, data on the comparison subjects' use of these grant-funded housing enhancements and of the other ACT-style programs were unavailable to adequately control for potential confounds in the analyses.

There are a variety of strengths and limitations to this study. It successfully used an experimental design and had low subject refusal and attrition rates. A standard battery of outcome measures was used, and we monitored both services and patient outcomes, thus providing an empirical validation that the 2 conditions differed on expected service variables as well as on outcomes. The major limitations of the study are that it involved a single demonstration city, thus limiting its generalizability; had a relatively short follow-up period, thus limiting its capacity to assess longer-term group differences, especially functional status; and experienced some contamination of the comparison condition, thus leaving open the possibility that the experiment underestimates the relative value of an ACT program for these homeless persons with SPMI. The study also does not provide information on the effectiveness of ACT relative to other model programs for the homeless with severe mental illness, nor does it permit a "dismantling" analysis of the ACT model to determine if some specific components of ACT explain the program's success.

At this time of major changes in the health care system that are driven by concerns about cost-effectiveness, it is critical to have access to data on interventions for high-risk subjects. Based on the results of this study, the ACT model appears effective for homeless persons with SPMI. An analysis comparing the costs of the ACT program with usual care is underway. The fact that the state of Maryland decided to continue to fund the ACT program after cessation of the federal demonstration attests to its credibility. The most critical remaining issues are how to enhance the ACT model for these subjects to improve functional outcomes and whether subjects need to continue indefinitely in this intense service program. Strategies to transfer patients to less intensive levels of service after an extended period of stability need to be explored.

Finally, it is useful to comment on the utility of this type of services research in the development of health care policies. Effectiveness research addresses the transfer into routine practice of technologies previously shown to be efficacious under standard research conditions. In this study, the research on the efficacy of ACT for domiciled persons with SPMI[4,5] was extended to the homeless in a large service system. More of this type of research is needed to inform rational management of health care resources.

Accepted for publication January 16, 1997.

This work was supported by grant R18 MH48070 from the Center for Mental Health Services, University of Maryland, Baltimore.

A version of this paper was presented at the Annual Meeting of the American Psychiatric Association, Miami, Fla, May 1995.

We are indebted to Baltimore Mental Health Systems Inc, and its director, Stephen Baron, MSW, who hosted this demonstration project. We also acknowledge the participation and support of Health Care for the Homeless of Baltimore and Project PLASE, Baltimore.

Reprints: Anthony F. Lehman, MD, Department of Psychiatry, University of Maryland, Center for Mental Health Sciences, 685 W Baltimore St, MSTF Suite 300, Baltimore, MD 21201-1549.

REFERENCES

1. Lamb HR, ed. *The Homeless Mentally Ill.* Washington, DC: American Psychiatric Association Press; 1984.
2. Lehman AF, Cordray DS. Prevalence of alcohol, drug, and mental disorders among the homeless: one more time. *Contemp Drug Prob.* 1993;20:355-383.
3. Lamb HR, Lamb DM. Factors contributing to homelessness among the chronically and severely mentally ill. *Hosp Comunm Psychiatry.* 1990;41:301-305.
4. Burns BJ, Santos AB. Assertive community treatment: an update of randomized trials. *Hosp Commun Psychiatry.* 1995;46:669-675.
5. Olfson M. Assertive community treatment: an evaluation of the experimental evidence. *Hosp Commun Psychiatry.* 1990;41:634-641.
6. Morse GA, Calsyn RJ, Allen G, Tempelhoff B, Smith R. Experimental comparison of the effects of three treatment programs for homeless mentally ill people. *Hosp Commun Psychiatry.* 1992;43:1005-1010.
7. Goldman HH, Gatozzi AA, Taube CA. Defining and counting the chronically mentally ill. *Hosp Commun Psychiatry.* 1981;32:21-27.
8. Schinnar AP, Rothbard AB, Kanter R, Jung YS. An empirical literature review of definitions of severe and persistent mental illness. *Am J Psychiatry.* 1990;147:1602-1608.
9. Lehman AF, Postrado LT, Roth D, McNary S, Goldman HH. Continuity of care and client outcomes in the Robert Wood Johnson Foundation Program on Chronic Mental Illness. *Milbank Q.* 1994;72:105-122.
10. American Psychiatric Association. *Diagnostic and Statistical Manual of Mental Disorders, Third Edition, Revised.* Washington, DC: American Psychiatric Association; 1987.
11. Morrissey JP, Dennis DL, eds. *Homelessness and Mental Illness: Toward the Next Generation of Research Studies.* Rockville, Md; National Institute of Mental Health: 1990.
12. Stein LI, Test MA. Alternative to mental hospital treatment, I: conceptual model, treatment program, and clinical evaluation. *Arch Gen Psychiatry.* 1980;37:392-397.
13. Dixon LB, Krauss N, Kernan E, Lehman AF, DeForge BR. Modifying the PACT model to serve homeless persons with severe mental illness. *Psychiatr Serv.* 1995; 46:684-688.
14. Goldman HH, Morrissey J, Ridgely S. Evaluating the Robert Wood Johnson Foundation Program on Chronic Mental Illness. *Milbank Q.* 1994;71:37-47.
15. Hargreaves WA. Measuring program practices. Presented at the Third Workshop on Costs and Assessment in Psychiatry; October 29, 1994; Venice, Italy.
16. McGrew JH, Bond GR, Dietzen LL, Salyers MP. Measuring the fidelity of implementation of a mental health program model. *J Consult Clin Psychol.* 1994;62: 670-678.
17. Teague GB, Drake RE, Ackerson TH. Evaluating use of continuous treatment teams for persons with mental illness and substance abuse. *Psychiatr Serv.* 1995;46: 689-695.
18. Spitzer RL, Williams JBW. *Structured Clinical Interview for DSM-III-R.* New York, NY: New York State Psychiatric Institute; 1987.
19. Lehman AF. A quality of life interview for the chronically mentally ill. *Evaluation Program Planning.* 1988;11:51-62.
20. Shern DL, Wilson NZ, Coen AS, Patrick DC, Foster M, Bartsch DA. Client outcomes, II: longitudinal client data from the Colorado Treatment Outcome Study. *Milbank Q.* 1994:72:123-148.
21. Ware JE, Sherbourne CD. The MOS 36 Item Short-Form Health Survey (SF-36). *Med Care.* 1992;30:473-483.
22. Heintze JL. *PASS.* Kaysville, Utah: NCSS; 1991.
23. SAS Institute Inc. *SAS/PC Statistical Software Version 6.04 for the Personal Computer.* Cary, NC: SAS Institute; 1990.
24. SPSS Inc. *SPSS/PC Statistical Software Version 5.01 for the Personal Computer.* Chicago, Ill: SPSS Inc; 1992.

ORIGINAL ARTICLE

Sex Differences in Posttraumatic Stress Disorder

Naomi Breslau, PhD; Glenn C. Davis, MD; Patricia Andreski, MA; Edward L. Peterson, PhD; Lonni R. Schultz, PhD

Background: Epidemiologic surveys in the general population documented a higher rate of posttraumatic stress disorder (PTSD) in women than in men. To date, the finding has received little scientific attention. This study examines the extent to which sex differences in PTSD might be explained by previously identified risk factors and whether the sex difference in PTSD varied by age at exposure to traumatic events.

Methods: The *NIMH-DIS* (*NIMH Diagnostic Interview Schedule, Version III Revised*) was used to measure *DSM-IIIR* disorders in a random sample of 1007 young adults. Cox proportional hazards models were used to estimate changes in the hazards ratio for PTSD associated with sex when potential risk factors were included.

Results: Lifetime prevalence of exposure to traumatic events and number of traumatic events did not vary by sex. The prevalence of PTSD was higher for women than for men exposed to traumatic events (hazards ratio, 2.3; 95% confidence interval, 1.5-3.6). Preexisting anxiety disorders or major depressive disorders played a part in the observed sex difference in PTSD. Family history of anxiety disorder and early separation from parents, although significant risk factors for PTSD in subjects of both sexes, were unrelated to the sex difference in PTSD. The sex difference in PTSD was markedly greater if exposure occurred in childhood than later on.

Conclusions: Posttraumatic stress disorder is more likely to develop in females than in males after exposure to a traumatic event. Susceptibility to PTSD in females might be greater in childhood than after age 15 years. Explanations of the sex difference might involve characteristics of individuals and of the traumatic experiences.

Arch Gen Psychiatry. 1997;54:1044-1048

From the Departments of Psychiatry (Dr Breslau and Ms Andreski) and Biostatistics and Research Epidemiology (Drs Breslau, Peterson, and Schultz) and the Office of Academic Affairs (Dr Davis), Henry Ford Health Sciences Center, Detroit, Mich; Department of Psychiatry, Case Western Reserve University, Cleveland, Ohio (Drs Breslau and Davis); and Department of Psychiatry, University of Michigan, Ann Arbor (Drs Breslau and Davis).

RECENT epidemiologic surveys in the general population have documented a higher rate of posttraumatic stress disorder (PTSD) for women than for men.[1-4] The sex difference in PTSD might reflect greater vulnerability of women to the PTSD-inducing effects of traumatic experiences.[3,4] To date, the finding has received little scientific attention. Previous research[3,5-7] has identified other risk factors for PTSD, but it has not examined the extent to which these factors might explain the sex difference in the rate of PTSD. Suspected risk factors might interact with sex, increasing susceptibility to PTSD more in women than in men. Even if their effects on PTSD did not vary between subjects of both sexes, factors that increase the susceptibility of exposed persons to PTSD might explain the sex difference in PTSD if these factors were more common in women than in men.

We examined the extent to which the sex difference in PTSD might be explained by previously identified risk factors and whether the sex difference in PTSD varied by age at exposure to traumatic events, specifically if an exposure in childhood resulted in a wider sex difference in PTSD than if an exposure occurred later in life.

Several personal characteristics have been identified as factors that increase the probability of PTSD after exposure to traumatic events. Chief of these are preexisting psychiatric disorders, family history of anxiety disorders (ADs), and prolonged early separation from parents.[3,5-7] Previous research has not examined whether preexisting vulnerabilities are distributed differently between the subjects of both sexes or whether they influence differentially the susceptibility of subjects of both sexes to the PTSD effects of traumatic experiences. In reference to 1 of these characteristics, ie, preexisting psychiatric disorders, especially ADs and major depressive disorders (MDDs), a higher prevalence in women than men can be expected, based on evidence of an excess in these disorders in women that emerges early in life.[8-12] In this study, we examined the extent to which a greater susceptibility of women to the PTSD effects of traumatic events might be explained by

SUBJECTS AND METHODS

STUDY SAMPLE

A random sample of 1200 was drawn from all 21- to 30-year-old members of a 400 000-member health maintenance organization in southeast Michigan, which includes the city of Detroit and surrounding communities. A total of 1007 subjects (84%) were interviewed in person in 1989. Follow-up personal interviews were conducted with 979 subjects in 1992 and with 974 subjects in 1994, in each case exceeding 97% of the target sample, with the exclusion of 3 persons who died during the follow-up intervals. Telephone follow-up interviews were conducted with respondents who moved out of the area. At baseline, the median age was 26 years. Approximately 80% of the respondents were white, and 62% were female.

METHODS

Data Collection

Information about common psychiatric disorders, including PTSD, was elicited by the use of the *NIMH Diagnostic Interview Schedule, Version III Revised*[13] (*NIMH-DIS*) (revised to measure *DSM-IIIR* disorders). The PTSD section of the revised *NIMH-DIS* opens with a question in which typical PTSD events are listed, and respondents are asked whether any of these events has ever happened to them. The description of traumatic events follows closely the *DSM-IIIR* text, using the examples it lists (eg, "being attacked or raped, being in a fire or flood or bad traffic accident, being threatened with a weapon, or watching someone being seriously injured or killed").[14] A report of a qualifying stressor is followed by questions about the occurrence of PTSD symptoms after the event. The inquiry begins with the worst event and continues up to 3 events and their PTSD sequelae. For each event, information is elicited on age at exposure and time of onset of symptoms. Age at exposure to traumatic events was defined as age at first exposure and age at onset of PTSD, as the earliest age at which PTSD has ever occurred.

The *NIMH-DIS* is a structured interview, designed to be administered by experienced interviewers without clinical training. Detailed description of the *NIMH-DIS* and information about its reliability and validity have been previously reported.[15-17] A validation study of the modified PTSD section of the *NIMH-DIS* in the National Comorbidity Survey (NCS) yielded high agreement with clinicians' diagnoses.[4] In this study, the interviewers had 3 years or more of prior interviewing experience. An extensive training program was used to ensure close adherence to the questionnaire and the sequence of follow-up probes.

The baseline interview also inquired about sociodemographic characteristics, psychiatric disorders in parents and siblings, and early separation from parents. Data about family history of psychiatric disorders were gathered by the set of questions developed and used in the St Louis site of wave II of the Epidemiologic Catchment Area survey.[1] A module on ADs in relatives was added in this study.[3] A positive reply to the question of whether the respondent was brought up by someone other than parents for a period of 4 months or more before age 16 years was used to indicate early separation from parents.

Statistical Analysis

The analysis was performed on the combined data from the baseline and follow-up interviews. The baseline interview covered lifetime history of psychiatric disorders, up to the time of the interview. Follow-up interviews covered the interval periods from baseline to the first follow-up and from the first to the second follow-up. Combining follow-up and baseline data provides lifetime information up to age 35 years, the upper age limit at the last interview. Estimates of exposure to traumatic events were calculated on the entire sample of 1007 subjects. The analysis of sex differences in PTSD was performed on the subset *exposed to traumatic events*. Preexisting psychiatric disorders were measured as a single binary variable, which includes all ADs other than PTSD or MDD (any AD or MDD).

Cox proportional hazards models for censored survival data were used,[18-21] employing the Statistical Analysis Systems procedure (SAS Institute Inc, Cary, NC) for proportional hazards regression.[22] Time was defined as chronologic age, and all persons who did not develop PTSD by the time of their last interview were censored. Three successive models were calculated. The first model estimated the unadjusted hazards ratio for PTSD in women vs men. The second model also included preexisting AD or MDD as a time-dependent covariate. Other risk factors for PTSD (ie, family history of AD, early separation from parents, race, and education) were added to the third model as fixed covariates. A comparison of the coefficient of women vs men (sex factor) in the first model with the partial (adjusted) coefficients of this variable in the second and third models would reveal the extent to which the sex difference in PTSD might be explained by preexisting AD or MDD and other risk factors. A model with an interaction term was used to test whether preexisting AD or MDD had a differential effect on the probability of PTSD in women vs men. Interactions between sex and other risk factors were also tested. No significant interactions were detected using $\alpha < .15$.

To examine whether the sex difference in PTSD was greater if exposure to traumatic events occurred in childhood than later in life, we used age 15 years as the cutoff. In the child development literature, the cutoff is typically set between 14 and 15 years or between 15 and 16 years, because by that age most children have entered adolescence.[23] This cutoff has been adopted in major official reporting systems, such as those of the World Health Organization or the National Center for Health Statistics, and has been widely used in psychiatric research and classification.

To estimate the hazards ratio for PTSD in women vs men, stratified by age at first exposure to traumatic events (≤ 15 vs >15 years), time at risk was redefined. Because age at exposure and age at onset of PTSD are highly correlated, the use of chronologic age would have violated the proportionality assumption of the hazards ratios. To avoid this, we defined time to event as chronologic age for those who were exposed to traumatic events at age 15 years or younger and as the number of years since age 15 years for those whose exposure occurred after age 15 years. Kaplan-Meier survival curves of PTSD in women and men by age at exposure to traumatic events were estimated, using the same approach to time at risk.

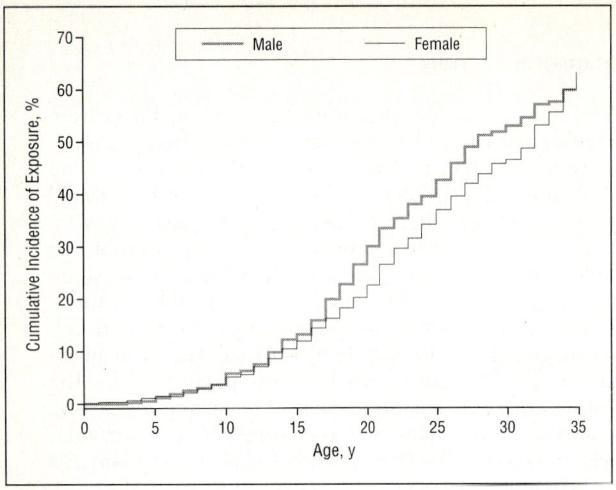

Figure 1. *Cumulative incidence of exposure to traumatic events by sex (n=1007).*

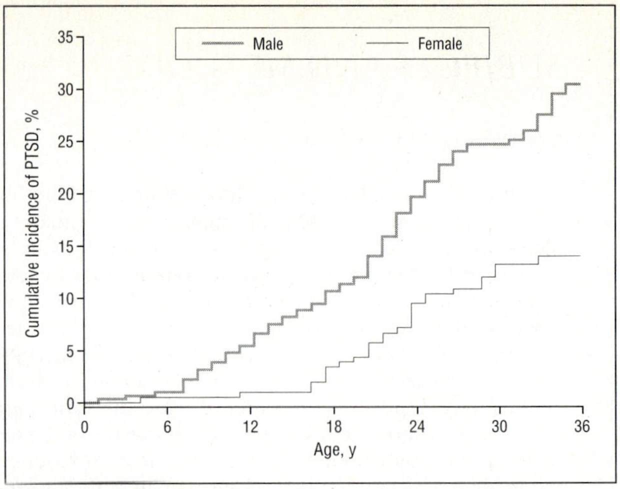

Figure 2. *Cumulative incidence of posttraumatic stress disorder (PTSD) in subjects exposed to traumatic events (n=540) by sex.*

preexisting psychiatric disorders, family history of AD, and early separation from parents.

RESULTS

TRAUMATIC EVENTS AND PTSD IN WOMEN VS MEN

The cumulative incidence of exposure to traumatic events, estimated in Kaplan-Meier survival analysis,[24] was 61.6% (95% confidence interval [CI], 57.5-65.7) and did not vary significantly between men and women (P=.17, log-rank test) (**Figure 1**). There was also no sex difference in the *number* of traumatic events in lifetime reported at baseline or in the combined data up to the last follow-up assessment. Although the *NIMH-DIS* restricts the inquiry to 3 traumatic events, 96.4% of subjects of either sex reported only 1 or 2 events at baseline, indicating that the limits on the number of events did not curtail materially women's and men's opportunity to report their complete history of traumatic events. The number of lifetime events in the combined data did not vary between subjects of both sexes. Mean numbers of traumatic events among the 216 exposed men and 324 exposed women were 1.87 and 1.75, respectively (P=.22).

The cumulative incidence of PTSD among persons exposed to traumatic events was significantly higher in women (30.2% [95% CI, 24.6-35.8]) than in men (13% [95% CI, 10.0-18.7]) (P<.001, log-rank test) (**Figure 2**). The hazards ratio of PTSD in exposed women vs men, calculated in a Cox proportional hazards model, was 2.3 (95% CI, 1.5-3.6). Additional analysis revealed that the higher risk of PTSD in women did not decrease when history of multiple traumatic events was controlled.

POTENTIAL EXPLANATIONS FOR THE SEX DIFFERENCE IN PTSD: PREEXISTING DISORDERS

Preexisting AD or MDD significantly increased the risk for subsequent PTSD (hazards ratio, 2.1; 95% CI, 1.4-3.1), with no significant interaction with sex (χ^2=1.83; P=<.18). Adjusting for preexisting any AD or MDD decreased the hazards ratio for PTSD in exposed women vs men from 2.3 to 1.8 (95% CI, 1.2-2.9; P=.006).

To illustrate these results more clearly, in **Figure 3**, we present the sex-specific cumulative incidence curves of PTSD in exposed subjects (n=540), according to the presence or absence of preexisting AD or MDD. These curves differ from the standard Kaplan-Meier curves in that the grouping variable is not fixed but, instead, can vary with time. Specifically, a person's status can change from "no prior AD or MDD" to "prior AD or MDD" at any age until the age at onset of PTSD or censoring. As can be seen in Figure 3, the incidence of PTSD in both males and females accumulated faster if any AD or MDD had occurred in the preceding years than if it had not. Additionally, the cumulative incidence of PTSD in females with and without preexisting AD or MDD was higher than in male counterparts.

OTHER RISK FACTORS

We tested the role of other potential risk factors on the observed excess risk of PTSD in women by adding to the model family history of AD early separation from parents, race, and education. Family history of AD increased significantly the hazards ratio for PTSD (2.4; 95% CI, 1.4-3.9). Early separation from parents also increased significantly the hazards ratio for PTSD (1.6; 95% CI, 1.1-2.4). Neither race nor education was associated significantly with PTSD. The *adjusted* hazards ratio for PTSD in women vs men was reduced only marginally, when these additional covariates were in the model (1.7; 95% CI, 1.1-2.7).

SEX DIFFERENCE IN PTSD AND AGE AT FIRST EXPOSURE

We tested whether the hazards ratio for PTSD in females vs males varied by age at first exposure to traumatic events, classified as childhood (at ≤15 years of age) vs later (at >15 years of age) exposure. The hazards ratio for PTSD in females vs males was markedly higher if exposure to traumatic events occurred by age 15 years than later (11.4; 95% CI, 2.7-47.9 vs 1.5; 95% CI, 0.9-2.5). The interaction term of age by sex was statistically

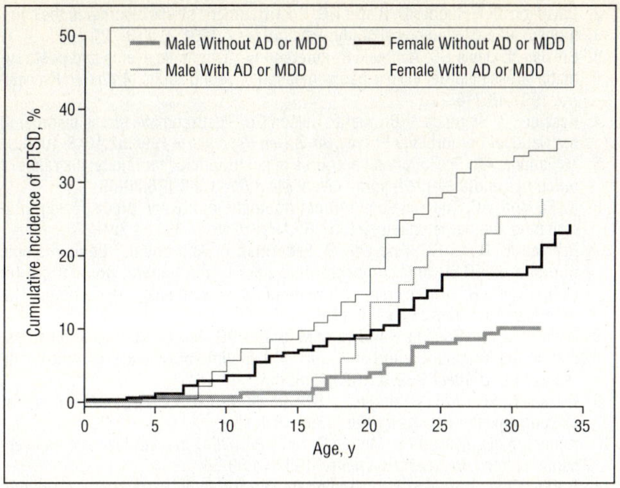

Figure 3. *Cumulative incidence of posttraumatic stress disorder (PTSD) in subjects exposed to traumatic events (n=540) by sex and preexisting anxiety disorder (AD) or major depressive disorder (MDD).*

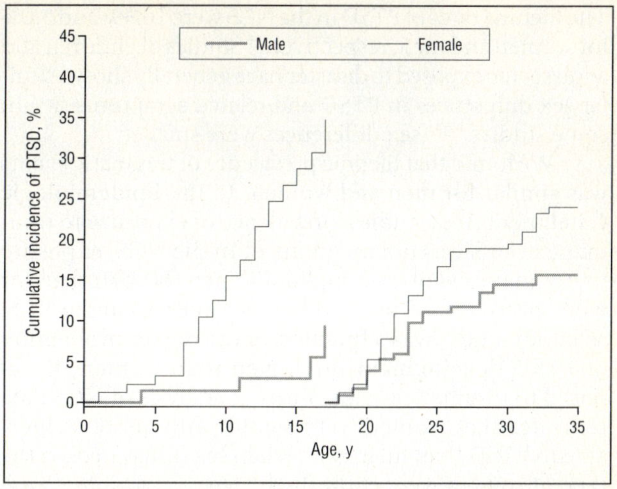

Figure 4. *Cumulative incidence of posttraumatic stress disorder (PTSD) in subjects exposed to traumatic events (n=540) by sex and age at exposure.*

significant ($P=.006$), indicating that the 2 hazards ratios were significantly different.

Figure 4 shows the Kaplan-Meier cumulative incidence curves of PTSD by sex and age at exposure. The sex gap in the cumulative incidence of PTSD was dramatic in the early-exposure groups ($P<.001$, log-rank test) but small in the late-exposure groups ($P=.08$, log-rank test).

SEX COMPARISON OF CHILDHOOD TRAUMATIC EVENTS: AN EXPLORATORY ANALYSIS

Similar proportions of men and women who reported lifetime exposure to traumatic events dated their earliest exposure at age 15 years or earlier (30.1% [n=50] and 31.3% [n=71], respectively). Among those with childhood exposure, a higher proportion of women (27%) than men (8%) reported rape, assault, or ongoing physical or sexual abuse. In contrast, a higher proportion of men (28%) than women (11%) with childhood exposure reported serious accidents or injury. Exposure to serious accidents or injury in childhood did not lead to PTSD in subjects of either sex. In contrast, the effects of exposure to the category that included rape, assault, or abuse differed by sex, yielding a high rate of early PTSD in women (63%) but no PTSD cases in men. Across other types of traumatic events in childhood, the PTSD rates were also higher in women than in men, including the 2 largest classes—news of sudden death or injury and witnessing violence—with 39.1% of the women vs 4.5% of the men who reported these experiences in childhood meeting PTSD criteria. Thus, the observed sex differences in traumatic events in childhood do not provide an explanation for the sex difference in PTSD.

COMMENT

The key findings of this study are as follows: (1) lifetime prevalence of exposure to traumatic events and number of traumatic events did not vary by sex; (2) the risk for PTSD after exposure to traumatic events was more than 2-fold higher in women than in men; (3) preexisting AD or MDD played a small part in the observed sex difference in PTSD after exposure; (4) family history of AD and early separation from parents, although significant risk factors for PTSD in men and women exposed to traumatic events, did not play a role in the observed sex difference in PTSD; and (5) sex difference in PTSD was markedly wider if exposure occurred in childhood than after age 15 years.

The interpretation of these findings should take into account 2 limitations. Although the study used a prospective design, the findings are based on the combined data from the baseline and follow-up interviews. The baseline interview covered lifetime history, when the respondents' age ranged from 21 to 30 years, and the follow-up interviewers added information about the subsequent 5-year period. Although prospective data are less likely to be subject to recall errors, lifetime data were essential in this study. As we have shown, sex differences in PTSD emerged early in life and women's vulnerability to the PTSD-inducing effects of traumatic events seems to be far greater if exposure occurred in childhood rather than later on. It is the availability of lifetime data that enabled us to detect these relationships. A general caveat on the accuracy of family history data is also in order, although the issue has little bearing on our key findings.

The generalizability of the results is limited by the age range of the sample. There is little in these data about sex differences in PTSD when first exposure to traumatic events occurred after the third decade of life. The generalizability is restricted also by the socioeconomic and geographic characteristics of the sample. Selected from a health maintenance organization membership, subscribers and their dependents, the sample does not represent the extremes of the socioeconomic range, especially the uninsured poor. However, whereas rates of exposure to typical PTSD events are likely to vary across socioeconomic strata, there is no evidence to suggest that the PTSD-inducing effects of exposure vary widely across strata.[25]

Our finding of a sex difference in PTSD replicates earlier reports. The lifetime prevalence of PTSD in the 2 sites of the Epidemiologic Catchment Area, St Louis and North Carolina, was approximately 2-fold higher for women than for men,[1,2] specifically rates for women vs men (1.3% vs 0.5% in St Louis and 1.7% vs 0.9% in North Carolina, respectively).

The lifetime rates of PTSD in the NCS were 10.4% and 5.0% for women and men, respectively.[4] Studies of children and adolescents exposed to disaster have generally shown similar sex differences in PTSD and related symptoms.[26-31] In some studies,[32,33] sex differences were smaller.

We found that lifetime prevalence of traumatic events was similar for men and women. In the Epidemiologic Catchment Area studies, prevalence of exposure to traumatic events was not ascertained. In the NCS, exposure to traumatic events was higher for men (60.7%) than for women (51.2%).[4] The sex difference in PTSD in the NCS, as in our study, was a function of the higher probability of PTSD development in women than in men, if exposed to traumatic events. Further analysis of NCS data indicates that women were significantly more vulnerable to PTSD than men, even when sex differences in the type of trauma were controlled.[4]

We found that the burden of exposure, as measured by the number of traumatic events in lifetime, did not vary between the sexes. The NCS, in which exposure to traumatic events was measured by a list of 12 specific events, reported a higher proportion (of 3 or 4 events) for exposed men than exposed women.[4] These observations suggest that women's higher rate of PTSD was unlikely to result from their higher number of traumatic events experienced in lifetime. Furthermore, we found that the higher risk of PTSD in women relative to that in men was not accounted for by history of multiple traumatic events. Women were neither more likely to report multiple events nor more likely to be affected by the cumulative effects of multiple events.

Three personal characteristics were found to be significant risk factors for PTSD in subjects of *both* sexes: preexisting ADs or MDDs, family history of AD, and early separation from parents. None of these factors differentially increased women's vulnerability to PTSD. The observed role of preexisting AD or MDD in the sex difference in PTSD was a function of the higher rate of preexisting AD or MDD for women than for men.

Our exploratory analysis of childhood events did not yield an explanation for the marked sex difference in the PTSD sequelae of childhood events. Across major event types, females had higher rates of PTSD than did males. Nonetheless, the question of childhood exposure and its consequences in women and men needs further examination. A detailed investigation of characteristics of events might shed light on the sex difference in PTSD after traumatic experiences in childhood.

Accepted for publication November 6, 1996.

This work was supported by grant MH 48802 from the National Institute of Mental Health, Bethesda, Md.

Reprints: Naomi Breslau, PhD, Department of Psychiatry, Henry Ford Health Sciences Center, One Ford Place, Detroit, MI 48202-3450.

REFERENCES

1. Helzer J, Robins L, McEvoy L. Post-traumatic stress disorder in the general population: findings of the Epidemiologic Catchment Area survey. *N Engl J Med.* 1987; 317:1630-1634.
2. Davidson JRT, Hughes D, Blazer DG. Post-traumatic stress disorder in the community: an epidemiological study. *Psychol Med.* 1991;21:713-721.
3. Breslau N, Davis GC, Andreski P, Peterson EL. Traumatic events and posttraumatic stress disorder in an urban population of young adults. *Arch Gen Psychiatry.* 1991;48:216-222.
4. Kessler RC, Sonnega A, Bromet E, Nelson CB. Posttraumatic stress disorder in the National Comorbidity Survey. *Arch Gen Psychiatry.* 1995;52:1048-1060.
5. McFarlane, AC. The longitudinal course of posttraumatic morbidity: the range of outcomes and their predictors. *J Nerv Ment Dis.* 1988;176:30-39.
6. McFarlane, AC. The aetiology of post-traumatic morbidity: predisposing, precipitating and perpetuating factors. *Br J Psychiatry.* 1989;54:221-228.
7. Breslau N, Davis GC, Andreski P, Federman B, Anthony JC. Epidemiologic findings on PTSD and comorbid disorders in the general population. In: Dohrenwend B, ed. *Adversity, Stress, and Psychopathology.* Washington, DC: American Psychiatric Press. In press.
8. Kessler RC, McGonagle KA, Swartz M, Blazer DG, Nelson CB. Sex and depression in the National Comorbidity Survey, I: lifetime prevalence, chronicity and recurrence. *J Affect Disord.* 1993;29:85-96.
9. Breslau N, Schultz L, Peterson EL. Sex differences in depression: a role for preexisting anxiety. *Psychiatry Res.* 1995;58:1-12.
10. Anderson JC, Williams S, McGee R, Silva PA. *DSM-III* disorders in preadolescent children. *Arch Gen Psychiatry.* 1987;44:69-76.
11. Burke JD Jr, Wittchen H-U, Regier DA, Sartorius N. Extracting information from diagnostic interviews on co-occurrence of symptoms of anxiety and depression. In: Maser JD, Cloninger CR, eds. *Comorbidity of Mood and Anxiety Disorders.* Washington, DC: American Psychiatric Press Inc; 1990:649-667.
12. Nolen-Hoeksema S, Girgus JS. The emergence of gender differences in depression during adolescence. *Psychol Bull.* 1994;115:424-443.
13. Robins LN, Helzer JE, Cottler L, Golding E. *NIMH Diagnostic Interview Schedule, Version III Revised.* St Louis, Mo: Washington University; 1989.
14. American Psychiatric Association. *Diagnostic and Statistical Manual of Mental Disorders, Third Edition, Revised.* Washington, DC: American Psychiatric Association; 1987.
15. Robins LN, Helzer JE, Ratcliff KS, Seyfried W. Validity of the *Diagnostic Interview Schedule, Version II: DSM-III* Diagnoses. *Psychol Med.* 1982;12:855-870.
16. Helzer JE, Robins LN, McEvoy LT, Spitznagel EL, Stoltzman RK, Farmer A, Brockington I. A comparison of clinician and *Diagnostic Interview Schedule* diagnoses. *Arch Gen Psychiatry.* 1985;42:657-666.
17. Anthony JC, Folstein M. Romanoski AJ, VonKorff MR, Hestadt GR, Chahal R, Merchant A, Brown CH, Shapiro S, Kramer M, Gruenberg EM. Comparison of the lay *Diagnostic Interview Schedule* and a standardized psychiatric diagnosis. *Arch Gen Psychiatry.* 1985;42:667-675.
18. Cox DR. Regression models and life tables. *J R Statist Soc Series B.* 1974;34: 187-220.
19. Cox DR. Partial likelihood. *Biometrika.* 1975;62:269-276.
20. Breslow N. Covariance analysis of censured survival data. *Biometrics.* 1974;30: 89-99.
21. Kay R. Proportional hazards regression models and the analysis of censored survival data. *Appl Statist.* 1977;26:227-237.
22. SAS Institute Inc. *SAS Technical Report p-217, SAS/STAT Software: The PHREG Procedure, Version 6.* Cary, NC: SAS Institute Inc; 1991.
23. Piaget J, Inhelder B. *The Psychology of the Child.* New York, NY: Basic Books Inc; 1969.
24. Kaplan EL, Meier P. Nonparametric estimation from incomplete observations. *J Am Statist Assoc.* 1958;53:457-481.
25. Breslau N, Davis GC, Peterson EL, Schultz LR. Psychiatric sequelae of posttraumatic stress disorder in women. *Arch Gen Psychiatry.* 1997;54:81-87.
26. Green BL, Korol M, Grace MC, Vary MG, Leonard AC, Gleser GC, Smitson-Cohen S. Children and disaster: age, gender, and parental effects on PTSD symptoms. *J Am Acad Child Adolesc Psychiatry.* 1991;30:945-951.
27. Green, BL, Grace, MC, Vary, MG, Kramer, TL, Gleser, GC, Leonard, AC. Children of disaster in the second decade: a 17-year follow-up of Buffalo Creek survivors. *J Am Acad Child Adolesc Psychiatry.* 1994;33:71-79.
28. Garrison CZ, Weinrich MW, Hardin SB, Weinrich S, Wang L. Post-traumatic stress disorder in adolescents after a hurricane. *Am J Epidemiol.* 1993;138:522-530.
29. Shannon MP, Lonigan CJ, Finch Jr AJ, Taylor CM. Children exposed to disaster, I: epidemiology of post-traumatic symptoms and symptom profiles. *J Consult Clin Psychol.* 1994;33:80-93.
30. Brent DA, Perper JA, Moritz G, Liotus L, Richardson D, Canobbio R, Schweers J, Roth C. Posttraumatic stress disorder in peers of adolescent suicide victims: predisposing factors and phenomenology. *J Am Acad Child Adolesc Psychiatry.* 1995;34:209-215.
31. Shaw JA, Applegate B, Schorr C. Twenty-one-month follow-up study of school-age children exposed to hurricane Andrew. *J Am Acad Child Adolesc Psychiatry.* 1996;35:359-685.
32. Shore JH, Vollmer WM, Tatum EL. Community patterns of posttraumatic stress disorders. *J Nerv Ment Dis.* 1989;177:681-685.
33. Norris, F. Epidemiology of trauma: frequency and impact of different potentially traumatic events on different demographic groups. *J Consult Clin Psychol.* 1992; 60:409-418.

A 'Second Life' Agenda

Psychiatric Research Issues Raised by Protease Inhibitor Treatments for People With the Human Immunodeficiency Virus or the Acquired Immunodeficiency Syndrome

Judith G. Rabkin, PhD, MPH; Stephen Ferrando, MD

Seldom in the history of medicine has an entire generation of patients with an incurable, progressive, and ultimately fatal disease suddenly been offered the prospect of extended survival and even, perhaps, a "second life." The relatively simultaneous appearance of 2 major treatment developments has created profound changes in therapeutic options and outlook. The first development is an assay of serum levels of human immunodeficiency virus viral copies, providing a critical tool for clinical decision making. The second is the marketing between December 1995 and April 1997 of 4 human immunodeficiency virus protease inhibitors that, combined with previously available antiviral medications, achieve a new level of efficacy. With the advent of these changes come multiple psychiatric research and policy issues. These include the development of strategies to establish and maintain medication adherence. This is a critical task, given the complexity of combination therapy regimens and the rapid onset of viral resistance to protease inhibitors within days to weeks of missed or suboptimal dosing. The psychological issues to be studied include the process of restructuring lives and expectations in the event of clinical benefit or managing the distress associated with clinical failure. Other research questions include the effects of restored health on the appraisal of human immunodeficiency virus risk behaviors, assessment of effect of neurocognitive functioning, and unanswered questions about psychotropic or protease inhibitor drug interactions due to their shared metabolic pathways. Behavioral scientists can inform provision of care to patients who may be considered difficult to treat, such as those with severe and persistent mental illness or active substance abuse or the homeless. This includes the provision of empirical data regarding individual and situational characteristics that are likely to promote or impede adherence, as well as innovative provision systems. Psychiatry can make notable contributions during this turning point in human immunodeficiency virus therapeutics and research.

Arch Gen Psychiatry. 1997;54:1049-1053

Seldom in the history of medicine has an entire generation of patients with an incurable, progressive, and ultimately fatal disease suddenly been offered the prospect of extended survival and even, perhaps, a "second life." We may have reached such a point for the estimated 1 million people in the United States infected with the human immunodeficiency virus (HIV) or the acquired immunodeficiency syndrome (AIDS). This has occurred because of the relatively simultaneous appearance of 2 important medical breakthroughs. The first is the HIV RNA viral load assay as a clinical marker of HIV illness progression and as a critical tool with which to make treatment decisions.[1-4] Viral quantification in the blood has been made possible by application of the polymerase chain reaction assay, which serves to directly amplify viral genetic material,[5] or an alternative method, branched DNA, which amplifies the signal generated by the viral genetic material.[6] Viral load does not replace $CD4^+$ cell counts as an index of immunosuppression but rather adds

From the Department of Psychiatry, Cornell University Medical College, New York, NY.

information. It has been said that the viral load tells how fast the train is going and that the CD4+ cell count tells how much track remains ahead.

The second medical breakthrough has been the development and Food and Drug Administration approval since December 1995 of HIV protease inhibitors, a new class of antiretroviral medications that attack the virus at a different point in the replicative cycle than previously available reverse transcriptase inhibitors such as zidovudine. There are 4 marketed protease inhibitors (saquinavir mesylate [Invirase], ritonavir [Norvir], indinavir sulfate [Crixivan], and nelfinavir mesylate [Viracept]), 5 nucleoside reverse transcriptase inhibitors (AZT, DDI, ddC, 3TC, and d4T, also known as zidovudine [Retrovir], didanosine [Videx], zalcitibane [Hivid], lamivudine [Epivir], and stavudine [Zerit], respectively), and 2 non–nucleoside reverse transcriptase inhibitors (nevirapine [Viramune] and delavirdine [Rescriptor]). At least 4 other promising protease inhibitors are in clinical trials.[7] Monotherapy (treatment with just one of these agents) is no longer recommended in most cases, and monotherapy with a nonnucleoside reverse transcriptase inhibitor or a protease inhibitor is never indicated because of the rapid development of viral resistance. Combination therapy has become the standard and typically includes 2 nucleoside reverse transcriptase inhibitors plus a protease inhibitor.[8] Ongoing studies are comparing 4- and 5-drug combinations.

Protease inhibitor use has increased from approximately 3000 patients enrolled in clinical trials and compassionate use protocols in the fall of 1995 to approximately 140 000 patients by the end of 1996. Indinavir was the most widely used before the release of nelfinavir in April 1997 (Thaddeus Grimes-Gruczka, oral communication, March 1997). Since the advent of protease inhibitors, physicians and patients are beginning to speak of the possibility of a "cure." The cover article of the *New York Times Magazine* in November 1996 was titled, "When Plagues End: Notes on the Twilight of an Epidemic."[9] Clinical stories are being told about patients with dramatic reductions in viral load, notable increases in CD4+ cell counts, and striking improvements in overall health. The declining census in AIDS units of hospitals also is being ascribed, in part, to the effects of combination therapies. In 1996, deaths from AIDS declined nationally by 15%; in New York City, they declined by 30%.[10]

On the other hand, in part due to the rapid approval and fast release of the protease inhibitors (setting new records for the Food and Drug Administration), questions remain about almost every aspect of the new treatments: when to initiate combination therapy, for whom, and whether to start "slow" with 2 drugs or to "hit hard" (as in treatment of tuberculosis) with 3 or more; and what the clinical outcomes will be for which patients over what period. To date, the double-blind clinical trials leading to Food and Drug Administration approval have been relatively brief (6 weeks to 6 months), with relatively few highly motivated patients, and have had few clinical end points. No data exist to show how to manage loss of efficacy, as indicated by viral load rebound after initial effect.

Despite notable gaps in our knowledge and experience with combination therapies, these treatment developments clearly are exciting from multiple perspectives. However, already their arrival has created a paradoxical crisis for patients who experience major improvement and devastating disappointment for those who do not.[11] Among those who thrive, many who had been in the workforce had gone on disability, cashed in their insurance policies, used up their personal credit, and had prepared themselves for a foreshortened life. Others, who may have spent much of their lives unemployed and who are receiving rent assistance, cash benefits, and other entitlements in an ironic twist of positive fate due to HIV may eventually face bureaucratic expectations that they give up their entitlements and go to work.[12]

Given these second life dilemmas, multiple psychiatric research and policy questions arise. These include medication adherence, restructuring lives and expectations, HIV risk behaviors, neuropsychiatric functioning, and drug interactions, as well as costs and access to the new tests and treatments.

RESEARCH ISSUES

Treatment Adherence

Because all members of the class of protease inhibitors have the unfortunate characteristic of early resistance after even a week of missed medication,[13] with partial or complete cross-resistance occurring to other protease inhibitors as well, failures of compliance can eliminate this treatment for the individual forever, as well as any people who he or she subsequently infects. The treatment regimen is extraordinarily demanding, requiring 10 to 20 pills a day in addition to other medications and meticulous timing every 8 (for saquinavir, indinavir, and nelfinavir) or 12 (for ritonavir) hours, indefinitely. Alterations of eating patterns are required because saquinavir, ritonavir, and nelfinavir must be taken with food but indinavir must be taken 1 hour before or 2 hours after eating. While the twice-daily schedule of ritonavir is simpler, the medication causes notable toxic effects, especially in the first few weeks, that many patients cannot tolerate.

There is extensive but inconclusive literature on assessment methods and interventions to promote medication adherence.[14-18] Methodological problems abound, and indeed there is no standard criterion outcome measure for adherence for even a single drug. For measuring adherence in general, and particularly for combination therapy, multiple outcome measures are required, including patient reports, behavioral measures such as pill counts, biological variables such as change in viral load, and perhaps genotypic and phenotypic assays to identify development of drug resistance, when these assays are sufficiently developed to be reliable research tools. Research challenges include designing feasible and acceptable interventions, in addition to demonstrating efficacy.

Effect on Primary Prevention Efforts

Media stories about the potential of protease inhibitors to cure HIV or AIDS, accompanied by beliefs that undetectable viral loads render the person noninfectious, pose a risk to primary prevention efforts. (Undetectable means the assay in question cannot detect viral copies below a specified threshold if indeed any are present.) Already physicians anecdotally report hearing from their patients about lapses in safer sex practices. Sexually transmitted diseases are being seen more commonly in infected patients, and drug use accompanying sex seems on the increase.[19] Uninfected people may be less concerned about seroconversion now that HIV or AIDS is "curable." In fact, no data exist to support any of these beliefs. Previous studies on the recovery of HIV from semen found that the presence and amount of HIV does not correlate with $CD4^+$ cell count or zidovudine therapy.[20] Whether protease inhibitors reduce or eliminate virus in semen and vaginal or cervical fluids is a largely unanswered question. Research is needed to address these issues and to modify public health messages so that they are taken into account.

Planning to Live

Another salient research area concerns "what to do with a second life." Will people on disability who respond to combination therapy actually return to their former lifestyles and occupations or will they make changes in their life trajectory? Will they return to their former employment, go to school, or change careers? For those who were formerly unable to work because of illness, but have improved and want to return to work, what are the criteria (physical, psychological, and especially cognitive) for fitness to work? Will there be practical incentives to return to work, or will there be implicit disadvantages such as the loss of disability policies or insurance benefits should they become ill in the future?[12]

The possibility of an extended life with HIV will inevitably raise novel personal and social issues, including decisions about personal relationships. Individuals may choose to enter relationships that had been avoided or dissolve relationships in which they had "settled for less" because of anticipated diminished life expectancy. Family roles may shift from dependency to greater responsibility. Decisions about geographic relocation (for better medical care) may change. These issues will have a profound effect on individuals and society, and they require research attention.

Failed Promises

There will be other patients whose hopes are raised but who fail to achieve or maintain benefit from the new combination therapies, despite every effort at adherence to their difficult regimens.[21] Treatment failure may take at least 3 forms. The patient's viral load may not decline meaningfully even after the available drug combinations are initiated, intolerable side effects to the available drug regimens may develop in the patient, or combination therapy may initially succeed but lose its effect. The psychological implications differ somewhat. Failure of the drugs to work at the outset may lead to a sense of injustice and external assignment of responsibility. In contrast, drug intolerance may lead to a sense of personal failure or the perception of betrayal by one's own body.

Other determinants of reaction to failure of combination treatment include such antecedents as a prior history of drug failure or intolerance (so that this failure is "the last straw") or the perception that failure was preventable in the case of patients who earlier had been given sequential antiviral monotherapies, developing resistance to each one at a time. At the time of failure, exacerbating factors may include a sense of guilt for not perfectly adhering to what is, in reality, an almost impossibly onerous schedule of drug adherence. Patients who had not been forewarned about the possibilities of treatment failure may be more upset than those who were aware of the uncertainties. Disappointment about treatment failure is often magnified by fears (often real) that there remain no known therapies to halt an unalterable decline. The distress of treatment failure may be magnified by seeing the success of friends and acquaintances, creating the sense of being the only one left out of the triumphant scientific achievement.

What does psychotherapeutic intervention have to offer in this context? What treatment models are appropriate? Strategies based on models of bereavement and mourning[22] may seem salient in several respects (grief, loss, and anger), but the fit is not exact. Treatment failure does not preclude the possibility of new drugs if they become available soon enough. While this is preferable to the finality of bereavement by death, it constitutes another layer of stress generated by ambiguity, by the absence of personal control over one's destiny, and by the fear that time is running out. An integrative model may be required, including but not limited to components of bereavement or acute stress interventions.[23,24] Research regarding appropriate components is needed, as is evaluation of the relative benefits of group compared with individual sessions or the conceptualization of interventions in terms of support groups or more formal psychotherapy.

Neuropsychiatric Issues

Human immunodeficiency virus enters the central nervous system (CNS) early during the course of HIV infection[25] and may produce a range of neuropsychiatric symptoms over time.[26] In the late stages of illness, HIV-associated dementia occurs, with a yearly incidence of 4% to 7%.[27-29] Structural and functional brain abnormalities have correlated with degree of immunosuppression, stage of disease, and neuropsychological impairment.[30] While functional impairment is by definition a feature of HIV-associated dementia, there is preliminary evidence that early neuropsychological impairment may be associated with subjectively impaired work performance and unemployment.[31]

The mechanism by which HIV itself produces neuropathological features is not completely understood. Evidence suggests that HIV is transported into the CNS across an intact blood-brain barrier (BBB) by infected macrophages. Neuronal dysfunction or loss and increased

BBB permeability may then be caused by various factors, including HIV envelope protein GP120, immune cytokines, and toxic metabolites.[32] With more advanced immunosuppression, the combination of increased BBB permeability, increased CNS viral burden, and the continued release of neurotoxic substances may accelerate HIV-related neuropathological features.[32]

The dynamics of CNS viral burden, its relationship to peripheral viral load, and its effect on the development of cognitive impairment remain unclear. This is an important issue for the protease inhibitors. Relative to zidovudine and stavudine, marketed protease inhibitors have minimal BBB penetration, so that infected cells in the CNS, such as macrophages, that have a longer half-life than $CD4^+$ cells may serve as a reservoir for HIV while the peripheral viral load is reduced.[33] If this is true, combination therapies could be expected to produce improvements in general health but allow for progression of cognitive impairment.

Pending the development of protease inhibitors that traverse the BBB, several research questions exist. What is the relationship between peripheral and CNS viral burden?[34] Does the relationship between these compartments change over time with progression of HIV illness and increased BBB permeability? What is the relationship between CNS viral load, neuropathological processes, neuropsychological measures, and actual functional impairment? Further clarification of CNS viral dynamics, coupling of viral load, neuroimaging and neuropsychological studies, and the inclusion of functional and neuropsychological end points in clinical trials of combination therapies will be essential areas of HIV-related neuropsychiatric research.

Drug Interactions

Protease inhibitors have the potential for interaction with psychotropic drugs. Protease inhibitors are all metabolized via the cytochrome P-450 oxidase system, primarily the 3A3/4 isoform, with the 2D6 isoform being a secondary metabolic pathway. These are common metabolic pathways shared by many psychotropic drugs.[35] Protease inhibitors and psychotropic drugs may interact in several ways. First, drugs that are inducers of cytochrome P-450 3A3/4, such as carbamazepine and phenobarbital, are likely to increase the clearance of protease inhibitors, reducing serum levels and therapeutic benefit.

Second, protease inhibitors slow the metabolism of several benzodiazepines, antidepressants, and antipsychotics, as well as methadone hydrochloride and recreational drugs such as methylenedioxymethamphetamine (MDMA or Exstasy), and may cause large increases in serum concentrations of these psychotropic drugs and, hence, toxic effects.

Third, other psychotropic drugs such as nefazodone hydrochloride may slow the metabolism of protease inhibitors, leading to increased protease inhibitor side effects, which may interfere with dosing regimens and adherence.

Finally, protease inhibitors may actually induce the metabolism of some psychotropic drugs, such as lorazepam and valproate sodium, that undergo only hepatic conjugation (per information on the package insert of ritonavir), leading to diminution of therapeutic benefit and possibly withdrawal syndromes. Similar concerns have been raised about oral contraceptives.

While many psychotropic drugs are listed as relatively or absolutely contraindicated in protease inhibitor package inserts, and dosage reduction of others is often recommended, presumptive drug interactions have not been systematically studied. Thus, the clinical significance of interactions between protease inhibitors and psychotropic drugs is largely unknown. Recommendations regarding dosage changes and contraindications may be too sweeping, depriving some HIV-positive patients with psychiatric problems of needed treatments. Other potentially troublesome interactions may not yet be known. Systematic studies of protease inhibitors combined with various classes of psychotropic drugs, and effects on serum concentrations of both classes of medication, are urgently needed.

POLICY ISSUES

These include practical and attitudinal barriers, financial effects, and the determination of selection criteria for the new combination treatments. The cost of a protease inhibitor per patient is between $4000 and $6000 a year, so that combination therapy costs approximately $15 000 a year per patient, not including laboratory tests, physician visits, or other expensive medications that the patient may need.

Prior research in the United States has shown that medications for minority patients and intravenous drug users have been less likely to be prescribed; if prescribed, these patients are less likely to take reverse transcriptase inhibitors such as zidovudine. Contributing factors include access to care,[36] inconsistent clinic attendance, psychiatric comorbidity and concurrent substance abuse,[37] and cultural differences in attitudes toward the medical system and conventional medications.[38,39] Patients who are homeless or have severe and persistent mental illnesses face even greater obstacles to medication adherence.[40,41] If they only have one chance at success, is it in the best interest of some patients to defer treatment until more "user friendly" protease inhibitors can be marketed? Who should decide, using what criteria? The task for behavioral scientists is to inform such decision-making with empirical data regarding individual and situational characteristics that are likely to promote adherence or that are almost certainly likely to prevent it.

CONCLUSIONS

Finally, the second life dilemma presumes that there is, indeed, a second life. Similar hope was engendered with the advent in 1987 of the first antiretroviral drug, zidovudine, to which viral resistance subsequently developed and which later showed no survival benefit.[42,43] From the time of this latter realization, around 1993, to the current era of protease inhibitors in 1996, physicians and patients shared a therapeutic nihilism regarding the likelihood of survival with AIDS. It will be important to follow the progress of the protease inhibitors in terms of long-term efficacy. If widespread viral resistance develops once again, or unanticipated side effects or interactions emerge over time, there may be a backlash against accepting new medical therapies for HIV in the future. Nevertheless, we believe that we are witnessing a radical turning point in HIV therapeutics and research.

Accepted for publication April 4, 1997.

This study was supported in part by grant 5 R01 MH42277 from the National Institute of Mental Health, Rockville, Md.

Reprints: Judith G. Rabkin, PhD, Department of Psychiatry, Cornell University Medical College, 445 E 68th St, Room 3K, New York, NY 10021.

REFERENCES

1. Henrad DR, Phillips JF, Muenz LR, Blattner WA, Wiesner D, Eyster ME, Goedert J. Natural history of HIV-1 cell-free viremia. *JAMA.* 1995;274:554-558.
2. O'Brien WA, Hartigan PM, Martin D, Esinhart J, Hill A, Benoit S, Rubin M, Simberkoff M, Hamilton JD. Changes in plasma HIV-1 RNA and CD4+ lymphocyte counts and the risk of progression to AIDS. *N Engl J Med.* 1996;334:426-431.
3. Ho DD. Viral counts count in HIV infection. *Science.* 1996;272:1123-1125.
4. Saag MS, Holodniy M, Kuritzkes D, O'Brien WA, Coombs R, Poscher ME, Jacobsen DM, Shaw GM, Richman DD, Volberding PA. HIV viral load markers in clinical practice. *Nat Med.* 1996;82:625-629.
5. Mulder J, McKinney N, Christopherson J, Sninsky J, Greenfield L, Kwok S. Rapid and simple PCR assay for quantitation of human immunodeficiency virus type 1 RNA in plasma. *J Clin Microbiol.* 1994;32:292-300.
6. Dewar RL, Highbarger H, Sarmiento MD, Todd J, Vasudevachari MB, Davey R, Kovacs JA, Salzman NP, Lane HC, Urdea MS. Application of branched DNA signal amplification to monitor human immunodeficiency virus type 1 in human plasma. *J Infect Dis.* 1994;170:1172-1179.
7. Steele FR. Optimism invades HIV conference. *Nat Med.* 1996;2:257-258.
8. Carpenter C, Fischl M, Hammer S, Hirsch M, Jacobsen D, Katzenstein D, Montaner JS, Richman D, Saag S, Schooley R, Thompson M, Vella S, Yeni P, Volberding P, for the International AIDS Society. Antiretroviral therapy for HIV infection in 1997: updated recommendations of the International AIDS Society—USA panel. *JAMA.* 1997;277:1962-1969.
9. Sullivan A. When plagues end: notes on the twilight of an epidemic. *New York Times Magazine.* November 10, 1996:23ff.
10. Altman L. US reporting sharp decrease in AIDS deaths. *The New York Times.* February 28, 1997: A1, A10.
11. Altman L. Discussing possible AIDS cure raises hope, anger and question: what exactly is meant by cure? *The New York Times.* July 16, 1996:C3.
12. Anders G. Able to work again, AIDS patients worry about disability pay. *Wall Street Journal.* November 18, 1996:1.
13. Roberts NA. Drug-resistance patterns of saquinavir and other HIV proteinase inhibitors. *AIDS.* 1995; 9(suppl 2):S27-S32.
14. Shafer RW, Edlin BR. Tuberculosis in patients infected with human immunodeficiency virus: perspective on the past decade. *Clin Infect Dis.* 1996; 22:683-704.
15. Curtis R, Friedman SR, Neaigus A, Jose B, Goldstein M, DesJarlais DC. Implications of directly observed therapy in tuberculosis control measures among IDUs. *Public Health Rep.* 1994;109:327-329.
16. Meichenbaum D, Turk D. *Facilitating Treatment Adherence.* New York, NY: Plenum Publishing Corp; 1987.
17. Sumartojo E. When tuberculosis treatment fails: a social behavioral account of patient adherence. *Am Rev Respir Dis.* 1993;147:1311-1320.
18. Wall TL, Sorensen JL, Batki SL, Delucchi KL, London JA, Chesney MA. Adherence to zidovudine (AZT) among HIV-infected methadone patients: a pilot study of supervised therapy and dispensing compared to usual care. *Drug Alcohol Depend.* 1995;37:261-269.
19. Green J. Flirting with suicide. *New York Times Magazine.* September 15, 1996:38ff.
20. Krieger JN, Coombs R, Collier A, Ross S, Chaloupka K, Cummings D, Murphy VL, Corey L. Recovery of human immunodeficiency virus type 1 from semen: minimal impact of stage of infection and current antiviral chemotherapy. *J Infect Dis.* 1991;163:386-388.
21. Gilden D. When HAART is not enough. *Gay Mens Health Crisis Treatment Issues.* 1996;10:1-3.
22. Rando T. *Treatment of Complicated Mourning.* Champaign, Ill: Research Press; 1993.
23. Horowitz M, Kaltreider N. Brief therapy of the stress response syndrome. *Psychiatr Clin North Am.* 1979;2:365-377.
24. Goodkin K, Blaney N, Feaster D, Burkhalter J, Leeds B, Tuttle R, Fletcher MA. A bereavement support group decreases distress in HIV-infected gay men. Presented at the 10th International Conference on AIDS; August 8, 1994; Yokohama, Japan.
25. Grant I, Atkinson J, Hesselink J, Kennedy CJ, Richman DD, Spector SA, McCutchan JA. Evidence for early central nervous system involvement in the acquired immunodeficiency syndrome (AIDS) and other human immunodeficiency virus (HIV) infections. *Ann Intern Med.* 1987;103:828-836.
26. Janssen RS, and the Working Group of the American Academy of Neurology AIDS Task Force. Nomenclature and research case definitions for neurologic manifestations of human immunodeficiency virus-type 1 (HIV-1) infection: report of a Working Group of the American Academy of Neurology AIDS Task Force. *Neurology.* 1991;41:778-785.
27. McArthur J, Harrison MJ. HIV-associated dementia. *Current Neurology.* St Louis, Mo: Mosby–Year Book Inc; 1994;14:chap 10.
28. Maj M, Janssen R, Starace F, Zaudig M, Satz P, Sughondhabirom B, Luabeya M, Riedel R, Ndetei D, Calil HM, Bing EG, St Louis M, Sartorius N. WHO Neuropsychiatric AIDS study, cross-sectional phase I. *Arch Gen Psychiatry.* 1994;51:39-49.
29. Bacellar H, Munoz A, Miller EN, Cohen BA, Besley D, Selnes OA, Becker JT, McArthur J. Temporal trends in the incidence of HIV-1–related neurologic diseases: Multicenter AIDS Cohort Study, 1985-1992. *Neurology.* 1994;44:1892-1900.
30. Heaton RK, Grant I, Butters N, White DA, Kirson D, Atkinson JH, McCutchan JA, Taylor MJ, Kelly MD, Ellis RJ, Wolfson T, Velin R, Marcotte TD, Hesselink JR, Jernigan TL, Chandler J, Wallace M, Abramson I, and the HNRC group. The HNRC 500: neuropsychology of HIV infection at different disease stages. *J Int Neuropsychol Soc.* 1995;1:231-251.
31. Heaton RK, Velin RA, McCutchan JA, Gulevich SJ, Atkinson JH, Wallace MR, Godfrey HPD, Kirson DA, Grant I, and the HNRC group. Neuropsychological impairment in human immunodeficiency virus-infection: implications for employment. *Psychosom Med.* 1994;56:8-17.
32. Power C, Kong P, Crawford TO, Wesselingh S, Glass JD, McArthur JC, Trapp BD. Cerebral white matter changes in acquired immunodeficiency syndrome dementia: alterations in the blood-brain barrier. *Ann Neurol.* 1993;34:339-350.
33. Deeks SG, Smith M, Holodniy M, Kahn JO. HIV-1 protease inhibitors: a review for clinicians. *JAMA.* 1997;277:145-153.
34. McCutchan JA, Ellis R, Hsia R. Relationship of cerebrospinal fluid HIV-1 RNA levels (CSF RNA) to plasma RNA, CSF pleocytosis, stage of HIV infection and cognitive functioning. Presented at the Fourth Conference on Retroviruses and Opportunistic Infections; January 24, 1997; Washington, DC.
35. Nemeroff CB, DeVane CL, Pollock BG. Newer antidepressants and the cytochrome P450 system. *Am J Psychiatry.* 1996;153:311-320.
36. Stein MD, Piette J, Mor V, Wachtel TJ, Fleishman J, Mayer KH, Carpenter CC. Differences in access to zidovudine (AZT) among symptomatic HIV-infected persons. *J Gen Intern Med.* 1991;6:35-40.
37. Ferrando SJ, Wall TW, Batki SL, Sorensen JL. Psychiatric morbidity, illicit drug use and adherence to zidovudine (AZT) among injection drug users with HIV disease. *Am J Drug Alcohol Abuse.* 1996; 22:475-487.
38. Reichman LB. Compliance with zidovudine therapy. *Ann Intern Med.* 1990;113:332-333.
39. Samet JH, Libman H, Steger KA, Dhawan RK, Chen J, Shevitz AH, Dewees-Dunk R, Levenson S, Kufe D, Craven DE. Compliance with zidovudine therapy in patients infected with human immunodeficiency virus, type 1: a cross-sectional study in a municipal hospital clinic. *Am J Med.* 1992;92: 495-502.
40. Adams SG, Howe TT. Predicting medication compliance in a psychotic population. *J Nerv Ment Dis.* 1993;181:558-560.
41. Banqsberg D, Tulsky JP, Hecht FM, Moss AR. Protease inhibitors in the homeless. *JAMA.* 1997; 278:63-65.
42. Volberding PA, Lagakos SW, Grimes JM, Stein DS, Balfour HH Jr, Reichman RC, Bartlett JA, Hirsch M, Phair JP, Mitsuyasu RT, Fischl M, Soeiro R. The duration of zidovudine benefit in persons with asymptomatic HIV infection: prolonged evaluation of protocol 019 of the AIDS Clinical Trials Group. *JAMA.* 1994;272:437-442.
43. Concorde Coordinating Committee. Concorde: MRC/ANR randomized double-blind controlled trial of immediate and deferred zidovudine in symptom-free HIV infection. *Lancet.* 1994;343:871-881.